S0-CMR-538

American
DRUG INDEX

43rd Edition

American DRUG INDEX

1999

43rd Edition

NORMAN F. BILLUPS, RPh, MS, PhD

Dean and Professor of Pharmacy
College of Pharmacy
The University of Toledo

Associate Editor

SHIRLEY M. BILLUPS, RN, LPC, MEd

Oncology Nurse
Licensed Professional Counselor

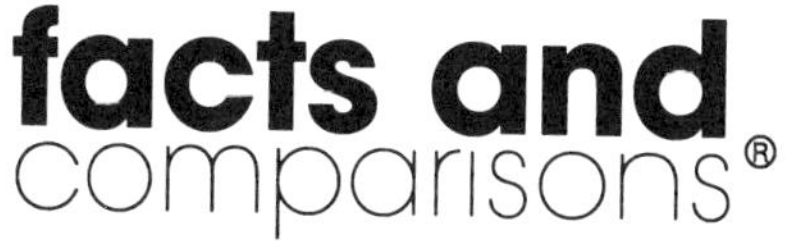

A Wolters Kluwer Company

Facts and Comparisons® Staff

Michael R. Riley
president and publisher

Steven K. Hebel, BS Pharm
director, editorial/production

Bernie R. Olin, PharmD
director of drug information

Heidi L. Meredith
business development

Noël A. Shamleffer
managing editor

Julie A. Scott
quality control editor

Jennifer B. Allen
Kimberly A. Faulhaber
Linda M. Jones
Susan H. Sunderman
Orlando L. Thomas
assistant editors

ISBN 1-57439-041-4

Library of Congress Catalog Card Number 55-6286

Printed in the United States of America

Published by
Facts and Comparisons®
A **Wolters Kluwer** Company
111 West Port Plaza, Suite 300
St. Louis, Missouri 63146-3098

Preface

The 43rd Edition of the *American Drug Index (ADI)* has been prepared for the identification, explanation and correlation of the many pharmaceuticals available to the medical, pharmaceutical and allied health professions. The need for this index has become even more acute as the variety and number of drugs and drug products have continued to multiply. Hence, *ADI* should be useful to pharmacists, nurses, healthcare administrators, physicians, medical transcriptionists, dentists, sales personnel, students and teachers in the fields incorporating pharmaceuticals.

Special note to medical transcriptionists: All generic names are in lowercase and all trade names are in upper/lowercase as appropriate to facilitate transcription. (Tradenames which happen to start with a lowercase letter have been set in uppercase for consistency.) The names for officially designated products (eg, United States Pharmacopeia or U.S.P.) are preceded by a bullet (•) and should appear in lowercase in transcription.

The organization of *ADI* falls into 18 major sections:

- Monographs of Drug Products
- Common Abbreviations Used in Medical Orders
- Common Systems of Weights and Measures
- Approximate Practical Equivalents
- International System of Units
- Normal Laboratory Values
- Trademark Glossary
- Medical Terminology Glossary
- Container Requirements for U.S.P. 23 Drugs
- Container and Storage Requirements for Sterile U.S.P. 23 Drugs
- Oral Dosage Forms that Should Not Be Crushed or Chewed
- Drug Names that Look Alike and Sound Alike
- Recommended Childhood Immunization Schedule
- Radio-Contrast Media
- Radio-Isotopes
- Agents for Imaging
- Pharmaceutical Company Labeler Code Index
- Pharmaceutical Manufacturer and Drug Distributor Listing

MONOGRAPHS: The organization of the monograph section of *ADI* is alphabetical with extensive cross-indexing. Names listed are generic (also called nonproprietary, public name or common name); brand (also called trademark, proprietary or specialty); and chemical. Synonyms that are in general use also are included. All names used for a pharmaceutical appear in alphabetical order with the pertinent data given under the brand name by which it is made available.

The monograph for a typical brand name product appears in upper/lowercase as appropriate, and consists of the manufacturer, generic name, composition and strength, pharmaceutical dosage forms available, package size and use; and appropriate legend designation (eg, *Rx, otc, c-v).*

Generic names appear in lowercase in alphabetical order, followed by the pronunciation and the corresponding recognition of the drug to the U.S.P. (United States Pharmacopeia), N.F. (National Formulary) and USAN (USP Dictionary of United States Adopted Names and International Drug Names). Each of these official generic names is preceded by a bullet (•) at the beginning of each entry. The information is in accord with the U.S.P. 23 and N.F. 18 which became official on January 1, 1995; Supplement 1 which became official on January 1, 1995 through Supplement 8 which became official May 15, 1998; and the 1998 USP Dictionary of USAN and International Drug Names.

Pronunciations have been included for many of the generic drugs. However, not every drug will have a corresponding pronunciation. Some of the most common names are not listed for every drug. The following list is included as a guide to very common names.

Acetate	ASS-eh-tate
Besylate	BESS-ih-late
Borate	BOE-rate
Bromide	BROE-mide
Butyrate	BYOO-tih-rate
Calcium	KAL-see-uhm
Chloride	KLOR-ide
Citrate	SIH-trate
Dipotassium	die-poe-TASS-ee-uhm
Disodium	die-SO-dee-uhm
Edetate	eh-deh-TATE
Fosfatex	foss-FAH-tex
Fumarate	FEW-mah-rate
Hydrobromide	HIGH-droe-BROE-mide
Hydrochloride	HIGH-droe-KLOR-ide
Iodide	EYE-oh-dide
Lactobionate	LACK-toe-BYE-oh-nate
Maleate	MAL-ee-ate
Mesylate	MEH-sih-LATE
Monosodium	MAHN-oh-SO-dee-uhm
Nitrate	NYE-trate
Pendetide	PEN-deh-TIDE
Pentetate	PEN-teh-tate
Phosphate	FOSS-fate
Potassium	poe-TASS-ee-uhm
Propionate	PRO-pee-oh-nate
Sodium	SO-dee-uhm
Succinate	SUCK-sih-nate
Sulfate	SULL-fate
Tartrate	TAR-trate
Trisodium	try-SO-dee-uhm

Because of the multiplicity of brand names used for the same therapeutic agent or the same combination of therapeutic agents, it was apparent that some correlation could be done. As an example of this, please turn to tetracycline HCl. Here under the generic name are listed the various brand names. Following are combinations of tetracycline HCl organized in a manner to point out relationships among the many products. Reference then is made to the brand name or names having the indicated composition. Under the brand name are given manufacturer, composition, available forms, sizes, dosage and use.

The multiplicity of generic names for the same therapeutic agent has complicated the nomenclature of these agents. Examples of multiple generic names for the same chemical substance are: (1) parabromdylamine, brompheniramine; (2) acetaminophen, p-hydroxy acetanilid, N-acetyl-p-aminophenol; (3) guaifenesin, glyceryl guaiacolate, glyceryl guaiacol ether, guaianesin, guaifylline, guaiphenesin, guayanesin, methphenoxydiol; (4) pyrilamine, pyranisamine, pyranilamine, pyraminyl, anisopyradamine.

The cross-indexing feature of *ADI* permits the finding of drugs or drug combinations when only one major ingredient is known. For example, a combination of aluminum hydroxide gel and magnesium trisilicate is available. This combination can be found by looking under the name of either of the two ingredients, and in each case the brand names are given. A second form of cross-indexing lists drugs under various therapeutic and pharmaceutical classes (ie, antacids, antihistamines, diuretics, laxatives, etc.).

ABBREVIATIONS: The listing of Common Abbreviations used in Medical Orders is included as an aid in interpreting medical orders. The Latin or Greek word and abbreviation are given with the meaning.

WEIGHTS AND MEASURES: Tables containing the Common Systems of Weights and Measures are included to aid the practitioner in calculating dosages in the metric, apothecary and avoirdupois systems, as well as the International System of Units.

CONVERSION FACTORS: A listing of Approximate Practical Equivalents is added as an aid in calculating and converting dosages among the metric, apothecary and avoirdupois systems.

INTERNATIONAL SYSTEM OF UNITS: A modernized version of the metric system listed in tables for rapid reference.

NORMAL LABORATORY VALUES: Tables containing normal reference values for commonly requested laboratory tests are included as a guideline for the healthcare practitioner.

TRADEMARK GLOSSARY: An alphabetical listing of trademarked dosage forms and package types is included to aid in the identification of drug products listed in *ADI*.

MEDICAL TERMINOLOGY GLOSSARY: Commonly used terms are listed and defined as an aid in interpreting the use given for drug monographs included in *ADI*.

CONTAINER AND STORAGE REQUIREMENTS FOR U.S.P. 23 DRUGS AND STERILE DRUGS: These sections on container and storage requirements specified by the U.S.P. 23 for compendial drugs have been added to aid the practitioner in storing and dispensing.

ORAL DOSAGE FORMS THAT SHOULD NOT BE CRUSHED OR CHEWED: This section has been added to alert the healthcare practitioner about oral dosage forms that should not be crushed, and to serve as an aid in consulting with patients. Examples of products falling into the "non-crush" category are extended-release, enteric-coated, encapsulated beads, wax matrix, sublingual dosage forms and encapsulated liquid formulations.

DRUG NAMES THAT LOOK ALIKE AND SOUND ALIKE: A listing of common drugs that look alike and sound alike. Familiarity with this list may save the prescriber from making a dispensing error.

RECOMMENDED CHILDHOOD IMMUNIZATION SCHEDULE: This section contains dosing and scheduling information for routine childhood vaccines.

RADIO-CONTRAST MEDIA AND ISOTOPES: These tables provide the generic and trade names, dose form and packaging, and manufacturer information as an aid to the healthcare provider.

AGENTS FOR IMAGING: This table provides the generic and trade names, dose form and packaging, and manufacturer information as an aid to the healthcare provider.

LABELER CODE INDEX: The Pharmaceutical Labeler Code Index is presented to aid in the identification of drug products. The codes are listed in numerical order followed by the name of the manufacturer.

MANUFACTURER ADDRESSES: The name, address and zip code of virtually every American pharmaceutical manufacturer and drug distributor are listed in alphabetical order in this section. Additionally, a pharmaceutical labeler code number appears before the address of each company as a further aid in identifying drug products.

Special appreciation and acknowledgment are given to my wife, Shirley, who served again this year as my Associate Editor – and to Dr. Bernie R. Olin, Director of Drug Information of Facts and Comparisons, for compiling the monograph section of this volume. Special thanks are also extended to the manufacturers who supplied product information, to Dr. Kenneth S. Alexander for organizing the Container and Storage Requirements information, to Dr. John F. Mitchell for the table on Oral Dosage Forms that Should Not Be Crushed or Chewed, and to Drs. Charles O. Wilson and Tony E. Jones for their earlier contributions to *ADI.*

Correspondence or communication with reference to a drug or drug products listed in *ADI* should be directed to Editorial/Production, Attn: ADI, Facts and Comparisons, 111 West Port Plaza, Suite 300, St. Louis, Missouri 63146, or call 1-800-223-0554.

Norman F. Billups, RPh, MS, PhD

Contents

[•] Denotes official name: Generic name or chemical name recognized by the U.S.P., N.F., or USAN.

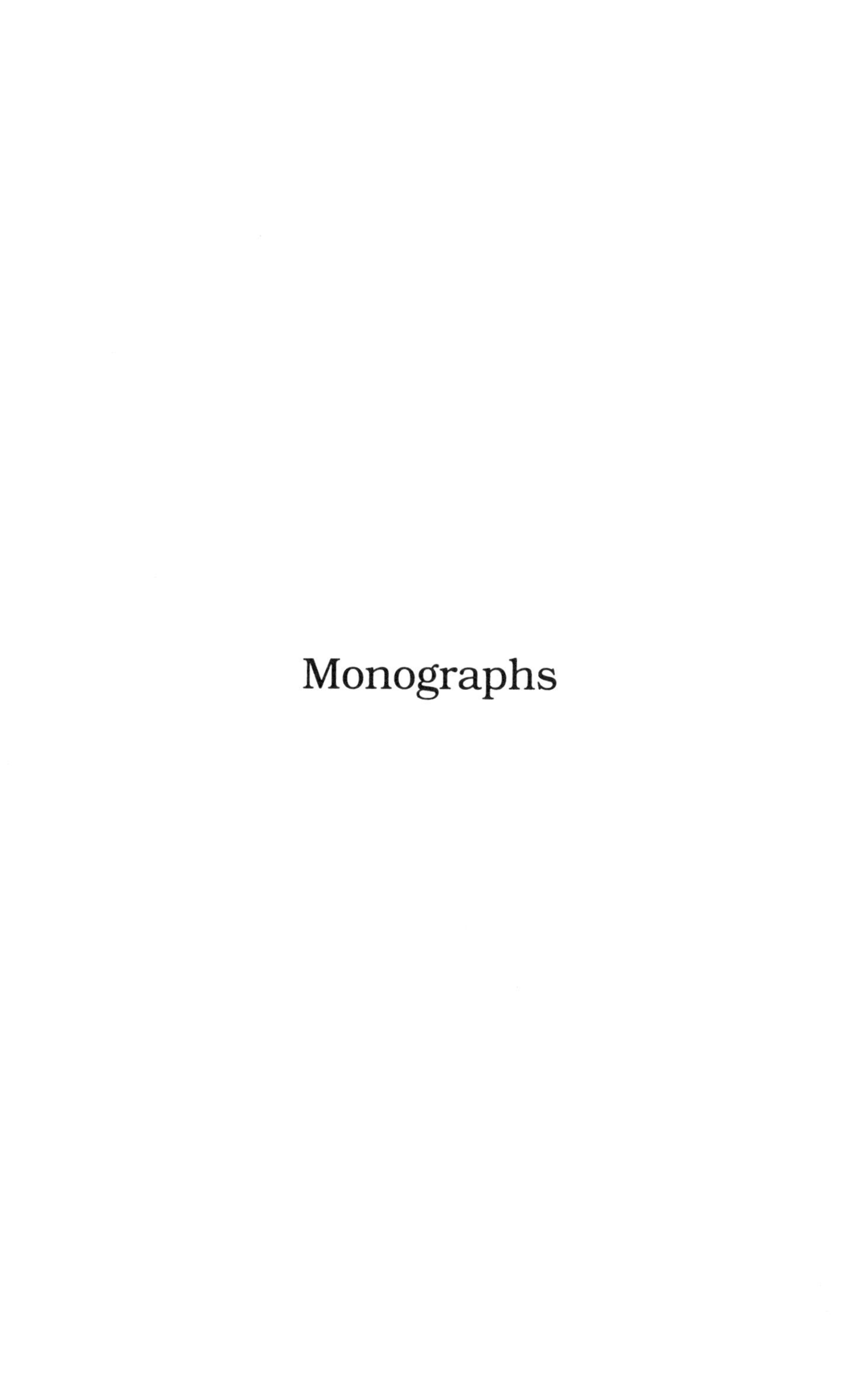

Monographs

A

AA-HC Otic. (Schein Pharmaceutical) Hydrocortisone 1%, acetic acid glacial 2%, propylene glycol diacetate 3%, benzethonium Cl 0.02%, sodium acetate 0.015%, citric acid 0.2%. Soln. Bot. 10 ml. *Rx.*
Use: Otic.

A and D Ointment. (Schering Plough) Fish liver oil, cholecalciferol. Tube 1.5 oz, 4 oz. Jar lb. *otc.*
Use: Emollient.

A & D Tablets. (Barth's) Vitamins A 10,000 IU, D 400 IU/Tab. Bot. 100s, 500s. *otc.*
Use: Vitamin supplement.

•**abacavir succinate.** (ab-ah-KAV-ear SUCK-sih-nate) USAN.
Use: Antiviral.

•**abafilcon a.** (ab-ah-FILL-kahn) USAN.
Use: Contact lens material (hydrophilic).

•**abamectin.** (abe-ah-MEK-tin) USAN.
Use: Antiparasitic.

Abbokinase. (Abbott Laboratories) Urokinase 250,000 IU/5 ml. Lyophilized pow. Vial 5 ml. *Rx.*
Use: Thrombolytic.

Abbokinase Open-Cath. (Abbott Laboratories) Urokinase for catheter clearance 5000 IU/ml. Univial 1 ml. *Rx.*
Use: Thrombolytic.

Abbott AFP-EIA. (Abbott Diagnostics) Enzyme immunoassay for the quantitative measurement of alpha-fetoprotein (AFP) in human serum and amniotic fluid. Test kits 100s.
Use: Diagnostic aid.

Abbott AFP-EIA Monoclonal. (Abbott Diagnostics) Enzyme immunoassay for the quantitative measurement of alpha-fetoprotein (AFP) in human serum and amniotic fluid.
Use: Diagnostic aid.

Abbott Anti-Delta. (Abbott Diagnostics) Radioimmunoassay for the detection of antibody to delta antigen (HDAg) in human serum or plasma. For research only. Not for use in diagnostic procedures.

Abbott Anti-Delta EIA. (Abbott Diagnostics) Enzyme immunoassay for the detection of antibody to hepatitis delta antigen in human serum or plasma. For research only. Not for use in diagnostic procedures.

Abbott β-HCG 15/15. (Abbott Diagnostics) Enzyme immunoassay for the quantitative determination of human chorionic gonadotropin in human serum.
Use: Diagnostic aid.

Abbott CA125-EIA. (Abbott Diagnostics) Enzyme immunoassay for the quantitative measurement of cancer antigen (CA) 125 in human serum. For research only. Not for use in diagnostic procedures.

Abbott CEA-EIA Monoclonal. (Abbott Diagnostics) Enzyme immunoassay for the quantitative measurement of carcinoembryonic antigen (CEA) in human serum or plasma to aid in the management of cancer patients and assessing prognosis.
Use: Diagnostic aid.

Abbott CEA-RIA. (Abbott Diagnostics) Solid phase radioimmunoassay for the quantitative measurement of carcinoembryonic antigen (CEA) in human serum or plasma to aid in the management of cancer patients and assessing prognosis.
Use: Diagnostic aid.

Abbott CMV Total AB EIA. (Abbott Diagnostics) Enzyme immunoassay for the detection of antibody to cytomegalovirus in human serum, plasma, and whole blood. Test kits 100s.
Use: Diagnostic aid.

Abbott Diagnostic Reagents. (Abbott Diagnostics) A series of diagnostic tests for cancer, cardiovascular, hepatitis, infectious disease and immunology, metabolic and digestive disease, OB/GYN, rubella and thyroid.
Use: Diagnostic aid.

Abbott ER-EIA Monoclonal. (Abbott Diagnostics) Enzyme immunoassay for the quantitative measurement of human estrogen receptor in tissue cytosol. For research only. Not for use in diagnostic procedures.

Abbott ER-ICA Monoclonal. (Abbott Diagnostics) Immunoassay for the detection of estrogen receptor. For research only. Not for use in diagnostic procedures.

Abbott-HB EIA. (Abbott Diagnostics) Enzyme immunoassay for the detection of hepatitis Be antigen or antibody to hepatitis Be antigen.
Use: Diagnostic aid.

Abbott-HBe Test. (Abbott Diagnostics) Radioimmunoassay or enzyme immunoassay for detection of hepatitis Be antigen or antibody to hepatitis Be antigen. Test kits 100s.

Use: Diagnostic aid.

Abbott HIVAB HIV-1 EIA. (Abbott Diagnostics) Enzyme immunoassay for the antibody to human immunodeficiency virus type 1 (HIV-1) in serum or plasma. Test kits 100s, 1000s.
Use: Diagnostic aid.

Abbott HIVAG-1. (Abbott Diagnostics) Enzyme immunoassay for the human immunodeficiency virus type 1 (HIV-1) antigens in serum or plasma. Test kits 100s, 1000s.
Use: Diagnostic aid.

Abbott HTLV I EIA. (Abbott Diagnostics) To detect antibody to Human T-Lymphotropic Virus Type I in serum or plasma. Test kits 100s.
Use: Diagnostic aid.

Abbott HTLV III Antigen EIA. (Abbott Diagnostics) Enzyme immunoassay for the detection of Human T-Lymphotropic Virus Type III (HIV) antigens. For research only. Not for use in diagnostic procedures.

Abbott HTLV III Confirmatory EIA. (Abbott Diagnostics) Enzyme immunoassay for confirmation of specimens found to be positive to antibody to HTLV III. Test kits 100s.
Use: Diagnostic aid.

Abbott HTLV III EIA. (Abbott Diagnostics) Enzyme immunoassay for the detection of antibody to Human T-Lymphotropic Virus Type III (HIV) in human serum or plasma. Test kits 1s.
Use: Diagnostic aid.

Abbott IGE EIA. (Abbott Diagnostics) Enzyme immunoassay for quantitative determination of IgE in human serum and plasma. Test kits 100s.
Use: Diagnostic aid.

Abbott PAP-EIA. (Abbott Diagnostics) Enzyme immunoassay for the measurement of prostatic acid phosphatase (PAP) in serum or plasma.
Use: Diagnostic aid.

Abbott RSV-EIA. (Abbott Diagnostics) Enzyme immunoassay for the detection of respiratory syncytial virus (RSV) in nasopharyngeal washes and aspirates.
Use: Diagnostic aid.

Abbott SCC-RIA. (Abbott Diagnostics) Radioimmunoassay for the quantitative measurement of squamous cell carcinoma associated antigen in human serum. For research only. Not for use in diagnostic procedures.

Abbott TdT EIA. (Abbott Diagnostics) Enzyme immunoassay for the quantitative measurement of terminal deoxynucleotidyl transferase (TdT), in extracts of human whole blood or isolated mononuclear cells.
Use: Diagnostic aid.

Abbott Testpack hCG-Serum. (Abbott Diagnostics) Monoclonal antibody, enzyme immunoassay for the qualitative determination of human chorionic gonadotropin (hCG) in serum. No instrumentation required.
Use: Diagnostic aid.

Abbott Testpak hCG-Urine. (Abbott Diagnostics) Monoclonal antibody, enzyme immunoassay for the qualitative determination of human chorionic gonadotropin (hCG) in urine. No instrumentation required.
Use: Diagnostic aid.

Abbott Testpack-Strep A. (Abbott Diagnostics) A rapid screening and confirmatory test for the detection of Group A beta-hemolytic streptococci from throat swabs. No instrumentation required.
Use: Diagnostic aid.

Abbott Toxo-G EIA. (Abbott Diagnostics) Enzyme immunoassay for the qualitative and quantitative determination of IgG antibody to toxoplasma gondii in human serum and plasma.
Use: Diagnostic aid.

Abbott Toxo-M EIA. (Abbott Diagnostics) Enzyme immunoassay for the qualitative determination of IgM antibody to toxoplasma gondii in human serum.
Use: Diagnostic aid.

ABC to Z. (NBTY) Iron 18 mg, Vitamins A 5000 IU, D 400 IU, E 30 IU, B_1 1.5 mg, B_2 1.7 mg, B_3 20 mg, B_5 10 mg, B_6 2 mg, B_{12} 6 mcg, C 60 mg, folic acid 0.4 mg, biotin 30 mcg, Ca, P, I, Mg, Cu, Mn, K, Cl, Cr, Mo, Se, Ni, Si, Sn, V, B, vitamin K, Zn 15 mg/Tab. Bot. 100s. *otc.*
Use: Mineral, vitamin supplement.

•**abciximab.** (ab-SICK-sih-mab) USAN.
Use: Monoclonal antibody (antithrombotic).
See: ReoPro (Eli Lilly).

Abelcet. (Liposome) Amphotericin B 100 mg/20 ml (as lipid complex)/Susp. for Inj. Single-use Vial w/5-micron filter needles. *Rx.*
Use: Invasive fungal infections. [Orphan drug]

Abitrexate. (International Pharm) Methotrexate sodium 25 mg/ml. Vial 2 ml, 4 ml, 8 ml. *Rx.*

Use: Antineoplastic.

•**ablukast.** (ab-LOO-kast) USAN.
Use: Antiasthmatic (leukotriene antagonist).

•**ablukast sodium.** (ab-LOO-kast) USAN.
Use: Antiasthmatic (leukotriene antagonist).
See: Ulpax (Roche Laboratories).

abortifacients.
See: Hemabate, Inj. (Pharmacia & Upjohn).
Prostin E_2, Supp. (Pharmacia & Upjohn).

absorbable cellulose cotton or gauze.
See: Oxidized Cellulose (Various Mfr.).

absorbable dusting powder.
Use: Lubricant.

absorbable gelatin film.
Use: Hemostatic, topical.
See: Gelfilm (Pharmacia & Upjohn).
Gelfilm Ophthalmic (Pharmacia & Upjohn).

absorbable gelatin powder.
Use: Hemostatic, topical.
See: Gelfoam, Pow. (Pharmacia & Upjohn).

absorbable gelatin sponge.
Use: Hemostatic.
See: Gelfoam (Pharmacia & Upjohn).

absorbable surgical suture.
Use: Surgical aid.

Absorbase. (Carolina Medical Products) Petrolatum, mineral oil, ceresin wax, wool wax, alcohol. Oint. Tube 114 g, 454 g. *otc.*
Use: Pharmaceutical aid, emollient base.

absorbent gauze.
Use: Surgical aid.

Absorbent Rub Relief Formula. (DeWitt) Green soap 11.64%, camphor 1.63%, menthol 1.63%, pine tar soap 0.87%, wintergreen oil 0.71%, sassafras oil 0.54%, benzocaine 0.48%, capsicum 0.03%, wormwood oil 0.6%, isopropyl alcohol 75%. Bot. 2 oz. *otc.*
Use: Analgesic, topical.

Absorbine Athlete's Foot Cream. (W.F. Young) Tolnaftate 1%, parabens. Cream. 21.3 g. *otc.*
Use: Antifungal, topical.

Absorbine FootCare. (W.F. Young) Tolnaftate 1%, menthol, acetone, chloroxylenol, wormwood oil. Spray Liq. Bot. 59.2 ml, 118.3 ml. *otc.*
Use: Antifungal, topical.

Absorbine Foot Powder. (W.F. Young) Zinc stearate, parachloroxylenol, aluminum chlorhydroxy, allantonate, benzethonium Cl, menthol. Plastic bot. 3 oz w/shaker top. *otc.*
Use: Antifungal, topical.

Absorbine, Jr. (W.F. Young) Wormwood, thymol, chloroxylenol, menthol, acetone, zinc stearate, parachloroxylenol, aluminum chlorhydroxy, allantonate, benzethonium Cl, menthol. Liq. Bot. 1 oz, 2 oz, 4 oz, 12 oz w/applicator. *otc.*
Use: Analgesic; antifungal, topical.

Absorbine Jr. Extra Strength Liniment. (W.F. Young) Natural menthol 4%, plant extracts of calendula, echinacea and wormwood, acetone, chloroxylenol iodine, potassium iodide, thymol, wormwood oil. Lot. Bot. 59 ml, 118 ml. *otc.*
Use: Liniment.

Absorbine Jr. Extra Strength Liquid. (W.F. Young) Menthol 4%. Liq. Bot. 59 ml, 118 ml. *otc.*
Use: Rub or liniment.

Absorbine Jr. Liniment. (W.F. Young) Menthol 1.27%, plant extracts of calendula, echinacea and wormwood, iodine, potassium iodide, thymol, acetone, chloroxylenol. Lot. Bot. 60 ml, 120 ml. *otc.*
Use: Liniment.

Abuscreen. (Roche Laboratories) An immunological and radiochemical assay for morphine and morphine glucuronide in nanogram levels. Utilizes I-125 labeled morphine requiring gamma scintillation equipment. Tests 100s.
Use: Diagnostic aid.

•**acacia.** (ah-KAY-shah) N.F. 18.
Use: Pharmaceutic aid (suspending, viscosity agent).

•**acadesine.** (ack-AH-dess-een) USAN.
Use: Platelet aggregation inhibitor.

•**acarbose.** (A-car-bose) USAN.
Use: Inhibitor (α-glucosidase).
See: Precose, Tab. (Bayer Corp).

Accolate. (Zeneca) Zafirlukast 20 mg/Tab. Bot. 60s, 100s. *Rx.*
Use: Treatment of asthma.

Accupep HPF. (Sherwood Medical) Hydrolyzed lactalbumin, maltodextrin, MCT oil, corn oil, mono- and diglycerides, vitamins A, B_1, B_2, B_3, B_5, B_6, B_{12}, C, D, E, K, Ca, Cl, Cu, Fe, I, Mg, Mn, P, Zn, biotin and choline. Pks. 128 g. *otc.*
Use: Nutritional supplement.

Accupril. (Parke-Davis) Quinapril 5 mg, 10 mg, 20 mg, 40 mg/Tab. Bot. Lactose. 90s and UD 100s. *Rx.*
Use: Antihypertensive.

Accurbron. (Hoechst Marion Roussel)

Theophylline, anhydrous 10 mg/ml. Bot. Pt. *Rx.*
Use: Bronchodilator.

Accusens T Taste Function Kit. (Westport) Test for ability to distinguish among salty, sweet, sour and bitter tastants. Kit contains 15 bottles (60 ml) tastants and 30 taste record forms.
Use: Diagnostic aid.

Accutane. (Roche Laboratories) Isotretinoin 10 mg, 20 mg, or 40 mg/Cap. Bot. UD 100s. *Rx.*
Use: Dermatologic, acne.

A-C-D Solution. Sodium citrate, citric acid and dextrose in sterile pyrogen-free solution. (Baxter) 600 ml bot. with 70 ml, 120 ml, 300 ml Soln.; 1000 ml Bot. with 500 ml Soln. (Cutter Biologicals) 500 ml Bot. with 75 ml, 120 ml Soln.; 650 ml bot. with 80 ml, 130 ml Soln. (Diamond) (Abbo-Vac) 250 ml, 500 ml. *Rx.*
Use: Anticoagulant for preparation of plasma or whole blood.

A-C-D Solution Modified. (Bristol-Myers Squibb) Acid citrate dextrose anticoagulant solution modified. *Rx.*
Use: Anticoagulant, radiolabeled.

•**acebutolol.** (ass-cee-BYOO-toe-lahl) USAN.
Use: Antiadrenergic (β-receptor).
See: Sectral, Cap. (Wyeth Ayerst).

•**acebutolol hydrochloride.** (ass-cee-BYOO-toe-lahl) U.S.P. 23.
Use: Antiadrenergic (β-receptor).
See: Sectral, Cap. (Wyeth Ayerst).

acebutolol hydrochloride. (ass-cee-BYOO-toe-lahl) (Mylan) 200, 400 mg/Cap. Bot. 100s. *Rx.*
Use: Antiadrenergic.

•**acecainide hydrochloride.** (ASS-eh-CANE-ide) USAN.
Use: Cardiovascular agent.
See: Napa (Medco Research/Parke-Davis).

•**aceclidine.** (ass-ECK-lih-DEEN) USAN.
Use: Cholinergic.
See: Glaucostat (Kingshill Pharmaceuticals Inc., Switzerland).

•**acedapsone.** (ASS-eh-DAP-sone) USAN.
Use: Antimalarial; antibacterial (leprostatic).

Acedoval. (Pal-Pak) Dover's powder 15 mg, ipecac 1.5 mg, aspirin 162 mg, caffeine anhydrous 8.1 mg/Tab. Bot. 1000s, 5000s. *otc.*
Use: Analgesic, antispasmodic, antiperistaltic.

•**aceglutamide aluminum.** (AH-see-GLUE-tah-mide ah-LOO-min-uhm) USAN.
Use: Antiulcerative.

Acel-Imune. (ESI Lederle Generics) Diphtheria toxoid 7.5 Lf units, tetanus toxoid 5 Lf units, acellular pertussis vaccine 300 hemagglutinating units and aluminum ≤ 0.85 mg/0.5 ml. With formaldehyde ≤ 0.02%, thimerosal final concentration of 1:10,000. Aluminum hydroxide and phosphate, thimerosal, gelatin, glycine, polysorbate 80. 5 ml/Vial for Inj. *Rx.*
Use: Immunization.

•**acemannan.** (ah-see-MAN-an) USAN.
Use: Antiviral; immunomodulator.
See: Carrisyn (Carrington).

Aceon. (Ortho McNeil) Perindopril erbumine 2 mg, 4 mg or 8 mg. Tab. Bot. 100s and UD blister packs. *Rx.*
Use: Antihypertensive.

Acephen. (G & W Laboratories) **Adult:** Acetaminophen 650 mg/Supp. Box 12s, 100s. **Pediatric:** Acetaminophen 120 mg/Supp. Box 12s, 100s. *otc.*
Use: Analgesic.

acepromazine. (ASS-ee-PRO-mah-zeen) (Wyeth Ayerst) *Rx.*
Use: Anxiolytic.

Acerola-C. (Barth's) Vitamin C 300 mg/Wafer. Bot. 30s, 90s, 180s, 360s. *otc.*
Use: Vitamin supplement.

Acerola-Plex. (Barth's) Vitamin C 100 mg, bioflavonoids 50 mg/Tab. Bot. 100s, 500s. *otc.*
Use: Vitamin supplement.

Aceta. (Century Pharm) Acetaminophen 325 mg or 500 mg/Tab. Bot. 100s, 1000s. *otc.*
Use: Analgesic.

Aceta w/Codeine. (Century Pharm) Acetaminophen 300 mg, codeine phosphate 30 mg/Tab. Bot. 100s. *c-III.*
Use: Analgesic combination-narcotic.

Aceta Elixir. (Century Pharm) Acetaminophen 160 mg/5 ml, alcohol 7%. Elix. Bot. 120 ml, 1 gal. *otc.*
Use: Analgesic.

Aceta-Gesic. (Rugby) Acetaminophen 325 mg, phenyltoloxamine citrate 30 mg/Tab. Bot. 100s, 1000s. *otc.*
Use: Analgesic, antihistamine.

•**acetaminophen.** (ass-cet-ah-MEE-noe-fen) U.S.P. 23. APAP.
Use: Analgesic, antipyretic.
See: Acephen, Supp. (G & W Laboratories).
Aceta, Tab., Elix., Supp. (Century Pharm).

Acetaminophen Uniserts, Supp. (Upsher-Smith Labs).
Actamin, Tab. (Buffington).
Actamin Extra, Tab. (Buffington).
Aminodyne, Elix. (Jones Medical Industries).
Anacin-3, Chew. tab., Tab., Elix., Drops (Whitehall Robins).
Anapap, Tab. (Forest Pharmaceutical).
Anexsia 5/500, Tab. (Mallinckrodt).
Anexsia 7.5/650, Tab. (Mallinckrodt).
Anexsia 10/660, Tab. (Mallinckrodt).
Apap, Cap., Tab. (Various Mfr.).
Children's Dynafed Jr., Chew. Tab. (BDI).
Dapa, Tab. (Ferndale Laboratories).
Datril 500, Tab. (Bristol-Myers).
Dorcol, Prods. (Novartis).
Dynafed Jr., Children's, Chew. Tab. (BDI).
Extra Strength Dynafed E.X., Tab. (BDI).
Fendon, Tab. (APC).
G-1 (Roberts Pharm).
Genapap, Chew. Tab. (Zenith Goldline).
Genebs, Tab., Cap. (Zenith Goldline).
Halenol, Tab., Elix. (Halsey).
Lestemp, Elix. (Solvay).
Liquiprin, Soln. (SmithKline Beecham Pharmaceuticals).
Meda Cap, Cap. (Circle).
Meda Tab, Tab. (Circle).
Neopap, Supp. (PolyMedica).
Panadol, Cap., Chew. tab., Tab., Liq. Drops (Bayer Corp).
Panex, Tab. (Roberts Pharm).
Parten, Tab. (Parmed).
Phenaphen, Cap., Tab. (Robins).
Proval, Cap., Elix., Drops, Tab. (Solvay).
Suppap-120, 325, 650, Supp. (Raway).
Tapanol Extra Strength, Tab. (Republic).
Temetan, Elix., Tab. (Nevin).
Tempra, Drops, Syr., (Bristol-Myers).
Ty-Caplets, Tab. (Major).
Ty-Caps, Cap. (Major).
Tylenol, Drops, Elix., Liq., Tab., Chew. tab. (Ortho McNeil).
Tylenol Extra-Strength, Tab., Cap. (Ortho McNeil).
Ty-Pap, Supp., Elix. (Major).
Ty-Tabs, Tab. (Major).

acetaminophen w/combinations.
See: Aceta w/Codeine, Tab. (Century Pharm).
Acid-X, Tab. (BDI).
Actifed Plus, Tab. (GlaxoWellcome).
Actifed Sinus Daytime/Nightime, Capl., (GlaxoWellcome).
Allerest Headache Strength, Tab. (Novartis).
Allergy-Sinus Comtrex, Capl., Tab. (Bristol-Myers).
Alumadrine, Tab. (Fleming).
Amaphen, Cap. (Trimen).
Anexsia, Tab. (Mallinckrodt).
Anodynos Forte, Tab. (Buffington).
Anoquan, Cap. (Roberts Pharm).
Apap w/Codeine, Tab. (Schwarz Pharma).
Aspirin Free Anacin P.M., Tab. (Robins).
Asprin-Free Bayer Select Head & Chest Cold, Capl. (Bayer).
Axocet, Cap. (Savage).
Bayer Select Flu Relief, Capl. (Bayer Corp).
Bayer Select Head Cold, Capl. (Bayer Corp).
Bayer Select Night Time Cold, Capl. (Bayer Corp).
BQ Cold, Tab. (Bristol-Myers).
Bromo-Seltzer, Gran. (Warner Lambert).
Bupap, Tab. (ECR).
Capital and Codeine, Susp. (Carnrick Labs).
Children's Cēpacol, Liq. (JB Williams).
Children's Dynafed Jr., Chew. Tab. (BDI).
Children's Tylenol Cold Plus Cough, Chew. Tab. (Ortho-McNeil).
Codimal, Tab. (Schwarz Pharma).
Comtrex Caplets (Bristol-Myers).
Comtrex Liquid (Bristol-Myers).
Comtrex Liqui-Gels (Bristol-Myers).
Comtrex Tablets (Bristol-Myers).
Contac Day & Night Allergy/Sinus Caplets (SmithKline Beecham Pharmaceuticals).
Contac Day & Night Colds & Flu Caplets (SmithKline Beecham Pharmaceuticals).
Coricidin, Tab. (Schering Plough).
Coricidin D, Tab. (Schering Plough).
Coricidin Sinus Headache, Tab. (Schering Plough).
Darvocet-N 100, Tab. (Eli Lilly).
DHC Plus, Cap. (Purdue Frederick).
Dristan Cold Multi-Symptom Formula, Tab. (Whitehall Robins).
Drixoral Cold & Flu, Tab. (Schering Plough).
Drixoral Cough & Sore Throat, Liquid caps. (Schering Plough).
Endolor, Cap. (Keene).
Esgic, Cap., Tab. (Gilbert).
Esgic-Plus, Tab. (Forest Pharm).

Excedrin Aspirin Free, Cap. (Bristol-Myers).
Excedrin Extra Strength, Geltab. (Bristol-Myers Squibb).
Excedrin Sinus, Capl., Tab. (Bristol-Myers).
Extra Strength Dynafed E.X., Tab. (BDI).
Femcet, Cap. (Russ).
Fem-1, Tab. (BDI).
Fioricet, Tab. (Novartis).
Fiorpap, Tab. (Creighton).
Histosal #2, Tab. (Ferndale Laboratories).
Hycomine Compound, Tab. (DuPont Merck Pharmaceuticals).
Hydrocet, Cap. (Carnrick Labs).
Hy-Phen, Tab. (B.F. Ascher).
Isocet, Tab. (Rugby).
Liquiprin, Soln. (Menley & James)
Lortab, Elix. (UCB Pharma).
Lortab 10/500, Tab. (UCB Pharma).
Mapap CF, Tab. (Major).
Margesic, Cap. (Marnel).
Maximum Strength Arthriten, Tab. (Alva-Amco).
Medigesic, Cap. (US Pharm).
Medipain 5, Cap. (Medi-Plex).
Midol Maximum Strength, Tab. (Bayer Corp).
Midol Teen, Cap. (Bayer Corp).
Midrin, Cap. (Carnrick Labs).
Multi-Symptom Tylenol Cough, Liq. (Ortho-McNeil).
Multi-Symptom Tylenol Cough with Decongestant (Ortho-McNeil).
Naldegesic, Tab. (Bristol-Myers Squibb).
N-D Gesic, Tab. (Hyrex).
Nyquil, Liq. (Procter & Gamble).
Ornex, (Menley & James).
Ornex Maximum Strength, Cap. (Menley & James).
Pamprin Prods. (Chattem Consumer Products).
Percocet, Tab. (Dupont).
Percogesic, Tab. (DuPont Merck Pharmaceuticals).
Phenaphen #2, #3, #4 (Robins).
Phrenilin, Tab. (Carnrick Labs).
Phrenilin Forte, Cap. (Carnrick Labs).
Prominol, Tab. (MCR American Pharm).
Propacet 100, Tab. (Teva USA).
Proval No. 3, Tab. (Solvay).
Quiet World, Tab. (Whitehall Robins).
Renpap, Tab. (Wren).
Repan, Tab. (Everett Laboratories).
Repan CF, Tab. (Everett).
Robitussin Night Relief, (Whitehall Robins).
Saleto, Tab. (Roberts Pharm).
Saleto-D, Tab. (Roberts Pharm).
Sedapap, Tab. (Merz).
Sinarest, Tab. (Novartis).
Sine-Aid Maximum Strength, Cap., Tab. (McNeil Consumer Products).
Sine-Off Maximum Strength No Drowsiness Formula, Capl. (SmithKline Beecham Pharmaceuticals).
Sine-Off Sinus Medicine, Capl. (SmithKline Beecham Pharmaceuticals).
Sinulin, Tab. (Carnrick Labs).
Sinutab, Prods. (Warner Lambert).
St. Joseph Cold Tablets for Children, Tab. (Schering Plough).
Sudafed Cold & Cough, Liq. Cap. (GlaxoWellcome).
Sudafed Severe Cold, Tab. (GlaxoWellcome).
Supac, Tab. (Mission Pharmacal).
Talacen, Cap. (Sanofi Winthrop).
Tencon, Cap. (Inter Ethical Labs).
Triad, Cap. (UAD)
Triaminic Sore Throat Formula, Liq. (Novartis).
Triaprin, Cap. (Dunhall Pharmaceuticals).
Two-Dyne, Tab. (Hyrex).
Tylenol Children's Chewable Tablets (Ortho McNeil).
Tylenol Children's Cold Tablets (Ortho McNeil).
Tylenol Children's Suspension (Ortho McNeil).
Tylenol Cold, Liq., Cap., Tab. (Ortho McNeil).
Tylenol Cold & Flu No Drowsiness, Pow. (Ortho McNeil).
Tylenol Cold Night Time, Liq. (Ortho McNeil).
Tylenol Cold No Drowsiness, Capl., Gelcap. (Ortho McNeil).
Tylenol Cough, Liq. (Ortho McNeil).
Tylenol Extended Relief, Capl. (Ortho McNeil).
Tylenol w/Codeine, Tab. (Ortho McNeil).
Tylenol, Preps. (Ortho McNeil).
Tylox, Cap. (Ortho McNeil).
Vanquish, Tab. (Bayer Corp).
Vicks NyQuil Multi-Symptom Cold and Flu Relief, Liq. (Procter & Gamble).
Vicodin, Tab. (Knoll Pharmaceuticals).
Vicodin HP, Tab. (Knoll).
Viro-Med, Tab. (Whitehall Robins).
Wygesic, Tab. (Wyeth Ayerst).
Zydone, Cap. (DuPont Merck Pharmaceuticals).

acetaminophen and aspirin tablets.
Use: Analgesic.

acetaminophen and caffeine capsules. Cap., Tab.
Use: Analgesic.

acetaminophen, aspirin and caffeine. Cap., Tab.
Use: Analgesic.

Acetaminophen w/Codeine. (ass-cet-ah-MEE-noe-fen) (Various Mfr.) **Tab.:** Codeine phosphate 15 mg, acetaminophen 300 mg/Tab. Bot. 100s, 500s, 1000s. Codeine phosphate 30 mg, acetaminophen 300 mg/Tab. Bot. 100s, 500s, 1000s, UD 100s, RN 100s. Codeine phosphate 60 mg, acetaminophen 300 mg/Tab. Bot. 100s, 500s, 1000s. *c-III.* **Soln.:** Codeine phosphate 12 mg, acetaminophen 120 mg/5 ml. Bot. 120 ml, 500 ml, pt, gal, UD 5 ml, 12.5 ml, 15 ml. *c-v.*
Use: Analgesic combination-narcotic.

acetaminophen and butalbital tablets.
Use: Analgesic.
See: Bupap, Tab. (ECR).

acetaminophen and codeine phosphate oral solution.
Use: Analgesic.

acetaminophen and diphenhydramine citrate tablets.
Use: Analgesic, antihistamine.
See: Excedrin PM, Prods. (Bristol-Myers Squibb).
Legatrin PM, Capl. (Columbia).
Midol PM, Capl. (Sterling Health).

acetaminophen and pamabrom tablets.
Use: Analgesic.
See: Fem-1, Tab. (BDI).

acetaminophen and pseudoephedrine hydrochloride tablets.
Use: Analgesic, decongestant.
See: Allerest No Drowsiness, Tab. (Ciba).
Coldrine, Tab. (Roberts).
Maximum Strength Dynafed Plus, Tab. (BDI).
Ornex No Drowsiness, Tab. (Menley & James).
Sinus Relief, Tab. (Major).

acetaminophen oral solution.
Use: Analgesic.

acetaminophen oral suspension.
Use: Analgesic.

acetaminophen suppositories.
Use: Analgesic.

acetaminophen uniserts. (Upsher-Smith Labs) Acetaminophen **120 mg or 325 mg/Supp.:** Ctn. 12s, 50s; **650 mg/ Supp.:** Ctn. 12s, 50s, 500s. *otc.*
Use: Analgesic.

acetaminophenol.
See: Acetaminophen.

acetanilid. (Various Mfr.) (Acetylaminobenzene, acetylaniline, antifebrin) N-phenylacetamide cry.
Use: Analgesic (former use).

Acetasol.
See: Acetarsone.

acetarsone. 3-Acetamido-4-hydroxyphenylarsonic acid. Acetasol, Acetphenarsine, Amarsan, Dynarsan, Ehrlich 594, Limarsol, Orarsan, Osarsal, Osvarsan, Paroxyl, Stovarsol.

acetarsone salt of arecoline.
See: Drocarbil.

Acetasol HC Otic. (Zenith Goldline) Hydrocortisone 1%, acetic acid 2%. Bot. 10 ml. *Rx.*
Use: Anti-infective; corticosteroid, otic.

Acetasol Otic. (Zenith Goldline) Acetic acid (non-aqueous) 2%. Bot. 5 ml. *Rx.*
Use: Anti-infective, otic.

•**acetazolamide.** (uh-seet-uh-ZOLE-uh-mide) U.S.P. 23.
Use: Carbonic anhydrase inhibitor.
See: Diamox (ESI Lederle Generics)

acetazolamide. (Various Mfr.) **Tab.:** 125 mg, Bot. 100s; 250 mg, Bot. 100s, 1000s, UD 100s. **Pow.:** 500 mg/vial.
Use: Carbonic anhydrase inhibitor.

•**acetazolamide sodium, sterile.** (uh-seet-uh-ZOLE-uh-mide) U.S.P. 23.
Use: Carbonic anhydrase inhibitor.

acet-dia-mer-sulfonamide. Sulfacetamide, sulfadiazine and sulfamerazine, Susp. *Rx.*
Use: Antibacterial, sulfonamide.

Acetest Reagent Tablets. (Bayer Corp) Sodium nitroprusside, disodium phosphate, aminoacetic acid, lactose. Tab. Bot. 100s, 250s.
Use: Diagnostic aid.

•**acetic acid.** (ah-SEE-tick) N.F. 18.
Use: Pharmaceutic aid (acidifying agent).
See: Otic Domeboro, Soln. (Bayer Corp).
Vosol Otic Solution, (Wallace Laboratories).

•**acetic acid, glacial.** U.S.P. 23.
Use: Pharmaceutic aid (acidifying agent).
See: Aci-Jel (Ortho McNeil).

acetic acid irrigation. 0.25% soln. (Abbott Laboratories) 250 ml glass cont.; 250 ml, 1000 ml.
Use: Irrigating solution.

Acetic Acid Otic. (Various Mfr.) Acetic acid 2% with propylene glycol diace-

tate 3%, benzethonium chloride 0.02% and sodium acetate 0.015%. Soln. Bot. 15 ml, 30 ml, 60 ml. *Rx.*
Use: Otic preparation.

acetic acid, potassium salt. Potassium Acetate, U.S.P. 23.

•**acetohexamide.** (uh-seet-toe-HEX-uh-mide) U.S.P. 23.
Use: Antidiabetic.

acetohexamide. (Various Mfr.) 250 or 500 mg/Tab. 100s. *Rx.*
Use: Antidiabetic.
See: Dymelor, Tab. (Eli Lilly).

•**acetohydroxamic acid.** (ass-EE-toe-high-drox-AM-ik) U.S.P. 23.
Use: Enzyme inhibitor (urease).
See: Lithostat (Mission Pharmacal).

acetomeroctol.
Use: Antiseptic, topical.

•**acetone.** (ASS-eh-tone) N.F. 18.
Use: Pharmaceutic aid (solvent).

acetone or diacetic acid test.
See: Acetest, Tab. (Bayer Corp).

acetophenetidin. Phenacetin, Ethoxy-acetanilide.
Use: Analgesic, antipyretic.

•**acetosulfone sodium.** (ah-SET-oh-SULL-fone) USAN.
Use: Antibacterial (leprostatic).

acetoxyphenylmercury.
See: Phenylmercuric acetate.

n-acetyl-p-aminophenol. Acetaminophen.

acetylaniline.
See: Acetanilid (Various Mfr.).

acetyl-bromo-diethylacetyl-carbamide.
See: Acetylcarbromal (Various Mfr.).

acetylcarbromal. Acetyladalin, acetyl-bromodiethylacetylcarbamide. Pow. for manufacturing.
Use: Sedative.
See: Paxarel, Tab. (Circle).
W/Bromisovalum, scopolamine aminoxide HBr.

•**acetylcholine chloride.** (ah-SEH-till-KOE-leen KLOR-ide) U.S.P. 23.
Use: Cardiovascular agent; cholinergic; miotic; vasodilator (peripheral).
See: Miochol Ophthalmic (Ciba Vision Ophthalmics).
Miochol-E (Ciba Vision Ophthalmics).

acetylcholine-like therapeutic agents.
See: Cholinergic agents.

•**acetylcysteine.** (ASS-cee-till-SIS-teen) U.S.P. 23.
Use: Mucolytic [Orphan drug].
See: Acetylcysteine (Various Mfr.).
Mucosil (Dey Labs).
Mucomyst, Soln. (Bristol-Myers Squibb).

acetylcysteine. (Various Mfr.) Soln: 10%, in 4, 10, and 30 ml vials; 20%, in 4, 10, 30 and 100 ml vials. *Rx.*
Use: Mucolytic.

acetylcysteine. (ASS-cee-till-sis-teen)
Use: Treatment for severe acetaminophen overdose. [Orphan drug]
See: Mucomyst (Apothecon).
Mucomyst 10 IV (Apothecon).

acetylcysteine and isoproterenol hydrochloride inhalation solution.
Use: Mucolytic.

acetylcysteine (Fluimucil). (Zambon). Phase I HIV, ARC, AIDS.
Use: Immunomodulator.

acetylin.
See: Acetylsalicylic Acid (Various Mfr.).

acetylphenylisatin. *Rx.*
See: Oxyphenisatin Acetate.

acetylprocainamide-n.
Use: Cardiovascular agent.
See: acecainide, NAPA.

acetylsalicylic acid. Aspirin.
Use: Analgesic; antipyretic; antirheumatic.
See: Aspirin Preps. (Various Mfr.).

acetyl sulfamethoxypyridazine. 3-(N-Acetylsulfanilamido)-6-methoxypyridazine.

n^1-acetylsulfanilamide. (Albucid; p-Aminobenzenesulfonacetamide; Sulfacet; Sulfacetamide, N-Sulfanilylacetamide). *Rx.*
Use: Sulfonamide therapy.

acetyl sulfisoxazole. Sulfisoxazole Acetyl, U.S.P. 23.

acetyltannic acid. Tannic acid acetate.
Use: Antiperistaltic.

AC Eye Drops. (Walgreens) Tetrahydrozoline HCl 0.05%, zinc sulfate 0.25%. Bot. 0.75 oz. *otc.*
Use: Decongestant combination, ophthalmic.

achlorhydria determination.
See: Diagnex Blue, Preps. (Bristol-Myers Squibb).

achlorhydria therapy.
See: Glutamic Acid HCl (Various Mfr.).

Achol. (Enzyme Process) Vitamin A 4000 units, ketocholanic acids 62 mg/Tab. Bot. 100s, 250s. *otc.*
Use: Vitamin supplement.

acid acriflavine.
See: Acriflavine HCl (Various Mfr.).

acid citrate dextrose anticoagulant solution modified.
See: A-C-D Solution Modified (Bristol-Myers Squibb).

acid citrate dextrose solution.
See: A.C.D. Soln. (Various Mfr.).

acidifiers.
See: Ammonium Cl (Various Mfr.).
K-Phos M.F. (Beach Pharmaceuticals).

Acid Mantle. (Doak) Water, cetearyl alcohol, sodium lauryl sulfate, sodium cetearyl sulfate, petrolatum, glycerin, synthetic beeswax, mineral oil, methlyparaben, aluminum sulfate, calcium acetate, white potato dextrin. Cream. Jar 4 oz. *otc.*
Use: Ointment, lotion base.

Acid Mantle. (Novartis) Aluminum sulfate, calcium acetate, cetearyl alcohol, glycerin, light mineral oil, methylparaben, sodium lauryl sulfate, synthetic beeswax, white petrolatum, ammonium hydroxide, citric acid. Cream. Jar 120 g. *otc.*
Use: Pharamceutic aid, emollient base.

Acid Mantle Creme. (Novartis) Aluminum acetate in specially prepared water-soluble hydrophilic cream at pH 4.2. Tube 1 oz, Jar 4 oz, lb. *otc.*
Use: Ointment, lotion base.

acidophilus.
See: Bacid (Medeva).
Lactinex (Becton Dickinson).
More-Dophilus (Freeda Vitamins).

acidophilus w/pectin. (Barth's) *Lactobacillus acidophilus* w/natural citrus pectin 100 mg/Cap. Bot. 100s. *otc.*
Use: Antidiarrheal.

acid trypaflavine.
See: Acriflavine HCl. (Various Mfr.).

Acidulated Phosphate Fluoride. (Scherer) Fluoride ion 0.31% in 0.1 molar phosphate. Soln. Bot. 64 oz. (Office Product).
Use: Dental caries agent.

Acid-X. (BDI) Acetaminophen 500 mg, calcium carbonate 250 mg/Tab. Bot. 36s. *otc.*
Use: Antacid.

•**acifran.** (ACE-ih-FRAN) USAN.
Use: Antihyperlipoproteinemic.

Aci-jel. (Ortho McNeil) Glacial acetic acid 0.921%, ricinoleic acid 0.7%, oxyquinoline sulfate 0.025%, glycerin 5%. Propylparaben. Tube 85 g w/dose applicator. *Rx.*
Use: Vaginal agent.

•**acitretin.** (ASS-ih-TREH-tin) USAN.
Use: Antipsoriatic.
See: Soriatane, Cap. (Roche Laboratories).

•**acivicin.** (ace-ih-VIH-sin) USAN.
Use: Antineoplastic.

•**aclarubicin.** (ack-lah-ROO-bih-sin) USAN. *Formerly Aclacinomycin A.*
Use: Antineoplastic.

Aclophen. (Nutripharm) Phenylephrine HCl 40 mg, chlorpheniramine maleate 8 mg, acetaminophen 500 mg/S.R. tab. Dye free. Bot. 100s. *Rx.*
Use: Analgesic, antihistamine, decongestant.

Aclovate. (GlaxoWellcome) Alclometasone dipropionate 0.05%. Cream or Oint. Tube 15 g, 45 g. *Rx.*
Use: Anti-inflammatory, topical.

A.C.N. (Person & Covey) Vitamin A 25,000 IU, ascorbic acid 250 mg, niacinamide 25 mg/Tab. Bot. 100s. *otc.*
Use: Vitamin supplement.

Acnaveen. (Rydelle)
See: Aveenobar Medicated (Rydelle).

Acna-Vite. (Cenci) Vitamins A 10,000 IU, C 250 mg, hesperidin 50 mg, niacinamide 25 mg/Cap. Bot. 75s. *otc.*
Use: Dermatologic, acne; vitamin supplement.

Acne-5. (Various Mfr.) Benzoyl peroxide 5%. Mask 30 ml. *otc.*
Use: Dermatologic, acne.

Acne-10. (Various Mfr.) Benzoyl peroxide 10%. Bot. 30 ml. *otc.*
Use: Dermatologic, acne.

Acno Cleanser. (Baker/Cummins) Isopropyl alcohol 60%, laureth-23, tetrasodium EDTA. Bot. 240 ml. *otc.*
Use: Dermatologic, acne.

Acno Lotion. (Baker/Cummins) Micronized sulfur 3%. Bot. 120 ml. *otc.*
Use: Dermatologic, acne.

Acnomel. (Menley & James) Resorcinol 2%, sulfur 8%, alcohol 11%. Cream Tube 28 g. *otc.*
Use: Dermatologic, acne.

Acnotex. (C & M Pharmacal) Sulfur 8%, resorcinol 2%, isopropyl alcohol 20%, acetone. In lotion base. Bot. 60 ml. *otc.*
Use: Dermatologic, acne.

•**acodazole hydrochloride.** (ah-KOE-dah-ZOLE) USAN.
Use: Antineoplastic.

aconiazide. (Lincoln Diagnostics)
Use: Antituberculous. [Orphan drug]

Acotus. (Whorton) Phenylephrine HCl 5 mg, guaiacol glyceryl ether 100 mg, menthol 1 mg, alcohol by volume 10%/5 ml. Bot. 4 oz, 12 oz, gal. *otc.*
Use: Antitussive, decongestant.

ACR. (Western Research) Ammonium Cl 7.5 gr/Tab. Handicount 28s (36 bags of 28 tab.). *Rx.*

Use: Diuretic.

acriflavine. (Eli Lilly) Tab. 1.5 gr. Bot. 100s.
Use: Antiseptic.

acriflavine hydrochloride. (Various Mfr.) Hydrochloride form of acriflavine. Acid acriflavine, acid trypaflavine, flavine, trypaflavine. National Aniline-Pow., Bot. (1 g, 5 g, 10 g, 25 g, 50 g). Tab. (1.5 gr). Bot. 50s, 100s. *Rx.*
Use: Anti-infective.

•**acrisorcin.** (ACK-rih-sahr-sin) USAN, U.S.P. XXII.
Use: Antifungal.
See: Akrinol (Schering Plough).

•**acrivastine.** (ACK-rih-VASS-teen) USAN.
Use: Antihistamine.
See: Semprex-D, Cap. (Glaxo-Wellcome)

•**acronine.** (ACK-row-neen) USAN.
Use: Antineoplastic.

ACT. Dactinomycin, U.S.P. 23.
Use: Antineoplastic.
See: Actinomycin D.

ACT. (J & J Merck Consumer Pharm) **Rinse:** 0.02% (from 0.05% sodium fluoride). **Mint:** Tartrazine, alcohol 8%. **Cinnamon:** Alcohol 7%. Bot. 360 ml, 480 ml. *otc.*
Use: Dentrifice.

A-C Tablet. (Century Pharm) Aspirin 6 gr, caffeine 0.5 gr/Tab. Bot. 100s, 1000s. *otc.*
Use: Analgesic.

Actacin-C Syrup. (Vangard) Codeine phosphate 10 mg, triprolidine HCl 2 mg, pseudoephedrine HCl 20 mg, guaifenesin 100 mg/5 ml. Bot. pt, gal. *c-v.*
Use: Antihistamine, antitussive, decongestant, expectorant.

Actacin Tablets. (Vangard) Triprolidine HCl 2.5 mg, pseudoephedrine HCl 60 mg/Tab. Bot. 100s, 1000s. *otc, Rx.*
Use: Antihistamine, decongestant.

Actagen Syrup. (Zenith Goldline) Triprolidine HCl 1.25 mg, pseudoephedrine HCl 30 mg/5 ml. Bot. 118 ml. *otc.*
Use: Antihistamine, decongestant.

Actagen Tablets. (Zenith Goldline) Triprolidine HCl 2.5 mg, pseudoephedrine HCl 60 mg/Tab. Bot. 100s, 1000s. *otc.*
Use: Antihistamine, decongestant.

Actagen-C Cough Syrup. (Zenith Goldline) Triprolidine HCl 1.25 mg, pseudoephedrine HCl 30 mg, codeine phosphate 10 mg/5 ml, alcohol 4.3%. Bot. 120 ml, pt, gal. *c-v.*
Use: Antihistamine, antitussive, decongestant.

Actal Plus Tablets. (Sanofi Winthrop) Aluminum hydroxide, magnesium hydroxide. *otc.*
Use: Antacid.

Actal Suspension. (Sanofi Winthrop) Aluminum hydroxide. *otc.*
Use: Antacid.

Actal Tablets. (Sanofi Winthrop) Aluminum hydroxide. *otc.*
Use: Antacid.

Actamin. (Buffington) Acetaminophen 325 mg/Tab. Dispens-A-Kit 100s, 200s, 500s. *otc.*
Use: Analgesic.

Actamin Extra. (Buffington) Acetaminophen 500 mg/Tab. Bot. 100s, 200s, 500s. *otc.*
Use: Analgesic.

Actamin Super. (Buffington) Acetaminophen 500 mg, caffeine. Sugar, salt, and lactose free. Tab. Dispens-A-Kit 500s, Medipak 200s. *otc.*
Use: Analgesic.

Actamine. (H.L. Moore) **Tab.:** Pseudoephedrine HCl 60 mg, triprolidine HCl 2.5 mg. Bot. 100s, 1000s. **Syr.:** Pseudoephedrine HCl 30 mg, triprolidine HCl 1.25 mg/5 ml. Bot. 120 ml, pt, gal. *otc, Rx.*
Use: Antihistamine, decongestant.

ACTH-Actest Gel. (Forest Pharmaceutical) Repository corticotropin 40 units or 80 units/ml. Vial 5 ml. *Rx.*
Use: Corticosteroid.

ACTH. Adrenocorticotropic hormone. Adrenocorticotropin. *Rx.*
Use: Corticosteroid.
See: Corticotropin, U.S.P.
(Hauck) (40 units/ml, 5 ml).
(Forest Pharmaceutical) 40 units or 80 units/ml, 5 ml.
(Parke-Davis) 25 units/vial; 40 units/vial.
(Pharmex) 40 units or 80 units/ml, 5 ml.

ACTH Gel, Purified. (Arcum) 40 or 80 units/ml, vial 5 ml. (Conal) 40 or 80 units/ml, vial 5 ml. (Hart Labs.) 40 units/ml, vial 5 ml. (Jones Medical Industries) Adrenocorticotropic hormone 40 units, aqueous gelatin 16%, phenol 0.5%/ml. Vial 5 ml. *Rx.*
Use: Repository corticotropin.
See: (Arcum) 40 or 80 units/ml, 5 ml.
(Bell) 40 or 80 units/ml, 5 ml.
(Jones Medical Industries) 40 units/ml, 5 ml.
(Hyrex) 40 or 80 units/ml, 5 ml.
(Jenkins) 40 or 80 units/ml, 5 ml.
(Wesley Pharmacal) 40 or 80 units/ml, vial 5 ml.

(Wyeth Ayerst) 40 or 80 units/ml or Tubex.

Acthar. (Centeon) Corticotropin for inj. Vial 25 units, 40 units/vial. (Lyophilized w/gelatin). *Rx.*
Use: Corticosteroid.

ActHIB. (Pasteur Merieux Connaught) Purified capsular polysaccharide of *Haemophilus influenzae* type b 10 mcg, tetanus toxoid 24 mcg/0.5 ml, sucrose 8.5%. Pow. for Inj. Equivalent to OmniHIB. In vials with 7.5 ml vials of diptheria and tetanus toxoids and pertussis vaccine as diluents. *Rx.*
Use: Vaccine against Haemophilus influenzae type b.

ActHIB/DTP. (Pasteur Merieux Connaught) Diphtheria and tetanus toxoids and pertussis and *Haemophilus influenzae* type b vaccines. One package consists of one 7.5 ml vial of Connaught's DTwP and 10 single-dose vials of ActHIB vaccine. *Rx.*
Use: Immunization.

Acthrel. (Ferring) Corticorelin ovine triflutata 100 mcg. Cake, lypholized. 5 ml single-dose vial w/diluent. *Rx.*
Use: Diagnostic aid.

ActiBath. (Jergens) Colloidal oatmeal 20%. Tab. Effervescent. Pkg. 4s. *otc.*
Use: Emollient.

Acticin. (Alpharma USPD) Permethrin 5%. Cream. Tube 60 g. *Rx.*
Use: Scabicide.

Acticort 100 Lotion. (Baker/Cummins) Hydrocortisone 1%. Bot. 60 ml. *Rx.*
Use: Corticosteroid, topical.

Actidose. (Paddock) Activated charcoal. Soln. 25 g/120 ml or 50 g/240 ml. *otc.*
Use: Antidote.

Actidose-Aqua. (Paddock) Activated charcoal. Aqueous susp. 25 g/120 ml or 50 g/240 ml. *otc.*
Use: Antidote.

Actidose w/Sorbitol. (Paddock) Activated charcoal. Liq: 25 g in 120 ml susp. w/sorbitol, 50 g in 240 ml susp. w/ sorbitol. *otc.*
Use: Antidote.

Actifed. (Warner Lambert Consumer Health Products) **Tab.:** Triprolidine HCl 2.5 mg, pseudoephedrine HCl 60 mg/ Tab. Pkg. 12s. Bot. 24s, 48s, 100s. *otc.* **Cap.:** Triprolidine HCl 2.5 mg, pseudoephedrine HCl 60 mg/Cap. Box 10s, 20s. *otc.*
Use: Antihistamine,decongestant.

Actifed Allergy. (Warner Lambert Consumer Health Products) **Daytime:** Pseudoephedrine 30 mg; **Nighttime:** Pseudoephedrine 30 mg, diphenhydramine HCl 25 mg/Capl. Pkg. 24 daytime, 8 nighttime. *otc.*
Use: Antihistamine, decongestant.

Actifed 12-Hour Capsules. (GlaxoWellcome) Triprolidine HCl 5 mg, pseudoephedrine HCl 120 mg/Cap. Box 10s, 20s. *otc.*
Use: Antihistamine, decongestant.

Actifed Plus. (Warner Lambert Consumer Health Products) Pseudoephedrine HCl 30 mg, triprolidine HCl 1.25 mg, acetaminophen 500 mg/Tab. or Cap. Bot. 20s, 40s. *otc.*
Use: Analgesic, antihistamine, decongestant.

Actifed Sinus Daytime/Nightime. (Warner Lambert Consumer Health Products) **Daytime:** Pseudoephedrine HCl 30 mg, acetaminophen 500 mg/ Capl. pk. 18s. **Nighttime:** Pseudoephedrine HCl 30 mg, diphenhydramine HCl 25 mg, acetaminophen 500 mg/ Capl. pk. 6s. *otc.*
Use: Analgesic, antihistamine, decongestant.

Actigall. (Novartis) Ursodiol (Ursodeoxycholic acid) 300 mg/Cap. Bot. 100s. *Rx.*
Use: Urolithic.

Actimmune. (Genentech) Interferon gamma-1b 100 mcg (3 million units)/ vial. *Rx.*
Use: Anti-infective.

Actinex. (Schwarz Pharma) Masoprocol 10%, isostearyl and stearyl alcohol, light mineral oil, parabens, polyethylene glycol 400, propylene glycol and sodium metabisulfite. Cream, Tube 30 g. *Rx.*
Use: Antineoplastic.

actinomycin c. Name previously used for Cactinomycin.

actinomycin d. Dactinomycin, U.S.P. 23. *Rx.*
Use: Antineoplastic.
See: Cosmegen (Merck).

•**actinoquinol sodium.** (ack-TIN-oh-kwih-nole) USAN.
Use: Ultraviolet screen.

actinospectocin. Name previously used for Spectinomycin.

Actisite. (Alza) Tetracycline HCl 12.7 mg/ 23 cm. Fiber. In 10s. *Rx.*
Use: Mouth and throat preparation.

•**actisomide.** (ackt-EYE-so-MIDE) USAN.
Use: Cardiovascular agent.

Activase. (Genentech) Alteplase recombinant. Inj. Vial 20 mg, 50 mg, 100 mg. *Rx.*

Use: Thrombolytic.

activated attapulgite.

W/Aluminum hydroxide, magnesium carbonate coprecipitate, compressed gel.
See: Hykasil, Cream (Roxane).

W/Polysorbate 80, colloidal sulfur, salicylic acid, propylene glycol. *otc.*
Use: Dermatologic, acne.
See: Sebasorb Lotion (Summers Labs.).

activated charcoal tablets. (Cowley) 5 gr/Tab. Bot. 1000s. *otc.*
Use: Antidote.

activated charcoal powder. (Various Mfr.) 15, 30, 40, 120 and 140 g. *otc.*
Use: Antidote.

activated charcoal liquid. (Various Mfr.) 12.5 g or 25 g with propylene glycol. 60 ml (12.5 g), 120 ml (25 g). *otc.*
Use: Antidote.

activated 7-dehydrocholesterol.
See: Vitamin D-3 (Various Mfr.).

activated ergosterol.
See: Calciferol.

•**actodigin.** (ACK-toe-dihj-in) USAN.
Use: Cardiovascular agent.

Actonel. (Procter & Gamble) Risedronate sodium 30 mg, lactose/Tab. 30s. *Rx.*
Use: Bone resorption inhibitor.

actoquinol sodium.
Use: Ultraviolet screen.

Acucron. (Seatrace) Acetaminophen 300 mg, salicylamide 200 mg, phenyltoloxamine 20 mg/Tab. Bot. 100s, 1000s, 5000s. *otc.*
Use: Analgesic, antihistamine.

Acu-Dyne. (Acme-United) **Douche:** Povidone-iodine. Pkt. 240 ml. **Oint.:** Povidone-iodine. Jar. lb. Pkt. 1.2, 2.7 (100s). **Perineal wash conc.:** Available iodine 1%. Bot. 40 ml. **Prep. Soln.:** Povidone-iodine. Bot. 240 ml, pt, qt, gal. Pkt. 30 ml, 60 ml. **Skin Cleanser:** Povidone-iodine. Bot. 60 ml, 240 ml, pt, qt, gal. **Soln, prep. swabs:** Available iodine 1%. Bot. 100s. **Soln, swabsticks:** Povidone-iodine. Pkt. 1 or 3 in 25s. **Whirlpool conc.:** Available iodine 1%. Bot. gal. *otc.*
Use: Antiseptic, antimicrobial.

Acular. (Allergan) Ketorolac tromethamine 0.5% Ophth. Soln. Drop. Bot. 5 ml. *Rx.*
Use: NSAID, ophthalmic.

Acutrim Maximum Strength. (Novartis Consumer Health) Phenylpropanolamine HCl 75 mg./Tab., precision release Bot. 20s, 40s. *otc.*
Use: Dietary aid.

Acutrim II, Maximum Strength. (Novartis Consumer Health) Phenylpropanolamine HCl 75 mg/Tab. precision release, Bot. 20s, 40s. *otc.*
Use: Dietary aid.

Acutrim 16 Hour. (Novartis Consumer Health) Phenylpropanolamine HCl 75 mg/Tab., precision release. Bot. 20s, 40s. *otc.*
Use: Dietary aid.

•**acyclovir.** (A-SIKE-low-vir) U.S.P. 23.
Use: Antiviral.
See: Zovirax Cap., Oint., Tab., Susp. (GlaxoWellcome).

acyclovir. (Various Mfr.) Acyclovir 400 mg, 800 mg/Tab. Bot. 100s, 500s, 1000s (400 mg only). Acyclovir 200 mg/Cap. Bot. 100s.
Use: Antiviral.

•**acyclovir sodium.** (A-SIKE-low-vir) USAN.
Use: Antiviral.
See: Zovirax Sterile Powder (GlaxoWellcome).

acyclovir sodium. (A-SIKE-low-vir) (Bedford) 50 mg/ml Inj. Cartons of 10. *Rx.*
Use: Antiviral.

Adagen. (Enzon) Pegademase bovine 250 units/ml. Vial 1.5 ml. *Rx.*
Use: Enzyme (ADA) replacement therapy.

Adalat. (Bayer Corp) Nifedipine 10 mg or 20 mg/Cap. Bot. 100s, 300s. UD 100s. *Rx.*
Use: Calcium channel blocker.

Adalat CC. (Bayer Corp) Nifedipine 30 mg, 60 mg or 90 mg. ER Tab. Bot. 100s, 1000s. *Rx.*
Use: Calcium channel blocker.

adamantanamine hydrochloride.
See: Amantadine HCl.
Symmetrel, Cap., Syr. (DuPont Merck Pharmaceuticals).

•**adapalene.** (ADE-ah-PALE-een) USAN.
Use: Dermatologic, acne.
See: Differin (Galderma).

Adapettes. (Alcon Laboratories) Povidone and other water-soluble polymers, sorbic acid, EDTA. Soln. Bot. 15 ml. *otc.*
Use: Contact lens care.

Adapettes for Sensitive Eyes. (Alcon Laboratories) Povidone and other water-soluble polymers, EDTA, sorbic acid. Pkg. 15 ml. *otc.*
Use: Contact lens care.

Adapin. (Lotus) Doxepin HCl **10 mg, 75 mg, 100 mg:** Cap. Bot. 100s, 1000s, UD 100s; **25 mg, 50 mg:** Cap. Bot. 100s, 1000s, 5000s, UD 100s; **150 mg:** Cap. Bot. 50s, 100s. *Rx.*
Use: Antidepressant.

•**adaprolol maleate.** (ad-AH-prole-ole) USAN.
Use: Antihypertensive (β-blocker, ophthalmic).

Adapt. (Alcon Laboratories) Povidone, EDTA 0.1%, thimerosal 0.004%. Bot. 15 ml. *otc.*
Use: Contact lens care.

Adapt Wetting Solution. (Alcon Laboratories) Adsorbobase with thimerosol 0.004%, EDTA 0.1%. Soln. Bot. 15 ml. *otc.*
Use: Contact lens care.

•**adatanserin hydrochloride.** (ahd-at-AN-ser-in) USAN.
Use: Antidepressant, anxiolytic.

AdatoSil 5000. (Escalon Ophthalmics) Polydimethylsiloxane oil. Inj. Vial 10 ml, 15 ml. *Rx.*
Use: Ophthalmic.

Adavite. (Hudson) Vitamins A 5000 IU, D 400 IU, E 30 mg, B_1 3 mg, B_2 3.4 mg, B_3 30 mg, B_5 10 mg, B_6 3 mg, B_{12} 9 mcg, C 90 mg, folic acid 0.4 mg, biotin 35 mcg, beta carotene 1250 IU/Tab. Bot. 130s. *otc.*
Use: Mineral, vitamin supplement.

Adavite. (NBTY) Vitamins A 5500 IU, D 400 IU, E 30 mg, B_1 3 mg, B_2 3.4 mg, B_3 30 mg, B_5 10 mg, B_6 3 mg, B_{12} 9 mcg, C 120 mg, folic acid 0.4 mg, biotin 15 mcg. Tab. Bot. 100s. *otc.*
Use: Vitamin supplement.

Adavite-M. (Hudson) Iron 27 mg, Vitamins A 5000 IU, D 400 IU, E 30 mg, B_1 3 mg, B_2 3.4 mg, B_3 20 mg, B_5 10 mg, B_6 3 mg, B_{12} 9 mcg, C 190 mg, folic acid 0.4 mg, Ca, Cl, Cr, Cu, I, K, Mg, Mn, Mo, P, Se, Zinc 15 mg, biotin 30 mcg/Tab. Bot. 130s. *otc.*
Use: Mineral, vitamin supplement.

ADC with Fluoride. (Various Mfr.) Drops: Flouride 0.5 mg, vitamins A 1500 IU, D 400 IU, C 35 mg, methylparaben/ml. Bot. 50 ml. *Rx.*
Use: Mineral, vitamin supplement.

Adderall. (Richwood) **5 mg:** Dextroamphetamine saccharate 1.25 mg, amphetamine aspartate 1.25 mg, dextroamphetamine sulfate 1.25 mg, amphetamine sulfate 1.25 mg/Tab. Bot. 100s. **10 mg:** Dextroamphetamine sulfate 2.5 mg, dextroamphetamine saccharate 2.5 mg, amphetamine aspartate 2.5 mg, amphetamine sulfate 2.5 mg/Tab. Bot. 100s. **20 mg:** Dextroamphetamine sulfate 5 mg, dextroamphetamine saccharide 5 mg, amphetamine aspartate 5 mg, amphetamine sulfate 5 mg/Tab. Bot. 100s. **30 mg:** Dextroamphetamine saccharate 7.5 mg, amphetamine aspartate 7.5 mg, dextroamphetamine sulfate 7.5 mg, amphetamine sulfate 7.5 mg/Tab. Bot. 100s. *c-II.*
Use: CNS stimulant.

Adeecon. (CMC) Vitamins A 5000 IU, D 1000 IU/Cap. Bot. 1000s. *otc.*
Use: Vitamin supplement.

Adeflor M Tablets. (Kenwood/Bradley) Vitamins A 6000 IU, D 400 IU, B_1 1.5 mg, B_2 2.5 mg, C 100 mg, B_3 20 mg, B_5 10 mg, B_6 10 mg, B_{12} 2 mcg, fluoride 1 mg, calcium 250 mg, iron 30 mg, sorbitol, sucrose/Tab. Bot. 100s, 500s. *Rx.*
Use: Dental caries agent, vitamin supplement.

•**adefovir.** (ah-DEF-fah-vihr) USAN.
Use: Antiviral.

•**adefovir dipivoxil.** (ah-DEF-fah-vihr) USAN.
Use: Antiviral (treatment of HIV and HBV infections.

ADEKs. (Scandipharm) Vitamins A 4000 IU, D 400 IU, E 150 IU, vitamin K, C 60 mg, B_1 1.2 mg, B_2 1.3 mg, B_3 10 mg, B_6 1.5 mg, B_{12} 12 mcg, B_5 10 mg, folic acid 0.2 mg, biotin 50 mcg, beta carotene 3 mg, Zn 1.1 mg, fructose. Tab. Bot. 60s. *otc.*
Use: Mineral, vitamin supplement.

ADEKs Pediatric Drops. (Scandipharm) Vitamin A 1500 IU, D 400 IU, E 40 IU, K_1 0.1 mg, C 45 mg, B_1 0.5 mg, B_2 0.6 mg, B_3 6 mg, B_5 3 mg, B_6 0.6 mg, B_{12} 4 mcg, biotin 15 mcg, Zn 5 mg, betacarotene 1 mg per ml/drop. 60 ml. *otc.*
Use: Vitamin supplement.

•**adenine.** U.S.P. 23.
Use: Vitamin.

adeno-associated viral-based vector cystic fibrosis gene therapy. (Targeted Genetics)
Use: Cystic fibrosis. [Orphan Drug]

Adeno Twelve Gel Injection. (Forest Pharmaceutical) Adenosine-5-monophosphate 25 mg, methionine 25 mg, niacin 10 mg/ml. Vial 10 ml. *Rx.*
Use: Anti-inflammatory.

Adenocard. (Fujisawa) Adenosine 6 mg/2 ml. NaCl 9 mg/ml. Preservative free. Inj. Vial 2 ml, 5 ml. *Rx.*

Use: Antiarrhythmic.

Adenolin Forte. (Lincoln) Adenosine-5-monophosphate 25 mg, methionine 25 mg, niacin 10 mg/ml. Vial 15 ml. *Rx.*
Use: Anti-inflammatory.

Adenoscan. (Fujisawa) Inj.: Adenosine 3 mg/ml. Vial 30 ml. *Rx.*
Use: Diagnostic aid.

•**adenosine.** (ah-DEN-oh-seen) USAN.
Use: Cardiovascular agent.
See: Adenocard, Inj. (Fujisawa).
Adenoscan, Inj. (Fujisawa).

adenosine. (ah-DEN-oh-seen) (Medco Research)
Use: Antineoplastic. [Orphan drug]

adenosine in gelatin. (Forest Pharmaceutical) **Forte:** Adenosine-5-monophosphate 50 mg/ml. **Super:** Adenosine-5-monophosphate 100 mg/ml. *Rx.*
Use: Varicosity.

•**adenosine phosphate.** (ah-DEN-oh-seen) USAN. Adenosine monophosphate, AMP.
Use: Nutritional supplement.
See: Cobalasine, Inj. (Keene Pharmaceuticals).

adenosine phosphate. (Various Mfr.) 25 mg/ml. May contain benzyl alcohol. 10 ml, 30 ml/Inj. *Rx.*
Use: Treatment of statis dermatitis.

adenovirus vaccine type 4. (Wyeth Ayerst) Adenovirus vaccine live type 4. At least 32,000 $TCID_{50}$ per Tab. Bot. 100s. *Rx.*
Use: Immunization.

adenovirus vaccine type 7. (Wyeth Ayerst) Adenovirus vaccine live type 7. At least 32,000 $TCID_{50}$ per Tab. Bot. 100s. *Rx.*
Use: Immunization.

adepsine oil.
See: Petrolatum Liquid (Various Mfr.).

AdGVCFTR 10. (GenVec)
Use: Cystic fibrosis. [Orphan drug]

•**adinazolam.** (AHD-in-AZE-oh-lam) USAN.
Use: Antidepressant, hypnotic, sedative.

•**adinazolam mesylate.** (AHD-in-AZE-oh-lam) USAN.
Use: Antidepressant.
See: Deracyn (Pharmacia & Upjohn).

Adipex-P. (Teva USA) **Cap.:** Phentermine HCl 37.5 mg. Bot. 100s, 400s. **Tab.:** Phentermine HCl 37.5 mg. Bot. 100s, 400s, 1000s. *c-IV.*
Use: Anorexiant.

•**adiphenine hydrochloride.** (ah-DIH-feh-neen) USAN.
Use: Muscle relaxant.

Adipost. (Jones Medical Industries) Phendimetrazine tartrate 105 mg/S.R. Cap. 100s. *c-III.*
Use: Anorexiant.

Adisol Tab. (Major) Disulfiram **250 mg/Tab:** Bot. 100s. **500 mg/Tab:** Bot. 50s. *Rx.*
Use: Antialcoholic.

Adlerika. (Last) Magnesium sulfate 4 g/15 ml. Bot. 12 oz. *otc.*
Use: Laxative.

Adlone. (Forest Pharmaceutical) Methylprednisolone acetate 40 mg, 80 mg/Inj. Vial 5 ml. *Rx.*
Use: Corticosteroid, topical.

Adolph's Salt Substitute. (Adolph's) Potassium Cl 2480 mg/5 g, silicon dioxide, tartaric acid. Gran. Bot. 99.2 g. *otc.*
Use: Salt substitute.

Adolph's Seasoned Salt Substitute. (Adolph's) Potassium Cl 1360 mg/5 g, silicon dioxide, tartaric acid. Gran. Bot. 92.1 g. *otc.*
Use: Salt substitute.

Adonidine. (City Chemical) Bot. g. *Rx.*
Use: Cardiovascular agent.

•**adozelesin.** (ADE-oh-ZELL-eh-sin) USAN.
Use: Antineoplastic.

Adprin-B. (Pfeiffer) Aspirin 325 mg w/calcium carbonate, magnesium carbonate, magnesium/Tab. Bot. 130s. *otc.*
Use: Analgesic.

Adprin-B, Extra Strength. (Pfeiffer) Aspirin 500 mg w/calcium carbonate, magnesium carbonate, magnesium oxide/Tab. Bot. 130s. *otc.*
Use: Analgesic.

ADR.
Use: Antineoplastic.
See: Doxorubicin HCl.

adrenalin(e).
See: Epinephrine. (Various Mfr.).

Adrenalin Chloride Solution. (Parke-Davis) Epinephrine HCl. Principle of the medullary portion of suprarenal glands. **Amp:** 1:1000-1 ml Epinephrine 1 mg/ml with not more than 0.1% sodium bisulfite as antioxidant. Amp. 10s. **Steri-Vial 1:1000:** Epinephrine 100 mg/ml in isotonic sodium Cl solution with 0.5% chlorobutanol as preservative and not more than 0.15% sodium bisulfite as antioxidant. Vial 30 ml. **Soln. 1:1000:** Bot. 30 ml. (Same as Steri-Vial). **Soln. 1:100:** Each 100 ml contains 1 g epinephrine HCl dissolved in sodium Cl citrate buffer soln w/

phemerol Cl 0.2 mg/ml as preservative, sodium bisulfite 0.2% as antioxidant. Bot. 0.25 oz. *Rx.*
Use: Sympathomimetic.

adrenaline hydrochloride.
See: Epinephrine Hydrochloride. (Various Mfr.)

•**adrenalone.** (ah-DREN-ah-lone) USAN.
Use: Adrenergic (ophthalmic).

adrenamine.
See: Epinephrine (Various Mfr.).

adrenergic agents.
See: Sympathomimetic agents.

adrenergic-blocking agents.
See: Sympatholytic agents.

adrenine.
See: Epinephrine (Various Mfr.).

adrenocorticotropic hormone. ACTH acts by stimulating the endogenous production of cortisone. *Rx.*
See: ACTH.
Corticotropin, U.S.P.

Adrenomist Inhalant and Nebulizers. (Nephron) Epinephrine 1%, Bot. 0.5 oz, 1.25 oz. *otc, Rx.*
Use: Bronchodilator.

Adrenucleo. (Enzyme Process) Vitamin C 250 mg, d-calcium pantothenate 12.5 mg, bioflavonoids 62.5 mg/Tab. Bot. 100s, 250s. *otc.*
Use: Vitamin supplement.

Adriamycin. (Pharmacia & Upjohn) Doxorubicin HCl 20 mg/vial. *Rx.*
Use: Antineoplastic.

Adriamycin PFS. (Pharmacia & Upjohn) Doxorubicin HCl 2 mg/ml. Inj. Vial: 5 ml, 10 ml, 25 ml. *Rx.*
Use: Antineoplastic.

Adriamycin RDF. (Pharmacia & Upjohn) Doxorubicin HCl. **10 mg:** Methylparaben 1 mg, lactose 50 mg/Vial. Pkg. 10s. **20 mg:** Methylparaben 2 mg, lactose 100 mg/Vial. Pkg. 5s. **50 mg:** Methylparaben 5 mg, lactose 250 mg/Vial. Ctn. 1s. **150 mg:** Methylparaben 15 mg, lactose 750 mg/multi-dose vial. Rapid dissolution formula. *Rx.*
Use: Antineoplastic.

Adrucil. (Pharmacia & Upjohn) Fluorouracil 50 mg/10 ml. Amp. 10 ml. *Rx.*
Use: Antineoplastic.

Adsorbocarpine. (Alcon Laboratories) Pilocarpine HCl 1%, 2% or 4%. Bot. 15 ml. *Rx.*
Use: Miotic.

Adsorbonac Ophth. Solution. (Alcon Laboratories) Sodium Cl 2% or 5%. Vial 15 ml. *otc.*
Use: Hyperosmolar preparation.

Adsorbotear. (Alcon Laboratories) Hydroxyethylcellulose 0.4%, povidone 1.67%, water-soluble polymers, thimerosal 0.004%, EDTA 0.1%. Soln. Bot. dropper 15 ml. *otc.*
Use: Artificial tears.

Advance. (Ross Laboratories) **Ready-to-Feed infant formula:** (16 cal/fl oz). Can 13 fl oz. **Conc. liq:** 32 fl oz. *otc.*
Use: Nutritional supplement.

Advance Pregnancy Test. (Advanced Care Products) Can be used as early as 3 days after a missed period. Gives results in 30 min. Test kit 1s.
Use: Diagnostic aid.

Advanced Care Cholesterol Test. (Johnson & Johnson Consumer Products)
Use: At home cholesterol test.

Advanced Formula Centrum Liquid. (ESI Lederle Generics) Vitamins A 2500 IU, E 30 IU, C 60 mg, B_1 1.5 mg, B_2 1.7 mg, B_3 20 mg, B_5 10 mg, B_6 2 mg, B_{12} 6 mcg, D 400 IU, iron 9 mg, biotin 300 mcg, I, Zn 3 mg, Mn, Cr, Mo, alcohol 6.7%, sucrose. Bot. 236 ml. *otc.*
Use: Mineral, vitamin supplement.

Advanced Formula Centrum Tablets. (ESI Lederle Generics) Iron 18 mg, vitamins A 5000 IU, D 400 IU, E 30 IU, B_1 1.5 mg, B_2 1.7 mg, B_3 20 mg, B_5 10 mg, B_6 2 mg, B_{12} 6 mcg, C 60 mg, folic acid 0.4 mg, biotin 30 mcg, B, Ca, Cl, Cr, Cu, I, K, Mg, Mn, Mo, Ni, P, Se, Si, Sn, V, Zn 15 mg, vitamin K/Tab. Bot. 60s, 130s, 200s. *otc.*
Use: Mineral, vitamin supplement.

Advanced Formula Oxy Sensitive. (SmithKline Beecham Pharmaceuticals) Benzoyl peroxide 2.5%, diazolidinyl urea, EDTA. Gel. 30 g. *otc.*
Use: Dermatologic, acne.

Advanced Formula Plax. (Pfizer) Tetrasodium pyrophosphate, alcohol, saccharin. Mouthwash. In 120 ml, 240 ml, 473 ml, 720 ml, 1740 ml. *otc.*
Use: Anti-infective.

Advanced Formula Tegrin. (Block Drug) Coal tar solution USP 7%, alcohol 7%, hydroxypropyl methylcellulose, parabens. Shampoo. Bot. 207 ml. *otc.*
Use: Antiseborrheic.

Advanced Formula Zenate. (Solvay) Vitamins A 4000 IU, D 400 IU, E 10 IU, C 70 mg, folic acid 1 mg, B_1 1.5 mg, B_2 1.6 mg, B_3 17 mg, B_6 2.2 mg, B_{12} 70 mg, Ca, I, Mg, Se, Zn 15 mg. Tab. Bot. 100s. *Rx.*
Use: Mineral, vitamin supplement.

Advantage 24. (Women's Health Institute) Nonoxynol-9 3.5%. Gel. 1.5 g (3s, 6s). *otc.*
Use: Contraceptive, spermicide.

Advera. Protein 14.2 g, fat 5.4 g, carbohydrate 51.2 g, l-carnitine 30 mg, taurine 50 mg, vitamins A 2550 IU, D 80 IU, E 9 IU, K 24 mcg, C 90 mg, folic acid 120 mcg, B_1 0.75 mg, B_2 0.68 mg, B_6 9.5 mg, B_{12} 12 mcg, niacin 6 mg, choline 50 mg, biotin 50 mcg, pantothenic acid 3 mg, sodium 250 mg, potassium 670 mg, chloride 350 mg, Ca 260 mg, P 260 mg, Mg 50 mg, I 30 mcg, Mn 1.3 mg, Cu 0.5 mg, Zn 2 mg, Fe 4.5 mg, Se 14 mcg, chromium 17 mcg, Md 54 mcg/240 ml. 1.28 calories/ml. Vanilla flavor. Bot. 273 ml. *otc.*
Use: Nutritional supplement-enteral.

Advil. (Whitehall Robins) Ibuprofen 200 mg, sucrose (Tab.), parabens (Capl.). In 8s, 24s, 50s, 100s, 165s, 250s (Tab.). *otc.*
Use: Analgesic, NSAID.

Advil, Children's. (Whitehall Robins) Ibuprofen Susp. 100 mg per 5 ml. Fruit flavor, sorbitol, sucrose, EDTA. Liq. Bot. 199 ml, 473 ml. *Rx.*
Use: Analgesic, NSAID.

Advil Cold & Sinus. (Whitehall Robins) Pseudoephedrine HCl 30 mg, ibuprofen 200 mg/Tab. Pkg. 20s. Bot. 40s, 75s. *otc.*
Use: Analgesic, decongestant.

A.E.R. (Birchwood) Hamamelis water (witch hazel) 50%, glycerin 12.5%, methylparaben, benzalkonium chloride. Pads. Jar 40s. *otc.*
Use: Dermatologic.

Aerdil. (Econo Med Pharmaceuticals) Triprolidine HCl 1.25 mg, pseudoephedrine HCl 30 mg/5 ml. Bot. pt, gal. *otc.*
Use: Antihistamine, decongestant.

Aeroaid. (Graham Field) Thimerosal 1:1000, alcohol 72%. Spray bot 90 ml.
Use: Antiseptic.

Aeroaid merthiolate. (Health & Medical Techniques) Merthiolate (Eli Lilly) 1:1000, alcohol 72%. Spray bot. 3 oz.
Use: Antiseptic.

AeroBid. (Forest Pharmaceutical) Flunisolide in an inhaler system ≈250 mcg/actuation. Canister 100 metered inhalations. *Rx.*
Use: Corticosteroid.

AeroBid M. (Forest Pharmaceutical) Flunisolide in an inhaler system ≈250 mcg/actuation. Canister 7 g, 100 metered inhalations. Menthol flavor. *Rx.*
Use: Corticosteroid.

AeroCaine. (Health & Medical Techniques) Benzocaine 13.6%, benzethonium Cl 0.5%. Spray bot. 0.5 oz, 2.5 oz. *otc.*
Use: Local anesthetic, topical.

Aerocell. (Health & Medical Techniques) Exfoliative cytology fixative spray. Bot. 3.5 oz.
Use: Exfoliative cytology fixative spray.

Aerodine. (Health & Medical Techniques) Povidone-iodine. Bot. 3 oz.
Use: Antiseptic.

Aerofreeze. (Graham Field) Trichloromonofluoromethane and dichlorodifluoromethane. 240 ml/Aerosol spray. Cont. 8 oz. (12s). *otc.*
Use: Anesthetic, local.

Aerolate-III. (Fleming) Theophylline 65 mg/T.D. Cap. Bot. 100s, 1000s. *Rx.*
Use: Bronchodilator.

Aerolate Sr. & Jr. (Fleming) **Cap.:** Theophylline 4 gr for Sr., 2 gr for Jr./Cap. Bot. 100s, 1000s. **Syr.:** 160 mg/15 ml. Bot. pt, gal. *Rx.*
Use: Bronchodilator.

Aeropin. Heparin, 2-0-desulfated.
Use: Cystic fibrosis. [Orphan drug]

Aeropure. (Health & Medical Techniques) Isopropanol 7.8%, triethylene glycol 3.9%, essential oils 3%, methyldodecyl benzyl trimethyl ammonium Cl 0.12%, methyldodecylxylene bis (trimethyl ammonium Cl) 0.03%, inert ingredients, 85.15%. Bot. 0.8 oz, 4.5 oz.
Use: Antiseptic, deodorant.

Aerosan. (Ulmer) Aerosol 16.6 oz.
Use: Antiseptic, deodorant.

Aeroseb-Dex. (Allergan) Dexamethasone 0.01%, alcohol 65.1%. Aerosol 58 g. *Rx.*
Use: Corticosteroid, topical.

Aerosil. (Health & Medical Techniques) Dimethylpolysiloxane. Bot. 4.5 oz.
Use: Lubricant, protectant.

aerosol ot.
See: Docusate Sodium, U.S.P.

aerosol talc, sterile. (Bryan Corp.)
Use: Malignant pleural effusion. [Orphan drug]

Aerosolv. (Health & Medical Techniques) Isopropyl alcohol, methylene Cl, silicone. Aerosol 5.5 oz.
Use: Adhesive remover.

Aerosporin Sterile Powder. (Glaxo-Wellcome) Polymyxin B sulfate 500,000 units/vial. Multidose vial 20 ml. *Rx.*
Use: Anti-infective.

AeroTherm. (Health & Medical Techniques) Benzethonium Cl 0.5%, benzo-

caine 13.6%. Spray bot. 5 oz. *otc.*
Use: Anesthetic, local.

AeroZoin. (Health & Medical Techniques) Comp. tr. of benzoin 30%, isopropyl alcohol 44.8%. Spray bot. 3.5 oz. *otc.*
Use: Dermatologic, protectant.

Afaxin Capsules. (Sanofi Winthrop) Vitamin A Palmitate 10,000 IU or 50,000 IU/Cap. *otc, Rx.*
Use: Vitamin supplement.

A-Fil. (GenDerm) Methyl anthranilate 5%, titanium dioxide 5% in vanishing cream base. Tube 45 g. Neutral or dark. *otc.*
Use: Sunscreen.

Afko-Lube. (APC) Docusate sodium 100 mg/Cap. Bot. 100s. *otc.*
Use: Laxative.

Afko-Lube Lax. (APC) Docusate sodium 100 mg, casanthranol 30 mg/Cap. Bot. 100s. *otc.*
Use: Laxative.

Afrikol. (Citroleum) Bot. 4 oz.
Use: Sunscreen.

Afrin. (Schering Plough) Oxymetazoline HCl 0.05%. **Nose Drops:** Drop. Bot. 20 ml. **Nasal Spray:** Reg.: Bot. 15 ml, 30 ml; Menthol: Bot. 15 ml. **Children's Nose Drops:** Oxymetazoline HCl 0.025%. Drop. Bot. 20 ml. *otc.*
Use: Decongestant.

Afrin Moisturizing Saline Mist. (Schering Plough) 0.64% sodium chloride, benzalkonium chloride, EDTA/Soln. Bot. 30 ml. *otc.*
Use: Decongestant.

Afrin Sinus. (Schering Plough) Oxymetazoline HCl 0.05%, benzyl alcohol. Spray. 15 ml. *otc.*
Use: Decongestant.

Afrinol Repetabs. (Schering Plough) Pseudoephedrine sulfate 120 mg/Repeat Action Tab. Box 12s. Bot. 100s, dispensary pack 48s. *otc.*
Use: Decongestant.

After Bite. (Tender) Ammonium hydroxide 3.5% in aqueous solution. Pen-like dispenser. *otc.*
Use: Analgesic; antipruritic, topical.

After Burn. (Tender) Lidocaine 0.5% in aloe vera 98% solution. *otc.*
Use: Anesthetic, local.

•**agar.** (AH-gahr) N.F. 18.
Use: Pharmaceutical aid (suspending agent).
W/Mineral oil.
See: Agoral, Emulsion (Parke-Davis). Petrogalar (Wyeth Ayerst).

Aggrastat. (Merck) Tirofiban HCl 250 mcg/ml, preservative free. Inj. for Soln. Vial 50 ml. Tirofiban 50 mcg/ml, preservative free. Inj. Single-dose *IntraVia* cont. 500 ml. *Rx.*
Use: Antiplatelet.

aglucerase injection. (Genzyme Corp)
Use: Treatment of Type II and III Gaucher's disease. [Orphan drug]

Agoral. (Parke-Davis) Phenolphthalein 0.2 g, mineral oil 4.2 g/15 ml in an emulsion containing agar, tragacanth, egg-albumin, acacia, glycerin. Raspberry flavor. Bot. 240 ml, 480 ml. *otc.*
Use: Laxative.

Agrylin. (Roberts Pharm) Anagrelide HCl 0.5 mg and 1 mg. Lactose/Cap. Bot. 100s. *Rx.*
Use: Thrombocythemia; polycythemia vera; essential thrombocythemia; thrombocytosis in chronic myelogenous leukemia. [Orphan drug]

A/G-Pro. (Miller) Protein hydrolysate 50 gr w/essential and nonessential amino acids 45%, l-lysine 300 mg, methionine 75 mg, Vitamins C, B_6, Fe, Cu, I, Mn, K, Zn, Mg/6 Tab. Bot. 180s. *otc.*
Use: Nutritional supplement.

agurin.
See: Theobromine Sodium Acetate (Various Mfr.).

AH-Chew. (WE Pharm) Chlorpheniramine maleate 2 mg, phenylephrine HCl 10 mg, methscopolamine nitrate 1.25 mg. Chew. tab. 100s. *Rx.*
Use: Antihistamine, decongestant.

AH-Chew D. (WE Pharm) Phenylephrine 10 mg/Tab. Chewable. Bot. 100s. *Rx.*
Use: Decongestant.

AHF.
See: Antihemophilic factor.

A-Hydrocort. (Abbott Hospital Prods) Hydrocortisone sodium succinate. 100 mg or 250 mg/2 ml Univial, with benzyl alcohol; 500 mg/4 ml Univial with benzyl alcohol; 1000 mg/8 ml Univial with benzyl alcohol. *Rx.*
Use: Corticosteroid.

AIDS vaccine. (MicroGeneSys/Genentech/Immuno AG/NIH/Wyeth Ayerst) Phase I-III AIDS, HIV prophylaxis and treatment. *Rx.*
Use: Immunization.

Airet. (Adams Labs) Albuterol sulfate 0.083%. Soln. for Inhalation. Vial. *Rx.*
Use: Bronchodilator.

•**air, medical.** U.S.P. 23.
Use: Gas, medicinal.

AI-RSA. (Autoimmune, Inc.)
Use: Autoimmune uveitis. [Orphan drug]

air & surface disinfectant. (Health &

Medical Techniques) Aerosol 16 oz.
Use: Antiseptic, deodorant.

Akarpine. (Akorn) Pilocarpine HCl 1%, 2% or 4%. Soln. Bot. 15 ml. *Rx.*
Use: Miotic.

AKBeta. (Akorn) Levobunolol HCl 0.25%. Ophthalmic Soln. 5 ml, 10 ml. Levobunolol HCl 0.5%. Soln. Bot. 5 ml, 10 ml, 15 ml. *Rx.*
Use: Antiglaucoma.

AK-Chlor. (Akorn) **Oint.:** Chloramphenicol 10 mg/g. Tube 3.5 g. **Soln.:** Chloramphenicol 5 mg/ml. Bot. 7.5 ml, 15 ml. *Rx.*
Use: Anti-infective, ophthalmic.

AK-Cide. (Akorn) **Susp.:** Prednisolone acetate 0.5%, sulfacetamide sodium 10%. Dropper bot. 5 ml. **Oint.:** Prednisolone acetate 0.5%, sodium sulfacetamide 10%. Tube 3.5 g. *Rx.*
Use: Anti-infective; corticosteroid, ophthalmic.

AK-Con. (Akorn) Naphazoline HCl 0.1%. Soln. Bot. 15 ml. *Rx.*
Use: Mydriatic, vasoconstrictor.

AK-Con-A. (Akorn) Naphazoline HCl 0.025%, pheniramine maleate 0.3%, benzalkonium Cl 0.01%, EDTA. Soln. Bot. 15 ml. *Rx.*
Use: Antihistamine; decongestant, ophthalmic.

AK-Dex. (Akorn) Dexamethasone phosphate (as sodium phosphate). **Oint.:** 0.05%. Tube 3.5 g. **Soln.:** 0.1%. Bot 5 ml. *Rx.*
Use: Corticosteroid, ophthalmic.

AK-Dilate. (Akorn) Phenylephrine HCl 2.5% or 10%. Bot. 2 ml, 5 ml (10%), 15 ml (2.5%). *Rx.*
Use: Mydriatic, vasoconstrictor.

AK-Fluor. (Akorn) Fluorescein sodium. **10%:** Amp. 5 ml, Vial 5 ml; **25%:** Amp. 2 ml, Vial 2 ml.
Use: Diagnostic aid, ophthalmic.

Akineton. (Knoll Pharmaceuticals) Biperiden HCl 2 mg/Tab. Bot. 100s, 1000s. *Rx.*
Use: Antiparkinsonian.

Akineton Lactate. (Knoll Pharmaceuticals) Biperiden lactate 5 mg in aqueous 1.4% sodium lactate soln/ml. Amp 1 ml, Box 10s. *Rx.*
Use: Antiparkinsonian.

AK-Mycin. (Akorn) Erythromycin 5 mg/g with white petrolatum, mineral oil. Oint. Tube 3.75 g. *Rx.*
Use: Anti-infective, ophthalmic.

AK-NaCl. (Akorn) **Oint.:** Sodium Cl hypertonic 5%. Tube 3.5 g. **Soln.:** Sodium Cl, hypertonic 5%. Bot. 15 ml. *otc.*
Use: Ophthalmic.

Akne Drying Lotion. (Alto Pharmaceuticals) Zinc oxide 12%, urea 10%, sulfur 6%, salicylic acid 2%, benzalkonium Cl 0.2%, isopropyl alcohol 70%, in a base containing menthol, silicon dioxide, iron oxide, perfume. Bot. ¾ oz, 2.25 oz. *otc.*
Use: Dermatologic, acne.

AK-Nefrin. (Akorn) Phenylephrine HCl. Soln. Bot. 15 ml. *otc.*
Use: Mydriatic, vasoconstrictor.

Akne-Mycin. (Hermal) Erythromycin. **Oint.:** 2%. Tube 25 g. **Soln.:** 2%. Bot. 60 ml. *Rx.*
Use: Dermatologic, acne.

AK-Neo-Dex. (Akorn) Dexamethasone sodium phosphate 0.1% and neomycin sulfate 0.35%. Ophth. Soln. 5 ml. *Rx.*
Use: Anti-infective; corticosteroid, ophthalmic.

Akne Scrub. (Alto Pharmaceuticals) Povidone iodine with polyethylene granules. Bot. ¾ oz. *otc.*
Use: Dermatologic, acne.

AK-Pentolate. (Akorn) Cyclopentolate HCl 1%, benzalkonium Cl 0.01%, EDTA. Soln. Bot. 2 ml, 15 ml. *Rx.*
Use: Cycloplegic, mydriatic.

AK-Poly-Bac. (Akorn) Polymyxin B sulfate 10,000 units, bacitracin zinc 500 units/g. Oint. Tube 3.5 g. *Rx.*
Use: Anti-infective, ophthalmic.

AK-Pred. (Akorn) Prednisolone sodium phosphate 0.125% or 1%. **0.125%:** Soln. Bot. 5 ml. **0.1%:** Soln. Bot. 5 ml, 15 ml. *Rx.*
Use: Corticosteroid, ophthalmic.

AKPro. (Akorn) Dipivefrin HCl 0.1%. Liq. 2, 5, 10, 15 ml. Liq. *Rx.*
Use: Antiglaucoma agent.

AK-Ramycin. (Akorn) Doxycycline hyclate 100 mg/Cap. Bot. 50s, 100s, 200s, 250s, 500s, UD 100s. *Rx.*
Use: Anti-infective, tetracycline.

AK-Ratabs. (Akorn) Doxycycline hyclate 100 mg/Tab. Bot. 50s. *Rx.*
Use: Anti-infective, tetracycline.

Akrinol. (Schering Plough) Acrisorcin.
Use: Antifungal.

AK-Rinse. (Akorn) Sodium carbonate, potassium Cl, boric acid, EDTA, benzalkonium Cl 0.01%. Soln. Bot. 30 ml, 118 ml. *otc.*
Use: Irrigant, ophthalmic.

AK-Spore. (Akorn) **Oint.:** Polymyxin B sulfate 10,000 units, neomycin (as sulfate) 3.5 mg, bacitracin zinc 400 units/

g. Tube 3.5 g. **Soln.:** Polymyxin B sulfate 10,000 units, neomycin sulfate 1.75 mg, gramicidin 0.025 mg/ml. Soln. Dropper bot. 2 ml, 10 ml. *Rx.*
Use: Anti-infective, ophthalmic.

AK-Spore H.C. ophthalmic. (Akorn) **Susp.:** Hydrocortisone 1%, neomycin sulfate 0.35%, polymyxin B sulfate 10,000 units. Soln. Bot. 7.5 ml. **Oint.:** Hydrocortisone 1%, neomycin sulfate 0.35%, bacitracin zinc 400 units, polymyxin B sulfate 10,000 units. Tube 3.5 g. *Rx.*
Use: Corticosteroid, anti-infective.

AK-Spore H.C. Otic. (Akorn) **Susp.:** Hydrocortisone 1%, neomycin sulfate 5 mg, polymyxin B sulfate 10,000 units/ ml. Bot. w/dropper 10 ml. **Soln.:** Hydrocortisone 1%, neomycin sulfate 5 mg, polymyxin B sulfate 10,000 units/ml. Bot. w/dropper 10 ml. *Rx.*
Use: Corticosteroid, anti-infective.

AK-Sulf. (Akorn) **Soln.:** Sodium sulfacetamide 10%. Dropper Bot. 2 ml, 5 ml, 15 ml; **Oint.:** Sodium sulfacetamide 10%. Tube 3.5 g. *Rx.*
Use: Anti-infective, ophthalmic.

AK-Taine. (Akorn) Proparacaine HCl 0.5%, glycerin, chlorobutanol, benzalkonium Cl. Dropper bot. 2 ml, 15 ml. *Rx.*
Use: Anesthetic, ophthalmic.

AK-Tate. (Akorn) Prednisolone acetate 1%, benzalkonium Cl, EDTA, polysorbate 80, polyvinyl alcohol, hydroxyethyl cellulose. Susp. Dropper bot. 5 ml, 10 ml, 15 ml. *Rx.*
Use: Corticosteroid, ophthalmic.

AKTob. (Akorn)Tobramycin 0.3%. Soln. Bot. 5 ml. *Rx.*
Use: Anti-infective, ophthalmic.

AK-Tracin. (Akorn) Bacitracin 500 units/ g. Oint. Tube 3.5 g. *Rx.*
Use: Anti-infective, ophthalmic.

AK-Trol. (Akorn) **Susp.:** Dexamethasone 0.1%, neomycin sulfate equivalent to 0.35% neomycin base, polymyxin B sulfate 10,000 units. Bot. 5 ml. **Oint.:** Dexamethasone 0.1%, neomycin sulfate equivalent to 0.35% neomycin base, polymyxin B sulfate 10,000 units. Tube 3.5 g. *Rx.*
Use: Anti-infective; corticosteroid, ophthalmic.

Akwa Tears. (Akorn) **Soln.:** Polyvinyl alcohol 1.4%, sodium Cl, sodium phosphate, benzalkonium Cl 0.01%, EDTA. Bot. 15 ml. **Oint.:** White petrolatum, mineral oil, lanolin. Tube 3.5 g. *otc.*
Use: Artificial tears.

AL-721. (Matrix Pharm) Phase I/II AIDS, ARC, HIV positive.
Use: Antiviral.

Ala-Bath. (Del-Ray) Bath oil. Bot. 8 oz. *otc.*
Use: Emollient.

Ala-Cort. (Del-Ray) Hydrocortisone 1%. **Cream:** Tube 1 oz, 3 oz. **Lot.:** Bot. 4 oz. *Rx.*
Use: Corticosteroid, topical.

Ala-Derm. (Del-Ray) Lot. Bot 8 oz, 12 oz.
Use: Emollient.

Aladrine. (Scherer) Ephedrine sulfate 8.1 mg, secobarbital sodium 16.2 mg/Tab. Bot. 100s. *c-II.*
Use: Decongestant, hypnotic, sedative.

Alamag. (Alphalma USPD) Magnesium-aluminum hydroxide gel. Susp. Bot. Pt. *otc.*
Use: Antacid.

W/Belladonna alkaloid. Susp. Bot. 8 oz.

Alamag Suspension. (Zenith Goldline) Aluminum hydroxide 225 mg, magnesium hydroxide 200 mg, sorbitol, sucrose, parabens. Bot. 355 ml. *otc.*
Use: Antacid.

Alamag Plus Antacid. (Zenith Goldline) Magnesium hydroxide 200 mg, aluminum hydroxide 225 mg, simethicone 25 mg/5 ml. Bot. 355 ml. *otc.*
Use: Antacid.

•**alamecin.** (al-ah-MEE-sin) USAN.
Use: Anti-infective.

•**alanine.** (AL-ah-NEEN) U.S.P. 23.
Use: Amino acid.

•**alaproclate.** (AL-ah-PRO-klate) USAN.
Use: Antidepressant.

Ala-Quin 0.5%. (Del-Ray) Hydrocortisone, iodochlorhydroxyquinoline cream. Tube 1 oz. *otc, Rx.*
Use: Corticosteroid, topical.

Ala-Scalp HP 2%. (Del-Ray) Hydrocortisone lotion. Bot. 1 oz. *Rx.*
Use: Corticosteroid, topical.

Ala-Seb Shampoo. (Del-Ray) Bot. 4 oz, 12 oz. *otc.*
Use: Antiseborrheic.

Ala-Seb T Shampoo. (Del-Ray) Bot. 4 oz, 12 oz. *otc.*
Use: Antiseborrheic.

Alasulf. (Major) Sulfanilamide 15%, aminacrine HCl 0.2%, allantoin 2%. Vaginal Cream Tube w/applicator 120 g. *Rx.*
Use: Anti-infective, vaginal.

Alatone. (Major) Spironolactone 25 mg/ Tab. Bot. 100s, 250s, 500s, 1000s, UD 100s. *Rx.*

Use: Antihypertensive.

•**alatrofloxacin mesylate.** (al-at-row-FLOX-ah-sin) USAN.
Use: Anti-infective.
See: Trovan, Inj. (Pfizer).

Alaxin. (Delta) Oxyethlene oxypropylene polymer 240 mg/Cap. Bot. 100s. *otc.*
Use: Laxative.

Al-Ay. (Jones Medical Industries) *otc.* **Green Oblong Tube:** Phenylephrine HCl 5 mg, chlorpheniramine maleate 2 mg, aspirin 162 mg, caffeine 15 mg, aminoacetic acid 162 mg/Tab. Bot. 100s, 1000s. **Dark Green S.C:** Phenylephrine HCl 5 mg, chlorpheniramine maleate 2 mg, acetaminophen 160 mg, caffeine 15 mg/Tab. Bot. 100s, 1000s. *otc.*
Use: Analgesic, antihistamine, decongestant.

alazanine trichlorphate. *Rx.*
Use: Anthelmintic.

Alazide Tabs. (Major) Spironolactone w/ hydrochlorothiazide. Bot. 250s, 1000s. *Rx.*
Use: Antihypertensive, diuretic.

Alazine Tabs. (Major) Hydralazine 10 mg, 25 mg or 50 mg/Cap. Bot. 100s, 1000s. *Rx.*
Use: Antihypertensive.

Albalon. (Allergan) Naphazoline HCl 0.1%. Bot. 15 ml. *Rx.*
Use: Vasoconstrictor, ophthalmic.

Albamycin. (Pharmacia & Upjohn) Novobiocin sodium 250 mg/Cap. Bot. 100s. *Rx.*
Use: Anti-infective.

Albay. (Bayer Corp) Freeze-dried venom and venom protein. Vials of 550 mcg for each of honey bee, white-faced hornet, yellow hornet, yellow jacket or wasp. Vials of 1,650 mcg for mixed vespids (white-faced hornet, yellow hornet, yellow jacket). 10 ml/Inj. *Rx.*
Use: Antivenin

•**albendazole.** (AL-BEND-ah-zole) U.S.P. 23.
Use: Anthelmintic.
See: Zentel (SmithKline Beecham Pharmaceuticals).

albendazole. (SmithKline Beecham Pharmaceuticals) 200 mg/Tab. Bot. 112s. *Rx.*
Use: Anthelmintic. Hydatid disease. [Orphan drug]
See: Albenza, Tab. (SmithKline Beecham Pharmaceuticals).

Albenza. (SmithKline Beecham Pharmaceuticals) Albendazole 200 mg/Tab. Bot. 112s. *Rx.*
Use: Anthelmintic. Hydatid disease. [Orphan drug]

Albolene Cream. (SmithKline Beecham Pharmaceuticals) Unscented or scented. Jar 6 oz, 12 oz.

Albuconn 25% Solution. (Cryosan) Normal serum albumin (human) 12.5 g in 50 ml solution for IV administration. Vial 50 ml. *Rx.*
Use: Treatment of plasma or blood volume deficit, acute hypoproteinemia, oncotic deficit.

•**albumin, aggregated.** (al-BYOO-min AGG-reh-GAY-tuhd) USAN.
Use: Diagnostic aid (lung-imaging).
See: Technescan MAA.

•**albumin, aggregated iodinated I 131 injection.** (al-BYOO-min AGG-reh-GAY-tuhd) U.S.P. 23.
Use: Radiopharmaceutical.

•**albumin, aggregated iodinated I 131 serum.** (al-BYOO-min AGG-reh-GAY-tuhd) USAN. Blood serum aggregates of albumin labeled with iodine-131.
Use: Radiopharmaceutical.
See: Albumotope-LS (Squibb).

•**albumin, chromated cr 51 serum.** USAN. Blood serum albumin labeled with chromium-51.
Use: Radiopharmaceutical.
See: Chromalbin (Bristol-Myers Squibb).

•**albumin human.** (al-BYOO-MIN human) U.S.P. 23. *Formerly Albumin, Normal Human Serum.*
Use: Plasma protein fraction; blood volume supporter.
See: Albunex, Inj. (Mallinckrodt).
Albutein 5%, Inj. (Alpha Therapeutics).
Albutein 25%, Inj. (Alpha Therapeutics).
Buminate, Soln. (Baxter).
Plasbumin-5 (Bayer Corp).
Plasbumin-25 (Bayer Corp).
Proserum 5, Inj. (Hoechst Marion Roussel).

albumin human, 5%. (al-BYOO-MIN human) (Immuno-U.S.) Normal serum albumin 5%. Inj. Vial 250 ml. *Rx.*
Use: Plasma protein fraction.
See: Albuminar-5, Inj. (Centeon).
Albutein 5%, Inj. (Alpha Therapeutics).
Buminate 5%, Inj. (Baxter).
Plasbumin-5, Inj. (Bayer Corp).

albumin human, 25%. (al-BYOO-MIN human) (Immuno-U.S.) Normal serum albumin 25%. Inj. Vial 10 ml, 50 ml. *Rx.*
Use: Plasma protein fraction.

See: Albuminar-25, Inj. (Centeon).
Albutein 25%, Inj. (Alliance Therapeutic).
Buminate 25%, Inj. (Baxter).
Plasbumin-25, Inj. (Bayer Corp).

•**albumin, iodinated I 125 injection.** U.S.P. 23. Albumin labeled with iodine-125.
Use: Diagnostic aid (blood volume determination); radiopharmaceutical.

•**albumin, iodinated I 125 serum.** USAN. U.S.P. XIX.
Use: Diagnostic aid (blood volume determination); radiopharmaceutical.

•**albumin, iodinated I 131 injection.** U.S.P. 23. Albumin labeled with iodine-131. Inj.
Use: Diagnostic aid (blood volume determination; intrathecal imaging); radiopharmaceutical.

albumin, iodinated I 131 serum. USAN. U.S.P. XIX.
Use: Diagnostic aid (Blood volume determination, intrathecal imaging); radioactive agent.

albumin, normal serum 5%. (Immuno-U.S.) Albumin human 5%. Inj. vial 120 ml. *Rx.*
Use: Plasma protein fraction.

albumin, normal serum 25%. (Immuno-U.S.) Albumin human 25%. Inj. vial 10 ml, 50 ml. *Rx.*
Use: Plasma protein fraction.

albumin-saline diluent. (Bayer Corp) Dilute allergenic extracts and venom products for patient testing and treating. Pre-measured vials 1.8 ml, 4 ml, 4.5 ml, 9 ml, 30 ml. Vial 2 ml, 5 ml, 10 ml, 30 ml.
Use: Pharmaceutical necessity, diluent.

Albuminar-5 and Albuminar-25. (Centeon) Albumin, (human) U.S.P. 5%: solution with administration set. Bot. 50 ml, 250 ml, 500 ml, 1000 ml. 25%: solution. Vial 20 ml, 50 ml, 100 ml with administration set. *Rx.*
Use: Plasma protein fraction.

Albumotope I-131. (Bristol-Myers Squibb) Albumin, Iodinated I-131 Serum (50 uCi).
Use: Diagnostic aid.

Albunex. (Mallinckrodt) Albumin (human) 5%, sonicated. Sodium acetyl tryptophanate 0.08 mmol, sodium caprylate 0.08 mmol/g albumin. Vial. 5 ml, 10 ml, 20 ml. 6s. *Rx.*
Use: Plasma protein fraction.

Albustix Reagent Strips. (Bayer Corp) Firm paper reagent strips impregnated with tetrabromphenol blue, citrate buffer and a protein-adsorbing agent. Bot. 50s, 100s.
Use: Diagnostic aid.

Albutein 5%. (Alpha Therapeutics) Normal serum albumin 5%. Inj. Vial w/IV set: 250 ml, 500 ml. *Rx.*
Use: Plasma protein fraction.

Albutein 25%. (Alpha Therapeutics) Normal serum albumin 25%. Inj. Vial w/IV set: 50 ml. *Rx.*
Use: Plasma protein fraction.

•**albuterol.** (al-BYOO-ter-ahl) U.S.P 23.
Use: Bronchodilator.
See: Proventil Inhaler (Schering Plough)
Ventolin, Inh. Aerosol (Glaxo-Wellcome).

albuterol inhalation aerosol. (Various Mfr.) Albuterol 90 mcg per actuation. 17 g (200 inhalations). *Rx.*
Use: Bronchodilator.

•**albuterol sulfate.** (al-BYOO-teh-rahl) U.S.P. 23.
Use: Bronchodilator.
See: Airet, Inhalation soln. (Adams Labs).
Proventil, Repetabs, Tab., Soln., Syr. (Schering Plough).
Ventolin, Inhalation Soln., Syr., Tab., Nebules (GlaxoWellcome).
Ventolin Rotacaps (GlaxoWellcome).
Volmax, ER Tab. (Muro).

albuterol sulfate and ipratropium bromide. (al-BYOO-ter-ahl and IH-pruh-TROE-pee-uhm)
Use: Chronic obstructive pulmonary disease (COPD).
See: Combivent, Aerosol (Boehringer Ingelheim).

albuterol tablets.
Use: Bronchodilator.

•**albutoin.** (al-BYOO-toe-in) USAN.
Use: Anticonvulsant.

Alcaine. (Alcon Laboratories) Proparacaine HCl 0.5%, glycerin, sodium Cl, benzalkonium Cl. Bot. 15 ml. *Rx.*
Use: Anesthetic, ophthalmic.

Alcare. (SmithKline Beecham Pharmaceuticals) Ethyl alcohol 62%. Foam Bot. 210 ml, 300 ml, 600 ml. *otc.*
Use: Antiseptic.

Alclear Eye Lotion. (Walgreens) Sterile isotonic fluid. Bot. 8 oz. *otc.*
Use: Anti-irritant, ophthalmic.

•**alclofenac.** (al-KLOE-feh-nak) USAN.
Use: Analgesic, anti-inflammatory.
See: Mervan (Continental Pharma, Belgium).

•**alclometasone dipropionate.** (al-kloe-MEH-tah-zone die-PRO-pee-oh-nate) U.S.P. 23.
Use: Anti-inflammatory, topical.
See: Aclovate, Cream, Oint. (Glaxo-Wellcome).

•**alcloxa.** (al-KLOX-ah) USAN.
Use: Astringent, keratolytic.

Alco-Gel. (Tweezerman) Ethyl alcohol 60%. Tube 60 g, 480 g. *otc.*
Use: Dermatologic, cleanser.

•**alcohol.** U.S.P. 23. Ethanol, ethyl alcohol.
Use: Anti-infective, topical; pharmaceutic aid (solvent).
See: Anbesol, Gel, Liq. (Whitehall Robins)
Anbesol Maximum Strength, Gel. Liq. (Whitehall Robins).
Ru-Tuss Expectorant (Knoll Pharmaceuticals). Ru-Tuss w/ Hydrocodone (Knoll Pharmaceuticals).
Ru-Tuss Liquid (Knoll Pharmaceuticals).

alcohol, dehydrated.
Use: Solvent, vehicle.

•**alcohol, diluted.** N.F. 18.
Use: Pharmaceutic aid (solvent).

•**alcohol, rubbing.** U.S.P. 23.
Use: Rubefacient.
See: Lavacol (Parke-Davis).

Alcohol 5% and Dextrose 5%. (Abbott Hospital Prods) Alcohol 5 ml, dextrose 5 g/100 ml. Bot. 1000 ml. *Rx.*
Use: Nutritional supplement, parenteral.

Alcojet. (Alconox) Biodegradable machine washing detergent and wetting agent. Ctn. 9 × 4 lb, 25 lb, 50 lb, 100 lb, 300 lb. *otc.*
Use: Detergent, wetting agent.

Alcolec. (American Lecithin) Lecithin w/ choline base, cephalin, lipositol. Cap. 100s. Gran. 8 oz, lb. *otc.*
Use: Nutritional supplement.

Alconefrin 12 and 50. (PolyMedica) Phenylephrine HCl 0.16% w/benzalkonium Cl. Dropper bot. 30 ml. *otc.*
Use: Decongestant.

Alconefrin 25. (PolyMedica) Phenylephrine HCl 0.25% w/benzalkonium Cl. Dropper bot. 30 ml. Spray Pkg. 30 ml. *otc.*
Use: Decongestant.

Alcon Enzymatic Cleaning Tablets for Extended Wear. (Alcon Lenscare) Pancreatin tablets. Pkg. 12s. *otc.*
Use: Contact lens care.

Alcon Lens Case. (Alcon Lenscare) Two lens cases. Ctn. 12s. *otc.*
Use: Contact lens care.

Alcon Opti-Pure Sterile Saline Solution. (Alcon Lenscare) Sterile unpreserved saline solution. Aerosol 8 oz. *otc.*
Use: Contact lens care.

Alcon Saline Solution for Sensitive Eyes. (Alcon Lenscare) Sodium Cl, edetate disodium, borate buffer system, sorbic acid. Bot. 360 ml. *otc.*
Use: Contact lens care.

Alconox. (Alconox) Biodegradable detergent and wetting agent. Box 4 lb, Container 25 lb, 50 lb, 100 lb, 300 lb. *otc.*
Use: Contact lens care, detergent; wetting agent.

Alcotabs. (Alconox) Tab. Box 6s, 100s.
Use: Cleanser.

•**alcuronium chloride.** (al-cure-OH-nee-uhm) USAN. Diallyldinortoxiferin dichloride.
Use: Muscle relaxant.
See: Alloferin (Roche Laboratories).

Aldactazide Tablets. (Searle) Spironolactone and hydrochlorothiazide. **25 mg/25 mg:** Bot. 100s, 500s, 1000s, 2500s, UD 100s. **50 mg/50 mg:** Bot. 100s, UD 32s, UD 100s. *Rx.*
Use: Antihypertensive, diuretic.

Aldactone Tablets. (Searle) Spironolactone. **25 mg/Tab.:** Bot. 100s, 500s, 1000s, UD 100s. **50 mg/Tab.:** Bot. 100s, UD 100s. **100 mg/Tab.:** Bot. 100s, UD 100s. *Rx.*
Use: Antihypertensive.

Aldara. (3M Pharm) Imiquimod 5%/ Cream Box. 12s. (In 250 mg single-use packets.) *Rx.*
Use: Treatment of external gential and perianal warts/condyloma.

•**aldesleukin.** (al-dess-LOO-kin) USAN. Recombinant form of interleukin-2.
Use: Biological response modifier; antineoplastic; immunostimulant.
See: Proleukin, Pow for Inj. (Chiron Therapeutics).

aldesleukin. (al-dess-LOO-kin)
Use: Metastatic renal cell carcinoma/ melanoma; primary immunodeficiency disease associated with T-cell defects.
See: Proleukin, Pow. for Inj. (Chiron).

aldinamide.

•**aldioxa.** (al-DIE-ox-ah) USAN. Aluminum dihydroxy allantoinate.
Use: Astringent, keratolytic.

Aldoclor 150. (Merck) Methyldopa 250 mg, chlorothiazide 150 mg/Tab. Bot. 100s. *Rx.*
Use: Antihypertensive.

Aldoclor 250. (Merck) Methyldopa 250 mg, chlorothiazide 250 mg/Tab. Bot. 100s. *Rx.*
Use: Antihypertensive.

Aldomet. (Merck) Methyldopa. **125 mg/Tab.:** Bot. 100s. **250 mg/Tab.:** Bot. 100s, 1000s, UD 100s, Unit-of-use 100s. **500 mg/Tab.:** Bot. 100s, 500s, UD 100s, Unit-of-use 60s, 100s. *Rx.*
Use: Antihypertensive.
W/Chlorothiazide.
See: Aldoclor, Tab. (Merck).
W/Hydrochlorothiazide.
See: Aldoril, Tab. (Merck).

Aldomet Ester Hydrochloride. (Merck) Methyldopate HCl 250 mg/5 ml, citric acid anhydrous 25 mg, sodium bisulfite 16 mg, disodium edetate 2.5 mg, monothioglycerol 10 mg, sodium hydroxide to adjust pH, methylparaben 0.15%, propylparaben 0.02% w/water for inj. q.s. to 5 ml. Vial 5 ml. *Rx.*
Use: Antihypertensive.

Aldomet Oral Suspension. (Merck) Methyldopa 250 mg/5 ml, alcohol 1%, benzoic acid 0.1%, sodium bisulfite 0.2%. Bot. 473 ml. *Rx.*
Use: Antihypertensive.

Aldoril-15. (Merck) Methyldopa 250 mg, hydrochlorothiazide 15 mg/Tab. Bot. 100s, 1000s. *Rx.*
Use: Antihypertensive.

Aldoril-25. (Merck) Methyldopa 250 mg, hydrochlorothiazide 25 mg/Tab. Bot. 100s, 1000s, UD 100s. *Rx.*
Use: Antihypertensive.

Aldoril D30 & D50. (Merck) Methyldopa 500 mg, hydrochlorothiazide 30 mg or 50 mg. Tab. Bot. 100s. *Rx.*
Use: Antihypertensive.

Aldosterone RIA Diagnostic Kit. (Abbott Diagnostics) Test kits 50s.
Use: Diagnostic aid.

ALEC. (Forum Products) Dipalmitoylphosphatidylcholine/phosphatidylglycerol.
Use: Neonatal respiratory distress syndrome. [Orphan drug]

•**alendronate sodium.** (al-LEN-droe-nate) USAN.
Use: Bone resorption inhibitor.
See: Fosamax, Tab. (Merck).

Alenic Alka Liquid. (Rugby) Aluminum hydroxide 31.7 mg, magnesium carbonate 137.3 mg, sodium alginate, EDTA, sodium 13 mg. Bot. 355 ml. *otc.*
Use: Antacid.

Alenic Alka Tablets. (Rugby) Aluminum Hydroxide 80 mg, magnesium trisilicate 20 mg, sodium bicarbonate, calcium stearate, sugar. Chew Tab. Bot. 100s. *otc.*
Use: Antacid.

Alenic Alka Tablets, Extra Strength. (Rugby) Aluminum hydroxide 160 mg, magnesium carbonate 105 mg, sodium 29.9 mg. Chew. Tab. Bot. 100s. *otc.*
Use: Antacid.

•**alentemol hydrobromide.** (al-EN-teh-mole) USAN
Use: Antipsychotic; dopamine agonist.

Alersule Capsules. (Misemer) Chlorpheniramine maleate 8 mg, phenylephrine HCl 20 mg/Cap. Bot. 100s. *otc, Rx.*
Use: Antihistamine, decongestant.

Alert-Pep. (Health for Life Brands) Caffeine 200 mg/Cap. Bot. 16s. *otc.*
Use: CNS stimulant.

Alesse-21. (Wyeth-Ayerst) Levonorgestrel 0.1 mg, ethinyl estradiol 0.02 mg, lactose/Tab. 21s. *Rx.*
Use: Contraceptive.

Alesse-28. (Wyeth-Ayerst) Levonorgestrel 0.1 mg, ethinyl estradiol 0.02 mg, lactose/Tab. 21s. Lactose/Inactive Tab. 7s. *Rx.*
Use: Contraceptive.

•**aletamine hydrochloride.** (al-ETT-ah-meen) USAN.
Use: Antidepressant.

Aleve. (Procter & Gamble) Naproxen sodium 220 mg (naproxen base 200 mg with sodium 20 mg) Tab. Bot. 24s, 50s, 100s. *otc.*
Use: NSAID.

•**alexidine.** (ah-LEX-ih-DEEN) USAN.
Use: Anti-infective.

alfa interferon-2a.
See: Roferon A (Roche Laboratories).

alfa interferon-2b.
See: Intron A (Schering Plough).

alfa interferon-n3.
See: Alferon N (Purdue Frederick).

Alfenta. (Janssen) Alfentanil 0.5 mg/ml. Amp. 2 ml, 5 ml, 10 ml, 20 ml. *c-II.*
Use: Analgesic, anesthetic-narcotic.

•**alfentanil hydrochloride.** (al-FEN-tuh-NILL) USAN.
Use: Analgesic, anesthetic-narcotic.
See: Alfenta, Inj. (Janssen).

•**alfuzosin hydrochloride.** (al-FEW-zoe-sin) USAN.
Use: Antihypertensive (α-blocker).

Algel. (Faraday) Magnesium trisilicate 0.5 g, aluminum hydroxide 0.25 g/Tab. Bot. 100s. Susp. Bot. gal. *otc.*
Use: Antacid.

•**algeldrate.** (AL-jell-drate) USAN.
Use: Antacid.

Algemin. (Thurston) Macrocystis pyrifera alga. Pow. Jar 8 oz. Tab. Bot. 300s. *otc.*
Use: Dietary aid.

Algenic Alka Improved Tablets. (Rugby) Aluminum hydroxide 240 mg, magnesium hydroxide 100 mg/Chew. tab. Bot. 100s, 500s. *otc.*
Use: Antacid.

Algenic Alka Liquid. (Rugby) Aluminum hydroxide 31.7 mg/ml, magnesium carbonate 137 mg/ml, sodium alginate, sorbitol. Bot. 355 ml. *otc.*
Use: Antacid.

•**algestone acetonide.** (al-JESS-tone ah-SEE-toe-nide) USAN.
Use: Anti-inflammatory.

•**algestone acetophenide.** (al-JESS-tone ah-SEE-toe-FEN-ide) USAN.
Use: Hormone, progestin.

Algex liniment. (Health for Life Brands) Menthol, camphor, methylsalicylate, eucalyptus. Bot. 4 oz. *otc.*
Use: Analgesic, topical.

algin.
See: Sodium Alginate, N.F. 18.

Algin-All. (Barth's) Sodium alginate from kelp. Tab. Bot. 100s, 500s.

•**alginic acid.** (al-JIN-ik) N.F. 18.
Use: Pharmaceutic aid (tablet binder, emulsifying agent).

alginic acid.
W/Aluminum hydroxide dried gel, magnesium trisilicate, sodium bicarbonate. *otc.*
Use: Antacid.
See: Gaviscon Foamtabs (Hoechst Marion Roussel).

alginic acid combinations. (al-JIN-ik)
See: Pretts Diet-Aid, Chew. Tab. (Mi-Lance).

•**alglucerase.** (al-GLUE-ser-ACE) USAN.
Formerly Macrophage-targeted β-glucocerebrosidase.
Use: Enzyme replenisher (glucocerebrosidase). [Orphan drug]
See: Ceredase, Inj. (Genzyme).

alglucerase. (al-GLUE-ser-ACE) Inj.
Use: Replacement therapy in Gaucher's disease type I, II, III. [Orphan drug]
See: Ceredase, Inj. (Genzyme).

alidine dihydrochloride or phosphate.
Anileridine, N.F.

•**aliflurane.** (al-IH-flew-rane) USAN.
Use: Anesthetic (inhalation).

Alikal Powder. (Sanofi Winthrop) Sodium bicarbonate, tartaric acid powder. *otc.*
Use: Antacid.

Alimentum. (Ross Laboratories) Casein hydrolysate, sucrose, tapioca starch, MCT (fractionated coconut oil), safflower oil, soy oil. Qt ready-to-use. *otc.*
Use: Nutritional supplement-enteral.

•**alipamide.** (al-IH-pam-ide) USAN.
Use: Antihypertensive, diuretic.

alisobumal.
See: Butalbital, U.S.P. 23.

•**alitame.** (AL-ih-TAME) USAN.
Use: Sweetener.

alkalinizers, minerals and electrolytes.
See: Polycitra (Baker Norton).
Oracit (Carolina Medical Products).
Bicitra (Baker Norton).

alkalinizers urinary tract products.
See: Sodium Bicarbonate (Various Mfr.).
Urocit-K (Mission Pharmacal).
Citrolith (Beach Pharm).
Polycitra (Baker Norton).
Bicitra (Baker Norton).

Alkalol. (Alkalol) Thymol, eucalyptol, menthol, camphor, benzoin, potassium alum, potassium chlorate, sodium bicarbonate, sodium Cl, sweet birch oil, spearmint oil, pine and cassia oil, alcohol 0.05%. Bot. Pt. Nasal douche cup pkg. 1s. *otc.*
Use: Eyes, nose, throat and all inflamed mucous membranes.

Alka-Med Liquid. (Halsey) Aluminum hydroxide 200 mg, magnesium hydroxide 200 mg/ 5 ml. Bot. 8 oz. *otc.*
Use: Antacid.

Alka-Med Tablets. (Halsey) Magnesium hydroxide, aluminum hydroxide. Bot. 60s. *otc.*
Use: Antacid.

Alka-Mints. (Bayer Corp) Calcium carbonate 850 mg/Chew. tab. Carton 30s. *otc.*
Use: Antacid.

Alka-Seltzer. (Bayer Corp) Heat treated sodium bicarbonate 1916 mg, citric acid 1000 mg, aspirin 325 mg, sodium 567 mg/Tab. Bot. 36s. *otc.*
Use: Analgesic, antacid.

Alka-Seltzer, Advanced Formula. (Bayer Corp) Heat treated sodium bicarbonate 465 mg, citric acid 900 mg, acetaminophen 325 mg, potassium bicarbonate 300 mg, calcium carbonate 280 mg/Tab. Foil pack 36s. *otc.*
Use: Analgesic, antacid.

Alka-Seltzer Effervescent, Gold Tablets. (Bayer Corp) Heat treated sodium bicarbonate 958 mg, citric acid 832 mg, potassium bicarbonate 312 mg, so-

dium 311 mg/Tab. Bot. 20s, 36s. *otc.*
Use: Analgesic, antacid.

Alka-Seltzer, Extra Strength. (Bayer Corp) Aspirin 500 mg, heat treated sodium bicarbonate 1985 mg, citric acid 1000 mg, sodium 588 mg/Tab. Bot. 12s, 24s. *otc.*
Use: Analgesic, antacid.

Alka-Seltzer Flavored Effervescent Antacid-Analgesic. (Bayer Corp) Aspirin 325 mg, sodium bicarbonate 1700 mg, citric acid 1000 mg, phenylalanine 9 mg, sodium 506 mg, aspartame, lemon-lime flavor. Tab. Bot. 24s. *otc.*
Use: Analgesic, antacid.

Alka-Seltzer Plus. (Bayer Corp) Chlorpheniramine maleate 2 mg, phenylpropanolamine bitartrate 24 mg, aspirin 324 mg, sodium 506 mg/Tab. Foil pack 20s, 36s. *otc.*
Use: Analgesic, antihistamine, decongestant.

Alka-Seltzer Plus Allergy Liqui-Gels. (Bayer Corp) Pseudoephedrine HCl 30 mg, brompheniramine maleate 2 mg, acetaminophen 500 mg/Tab. Pkg. 12s. *otc.*
Use: Analgesic, antihistamine, decongestant.

Alka-Seltzer Plus Cold and Cough Liqui-Gels. (Bayer Corp) Dextromethorphan HBr 10 mg, pseudoephedrine HCl 30 mg, chlorpheniramine maleate 2 mg, acetaminophen 250 mg/Cap. Pkg. 12s, 20s. *otc.*
Use: Analgesic, antihistamine, antitussive, decongestant.

Alka-Seltzer Plus Cold & Cough Tablets. (Bayer Corp) Phenylpropanolamine bitartrate 20 mg, chlorpheniramine maleate 2 mg, dextromethorphan HBr 10 mg, aspirin 325 mg, phenylalanine 11.2 mg/Tab. 12s, 20s, 36s. *otc.*
Use: Analgesic, antitussive, antihistamine, decongestant.

Alka-Seltzer Plus Cold Liqui-Gels. (Bayer Corp) Chlorpheniramine maleate 2 mg, pseudoephedrine HCl 30 mg, acetaminophen 250 mg/Cap. Pkg. 12s, 20s. *otc.*
Use: Analgesic, antihistamine, decongestant.

Alka-Seltzer Plus Cold Medicine. (Bayer Corp) Phenylpropanolamine bitartrate 20 mg, chlorpheniramine maleate 2 mg, aspirin 325 mg/Tab. 12s, 20s, 36s, 48s. *otc.*
Use: Analgesic, antihistamine, decongestant.

Alka-Seltzer Plus Cold Tablets. (Bayer Corp) Phenylpropanolamine bitartrate 24.08 mg, chlorpheniramine maleate 2 mg, aspirin 325 mg/Tab. Pkg. 12s, 20s. Bot. 36s, 48s. *otc.*
Use: Analgesic, antihistamine, decongestant.

Alka-Seltzer Plus Flu & Body Aches Non-Drowsy Liqui-Gels. (Bayer Corp) Pseudoephedrine HCl 30 mg, dextromethorphan HBr 10 mg, acetaminophen 250 mg/Tab. Pkg. 12s. *otc.*
Use: Analgesic, antitussive, decongestant.

Alka-Seltzer Plus Nighttime Cold Liqui-Gels. (Bayer Corp) Pseudoephedrine HCl 30 mg, dextromethorphan HBr 10 mg, doxylamine succinate 6.25 mg, acetaminophen 250 mg/Cap. Pkg. 20s. *otc.*
Use: Antihistamine, antitussive, decongestant.

Alka-Seltzer Plus Night-Time Cold Tablets. (Bayer Corp) Phenylpropanolamine bitartrate 20 mg, doxylamine succinate 6.25 mg, dextromethorphan HBr 15 mg, aspirin 500 mg, phenylalanine 16.2 mg/Tab. Bot. 12s, 20s, 36s. *otc.*
Use: Analgesic, antihistamine, decongestant.

Alka-Seltzer Plus Sinus. (Bayer Corp) Phenylpropanolamine bitartrate 20 mg, aspirin 325 mg, aspartame, phenylalanine 8.98 mg/Tab. Pkg. 20s. *otc.*
Use: Analgesic, decongestant.

Alka-Seltzer Plus Sinus Allergy. (Bayer Corp) Phenylpropanolamine bitartrate 24.08 mg, brompheniramine maleate 2 mg, aspirin 500 mg, aspartame, phenylalanine 9 mg/Tab. Bot. 16s, 32s. *otc.*
Use: Analgesic, antihistamine, decongestant.

Alka-Seltzer Special Effervescent Antacid. (Bayer Corp) Heat treated sodium bicarbonate 958 mg, citric acid 832 mg, potassium bicarbonate 312 mg, sodium 284 mg/Tab. Foil pack 12s, 20s, 36s. *otc.*
Use: Effervescent antacid.

Alka-Seltzer Tablets. (Bayer Corp) Aspirin 325 mg, citric acid 1000 mg, phenylalanine 9 mg, sodium 506 mg/Tab. Bot. 24s. *otc.*
Use: Analgesic, antacid.

Alka-Seltzer w/Aspirin. (Bayer Corp) Sodium bicarbonate 1916 mg, citric acid 1000 mg, aspirin 325 mg and sodium 567 mg. 17.2 mEq acid neutralizing capacity. Foil pack 8s, 12s, 24s, 26s and 36s. *otc.*

Use: Analgesic, antacid.

Alkeran. (GlaxoWellcome) Melphalan; 50 mg/Pow. for Inj. Single-use vial w/ 10 ml of sterile diluent. *Rx.*
Use: Antineoplastic.

Alkets. (Roberts Pharm) Calcium carbonate 500 mg, dextrose, peppermint flavor. Chew. tab. Bot. 36s, 96s, 150s. *otc.*
Use: Antacid.

alkylbenzyldimethylammonium chloride. Benzalkonium Cl, N.F. 18.
W/Methylrosaniline Cl, polyoxyethylenenonylphenol, polyethylene glycol tertdodecylthioether.
See: Hyva, Tab. (Holland-Rantos).

•**alkyl (C12-15) benzoate, N.F. 18.**
Use: Pharmaceutical aid (oleaginous vehicle emollient).

•**allantoin.** (al-AN-toe-in) USAN.
Use: Vulnerary (topical).
See: Cutemol (Summers).
W/Aminacrine, sulfanilamide.
See: Par Cream (Parmed).
Vagidine, Cream (Zeneca).
Vagitrol, Cream (Syntex).
W/Balsam, Lano-sil, silicone.
See: Balmex Med. Lot. (Macsil).
W/p-Chloro-m-xylenol.
See: Cebum, Shampoo (Dermik Laboratories).
W/Coal tar extract, hexachlorophene, glycerin, lanolin.
See: Pso-Rite, Cream (DePree).
W/Coal tar in cream base.
See: Tegrin Cream (Block Drug).
W/Coal tar solution, isopropyl myristate, psorilan.
See: Psorelief, Soln. (Quality Formulations).
W/Dienestrol, sulfanilamide, aminacrine HCl.
See: AVC/Dienestrol Cream, Supp. (Hoechst Marion Roussel).
W/Hydrocortisone.
See: Tarcortin, Cream (Schwarz Pharma).
W/Nitrofurazone.
See: Eldezol, Oint. (Zeneca).
W/Pramoxine HCl, benzalkonium Cl.
See: Perifoam, Aerosol (Solvay).
W/Resorcinol, hexachlorophene, menthol.
See: Tackle, Gel. (Colgate Oral).
W/Salicylic acid, sulfur.
See: Neutrogena Disposables (Neutrogena).
W/Sulfanilamide, 9-aminoacridine HCl.
Nil Vaginal Cream (Century Pharm).
Vagisan, Creme (Sandia).
Vagisul, Creme (Sheryl).
W/Sulfisoxazole, Aminoacridine.
Use: Topically, aid in the promotion of granulation.
See: Vagilia, Cream, Supp. (Teva USA).
W/Tarbonis.
See: Sebical, Shampoo (Schwarz Pharma).
W/Vitamins A, D.
See: A-D Dressing (LaCrosse).

Allay. (LuChem) Acetaminophen 650 mg, hydrocodone bitartrate 7.5 mg/ Cap. Bot. 100s. *c-III.*
Use: Analgesic combination, narcotic.

Allbee C-800. (Robins) Vitamins E 45 IU, C 800 mg, B_1 15 mg, B_2 17 mg, B_3 100 mg, B_5 25 mg, B_{12} 12 mcg/Tab. Bot. 60s. *otc.*
Use: Vitamin supplement.

Allbee C-800 Plus Iron. (Robins) Vitamins E 45 IU, C 800 mg, B_1 15 mg, B_2 17 mg, niacin 100 mg, B_6 25 mg, B_{12} 12 mcg, pantothenic acid 25 mg, iron 27 mg, folic acid 0.4 mg/Tab. Bot. 60s. *otc.*
Use: Mineral, vitamin supplement.

Allbee w/C. (Robins) Vitamins B_1 15 mg, B_6 5 mg, B_2 10.2 mg, B_3 50 mg, B_5 10 mg, C 300 mg/Cap. Bot. 30s. *otc.*
Use: Vitamin supplement.

Allbee-T. (Robins) Vitamins B_1 15.5 mg, B_2 10 mg, B_6 8.2 mg, B_5 23 mg, B_3 100 mg, C 500 mg, B_{12} 5 mcg/Tab. Bot. 100s, 500s. *otc.*
Use: Vitamin supplement.

Allbex. (Health for Life Brands) Vitamins B_1 5 mg, B_2 2 mg, B_6 0.25 mg, calcium pantothenate 3 mg, niacinamide 20 mg, ferrous sulfate 194.4 mg, inositol 10 mg, choline 10 mg, B_{12} (concentrate) 3 mcg/Cap. Bot. 100s, 1000s. *otc.*
Use: Mineral, vitamin supplement.

All-Day-C. (Barth's) Vitamin C 200 mg/ Cap. or 500 mg/Tab. with rose hip extract. Bot. 30s, 90s, 180s, 360s. *otc.*
Use: Vitamin supplement.

All-Day Iron Yeast. (Barth's) Iron 20 mg, Vitamins B_1 2 mg, B_2 4 mg, niacin 0.57 mg/Cap. Bot. 30s, 90s, 180s. *otc.*
Use: Mineral, vitamin supplement.

All-Day-Vites. (Barth's) Vitamins A 10,000 IU, D 400 IU, B_1 3 mg, B_2 6 mg, niacin 1 mg, C 120 mg, B_{12} 10 mcg, E 30 IU/Cap. Bot. 30s, 90s, 180s, 360s. *otc.*
Use: Vitamin supplement.

Allegra. (Hoechst Marion Roussel) Fexofenadine HCl 60 mg, lactose/Cap. Bot. 60s, 100s, 500s, UD 100s. *Rx.*
Use: Antihistamine.

Allegra-D. (Hoechst-Marion Roussel) Fexofenadine 60 mg, pseudoephedrine HCl 120 mg/ER Tab. Bot. 60s, 100s, 500s, UD 100s. *Rx.*
Use: Antihistamine.

allegron. Nortriptyline.
Use: Antidepressant.

Allent. (B.F. Ascher) Pseudoephedrine HCl 120 mg, brompheniramine maleate 12 mg. Slow-release cap. Bot. 100s. *Rx.*
Use: Antihistamine, decongestant.

Allerben Injection. (Forest Pharmaceutical) Diphenhydramine 10 mg/ml. Vial 30 ml. *Rx.*
Use: Antihistamine.

Allerchlor injection. (Forest Pharmaceutical) Chlorpheniramine maleate 10 mg/ml. Vial 30 ml. *Rx.*
Use: Antihistamine.

Aller-Chlor. (Rugby) Chlorpheniramine maleate. **Tab.:** 4 mg. Bot. 100s. **Syr.:** 2 mg/5 ml. Alcohol 5%, menthol parabens, sugar. Bot. 118 ml. *otc.*
Use: Antihistamine.

Allercon. (Parmed) Pseudoephedrine HCl 60 mg, triprolidine HCl 2.5 mg/Tab. Bot. 24s, 100s and 1000s. *otc.*
Use: Antihistamine, decongestant.

Allercreme Skin Lotion. (Galderma) Mineral oil, petrolatum, lanolin, lanolin oil, lanolin alcohols, glycerin, triethanolamine, cetyl alcohol, stearic acid, parabens. Lot. Bot. 240 ml. *otc.*
Use: Emollient.

Allercreme Ultra Emollient. (Galderma) Mineral oil, petrolatum, lanolin, lanolin alcohol, lanolin oil, glycerin, glyceryl stearate, PEG-100 stearate, squalane, cetyl alcohol, sorbitan laurate, quaternium-15, parabens. Cream Bot. 60 g. *otc.*
Use: Emollient.

Allerdec Capsules. (Towne) Phenylpropanolamine HCl 25 mg, chlorpheniramine maleate 1 mg, pyrilamine maleate 5 mg/Cap. Bot. 25s, 50s. *otc.*
Use: Antihistamine, decongestant.

Allerest. (Novartis Consumer Health) **Tab.:** Phenylpropanolamine HCl 18.7 mg, chlorpheniramine maleate 2 mg/Tab. Sleeve Pack 24s, 48s. Bot. 72s. **Chew. tab. for Children:** Phenylpropanolamine HCl 9.4 mg, chlorpheniramine maleate 1 mg/Tab. Sleeve Pack 24s. **Eye Drops:** Naphazoline HCl 0.012%. Bot. 0.5 oz. **Headache Strength Tab.:** Acetaminophen 325 mg, pseudoephedrine HCl 30 mg, chlorpheniramine maleate 2 mg/Tab. Pkg. 24s. **Nasal Spray:** Oxymetazoline HCl 0.05%. Bot. 0.5 oz. *otc.*
Use: Analgesic (Headache Strength Tab. only), antihistamine, decongestant.

Allerest 12-Hour. (Novartis) Phenylpropanolamine HCl 75 mg, chlorpheniramine maleate 8 mg/Cap. Sleeve pak 10s. *otc.*
Use: Antihistamine, decongestant.

Allerest, Children's. (Novartis) Phenylpropanolamine HCl 94 mg, chlorpheniramine maleate 6 mg. Chew. tab. Bot. 24s. *otc.*
Use: Antihistamine, decongestant.

Allerest Maximum Strength. (Medeva) Pseudoephedrine 30 mg, chlorpheniramine maleate 2 mg/Tab. Bot. 24s, 48s, 72s. *otc.*
Use: Antihistamine, decongestant.

Allerest Maximum Strength 12-Hour Caplets. (Novartis) Phenylpropanolamine HCl 75 mg, chlorpheniramine maleate 12 mg/Capl. Pkg. 10s. *otc.*
Use: Antihistamine, decongestant.

Allerest No Drowsiness. (Novartis) Pseudoephedrine 30 mg, acetaminophen 325 mg/Tab. Bot. 20s. *otc.*
Use: Analgesic, decongestant.

Allerest Sinus Pain Formula. (Novartis) Acetaminophen 500 mg, pseudoephedrine HCl 30 mg, chlorpheniramine maleate 2 mg/Tab. Pkg. 20s. *otc.*
Use: Analgesic, antihistamine, decongestant.

Allerfrim. (Rugby) **Tab.:** Pseudoephedrine HCl 60 mg, triprolidine HCl 2.5 mg. Bot. 24s, 100s, 1000s. **Syr.:** Pseudoephedrine HCl 30 mg, triprolidine HCl 1.25 mg. Bot. 118 ml, 473 ml. *otc.*
Use: Antihistamine, decongestant.

Allerfrin OTC Syrup. (Rugby) Pseudoephedrine 30 mg, triprolidine 1.25 mg. Syr. Bot. Pt. *otc.*
Use: Antihistamine, decongestant.

Allerfrin w/Codeine. (Rugby) Pseudoephedrine HCl 30 mg, triprolidine HCl 1.25 mg, codeine phosphate 10 mg, alcohol 4.3%. Syr. Bot. 120 ml, pt, gal. *c-v.*
Use: Antihistamine, antitussive, decongestant.

Allergan Enzymatic. (Allergan) Papain, sodium Cl, sodium carbonate, sodium borate, edetate disodium. Kits 12s, 24s, 36s, 48s. *otc.*
Use: Contact lens care.

Allergan Hydrocare Cleaning & Disin-

fecting Solution. (Allergan) tris(2-hydroxyethyl)tallow ammonium Cl 0.013%, thimerosal 0.002%, bis(2-hydroxyethyl)tallow ammonium Cl, sodium bicarbonate, dibasic, monobasic and anhydrous sodium phosphate, hydrochloric acid, propylene glycol, polysorbate 80, special soluble polyhema. Bot. 4 oz, 8 oz, 12 oz. *otc.*
Use: Contact lens care.

Allergan Hydrocare Preserved Saline Solution. (Allergan) Sodium Cl, sodium hexametaphosphate, sodium hydroxide, boric acid, sodium borate, EDTA 0.01%, thimerosal 0.001%. Bot. 8 oz, 12 oz. *otc.*
Use: Contact lens care.

Allergen Ear Drops. (Zenith Goldline) Benzocaine 1.4%, antipyrine 5.4%, glycerin, oxyquinoline sulfate. Bot. 0.5 oz. *Rx.*
Use: Otic.

Allergen Patch Test Kit. (Hermal) Box of tubes of semi-solid pastes or solutions. Allergens are either suspended in 4.5 g petrolatum, USP, or dissolved in 5.5 g water. Kit includes 20 reclosable syringes for topical use only (not for injection), each exuding sufficient allergen to test 150 patients, housed in a plastic case with two drawers. Allergens include benzocaine, mercaptobenzothiazole, colophony, p-phenylenediamine, imidazolidinyl urea (Germall 115), cinnamin aldyhyde, lanolin alcohol (wool wax alcohols), carba rubber mix, neomycin sulfate, thiuram rubber mix, formaldehyde, ethylenediamine dihydrochloride, epoxy resin, quaternium 15, p-tert-butylphenol formaldehyde resin, mercapto rubber mix, black rubber p-phenylenediamine mix, potassium dichromate, balsam of Peru and nickel sulfate.

allergen test patches.
Use: Diagnostic aid, allergic dermatitis.
See: T.R.U.E. Test (GlaxoWellcome).

Allergenic Extracts. (Various Mfr.) Allergenic extracts of pollen, mold, house dust, inhalants, epidermals, insects in saline 0.9% and phenol 0.4% up to 1:10 w/v or 40,000 PNU/ml in sets or vials up to 30 ml.
Use: Diagnostic aid, allergens.

Allergenic Extracts. (Bayer Corp) Allergenic extracts of pollens, foods, inhalants, epidermals, fungi, insects, miscellaneous antigens.
Use: Diagnostic aid, allergens.

allergenic extracts, alum-precipitated.
See: Allpyral (Bayer Corp).
Center-Al (Center Laboratories).

Allergex. (Bayer Corp) Silicones, polyethylene and triethylene glycol, antioxidants, mineral oil concentrate. Bot. Pt. Aerosol pt.
Use: Antiallergic.

Allergy. (Major) Chlorpheniramine maleate 4 mg, lactose/Tab. Bot. 24s, 100s. *otc.*
Use: Antihistamine.

Allergy Drops. (Bausch & Lomb) Naphazoline HCl 0.012%. Bot. 15 ml. *otc.*
Use: Mydriatic, vasoconstrictor.

allergy preparations.
See: Antihistamine Preparations.

allergy relief medicine.
Use: Antihistamine, decongestant.
See: A.R.M. Caplets (SmithKline Beecham Pharmaceuticals).

Allergy-Sinus Comtrex. (Bristol-Myers) Pseudoephedrine HCl 30 mg, chlorpheniramine maleate 2 mg, acetaminophen 500 mg/Capl. or Tab. Bot. 50s, UD 24s. *otc.*
Use: Analgesic, antihistamine, decongestant.

Allergy Tablets. (Weeks & Leo) Phenylpropanolamine HCl 37.5 mg, chlorpheniramine 4 mg/Tab. Bot. 30s. *otc.*
Use: Antihistamine, decongestant.

AllerMax. (Pfeiffer) Diphenhydramine HCl 50 mg, lactose/Capl. Pkg. 24s. *otc.*
Use: Antihistamine.

AllerMax Allergy & Cough Formula. (Pfeiffer) Diphenhydramine HCl 6.25 mg/5 ml, alcohol 0.5%, raspberry flavor, menthol, sucrose, glucose, saccharin, sorbitol. 118 ml. *otc.*
Use: Antihistamine.

Allerphed Syrup. (Great Southern) Pseudoephedrine HCl 30 mg, triprolidine HCl 1.25 mg/5 ml. Syr. Bot. 118 ml. *otc.*
Use: Antihistamine, decongestant.

Allersone. (Roberts Pharm) Hydrocortisone 0.5%, diperodon HCl 0.5%, zinc oxide 5%, sodium lauryl sulfate, propylene glycol, cetyl alcohol, petrolatum, methyl and propyl parabens. Oint. Tube 15 g. *otc, Rx.*
Use: Corticosteroid, topical.

Allersule Forte. (Misemer) Phenylephrine HCl 20 mg, chlorpheniramine maleate 8 mg, methscopolamine nitrate 2.5 mg/Cap. Bot. 100s. *otc, Rx.*
Use: Anticholinergic, antihistamine, decongestant.

All-Nite Cold Formula. (Major) Pseudo-

ephedrine HCl 10 mg, doxylamine succinate 1.25 mg, dextromethorphan HBr 5 mg, acetaminophen 167 mg/5 ml. Liq. Bot. 177 ml. *otc.*
Use: Analgesic, antihistamine, antitussive, decongestant.

•**allobarbital.** (AL-low-BAR-bih-tal) USAN.
Formerly Diallybarbituric acid.
Use: Hypnotic, sedative.
W/Acetaminophen, salicylamide, caffeine.
See: Allylvon, Cap. (Zeneca).
W/Aspirin, acetaminophen, aluminum aspirin.
See: Allylgesic, Tab. (Zeneca).
W/Ergotamine tartrate.
See: Allylgesic w/Ergotamine, Cap. (Zeneca).

allobarbitone.
See: Diallylbarbituric Acid (Various Mfr.).

•**allopurinol.** (AL-oh-PURE-ee-nahl) U.S.P. 23.
Use: Antigout, xanthine oxidase inhibitor.
See: Lopurin, Tab. (Knoll Pharmaceuticals).
Zyloprim, Tab. (GlaxoWellcome).

allopurinol riboside.
Use: Antiprotozoal.

allopurinol sodium. (AL-oh-PURE-ee-nal) Inj.
Use: Ex vivo preservation of cadaveric kidneys for transplantation; antineoplastic. [Orphan drug]
See: Zyloprim, Inj. (Glaxo Wellcome).

Allpyral. (Bayer Corp) Allergenic extracts, alum-precipitated. For subcutaneous inj. pollens, molds, epithelia, house dust, other inhalants, stinging insects.
Use: Diagnostic aid, allergens.

allylbarbituric acid. Allylisobutyl-barbituric acid, butalbital. Tab. (Various Mfr.).
Use: Sedative.
W/A.P.C.
See: Anti-Ten, Tab. (Century Pharm).
Fiorinal, Cap., Tab. (Novartis).
Tenstan (Standex).
W/Acetaminophen, homatropine methylbromide.
See: Panitol H.M.B., Tab. (Wesley Pharmacal).
W/Acetaminophen, salicylamide, caffeine.
See: Renpap, Tab. (Wren).

allylestrenol.

allyl-isobutylbarbituric acid.
See: Allylbarbituric Acid.

allylisopropylmalonylurea.
See: Aprobarbital.

•**allyl isothiocyanate.** U.S.P. 23.
Use: Counterirritant in neuralgia.

4-allyl-2-methoxyphenol. U.S.P. 23.

n-allylnoroxymorphone hcl. U.S.P. 23.

5-allyl-sec-butylbarbituric acid.
See: Talbutal.

Almacone. (Rugby) **Chew tab.:** Aluminum hydroxide 200 mg, magnesium hydroxide 200 mg, simethicone 20 mg/ Bot. 100s, 1000s. **Liq.:** Aluminum hydroxide 200 mg, magnesium hydroxide 200 mg, simethicone 20 mg, sodium 0.75 mg/5 ml. Bot. 360 ml, gal. *otc.*
Use: Antacid.

Almacone II Double Strength Liquid. (Rugby) Aluminum hydroxide 400 mg, magnesium hydroxide 400 mg, simethicone 40 mg/5 ml. Bot. 360 ml, gal. *otc.*
Use: Antacid.

•**almadrate sulfate.** (AL-ma-drate) USAN. Aluminum magnesium hydroxide-oxide-sulfate-hydrate.
Use: Antacid.

•**almagate.** (AL-mah-gate) USAN.
Use: Antacid.

almagucin. Gastric mucin, dried aluminum hydroxide gel, magnesium trisilicate. *otc.*
Use: Antacid.

Almebex Plus B_{12}. (Dayton) Vitamins B_1 1 mg, B_2 2 mg, B_3 5 mg, B_6 0.4 mg, B_{12} 5 mcg, choline 33 mg/5 ml. 473 ml (with B_{12} in separate container). *otc.*
Use: Vitamin supplement.

•**almond oil.** N.F. 18.
Use: Pharmaceutic aid (emollient, oleaginous vehicle, perfume).

Almora. (Forest Pharmaceutical) Magnesium gluconate 0.5 g/Tab. Pkg. 100s. *otc.*
Use: Mineral supplement.

•**almotriptan.** (al-moe-TRIP-tan) USAN.
Use: Antimigraine.

•**alniditan dihydrochloride.** (al-nih-DIH-tan die-HIGH-droe-KLOR-ide) USAN.
Use: Antimigraine.

Alnyte. (Mayer) Scopolamine aminoxide HBr 0.2 mg, salicylamide 250 mg/Tab. Pkg. 16s. *Rx.*
Use: Analgesic, anticholinergic.

Alocass Laxative. (Western Research) Aloin 0.25 gr, cascara sagrada 0.5 gr, rhubarb 0.5 gr, ginger 1/32 gr, powdered extract of belladonna gr/Tab. Bot. 1000s. Pak 28s. *otc.*
Use: Laxative.

Alodopa-15 Tablets. (Major) Hydrochlorothiazide 15 mg, methyldopa 250 mg. Bot. 100s. *Rx.*
Use: Antihypertensive.

Alodopa-25 Tablets. (Major) Hydrochlorothiazide 25 mg, methyldopa 250 mg. Bot. 100s. *Rx.*
Use: Antihypertensive.

•**aloe.** U.S.P. 23.
Use: See Compound Benzoin Tincture.

Aloe Grande Creme. (Gordon Laboratories) Aloe, vitamins E 1500 IU, A 100,000 units/oz in cream base. Jar 2.5 oz. *otc.*
Use: Emollient.

aloe vera active principle.
See: Alvagel, Oint. (Kenyon).

Aloe Vesta Perineal. (SmithKline Beecham Pharmaceuticals) Solution of sodium C14-16 olefin sulfonate, propylene glycol, aloe vera gel, hydrolyzed collagen. Bot. 118 ml, 236 ml, gal. *otc.*
Use: Perianal hygiene.

•**alofilcon a.** (AL-oh-FILL-kahn) USAN.
Use: Contact lens material (hydrophilic).

aloin. (Baker, J.T.) A mixture of crystalline pentosides from various aloes. Bot. oz. *otc.*
Use: Laxative.

W/Ox bile (desiccated), phenolphthalein, cascara sagrada extract, podophyllin.
See: Bilgon (Solvay).

Alomide. (Alcon Laboratories) Lodoxamide tromethamine 0.1%. Soln. Droptainers 10 ml. *Rx.*
Use: Antiallergic, ophthalmic.

•**alonimid.** (ah-LAHN-ih-mid) USAN.
Use: Hypnotic, sedative.

Alor 5/500. (Atley Pharmaceuticals) Hydrocodone bitartrate 5 mg, aspirin 500 mg/Tab. Bot. 100s. *c-III.*
Use: Analgesic, narcotic.

Alora. (Procter & Gamble) Estradiol 1.5 mg (0.05 mg/day), 2.3 mg (0.1 mg/day) and 3 mg (0.075 mg/day)/Patch. Calendar packs, 48 and 24 systems. *Rx.*
Use: Estrogen.

•**alosetron hydrochloride.** (al-OH-seh-trahn) USAN.
Use: Antiemetic.

Alotone. (Major) Triamcinolone 4 mg/Tab. Bot. 100s. *Rx.*
Use: Corticosteroid.

•**alovudine.** (al-OHV-you-deen) USAN.
Use: Antiviral.

•**alpertine.** (al-PURR-teen) USAN.
Use: Antipsychotic.

l-alpha-acetyl-methadol (LAAM). (Biodevelopment) *Rx.*
Use: Treatment of heroin addicts.

•**alpha amylase.** (AL-fah AM-ih-lace) USAN. A concentrated form of alpha amylase produced by a strain of nonpathogenic bacteria.
Use: Digestive aid; anti-inflammatory.
See: Kutrase, Cap. (Schwarz Pharma). Ku-Zyme, Cap. (Schwarz Pharma).

alpha-amylase w-100. W/Proteinase W-300, cellase W-100, lipase, estrone, testosterone, vitamins, minerals. *Rx.*
Use: Digestive aid.
See: Geramine, Tab. (Zeneca).

alpha-1-adrenergic blockers.
Use: Antihypertensive.
See: Cardura (Roerig).

alpha-1-antitrypsin (recombinant DNA origin).
Use: Supplementation therapy for alpha$_1$-antitrypsin deficiency in the ZZ phenotype population. [Orphan drug]

alpha/beta-adrenergic blocker.
See: Normodyne (Schering Plough). Trandate (Allen & Hanburys).

alpha-chymotrypsin.
See: Alpha Chymar, Vial (Centeon). Zolyse, Vial (Alcon Laboratories).

Alphaderm. (Teva USA) Hydrocortisone 1%. Cream 30 g, 100 g. *otc, Rx.*
Use: Corticosteroid, topical.

alpha-d-galactosidase.
Use: Antiflatulent.

Alpha-E. (Barth's) d-Alpha tocopherol. **50 IU or 100 IU:** Cap. Bot. 100s, 500s, 1000s. **200 IU:** Cap. Bot. 100s, 250s. **400 IU:** Cap. Bot. 100s, 250s, 500s. *otc.*
Use: Vitamin supplement.

alpha-estradiol. Known to be beta-estradiol.
See: Estradiol (Various Mfr.).

alpha-estradiol benzoate.
See: Estradiol benzoate (Various Mfr.).

Alpha Fast. (Eastwood) Bath oil. Bot. 16 oz. *otc.*
Use: Emollient.

alpha-fetoprotein w/tc-99m. USAN.
Use: Diagnostic aid.

•**alphafilcon a.** (al-fah-FILL-kahn) USAN.
Use: Contact lens material (hydrophilic).

alpha-galactosidase.
See: Aspergillus niger enzyme.

alpha-galactosidase a.
Use: Fabry's disease. [Orphan drug]

alpha-galactoside a. USAN.
Use: Treatment of Fabry's disease.

Alphagan. (Allergan) Brimonidine tartrate 0.2%, polyvinyl alcohol/Soln. Dropper Bot. 5 ml, 10 ml. *Rx.*
Use: Agent for glaucoma.

alpha-hypophamine.
See: Oxytocin Inj.

alpha interferon-2a.
See: Roferon-A (Roche Laboratories).

alpha interferon-2b.
See: Intron A (Schering Plough).

alpha interferon-N3.
See: Alferon-N (Purdue Frederick).

Alpha-Keri. (Westwood Squibb) **Therapeutic Bath:** Mineral oil, lanolin oil, PEG-4-dilaurate, benzophenone-3, D & C green #6, fragrance. Bot. 4 oz, 8 oz, 16 oz. **Cleansing Bar:** Bar containing sodium tallowate, sodium cocoate, water, mineral oil, fragrance, PEG-75, glycerin, titanium dioxide, lanolin oil, sodium Cl, BHT, EDTA, D & C green #5, D & C yellow # 10. 120 g. *otc.*
Use: Emollient.

alpha-methyldopa. Name previously used for Methyldopa.

Alphanate. (Alliance Therapeutic) ≥ 10 IU FVIII: C/mg total protein. 0.05 to 1 g albumin (human), ≤ 10 mmol Ca/ml, ≤ 750 mcg glycine/IU FVIII: C, ≤ 2 IU heparin/ml, ≤ 300 mmol arginine/L, ≤ 2.5 mg PEG, 80/IU FVIII: C, ≤ 10 mEq Na/vial after reconstitution. Pow. Lypholized. Single-dose vials with diluent. *Rx.*
Use: Antihemophilic, treatment for Von Willebrand's disease. [Orphan drug]

AlphaNine. (Alpha Therapeutics) Purified heat-treated/solvent preparation of coagulation Factor IX from human plasma. With ≥ 50 units Factor IX per mg protein, < 5 units each Factor II (prothrombin) and Factor VII (proconvertin) per 100 IU Factor IX and < 20 units Factor X (Stuart-Power Factor) per 100 IU Factor IX. In single-dose vials with diluent, double-ended needle and microaggregated filter. Pow. for Inj. *Rx.*
Use: Antihemophilic.

Alphanine SD. (Alpha Therapeutics) ≥ 150 IU Factor IX/mg. Pow., lyophilized. In a single-dose vial with 10 ml diluent, double-ended needle and filter. *Rx.*
Use: Antihemophilic.

alpha-phenoxyethyl penicillin, potassium.
See: Phenethicillin Potassium.

alpha-1-antitrypsin (recombinant DNA origin). (Chiron)
Use: Treatment of alpha-1-antitrypsin deficiency. [Orphan drug]

alpha-1-proteinase inhibitor.
Use: Treatment of Alpha-1-antitrypsin deficiency. [Orphan drug]
See: Prolastin (Miles).

alpha-galactosidase A.
Use: Fabry's disease. [Orphan drug]
See: Fabrase CC-Galactosidase.

alphasone acetophenide. Name previously used for Algestone acetonide.

alpha-tocopherol.
See: Dalfatol, Cap. (Solvay).
Tocopherol, Alpha (Various Mfr.).

dl-alpha-tocopherol succinate.
See: DAlpha-E, Cap. (Alto Pharmaceuticals).

Alphatrex. (Savage) **Cream and Oint.:** Betamethasone dipropionate 0.05%. Tube 15 g, 45 g. **Lot.:** Betamethasone dipropionate 0.05%. Bot. 60 ml. *Rx.*
Use: Corticosteroid, topical.

Alpha Vee-12. (Schlicksup) Hydroxocobalamin 1000 mcg/ml. Vial 10 ml. *Rx.*
Use: Vitamin supplement.

Alphosyl. (Schwarz Pharma) Allantoin 1.7%, special crude coal tar extracts 5%. **Lot.:** Bot. 8 fl oz. **Cream:** 2 oz. *otc.*
Use: Antipruritic.

•**alpidem.** (AL-PIH-dem) USAN.
Use: Antianxiety (anxiolytic).

•**alprazolam.** (al-PRAY-zoe-lam) U.S.P. 23.
Use: Hypnotic, sedative.
See: Xanax, Tab. (Pharmacia & Upjohn).

alprazolam. (Various Mfr.) Alprazolam **0.25 mg, 0.5 mg, 1 mg:** Tab. Bot. 30s, 100s, 500s, 1000s, UD 100s; **2 mg:** Tab. Bot. 100s, 500s. *c-IV.*
Use: Management of anxiety disorders.

alprazolam. (Roxane) **Oral Soln.:** Alprazolam 0.5 mg/5 ml, sorbitol, saccharin, fruit-mint flavor. Bot. 500 ml, UD 2.5 ml, UD 5 ml, UD 10 ml. **Intensol Soln.:** Alprazolam 1 mg/ml. Dropper. Bot. 30 ml. *c-IV.*
Use: Anxiolytic.

•**alprenolol hydrochloride.** (al-PREH-no-lole) USAN.
Use: Antiadrenergic (β-receptor).

•**alprenoxime hydrochloride.** (al-PREN-ox-eem) USAN.
Use: Antiglaucoma agent.

•**alprostadil.** (al-PRAHST-uh-dill) U.S.P. 23. *Formerly Prostaglandin* E_1, *PGE*$_1$.
Use: Vasodilator, antiimpotence agent, arterial patency agent.
See: Caverject (Pharmacia & Upjohn).
Edex, Inj. (Schwarz Pharma).
Muse (Vivus).
Prostin VR, Inj. (Pharmacia & Upjohn).
Prostin VR Pediatric, Inj. (Pharmacia & Upjohn).

alprostadil. (al-PRAHST-uh-dill) (Schwarz Pharma)
Use: Severe peripheral arterial occlusive disease. [Orphan drug]

Alramucil. (Alra Laboratories) Psyllium hydrophilic mucoloid 3.6 g, citric acid, sucrose, saccharin, potassium bicarbonate, sodium bicarbonate, 4 calories and < 0.01 g sodium per packet. Pow. effervescent Pkg. 30s. *otc.*
Use: Laxative.

Alredase. (Wyeth Ayerst). Tolrestat. *Rx.*
Use: Aldose reductase inhibitor.

•**alrestatin sodium.** (AHL-reh-STAT-in) USAN.
Use: Enzyme inhibitor (aldose reductase).

Alrex. (Bausch & Lomb) Loteprednol etabonate 2 mg/ml, EDTA, glycerin, povidone, tyloxapol. Ophth. Susp. 5 ml, 10 ml. *Rx.*
Use: Conjunctivitis, allergic.

Alsorb Gel. (Standex) Magnesium and aluminum hydroxide. Colloidal Susp. *otc.*
Use: Antacid.

Alsorb Gel, C.T. (Standex) Calcium carbonate 2 gr, glycine 3 gr, magnesium trisilicate 3 gr/Tab. *otc.*
Use: Antacid.

Altace. (Hoechst Marion Roussel/Pharmacia & Upjohn) Ramipril 1.25 mg, 2.5 mg, 5 mg or 10 mg/Cap. Bot. 100s, UD 100s. *Rx.*
Use: Antihypertensive; congestive heart failure.

•**altanserin tartrate.** (AL-TAN-ser-in) USAN.
Use: Serotonin antagonist.

•**alteplase.** (AL-teh-PLACE) U.S.P. 23
Use: Plasminogen activator.
See: Activase, Inj. (Genentech).

AlternaGEL. (J & J Merck Consumer Pharm) Aluminum hydroxide 600 mg/5 ml. Liq. Bot. 150 ml, 360 ml. *otc.*
Use: Antacid.

•**althiazide.** (al-THIGH-azz-ide) USAN.
Use: Antihypertensive; diuretic.

Altracin. (AL Labs) Bacitracin.
Use: Antibiotic. [Orphan drug]

•**altretamine.** (ahl-TRETT-uh-meen) USAN.
Use: Antineoplastic. [Orphan drug]
See: Hexalen (US Bioscience).

altretamine. (ahl-TRETT-uh-meen)
Use: Antineoplastic. [Orphan drug]
See: Hexalen, (US Bioscience).

Alu-Cap. (3M Pharm) Aluminum hydroxide gel 400 mg/Cap. Bot. 100s. *otc.*
Use: Antacid.

Al-U-Creme. (MacAllister) Aluminum hydroxide equivalent to 4% aluminum oxide. Susp. Bot. pt, gal. *otc.*
Use: Antacid.

Aludrox. (Wyeth Ayerst) Aluminum hydroxide gel 307 mg, magnesium hydroxide 103 mg/5 ml. Susp. Bot. 355 ml. *otc.*
Use: Antacid.

alukalin. Activated kaolin.
Use: Antidiarrheal.
See: Lusyn, Tab. (Medeva).

Alulex. (Lexington) Magnesium trisilicate 3.25 gr, aluminum hydroxide gel 3.5 gr, phenobarbital 1/8 gr, homatropine methylbromide gr/Tab. Bot. 100s. *Rx.*
Use: Agent for peptic ulcer.

alum. Sulfuric acid, aluminum ammonium salt (2:1:1), dodecahydrate. Sulfuric acid, aluminum potassium salt (2:1:1), dodecahydrate.
Use: Astringent.

•**alum, ammonium.** U.S.P. 23.
Use: Astringent.

•**alum, potassium.** U.S.P. 23.
Use: Astringent.

alum-precipitated allergenic extracts.
See: Allpyral (Bayer Corp).
Center-Al (Center Laboratories).

Alumadrine. (Fleming) Acetaminophen 500 mg, phenylpropanolamine HCl 25 mg, chlorpheniramine maleate 4 mg/Tab. Bot. 100s, 1000s. *Rx.*
Use: Analgesic, antihistamine, decongestant.

Alumate-HC. (Dermco) Hydrocortisone 0.125%, 0.25%, 0.5% or 1%/Cream. Pkg. 0.5 oz, 1 oz, 4 oz. *otc.*
Use: Corticosteroid, topical.

Alumate Mixture. (Schlicksup) Aluminum hydroxide gel, milk of magnesia/5 ml. Bot. 12 oz, gal. *otc.*
Use: Antacid.

alumina hydrated powder.
W/Activated attapulgite, pectin. *otc.*
Use: Antidiarrheal.
See: Polymagma, Plain, Tab. (Wyeth Ayerst).

alumina, magnesia and calcium carbonate tablets.
Use: Antacid.

alumina, magnesia, calcium carbonate and simethicone tablets.
Use: Antacid.

alumina, magnesia and calcium chloride oral suspension.
Use: Antacid.

alumina and magnesia oral suspension.
Use: Antacid.

alumina and magnesia tablets.
Use: Antacid.

alumina, magnesia and simethicone.
Use: Antacid, antiflatulent.

alumina, magnesia and simethicone suspension. (Roxane) Aluminum hydroxide 213 mg, magnesium hydroxide 200 mg, simethicone 20 mg, parabens, sorbitol/5 ml. Susp. Bot. UD 15, 30 ml. *otc.*
Use: Antacid.

alumina and magnesium carbonate oral suspension.
Use: Antacid.

alumina, magnesium carbonate and magnesium oxide tablets.
Use: Antacid.

alumina and magnesium trisilicate oral suspension.
Use: Antacid.

alumina and magnesium trisilicate tablets.
Use: Antacid.

Aluminostomy. (Richards Pharm) Aluminum pow. 18%, zinc oxide, zinc stearate in a bland water repellent ointment. Jar 2 oz, 6 oz, lb.
Use: Dermatologic, protectant.

aluminum. (uh-LOO-min-uhm)
See: Aluminostomy (Richards Pharm).

aluminum acetate.
Use: Astringent.
See: Acid Mantle Creme (Novartis).
Buro-Sol, Pow., Sol. (Doak Dermatologics).
W/Salicylic acid, boric acid.

•**aluminum acetate topical solution.** U.S.P. 23.
Use: Astringent.
See: Bluboro Powder (Allergan).
Buro-Sol Antiseptic Powder Conc. (Doak Dermatologics).
Burotor, Emul. (Torch).
Domeboro, Pow., Tab. (Bayer Corp).
Domeboro Otic, Soln. (Bayer Corp).

aluminum aminoacetate, dihydroxy.
See: Dihydroxy aluminum aminoacetate (Various Mfr.)

aluminum carbonate basic.
Use: Antacid.
See: Basaljel, Susp. (Wyeth Ayerst).

aluminum carbonate, dried basic, gel. Cap., Tab.
Use: Antacid.

•**aluminum carbonate, basic.** USAN. U.S.P. XXII.
Use: Antacid.
See: Basaljel, Susp., Cap., Tab. (Wyeth Ayerst).

aluminum chlorhydroxy allantoinate.
See: Alcloxa (Schuylkill).

•**aluminum chloride.** U.S.P. 23. Aluminum Cl hexahydrate.
Use: Astringent.
Drysol (Person & Covey).
Xerac AC (Person & Covey).
W/Oxyquinoline sulfate, benzalkonium Cl.

aluminum chloride hexahydrate.
Use: Astringent.
See: Drysol (Person & Covey).

•**aluminum chlorohydrate.** (ah-LOO-min-uhm) U.S.P. 23. *Formerly Aluminum chlorhydroxide, aluminum hydroxychloride.*
Use: Anhidrotic.
See: Ostiderm, Lot., Roll-On (Pedinol).

•**aluminum chlorohydrex.** (ah-LOO-min-uhm) USAN. *Formerly Aluminum chlorhydroxide alcohol soluble complex, aluminum chlorohydrol propylene glycol complex.*
Use: Astringent.

•**aluminum chlorohydrex polyethylene glycol.** U.S.P. 23.
Use: Anhidrotic.

•**aluminum chlorohydrex propylene glycol.** U.S.P. 23.
Use: Anhidrotic.

•**aluminum dichlorohydrate.** U.S.P. 23.
Use: Anhidrotic.

•**aluminum dichlorohydrex polyethylene glycol.** U.S.P. 23.
Use: Anhidrotic.

•**aluminum dichlorohydrex propylene glycol.** U.S.P. 23.
Use: Anhidrotic.

aluminum dihydroxyaminoacetate.
See: Dihydroxy Aluminum Aminoacetate, U.S.P. 23. (Various Mfr.).

aluminum glycinate, basic.
See: Dihydroxy Aluminum Aminoacetate, U.S.P. 23.
W/Aspirin, Magnesium carbonate.
See: Bufferin, Tab. (Bristol-Myers).

•**aluminum hydroxide gel.** U.S.P. 23.
Use: Antacid.
See: Alterna GEL, Liq. (J & J Merck Consumer Pharm).
Alu-Cap, Cap. (3M Pharm).
Al-U-Creme, Susp. (MacAllister).
Alu-Tab, Tab. (3M Pharm).
Amphojel, Susp., Tab. (Wyeth Ayerst).
Gelusil, Chew. tab. (Parke-Davis).
Maalox HRF, Liq. (Rhone-Poulenc Rorer).

Maalox Plus, Tab. (Rhone-Poulenc Rorer).
Nutrajel (Cenci).
W/Aminoacetic acid, magnesium trisilicate.
See: Maracid-2, Tab. (Marin).
W/Belladonna extract, magnesium hydroxide.
See: Trialka, Liq., Tab. (Del Pharmaceuticals).
W/Calcium carbonate.
See: Alkalade, Susp., Tab. (DePree).
W/Calcium carbonate, magnesium carbonate, magnesium trisilicate.
See: Marblen, Susp., Tab. (Fleming).
W/Clioquinol, methylcellulose, atropine sulfate, hyoscine HBr, hyoscyamine sulfate.
See: Enterex, Tab. (Person & Covey).
W/Dicyclomine HCl, magnesium hydroxide, methylcellulose.
See: Triactin Liq., Tab. (Procter & Gamble).
W/Gastric mucin, magnesium glycinate.
See: Mucogel, Liq., Tab. (Inwood).
W/Kaolin, pectin.
See: Metropectin, Liq. (Medeva).
W/Magnesium carbonate.
See: Algicon, Tab. (Rhone-Poulenc Rorer).
Estomul-M Liq., Tab. (3M Pharm).
W/Magnesium carbonate, calcium carbonate, amino-acetic acid.
See: Glycogel Tab., Susp. (Schwarz Pharma).
W/Magnesium hydroxide.
See: Alsorb Gel (Standex).
Aludrox, Susp., Tab. (Wyeth Ayerst).
Delcid, Liq. (Hoechst Marion Roussel).
Gas-Ban DS, Liq. (Roberts Pharm).
Kolantyl, Gel, Wafer (Hoechst Marion Roussel).
Maalox, Susp. (Rhone-Poulenc Rorer).
Mylanta, Tab. (Zeneca).
Mylanta II, Tab. (Zeneca).
Neutralox, Susp. (Teva USA).
WinGel, Liq., Tab. (Sanofi Winthrop).
W/Magnesium hydroxide, aspirin.
See: Ascriptin, Tab. (Rhone-Poulenc Rorer).
Ascriptin Extra Strength, Tab. (Rhone-Poulenc Rorer).
Calciphen, Tab. (Westerfield).
Cama, Tab. (Novartis).
Cama Inlay-Tab. (Novartis).
W/Magnesium hydroxide, belladonna extract
W/Magnesium hydroxide, calcium carbonate.
See: Camalox, Susp. (Rhone-Poulenc Rorer).
W/Magnesium hydroxide, glycine, magnesium trisilicate, belladonna extract.
W/Magnesium hydroxide and simethicone.
See: DI-GEL, Liq. (Schering Plough).
Maalox Plus, Susp. (Rhone-Poulenc Rorer).
Mylanta, Liq. (Zeneca).
Mylanta-II, Liq. (Zeneca).
Silain-Gel, Liq., Tab. (Robins).
Simeco, Liq. (Wyeth Ayerst).
W/Magnesium trisilicate.
See: Antacid G, Tab. (Walgreens).
Antacid Tablets, Tab. (Panray).
Arcodex Antiacid, Tab. (Arcum).
Gacid, Tab. (Arcum).
Malcogel, Susp. (Pharmacia & Upjohn).
Malcotabs (Pharmacia & Upjohn).
Manalum, Tab. (Paddock).
W/Phenindamine tartrate, phenylephrine HCl, aspirin, caffeine, magnesium carbonate.
See: Dristan, Tab. (Whitehall Robins).
W/Phenol, zinc oxide, camphor, eucalyptol, ichthammol.
See: Almophen, Oint. (Jones Medical Industries).
W/Prednisolone.
See: Fernisolone-B (Ferndale Laboratories).
Predoxine, Tab. (Roberts Pharm).
W/Sodium salicylate, acetaminophen, vitamin C.
See: Gaysal-S., Tab. (Roberts Pharm).

aluminum hydroxide gel. (Various Mfr.) 320 mg/5 ml. Susp. Bot. 360 ml, 480 ml, UD 15 and 30 ml. *otc.*
Use: Antacid.

aluminum hydroxide gel, concentrated. (Various Mfr.) 600 mg/5 ml. Liq. Bot. 30 ml, 180 ml, 480 ml. *otc.*
Use: Antacid.

aluminum hydroxide gel, concentrated. (Roxane) Susp. **450 mg/5 ml:** Bot. 500 ml, UD 30 ml; **675 mg/5 ml:** Bot. 180 ml, 500 ml, UD 20 ml and 30 ml. *otc.*
Use: Antacid.

•**aluminum hydroxide gel, dried.** U.S.P. 23.
Use: Antacid.
See: ALterna GEL, Liq. (J & J Merck Consumer Pharm)
Alu-Cap, Cap. (3M Pharm)
Amphojel, Tab. (Wyeth Ayerst)
Ascriptin, Tab. (Rhone-Poulenc Rorer)
Di-Gel, Liq. (Schering Plough)

Mylanta, Liq., Tab. (J & J Merck Consumer Pharm).

aluminum hydroxide gel, dried w/combinations.
Use: Antacid.
See: Aludrox, Susp., Tab. (Wyeth Ayerst).
Alurex, Tab. (Rexall).
Banacid, Tab. (Buffington).
Camalox, Tab. (Rhone-Poulenc Rorer).
Delcid, Liq. (Hoechst Marion Roussel).
Eulcin, Tab. (Leeds).
Fermalox, Tab. (Rhone-Poulenc Rorer).
Gaviscon, Foamtab (Hoechst Marion Roussel).
Gelusil, Preps. (Parke-Davis).
Kolantyl, Wafers (Hoechst Marion Roussel).
Maalox, Tab. (Rhone-Poulenc Rorer).
Maalox Plus, Tab. (Rhone-Poulenc Rorer).
Malcotabs, Tab. (Pharmacia & Upjohn).
Mylanta, Tab., Liq. (Zeneca).
Mylanta II, Tab., Liq. (Zeneca).
Phencaset Improved, Tab. (Zeneca).
Presalin, Tab. (Roberts Pharm).
Spasmasorb, Tab. (Roberts Pharm).

aluminum hydroxide glycine.
See: Dihydroxy aluminum aminoacetate.

aluminum hydroxide magnesium carbonate.
Use: Antacid.
See: Aloxine (Forest Pharmaceutical).
DI-GEL, Tab. (Schering Plough).
Magnagel, Susp., Tab. (Roberts Pharm).
W/Aminoacetic acid, calcium carbonate.
See: Eugel, Tab., Liq. (Solvay).
W/Dicyclomine HCl, magnesium trisilicate, methylcellulose.
See: Triactin, Liq., Tab. (Procter & Gamble).
W/Magnesium trisilicate.
See: Escot, Cap. (Solvay).
W/Magnesium trisilicate, bismuth alum.
See: Escot, Cap. (Solvay).

•**aluminum monostearate.** N.F. 18.
Use: Pharmaceutic necessity for preparation of penicillin G procaine w/aluminum stearate suspension.
See: Penicillin G procaine w/aluminum stearate suspension.

aluminum oxide.
See: Epi-Clear Scrub Cleanser (Bristol-Myers Squibb).

Aluminum Paste. (Paddock) Metallic aluminum 10%. Oint. Jar lb. *otc.*
Use: Dermatologic, protectant.

aluminum phenosulfonate.
See: AR-EX Cream Deodorant (Ar-Ex).

•**aluminum phosphate gel.** U.S.P. 23.
Use: Antacid.
See: Phosphaljel, Susp. (Wyeth Ayerst).

•**aluminum sesquichlorohydrate.** (ah-LOO-min-uhm sess-kwih-KLOR-oh-HIGH-drate) U.S.P. 23.
Use: Anhidrotic.

•**aluminum sesquichlorohydrex polyethylene glycol.** U.S.P. 23.
Use: Anhidrotic.

•**aluminum sesquichlorohydrex propylene glycol.** U.S.P. 23.
Use: Anhidrotic.

aluminum sodium carbonate hydroxide.
See: Dihydroxyaluminum Sodium Carbonate.

•**aluminum subacetate topical solution.** U.S.P. 23.
Use: Astringent.

•**aluminum sulfate.** U.S.P. 23.
Use: Pharmaceutic necessity for preparation of aluminum subacetate solution.
See: Aluminum Subacetate, Soln.
Bluboro, Pow. (Allergan).
Ostiderm, Roll-on (Pedinol).

•**aluminum zirconium octachlorohydrate.** U.S.P. 23.
Use: Anhidrotic.

•**aluminum zirconium octachlorohydrex gly.** U.S.P. 23.
Use: Anhidrotic.

•**aluminum zirconium pentachlorohydrate.** U.S.P. 23.
Use: Anhidrotic.

•**aluminum zirconium pentachlorohydrex gly.** U.S.P. 23.
Use: Anhidrotic.

•**aluminum zirconium tetrachlorohydrate.** U.S.P. 23.
Use: Anhidrotic.

•**aluminum zirconium tetrachlorohydrex gly.** (ah-LOO-min-uhm zihr-KOE-nee-uhm teh-trah-KLOR-oh-HIGH-drex Gly) U.S.P. 23.
Use: Anhidrotic.

•**aluminum zirconium trichlorohydrate.** U.S.P. 23.
Use: Anhidrotic.

•**aluminum zirconium trichlorohydrex gly.** (ah-LOO-min-uhm zihr-KOE-nee-uhm try-KLOR-oh-HIGH-drex Gly) U.S.P. 23.

Use: Anhidrotic.

Alupent. (Boehringer Ingelheim) Metaproterenol sulfate. **Metered dose inhaler:** 225 mg in 15 ml. **Tab.:** 10 mg or 20 mg. Bot. 100s. **Syr.:** 10 mg/5 ml. Bot. Pt. **Inhalant Soln.: 0.4%:** 2.5 ml UD vial. **0.6%:** 2.5 ml UD vial. **5%:** Bot. 10 ml, 30 ml UD. *Rx.*
Use: Bronchodilator.

Alurate. (Roche Laboratories) Aprobarbital 40 mg/5 ml. Alcohol 20%. Elix. Bot. Pt. *c-III.*
Use: Hypnotic, sedative.

Alurex. (Rexall) Magnesium-aluminum hydroxide. **Susp.:** (200 mg-150 mg/5 ml) Bot. 12 oz. **Tab:** (400 mg-300 mg) Box 50s. *otc.*
Use: Antacid.

Alu-Tab. (3M Pharm) Aluminum hydroxide gel 500 mg/Tab. Bot. 250s. *otc.*
Use: Antacid.

Alvedil Caps. (Luly-Thomas) Theophylline 4 gr, pseudoephedrine HCl 50 mg, butabarbital 15 mg/Cap. Bot. 100s. *Rx.*
Use: Bronchodilator, decongestant, hypnotic, sedative.

•**alverine citrate.** (AL-ver-een) USAN. N.F. XIII.
Use: Anticholinergic.

•**alvircept sudotox.** (AL-vihr-sept SOOD-ah-tox) USAN.
Use: Antiviral.

Alzapam. (Major) Lorazepam 0.5 mg, 1 mg or 2 mg/Tab. Bot. 100s, 500s. *c-IV.*
Use: Antianxiety.

Ama. (Wampole Laboratories) Antimitochondrial antibodies test by IFA. Test 48s.
Use: Diagnostic aid.

amacetam sulfate.
Use: Cognition adjuvant.

•**amadinone acetate.** (aim-AD-ih-nohn) USAN.
Use: Hormone, progestin.

amanozine hydrochloride.

•**amantadine hydrochloride.** (uh-MAN-tuh-deen) U.S.P. 23.
Use: Antiviral.

amantadine hydrochloride. (uh-MAN-tuh-deen) (Various Mfr.) **Cap.:** 100 mg. Bot. 100s, 250s, 500s, UD 100s. **Syrup:** 50 mg/5 ml Bot. pint.
Use: Antiviral, treatment of Parkinson's disease.
See: Symmetrel, Cap., Syr. (DuPont Merck Pharmaceuticals).

Amaphen. (Trimen) Acetaminophen 325 mg, caffeine 40 mg, butalbital 50 mg/Cap. Bot. 100s. *Rx.*
Use: Analgesic, hypnotic, sedative.

amaranth.
Use: Color (Not for internal use).

Amaryl. (Hoechst Marion Roussel) Glimepiride 1, 2 or 4 mg, lactose/Tab. 100s, UD 100s. *Rx.*
Use: Antidiabetic.

Amatine. (Roberts Pharm) Midodrine HCl.
Use: Orthostatic hypotension. [Orphan drug]

amazone.

ambenonium chloride.
Use: Cholinergic for treatment of myasthenia gravis.
See: Mytelase, Cap. (Sanofi Winthrop).

Ambenyl Cough Syrup. (Forest Pharmaceutical) Codeine phosphate 10 mg, bromodiphenhydramine HCl 12.5 mg/5 ml, alcohol 5%. Bot. 4 oz, pt, gal. *c-V.*
Use: Antihistamine, antitussive.

Ambenyl-D Liquid. (Forest Pharmaceutical) Guaifenesin 100 mg, pseudoephedrine HCl 30 mg, dextromethorphan HBr 15 mg/10 ml, alcohol 9.5%. Bot. 4 oz. *otc.*
Use: Antitussive, decongestant, expectorant.

Amberlite. I.R.P.-64. (Rohm and Haas). Polacrilin.

Amberlite. I.R.P.-88. (Rohm and Haas). Polacrilin potassium.

Ambi 10 Cream. (Kiwi Brands) Benzoyl peroxide 10%, parabens. Cream. Tube 28.3 g. *otc.*
Use: Antiacne.

Ambi 10 Soap. (Kiwi Brands) Triclosan, sodium tallouate, PEG-20, titanium dioxide. Soap, Bar 99 g. *otc.*
Use: Antiacne.

Ambien. (Searle) Zolpidem tartrate 5 mg, 10 mg/Tab. Bot. 100s, 500s, UD 100s. *c-IV.*
Use: Hypnotic, sedative.

Ambi Skin Tone. (Kiwi Brands) Hydroquinone, padimate O, sodium metabisulfite, parabens, EDTA, vitamin E. Cream. Tube 57 g, 28.4 g. *otc.*
Use: Dermatologic.

•**ambomycin.** (AM-boe-MY-sin) USAN. Isolated from filtrates of *Streptomyces ambofaciens.*
Use: Antineoplastic.

•**ambruticin.** (am-brew-TIE-sin) USAN.
Use: Antifungal.

ambucaine. Ambutoxate HCl.

ambucetamide.

•**ambuphylline.** (AM-byoo-fill-in) USAN. *Formerly Bufylline.*

Use: Diuretic, muscle relaxant.

•**ambuside.** (AM-buh-SIDE) USAN.
Use: Diuretic.
See: Novohydrin.

ambutonium bromide.
Use: Antispasmodic.

ambutoxate hydrochloride.

AMC. (Schlicksup) Ammonium Cl 7.5 gr/Tab. Bot. 1000s. *Rx.*
Use: Diuretic, expectorant.

Amcill. (Parke-Davis) **Cap.:** Ampicillin trihydrate 250 mg or 500 mg/Cap. Bot. 100s, 500s, UD pkg 100s. **Oral Susp.:** 125 mg or 250 mg/5 ml. Bot. 100 ml, 200 ml.
Use: Anti-infective, penicillin.

•**amcinafal.** (am-SIN-ah-fal) USAN.
Use: Anti-inflammatory.

•**amcinafide.** (am-SIN-ah-fide) USAN.
Use: Anti-inflammatory.

•**amcinonide.** (am-SIN-oh-nide) U.S.P. 23.
Use: Corticosteroid, topical.
See: Cyclocort, Cream, Oint. (ESI Lederle Generics).

Amcort. (Keene Pharmaceuticals) Triamcinolone diacetate 40 mg/ml. Vial 5 ml. *Rx.*
Use: Corticosteroid.

•**amdinocillin.** (am-DEE-no-SILL-in) U.S.P. 23.
Use: Anti-infective.

•**amdinocillin pivoxil.** (am-DEE-no-SILL-in pihv-OX-ill) USAN.
Use: Anti-infective.

ameban.
See: Carbarsone.

amebicides.
See: Acetarsone (Various Mfr.).
Aralen HCl, Inj. (Sanofi Winthrop).
Aralen Phosphate, Tab. (Sanofi Winthrop).
Carbarsone, Pulv., Tab. (Eli Lilly).
Chiniofon, Tab. (Various Mfr.).
Chloroquine Phosphate, Tab. (Various Mfr.).
Diiodohydroxyquin (Various Mfr.).
Diodoquin, Tab. (Searle).
Emetine HCl (Various Mfr.).
Flagyl, Tab. (Searle).
Humatin, Kapseal, Syr. (Parke-Davis).
Yodoxin, Tab. (Glenwood).

Amechol.
Use: Diagnostic aid.
See: Methacholine Cl.

•**amedalin hydrochloride.** (ah-MEH-dah-lin) USAN.
Use: Antidepressant.

•**ameltolide.** (AH-mell-TOE-lide) USAN.
Use: Anticonvulsant.

Amen. (Carnrick Labs) Medroxyprogesterone acetate 10 mg, lactose/Tab. Bot. 50s, 100s, 1000s. *Rx.*
Use: Hormone, progestin.

Amerge. (Glaxo Wellcome) Naratriptan HCl 1 mg, 2.5 mg, lactose/Tab. Blister pack 9s. *Rx.*
Use: Antimigraine.

Americaine Aerosol. (Novartis) Benzocaine 20% in a water-soluble vehicle. In 60 ml Bot. 0.67 oz, 2 oz, 4 oz. *otc.*
Use: Anesthetic, local.

Americaine. (Ciba Consumer) Benzocaine 20%. Spray 60 ml. *otc.*
Use: Anesthetic, local.

Americaine First Aid Burn Ointment. (Novartis) Benzocaine 20%, benzethonium Cl 0.1% in a water-soluble polyethylene glycol base. Tube 0.75 oz. *otc.*
Use: Anesthetic, local.

Americaine Hemorrhoidal Ointment. (Novartis) Benzocaine 20%. Tube 22.5 g w/rectal applicator. *otc.*
Use: Anesthetic, local.

Americaine Otic. (Novartis) Benzethonium Cl 0.1%, benzocaine 20% in a water-soluble base of 1% (w/w) glycerin, polyethylene glycol 300. Bot. 0.5 oz. *Rx.*
Use: Otic.

Ames Dextro System Lancets. (Bayer Corp) Sterile disposable lancet. Box 100s.
Use: Diagnostic aid.

•**amesergide.** (am-eh-SIR-jide) USAN.
Use: Serotonin antagonist.

•**ametantrone acetate.** (am-ETT-an-TRONE) USAN.
Use: Antineoplastic.

A-Methapred Univial. (Abbott Hospital Prods) Methylprednisolone sodium succinate. **40 mg/ml:** Pkg. 1s, 25s, 50s, 100s; 125 mg/2 ml Pkg. 1s, 5s, 25s, 50s, 100s; **500 mg/4 ml:** Pkg. 1s, 5s, 25s, 100s; **1000 mg/8 ml:** Pkg. 1s, 5s, 25s, 100s. *Rx.*
Use: Corticosteroid.

amethocaine hydrochloride.
Use: Anesthetic, local.
See: Tetracaine HCl.

amethopterin.
Use: Antineoplastic.
See: Methotrexate (ESI Lederle Generics).

•**amfenac sodium.** (AM-fen-ack SO-dee-uhm) USAN.
Use: Anti-inflammatory.

•**amfilcon a.** (AM-FILL-kahn A) USAN.
Use: Contact lens material (hydrophilic).

•**amflutizole.** (am-FLEW-tih-zole) USAN.
Use: Treatment of gout.

amfodyne.
See: Imidecyl iodine.

•**amfonelic acid.** (am-fah-NEH-lick Acid) USAN.
Use: Central nervous system stimulant.

Amgenal Cough Syrup. (Zenith Goldline) Bromodiphenhydramine HCl 12.5 mg, codeine phosphate 10 mg/5 ml, alcohol 5%. Bot. 120 ml, pt, gal. *c-v.*
Use: Antihistamine, antitussive.

amibiarson.
See: Carbarsone (Various Mfr.).

Amicar. (Immunex) **Tab.:** Aminocaproic acid 500 mg. In 100s. **Syr.:** Aminocaproic acid 250 mg/ml, sorbitol, saccharin. In 480 ml. **Inj.:** Aminocaproic acid 250 mg/ml, benzyl alcohol 0.9%. In 20 or 96 ml. *Rx.*
Use: Hemostatic, systemic.

•**amicycline.** (AM-ee-SIGH-kleen) USAN.
Use: Anti-infective.

Amidate. (Abbott Hospital Prods) Etomidate 2 mg/ml, propylene glycol 35%. Single dose Amp 20 mg/10 ml or 40 mg/20 ml; Abboject syringe 40 mg/20 ml. *Rx.*
Use: Anesthetic, general.

•**amidephrine mesylate.** (AM-ee-DEH-frin MEH-sih-LATE) USAN.
Use: Adrenergic.

amidofebrin.
See: Aminopyrine (Various Mfr.).

amidone hydrochloride.
Use: Analgesic, narcotic.
See: Methadone HCl (Various Mfr.).

amidopyrazoline.
See: Aminopyrine (Various Mfr.).

amidotrizoate, sodium.
See: Diatrizoate sodium.

•**amifloxacin.** (am-ih-FLOX-ah-SIN) USAN.
Use: Anti-infective.

•**amifloxacin mesylate.** (am-ih-FLOX-ah-SIN MEH-sih-LATE) USAN.
Use: Anti-infective.

•**amifostine.** (am-ih-FOSS-teen) USAN.
Formerly Ethiofos.
Use: Protectant (topical); radioprotector.
See: Ethyol (Alza/US Bioscience).

amifostine. (am-ih-FOSS-teen)
Use: Chemoprotective. [Orphan drug]
See: Ethyol (US Bioscience).

Amigen. (Baxter) Protein hydrolysate. *Rx.* **5%:** Bot. 500 ml, 1000 ml; **10%:** Bot. 500 ml, 1000 ml. **5% w/dextrose 5%:** Bot. 500 ml, 1000 ml. **5% w/dextrose 5%, alcohol 5%:** Bot. 1000 ml. **5% w/fructose 10%:** Bot. 1000 ml. **5% w/fructose 12.5%, alcohol 2.4%:** Bot. 1000 ml.
Use: Nutritional supplement.

Amigesic. (Amide Pharmaceuticals) Salsalate 500 mg/Cap or Tab. Salsalate 75 mg/capl. Bot. 100s, 500s. *Rx.*
Use: Analgesic.

•**amikacin.** (am-ih-KAE-sin) U.S.P. 23.
Use: Anti-infective.

amikacin. (Bedford Labs) Amikacin sulfate 250 mg, sodium metabisulfite 0.66%, sodium citrate dihydrate 2.5%/ml. Inj. Vial 2 ml, 4 ml. *Rx.*
Use: Anti-infective.

amikacin. (Gensia) 50 mg (as sulfate) per ml, sodium metabisulfite 0.13%, sodium citrate dihydrate 0.5%. Inj. Vial 2, 4 ml (10s). *Rx.*
Use: Anti-infective.

•**amikacin sulfate.** (am-ih-KAE-sin) U.S.P. 23.
Use: Anti-infective.

amikacin sulfate injection. (Various Mfr.) Amikacin sulfate 50 mg/ml. Vial 2 ml, 4 ml (10s).
Use: Anti-infective.
See: Amikin, Inj. (Bristol-Myers Squibb).

Amikin. (Bristol-Myers Squibb) Amikacin sulfate. Inj. Vial 100 mg, 500 mg, 1 g, disposable syringes 500 mg. *Rx.*
Use: Anti-infective, aminoglycoside.

•**amiloride hydrochloride.** (uh-MILL-oh-ride) U.S.P. 23.
Use: Diuretic.
See: Midamor, Tab. (Merck).

amiloride hydrochloride solution for inhalation. (GlaxoWellcome)
Use: Cystic fibrosis. [Orphan drug]

amiloride hydrochloride and hydrochlorthiazide tablets.
Use: Antihypertensive, diuretic.
See: Moduretic, Tab. (Merck).

Amina-21. (Miller) L-form amino acids 600 mg/Cap. Bot. 100s, 300s.
Use: Dermatologic, wound therapy.

aminacrine. F.D.A. 9-Aminoacridine.
Use: Anti-infective, topical.

•**aminacrine hydrochloride.** (ah-MEE-nah-kreen) USAN.
Use: Anti-infective, topical.
W/Dienestrol, sulfanilamide, allantoin.
See: AVC/Dienestrol Cream, Supp. (Hoechst Marion Roussel).
Use: Bacteriostatic agent.
W/Oxyquinoline benzoate.
See: Triva, Vaginal Jelly (Boyle).
W/Sulfanilamide, allantoin.

See: AVC, Cream, Supp. (Hoechst Marion Roussel).
Femguard Vaginal Cream (Solvay)
Vagidine, Cream (Zeneca).
Vagitrol, Cream, Supp. (Teva USA).

aminarsone.
See: Carbarsone (Various Mfr.).

amine resin.
See: Polyamine Methylene Resin.

Aminess. (Clintec Nutrition) Essential amino acids. 10 Tab. = adult amino acid MDR. Jar 300s. *Rx.*
Use: Parenteral nutritional supplement.

Aminess 5.2%. (Clintec Nutrition) Amino acids and electrolytes, Inj. *Rx.*
Use: Nutritional supplement, parenteral.

Aminicotin.
Use: Vitamin supplement.
See: Nicotinamide (Various Mfr.).

aminoacetic acid. Glycerine, U.S.P. 23. (Various Mfr.) (Glycine, glycocoll) available as elix., pow., tab.
Use: Myasthenia gravis, irrigant.
W/Aluminum hydroxide, magnesium hydroxide, calcium carbonate.
See: Eugel, Tab., Liq. (Solvay).
W/Calcium carbonate.
See: Antacid pH, Tab. (Towne).
Eldamint, Tab. (Zeneca).
W/Calcium carbonate, aluminum hydroxide, magnesium carbonate.
See: Glytabs, Tab. (Pharmics).
W/Calcium carbonate, magnesium carbonate, bismuth subcarbonate, dried aluminum hydroxide gel.
See: Buffer-Tabs (Forest Pharmaceutical).
W/Magnesium trisilicate, aluminum hydroxide.
See: Maracid-2, Tab. (Marin).
W/Phenylephrine HCl, pyrilamine maleate, acetylsalicylic acid, caffeine.
See: Al-Ay, Tab. (Jones Medical Industries).
W/Phenylephrine HCl, chlorpheniramine maleate, acetaminophen, caffeine.
See: Codimal, Tab. (Schwarz Pharma).

aminoacetic acid & calcium carbonate.
W/Lysine.
See: Lycolan, Elix. (Lannett).

amino acid & protein prep.
See: Aminoacetic Acid, U.S.P. 23.
Glutamic Acid.
Histidine HCl.
Lysine.
Phenylalanine.
Thyroxine.

amino acids.
Use: Amino acid supplement.
See: Aminosol, Soln. (Abbott Laboratories).
Aminosyn, Soln. (Abbott Laboratories).
W/Estrone, testosterone, vitamins, minerals.
See: Geramine, Tab., Inj. (ICN Pharmaceuticals).
W/Vitamin B_{12}.
See: Stuart Amino Acids and B_{12}, Tab. (Zeneca).

amino acid combinations.
See: Dequasine (Miller).
NeuRecover-LT (NeuroGenesis).
NeuroSlim (NeuroGenesis/Matrix).
NeuRecover-DA (NeuroGenesis/Matrix).
NeuRecover-SA (NeuroGenesis/Matrix).
Herpetrol (Alva).
A/G-Pro (Miller).
Jets (Freeda Vitamins).
PDP Liquid Protein (Wesley Pharmacal).

Amino-Min-D Capsules. (Tyson and Associates) Ca 250 mg, D 100 IU, Fe 7.5 mg, Zn 5.6 mg, Mg, I, Mn, Cu, K, Cr, Se, betaine HCl, glutamic acid HCl. Cap. Bot. 100s. *otc.*
Use: Mineral, vitamin supplement.

aminoacridine. (ah-MEE-no-ACK-rih-deen)
Use: Bacteriostatic agent.
See: 9-aminoacridine.

9-aminoacridine hydrochloride. (9-ah-MEE-no-ACK-rih-deen) (Various Mfr.) Aminacrine HCl.
Use: Anti-infective, vaginal.
See: Vagisec Plus (Schmid).
W/Hydrocortisone acetate, tyrothricin, phenylmercuric acetate, polysorbate-80, urea, lactose.
See: Aquacort, Vaginal Supp. (Poly-Medica).
W/Iodoquinol.
See: Vagitric, Oint. (Zeneca).
W/Phenylmercuric acetate, tyrothricin, urea, lactose.
See: Trinalis, Vaginal Supp. (Poly-Medica).
W/Polyoxyethylene nonyl phenol, sodium edetate, docusate sodium.
See: Vagisec Plus, Supp. (Schmid).
W/Pramoxine HCl, acetic acid, parachlorometa-xylenol, methyl-dodecylbenzyltrimethyl ammonium Cl.
See: Drotic No. 2, Drops (B.F. Ascher).
W/Sulfanilamide, allantoin.
See: AVC Cream, Supp. (Hoechst Marion Roussel).
Nil Vaginal Cream (Century Pharm).
Par Cream (Parmed).

Vagisan, Creme (Sandia).
Vagisul, Creme (Sheryl).
W/Sulfisoxazole, allantoin.
See: Vagilia, Cream (Teva USA).

p-aminobenzene-sulfonylacetylimide.
See: Sulfacetamide.

•**aminobenzoate potassium.** (ah-MEE-no-BEN-zoe-ate) U.S.P. 23.
Use: Analgesic.
See: Potaba, Pow., Tab. (Glenwood).
W/Hydrocortisone, ammonium salicylate, ascorbic acid.
See: Neocylate sodium free, Tab. (Schwarz Pharma).
W/Potassium salicylate.
See: Pabalate-SF, Tab. (Robins).

•**aminobenzoate sodium.** U.S.P. 23.
Use: Analgesic.
See: PABA sodium, Tab. (Various Mfr.).
W/Phenobarbital, colchicine salicylate, Vitamin B_1, aspirin.
See: Doloral, Tab. (Alamed).
W/Salicylamide, ascorbic acid.
W/Salicylamide, sodium salicylate, ascorbic acid, butabarbital sodium.
See: Bisalate, Tab. (Allison Lab).
W/Sodium salicylate.
See: Pabalate, Tab. (Robins).

•**aminobenzoic acid.** U.S.P. 23. *Formerly Para-aminobenzoic acid.*
Use: Ultraviolet screen.
See: Pabafilm (Galderma).
Pabanol, Lot. (Zeneca).
W/Mephenesin, salicylamide.
See: Sal-Phenesin, Tab. (Hoechst Marion Roussel).
W/Sodium salicylate, ascorbic acid.
See: Nucorsal, Tab. (Westerfield).

p-aminobenzoic acid, salts.
See: p-Aminobenzoate potassium and p-Aminobenzoate sodium.

•**aminocaproic acid.** (uh-mee-no-kuh-PRO-ik) U.S.P. 23.
Use: Hemostatic.
See: Amicar, Syr., Tab., Vial (Immunex).

aminocaproic acid. (uh-mee-no-kuh-PRO-ik) (Orphan Medical)
Use: Topical treatment of traumatic hyphema of the eye.

aminocaproic acid. (Various Mfr.) 250mg/ml. 20 ml/Inj. *Rx.*
Use: Antifibrinolytic.

aminocardol.
Use: Bronchodilator.
See: Aminophylline (Various Mfr.).

Amino-Cerv pH 5.5. (Milex) Urea 8.34%, sodium propionate 0.5%, methionine 0.83%, cystine 0.35%, inositol 0.83%, benzalkonium Cl, water miscible base. Tube with applicator 82.5 g. *Rx.*
Use: Vaginal agent.

Aminodyne Compound. (Jones Medical Industries) Acetaminophen 2.5 gr, aspirin 3.5 gr, caffeine 0.5 gr/Tab. Bot. 100s, 1000s. *otc.*
Use: Analgesic combination.

2-aminoethanethiol. USAN.
Use: Urinary tract agent.

amino-ethyl-propanol.
See: Aminoisobutanol.
W/Bromotheophyllin.
See: Pamabrom (Various Mfr.).

Aminofen. (Dover Pharmaceuticals) Acetaminophen 325 mg/Tab. Sugar, lactose and salt free. UD Box 500s. *otc.*
Use: Analgesic.

Aminofen Max. (Dover Pharmaceuticals) Acetaminophen 500 mg/Tab. Sugar, lactose and salt free. UD Box 500s. *otc.*
Use: Analgesic.

aminoform.
Use: Anti-infective, urinary.
See: Methenamine (Various Mfr.).

Aminogen. (Christina) Vitamin B complex, folic acid. Amp. 2 ml Box 12s, 24s, 100s. Vial 10 ml. *Rx.*
Use: Vitamin supplement.

•**aminoglutethimide.** (ah-MEE-no-glue-TETH-ih-mide) U.S.P. 23.
Use: Treatment of Cushing's syndrome; adrenocortical suppressant; antineoplastic.
See: Cytadren, Tab. (Novartis).

•**aminohippurate sodium injection.** (ah-MEE-no-HIP-your-ate) U.S.P. 23.
Use: Diagnostic aid (renal function determination).

aminohippurate sodium. (Merck) 0.2g/10 ml. Amp 10 ml, 50 ml.
Use: I.V., diagnostic aid for renal plasma flow and function determination.

•**aminohippuric acid.** (ah-MEE-no-hip-YOUR-ik) U.S.P. 23.
Use: Component of aminohippurate sodium (Inj.); diagnostic aid (renal function determination).

aminoisobutanol.
See: Butaphyllamine.
Pamabrom for combinations.

aminoisometradine.
See: Methionine.

Aminonat. Protein hydrolysates (oral).

aminonitrozole. N-(5-Nitro-2-thiazolyl) acetamide.
Use: Antitrichomonal.

Amino-Optic-C. (Tyson and Associates) Lemon bioflavonoids 250 mg, rutin, hesperidin, vitamin C and rose hips powder 1000 mg/SR Tab. Bot. 100s. *otc.*
Use: Vitamin supplement.

Amino-Opti-E. (Tyson and Associates) 165 mg/Cap. Bot. 100s. *otc.*
Use: Vitamin supplement.

aminopentamide sulfate.
Use: Anticholinergic.

Aminophyllin. (Searle) Trademark for Aminophylline. **100 mg/Tab.** Bot. 100s, 1000s, UD 100s. **200 mg/Tab.** Bot. 100s, 1000s, UD 100s. *Rx.*
Use: Bronchodilator.

Aminophyllin Injection. (Searle) Trademark for Aminophylline. Amp. **250 mg:** 10 ml; 25s, 100s; **500 mg:** 20 ml; 25s, 100s. *Rx.*
Use: Bronchodilator.

•**aminophylline.** (am-in-AHF-ih-lin) U.S.P. 23. *Formerly Theophylline ethylenediamine.*
Use: Muscle relaxant.
See: Aminodur, Dura-Tab. (Berlex).
Lixaminol, Elix. (Ferndale Laboratories).
Phyllocontin, Tab. (Purdue Frederick).
Rectalad-Aminophylline (Wallace Laboratories).
Somophyllin Oral Liq. (Medeva).
Somophyllin Rectal Soln. (Medeva).

aminophylline combinations.
Amesec, Cap. (GlaxoWellcome).
Amphedrine Compound, Cap. (Lannett).
Asminorel, Tab. (Solvay).
B.M.E., Elix. (Brothers).
Lixaminol AT/5 ml (Ferndale Laboratories).
Mudrane GG-2, Tab. (ECR Pharmaceuticals).
Orthoxine and Aminophylline, Cap. (Pharmacia & Upjohn).
Quinamm, Tab. (Hoechst Marion Roussel).
Quinite, Tab. (Solvay).
Strema, Cap. (Foy).

aminophylline injection. (Abbott Laboratories) Amp. 250 mg/10 ml, 500 mg/20 ml; Fliptop vial 10 mg/20 ml, 20 mg/50 ml.
Use: Bronchodilator.

aminophylline injection. Theophylline ethylenediamine. Amp. 3¾ gr, 7.5 gr (Various Mfr.).
Use: Muscle relaxant.

aminophylline suppositories. 3⅜ gr, 7.5 gr (Various Mfr.).
Use: Muscle relaxant.

aminophylline tablets. Plain or enteric coated 1.5 gr, 3 gr (Various Mfr.).
Use: Muscle relaxant.

aminophylline with phenobarbital combinations.
Amodrine, Tab. (Searle).
Mudrane, Tab. (ECR Pharmaceuticals).
Mudrane GG, Tab. (ECR Pharmaceuticals)).

Aminoprel. (Taylor Pharmaceuticals) L-lysine 60 mg, dl-methionine 15 mg, hydrolyzed protein 750 mg, iron 2 mg, Cu, I, K, Mg, Mn, Zn. Cap. Bot. 180s.
Use: Nutritional supplement.

aminopromazine. (I.N.N.). Proquamezine.

4-aminopyridine.
Use: Relief of symptoms of multiple sclerosis. [Orphan drug]

aminopyrine. Amidofebrin, Amidopyrazoline, Anafebrina, Novamidon, Pyradone.
Use: Antipyretic, analgesic.
See: Dipyrone, Vial (Maurry).

aminoquin naphthoate.
See: Pamaquine Naphthoate.

4-aminoquinoline derivatives.
Use: Antimalarial.
See: Aralen HCl (Sanofi Winthrop).
Chloroquine Phosphate (Various Mfr.).
Plaquenil Sulfate (Sanofi Winthrop).

8-aminoquinoline derivatives.
Use: Antimalarial.
See: Primaquine Phosphate, U.S.P.
Primaquine Phosphate (Sanofi Winthrop).

•**aminorex.** (am-EE-no-rex) USAN.
Use: Anorexic.
See: Apiquel fumarate.

aminosalicylate calcium. U.S.P. XXI. (Dumas-Wilson) 7.5 gr, Bot. 1000s.
Use: Tuberculosis therapy.
W/Isoniazid, pyridoxine HCl.
See: Calpas-Inah-6, Tab. (Amer. Chem. & Drug).

aminosalicylate potassium. Monopotassium 4-aminosalicylate.
Use: Antibacterial (tuberculostatic).
See: Paskalium, Tab., Pow. (Glenwood).

•**aminosalicylate sodium.** (uh-MEE-no-suh-LIS-ih-LATE) U.S.P. 23.
Use: Anti-infective (tuberculostatic).

aminosalicylate sodium. (uh-MEE-no-suh-LIS-ih-LATE) (Syncom)
Use: Crohn's disease. [Orphan drug]

•**aminosalicylic acid.** (ah-MEE-no-sal-ih-SILL-ik) U.S.P. 23.

Use: Anti-infective (tuberculostatic).

aminosalicylic acid. (ah-MEE-no-SAL-ih-sill-ik)
Use: Tuberculosis infection treatment.
See: Pasar, Gran. (Jacobus).

4-aminosalicylic acid.
Use: Treatment of ulcerative colitis in patients intolerant to sulfasalazine. [Orphan drug]
See: Pamisyl (Parke-Davis).
Rezipas (Bristol-Myers Squibb).

5-aminosalicylic acid.
See: Mesalamine.

p-aminosalicylic acid salts.
See: Aminosalicylate Calcium.
Aminosalicylate Potassium.
Aminosalicylate Sodium.

aminosidine.
Use: Mycobacterium avium complex; tuberculosis; visceral leishmaniasis (KALA-AZAR). [Orphan drug]
See: Gabbromicina.
Paromomycin.

Aminosyn. (Abbott Hospital Prods) Crystalline amino acid solution. **3.5%:** 1000 ml; **5%:** Container 250 ml, 500 ml, 1000 ml; **7%:** 500 ml; 7% kit (cs/3); **8.5%:** Single dose container 500 ml, 1000 ml. **10%:** 500 ml, 1000 ml. *Rx.*
W/Dextrose.
W/Electrolytes.
7%: 500 ml; **8.5%:** 500 ml.
Use: Nutritional supplement, parenteral.

Aminosyn (pH6). (Abbott Laboratories) Crystalline amino acid infusion. 10%: 500 ml, 1000 ml. *Rx.*
Use: Nutritional supplement, parenteral.

Aminosyn-HBC 7%. (Abbott Laboratories) Crystalline amino acid infusion for high metabolic stress. 500 ml, 1000 ml. *Rx.*
Use: Nutritional supplement, parenteral.

Aminosyn M 3.5%. (Abbott Laboratories) Crystalline amino acid infusion with electrolytes. 1000 ml. *Rx.*
Use: Nutritional supplement, parenteral.

Aminosyn-PF. (Abbott Laboratories) Crystalline amino acid infusions for pediatric use. **7%:** 250 ml, 500 ml; **10%:** 1000 ml. *Rx.*
Use: Nutritional supplement, parenteral.

Aminosyn-RF. (Abbott Laboratories) Crystalline amino acid infusion for renal failure patients. **5.2%:** 300 ml. *Rx.*
Use: Nutritional supplement, parenteral.

Aminosyn II. (Abbott Laboratories) Crystalline amino acid infusion. **3.5%:** 1000 ml; **5%:** 1000 ml; **7%:** 500 ml; **8.5%:** 500 ml, 1000 ml; **10%:** 500 ml, 1000 ml. *Rx.*
W/Dextrose:
3.5% in 5% dextrose: 1000 ml; **3.5% in 25% dextrose:** 1000 ml; **5% in 25% dextrose:** 1000 ml. *Rx.*
W/Dextrose and electrolytes.
3.5% in 5% dextrose: 1000 ml; **3.5% in 25% dextrose:** 1000 ml; **4.25% in 10% dextrose:** 1000 ml; **4.25% in 25% dextrose:** 1000 ml. *Rx.*
W/Electrolytes.
7%: 1000 ml; **8.5%:** 1000 ml; **10%:** 1000 ml. *Rx.*
Use: Nutritional supplement, parenteral.

Aminosyn II M. (Abbott Laboratories) Crystalline amino acid infusion with maintenance electrolytes, 10% dextrose. Soln. 1000 ml. *Rx.*
Use: Nutritional supplement, parenteral.

Amino-Thiol. (Marcen) Sulfur 10 mg, casein 50 mg, sodium citrate 5 mg, phenol 5 mg, benzyl alcohol 5 mg/ml. Vial 10 ml, 30 ml. *Rx.*
Use: Treatment of arthritis, neuritis.

aminotrate phosphate. Trolnitrate phosphate.
See: Triethanolamine, Preps.

aminoxytropine tropate hydrochloride. Atropine-N-oxide HCl.

Amio-Aqueous. (Academic Pharm) Amiodarone.
Use: Antiarrhythmic. [Orphan drug]

•**amiodarone.** (A-MEE-oh-duh-rone) USAN.
Use: Cardiovascular agent (antiarrhythmic, ventricular).

amiodarone hydrochloride.
Use: Antiarrhythmic. [Orphan drug]
See: Amio-Aqueous (Academic Pharm).
Cordarone, Tab., Inj. (Wyeth Ayerst).

Amipaque. (Sanofi Winthrop) Metrizamide 18.75%/20 ml Vial.
Use: Radiopaque agent.

amiphenazole hydrochloride.

•**amiprilose hydrochloride.** (ah-MIH-prih-LOHS) USAN.
Use: Anti-infective, antifungal, anti-inflammatory, antineoplastic, antiviral, immunomodulator.

•**amiquinsin hydrochloride.** (AM-ih-KWIN-sin) USAN. Under study.
Use: Antihypertensive.

Ami-Tex LA. (Amide Pharmaceuticals) Phenylpropanolamine HCl 75 mg, guaifenesin 400 mg/tab. Bot. 100s, 500s, 1000s. *Rx.*
Use: Decongestant, expectorant.

Amitin. (Thurston) Vitamin C 200 mg, lemon bioflavonoid 100 mg, niacinamide 60 mg, methionine 100 mg/Tab.

Bot. 100s, 500s. *Rx.*
Use: Vitamin supplement.

Amitone. (Menley & James) Calcium carbonate 350 mg/Chew. tab. Bot. 100s. *otc.*
Use: Antacid.

•**amitraz.** (AM-ih-trazz) U.S.P. 23.
Use: Scabicide.

•**amitriptyline hydrochloride.** (am-ee-TRIP-tih-leen) U.S.P. 23.
Use: Antidepressant.
See: Amitril, Tab. (Parke-Davis).
Elavil HCl, Tab., Inj. (Merck).
Emitrip, Tab. (Major).
Endep, Tab. (Roche Laboratories).
W/Chlordiazepoxide.
See: Limbitrol, Tab. (Roche Laboratories).
W/Perphenazine.
See: Etrafon, Prods. (Schering Plough).
Triavil, Tab. (Merck).

AmLactin. (Upsher-Smith) Ammonium lactate 12%/Cream, Lot. 140 g, 225 g, 400 g. *otc.*
Use: Emollient.

•**amlexanox.** (am-LEX-an-ox) USAN.
Use: Treatment of mouth ulcers; antiallergic.
See: Aphthasol.

•**amlintide.** (AM-lin-tide) USAN.
Use: Treatment of insulin-dependent diabetes mellitus; antidiabetic.

amlodipine. (am-LOW-dih-PEEN)
Use: Calcium channel blocker.
See: Norvasc (Pfizer).

amlodipine and benazepril HCl. (am-LOW-dih-PEEN and BEN-AZE-eh-prill)
See: Lotrel, Cap. (Ciba-Geigy).

•**amlodipine besylate.** (am-LOW-dih-PEEN) USAN.
Use: Antianginal; antihypertensive.
See: Norvasc (Pfizer).

•**amlodipine maleate.** (am-LOW-dih-PEEN) USAN.
Use: Antianginal, antihypertensive.

Ammens Medicated Powder. (Bristol-Myers) Boric acid 4.55%, zinc oxide 9.10%, talc, starch. Can 6.25 oz, 11 oz. *otc.*
Use: Dermatologic, protectant.

ammoidin. Methoxsalen.
Use: Psoralen.

•**ammonia N 13 injection.** (ah-MOE-nee-ah N13) U.S.P. 23.
Use: Diagnostic aid (cardiac imaging, liver imaging); radiopharmaceutical.

•**ammonia solution, strong.** (ah-MOE-nee-ah) N.F. 18.
Use: Pharmaceutic aid (solvent; source of ammonia).

•**ammonia spirit, aromatic.** (ah-MOE-nee-ah) U.S.P. 23.
Use: Respiratory.

ammoniated mercury. (Various Mfr.)
Use: Anti-infective, topical.
See: Mercuronate 5% Oint. (Jones Medical Industries).
W/Salicylic acid.
See: Emersal, Lot. (Medco Research).

•**ammonio methacrylate copolymer.** (ah-MOE-nee-oh meth-ah-KRILL-ate koe-PAHL-ih-mer) N.F. 18.
Use: Pharmaceutic aid (coating agent).

ammonium benzoate.
Use: Antiseptic, urinary.

ammonium biphosphate, sodium biphosphate and sodium acid pyrophosphate.
Use: Genitourinary.
See: pHos-pHaid (Guardian Laboratories).

•**ammonium carbonate.** (ah-MOE-nee-uhm) N.F. 18.
Use: Pharmaceutic aid (source of ammonia).

•**ammonium chloride.** (ah-MOE-nee-uhm) U.S.P. 23.
Use: Acidifier; diuretic.
See: Nodema, Tab. (Towne).

ammonium chloride. (Various Mfr.) **Delayed Release Tab.:** Plain or E.C. 5 gr, 7.5 gr. (Bayer Corp) **Inj.:**120 mEq/30 ml. Vial.
Use: Acidifier; diuretic; expectorant; alkalosis.

Ammonium Chloride, Enseals. (Eli Lilly) Ammonium Cl. Tab. Enseal 7.5 gr. Bot. 100s. *Rx.*
Use: Acidifier, urinary.

•**ammonium lactate.** (ah-MOE-nee-uhm LACK-tate) USAN.
Use: Antipruritic (topical).
See: AmLactin, Cream, Lot. (Upsher-Smith).
Lac-Hydrin, Lot. (Westwood-Squibb).

ammonium mandelate. Ammonium salt of mandelic acid. Syr. 8 g/fl oz. Bot. pt, gal.
Use: Urinary antiseptic, oral.

•**ammonium molybdate.** (ah-MOE-nee-uhm) U.S.P. 23.

ammonium nitrate.
See: Reditemp-C, Cold Pack (Wyeth Ayerst).

•**ammonium phosphate.** (ah-MOE-nee-uhm) N.F. 18. Phosphoric acid diammonium salt. Diammonium phosphate.
Use: Pharmaceutic aid.

ammonium tetrathiomolybdate.

Use: Treatment of Wilson's disease. [Orphan drug]

ammonium valerate.
Use: Sedative.

ammophyllin.
Use: Bronchodilator.
See: Aminophylline, U.S.P. 23. (Various Mfr.).

amobarbital. (am-oh-BAR-bih-tahl) (Various Mfr.) Tab. Elix.
Use: Hypnotic of intermediate duration.
See: Amytal, Elix., Pulv. (Eli Lilly).

amobarbital w/combinations.
See: Amodex, Cap. (Forest Pharmaceutical).
Ectasule, Cap. (Fleming). (Lannett).

•**amobarbital sodium.** (am-oh-BAR-bih-tahl) U.S.P. 23.
Use: Hypnotic, sedative.

amobarbital sodium. (Various Mfr.)
Cap. **1 gr:** Bot. 100s, 500s; **3 gr:** Bot. 100s, 500s, 1000s (Various Mfr.).
Tab. **30 mg:** Bot. 100s; **50 mg:** Bot. 100s; **100 mg:** Bot. 100s. (Eli Lilly).
Vial 250 mg, 500 mg. (Eli Lilly).
Use: Hypnotic of intermediate tion, sedative.
See: Amytal sodium (Eli Lilly).
W/Ephedrine HCl, theophylline, chlorpheniramine maleate.
See: Theo-Span, Cap. (Scrip).
W/Secobarbital sodium.
See: Compobarb, Cap. (Eon Labs Manufacturing).
Dusotal, Cap. (Harvey).
Tuinal, Cap. (Eli Lilly).

AMO Endosol. (Allergan) Sodium chloride 0.64%, potassium chloride 0.075%, calcium chloride dihydrate 0.048%, magnesium chloride hexahydrate 0.03%, sodium acetate trihydrate 0.39%, sodium citrate dihydrate 0.17%. Preservative free. Soln. 18,500 ml. *Rx.*
Use: Physiological irrigating solution.

AMO Endosol Extra. (Allergan) **Part I:** water for injection with sodium chloride 7.14 mg, potassium chloride 0.38 mg, calcium chloride dihydrate 0.154 mg, magnesium chloride hexahydrate 0.2 mg, dextrose 0.92 mg, sodium hydroxide or hydrochloric acid/ml. Soln. Bot. 515 ml. **Part II:** Sodium bicarbonate 1081 mg, dibasic sodium phosphate anhydrous 216 mg, glutathione disulfide 95 mg. Soln. Bot. 60 ml. *Rx.*
Use: Ophthalmic irrigation solution.

•**amodiaquine.** (am-oh-DIE-ah-kwin) U.S.P. 23.
Use: Antiprotozoal.

•**amodiaquine hydrochloride.** U.S.P. 23.
Use: Antimalarial.

Amodopa. (Major) Methyldopa 125 mg, 250 mg or 500 mg. **125 mg:** 100s, UD 100s. **250 mg:** 100s, 1000s, UD 100s. **500 mg:** 100s, 500s, UD 100s. *Rx.*
Use: Antihypertensive.

AMO Endosol. (Allergan) Sodium chloride 0.64%, potassium chloride 0.075%, calcium chloride dihydrate 0.048%, magnesium chloride hexahydrate 0.03%, sodium acetate trihydrate 0.39%, sodium citrate dihydrate 0.17%, preservative free. Sol. 18 ml, 500 ml. *Rx.*
Use: Ophthalmic irrigant.

Amol. Mono-n-amyl-hydroquinone ether.
See: B-F-I, Pow. (SmithKline Beecham Pharmaceuticals).

Amoline. (Major) Aminophylline 100 mg or 200 mg/Tab. Bot. 100s, 1000s, UD 100s. *otc, Rx.*
Use: Bronchodilator.

amopyroquin hydrochloride.
See: Propoquin.

•**amorolfine.** (am-OH-role-feen) USAN.
Use: Antimycotic.

Amosan. (Oral-B Laboratories) Sodium perborate, saccharin. 1.76 g single-dose packet box. 20s, 40s. *otc.*
Use: Mouth and throat preparation.

Amotriphene. *Rx.*
Use: Coronary vasodilator.

AMO Vitrax. (Allergan) Sodium hyaluronate 30 mg/ml. Inj. Disp. syringe 0.65 ml. *Rx.*
Use: Viscoelastic, ophthalmic.

•**amoxapine.** (am-OX-uh-peen) U.S.P. 23.
Use: Antidepressant.
See: Asendin, Tab. (ESI Lederle Generics).

amoxapine tablets.
Use: Antidepressant.

•**amoxicillin.** (a-MOX-ih-sil-in) U.S.P. 23.
Use: Anti-infective.
See: Amoxil, Preps. (SmithKline Beecham Pharmaceuticals).
Polymox, Preps. (Bristol-Myers Squibb).

amoxicillin. (Various Mfr.) Chew. tab. 250 mg. Lactose, sucrose. 100s, 500s. *Rx.*
Use: Anti-infective.

amoxicillin and clavulanate potassium for oral suspension. (a-MOX-ih-sil-in and CLAV-you-lon-ate poe-TASS-ee-uhm)
Use: Anti-infective, inhibitor (β-*lactamase*).
See: Augmentin (SmithKline Beecham Pharmaceuticals).

amoxicillin and clavulanate potassium tablets. (a-MOX-ih-sil-in and CLAV-you-lon-ate poe-TASS-ee-uhm)
Use: Anti-infective, inhibitor (β-*lactamase*).
See: Augmentin, Tab., Chew Tab., Pow for Susp. (SmithKline Beecham Pharmaceuticals).

amoxicillin intramammary infusion.
Use: Anti-infective, penicillin.

amoxicillin trihydrate.
Use: Anti-infective, penicillin.
See: Amoxil Chew. tab. (SmithKline Beecham Pharmaceuticals).
Polymox, Cap., Susp. (Bristol-Myers Squibb).
Trimox, Preps. (Squibb Diagnostic)
Utimox, Cap, Susp. (Parke-Davis).
Wymox, Cap, Liq. (Wyeth Ayerst).
W/Clavulanate Potassium.
See: Augmentin, Tab., Chew. tab., Pow. for susp. (SmithKline Beecham Pharmaceuticals).

Amoxil. (SmithKline Beecham Pharmaceuticals) Amoxicillin. **Cap.:** 250 mg. Bot. 100s, 500s, UD 10 × 10; 500 mg Bot. 50s, 500s. UD 10 × 10; **Pow. for Oral Susp.:** 125 mg or 250 mg/5 ml. Bot. 80 ml, 100 ml, 150 ml, UD 5 ml. *Rx.*
Use: Anti-infective, penicillin.

Amoxil Chewable Tablets. (SmithKline Beecham Pharmaceuticals) Amoxicillin trihydrate. 125 mg or 250 mg/Tab. Bot. 60s. *Rx.*
Use: Anti-infective, penicillin.

Amoxil Pediatric Drops. (SmithKline Beecham Pharmaceuticals) Amoxicillin 50 mg/ml. Bot. 15 ml, 30 ml. *Rx.*
Use: Anti-infective, penicillin.

d-AMP. (Dunhall Pharmaceuticals) Ampicillin trihydrate 500 mg. Cap. Bot. 100s. *Rx.*
Use: Anti-infective, penicillin.

AMP. Adenosine Phosphate, USAN.
Use: Nutrient.

amperil. (Armenpharm) Ampicillin trihydrate 250 mg or 500 mg/Cap. Bot. 100s, 500s. *Rx.*
Use: Anti-infective, penicillin.

•**amphecloral.** (AM-feh-klahr-ahl) USAN.
Use: Sympathomimetic; anorexic.

amphenidone.
Use: CNS stimulant.

amphetamine aspartate combinations. (am-FET-uh-meen)
See: Adderall, Tab. (Richwood).

amphetamine hydrochloride. (am-FET-uh-meen) **Amp:** 20 mg/ml, 1 ml (Various Mfr.). **Cap:** (Various Mfr.) *Rx.*
Use: Vasoconstrictor, CNS stimulant.

amphetamine, levo.
Use: CNS stimulant.
See: Levamphetamine.

amphetamine phosphate.
Use: CNS stimulant.

amphetamine phosphate, dextro. Tab. Dextroamphetamine phosphate. (Various Mfr.).
Use: CNS stimulant.

amphetamine phosphate, dibasic. (Various Mfr.) Racemic amphetamine phosphate. **Cap:** 5 mg or 10 mg. **Tab:** 5 mg or 10 mg. *Rx.*
Use: CNS stimulant.

amphetamines.
See: Amphetamine Sulfate, Tab. (Lannett).
Biphetamine, Cap. (Medeva).
Desoxyn, Tab. (Abbott Laboratories).
Desoxyn Gradumets, Long-acting tab. (Abbott Laboratories).
Dexampex, Cap., Tab. (Teva USA).
Dexedrine, Elix., Tab., S.R. Cap. (SmithKline Beecham Pharmaceuticals).
Dextroamphetamine Sulfate, Tab., S.R. Cap. (Various Mfr.).
Ferndex, Tab. (Ferndale Laboratories).
Methampex, Tab. (Teva USA).

•**amphetamine sulfate.** U.S.P. 23.
Use: CNS stimulant.

amphetamine sulfate. (Various Mfr.) 5 mg, 10 mg/Cap. Tab; 20 mg/ml Vial
Use: CNS stimulant.

amphetamine sulfate combinations. (am-FET-uh-meen)
See: Adderall, Tab. (Richwood).

amphetamine sulfate, dextro.
Use: CNS stimulant.
See: Dextroamphetamine Sulfate, U.S.P. 23.

amphetamine with dextroamphetamine as resin complexes.
Use: Appetite depressant.
See: Biphetamine, Cap. (Medeva).

Amphocaps. (Halsey) Ampicillin 250 mg or 500 mg/Cap. Bot. 100s. *Rx.*
Use: Anti-infective, penicillin.

Amphojel. (Wyeth Ayerst) Aluminum hydroxide gel. **Susp.:** 320 mg/5 ml. Bot. 355 ml; **Tab.:** 300 mg or 600 mg. Bot. 100s. *otc.*
Use: Antacid.

•**amphomycin.** (AM-foe-MY-sin) USAN. An antibiotic produced by *Streptomyces canus.*
Use: Anti-infective.

See: Ecomytrin.

Amphotec. (Sequus Pharmaceuticals) Amphotericin B (as cholesteryl) 50 mg and 100 mg/Pow. for Inj. Vial 20 ml, 50 ml. *Rx.*
Use: For treatment of certain fungal infections.

amphotericin.
Use: Antifungal.
See: Fungizone, Preps. (Bristol-Myers Squibb).

•**amphotericin b.** (am-foe-TER-ih-sin B) U.S.P. 23.
Use: Antifungal.
See: Abelcet, Susp. for Inj. (Liposome Co.).
AmBisome, Pow. for Inj. (Fujisawa).
Amphotec, Pow. for Inj. (Sequus Pharmaceuticals).
Amphotericin B (PharmaTek).
Fungizone, Preps. (Bristol-Myers Squibb).
W/Tetracycline and K metaphosphate.
See: Mysteclin-F, Preps. (Bristol-Myers Squibb).

amphotericin B. (Pharmos) 50 mg as desoxycholate/Inj. Vial. *Rx.*
Use: Antifungal.

amphotericin B lipid complex. (Bristol-Myers Squibb)
Use: Anti-infective.

amphotericin b lipid complex. (am-foe-TER-ih-sin B)
Use: Invasive fungal infections. [Orphan drug]
See: Abelcet, Inj. (Liposome).

•**ampicillin.** (am-pih-SILL-in) U.S.P. 23.
Use: Anti-infective.
See: Omnipen, Preps. (Wyeth Ayerst).
Polycillin, Preps. (Bristol-Myers Squibb).
Principen, Preps. (Squibb Diagnostic).
Totacillin, Preps. (SmithKline Beecham Pharmaceuticals).
W/Probenecid.
See: Polycillin-PRB, UD (Bristol-Myers Squibb).
Principen W/Probenecid Cap. (Bristol-Myers Squibb).

ampicillin with probenecid. Cap., Oral Susp.
Use: Anti-infective, penicillin.
See: Principen w/Probenecid (Bristol-Myers Squibb).

•**ampicillin sodium.** (am-pih-SILL-in) U.S.P. 23.
Use: Anti-infective.
See: Omnipen-N, Inj. (Wyeth Ayerst).
Totacillin-N, Vial (SmithKline Beecham Pharmaceuticals).

ampicillin sodium/sulbactam sodium. (am-pih-SILL-in/sull-BAK-tam)
Use: Anti-infective, penicillin.
See: Unasyn (Roerig).

ampicillin trihydrate. (Various Mfr.) Cap., Oral Susp. *Rx.*
Use: Anti-infective, penicillin.
See: Amcil, Cap., Susp. (Parke-Davis).
D-Amp, Cap., Susp. (Dunhall Pharmaceuticals).
Marcillin, Cap., Susp. (Marnel).
Omnipen, Cap., Susp. (Wyeth Ayerst).
Polycillin Preps. (Bristol-Myers Squibb).
Principen, Cap., Susp. (Bristol-Myers Squibb).
Totacillin, Cap., Susp. (SmithKline Beecham Pharmaceuticals).

Amplicor. (Roche Laboratories) Kits 10s, 96s, 100s.
Use: Diagnostic aid, chlamydia. *Rx.*

Amplicor HIV-1 Monitor. (Roche Laboratories) Kit. 24 tests.
Use: Test kit for plasma HIV-1 tests.

Ampligen. (HEM Pharmaceutical) Poly I: Poly C12U. Phase II/III HIV.
Use: Immunomodulator.

amprotropine phosphate.

•**ampyzine sulfate.** (AM-pih-zeen) USAN.
Use: Central nervous system stimulant.

•**amquinate.** (am-KWIN-ate) USAN.
Use: Antimalarial.

•**amrinone.** (AM-rih-nohn) U.S.P. 23.
Use: Cardiovascular agent.
See: Inocor Lactate Inj. (Sanofi Winthrop).

amrinone lactate. (AM-rih-nohn LAK-tate)
See: Inocor (Sanofi Winthrop).

•**amsacrine.** (AM-sah-KREEN) USAN.
Use: Antineoplastic. [Orphan drug]

Am-Tuss Elixir. (T.E. Williams) Codeine phosphate 10 mg, phenylephrine HCl 10 mg, phenylpropanolamine HCl 5 mg, prophenpyridamine maleate 12.5 mg, guaifenesin 44 mg, fluid extract of ipecac 0.17 min., citric acid 60 mg, sodium citrate 197 mg/5 ml, alcohol 5%. Bot. pt, gal. *c-v.*
Use: Antihistamine, antitussive, decongestant, expectorant.

Amvisc. (Chiron Therapeutics) **Inj.:** Sodium hyaluronate 12 mg/ml. Disp. syringe 0.5 ml, 0.8 ml. *Rx.*
Use: Viscoelastic.

Amvisc Plus. (Chiron Therapeutics) **Inj.:** Sodium hyaluronate 16 mg/ml. Disp. syringe: 0.5 ml, 0.8 ml. *Rx.*

Use: Viscoelastic.

Am-Wax. (Amlab) Urea, benzocaine, propylene glycol, glycerin. Bot. 10 ml. *otc.*
Use: Otic.

amyl. Phenyl phenol, phenyl mercuric nitrate.
See: Lubraseptic Jelly (Guardian Laboratories).

•**amyl nitrite.** (A-mill NYE-trite) U.S.P. 23.
Use: Vasodilator.

amyl nitrite. Isoamyl nitrite. Isopentyl nitrite. (GlaxoWellcome). Vaporole 0.18 ml or 0.3 ml. Box 12s. (Eli Lilly). Aspirols 0.3 ml. Box 12s.
Use: Inhalation, coronary vasodilator in angina pectoris.
W/Sodium nitrite, sodium thiosulfate.
See: Cyanide Antidote Pkg. (Eli Lilly).

α**amylase.**
W/Calcium carbonate, glycine, belladonna extract.
See: Trialka, Tab. (Del Pharmaceuticals).
W/Pancreatin, protease, lipase.
See: Dizymes, Cap. (Recsei).
W/Pepsin, homatropine methyl bromide, lipase, protease, bile salts.
See: Digesplen, Tab., Elix. (Med. Prod. Panamericana).
W/Pepsin, pancreatin, ox bile extract.
See: Gourmase, Cap. (Solvay).
W/Phenobarbital, belladonna, pepsin, amylase, pancreatin, ox bile extract.
See: Gourmase-PB, Cap. (Solvay).

•**amylene hydrate.** N.F. 18. (AM-ih-leen HIGH-drate)
Use: Pharmaceutic aid (solvent).

amylolytic enzyme.
W/Butabarbital sodium, belladonna extract, cellulolytic enzyme, proteolytic enzyme, lipolytic enzyme, iron ox bile.
See: Butibel-Zyme, Tab. (Ortho McNeil).
W/Calcium carbonate, glycine, proteolytic and cellulolytic enzymes.
See: Co-Gel, Tab. (Arco).
W/Cellulolytic, proteolytic and lipolytic enzymes, hyoscyamine sulfate.
See: Converspaz, Tab. (B.F. Ascher).
W/Lipase, proteolytic, cellulolytic enzymes, phenobarbital, hyoscyamine sulfate, atropine sulfate.
See: Arco-Lipase Plus, Tab. (Arco).
W/Proteolytic, cellulolytic, lipolytic enzymes, iron, ox bile.
See: Spaszyme, Tab. (Dooner).
W/Proteolytic enzyme, d-sorbitol.
See: Kuzyme, Cap. (Schwarz Pharma).
W/Proteolytic, cellulolytic, lipolytic enzymes.
See: Arco-Lase, Tab. (Arco).
Zymme, Tab. (Scrip).
W/Proteolytic enzyme (Papain), homatropine methylbromide, d-sorbitol.
See: Converzyme, Liq. (B.F. Ascher).
W/Proteolytic enzyme, lipolytic enzyme, cellulolytic enzyme, belladonna extract.
See: Mallenzyme Improved, Tab. (Roberts Pharm).

Amytal Sodium. (Eli Lilly) Amobarbital sodium. Pow. for Inj.: 15 g, 30 g. Vial: 250 mg/vial or 500 mg/vial. Traypak 10s, 25s. *c-II.*
Use: Hypnotic, sedative.

Ana. (Wampole Laboratories) Antinuclear antibodies test by IFA. Test 54s.
Use: Diagnostic aid.

Ana Hep-2. (Wampole Laboratories) Antinuclear antibodies test by IFA. Tests 60s.
Use: Diagnostic aid.

anabolic agents. These agents stimulate constructive processes leading to retention of nitrogen and increasing the body protein.
See: Adroyd, Tab. (Parke-Davis).
Anabolin-IM, Vial (Alto Pharmaceuticals).
Anadrol, Tab. (Syntex).
Anavar, Tab. (Searle).
Android, Tab. (Zeneca).
Androlone, Vial (Keene Pharmaceuticals).
Crestabolic, Vial (Nutrition).
Deca-Durabolin, Amp., Vial (Organon Teknika).
Dianabol, Tab. (Novartis).
Di Genik, Vial (Savage).
Drolban, Vial (Eli Lilly).
Durabolin, Amp., Vial (Organon Teknika).
Halotestin, Tab. (Pharmacia & Upjohn).
Hybolin, Vial (Hyrex).
Maxibolin, Elix., Tab. (Organon Teknika).
Nandrobolic, Vial (Forest Pharmaceutical).
Ora-Testryl, Tab. (Bristol-Myers Squibb).
Os-Cal-Mone, Tab. (Hoechst Marion Roussel).
Winstrol, Tab. (Sanofi Winthrop).
W/Vitamins and minerals.
See: Dumogran, Tab. (Bristol-Myers Squibb).

Anabolin. (Alto Pharmaceuticals) Nandrolone phenpropionate 50 mg, benzyl alcohol 2%, sesame oil q.s./ml. Vial 2 ml. *Rx.*

Use: Anabolic steroid.

Anabolin-IM. (Alto Pharmaceuticals) Nandrolone phenpropionate 50 mg, benzyl alcohol 2%, sesame oil q.s./ml. Vial 2 ml. *Rx.*
Use: Anabolic steroid.

Anabolin LA-100. (Alto Pharmaceuticals) Nandrolone decanoate 100 mg/ml. Vial 2 ml. *Rx.*
Use: Anabolic steroid.

Anacaine. (Gordon Laboratories) Benzocaine 10%. Jar oz, lb. *otc.*
Use: Anesthetic, local.

Anacin Tablets. (Whitehall Robins) Aspirin 400 mg, caffeine 32 mg. **Tab.:** Tin 12s, bot. 30s, 50s, 100s, 200s. **Cap.:** Bot. 30s, 50s, 100s. *otc.*
Use: Analgesic.

Anacin Maximum Strength. (Whitehall Robins) Aspirin 500 mg, caffeine 32 mg/ Tab. Bot. 12s, 20s, 24s, 40s, 72s, 75s, 150s. *otc.*
Use: Analgesic.

Anadrol-50. (Syntex) Oxymetholone 50 mg/Tab. Bot. 100s. *c-III.*
Use: Anabolic steroid.

anafebrina.
See: Aminopyrine (Various Mfr.).

Anafranil. (Novartis) Clomipramine HCl 25 mg, 50 mg or 75 mg/Cap. Bot. 100s, UD 100s. *Rx.*
Use: Antidepressant.

•**anagestone acetate.** (AN-ah-JEST-ohn) USAN.
Use: Hormone, progestin.
See: Anatropin (Ortho McNeil).

anagrelide. (AN-AGG-reh-lide)
Use: Polycythemia vera; essential thrombocythemia; thrombocytosis in chronic myelogenous leukemia. [Orphan drug]
See: Agrylin, Cap. (Roberts Pharm).

•**anagrelide hydrochloride.** (AN-AGG-reh-lide) USAN.
Use: Antithrombotic.
See: Agrylin, Cap. (Roberts Pharm).

Ana-Guard Epinephrine. (Bayer Corp) Epinephrine 1:1000, chlorobutanol < 5 mg and sodium bisulfite 1.5 mg per ml. In 1 ml syringes designed to deliver 2 doses of 0.3 ml each. *Rx.*
Use: Anaphylaxis or severe allergy treatment.

•**anakinra.** (an-ah-KIN-rah) USAN. Interleukin-1 receptor antagonist (recombinent).
Use: Anti-inflammatory (nonsteroidal); suppressant (inflammatory bowel disease).

Ana-Kit. (Bayer Corp) Syringe, epinephrine 1:1000 in 1 ml; four (each 2 mg) chlorpheniramine maleate; two sterilized swabs, tourniquet, instructions/kit. *Rx.*
Use: Anaphylactic therapy.

Analbalm Improved Formula. (Schwarz Pharma) Methyl salicylate 10%, menthol 1.25%, camphor 3%. Liq. Bot. **Green:** 4 oz, gal. **Pink:** 4 oz, pt, gal. *otc.*
Use: Counterirritant.

analeptics. Usually a term applied to agents with stimulant action, particularly on the central nervous system. See also central nervous system stimulants.
See: Amphetamine salts (Various Mfr.).
Caffeine (Various Mfr.).
Cylert, Tab. (Abbott Laboratories).
Dextroamphetamine salts (Various Mfr.).
Dopram, Vial (Robins).
Ephedrine Salts (Various Mfr.).
Methamphetamine salts (Various Mfr.).
Ritalin HCl, Tab. (Novartis).
Sodium Succinate (Various Mfr.).

Analgesia Creme. (Rugby) Trolamine sulfate 10%. Cream, Tube 85 g. *otc.*
Use: Liniment.

analgesic balm. (Various Mfr.) Menthol w/methyl salicylate in a suitable base. *otc.*
Use: Counterirritant.
See: A.P.C., 1.5 oz, lb.
Fougera, oz.
Horton & Converse, oz, lb.
Lilly, oz.
Musterole (Schering Plough).
Stanlabs, oz, pt.
Wisconsin, 1 lb, 5 lb.

Analgesic Liquid. (Weeks & Leo) Triethanolamine salicylate 20% in an alcohol base. Bot. 4 oz. *otc.*
Use: Analgesic, topical.

Analgesic Lotion. (Weeks & Leo) Methyl nicotinate 1%, methyl salicylate 10%, camphor 0.1%, menthol 0.1%. Bot. 4 oz. *otc.*
Use: Analgesic, topical.

Analpram-HC. (Ferndale Laboratories) Hydrocortisone acetate 1% or 2%, pramoxine HCl 1%. Cream Tube 30 g. *Rx.*
Use: Anesthetic; corticosteroid, local.

Analval Tablets. (Pal-Pak) Aspirin 227 mg, acetaminophen 162 mg, caffeine 32 mg/Tab. Bot. 1000s. *otc.*
Use: Analgesic combination.

Anamine. (Merz) Pseudoephedrine HCl 30 mg, chlorpheniramine maleate 2 mg/5 ml. Syr. Bot. 473 ml. *Rx.*
Use: Antihistamine, decongestant.

Anamine HD Syrup. (Merz) Phenylephrine HCl 5 mg, chlorpheniramine maleate 2 mg, hydrocodone bitartrate 1.67 mg. 10 ml tid or qid. *c-III.*
Use: Antihistamine, antitussive, decongestant.

Anamine T.D. Capsules. (Merz) Chlorpheniramine maleate 8 mg, pseudoephedrine HCl 120 mg/T.D. Cap. Bot. 100s. *Rx.*
Use: Antihistamine, decongestant.

Ananain, Comosain.
Use: Burn therapy. [Orphan drug]
See: Vianain (Genzyme).

Anaplex. (ECR Pharmaceuticals) Pseudoephedrine HCl 30 mg, chlorpheniramine maleate 2 mg/5 ml. Syr. Bot. 473 ml. *Rx.*
Use: Antihistamine, decongestant.

Anaplex HD Syrup. (ECR Pharmaceuticals) Hydrocodone bitartrate 1.7 mg, phenylephrine HCl 5 mg, chlorpheniramine maleate 2 mg. Bot. 120 ml, 480 ml. *c-III.*
Use: Antihistamine, antitussive, decongestant.

Anaprox. (Syntex) Naproxen sodium 275 mg (naproxen base 250 mg with sodium 25 mg), lactose/Tab. Bot. 100s, 500s. UD 100s. *Rx.*
Use: NSAID.

Anaprox DS. (Syntex) Naproxen sodium 550 mg (naproxen base 500 mg with sodium 50 mg)/Tab. Bot. 100s, 500s, UD 100s. *Rx.*
Use: NSAID.

anarel. Guanadrel sulfate.

•**anaritide acetate.** (an-NAR-ih-TIDE) USAN.
Use: Antihypertensive, diuretic.

anaritide acetate. (an-NAR-ih-TIDE)
Use: Improvement of early renal allograft function following renal transplantation; acute renal failure.
See: Auriculin (Scios).

Anaspaz. (B.F. Ascher) l-Hyoscyamine sulfate 0.125 mg/Tab. Bot. 100s, 500s. *Rx.*
Use: Anticholinergic, antispasmodic.

•**anastrozole.** (an-ASS-troe-zole) USAN.
Use: Antineoplastic.
See: Arimidex, Tab. (Zeneca).

Anatrast. (Lafayette Pharm) GI contrast agent, 100% paste. Tube 500 g.

Anatuss DM. (Merz) **Syrup:** Guaifenesin 100 mg, pseudoephedrine HCl 30 mg, dextromethorphan HBr 10 mg, cherry flavor/5 ml. Bot. 480 ml; **Tab.:** Guaifenesin 400 mg, pseudoephedrine HCl 60 mg, dextromethorphan HBr 20 mg. Bot. 100s. *otc.*
Use: Antitussive, decongestant, expectorant.

Anatuss LA. (Merz) Guaifenesin 400 mg, pseudoephedrine HCl 120 mg. Tab. Bot. 100s. *Rx.*
Use: Decongestant, expectorant.

Anatuss Syrup. (Merz) Dextromethorphan HBr 15 mg, phenylpropanolamine HCl 25 mg, guaifenesin 100 mg/10 ml. Bot. 120 ml, 480 ml. *otc.*
Use: Antitussive, decongestant, expectorant.

Anatuss Tabs. (Merz) Guaifenesin 100 mg, acetaminophen 325 mg, dextromethorphan HBr 15 mg, phenylpropanolamine HCl 25 mg/Tab. Bot. 100s, 500s. *Rx.*
Use: Analgesic, antitussive, decongestant, expectorant.

Anatuss w/Codeine. (Merz) **Syr.:** Phenylpropanolamine HCl 25 mg, codeine phosphate 10 mg, guaifenesin 100 mg/5 ml. Bot. 120 ml, 480 ml. *c-v.* **Tab.:** Phenylpropanolamine HCl 25 mg, codeine phosphate 10 mg, guaifenesin 100 mg, acetaminophen 300 mg. Bot. 100s. *c-III.*
Use: Analgesic (Tab. only), antitussive, decongestant, expectorant.

Anavar. (Searle) Oxandrolone 2.5 mg/Tab. Bot. 100s. *Rx.*
Use: Anabolic steroid.

anayodin.
See: Chiniofon.

•**anazolene sodium.** (an-AZZ-oh-leen) USAN. Sodium Anoxynaphthonate.
Use: Diagnostic aid (blood volume, cardiac output determination).
See: Coomassie Blue (Wyeth Ayerst).

Anbesol Baby Gel. (Whitehall Robins) Benzocaine 7.5%. Tube 0.25 oz. *otc.*
Use: Anesthetic, local.

Anbesol Gel. (Whitehall Robins) Benzocaine 6.3%, phenol 0.5%, alcohol 70%. Tube 7.5 g. *otc.*
Use: Anesthetic, topical combination.

Anbesol Liquid. (Whitehall Robins) Benzocaine 6.3%, phenol 0.5%, povidone-iodine 0.04%, alcohol 70%. Bot. 9 ml, 22 ml. *otc.*
Use: Anesthetic combination, topical.

Anbesol Maximum Strength. (Whitehall Robins) **Gel:** Benzocaine 20%, alcohol

60%, carbomer 934P, polyethylene glycol, saccharin. Tube 7.2 g. **Liq.:** Benzocaine 20%, alcohol 60%, saccharin, polyethylene glycol. Bot. 9 ml. *otc.*
Use: Anesthetic, local.

Ancef. (SmithKline Beecham Pharmaceuticals) Cefazolin sodium. **Vial:** Equivalent to 500 mg or 1 g of cefazolin. **Multi Pack:** 500 mg or 1 g/Pack. 25s. **Bulk Vial:** 5 g, 10 g. **Piggyback Vial:** 500 mg or 1 g/100 ml. **Minibag:** 500 mg/50 ml, 1 g/50 ml w/5% dextrose inj. (D5W). 500 mg/50 ml D5W. *Rx.*
Use: Anti-infective, cephalosporin.

Ancid Tablet and Suspension. (Sheryl) Calcium aluminum carbonate, di-amino acetate complex. Tab. 100s. Susp. pt. *otc.*
Use: Antacid.

Ancobon. (Roche Laboratories) Flucytosine 250 mg or 500 mg/Cap. Bot. 100s. *Rx.*
Use: Anti-infective.

•**ancrod.** (AN-krahd) USAN. An active principle obtained from the venom of the Malayan pit viper *Agkistrodon rhodostoma.*
Use: Anticoagulant.

ancrod. (AN-krahd) (Knoll Pharm)
Use: Antithrombotic in patients with heparin-induced thrombocytopenia or thrombosis who require immediate and continued anticoagulation.

Andesterone Suspension. (Lincoln) Estrone 2 mg, testosterone 6 mg/ml. Vial 15 ml. **Forte:** Estrone 1 mg, testosterone 20 mg/ml. Inj. Vial 15 ml. *Rx.*
Use: Androgen, estrogen combination.

Andrest 90-4. (Seatrace) Testosterone enanthate 90 mg, estradiol valerate 4 mg/ml. Vial 10 ml. *Rx.*
Use: Androgen, estrogen combination.

Andro 100. (Forest Pharmaceutical) Testosterone 100 mg/ml. Vial 10 ml. *c-III.*
Use: Androgen.

Androcur. Cyproterone acetate.
Use: Hirsutism, severe. [Orphan Drug] Sponsor: Berlex.

Andro-Cyp 100. (Keene Pharmaceuticals) Testosterone cypionate 100 mg/ml. Vial 10 ml. *c-III.*
Use: Androgen.

Andro-Cyp 200. (Keene Pharmaceuticals) Testosterone cypionate 200 mg/ml. Vial 10 ml. *c-III.*
Use: Androgen.

Androderm. (SmithKline Beecham) 12.2 mg testosterone USP. 37 cm^2. Transdermal patch, releases 2.5 mg or 5 mg/day. 30s, 60s. *c-III.*
Use: Hormone, testosterone.

Andro-Estro 90-4. (Rugby) Estradiol valerate 4 mg, testosterone enanthate 90 mg/ml with chlorobutanol in sesame oil. Inj. Vial. 10 ml. *Rx.*
Use: Androgen, estrogen combination.

Androgel. (Unimed) Testosterone.
Use: AIDS. [Orphan drug]

Androgel-DHT. (Unimed) Dihydrotestosterone.
Use: AIDS. [Orphan drug]

androgens. Substances which possess masculinizing activities.
See: Methyltestosterone.
Testosterone.
Testosterone cyclopentylpropionate.
Testosterone enanthate.
Testosterone heptanoate.
Testosterone phenylacetate.
Testosterone propionate.

androgen-estrogen therapy.
See: Dienestrol with Methyltestosterone.
Estradiol Esters with Methyltestosterone.
Estradiol Esters with Testosterone.
Estrogenic Substance, Conjugated with Methyltestosterone.
Estrogenic Substance Mixed with Methyltestosterone.
Estrogenic Substance Mixed with Testosterone.
Estrone with Testosterone.
Gynetone, Tab. (Schering Plough).

androgen hormone inhibitor.
See: Proscar (Merck).

Android-10 and 25. (Zeneca) Methyltestosterone 5 mg/Buccal Tab., 10 mg/Tab. or 25 mg/Tab. Bot. 60s. *c-III.*
Use: Androgen.

Andro L.A. 200. (Forest Pharmaceutical) Testosterone enanthate 200 mg/ml. Inj. vial 10 ml. *c-III.*
Use: Androgen.

Androlin. (Lincoln) Testosterone 100 mg/ml. Vial 10 ml. *c-III.*
Use: Androgen.

Androlone. (Keene Pharmaceuticals) Nandrolone phenpropionate 25 mg/ml in sesame oil. Vial 5 ml. *c-III.*
Use: Anabolic steroid.

Androlone-D 200. (Keene Pharmaceuticals) Nandrolone decanoate w/benzyl alcohol, 200 mg/ml. Inj. Vial 1 ml. *c-III.*
Use: Anabolic steroid.

Andronaq-50. (Schwarz Pharma) Testo-

sterone 50 mg/ml, sodium carboxymethylcellulose, methylcellulose, povidone, DSS, thimerosal. Inj. Vial. 10 ml. *c-III.*
Use: Androgen.

Andronaq LA. (Schwarz Pharma) Testosterone cypionate 100 mg, benzyl alcohol 0.9% in cottonseed oil. Vial 10 ml. Bot. 12s. *c-III.*
Use: Androgen.

Andronate 100. (Taylor Pharmaceuticals) Testosterone cypionate 100 mg/ml with benzyl alcohol in cottonseed oil. Vial 10 ml. *c-III.*
Use: Androgen.

Andronate 200. (Taylor Pharmaceuticals) Testosterone cypionate 200 mg/ml with benzyl alcohol, benzyl benzoate in cottonseed oil. Vial 10 ml. *c-III.*
Use: Androgen.

Andropository 200. (Rugby) Testosterone enanthate 200 mg/ml in sesame oil with chlorobutanol. Inj. Vial 10 ml. *c-III.*
Use: Androgen.

androstanazole.
See: Stanozolol.

androstane-17-(beta)-ol-3-one.
See: Stanolone.

androstanolone. (I.N.N.) Stanolone.

androstenopyrazole. Anabolic steroid; pending release.

Androtest P.
See: Testosterone propionate.

Androvite. (Optimox) Tab.: Iron 3 mg, vitamins A 4167 IU, D 67 IU, E 67 IU, B_1 8.3 mg, B_2 8.3 mg, B_3 8.3 mg, B_5 16.7 mg, B_6 16.7 mg, B_{12} 20.8 mcg, C 167 mg, folic acid 0.06 mg, PABA, inositol, biotin, betaine, B, Cr, Cu, I, Mg, Mn, Se, Zn 8.3 mg, pancreatin, hesperidin, rutin. Bot. 180s. *otc.*
Use: Vitamin/mineral supplement.

Andryl 200. (Keene Pharmaceuticals) Testosterone enanthate 200 mg/ml. Vial 10 ml. *c-III.*
Use: Androgen.

Andylate Forte. (Vita Elixir) Acetaminophen 3 gr, salicylamide 3 gr, caffeine 0.25 gr/Tab. *otc.*
Use: Analgesic combination.

Andylate Rub. (Vita Elixir) Methylnicotinate, methylsalicylate, camphor, dipropyleneglycol salicylate, oil of cassia, oleoresin of capsicum, oleoresin of ginger. *otc.*
Use: Analgesic, topical.

Andylate Tablets. (Vita Elixir) Sodium salicylate 10 gr/Tab. *otc.*
Use: Analgesic.

Anectine. (GlaxoWellcome) Succinylcholine Cl. Soln. 20 mg/ml. Multidose Vial 10 ml. Sterile Pow. Flo-Pak 500 mg or 1000 mg. Box 12s. *Rx.*
Use: Muscle relaxant.

Anefrin Nasal Spray, Long Acting. (Walgreens) Oxymetazoline HCl 0.05%. Bot. 0.5 oz. *otc.*
Use: Decongestant.

Anergan 50. (Forest Pharmaceutical) Promethazine HCl 50 mg/ml EDTA, phenol. Vial 10 ml. *Rx.*
Use: Antihistamine.

anertan.
See: Testosterone propionate.

Anestacon. (PolyMedica) Lidocaine HCl 20 mg/ml. Jelly, 15 ml, 240 ml. *Rx.*
Use: Anesthetic, local.

Anesthesin. Ethyl-p-aminobenzoate.
Use: Anesthetic, local.
See: Benzocaine, U.S.P. 23.

anethaine.
See: Tetracaine HCl.

•**anethole.** (AN-eh-thole) N.F. 18.
Use: Pharmaceutic aid (flavor).

aneurine hydrochloride.
See: Thiamine HCl, Preps. (Various Mfr.).

Anexsia 5/500. (Mallinckrodt) Hydrocodone bitartrate 5 mg, acetaminophen 500 mg/Tab. Bot. 100s. *c-III.*
Use: Analgesic combination, narcotic.

Anexsia 7.5/650. (Mallinckrodt) Hydrocodone bitartrate 7.5 mg, acetaminophen 650 mg/Tab. Bot. 100s. *c-III.*
Use: Analgesic combination, narcotic.

Anexsia 10/660. (Mallinckrodt) Hydrocodone bitartrate 10 mg, acetaminophen 660 mg/Tab. Bot. 100s and 1000s. *c-III.*
Use: Analgesic combination, narcotic.

Angel Sweet. (Garrett) Vitamins A and D_2. Cream 90 g. *otc.*
Use: Dermatologic, protectant.

Angen. (Davis & Sly) Estrone 2 mg, testosterone 25 mg/ml Aqueous susp. Vial 10 ml. *Rx.*
Use: Androgen, estrogen combination.

Angerin. (Kingsbay) Nitroglycerin 1 mg/Cap. Bot. 60s. *Rx.*
Use: Coronary vasodilator.

Angex. (Janssen) Lidoflazine. *Rx.*
Use: Coronary vasodilator.

Angio-Conray. (Mallinckrodt) Iothalamate sodium 80% (48% iodine), EDTA. Inj. Vial 50 ml.
Use: Radiopaque agent.

•**angiotensin amide.** (an-JEE-oh-TEN-sin AH-mid) USAN. N.F. XIII.
Use: Vasoconstrictor.
See: Hypertensin (Novartis).

angiotensin-converting enzyme inhibitors.
Use: Antihypertensive; congestive heart failure.
See: Accupril, Tab. (Parke-Davis).
Altace, Cap. (Hoechst Marion Roussel).
Capoten, Tab. (Bristol-Myers Squibb).
Lotensin, Tab. (Novartis).
Monopril, Tab. (Bristol-Myers).
Prinivil, Tab. (Merck).
Univasc, Tab. (Schwarz Pharma).
Vasotec, Tab. (Merck).
Vasotec I.V., Inj. (Merck).
Zestril, Tab. (Zeneca).

Angiovist 282. (Berlex) Diatrizoate meglumine 60% (iodine 28%). Vial 50 ml, 100 ml or 150 ml. Box 10s.
Use: Radiopaque agent.

Angiovist 292. (Berlex) Diatrizoate meglumine 52%, diatrizoate sodium 8% (iodine 29.2%). Vial 30 ml, 50 ml or 100 ml. Box 10s.
Use: Radiopaque agent.

Angiovist 370. (Berlex) Diatrizoate meglumine 66%, diatrizoate sodium 10%, (iodine 37%). Vial 50 ml, 100 ml, 150 ml or 200 ml. Box 10s.
Use: Radiopaque agent.

anhydrohydroxyprogesterone. Ethisterone.

•**anidoxime.** (AN-ih-DOX-eem) USAN.
Use: Analgesic.
See: Bamoxine (U.S.V. Pharm).

A-Nil. (Vangard) Codeine phosphate 10 mg, bromodiphenhydramine HCl 3.75 mg, diphenhydramine HCl 8.75 mg, ammonium Cl 80 mg, potassium guaiacolsulfonate 80 mg, menthol 0.5 mg/5 ml, alcohol 5%. Bot. Pt. gal. *c-v.*
Use: Antitussive, expectorant.

•**anileridine.** (an-ih-LURR-ih-deen) U.S.P. 23.
Use: Analgesic (narcotic).

•**anileridine hydrochloride.** U.S.P. 23.
Use: Analgesic (narcotic).
See: Leritine HCl, Tab. (Merck).

•**anilopam hydrochloride.** (AN-ih-low-pam) USAN.
Use: Analgesic.

Animal Shapes. (Major) Vitamin A 2500 IU, D 400 IU, E 15 IU, C 60 mg, B_1 1.05 mg, B_2 1.2 mg, B_3 13.5 mg, B_6 1.05 mg, B_{12} 4.5 mcg, folic acid 0.3 mg. Chew. tab. Bot. 100s, 250s. *otc.*
Use: Vitamin supplement.

Animal Shapes + Iron. (Major) Vitamin A 2500 IU, D 400 IU, E 15 IU, C 60 mg, B_1 1.05 mg, B_2 1.2 mg, B_3 13.5 mg, B_6 1.05 mg, B_{12} 4.5 mcg, folic acid 0.3 mg, iron 15 mg. Chew. tab. Bot. 100s, 250s. *otc.*
Use: Mineral, vitamin supplement.

anion exchange resins.
See: Polyamine-Methylene Resin.

•**aniracetam.** (AN-ih-RASS-eh-tam) USAN.
Use: Mental performance enhancer.

•**anirolac.** (ah-NIH-role-ACK) USAN.
Use: Analgesic, anti-inflammatory.

anise oil. N.F. XVI.
Use: Flavoring.

anisindione.
See: Miradon (Schering Plough).

anisopyradamine.
See: Pyrilamine Maleate.

anisotropine. F.D.A. Tropine 2-propylvalerate.

•**anisotropine methylbromide.** (ah-NIH-so-TROE-peen meth-ill-BROE-mide) USAN.
Use: Anticholinergic.
See: Valpin 50, Tab. (DuPont).

•**anistreplase.** (uh-NISS-truh-place) USAN.
Use: Fibrinolytic, thrombolytic.
See: Eminase (SmithKline Beecham Pharmaceuticals).

•**anitrazafen.** (AN-ih-TRAY-zaff-en) USAN.
Use: Anti-inflammatory, topical.

anodynon.
See: Ethyl Cl.

Anodynos. (Buffington) Aspirin 420.6 mg, salicylamide 34.4 mg caffeine 34.4 mg/Tab. Sugar, lactose and salt free. Dispens-A-Kit 500s, Bot. 100s, 500s, Medipak 200s. *otc.*
Use: Analgesic combination.

Anodynos-DHC Tablets. (Forest Pharmaceutical) Hydrocodone bitartrate 5 mg, acetaminophen 500 mg/Tab. Bot. 100s. *c-III.*
Use: Analgesic combination, narcotic.

Anodynos Forte. (Buffington) Chlorpheniramine maleate, phenylephrine HCl, salicylamide, acetaminophen, caffeine/Tab. Sugar, lactose and salt free. Dispens-A-Kit 500s, Bot. 100s. *Rx.*
Use: Analgesic, antihistamine, decongestant.

Anoquan. (Roberts Pharm) Butalbital 50 mg, caffeine 40 mg, acetaminophen 325 mg/Cap. Bot. 100s, 1000s. *Rx.*

Use: Analgesic, hypnotic, sedative.

Anorex. (Dunhall Pharmaceuticals) Phendimetrazine 35 mg/Tab. Bot. 100s. *c-III.*
Use: Anorexiant.

anorexigenic agents. Appetite depressants.
See: Amphetamine Preps.
Didrex, Tab. (Pharmacia & Upjohn).
Plegine, Tab. (Wyeth Ayerst).
Preludin HCl (Boehringer Ingelheim).
Sanorex, Tab. (Novartis).
Tenuate (Hoechst Marion Roussel).
Tepanil, Tab. (3M Pharm).
Wilpo, Tab. (Novartis).

anovlar. Norethindrone plus ethinyl estradiol. *Rx.*
Use: Contraceptive.

•**anoxomer.** (an-OX-ah-MER) USAN.
Use: Pharmaceutic aid (antioxidant); food additive.

anoxynaphthonate sodium. Anazolene Sodium.

Ansaid. (Pharmacia & Upjohn) Flurbiprofen 50 mg or 100 mg. Tab. 100s, 500s, UD 100s. *Rx.*
Use: Analgesic, NSAID.

Anspor. (SmithKline Beecham Pharmaceuticals) Cephradine (a semisynthetic cephalosporin) **Cap.:** 250 mg. Bot. 100s, UD 100s; 500 mg. Bot. 20s, 100s, UD 100s. **Oral Susp.:** 125 mg or 250 mg/5 ml. Bot. 100 ml.
Use: Anti-infective, cephalosporin.

Answer. (Carter Products) Reagent in-home pregnancy test kit for urine testing. Test kit box 1s.
Use: Diagnostic aid.

Answer 2. (Carter Products) Reagent in-home pregnancy test kit for urine testing. Test kit box 2s.
Use: Diagnostic aid.

Answer Ovulation. (Carter Products) Home test to predict time of ovulation. In 6 day test kits.
Use: Diagnostic aid, ovulation.

Answer Plus. (Carter Products) Reagent in-home pregnancy test kit for urine testing. Test kit box 1s.
Use: Diagnostic aid.

Answer Plus 2. (Carter Products) Reagent in-home pregnancy test kit for urine testing. Test kit box 2s.
Use: Diagnostic aid.

Answer Quick & Simple. (Carter Products) Reagent in-home kit for urine testing. Test kit box 1s.

Antabuse. (Wyeth Ayerst) Disulfiram. **250 mg/Tab.** Bot. 100s; **500 mg/Tab.** Bot. 50s, 1000s. *Rx.*
Use: Antialcoholic.

Antacid. (Walgreens) Calcium carbonate 500 mg/Tab. Bot. 75s. *otc.*
Use: Antacid.

Antacid #2. (Global Source) Calcium carbonate 5.5 gr, magnesium carbonate 2.5 gr/Tab. Bot. 100s. *otc.*
Use: Antacid.

Antacid M Liquid. (Walgreens) Aluminum oxide 225 mg, magnesium hydroxide 200 mg/5 ml. Bot. 12 oz, 26 oz. *otc.*
Use: Antacid.

Antacid No. 6. (Jones Medical Industries) Calcium carbonate 0.42 g, glycine 0.18 g/Tab. Bot. 100s. *otc.*
Use: Antacid.

Antacid Relief Tablets. (Walgreens) Dihydroxyaluminum sodium carbonate 334 mg/Tab. Bot. 75s. *otc.*
Use: Antacid.

antacids. Drugs that neutralize excess gastric acid.
See: Alka-Seltzer, Tab. (Bayer Corp).
Alka-Seltzer Plus, Tab. (Bayer Corp).
Alka-Seltzer Special Effervescent Antacid, Tab. (Bayer Corp).
Alka-2 Chewable Antacid, Tab. (Bayer Corp).
Aluminum Hydroxide Gel (Various Mfr.).
Aluminum Hydroxide Gel w/Combinations (Various Mfr.).
Aluminum Hydroxide Gel Dried (Various Mfr.).
Aluminum Hydroxide Gel Dried w/ Combinations (Various Mfr.).
Aluminum Hydroxide Magnesium Carbonate, Tab. (Various Mfr.).
Aluminum Phosphate Gel (Wyeth Ayerst).
Aluminum Proteinate, Tab. (Solvay).
Amitone, Tab. (SmithKline Beecham).
Calcium Carbonate, Precipitated (Various Mfr.).
Calcium Carbonate Tab. (Various Mfr.).
Carbamine (Key Pharm).
Ceo-Two, Supp. (Beutlich).
Chooz, Gum Tab. (Schering Plough).
Citrocarbonate, Liq. (Pharmacia & Upjohn).
Dicarbosil, Tab. (Arch).
Di-Gel, Liq., Tab. (Schering Plough).
Dihydroxyaluminum Aminoacetate (Various Mfr.).
Dihydroxyaluminum Sodium Carbonate Tab. (Warner Lambert).
Magaldrate, Tab., Susp. (Wyeth Ayerst).

Magnesium Carbonate (Various Mfr.).
Magnesium Glycinate, Tab. (Various Mfr.).
Magnesium Hydroxide (Various Mfr.).
Magnesium Oxide, Tab., Cap. (Various Mfr.).
Magnesium Trisilicate (Various Mfr.).
Neutralox, Susp. (Teva USA).
Oxaine, Susp. (Wyeth Ayerst).
Ratio, Tab. (Pharmacia & Upjohn).
Rolaids, Tab. (Warner Lambert).
Romach, Tab. (ROR Pharmacal).
Sodium Bicarbonate, Inj., Tab. (Various Mfr.).
Tums, Tab. (SmithKline Beecham).

Antacid Suspension. (Geneva Pharm) Aluminum hydroxide 225 mg, magnesium hydroxide 200 mg/5 ml. Bot. 360 ml. *otc.*
Use: Antacid.

Antacid Tablets. (Zenith Goldline) Calcium carbonate 500 mg/Chew. tab. Bot. 150s. *otc.*
Use: Antacid.

Antacid Extra Strength. (Various Mfr.) Calcium carbonate 750 mg/Tab. Bot. 96s. *otc.*
Use: Antacid.

Anta-Gel. (Halsey) Aluminum hydroxide 200 mg, magnesium hydroxide 200 mg, simethicone 20 mg/5 ml. Bot. 12 oz. *otc.*
Use: Antacid, antiflatulent.

antagonists of curariform drugs.
See: Neostigmine Methylsulfate.
Tensilon Cl (Roche Laboratories).

antastan.
See: Antazoline Hydrochloride, U.S.P. 23.

antazoline hydrochloride. Antastan.
See: Arithmin, Tab. (Lannett).

•**antazoline phosphate.** U.S.P. 23.
Use: Antihistamine.
W/Naphazoline, boric acid, phenylmercuric acetate, sodium Cl, sodium carbonate anhydrous.
See: Vasocon-A Ophthalmic, Soln. (Smith, Miller & Patch).
W/Naphazoline HCl, polyvinyl alcohol.
See: Albalon-A Liquifilm, Ophth. Soln. (Allergan).

Antazoline-V. (Rugby) Naphazoline HCl 0.05%, antazoline phosphate 0.5%, PEG 8000, polyvinyl alcohol, EDTA, benzalkonium chloride 0.01%. Soln. Drop. Bot. 5 ml, 15 ml. *Rx.*
Use: Ophthalmic decongestant combination.

anterior pituitary.
See: Pituitary, anterior.

anthelmintic. A remedy for worms.
See: Antiminth, Susp. (Roerig).
Atabrine, Tab. (Sanofi Winthrop).
Betanaphthol Benzoate (Various Mfr.).
Biltricide, Tab. (Bayer Corp).
Carbon Tetrachloride (Various Mfr.).
Gentian Violet (Various Mfr.).
Jayne's PW Vermifuge (Bayer Corp).
Jayne's RW, Tab. (Bayer Corp).
Mintezol, Tab., Susp. (Merck).
Niclocide, Chew. tab. (Bayer Corp).
Piperazine Preps. (Various Mfr.).
Povan, Tab., Susp. (Parke-Davis).
Terramycin (Various Mfr.).
Tetrachloroethylene.
Vansil, Cap. (Pfipharmecs).
Vermox, Chew tab., Oral Susp. (Merck).

•**anthelmycin.** (AN-thell-MY-sin) USAN.
Use: Anthelmintic.

Anthelvet. Tetramisole HCl.

•**anthralin.** (AN-thrah-lin) U.S.P. 23.
Use: Antipsoriatic.
Lasan, Cream, Oint. (Stiefel).
W/Mineral oil.
See: Lasan Pomade (Stiefel).

•**anthramycin.** (an-THRAH-MY-sin) USAN.
Use: Antineoplastic.

anthraquinone of cascara.
See: Cascara Sagrada, Prods.

anthrax vaccine. (Michigan Biological Products Institute) Vial 5 ml. *Rx.*
Use: Immunization.

anti-a blood grouping serum.
Use: Diagnostic aid (blood in vitro).

anti-b blood grouping serum.
Use: Diagnostic aid (blood in vitro).

Antiacid. (Hillcrest North) Aluminum hydroxide, magnesium trisilicate, calcium carbonate/Tab. Bot. 100s. *otc.*
Use: Antacid.

Antialcoholic.
See: Disulfiram (Various Mfr.).
Antabuse (Wyeth Ayerst).

Anti-Allergy tablet. (Walgreens) Phenylpropanolamine HCl 18.7 mg, chlorpheniramine maleate 2 mg/Tab. Bot. 24s. *otc.*
Use: Antihistamine, decongestant.

antiandrogen.
See: Eulexin (Schering Plough).

antiasthmatic combinations.
See: Cromolyn Sodium, Cap. (Various Mfr.).
Decadron Respihaler, Aerosol. (Merck).
Ephedrine HCl (Various Mfr.).
Ephedrine Sulfate (Various Mfr.).

Isoephedrine HCl (Various Mfr.).
Isoetharine (Sanofi Winthrop).
Isoetharine HCl (Sanofi Winthrop).
Isoetharine Mesylate (Sanofi Winthrop).
Isoproterenol HCl (Various Mfr.).
Isoproterenol Sulfate (Various Mfr.).
Methoxyphenamine HCl (Various Mfr.).
Phenylephrine HCl (Various Mfr.).
Phenylpropanolamine HCl (Various Mfr.).
Pseudoephedrine HCl (Various Mfr.).
Racephedrine HCl (Various Mfr.).

antiasthmatic inhalant.
See: AsthmaHaler (SmithKline Beecham).
AsthmaNefrin, Soln. (SmithKline Beecham).

antibacterial antibodies.
See: Botulinum antitoxin.
Diphtheria antitoxin.
Immune globulin IM.
Immune globulin IV.
Tetanus immune globulin.

antibason.
See: Methylthiouracil (Various Mfr.).

Antibiotic. (Parnell) **Otic susp.:** Polymyxin B sulfate 10,000 units, neomycin (as sulfate) 3.5 mg, hydrocortisone 10 mg/ml, thimerosal 0.01%. Bot. 10 ml w/dropper. **Otic soln.:** Polymyxin B sulfate 10,000 units, neomycin (as sulfate) 3.5 mg, hydrocortisone 10 mg/ml. Bot. 10 ml w/dropper. *Rx.*
Use: Anti-infective, anti-inflammatory.

antibiotics/anti-infectives.
See: Amebicides, general.
Amikacin Sulfate, vial (Various Mfr.).
Amoxicillin (Various Mfr.).
Amoxicillin and Potassium Clavulanate (SmithKline Beecham Pharmaceuticals).
Amoxicillin w/Comb. (Various Mfr.).
Ampicillin (Various Mfr.).
Ampicillin w/Comb. (Various Mfr.).
Anthelmintic agents, general.
Antimalarial agents, general.
Antiprotozoan agents, general.
Antituberculosis agents, general.
Antiviral agents, general.
Azithromycin, Caps. (Pfizer).
Aztreonam, Vial (Bristol-Myers Squibb).
Bacampicillin HCl (Roerig).
Bacitracin (Various Mfr.).
Carbenicillin (Various Mfr.).
Cefaclor (Various Mfr.).
Cefadroxil (Various Mfr.).
Cefamandole Nafate (Eli Lilly).
Cefazolin Sodium, Vial (Various Mfr.).
Cefixime (ESI Lederle Generics).
Cefmetazole Sodium (Pharmacia & Upjohn).
Cefonicid Sodium, Vial (SmithKline Beecham Pharmaceuticals).
Cefoperazone Sodium, Vial (Roerig).
Cefotaxime Sodium, Vial (Hoechst Marion Roussel).
Cefotetan Disodium, Vial (Zeneca).
Cefoxitin Sodium, Vial (Merck).
Cefpodoxime Proxetil (Pharmacia & Upjohn).
Cefprozil (Bristol-Myers).
Ceftazidime, Vial (Various Mfr.).
Ceftizoxime Sodium, Vial (Fujisawa).
Ceftriaxone Sodium, Vial (Roche Laboratories).
Cefuroxime (Various Mfr.).
Cephalexin (Various Mfr.).
Cephalexin Monohydrate, Pulv., Susp. (Various Mfr.).
Cephalothin, Sodium, Vial (Various Mfr.).
Cephradine (Various Mfr.).
Chloramphenicol (Various Mfr.).
Cinoxacin, Cap. (Various Mfr.).
Ciprofloxacin (Bayer Corp).
Clarithromycin (Abbott Laboratories).
Clindamycin (Various Mfr.).
Clofazimine, Cap. (Novartis).
Cloxacillin Sodium (Various Mfr.).
Colistimethate Sodium, Inj. (Parke-Davis).
Colistin Sulfate (Various Mfr.).
Dapsone, Tab. (Jacobus).
Demeclocycline (ESI Lederle Generics).
Dicloxacillin, Cap., Susp. (Various Mfr.).
Doxycycline (Various Mfr.).
Enoxacin, Tab. (Rhone-Poulenc Rorer).
Erythromycin (Various Mfr.).
Erythromycin w/Comb. (Various Mfr.).
Fungicides, general.
Furazolidone (Procter & Gamble).
Gentamicin Sulfate (Various Mfr.).
Imipenem-Cilastatin, Vial (Merck).
Kanamycin Sulfate (Various Mfr.).
Lincomycin (Various Mfr.).
Lomefloxacin HCl, Tab. (Searle).
Loracarbef (Eli Lilly).
Methacycline HCl, Cap., Syr. (Wallace Laboratories).
Methenamine (Various Mfr.).
Methenamine w/Comb. (Various Mfr.).
Methicillin Sodium, Vial, Pow. (Various Mfr.).
Methylene Blue, Tab. (Various Mfr.).
Metronidazole (Various Mfr.).

Mezlocillin Sodium, Vial (Bayer Corp).
Minocycline (ESI Lederle Generics).
Nafcillin Sodium, Vial, Cap., Pow. (Wyeth Ayerst).
Nalidixic Acid (Sanofi Winthrop).
Netilmicin Sulfate, Vial (Schering Plough).
Neomycin Sulfate (Various Mfr.).
Nitrofurantion (Various Mfr.).
Norfloxacin, Tab. (Roberts Pharm).
Novobiocin (Various Mfr.).
Ofloxacin (Ortho McNeil).
Oxacillin, Sodium (Various Mfr.).
Oxytetracycline (Various Mfr.).
Paromomycin, Cap., Syr. (Parke-Davis).
Penicillin G Benzathine (Various Mfr.).
Penicillin G Benzathine w/ Comb. (Various Mfr.).
Penicillin G, Potassium (Various Mfr.).
Penicillin G Potassium w/Comb. (Various Mfr.).
Penicillin G Procaine (Various Mfr.).
Penicillin G Procaine w/Comb. (Various Mfr.).
Penicillin G Sodium (Various Mfr.).
Penicillin V Potassium (Various Mfr.).
Pentamidine Isethionate (Fujisawa).
Phenoxymethyl Penicillin (Various Mfr.).
Piperacillin Sodium, Vial (ESI Lederle Generics)
Piperacillin Sodium w/Comb. (Various Mfr.).
Polymyxin B Sulfate (Various Mfr.).
Spectinomycin, Vial (Pharmacia & Upjohn).
Streptomycin Sulfate (Various Mfr.).
Sulfadiazine (Various Mfr.).
Sulfamethizole, Tab. (Wyeth Ayerst).
Sulfamethoxazole (Various Mfr.).
Sulfamethoxazole w/Comb. (Various Mfr.).
Sulfasalazine (Various Mfr.).
Sulfasalazine w/Comb. (Various Mfr.).
Sulfisoxazole (Various Mfr.).
Tetracycline HCl (Various Mfr.).
Ticarcillin w/Comb. (Various Mfr.).
Ticarcillin Disodium, Vial (SmithKline Beecham Pharmaceuticals).
Tobramycin Sulfate (Various Mfr.).
Triacetyloleandomycin (Various Mfr.).
Trimethoprim (Various Mfr.).
Trimethoprim w/Comb. (Various Mfr.).
Trimetrexate Glucuronate, Vial (US Bioscience).
Troleandomycin, Cap. (Roerig).
Vancomycin HCl (Eli Lilly).

anticholinergic agents. Parasympatholytic agents.
See: Akineton (Knoll Pharmaceuticals).
Antrenyl Bromide (Novartis).
Artane HCl (ESI Lederle Generics).
Atropine Preps.
Atrovent, Spray (Boehringer Ingelheim).
Banthine Bromide (Searle).
Belladonna Preps.
Cantil Preps. (Hoechst Marion Roussel).
Cogentin (Merck).
Daricon, Tab. (SmithKline Beecham Pharmaceuticals).
Dicyclomine HCl (Various Mfr.).
Disipal (3M Pharm).
Donabarb Sr., Cap. (Zeneca).
Homatropine methylbromide.
Hybephen, Prods. (SmithKline Beecham Pharmaceuticals).
Kemadrin, Tab. (GlaxoWellcome).
Kinesed, Tab. (Zeneca).
L-Hyoscyamine, Tab. (Schwarz Pharma).
Murel, Amp. (Wyeth Ayerst).
Norflex, Inj., Tab. (3M Pharm).
Oxyphencyclimine HCl (Various Mfr.).
Pagitane HCl, Tab. (Eli Lilly).
Pamine Bromide, Tab., Soln. (Pharmacia & Upjohn).
Panparnit HCl.
Parsidol HCl, Tab. (Parke-Davis).
Pathilon (ESI Lederle Generics).
Phenoxine HCl (Hoechst Marion Roussel).
Prantal Methylsulfate, Tab. (Schering Plough).
Pro-Banthine Bromide, Preps. (Searle).
Robinul, Tab., Inj. (Robins).
Scopolamine methylbromide.
Scopolamine methylbromide HBr.
Tral, Preps. (Abbott Laboratories).
Trihexyphenidyl HCl (Various Mfr.).
Valpin 50, Tab. (DuPont Merck Pharmaceuticals).
Valpin 50-PB, Tab. (DuPont Merck Pharmaceuticals).

•**anticoagulant citrate dextrose solution.** U.S.P. 23.
Use: Anticoagulant (for storage of whole blood).
See: A.C.D. Solution. (Various Mfr.).

•**anticoagulant citrate phosphate dextrose adenine solution.** U.S.P. 23.
Use: Anticoagulant (for storage of whole blood).

•**anticoagulant citrate phosphate dextrose solution.** U.S.P. 23.
Use: Anticoagulant (for storage of whole blood).

•**anticoagulant heparin solution.** U.S.P. 23.

Use: Anticoagulant (for storage of whole blood).

anticoagulants.

See: Acenocoumarin.
Anisindione.
Calciparine, Inj. (DuPont Merck Pharmaceuticals).
Coumadin, Amp., Tab. (DuPont Merck Pharmaceuticals).
Dalteparin Sodium.
Depo-Heparin, Sodium (Pharmacia & Upjohn).
Dipaxin, Tab. (Pharmacia & Upjohn).
Diphenadione.
Eridione, Tab. (Eric, Kirk & Gary).
Enoxaparin Sodium.
Ethyl Biscoumacetate, Tab.
Fragmin (Pharmacia & Upjohn).
Hedulin, Tab. (Hoechst Marion Roussel).
Heparin Calcium.
Heparin, Sodium (Various Mfr.).
Liquaemin Sodium, Vial (Organon Teknika).
Liquamar, Tab. (Organon Teknika).
Lovenox, Inj. (Rhone-Poulenc Rorer).
Miradon, Tab. (Schering Plough).
Panheprin, Amp., Vial (Abbott Laboratories).
Panwarfin, Tab. (Abbott Laboratories).
Phenindione, Tab. (Various Mfr.).
ReoPro (Eli Lilly).
Sofarin (Teva USA).
Warfarin (Various Mfr.).

•**anticoagulant sodium citrate solution.** U.S.P. 23.

Use: Anticoagulant (for plasma and blood fractionation).

anticonvulsants.

See: Acetazolamide, Tab. (Various Mfr.).
Amytal Sodium, Amp. (Eli Lilly).
Carbamazepine, Tab. (Various Mfr.).
Celontin Kapseals (Parke-Davis).
Clorazepate, Tab. (Various Mfr.).
Depakene (Abbott Laboratories).
Diamox, Tab., Inj. (ESI Lederle Generics).
Diazepam, Tab., Soln. (Various Mfr.).
Diazepam Intensol, Soln. (Roxane).
Dilantin, Preps. (Parke-Davis).
Epitol, Tab. (Teva USA).
Felbatol, Tab., Susp. (Wallace Laboratories).
Gen-Xene, Tab. (Alra Laboratories).
Klonopin, Tab. (Roche Laboratories).
Lamictal, Tab. (GlaxoWellcome).
Magnesium sulfate (Various Mfr.).
Mephobarbital, Tab. (Sanofi Winthrop).
Mesantoin, Tab. (Novartis).
Milontin, Kapseals (Parke-Davis).
Mysoline, Tab., Susp. (Wyeth Ayerst).
Neurontin, Cap. (Parke-Davis).
Peganone, Tab. (Abbott Laboratories).
Phenobarbital (Various Mfr.).
Phenurone, Tab. (Abbott Laboratories).
Phenytoin, Susp., Tab. (Various Mfr.).
Phenytoin Sodium, Cap. (Various Mfr.).
Primidone, Tab. (Various Mfr.).
Tegretol, Tab. (Novartis).
Tranxene, Tab. (Abbott Laboratories).
Tranxene-SD, Tab. (Abbott Laboratories).
Tranxene-T, Tab. (Abbott Laboratories).
Tridione (Abbott Laboratories).
Valium, Tab. (Roche Laboratories).
Valrelease, Cap. (Roche Laboratories).
Zarontin, Cap., Syr. (Parke-Davis).

anti-cytomegalovirus monoclonal antibodies.

Use: Treatment of cytomegalovirus.

antidepressants.

See: Adapin, Cap. (Lotus).
Amitriptyline HCl (Various Mfr.).
Amoxapine, Tab. (Various Mfr.).
Anafranil, Cap. (Novartis).
Asendin, Tab. (ESI Lederle Generics).
Aventyl HCl, Pulv., Liq. (Eli Lilly).
Deprol, Tab. (Wallace Laboratories).
Desipramine HCl, Cap., Tab. (Various Mfr.).
Desyrel, Tab. (Bristol-Myers).
Effexor, Tab. (Wyeth Ayerst).
Elavil Tab., Inj. (Merck).
Endep, Tab. (Roche Laboratories).
Imipramine HCl, Amp., Tab. (Various Mfr.).
Imipramine Pamoate, Cap. (Novartis).
Janimine, Tab. (Abbott Laboratories).
Ludiomil, Tab. (Novartis).
Luvox, Tab. (Solvay).
Maprotiline HCl, Tab. (Various Mfr.).
Monoamine oxidase inhibitors.
Nardil, Tab. (Parke-Davis).
Norpramin, Preps. (Hoechst Marion Roussel).
Pamelor, Cap., Liq. (Novartis).
Parnate Sulfate, Tab. (SmithKline Beecham Pharmaceuticals).
Paxil, Tab. (SmithKline Beecham Pharmaceuticals).
Pertofrane, Cap. (Rhone-Poulenc Rorer).

Protriptyline HCl (Merck).
Prozac, Liq., Pulv. (Eli Lilly).
Serzone, Tab. (Bristol-Myers Squibb).
Sinequan, Cap. (Pfizer).
Surmontil, Cap. (Wyeth Ayerst).
Tofranil, Amp., Tab. (Novartis).
Tofranil-PM, Cap. (Novartis).
Trazodone HCl, Tab. (Various Mfr.).
Triavil, Tab. (Merck).
Vivactil, Tab. (Merck).
Wellbutrin, Tab. (GlaxoWellcome).
Zoloft, Tab. (Roerig).

antidiarrheals.
See: Attapulgite, Activated (Various Mfr.).
Bismatrol, Tab. (Major).
Cantil, Liq., Tab. (Hoechst Marion Roussel).
Coly-Mycin S, Oral Susp., (Parke-Davis).
DIA-Quel Liq. (Inter. Pharm. Corp.).
Diasorb, Liq., Tab. (Columbia).
Diphenoxylate HCl w/atropine sulfate, Tab., Liq. (Various Mfr.).
Donnagel, Chew. tab., Liq., Susp. (Wyeth Ayerst).
Furoxone Liq., Tab. (Eaton Medical).
Imodium, Cap. (Janssen).
Imodium A-D, Tab., Liq. (McNeil Consumer Products).
Kaodene Non-Narcotic, Liq. (Pfeiffer).
Kaolin (Various Mfr.)
Kaolin Colloidal (Various Mfr.).
Kaopectate, Prods. (Pharmacia & Upjohn).
Kao-Spen, Susp. (Century Pharm).
Kapectolin (Various Mfr.).
K-C, Susp. (Century Pharm).
K-Pek, Susp. (Rugby).
Lactinex, Tab., Gran. (Becton Dickinson).
Lactobacillus acidophilus & bulgaricus mixed culture, Tab. (Becton Dickinson).
Lactobacillus acidophilus, viable culture (Various Mfr.).
Logen, Tab. (Zenith Goldline).
Lomanate, Liq. (Various Mfr.).
Lomotil, Liq., Tab., (Searle).
Lonox, Liq. (Geneva Pharm).
Loperamide, Cap., Liq. (Various Mfr.).
Maalox Antidiarrheal, Capl. (Rhone-Poulenc Rorer).
Milk of Bismuth (Various Mfr.).
Motofen, Tab. (Carnrick Labs).
Mycifradin Sulfate, Soln., Tab. (Pharmacia & Upjohn).
Parepectolin, Susp. (Rhone-Poulenc Rorer).
Pepto-Bismol, Liq., Tab. (Procter & Gamble).
Pepto Diarrhea Control, Liq. (Procter & Gamble).
Pink Bismuth, Liq. (Various Mfr.).
Rheaban Maximum Strength, Capl. (Pfizer).

antidiuretics.
See: Pitressin, Amp. (Parke-Davis).
Pitressin Tannate In Oil, Amp. (Parke-Davis).
Pituitary Post. Inj. (Various Mfr.).

antiemetic/antivertigo agents.
See: Antivert, Tab. (Roerig).
Antrizine, Tab. (Major).
Arrestin, Inj. (Vortech).
Atarax, Tab., Syr. (Roerig).
Bonine, Tab. (Pfizer).
Bucladin-S, Softab Tab. (Zeneca).
Calm-X, Tab. (Republic Drug).
Compazine, Preps. (SmithKline Beecham Pharmaceuticals).
Dimenhydrinate, Tab., Inj., Liq. (Various Mfr.).
Dimetabs, Tab. (Jones Medical Industries).
Dinate, Inj. (Seatrace).
Dizmiss, Tab. (Jones Medical Industries).
Dramamine, Preps. (Searle).
Dramanate, Inj. (Taylor Pharmaceuticals).
Dramilin, Inj. (Kay Pharm).
Dramoject, Inj. (Merz).
Dymenate, Inj. (Keene Pharmaceuticals).
Emecheck, Liq. (Savage).
Emetrol, Liq. (Rhone-Poulenc Rorer).
Hydrate, Inj. (Hyrex).
Kytril, Tab., Inj. (SmithKline Beecham Pharmaceuticals).
Marezine, Tab. (GlaxoWellcome).
Marinol, Cap. (Roxane).
Maxolon, Tab. (SmithKline Beecham Pharmaceuticals).
Meclizine HCl, Tab. (Various Mfr.).
Meni-D, Cap. (Seatrace).
Mepergan, Inj. (Wyeth Ayerst).
Metoclopramide, Tab. (Various Mfr.).
Naus-A-Tories, Supp. (Table Rock).
Naus-A-Way, Soln. (Roberts Pharm).
Nausetrol, Syr. (Medical Chemicals).
Octamide, Tab. (Pharmacia & Upjohn).
Phenergan, Preps. (Wyeth Ayerst).
Prochlorperazine, Supp. (Various Mfr.).
Reclomide, Tab. (Major).
Reglan, Inj., Syr., Tab. (Robins).
Ru-Vert-M, Tab. (Solvay).
Tebamide, Supp. (G & W Labs).
T-Gen, Supp. (Zenith Goldline).
Thorazine, Preps. (SmithKline

Beecham Pharmaceuticals).
Ticon, Inj. (Roberts Pharm).
Tigan, Preps. (SmithKline Beecham Pharmaceuticals).
Torecan Amp., Supp., Tab. (Novartis).
Transderm-Scop, Transdermal Therapeutic System (Novartis).
Trilafon, Preps. (Schering Plough).
Trimazide, Cap., Supp. (Major).
Trimethobenzamide HCl, Cap., Inj., Supp. (Various Mfr.).
Triptone, Capl. (Del Pharmaceuticals)
Vesprin, Inj. (Bristol-Myers).
Vistaril, Cap., Susp., Soln. (Pfizer).
Vontrol, Tab. (SmithKline Beecham Pharmaceuticals).
Zofran, Inj., Tab. (GlaxoWellcome).

antiepilepsirine.
Use: Treatment for drug-resistant generalized tonic-clonic epilepsy. [Orphan drug]

antiepileptic agents.
See: Anticonvulsant.

antiestrogen. Tamoxifen citrate.
Use: Hormone for cancer therapy.
See: Nolvadex (Zeneca).
Tamoxifen (Barr Laboratories).

antifebrin.
See: Acetanilid (Various Mfr.).

antiflatulents.
See: Di-Gel, Prods. (Schering Plough).
Silain, Tab., Gel (Robins).
Simethicone Prods.

Antifoam A Compound. (Hoechst Marion Roussel).
Use: Antiflatulent.
See: Simethicone, U.S.P. 23.

antifolic acid.
See: Methotrexate, Tab. (ESI Lederle Generics).

Antiformin. Sodium hypochlorite in sodium hydroxide 7.5%, available chlorine 5.2%; may be colored with meta cresol purple.
Use: Antiseptic, antimicrobial.

antifungal agents.
See: Fungicides.

•**antihemophilic factor.** U.S.P. 23.
Use: Antihemophilic.

antihemophilic factor. (Baxter & Alpha Therapeutics) Antihemophilic Factor, human. Method for Syringe Administration 10 ml 450 A.H.F. or 300 A.H.F. units/Pkg. W/Syringe 30 ml or 900 A.H.F. units/Pkg.
Use: Antihemophilic.
See: Alphanate, Inj. (Alpha Therapeutics).
Bioclate, Inj. (Centeon).
Helixate, Inj. (Centeon).
Hemofil, Vial (Baxter).
Humate-P, Inj. (Centeon).
Koate HP, Inj. (Bayer Corp).
Kogenate, Inj. (Bayer Corp).
Monoclate-P, Inj. (Centeon).
Profilate HP. Inj. (Alpha Therapeutics).
Recombinate, Inj. (Baxter).

antihemophilic factor, human.
Use: Treatment of Von Willebrand's disease. [Orphan drug]
See: Alphanate (Alpha Therapeutics).
Humate P (Behringwerke Aktiengesellschaft).

Antihemophilic Factor (Porcine) Hyate: C. (Speywood) Freeze-dried concentrate of Antihemophilic Factor, 400 to 700 porcine units of Factor VIII:C. Pow. for Inj. Vials. *Rx.*
Use: Antihemophilic.

antihemophilic factor (recombinant).
Use: Prophylaxis/treatment of bleeding in hemophilia A. [Orphan drug]
See: Kogenate (Miles).

antiheparin.
See: Protamine Sulfate.

Antihist-D. (Goldline) Clemastine fumarate (immediate release) 1.34 mg, phenylpropanolamine (extended release) 75 mg, lactose/Tab. 16s. *otc.*
Use: Antihistamine, decongestant.

Antihist-1. (Various Mfr.) Clemastine fumarate 1.34 mg/Tab. Pkg. 16s. *otc.*
Use: Antihistamine.

Antihistamine Cream. (Towne) Methapyrilene HCl 10 mg, pyrilamine maleate 5 mg, allantoin 2 mg, diperodon HCl 2.5 mg, benzocaine 10 mg, menthol 2 mg/g. Cream Jar 2 oz. *otc.*
Use: Antihistamine, topical.

antihistamines.
See: Aller-Chlor, Syr., Tab. (Rugby).
AllerMax, Capl. (Pfeiffer).
Anergan, Inj. (Forest Pharmaceutical).
Astelin, Nasal Spray (Wallace).
Allegre, Cap. (Hoechst-Marion Roussel).
Banophen, Cap., Capl. (Major).
Belix, Elix. (Halsey).
Benadryl, Preps. (Parke-Davis).
Bena-D, Inj. (Seatrace).
Benahist, Inj. (Keene Pharmaceuticals).
Ben-Allergin-50, Inj. (Dunhall Pharmaceuticals).
Benoject, Inj, (Merz).
Benylin Cough, Syr. (Parke-Davis).
Brompheniramine, Tab., Elix. (Various Mfr.).

Bromphen, Elix. (Various Mfr.).
Bydramine, Syr. (Major).
Chlo-Amine, Tab. (Bayer Corp).
Chlorate, Tab. (Major).
Chlorpheniramine Maleate (Various Mfr.).
Chlor-Pro, Inj. (Schein Pharmaceutical).
Chlortab, Tab. (Vortech).
Chlor-Trimeton, Inj., Syr., Tab. (Schering Plough).
Claritin, Tab. (Schering Plough).
Cophene-B, Inj. (Dunhall Pharmaceuticals).
Co-Pyronil 2, Pulv., Susp. (Eli Lilly).
Cyproheptadine HCl, Syr., Tab. (Various Mfr.).
Dexchlor, Tab. (Schein Pharmaceutical).
Dexchlorpheniramine Maleate, Tab. (Various Mfr.).
Dimetane, Preps. (Robins).
Diphen Cough, Syr. (Rosemont).
Diphenhydramine HCl (Various Mfr.).
Diphenylpyraline HCl (Various Mfr.).
Disophrol, Prods. (Schering Plough).
Doxylamine Succinate (Various Mfr.).
Drixoral, Prods. (Schering Plough).
Diphen Cough, Syr. (Rosemont).
Genahist, Cap., Tab., Elix. (Zenith Goldline).
Hismanal, Tab. (Janssen).
Histaject, Inj. (Merz).
Hydramyn, Syr. (HN Norton).
Hyrexin-50, Inj. (Hyrex).
Myidyl, Syr. (Rosemont).
Nasahist B, Inj. (Keene Pharmaceuticals).
ND Stat, Inj. (Hyrex).
Nidryl, Elix. (Geneva Pharm).
Nolahist, Tab. (Carnrick Labs).
Optimine, Tab. (Schering Plough).
Oraminic, Inj. (Vortech).
PBZ, Tab. (Novartis).
PBZ-SR, Tab. (Novartis).
Pelamine, Tab. (Major).
Pentazine, Inj. (Century Pharm).
Periactin, Syr., Tab. (Merck).
Pfeiffer's Allergy, Tab. (Pfeiffer).
Phenameth, Tab. (Major).
Phenazine, Inj. (Keene Pharmaceuticals).
Phendry, Prods. (HN Norton).
Phenergan, Prods .(Wyeth Ayerst).
Phenoject-50, Inj. (Merz).
Poladex, Tab. (Major).
Polaramine, Syr., Tab. (Schering Plough).
Poly-Histine, Elix. (Sanofi Winthrop).
Pro-50, Inj. (Dunhall Pharmaceuticals).
Prometh-50, Inj. (Seatrace).
Promethazine HCl (Various Mfr.).
Prophenpyridamine Maleate (Various Mfr.).
Prorex, Inj. (Hyrex).
Prothazine, Prods. (Vortech).
Pyrilamine Maleate (Various Mfr.).
Tacaryl, Tab., Syr. (Westwood Squibb).
Tavist, Tab. Syr. (Novartis).
Telachlor, Cap. (Major).
Teldrin, Cap. (SmithKline Beecham Pharmaceuticals).
Temaril, Tab., Span., Syr. (Allergan).
Tripelennamine HCl (Various Mfr.).
Triprolidine HCl (Various Mfr.).
Tusstat, Syr. (Century Pharm).
V-Gan, Inj. (Roberts Pharm).
Wehydryl, Inj. (Roberts Pharm).

antihyperlipidemics.
See: Atromid-S, Cap. (Wyeth Ayerst).
Choloxin, Tab. (Knoll Pharmaceuticals).
Clofibrate, Cap. (Various Mfr.).
Mevacor, Tab. (Merck).
Niacin, Prods. (Various Mfr.).
Pravachol, Tab. (Bristol-Myers Squibb).
Questran, Prods. (Bristol-Myers).
Zocor, Tab. (Merck).

antihypertensives.
See: Accupril, Tab. (Parke-Davis).
Acebutolol hydrochloride.
Aceon, Tab. (Ortho McNeil).
Adaprolol maleate.
Alazide, Tab. (Major).
Alazine, Tab. (Major).
Aldactazide, Tab. (Searle).
Aldactone, Tab. (Searle).
Aldoclor 250, Tab. (Merck).
Aldomet, Tab. (Merck).
Aldoril, Tab. (Merck).
Alfuzosin hydrochloride.
Aldopa, Tab. (Major).
Alpha 1-adrenergic blockers.
Altace, Cap. (Hoechst Marion Roussel, Pharmacia & Upjohn).
Althiazide.
Amiquinsin hydrochloride.
Amlodipine besylate.
Amlodipine maleate.
Amodopa (Major).
Anaritide acetate.
ACE inhibitors.
Apresazide, Cap. (Novartis).
Apresodex, Tab. (Rugby).
Apresoline, Amp., Tab. (Novartis).
Aprozide, Cap. (Major).
Arcum R-S, Tab. (Arcum).
Arlix (Hoechst Marion Roussel).
Artarau, Tab. (Archer-Taylor).

Atenolol/chlorthalidone, Tab. (Various Mfr.).
Atiprosin maleate.
Belfosdil.
Bendacalol mesylate.
Bendroflumethiazide.
Benzthiazide.
Betaxolol hydrochloride.
Bethanidine sulfate.
Bevantolol hydrochloride.
Biclodil hydrochloride.
Bosoprolol.
Bisoprolol fumarate.
Bucindolol hydrochloride.
Cam-Ap-Es, Tab. (Camall).
Candoxatril.
Candoxatrilat.
Capoten, Tab. (Bristol-Myers Squibb).
Capozide, Tab. (Bristol-Myers Squibb).
Captopril.
Cardura, Tab. (Roerig).
Carvedilol.
Catapres, Tab. (Boehringer Ingelheim).
Ceronapril.
Chlorothiazide sodium.
Chlorthalidone, Tab. (Various Mfr.).
Cicletanine.
Cilazapril.
Cithal, Cap. (Table Rock).
Citrin, Cap. (Table Rock).
Clentiazem maleate.
Clonidine.
Clonidine hydrochloride.
Clonidine hydrochloride and Chlorthalidone, Tab. (Various Mfr.).
Clopamide.
Combipres, Tab. (Boehringer Ingelheim).
Coreg, Tab., (SmithKline Beecham Pharmaceuticals).
Cyclothiazide.
Debrisoquin sulfate.
Delapril hydrochloride.
Demser, Cap. (Merck).
De Serpa, Tab. (de Leon).
Diaserp, Tab. (Major).
Diazoxide.
Diazoxide parenteral.
Dibenzyline, Cap. (SmithKline Beecham Pharmaceuticals).
Dilevalol hydrochloride.
Diovan, Cap. (Novartis).
Ditekiren.
Diucardin, Tab. (Wyeth Ayerst).
Diulo, Tab. (Searle).
Diurigen w/Reserpine, Tab. (Zenith Goldline).
Diuril, Tab., Susp. (Merck).
Diuril sodium, I.V., (Merck).
Diutensen-R, Tab. (Wallace Laboratories).
Doxazosin mesylate.
Elserpine, Tab. (Canright).
Enalapril maleate.
Enalaprilat.
Enalkiren.
Endralazine mesylate.
Enduronyl, Tab. (Abbott Laboratories).
Enduronyl forte, Tab. (Abbott Laboratories).
Eprosartan.
Eprosartan mesylate.
Eserdine, Tab. (Major).
Eserdine forte, Tab. (Major).
Esidrix, Tab. (Novartis).
Esimil, Tab. (Novartis).
Exna, Tab. (Robins).
Fenoldopam mesylate.
Flavodilol maleate.
Flolan, Pow. for Inj. (Glaxo-Wellcome).
Flordipine.
Flosequinan.
Forasartan.
Fosinopril.
Fosinopril sodium.
Fosinoprilat.
Guanabenz.
Guanabenz acetate.
Guanacline sulfate.
Guanadrel sulfate.
Guancydine.
Guanethidine monosulfate.
Guanethidine sulfate.
Guanfacine hydrochloride.
Guanisoquin.
Guanisoquin sulfate.
Guanoclor sulfate.
Guanocitine hydrochloride.
Guanoxabenz.
Guanoxan sulfate.
Guanoxyfen sulfate.
Harbolin, Tab. (Arcum).
H.H.R., Tab. (Geneva Pharm).
Hiwolfia, Tab. (Jones Medical Industries).
Hydralazine, Inj. (Solopak).
Hydralazine hydrochloride, Tab. (Various Mfr.).
Hydralazine polistirex.
Hydrap-ES, Tab. (Parmed).
Hydraserp, Tab. (Zenith Goldline).
Hydrazide, Cap. (Zenith Goldline).
Hydra-Zide, Cap. (Par Pharm).
Hydrochloroserpine, Tab. (Freeport).
Hydrochlorothiazide/hydralazine, Cap. (Various Mfr.).
Hydroflumethiazide.
Hydromox-R, Tab. (ESI Lederle Generics).

Hydropine, Tab. (Rugby).
Hydropine H.P., Tab. (Rugby).
Hydropres-50, Tab. (Merck).
Hydroserp, Tab. (Zenith Goldline).
Hydroserp-50, Tab. (Freeport).
Hydroserpine #1, #2 (Various Mfr.).
Hydrosine 25, 50, Tab. (Major).
Hydrotensin-50, Tab. (Merz).
Hydroxyisoindolin.
Hylorel, Tab. (Hyrex).
Hyperstat, I.V. Inj. (Schering Plough).
Hytrin, Tab., Cap. (Abbott Laboratories).
Hyzaar, Tab. (Merck).
Indacrinone.
Indapamide.
Inderide, Tab. (Wyeth Ayerst).
Inderide LA, Cap. (Wyeth Ayerst).
Indolapril hydrochloride.
Indoramin.
Indoramin hydrochloride.
Indorenate hydrochloride.
Ingadine, Tab. (Major).
Inhibace (Roche/Glaxo Wellcome).
Inversine, Tab. (Merck).
Irbesartan.
Ismelin, Tab. (Novartis).
Labetalol hydrochloride.
Leniquinsin.
Levcromakalim.
Lexxel, ER Tab. (Astra Merck).
Lofexidine hydrochloride.
Loniten, Tab. (Pharmacia & Upjohn).
Lopressor HCT, Tab. (Novartis).
Losartan potassium.
Losulazine hydrochloride.
Lotensin, Tab. (Novartis).
Lotrel, Cap. (Novartis).
Lozol, Tab. (Rhone-Poulenc Rorer).
Marpres, Tab. (Marnel).
Mavik, Tab. (Knoll Pharmaceuticals).
Maxzide, Tab. (ESI Lederle Generics).
Mebutamate.
Mecamylamine hydrochloride.
Medroxalol.
Medroxalol hydrochloride.
Metatensin, Tab. (Hoechst Marion Roussel).
Methalthiazide.
Methyclodine, Tab. (Rugby).
Methyclothiazide.
Methyldopa.
Methyldopa and Chlorothiazide, Tab.
Methyldopa and Hydrochlorothiazide, Tab. (Various Mfr.).
Methyldopate hydrochloride, Inj. (Fujisawa).
Metipranolol.
Metipranolol hydrochloride.
Metolazone.
Metoprolol fumarate.
Metoprolol succinate.
Metoprolol tartrate and Hydrochlorothiazide.
Metyrosine.
Midamor, Tab. (Merck).
Minipress, Cap. (Pfizer).
Minizide, Cap. (Pfizer).
Minoxidil, Tab. (Rugby).
Moduretic, Tab. (Merck).
Moexipril hydrochloride.
Monopril, Tab. (Bristol-Myers).
Muzolimine.
Nadolol, Tab. (Various Mfr.).
Nadolol and Bendroflumethiazide.
Natrico, Pulvoid (Drug Products).
Nebivolol.
Nitrendipine.
Nitropress, Vial (Abbott Laboratories).
Nitroprusside sodium.
Normodyne, Inj., Tab. (Schering Plough).
Normotensin, Inj. (Marcen).
Pargyline hydrochloride.
Pelanserin hydrochloride.
Pentina, Tab. (Freeport).
Pentolinium tartrate.
Perindopril erbumine.
Pheniprazine hydrochloride.
Phenoxybenzamine hydrochloride.
Phentolamine hydrochloride.
Pinacidil.
Pivopril.
Prazosin hydrochloride, Cap. (Various Mfr.).
Prinivil, Tab. (Merck).
Prinzide, Tab. (Merck).
Priscoline, Vial (Novartis).
Prizidilol hydrochloride.
Propranolol hydrochloride and Hydrochlorothiazide, Tab. (Various Mfr.).
Quinapril hydrochloride.
Quinaprilat.
Quinazosin hydrochloride.
Quinelorane hydrochloride.
Quinuclium bromide.
Ramipril.
Rauneed, Tab. (Hanlon).
Raunescine (Penick).
Raurine, Tab., Cap. (New Eng. Phr. Co.).
Rautina, Tab. (Fellows).
Rauval, Tab. (Pal-Pak).
Rauwolfia/bendroflumethiazide, Tab. (Various Mfr.).
Rauwolfia serpentina.
Rauwolscine.
Rauzide, Tab. (Bristol-Myers Squibb).
Rawfola, Tab. (Foy).
Regroton, Tab. (Rhone-Poulenc Rorer).

Regroton Demi, Tab. (Rhone-Poulenc Rorer).
Renese, Tab. (Pfizer).
Renese-R, Tab. (Pfizer).
Reserpaneed, Tab. (Hanlon).
Reserpine.
Reserpine and Chlorothiazide, Tab.
Reserpine and Hydrochlorothiazide, Tab. (Various Mfr.).
Reserpine, hydralazine hydrochloride and Hydrochlorothiazide, Tab. (Various Mfr.).
R-HCTZ-H, Tab. (ESI Lederle Generics).
Salazide, Tab. (Major).
Salazide-Demi, Tab. (Major).
Salutensin, Tab. (Roberts Pharm).
Salutensin-Demi, Tab. (Bristol-Myers).
Saprisartan potassium.
Saralasin acetate.
Sectral, Cap. (Wyeth Ayerst).
Ser-A-Gen, Tab. (Zenith Goldline).
Ser-Ap-Es, Tab. (Novartis).
Serpasil-Apresoline, Tab. (Novartis).
Serpasil-Esidrix, Tab. (Novartis).
Serpazide, Tab. (Major).
Sertabs, Tab. (Table Rock).
Sertina, Tab. (Fellows).
Sodium nitroprusside, Pow. for Inj. (ESI Lederle Generics).
Sulfinalol hydrochloride.
Tarka, Tab. (Knoll Pharmaceuticals).
Teludipine hydrochloride.
Temocapril hydrochloride.
Tenex, Tab. (Robins).
Tenoretic, Tab. (Zeneca).
Tenormin, Amp, Tab. (Zeneca).
Terazosin hydrochloride.
Tiamenidine hydrochloride.
Ticrynafen.
Timolide 10-25, Tab. (Merck).
Timolol maleate
Timolol maleate and Hydrochloride, Tab.
Tinabinol.
Tipentosin hydrochloride.
Tolazoline hydrochloride.
Toprol XL, Tab. (Astra USA).
Trandate, Tab., Inj. (Allen & Hanburys).
Trandate hydrochlorothiazide, Tab. (Allen & Hanburys).
Tri-Hydroserpine, Tab. (Rugby).
Trimazosin hydrochloride.
Trimethamide.
Trimethaphan camsylate.
Trimoxamine hydrochloride.
T-Sert, Tab. (Tennessee Pharmaceutic).
Univasc, Tab. (Schwarz Pharma).
Valsartan.
Vaseretic, Tab. (Merck).
Vasotec, Tab., Inj. (Merck).
Visken, Tab. (Novartis).
Xipamide.
Zankiren hydrochloride.
Zepine, Tab. (Foy).
Zestoretic, Tab. (Zeneca).
Zestril, Tab. (Zeneca).
Ziac, Tab. (ESI Lederle Generics).
Zofenoprilat arginine.

anti-infectives.
See: antibiotics/anti-infectives.

anti-inhibitor coagulant complex.
Use: Antihemophilic.
See: Autoplex T. (Baxter).
Feiba VH. (Immuno-U.S.).

Anti-Itch Cream. (Rugby) Burow's solution 5%, phenol 0.5%, menthol 0.5%, camphor 1% in washable base. Tube oz. *otc.*
Use: Antipruritic, counterirritant.

Antilerge. (Metz) Chlorpheniramine maleate 8 mg, phenylephrine HCl 12 mg/Tab. Bot. 30s. *otc.*
Use: Antihistamine, decongestant.

antileukemia.
See: Antineoplastic agents.

Antilirium. (Forest Pharmaceutical) Physostigmine salicylate 1 mg/ml, benzyl alcohol 2%, sodium bisufite 0.1%. 2 ml. *Rx.*
Use: Antidote. [Orphan drug]
See: Ataxia.

antimalarial agents.
See: Amodiaquin HCl.
Aralen HCl, Inj. (Sanofi Winthrop).
Aralen Phosphate (Sanofi Winthrop).
Aralen Phosphate w/Primaquine (Sanofi Winthrop).
Atabrine HCl, Tab. (Sanofi Winthrop).
Chloroguanide HCl.
Daraprim Tab. (GlaxoWellcome).
Hydroxychloroquine Sulfate.
Paludrine HCl, Tab. (Wyeth Ayerst).
Pamaquine Naphthoate.
Plaquenil Sulfate, Tab. (Sanofi Winthrop).
Plasmochin Naphthoate.
Primaquine Phosphate, Tab. (Sanofi Winthrop).
Pyrimethamine.
Quinacrine HCl, Tab.
Quinine Salts (Various Mfr.).
Quinine Sulfate (Various Mfr.).
Totaquine, Pow.

Antiminth. (Pfizer) Pyrantel pamoate 250 mg/5 ml. Oral susp. Bot. 60 ml. *otc.*
Use: Anthelmintic.

•**antimony potassium tartrate.** U.S.P. 23.
Use: Antischistosomal, leishmaniasis,

expectorant, emetic.
W/Cocillana, euphorbia pilulifera, squill, senega.
See: Cylana, Syr. (Jones Medical Industries).
W/Guaifenesin, codeine phosphate.
See: Cheracol, Syr. (Pharmacia & Upjohn).
W/Guaifenesin, dextromethorphan HBr.
See: Cheracol-D, Syr. (Pharmacia & Upjohn).
W/Paregoric, glycyrrhiza fluid extract.
See: Brown Mixture (Eli Lilly).
W/Thenylpyramine HCl, ammonium Cl, sodium citrate, menthol, aromatics.
See: Histacomp, Syr., Tab. (Health for Life Brands).

antimony preparations.
See: Antimony Potassium Tartrate (Various Mfr.).
Antimony Sodium Thioglycollate (Various Mfr.).
Tartar Emetic (Various Mfr.).

•**antimony sodium tartrate.** U.S.P. 23.
Use: Antischistosomal.

antimony sodium thioglycollate. (Various Mfr.) *Rx.*
Use: Schistosomiasis, leishmaniasis, filariasis.

•**antimony trisulfide colloid.** USAN.
Use: Pharmaceutic aid.

antimonyl potassium tartrate.
See: Antimony Potassium Tartrate, U.S.P. 23.

anti-my9-blocked ricin. USAN.
Use: Leukemia treatment.

antinauseants.
See: Antiemetic, antivertigo.

antineoplastic agents.
See: Adriamycin, Vial (Pharmacia & Upjohn & Pharmacia & Upjohn).
Alkeran, Tab. (GlaxoWellcome).
Amsacrine.
Azacitidine
Blenoxane, Amp. (Bristol-Myers Squibb).
Cosmegen, Inj. (Merck).
Elspar, Inj. (Merck).
Emcyt, Cap. (Pharmacia & Upjohn).
Estinyl, Tab. (Schering Plough).
5-Fluorouracil, Amp. (Roche Laboratories).
FUDR, Vial (Roche Laboratories).
Hexalen (US Bioscience).
Hydrea, Cap. (Bristol-Myers Squibb).
Idamycin (Pharmacia & Upjohn).
Leukeran, Tab. (GlaxoWellcome).
Lysodren, Tab. (Bristol-Myers Oncology/Immunology).
Matulane, Cap. (Roche Laboratories).
Medroxyprogesterone Acetate Tab., Vial (Various Mfr.).
Megace, Tab. (Bristol-Myers).
Mercaptopurine, Tab.
Methotrexate, Tab. (ESI Lederle Generics).
Methotrexate Sodium, Vial (ESI Lederle Generics).
Mithracin, Vial (Pfizer).
Mustargen, Inj. (Merck).
Myleran, Tab. (GlaxoWellcome).
Nolvadex, Tab. (Zeneca).
Oncovin, Amp. (Eli Lilly).
Purinethol, Tab. (GlaxoWellcome).
TACE, Cap. (Hoechst Marion Roussel).
Tamoxifen, Tab. (Barr Laboratories).
Thioguanine, Tab. (GlaxoWellcome).
Thio Tepa, Vial (ESI Lederle Generics).
Uracil Mustard, Cap. (Pharmacia & Upjohn).
Velban, Amp. (Eli Lilly).

antiobesity agents.
See: Acutrim, Prods. (Novartis).
Adderall (Richwood).
Adipex-P, Tab., Cap. (Teva USA).
Amphetamine Preps. (Various Mfr.).
Anorex, Cap. (Dunhall Pharmaceuticals).
Bontril, Prods. (Carnrick Labs).
Control, Cap. (Thompson Medical).
Dexatrim Pre-Meal, Cap. (Thompson Medical).
Dextroamphetamine Preps. (Various Mfr.).
Didrex, Tab. (Pharmacia & Upjohn).
Diethylpropion HCl.
Dieutrim T.D., Cap. (Legere).
Fastin, Cap. (SmithKline Beecham Pharmaceuticals).
Ionamin, Cap. (Medeva).
Levo-Amphetamine.
Maximum Strength Dexatrim, Cap. (Thompson Medical).
Mazanor, Tab. (Wyeth Ayerst).
Melfiat-105 Unicelles, Cap. (Solvay)
Methamphetamine Preps. (Various Mfr.).
Obe-Nix 30, Cap. (Holloway).
Obephen, Cap. (Roberts Pharm).
Obestin-30, Cap. (Ferndale Laboratories).
Phendimetrazine Tartrate, Cap., Tab. (Various Mfr.).
Phentermine HCl, Tab., Cap. (Various Mfr.)
Phentermine Resin, Cap. (Various Mfr.).
Phenyldrine, Tab. (Rugby).
Pondimin, Tab. (Robins).

Prelu-2, Cap. (Boehringer Ingelheim).
Sanorex, Tab. (Novartis).
Slim-Mint, Gum (Thompson Medical).
Tenuate, Tab. (Hoechst Marion Roussel).
Tenuate Dospan, Tab. (SmithKline Beecham Pharmaceuticals).
Tepanil, Tab. (3M Pharm).
Trimstat, Tab. (Laser).
Wehless Timecelles, Cap. (Roberts Pharm).

Antiox. (Merz) Vitamin C 120 mg, vitamin E 100 IU, beta carotene 25 mg. Cap. Bot. 60s. *otc.*
Use: Vitamin supplement.

Anti-Pak Compound. (Lowitt) Phenylephrine HCl 5 mg, salicylamide 0.23 g, acetophenetidin 0.15 gr, caffeine 0.03 g, ascorbic acid 50 mg, hesperidin complex 50 mg, chlorprophen-pyridamine maleate 2 mg/Tab. Bot. 30s, 100s. *otc.*
Use: Analgesic, antihistamine, decongestant combination.

antiparasympathomimetics.
See: Parasympatholytic agents.

anti-pellagra vitamin.
See: Nicotinic acid.

anti-pernicious anemia principle.
See: Vitamin B_{12}.

Antiphlogistine. (Denver Chemical) Medicated poultice. Jar 5 oz, lb. Tube 8 oz. Can 5 lb.

antiplatelet antibodies.
See: ReoPro (Eli Lilly).

antiprotozoan agents.
See: Antimony Preps.
Arsenic Preps.
Bismuth Preps.
Chiniofon (Various Mfr.).
Diiodohydroxyquinoline.
Emetine HCl (Various Mfr.).
Furazolidone.
Iodochorhydroxyquinoline.
Iodohydroxyquinoline Sulfonate Sodium.
Levofuraltadone.
Ornidyl (Hoechst Marion Roussel).
Quinoxyl.
Suramin Sodium.

•**antipyrine.** U.S.P. 23.
Use: Analgesic, antipyretic.
W/Benzocaine, chlorobutanol.
See: G.B.A., Drops (Scrip).
W/Carbamide, benzocaine, cetyldimethylbenzylammonium HCl.
See: Auralgesic, Liq. (ICN Pharmaceuticals).
W/Phenylephrine HCl, benzocaine.
See: Tympagesic, Liq. (Pharmacia & Upjohn).
W/Pyrilamine maleate, phenylephrine, benzalkonium.
See: Prefrin-A Ophthalmic (Allergan).

antipyrine and benzocaine otic solution.
Use: Anesthetic, local.
See: Auro Ear Drops (Del Pharmaceuticals).
Lanaurine, Drops (Lannett).

antipyrine, benzocaine and phenylephrine hydrochloride otic solution.
Use: Anesthetic, local; decongestant eardrop.

•**antirabies serum.** U.S.P. 23.
Use: Immunization.

antirickettsial agents.
See: p-Aminobenzoic Acid (Various Mfr.).
p-Aminobenzoate Sodium (Various Mfr.).
Aureomycin, Preps. (ESI Lederle Generics).
Chloromycetin, Preps. (Parke-Davis).
Terramycin, Preps. (Pfizer).

antiscorbutic vitamin.
See: Ascorbic Acid.

antiseptic, chlorine, active.
See: Antiseptic, N-Chloro Compounds, Hypochlorite Preps.

antiseptic, dyes.
See: Acriflavine (Various Mfr.).
Aminoacridine HCl.
Bismuth Violet, Preps. (Table Rock).
Brilliant Green.
Crystal Violet.
Fuchsin.
Gentian Violet (Various Mfr.).
Methylrosaniline Cl (Various Mfr.).
Methyl Violet.
Pyridium, Tab. (Parke-Davis).

antiseptic, mercurials.
See: Mercresin (Pharmacia & Upjohn).
Merthiolate, Preps. (Eli Lilly).
Phenylmercuric Acetate (Various Mfr.).
Phenylmercuric Borate (Various Mfr.).
Phenylmercuric Nitrate (Various Mfr.).
Phenylmercuric Picrate (Various Mfr.).
Thimerosal.

antiseptic, n-chloro compounds.
See: Chloramine-T (Various Mfr.).
Chlorazene, Pow., Tab. (Badger).
Dichloramine-T (Various Mfr.).
Halazone, Tab. (Abbott Laboratories).

antiseptic, phenols.
See: Anthralin (Various Mfr.).
Bithionol.
Coal Tar Products (Various Mfr.).
Creosote (Various Mfr.).

Cresols (Various Mfr.).
Guaiacol (Various Mfr.).
Hexachlorophene (Various Mfr.).
Hexylresorcinol (Various Mfr.).
Methylparaben (Various Mfr.).
o-Phenylphenol (Various Mfr.).
Oxyquinoline Salts (Various Mfr.).
Parachlorometaxylenol (Various Mfr.).
Phenol (Various Mfr.).
Picric Acid (Various Mfr.).
Propylparaben (Various Mfr.).
Pyrogallol (Various Mfr.).
Resorcinol (Various Mfr.).
Resorcinol Monoacetate (Various Mfr.).
Thymol (Various Mfr.).
Trinitrophenol (Various Mfr.).

antiseptics.
See: Furacin, Preps. (Eaton Medical).
Iodine Products.
Mercurials.
N-Chloro Compounds.
Phenols.
Surface-Active Agents.

antiseptic, surface-active agents.
See: Bactine, Preps. (Bayer Corp).
Benzalkonium Cl (Various Mfr.).
Benzethonium Cl (Various Mfr.).
Ceepryn (Hoechst Marion Roussel).
Cēpacol Preps. (Hoechst Marion Roussel).
Cetylpyridinium Cl (Various Mfr.).
Diaparene Cl, Preps. (Bayer Corp).
Methylbenzethonium Cl (Various Mfr.).
Zephiran Cl, Preps. (Sanofi Winthrop).

Antispas. (Keene Pharmaceuticals) Dicyclomine HCl 10 mg/ml. Vial 10 ml. *Rx.*
Use: Antispasmodic.

antispasmodics. Parasympatholytic agents.
See: Anticholinergic Agents.
Spasmolytic Agents.

Antispasmodic Capsules. (Teva USA) Phenobarbital 16.2 mg, hyoscyamine sulfate 0.1037 mg, atropine sulfate 0.0194 mg, scopolamine HBr 0.0065 mg/Cap. Bot. 1000s. *Rx.*
Use: Anticholinergic, antispasmodic, hypnotic, sedative.

Antispasmodic Elixir. (Various Mfr.) Atropine sulfate 0.0194 mg, scopolamine HBr 0.0065 mg, hyoscyamine HBr or SO_4 0.1037 mg, phenobarbital 16.2 mg/ml w/alcohol 23%. Elix. Bot. 120 ml, pt, gal and UD 5 ml. *Rx.*
Use: Anticholinergic, antispasmodic, hypnotic, sedative.

antistreptolysin-O. Titration procedure.
See: Also (Wampole Laboratories).

antisterility vitamin.
See: Vitamin E.

anti-t lymphocyte immunotoxin xmmly-h65-rta. (Xoma)
See: Anti Pan T Lymphocyte Monoclonal Antibody.

Anti-Tac, Humanized. (Roche Laboratories)
Use: Prevention of acute renal allograft rejection. [Orphan drug]

Anti-Ten. (Century Pharm) Allylisobutylbarbituric acid ¾ gr, aspirin 3 gr, phenacetin 2 gr, caffeine gr/Tab. Bot. 100s, 1000s. *Rx.*
Use: Analgesic, sedative, stimulant.

antithrombin III concentrate IV.
Use: Prophylaxis/treatment of thromboembolic episodes in AT-III deficiency. [Orphan drug]
See: Kybernin (Centeon).

antithrombin III human.
Use: Thromboembolic. [Orphan drug]
See: ATnativ (Kabivitrum).
Thrombate III (Miles).

antithrombin III human. (Red Cross)
Use: Thromboembolic. [Orphan drug]

antithymocyte globulin.
Use: Immunosuppressant. [Orphan drug]

Nashville Rabbit Antithymocyte. (Applied Medical Research) Antithymocyte serum.
Use: Immunosuppressant.

antithyroid agents.
See: Iothiouracil Sodium.
Methimazole.
Methylthiouracil (Various Mfr.).
Propylthiouracil (Various Mfr.).
Tapazole, Tab. (Eli Lilly).

antitoxins.
See: Botulism Antitoxin.
Diphtheria Antitoxin.
Tetanus Immune Globulin.

antitrypsin, alpha 1.
See: alpha-1-antitrypsin.

antituberculosis agents.
See: Aminosalicylates (Na, Ca, K) (Various Mfr.).
Benzoylpas Calcium (Various Mfr.).
Capastat Sulfate, Amp. (Eli Lilly).
Cycloserine.
Dihydrostreptomycin (Various Mfr.).
Isoniazid (Various Mfr.).
Myambutol, Tab. (ESI Lederle Generics).
Niconyl, Tab. (Parke-Davis).
P.A.S. Acid, Tab. (Kasar).
Pasdium, Tab. (Kasar).

Pyrazinamide, Tab. (ESI Lederle Generics).
Rifadin, Cap., Inj. (Hoechst Marion Roussel).
Rimactane, Cap. (Novartis).
Rimactane/INH (Novartis).
Seromycin, Pulv. (Eli Lilly).
Streptomycin (Various Mfr.).
Trecator-SC, Tab. (Wyeth Ayerst).
Triniad, Tab. (Kasar).
Triniad Plus 30 (Kasar).
Uniad, Tab. (Kasar).
Uniad-Plus 5,10, Tab. (Kasar).

Anti-Tuss. (Century Pharm) Guaifenesin 100 mg/5 ml. Bot. 4 oz, gal. *otc.*
Use: Expectorant.

Anti-Tuss D.M. (Century Pharm) Guaifenesin 100 mg, dextromethorphan HBr 15 mg/5 ml. Bot. 4 oz, pt, gal. *otc.*
Use: Antitussive, expectorant.

Anti-Tussive. (Canright) Dextromethorphan HBr 10 mg, potassium guaiacol sulfonate 125 mg, terpin hydrate 100 mg, phenylpropanolamine HCl 12.5 mg, pyrilamine maleate 12.5 mg/Tab. Bot. 60s. *otc.*
Use: Antihistamine, antitussive, decongestant, expectorant.

Antitussive Cough Syrup. (Weeks & Leo) Chlorpheniramine 2 mg, phenylephrine HCl 5 mg, dextromethorphan 15 mg, ammonium Cl 50 mg/5 ml. *otc.*
Use: Antihistamine, antitussive, decongestant, expectorant.

Antitussive Cough Syrup with Codeine. (Weeks & Leo) Chlorpheniramine maleate 2 mg, phenylephrine HCl 5 mg, codeine phosphate 10 mg, ammonium Cl 50 mg/5 ml. Bot. 4 oz. *c-v.*
Use: Antihistamine, antitussive, decongestant, expectorant.

antitussive-decongestant.
See: St. Joseph Cough Syrup for Children (Schering Plough).
Tussend, Tab., Liq. (Hoechst Marion Roussel).

•**antivenin (latrodectus mactans).** U.S.P. 23. *Formerly Widow spider species antivenin (Latrodectus mactans).*
Use: Immunization.

antivenin (latrodectus mactans). Black widow spider antivenin. Each vial contains not less than 6000 antivenin units. Thimerosal (mercury derivative) 1:10,000 added as preservative. Vial 2.5 ml of Sterile Water for Injection and a 1 ml vial of normal horse serum for sensitivity testing.
Use: Treatment of black widow spider bites.

•**antivenin (micrurus fulvius).** U.S.P. 23.
Use: Immunization.

antivenin (micrurus fulvius). North American coral snake antivenin. Lyophilized antivenin of animal origin (*Micrurus fulvius*) with phenol 0.25% and thimerosal 0.005% as preservatives. Bacteriostatic water w/phenylmercuric nitrate 1:100,000 as preservative. Combination package. Vial 10 ml.
Use: Bites of North American coral snake and Texas coral snake.

antivenin Centruroides sculpturatus. (Arizona State University) Available in Arizona only. 5 ml vials.
Use: Antivenin.

•**antivenin (crotalidae) polyvalent.** U.S.P. 23.
Use: Immunization.

antivenin (crotalidae) polyvalent. (Wyeth Ayerst) Rattlesnake, copperhead and cottonmouth moccasin antitoxic serum. One vial lyophilized serum with 0.25% phenol and 0.005% thimerosal. One vial, 10 ml of bacteriostatic water for inj. w/phenyl mercuric nitrate 0.001%; one vial normal horse serum 1:10, as sensitivity testing material w/ thimerosal 0.005% and phenol 0.35%.
Use: Bites of crotalid snakes of North, Central and South America.

antivenin, polyvalent crotalid (ovine) fab.
Use: Bites of North American crotalid snakes. [Orphan drug]
See: Crotab (Therapeutic Antibodies).

antivenom (crotalidae) purified (avian). (Ophidian)
Use: Bites of snakes of the crotalidae family. [Orphan drug]

Antivert. (Roerig) Meclizine HCl 12.5 mg, 25 mg or 50 mg/Tab. **12.5 mg:** Bot. 100s, 1000s, UD 100s; **25 mg:** Bot. 100s, 1000s, UD 100s. **50 mg:** Bot. 100s. *Rx.*
Use: Antiemetic, antivertigo.

antiviral agents.
See: Cytovene, Inj. (Syntex).
Famvir, Tab. (SmithKline Beecham Pharmaceuticals).
Foscavir, Inj. (Astra Merck).
Hivid, Tab. (Roche Laboratories).
Retrovir, Preps. (GlaxoWellcome).
Symmetrel, Cap., Syr. (DuPont Merck Pharmaceuticals).
Videx, Pow., Tab. (Bristol-Myers Squibb).
Vira-A, Inj. (Parke-Davis).
Virazole, Pow. for Reconstitution for aerosol (ICN Pharmaceuticals).

Zerit, Cap. (Bristol-Myers Squibb).
Zovirax, Cap, Inj. (GlaxoWellcome).

antiviral antibodies.
See: Cytomegalovirus immune globulin.
Immune globulin IM.
Immune globulin IV.
Hepatitis B immune globulin.
Rabies immune globulin.
Vaccinia immune globulin.
Varicella-zoster immune globulin.

antixerophthalmic vitamin.
See: Vitamin A.

Antizol. (Orphan Medical) Fomepizole 1 g/ml. Preservative free. Inj. Conc. Vial 1.5 ml. *Rx.*
Use: Antidote.

Antril. (Amgen) Interleukin-1 receptor antagonist (human recombinant).
Use: Arthritis, organ rejection. [Orphan drug]

Antrizine Tabs. (Major) Meclizine 12.5 mg, 25 mg or 50 mg/Tab. **12.5 mg:** 100s, 500s, 1000s. **25 mg:** 100s, 500s, 1000s, UD 100s. **50 mg:** 100s. *Rx.*
Use: Antiemetic, antivertigo.

Antrocol Elixir. (ECR Pharmaceuticals) Atropine sulfate 0.195 mg, phenobarbital 16 mg, alcohol 20%/5 ml. Sugar free. Bot. Pt. *Rx.*
Use: Anticholinergic, antispasmodic, hypnotic, sedative.

Antrypol. Suramin. *Rx.*
Use: CDC anti-infective agent.

Anturane. (Novartis) Sulfinpyrazone, U.S.P. **100 mg/Tab.:** Bot 100s. **200 mg/Cap.:** Bot. 100s. *Rx.*
Use: Antigout agent.

Anucaine. (Calvin) Procaine 50 mg, butyl-p-aminobenzoate 200 mg, benzyl alcohol 265 mg in sweet almond oil/5 ml. Amp. 5 ml. Box 6s, 24s, 100s. *otc.*
Use: Anorectal preparation.

Anucort-HC. (G & W Laboratories) Hydrocortisone acetate 25 mg in a hydrogenated vegetable oil base. Supp. Box 12s, 24s, 100s. *Rx.*
Use: Anorectal preparation.

Anuject. (Roberts Pharm) Procaine. Soln. Vial 5 ml or 10 ml. *Rx.*
Use: Anorectal preparation.

Anumed. (Major) Bismuth subgallate 2.25%, bismuth resorcin compound 1.75%, benzyl benzoate 1.2%, zinc oxide 11%, balsam Peru 1.8% in a hydrogenated vegetable oil base. Supp. Box 12s. *otc.*
Use: Anorectal preparation.

Anumed HC. (Major) Hydrocortisone acetate 10 mg. Supp. Box 12s. *Rx.*
Use: Anorectal preparation.

Anuprep HC. (Great Southern) Hydrocortisone acetate 25 mg. Supp. Box 12s.
Use: Anorectal preparation.

Anuprep Hemorrhoidal. (Great Southern) Bismuth subgallate 2.25%, bismuth resorcin compound 1.75%, benzyl benzoate 1.2%, peruvian balsam 1.8% and zinc oxide 11% in a hydrogenated vegetable oil base. Supp. Box 12s, 24s. *Rx.*
Use: Anorectal prepration.

Anusol. (GlaxoWellcome) Topical starch 51%, benzyl alcohol, soybean oil, tocopheryl acetate. Supp. 12s. *otc.*
Use: Anorectal preparation.

Anusol-HC 2.5%. (Monarch) Hydrocortisone 2.5%. Cream Tube 30 g. *Rx.*
Use: Corticosteroid, topical.

Anusol HC-1. (Monarch) Hydrocortisone 1%, diazolidinyl urea, parabens, mineral oil, sorbitan sesquioleate, white petrolatum. Oint. Tube 21 g. *otc.*
Use: Corticosteroid, topical.

Anusol Ointment. (Monarch) Pramoxine HCl 1%, zinc oxide 12.5%/g, benzyl benzoate 1.2%, pramoxine HCl 1% in a mineral oil and cocoa butter. Tube. 30 g. *otc.*
Use: Anorectal preparation.

Anzemet. (Hoechst-Marion Roussel) Dolasetron mesylate 50 mg, 100 mg, lactose/Tab. 5s, UD 5s, 10s. Dolasetron mesylate 20 mg/ml, mannitol 38.2 mg/ml/Inj. Single-use Amp. 0.625 ml, single-use Vial 5 ml. *Rx.*
Use: Antiemetic.

AOSEPT. (Ciba Vision Ophthalmics) Hydrogen peroxide 3%, sodium Cl 0.85%, phosphonic acid, phosphate buffer. Soln. Bot. 120 ml, 240 ml, 360 ml. *otc.*
Use: Contact lens care.

Apacet. (Parmed) Acetaminophen 80 mg/Chew. tab. Bot. 100s. *otc.*
Use: Analgesic.

•**apalcillin sodium.** (APE-al-SIH-lin) USAN.
Use: Anti-infective.

APAP.
See: Acetaminophen.

Apatate w/Fluoride. (Kenwood/Bradley) Vitamins B_1 15 mg, B_6 0.5 mg, B_{12} 25 mcg, F 0.5 mg/5 ml. Liq. Bot. 120 ml. *Rx.*
Use: Mineral, vitamin supplement.

Apatate Liquid. (Kenwood/Bradley) Vitamins B_1 15 mg, B_{12} 25 mcg, B_6 0.5 mg/

5 ml. Liq. Bot. 120 ml, 240 ml. *otc.*
Use: Vitamin supplement.

Apatate Tablets. (Kenwood/Bradley) Vitamins B_1 15 mg, B_{12} 25 mcg, B_6 0.5 mg/Tab. Bot. 50s. *otc.*
Use: Vitamin supplement.

•**apaxifylline.** (A-pock-SIH-fih-leen) USAN.
Use: Selective adenosine A_1 antagonist.

•**apazone.** (APP-ah-zone) USAN.
Use: Anti-inflammatory.

A.P.C. (Various Mfr.) Aspirin, phenacetin, caffeine. Cap., Tab.
Use: Analgesic combination.
See: A.S.A. Compound, Preps. (Eli Lilly).
P.A.C. Compound, Cap., Tab. (Pharmacia & Upjohn).
Pan-APC, Tab. (Panray).
Phensal, Tab. (Hoechst Marion Roussel).
W/Codeine phosphate. (Various Mfr.).
See: Anexsia w/Codeine, Tab. (SmithKline Beecham Pharmaceuticals).
Anexsia D, Tab. (SmithKline Beecham Pharmaceuticals).

A.P.C. w/gelsemium combinations.
See: Aidant, Tab. (Noyes).
Ansemco, No. 2, Tab. (Zeneca).
Asphac-G, Tab. (Schwarz Pharma).
Valacet, Tab. (Pal-Pak).

Apcogesic. (Apco) Sodium salicylate 5 gr, colchicine 1/320 gr, calcium carbonate 65 mg, dried aluminum hydroxide gel 130 mg, phenobarbital ⅛ gr/Tab. Bot. 100s. *Rx.*
Use: Antigout agent, hypnotic, sedative.

Apcohist. (APC) Phenylpropanolamine HCl 25 mg, chlorpheniramine maleate 1 mg/Tab. Bot. 100s. *otc.*
Use: Antihistamine, decongestant.

Apcoretic. (APC) Caffeine anhydrous 100 mg, ammonium Cl 325 mg/Tab. Bot. 90s. *Rx.*
Use: Diuretic.

Ap Creme. (T.E. Williams) Hydrocortisone 0.5%, iodochlorhydroxyquin 3%. Tube oz. *otc, Rx.*
Use: Antifungal; corticosteroid, topical.

Apetil. (Kenwood/Bradley) B_1 1.7 mg, B_2 0.3 mg, B_3 6.7 mg, B_6 2.5 mg, B_{12} 5 mcg, Zn 14.6 mg, Mg, Mn, l-lysine. Liq. Bot. 237 ml. *otc.*
Use: Mineral, vitamin supplement.

APF. (Whitehall Robins).
Use: Analgesic.
See: Arthritis Pain Formula. (Whitehall Robins).

Aphco Hemorrhoidal Combination. (APC) Combination package of Aphco Hemorrhoidal Ointment 1.5 oz tube, Aphco Hemorrhoidal Supp. Box 12s, 1000s. *otc.*
Use: Anorectal preparation.

Aphen Tabs. (Major) Trihexyphenidyl 2 mg or 5 mg/Tab. Bot. 250s, 1000s. *Rx.*
Use: Antiparkinsonian.

Aphrodyne. (Star) Yohimbine HCl 5.4 mg/Tab. Bot. 100s, 1000s. *Rx.*
Use: Alpha-adrenergic blocker.

Aphthasol. (Block Drug) Amlexanox 5%, benzyl alcohol, glyceryl monostearate, mineral oil, petrolatum/Paste. Tube. 5 g. *Rx.*
Use: Treatment of mouth ulcers.

Apicillin. D-(-)-α-Aminobenzyl penicillin.
See: Ampicillin.

A.P.L. (Wyeth Ayerst) Chorionic Gonadotropin for Injection. 5000 units, 10,000 units or 20,000 units, sterile diluent, w/ benzyl alcohol, phenol, lactose. *Rx.*
Use: Hormone, chorionic gonadotropin.

APL 400-020. (Apollon)
Use: Treatment of cutaneous t-cell lymphoma. [Orphan drug]

Aplisol. (Parke-Davis) Tuberculin purified protein derivative diluted 5 units/0.1 ml, polysorbate 80, potassium and sodium phosphates, phenol. Vial 1 ml (10 tests), 5 ml (50 tests). *Rx.*
Use: Diagnostic aid.

Aplitest. (Parke-Davis) Purified tuberculin protein derivative buffered with potassium and sodium phosphates, phenol 0.5%/single-use, multipuncture unit. 25s. *Rx.*
Use: Diagnostic aid.

•**apomorphine hydrochloride.** (ah-poh-MORE-feen) U.S.P. 23.
Use: Treatment of Parkinson's disease; emetic.

apomorphine hydrochloride. (ah-poh-MORE-feen) (Forum Products) (Pentec Pharm)
Use: Treatment of Parkinson's disease.

aporphine-10, 11-diol hydrochloride.
See: Apomorphine HCl.

appetite-depressants.
See: Anorexiants.

APPG.
See: Penicillin G, Procaine, Aqueous.

•**apraclonidine hydrochloride.** (app-rah-KLOE-nih-deen) U.S.P. 23.
Use: Adrenergic (α_2-agonist).
See: Iopidine (Alcon Laboratories).

•**apramycin.** (APP-rah-MY-sin) USAN.
Use: Anti-infective.

Aprazone. (Major) Sulfinpyrazone. **Cap.:** 200 mg. Bot. 100s, 500s, 1000s. **Tab.:** 100 mg. Bot. 100s. *Rx.*
Use: Antigout agent.

Apresazide. (Novartis) **25/25:** Hydralazine HCl 25 mg, hydrochlorothiazide 25 mg/Cap. **50/50:** Hydralazine HCl 50 mg, hydrochlorothiazide 50 mg/Cap. **100/50:** Hydralazine 100 mg, hydrochlorothiazide 50 mg/Cap. Bot. 100s. *Rx.*
Use: Antihypertensive.

Apresodex. (Rugby) Hydrochlorothiazide 15 mg, hydralazine HCl 25 mg. Tab. Bot. 100s, 1000s. *Rx.*
Use: Antihypertensive.

Apresoline. (Novartis) Hydralazine HCl. **Amp.:** 20 mg w/propylene glycol, methyl and propyl parabens/ml. Pkg. 5s. **Tab.:** 10 mg Bot. 100s, 1200s; 25 mg or 50 mg Bot. 100s, 1000s; 100 mg Bot. 100s. Consumer pack 100s. *Rx.*
Use: Antihypertensive.
W/Serpasil.
See: Serpasil Prods., Preps. (Novartis).

Apresoline-Esidrix. (Novartis) Hydralazine HCl 25 mg, hydrochlorothiazide 15 mg/Tab. Bot. 100s. *Rx.*
Use: Antihypertensive.

•**aprindine.** (APE-rin-deen) USAN.
Use: Cardiovascular agent.

•**aprindine hydrochloride.** (APE-rin-deen) USAN.
Use: Cardiovascular agent.

aprobarbital. Pow. *c-III.*
Use: Hypnotic, sedative.
See: Alurate, Elix. (Roche Laboratories).

Aprobee w/C. (Health for Life Brands) Vitamins B_1 15 mg, B_2 10 mg, B_6 5 mg, niacinamide 50 mg, calcium pantothenate 10 mg, C 250 mg/Cap. or Tab. **Cap.:** Bot. 100s, 1000s. **Tab.:** Bot. 50s, 100s, 1000s. *otc.*
Use: Mineral, vitamin supplement.

Aprodine. (Major) **Tab.:** Pseudoephedrine HCl 60 mg, triprolidine HCl 2.5 mg. Bot. 24s, 100s, 1000s, UD 100s. **Syr.:** Pseudoephedrine HCl 30 mg, triprolidine HCl 1.25 mg/5 ml. Bot. 120 ml, pt. *otc.*
Use: Antihistamine, decongestant.

Aprodine w/Codine. (Major) Pseudoephedrine HCl 30 mg, triprolidine HCl 1.25 mg, codeine phosphate 10 mg. Syr. Bot. pt, gal. *c-v.*
Use: Antihistamine, decongestant.

•**aprotinin.** (app-row-TIE-nin) USAN.
Use: Enzyme inhibitor (proteinase).
See: Trasylol, Inj. (Bayer Corp).

aprotinin. (app-row-TIE-nin)
Use: Blood loss prophylaxis and homologous blood transfusion in coronary artery bypass graft surgery. (CABG).
See: Trasylol (Miles).

Aprozide 25/25 capsules. (Major) Hydralazine 25 mg, hydrochlorothiazide 25 mg/Cap. Bot. 100s, 250s. *Rx.*
Use: Antihypertensive.

Aprozide 50/50 capsules. (Major) Hydrochlorothiazide 50 mg, hydralazine 50 mg/Cap. Bot. 100s, 250s. *Rx.*
Use: Antihypertensive.

A.P.S. Aspirin, phenacetin and salicylamide.

•**aptazapine maleate.** (app-TAZZ-ah-PEEN MAL-ee-ate) USAN.
Use: Antidepressant.

•**aptiganel hydrochloride.** (app-tih-GAN-ehl) USAN.
Use: Stroke and traumatic brain injury treatment (NMDA ion channel blocker).

APSAC. Thrombolytic enzyme.
See: Eminase (SmithKline Beecham Pharmaceuticals).

apyron.
See: Magnesium acetylsalicylate.

AQ-4B. (Western Research) Trichlormethiazide 4 mg/Tab. Bot. 1000s. *Rx.*
Use: Diuretic.

Aqua-Ban. (Thompson Medical) Caffeine 100 mg, ammonium Cl 325 mg/Tab. Bot. 60s. *otc.*
Use: Diuretic.

Aqua-Ban, Maximum Strength.
See: Maximum Strength Aqua-Ban, Tab. (Thompson).

Aqua-Ban Plus. (Thompson Medical) Ammonium Cl 650 mg, caffeine 200 mg, iron 6 mg/Tab. Bot. 30s. *otc.*
Use: Diuretic, mineral supplement.

Aquabase. (Pal-Pak) Cetyl alcohol, propylene glycol, sodium lauryl sulfate, white wax, purified water. Jar lb. *otc.*
Use: Pharmaceutic aid, ointment base.

Aquacare Cream. (Allergan) Urea 2%, benzyl alcohol, carbomer 934, cetyl esters wax, fragrance, glycerin, oleth-3 phosphate, petrolatum, phenyl dimethicone, water, sodium hydroxide. Tube 2.5 oz. *otc.*
Use: Emollient.

Aquacare/HP. (Allergan) Urea 10%, benzyl alcohol. **Cream:** Tube 2.5 oz. **Lot.:** Bot. 8 oz, 16 oz. *otc.*

Use: Emollient.

Aquacare Lotion. (Allergan) Benzyl alcohol, oleth-3 phosphate, phenyl dimethicone, fragrance. Bot. 8 oz. *otc.*
Use: Emollient.

Aquachloral. (PolyMedica) Chloral hydrate, polyethylene glycol, spreading agent. Supp. 5 gr, 10 gr. Strip 12s. *c-iv.*
Use: Hypnotic, sedative (rectal).

Aquacillin G. (Armenpharm) Penicillin G. *Rx.*
Use: Anti-infective, penicillin.

Aquacycline. (Armenpharm) Tetracycline HCl. *Rx.*
Use: Anti-infective, tetracycline.

Aquaderm. (C & M Pharmacal) Purified water, glycerin 25%, salicylic acid 0.1%, octoxynol-9 0.03%, FD & C; Red #40 0.0001%. Bot. 2 oz. *otc.*
Use: Emollient.

Aquaderm. (Baker Norton). Octyl methoxycinnamate 7.5%, oxybenzone 6%. SPF 15. Cream 105 g. *otc.*
Use: Sunscreen.

Aquaflex Ultrasound Gel Pad. (Parker) Clear, solid, flexible, moist, standoff gel pad for use where transducer movement is impeded by bony or irregular body surfaces. 2 cm × 9 cm.
Use: Ultrasound aid.

Aquafuren. (Armenpharm) Nitrofurantoin. *Rx.*
Use: Anti-infective, urinary.

Aquagen. (ALK Laboratories) Allergenic extracts. Vials.

aquakay.
See: Menadione (Various Mfr.).

Aqua Lacten Lotion. (Herald Pharmacal) Demineralized water, urea, petrolatum, propylene glycol monostearate, sorbitan monostearate, lactic acid. Bot. 8 oz. *otc.*
Use: Emollient.

AquaMEPHYTON Injection. (Merck) Phytonadione 2 mg/ml or 10 mg/ml, vitamin K-1, w/polyoxyethylated fatty acid derivative 70 mg, dextrose 37.5 mg, benzyl alcohol 0.9%, water for injection q.s. to 1 ml. Inj. Amp. 1 mg/0.5 ml Box 25s; 10 mg/1 ml Box 6s, 25s. Vial 10 mg/ml 2.5 ml, 5 ml. *Rx.*
Use: Coagulant.

Aqua Mist. (Faraday) Nasal spray. Squeeze Bot. 20 ml.

Aquamycin. (Armenpharm) Erythromycin. *Rx.*
Use: Anti-infective, erythromycin.

Aquanil. (Sigma-Tau Pharmaceuticals) Mersalyl 100 mg, theophylline (hydrate) 50 mg, methylparaben 0.18%, propylparaben 0.02%. Vial 10 ml. *otc.*
Use: Bronchodilator, diuretic.

Aquanil Cleanser. (Person & Covey) Glycerin, cetyl, stearyl and benzyl alcohol, sodium laureth sulfate, xanthan gum. Lipid free. Lot. Bot. 240 ml, 480 ml. *otc.*
Use: Dermatologic, cleanser.

Aquanine. (Armenpharm) Quinine HCl. *Rx.*
Use: Antimalarial.

Aquaoxy. (Armenpharm) Oxytetracycline HCl. *Rx.*
Use: Anti-infective, tetracycline.

Aquaphenicol. (Armenpharm) Chloramphenicol. *Rx.*
Use: Anti-infective.

Aquaphilic Ointment. (Medco Lab) Hydrated hydrophilic oint. Jar 16 oz. *otc.*
Use: Emollient, ointment base.

Aquaphilic Ointment with Carbamide 10% and 20%. (Medco Lab) Stearyl alcohol, white petrolatum, sorbitol, propylene glycol, sodium lauryl sulfate, lactic acid, methylparaben, propylparaben.
Use: Prescription compounding, emollient.

Aquaphor Natural Healing. (Beiersdorf) Petrolatum, mineral oil, mineral wax, woolwax alcohol, panthenol, glycerin, chamomile essense. Oint. Tube 52.5 g. *otc.*
Use: Emollient.

Aquaphor. (Beiersdorf) Cholesterolized anhydrous petrolatum ointment base. Tube 1.75 oz, 3.25 oz, 16 oz, Jar 5 lb, Bar 3 oz. *otc.*
Use: Pharmaceutic aid, ointment base.
See: Eucerin, Emulsion (Duke).

Aquaphor Antibiotic. (Beiersdorf) 10,000 units polymyxin B sulfate and 500 units bacitracin zinc/g in a cholesterolized ointment base. Oint. Tube 15 g. *otc.*
Use: Anti-infective, topical.

Aquaphyllin Syrup. (Ferndale Laboratories) Theophylline anhydrous 80 mg/15 ml UD pk. 15 ml, 30 ml. Bot. 16 oz, gal. *Rx.*
Use: Bronchodilator.

Aquapool Concentrate. (Parker) Color additive for hydrotherapy to control foaming. Bot. pt, gal.

AquaSite. (Ciba Vision Ophthalmics) PEG-400 0.2%, dextran 70, polycarbophil, NaCl, EDTA, sodium hydroxide. Preservative free. Soln. Single-use vi-

Arava

als 0.6 ml, 15 ml. *otc.*
Use: Artificial tears.

Aquasol A. (Astra Merck) Water-miscible Vitamin A. Chlorobutanol 0.5%, polysorbate 80, butylated hydroxyanisole, butylated hydroxytoluene. **Inj.:** 50,000 U.S.P. units/ml. Vial 2 ml Box 10s. **Cap.:** 25,000 U.S.P. units/Cap. Bot. 100s. 50,000 U.S.P. units/Cap. Bot. 100s, 500s. **Drops:** 5000 U.S.P. units/0.1 ml. Bot. 30 ml w/dropper. *otc, Rx.*
Use: Vitamin supplement.

Aquasol E. (Astra Merck) Vitamin E. **Cap.:** 73.5 mg Bot. 100s; 400 IU Bot. 30s. **Drops:** 50 mg/ml Bot. 12 ml, 30 ml w/dropper. *otc.*
Use: Vitamin supplement.

Aquasonic 100. (Parker) Water-soluble, viscous, contact medium gel for ultrasonic transmission. Bot. 250 ml, 1 L, 5 L.
Use: Ultrasound aid.

Aquasonic 100 sterile. (Parker) Water-soluble, sterile gel for ultrasonic transmission. Overwrapped Foil Pouches 15 g, 50 g.
Use: Ultrasound aid.

Aquasulf. (Armenpharm) Triple sulfa tablet. *Rx.*
Use: Anti-infective.

Aquatensen. (Wallace Laboratories) Methyclothiazide 5 mg/Tab. Bot. 100s, 500s. *Rx.*
Use: Antihypertensive, diuretic.

Aquavite. (Armenpharm) Soluble multivitamin.
Use: Vitamin supplement.

Aquavite-E. (Cypress) Di-Alpha tocopheryl acetate 15 IU/0.3 ml. Sol., Oral. 30 ml. *Rx.*
Use: Vitamin supplement.

Aquazide. (Western Research) Trichlormethiazide 4 mg/Tab. Bot. 100s. *Rx.*
Use: Antihypertensive, diuretic.

Aquazide H. (Western Research) Hydrochlorothiazide 50 mg/Tab. Bot. 1000s. *Rx.*
Use: Diuretic.

Aquazol. (Armenpharm) Sulfisoxazole.
Use: Anti-infective.

Aqueous Allergens. (Bayer Corp).
Use: Antiallergic.

aquinone.
See: Menadione, U.S.P. 23.

Aquol Bath Oil. (Lamond) Vegetable oil, olive oil. Bot. 4 oz, 6 oz, 16 oz, qt, gal. *otc.*
Use: Antipruritic, emollient.

AR-121. (Argus) Phase I/II HIV. *Rx.*
Use: Antiviral.

ARA-A.
See: Vidarabine.

ARA-C.
See: Cytarabine.

Aralen Hydrochloride. (Sanofi Winthrop) Chloroquine HCl 50 mg/ml. Amp 5 ml. *Rx.*
Use: Amebicide, antimalarial.

Aralen Phosphate. (Sanofi Winthrop) Chloroquine phosphate 500 mg/Tab. Bot. 25s. *Rx.*
Use: Amebicide, antimalarial.

Aralis Tablets. (Sanofi Winthrop) Glycobiarsol, chloroquine phosphate. *Rx.*
Use: Amebicide.

Aramine. (Merck) Metaraminol bitartrate (equivalent to metaraminol) 10 mg/ml, sodium Cl 4.4 mg, water for injection q.s. ad. 1 ml, methylparaben 0.15%, propylparaben 0.02%, sodium bisulfite 0.2%. Vial 10 ml. *Rx.*
Use: Antihypotensive.

•**aranotin.** (AR-ah-NO-tin) USAN.
Use: Antiviral.

•**arbaprostil.** (ahr-bah-PRAHST-ill) USAN.
Use: Antisecretory (gastric).

Arbolic. (Burgin-Arden) Methandriol dipropionate 50 mg/ml. Vial 10 ml. *Rx.*
Use: Anabolic steroid.

Arbutal. (Arcum) Butalbital ¾ gr, phenacetin 2 gr, aspirin 3 gr, caffeine gr/Tab. Bot. 100s, 1000s. *Rx.*
Use: Analgesic, hypnotic, sedative.

•**arbutamine hydrochloride.** (ahr-BYOO-tah-meen) USAN.
Use: Cardiovascular agent.
See: GenESA, Inj. (Gensia Automedics).

Arcet. (Econo Med Pharmaceuticals) Butalbital 50 mg, acetaminophen 325 mg, caffeine 40 mg/Tab. Bot. 100s. *Rx.*
Use: Analgesic, hypnotic, sedative.

•**arcitumomab.** (ahr-sigh-TOO-moe-mab) USAN.
Use: Monoclonal antibody.
See: CEA-Scan (Immunomedics, Mallinckrodt).

arcitumomab. (ahr-sigh-TOO-moe-mab)
Use: Diagnosis and localization of thyroid carcinoma.
See: 99 m Tc-labeled CEA-Scan (Immunomedics).

•**arclofenin.** (AHR-kloe-FEN-in) USAN.
Use: Diagnostic aid for hepatic function determination.

Arcoban Tablets. (Arcum) Meprobamate 400 mg/Tab. Bot. 50s, 1000s. *Rx.*
Use: Anxiolytic.

Arcobee w/C. (NBTY) Vitamins B_1 15 mg, B_2 10.2 mg, B_3 50 mg, B_5 10 mg, B_6 5 mg, C 300 mg, tartrazine. Cap. Box 100s. *otc.*
Use: Vitamin supplement.

Arcobex Extra Strength Caps. (Arcum) Vitamins B_1 100 mg, B_2 2 mg, B_6 5 mg, niacinamide 125 mg, panthenol 10 mg, B_{12} 30 mcg, benzyl alcohol 1%, gentisic acid ethanolamide 2.5%/ml. Vial 30 ml. *Rx.*
Use: Vitamin supplement.

Arcodex Antacid Tablets. (Arcum) Magnesium trisilicate 500 mg, aluminum hydroxide 250 mg/Tab. Bot. 100s, 1000s. *otc.*
Use: Antacid.

Arco-Lase. (Arco) Trizyme 38 mg (amylase 30 mg, protease 6 mg, cellulase 2 mg), lipase 25 mg/Tab. Bot. 50s. *Rx.*
Use: Digestive aid.

Arcosterone. (Arcum) Methyltestosterone. **Oral:** 10 mg or 25 mg/Tab. Bot. 100s, 1000s. **Sublingual:** 10 mg/Tab. Bot. 100s, 1000s. *Rx.*
Use: Androgen.

Arco-Thyroid. (Arco) Thyroid 1.5 gr/Tab. Bot. 1000s. *Rx.*
Use: Hormone, thyroid.

Arcotrate. (Arcum) Pentaerythritol tetranitrate 10 mg/Tab. **No. 2:** Pentaerythritol tetranitrate 20 mg/Tab. **No. 3:** Pentaerythritol tetranitrate 20 mg, phenobarbital ⅛ gr/Tab. Bot. 100s, 1000s. *Rx.*
Use: Antianginal.

Arcoval Improved. (Arcum) Vitamin A palmitate 10,000 IU, D 400 IU, thiamine mononitrate 15 mg, B_2 10 mg, nicotinamide 150 mg, B_6 5 mg, calcium pantothenate 10 mg, B_{12} 5 mcg, C 150 mg, E 5 IU/Cap. Bot. 100s, 1000s. *otc.*
Use: Mineral, vitamin supplement.

Arcum R-S. (Arcum) Reserpine 0.25 mg/Tab. Bot. 100s, 1000s. *Rx.*
Use: Antihypertensive.

Arcum V-M. (Arcum) Vitamin A palmitate 5000 IU, D 400 IU, B_1 2.5 mg, B_2 2.5 mg, B_6 0.5 mg, B_{12} 2 mcg, C 50 mg, niacinamide 20 mg, calcium pantothenate 5 mg, iron 18 mg/Cap. Bot. 100s, 1000s. *otc.*
Use: Mineral, vitamin supplement.

A-R-D. (Birchwood) Anatomically shaped dressing. Dispenser 24s.
Use: Antipruritic; counterirritant, rectal.

Ardeben. (Burgin-Arden) Diphenhydramine HCl 10 mg, chlorobutanol 0.5%. Inj. Vial 30 ml. *Rx.*
Use: Antihistamine.

Ardecaine 1%. (Burgin-Arden) Lidocaine HCl 1%. Inj. Vial 30 ml. *Rx.*
Use: Anesthetic, local.

Ardecaine 2%. (Burgin-Arden) Lidocaine HCl 2%. Inj. Vial 30 ml. *Rx.*
Use: Anesthetic, local.

Ardecaine 1% w/Epinephrine. (Burgin-Arden) Lidocaine HCl 1%, epinephrine. Inj. Vial 30 ml. *Rx.*
Use: Anesthetic, local.

Ardecaine 2% w/Epinephrine. (Burgin-Arden) Lidocaine HCl 2%, epinephrine. Inj. Vial 30 ml. *Rx.*
Use: Anesthetic, topical.

Ardefem 10. (Burgin-Arden) Estradiol valerate 10 mg/ml. Vial 10 ml. *Rx.*
Use: Estrogen.

Ardefem 20. (Burgin-Arden) Estradiol valerate 20 mg/ml. Vial 10 ml. *Rx.*
Use: Estrogen.

Ardefem 40. (Burgin-Arden) Estradiol valerate 40 mg/ml. Vial 10 ml. *Rx.*
Use: Estrogen.

•**ardeparin sodium.** (ahr-dee-PA-rin) USAN.
Use: Anticoagulant.
See: Normiflo, Inj. (Wyeth-Ayerst).

Ardepred Soluble. (Burgin-Arden) Prednisolone 20 mg, niacinamide 25 mg, disodium edetate 0.5 mg, sodium bisulfite 1 mg, phenol 5 mg/ml. Vial 10 ml. *Rx.*
Use: Corticosteroid combination.

Arderone 100. (Burgin-Arden) Testosterone enanthate 100 mg/ml. Vial 10 ml. *c-III.*
Use: Androgen.

Arderone 200. (Burgin-Arden) Testosterone enanthate 200 mg/ml. Vial 10 ml. *c-III.*
Use: Androgen.

Ardevila tablets. (Sanofi Winthrop) Inositol hexanicotinate. *Rx.*
Use: Vasodilator.

Ardiol 90/4. (Burgin-Arden) Testosterone enanthate 90 mg, estradiol valerate 4 mg/ml. Vial 10 ml. *Rx.*
Use: Androgen, estrogen combination.

Arduan. (Organon Teknika) Pipecuronium Br 10 mg/10 ml. Vial. *Rx.*
Use: Neuromuscular blocker.

arecoline acetarsone salt.
See: Drocarbil.

Aredia. (Novartis) Pamidronate disodium 30 mg (470 mg mannitol), 60 mg (400 mg mannitol), 90 mg (375 mg mannitol). Pow. for Inj., lyophilized. Vial. *Rx.*
Use: Antihypercalcemic.

•**argatroban.** (ahr-GAT-troe-ban) USAN.
Use: Anticoagulant.

Argesic. (Econo Med Pharmaceuticals) Methyl salicylate and triethanolamine in a nongreasy vanishing cream base. Jar 60 g. *otc.*
Use: Analgesic, topical.

Argesic-SA. (Econo Med Pharmaceuticals) Disalicylic acid 500 mg/Tab. Bot. 100s. *Rx.*
Use: Analgesic, topical.

•**arginine.** (AHR-jih-neen) U.S.P. 23.
Use: Ammonia detoxicant; diagnostic aid (pituitary function determination).

arginine butyrate. (AHR-jih-neen)
Use: Sickle cell disease, beta-thalassemia. [Orphan drug]

•**arginine glutamate.** (AHR-jih-neen GLUE-tah-mate) USAN.
Use: Ammonia detoxicant.
See: Modumate (Abbott Laboratories).

arginine hydrochloride. (AHR-jih-neen)
Use: Diagnostic aid.
See: R-Gene 10, Inj. (Pharmacia & Upjohn).

•**arginine hydrochloride.** (AHR-jih-neen) U.S.P. 23.
Use: Ammonia detoxicant.

8-arginine-vasopressin.
See: Vasopressin.

•**argipressin tannate.** (AHR-JIH-press-in TAN-ate) USAN.
Use: Antidiuretic.

argyn.
See: Mild Silver Protein (Various Mfr.).

Aricept. (Eisai/Pfizer) Donepezil HCl 5 mg and 10 mg/Tab. Blister pack. 30s and 100s. *Rx.*
Use: Treatment of mild to moderate dementia associated with Alzheimer's disease.

Aridol. (MPL) Pamabrom 52 mg, pyrilamine maleate 30 mg, homatropine methylbromide 1.2 mg, hyoscyamine sulfate 0.10 mg, scopolamine HBr 0.02 mg, methamphetamine HCl 1.5 mg/Tab. Bot. 100s. *Rx.*
Use: Anticholinergic, antispasmodic, diuretic, stimulant.

•**arildone.** (AR-ill-dohn) USAN.
Use: Antiviral.

Arimidex. (Zeneca) Anastrozole 1 mg, lactose/Tab. 30s *Rx.*
Use: Aromatase inhibitor.

•**aripiprazole.** (A-rih-PIP-ray-zole) USAN.
Use: Antipsychotic, antischizophrenic.

Aris Phenobarbital Reagent Strips. (Bayer Corp) Box 25s.
Use: Diagnostic aid.

Aris Phenytoin Reagent Strips. (Bayer Corp) Box 25s.
Use: Diagnostic aid.

Aristocort. (ESI Lederle Generics) Triamcinolone. **Tab.:** 1 mg Bot. 50s; 2 mg Bot. 100s; 4 mg Bot. 30s, 100s; 8 mg Bot. 50s. **Syr.:** Diacetate (w/methylparaben 0.08%, propylparaben 0.02%) 2 mg/5 ml. Bot. 4 oz. *Rx.*
Use: Corticosteroid.

Aristocort A Cream. (Fujisawa) Triamcinolone acetonide w/emulsifying wax, isopropyl palmitate, glycerin, sorbitol, lactic acid, benzyl alcohol. **0.025% w/Aquatain:** Tube 15 g, 60 g. **0.1%:** Tube 15 g, 60 g, Jar 240 g. **0.5%:** Tube 15 g. *Rx.*
Use: Corticosteroid, topical.

Aristocort Acetonide, Sodium Phosphate Salt. (ESI Lederle Generics)
Use: Corticosteroid, topical.
See: Aristocort Preps.
Sodium Phosphate Triamcinolone Acetonide.

Aristocort A Ointment. (Fujisawa) Triamcinolone acetonide 0.1%. Tube 15 g, 60 g. *Rx.*
Use: Corticosteroid, topical.

Aristocort Cream. (Fujisawa) Triamcinolone acetonide w/emulsifying wax, polysorbate 60, mono and diglycerides, squalane, sorbitol soln., sorbic acid, potassium sorbate. **LP: 0.025%:** Tube 15 g, 60 g, Jar 240 g, 480 g; **R: 0.1%:** Tube 15 g, 60 g, Jar 240 g, 480 g; **HP: 0.5%:** Tube 15 g, Jar 240 g. *Rx.*
Use: Corticosteroid, topical.

Aristocort Forte. (ESI Lederle Generics) Triamcinolone diacetate 40 mg/ml. Vial 1 ml, 5 ml. *Rx.*
Use: Corticosteroid.

Aristocort Intralesional. (ESI Lederle Generics) Triamcinolone diacetate 25 mg/ml. Vial 5 ml. *Rx.*
Use: Corticosteroid.

Aristocort Ointment. (Fujisawa) Triamcinolone acetonide. **R: 0.1%:** Tube 15 g, 60 g, Jar 240 g. **HP: 0.5%:** Tube 15 g, Jar 240 g. *Rx.*
Use: Corticosteroid, topical.

Aristo-Pak. (ESI Lederle Generics) Triamcinolone 4 mg/Tab. 16s. *Rx.*
Use: Corticosteroid.

Aristospan Intra-articular. (ESI Lederle Generics) Triamcinolone hexacetonide 20 mg/ml micronized susp., polysorbate 80 0.4% w/v, sorbitol soln. 64% w/v, water q.s., benzyl alcohol 0.9% w/v. Vial 1 ml, 5 ml. *Rx.*
Use: Corticosteroid.

Aristospan Intralesional. (ESI Lederle Generics) Triamcinolone hexacetonide 5 mg/ml, polysorbate 80 0.2% w/v, sorbitol soln. 64% w/v, water q.s., benzyl alcohol 0.9% w/v. Vial 5 ml. *Rx.*
Use: Corticosteroid.

Arlacel 83. (Zeneca) Sorbitan Sesquioleate.
Use: Surface active agent.

Arlacel 165. (Zeneca) Glyceryl monostearate, PEG-100 stearate nonionic self-emulsifying.
Use: Surface active agent.

Arlacel C. (Zeneca) Sorbitan Sesquioleate. Mixture of oleate esters of sorbitol and its anhydrides.
Use: Surface active agent.

Arlamol E. (Zeneca) Polyoxypropylene (15), stearyl ether, BHT 0.1%.
Use: Emollient.

Arlatone 507. (Zeneca) Padimate O. *otc.*
Use: Sunscreen.

Arlix. (Hoechst Marion Roussel) Piretanide HCl. *Rx.*
Use: Antihypertensive, diuretic.

Arm-a-Med Metaproterenol Sulfate. (Centeon) Soln. for nebulization: Metaproterenol sulfate 0.4% or 0.6% with sodium Cl, EDTA. Vial UD 2.5 ml for use with IPPB device. *Rx.*
Use: Bronchodilator.

Arm-a-Vial. (Centeon) Sterile water, sodium Cl 0.45% or 0.9%. Box 100s. Plastic vial 3 ml, 5 ml.
Use: Electrolyte supplement.

A.R.M. Caplets. (Menley & James) Chlorpheniramine maleate 4 mg, phenylpropanolamine HCl 25 mg/Capl. Pkg. 20s, 40s. *otc.*
Use: Antihistamine, decongestant.

Aromatic Ammonia Vaporole. (Glaxo-Wellcome) Inhalant. Vial 5 min. Box 10s, 12s, 100s. *Rx.*
Use: Respiratory.

•**aromatic elixir.** N.F. 18.
Use: Pharmaceutic aid (vehicle; flavored, sweetened).

aromatic elixir. (Eli Lilly) Alcohol 22%. Bot. 16 fl. oz.
Use: Pharmaceutic aid, flavoring.

Arnica Tincture. (Eli Lilly) Arnica 20% in alcohol 66%. Bot. 120 ml, 480 ml. *otc.*
Use: Analgesic, topical.

•**arprinocid.** (ahr-PRIN-oh-sid) USAN.
Use: Coccidiostat.

arseclor.
See: Dichlorophenarsine HCl (Various Mfr.).

arsenic compounds.
Use: Rarely employed in modern medicine; there are no longer any official compounds.
See: Acetarsone.
Arsphenamine.
Carbarsone (Various Mfr.).
Dichlorophenarsine HCl.
Ferric Cacodylate.
Glycobiarsol.
Neoarsphenamine.
Oxophenarsine HCl.
Sodium Cacodylate (Various Mfr.).
Tryparsamide.

arsenobenzene.
See: Arsphenamine.

arsenphenolamine.
See: Arsphenamine.

Arsobal. Melarsoprol (Mel B).
Use: CDC anti-infective agent.

arsphenamine. Arsenobenzene, arsenobenzol, arsenphenolamine, Ehrlich 606, salvarsan.
Use: Formerly used as antisyphilitic.

arsthinol. Cyclic.
Use: Antiprotozoal.

Artane. (ESI Lederle Generics) Trihexyphenidyl HCl. **Elix.:** 2 mg/5 ml w/methylparaben 0.08%, propylparaben 0.02%, Bot. Pt. **Tab.:** 2 mg or 5 mg, Bot. 100s, 1000s, UD 10×10 in 10s. **Sequel:** 5 mg Bot. 60s, 500s. *Rx.*
Use: Antiparkinsonian.

Artarau. (Archer-Taylor) Rauwolfia serpentina 50 mg or 100 mg/Tab. Bot. 100s, 1000s. *Rx.*
Use: Antihypertensive.

Arta-Vi-C. (Archer-Taylor) Multivitamins with Vitamin C 100 mg/Tab. Bot. 100s. *otc.*
Use: Vitamin supplement.

Artazyme. (Archer-Taylor) Bot. 13 ml.
Use: Autolyzed proteolytic enzyme.

•**arteflene.** (AHR-teh-fleen) USAN.
Use: Antimalarial.

•**artegraft.** (AHR-teh-graft) USAN. Arterial graft composed of a section of bovine carotid artery that has been subjected to enzymatic digestion with ficin and tanned with dialdehyde starch.
Use: Prosthetic aid (arterial).

arterenol.
See: Norepinephrine bitartrate.

Artha-G. (T.E. Williams) Salsalate 750 mg/Tab. Bot. 120s. *Rx.*
Use: Analgesic.

Arthralgen. (Robins) Salicylamide 250 mg, acetaminophen 250 mg/Tab. Bot. 30s, 100s, 500s. *otc.*

Use: Analgesic combination.

Arthricare Daytime Formula. (Del Pharmaceuticals) Menthol 1.25%, methyl nicotinate 0.25%, capsaicin 0.025%, with aloe vera gel, carbomer 940, DMDM hydantoin, glyceryl stearate SE, myristyl propionate, propylparaben, triethanolamine. Cream. Jar 90 g. *otc.*
Use: Analgesic, topical.

ArthriCare Double Ice. (Del Pharmaceuticals) Menthol 4%, camphor 3.1%, with aloe vera gel, carbomer 940, dioctyl sodium sulfosuccinate, propylene glycol, triethanolamine. Gel. Jar 90 g. *otc.*
Use: Analgesic, topical.

ArthriCare Odor Free Rub. (Del Pharmaceuticals) Menthol 1.25%, methyl nicotinate 0.25%, capsaicin 0.025%, aloe vera gel, carbomer 940, DMDM hydantoin, emulsifying wax, glyceryl stearate SE, isopropyl alcohol, myristyl propionate, propylparaben, triethanolamine. Oint. Jar 90 g. *otc.*
Use: Liniment.

ArthriCare Triple Medicated. (Del Pharmaceuticals) Methylsalicylate 30%, menthol 1.25%, methyl nicotinate 0.7%, dioctyl sodium sulfosuccinate, hydroxypropylmethylcellulose, isopropyl alcohol, propylene glycol. Gel. Tube 3 oz. *otc.*
Use: Analgesic, topical.

Arthritic Pain Lotion. (Walgreens) Triethanolamine salicylate 10%. Bot. 6 oz. *otc.*
Use: Analgesic, topical.

Arthriten, Maximum Strength. (Alva-Amco) Acetaminophen 250 mg, magnesium salicylate 250 mg, caffeine anhydrous 32.5 mg. Buffered with magnesium carbonate, magnesium oxide, calcium carbonate. 40s. *otc.*
Use: Analgesic.

Arthritis Bayer Timed Release Aspirin. (Bayer Corp) Aspirin 650 mg/TR Tab. Bot. 30s, 72s, 125s. *otc.*
Use: Analgesic.

Arthritis Hot Creme. (Thompson Medical) Methyl salicylate 15%, menthol 10%, glyceryl stearate, carbomer 934, lanolin, PEG-100 stearate, propylene glycol, trolamine, parabens. Cream Jar 90 g. *otc.*
Use: Liniment.

Arthritis Pain Formula. (Whitehall Robins) Aspirin 486 mg, aluminum hydroxide gel 20 mg, magnesium hydroxide 60 mg/Tab. Bot. 40s, 100s, 175s. *otc.*
Use: Analgesic combination.

Arthritis Pain Formula, Aspirin Free. (Whitehall Robins) Acetaminophen 500 mg/Tab. Bot. 30s, 75s. *otc.*
Use: Analgesic.

Arthropan Liquid. (Purdue Frederick) Choline salicylate 870 mg/5 ml. Bot. 8 oz, 16 oz. *Rx.*
Use: Analgesic.

Arthrotec. (Searle) Diclofenac sodium 50 mg/misoprostol 200 mcg or diclofenac sodium 75 mg/misoprostol 200 mcg, lactose/Tab. Bot. 60s, 90s. *Rx.*
Use: Analgesic.

Arthrotrin Tablets. (Whiteworth Towne) Enteric coated aspirin 325 mg/Tab. Bot. 100s.
Use: Analgesic.

Articulose L. A. (Seatrace) Triamcinolone diacetate 40 mg/ml. Vial 5 ml. *Rx.*
Use: Corticosteroid.

artificial tanning agent.
See: QT, Prods. (Schering Plough).
Sudden Tan, Prods. (Schering Plough).

artificial tear insert.
See: Lacrisert (Merck).

artificial tears. (Various Mfr.) Benzalkonium Cl 0.01%. May also contain EDTA, NaCl, polyvinyl alcohol. Sol. Bot. 15 ml or 30 ml. *otc.*
Use: Lubricant, ophthalmic.

Artificial Tears Ointment. (Rugby) White petrolatum, anhydrous liquid lanolin, mineral oil. Ophth. Oint. Tube 3.5 g. *otc.*
Use: Lubricant, ophthalmic.

Artificial Tears Plus. (Various Mfr.) Polyvinyl alcohol 1.4%, povidone 0.6%, chlorobutanol 0.5%, NaCl. Soln. Bot. 15 ml. *otc.*
Use: Lubricant, ophthalmic.

•**artilide fumarate.** (AHR-tih-lide) USAN.
Use: Cardiovascular agent.

Artra Beauty Bar. (Schering Plough) Triclocarban 1% in soap base. Cake 3.6 oz. *otc.*
Use: Dermatologic, cleanser.

Artra Skin Tone Cream. (Schering Plough) Hydroquinone 2%. Oint. Tube 1 oz. (normal only), 2 oz, 4 oz.
Use: Dermatologic.

AS-101. (Wyeth Ayerst) Phase I/II ARC, AIDS. *Rx.*
Use: Immunomodulator.

5-asa. Mesalamine.
See: Asacol (Procter & Gamble Pharm).
Rowasa (Solvay).

ASA. (Wampole Laboratories) Anti-skin antibodies test by IFA. Test 48s.
Use: Diagnostic aid.

A.S.A. (Eli Lilly) Aspirin. Acetylsalicylic acid. **Enseal:** 5 gr or 10 gr. Bot. 100s, 1000s. **Supp.:** 5 gr or 10 gr. Pkg. 6s, 144s. *otc.*
Use: Analgesic.

Asacol. (Procter & Gamble Pharm) Mesalamine 400 mg/Tab. DR Bot. 100s. *Rx.*
Use: Anti-inflammatory.

asafetida, emulsion of. Milk of Asafetida.

Asaped Tablets. (Sanofi Winthrop) Acetylsalicylic acid. *otc.*
Use: Analgesic.

Asawin Tablets. (Sanofi Winthrop) Acetylsalicylic acid. *otc.*
Use: Analgesic.

A.S.B. (Femco) Calcium carbonate, magnesium carbonate, bismuth subcarbonate, sodium bicarbonate, kaolin. Pow., Can 3 oz. Tabs. 50s. *otc.*
Use: Antacid.

Asclerol. (Spanner) Liver injection crude (2 mcg/ml) 50%, Vitamins B_1 20 mg, B_2 3 mg, B_6 1 mg, B_{12} 30 mcg, niacinamide 100 mg, panthenol 2.8 mg, choline Cl 20 mg, inositol 10 mg/ml. Multiple dose vial 10 ml. *Rx.*
Use: Vitamin supplement.

ascorbate sodium. Antiscorbutic vitamin.

•**ascorbic acid.** (ASS-kor-bik) U.S.P. 23.
Use: Vitamin (antiscorbutic); acidifier (urinary).

ascorbic acid. (ASS-kor-bik) (Various Mfr.) Antiscorbutic vitamin; Vitamin C. **Cap.:** 25 mg, 100 mg, 250 mg, 500 mg. **Inj.:** Amp. (100 mg/ml) 1 ml, 2 ml, 5 ml; (200 mg/ml) 5 ml, (500 mg) 2 ml, 5 ml, 10 ml, 30 ml, (250 mg/ml) 10 ml; (1000 mg/ml) 10 ml. **Tab.:** 50 mg, 100 mg, 250 mg, 500 mg. **Chew. tab.:** 100 mg, 250 mg, 500 mg. **SR Tab.:** 500 mg, 1500 mg. **SR Cap.:** 500 mg. **Pow.:** 4 g/5 ml. **Soln.:** 35 mg/0.6 ml or 100 mg/ml.
Use: Vitamin supplement.
See: Ascorbicap, Cap. (ICN Pharmaceuticals).
Ascorbineed, Cap. (Hanlon).
C-Caps 500 (Drug Industries).
Cecon, Soln. (Abbott Laboratories).
Cenolate, Amp. (Abbott Laboratories).
Cetane, Cap., Vial (Forest Pharmaceutical).
Cevalin, Tab., Amp. (Eli Lilly).
Cevi-Bid, Cap. (Roberts Pharm).
Ce-Vi-Sol, Drops (Bristol-Myers).
Neo-Vadrin, Preps. (Scherer).
Sunkist Vitamin C, Capl., Chew. tab. (Novartis).

ascorbic acid injection.
Use: Vitamin supplement.
See: Cevalin, Amp. (Eli Lilly).

ascorbic acid salts.
See: Bismuth Ascorbate.
Calcium Ascorbate.
Sodium Ascorbate.

Ascorbicap. (ICN Pharmaceuticals) Ascorbic acid 500 mg/S.R. Cap. Bot. 50s. *otc.*
Use: Vitamin supplement.

Ascorbin/11. (Taylor Pharmaceuticals) Lemon bioflavonoids 110 mg, Vitamin C 1 g, rose hips powder 50 mg, rutin 25 mg/S.R. Tab. Bot. 100s. *otc.*
Use: Vitamin supplement.

Ascorbineed. (Hanlon) Vitamin C 500 mg/T-Cap. Bot. 100s. *otc.*
Use: Vitamin supplement.

Ascorbocin Powder. (Paddock) Vitamin C 500 mg, niacin 500 mg, B_1 50 mg, B_6 50 mg, d-α-tocopheryl, polyethylene glycol 1000 succinate 50 IU, lactose/3 g. Bot. lb. *otc.*
Use: Vitamin supplement.

•**ascorbyl palmitate.** (ah-SCORE-bill PAL-mih-tate) N.F. 18. L-Ascorbic acid 6-palmitate.
Use: Preservative; pharmaceutic aid (antioxidant).

Ascorvite S.R. (Eon Labs Manufacturing) Vitamin C 500 mg/S.R. Cap. *otc.*
Use: Vitamin supplement.

Ascriptin. (Rhone-Poulenc Rorer) Aspirin 325 mg, magnesium hydroxide 50 mg, aluminum hydroxide 50 mg/Tab. Bot. 50s, 100s, 225s, 500s. *otc.*
Use: Analgesic, antacid.

Ascriptin A/D. (Rhone-Poulenc Rorer) Acetylsalicylic acid 325 mg with magnesium hydroxide 75 mg, aluminum hydroxide and calcium carbonate 75 mg/Capsule shape coated tabs. Bot. 225s. *otc.*
Use: Analgesic, antacid.

Ascriptin Extra Strength. (Rhone-Poulenc Rorer) Aspirin 500 mg with magnesium hydroxide 80 mg, aluminum hydroxide and calcium carbonate 80 mg. Capsule shape coated tabs. Bot. 50s. *otc.*
Use: Analgesic, antacid.

Asendin. (ESI Lederle Generics) Amoxapine. Tab.:**25 mg** Bot. 100s; **50 mg** Bot. 100s, 500s, UD 100s; **100 mg** Bot. 100s, UD 100s; **150 mg** Bot. 30s. *Rx.*
Use: Antidepressant.

aseptichrome.
See: Merbromin (Various Mfr.).

Aslum. (Drug Products) Carbolic acid 1%, aluminum acetate, ichthammol, zinc oxide, aromatic oils in a petrolatum-stearin base. Tube oz. Jar lb.
Use: Astringent.

Asma. (Wampole Laboratories) Anti-smooth muscle antibody test by IFA. Test 48.
Use: Diagnostic aid.

Asmalix. (Century Pharm) Theophylline 80 mg, alcohol 20%/15 ml. Bot. qt, gal. *Rx.*
Use: Bronchodilator.

Asma-Tuss. (Halsey) Phenobarbital 4 mg, theophylline 15 mg, ephedrine sulfate 12 mg, guaifenesin 50 mg/5 ml. Bot. 4 oz. *Rx.*
Use: Bronchodilator.

Asolectin. (Associated Concentrates) Chemical lecithin 25%, chemical cephalin 22%, inositol phosphatides 16%, soybean oil 2.5%, other miscellaneous sterols and lipids 34.5%. *otc.*
Use: Diet supplement.

•**asparaginase.** (ass-PAR-uh-jin-aze) USAN.
Use: Antineoplastic.
See: Elspar, Inj. (Merck).

•**aspartame.** (ass-PAR-tame) N.F. 18.
Use: Sweetener.

•**aspartic acid.** (ass-PAR-tick Acid) USAN. Aspartic acid; aminosuccinic acid.
Use: Management of fatigue; amino acid.

•**aspartocin.** (ass-PAR-toe-sin) USAN.
Use: Anti-infective.

A-Spas. (Hyrex) Dicyclomine HCl 10 mg/ml. Vial 10 ml. *Rx.*
Use: Antispasmodic.

A-Spas S/L. (Hyrex) Hyoscyamine sulfate 0.125 mg/Tab., sublingual. 100s. *Rx.*
Use: Antispasmodic.

Aspercreme. (Thompson Medical) Triethanolamine salicylate 10% in cream base. *otc.*
Use: Analgesic, topical.

aspergillus niger enzyme. Alpha-galactosidase. *otc.*
See: Beano, Tab. (AK-Pharma).

aspergillus oryzae enzyme. Diastase.
See: Taka-Diastase, Preps. (Parke-Davis).

Aspergum. (Schering Plough) Aspirin 227.5 mg/1 Gum. Tab. Orange or Cherry flavor. Box 16s, 40s. *otc.*
Use: Analgesic.

asperkinase. Proteolytic enzyme mixture derived from aspergillus oryzae.

•**asperlin.** (ASS-per-lin) USAN.
Use: Anti-infective, antineoplastic.

Aspermin. (Buffington) Aspirin 325 mg/Tab. Sugar, caffeine, lactose, and salt free. Dispens-A-Kit 500s. *otc.*
Use: Analgesic.

Aspermin Extra. (Buffington) Aspirin 500 mg/Tab. Sugar, caffeine, lactose, and salt free. Dispens-A-Kit 500s. *otc.*
Use: Analgesic.

•**aspirin.** (ASS-pihr-in) U.S.P. 23. Acetophen, Acetol, Acetasol, Acetosalin, Aceticyl, Acetylin, Acetylsal, Empirin, Saletin. Acetylsalicylic acid, Benzoic acid, 2-(acetyloxy)-., Salicyclic acid acetate.
Use: Analgesic, antipyretic, antirheumatic. Prophylactic to reduce risk of death or non-fatal MI in patients with a previous infarction or unstable angina pectoris.
See: A.S.A., Preps. (Eli Lilly).
Aspergum, Gum, Tab. (Schering Plough).
Bayer Children's Aspirin, Tab. (Bayer Corp).
Bayer, 8-Hour Timed-Release, Tab. (Bayer Corp).
Easprin, Tab. (Parke-Davis).
Ecotrin, Tab. (SmithKline Beecham Pharmaceuticals).
Ecotrin Maximum Strength, Capl., Tab. (SmithKline Beecham Pharmaceuticals).
Genprin, Tab. (Zenith Goldline).
Genuine Bayer Aspirin, Tab., Capl. (Bayer Corp).
Halfprin 81, EC Tab. (Kramer).
Heartline, Tab. Enteric Coated (BDI).
Maximum Bayer Aspirin, Tab., Capl. (Bayer Corp).
Norwich Aspirin, Tab. (Procter & Gamble).
St. Joseph, Prods. (Schering Plough).
ZORprin, Tab. (Knoll Pharmaceuticals).

aspirin, alumina, and magnesia tablets.
Use: Analgesic, antacid.

aspirin, alumina, and magnesium oxide tablets.
Use: Analgesic, antacid.

aspirin-barbiturate combinations.
Use: Analgesic, sedative, hypnotic.
See: BA-C, Tab. (Merz).
Butalbital, Tab., Cap. (Various Mfr.).
Fiorgen, Tab. (Zenith Goldline).
Fiorinal, Cap., Tab. (Novartis).
Fiortal, Cap. (Geneva).
Isollyl, Tab. (Rugby).

Lanorinal, Cap., Tab. (Lannett)
Marnal, Tab., Cap. (Vortech).

aspirin, caffeine and dihydrocodeine bitartrate capsules.
Use: Analgesic.

aspirin w/codeine no. 3. (Various Mfr.) Codeine phosphate 30 mg, aspirin 325 mg Tab. Bot. 100s, 1000s. *c-III.*
Use: Analgesic combination, narcotic.

aspirin w/codeine no. 4. (Various Mfr.) Codeine phosphate 60 mg, aspirin 325 mg Tab. Bot. 100s, 500s, 1000s. *c-III.*
Use: Analgesic combination, narcotic.

aspirin, codeine, phosphate alumina, and magnesia tablets.
Use: Analgesic.

aspirin and codeine phosphate tablets.
Use: Analgesic.

aspirin delayed-release capsules.
Use: Analgesic.

aspirin delayed-release tablets.
Use: Analgesic.
See: Bayer Low Adult Strength (Bayer Corp).

aspirin, enteric coated.
Use: Analgesic.
See: A.S.A., Preps. (Eli Lilly).
Ecotrin, Tab. (SmithKline Beecham Pharmaceuticals).

Aspirin Free Anacin Maximum Strength. (Whitehall Robins) Acetaminophen 500 mg. **Capl., Gel Capl.:** Bot. 100s; **Tab.:** Bot. 60s. *otc.*
Use: Analgesic.

Aspirin Free Anacin P.M. (Robins) Diphenhydramine HCl 25 mg, acetaminophen 500 mg/Tab. Bot. 20s. *otc.*
Use: Sleep aid.

Aspirin-Free Bayer Select Allergy Sinus. (Bayer Corp) Pseudoephedrine HCl 30 mg, chlorpheniramine maleate 2 mg, acetaminophen 500 mg/Cap. Pkg. 16s. *otc.*
Use: Analgesic, antihistamine, decongestant.

Aspirin-Free Bayer Select Head & Chest Cold. (Bayer Corp) Pseudoephedrine HCl 30 mg, dextromethorphan HBr 10 mg, guaifenesin 100 mg, acetaminophen 325 mg. Cap. Bot. 16s. *otc.*
Use: Analgesic, decongestant, expectorant.

Aspirin-Free Bayer Select Headache. (Bayer Corp) Acetaminophen 500 mg, caffeine 65 mg. Cap. Bot. 50s. *otc.*
Use: Analgesic combination.

Aspirin Free Excedrin. (Bristol-Myers) Acetaminophen 500 mg, caffeine 65 mg/Tab., Capl. Bot. 20s, 40s, 80s. *otc.*
Use: Analgesic combination.

Aspirin-Free Excedrin Dual. (Bristol-Myers Squibb) Acetaminophen 500 mg, calcium carbonate 111 mg, magnesium carbonate 64 mg, magnesium oxide 30 mg/Capl. Bot. 100s. *otc.*
Use: Analgesic combination.

Aspirin Free Pain Relief. (Hudson) Acetaminophen 325 mg/Tab. Bot. 100s. *otc.*
Use: Analgesic.

aspirin-narcotic combinations.
See: Alor 5/500, Tab. (Atley).

aspirin w/o.t.c. combinations.
See: Adprin-B, Tab. (Pfeiffer).
Alka Seltzer, Tab. (Bayer Corp).
Alka Seltzer Plus, Tab. (Bayer Corp).
Anacin, Cap., Tab. (Whitehall Robins).
A.P.C., Tab., Cap. (Various Mfr.).
Arthritis Foundation Pain Reliever, Tab. (McNeil-PPC).
Arthritis Strength BC Powder (Block Drug).
Ascriptin, Tab. (Rhone-Poulenc Rorer).
Ascriptin A/D, Tab. (Rhone-Poulenc Rorer).
Ascriptin, Extra Strength, Tab. (Rhone-Poulenc Rorer).
Asprimox Extra Protection for Arthritis Pain, Capl. (Invamed).
Bayer Aspirin Preps. (Bayer Corp).
Bayer Buffered Aspirin, Tab. (Sterling Health).
Bayer Low Adult Strength, DR Tab. (Sterling Health).
BC, Powder, Tab. (Block Drug).
Buffaprin, Tab. (Buffington).
Buffets, Tab. (Jones Medical Industries).
Cama, Tab. (Novartis).
Cope, Tab. (Mentholatum).
Ecotrin Adult Low Strength, EC Tab. (SmithKline Beecham).
Excedrin, Cap., Tab. (Bristol-Myers).
4-Way, Tab., Spray (Bristol-Myers).
Gelpirin, Tab. (Alra Laboratories).
Gensan, Tab. (Zenith Goldline).
Goody's Headache Powders (Goody).
Halfprin 81, EC Tab. (Kramer).
Heartline, EC Tab. (BDI).
Midol, Cap., Spray (Bayer Corp).
Momentum, Cap. (Whitehall Robins).
Night-Time Effervescent, Tab. (Zenith Goldline).
Pain Reliever, Tab. (Rugby).
Presalin, Tab. (Roberts Pharm).

St. Joseph Adult Chewable Aspirin, Chew. Tab. (Schering-Plough).
Saleto, Preps. (Roberts Pharm).
Salocol, Tab. (Roberts Pharm).
Sine-Off Tablets (Menley & James).
Stanback, Pow., Tab. (Stanback).
St. Joseph Cold Tablets For Children (Schering Plough).
Supac, Tab. (Mission Pharmacal).
Vanquish, Cap. (Bayer Corp).

aspirin & oxycodone. (Various Mfr.) Oxycodone HCl 4.5 mg, oxycodone terephthalate 0.38 mg, aspirin 325 mg/ Tab. Bot. 100s, 500s, 1000s, UD 25s. *c-II.*
Use: Analagesic combination, narcotic.

Aspirin Plus. (Walgreens) Aspirin 400 mg, caffeine 32 mg/Tab. Bot. 100s. *otc.*
Use: Analgesic combination.

aspirin salts.
See: Calcium Acetylsalicylate.

aspirin tablets, buffered.
Use: Analgesic.

Aspirin Uniserts. (Upsher-Smith Labs) Aspirin 125 mg, 300 mg or 650 mg/ supp. Ctn. 12s, 50s. *otc.*
Use: Analgesic.

Aspirtab. (Dover Pharmaceuticals) Aspirin 325 mg/Tab. Sugar, lactose and salt free. UD Box 500s. *otc.*
Use: Analgesic.

Aspirtab Max. (Dover Pharmaceuticals) Aspirin 500 mg/Tab. Sugar, lactose and salt free. UD Box 500s. *otc.*
Use: Analgesic.

Aspogen. Dihydroxyaluminum aminoacetate.

Asprimox Extra Protection for Arthritis Pain. (Invamed) Aspirin (buffered) 325 mg/Capl. Bot. 100s, 500s. *otc.*
Use: Analgesic.

Astaril tablets. (Sanofi Winthrop) Theophylline anhydrous, ephedrine sulphate. *Rx.*
Use: Bronchodilator.

Astelin. (Wallace Laboratories) Azelatine HCl 125 mcg, benzalkonium chloride, EDTA/Spray. Bot. 17 mg (100 actuations) per bottle. 2s. *Rx.*
Use: Antihistamine.

•**astemizole.** (ASS-TEM-ih-zole) USAN.
Use: Antihistamine; antiallergic
See: Hismanal, Tab. (Janssen).

asterol.
Use: Antifungal.

AsthmaHaler Mist. (SmithKline Beecham Pharmaceuticals) Epinephrine bitartrate 0.3 mg/ml in an inert propellant. Oral inhaler, 15 ml with mouthpiece; 15 ml refills. *otc.*
Use: Bronchodilator.

Asthmalixir. (Reese Pharmaceutical) Theophylline 45 mg, ephedrine sulfate 36 mg, guaifenesin 150 mg, phenobarbital 12 mg/ 15 ml. Alcohol 19%. Bot. *Rx.*
Use: Bronchodilator, expectorant, hypnotic, sedative.

AsthmaNefrin. (Menley & James) Racepinephrine HCl 2.25%. Soln. Nebulizer 15 ml, 30 ml. *otc.*
Use: Sympathomimetic.

AsthmaNefrin Solution & Nebulizer. (SmithKline Beecham Pharmaceuticals) Racepin (racemic epinephrine) as HCl equivalent to epinephrine base 2.25%, chlorobutanol 0.5%. Bot. 0.5 fl oz. With sodium bisulfite. Bot. 1 fl oz. *otc.*
Use: Bronchodilator.

•**astifilcon a.** (ASS-tih-FILL-kahn) USAN.
Use: Contact lens material (hydrophilic).

Astramorph PF. (Astra Merck) Morphine sulfate 0.5 mg/ml or 1 mg/ml preservative free. Amp. 10 ml, Vial 10 ml. *c-II.*
Use: Analgesic, narcotic.

Astroglide. (BioFilm) Purified water, glycerin, propylene glycol and parabens. Vaginal gel. Bot 66.5 ml. Travel pks. 5 ml. *otc.*
Use: Lubricant.

•**astromicin sulfate.** (ASS-troe-MY-sin) USAN.
Use: Anti-infective.

Astro-Vites. (Faraday) Vitamins A 3500 IU, D 400 IU, C 60 mg, B_1 0.8 mg, B_2 1.3 mg, niacinamide 14 mg, B_6 1 mg, B_{12} 2.5 mcg, folic acid 0.05 mg, pantothenic acid 5 mg, iron 12 mg/Tab. Bot. 100s, 250s. *otc.*
Use: Mineral, vitamin supplement.

AST/SGOT Reagent Strips. (Bayer Corp) Seralyzer reagent strip. A quantitative strip test for aspartate transaminase/serum glutamic oxaloacetic transaminase in serum or plasma. Bot. Strip 25s.
Use: Diagnostic aid.

Asupirin. (Suppositoria) Aspirin 60 mg, 120 mg, 200 mg, 300 mg, 600 mg or 1.2 g/Supp. Box 12s, 100s, 1000s. *otc.*
Use: Analgesic.

A.T. 10.
See: Dihydrotachysterol.

Atabee TD. (Defco) Vitamins C 500 mg, B_1 15 mg, B_2 10 mg, B_6 2 mg, nicotinamide 50 mg, calcium pantothenate 10 mg/Cap. Bot. 30s, 1000s. *otc.*

Use: Vitamin supplement.

Atarax. (Pfizer) Hydroxine HCl. **Tab.:** 10 mg or 25 mg Bot. 100s, 500s, UD 100s, 40s; 50 mg Bot. 100s, 250s, 500s, 1000s, UD 100s. **Syr.:** 10 mg/5 ml, alcohol 0.5%. Bot. Pt. *Rx.*
Use: Anxiolytic.
W/Ephedrine sulfate, theophylline.
See: Marax, Tab., Syr. (Roerig).
W/Penta-erythrityltetranitrate.
See: Cartrax, Tab. (Roerig).

Atarax 100. (Pfizer) Hydroxyzine HCl 100 mg, lactose/Tab. Bot. 100s, UD 100s. *Rx.*
Use: Antihistamine.

atarvet. Acepromazine.

•**atenolol.** (ah-TEN-oh-lahl) U.S.P. 23.
Use: Beta-adrenergic blocker.
See: Tenormin, Tab. (Zeneca).

atenolol/chlorthalidone. (ah-TEN-oh-lahl/klor-THAL-ih-dohn) (Various Mfr.) Atenolol 50 mg or 100 mg, chlorthalidone 25 mg/Tab. Bot. 50s, 100s, 250s, 500s, 1000s. *Rx.*
Use: Antihypertensive.

•**atevirdine mesylate.** (at-TEH-vihr-DEEN) USAN.
Use: Antiviral.

Atgam. (Pharmacia & Upjohn) Lymphocyte immune globulin, antithymocyte globulin 250 mg protein (50 mg/ml). Amp. 5 ml. *Rx.*
Use: Immunosuppressant.

Athlete's Foot Ointment. (Walgreens) Zinc undecylenate 20%, undecylenic acid 5%. Tube 1.5 oz. *otc.*
Use: Antifungal, topical.

•**atipamezole.** (AT-ih-pam-EH-zole) USAN.
Use: Antagonist (α_2-receptor).

•**atiprimod dihydrochloride.** (at-TIH-prih-mahd) USAN.
Use: Antiarthritic (immunomodulator, suppressor cell inducing agent), anti-inflammatory, antirheumatic (disease modifying).

•**atiprimod dimaleate.** USAN.
Use: Antiarthritic; anti-inflammatory; immunomodulator; antirheumatic, disease-modifying.

•**atiprosin maleate.** (ah-TIH-pro-SIN) USAN.
Use: Antihypertensive.

Ativan Injection. (Wyeth Ayerst) Lorazepam in 2 mg/ml or 4 mg/ml. Vial 1 ml, 10 ml/2 ml Tubex (w/1 ml fill). Pkg. 10s. *c-IV.*
Use: Anxiolytic.

Ativan Tablets. (Wyeth Ayerst) Lorazepam 0.5 mg, 1 mg or 2 mg/Tab. Bot. 100s, 500s, 1000s, Redipak 25s. *c-IV.*
Use: Anxiolytic.

•**atlafilcon a.** (at-LAH-FILL-kahn A) USAN.
Use: Contact lens material (hydrophilic).

ATnativ. (Miles) Antithrombin III (human), lyophilized powder/500 IU. Inj. Bot. 50 ml w/10 l sterile water. *Rx.*
Use: Thromboembolic. [Orphan drug]

•**atolide.** (ATE-oh-lide) USAN. Under study.
Use: Anticonvulsant.

Atolone. (Major) Triamcinolone 4 mg/Tab. Bot. 100s, Uni-Pak 16s. *Rx.*
Use: Corticosteroid.

•**atorvastatin calcium.** USAN.
Use: HMG-CoA reductase inhibitor; antihyperlipidemic.
See: Lipitor, Tab. (Parke-Davis).

•**atosiban.** (at-OH-sih-ban) USAN.
Use: Antagonist, oxytocin.

•**atovaquone.** (uh-TOE-vuh-KWONE) USAN.
Use: Antipneumocystic.
See: Mepron (GlaxoWellcome).

atovaquone. (uh-TOE-vuh-KWONE)
Use: Treatment and prevention of AIDS-associated *Pneumocystis carinii,* pneumonia (PCP), and *toxoplasma gondii encephalitis.*
See: Mepron (GlaxoWellcome).

Atozine Tabs. (Major) Hydroxyzine HCl 10 mg, 25 mg or 50 mg/Tab; **10 and 25 mg:** Bot. 100s, 250s, 1000s, UD 100s; **50 mg:** Bot. 100s, 250s, 500s, UD 100s. *Rx.*
Use: Anxiolytic.

Atpeg. (Zeneca) Polyethylene glycol available as 300, 400, 600 or 4000.
Use: Humectant, surfacant.

•**atracurium besylate.** (AT-rah-CUE-ree-uhm BESS-ih-late) USAN.
Use: Neuromuscular blocker; muscle relaxant.
See: Tracrium (GlaxoWellcome).

Atragen. (Hannan Ophthalmic) Tretinoin.
Use: Antineoplastic. [Orphan drug]

Atretol. (Athena Neurosciences) Carbamazepine 200 mg, lactose/Tab. 100s. *Rx.*
Use: Antiepileptic.

Atridine. (Henry Schein) Triprolidine 2.5 mg, pseudoephedrine HCl 60 mg/Tab. Bot. 100s, 1000s. *otc.*
Use: Antihistamine, decongestant.

Atrocap. (Freeport) Atropine sulfate 0.06 mg, hyoscyamine sulfate 0.3 mg, hyoscine hydrobromide 0.02 mg, pheno-

barbital 50 mg/T.R. Cap. Bot. 1000s. *Rx.*
Use: Anticholinergic, antispasmodic, hypnotic, sedative.

Atrocholin Tablets. (GlaxoWellcome) Dehydrocholic acid 130 mg/Tab. Bot. 100s. *otc.*
Use: Laxative.

Atrofed. (Genetco) Pseudoephedrine HCl 60 mg, triprolidine HCl 2.5 mg. Tab. Bot. 24s, 100s, 1000s. *otc.*
Use: Antihistamine, decongestant.

Atrohist LA. (Adams Labs) Pseudoephedrine HCl 120 mg, brompheniramine maleate 4 mg, phenyltoloxamine citrate 50 mg/SR Tab with atropine sulfate 0.0242 mg available for immediate release. Bot. 100s. *Rx.*
Use: Antihistamine, decongestant.

Atrohist Pediatric Capsules. (Adams Labs) Chlorpheniramine maleate 4 mg, pseudoephedrine HCl 60 mg/SR Cap. Bot. 100s. *Rx.*
Use: Antihistamine, decongestant.

Atrohist Pediatric Suspension. (Adams Labs) Phenylephrine tannate 5 mg, chlorpheniramine tannate 2 mg, pyrilamine tannate 12.5 mg. Susp. Bot. 473 ml. Unit-of-use 118 ml. *Rx.*
Use: Antihistamine, decongestant.

Atrohist Plus Tablets. (Adams Labs) Phenylephrine HCl 25 mg, phenylpropanolamine HCl 50 mg, chlorpheniramine maleate 8 mg, hyoscyamine sulfate 0.19 mg, atropine sulfate 0.04 mg, scopolamine HBr 0.01 mg/SR Tab. Bot. 100s. *Rx.*
Use: Anticholinergic, antihistamine, decongestant.

Atrohist Sprinkle. (Adams Labs) Pseudoephedrine HCl 120 mg, brompheniramine maleate 2 mg, phenytoloxamine citrate 25 mg/SR Cap. Bot. 100s. *Rx.*
Use: Antihistamine, decongestant.

Atromid-S. (Wyeth Ayerst) Clofibrate 500 mg/Cap. Bot. 100s. *Rx.*
Use: Antihyperlipidemic.

AtroPen Auto-Injecter. (Survival Technology) Atropine sulfate, phenol 2 mg. In prefilled automatic injection device. *Rx.*
Use: Antidote, cholinergics.

•**atropine.** (AT-troe-peen) U.S.P. 23.
Use: Anticholinergic.

Atropine-1. (Optopics) Atropine sulfate 1% soln. Bot. 2, 5, 15 ml. *Rx.*
Use: Cycloplegic, mydriatic.

Atropine Care. (Akorn) Atropine sulfate 1%. Soln. Bot. 2 ml, 5 ml, 15 ml. *Rx.*
Use: Cycloplegic, mydriatic.

atropine and demerol injection. (Sanofi Winthrop) Atropine sulfate 0.4 mg, meperidine HCl 50 mg or 75 mg/Carpuject. *c-II.*
Use: Sedative.

atropine-hyoscine-hyoscyamine combinations. (See also Belladonna Products)
See: Barbella, Tab., Elix. (Forest Pharmaceutical).
Barbeloid, Tab. (Pal-Pak).
Bar-Don, Tab., Elix. (Warren-Teed).
Belakoids TT, Tab. (Roxane).
Belbutal No. 2 Kaptabs. (Churchill).
Brobella-P.B., Tab. (Brothers).
Buren, Tab. (B.F. Ascher).
Donnagel, Susp. (Robins).
Donnamine, Elix., Tab. (Tennessee Pharmaceutic).
Donnatal, Cap., Elix., Tab. (Robins).
Donnatal #2, Tab. (Robins).
Donnatal Extentabs, Tab. (Robins).
Donnazyme, Tab. (Robins).
Eldonal, Preps. (Canright).
Hyatal, Elix. (Winsale).
Hybephen, Preps. (SmithKline Beecham Pharmaceuticals).
Hyonal, Preps. (Paddock).
Hyonatol B, Preps. (Jones Medical Industries).
Hytrona, Tab. (PolyMedica).
Kinesed, Tab. (Zeneca).
Koryza, Tab. (Forest Pharmaceutical).
Maso-Donna, Elix., Tab. (Mason).
Nilspasm, Tab. (Parmed).
Sedamine, Tab. (Dunhall Pharmaceuticals).
Sedapar, Tab. (Parmed).
Seds, Tab. (Taylor Pharmaceuticals).
Spabelin, Elix. (Arcum).
Spasdel, Cap. (Marlop Pharm).
Spasmolin, Tab. (Bell).
Spasquid, Elix. (Geneva Pharm).
Urogesic, Tab. (Edwards Pharmaceuticals).

atropine methylnitrate. (Various Mfr.) dl-Hyoscyamine methylnitrate.
See: Harvatrate, Tab. (Forest Pharmaceutical).
W/Hyoscine HBr, hyoscyamine sulfate, amobarbital sodium.
See: Amocine, Tab. (Roberts Pharm).
W/Methenamine mandelate and phenylazo diamino pyridine HCl.
See: Uritral, Cap. (Schwarz Pharma).
W/Phenobarbital and dihydroxyaluminum aminoacetate.
See: Atromal, Tab. (Blaine).

Harvatrate A, Tab. (Forest Pharmaceutical).

atropine-n-oxide hydrochloride.
See: Atropine Oxide HCl.

•**atropine oxide hydrochloride.** (AT-row-peen OX-ide) USAN. Atropine N-oxide HCl.
Use: Anticholinergic.
See: X-Tro (Xttrium).

•**atropine sulfate.** (AT-row-peen) U.S.P. 23.
Use: Anticholinergic (ophthalmic).

atropine sulfate. (Various Mfr.) **Pediatric Inj.:** 0.05 mg/ml 5 ml Abboject. **Tab, Hypodermic:** 0.3 mg, 0.4 mg and 0.6 mg/Tab. Bot. 100s. **Tab, Oral:** 0.4 mg/Tab. Bot. 100s. **Inj.:** 0.1 mg/ml 5 ml and 10 ml Abboject 0.3 mg/ml. Vial 1 ml; 0.4 mg/ml. Amp. 1 ml, vial 20 ml; 0.8 mg/ml. Amp. 1 ml, dosette 0.5 ml; 1 mg/ml. Amp., vial 1 ml, syringe 10 ml; 1.2 mg/ml. Vial 1 ml syringe. **Lyophilized:** Lyopine (Hyrex). **Ophth. Oint:** 1%. Tube 3.5 g., UD 1 g. **Ophth. Soln:** 1%. Bot. UD 1 ml, 2 ml, 5 ml, 15 ml; 2%. Bot. 2 ml.
Use: Anticholinergic (ophthalmic).
See: Atropine-1, Soln., (Optopics).
Atropine Care, Soln., (Akorn).
Atropine Sulfate S.O.P., Oint., (Allergan).
Atropisol, Soln., (Ciba Vision Ophthalmics).
Isopto-Atropine (Alcon Laboratories).
Lyopine, Inj. (Hyrex).
Parasympatholytic and antispasmodic.
Sal-Tropine, Tab. (Hope Pharm).
W/Ephedrine sulfate.
See: Enuretrol, Tab. (Berlex).

atropine sulfate/edrophonium chloride. Anticholinesterase muscle stimulant.
See: Enlon-Plus (Ohmeda Pharmaceuticals).

atropine sulfate and meperidine hcl.
See: Atropine and Demerol. (Sanofi Winthrop).

atropine sulfate and morphine sulfate.
See: Morphine and Atropine Sulfates. (SmithKline Beecham Pharmaceuticals).

atropine sulfate S.O.P. (Allergan) 0.5%, 1%. Oint. Tube 3.5 g. *Rx.*
Use: Cycloplegic, mydriatic.

atropine sulfate combinations.
See: Bellatal, Tab. (Richwood).

atropine sulfate w/phenobarbital.
See: Antrocol, Tab., Cap. (ECR Pharmaceuticals).
Arco-Lase Plus, Tab. (Arco).
Barbeloid, Tab. (Pal-Pak).
Briabell, Tab. (Briar).
Brobella-P.B., Tab. (Brothers).
Donnatal, Cap., Extentab, Tab., Elix. (Robins).
Donnatal #2, Tab. (Robins).
Hyatal Elix. (Winsale).
Palbar No. 2, Tab. (Roberts Pharm).
Seds, Tab. (Taylor Pharmaceuticals).
Spabelin, Elix. (Arcum).
Spasdel, Cap. (Marlop Pharm).
Stannitol (Standex).

Atropisol. (Ciba Vision Ophthalmics) Atropine sulfate 1%. Soln. Dropperette 1 ml. *Rx.*
Use: Cycloplegic, mydriatic.

Atrosed. (Freeport) Atropine sulfate 0.0195 mg, hyoscine HBr 0.0065 mg, hyoscyamine sulfate 0.104 mg, phenobarbital 0.25 gr/Tab. Bot. 1000s, 5000s. *Rx.*
Use: Anticholinergic, antispasmodic, hypnotic, sedative.

Atrosept. (Geneva Pharm) Methenamine 40.8 mg, phenyl salicylate 18.1 mg, atropine sulfate 0.03 mg, hyoscyamine 0.03 mg, benzoic acid 4.5 mg, methylene blue 5.4 mg/Tab. Bot. 100s, 1000s. *Rx.*
Use: Anti-infective, urinary.

Atrovent. (Boehringer Ingelheim) Ipratropium bromide. **Aerosol:** 18 mcg/dose. 14 g; **Soln.:** 0.02% (500 mg/vial) 25s. **Spray:** 0.03% in 30 ml vials; 0.06% in 15 ml vials. *Rx.*
Use: Bronchodilator.

A/T/S. (Hoechst Marion Roussel) Erythromycin 2%. Gel. Tube 30 g. *Rx.*
Use: Dermatologic, acne.

A/T/S Topical Solution. (Hoechst Marion Roussel) Erythromycin 2% topical soln. Bot. 60 ml. *Rx.*
Use: Dermatologic, acne.

AT-Solution. (Sanofi Winthrop) Dihydrotachysterol solution.
Use: Antihypocalcemic.

Attain Liquid. (Sherwood Medical). Sodium caseinate, calcium caseinate, maltodextrin, corn oil, soy lecithin. Can 250 ml and 1000 ml closed system. *otc.*
Use: Nutritional supplement.

•**attapulgite, activated.** (at-ah-PULL-gyte) U.S.P. 23.
Use: Antidiarrheal; pharmaceutic aid (suspending agent).
W/Pectin, hydrated alumina powder.
See: Polymagma Plain Tab. (Wyeth Ayerst).

W/Polysorbate 80, salicylic acid, propylene glycol.
See: Sebasorb Lot. (Summer).

Attenuvax. (Merck) Measles virus vaccine, live, attenuated w/neomycin 25 mcg/Vial. Single-dose vial w/diluent. Pkg. 1s, 10s. *Rx.*
Use: Immunization.
W/Meruvax.
See: M-R-Vax-II, Vial (Merck).
W/Mumpsvax, Meruvax.
See: M-M-R II, Vial (Merck).

Atuss DM. (Atley Pharmaceuticals) Dextromethorphan 15 mg, phenylephrine HCl 5 mg, chlorpheniramine maleate 2 mg, sucrose, saccharin, menthol, methylparaben, strawberry flavor/Syr. Bot. 480 ml. *Rx.*
Use: Antihistamine, antitussive, decongestant.

Atuss EX. (Atley Pharmaceuticals) Hydrocodone bitartrate 5 mg, guaifenesin 100 mg, parabens, menthol, saccarhin, sorbitol, cherry flavor/Syr. Bot. 473 ml. *c-III.*
Use: Expectorant, narcotic.

Atuss G. (Atley Pharmaceuticals) Hydrocodone bitartrate 2 mg, phenylephrine HCl 10 mg, guaifenesin 100 mg, sucrose, saccarhin, grape flavor/Syr. Bot. 480 ml. *c-III.*
Use: Narcotic decongestant expectorant.

Atuss HD. (Atley Pharmaceuticals) Hydrocodone bitartrate 2.5 mg, phenylephrine HCl 5 mg, chlorpheniramine maleate 2mg/5ml. Menthol, sucrose, alcohol, cherry flavor. Liq. Bot. 480 ml. *Rx.*
Use: Antihistamine, antitussive, decongestant.

Augmented Betamethasone Dipropionate.
Use: Corticosteroid, topical.
See: Diprolene (Schering Plough).

Augmentin Chewable Tablets. (SmithKline Beecham Pharmaceuticals) **125:** Amoxicillin 125 mg, clavulanic acid 31.25 mg, saccharin/Tab. Ctn. 30s. **250:** Amoxicillin 250 mg, clavulanic acid 62.5 mg, saccharin/Tab. Ctn. 30s. *Rx.*
Use: Anti-infective, penicillin.

Augmentin Oral Suspension. (SmithKline Beecham Pharmaceuticals) **125:** Amoxicillin 125 mg, clavulanic acid (as potassium salt) 31.25 mg/5 ml. Bot. 75 ml, 150 ml. **200:** Amoxicillin 200 mg, clavulanic acid/5ml. Mannitol, aspartame/Pow. Bot. 50 ml, 75 ml, 100 ml. **250:** Amoxicillin 250 mg, clavulanic acid (as potassium salt) 62.5 mg/5 ml. Bot. 75 ml, 150 ml. **400:** Amoxicillin 400 mg, clavulanic acid 28.5 mg/5ml. Mannitol, aspartame/Pow. Bot. 50 ml, 75 ml, and 100 ml. *Rx.*
Use: Anti-infective, penicillin.

Augmentin Tablets. (SmithKline Beecham Pharmaceuticals) Amoxicillin trihydrate 250 mg, 500 mg or 850 mg, clavulanic acid (as potassium salt) 125 mg/Tab. **250:** Bot. 30s, UD 100s. **500:** Bot. 30s, 100s. **850:** 20s, UD 100s. *Rx.*
Use: Anti-infective, penicillin.

Auralgan Otic Solution. (Wyeth Ayerst) Antipyrine 54 mg, benzocaine 14 mg/ml w/oxyquinoline sulfate in dehydrated glycerin (contains not more than 0.6% moisture). Bot. Dropper 15 ml. *Rx.*
Use: Otic.

Auralgesic. (Wesley Pharmacal) Carbamide 10%, antipyrine 5%, benzocaine 2.5%, cetyldimethylbenzylammonium HCl 0.2%. Bot. 0.5 oz. *Rx.*
Use: Otic.

•**auranofin.** (or-RAIN-oh-fin) USAN.
Use: Antirheumatic.
See: Ridaura, Cap. (SmithKline Beecham Pharmaceuticals).

aureomycin preparations. (Storz Ophthalmics) Chlortetracycline HCl. **Ophth. Oint.:** 1% (10 mg/g) Tube 0.125 oz. **Topical Oint.:** 3% (30 mg/g) in white petrolatum, anhydrous lanolin base. Tube 0.5 oz, 1 oz. *Rx.*
Use: Anti-infective.

Aureoquin Diamate. Name previously used for Quinetolate.

Auriculin. (Scios) Anaritide acetate.
Use: Improvement of early renal allograft function following renal transplantation; acute renal failure.

Aurinol Ear Drops. (Various Mfr.) Chloroxylenol and acetic acid, w/benzalkonium chloride and glycerin. Soln. Bot. 15 ml. *Rx.*
Use: Otic.

Aurocein. (Christina) Gold naphthyl sulfhydryl derivative. 5% or 12.5% Amp. 10 ml. *Rx.*
Use: Antirheumatic.

Auro-Dri. (Del Pharmaceuticals) Boric acid 2.75% in isopropyl alcohol. Bot. oz. *otc.*
Use: Otic.

Auro Ear Drops. (Del Pharmaceuticals) Carbamide peroxide 6.5% in a specially prepared base. Bot. 15 ml. *otc.*
Use: Otic.

Aurolate. (Taylor Pharmaceuticals) Gold

sodium thiomalate 50 mg, benzyl alcohol 0.5%/ml. Inj. Vial 2 ml, 10 ml. *Rx.*
Use: Antirheumatic.

aurolin.
See: Gold sodium thiosulfate.

auropin.
See: Gold sodium thiosulfate.

aurosan.
See: Gold sodium thiosulfate.

aurothioblycanide.
Use: Antirheumatic.

•**aurothioglucose.** (or-oh-THIGH-oh-GLUE-kose) U.S.P. 23.
Use: Antirheumatic.

aurothioglucose injection.
See: Sterile aurothioglucose suspension.

aurothiomalate, sodium.
See: Gold Sodium Thiomalate, U.S.P. 23.

Auroto Otic. (Alphalma USPD) Benzocaine 1.4%, antipyrine 5.4%, glycerin and oxyquinoline sulfate/Soln. Bot. 15 ml w/dropper. *Rx.*
Use: Otic preparation.

Ausab. (Abbott Diagnostics) Radioimmunoassay or enzyme immunoassay for detection of antibody to hepatitis B surface antigen. Test kit 100s.
Use: Diagnostic aid.

Ausab EIA. (Abbott Diagnostics) Enzyme immunoassay for the detection of antibody to hepatitis B surface antigen.
Use: Diagnostic aid.

Auscell. (Abbott Diagnostics) Reverse passive hemagglutination test for hepatitis B surface antigen. Test kit 110s, 450s, 1800s.
Use: Diagnostic aid.

Ausria II-125. (Abbott Diagnostics) Radioimmunoassay for detection of hepatitis B surface antigen. Test kit 100s, 500s, 600s, 700s, 800s, 900s, 1000s.
Use: Diagnostic aid.

Auszyme II. (Abbott Diagnostics) Enzyme immunoassay for detection of hepatitis B surface antigen (HBsAg) in human serum or plasma. Test kit 100s, 500s.
Use: Diagnostic aid.

Auszyme Monoclonal. (Abbott Diagnostics) Qualitative third generation enzyme immunoassay for the detection of hepatitis B surface antigen (HBsAg) in human serum or plasma.
Use: Diagnostic aid.

Autoantibody Screen. (Wampole Laboratories) Autoantibody screening system. To screen serum for the presence of a variety of autoantibodies. Test 48s.
Use: Diagnostic aid.

Autolet Kit. (Bayer Corp) Automatic blood letting spring-loaded device to obtain capillary blood samples from fingertips, earlobes or heels.
Use: Diagnostic aid.

autolymphocyte therapy; ALT. (Cellcor)
Use: Treatment of renal cancer. [Orphan drug]

Autoplex. (Baxter) Anti-inhibitor coagulant complex prepared from pooled human plasma. Vial 30 ml.
Use: Diagnostic aid.

Autoplex T. (Baxter) Dried anti-inhibitor coagulant complex. With a maximum of heparin 2 units and polyethylene glycol 2 mg per ml reconstituted material. Inj. Vial with diluent and needles. *Rx.*
Use: Diagnostic aid.

Autrinic. Intrinsic factor concentrate. *Rx.*
Use: To increase absorption of Vitamin B_{12}.

Auxotab Enteric 1 & 2. (Colab) Rapid identification of enteric bacteria and *pseudomonas.* Test contains capillary units with selective biochemical reagents.
Use: Diagnostic aid.

Avail. (Menley & James) Iron 18 mg, vitamin A 5000 IU, D 400 IU, E 30 mg, B_1 2.25 mg, B_2 2.55 mg, B_3 20 mg, B_6 3 mg, B_{12} 9 mcg, C 90 mg, folic acid 0.4 mg, Ca, Cr, I, Mg, Se and zinc 22.5 mg/Tab. Bot. 60s. *otc.*
Use: Mineral, vitamin supplement.

Avalgesic Lotion. (Various Mfr.) Methyl salicylate, menthol, camphor, methyl nicotinate, dipropylene glycol salicylate, oil of cassia, oleoresins capsicum and ginger. Bot. 120 ml, pt, gal. *otc.*
Use: Analgesic, topical.

A-Van. (Stewart-Jackson) Dimenhydrinate 50 mg/Cap. Bot. 100s.
Use: Antivertigo.

Avapro. (Sanofi Winthrop) Irbesartan 75 mg, 150 mg, 300 mg, lactose/Tab. Bot. 30s, 90s, 500s, blister 100s. *Rx.*
Use: Antihypertensive.

AVC Cream. (Hoechst Marion Roussel) Sulfanilamide 15% in a water-miscible base of propylene glycol, stearic acid, diglycol stearate to acid pH. Tube 4 oz. w/applicator. *Rx.*
Use: Anti-infective, vaginal.

AVC Suppositories. (Hoechst Marion Roussel) Sulfanilamide 1.05 g in a base made from polyethylene glycol

400, polysorbate 80, polyethylene glycol 3350, glycerin, inert glycerin-gelatin covering. Box 16s w/inserter. *Rx.*
Use: Anti-infective, vaginal.

Aveeno Anti-Itch. (Rydelle) Calamine 3%, pramoxine HCl, camphor 0.3% in a base of glycerin, distearyldimonium chloride, petrolatum, oatmeal flour, isopropyl palmitate, cetyl alcohol, dimethicone and sodium chloride. Cream 30 g, Lotion 120 ml. *otc.*
Use: Antipruritic.

Aveenobar Medicated. (Rydelle) Aveeno colloidal oatmeal 50%, sulfur 2%, salicylic acid 2%, in soap-free cleansing bar. Formerly Acnaveen. Bar 3.5 oz. *otc.*
Use: Antipruritic.

Aveenobar Oilated. (Rydelle) Vegetable oils, lanolin derivative, glycerine 29%, aveeno colloidal oatmeal 30% in soap-free base. Formerly Emulave. Bar. 3 oz. *otc.*
Use: Emollient.

Aveenobar Regular. (Rydelle) Colloidal oatmeal 50%, anionic sulfonate, hypoallergenic lanolin. Formerly Aveeno Bar. Bar 3.2 oz, 4.4 oz. *otc.*
Use: Dermatologic, cleanser.

Aveeno Bath. (Rydelle) Colloidal oatmeal. Box 1 lb, 4 lb. *otc.*
Use: Emollient.

Aveeno Cleansing for Acne Prone Skin. (Rydelle) Sulfur 2%, salicylic acid 2%, colloidal oatmeal 50%, glycerin, titanium dioxide. Soap Bar 90 g. *otc.*
Use: Antiacne.

Aveeno Cleansing Bar. (Rydelle) **Combination Skin:** Soap free. Colloidal outmeal 51%, sodium cocoyl isethionate, glycerin, lactic acid, sodium lactate, petrolatum, magnesium aluminum silicate, potassium sorbate, titanium dioxide, PEG 14M. Bar 90 g. **Dry Skin:** Soap free. Colloidal oatmeal 51%, sodium cocoyl isethionate, vegetable oil and shortening, glycerin, PEG-75, lauramide DEA, lactic acid, sodium lactate, sorbic acid, titanium dioxide. Bar 90 g. *otc.*
Use: Dermatologic, cleanser.

Aveeno Colloidal Oatmeal. (Rydelle) Colloidal oatmeal. Box 1 lb, 4 lb. *otc.*
Use: Emollient.

Aveeno Dry. (Rydelle) Dry skin formula, soap free, emollient colloidal oatmeal, vegetable oils, lanolin derivative and glycerin 29% in mild surfactant base. Cleansing bar 90 g. *otc.*
Use: Dermatologic, cleanser.

Aveeno Lotion. (Rydelle) Colloidal oatmeal 1%. Glycerin, petrolatum, dimethicone, phenylcarbinol. 240 ml. *otc.*
Use: Emollient.

Aveeno Moisturizing Cream. (Rydelle) Colloidal oatmeal, glycerin, petrolatum, dimethicone, phenylcarbinol. Cream Tube 120 g. *otc.*
Use: Emollient.

Aveeno Normal. (Rydelle) Normal to oily skin formula, soap free. Colloidal oatmeal 50%, lanolin derivative and mild surfactant. Cleansing bar 96 g, 132 g. *otc.*
Use: Dermatologic, cleanser.

Aveeno Oilated. (Rydelle) Aveeno colloidal oatmeal impregnated with 35% liquid petrolatum, refined olive oil. Box 8 oz, 2 lb. *otc.*
Use: Emollient.

Aveeno Shave. (Rydelle) Oatmeal flour. Gel. Can 210 g. *otc.*
Use: Emollient.

Aveeno Shower & Bath. (Rydelle) Colloidal oatmeal, 5% mineral oil, glyceryl stearate, PEG 100 stearate, laureth-4, benzyl alcohol, silica benzaldehyde. Oil. Bot. 240 ml. *otc.*
Use: Emollient.

Aventyl Hydrochloride. (Eli Lilly) Nortriptyline HCl. **Liq.:** Equivalent to 10 mg base/5 ml in alcohol 4%. Bot. 16 fl. oz. **Pulv.:** Equivalent to 10 mg base or 25 mg base/Cap. Bot. 100s, 500s, Blisterpak 10 × 10s. *Rx.*
Use: Antidepressant.

Avertin. Tribromoethanol (Various Mfr.).

•**avilamycin.** (ah-VILL-ah-MY-sin) USAN.
Use: Anti-infective.

Avinar. Uredepa.
Use: Antineoplastic.

Avita. (DPT) Tretinoin 0.025%. Cream 20, 45 g. *Rx.*
Use: Dermatologic, acne.

Avitene Hemostat. (Med Chem) Hydrochloric acid salt of purified bovine corium collagen. **Fibrous Form:** Jar 1 g, 5 g. **Web Form:** Blister Pak. Sheets of 70 mm × 70 mm, 70 mm × 35 mm, 35 mm × 35 mm. *Rx.*
Use: Hemostatic, topical.

•**avitriptan fumarate.** (av-ih-TRIP-tan FEW-mah-rate) USAN.
Use: Antimigraine.

•**avobenzone.** (AV-ah-BENZ-ohn) USAN.
Use: Sunscreen.

avobenzone w/combinations. (AV-ah-BENZ-ohn)
See: PreSun Ultra, Lot., Clear Gel

(Westwood Squibb).

Avonex. (Biogen) Interferon Beta-1a 33 mcg (6.6 million IU) albumin human 15 mg, sodium chloride and sodium phosphates. Pow. for inj. Vials. Single-use vial w/ 10 ml vial of diluent, swabs, syringe, access pin, needle and bandage. *Rx.*
Use: Multiple sclerosis agent, hepatitis, brain tumor. [Orphan drug]

Avonique. (Armenpharm) Vitamins A 4000 IU, D 400 IU, B_1 1 mg, B_2 1.2 mg, B_6 2 mg, B_{12} 2 mcg, calcium pantothenate 5 mg, B_3 10 mg, C 30 mg, calcium 100 mg, phosphorous 76 mg, iron 10 mg, manganese 1 mg, magnesium 1 mg, zinc 1 mg. *otc.*
Use: Mineral, vitamin supplement.

•**avoparcin.** (AVE-oh-PAR-sin) USAN.
Use: Anti-infective.

•**avridine.** (AV-rih-deen) USAN.
Use: Antiviral.

Awake. (Walgreens) Caffeine 100 mg/Tab. Bot. 36s. *otc.*
Use: CNS stimulant.

axerophthol.
See: Vitamin A.

Axid. (Eli Lilly) Nizatidine 150 mg or 300 mg/Cap. Bot. 30s, 60s. *Rx.*
Use: H_2 antagonist.

Axid AR. (Whitehall Robins) Nizatidine 75 mg/Tab. Bot. 6s, 12s, 18s, 30s. *otc.*
Use: Gastrointestinal.

Axocet. (Savage) Butalbital 50 mg, acetaminophen 650 mg, parabens/Cap. Bot. 100s. *Rx.*
Use: Analgesic, hypnotic, sedative.

Axsain.
See: Zostrix (GenDerm).

Ayds Appetite Suppressant Candy. (DEP) Benzocaine 5 mg in chewy candy base w/25 cal./Cube. Ctn. 12s, 48s, 96s. *otc.*
Use: Dietary aid.

Aygestin. (ESI Lederle) Norethindrone acetate 5 mg, lactose/Tab. Bot. 50s. *Rx.*
Use: Hormone, progestin.

Ayr Saline Nasal Drops. (B.F. Ascher) Sodium Cl 0.65% adjusted with phosphate buffers to proper tonicity and pH to prevent nasal irritation. **Drops:** Bot. 20 ml. **Mist:** Bot. 50 ml. *otc.*
Use: Dermatologic, moisturizer.

•**azabon.** (AZE-ah-bahn) USAN.
Use: CNS stimulant.

•**azacitidine.** (AZE-ah-SIGH-tih-deen) USAN. *Formerly Ladakamycin.*
Use: Antineoplastic.

•**azaclorzine hydrochloride.** (AZE-ah-KLOR-zeen) USAN. *Formerly Nonachlazine.*
Use: Coronary vasodilator.

•**azaconazole.** (AZE-ah-CONE-ah-zole) USAN. *Formerly Azoconazole.*
Use: Antifungal.

AZA-CR. NCI Investigational agent.
See: Azacitidine.

Azactam for Injection. (Bristol-Myers Squibb) L-arginine 780 mg/g aztreonam. **Single dose 15 ml vial:** 500 mg/Vial Pkg. 10s, 25s. 1 g/Vial Pkg. 10s, 25s. 2 g/vial Pkg. 10s, 25s. **Single dose 100 ml IV infusion bottle w/ball bands:** 500 mg/Bot. Pkg. 10s. 1 g/vial Pkg. 10s. 2 g/vial Pkg. 10s. *Rx.*
Use: Anti-infective.

azacyclonol hydrochloride.

5-aza-2 deoxycytidine.
Use: Treatment of acute leukemia.

•**azalanstat dihydrochloride.** (aze-ah-LAN-stat die-HIGH-droe-KLOR-ide) USAN.
Use: Hypolipidemic.

Azaline Tabs. (Major) Sulfasalazine 500 mg/Tab. Bot. 100s, 500s, 1000s.
Use: Anti-inflammatory.

•**azaloxan fumarate.** (aze-ah-LOX-ahn) USAN.
Use: Antidepressant.

azamethonium bromide. (Novartis) *Rx.*
Use: Ganglionic blocking.

•**azanator maleate.** (AZE-an-nay-tore) USAN.
Use: Bronchodilator.

•**azanidazole.** (AZE-ah-NIH-dah-zole) USAN.
Use: Antiprotozoal.

•**azaperone.** (AZE-app-eh-RONE) U.S.P. 23.
Use: Antipsychotic.

azapetine phosphate.

•**azaribine.** (aze-ah-RYE-bean) USAN.
Use: Dermatologic.

•**azarole.** (AZE-ah-role) USAN.
Use: Immunoregulator.

•**azaserine.** (AZE-ah-SER-een) USAN.
Use: Antifungal.

•**azatadine maleate.** (aze-AT-ad-EEN) U.S.P. 23.
Use: Antihistamine.
See: Optimine, Tab. (Key).
Trinalin, Tab. (Schering Plough).

•**azathioprine.** (AZE-uh-THIGH-oh-preen) U.S.P. 23.
Use: Immunosuppressant.
See: Imuran, Inj. Tab. (Glaxo-Wellcome).

•**azathioprine sodium for injection.** (AZE-uh-THIGH-oh-preen) U.S.P. 23.
Use: Immunosuppressant.

azathioprine sodium. (Bedford Labs) Pow. for Inj. 100 mg. Vial. 20 ml. *Rx.*
Use: Antileukemic.

5-azc.
See: Azacitidine.

Azdone. (Schwarz Pharma) Hydrocodone bitartrate 5 mg, aspirin 500 mg/Tab. Bot. 100s, 1000s. *c-III.*
Use: Analgesic combination, narcotic.

•**azelaic acid.** (aze-eh-LAY-ik) USAN.
Use: Dermatologic, acne.
See: Azelex, cream. (Allergan).

•**azelastine hydrochloride.** (ah-ZELL-ass-teen) USAN.
Use: Antiallergic, antiasthmatic.
See: Astelin, Nasal Spray (Wallace Laboratories).

Azelex. (Allergan) Azelaic acid 20%, glycerin, cetearyl, alcohol, benzoic acid. Cream 30 g. *Rx.*
Use: Dermatologic, acne.

•**azepindole.** (AZE-eh-PIN-dole) USAN.
Use: Antidepressant.

•**azetepa.** (AZE-eh-teh-pah) USAN.
Use: Antineoplastic.

•**3-azido-2, 3 dideoxyuridine.** USAN.
Use: Antiviral, HIV.

azidothymidine.
See: Zidovudine.

Azidouridine. (Berlex) Phase I HIV positive symptomatic, ARC, AIDS. *Rx.*
Use: Antiviral.

•**azimilide dihydrochloride.** (azz-IM-ih-lide die-HIGH-droe-KLOR-ide) USAN.
Use: Cardiovascular agent.

•**azipramine hydrochloride.** (aze-IPP-RAH-meen) USAN.
Use: Antidepressant.

•**azithromycin.** (UHZ-ith-row-MY-sin) U.S.P. 23.
Use: Anti-infective.
See: Zithromax, Tab., Pow. for Inj., Pow. for Oral Susp. (Pfizer).

Azlin. (Bayer Corp) Azlocillin sodium. Vial 2 g, 3 g, 4 g.
Use: Anti-infective, penicillin.

•**azlocillin.** (AZZ-low-SILL-in) USAN.
Use: Anti-infective.
See: Azlin, Inj. (Bayer Corp).

•**azlocillin sodium.** (AZZ-low-SILL-in) U.S.P. 23.
Use: Anti-infective.

Azma-Aid. (Purepac) Theophylline 118 mg, ephedrine 24 mg, phenobarbital 8 mg/Tab. Bot. 100s, 250s, 1000s. *Rx.*
Use: Bronchodilator.

Azmacort. (Rhone-Poulenc Rorer) Triamcinolone acetonide in an inhaler system ≈ 100 mcg/actuation. Canister 20 g, 240 metered doses. *Rx.*
Use: Corticosteroid.

AZO-100. (Scruggs) Phenylazodiaminopyridine HCl 100 mg/Tab. Bot. 100s, 1000s. *otc.*
Use: Analgesic, urinary.

azoconazole.
Use: Antifungal.

Azodyne.
W/Sulfadiazine, sulfamethizole

Azodyne Hydrochloride.
See: Pyridium, Tab. (Parke-Davis).

•**azolimine.** (aze-OLE-ih-meen) USAN.
Use: Diuretic.

AZO Negacide Tablets. (Sanofi Winthrop) Nalidixic acid, phenazopyridine HCl. *Rx.*
Use: Anti-infective, urinary.

Azopt. (Alcon) Brinzolamide 1%/Ophth. Susp. 2.5 ml, 5 ml, 10 ml, 15 ml. *Rx.*
Use: Glaucoma treatment.

•**azosemide.** (AZE-oh-SEH-mide) USAN.
Use: Diuretic.

AZO-Standard. (PolyMedica) Phenazopyridine HCl 100 mg/Tab. Bot. 360s. *otc.*
Use: Analgesic, urinary.

Azostix Reagent Strips. (Bayer Corp) Bromthymol blue, urease, buffers. Colorimetric test for blood urea nitrogen level. Bot 25 strips.
Use: Diagnostic aid.

azo-sulfisoxazole. (Various Mfr.) Sulfisoxazole 500 mg, phenazopyridine HCl 50 mg/Tab. Bot. 100s, 1000s. *Rx.*
Use: Anti-infective, urinary.

•**azotomycin.** (aze-OH-toe-MY-sin) USAN. Antibiotic isolated from broth filtrates of *Streptomyces ambofaciens.*
Use: Antineoplastic.

Azovan Blue.
See: Evans Blue Dye, Amp. (City Chemical; Harvey).

AZO Wintomylon. (Sanofi Winthrop) Nalidixic acid, phenazopyridine HCl. *Rx.*
Use: Anti-infective, urinary.

AZT.
See: Zidovudine.

AZT-P-ddi. (Baker Norton) Phase I AIDS.
Use: Antiviral.

•**aztreonam.** (AZZ-TREE-oh-nam) U.S.P. 23.
Use: Antimicrobial.
See: Azactam, Vial (Bristol-Myers Squibb).

Azulfidine. (Pharmacia & Upjohn) Sulfasalazine. 500 mg/Tab. Bot. 100s, 300s, UD 100s. *Rx.*
Use: Anti-inflammatory.

Azulfidine EN-tabs. (Pharmacia & Upjohn) Sulfasalazine. Enteric coated. 500 mg/Tab. Bot. 100s, 300s. *Rx.*
Use: Anti-inflammatory.

•**azumolene sodium.** (AH-ZUH-moe-leen) USAN.
Use: Muscle relaxant.

B

B_1. Thiamine HCl.

B_2. Riboflavin.

B_3. Niacin, nicotinamide.

B_5. Calcium pantothenate.

B_6. Pyridoxine HCl.

B_6 50. (Western Research) Vitamin B_6 50 mg/Tab. Bot. 1000s. *otc.*
Use: Vitamin supplement.

B_{12}. Cyanocobalamin. *otc.*

B-50. (NBTY) Vitamins B_1 50 mg, B_2 50 mg, B_3 50 mg, B_5 50 mg, B_6 50 mg, B_{12} 50 mcg, folic acid 0.1 mg, d-biotin 50 mcg, PABA, choline bitartrate, inositol/Tab. Bot. 50s, 100s. *otc.*
Use: Mineral, vitamin supplement.

B-50 Time Release. (NBTY) Vitamins B_1 50 mg, B_2 50 mg, B_3 50 mg, B_5 50 mg, B_6 50 mg, B_{12} 50 mcg, folic acid 0.1 mg, d-biotin 50 mcg, PABA 50 mg, choline bitartrate 50 mg, inositol 50 mg, lecithin/Tab. Bot. 100s. *otc.*
Use: Mineral, vitamin supplement.

B 100. (Fibertone) B_1 100 mg, B_2 100 mg, B_3 100 mg, B_5 100 mg, B_6 100 mg, B_{12} 100 mcg, FA 0.4 mg, biotin 50 mcg, PABA 100 mg, choline bitartrate 100 mg, inositol 100 mg/ SR Tab. Bot. 100s. *otc.*
Use: Vitamin supplement.

B-100. (NBTY) Vitamins B_1 100 mg, B_2 100 mg, B_3 100 mg, B_5 100 mg, B_6 100 mg, B_{12} 100 mcg, folic acid 0.1 mg, d-biotin 100 mcg, PABA 100 mg, choline bitartrate, inositol, lecithin. Tab. Bot. 50s, 100s. *otc.*
Use: Mineral, vitamin supplement.

B125. (NBTY) Vitamins B_1 125 mg, B_2 125 mg, B_3 125 mg, B_5 125 mg, B_6 125 mg, B_{12} 125 mcg, folic acid 0.1 mg, d-biotin 125 mcg, PABA 125 mg, choline bitartrate 125 mg, inositol 125 mg, lecithin. Tab. Bot. 100s. *otc.*
Use: Mineral, vitamin supplement.

B150. (NBTY) Vitamins B_1 150 mg, B_2 150 mg, B_3 150 mg, B_5 150 mg, B_6 150 mg, B_{12} 150 mcg, folic acid 0.1 mg, d-biotin 150 mcg, PABA 150 mg, choline bitartrate 150 mg, inositol 150 mg, lecithin. Tab. Bot. 100s. *otc.*
Use: Mineral, vitamin supplement.

B & A. (Eastern Research) Sodium bicarbonate, potassium, aluminum, borax. Hygienic pow. Jar. 8 oz, 5 lb. *Rx.*
Use: Vaginal agent.

B.A. Gradual. (Federal) Theophylline 260 mg, pseudoephedrine HCl 50 mg, butabarbital 15 mg/Gradual. Bot. 50s, 1000s. *Rx.*
Use: Bronchodilator, decongestant, hypnotic, sedative.

Babee Teething. (Pfeiffer) Benzocaine 2.5%, cetalkonium Cl 0.02%, alcohol, eucolyptol, menthol, camphor. Soln. Bot. 15 ml. *otc.*
Use: Anesthetic, local.

Baby Anbesol. (Whitehall Robins) Benzocaine 7.5%, saccharin. Gel Tube 7.2 g. *otc.*
Use: Mouth and throat preparation.

Baby Cough Syrup. (Towne) Ammonium Cl 300 mg, sodium citrate 600 mg/oz w/citric acid. Bot. 4 oz.
Use: Antitussive.

Baby Orajel. (Del Pharmaceuticals) Benzocaine 7.5%, saccharin, sorbitol, alcohol free. Gel. Tube 9.45 g. *otc.*
Use: Mouth and throat preparation.

Baby Orajel Nighttime Formula. (Del Pharmaceuticals) Benzocaine 10%, saccharin, sorbitol, alcohol free. Gel. Tube 6 g. *otc.*
Use: Mouth and throat preparation.

Baby Oragel Teeth & Gum Cleanser. (Del Pharmaceuticals) Poloxamer 407 2%, simethicone 0.12%, parabens, saccharin, sorbitol. Gel Tube 14.2 g. *otc.*
Use: Mouth and throat preparation.

Baby Vitamin Drops. (Zenith Goldline) Vitamins A 1500 IU, D 400 IU, E 5 IU, B_1 0.5 mg, B_2 0.6 mg, B_3 8 mg, B_6 0.4 mg, B_{12} 2 mcg, C 35 mg/ml/ Drop. Bot. 50 ml. *otc.*
Use: Vitamin supplement.

Baby Vitamin Drops with Iron. (Zenith Goldline) Iron 10 mg, vitamins A 1500 IU, D 400 IU, E 5 IU, B_1 0.5 mg, B_2 0.6 mg, B_3 8 mg, B_6 0.4 mg, C 35 mg/ml/ Bot. 50 ml. *otc.*
Use: Mineral, vitamin supplement.

BAC. Benzalkonium Cl.

•**bacampicillin HCl.** (BACK-am-PIH-sill-in) U.S.P. 23.
Use: Anti-infective.
See: Spectrobid (Roerig). B-C Bid. [NAME] [/NAME](Roberts Pharm) Vitamins C 300 mg, B_1 15 mg, B_2 10.2 mg, B_3 50 mg, B_6 5 mg, B[SUB]5[/Sub] 10 mg/Caplets. Bot. 100s.*otc.*
Use: Vitamin supplement.

Bacco-Resist. (Vita Elixir) Lobeline sulfate 1/64 gr.
Use: Smoking deterrent.

Bacid. (Novartis Nutrition) A specially cultured strain of human *Lactobacillus acidophilus*, sodium carboxymethylcellulose 100 mg, sodium 0.5 mEq/Cap. Bot. 50s, 100s. *otc.*

Use: Antidiarrheal, nutritional supplement.

Baciguent Antibiotic Ointment. (Pharmacia & Upjohn) Bacitracin 500 units/g. Oint. Tube 0.5 oz, 1 oz, 4 oz. *otc.*
Use: Anti-infective, topical.

Bacillus Calmette-Guerin.
See: BCG Vaccine.

bacitracin. (Various Mfr.). An antibiotic produced by a strain of *Bacillus subtilis.*
Diagnostic Tabs. Oint., Ophthalmic Oint. 500 units/Gm. Tube 3.5 g, 3.75 g.
Soluble Tab., Systemic Use, Vial., Topical Use, Vial., Troche. Vaginal Tab.
Use: Anti-infective. [Orphan drug]

•**bacitracin.** (bass-ih-TRAY-sin) U.S.P. 23.
Use: Anti-infective.
See: AK-Tracin, Oint. (Akorn).
Altracin (AL Labs).
Baciguent, Oint. (Pharmacia & Upjohn).
W/Neomycin sulfate.
See: Bacimycin, Oint. (Hoechst Marion Roussel).
Bacitracin-Neomycin, Oint., Ophth. Oint. (Various Mfr.).
W/Neomycin, polymyxin B sulfate.
See: Baximin, Oint. (Quality Generics).
BPN Ointment (Procter & Gamble).
Mycitracin, Oint., Ophth. Oint. (Pharmacia & Upjohn).
Neosporin, Oint., Ophth. Oint., Aerosol, Pow. (GlaxoWellcome).
Neo-Thrycex, Oint. (Del Pharmaceuticals).
Tigo, Oint. (Burlington).
Tri-Biotic Oint. (Burgin-Arden).
Tri-Biotic, Oint. (Standex).
Tri-Bow Oint. (Jones Medical Industries).
Triple Antibiotic Oint. (Towne).
W/Neomycin sulfate, polymyxin B sulfate, diperodon HCl.
See: Epimycin A, Oint. (Delta).
Mity-Mycin, Oint. (Solvay).
W/Neomycin sulfate, polymyxin B sulfate, hydrocortisone acetate.
See: Neopolycin-HC, Oint., Ophth. Oint. (Hoechst Marion Roussel).
W/Polymyxin B sulfate.
See: Polysporin, Oint., Ophth. Oint. (GlaxoWellcome).
W/Polymyxin B Sulfate, neomycin sulfate, lidocaine.
See: Clomycin, Oint. (Roberts Pharm).
Triliotic Plus, Oint. (Thompson).
W/Polymyxin B sulfate and neomycin sulfate.
See: Trimixin, Oint. (Hance).
W/Polymyxin B sulfate, neomycin sulfate and hydrocortisone-free alcohol.
See: Biotic-Ophth.
W/HC, Oint. (Scrip).
Cortisporin, Preps. (GlaxoWellcome).

bacitracin-neomycin ointment. (Various Mfr.) Neomycin sulfate equivalent to 3.5 mg base, bacitracin 500 units/Gm. Topical Oint. Tube 0.5 oz, 1 oz, Ophth. Oint. 1/8 oz. *otc.*
Use: Anti-infective, topical.

bacitracin/neomycin/polymyxin B ointment. (Various Mfr.) Polymyxin B sulfate 10,000 units/g, neomycin sulfate 3.5 mg/g, bacitracin zinc 400 units/g. Tube 3.5 g. *Rx.*
Use: Anti-infective, ophthalmic.

bacitracin and polymyxin b sulfate. Topical Aerosol.
Use: Anti-infective, topical.
See: Polysporin Oint., Pow. (GlaxoWellcome).

bacitracin zinc. (Pharmacia & Upjohn) Sterile pow. 10,000 units, 50,000 units/Vial.
Use: Anti-infective.

•**bacitracin zinc,** U.S.P. 23.
Use: Anti-infective.
W/Neomycin sulfate, polymyxin B sulfate
See: AK-Spore Ophth. Oint. (Akorn).
Neomixin, Oint. (Roberts Pharm)
Neosporin, Prods. (GlaxoWellcome)
Neotal, Oint. (Roberts Pharm)
Ocutricin Ophth. Oint. (Bausch & Lomb)
Triple Antibiotic Ophth. Oint. (Various Mfr.).
W/Neomycin sulfate, polymyxin B, benzalkonium Cl.
See: Biotres, Oint. (Schwarz Pharma)
W/Neomycin sulfate, polymyxin B sulfate, hydrocortisone acetate
See: Biotres HC, Cream (Schwarz Pharma).
Coracin, Oint. (Roberts Pharm).
W/Polymyxin B sulfate, neomycin sulfate.
See: Ophthel, Ophth. Oint. (ICN Pharmaceuticals).

bacitracin zinc/neomycin sulfate/polymixin B sulfate/hydrocortisone. (Various Mfr.) Hydrocortisone 1%, neomycin sulfate 0.35%, bacitracin zinc 400 units, polymyxin B sulfate 10,000 units. Tube 3.5 g*Rx.*
Use: Anti-infective, corticosteroid ophthalmic.

bacitracin zinc ointment. Bacitracin zinc is an anhydrous ointment base. (Al-Pharma) Polymyxin B sulfate 10,000

units, bacitracin zinc 500 units. Tube 3.5 g.
Use: Anti-infective, topical.

Bacit White. (Whiteworth Towne) Bacitracin. Oint. Tube 0.5 oz, 1 oz. *otc.*
Use: Anti-infective, topical.

Backache Maximum Strength Relief. (Bristol-Myers Squibb) Magnesium salicylate anhydrous (as tetrahydrate) 467 mg. Capl. Bot. 24s, 50s.*otc.*
Use: Analgesic.

baclofen. (BACK-low-fen) **Tab.** Bot. 10 mg, 20 mg. 100s, UD 100s; **Intrathecal.** 10 mg/20 ml, 10 mg/5 ml. Single use amps 1 amp refill kit (10 mg/20 ml), 2 or 4 amp refill kit (10 mg/5 ml).
Use: Muscle relaxant.

•**baclofen.** U.S.P. 23.
Use: Muscle relaxant.
See: Baclofen, Tab. (Eon Labs Manufacturing).
Lioresal, Tab., Intrathecal. (Novartis Pharmaceuticals).

baclofen, l-baclofen. *Rx.*
Use: Treatment of muscle spasticity. [Orphan Drug]
See: Neuralgon.

Bacmin. (Marnel) Iron 27 mg, Vitamin A 5000 IU, E 30 IU, C 500 mg, B_1 20 mg, B_2 20 mg, B_3 100 mg, B_5 25 mg, B_6 25 mg, B_{12} 50 mcg, biotin 0.15 mg, folic acid 0.8 mg, Cr, Cu Mg, Mn, Zn 22.5 mg/Tab. Bot. 100s*Rx.*
Use: Mineral, vitamin supplement.

Bac-Neo-Poly Ointment. (Burgin-Arden) Bacitracin 400 units, neomycin sulfate 5 mg, polymyxin B sulfate 5000 units/Gm. Tube 5 oz.*otc.*
Use: Anti-infective, topical.

Bactal Soap. (Whittaker General) Triclosan 0.5% and anhydrous soap 10%. Liq. 240 ml, 1/2 gal.*otc.*
Use: Antiseptic, cleaner.

bacteriostatic sodium chloride. (Various Mfr.) Sodium Cl 0.9%. Also contains benzyl alcohol or parabens. Inj. Bot. 10 ml, 20 ml, 30 ml. *Rx.*
Use: Parenteral diluent.

bacteriostatic water for injection. U.S.P. 23. (Abbott Laboratories) 30 ml. Multiple-dose Fliptop vial (plastic).
Use: Pharmaceutic aid for diluting and dissolving drugs for injection.

bacteriuria tests. In vitro diagnostic aids.
See: Isocult for bacteriuria (SmithKline Diagnostics)
Microstix-3 strips (Bayer Corp)
Uricult (Orion Diagnostica).

Bacti-Cleanse. (Pedinol) Benzylkonium Cl, mineral oil, isopropyl palmitate, cetyl alcohol, glycerine, glyceryl stearate, PEG-100 stearate, dimethicone, diazolidinyl urea, parabens, DMDM hydantion, EDTA. Liq. Bot. 453.6 ml. *otc.*
Use: Dermatolgic cleanser.

Bacticort. (Rugby) Hydrocortisone 1%, neomycin sulfate equivalent to 0.35% neomycin base, polymyxin B sulfate 10,000 units/ml, benzalkonium Cl, cetyl alcohol, glyceryl monostearate, mineral oil, polyoxyl 40 stearate, propylene glycol. Ophth. Soln. Bot. 7.5 ml.*Rx.*
Use: Anti-infective, corticosteroid, ophthalmic.

Bactigen Group A Streptococcus. (Wampole Laboratories) Latex agglutination slide test for the qualitative detection of group A streptococcal antigen directly from throat swabs. Test kit 60s.
Use: Diagnostic aid.

Bactigen Group A Streptococcus with Gast Trak Slides. (Wampole Laboratories) Latex agglutination slide test for qualitative detection of group A streptococcal antigen directly from throat swabs. Test 24s. Test kit 48s.
Use: Diagnostic aid.

Bactigen H. Influenzae. (Wampole Laboratories) Rapid latex agglutination slide test for the qualitative detection of *Haemophilus influenzae*, type b antigen in cerebrospinal fluid, serum and urine. Test kit 15s, 30s.
Use: Diagnostic aid.

Bactigen Meningitis Panel. (Wampole Laboratories) Rapid latex agglutination slide test for the qualitative detection of *Haemophilus influenzae* type b, *Neisseria meningitidis* A/B/C/Y/W135 and Streptococcus pneumoniae antigens in cerebrospinal fluid, serum and urine. Test kit 18.
Use: Diagnostic aid.

Bactigen N. Meningitidis. (Wampole Laboratories) Rapid latex agglutination slide test for the qualitative detection of *Neisseria meningitidis*, serogroups A/B/C/Y/W135 antigens in cerebrospinal fluid, serum and urine. Test kit 15s, 30s.
Use: Diagnostic aid.

Bactigen Salmonella-Shigella. (Wampole Laboratories) Latex agglutination slide test for the qualitative detection of *Salmonella* or *Shigella* from cultures. 96s.
Use: Diagnostic aid.

Bactine Antiseptic/Anesthetic First Aid Spray. (Bayer Corp) Benzalkonium Cl

0.13%, lidocaine 2.5%. **Squeeze Bot.:** 2 oz, 4 oz. **Liq.:** 16 oz. **Aerosol:** 3 oz. *otc.*
Use: Anesthetic, antiseptic, topical.

Bactine First Aid Antibiotic. (Bayer Corp) Polymyxin B sulfate 5,000 units, bacitracin 500 units, neomycin sulfate 5 mg/g in mineral oil, white petrolatum. Oint. Tube 15 g. *otc.*
Use: Anti-infective, topical.

Bactine First Aid Antibiotic Plus Anesthetic. (Bayer Corp) Polymyxin B sulfate 5,000 units, neomycin 3.5 mg/g, bacitracin 400 units, diperodon HCl 10 mg, in mineral oil and white petrolatum. Oint. Tube 15 g. *otc.*
Use: Anti-infective, topical.

Bactine Hydrocortisone Skin Cream. (Bayer Corp) Hydrocortisone 0.5%. Tube 0.5 oz. *otc.*
Use: Corticosteroid, topical.

Bactine Maximum Strength. (Bayer Corp) Hydrocortisone 1%, glycerin, mineral oil, methylparaben, white petrolatum. Cream tube 30 g. *otc.*
Use: Corticosteroid, topical.

Bactocill. (SmithKline Beecham Pharmaceuticals) Oxacillin sodium. **Vial:** (w/ dibasic sodium phosphate 40 mg, methylparaben 3.6 mg, propylparaben 0.4 mg, sodium 3.1 mEq/Gm) 500 mg, 1 g, 2 g or 4 g/Vial; 10s. Piggyback vial 1 g, 2 g; 25s. Bulk pharm pkg 10 g; Box 25s. *Rx.*
Use: Anti-infective; penicillin.

Bacto Shield Foam. (Steris Laboratories) Chlorhexidine gluconate 4%, isopropyl alcohol 4%/Foam. Aerosol. 180 ml. *otc.*
Use: Dermatologic, cleanser.

Bacto shield Solution. (Steris Laboratories) Chlorhexidine gluconate 4%/Soln. Bot. 960 ml. *otc.*
Use: Dermatologic, cleanser.

Bacto shield 2. (Steris Laboratories) Chlorhexidine glyconate 2%, isorpropyl alcohol 4%. Soln. Bot. 960 ml. *otc.*
Use: Pre-operative skin preparation/ cleanser.

Bactrim. (Roche Laboratories) Sulfamethoxazole 400 mg, trimethoprim 80 mg/Tab. Bot. 100s. *Rx.*
Use: Anti-infective.

Bactrim DS. (Roche Laboratories) Trimethoprim 160 mg, sulfamethoxazole 800 mg/Tab. Bot. 100s, 200s, 500s. *Rx.*
Use: Anti-infective.

Bactrim IV Infusion. (Roche Laboratories) Sulfamethoxazole 400 mg, trimethoprim 80 mg/5 ml. Multidose vials. 10ml, 30ml. *Rx.*
Use: Anti-infective.

Bactrim Pediatric Suspension. (Roche Laboratories) Trimethoprim 40 mg, sulfamethoxazole 200 mg/5 ml. Bot. 480 ml. *Rx.*
Use: Anti-infective combination.

Bactrim Suspension. (Roche Laboratories) Sulfamethoxazole 200 mg, trimethoprim 40 mg/5 ml. Bot. 16 oz. *Rx.*
Use: Anti-infective.

Bactroban. (SmithKline Beecham Pharmaceuticals) Mupirocin 2% in a polyethylene glycol base/Oint (Topical). Tube 15 g. Mupirocin calcium 2%/Oint (Intranasal). Tube 1 g. Mupirocin Calcium 2%, alcohols. Cream Tube 15g, 30 g. *Rx.*
Use: Anti-infective, topical; anti-infective used in adult patients and healthcare workers during institutional outbreaks (intranasal).

Bacturcult. (Wampole Laboratories) A urinary bacteria culture medium diagnostic urine culture system for urine collection, bacteriuria screening and presumptive bacterial identification. Test kit 10s, 100s.
Use: Diagnostic aid.

Bain de Soleil All Day For Kids SPF 30. (Procter & Gamble) Ethylhexyl p-methoxycinnamate, 2-ethylhexyl 2-cyano-3, 3 diphenyl acrylate, oxybenzone, titanium dioxide, stearyl alcohol, tocopheryl acetate, EDTA. PABA free. Waterproof. Lot. Bot. 120 ml. *otc.*
Use: Sunscreen.

Bain de Soleil All Day Waterproof Sunblock. (Procter & Gamble) SPF 15, 30. Ethylhexyl p-methoxycinnamate, 2-ethylhexyl 2-cyano-3, 3-diphenyl acrylate, oxybenzone, titanium dioxide, stearyl alcohol, vitamin E, EDTA. Lot. Bot. 120 m/g. *otc.*
Use: Sunscreen.

Bain de Soleil All Day Waterproof Sunfilter. (Procter & Gamble) SPF 4, 8. 2-ethylhexyl 2-cyano-3, 3 diphenyl acrylate, ethylhexyl p-methoxycinnamate, titanium dioxide, stearyl alcohol, vitamin E, EDTA. Lot. Bot. 120 ml. *otc.*
Use: Sunscreen.

Bain de Soleil Body Silkening Creme. (Procter & Gamble) Padimate O, ethylhexyl p-methoxycinnamate, oxybenzone, benzyl alcohol. Waterproof cream. Bot. 94 g. *otc.*
Use: Sunscreen.

Bain de Soleil Body Silkening Spray. (Procter & Gamble) Padimate O, oxybenzone, ethylhexyl p-methoxycinnamate. Waterproof lotion. Bot. 240 ml. *otc.*
Use: Sunscreen.

Bain de Soleil Body Silkening Stick. (Procter & Gamble) Padimate O, ethylhexyl p-methoxycinnamate, oxybenzone, dioxybenzone. Stick 53 g. *otc.*
Use: Sunscreen.

Bain de Soleil Face Creme. (Procter & Gamble) Padimate O, ethylhexyl p-methoxycinnamate, oxybenzone. Waterproof cream. Bot. 60 g. *otc.*
Use: Sunscreen.

Bain de Soleil Kids Sport. (Procter & Gamble) SPF 25. Ethylhexyl-p-methoxycinnamate, 2-ethylhexyl 2-cyano-3, 3-diphenyl acrylate, titanium dioxide, PVP/eicosene copolymer, dimethicone, cyclomethicone, triethanolamine, glyceryl tribehenate, tocopheryl acetate, carbomer, EDTA, DMDM hydantoin. PABA free. Waterproof, all day protection. Lot. Bot. 120 ml. *otc.*
Use: Sunscreen.

Bain de Soleil Lip Protecteur. (Procter & Gamble) Ethylhexyl p-methoxycinnamate, oxybenzone, 2-ethylhexyl salicylate, oleyl alcohol, petrolatum. PABA free lip balm, 3 g. *otc.*
Use: Sunscreen.

Bain de Soleil Megatan. (Procter & Gamble) Ethylhexyl p-methoxycinnamate, 2-ethylhexyl salicylate, lanolin, cocoa butter, palm oil, aloe, DMDM hydantoin, xanthan gum, shea butter, EDTA. Lot. Bot. 120 ml. *otc.*
Use: Sunscreen.

Bain de Soleil Orange Gelee SPF 4. (Procter & Gamble) Ethylhexyl p-methoxycinnamate, 2-ethylhexyl salicylate. PABA free. Gel Tube 93.75 g. *otc.*
Use: Sunscreen.

Bain de Soleil SPF 8 + Color. (Procter & Gamble) Octyl methoxycinnamate, octocrylene, mineral oil, cetyl alcohol, EDTA. Lot. Bot. 118 ml. *otc.*
Use: Sunscreen.

Bain de Soleil SPF 15 + Color. (Procter & Gamble) Octyl methoxycinnamate, octocrylene, oxybenzone, mineral oil, cetyl alcohol, EDTA. Lot. Bot. 118 ml. *otc.*
Use: Sunscreen.

Bain de Soleil SPF 30 + Color. (Procter & Gamble). Octocrylene, octyl methoxycinnamate, oxybenzone, mineral oil, cetyl alcohol, EDTA. Lot. Bot. 118 ml. *otc.*
Use: Sunscreen.

Bain de Soleil Sport. (Procter & Gamble). SPF 15. 2-ethylhexyl 2-cyan-3, 3 diphenyl acrylate, ethylhexyl-p-methoxycinnamate, titanium dioxide, dimethicone, cyclomethicone, panthenol, tocopheryl acetate, carbomer, EDTA, DMDM hydantoin. PABA free. Waterproof, sweatproof, all day protection. Lot. Bot. 180 ml. *otc.*
Use: Sunscreen.

Bain de Soleil Tropical Deluxe SPF 4. (Procter & Gamble) Ethylhexyl p-methoxycinnamate, 2-ethylhexyl salicylate, cetyl alcohol, EDTA. PABA free. Waterproof. Lot. Bot. 240 ml. *otc.*
Use: Sunscreen.

Bain de Soleil Under Eye. (Procter & Gamble) Ethylhexyl p-methoxycinnamate, oxybenzone, 2-ethylhexyl salicylate. Stick 1.5 g. *otc.*
Use: Sunscreen.

Bakers Best. (Scherer) Water, alcohol 38%, propylene glycol, extract of capsicum, glycerin, boric acid, Tween 80, diethylphthalate, rose oil, pyrilamine maleate, glacial acetic acid, Uvinul MS 40, hexetidine, benzalkonium Cl 50%, sodium hydroxide 76%. Bot. 8 oz. *otc.*
Use: Antipruritic, antiseborrheic, topical.

•**balafilcon A.** (ba-lah-FILL-kahn A) USAN.
Use: Contact lens material (hydrophilic).

Balanced B_{100}. (Fibertone) Vitamins B_1 100 mg, B_2 100 mg, B_3 100 mg, B_5 100 mg, B_6 100 mg, B_{12} 100 mcg, folic acid 0.1 mg, PABA 100 mg, inositol 100 mg, d-biotin 100 mcg/SR Tab. Bot. 50s.
Use: Mineral, vitamin supplement.

Balanced Salt Solution. (Various Mfr.) Sodium Cl 0.64%, potassium Cl, 0.075%, calcium Cl 0.048%, magnesium Cl 0.03%, sodium acetate 0.39%, sodium citrate 0.17%, sodium hydroxide or hydrochloric acid. Soln. Droptainer 18 ml, 500 ml.
Use: Irrigant, ophthalmic.

Baldex Ophthalmic Ointment. (Bausch & Lomb) Dexamethasone phosphate 0.05%. 3.75 g. *Rx.*
Use: Corticosteroid, ophthalmic.

Baldex Ophthalmic Solution. (Bausch & Lomb) Dexamethasone phosphate 0.01%. Dropper Bot. 5 ml. *Rx.*
Use: Corticosteroid, ophthalmic.

BAL in Oil. (Becton Dickinson) 2,3-dimercaptopropanol 100 mg, benzyl benzoate 210 mg, peanut oil 680 mg/ml. Amp. 3 ml Box 10s. *Rx.*

Use: Antidote.

Balmex Baby Powder. (Macsil) Specially purified balsam Peru, zinc oxide, starch, calcium carbonate. Shaker top can. 4 oz. *otc.*
Use: Adsorbent, emollient.

Balmex Ointment. (Macsil) Specially purified balsam Peru, Vitamins A and D, zinc oxide, bismuth subnitrate in a base w/silicone. Tube 1 oz, 2 oz, 4 oz. Jar lb. *otc.*
Use: Emollient.

Balneol Perianal Cleansing. (Solvay) Mineral oil, lanolin oil, methylparaben. Bot. 120 ml. *otc.*
Use: Anorectal preparation.

Balnetar. (Westwood Squibb) Tar equivalent to 2.5% coal tar, U.S.P. Bot. 8 oz. *otc.*
Use: Dermatologic.

•**balsalazide disodium.** (bahl-SAL-ah-zide) USAN.
Use: Anti-inflammatory (gastrointestinal).

Balsan. Specially purified balsam Peru.
See: Balmex Prods. (Macsil).

•**bambermycins.** (BAM-ber-MY-sinz) USAN.
Use: Anti-infective.

•**bamethan sulfate.** (BAM-eth-an) USAN.
Use: Vasodilator.

•**bamifylline hydrochloride.** (BAM-ih-FILL-in) USAN.
Use: Bronchodilator.

•**bamnidazole.** (bam-NIH-DAH-zole) USAN.
Use: Antiprotozoal (trichomonas).

Banacid Tablets. (Buffington) Magnesium trisilicate 220 mg. Bot. 100s, 200s, 500s. *otc.*
Use: Antacid.

Banadyne-3. (Norstar) Lidocaine 4%, menthol 1%, alcohol 45%. Soln. Bot. 7.5 ml. *otc.*
Use: Mouth and throat preparation.

Banalg. (Forest Pharmaceutical) Methyl salicylate 4.9%, camphor 2%, menthol 1%. Lot. Bot. 60 ml and 480 ml. *otc.*
Use: Analgesic, topical.

Banalg Hospital Strength Liniment. (Forest Pharmaceutical) Methyl salicylate 14%, menthol 3%. Bot. 60 ml. *otc.*
Use: Analgesic, topical.

Bancap HC. (Forest Pharmaceutical) Acetaminophen 500 mg, hydrocodone bitartrate 5 mg/Cap. Bot. 100s, 500s. *c-III.*
Use: Analgesic combination, narcotic.

•**bandage, adhesive.** U.S.P. 23.
Use: Surgical aid.

•**bandage, gauze.** U.S.P. 23.
Use: Surgical aid.

Banex Capsules. (LuChem) Phenylpropanolamine HCl 45 mg, phenylephrine HCl 5 mg, guaifenesin 200 mg. Bot. 100s, 500s. *otc.*
Use: Decongestant, expectorant.

Banex-LA Tablets. (LuChem) Phenylpropanolamine HCl 75 mg, guaifenesin 400 mg. Bot. 100s, 500s. *otc.*
Use: Decongestant, expectorant.

Banflex. (Forest Pharmaceutical) Orphenadrine citrate 30 mg/ml. Inj. Vial 10 ml. *Rx.*
Use: Muscle relaxant.

Bangesic. (H.L. Moore) Menthol, camphor, methyl salicylate, eucalyptus oil in non-greasy base. Bot. 2 oz, gal. *otc.*
Use: Analgesic, topical.

Banocide.
See: Diethylcarbamazine Citrate, U.S.P.

Baophen. (Major) Diphenhydramine HCl 25 mg, lactose, parabens. Cap. Bot. 100s. *otc.*
Use: Antihistamine.

Bansmoke. (Thompson Medical) Benzocaine 6 mg, corn syrup, dextrose, lecithin, sucrose. Gum Pack 24s. *otc.*
Use: Smoking deterrent.

Banthine. (Schiapparelli Searle) Methantheline bromide 50 mg/Tab. Bot. 100s. *Rx.*
Use: Anticholinergic.

Bantron Smoking Deterrent Tablets. (DEP) Magnesium carbonate 129.6 mg, lobeline sulfate 2 mg, tribasic calcium phosphate 129.6 mg/Tab. Carton 18s, 36s. *otc.*
Use: Smoking deterrent.

Barbased. (Major) **Tab.:** Butabarbital 0.25 gr or 0.5 gr/Tab. Bot. 1000s. **Elix.:** Butabarbital- 30 mg/5 ml, alcohol 7%. Bot. 480 ml. *Rx.*
Use: Hypnotic, sedative.

Barbatose No. 2 Tablets. (Pal-Pak) Barbital 64.8 mg/Tab. w/hyoscyamus sulfate, passiflora, valerian. Bot. 1000s. *Rx.*
Use: Sedative.

Barbella Elixir. (Forest Pharmaceutical) Phenobarbital 0.25 gr, hyoscyamine sulfate 0.1037 mg, atropine sulfate 0.0194 mg, scopolamine HBr 0.0065 mg, alcohol 23%/5 ml. Bot. 4 oz, gal. *Rx.*
Use: Anticholinergic, antispasmodic, hypnotic, sedative.

Barbella Tablets. (Forest Pharmaceutical) Phenobarbital 16.2 mg, atropine sulfate 0.0194 mg, hyoscyamine sulfate 0.1037 mg, hyoscine HBr 0.0065 mg/Tab. Bot. 100s, 1000s, 5000s. *Rx.*
Use: Anticholinergic, antispasmodic, hypnotic, sedative.

Barbeloid. (Pal-Pak) Phenobarbital 16.2 mg, hyoscyamine sulfate 0.1037 mg, atropine sulfate 0.0194 mg, scopolamine HBr 0.0065 mg/Tab. Bot. 100s, 1000s. *Rx.*
Use: Anticholinergic, antispasmodic, hypnotic, sedative.

Barbenyl.
See: Phenobarbital.

Barbidonna. (Wallace Laboratories) Phenobarbital 16 mg, hyoscyamine sulfate 0.1286 mg, atropine sulfate 0.025 mg, scopolamine HBr 0.0074 mg, lactose. Tab. Bot. 100s, 500s. *Rx.*
Use: Anticholinergic, antispasmodic, hypnotic, sedative.

Barbidonna No. 2. (Wallace Laboratories) Phenobarbital 32 mg, hyoscyamine sulfate 0.1286 mg, atropine sulfate 0.025 mg, scopolamine HBr 0.0074 mg, lactose. Tab. Bot. 100s. *Rx.*
Use: Anticholinergic, antispasmodic, hypnotic, sedative.

Barbiphenyl.
See: Phenobarbital.

barbital. Barbitone, Deba, Dormonal, Hypnogene, Malonal, Sedeval, Uronal, Veronal, Vesperal, diethylbarbituric acid, diethylmalonylurea.
Use: Hypnotic, sedative.

W/Aspirin, caffeine, niacinamide.
See: Mentran, Tab. (Taylor Pharmaceuticals).

barbital sodium. Barbitone Sodium, diethylbarbiturate monosodium, diethylmalonylurea sodium, Embinal, Medinal, Veronal Sodium.
Use: Hypnotic, sedative.

barbitone.
See: Barbital.

barbitone sodium.
See: Barbital Sodium.

barbiturate-aspirin combinations.
See: Aspirin-Barbiturate Combination.

barbiturates, intermediate duration.
See: Butabarbital (Various Mfr.).
Butethal (Various Mfr.).
Diallylbarbituric Acid (Various Mfr.).
Lotusate, Cap. (Sanofi Winthrop).

barbiturates, long duration.
See: Barbital (Various Mfr.).
Mebaral, Tab. (Sanofi Winthrop).
Mephobarbital (Various Mfr.).
Phenobarbital (Various Mfr.).
Phenobarbital Sodium (Various Mfr.).

barbiturates, short duration.
See: Amobarbital (Various Mfr.).
Amobarbital Sodium (Various Mfr.).
Butalbital (Various Mfr.).
Butallylonal (Various Mfr.).
Cyclobarbital (Various Mfr.).
Cyclopal.
Pentobarbital Salts (Various Mfr.).
Sandoptal.
Secobarbital (Various Mfr.).

barbiturates, triple.
See: Butseco, S.C.T., Tab. (Jones Medical Industries).
Ethobral, Cap. (Wyeth Ayerst).

barbiturates, ultrashort duration.
See: Hexobarbital.
Neraval.
Pentothal Sodium, Amp. (Abbott Laboratories).
Surital Sodium, Amp., Vial (Parke-Davis).
Thiopental Sodium (Various Mfr.).

Barc Gel. (Del Pharmaceuticals) Pyrethrins 0.18%, piperonyl butoxide technical 2.2%, petroleum distillate 4.8% in gel base. Tube oz. *otc.*
Use: Pediculicide.

Barc Non-Body Lice Control Spray. (Del Pharmaceuticals) Spray can 5 oz. *otc.*
Use: Pediculicide.

Baricon. (Lafayette Pharm) Barium sulfate 95% pow. for susp. In UD 340 g. *Rx.*
Use: Radiopaque agent, gastrointestinal.

Baridium. (Pfeiffer) Phenazopyridine HCl 100 mg/Tab. Bot.32s. *otc.*
Use: Analgesic, urinary.

Bari-Stress M. (Alphalma USPD) Vitamins B_1 10 mg, B_2 10 mg, niacinamide 100 mg, C 300 mg, B_6 2 mg, B_{12} 4 mcg, folic acid 1.5 mg, calcium pantothenate 20 mg/Cap or Tab. **Cap.:** Bot. 30s, 100s, 1000s. **Tab.:** Bot. 100s, 1000s. *Rx.*
Use: Mineral, vitamin supplement.

•**barium hydroxide lime.** (BA-ree-uhm) U.S.P. 23.
Use: Carbon dioxide absorbant.

•**barium sulfate,** U.S.P. 23.
Use: Diagnostic aid (radiopaque medium).

barium sulfate preparation.
See: Barotrast, Pow., Cream (PBH Wesley Jessen).

Fleet.
Redi-Flow, Susp. (Berlex).

Barlevite. (Barth's) Vitamins B_6 0.6 mg, B_{12} 3 mcg, pantothenic acid 0.6 mg, D 3 IU, l-lysine 20 mg/0.6 ml. 100-Day Supply. *otc.*
Use: Vitamin/mineral supplement.

•**barmastine.** (BAR-mast-een) USAN.
Use: Antihistamine.

BarnesHind Cleaning and Soaking Solution. (PBH Wesley Jessen) Cleaning and buffering agents, benzalkonium Cl 0.01%, disodium edetate 0.2%. Bot. 1.2 oz, 4 oz. *otc.*
Use: Contact lens care.

BarnesHind Saline for Sensitive Eyes. (PBH Wesley Jessen) Potassium sorbate 0.13%, EDTA 0.025%. Soln. Bot. 360 ml (2s). *otc.*
Use: Contact lens care.

BarnesHind Wetting & Soaking Solution. (PBH Wesley Jessen) Polyvinyl alcohol, povidone, hydroxyethyl cellulose, octylphenoxy (oxyethylene) ethanol, benzalkonium Cl, edetate disodium. Bot. 4 oz. *otc.*
Use: Contact lens care.

BarnesHind Wetting Solution. (PBH Wesley Jessen) Polyvinyl alcohol, edetate disodium 0.02%, benzalkonium Cl 0.004%. Bot. 35 ml, 60 ml. *otc.*
Use: Contact lens care.

Baro-Cat. (Lafayette Pharm) Barium sulfate 1.5% susp. 300 ml, 900 ml.
Use: Radiopaque agent, gastrointestinal.

Baros. (Lafayette Pharm) Sodium bicarbonate 460 mg (sodium 126 mg) and tartaric acid 420 mg/g with simethicone. Granules, effervescent. Plastic amp. 3 g. *Rx.*
Use: Diagnostic aid.

Baroset. (Lafayette Pharm) Air contrast stomach. Unit-of-use kit. Case 12s.
Use: Radiopaque agent.

barosmin.
See: Diosmin.

Barosperse. (Lafayette Pharm) Barium sulfate 95%, suspending agent. Susp. 25 lb.
Use: Radiopaque agent.

Barosperse 110. (Lafayette Pharm) Barium sulfate 95%. Susp. 900 g.
Use: Radiopaque agent.
W/Iron. Ferric pyrophosphate 250 mg/5 ml plus Barovite liquid formula.

Basa. (Freeport) Acetylsalicylic acid 324 mg/Tab. Bot. 1000s. *otc.*
Use: Analgesic.

Basaljel. (Wyeth Ayerst) Aluminum carbonate gel. **Susp.:** Equivalent to aluminum hydroxide 400 mg/5 ml. Bot. 355 ml. **Cap.:** Equivalent to 608 mg dried aluminum hydroxide gel or 500 mg aluminum hydroxide. Bot. 100s, 500s. **Tab.:** Equivalent to 608 mg dried aluminum hydroxide gel or 500 mg aluminum hydroxide. Bot. 100s. *otc.*
Use: Antacid.

basic aluminum aminoacetate.
See: Dihydroxyaluminum Aminoacetate.

basic aluminum carbonate.
See: Basaljel, Susp. (Wyeth Ayerst).

basic aluminum glycinate.
See: Dihydroxyaluminum aminoacetate.

basic bismuth carbonate.
See: Bismuth Subcarbonate.

basic bismuth gallate.
See: Bismuth Subgallate (Various Mfr.).

basic bismuth nitrate.
See: Bismuth Subnitrate (Various Mfr.).

basic bismuth salicylate.
See: Bismuth Subsalicylate,

basic fuchsin.
See: Carbol-Fuchsin Topical Soln., U.S.P. 23.

•**basifungin.** (bass-ih-FUN-jin) USAN.
Use: Antifungal.

Basis, Glycerin Soap. (Beiersdorf) **Bar:** Tallow, coconut oil, glycerin. **Sensitive:** Bar 90 g, 150 g. **Normal to dry:** Bar 90 g, 150 g. *otc.*
Use: Dermatologic, cleanser.

Basis, Superfatted Soap. (Beiersdorf) **Bar:** Sodium tallowate, sodium cocoate, petrolatum, glycerin, zinc oxide, sodium Cl, titanium dioxide, lanolin, alcohol, beeswax, BHT, EDTA. Bar 99 g, 225 g. *otc.*
Use: Dermatologic, cleanser.

•**batanopride hydrochloride.** (bah-TAN-oh-pride) USAN.
Use: Antiemetic.

•**batelapine maleate.** (bat-EH-lap-EEN) USAN.
Use: Antipsychotic.

•**batimastat.** (bat-IM-ah-stat) USAN.
Use: Antineoplastic.

Baycol. (Bayer) Cerivastatin sodium 0.2 mg, 0.3 mg, mannitol. Tab. Bot. 100s. *Rx.*
Use: Antihyperlipidemic.

Bayer 8-Hour Timed-Release Aspirin. (Bayer Corp) Aspirin 10 gr (650 mg)/ T.R. Tab. Bot. 30s, 72s, 125s. *otc.*
Use: Analgesic.

Bayer 205.
See: Suramin Sodium. (No Mfr. currently listed.).

Bayer 2502.
See: Nifurtimox. (No Mfr. currently listed.).

Bayer Aspirin, Genuine. (Bayer Corp) Aspirin 325 mg/Tab. Bot. 50s, 100s, 200s, 300s. Pkg. 12s, 24s. *otc.*
Use: Analgesic.

Bayer Aspirin, Maximum. (Bayer Corp) Aspirin 500 mg/Tab. Bot. 30s, 60s, 100s. *otc.*
Use: Analgesic.

Bayer Buffered Aspirin. (Bayer Corp) Buffered aspirin 325 mg. Tab. Bot. 100s. *otc.*
Use: Analgesic.

Bayer Children's Chewable Aspirin. (Bayer Corp) Aspirin 1.25 gr (81 mg)/Tab. Bot. 30s. *otc.*
Use: Analgesic.

Bayer Children's Cold Tablets. (Bayer Corp) Phenylpropanolamine HCl 3.125 mg, aspirin 1.25 gr (81 mg)/Tab. Bot. 30s. *otc.*
Use: Analgesic, decongestant.

Bayer Cough Syrup for Children. (Bayer Corp) Phenylpropanolamine HCl 9 mg, dextromethorphan HBr 7.5 mg/5 ml w/alcohol 5%. Bot. 3 oz. *otc.*
Use: Antitussive, decongestant.

Bayer Enteric 500 Aspirin, Extra Strength. (Bayer Corp) Aspirin 500 mg. Tab. Enteric coated. Bot. 60s. *otc.*
Use: Analgesic.

Bayer Enteric Coated Caplets, Regular Strength. (Bayer Corp) Aspirin 325 mg. Tab. Enteric coated. Bot. 50s, 100s, *otc.*
Use: Analgesic.

Bayer Low Adult Strength. (Bayer Corp) Aspirin 81 mg, lactose. DR Tab. Bot. 120s. *otc.*
Use: Analgesic.

Bayer Plus Extra Strength. (Bayer Corp) Aspirin 500 mg buffered with calcium carbonate, magnesium carbonate, magnesium oxide. Cap. Bot. 30s, 60s. *otc.*
Use: Analgesic.

Bayer Select Chest Cold. (Bayer Corp) Dextromethorphan HBr 15 mg, acetaminophen 500 mg. Caplets in Pkg. 16s. *otc.*
Use: Analgesic, antitussive.

Bayer Select Flu Relief. (Bayer Corp) Acetaminophen 500 mg, pseudoephedrine HCl 30 mg, dextromethorphan HBr 15 mg, chlorpheniramine maleate 2 mg. Capl. Blister-pack 16s. *otc.*
Use: Analgesic, antihistamine, antitussive, decongestant.

Bayer Select Head Cold. (Bayer Corp) Pseudoephedrine HCl 30 mg, acetaminophen 500 mg. Capl. Pkg. 16s. *otc.*
Use: Analgesic, decongestant expectorant.

Bayer Select Maximum Strength Backache. (Bayer Corp) Magnesium salicylate tetrahydrate 580 mg. Capl. Bot. 24s, 50s. *otc.*
Use: Analgesic.

Bayer Select Maximum Strength Headache. (Bayer Corp) Acetaminophen 500 mg, caffeine 65 mg/Cap. Bot. 36s. *otc.*
Use: Analgesic combination.

Bayer Select Maximum Strength Menstrual. (Bayer Corp) Acetaminophen 500 mg, pamabrom 25 mg/Capl. Bot. 24s, 50s. *otc.*
Use: Analgesic, diuretic.

Bayer Select Maximum Strength Night Time Pain Relief. (Bayer Corp) Acetaminophen 500 mg, diphenhydramine HCl/Tab. Bot. 24s, 50s. *otc.*
Use: Antihistamine.

Bayer Select Maximum Strength Sinus Pain Relief. (Bayer Corp) Acetaminophen 500 mg, pseudoephedrine HCl 30 mg/Tab. Bot. 50s. *otc.*
Use: Analgesic, decongestant.

Bayer Select Night Time Cold. (Bayer Corp) Acetaminophen 500 mg, pseudoephedrine HCl 30 mg, dextromethorphan HBr 15 mg, triprolidine HCl 1.25 mg. Capl. Blister-pack 16s. *otc.*
Use: Analgesic, antihistamine, antitussive, decongestant.

BayHep B. (Bayer Corp) Hepatitis B immune globulin (Human). Vial 250 unit, prefilled syringe 250 unit. Vial 1 ml. *Rx.*
Use: Immunization.

Baylocaine 2% Viscous. (Bay Labs) Lidocaine 2% w/sodium carboxymethylcellulose. Soln. Bot. 100 ml. *otc.*
Use: Local anesthetic, topical.

Baylocaine 4%. (Bay Labs) Lidocaine 4% w/methylparaben. Soln. Bot. 50 ml, 100 ml.
Use: Anesthetic, local.

Baypress. Type II calcium channel blocking agent. *Rx.*
See: Nitrendipine.

Bayrab. (Bayer Corp) Rabies immune globulin (Human) 150 IU/ml. Vial 2 ml, 10 ml. *Rx.*
Use: Immunization.

BayRho D. (Bayer Corp) Rh_o (D) immune globulin (Human). Prefilled single dose syringe. Single dose syringe. Single dose vial. Pkg. *Rx.*
Use: Immunization.

Baytet. (Bayer Corp) Tetanus immune globulin (Human). Vial 250 units, Disp. Syringe 250 units. *Rx.*
Use: Immunization.

BC-1000. (Solvay) Vitamins B_1 50 mg, B_2 5 mg, B_{12} 1000 mcg, B_6 5 mg, d-panthenol 6 mg, niacinamide 125 mg, ascorbic acid 50 mg, benzyl alcohol 1%/ml. Vial 10 ml. *otc.*
Use: Vitamin supplement.

BC Arthritis Strength. (Block Drug) Aspirin 742 mg, salicylamide 222 mg, caffeine 36 mg/Pow. Bot. 6s, 24s, 50s. *otc.*
Use: Analgesic combination.

B-C-Bid. (Roberts Pharm) Vitamins B_1 15 mg, B_2 10 mg, B_3 50 mg, B_5 10 mg, B_6 5 mg, vitamin C 300 mg, B_{12} 5 mcg /Cap. Bot. 30s, 100s, 500s. *otc.*
Use: Mineral, vitamin supplement.

B-C Bid Caplets. (Roberts Pharm) Vitamin C 300 mg, B_1 15 mg, B_2 10.2 mg, B_3 50 mg, B_5 10 mg B_6 5 mg/Cap. Bot. 100s. *otc.*
Use: Vitamin supplement.

BC Cold-Sinus-Allergy Powder. (Block Drug) Phenylpropanolamine HCl 25 mg, chlorpheniramine maleate 4 mg, aspirin 650 mg, lactose. Pow. Pck. 6s, 24s. *otc.*
Use: Analgesic, antihistamine, decongestant.

BC Cold-Sinus Powder. (Block Drug) Phenylpropanolamine HCl 25 mg, aspirin 650 mg, lactose. Pkg. 6s.*otc.*
Use: Decongestant combination.

B-Complex-50. (Nion) Vitamins B_1 50 mg, B_2 50 mg, B_3 50 mg, B_5 50 mg, B_6 50 mg, B_{12} 50 mcg, FA 0.4 mg, biotin 50 mcg, PABA 50 mg, choline bitartrate 50 mg, inositol 50 mg/SR Tab. Bot. 100s. *otc.*
Use: Mineral, vitamin supplement.

B-Complex-150. (Nion) Vitamins B_1 150 mg, B_2 150 mg, B_3 150 mg, B_5 150 mg, B_6 150 mg, B_{12} 1 mcg, FA 0.4 mg, biotin 150 mcg, PABA 100 mg, choline bitartrate 150 mg, inositol 150 mg. SR Tab. Bot. 30s. *otc.*
Use: Mineral, vitamin supplement.

B-Complex Elixir. (Nion) B_1 2.3 mg, B_2 1 mg, B_3 6.7 mg, B_6 0.3 mg, alcohol 10%. Elix. Bot. 240 ml, 480 ml.*otc.*
Use: Mineral, vitamin supplement.

•**BCG vaccine,** U.S.P. 23.
Use: Immunization.

BCG vaccine. (Organon) Prepared from Tice strain of BCG bacillus. Amp. 2 ml. *Rx.*
Use: Immunization against tuberculosis, active.
See: Tice BCG (Organon)

BCG for Intravesicular Use.
Use: Antineoplastic.
See: TheraCys (Pasteur Merieux Connaught).
TICE BCG, Pow. for Susp. (Organon).

BCNU.
Use: Antineoplastic.
See: BiCNU, Inj. (Bristol-Myers Squibb).

BCO. (Western Research) Vitamins B_1 10 mg, B_2 2 mg, B_6 1.5 mg, B_{12} 25 mcg, niacinamide 50 mg/Tab. Bot. 1000s. *otc.*
Use: Vitamin supplement.

B-Com. (Century Pharm) Vitamins B_1 3 mg, B_2 3 mg, B_6 0.5 mg, niacinamide 20 mg, calcium pantothenate 5 mg, B_{12} 1 mcg, desiccated liver (undefatted) 60 mg, debittered brewer's dried yeast 60 mg/Cap. Bot. 100s, 1000s. *otc.*
Use: Mineral, vitamin supplement.

B-Complex 25-25 Inj. (Forest Pharmaceutical) Niacinamide 100 mg, Vitamins B_1 25 mg, B_2 1 mg, B_6 2 mg, pantothenic acid 2 mg/ml. Vial 30 ml. *Rx.*
Use: Vitamin supplement.

B-Complex "50". (Vitaline) Vitamins B_1 50 mg, B_2 50 mg, B_3 50 mg, B_4 50 mg, B_5 50 mg, B_6 50 mg, B_{12} 50 mcg, FA 0.1 mg, PABA 30 mg, inositol 50 mg, biotin 50 mcg, choline bitartrate 50 mg. Reg. or TR tabs. Bot. 90s, 1000s. *otc.*
Use: Vitamin supplement.

B-Complex #100. (Medical Chem) Vitamins B_1 100 mg, B_2 2 mg, B_6 4 mg, d-panthenol 4 mg, niacinamide 100 mg/ml. Vial 30 ml. *Rx.*
Use: Vitamin supplement.

B-Complex 100. (Rabin-Winters) Vitamins B_1 100 mg, B_2 2 mg, B_6 2 mg, niacinamide 125 mg, panthenol 10 mg/ml. Vial 30 ml. *Rx.*
Use: Vitamin supplement.

B-Complex 100/100. (Sandia) Vitamins B_1 100 mg, B_2 2 mg, B_6 2 mg, niacinamide 100 mg/ml. Inj. Vial 30 ml. *Rx.*
Use: Vitamin supplement.

B-Complex and B_{12}. (NBTY) Vitamins B_1 7 mg, B_2 14 mg, B_3 4.5 mg, B_{12} 25 mcg, protease 10 mg/Tab. Bot. 90s. *otc.*
Use: Vitamin supplement.

B-Complex with B-12. (Zenith Goldline) B_1 1.5 mg, B_2 1.7 mg, B_3 20 mg, B_5 10 mg, B_6 2 mg, B_{12} 6 mcg, FA 0.4 mg/ Tab. Bot. 100s *otc.*
Use: Mineral, vitamin supplement.

B-Complex Capsules. (Arcum) Vitamins B_1 1.5 mg, B_2 2 mg, niacinamide 10 mg, B_6 0.1 mg, calcium pantothenate 1 mg, desiccated liver 70 mg, dried yeast 100 mg/Cap. Bot. 100s, 1000s. *otc.*
Use: Mineral, vitamin supplement.

B-Complex Capsules J.F. (Bryant) Vitamins B_1 1 mg, B_2 0.3 mg, nicotinic acid 0.3 mg, B_6 0.25 mg, desiccated liver 0.15 g, yeast powder, dried 0.15 g/Cap. Bot. 100s, 1000s. *otc.*
Use: Mineral, vitamin supplement.

B-Complex Injection with Vitamin C.
Use: Vitamin supplement.
See: Cplex Cap. (Arcum).

B Complex with B_{12} Capsules. (Bryant) Vitamins B_1 2 mg, B_2 2 mg, B_6 0.5 mg, niacinamide 10 mg, B_{12} 2 mcg, biotin 10 mcg, calcium pantothenate 1.5 mg, choline dihydrogen citrate 40 mg, inositol 30 mg, desiccated liver 1 gr, brewer's yeast 3 gr/Cap. Bot. 100s, 1000s. *otc.*
Use: Mineral, vitamin supplement.

B-Complex/Vitamin C Caplets. (Geneva Pharm) Vitamins B_1 15 mg, B_2 10.2 mg, B_3 50 mg, B_5 10 mg, B_6 5 mg, C 300 mg/Capl. Bot. 100s. *otc.*
Use: Vitamin supplement.

B-Complex with Vitamin C and B_{12}-10,000. (Fujisawa) Vitamins B_1 20 mg, B_2 3 mg, B_3 75 mg, B_5 5 mg, B_6 5 mg, B_{12} 1000 mcg, C 100 mg. Covial. 10 ml multiple dose. *Rx.*
Use: Vitamin supplement.

B Complex + C. (Various Mfr.) Vitamins B_1 15 mg, B_2 10 mg, B_3 100 mg, B_5 20 mg, B_6 5 mg, B_{12} 10 mcg, C 500 mg/ Tab. Bot. 100s. *otc.*
Use: Vitamin supplement

B-Complex + C. (NBTY) C 200 mg, B_1 10 mg, B_2 10 mg, B_3 50 mg, B_5 10 mg, B_6 5 mg/Tab. Bot. 100s. *otc.*
Use: Vitamin supplement.

B Complex with C and B-12 Injection. (Zenith Goldline) B_1 50 mg, B_2 5 mg, B_3 125 mg, B_5 6 mg, B_6 5 mg, B_{12} 1000 mcg, C 50 mg/Inj. 10 ml. *Rx.*
Use: Vitamin supplement.

BC Powder. (Block Drug) Aspirin 650 mg, salicylamide 145 mg, caffeine 32 mg/ Pow. Pkg. 2s, 6s, 24s, 50s. *otc.*
Use: Analgesic combination.

BC Powder, Arthritis Strength. (Block Drug) Aspirin 742 mg, salicylamide 222 mg, caffeine 36 mg/Powder. Pkg. 6s, 24s, 50s. *otc.*
Use: Analgesic combination.

BC Tablets. (Block Drug) Aspirin 325 mg, salicylamide 95 mg, caffeine 16 mg/ Tab. Pkg 4s. Bot. 50s, 100s. *otc.*
Use: Analgesic combination.

B-C with Folic Acid. (Geneva Pharm) Vitamins B_1 15 mg, B_2 15 mg, B_3 100 mg, B_5 18 mg, B_6 4 mg, B_{12} 5 mcg, C 500 mg, folic acid 0.5 mg/Tab. Bot. 100s. *Rx.*
Use: Mineral, vitamin supplement.

B-C w/Folic Acid Plus. (Geneva Pharm) Fe 27 mg, vitamins A 5000 IU, E 30 IU, B_1 20 mg, B_2 20 mg, B_3 100 mg, B_5 25 mg, B_6 25 mg, B_{12} 50 mcg, C 500 mg, FA 0.8 mg, biotin 0.15 mg, Cr, Cu, Mg, Mn, Zn 22.5 mg. Tab. Bot. 100s. *Rx.*
Use: Mineral, vitamin supplement.

B-Day Tablets. (Barth's) Vitamins B_1 7 mg, B_2 14 mg, niacin 4.67 mg, B_{12} 5 mcg/Tab. Bot. 100s, 500s. *otc.*
Use: Vitamin supplement.

B-D Glucose. (Becton Dickinson) Glucose 5 g. Chew. Tab. Bot. 36s. *otc.*
Use: Hyperglycemic.

bdep.
See: Benzathine Penicillin G.

B Dozen. (Standex) Vitamin B_{12} 25 mcg Tab. Bot. 1000s. *otc.*
Use: Vitamin supplement.

B-Dram w/C Computabs. (Dram) Vitamins B_1 5mg, B_2 10 mg, B_6 5 mg, nicotinamide 50 mg, calcium pantothenate 20 mg/Tab. Bot. 100s. *otc.*
Use: Mineral, vitamin supplement.

Beano. (Akpharma) alpha-D-galactosidase derived from *Aspergillus niger*, a fungal source in carrier of water and glycerol. Liq. Bot. 75 serving size at 5 drops per dose. Tab. Pkg. 12s. Bot. 30s, 100s. *otc.*
Use: Antiflatulent.

Bebatab No. 2. (Freeport) Belladonna ⅙ gr, phenobarbital 0.25 gr/Tab. Bot. 1000s. *Rx.*
Use: Anticholinergic, antispasmodic, hypnotic, sedative.

•**becanthone hydrochloride.** (BEE-kan-thone) USAN.
Use: Antischistosomal.

•**becaplermin.** (beh-kah-PLER-min) USAN.
Use: Chronic dermal ulcers treatment.
See: Regranex, Gel. (Ortho-McNeil).

Beceevite Capsules. (Halsey) Vitamins C 300 mg, B_1 15 mg, B_2 10 mg, nia-

cin 50 mg, B_6 5 mg, pantothenic acid 10 mg/Tab. Bot. 100s. *otc.*
Use: Vitamin supplement.

•**beclomethasone dipropionate.** (BEK-low-METH-uh-zone die-PRO-peo-uh-NATE) U.S.P. 23.
Use: Corticosteroid, topical.
See: Beclovent Inhalation Aerosol (Allen & Hanburys).
Beconase Prods. (Allen & Hanburys).
Vancenase Prods. (Schering Plough).
Vanceril Inhaler (Schering Plough).

beclomycin dipropionate.
Use: Corticosteroid.

Beclovent Inhalation Aerosol. (Glaxo-Wellcome) Beclomethasone dipropionate 42 mcg/actuation. Canister 6.7 g (80 metered doses), 16.8 (200 metered doses), adapter. Refill canister 16.8 g. *Rx.*
Use: Corticosteroid.

Becomp-C. (Cenci) Vitamins C 250 mg, B_1 25 mg, B_2 10 mg, nicotinamide 50 mg, B_6 2 mg, calcium pantothenate 10 mg, hesperidin complex 50 mg/Cap. Bot. 100s, 500s. *otc.*
Use: Mineral, vitamin supplement.

Beconase AQ Nasal Spray. (Glaxo-Wellcome)) Beclomethasone dipropionate 42 mcg/metered spray. Pump aerosol bot. 25 g (200 metered inhalations). *Rx.*
Use: Corticosteroid.

Beconase Inhalation Aerosol. (Glaxo-Wellcome)) Beclomethasone dipropionate 42 mcg/actuation. Aerosol canister (16.8 g) containing 200 metered inhalations. Canister 16.8 g. *Rx.*
Use: Corticosteroid.

Becotin-T. (Eli Lilly) Vitamins B_1 15 mg, B_2 10 mg, B_6 5 mg, niacinamide 100 mg, pantothenic acid 20 mg, B_{12} 4 mcg, C 300 mg/Tab. Bot. 100s, 1000s, Blister pkg. 10 × 10s. *otc.*
Use: Vitamin supplement.

•**bectumomab.** (beck-TYOO-moe-mab) USAN.
Use: Monoclonal antibody (diagnosis of non-Hodgkin's lymphoma and detection of AIDS-related lymphoma).

Bedoce. (Lincoln) Crystalline anhydrous vitamin B_{12} 1000 mcg/ml. Vial 10 ml. *Rx.*
Use: Vitamin supplement.

Bedoce-Gel. (Lincoln) Vitamin B_{12} 1000 mcg/ml in 17% gelatin soln. Vial 10 ml. *Rx.*
Use: Vitamin supplement.

Bedside Care. (Sween) Bot. 8 oz, gal.
Use: Dematologic.

Beeceevites Capsules. (Halsey)
Use: Vitamin supplement.

beechwood creosote.
See: Creosote, N.F.

Bee-Forte w/C. (Rugby) Vitamins B_1 25 mg, B_2 12.5 mg, B_3 50 mg, B_5 10 mg, B_6 3 mg, B_{12} 2.5 mcg, C 250 mg/Cap. Bot. 100s. *otc.*
Use: Vitamin supplement.

beef peptones. (Sandia) Water soluble peptones derived from beef 20 mg/2 ml. Inj. Vial 30 ml. *Rx.*
Use: Nutritional supplement, parenteral.

Beelith. (Beach Pharmaceuticals) Pyridoxine HCl 20 mg, magnesium oxide 600 mg/Tab. Bot. 100s. *otc.*
Use: Mineral, vitamin supplement.

Beepen-VK. (SmithKline Beecham Pharmaceuticals) Penicillin VK. **Tab.:** 250 mg. Bot. 1000s; 500 mg. Bot. 500s. **Oral Susp.:** 125 mg/5 ml Bot. 100 ml, 200 ml; 250 mg/5 ml Bot. 100 ml, 200 ml. *Rx.*
Use: Anti-infective; penicillin.

Bee-Thi. (Burgin-Arden) Cyanocobalamin 1000 mcg, thiamine HCl 100 mg in isotonic soln. of sodium Cl/ml. Vial 10 ml, 20 ml. *Rx.*
Use: Vitamin supplement.

Bee-Twelve 1000. (Burgin-Arden) Cyanocobalamin 1000 mcg /ml. Vial 10 ml, 30 ml. *Rx.*
Use: Vitamin supplement.

Bee-Zee. (Rugby) Vitamins E 45 mg, B_1 15 mg, B_2 10.2 mg, B_3 100 mg, B_5 25 mg, B_6 10 mg, B_{12} 6 mcg, C 600 mg, zinc 5.2 mg/Tab. Bot. 60s. *otc.*
Use: Mineral, vitamin supplement.

Behepan.
See: Vitamin B_{12}.

Belatol No. 1; No. 2. (Cenci) **No. 1:** Belladonna leaf extract ⅛ gr, phenobarbital 0.25 gr/Tab. 100s, 1000s. **No. 2:** Belladonna leaf extract gr, phenobarbital 0.5 gr/Tab. Bot. 100s, 1000s. *Rx.*
Use: Anticholinergic, antispasmodic, hypnotic, sedative.

Belatol Elixir. (Cenci) Phenobarbital 20 mg, belladonna 6.75 min./5 ml w/ alcohol 45%. Elix. Bot. pt, gal. *Rx.*
Use: Anticholinergic, antispasmodic, hypnotic, sedative.

Belbutal No. 2 Kaptabs. (Churchill) Phenobarbital 32.4 mg, hyoscyamine sulfate 0.1092 mg, atropine sulfate 0.0215 mg, hyoscine HBr 0.0065 mg/Tab. Bot. 100s. *Rx.*

Use: Anticholinergic, antispasmodic, hypnotic, sedative.

Beldin. (Halsey) Diphenhydramine HCl 12.5 mg/5 ml w/alcohol 5%. Bot. gal. *otc.*
Use: Antihistamine.

Belexal. (Pal-Pak) Vitamins B_1 1.5 mg, B_2 2 mg, B_6 0.167 mg, calcium pantothenate 1 mg, niacinamide 10 mg/Tab. w/brewer's yeast. Bot. 1000s, 5000s. *otc.*
Use: Mineral, vitamin supplement.

Belexon Fortified Improved. (APC) Liver fraction No. 2, 3 gr, yeast extract 3 gr, vitamins B_1 5 mg, B_2 6 mg, niacinamide 10 mg, calcium pantothenate 2 mg, cyanocobalamin 1 mcg, iron 10 mg/Cap. Bot. 100s. *otc.*
Use: Mineral, vitamin supplement.

Belfer. (Forest Pharmaceutical) Vitamins B_1 2 mg, B_2 2 mg, B_{12} 10 mcg, B_6 2 mg, C 50 mg, iron 17 mg/Tab. Bot. 100s. *otc.*
Use: Mineral, vitamin supplement.

•**belfosdil.** (bell-FOSE-dill) USAN.
Use: Antihypertensive (calcium channel blocker).

Belganyl. CDC anti-infective agent. *Rx.*
See: Suramin.

belladonna alkaloids.
Use: Anticholinergic, antispasmodic.
W/Combinations.
See: Accelerase-PB, Cap. (Organon Teknika).
Belphen Timed Cap. (Robinson).
Coryztime, Cap. (ICN Pharmaceuticals).
Fitacol Stankaps (Standex).
Nilspasm, Tab. (Parmed).
Ultabs, Tab. (Burlington).
Urised, Tab. (PolyMedica).
U-Tract, Tab. (Jones Medical Industries).
Wigraine, Tab., Supp. (Organon Teknika).
Wyanoids, Supp. (Wyeth Ayerst).

belladonna alkaloids w/phenobarbital. (Various Mfr.) Atropine sulfate 0.0194 mg, scopolamine HBr 0.0065 mg, hyoscyamine HBr or SO_4 0.1037 mg, phenobarbital 16.2 mg/Tab. Bot. 20s, 1000s, UD 100s. *Rx.*
Use: Anticholinergic, antispasmodic, hypnotic, sedative.

•**belladonna extract.** U.S.P.23.
Use: Antispasmodic.

belladonna extract. (Eli Lilly) 15 mg (0.187 mg belladonna)/Tab.
Use: Antispasmodic.

belladonna extract combinations.
Use: Anticholinergic, antispasmodic.
See: Amobell, Cap. (Sanofi Winthrop).
Amsodyne, Tab. (ICN Pharmaceuticals).
B & O Supprettes (PolyMedica).
Belap, Tab. (Teva USA).
Bellkatal, Tab. (Ferndale Laboratories).
Butibel, Tab., Elix. (Ortho McNeil).
Gelcomul, Liq. (Del Pharmaceuticals).
Hycoff Cold, Cap. (Saron).
Phebe (Western Research).
Rectacort, Supp. (Century Pharm).

belladonna leaf.
Use: Antispasmodic.
W/Phenobarbital and benzocaine.
Use: Anticholinergic.
See: Gastrolic, Tab. (Roberts Pharm).

belladonna products and phenobarbital combinations.
Use: Anticholinergic, antispasmodic, hypnotic, sedative.
See: Accelerase-PB, Cap. (Organon Teknika).
Alised, Tab. (ICN Pharmaceuticals).
Atrocap, Cap. (Freeport).
Atrosed, Tab. (Freeport).
Bebatab, Tab. (Freeport).
Belap, Tab., Elix. (Teva USA).
Belatol, Tab., Elix. (Cenci).
Bellergal, Tab., Spacetab. (Novartis).
Bellkatal, Tab. (Ferndale Laboratories).
Bellophen, Tab. (Richlyn).
B-Sed, Tab. (Scrip).
Chardonna, Tab. (Rhone-Poulenc Rorer).
Donabarb, Tab., Elix. (ICN Pharmaceuticals).
Donnafed Jr., Tab. (Jenkins).
Donnatal, Tab., Extentab, Cap., Elix. (Robins).
Donnatal #2, Tab. (Robins).
Donnazyme, Tab. (Robins).
Gastrolic, Tab. (Roberts Pharm).
Hypnaldyne, Tab. (Vortech).
Kinesed, Tab. (Zeneca).
Mallenzyme, Tab. (Roberts Pharm).
Medi-Spas, Elix. (Medical Chemicals).
Phenobarbital and Belladonna, Tab. (Eli Lilly).
Sedapar, Tab. (Parmed).
Spabelin, Tab. (Arcum).
Spabelin No. 2, Tab.

belladonna tincture. (Eli Lilly) Bot. 4 oz, 16 oz.
Use: Antispasmodic.

Bellaneed. (Hanlon) Belladonna, phenobarbital 16 mg/Cap. Bot. 100s. *Rx.*

Use: Anticholinergic, antispasmodic, hypnotic, sedative.

Bell/ans. (C.S. Dent) Sodium bicarbonate 520 mg, sodium content 144 mg/Tab. Bot. 30s, 60s. *otc.*
Use: Antacid.

Bellastal. (Wharton) Atropine sulfate 0.0194 mg, scopolamine HBr 0.0065 mg, hyoscyamine HBr or SO_4 0.1037 mg, phenobarbital 16.2 mg Cap. Bot. 1000s. *Rx.*
Use: Anticholinergic, antispasmodic.

Bellatal. (Richwood) Phenobarbital 16.2 mg (hyoscyamine sulfate 0.1037 mg, atropine sulfate 0.0194 mg, scopolamine HBr 0.0065 mg), Lactose/Tab. Bot. 100s, 500s. *Rx.*
Use: Hypnotic, sedative.

Bellergal-S. (Novartis) Ergotamine tartrate 0.6 mg, bellafoline 0.2 mg, phenobarbital 40 mg, tartrazine, lactose, sucrose. SR Tab. Bot. 100s. *Rx.*
Use: Anticholingergic, antispasmodic, hypnotic, sedative.

•**beloxamide.** (bell-OX-ah-mid) USAN.
Use: Antihyperlipoproteinemic.

Bel-Phen-Ergot SR. (Zenith Goldline) Phenobarbital 40 mg, ergotamine tartrate 0.6 mg, l-alkaloids of belladonna 0.2 mg. Tab. Bot. 100s. *Rx.*
Use: Anticholingergic.

Bel-Phen-Ergot SR. (Zenith Goldline) l-alkaloids of belladonna 0.2 mg, phenobarbital 40 mg, ergotamine tartrate 0.6 mg, lactose/SR Tabs. Bot. 100s. *Rx.*
Use: Anticholinergic.

•**bemarinone hydrochloride.** (BEH-mah-rih-NOHN) USAN.
Use: Cardiovascular agent (positive inotropic, vasodilator).

•**bemesetron.** (beh-meh-SET-rone) USAN.
Use: Antiemetic.

Beminal 500. (Whitehall Robins) Vitamins B_1 25 mg, B_2 12.5 mg, B_3 100 mg, B_6 10 mg, B_5 20 mg, C 500 mg, B_{12} 5 mcg/Tab. Bot. 100s. *otc.*
Use: Vitamin supplement.

Beminal Forte w/Vit. C. (Wyeth Ayerst) Vitamins B_1 25 mg, B_2 12.5 mg, niacinamide 50 mg, B_6 3 mg, calcium pantothenate 10 mg, C 250 mg, B_{12} 2.5 mcg/Cap. Bot. 100s. *otc.*
Use: Mineral, vitamin supplement.

Beminal Stress Plus Iron. (Wyeth Ayerst) Vitamins B_1 25 mg, B_2 12.5 mg, B_3 100 mg, B_5 20 mg, B_6 10 mg, B_{12} 25 mcg, folic acid 400 mcg, C 700 mg, E 45 IU, iron 27 mg. Dye-free. Tab. Bot. 60s. *otc.*
Use: Mineral, vitamin supplement.

Beminal Stress Plus Zinc. (Wyeth Ayerst) Vitamins B_1 25 mg, B_2 12.5 mg, B_3 100 mg, B_5 20 mg, B_6 10 mg, B_{12} 25 mcg, C 700 mg, E 45 IU, zinc 45 mg/Tab. Bot. 60s, 250s. *otc.*
Use: Mineral, vitamin supplement.

•**bemitradine.** (beh-MIH-trah-DEEN) USAN.
Use: Antihypertensive, diuretic.

•**bemoradan.** (beh-MOE-rah-DAN) USAN.
Use: Cardiovascular agent.

Benacen. (Cenci) Probenecid 0.5 g/Tab. Bot. 100s, 1000s. *Rx.*
Use: Anitgout.

Benacol. (Cenci) Dicyclomine HCl 20 mg/Tab. Bot. 100s, 1000s. *Rx.*
Use: Anticholinergic, antispasmodic.

benactyzine hydrochloride. 2-Diethylaminoethyl benzilate HCl.
Use: Anxiolytic.
W/Meprobamate.
See: Deprol, Tab. (Wallace Laboratories).

benactyzine/meprobamate. Psychotherapeutic combination.
See: Deprol (Wallace Laboratories).

Benadryl. (Parke-Davis) Diphenhydramine HCl. *otc, Rx.* **Cream:** 1%. Tube 1 oz. **Elix. (w/alcohol 14%):** 12.5 mg/5 ml. Bot. 4 oz, pt, gal, UD 5 ml 100s. **Spray:** 1%. Bot. 2 oz. **Tab.:** 25 mg. Bot. 100s.
Use: Antihistamine.

Benadryl Allergy. (Warner Lambert Consumer Health Products) Diphenhydramine HCl, phenylalanine 4.2 mg. **Chew. Tab.:** 12.5 mg/Tab. Pkg. 24s. **Liq.:** 6.25 mg/5 ml. Liq. Bot. 118 ml. *otc.*
Use: Antihistamine.

Benadryl Allergy Decongestant Liquid. (Warner Lambert Consumer Health Products) Pseudoephedrine HCl 30mg, diphenhydramine HCl 12.5 mg/5ml. Liq. Bot. 118 ml. *otc.*
Use: Antihistamine, decongestant.

Benadryl Allergy/Sinus Headache Caplets. (Warner Lambert Consumer Health Products) Pseudoephedrine HCl 30 mg, diphenhydramine HCl 12.5 mg, acetaminophen 500 mg/Capl. Bot. 24s. *otc.*
Use: Analgesic, antihistamine, decongestant.

Benadryl Allergy Ultratabs. (Warner Lambert Consumer) Diphenhydramine HCl 25 mg. Tab. 24s, 48s. *otc.*
Use: Antihistamine.

Benadryl Cold Liquid. (Parke-Davis)

Pseudoephedrine HCl 10 mg, diphenhydramine HCl 8.3 mg, acetaminophen 167 mg, alcohol 10%, saccharin. Liq. Bot. 180 ml. *otc.*
Use: Antihistamine, decongestant.

Benadryl Cough Preparation.
See: Benylin Cough Syrup (Parke-Davis).

Benadryl Decongestant Allergy Capsules. (Warner Lambert Consumer Health Products) Diphenhydramine HCl 25 mg, pseudoephedrine HCl 60 mg/Cap. Box 24s. *otc.*
Use: Antihistamine, decongestant.

Benadryl Dye Free. (Warner Lambert Consumer Health Products) Diphenhydramine HCl 6.25 mg/5 ml. Liq. 236 ml. *otc.*
Use: Antihistamine.

Benadryl Dye-Free Allergy Liqui Gels. (Parke-Davis) Diphenhydramine HCl 25 mg, sorbitol/Softgel Cap/Bot. 24s. *otc.*
Use: Antihistamine.

Benadryl Dye Free LiquiGels. (Glaxo-Wellcome) Diphenhydramine HCl 25 mg/Cap. Pkg. 24s. *otc.*
Use: Antihistamine.

Benadryl Elixir. (Parke-Davis) Diphenhydramine HCl 12.5 mg/5 ml w/alcohol 14%. Bot. 4 oz, pt, gal, UD (5 ml) 100s. *otc.*
Use: Antihistamine.

Benadryl Injection. (Parke-Davis) Diphenhydramine HCl. 50 mg/ml Inj. Amp. 1 ml, Steri-Vials 10ml, Steri-dose syringe 1 ml. *Rx.*
Use: Antihistamine.

Benadryl Itch Relief. (GlaxoWellcome) Diphenhydramine HCl 1%, zinc acetate 0.1%, alcohol 73.6%, aloe vera. Spray. 59 ml. *otc.*
Use: Antihistamine.

Benadryl Itch Relief Children's. (Glaxo-Wellcome) **Cream:** Diphenhydramine HCl 1%, zinc acetate 0.1%, aloe vera, cetyl alcohol, parabens. Jar 14.2 g. **Spray:** Diphenhydramine HCl 1%, zinc acetate 0.1%, alcohol 73.6%, aloe vera, povidone. Can. 59 ml. *otc.*
Use: Antihistamine.

Benadryl Itch Relief, Maximum Strength. (GlaxoWellcome) **Cream:** Diphenhydramine HCl 2%, zinc acetate 0.1%, parabens, aloe vera. 14.2 g. **Stick:** Diphenhydramine HCl 2%, zinc acetate 0.1%, alcohol 73.5%, aloe vera. 14 ml.

Benadryl Itch Stopping Gel Children's Formula. (GlaxoWellcome) Diphenhydramine HCl 1%, zinc acetate 1%. Tube 118 ml. *otc.*
Use: Antihistamine.

Benadryl Itch Stopping Gel Maximum Strength. (GalxoWellcome) Diphenhydramine HCl 2%, zinc acetate 1%. Tube 118 g. *otc.*
Use: Antihistamine.

Benadryl Maximum Strength. (Parke-Davis) **Cream:** Diphenhydramine HCl 2% and parabens in a greaseless base in 15 g. **Non-aerosol spray:** Diphenhydramine HCl 2%, alcohol 85% in 60 ml. *otc.*
Use: Dermatologic.

Benadryl Plus. (Parke-Davis) Pseudoephedrine 30 mg, diphenhydramine 12.5 mg, acetaminophen 500 mg/Tab. 24s. *otc.*
Use: Analgesic, antihistamine, decongestant.

Benadryl Plus Nighttime. (Parke-Davis). Pseudoephedrine 30 mg, diphenhydramine 25 mg, acetaminophen 500 mg/5 ml. 180 ml, 300 ml. *otc.*
Use: Analgesic, antihistamine, decongestant.

Benahist 10. (Keene Pharmaceuticals) Diphenhydramine 10 mg/ml. Vial 30 ml. *Rx.*
Use: Antihistamine.

Benahist 50. (Keene Pharmaceuticals) Diphenhydramine 50 mg/ml. Vial 10 ml. *Rx.*
Use: Antihistamine.

benanserin hydrochloride.
Use: Serotonin antagonist.

Benapen.
See: Benethamine.

Benaphen Caps. (Major) Diphenhydramine 25 mg or 50 mg/Cap. Bot. 100s, 1000s. *otc, Rx.*
Use: Antihistamine.

•**benapryzine hydrochloride.** (BEN-ah-PRY-zeen) USAN.
Use: Anticholinergic.

Benase. (Ferndale Laboratories) Proteolytic enzymes extracted from Carica papaya 20,000 units enzyme activity. Tab. Bot. 1000s. *Rx.*
Use: Reduction of edema, relief of episiotomy.

Benat-12. (Roberts Pharm) Cyanocobalamin 30 mcg, liver injection 0.5 ml, vitamins B_1 10 mg, B_2 2 mg, niacinamide 50 mg, d-panthenol 1 mg, B_6 1 mg/ml, benzyl alcohol 4%, phenol 0.5%. Vial 10 ml. *Rx.*

Use: Mineral, vitamin supplement.

•**benazepril hydrochloride.** (BEN-AZE-eh-prill) USAN.
Use: ACE inhibitor.
See: Lotensin (Novartis Pharmaceuticals).

•**benazeprilat.** (BEN-AZE-eh-prill-at) USAN.
Use: ACE inhibitor.

•**bendacalol mesylate.** (ben-DACK-ah-LOLE) USAN.
Use: Antihypertensive.

•**bendazac.** (BEN-dah-ZAK) USAN.
Use: Antiinflammatory.

•**bendroflumethiazide,** U.S.P. 23.
Use: Antihypertensive, diuretic.
See: Naturetin, Tab. (Bristol-Myers Squibb).
W/Potassium Cl.
See: Naturetin W-K, Tab. (Bristol-Myers Squibb).
W/Rauwolfia serpentina.
See: Rauzide, Tab. (Bristol-Myers Squibb)
W/Rauwolfia serpentina, potassium Cl.
See: Rautrax-N, Tab. (Bristol-Myers Squibb).
Rautrax-N Modified, Tab. (Bristol-Myers Squibb).

BeneFix. (Genetics Inst) Non-pyrogenic lyophilized powder preparation. Purified protein produced by recombinant DNA. Single dose vial with diluent needle, filter, infusion set and alcohol swabs. 250, 500 and 1000 IU. *Rx.*
Use: For use in therapy of Factor IX deficiency.

Benemid. (Merck) Probenecid 0.5 g/Tab. Bot. 100s, 1000s, UD 100s. *Rx.*
Use: Antigout.
W/Colchicine.
See: Colbenemid, Tab. (Merck).

Benephen Antiseptic Medicated Powder. (Halsted) Methylbenzethonium Cl 1:1800, magnesium carbonate in cornstarch base. Shaker can 3.56 oz. *otc.*
Use: Antiseptic, deodorant.

Benephen Antiseptic Ointment w/Cod Liver Oil. (Halsted) Methylbenzethonium Cl 1:1000, water-repellent base of zinc oxide, cornstarch. Tube 1.5 oz, jar lb. *otc.*
Use: Antiseptic.

Benephen Antiseptic Vitamin A & D Cream. (Halsted) Methylbenzethonium Cl 1:1000, cod liver oil w/vitamins A and D in petrolatum and glycerin base. Tube 2 oz, jar lb. *otc.*
Use: Antiseptic.

Benepro Tabs. (Major) Probenecid 500 mg/Tab. Bot. 100s, 1000s. *Rx.*
Use: Antigout.

bengal gelatin.
See: Agar.

Ben-Gay Children's Vaporizing Rub. (Pfizer) Camphor, menthol, w/oils of turpentine, eucalyptus, cedar leaf, nutmeg, thyme in stainless white base. Jar 1.125 oz. *otc.*
Use: Analgesic, topical.

Ben-Gay Extra Strength Balm. (Pfizer) Methylsalicylate 30%, menthol 8%. Jar 3.75 oz. *otc.*
Use: Analgesic, topical.

Ben-Gay Extra Strength Sports Balm. (Pfizer) Methylsalicylate 28%, menthol 10%. Tube 1.25 oz, 3 oz. *otc.*
Use: Analgesic, topical.

Ben-Gay Gel. (Pfizer) Methylsalicylate 15%, menthol 7%, alcohol 40%. Tube 1.25 oz, 3 oz. *otc.*
Use: Analgesic, topical.

Ben-Gay Greaseless Ointment. (Pfizer) Methylsalicylate 18.3%, menthol 16%. Tube 1.25 oz, 3 oz, 5 oz. *otc.*
Use: Analgesic, topical.

Ben-Gay Lotion. (Pfizer) Methylsalicylate 15%, menthol 7% in lotion base. Bot. 2 oz, 4 oz. *otc.*
Use: Analgesic, topical.

Ben-Gay Original. (Pfizer) Methyl salicylate 18.3% and menthol 16%. Oint. Tube. 37.5 g, 90 g, 150 g. *otc.*
Use: Analgesic, topical.

Ben-Gay Ointment. (Pfizer) Methylsalicylate 15%, menthol 10% in ointment base. Tube 1.25 oz, 3 oz, 5 oz. *otc.*
Use: Analgesic, topical.

Ben-Gay Sportsgel. (Pfizer) Methylsalicylate, menthol, alcohol 40%. Tube 1.25 oz, 3 oz. *otc.*
Use: Analgesic, topical.

Benoquin. (ICN Pharmaceuticals) Monobenzone 20% in cream base. Tube 35 g, 453.6 g. *Rx.*
Use: Dermatologic.

•**benorterone.** (bee-NAHR-ter-ohn) USAN.
Use: Antiandrogen.

•**benoxaprofen.** (ben-OX-ah-PRO-fen) USAN.
Use: Anti-inflammatory, analgesic.

•**benoxinate hydrochloride,** (ben-OX-ih-nate) U.S.P. 23.
Use: Anesthetic (topical).
See: Flurate, Soln. (Bausch & Lomb).
Fluress (PBH Wesley Jessen).

Benoxyl Lotion. (Stiefel) Benzoyl per-

oxide 5% or 10% in mild lotion base. Bot. 30 ml, 60 ml. *otc.*
Use: Antiacne.

•**benperidol.** (BEN-peh-rih-dahl) USAN.
Use: Antipsychotic.
See: Anquil.

•**bensalan.** (BEN-sal-an) USAN. Under study.
Use: Disinfectant.

•**benserazide.** (ben-SER-ah-zide) USAN.
Use: Inhibitor (decarboxylase); antiparkinson.

Bensulfoid. (ECR Pharmaceuticals) Sulfur 8%, resorcinol 2%, alcohol 12%. Cream 15 g. *otc.*
Use: Antiacne.

•**bentazepam.** (BEN-tay-zeh-pam) USAN.
Use: Hypnotic, sedative.

Bentical. (Lamond) Bentonite, zinc oxide, zinc carbonate, titanium dioxide. Bot. 4 oz, 6 oz, 8 oz, 16 oz, 32 oz, 0.5 gal, gal.
Use: Emollient.

•**bentiromide.** (ben-TIRE-oh-mide) USAN.
Use: Diagnostic aid (pancreas function determination).
See: Chymex, Soln. (Pharmacia & Upjohn).

•**bentonite,** N.F. 18.
Use: Pharmaceutic aid (suspending agent).

bentonite magma.
Use: Pharmaceutic aid (suspending agent).

bentonite, purified.
Use: Pharmaceutic aid.

•**bentoquatam.** (BEN-toe-KWAH-tam) USAN.
Use: Barrier for prevention of allergic contact dermatitis.

Bentyl. (SmithKline Beecham Pharmaceuticals) Dicyclomine HCl. **Cap.:** 10 mg. Bot. 100s, 500s, UD 100s. **Tab.:** 20 mg. Bot. 100s, 500s, 1000s, UD 100s. **Syr.:** 10 mg/5 ml. Bot. pt. **Inj.:** 10 mg/ml. Amp. 2 ml, syringe 2 ml. Vial 10 ml (also contains chlorobutanol). *Rx.*
Use: Anticholinergic, antispasmodic.

•**benurestat.** (BEN-YOU-reh-stat) USAN.
Use: Enzyme inhibitor (urease).

Benylin Adult. (Warner Lambert Consumer Health Products) Dextromethorphan HBr 15 mg/5 ml. Liq. Bot. 118 ml. *otc.*
Use: Antitussive.

Benylin DM Cough Syrup. (Parke-Davis) Dextromethorphan HBr 10 mg/5 ml, alcohol 5%. Bot. 4 oz, 8 oz. *otc.*
Use: Antitussive.

Benylin DME. (Parke-Davis) **Liq.:** Dextromethorphan HBr 5 mg, guaifenesin 100 mg, alcohol 5%, saccharin, menthol. Bot. 240 ml. *otc.*
Use: Antitussive, expectorant.

Benylin Expectorant Liquid. (Glaxo-Wellcome) Dextromethorphan HBr 5 mg, guaifenesin 100 mg, saccharin, menthol, sucrose, alcohol free. Bot. Liq. 118, 236 ml. *otc.*
Use: Antitussive, expectorant.

Benylin Multi-Symptom. (Glaxo-Wellcome) Dextromethorphan HBr 5 mg, pseudoephedrine HCl 15 mg, guaifenesin 100 mg/5 ml. Liq. Bot. 118 ml. *otc.*
Use: Antitussive, decongestant, expectorant.

Benylin Pediatric. (Warner Lambert Consumer Health Products) Dextromethorphan HBr 7.5 mg/5 ml, EDTA, saccharin, sorbitol, alcohol free. Liq. Bot. 118 ml. *otc.*
Use: Antitussive.

Benza. (Century Pharm) Benzalkonium Cl 1:5000 and 1:750. Bot. 2 oz, 4 oz.
Use: Antimicrobial, antiseptic.

Benzac 5 & 10. (Galderma) Benzoyl peroxide 5% or 10%, alcohol 12%. Tube 60 g, 90 g. *Rx.*
Use: Antiacne.

Benzac w/ 2.5, 5 & 10. (Galderma) Benzoyl peroxide 2.5%, 5%, 10%. Tube 60 g, 90 g. *Rx.*
Use: Antiacne.

Benzac AC 2.5, 5, & 10. (Galderma) Benzoyl peroxide 2.5%, 5% or 10%, glycerine and EDTA in water base. Gel. Tube. 60 g, 90 g. *Rx.*
Use: Antiacne.

Benzac AC Wash 2.5, 5, & 10. (Galderma) Benzoyl peroxide 2.5%, 5%, 10%, glycerin. Liq. Bot. 240 ml. *Rx.*
Use: Antiacne.

Benzac w Wash 5, & 10. (Galderma) Benzoyl peroxide 5% or 10%. **5%:** Bot. 120 ml, 240 ml. **10%:** Bot. 240 ml. *Rx.*
Use: Antiacne.

5- & 10-Benzagel. (Dermik Laboratories) Benzoyl peroxide 5% or 10% in gel base of water, alcohol 14%, laureth-4 6% (10% only). Tube 42.5 g, 85 g. *Rx.*
Use: Antiacne.

benzalkonium chloride. (benz-al-KOE-nee-uhm) N.F. 18.
Use: Surface antiseptic; pharmaceutical aid (preservatitive).
See: Benz-All, Liq. (Xttrium).
Econopred, Susp. (Alcon Laboratories).

Eye-Stream (Alcon Laboratories).
Germicin, Soln. (Consolidated Mid.).
Hyamine 3500 (Rohm and Haas).
Otrivin Spray (Novartis Pharmaceuticals).
Ultra Tears (Alcon Laboratories).
Zephiran Chloride Preps. (Sanofi Winthrop).

W/Aluminum Cl, oxyquinoline sulfate.
See: Alochor Styptic, Liq. (Gordon Laboratories).

W/Bacitracin zinc, polymyxin B, neomycin sulfate.
See: Biotres, Oint. (Schwarz Pharma).

W/Benzocaine, benzyl alcohol.
See: Aerocaine, Oint. (Aeroceuticals).

W/Benzocaine, orthohydroxyphenyl-mercuric Cl, parachlorometaxylenol.
See: Unguentine, Aerosol (Procter & Gamble).

W/Berberine HCl, sodium borate, phenylephrine HCl, sodium Cl, boric acid.
See: Ocusol, Eye Lotion, Drops (Procter & Gamble).

W/Boric acid, potassium Cl, sodium carbonate anhydrous, disodium edetate.
See: Swim-Eye, Drops (Savage).

W/Chlorophyll.
See: Mycomist, Spray Liq. (Gordon Laboratories).

W/Hydrocortisone.
See: Barseb Thera-Spray, Soln. (PBH Wesley Jessen).

W/Diperodon HCl, carbolic acid, ichthammol, thymol, camphor, juniper tar.
See: Boro Oint. (Scrip).

W/Disodium edetate, potassium Cl, isotonic boric acid.
See: Dacriose (Smith, Miller & Patch).

W/Epinephrine.
See: Epinal, Soln. (Alcon Laboratories).

W/Epinephrine bitartrate, pilocarpine HCl, mannitol.
See: E-Pilo Ophth., Preps. (Smith, Miller & Patch).

W/Ethoxylated lanolin, methylparaben, hamamelis water, glycerin.
See: Medicone, clothwipes. (Medicone).

W/Gentamicin sulfate disodium phosphate, monosodium, phosphate, sodium Cl.
See: Garamycin Ophth. Soln., Preps. (Schering Plough).

W/Hydroxypropyl methylcellulose.
See: Isopto Plain & Tears (Alcon Laboratories).

W/Hydroxypropyl methylcellulose, disodium edetate.
See: Goniosol (Smith, Miller & Patch).

W/Isopropyl alcohol, methyl salicylate.
See: Cydonol Massage Lotion (Gordon Laboratories).

W/Lidocaine, phenol.
See: Unguentine, spray (Procter & Gamble).

W/Methylcellulose.
See: Tearisol (Smith, Miller & Patch).

W/Methylcellulose, phenylephrine HCl.
See: Efricel % (Professional Pharmacal).

W/Oxyquinolin sulfate, distilled water.
See: Oxyzal Wet Dressing, Soln. (Gordon Laboratories).

W/Phenylephrine, pyrilamine maleate, antipyrine.
See: Prefrin-A, Ophth. (Allergan).

W/Pilocarpine HCl, epinephrine bitartrate, mannitol.
See: E-Pilo Ophth., Preps. (Smith, Miller & Patch).

W/Polymyxin B, neomycin sulfate, zinc bacitracin.
See: Biotres, Oint. (Schwarz Pharma).

W/Polyoxyethylene ethers.
See: Ionax, Aerosol Can (Galderma).

W/Polyvinyl alcohol.
See: Contique Artificial Tears (Alcon Laboratories).

W/Pramoxine.

benzalkonium chloride.
Use: Antiseptic.
See: Ony-Clear, Soln. (Pedinol).
Bacti-Cleanse, Liq. (Pedinol).
Mycocide NS, Sol. (Woodward).

•**benzbromarone.** (BENZ-brome-ah-rone) USAN.
Use: Uricosuric.

•**benzethonium chloride,** (benz-eth-OH-nee-uhm) U.S.P. 23.
Use: Anti-infective, topical, pharmaceutic aid (preservative).

•**benzetimide hydrochloride.** (benz-ETT-ih-mide HIGH-droe-klor-ide) USAN.
Use: Anticholinergic.

•**benzilonium bromide.** (BEN-zill-oh-nih-uhm-BROE-mide) USAN.
Use: Anticholinergic.

•**benzindopyrine hydrochloride.** (BENZ-in-doe-pie-reen HIGH-droe-KLOR-ide) USAN.
Use: Antipsychotic.

benzoate and pheylacetate.
Use: Treatment of hyperammonemia. [Orphan drug]
See: Ucephan (Kendall McGraw).

Benzo-C. (Freeport) Benzocaine 5 mg, cetalkonium Cl 5 mg, ascorbic acid 50 mg/Troche. Bot. 1000s, cello-packed boxes 1000s. *otc.*
Use: Anesthetic, local.

•**benzocaine.** U.S.P. 23. Ethyl-p-aminobenzoate. Anesthesin, orthesin, parathesin.
Use: Anesthetic, topical.
See: BanSmoke, Gum (Thompson Medical).
Trocaine, Loz. (Roberts Pharm).
SensoGARD, Gel. (Block).
Cēpacol Maximum Strength, Loz. (JB Williams).
W/Combinations.
See: Aerocaine, Oint. (Aeroceuticals).
Aerotherm, Oint. (Aeroceuticals).
Americaine, Oint., Aerosol (DuPont Merck Pharmaceuticals).
Anacaine, Oint. (Gordon Laboratories).
Auralgan, Otic Drops (Wyeth Ayerst).
Auralgesic, Liq. (ICN Pharmaceuticals).
Benadex, Oint. (Fuller).
Benzo-C, Troche (Freeport).
Benzocol, Oint. (Roberts Pharm).
Benzodent, Oint. (Procter & Gamble).
Bicozene, Cream. (Novartis).
Boil-Ease Anesthetic, Oint (Del Pharmaceuticals).
Bowman Drawing Paste, Oint. (Jones Medical Industries).
20-Cain Burn Relief, (Alto Pharmaceuticals).
Calamatum, Preps. (Blair).
Cetacaine, Preps. (Cetylite Industries).
Chiggerex, Oint. (Scherer).
Chigger-Tox, Liq. (Scherer).
Chloraseptic Children's Lozenges (Procter & Gamble).
Cēpacol, Troches (Hoechst Marion Roussel).
CPI Hemorrhoidal, Supp. (Century Pharm).
Culminal, Cream (Culminal).
D.D.D. Cream (Campana).
Dent's Dental Poultice (C.S. Dent).
Dent's Lotion, Jel (C.S. Dent).
Dent's Toothache Gum (C.S. Dent).
Derma Medicone (Medicone).
Derma Medicone-HC (Medicone).
Dermoplast, Lot (Wyeth Ayerst).
Detane, Gel (Del Pharmaceuticals).
Diplan, Cap. (Solvay).
Dulzit, Cream (Del Pharmaceuticals).
Epinephricaine, Oint. (Pharmacia & Upjohn).
Erase, Supp. (LaCrosse).
E.R.O. Forte, Liq. (Scherer).
Foille, Preps. (Carbisulphoil).
Foille, Spray (Blistex).
Foille Medicated First Aid, Oint, Spray. (Blistex).
Foille Plus, Spray (Blistex)
Formula 44 Cough Control Discs, Loz. (Procter & Gamble).
Fung-O-Spray (Scrip).
G.B.A. Drops (Scrip).
Hemocaine, Oint. (Roberts Pharm).
Hurricaine, Liq, Spray or Gel (Beutlich).
Isodettes Loz. (SmithKline Beecham Pharmaceuticals).
Jiffy, Drops (Block Drug).
Lanacane, Spray, Cream (Whitehall Robins).
Listerine Cough Control Lozenges (Warner Lambert).
Maximum Strength Anbesol, Liq, Gel (Whitehall Robins).
Medicone Dressing (Medicone).
Meditrating Throat Lozenge, Loz. (Procter & Gamble).
My-Cort Drops (Scrip).
Myringacaine, Liq. (Pharmacia & Upjohn).
Nilatus, Loz. (Jones Medical Industries).
Off-Ezy Corn Remover, Liq. (Del Pharmaceuticals).
Oracin, Loz. (Procter & Gamble).
Orabase Gel (Colgate-Palmolive).
Oradex-C, Troche (Del Pharmaceuticals).
Orajel Mouth-Aid, Liq, Gel (Del Pharmaceuticals).
Ora-Jel, Gel. (Del Pharmaceuticals).
Pazo, Oint., Supp. (Bristol-Myers).
Pyrogallic Acid Oint. (Gordon Laboratories).
Rectal Medicone (Medicone).
Rectal Medicone-HC, Supp. (Medicone).
Rectal Medicone Unguent (Medicone).
Scrip, Preps. (Scrip).
Solarcaine, Lot, Spray (Schering Plough).
Spec-T Sore Throat-Cough Suppressant Loz. (Bristol-Myers Squibb).
Spec-T Sore Throat-Decongestant Loz. (Bristol-Myers Squibb).
Sucrets Cold Decongestant Lozenge (SmithKline Beecham Pharmaceuticals).
Sucrets Cough Control Lozenge (SmithKline Beecham Pharmaceuticals).
Tanac, Liq. (Del Pharmaceuticals).
Toothache Gel (Roberts Pharm).
Tympagesic, Liq. (Pharmacia & Upjohn).
Unguentine Aerosol (Procter & Gamble).

Vicks Cough Silencers, Loz. (Procter & Gamble).
Vicks Formula 44 Cough Control Discs, Loz. (Procter & Gamble).
Vicks Medi-Trating Throat Lozenges, Loz. (Procter & Gamble).
Vicks Oracin, Loz. (Procter & Gamble).
Zilactin-B Medicated, Gel (Zila).

benzochlorophene sodium. The sodium salt of ortho-benzyl-para-chlorophenol.

•**benzoctamine hydrochloride.** (benz-OCK-tah-meen) USAN.
Use: Hypnotic, muscle relaxant, sedative.

Benzodent. (Procter & Gamble) Benzocaine 20%. Tube 30 g. *otc.*
Use: Anesthetic, local.

•**benzodepa.** (BEN-zoe-DEH-pah) USAN.
Use: Antineoplastic.

benzoic acid. (Various Mfr.) Pkg. 0.25 lb, 1 lb. *otc.*
Use: Antifungal, fungistatic.

•**benzoic acid,** (ben-ZOE-ik) U.S.P. 23.
Use: Pharmaceutic aid (antifungal).
W/Boric acid, zinc oxide, zinc stearate.
See: Ting, Cream, Pow. (Novartis Pharmaceuticals).
W/Salicylic acid.
See: Whitfield's Oint. (Various Mfr.).

benzoic acid, 2-hydroxy. Salicylic Acid.

benzoic and salicylic acids ointment.
Use: Antifungal, topical.
See: Whitfield's Oint. (Various Mfr.).

•**benzoin,** (BEN-zoyn) U.S.P. 23.
Use: Topical protectant, expectorant.
See: Arcum–Bot. 2 oz, 4 oz, pt, gal.
Lilly–Bot. 4 fl oz, pt.
Rals–Aerosol 12 oz.
Stanlabs–Bot. 2 oz, 4 oz, pt, Compound. Bot. 1 oz, 4 oz, pt.
W/Methyl salicylate, guaiacol.
See: Methagual, Oint. (Gordon Laboratories).
W/Podophyllum resin.
See: Podoben, Liq. (Maurry).
W/Polyoxyethylene dodecanol, aromatics.
See: Vicks Vaposteam, Liq. (Procter & Gamble).

Benzoin Spray. (Morton International) Benzoin, tolu balsam, styrax, alcohol w/propellant. Aerosol can 7 oz. *otc.*
Use: Skin protectant.

benzol. Usually refers to benzene.

Benzo-Menth Tablets. (Pal-Pak) Benzocaine 2.2 mg/Tab. Bot. 1000s. *otc.*
Use: Anesthetic, topical.

•**benzonatate.** (ben-ZOE-nah-tate) U.S.P. 23.
Use: Antitussive.
See: Tessalon, Perles (DuPont Merck Pharmaceuticals).

benzonatate softgels. (Various Mfr.) Benzonatate 100 mg. Cap. Bot. 100s, 1000s. *Rx.*
Use: Antitussive.

benzophenone.
See: Pan Ultra, Lot., Lipstick (Baker Norton).
W/Oxybenzone, dioxybenzone.
See: Solbar Lotion (Person & Covey).

benzopyrrolate.
See: Benzopyrronium.

benzoquinolimine.
See: Emete-Con (Pfizer).

benzoquinonium chloride. (Various Mfr.) *Rx.*
Use: Muscle relaxant.

benzosulfimide.
See: Saccharin, U.S.P. 23.

benzosulphinide sodium. Name previously used for Saccharin Sodium.

•**benzoxiquine.** (benz-OX-ee-kwine) USAN.
Use: Disinfectant.

benzoyl p-aminosalicylic. (BEN-zoyl)
See: Benzapas, Pow., Tab. (Novartis).

•**benzoylpas calcium.** (benz-oe-ILL-pass) USAN.
Use: Anti-infective (tuberculostatic).
See: Benzapas, Tab., Pow. (Novartis).

benzoyl peroxide, hydrous, (BEN-zoyl per-OX-ide) Peroxide, dibenzoyl. (Various) **Mask:** 5%. In 30 ml. **Lotion:** 5%, 10%. Bot. 30 ml. **Gel:** 5%, 10%. 45 g, 90 g (10% only).
Use: Keratolytic.

•**benzoyl peroxide, hydrous,** (BEN-zoyl per-OX-ide) U.S.P. 23.
Use: Keratolytic.
See: Benoxyl, Lot. (Stiefel)
Benzac AC, Gel, Liq. (Galderma).
Benzagel-5 & 10, Oint. (Dermik Laboratories).
Brevoxyl, Gel (Stiefel).
Clearasil Acne Treatment, Cream (Procter & Gamble).
Clearasil Antibacterial Acne Lotion (Procter & Gamble).
Dermoxyl, Gel (Zeneca).
Epi-Clear Antiseptic Lotion, Scrub (Bristol-Myers Squibb).
Exact, Cream (Advanced Polymer Systems).
Oxy Wash Antibacterial Skin Wash (SmithKline Beecham Pharmaceuticals).

Panoxyl, Bar (Stiefel).
Peroxin A5, A10, Gel (Dermol).
Persadox, Cream, Lot. (Ortho McNeil).
Persadox HP, Cream, Lot. (Galderma).
Persa-Gel, Gel (Ortho McNeil).
Theroxide, Liq., Lot. (Medicis Dermatologics).
Triaz, Gel (Medicus Dermatologics).
W/Chlorhydroxyquinoline, hydrocortisone.
See: Loroxide-HC, Lot. (Dermik Laboratories).
Vanoxide-HC, Lot. (Dermik Laboratories).
W/Polyoxyethylene lauryl ether.
See: Benzac 5 & 10, Gel (Galderma).
Desquam-X, Gel (Westwood Squibb).
W/Sulfur.
See: Sulfoxyl Lotion (Stiefel).

Benzoyl Peroxide Wash, 5% & 10%. (Glades) Benzoyl peroxide 5%. Liq. Bot. 120 ml, 150 ml, 240 ml. 10%. Liq. Bot. 150 ml, 240 ml. *Rx.*
Use: Keratolytic.

n'-benzoylsulfanilamide.
See: Sulfabenzamide.
W/Sulfacetamide, sulfathiazole, urea.
See: Sultrin, Tab, Cream (Ortho McNeil).

benzphetamine hydrochloride. (benz-FET-uh-meen) N-Benzyl-N-α-dimethylphenethylamine HCl, dextro. *c-III.*
Use: Anorexiant.
See: Didrex, Tab. (Pharmacia & Upjohn).

benzpyrinium bromide.

•**benzquinamide.** (benz-KWIN-ah-mid) USAN.
Use: Antiemetic.
See: Emete-Con, Vial (Roerig).

benzquinamide hydrochloride.
See: Emete-Con. (Roerig).

benzthianide.

•**benzthiazide,** (benz-THIGH-ah-zide) U.S.P. 23.
Use: Antihypertensive, diuretic.
See: Aquatag, Tab. (Solvay).
Exna, Tab. (Robins).
Hydrex, Tab. (Trimen).
Proaqua, Tab. (Solvay).
W/Reserpine.
See: Exna-R, Tab. (Robins).

•**benztropine mesylate,** (BENZ-troe-peen) U.S.P. 23.
Use: Parasympatholytic, antiparkinsonian.
W/sodium Cl.
See: Cogentin, Tab., Amp. (Merck).

benztropine methanesulfonate.
See: Benztropine mesylate.

•**benzydamine hydrochloride.** (ben-ZIH-dah-meen) USAN.
Use: Analgesic, anti-inflammatory, antipyretic.

benzydroflumethiazide.
See: Bendroflumethiazide.

benzyhydryl-n-methylpiperazine hydrochloride.
See: n-benzyhydryl-n-methylpiperazine HCl.

•**benzyl alcohol.** N.F. 18. Phenylcarbinol.
Use: Anesthetic, antiseptic, topical, pharmaceutic aid (antimicrobial).
See: Topic, Gel (Ingram).
Vicks Blue Mint, Regular & Wild Cherry Medicated Cough Drops (Procter & Gamble).

•**benzyl benzoate,** U.S.P. 23.
Use: Pharmaceutical necessity for Dimercaprol Inj.

benzyl benzoate saponated. Triethanolamine 20 g, oleic acid 80 g, benzyl benzoate q.s. 1000 ml.

benzyl carbinol.
See: Phenylethyl Alcohol, U.S.P. 23.

benzylpenicillin, benzylpenicilloic, benzylpenilloic acid. (Kremers Urban)
Use: Assessment of penicillin sensitivity. [Orphan drug]
See: Pre-Pen/MDM.

benzyl penicillin-C-14. (Nuclear-Chicago) Carbon-14 labelled penicillin. Vacuum-sealed glass vial 50 microcuries, 0.5 millicuries.
Use: Radiopharmaceutical.

benzyl penicillin G, potassium.
See: Penicillin G Potassium.

benzyl penicillin G, sodium.
See: Penicillin G Sodium.

•**benzylpenicilloyl polylysine concentrate.** U.S.P. 23.
Use: Diagnostic aid (penicillin sensitivity).
See: Pre-Pen (Kremers Urban).

bepanthen.
See: Panthenol.

bephedin. Benzyl ephedrine.

bephenium bromide.

bephenium hydroxynaphthoate, U.S.P. XXI.
Use: Anthelmintic (hookworms).

•**bepridil hydrochloride.** USAN.
Use: Vasodilator.
See: Vascor (Ortho McNeil).

•**beractant.** (ber-ACT-ant) USAN.
Use: Lung surfactant. [Orphan drug]
See: Survanta (Ross Laboratories).

beractant intrathecal suspension.
Use: Lung surfactant. [Orphan drug]
See: Survanta.

•**beraprost.** USAN.
Use: Platelet aggregation inhibitor, improves ischemic syndromes.

•**beraprost sodium.** (BEH-reh-prahst) USAN.
Use: Platelet aggregation inhibitor, improves ischemic action.

berberine.
W/Hydrastine, glycerin.
See: Murine, Ophth. Soln.

berberine hydrochloride.
W/Borax, sodium Cl, boric acid, camphor water, cherry laurel water, rose water, thimerosol.
See: Lauro, eye irrigator and drops (Otis Clapp).

•**berefrine.** (BEH-reh-FREEN) USAN. Formerly Burefrine.
Use: Mydriatic.

Ber-Ex. (Dolcin) Calcium succinate 2.8 gr, acetylsalicylic acid 3.7 gr/Tab. Bot. 100s, 500s. *otc.*
Use: Antiarthritic, antirheumatic.

Berinert P. (Behringwerke Aktiengesellschaft). C1-Esterase-inhibitor, human, pasteurized.
Use: Hereditary angioedema. [Orphan drug]

Berocca Plus Tablets. (Roche Laboratories) Vitamins A 5000 IU, E 30 IU, C 500 mg, B_1 20 mg, B_2 20 mg, B_3.

•**berythromycin.** (beh-RITH-row-MY-sin) USAN.
Use: Antiamebic, anti-infective.

Beserol Tablets. (Sanofi Winthrop) Acetaminophen, chlormezanone. *Rx.*
Use: Analgesic, tranquilizer, muscle relaxant.

•**besipirdine hydrochloride.** (beh-SIH-pihr-deen) USAN.
Use: Cognition enhancer (Alzheimer's disease).

Besta Capsules. (Roberts Pharm) Vitamins B_1 20 mg, B_2 15 mg, niacinamide 100 mg, calcium pantothenate 20 mg, E 50 IU, magnesium sulfate 70 mg, zinc 18.4 mg, B_{12} 4 mcg, B_6 25 mg, C 300 mg/Cap. Bot. 100s. *otc.*
Use: Vitamin/mineral supplement.

Best C Caps. (Roberts Pharm) Ascorbic acid 500 mg/TR Cap. Bot. 100s. *otc.*
Use: Vitamin supplement.

Bestrone Injection. (Bluco) Estrone in aqueous susp. 2 mg or 5 mg/ml. Vial 10 ml. *Rx.*
Use: Hormone, estrogen.

Beta-2. (Nephron) Isoetharine HCl 1% with glycerin, sodium bisulfite, parabens. Bot. 10 ml, 30 ml. *Rx.*
Use: Respiratory.

beta-adrenergic blockers.
See: Blocadren, Tab. (Merck).
Brevibloc, Inj. (DuPont Merck Pharmaceuticals).
Cartrol, Tab. (Abbott Laboratories).
Corgard, Tab. (Bristol-Myers).
Inderal, Tab., Inj. (Wyeth Ayerst).
Inderal LA, Sustained Release Cap. (Wyeth Ayerst).
Kerlone, Tab. (Searle).
Levatol, Tab. (Schwarz Pharma).
Lopressor, Tab., Inj. (Novartis Pharmaceuticals).
Nadolol, Tab. (Various Mfr.)
Propranolol HCl, Tab. (Various Mfr.).
Propranolol HCl, Inj. (SoloPak).
Sectral, Cap. (Wyeth Ayerst).
Tenormin, Tab. (ICI Pharm).
Timolol, Tab. (Various Mfr.).
Visken, Tab. (Novartis).

beta-adrenergic blockers, ophthalmic.
See: Betagan Liquifilm, Soln. (Allergan).
Betoptic, Soln. (Alcon Laboratories).
Ocupress, Soln. (Otsuka).
OptiPranolol, Soln. (Bausch & Lomb).
Timoptic in Ocudose, Soln. (Merck).
Timoptic, Soln. (Merck).

beta alethine. .
Use: Antineoplastic. [Orphan drug]
See: Betathine (Dovetail Tech).

•**beta carotene,** (BAY-tah CARE-oh-teen) U.S.P. 23.
Use: Ultraviolet screen.
See: Max-Caro (Marlyn).
Provatene (Solgar).
Solatene (Roche Laboratories).

Betachron E-R. (Inwood) Propranolol HCl 60 mg, 80 mg, 120 mg, 160 mg. ER Cap. **60 mg, 120mg, 160 mg:** Bot. 100s. **80 mg:** Bot. 100s, 250s (80 mg only). *Rx.*
Use: Beta-adrenergic blockers.

•**beta cyclodextrin.** (BAY-tah-sigh-kloe-DEX-trin) N.F. 18.
Use: Pharmaceutic aid (sequestering agent).

Betadine. (Purdue Frederick) Povidone-iodine. *otc.*
Aerosol Spray, Bot. 3 oz.
Antiseptic Gz. Pads 3"×9". Box 12s.
Antiseptic Lubricating Gel, Tube 5 g.
Disposable Medicated Douche, concentrated packette w/cannula and 6 oz water.

Douche, Bot. 1 oz, 4 oz, 8 oz.
Douche Packette, 0.5 oz (6 per carton).
Helafoam Solution Canister 250 g.
Mouthwash/Gargle, Bot. 6 oz.
Oint., Tube 1 oz, Jar 1 lb, 5 lb.
Oint., packette oz, oz.
Perineal Wash Conc. Kit, Bot. 8 oz w/ dispenser.
Skin Cleanser, Bot. 1 oz, 4 oz.
Skin Cleanser Foam, Canister 6 oz.
Solution, 0.5 oz, 8 oz, 16 oz, 32 oz, gal.
Solution Packette, oz.
Solution Swab Aid, 100s.
Solution Swabsticks, 1s Box 200s; 3s Box 50s.
Surgical Scrub, Bot. pt, pt w/dispenser, qt, gal, packette 0.5 oz.
Surgi-prep Sponge-Brush 36s.
Vaginal Suppositories, Box 7s w/vaginal applicator.
Viscous Formula Antiseptic Gauze Pads: 3"×9", 5"×9". Box 12s.
Whirlpool Concentrate, Bot. gal.
Use: Antiseptic.

Betadine Antiseptic. (Purdue Frederick) Povidone-iodine 10%. Vaginal gel. 18 g with applicator. *otc.*
Use: Vaginal agent.

Betadine Cream. (Purdue Frederick) Povidone-iodine 5% mineral oil, polyoxyethylene stearate, polysorbate, sorbitan monostearate, white petrolatum. Cream Tube 14 g. *otc.*
Use: Antimicrobial, antiseptic.

Betadine First Aid Antibiotics & Moisturizer. (Purdue Frederick) Polymyxin B sulfate 10,000 IU, bacitracin zinc 500 IU. Oint. 14 g. *otc.*
Use: Anti-infective, topical.

Betadine 5% Sterile Ophthalmic Prep Solution. (Akorn) Povidone iodine 5%. Soln. Bot. 50 ml. *Rx.*
Use: Antiseptic, ophthalmic.

Betadine Medicated Disposable Douche. (Purdue Frederick) Povidone-iodine 10% Soln (0.3% when diluted). Vial 5.4 ml with 180 ml bot. Sanitized water. 1 and 2 packs. *otc.*
Use: Vaginal agent.

Betadine Medicated Douche. (Purdue Frederick) Povidone-iodine 10% (0.3% when diluted). Soln. In 15 ml (6s) packettes and 240 ml. *otc.*
Use: Vaginal agent.

Betadine Medicated Premixed Disposable Douche. (Purdue Frederick) Povidone-iodine 10% soln (0.3% when diluted). Bot. 180 ml. 1s, 2s. *otc.*
Use: Vaginal agent.

Betadine Medicated Vaginal Gel and Suppositories. (Purdue Frederick) **Gel:** Povidone-iodine 10%. Tube 18 g, 85 g w/applicator. **Supp:** Povidone-iodine 10%. In 7s w/applicator. *otc.*
Use: Vaginal agent.

Betadine Plus First Antibiotics and Pain Reliever. (Purdue Frederick) Polymyxin B sulfate 10,000 IU, bacitracin zinc 500 IU, pramoxine 10 mg/g. Oint.
Use: Anti-infective, topical.

Betadine Shampoo. (Purdue Frederick) Povidone-iodine 7.5%. Shampoo Bot. 118 ml. *otc.*
Use: Antiseborrheic.

beta-estradiol.
See: Estradiol, U.S.P. 23.

betaeucaine hydrochloride. Name previously used for Eucaine HCl.

Betagan Liquifilm. (Allergan) Levobunolol HCl 0.25% or 0.5%. Bot. 2 ml (0.5%), 5 ml, 10 ml (0.25%) w/ B.I.D. C Cap and Q.D. C Cap (0.5%). *Rx.*
Use: Beta-adrenergic blocker.

Betagen. (Enzyme Process) Vitamins B_1 1 mg, B_2 1.2 mg, niacin 15 mg, B_6 18 mg, pantothenic acid 18 mg, choline 1.8 g, betaine 96 mg/6 Tab. Bot. 100s, 250s. *otc.*
Use: Mineral, vitamin supplement.

Betagen Ointment. (Zenith Goldline) Povidone iodine. Oint. Tube oz. Jar lb. *otc.*
Use: Antiseptic.

Betagen Solution. (Zenith Goldline) Povidone iodine. Bot. pt, gal. *otc.*
Use: Antiseptic.

Betagen Surgical Scrub. (Zenith Goldline) Povidone iodine. Bot. pt, gal. *otc.*
Use: Antiseptic.

•**betahistine hydrochloride.** (BEE-tah-HISS-teen) USAN.
Use: Vasodilator. Meniere's disease. A diamine oxidase inhibitor. Increase microcirculation.

beta-hypophamine.
See: Vasopressin.

betaine anhydrous. (Orphan Medical)
Use: Treatment of homocystinuria. [Orphan drug]
See: Cystadane (Orphan Medical).

•**betaine hydrochloride.** (BEE-tane) U.S.P. 23. Acidol HCl, lycine HCl.
Use: Replenisher adjunct (electrolyte).
W/Ferrous fumarate, docusate sodium, desiccated liver, vitamins, minerals.
See: Hemaferrin, Tab. (Western Research).
W/Pancreatin, pepsin, ammonium Cl.

See: Zypan, Tab. (Standard Process).
W/Pepsin.
See: Normacid, Tab. (Zeneca).

Betalin S. (Eli Lilly) Thiamine HCl 50 mg or 100 mg. Tab. Bot. 100s. *otc.*
Use: Vitamin supplement.

•**betamethasone.** (BAY-tuh-METH-uh-zone) U.S.P. 23.
Use: Corticosteroid, topical.
See: Celestone, Inj., Syr., Tab. (Schering Plough).

•**betamethasone acetate.** (BAY-tuh-METH-uh-zone) U.S.P. 23.
Use: Corticosteroid, topical.

•**betamethasone dipropionate.** (BAY-tah-METH-ah-zone die-PRO-pee-oh-nate) U.S.P. 23.
Use: Corticosteroid, topical.
See: Alphatrex Prods. (Savage).
Diprolene Prods. (Schering Plough).
Diprosone Prods. (Schering Plough).
Psorion Cream (Zeneca).

•**betamethasone sodium phosphate.** (BAY-tah-METH-ah-zone) U.S.P. 23.
Use: Corticosteroid, topical.
See: Celestone Phosphate Inj. (Schering Plough).

betamethasone sodium phosphate and betamethasone acetate suspension, sterile,
See: Celestone Soluspan (Schering Plough).

•**betamethasone valerate.** (BAY-tah-METH-ah-zone VAL-eh-rate) U.S.P. 23.
Use: Corticosteroid, topical.
See: Betatrex Prods. (Savage).
Beta-Val Prods. (Teva USA).
Valisone Prods. (Schering Plough).
Valnac Prods. (Schering Plough).

•**betamicin sulfate.** (bay-tah-MY-sin) USAN.
Use: Anti-infective.

betanaphthol. 2-Naphthol.
Use: Parasiticide.

Betapace. (Berlex) Sotalol HCl 80 mg, 120 mg, 160 mg, 240 mg/Tab. Bot. 100s, UD 100s. *Rx.*
Use: Beta-adrenergic blocker.

Betapen-VK. (Bristol-Myers Squibb) Penicillin V potassium. **Oral Soln.:** 125 mg/ml Bot. 100 ml. 250 mg/5 ml Bot. 100 ml, 200 ml. **Tab.:** 250 mg/Tab. Bot. 100s, 1000s; 500 mg/Tab. Bot. 100s. *Rx.*
Use: Anti-infective, penicillin.

beta-phenyl-ethyl-hydrazine. Phenelzine dihydrogen sulfate.
See: Nardil, Tab. (Parke-Davis).

beta-propiolactone.
See: Betaprone, Vial (Forest Pharmaceutical).

beta-pyridyl-carbinol. Nicotinyl alcohol. Alcohol corresponding to nicotinic acid.
See: Roniacol, Elix., Tab. (Roche Laboratories).

BetaRx. (Vivo Rx). Encapsulated porcine islet preparation.
Use: Type I diabetic patients already on immunosuppression. [Orphan drug]

Betasept. (Purdue Frederick) Chlorhexidine gluconate 4%, isopropyl 4%, alcohol/Liq. Bot. 946 ml. *otc.*
Use: Dermatologic.

Betaseron. (Berlex) Interferon beta 1b 0.3 mg, (9.6 million IU per vial, albumin human 15 mg, dextrose 15 mg. Pow. for Inj. Single-use Vial w/2 ml vial of diluent. *Rx.*
Use: Multiple sclerosis agent.

Betathine. (Dovetail Tech) Beta alethine.
Use: Antineoplastic. [Orphan drug]

Betatrex. (Savage) Betamethasone valerate 0.1%. Cream, Oint. Tube 15 g, 45 g; Lot. Bot. 60 ml. *Rx.*
Use: Corticosteroid, topical.

Beta-Val Cream. (Teva USA) Betamethasone valerate equivalent to 0.1% betamethasone base in cream base. Tube 15 g, 45 g. *Rx.*
Use: Corticosteroid, topical.

•**betaxolol hydrochloride.** (BAY-TAX-oh-lahl) U.S.P. 23.
Use: Antianginal, antihypertensive.
See: Betoptic, Ophth. (Alcon Laboratories).
Kerlone (Searle).

betaxolol ophthalmic solution.
Use: Beta-adrenergic blocker.

•**bethanechol chloride.** (beth-AN-ih-kole) U.S.P. 23.
Use: Cholinergic.
See: Duvoid, Tab. (Procter & Gamble).
Myotonachol, Tab., Amp. (Glenwood).
Urabeth, Tab. (Major).
Urecholine, Tab., Amp. (Merck).

bethanidine.
Use: Hypotensive.

•**bethanidine sulfate.** (beth-AN-ih-deen) USAN.
Use: Antihypertensive.

Bethaprim. (Major) Trimethoprim 40 mg, sulfamethoxazole 200 mg/5 ml, alcohol 0.26%, saccharin and sorbitol. Susp. *Rx.*
Use: Anti-infective.

Bethaprim DS Tabs. (Major) Trimethoprim 160 mg, sulfamethoxazole 800

mg/Tab. Bot. 100s, 500s, UD 100s. *Rx.*
Use: Anti-infective.

Bethaprim SS Tabs. (Major) Trimethoprim 80 mg, sulfamethoxazole 400 mg/Tab. Bot. 100s, 500s. *Rx.*
Use: Anti-infective.

•**betiatide.** (BEH-tie-ah-tide) USAN.
Use: Pharmaceutic aid.

Betimol. (Ciba Vision Ophthalmics) Timolol 0.25% or 0.5%, benzalkonium Cl 0.01%/Soln. Bot. 2.5 ml, 5 ml, 10 ml, 15 ml. *Rx.*
Use: Antiglaucoma agent.

Betoptic. (Alcon Laboratories) Betaxolol HCl 0.5%. Bot. 2.5 ml, 5 ml, 10 ml, 15 ml. *Rx.*
Use: Beta-adrenergic blocking agent, ophthalmic.

Betoptic S. (Alcon Laboratories) Betaxalol HCl 0.25%. Bot. 2.5 ml, 5 ml, 10 ml, 15 ml. *Rx.*
Use: Beta-adrenergic blocking agent, ophthalmic.

•**bevantolol hydrochloride.** (beh-VAN-toe-LOLE) USAN.
Use: Antianginal, antihypertensive, cardiac depressant (antiarrhythmic).

Bexomal-C. (Roberts Pharm) Vitamins B_1 6 mg, B_2 7 mg, B_3 80 mg, B_5 10 mg, B_6 5 mg, B_{12} 6 mcg, C 250 mg/Tab. Bot. 50s. *otc.*
Use: Vitamin supplement.

•**bezafibrate.** (BEH-zah-FIE-brate) USAN.
Use: Antihyperlipoproteinemic.
See: Bezalip (Procter & Gamble).

Bezon. (Whittier) Vitamins B_1 5 mg, B_2 3 mg, niacinamide 20 mg, pantothenic acid 3 mg, B_6 0.5 mg, C 50 mg, B_{12} 1 mcg/Cap. Bot. 30s, 100s. *otc.*
Use: Vitamin supplement.

Bezon Forte. (Whittier) Vitamins B_1 25 mg, B_2 12.5 mg, niacinamide 50 mg, pantothenic acid 10 mg, B_6 5 mg, C 250 mg/Cap. Bot. 30s, 100s. *otc.*
Use: Vitamin supplement.

B-F-I Powder. (SmithKline Beecham Pharmaceuticals) Bismuth-formic-iodide, zinc phenolsulfonate, bismuth subgallate, amol, potassium alum, boric acid, menthol, eucalyptol, thymol and inert diluents. Can 0.25 oz, 1.25 oz, 8 oz. *otc.*
Use: Antiseptic, topical.

B.G.O. (Calotabs) Iodoform, salicylic acid, sulfur, zinc oxide, phenol (liquefied) 1%, calamine, menthol, petrolatum, lanolin, mineral oil, undecylenic acid 1%. Jar ⅞ oz, Tube 1 oz. *otc.*
Use: Antifungal, topical, antiseptic.

•**bialamicol hydrochloride.** (bye-AH-lam-IH-KAHL) USAN.
Use: Antiamebic.

•**biapenem.** (bye-ah-PEN-en) USAN.
Use: Anti-infective.

biaphasic insulin injection. A suspension of insulin crystals in a solution of insulin buffered at pH 7. Insulin Novo Rapitard.

Biavax-II. (Merck) Rubella and mumps virus vaccine, live. See details under Meruvax-II and Mumpsvax. Single-dose vial w/diluent. Pkg. 1s, 10s. *Rx.*
Use: Immunization.

Biaxin. (Abbott Laboratories) Clarithromycin 125 mg, 250 mg/Tab. Bot. 60s, UD 100s. Clarithromycin 125 mg/5 ml and 250 mg/5 ml 1250 mg, 2500 mg, 5000 mg (50 ml, 100 ml after reconstitution). Gran for Oral Susp. Bot. sucrose, fruit punch flavor. *Rx.*
Use: Anti-infective, erythromycin.

•**bicalutamide.** (bye-kah-LOO-tah-mide) USAN.
Use: Antineoplastic.
See: Casodex, Tab (Zeneca).

•**bicifadine hydrochloride.** (bye-SIGH-fah-deen) USAN.
Use: Analgesic.

Bicillin. (Wyeth Ayerst) Penicillin G benzathine 200,000 units/Tab. Bot. 36s. *Rx.*
Use: Anti-infective, penicillin.

Bicillin C-R. (Wyeth Ayerst) Penicillin G benzathine 150,000 units, penicillin G procaine 150,000 units/ml w/lecithin, povidone, methyl and propylparabens. Vial 10 ml. Bicillin 300,000 units, penicillin G procaine 300,000 units/1 ml w/lecithin, povidone, methyl and propylparaben. Pkg. 10s. Bicillin 1,200,000 units, penicillin G procaine 1,200,000 units with parabens, lecithin and povidone/4 single-dose disposable syringe, 10s, 4 ml. *Rx.*
Use: Anti-infective, penicillin.

Bicillin C-R 900/300 Injection. (Wyeth Ayerst) Penicillin G benzathine 900,000 units, penicillin G procaine 300,000 units with parabens, lecithin and povidone/2 ml. Tubex. Pkg. 10s. *Rx.*
Use: Anti-infective, penicillin.

Bicillin Long-Acting. (Wyeth Ayerst) Penicillin G benzathine 300,000 units/ml w/lecithin, povidone, methyl and propylparabens. 300,000 units/ml. Vial 10 ml 600,000 units/Tubex. 1,200,000 units/2 ml Tubex 10s. 2,400,000 units/4 ml single dose disposable syringe, 10s. *Rx.*

Use: Anti-infective, penicillin.

•**biciromab.** (bye-SIH-rah-mab) USAN
Use: Monoclonal antibody (antifibrin).

Bicitra. (Baker Norton) Sodium citrate dihydrate 500 mg, citric acid monohydrate 334 mg, 5 mEq sodium ion/5 ml. Shohl's Solution. Bot. 4 oz, pt, gal, Unit-dose 15 ml, 30 ml. *Rx.*
Use: Systemic alkalinizer.

•**biclodil hydrochloride.** (BYE-kloe-DILL) USAN.
Use: Antihypertensive (vasodilator).

BiCNU. (Bristol-Myers Oncology) Carmustine (BCNU) 100 mg, sterile diluent 3 ml Pow. for Inj. Vial. *Rx.*
Use: Antineoplastic.

Bicozene Cream. (Novartis) Benzocaine 6%, resorcinol 1.66% in cream base/ Cream. Tube 30 g. *otc.*
Use: Anesthetic, topical.

Bicycline. (Knight) Tetracycline HCl 250 mg/Cap. Bot. 100s.
Use: Anti-infective.

•**bidisomide.** USAN. (bye-DIH-so-mide)
Use: Cardiovascular agent (antiarrhythmic).

•**bifonazole.** (BYE-FONE-ah-zole) USAN.
Use: Antifungal.

bile acids, oxidized. Note also dehydrocholic acid.
W/Atropine methyl nitrate, ox and hog bile extract, phenobarbital.
See: G.B.S., Tab. (Forest Pharmaceutical).
W/Bile whole (desiccated), dessicated whole pancreas, homatropine methylbromide.
See: Pancobile, Tab. (Solvay).
W/Ox bile, steapsin, phenobarbital, homatropine methylbromide.
See: Oxacholin, Tab. (Roxane).

bile acid suquestrants. *Rx.*
See: Cholybar (Parke-Davis)
Questran (Bristol-Myers)
Questran Light (Bristol-Myers)
Colestid (Pharmacia & Upjohn)

bile extract. (Various Mfr.) Pow. 0.25 lb, 1 lb.
W/Cascara sagrada, dandelion root, podophyllin, nux vomica.
See: Oxachol, Liq. (Roxane).
W/Dehydrocholic acid, homatropine methylbromide, phenobarbital.
See: Neocholan, Tab. (Hoechst Marion Roussel).
W/Pancreatic substance, dl-methionine, choline bitartrate.
See: Licoplex, Tab. (Mills).

bile extract, ox. Purified ox gall. (Eli Lilly) Enseal 5 gr, Bot. 100s, 500s, 1000s. C. D. Smith–Tab. 5 gr, Bot. 1000s. Stoddard–Tab. 3 gr, Bot. 100s, 500s, 1000s.
W/Cellulase, pepsin, glutamic acid HCl, pancreatin.
See: Kanulase, Tab. (Novartis).
W/Cellulase, pepsin, glutamic acid HCl, pancreatin, methscopolamine nitrate, pentobarbital.
See: Kanumodic, Tab. (Novartis).
W/Colcynth compound extract, cascara sagrada extract, podophyllin, hyoscyamus extract.
W/Dehydrocholic acid, homatropine methylbromide, phenobarbital.
See: Bilamide, Tab. (Norgine).
W/Dehydrocholic acid, pepsin, homatropine methylbromide.
See: Biloric, Cap. (Arcum).
W/Desoxycholic acid, oxidized bile acids, pancreatin.
See: Bilogen, Tab. (Organon Teknika).
W/Enzyme concentrate, pepsin, dehydrocholic acid, belladonna extract.
See: Ro-Bile, Tab. (Solvay).
W/Oxidized bile acids, steapsin, phenobarbital, homatropine methylbromide.
See: Oxacholin, Tab. (Philips).
W/Pepsin, pancreatic enzyme concentrate.
See: Konzyme, Tab. (Brunswick).
Nu'Leven, Tab. (Teva USA).
Nu'Leven Plus, Tab. (Teva USA).
W/Sodium salicylate, phenolphthalein, chionanthus extract, cascara sagrada extract, sodium glycocholate, sodium taurocholate.
See: Glycols, Tab. (Jones Medical Industries).

bilein. Bile salts obtained from ox bile.

bile-like products. .[/NAME]
See: Bile Salts.
Dehydrocholic Acid.
Desoxycholic Acid.
Ketocholanic Acid.

bile salts. Sodium glycocholate and taurocholate. Note also Bile Extract, Ox and oxidized bile acids. (Eli Lilly) Enseal 5 gr, Bot. 100s.
See: Bilein.
Bisol, Tab. (Paddock).
Ox Bile Extract.
Oxidized Bile Acids.
W/Belladonna, nux vomica compound Bile salts 60 mg, belladonna leaf extract 5 mg, nux vomica extract 2 mg, phenolphthalein 30 mg, sodium salicylate 15 mg, aloin 15 mg/Tab. Bot. 1000s.

Use: Laxative, antispasmodic.
W/Cascara sagrada, phenolphthalein, capsicum oleoresin, peppermint oil.
See: Torocol, Tab. (Plessner).
W/Cellulase, calcium carbonate, pancrelipase.
See: Accelerase, Cap. (Organon Teknika).
W/Cellulase, pancrelipase, calcium carbonate, belladonna alkaloids, phenobarbital.
See: Accelerase-PB, Cap. (Organon Teknika).
W/Dehydrocholic acid, pancreatic substance.
See: Depancol, Tab. (Parke-Davis).
W/Dehydrocholic acid, pepsin, pancreatin.
See: Progestive, Tab. (NCP).
W/Pancrelipase, cellulase.
See: Cotazym-B, Tab. (Organon Teknika).
W/Papain, cascara sagrada extract, phenolphthalein, capsicum oleoresin.
See: Torocol Compound, Tab. (Plessner).
W/Pepsin, homatropine, methylbromide, amylase, lipase, protease.
See: Digesplen, Tab., Elix., Drops (Med. Prod.).
W/Phenolphthalein, chionanthus extract.
See: Bile Anthus Compound, Cap. (Scrip).
W/Sodium salicylate, phenolphthalein, chionanthus extract, bile extract, cascara sagrada extract.
See: Glycols, Tab. (Jones Medical Industries).

bile, whole desiccated.
W/Pancreatin, mycozyme diastase, pepsin, nux vomica extract.
See: Enzobile, Tab. (Roberts Pharm).

Bili-Labstix Reagent Strips. (Bayer Corp) Reagent strips. Bot. 100s. Test for pH, protein, glucose, ketones, bilirubin and blood in urine.
Use: Diagnostic aid.

Bili-Labstix SG Reagent Strips. (Bayer Corp) Bot. 100s. Urinalysis reagent strip test for specific gravity, pH, protein, glucose, ketone, bilirubin, and blood.
Use: Diagnostic aid.

Bilirubin Reagent Strips. (Bayer Corp) Seralyzer reagent strip. Bot. 25s. Quantitative strip test for total bilirubin in serum or plasma.
Use: Diagnostic aid.

Bilirubin Test.
See: Ictotest. (Bayer Corp).

Bilivist. (Berlex) Ipodate sodium 500 mg/Cap. Bot. 120s. *Rx.*
Use: Radiopaque agent.

Bilopaque. (Sanofi Winthrop) Tyropanoate sodium 750 mg/Cap. Catchcovers of 4 cap. Box 20s, Bot. 100s, 500s. *Rx.*
Use: Radiopaque agent.

Biloric. (Arcum) Pepsin 9 mg, ox bile 160 mg/Cap. Bot. 100s, 1000s. *otc, Rx.*
Use: Antispasmodic.

Bilstan. (Standex) Bile salts 0.5 gr, cascara sagrada powder extract 0.5 gr, phenolphthalein 0.5 gr, aloin ⅛ gr, podophyllin gr/Tab. Bot. 100s. *otc.*
Use: Laxative.

Biltricide. (Bayer Corp) Praziquantel 600 mg/Tab. Bot. 6s. *Rx.*
Use: Anthelmintic.

bimethoxycaine lactate.

•**bindarit.** (BIN-dah-rit) USAN.
Use: Antirheumatic.

•**biniramycin.** (bih-NEER-ah-MY-sin) USAN.
Use: Anti-infective.

•**binospirone mesylate.** (bih-NO-spy-rone) USAN.
Use: Anxiolytic.

Bintron Tablets. (Madland) Liver fraction 4.6 gr, ferrous sulfate 5 gr, vitamins B_1 3 mg, B_2 0.5 mg, B_6 0.15 mg, C 20 mg, calcium pantothenate 0.3 mg, niacinamide 10 mg/Tab. Bot. 100s, 1000s. *otc.*
Use: Mineral, vitamin supplement.

Bio-Acerola C Complex. (Solgar) Vitamin C 500 mg, citrus bioflavonoids 10 mg, rutin 5 mg in a natural base of acerola, rose hips, buckwheat, black currant and green pepper concentrate powders, cherry flavored. Wafers. Bot. 50s, 100s. *otc.*
Use: Vitamin supplement.

Biobrane. (Sanofi Winthrop) A temporary skin substitute available in various sizes. *otc.*
Use: Dermatologic.

Biocal 250. (Bayer Corp) Calcium 250 mg/Chew. Tab. Bot. 75s. *otc.*
Use: Calcium supplement.

Biocal 500. (Bayer Corp) Calcium 500 mg/Tab. Bot. 75s. *otc.*
Use: Mineral supplement.

Biocef. (Inter. Ethical Labs) Cephalexin monohydrate 500 mg/Cap. Bot. 100s. Cephalexin monohydrate 125 mg/ml and 250 mg/ml/Pow. for susp. Bot. 100 ml. *Rx.*
Use: Anti-infective, cephalosporin.

Bioclate. (Centeon) Concentrated

recombinant hemophilic factor. After reconstitution, also contains albumin (human) 12.5 mg/ml, PEG-3350 1.5 mg/ml, sodium 180 mEq/L, histidine 55 mM, polysorbate 80 1.5 mcg/AHF IU, calcium 0.2 mg/ml. Bot. IU 250, 500, 1000. *Rx.*
Use: Antihemophilic.

Biocult-GC. (Orion Diagnostica) Swab Test for gonorrhea. For endocervical, urethral, rectal and pharyngeal cultures. Box 1 test per kit.
Use: Diagnostic aid.

biodegradable polymer implant containing carmustine.
Use: Antineoplastic. [Orphan drug]
See: Biodel Implant/BCNU.

Biodel Implant/BCNU. (Scios Nova) Biodegradable polymer implant containing carmustine. *Rx.*
Use: Antineoplastic.

Biodine. (Major) Iodine 1%. Soln. Bot. pt, gal. *otc.*
Use: Antimicrobial, antiseptic.

bio-flavonoid compounds. Vitamin P.

bio-flavonoid compound, citrus. W/Vitamin C.
See: C.V.P. Syr., Cap. (Rhone-Poulenc Rorer).
Mevanin-C, Cap. (Beutlich).
Mevatinic-C, Tab. (Beutlich).
Peridin-C, Tab. (Beutlich).
Pregent, Tab. (Beutlich).

Biogastrone.
See: Carbenoxolone.

Biohist-LA. (Wakefield Pharm) Carbinoxamine maleate 8 mg, pseudoephedrine HCl 120 mg/TR Tab. Bot. 100s. *Rx.*
Use: Antihistamine, decongestant.

•**biological indicator for dry-heat sterilization, paper strip.** U.S.P. 23.
Use: Biological indicator, sterilization.

•**biological indicator for ethylene oxide sterilization, paper strip.** U.S.P. 23.
Use: Biological indicator, sterilization.

•**biological indicator for steam sterilization, paper strip.** U.S.P. 23.
Use: Biological indicator, sterilization.

•**biological indicator for steam sterilization, self-conatined.** U.S.P. 23.
Use: Biological indicator, sterilization.

Bion Tears. (Alcon Laboratories) Dextran 70 0.1%, hydroxypropyl methylcellulose 2910 0.3%, NaCl, KCl, sodium bicarbonate. Preservative free. Soln. In single-use 0.45 ml containers (28s). *otc.*
Use: Artificial tears.

Bionate 50-2. (Seatrace) Testosterone cypionate 50 mg, estradiol cypionate 2 mg/ml. Vial 10 ml. *Rx.*
Use: Androgen, estrogen combination.

Bioral.
See: Carbenoxolone.

Bio-Rescue. (Biomedical Frontiers) Dextran and deferoxamine.
Use: Acute iron poisoning. [Orphan drug]

Bios I.
See: Inositol.

Biosynject. (Chembiomed) Trisaccharides A and B.
Use: Hemolytic disease of the newborn. [Orphan drug]

Bio-Tab. (Inter. Ethical Labs) Doxycycline hyclate 100 mg, film coated. Tab. Bot. 50s, 100s, 500s. *Rx.*
Use: Anti-infective, tetracycline.

Biotel Diabetes. (Biotel) In vitro diagnostic test for diabetes and other metabolic disorders by screening for glucose in the urine. Test Kit 12s.
Use: Diagnostic aid.

Biotel kidney. (Biotel) In vitro diagnostic test for early detection of diseases of the kidneys, bladder and urinary tract by screening for hemoglobin, red blood cells and albumin in the urine. Test Kit 12s.
Use: Diagnostic aid.

Biotel U.T.I. (Biotel) In vitro diagnostic home test to detect urinary tract infections by screening for nitrate in urine. Test Kit 12s.
Use: Diagnostic aid.

Biotexin.
See: Novobiocin.

Biothesin. (Pal-Pak). Phosphorated carbohydrate solution cerium oxalate 120 mg, bismuth subnitrate 120 mg, benzocaine 15 mg, aromatics/Tab. 1000s. *otc.*
Use: Antiemetic antivertigo.

Bio-Tytra. (Health for Life Brands) Neomycin sulfate 2.5 mg, gramicidin 0.25 mg, benzocaine 10 mg/Troche. Box 10s. *Rx.*
Use: Anti-infective.

•**bipenamol hydrochloride.** (bye-PEN-ah-MAHL) USAN.
Use: Antidepressant.

•**biperiden.** (by-PURR-ih-den) U.S.P. 23.
Use: Anticholinergic; antiparkinson.

•**biperiden hydrochloride.** (by-BURR-ih-den) U.S.P. 23.
Use: Anticholinergic, antiparkinson.

biperiden hydrochloride and lactate.
Use: Anticholinergic, antiparkinson.

See: Akineton, Amp., Tab. (Knoll Pharmaceuticals).

•**biperiden lactate, injection.** (by-PURR-ih-den) U.S.P. 23.
Use: Anticholinergic, antiparkinsonian.

•**biphenamine hydrochloride.** (bye-FEN-ah-meen) USAN.
Use: Anesthetic, local, anti-infective, antimicrobial.

Bipole-S. (Spanner) Testosterone 25 mg, estrone 2 mg/ml/Inj. Vial. 10 ml. *Rx.*
Use: Androgen, estrogen combination.

bis (acetoxphenyl oxindol.
See: Oxyphenisatin.

•**bisacodyl.** (BISS-uh-koe-dill) U.S.P. 23.
Use: Laxative.
See: Bisacodyl Uniserts, Supp. (Upsher-Smith Labs).
Dacodyl, Tab. Supp. (Major).
Deficol, Tab., Supp. (Vangard).
Delco-Lax, Tab (Delco).
Dulcagen, Tab., Supp. (Zenith Goldline).
Dulcolax, Tab. Supp. (Novartis Self-Medication)
Fleet Bisacodyl, Tab. Supp. (C.B. Fleet Co.).

•**bisacodyl tannex.** (BISS-uh-koe-dill) USAN. Water-soluble complex of bisacodyl and tannic acid.
Use: Laxative.
See: Clysodrast, packet (PBH Wesley Jessen).

Bisacodyl Uniserts. (Upsher-Smith Labs) Bisacodyl 5 mg and 10 mg/Supp. Pack. 12, 50s, 500s. *otc.*
Use: Laxative.

Bisalate. (Allison) Sodium salicylate 5 gr, salicylamide 2.5 gr, sodium paraminobenzoate 5 gr, ascorbic acid 50 mg, butabarbital sodium 1/8 gr/Tab. Bot. 100s and 1000s. *Rx.*
Use: Antirheumatic.

•**bisantrene hydrochloride.** (BISS-an-TREEN HIGH-droe-KLOR-ide) USAN.
Use: Antineoplastic.

bisatin.
See: Oxyphenisatin.

bishydroxycoumarin.
See: Dicumarol, U.S.P. 23.

Bismapec Tablets. (Pal-Pak) Bismuth hydroxide 137.7 mg, colloidal kaolin 648 mg, citrus pectin 129.6 mg/Tab. Bot. 1000s. *otc.*
Use: Antidiarrheal.

Bismu-Kino. (Denver) Bismuth oxycarbonate 10 gr, eucalyptus gum 6 gr, phenyl salicylate, camphor, menthol, carminative oils of nutmeg and clove in soothing, demulcent base w/alcohol 2%/fl oz. Bot. 4 oz, pt. *otc.*
Use: Gastrointestinal.

•**bismuth aluminate.** (BISS-muth) USAN. Aluminum bismuth oxide.
See: Escot, Cap. (Solvay).

•**bismuth carbonate.** (BISS-muth) USAN.
Use: Protectant, topical.

bismuth glycolylarsanilate. (BISS-muth)
Use: Antiamebic.
See: Glycobiarsol, N.F. 18.

bismuth hydroxide.
See: Milk of Bismuth, U.S.P. 23.

bismuth, insoluble products.
See: Bismuth Subgallate (Various Mfr.).
Bismuth Subsalicylate (Various Mfr.).
Bismuth Tribromophenate (N.Y. Quinine).

bismuth, magma. Name previously used for Milk of Bismuth.

•**bismuth, milk of.** (BISS-muth) U.S.P. 23.
Formerly Bismuth Magma
Use: Astringent, antacid.

bismuth oxycarbonate.
See: Bismuth Subcarbonate.

bismuth potassium tartrate. Basic bismuth potassium bismuthotartrate. (Brewer) 25 mg/ml Amp. 2 ml. (Miller) 0.016 g/ml Amp. 2 ml, Box 12s, 100s; Bot. 30 ml, 60 ml. (Raymer) 2.5% Amp. 2 ml, Box 12s, 100s. *Rx.*
Use: Agent for syphilis.

bismuth resorcin compound.
W/Bismuth subgallate, balsam Peru, benzocaine, zinc oxide, boric acid.
See: Bonate, Supp. (Suppositoria).
W/Bismuth subgallate, balsam Peru, zinc oxide, boric acid.
See: Versal, Supp. (Suppositoria).
W/Bismuth subgallate, zinc oxide, boric acid, balsam Peru.
See: Anulan, Supp. (Lannett).

bismuth sodium tartrate. (BISS-muth)
Use: I.M., syphilis.

bismuth subbenzoate. (BISS-muth)
Use: Dusting powder for wounds.

•**bismuth subcarbonate.** (BISS-muth) U.S.P. 23.
Use: Protectant (topical).

bismuth subcarbonate. (BISS-muth)
Use: Gastroenteritis, diarrhea.
W/Benzocaine, zinc oxide, boric acid.
See: Aracain Rectal Supp. (Del Pharmaceuticals).
W/Calcium carbonate, magnesium carbonate, aminoacetic acid, dried aluminum hydroxide gel.
See: Buffertabs, Tab. (Forest Pharmaceutical).

W/Charcoal and ginger.
See: Harv-a-carbs, Tab. (Forest Pharmaceutical).
W/Hydrocortisone acetate, belladonna extract, ephedrine sulfate, zinc oxide, boric acid, balsam Peru, cocoa butter.
See: Rectacort, Supp. (Century Pharm).
W/Kaolin, pectin.
See: K-C, Liq. (Century Pharm).
W/Pectin, kaolin, opium powder.
See: KBP/O, Cap. (Cole).
W/Phenyl salicylate, zinc phenolsulfonate, pepsin.
See: Bismuth, salol, zinc compound (Jones Medical Industries).
W/Phenyl salicylate, chloroform, eucalyptus gum, camphor.
See: Bismu-Kino, Liq. (Denver Chem.).
W/Ephedrine sulfate, belladonna extract, zinc oxide, boric acid, bismuth oxyiodide, balsam Peru.
See: Wyanoids, Preps. (Wyeth Ayerst).

bismuth subgallate, (BISS-muth) (Various Mfr.) Dermatol.
Use: Topically for skin conditions; orally as an antidiarrheal.
See: Devrom, Tab (Parthenon).
W/Benzocaine, resorcin, cod liver oil, lanolin, zinc oxide.
See: Biscolan, Supp. (Lannett).
W/Benzocaine, zinc oxide, boric acid, balsam Peru.
See: Anocaine, Supp. (Roberts Pharm).
W/Bismuth oxyiodide, bismuth resorcin compound, benzocaine, boric acid.
See: Bonate, Supp. (Suppositoria).
W/Bismuth resorcin compound, balsam Peru, benzocaine, zinc oxide, boric acid.
See: Bonate, Supp. (Suppositoria).
W/Bismuth resorcin compound, zinc oxide, boric acid, balsam Peru.
See: Anulan, Supp. (Lannett).
Versal, Supp. (Suppositoria).
W/Cod liver oil, benzocaine, lanolin, zinc oxide, resorcin, balsam Peru, hydrocortisone.
See: Doctient HC, Supp. (Suppositoria).
W/Hydrocortisone acetate, bismuth resorcin compound, zinc oxide, balsam Peru, benzyl benzoate.
See: Anusol-HC, Supp. (Parke-Davis).
W/Diethylaminoacet-2,6-xylidide, zinc oxide, aluminum subacetate, balsam Peru.
See: Xylocaine Suppositories (Astra).
W/Kaolin, colloidal.
See: Diastop, Liq. (ICN Pharmaceuticals).
W/Kaolin colloidal, calcium carbonate, magnesium trisilicate, papain, atropine sulphate.
See: Kaocasil, Tab. (Jenkins).
W/Kaolin, opium, zinc phenolsulfonate, pectin.
See: Cholactabs, Tab. (Roxane).
W/Kaolin, pectin, zinc phenolsulfonate, opium powder.
See: Diastay, Tab. (ICN Pharmaceuticals).
W/Opium powder, pectin, kaolin, zinc phenolsulfonate.
See: Bismuth, Pectin, Paregoric (Teva USA).
W/Zinc oxide, bismuth resorcin compound, balsam Peru, benzyl benzoate.
See: Anugesic, Supp., Oint. (Parke-Davis).
Anusol, Supp., Oint. (Parke-Davis).

bismuth subiodide.
See: Bismuth oxyiodide.

•**bismuth subnitrate.** (BISS-muth) U.S.P. 23.
Use: Pharmaceutic necessity, gastroenteritis, amebic dysentery, locally for wounds.
W/Calcium carbonate, magnesium carbonate.
See: Antacid No. 2, Tab. (Jones Medical Industries).
Maygel, Tab. (Century Pharm).
W/Sodium bicarbonate, magnesium carbonate, diastase, papain.
Panacarb, Tab. (Lannett).

•**bismuth subsalicylate.** (BISS-muth) U.S.P. 23.
Use: Anitdiarrheal, antacid, antiulcerative. Basic bismuth salicylate. Agent for syphilis. Used in combination with metronidazole and tetracycline HCl to treat active duodenal ulcer associated with *H. pylori* infection.
W/Calcium carbonate, glycocoll.
See: Pepto-Bismol, Tab. (Procter & Gamble).
W/Pectin, salol, kaolin, zinc sulfocarbolate, aluminum hydroxide.
See: Wescola Antidiarrheal-Stomach Upset (Western Research).
W/Phenylsalicylate, zinc phenolsulfonate, methylcellulose, magnesium aluminum silicate.
See: Pepto-Bismol, Liq. (Procter & Gamble).

bismuth tannate. (BISS-muth) (Various Mfr.) Tanbismuth. *otc.*
Use: Astringent and protective in GI disorders.

bismuth tribromophenate. (BISS-muth)
Use: Intestinal antiseptic.

bismuth violet. (BISS-muth) (Table Rock) Bismuth Violet. **Oint.** 1%. Jar oz, lb. **Soln.** 0.5%. Bot. 0.5 oz, 6 oz, pt, gal. **Tr.** 0.5%. Bot. 6 oz, pt, also 1% w/ benzoic and salicylic acid. Bot. 0.5 oz, 6 oz, pt. *otc.*
Use: Anti-infective, topical.

bismuth, water-soluble products.
See: Bismuth Potassium Tartrate (Various Mfr.).

•**bisnafide dimesylate.** (BISS-nah-fide die-MEH-sih-late) USAN.
Use: Antineoplastic.

•**bisobrin lactate.** (BISS-oh-brin LACK-tate) USAN.
Use: Fibrinolytic.

•**bisoprolol.** (bih-SO-pro-lahl) USAN.
Use: Antihypertensive (β blocker).

•**bisoprolol fumarate.** USAN.
Use: Antihypertensive (β blocker).
See: Zebeta (ESI Lederle Generics).
Ziac, Tab. (ESI Lederle Generics).

•**bisoxatin acetate.** (biss-OX-at-in) USAN.
Use: Laxative.

bispecific antibody 520C9x22. (Medarex)
Use: Antineoplastic, serotherapy. [Orphan drug]

bisphosphonates.
Use: Antihypercalcomic, bone resorption inhibitor.
See: Aredia, Pow. for Inj. (Novartis).
Skelid, Tab. (Sanogi Winthrop).
Actonel, Tab. (Procter & Gamble).
Didronel (Procter & Gamble).
Didronel IV (MGI Pharma).
Aredia, Inj (Novartis Pharmaceuticals).
Fosamax, Tab (Merck).

•**bispyrithione magsulfex.** (BISS-PIHR-ih-thigh-ohn mag-sull-fex) USAN.
Use: Antidandruff, anti-infective, antimicrobial.

bisquadine. (Sterwin) Alexidine.

bis-tropamide. Tropicamide.
See: Mydriacyl, Soln. (Alcon Laboratories).

Bite & Itch Lotion. (Weeks & Leo) Pramoxine HCl 1%, pyrilamine maleate 2%, pheniramine maleate 0.2%, chlorpheniramine maleate 0.2%. Bot. 4 oz. *otc.*
Use: Dermatologic, topical.

•**bithionolate, sodium.** (bye-THIGH-oh-noe-late) USAN.
Use: Topical anti-infective.

Bitin. CDC Anti-infective agent.
See: Bithionol.

•**bitolterol mesylate.** (by-TOLE-tor-ole) USAN.
Use: Bronchodilator.
See: Tornalate, Inhalation soln. (Dura Pharm).

Bitrate. (Arco) Phenobarbital 15 mg, pentaerythritol tetranitrate 20 mg/Tab. Bot. 100s. *Rx.*
Use: Antianginal, hypnotic, sedative.

•**bivalirudin.** (bye-VAL-ih-ruh-din) USAN.
Use: Anticoagulant, antithrombotic.

•**bizelesin.** (bye-ZELL-eh-sin) USAN.
Use: Antineoplastic.

B-Ject-100. (Hyrex) Vitamins B_1 100 mg, B_2 2 mg, B_3 100 mg, B_5 2 mg, B_6 2 mg/ml. Inj. Vial 10 ml, 30 ml. *Rx.*
Use: Vitamin supplement.

Black and White Bleaching Cream. (Schering Plough) Hydroquinone 2%. Tube 0.75 oz, 1.5 oz. *Rx.*
Use: Dermatologic.

Black and White Ointment. (Schering Plough) Resorcinol 3%. Tube 0.62 oz, 2.25 oz.
Use: Antiseptic, dermatologic, topical.

Black-Draught. (Chattem Consumer Products) Powdered senna extract. **Tab.:** 600 mg. Bot. 30s. **Gran.:** 1.65 g/0.5 tsp. Jar 22.5 g. *otc.*
Use: Laxative.

Black-Draught Syrup. (Chattem Consumer Products) Casanthranol 90 mg w/senna, rhubarb, anise, methyl salicylate, ginger, peppermint oil, spearmint oil, menthol, alcohol 5%, tartrazine/Tbsp. Bot. 2 oz, 5 oz. *otc.*
Use: Laxative.

black widow spider, antivenin.
See: Antivenin (Lactrodectus mactens), Inj. (Merck).

Blairex Hard Contact Lens Cleaner. (Blairex Labs) Anionic detergent. Liq. Bot. 60 ml. *otc.*
Use: Contact lens care.

Blairex Lens Lubricant. (Blairex Labs) Isotonic. Sorbic acid 0.25%, EDTA 0.1%, borate buffer, NaCl, hydroxypropylmethylcellulose, glycerin. Soln. Bot. 15 ml. *otc.*
Use: Contact lens care.

Blairex Sterile Saline Solution. (Blairex Labs) Sodium Cl, boric acid, sodium borate. Aerosol. 90 ml, 240 ml, 360 ml. *otc.*
Use: Contact lens care.

Blairex System. (Blairex Labs) Sodium Cl 135 mg/Tab. 200s, 365s w/15 ml bot. *otc.*
Use: Contact lens care.

Blairex System II. (Blairex Labs) Sodium Cl 250 mg/Tab. 90s, 180s w/27.7 ml bot. *otc.*

Use: Contact lens care.

Blaud Strubel. (Strubel) Ferrous sulfate 5 gr/Cap. Bot. 100s. *otc.*
Use: Mineral supplement.

Blefcon. (Madland) Sodium sulfacetamide 30%. Oint. Tube ⅛ oz. *Rx.*
Use: Anti-infective, ophthalmic.

Blenoxane. (Bristol-Myers Oncology/Immunology) Bleomycin sulfate 15 units, 30 unites Pow. for Inj. Vial. *Rx.*
Use: Antineoplastic.

•**bleomycin sulfate, sterile.** (BLEE-oh-MY-sin) U.S.P. 23. Antibiotic obtained from cultures of *Streptomyces verticillus.*
Use: Antineoplastic.
See: Blenoxane, Inj. (Bristol-Myers Squibb).

Bleph-10. (Allergan) Sulfacetamide sodium 10%. Dropper Bot. 2.5 ml, 5 ml, 15 ml. *Rx.*
Use: Anti-infective, ophthalmic.

Bleph-10 Sterile Ophthalmic Ointment. (Allergan) Sulfacetamide sodium 10%. Tube 3.5 g. *Rx.*
Use: Anti-infective, ophthalmic.

Blephamide. (Allergan) Sulfacetamide sodium 10%, prednisolone acetate 0.2%. Bot. 2.5 ml, 5 ml, 10 ml. *Rx.*
Use: Anti-inflammatory, anti-infective, ophthalmic.

Blephamide Ophthalmic Ointment. (Allergan) Prednisolone acetate 0.2%, sulfacetamide sodium 10%. Tube 3.5 g. *Rx.*
Use: Anti-inflammatory, anti-infective, ophthalmic.

Blinx. (Akorn) Sodium Cl, potassium Cl, sodium phosphate, benzalkonium Cl 0.005%, EDTA 0.02%. Soln. Bot. 120 ml. *otc.*
Use: Irrigant, ophthalmic.

Blis. (Del Pharmaceuticals) Boric acid 47.5%, salicylic acid 17%. Bot. 7 oz. *otc.*
Use: Antifungal, topical.

BlisterGard. (Medtech) Alcohol 6.7%, pyroxylin solution, oil of cloves, B-hydroxyquinolone. Liq. Bot. 30 ml. *otc.*
Use: Dermatologic, protectant.

Blistex. (Blistex) Camphor 0.5%, phenol 0.5%, allantoin 1%, lanolin, mineral oil. Tube 4.2 g, 10.5 g. *otc.*
Use: Lip protectant.

Blistex Lip Balm. (Blistex) SPF 10. Camphor 0.5%, phenol 0.5%, allantoin 1%, dimethicone 2%, pamidate 0.25%, oxybenzone, parabens, petrolatum. Tube. 4.5 g. *otc.*
Use: Lip protectant.

Blistex Ultra Protection. (Blistex) Octyl methoxycinnamate, oxybenzone, octyl salicylate, menthyl anthranilate, homosalate, dimethicone. Tube 4.2 g. *otc.*
Use: Lip protectant.

Blistik. (Blistex) Padimate O 6.6%, oxybenzone 2.5%, dimethicone 2%. Lip balm stick 4.5 g. *otc.*
Use: Lip protectant.

Blis-To-Sol. (Chattem Consumer Products) **Liq.:** Tolnaftate 1%. Bot. 30 ml. **Pow.:** Zinc undecylenate 12%. Bot. 60 g. **Soln:** Tolnaftate 1% Bot. 30 ml and 55.5 ml. *otc.*
Use: Antifungal, topical.

BLM.
See: Bleomycin sulfate.

Blocadren. (Merck) Timolol maleate 5 mg, 10 mg or 20 mg/Tab. **5 mg:** Bot. 100s; **10 mg:** Bot. 100s, UD 100s; **20 mg:** Bot. 100s. *Rx.*
Use: Beta-adrenergic blocker.

Block Out By Sea & Ski. (Carter Products) Padimate O, octyl methoxycinnamate, oxybenzone. Cream. Tube 120 g. *otc.*
Use: Sunscreen.

Block Out Clear By Sea & Ski. (Carter Products) Padimate O, octyl methoxycinnamate, octyl salicylate, SD alcohol 40. Lot. Bot. 120 ml. *otc.*
Use: Sunscreen.

blood, anticoagulants.
See: Anticoagulants.

•**blood cells, red.** U.S.P. 23. *Formerly Blood cells, human red.*
Use: Blood replenisher.

blood coagulation.
See: Hemostatics.

blood fractions.
See: Albumin (Human) Salt-Poor (Armour; Baxter).

blood glucose concentrator.
See: Glucagon (Eli Lilly).

blood glucose test.
See: Chemstrip bG Strips. (Boehringer Mannheim).
Dextrostix Reagent Strips. (Bayer Corp).
First Choice, Strips (Polymer Technology, Int.).
Glucostix Strips. (Bayer Corp).

•**blood grouping serum, anti-A.** U.S.P. 23.
Use: Diagnostic aid (blood, in vitro).

•**blood grouping serum, anti-B.** U.S.P. 23.
Use: Diagnostic aid (blood, in vitro).

•**blood grouping serums anti-D, anti-C, anti-E, anti-c, anti-e.** U.S.P. 23. *Formerly Anti-Rh typing serums.*
Use: Diagnostic aid (blood, in vitro).

•**blood group specific substances a, b and ab.** U.S.P. 23. *Formerly Blood Grouping specific substances A and B.*
Use: Blood neutralizer.

•**blood, whole.** U.S.P. 23. *Formerly Blood, whole human.*
Use: Blood replenisher.

Blu-12 100. (Bluco) Cyanocobalamin 100 mcg /ml. Vial 30 ml. *Rx.*
Use: Vitamin supplement.

Blu-12 1000. (Bluco) Cyanocobalamin 1000 mcg /ml. Vial 30 ml. *Rx.*
Use: Vitamin supplement.

Bluboro Powder. (Allergan) Aluminum sulfate 53.9%, calcium acetate 43% w/boric acid, FD&C; Blue 1. Packet 1.9 g. Box 12s. *otc.*
Use: Astringent.

Bludex. (Burlington) Methenamine 40.8 mg, methylene blue 5.4 mg, phenyl salicylate 18.1 mg, atropine sulfate 0.03 mg, hyoscyamine 0.03 mg, benzoic acid 4.5 mg/Tab. Bot. 100s, 1000s. *Rx.*
Use: Antiseptic, antispasmodic, urinary.

Blue. (Various Mfr.) Pyrethrins 0.3%, piperonyl butoxide 3%, petroleum distillate 1.2%. Gel Bot. 30 g, 480 g. *otc.*
Use: Pediculicide.

Blue Gel Muscular Pain Reliever. (Rugby) Menthol in a specially formulated base. Gel. Tube 240 g. *otc.*
Use: Liniments.

Blue Star Ointment. (McCue Labs.) Salicylic acid, benzoic acid, methyl salicylate, camphor, lanolin, petrolatum. Jar 2 oz. *otc.*
Use: Dermatologic, counterirritant.

blutene chloride.

B-Major. (Barth's) Vitamins B_1 7 mg, B_2 14 mg, niacin 2.35 mg, B_{12} 7.5 mcg, B_6 0.15 mg, pantothenic acid 0.37 mg, choline 85 mg, inositol 6 mg, biotin, folic acid, aminobenzoic acid/Cap. Bot. 1s, 3s, 6s, 12s. *otc, Rx.*
Use: Mineral, vitamin supplement.

B.M.E. (Brothers) Aminophylline 32 mg, ephedrine sulfate 8 mg, phenobarbital 8 mg, chlorpheniramine maleate 2 mg, alcohol 15%/5 ml. Bot. pt. *Rx.*
Use: Antihistamine, bronchodilator, decongestant, hypnotic, sedative.

B-N. (Eric, Kirk & Gary). Bacitracin 500 units, neomycin sulfate 5 mg. Oint. Tube 0.5 oz. *otc.*
Use: Anti-infective, topical.

b-naphthyl salicylate. Betol, Naphthosalol, Salinaphthol.
Use: G.I. & G.U., antiseptic.

B-Nutron Tablets. (Nion) Vitamins B_1 2 mg, niacinamide 18 mg, B_2 3 mg, B_6 2.2 mg, cyanocobalamin 3 mcg, folic acid 0.4 mg, iron 6 mg, pantothenic acid 3.3 mg, B complex as provided by 150 mg Brewer's yeast/Tab. Bot. 100s, 500s. *otc.*
Use: Mineral, vitamin supplement.

B and O Supprettes No. 15A & No. 16A. (PolyMedica) Opium 30 mg or 60 mg, belladonna extract 16.2 mg/Supp. Jar 12s. *c-II.*
Use: Analgesic, antispasmodic, narcotic.

Bobid. (Boyd) Phenylpropanolamine HCl 50 mg, chlorphenlramine maleate 8 mg, methscopolamine bromide 2.5 mg/Cap. Bot. 100s. *otc.*
Use: Antihistamine, anticholinergic, decongestant.

Bo-Cal. (Fibertone) Calcium 250 mg, magnesium 125 mg, vitamin D_3 100 IU, boron 0.75 mg/Tab. Bot. 120s. *otc.*
Use: Mineral, vitamin supplement.

Boil-Ease Salve. (Del Pharmaceuticals) Benzocaine 20%, camphor, eucalyptus oil, menthol, petrolatum, phenol. Oint. 30 g. *otc.*
Use: Anesthetic drawing salve.

BoilnSoak. (Alcon Laboratories) Sodium Cl 0.7%, boric acid, sodium borate, thimerosal 0.001%, disodium edetate 0.1%. Bot. 8 oz, 12 oz. *otc.*
Use: Contact lens care.

•**bolandiol dipropionate.** (bole-AN-die-ole die-PRO-pee-oh-nate) USAN.
Use: Anabolic.

•**bolasterone.** (BOLE-ah-STEE-rone) USAN.
Use: Anabolic.

Bolax. (Boyd) Docusate sodium 240 mg, phenolphthalein 30 mg, dihydrocholic acid ¾ gr/Cap. Bot. 100s. *otc.*
Use: Laxative.

•**boldenone undecylenate.** (BOLE-deen-ohn uhn-deh-sih-LEN-ate) USAN. Parenabol. Under study.
Use: Anabolic.

•**bolenol.** (BOLE-ee-nahl) USAN.
Use: Anabolic.

•**bolmantalate.** (BOLE-MAN-tah-late) USAN.
Use: Anabolic.

Bonacal Plus Tablets. (Kenwood Labs) Vitamins A 5000 IU, D 400 IU, C 100 mg, B_1 3 mg, B_2 3 mg, B_6 10 mg, B_{12} 4

mcg, niacinamide 20 mg, d-calcium pantothenate 3.3 mg, iron 42 mg, calcium 350 mg, manganese 0.33 mg, zinc 0.1 mg, magnesium 1.67 mg, potassium 1.67 mg/Tab. Bot. 100s. *otc.*
Use: Mineral, vitamin supplement.

Bonamil Infant Formula with Iron. (Wyeth Ayerst) Protein 2.3 g (from nonfat milk, taurine), fat 5.4 g (from soybean and coconut oils, soy lecithin), carbohydrase 10.7 g (from lactose), linoleic acid 1300 mg, vitamin A 300 IU, D 60 IU, E 2.85 IU, K 8 mcg, B_1 100 mcg, B_2 150 mcg, B_6 63 mcg, B_{12} 0.2 mcg, B_3 750 mcg, folic acid 7.5 mcg, B_5 315 mcg, biotin 2.2 mcg, vitamin C 8.3 mg, choline 15 mg, Ca 69 mg, P 54 mg, Mg 6 mg, Fe 1.8 mg, Zn 0.75 mg, Mn 15 mcg, Cu 70 mcg, I 5 mcg, Na 27 mg, K 93 mg, Cl 63 mg/100 cal (5.3 cal/g). Conc., Liq. Bot. 453 g Conc. 384 ml. Ready-to-feed liq. 946 ml. *otc.*
Use: Nutritional supplement, enteral.

Bonate. (Suppositoria) Bismuth subgallate, balsam Peru, benzocaine, zinc oxide/Supp. Box 12s, 100s, 1000s. *otc.*
Use: Anorectal preparation.

Bonefos. (Leiras) Disodium Clodronate tetrahydrate.
Use: Bone resorption inhibitor. [Orphan drug]

Bone Meal w/ Vitamin D. (Natures Bounty) Calcium 220 mg, vitamin D 100 IU, phosphorus 100 mg, iron 0.45 mg, copper 3.25 mg, zinc 20 mcg, manganese 2.75 mcg, magnesium 0.925 mg. Tab. Bot. 100s, 250s. *otc.*
Use: Mineral, vitamin supplement.

Bonine. (Pfizer US Pharmaceutical Group) Meclizine HCl 25 mg/Chew. tab. Pkg. 8s, 48s. *otc.*
Use: Antiemetic, antivertigo.

Bontril PDM. (Schwarz Pharma) Phendimetrazine tartrate 35 mg/3 layer Tab. Bot. 100s, 1000s. *c-III.*
Use: Anorexiant.

Bontril Slow Release Capsules. (Schwarz Pharma) Phendimetrazine tartrate 105 mg/Cap. Bot. 100s, 1000s *c-III.*
Use: Anorexiant.

Boost. (Bristol-Myers Squibb) Protein 10 mg, fat 7 g, carbohydrate 35 g, sodium 130 mg, potassium 400 mg, vitamins A, C, D, E, B_1, B_2, B_3, B_5, B_6, B_9, B_{12}, biotin, Ca, P, I, Mg, Zn, Cu, sugar, corn syrup. Liq. Bot. 237 ml. *otc.*
Use: Nutritional supplement, enteral.

Bopen-VK. (Boyd) Potassium phenoxymethyl penicillin 400,000 units/Tab. Bot. 100s.
Use: Anti-infective, penicillin.

borax. Sodium Borate, N.F. 18.

•**boric acid.** N.F. 18.
Use: Antiseptic, pharmaceutic necessity.
See: Borofax, Oint. (GlaxoWellcome)).
W/Combinations.
See: Saratoga Ointment (Blair).

boric acid ointment. (Various Mfr.) Topical ointment 5% or 10%. Tube, Jar 30 g, 52.5 g, 60 g, 120 g, 454 g. Ophth. oint. 0.5% or 10%. Tube, Jar. 3.5 g, 3.75 g, 30 g, 60 g, 480 g. *otc, Rx.*
Use: Dermatologic, counterirritant.

2-bornanone. Camphor, U.S.P. 23.

•**bornelone.** (BORE-neh-LONE) USAN.
Use: Ultraviolet screen.

•**bornyl acetate.** USAN.

•**borocaptate sodium 10.** (bore-oh-CAP-tate) USAN.
Use: Antineoplastic, radiopharmaceutical.

Borocell. (Neutron Technology) Sodium monomercaptoundecahdrocloso-dodecaborate.
Use: Boron neutron capture therapy (BNCT) in glioblastoma multiforme.

Borofair Otic. (Major) Acetic acid 2% in aluminum acetate Soln. Bot. 60 ml. *Rx.*
Use: Otic.

Borofax Skin Protectant. (Warner Lambert Consumer Health Products) Zinc oxide 15%, petrolatum 68.6%, lanolin, mineral oil. Oint. Tube 50 g. *otc.*
Use: Dermatologic, counterirritant.

Boroglycerin. Glycerol borate. (Emerson) Bot. pt.

boroglycerin glycerite. Boric acid 31 parts, glycerin 96 parts.
Use: Agent for dermatitis.

Boropak Powder. (Glenwood) Aluminum sulfate and calcium acetate. One packet dissolved in a pint of water yields a 1:40 dilution. Pcks 2.4 g. 100s. *otc.*
Use: Anti-inflammatory, topical.

borotannic complex. Boric acid 31 mg, tannic acid 50 mg.
W/salicylic acid, ethyl alcohol.
See: Onycho-Phytex, Liq. (Unimed).

•**bosentan.** (boe-SEN-tan) USAN.
Use: Antagonist (endothelin receptor).

Boston Advance Cleaner. (Polymer Technology International) Concentrated homogenous surfactant with friction-enhancing agents. Soln. Bot. 30 ml. *otc.*
Use: Contact lens care.

Boston Advance Comfort Formula. (Polymer Technology International) Buffered, slightly hypertonic. Polyamino-

propyl biguanide 0.00015%, EDTA 0.05%, cationic cellulose derivative polymer. Soln. Bot. 120 ml. *otc.*
Use: Contact lens care.

Boston Advance Conditioning Solution. (Polymer Technology International) Sterile, buffered, slightly hypertonic. Polyaminopropyl biguanide 0.0015%, EDTA 0.05%. Bot. 120 ml or with cleaner in a convenience pack. *otc.*
Use: Contact lens care.

Boston Advance Rewetting Drops. (Polymer Technology International) Buffered, slightly hypertonic. Polyaminopropyl biguanide 0.0015%, EDTA 0.05%. Bot. 10 ml. *otc.*
Use: Contact lens care.

Boston Cleaner. (Polymer Technology International) Concentrated homogenons surfactant with friction-enhancing agents, sodium Cl. Soln. Bot. 30 ml. *otc.*
Use: Contact lens care.

Boston Conditioning Solution. (Polymer Technology International) Sterile, buffered, slightly hypertonic, low viscosity. EDTA 0.05%, chlorhexidine gluconate 0.006%. Bot. 120 ml. *otc.*
Use: Contact lens care.

Boston Reconditioning Drops. (Polymer Technology International) Hydrophilic polyelectrolyte, polyvinyl alcohol, hydroxyethylcellulose, chlorhexidine gluconate, EDTA. Soln. Bot. 120 ml. *otc.*
Use: Contact lens care.

Boston Rewetting Drops. (Polymer Technology International) Buffered, slightly hypertonic. Chlorhexidine gluconate 0.006%, EDTA 0.05%, cationic cellulose derivative polymer. Soln. Bot. 10 ml. *otc.*
Use: Contact lens care.

Botox. (Allergan) Botulinum toxin type A 100 units, albumin 0.05 mg, sodium chloride 0.9mg. Pow. for Inj. (lyophilized). Vials. *Rx.*
Use: Opthalmic.

Bottom Better. (Inno Visions) Petrolatum 49%, lanolin 15.5%, beeswax, sodium borate, lanolin alcohols, methylsalicylate, sorbitan sesquioleate, parabens, oxyquinolone, EDTA. Oint. Pkg. 18s. *otc.*
Use: Diaper rash preparation.

botulinum toxin type A.
Use: Ophthalmic. [Orphan drug]
See: Dysport (Porton).
Botox (Allergan).

botulinum toxin type B. (Athena Neurosciences).
Use: Cervical dystonia [Orphan drug]

botulinum toxin type F. (Porton)
Use: Cervical dystonia; essential blepharospasm. [Orphan drug]

•**botulism antitoxin.** U.S.P. 23.
Use: Prophylaxis and treatment of the toxins of C. botulinum, Types A or B; passive immunizing agent.

botulism immune globulin.
Use: Infant botulism. [Orphan drug]

Bounty Bears. (NBTY) Vitamins A 2500 IU, D 400 IU, E 15 IU, C 60 mg, B_1 1.05 mg, B_2 1.2 mg, B_3 13.5 mg, B_6 1.05 mg, B_{12} 4.5 mcg, folic acid 0.3 mg/Tab. Bot. 100s. *otc.*
Use: Mineral, vitamin supplement.

Bounty Bears Plus Iron. (NBTY) Vitamins A 2500 IU, D 400 IU, E 15 IU, C 60 mg, B_1 1.05 mg, B_2 1.2 mg, B_3 13.5 mg, B_6 1.05 mg, B_{12} 4.5 mcg, folic acid 0.3 mg, iron 15 mg/Tab. Bot. 100s. *otc.*
Use: Mineral, vitamin supplement.

bourbonal.
See: Ethyl Vanillin, N.F. 18.

bovine colostrum.
Use: AIDS-related diarrhea. [Orphan drug]

bovine immunoglobulin concentrate, cryptosporidium parvum.
Use: Anti-infective. [Orphan drug]
See: Sporidin-G (GalaGen).

bovine whey protein concentrate.
Use: Treatment of cryptosporidiosis. [Orphan drug]
See: Immuno-C (Biomune Systems).

Bowman Cold Tabs. (Jones Medical Industries) Acetaminophen 324 mg, phenylpropanolamine HCl 24.3 mg, caffeine 16.2 mg/Tab. Bot. 1000s, 5000s. *otc.*
Use: Analgesic, decongestant.

Bowman's Poison Antidote Kit. (Jones Medical Industries) Syrup of ipecac 1 oz, 1 bottle; activated charcoal liquid 2 oz, 3 bottles. *otc.*
Use: Antidote.

Bowsteral. (Jones Medical Industries) Isopropanol 60%. Bot. pt, gal.
Use: Disinfectant.

•**boxidine.** (BOX-ih-deen) USAN.
Use: Adrenal steroid blocker, antihyperlipoproteinemic.

Boylex. (Health for Life Brands) Diperodon, hexachlorophene, rosin cerate, ichthammol, carbolic acid, thymol, camphor, juniper tar. Tube oz. *otc.*
Use: Drawing salve.

B-Pap. (Wren) Acetaminophen 120 mg, sodium butabarbital 15 mg/5 ml. Bot. pt, gal. *Rx.*
Use: Analgesic, sedative.

b-pas.
See: Calcium Benzoyl PAS.

B-Plex. (Zenith Goldline) Vitamins B_1 15 mg, B_2 15 mg, B_3 100 mg, B_5 18 mg, B_6 4 mg, B_{12} 5 mcg, C 500 mg, folic acid 0.5 mg/Tab. Bot. 100s. *Rx.*
Use: Mineral, vitamin supplement.

BP-Papaverine. (Burlington) Papaverine HCl 150 mg/S.R. Cap. Bot. 50s. *Rx.*
Use: Vasodilator.

BP Cold Tablets. (Bristol-Myers) Acetaminophen 325 mg, phenylpropanolamine HCl 12.5 mg, chlorpheniramine maleate 2 mg/Tab. Card 16s, Bot. 16s, 30s, 50s. *otc.*
Use: Analgesic, antihistamine, decongestant.

Brace. (SmithKline Beecham Pharmaceuticals) Denture adhesive. Tube 1.4 oz, 2.4 oz.

Bradosol Bromide. (Novartis Pharmaceuticals) Domiphen bromide.

BranchAmin 4%. (Baxter) Isoleucine 1.38 g, leucine 1.38 g, valine 1.25 g, phosphate 31.6 mOsm/100 ml. Bot. 500 ml. *Rx.*
Use: Adjunct to regular TPN therapy for highly stressed or traumatized patients.

branched chain amino acids.
Use: Nutritional supplement; amyotrophic lateral sclerosis agent. [Orphan drug]

Brasivol Fine, Medium and Rough. (Stiefel) Aluminum oxide scrub particles in a surfactant cleansing base. **Fine:** Jar 153 g. **Medium:** Jar 180 g. **Rough:** Jar 195 g. *otc.*
Use: Scrub cleanser.

Breacol Decongestant Cough Medication. (Bayer Corp) Dextromethorphan HBr 10 mg, phenylpropanolamine HCl 37.5 mg, alcohol 10%, chlorpheniramine maleate 4 mg/5 ml. Bot. 3 oz, 6 oz. *otc.*
Use: Antihistamine, antitussive, decongestant.

Breatheasy. (Pascal) Racemic epinephrine HCl soln. 2.2% inhaled by use of nebulizer. Bot. 0.25 oz, 0.5 oz, 1 oz. *otc.*
Use: Bronchodilator.

Breezee Mist. (Pedinol) Aluminum chlorhydrate, undecylenic acid, menthol. Aerosol Bot. 4 oz. *otc.*
Use: Antifungal, deodorant, antiperspirant, foot powder.

Breezee Mist Foot Powder. (Pedinol) Isobutane, talc, aluminium chlorhydrate, cyclomethicone, isopropyl myristate, propylene carbonate, stearalkonium hectorite, underglenic acid, fragrance, menthol. Pow. 113 g. *otc.*
Use: Antifungal, topical.

Breonesin. (Sanofi Winthrop) Guaifenesin 200 mg/Cap. Bot. 100s. *otc.*
Use: Expectorant.

•**brequinar sodium.** (BREh-kwih-NAHR) USAN.
Use: Antineoplastic.

•**bretazenil.** (bret-AZZ-eh-nill) USAN
Use: Anxiolytic.

Brethaire. (Novartis) Terbutaline sulfate inhaler 7.5 ml. (10.5 g) w/mouthpiece. *Rx.*
Use: Bronchodilator.

Brethancer. (Novartis) Inhaler (complete unit to be used with Brethaire).

Brethine. (Novartis) Terbutaline sulfate. **Tab.:** 2.5 mg. Bot. 100s, 1000s, UD 100s, Gy-Pak 90s, 100s. 5 mg. Bot. 100s, 1000s, UD 100s, Gy-Pak 90s, 100s. **Amp.:** 1 mg/ml. Box 10s, 100s. *Rx.*
Use: Bronchodilator.

•**bretylium tosylate.** (bre-TILL-ee-uhm TAH-sill-ate) U.S.P. 23.
Use: Hypotensive, antiadrenergic, cardiovascular agent (antiarrhythmic).
See: Bretylol, Inj. (DuPont Merck Pharmaceuticals).

bretylium tosylate in 5% dextrose. (Various Mfr.) Bretylium tosylate 500 mg or 1000 mg/Vial. Inj. Vial 250 ml. *Rx.*
Use: Antiarrhythmic.

Brevibloc. (Ohmeda Pharmaceuticals) Esmolol HCl 10 mg/ml or 250 mg/ml, propylene glycol 25%. **10 mg/ml:** Vial 10 ml. **250 mg/ml:** Amp 10 ml. *Rx.*
Use: Beta-adrenergic blocker.

Brevicon. (Syntex) Norethindrone 0.5 mg, ethinyl estradiol 0.035 mg/Tab. 21 and 28 day (7 inert tabs) Wallette. *Rx.*
Use: Contraceptive.

Brevital Sodium. (Eli Lilly) Methohexital sodium. **Vial:** 500 mg/50 ml, 500 mg/ 50 ml w/diluent, 2.5 g/250 ml, 5 g/500 ml. **Amp.:** 2.5 g, 5 g. *Rx.*
Use: Anesthetic, general.

Brevoxyl. (Stiefel) Benzyol peroxide 4%, cetyl and stearyl alcohol. Gel. Tube 42.5 g, 90 g. *Rx.*
Use: Antiacne.

brewer's yeast. (NBTY) Vitamins B_1 0.06 mg, B_2 0.02 mg, B_3 0.2 mg/Tab. Bot 250s. *otc.*

Use: Vitamin supplement.

Brexin EX Liquid. (Savage) Pseudoephedrine HCl 30 mg, guaifenesin 200 mg/5 ml. *otc.*
Use: Decongestant, expectorant.

Brexin EX Tablet. (Savage) Pseudoephedrine HCl 60 mg, guaifenesin 400 mg/Tab. Bot. 100s. *otc.*
Use: Decongestant, expectorant.

Brexin L.A. (Savage) Chlorpheniramine maleate 8 mg, pseudoephedrine HCl 120 mg/L.A. Cap. Bot. 100s. *otc.*
Use: Antihistamine, decongestant.

Bricanyl Injection. (SmithKline Beecham Pharmaceuticals) Terbutaline sulfate 1 mg/Amp. 1 ml. 10s. *Rx.*
Use: Bronchodilator.

Bricanyl Tablets. (SmithKline Beecham Pharmaceuticals) Terbutaline sulfate 2.5 mg or 5 mg/Tab. Bot. 100s, 1000s, UD 100s. *Rx.*
Use: Bronchodilator.

•**brifentanil hydrochloride.** (brih-FEN-tah-NILL) USAN.
Use: Analgesic, narcotic.

Brigen-G. (Grafton) Chlordiazepoxide 5 mg, 10 mg or 25 mg/Tab. Bot. 500s. *c-iv.*
Use: Anxiolytic.

Brij 96 and 97. (ICI Americas) Polyoxyl 10 oleyl ether available as 96 and 97.
Use: Surface active agent.

Brij-721. (ICI Americas) Polyoxyethylene 21 stearyl ether (100% active).
Use: Surface active agent.

•**brimonidine tartrate.** (brih-MOE-nih-DEEN) USAN.
Use: Adrenergic (ophthalmic).
See: Alphagan (Allergan).

•**brinolase.** (BRIN-oh-laze) USAN. Fibrinolytic enzyme produced by *Aspergillus oryzae.*
Use: Fibrinolytic.

•**brinzolamide.** (brin-ZOE-lah-mide) USAN.
Use: Antiglaucoma agent.
See: Azopt, Ophth. Susp. (Alcon).

Brirel w/Superinone. (Sanofi Winthrop) Hexahydropyrazine, hexahydrate. *Rx.*
Use: Anthelmintic.

Bristoject. (Bristol-Myers Squibb) Prefilled disposable syringes w/needle.
Aminophylline: 250 mg/10 ml.
Atropine Sulfate: 5 mg/5 ml or 1 mg/ml. 10s.
Calcium Cl: 10%. 10 ml. 10s.
Dexamethasone: 20 mg/5 ml.
Dextrose: 50%. 50 ml. 10s.
Diphenhydramine: 50 mg/5 ml.
Dopamine HCl: 200 mg/5 ml, 400 mg/10 ml.
Ephedrine: 50 mg/10 ml.
Epinephrine: 1:10,000. 10 ml. 10s.
Lidocaine HCl.: 1%: 5 ml, 10 ml; 2%: 5 ml; 4%: 25 ml, 50 ml; 20%: 5 ml, 10 ml.
Magnesium Sulfate: 5 g/10 ml. 10s.
Metaraminol: 1%. 10 ml.
Sodium Bicarbonate: 7.5%: 50 ml; 8.4%: 50 ml. 10s.

british anti-lewisite. Dimercaprol.
See: BAL.

Brobella-P.B. (Brothers) Atropine sulfate 0.0195 mg, hyoscine HBr 0.0065 mg, hyoscyamine sulfate 0.1040 mg, phenobarbital 0.25 gr/Tab. Bot. 100s, 1000s. *Rx.*
Use. Anticholinergic, antispasmodic, hypnotic, sedative.

•**brocresine.** (broe-KREE-seen) USAN.
Use: Histidine decarboxylase inhibitor.
See: Contramine phosphate.

•**brocrinat.** (BROE-krih-NAT) USAN.
Use: Diuretic.

Brocycline. (Brothers) Tetracycline HCl 250 mg/Cap. Bot. 100s, 1000s. *Rx.*
Use: Anti-infective; tetracycline.

Brofed. (Marnel) Pseudoephedrine HCl 30 mg, brompheniramine maleate 4 mg/5 ml. Elix. Bot. 473 ml. *otc.*
Use: Antihistamine, decongestant.

•**brofoxine.** (BROE-fox-een) USAN.
Use: Antipsychotic.

Brolade. (Brothers) Chlorpheniramine maleate 8 mg, phenylephrine HCl 20 mg, methscopolamine nitrate 2.5 mg/Cap. Bot. 50s, 500s. *Rx.*
Use: Anticholinergic, antihistamine, decongestant.

Brolene. (Bausch & Lomb) Propamidine isethionate 0.1% Ophth. Soln.
Use: Acanthamoeba Keratitis. [Orphan drug]

bromacrylide.

Bromadine-DM. (Cypress) Brompheniramine maleate 2 mg, pseudophedrine 130 mg, dextrometherphan HBr 10mg/5 ml, cherry flavor, Syr. Bot. 473 ml. *Rx.*
Use: Antihistamine, antitussive, decongestant.

•**bromadoline maleate.** (BROE-mah-DOE-leen) USAN.
Use: Analgesic.

bromaleate.
See: Pamabrom.

Bromaline Elixir. (Rugby) Phenylpropanolamine HCl 12.5 mg, bromphenir-

amine maleate 2 mg, alcohol 2.3%. Elix. Bot. 118 ml, 473 ml and gal. *otc.*
Use: Antihistamine, decongestant.

Bromaline Plus. (Rugby) Phenylpropanolamine HCl 12.5 mg, brompheniramine maleate 2 mg, acetaminophen 500 mg. Captabs. Bot. 24s. *otc.*
Use: Analgesic, antihistamine, decongestant.

Bromalix. (Century Pharm) Brompheniramine maleate 4 mg, phenylephrine HCl 5 mg, phenylpropanolamine HCl 5 mg, alcohol 2.3%/5 ml. Bot. 4 oz, pt, gal. *otc.*
Use: Antihistamine, decongestant.

Bromanate DC Cough Syrup. (Various Mfr.) Phenylpropanolamine HCl 12.5 mg, brompheniramine maleate 2 mg, codeine phosphate 10 mg, alcohol 0.95%. Syr. Bot. 120 ml, pt, gal. *c-v.*
Use: Antihistamine, antitussive, decongestant.

Bromanate Elixir. (Alphalma USPD) Phenylpropanolamine HCl 12.5 mg, brompheniramine maleate 2 mg/5 ml. Elix. Bot. 118 ml, 237 ml, 473 ml, gal. *otc.*
Use: Antihistamine, decongestant.

Bromanyl. (Various Mfr.) Bromodiphenhydramine HCl 12.5 mg, codeine phosphate 10 mg, alcohol 5%. Syr. Bot. pt, gal. *c-v.*
Use: Antihistamine, antitussive.

Bromarest DX. (Warner Chilcott) Pseudoephedrine HCl 30 mg, brompheniramine maleate 2 mg, dextromethorphan HBr 10 mg, alcohol 0.95%. Butterscotch favor. Syr. Bot. 480 ml. *Rx.*
Use: Antihistamine, antitussive, decongestant.

Bromatane D.C. Cough Syrup. (Zenith Goldline) Brompheniramine maleate, phenylpropanolamine HCl, codeine phosphate. Bot. gal. *c-v.*
Use: Antihistamine, antitussive, decongestant.

Bromatane DX Cough Syrup. (Zenith Goldline) Pseudoephedrine HCl 30 mg, brompheniramine maleate 2 mg, dextromethorphan HBr 10 mg. Bot. 480 ml. *Rx.*
Use: Antihistamine, antitussive, decongestant.

Bromatap Elixir. (Zenith Goldline) Brompheniramine maleate 2 mg, phenylephrine HCl 12.5 mg, alcohol 2.3%/5 ml. Bot. 4 oz, 8 oz, pt, gal. *otc.*
Use: Antihistamine, decongestant.

Bromatapp Tablets. (Copley) Brompheniramine maleate 12 mg, phenylpropanolamine HCl 75 mg/Tab. Bot. 100s. *otc.*
Use: Antihistamine, decongestant.

bromauric acid. Hydrogen tetrabromoaurate.

•**bromazepam.** (broe-MAY-zeh-pam) USAN.
Use: Anxiolytic.

bromazine.
See: Ambodryl HCl, Elix., Kapseal (Parke-Davis).

Brombay Elixir. (Rosemont) Brompheniramine maleate 2 mg/5 ml, alcohol 3%. Bot. 4 oz, pt, gal. *otc.*
Use: Antihistamine.

•**bromchlorenone.** (brome-KLOR-ee-nohn) USAN.
Use: Anti-infective, topical.

•**bromelains.** (BROE-meh-lanes) USAN.
Use: Anti-inflammatory.
See: Dayto-Anase, Tab. (Dayton).

Bromenzyme. (Barth's) Bromelain 40 mg/Tab. Bot. 100s, 250s, 500s. *otc, Rx.*
Use: Digestive aid.

Bromezyme. (Barth's) Bromelain 40 mg, papaya fruit, papain enzyme/Tab. Bot. 100s, 250s, 500s. *otc, Rx.*
Use: Digestive aid.

bromethol.
See: Avertin.

Bromfed Capsules. (Muro) Brompheniramine maleate 12 mg, pseudoephedrine HCl 120 mg/TR Cap. Bot. 100s, 500s. *Rx.*
Use: Antihistamine, decongestant.

Bromfed-DM Syrup. (Muro) Brompheniramine maleate 2 mg, pseudoephedrine HCl 30 mg, dextromethorphan HBr 10 mg/5 ml. Bot. 120 ml, 240 ml, 480 ml. *Rx.*
Use: Antihistamine, antitussive, decongestant.

Bromfed-PD Capsules. (Muro) Brompheniramine maleate 6 mg, pseudoephedrine HCl 60 mg/TR Cap. Bot. 100s, 500s. *Rx.*
Use: Antihistamine, decongestant.

Bromfed Syrup. (Muro) Brompheniramine maleate 2 mg, pseudoephedrine HCl 30 mg/5 ml. Bot. 120 ml, 473 ml. *otc.*
Use: Antihistamine, decongestant.

Bromfed Tablets. (Muro) Brompheniramine maleate 4 mg, pseudoephedrine HCl 60 mg/Tab. Bot. 100s. *Rx.*
Use: Antihistamine, decongestant.

Bromfenex. (Ethex) Brompheniramine maleate 12 mg, pseudoephedrine HCl 120 mg/ER Cap. Bot. 100s, 500s. *Rx.*

Use: Antihistamine, decongestant.

Bromfenex PD. (Ethex) Brompheniramine maleate 6 mg, pseudoephedrine HCl 60 mg, sucrose/ER Cap. Bot. 100s, 500s. *Rx.*
Use: Antihistamine, decongestant.

•**bromhexine hydrochloride.** (brome-HEX-een) USAN.
Use: Expectorant, mucolytic.
See: Bisolvon (Boehringer Ingelheim).

bromhexine. (Boehringer Ingelheim)
Use: Mild/moderate keratoconjunctivitis sicca. [Orphan drug]

bromides.
See: Lanabrom, Elix. (Lannett).
Peacocks Bromides, Liq. (Natcon).

bromide salts.
See: Calcium Bromide.
Ferrous Bromide.
Potassium Bromide.
Sodium Bromide.
Strontium Bromide.

Bromi-Lotion. (Gordon Laboratories) Aluminum hydroxychloride 20%, emollient base. Bot. 1.5 oz, 4 oz. *otc.*
Use: Antiperspirant.

•**bromindione.** (BROME-in-die-ohn) USAN.
Use: Anticoagulant.
See: Circladin.

Bromi-Talc. (Gordon Laboratories) Potassium alum, bentonite, talc. Shaker can 3.5 oz, 1 lb, 5 lb. *otc.*
Use: Bromidrosis, hyperhidrosis.

•**bromocriptine.** (BROE-moe-KRIP-teen) USAN.
Use: Enzyme inhibitor (prolactin).

•**bromocriptine mesylate.** (BROE-moe-KRIP-teen) U.S.P. 23.
Use: Enzyme inhibitor (prolactin).
See: Parlodel, Tab. (Novartis).

bromodeoxyuridine. (Neopharm)
Use: Radiation sensitizer in treatment of primary brain tumors. [Orphan drug]

bromodiethylacetylurea.
See: Carbromal.

•**bromodiphenhydramine hydrochloride.** (BROE-moe-die-feu-HIGH-drahmeen) U.S.P. 23.
Use: Antihistamine.

bromodiphenhydramine HCl/codeine phosphate. (Rosemont) Bromodiphenhydramine HCl 12.5 mg, codeine phsophate 10 mg. Syr. Bot. 480 ml. *c-v.*
Use: Antitussive combination.

bromofrom. Tribromomethane.

bromoisovaleryl urea. Alpha, bromoisovaleryl urea.
See: Bromisovalum.

Bromophen T.D. (Rugby) Phenylpropanolamine HCl 15 mg, phenylephrine HCl 15 mg, brompheniramine maleate 12 mg/Tab. Bot. 100s, 1000s. *Rx.*
Use: Antihistamine, decongestant.

Bromophin.
See: Apomorphine HCl (Various Mfr.).

Bromo Quinine Cold Tablets.
See: BQ Cold Tablets (Bristol-Myers).

Bromo Seltzer. (Warner Lambert) Acetaminophen 325 mg, sodium bicarbonate 2.78 g, citric acid 2.22 g (when dissolved, forms sodium citrate 2.85 g)/ Dose. Large (2⅝ oz), King (4.25 oz), Giant (9 oz), Foil pack, single dose 48s. *otc.*
Use: Antacid, analgesic.

8-bromotheophylline.
See: Pamabrom.

bromotheophyllinate aminoisobutanol.
See: Pamabrom.

bromotheophyllinate pyranisamine.
See: Pyrabrom.

bromotheophyllinate pyrilamine.
See: Pyrabrom.

Bromotuss W/ Codeine. (Rugby) Bromodiphenhydramine HCl 12.5 mg, codeine phosphate 10 mg, alcohol 5 %. Syr. Bot. 120 ml, pt, gal. *c-v.*
Use: Antihistamine, antitussive.

•**bromoxanide.** (broe-MOX-ah-nide) USAN.
Use: Anthelmintic.

•**bromperidol.** (brome-PURR-ih-dahl) USAN.
Use: Antipsychotic.

•**bromperidol decanoate.** (brome-PURR-ih-dole deh-KAN-oh-ate) USAN.
Use: Antipsychotic.

Bromphen DC w/ Codeine Cough Syrup. (Various Mfr.) Phenylpropanolamine HCl 12.5 mg, brompheniramine maleate 2 mg, codeine phosphate 10 mg, alcohol 0.95%. Syr. Bot. 120 ml, pt, gal. *c-v.*
Use: Antihistamine, antitussive, decongestant.

Bromphen DX. (Rugby) Pseudoephedrine HCl 30 mg, brompheniramine maleate 2 mg, dextromethorphan HBr 10 mg, alcohol 0.95%. Syr. Bot. 480 ml. *Rx.*
Use: Antihistamine, antitussive, decongestant.

Bromphen Expectorant. (Various Mfr.) Phenylpropanolamine HCl 5 mg, phenylephrine HCl 5 mg, bromphenir-

amine maleate 2 mg, guaifenesin 100 mg, alcohol 3.5%. Liq. Bot. 120 ml, pt, gal. *otc.*
Use: Antihistamine, decongestant, expectorant.

Brompheniramine Cough Syrup. (Geneva Pharm) Pseudoephedrine HCl 30 mg, brompheniramine maleate 2 mg, dextromethorphan HBr 10 mg, alcohol 0.95%. Bot. 480 ml. *Rx.*
Use: Antihistamine, antitussive, decongestant.

Brompheniramine DC. (Geneva Pharm) Phenylpropanolamine HCl 12.5 mg, brompheniramine maleate 2 mg, codeine phosphate 10 mg, alcohol 0.95%. Syr. Bot. 120 ml. *c-v.*
Use: Antihistamine, antitussive, decongestant.

•**brompheniramine maleate.** (brome-fen-AIR-uh-meen) U.S.P. 23.
Use: Antihistamine.
See: Dimetane, Tab., Elix., Inj. (Robins).
Dimetapp Allergy, Liquigels (Att Robins).
Symptom 3, Liq. (Parke-Davis).
Veltane (Lannett).

brompheniramine maleate. (Various Mfr.) Brompheniramine maleate 10 mg/ml, parabens. Inj. Multi-dose vial 10 ml. *Rx.*
Use: Antihistamine.

brompheniramine maleate w/combinations.
See: Bro-Expectorant W/Codeine, Liq. (Solvay).
Bromadine-DM, Syr. (Cypress).
Bromepaph, Preps. (Quality Generics).
Bromfenex, ER Cap. (Ethex).
Cortane, Preps. (Standex).
Cortapp, Elix. (Standex).
Dimetane Decongestant, Tab., Elix. (Robins).
Dimetane Expectorant, Liq. (Robins).
Dimetane Expectorant-DC, Liq. (Robins).
Dimetapp Extentabs, Elix. (Robins).
Eldatapp, Tab., Liq. (ICN Pharmaceuticals).
Iofed, ER Cap. (Iomed).
Iofed PD, ER Cap. (Iomed).
Iohist DM, Syr. (Iomed).
Liqui-Histine DM, Syr. (Liquipharm).
Rondex, Chew. Tab. (Dura).

Brompton's Cocktail. Heroin or morphine 10 mg, cocaine 10 mg, alcohol, chloroform water, syrup. *c-II.*
Use: Analgesic, narcotic.

Bromtapp. (Halsey) Brompheniramine maleate 4 mg, phenylephrine HCl 5 mg, phenylpropanolamine HCl 5 mg/5 ml. Bot. 16 oz, gal. *otc.*
Use: Antihistamine, decongestant.

Bronchial Capsules. (Various Mfr.) Theophylline 150 mg, guaifenesin 90 mg. Cap. Bot. 100s, 1000s. *Rx.*
Use: Antiasthmatic, expectorant.

Broncholate Capsules. (Sanofi Winthrop) Ephedrine HCl 12.5 mg, guaifenesin 200 mg/Cap. Bot. 100s, 1000s. *Rx.*
Use: Bronchodilator, expectorant.

Broncholate Softgels. (Sanofi Winthrop) Ephedrine HCl 12.5 mg, guaifenesin 200 mg. Cap. Bot. 100s. *Rx.*
Use: Bronchodilator, expectorant.

Broncholate Syrup. (Sanofi Winthrop) Ephedrine HCl 6.25 mg, guaifenesin 100 mg/5 ml. Bot. pt. *Rx.*
Use: Bronchodilator, expectorant.

Broncho Saline. (Blairex Labs) 0.9% sodium Cl for diluting bronchodilator solutions for inhalation. Soln. 90 ml, 240 ml w/metered dispensing valve. *otc.*
Use: Diluent.

Brondecon. (Parke-Davis) **Tab.:** Oxtriphylline 200 mg, guaifenesin 100 mg/Tab. Bot. 100s. **Elix.:** Oxtriphylline 100 mg, guaifenesin 50 mg/5 ml w/alcohol 20%. Bot. 8 oz, 16 oz. *Rx.*
Use: Bronchodilator, expectorant.

Brondelate. (Various Mfr.) Oxtriphylline 300 mg, guaifenesin 150 mg/5 ml. Elix. Bot. 480 ml, gal. *Rx.*
Use: Bronchodilator, expectorant.

Bronitin. (Whitehall Robins) Theophylline hydrous 120 mg, guaifenesin 100 mg, ephedrine HCl 24.3 mg, pyrilamine maleate 16.6 mg/Tab. Bot. 24s, 60s. *otc.*
Use: Bronchodilator.

Bronitin Mist. (Whitehall Robins) Epinephrine bitartrate in inhalation aerosol. Each spray releases 0.3 mg epinephrine bitartrate equivalent to 0.16 mg epinephrine base. Bot 15 ml or 15 ml refills. *otc.*
Use: Bronchodilator.

Bronkaid Dual Action. (Bayer Corp) Ephedrine sulfate 25 mg, guaifenesin 400 mg. Capl. Bot. 24s. *otc.*
Use: Bronchodilator, expectorant.

Bronkodyl. (Sanofi Winthrop) Theophylline 100 mg or 200 mg/Cap. Bot. 100s. Theophylline 300 mg/SR Cap. Bot. 100s. *Rx.*
Use: Bronchodilator.

Bronkometer. (Sanofi Winthrop) Isoetharine mesylate 0.61%, saccharin, menthol, alcohol 30%. Metered dose of 340 mcg isoetharine in fluoro hydrocarbon propellant. Bot. w/nebulizer 10 ml, 15 ml. Refill 10 ml, 15 ml. *Rx.*
Use: Bronchodilator.

Bronkosol. (Sanofi Winthrop) Isoetharine HCl 1% w/glycerin, sodium bisulfite, parabens for oral inhalation. Bot. 10 ml, 30 ml. *Rx.*
Use: Bronchodilator.

Bronkotuss. (Hyrex) Chlorpheniramine maleate 4 mg, guaifenesin 100 mg, ephedrine sulfate 8.216 mg, hydriodic acid syrup 1.67 mg/5 ml w/alcohol 5%. Bot. pt, gal. *Rx.*
Use: Antihistamine, decongestant, expectorant.

Brontex Liquid. (Procter & Gamble) Codeine phosphate 2.5 mg, guaifenesin 75 mg per 5 ml, methylparaben, saccharin, sucrose/Liq. Bot. 473 ml. *c-v.*
Use: Antitussive expectorant, narcotic.

Brontex Tablets. (Procter & Gamble) Codeine phosphate 10 mg, guaifenesin 300 mg/Tab. Bot. 100s. *c-III.*
Use: Antitussive expecotrant, narcotic.

•**broperamole.** (BROE-PURR-ah-mole) USAN.
Use: Anti-inflammatory.

•**bropirimine.** (broe-PIE-rih-MEEN) USAN.
Use: Antineoplastic, antiviral.

Broserpine. (Brothers) Reserpine 0.25 mg/Tab. Bot. 250s, 100s.
Use: Antihypertensive.

Brotane Expectorant. (Halsey) Guaifenesin 100 mg, brompheniramine maleate 2 mg, phenylephrine HCl 5 mg, phenylpropanolamine HCl 5 mg/5 ml, alcohol 3.5%. Bot. 16 oz. *otc.*
Use: Antihistamine, decongestant, expectorant.

•**brotizolam.** (broe-TIE-zoe-LAM) USAN.
Use: Hypnotic, sedative.

Bro-T's. (Brothers) Bromisovalum 0.12 g, carbromal 0.2 g/Tab. Bot. 100s, 1000s. *Rx.*
Use: Sedative, anxiolytic.

Bro-Tuss. (Brothers) Dextromethorphan HBr 15 mg, chlorpheniramine maleate 2 mg, phenylephrine HCl 5 mg, ammonium Cl 100 mg, sodium citrate 150 mg, vitamin C 30 mg/10 ml. Bot. 4 oz, pt, gal. *otc.*
Use: Antihistamine, antitussive, decongestant, expectorant.

Bro-Tuss A.C. (Brothers) Acetaminophen 120 mg, codeine phosphate 10 mg, phenylephrine HCl 5 mg, chlorpheniramine maleate 2 mg, menthol 1 mg, alcohol 10%/5 ml. Bot. pt, gal. *c-v.*
Use: Analgesic, antihistamine, antitussive, decongestant.

Bryrel Syrup. (Sanofi Winthrop) Piperazine citrate anhydrous 110 mg/ml. Bot. oz. *Rx.*
Use: Anthelmintic.

B-Salt Forte. (Akorn) **Part I:** Sodium Cl 7.14 mg, potassium Cl 0.38 mg, calcium chloride dihydrate 0.154 mg, magnesium chloride hexahydrate 0.2 mg, dextrose 0.92 mg, hydrochloric acid or sodium hydroxide/ml. Soln. Bot. 515 ml. **Part II:** Sodium bicarbonate 1081 mg, dibasic sodium phosphate (anhydrous) 216 mg, glutathione disulfide 95 mg/vial. Soln. Bot. 60 ml. *Rx.*
Use: Irrigant, ophthalmic.

B-Scorbic. (Pharmics) Vitamins C 300 mg, B_1 25 mg, B_2 10 mg, calcium pantothenate 10 mg, niacinamide 50 mg, lemon flavored complex 200 mg/Tab. Bot. 100s, 1000s. *otc.*
Use: Mineral, vitamin supplement.

BSS. (Alcon Laboratories) Sodium Cl 0.64%, potassium Cl 0.075%, magnesium Cl 0.03%, calcium Cl 0.048%, sodium acetate 0.39%, sodium citrate 0.17%, sodium hydroxide or hydrochloric acid. Bot. 15 ml, 30 ml, 250 ml, 500 ml. *Rx.*
Use: Irrigant, ophthalmic.

BSS Plus. (Alcon Laboratories) **Part I:** Sodium Cl 7.44 mg, potassium Cl 0.395 mg, dibasic sodium phosphate 0.433 mg, sodium bicarbonate 2.19 mg, hydrochloric acid or sodium hydroxide/ml. Soln. Bot. 240 ml. **Part II:** Calcium chloride dihydrate 3.85 mg, magnesium chloride hexahydrate 5 mg, dextrose 23 mg, glutathione disulfide 4.5 mg/ml. Soln. Bot. 10 ml. *Rx.*
Use: Irrigant, ophthalmic.

BTA Rapid Urine Test. (Bard) Reagent kit for detection of bladder tumor associated analytes in urine to aid in management of bladder cancer. In kits of 15 and 30 tests. *Rx.*
Use: Diagnostic aid.

•**bucainide maleate.** (byoo-CANE-ide) USAN.
Use: Cardiovascular agent (antiarrhythmic).

Bucet. (Forest Pharmaceutical) Butalbital 50 mg, acetaminophen 650 mg. Cap. Bot. 100s. *Rx.*
Use: Analgesic.

buchu.
See: Barosmin.

•**bucindolol hydrochloride.** (BYOO-SIN-doe-lole) USAN.
Use: Investigative, antihypertensive.

Bucladin-S. (Zeneca) Buclizine HCl 50 mg. Softab. Tab. Bot. 100s. *Rx.*
Use: Antiemetic, antivertigo.

•**buclizine hydrochloride.** (BYOO-klih-zeen) USAN.
Use: Antiemetic, antinauseant.
See: Bucladin-S, Tab. (Zeneca).

•**bucromarone.** (byoo-KROE-mah-rone) USAN.
Use: Cardiovascular agent (antiarrhythmic).

•**bucrylate.** (BYOO-krih-late) USAN.
Use: Surgical aid (tissue adhesive).

•**budesonide.** (BYOO-DESS-oh-nide) USAN.
Use: Anti-inflammatory.
See: Pulmicort Turbuhaler, Drug Pow. for Inhalation (Astra).

Buf Acne Cleansing Bar. (3M Products) Salicylic acid 1%, sulfur 1% in detergent cleansing bar. 3.5 oz. *otc.*
Use: Antiacne.

Buf-Bar. (3M Products) Sulphur 3% and titanium dioxide. Bar 105 g. *otc.*
Use: Antiacne.

Buf Body Scrub. (3M Products) Round cleansing sponge on plastic handles. *otc.*
Use: Cleansing sponge.

Buff-A. (Merz) Aspirin acid 5 gr. buffered w/magnesium hydroxide, aluminum hydroxide dried gel. Tab. Bot. 100s, 1000s. *otc.*
Use: Analgesic, antacid.

Buffaprin. (Buffington) Aspirin 325 mg. buffered with magnesium oxide. Sugar, caffeine, lactose, salt free. Tab. Dispens-A-Kit 500s. *otc.*
Use: Analgesic.

Buffasal. (Dover Pharmaceuticals) Aspirin 325 mg/Tab. w/ magnesium oxide. Sugar, lactose, salt free. UD Box 500s. *otc.*
Use: Analgesic.

Buffasal Max. (Dover Pharmaceuticals) Aspirin 500 mg/Tab w/magnesium oxide. Sugar, lactose, salt free. *otc.*
Use: Analgesic.

Bufferin AF Nite Time. (Bristol-Myers Squibb) Acetaminophen 500 mg, diphenhydramine citrate 38 mg, simethicone. Cap shaped tab. Bot. 24s and 50s. *otc.*
Use: Analgesic, sedative.

Buffered Aspirin. (Various Mfr.) Aspirin 325 mg with buffers. Tab. Bot. 100s, 500s, 1000s and UD 100s and 200s. *otc.*
Use: Analgesic.

buffered intrathecal electrolyte/dextrose injection.
Use: Diluent. [Orphan drug]
See: Elliots B Solution.

Buffets II. (Jones Medical Industries) Aspirin 227 mg, acetaminophen 162 mg, caffeine 32.4 mg, aluminum hydroxide 50 mg/Tab. Bot. 1000s. *otc.*
Use: Analgesic combination.

Buffex. (Roberts Pharm) Aspirin 325 mg w/dihydroxyaluminum aminoacetate. Tab. Bot. 1000s, Sanipack 1000s. *otc.*
Use: Analgesic.

Buf Foot Care Kit. (3M Products) Cleansing system for the feet. *otc.*
Use: Foot preparation.

Buf Foot Care Lotion. (3M Products) Moisturizing lotion for feet. *otc.*
Use: Foot preparation.

Buf Foot Care Soap. (3M Products) Bar 3.5 oz. *otc.*
Use: Foot preparation.

•**bufilcon a.** (BYOO-fill-kahn A) USAN.
Use: Contact lens material (hydrophilic).

Buf Kit for Acne. (3M Products) Cleansing sponge, cleansing bar. 3.5 oz w/ booklet, holding tray. *otc.*
Use: Antiacne.

Buf Lotion. (3M Products) Moisturizing lotion. *otc.*
Use: Emollient.

•**buformin.** (BYOO-FORE-min) USAN.
Use: Antidiabetic.

Bufosal. (Table Rock) Sodium salicylate 15 gr/dram w/calcium carbonate, sodium bicarbonate as granulated effervescent powder. Bot. 4 oz. *otc.*
Use: Analgesic, antacid.

Buf-Ped Non Medicated Cleansing Sponge. (3M Products) Abrasive cleansing sponge. *otc.*
Use: Cleansing skin on feet.

Buf Puf Bodymate. (3M Products) Oval two-sided cleansing sponge. Abrasive/gentle. *otc.*
Use: Cleansing all areas of the body.

Buf-Puf Medicated. (3M Products) Water-activated. Salicylic acid 0.5% (reg. strength), alcohols benzoate, EDTA, triethanolamine and vitamin E acetate. Salicylic acid 2% (max. strength). Pads. Jar 30s. *otc.*
Use: Antiacne.

Buf-Puf Non-Medicated cleansing sponge. (3M Products) Abrasive cleansing sponge. *otc.*
Use: Skin cleansing.

Buf-Sul Tablets and Suspension. (Sheryl) Sulfacetamide 167 mg, sulfadiazine 167 mg, sulfamerazine 167 mg. Tab. 100s. Susp. pt. *Rx.*
Use: Anti-infective, sulfonamide.

Buf-Tabs. (Halsey) Aspirin 5 gr/Tab. w/ aluminum hydroxide, glycine magnesium carbonate. Bot. 100s. *otc.*
Use: Analgesic, antacid.

Bug-Pruf. (Scherer) n, n diethyl-m-toluamide (DEET) 94.525%, other isomers 4.975%, fragrance 0.5%. Bot. 2 oz.
Use: Insect repellent.

Bugs Bunny Chewable Vitamins and Minerals. (Bayer Corp) Vitamins A 5000 IU, D 400 IU, E 30 IU, C 60 mg, folic acid 0.4 mg, B_1 1.5 mg, B_2 1.7 mg, niacin 20 mg, B_6 2 mg, B_{12} 6 mcg, biotin 40 mcg, pantothenic acid 10 mg, iron 18 mg, calcium 100 mg, phosphorus 100 mg, iodine 150 mcg, magnesium 20 mg, copper 2 mg, zinc 15 mg/Tab. Bot 60s. *otc.*
Use: Mineral, vitamin supplement.

Bugs Bunny Complete. (Bayer Corp) Ca 100 mg, iron 18 mg, vitamins A 5000 IU, D 400 IU, E 30 mg, B_1 1.5 mg, B_2 1.7mg, B_3 20 mg, B_5 10 mg, B_6 mcg, C 60 mg, folic acid 0.4 mg, biotin 40 mcg, Cu, I, Mg, P, aspartame, phenylalanine, Zn 15 mg/Tab. Bot 60s. *otc.*
Use: Mineral, vitamin supplement.

Bugs Bunny Plus Iron. (Bayer Corp) Vitamins A 2500 IU, E 15 IU, C 60 mg, folic acid 0.3 mg, B_1 1.05 mg, B_2 1.2 mg, niacin 13.5 mg, B_6 1.05 mg, B_{12} 4.5 mcg, D 400 IU, iron 15 mg/Chew. tab. Bot. 60s. *otc.*
Use: Mineral, vitamin supplement.

Bugs Bunny With Extra C. (Bayer Corp) Vitamins A 2500 IU, D 400 IU, E 15 IU, C 250 mg, folic acid 0.3 mg, B_1 1.05 mg, B_2 1.2 mg, niacin 13.5 mg, B_6 1.05 mg, B_{12} 4.5 mcg/Tab. Bot. 60s. *otc.*
Use: Mineral, vitamin supplement.

bulkogen. A mucin extracted from the seeds of *Cyanopsis tetragonaloba.*

Bullfrog. (Chattem Consumer Products) Benzophenone-3, octyl methoxycinnamate, isostearyl alcohol, aloe, hydrogenated vegetable oil, vitamin E. Waterproof. Stick 16.5 g. *otc.*
Use: Sunscreen.

Bullfrog Extra Moisturizing Gel. (Chattem Consumer Products) Benzophenone-3, octocrylene, octyl methoxycinnamate, vitamin E, aloe. SPF 18. Tube 90 g. *otc.*
Use: Sunscreen.

Bullfrog for Kids. (Chattem Consumer Products). SPF 18. Octocrylene, octyl methoxycinnamate, octyl salicylate, vitamin E, aloe, alcohols benzoate. Gel Tube 60 g. *otc.*
Use: Sunscreen.

Bullfrog Sport Lotion. (Chattem Consumer Products) SPF 18. Benzophenone-3, octocrylene, octyl methoxycinnamate, octyl salicylate, titanium dioxide, diazolidinyl urea, EDTA, parabens, vitamin E, aloe. Bot. 120 ml. *otc.*
Use: Sunscreen.

Bullfrog Sunblock. (Chattem Consumer Products) SPF 18, 36. Benzophenone-3, octocrylene, octyl methoxycinnamate, aloe, vitamin E, isostearyl alcohol. PABA free. Waterproof. Gel Tube 120 g. *otc.*
Use: Sunscreen.

•**bumetanide.** (BYOO-MET-uh-hide) U.S.P. 23.
Use: Diuretic.
See: Bumex, Inj., Tab. (Roche Laboratories).

bumetanide. (BYOO-MET-uh-nide) (Various) (Mylan) **Tab:** 0.5 mg, 1 mg, 2 mg/Tab. Bot. 100s. (Various Mfr.) **Inj.:** 0.25 mg/ml. Amp. 2 ml. Vial 2 ml, 4 ml, 10 ml; 4 ml fill in 5 ml. *Rx.*
Use: Diuretic.

•**bumetrizole.** (BYOO-meh-TRY-zole) USAN.
Use: Ultraviolet screen.

Bumex. (Roche Laboratories) Bumetanide 0.5 mg, 1 mg or 2 mg/Tab. 0.5 mg and 1 mg Bot. 100s, 500s, UD 100s. 2 mg Bot. 100s, UD 100s. Inj. Amp 2 ml, 0.25 mg/ml. Box 10s. Vial 2 ml, 4 ml or 10 ml, 0.25 mg/ml. Box 10s. *Rx.*
Use: Diuretic.

Buminate. (Baxter) Normal serum albumin (human) **25%** soln. in 20 ml w/o administration set; 50 ml and 100 ml w/ administration set. **5%** soln. in 250 ml and 500 ml w/administration set. *Rx.*
Use: Albumin replacement.

•**bunamide hydrochloride.** (BYOO-NAm-ih-deen) USAN.
Use: Anthelmintic.

bunamiodyl sodium.
Use: Diagnostic aid (radiopaque medium).

•**bunaprolast.** (BYOO-nah-PROLE-ast) USAN.
Use: Antiasthmatic.

•**bunolol hydrochloride.** (BYOO-no-lole) USAN.
Use: Antiadrenergic (β-receptor).

Bun Reagent Strips. (Bayer Corp) Seralyzer reagent strips. A quantitative strip test for BUN in serum or plasma. Bot 25s.
Use: Diagnostic aid.

Bupap. (ECR) Butalbital 50 mg, acetaminophen 650 mg. Tab. Bot. 100s. *Rx.*
Use: Analgesic.

Buphenyl. (Ucyclyd Pharma) Sodium phenylbutyrate 500 mg/Tab. Bot. 250s, 500s. 3.2 g (3 g sodium phenylbutyrate)/tsp. and 9.1 g (8.6 g sodium phenylbutyrate)/tsp/Pow. for inj. Bot. 500 ml and 950 ml. *Rx.*
Use: Antihyperammonemic.

•**bupicomide.** (byoo-PIH-koe-mide) USAN.
Use: Antihypertensive.

•**bupivacaine hydrochloride.** (byoo-PIH-vah-cane) U.S.P. 23.
Use: Anesthetic, local.

Bupivacaine HCl. (Abbott Laboratories) Bupivacaine 0.25%/Inj. Vial. 20 ml, 50 ml. Bupivacaine HCl 0.5%/Inj. Vial. 20 ml, 30 ml. Bupivacaine HCl 0.75%/Inj. Vial. 20 ml. *Rx.*
Use: Anesthetic, local.

bupivacaine in dextrose injection.
Use: Anesthetic, local.

bupivacaine and epinephrine injection.
Use: Anesthetic, local.
See: Marcaine w/Epinephrine, Inj. (Sanofi Winthrop).

bupivacaine hydrochloride.
Use: Anesthetic, local.
See: Marcaine, Inj (Astra).
Marcaine w/Epinephrine, Inj. (Cook-Waite).
Marcaine Spinal, Inj (Astra).
Sensorcaine MPF, Inj (Astra).
Sensorcaine MPF Spinal, Inj (Astra).
Bupivacaine HCl, Inj (Abbott Laboratories).
Sensorcaine, Inj. (Astra).

Buprenex Injection. (Reckitt & Colman) Buprenorphine HCl 0.3 mg/ml w/50 mg anhydrous dextrose. Amp. 1 ml. [c-v] c-v.
Use: Analgesic, narcotic.

•**buprenorphine hydrochloride,** (BYOO-preh-NAHR-feen) U.S.P. 23.
Use: Analgesic.

buprenorphine HCl.

•**bupropion hydrochloride.** (Reckitt and Coleman).
Use: Treatment of opiate addiction. [Orphan drug] (byoo-PRO-pee-ahn) USAN.
Use: Antidepressant; smoking deterrent.
See: Wellbutrin (GlaxoWellcome).
Zyban, SR Tab. (GlaxoWellcome).

•**buramate.** (BYOO-rah-mate) USAN.
Use: Anticonvulsant, antipsychotic, anxiolytic.
See: Hyamate (Xttrium).

Burdeo. (Hill) Aluminum subacetate 100 mg, boric acid 300 mg/oz. Bot. 3 oz. Roll-on 8 oz. *otc.*
Use: Deodorant.

Burn-a-Lay. (Ken-Gate) Chlorobutanol 0.75%, oxyquinoline benzoate 0.025%, zinc oxide 2%, thymol 0.5%. Cream. Tube oz. *otc.*
Use: Burn therapy.

Burnate. (Burlington) Vitamins A 4000 IU, D-2 400 IU, thiamine HCl 3 mg, riboflavin 2 mg, niacinamide 10 mg, pyridine HCl 2 mg, cyanocobalamin 5 mcg, calcium pantothenate 0.5 mg, folic acid 0.4 mg, ascorbic acid 50 mg, ferrous fumarate 300 mg, calcium 200 mg, iodine 0.15 mg, copper 1 mg, magnesium 5 mg, zinc 1.5 mg/Tab. Bot. 100s. *otc.*
Use: Mineral, vitamin supplement.

burn therapy.
See: Americaine, Preps. (DuPont Merck Pharmaceuticals).
Amertan, Jelly (Eli Lilly).
Burn-A-Lay, Cream (Ken-Gate).
Burnicin, Oint. (Quality Generics).
Burn-Quel, Aerosol (Halperin).
Butesin Picrate Oint. (Abbott Laboratories).
Foille, Preps. (Carbisulphoil).
Kip, Preps. (Youngs Drug Prod.).
Nupercainal, Oint. (Novartis Pharmaceuticals).
Silvadene, Cream (Hoechst Marion Roussel).
Solarcaine, Preps. (Schering Plough).
Sulfamylon, Cream (Sanofi Winthrop).
Unguentine, Preps. (Procter & Gamble).

Burn-Quel. Halperin aerosol dispenser. 1 oz, 2 oz.
Use: Burn therapy.

Buro-Sol Antiseptic Powder. (Doak Dermatologics) Contents make a diluted Burow's Solution. Aluminum acetate topical soln. plus benzethonium Cl. Pkg. (2.36 g) 12s, 100s. Bot. Pow. 4 oz, 1 lb, 5 lb. *otc.*

Use: Astringent.

Buro-Sol Solution. (Doak Dermatologics) Aluminum acetate 0.23%. Soln. Pkt. 12s.
Use: Astringent.

Bursul. (Burlington) Sulfamethizole 500 mg/Tab. Bot. 100s. *Rx.*
Use: Anti-infective; sulfonamide.

Bur-Tuss. (Burlington) Chlorpheniramine maleate 2 mg, phenylephrine HCl 5 mg, phenylpropanolamine HCl 5 mg, guaifenesin 100 mg, alcohol 2.5%/5 ml. Bot. pt, gal. *otc.*
Use: Antihistamine, decongestant, expectorant.

Bur-Zin. (Lamond) Aluminum acetate solution 2%, zinc oxide 10%. Bot. 4 oz, 8 oz, pt, qt, gal. Also w/o lanolin. *otc.*
Use: Antipruritic, counterirritant.

•**buserelin acetate.** (BYOO-seh-REH-lin ASS-eh-tate) USAN.
Use: Gonad-stimulating principle.

BuSpar Tablets. (Bristol-Myers) Buspirone HCl 5 mg or 10 mg/Tab. *Rx.*
Use: Anxiolytic.

•**buspirone hydrochloride.** (byoo-SPY-rone) U.S.P. 23.
Use: Anxiolytic.
See: BuSpar, Tab. (Bristol-Myers).

•**busulfan.** (byoo-SULL-fate) U.S.P. 23.
Use: Antineoplastic, chronic myeloid leukemia. [Orphan drug]
See: Busulfanex (Orphan Medical).
Myleran, Tab. (GlaxoWellcome).

Busulfanex. (Orphan Medical). Busulfan.
Use: Antineoplastic. [Orphan drug]

•**butabarbital.** (byoo-tah-BAR-bih-tahl) U.S.P. 23
Use: Hypnotic, sedative.
See: BBS, Tab. (Solvay).
Butisol, Prods. (Wallace Laboratories).
Da-Sed, Tab. (Sheryl).
Expansatol, Cap. (Merit).
Medarsed, Elix., Tab. (Medar).
W/Acetaminophen.
See: G-3, Tab. (Roberts Pharm).
Sedapap, Elix. (Merz).
Sedapap-10, Tab. (Merz).
W/Acetaminophen, codeine phosphate.
See: G-3, Cap. (Roberts Pharm).
W/Acetaminophen, mephenesin.
See: See:T-Caps, Cap. (Burlington).
W/Acetaminophen, phenacetin, caffeine.
W/Acetaminophen, salicylamide, phenyltoloxamine citrate.
See: Dengesic, Tab. (Scott-Alison).
Scotgesic, Cap., Elix. (Scott/Cord).
W/Ambutonium bromide, aluminum hydroxide, magnesium hydroxide.
See: Aludrox, Susp., Tab. (Wyeth Ayerst).
W/Aminophylline, phenylpropanolamine HCl, chlorpheniramine maleate, aluminum hydroxide, magnesium trisilicate.
See: Asmacol, Tab. (Pal-Pak).
W/Carboxyphen.
See: Bontril Timed No. 2, Tab. (G. W. Carnrick).
W/Chlorpheniramine maleate, hyoscine HBr.
See: Pedo-Sol, Tab., Elix. (Warren Pharmacal).
W/Dihydroxypropyl theophylline, ephedrine HCl.
See: Airet R, Tab. (Baylor).
W/Ephedrine sulfate, theophylline.
See: Airet Y, Tab., Elix. (Baylor).
W/Ephedrine HCl, theophylline, guaifenesin.
See: Quibron Plus, Cap., Elix. (Bristol-Myers Squibb).
W/Ephedrine HCl, theophylline, isoproterenol.
W/Ephedrine sulfate, theophylline, guaifenesin.
See: Broncholate, Cap., Elix. (Sanofi Winthrop).
W/l-Hyoscyamine.
See: Cystospaz-SR, Cap. (PolyMedica).
W/Hyoscyamine sulfate, atropine sulfate, hyoscine HBr, homatropine methylbromide.
See: Butabell HMB, Tab., Elix. (Saron).
W/Hyoscyamine sulfate, scopolamine methylnitrate, atropine sulfate.
See: Banatil, Cap., Elix. (Trimen).
W/Nitroglycerin.
See: Nitrodyl-B, Cap. (Sanofi Winthrop).
W/Pentaerythritol tetranitrate.
See: Petn Plus (Saron).
W/Pentobarbital, phenobarbital.
See: Quiess, Tab. (Forest Pharmaceutical).
W/Phenazopyridine, hyoscyamine HBr.
See: Pyridium Plus, Tab. (Parke-Davis).
W/Phenazopyridine, scopolamine HBr, atropine sulfate, hyoscyamine sulfate.
See: Buren, Tab. (B.F. Ascher).
W/Phenobarbital, pentobarbital, hyoscyamine sulfate, hyoscine HBr, atropine sulfate.
See: Neoquess, Tab. (Forest Pharmaceutical).
W/Salicylamide.
See: Dapco, Tab. (Mericon).
W/Secobarbital.
See: Monosyl, Tab. (Arcum).
W/Secobarbital, pentobarbital, phenobarbital.

See: Quad-Set, Tab. (Kenyon).
W/Theophylline.
See: Theobid, Cap. (Meyer).
W/Theophylline, pseudoephedrine HCl.
See: Asmadil, Cap. (Solvay).
Ayr, Liq. (B.F. Ascher).
Ayrcap, Cap. (B.F. Ascher).
Az-Kap, Cap. (Keene Pharmaceuticals).
B. A., Prods. (Federal).
Bronchobid, Duracap (Meyer).

•**butabarbital sodium.** (byoo-tah-BAR-bih-tahl) U.S.P. 23.
Use: Hypnotic, sedative.
See: BBS, Tab. (Solvay).
Butalan, Elix. (Lannett).
Butisol Sodium, Elix., Tab. (Wallace Laboratories).
Expansatol, Cap. (Merit).
Quiebar, Spantab, Tab (Nevin).
Renbu, Tab. (Wren).
W/Acetaminophen.
See: Amino-Bar, Tab. (Jones Medical Industries).
Minotal, Tab. (Schwarz Pharma).
W/Acetaminophen, aspirin, caffeine.
See: Dolor Plus, Tab. (Roberts Pharm).
W/Acetaminophen, caffeine.
See: Dularin-TH, Tab. (Donner).
Phrenilin, Tab. (Schwarz Pharma).
W/Acetaminophen, mephenesin, codeine phosphate.
See: Bancaps-C, Cap. (Westerfield).
W/Acetaminophen, salicylamide.
See: Banesin Forte, Tab. (Westerfield).
Indogesic, Tab. (Century Pharm).
W/Acetaminophen, salicylamide, d-amphetamine sulfate, hexobarbital, secobarbital sodium, phenobarbital.
W/d-Amphetamine sulfate.
See: Bontril, Tab. (Schwarz Pharma).
W/Ascorbic acid, sodium p-aminobenzoate, salicylamide, sodium salicylate.
See: Bisalate, Tab. (Allison).
W/Atropine sulfate, hyoscyamine HBr, alcohol, hyoscine HBr.
See: Hyonatol Tab., Hyonatol B Elix., Hexett, Tab. (Jones Medical Industries).
W/Belladonna extract
See: Butibel, Tab., Elix. (Ortho McNeil).
Quiebel, Elix., Cap. (Nevin).
W/Dehydrocholic acid, belladonna extract.
See: Decholin-BB, Tab. (Bayer Corp).
W/Methscopolamine bromide, aluminum hydroxide gel, dried, magnesium trisilicate.
See: Eulcin, Tab. (Leeds).
W/Pentobarbital sodium, phenobarbital sodium.
See: Trio-Bar, Tab. (Jenkins).
W/Salicylamide, mephenesin.
See: Metrogesic, Tab. (Lexis).
W/Secobarbital sodium.
See: Monosyl, Tab. (Arcum).
W/Secobarbital sodium, pentobarbital sodium, phenobarbital.
See: Nidar, Tab. (Centeon).
W/Secobarbital sodium, phenobarbital.
See: S.B.P., Tab. (Teva USA).
W/Simethicone, hyoscyamine sulfate, atropine sulfate, hyoscine HBr.
See: Sidonna, Tab. (Schwarz Pharma).
W/Theophylline, pseudoephedrine HCl.
See: Dilorbron, Cap. (Roberts Pharm).

butabarbital sodium. (Various Mfr.) **Tab.:** 15 mg. Bot. 1000s; 30 mg Bot. 100s, 1000s. **Elixir:** 30 mg/5ml Bot. pt.
Use: Sedative, hypnotic.

butacaine.
Use: Anesthetic, local.

•**butacetin.** (byoot-ASS-ih-tin) USAN.
Use: Analgesic, antidepressant.

•**butaclamol hydrochloride.** (byoo-tah-KLAM-ole) USAN.
Use: Antipsychotic.

Butagen Caps. (Zenith Goldline) Phenylbutazone 100 mg/Cap. Bot. 100s, 500s. *Rx.*
Use: Antirheumatic.
Use: Hypnotic, sedative.

•**butalbital,** (BYOO-TAL-bih-tuhl) U.S.P. 23. *Formerly Allybarbituric acid.*
Use: Hypnotic, sedative.
See: Buff-A-Comp #3 (Merz).
Lotusate, Cap. (Sanofi Winthrop).
Sandoptal, Preps. (Novartis).
W/Acetaminophen.
See: Axocet, Cap. (Savage Labs).
Bupap, Tab. (ECR). Phrenilin, Tab. (Schwarz Pharma).
Phrenilin Forte, Cap. (Schwarz Pharma).
Prominol, Tab. (MCR American Pharm).
Repan CF, Tab. (Everett).
Tencon, Cap. (Inter. Ethical Labs).
W/Acetaminophen, codeine.
See: Phrenilin w/Codeine, Cap. (Schwarz Pharma).
W/Acetaminophen, caffeine.
See: Arbutal, Tab. (Arcum).
Buff-A-Comp, Tab., Cap. (Merz).
Esgic, Tab. (Gilbert).
Cefinal, Tab. (Alto Pharmaceuticals).
Protension, Tab. (Blaine).
Repan, Tab. (Everett Laboratories).
W/Aspirin, caffeine.
See: Duogesic, Cap. (Western Research).

Fiorinal, Cap., Tab. (Novartis).
W/Aspirin, caffeine, codeine phosphate.
See: Buff-A-Comp, Tab w/Codeine. (Merz).
Fiorinal With Codeine, Cap. (Novartis).
W/Caffeine, aspirin, acetaminophen.
See: Anaphen, Cap. (Roberts Pharm).

butalbital, acetaminophen and caffeine tablets. (BYOO-TAL-bih-tuhl, us-seet-uh-min-oh-fen and kaff-EEN) (Various Mfr.) Acetaminophen 325 mg, caffeine 40 mg, butalbital 50 mg, Tab. Bot. 100s, 500s. *Rx.*
Use: Analgesic.
See: Esgic-Plus, Tab. (Forest Pharm).
Fiorpap, Tab. (Creighton).
Isocet, Tab. (Rugby).
Margesic, Cap. (Marnell).
Triad, Cap. (UAD).

butalbital, aspirin & caffeine. (Various Mfr.) (BYOO-TAL-bih-tuhl, ass-pihr-in and kaff-EEN) **Tab.:** Aspirin 325 mg, caffeine 40 mg, butalbital 50 mg. Bot. 20s, 30s, 50s, 100s, 500s, 1000s, UD 100s. **Cap.:** Aspirin 325 mg, caffeine 40 mg, butalbital 50 mg. Bot. 100s, 1000s. *c-III.*
Use: Analgesic combination.

butalbital and aspirin tablets.
Use: Analgesic, sedative.

butalbital compound. (Various Mfr.) Tab., Cap. Bot. 15s, 30s, 100s, 500s, 1000s. *c-III.*
Use: Analgesic.
W/Acetaminophen, butalbital.
See: Phrenilin (Schwarz Pharma).
Bancap (Forest Pharmaceutical).
Bucet, Cap. (Forest Pharmaceutical).
Sedapap-10 (Merz).
Tencon, Cap. (Inter. Ethical Labs).
Triaprin (Dunhall Pharmaceuticals).
W/Acetaminophen, caffeine, butalbital.
See: Arcet, Tab. (Econo Med Pharmaceuticals).
Amaphen (Trimen).
Endolor (Keene Pharmaceuticals).
Esgic (Forest Pharmaceutical).
Esgic-Plus, Tab. (Forest Pharmaceutical).
Fioricet (Novartis).
G-1 (Roberts Pharm).
Isocet, Tab. (Rugby).
Margesic, Cap. (Marnel).
Medigesic Plus (US Pharmaceutical).
Phrenilin Forte (Schwarz Pharma).
Repan (Everett Laboratories).
Sedapap-10 (Merz).
Triad, Cap. (Forest Pharmaceutical).
W/Aspirin, butalbital. Aspirin 325 mg, caffeine 40mg, butalbital 50 mg.
See: Axotal (Pharmacia & Upjohn).
W/Aspirin, caffeine, butalbital.
See: Fiorgen PF (Zenith Goldline).
Fiorinal (Novartis).
Isollyl Improved (Rugby).
Lanorinal (Lannett).
Lorprn (UCB Pharmaceuticals).
B-A-C (Merz).

Butalan Elixir. (Lannett) Sodium butabarbital 0.2 g/30 ml. Bot. pt, gal.
Use: Hypnotic, sedative.

butalgin.
See: Methadone HCl (Various Mfr.).

butallylonal. (Pernocton).
Use: Hypnotic.

•**butamben.** (BYOO-tam-ben) U.S.P. 23.
Use: Anesthetic, local. *Formerly Butyl aminobenzoate.*

•**butamben picrate.** (BYOO-tam-ben PIC-rate) USAN.
Use: Anesthetic, local.
See: Butesin Picrate, Oint. (Abbott Laboratories).

•**butamirate citrate.** (byoo-tah-MY-rate SIH-trate) USAN.
Use: Antitussive.

•**butane,** N.F. 18.
Use: Aerosol propellant.

butanisamide.

•**butaperazine.** (BYOO-tah-PURR-ah-zeen) USAN.
Use: Antipsychotic.

•**butaperazine maleate.** USAN.
Use: Antipsychotic.

butaphyllamine. Ambuphylline. Theophylline aminoisobutanol. Theophylline with 2-amino-2-methyl-1-propanol.

Butapro Elixir. (Health for Life Brands) Butabarbital sodium 0.2 g/30 ml. Bot. pt, gal. *c-v.*
Use: Hypnotic, sedative.

•**butaprost.** (BYOO-tah-PRAHST) USAN.
Use: Bronchodilator.

Butazone. (Major) Phenylbutazone. **Cap.:** 100 mg. Bot. 100s, 500s. **Tab.:** 100 mg. Bot. 500s. *Rx.*
Use: Antirheumatic.

•**butedronate tetrasodium.** (BYOO-teh-DROE-nate TET-rah-SO-dee-uhm) USAN.
Use: Diagnostic aid (bone imaging).

butelline.
See: Butacaine Sulfate (Various Mfr.).

•**butenafine hydrochloride.** (byoo-TEN-ah-feen) USAN.
Use: Antifungal.

butenafine hydrochloride. (Penederm).
Use: Treatment of interdigital tinea pedis (athlete's foot).

See: Mentax (Penederm).

•**buterizine.** (byoo-TER-ih-ZEEN) USAN.
Use: Vasodilator (peripheral).

Butesin Picrate. (Abbott Laboratories) n-Butyl-p-aminobenzoate. Lidocaine 1%, lanolin, parabens, mineral oil/Oint. Jar. 28.4 g. *otc.*
Use: Anesthetic, local.

Butesin Picrate Ointment. (Abbott Laboratories) Butamben picrate 1%. Tube oz. *otc.*
Use: Anesthetic, local.

butethal. (Various Mfr.) *Rx.*
Use: Hypnotic, sedative.

butethamine formate.

butethamine hydrochloride.
See: Dentocaine (Amer. Chem. & Drug).

butethanol.
See: Tetracaine.

•**buthiazide.** (byoo-THIGH-azz-IDE) USAN.
Use: Antihypertensive, diuretic.

Butibel. (Wallace Laboratories) Butabarbital sodium 15 mg, belladonna extract 15 mg/Tab or 5 ml. **Tab.** Bot. 100s. **Elix.:** (w/alcohol 7%) Bot. pt. *Rx.*
Use: Anticholinergic, antispasmodic, hypnotic, sedative.

•**butikacin.** (BYOO-tih-KAY-sin) USAN.
Use: Anti-infective.

•**butilfenin.** (BYOO-till-FEN-in) USAN.
Use: Diagnostic aid (hepatic function determination).

•**butirosin sulfate.** (byoo-TIHR-oh-sin) USAN. A mixture of the sulfates of the A and B forms of an antibiotic produced by *Bacillus circularis.*
Use: Anti-infective.

Butisol Sodium. (Wallace Laboratories) Butabarbital sodium. **Elix.:** 30 mg/5 ml. Bot pt, gal. **Tab.:** 15 mg, 30 mg. Bot. 100s, 1000s. 50 mg or 100 mg. Bot. 100s. *c-III.*
Use: Hypnotic, sedative.
See: Buticaps, Cap. (Wallace Laboratories).
W/Belladonna extract.
See: Butibel, (Wallace Laboratories).

•**butixirate.** (BYOO-TIX-ih-rate) USAN.
Use: Analgesic, antirheumatic.

•**butoconazole nitrate.** (BYOO-toe-KOE-nuh-zole) U.S.P. 23.
Use: Antifungal.
See: Femstat, Cream (Procter-Syntex). Femstat 3, cream (Procter-Syntex).

butolan. Benzylphenyl carbamate.

•**butonate.** (BYOO-tahn-ate) USAN.
Use: Anthelmintic.

•**butopamine.** (BYOO-TOE-pah-meen) USAN.
Use: Cardiovascular agent.

•**butoprozine hydrochloride.** (byoo-TOE-pro-ZEEN) USAN.
Use: Cardiovascular agent (antiarrhythmic), antianginal.

butopyronoxyl. (Indalone) Butylmesityl oxide.
Use: Insect repellant.

•**butorphanol.** (BYOO-TAR-fan-ahl) USAN.
Use: Analgesic, antitussive.

•**butorphanol tartrate.** (BYOO-TAR-fan-ahl) U.S.P. 23.
Use: Analgesic, antitussive.
See: Stadol, Inj. (Bristol-Myers Squibb).

•**butoxamine hydrochloride.** (byoo-TOX-ah-meen) USAN.
Use: Antidiabetic, antihyperlipoproteinemic.

•**butriptyline hydrochloride.** (BYOO-TRIP-till-een) USAN.
Use: Antidepressant.

•**butyl alcohol.** N.F. 18. Butyl alcohol is n-butyl alcohol.
Use: Pharmaceutic aid (solvent).

butyl aminobenzoate. n-Butyl p-Aminobenzoate. Scuroforme.
Use: Anesthetic, local.
W/Benzocaine, tetracaine HCl.
See: Cetacaine, Preps. (Cetylite Industries).
W/Benzyl alcohol, phenylmercuric borate, benzocaine.
See: Dermathyn, Oint. (Davis & Sly).
W/Procaine, benzyl alcohol, in sweet almond oil.
See: Anucaine, Amp. (Calvin).
W/Tetracaine.
See: Pontocaine, Oint. (Sanofi Winthrop).

•**butylated hydroxyanisole.** N.F. 18.
Use: Pharmaceutic aid (antioxidant).

•**buylated hydroxytoluene.** N.F. 18.
Use: Pharmaceutic aid (antioxidant).

•**butylparaben,** (byo-till-PAR-ah-ben) N.F. 18.
Use: Pharmaceutic aid (antifungal).

butylphenamide.

butylphenylsalicylamide.
See: Butylphenamide.

butyrophenone. Class of antipsychotic agents. *Rx.*
See: Haloperidol.

butyrylcholinesterase. (Pharmavene)
Use: Treat cocaine overdose; post-surgical apnea. [Orphan drug]

B vitamins, parenteral.
See: B-Ject-100 (Hyrex)
Becomject-100 (Merz)

B vitamins with vitamin C, parenteral.
See: Key-Plex Injection (Hyrex)
Neurodep Injection (Medical Products)
Vicam Injection (Keene Pharmaceuticals)

B-Vite Injection. (Bluco) Vitamins B_1 50 mg, B_2 5 mg, B_6 5 mg, niacinamide 125 mg, B_{12} 1000 mcg, dexpanthenol 6 mg, C 50 mg/10 ml. Mono vial w/benzyl alcohol 1% in water for injection. *Rx.*
Use: Vitamin supplement.

BVU.
See: Bromisovalum.

Byclomine w/Phenobarbital. (Major) **Cap.:** Dicyclomine HCl 10 mg, phenobarbital 15 mg. Bot. 250s, 1000s. **Tab.:** Dicyclomine HCl 20 mg, phenobarbital 15 mg. Bot. 100s, 250s, 1000s. *Rx.*
Use: Antispasmodic, sedative, hypnotic.

Bydramine. (Major) Diphenhydramine HCl 12.5 mg/5 ml, alcohol 5%. Syr. Bot. 118 ml, pt, gal. *otc.*
Use: Antihistamine.

C

c1-esterase-inhibitor, human, pasteurized. (Alpha Ther)
Use: Prevention/treatment of angioedema [Orphan Drug]

c1-esterase-inhibitor, human, pasteurized.
Use: Prevention/treatment of angioedema.
See: Berinert P (Behring Werke Aktiengesellschaft).

c1 inhibitor. (Osterreichisches)
Use: Treatment of angioedema. [Orphan drug]

c1-inhibitor (human) vapor heated. (Immuno)
Use: Treatment of angioedema. [Orphan drug]

c vitamin.
See: Ascorbic Acid, Prep.

•**cabergoline.** (cab-ERR-go-leen) USAN.
Use: Antidyskinetic; antihyperprolactinemic; antiparkinsonian; dopamine agonist; hyperolactinemic disorders treatment.
See: Dostinex, Tab. (Pharmacia & Upjohn).

•**cabufocan a.** USAN.
Use: Contact lens material (hydrophobic).

•**cabufocon b.** (cab-YOU-FOE-kahn B) USAN.
Use: Contact lens material (hydrophobic).

Cachexon. (Telluride Pharm) L-Glutathione.
Use: AIDS-associated cachexila. [Orphan drug]

cacodylic acid salts.
Ferric Salt.
Iron Salt.
Sodium Salt.

•**cactinomycin.** (KACK-tih-no-MY-sin) USAN. Antibiotic produced by *Streptomyces chrysomallus. Formerly Actinomycin c.*
Use: Antineoplastic.

cade oil.
See: Juniper Tar.

•**cadexomer iodine.** (kad-EX-oh-mer) USAN.
Use: Antiseptic, antiulcerative.

C & E Softgels. (NBTY) E 400 mg, C 500 mg/Cap. Bot. 50s. *otc.*
Use: Vitamin supplement.

Cafatine Supps. (Major) Ergotamine tartrate 2 mg, caffeine 100 mg. Supp. Box 12s. *Rx.*
Use: Antimigraine.

Cafatine-PB. (Major) Ergotamine tartrate 2 mg, caffeine 100 mg, belladonna alkaloids 0.25 mg, pentobarbital 60 mg/Supp. Box foil 10s. *Rx.*
Use: Antimigraine.

Cafenol. (Sanofi Winthrop) Aspirin, caffeine. *otc.*
Use: Analgesic combination.

Cafergot P-B Suppositories. (Novartis) Ergotamine tartrate 2 mg, caffeine 100 mg, bellafoline 0.25 mg, pentobarbital 60 mg/Supp. Box 12s. *Rx.*
Use: Antimigraine.

Cafergot P-B Tablets. (Novartis) Ergotamine tartrate 1 mg, caffeine 100 mg, bellafoline 0.125 mg, pentobarbital sodium 30 mg/Tab. SigPak dispensing pkg. of 90s, 250s. *c-IV.*
Use: Antimigraine.

Cafergot Suppositories. (Novartis) Ergotamine tartrate 2 mg, caffeine 100 mg in cocoa butter base. Supp. Box 12s. *Rx.*
Use: Antimigraine.

Cafergot Tablets. (Novartis) Ergotamine tartrate 1 mg, caffeine 100 mg/S.C. Tab. Bot. 250s. SigPak dispensing pkg. of 90s. *Rx.*
Use: Antimigraine.

Caffedrine. (Thompson Medical) Caffeine 200 mg, lactose. Tab. Pkg. 16s. *otc.*
Use: CNS stimulant.

•**caffeine.** U.S.P. 23.
Use: CNS stimulant; apnea of prematurity. [Orphan drug]
See: Caffedrine, Tab. (Thompson).
Enerjets, Loz. (Chilton).
Femicin, Tab. (SmithKline Beecham Pharmaceuticals).
Neocaf (OPR Development).
NoDoz, Tab. (Bristol-Myers).
Quick Pep, Tab. (Thompson).
Stim 250, Cap. (Scrip).
Tirend (SmithKline Beecham Pharmaceuticals).
Vivarin, Tab. (J.B. Williams).

caffeine citrated.
Use: CNS stimulant.

caffeine sodio-benzoate.
See: Caffeine sodium benzoate.

caffeine and sodium benzoate injection. Caffeine and sodium benzoate 250 mg/ml (121. 25 mg caffeine, 128.75 mg sodium benxoate). Inj. Amp. 2 ml. *Rx.*
Use: Oral, IM CNS stimulant.

caffeine sodium salicylate. (Various

Mfr.) Bot. 1 oz; Pkg. 0.25 lb, 1 lb. *otc.*
Use: See caffeine.

caffeine-theophylline compound.

Cagol. (Harvey) Guaiacol 0.1 g, eucalyptol 0.08 g, iodoform 0.2 g, camphor 0.05 g/2 ml in olive oil. Vial 30 ml. *Rx.*
Use: Expectorant.

Caladryl. (Parke-Davis) Calamine 8%, pramoxine HCl 1%, alcohol 2.2%, camphor, diazolidinyl urea, parabens. Lot. Bot. 180 ml. *otc.*
Use: Antipruritic-topical.

Caladryl Clear. (Parke-Davis) Pramoxine HCl 1%, zinc acetate 0.1%, alcohol 2%, camphor, diazolidinyl urea, parabens. Lot. Bot. 180 ml. *otc.*
Use: Antipruritic, topical.

Caladryl for Kids. (Parke-Davis) Calamine 8%, pramoxine HCl 1%, camphor, cetyl alcohol, diazolidinyl urea, parabens. Cream. Tube 45 g. *otc.*
Use: Antipruritic, topical.

Calaformula. (Eric, Kirk & Gary) Ferrous gluconate 130 mg, calcium lactate 130 mg, vitamins A 1000 IU, D 400 IU, B_1 2 mg, B_2 2 mg, niacinamide 5 mg, ascorbic acid 20 mg, folic acid 0.13 mg, magnesium 0.25 mg, copper 0.25 mg, zinc 0.25 mg, manganese 0.25 mg, potassium 0.075 mg/Cap. Bot. 50s, 100s, 500s, 1000s, 5000s. *otc.*
Use: Mineral, vitamin supplement.

Calaformula F. (Eric, Kirk & Gary) Calaformula plus fluorine 0.333 mg/Tab. Bot. 100s. *Rx.*
Use: Mineral, vitamin supplement, dental caries agent.

Cala-Gen. (Zenith Goldline) Diphenhydramine HCl 1%, camphor, alcohol 2%. Lot. Bot. 178 ml. *otc.*
Use: Antipruritic-topical.

Calahist Lotion. (Walgreens) Diphenhydramine HCl 1%, calamine 8.1%, camphor 0.1%. Lot. Bot. 6 oz. *otc.*
Use: Antipruritic, topical.

Calamatum. (Blair Laboratories) **Lot.:** Calamine, zinc oxide, phenol, camphor, benzocaine 3%, nongreasy base. Bot. 1125 ml. **Oint:** Calamine, zinc oxide, phenol, camphor, benzocaine. Tube 45 g. *otc.*
Use: Dermatologic, counterirritant.

Calamatum Aerosol Spray. (Blair Laboratories) Benzocaine 3%, zinc oxide, calamine, phenol, camphor. Spray can 3 oz. *otc.*
Use: Anesthetic, local.

•**calamine.** U.S.P. 23.
Use: Protectant, topical.
See: Caladryl, Prods. (Parke-Davis)

calamine. (Various Mfr.) Calamine 8%, zinc oxide 8%, glycerin 2%, bentonite maga, calcium hydroxide soln. Lot. Bot. 120 ml, 240 ml, pt, gal.
Use: Antiseptic, astringent.

Calamine, Phenolated. (Humco Holding Group) Calamine 8%, zinc oxide 8%, glycerin 2%, bentonite maga and phenol 1% in calcium hydroxide solution. Lot. Bot. 120, 240 ml. *otc.*
Use: Antiseptic, astringent.

Calamox. (Roberts Pharm) Prepared calamine 0.17 g. Oint. Tube 60 g. *otc.*
Use: Antiseptic, astringent.

Calamycin. (Pfeiffer) Pyrilamine maleate, zinc oxide 10%, calamine 10%, benzocaine, chloroxylenol, zirconium oxide, isopropyl alcohol 10%. Lot. Bot. 120 ml. *otc.*
Use: Antipruritic, topical.

Calan. (Searle) Verapamil HCl 40 mg, 80 mg or 120 mg/Tab. Bot. 100s, 500s, 1000s, UD 100s. *Rx.*
Use: Calcium channel blocker.

Calan SR. (Searle) Verapamil HCl **120 mg, 180 mg/SR Tab.** Bot. 100s, UD 100s. **240 mg/SR Tab:** Bot. 100s, 500s, UD 100s. *Rx.*
Use: Calcium channel blocker.

Cal-Bid. (Roberts Pharm) Elemental calcium 250 mg, ascorbic acid 100 mg, vitamin D 125 IU/Tab. Bot. 100s. *otc.*
Use: Mineral, vitamin supplement.

Cal Carb-HD. (Konsyl Pharm) Calcium 6.5 g per packet, simethicone. Pow. 7 g packets, Bot. 210 g. *otc.*
Use: Antacid.

Calcet. (Mission Pharmacal) Elemental calcium 153 mg, vitamin D 100 units/ Tab. Bot. 100s. *otc.*
Use: Mineral, vitamin supplement.

Calcet Plus. (Mission Pharmacal) Elemental calcium 152.8 mg, elemental iron 18 mg, vitamins A 5000 IU, D 400 IU, E 30 mg, B_1 2.25 mg, B_2 2.55 mg, B_3 30 mg, B_5 15 mg, B_6 3 mg, B_{12} 9 mcg, C 500 mg, folic acid 0.8 mg, zinc 15 mg, sugar/Tab. Bot 60s. *otc.*
Use: Mineral, vitamin supplement.

Calcibind. (Mission Pharmacal) Inorganic phosphate content 34%, sodium content 11%. Packets: Cellulose sodium phosphate 25 g. Single dose 90 packets, 300 g bulk pack. *Rx.*
Use: Genitourinary.

CalciCaps. (Nion) Calcium (dibasic calcium phosphate, calcium gluconate, calcium carbonate) 125 mg, vitamin D

67 IU, phosphorus 60 mg/Tab. Bot. 100s, 500s. *otc.*
Use: Mineral, vitamin supplement.

CalciCaps with Iron. (Nion) Calcium 125 mg, phosphorus 60 mg, vitamin D 67 IU, ferrous gluconate 7 mg, tartrazine/ Tab. Bot. 100s, 500s. *otc.*
Use: Mineral, vitamin supplement.

CalciCaps M-Z. (Nion) Ca 400 mg, Mg 133 mg, Zn 5 mg, vitamin A 1667 mg, D 133 IU, Se. Tab. Bot. 90s. *otc.*
Use: Mineral, vitamin supplement.

CalciCaps, Super. (Nion) Calcium 400 mg, phosphorus 41.7 mg, vitamin D 100 IU/Tab. Bot. 90s. *otc.*
Use: Mineral, vitamin supplement.

Calci-Chew. (R & D) Calcium carbonate 1.25 g (500 mg calcium)/Chew. Tab. Bot. 100s. *otc.*
Use: Mineral supplement.

Calciday-667. (NBTY) Calcium carbonate 667 mg (266.8 mg calcium)/Tab. Bot. 60s. *otc.*
Use: Calcium supplement.

Calcidrine syrup. (Abbott Laboratories) Codeine 8.4 mg, calcium iodide anhydrous 152 mg, alcohol 6%/5 ml. Bot. 120 ml, 480 ml. *c-v.*
Use: Antitussive, expectorant.

•**calcifediol.** (KAL-sih-feh-DIE-ahl) U.S.P. 23.
Use: Calcium regulator.
See: Calderol (Organon Teknika).

calciferol. Ergosterol. (D_2) **Liq:** 8000 IU/ ml. Bot. 60 ml. **Tab:** 50,000 IU. Bot. 100s. **Inj:** 500,000 IU/ml. Amp. 1 ml. *Rx. otc.*
Use: Refractory rickets, familial hypophosphatemia, hypoparathyroidism.

Calcijex. (Abbott Laboratories) Calcitriol injection 1 mcg or 2 mcg/ml. Amp. 1 ml. *Rx.*
Use: Antihypocalcemic, antihypoparathyroid.

Calcimar Injection, Synthetic. (Rhone-Poulenc Rorer) Calcitonin solution (Salmon origin), phenol/200 IU/ml. Vial 2 ml. *Rx.*
Use: Treatment of Paget's disease.

Calci-Mix. (R & D Laboratories) Calcium carbonate 1250 mg. Cap. Bot. 100s. *otc.*
Use: Mineral supplement.

•**calcipotriene.** (kal-sih-POE-try-een) USAN.
Use: Antipsoriatic.
See: Dovonex Prods. (Westwood Squibb).

•**calcitonin.** (kal-sih-TOE-nin) USAN.
Use: Treatment of Paget's disease, calcium regulator.
See: Calcimar (Rhone-Poulenc Rorer).
Cibacalcin (Novartis).
Miacalcin (Novartis).

calcitonin-human for injection. (kal-sih-TOE-nin human) Hormone from thyroid gland.
Use: Plasma hypocalcemic hormone; symptomatic Paget's disease of bone. [Orphan drug]
See: Cibacalcin (Novartis).

calcitonin-salmon. (kal-sih-TOE-nin salmon)
Use: Antihypercalcemic.
See: Calcimar (Rhone-Poulenc Rorer).
Miacalcin (Novartis).
Osteocalcin, Inj. (Arcola Laboratories).

calcitonin salmon nasal spray.
Use: Symptomatic Paget's disease of bone. [Orphan drug]
See: Miacalcin (Novartis).

•**calcitriol.** (KAL-sih-TRY-ole) USAN.
Use: Anti hypocalcemia; calcium regulator.
See: Calcijex, Inj. (Abbott Laboratories).
Rocaltrol, Cap. (Roche Laboratories).

Calcium-600. (Schein Pharmaceutical) Calcium 600 mg. Tab. Bot. 60s. *otc.*
Use: Mineral supplement.

Calcium 600/Vitamin D. (Schein Pharmaceutical) Ca 600 mg, D 125 IU. Tab. Bot. 60s. *otc.*
Use: Mineral, vitamin supplement.

•**calcium acetate.** (KAL-see-uhm) U.S.P. 23.
Use: Pharmaceutic aid (buffering agent). Hyperphosphatemia [Orphan drug].

calcium acetate mineral/electrolytes.
See: Calphron, Tab. (Nephro-Tec).
Phos-Ex 62.5 Mini-Tabs (Vitaline).
Phos-Ex 167 (Braintree Laboratories).
Phos-Ex 250 (Vitaline).
Phos-Ex 125 (Vitaline).
PhosLo (Braintree Laboratories).

calcium acetylsalicylate. Kalmopyrin, kalsetal, soluble aspirin, tylcalsin.
Use: Analgesic.

calcium aluminum carbonate. W/Dl-Amino acetate complex.
See: Ancid Tab., Susp. (Sheryl).

calcium aminosalicylate. Aminosalicylate calcium, N.F. 18.

calcium amphomycin.
See: Amphomycin.

calcium and magnesium carbonates

tablets.
Use: Antacid.

•**calcium ascorbate.** U.S.P. 23.
Use: Nutritional supplement.

calcium ascorbate. (Freeda Vitamins) **Tab.:** Calcium ascorbate 610 mg (equivalent to 500 mg ascorbic acid). Bot. 100s, 250s, 500s. **Pow.:** Calcium ascorbate 1 g (equivalent to 826 mg ascorbic acid) per 1/4 tsp. Bot. 120 g, 448 g. *otc.*
Use: Mineral supplement.

calcium 4-benzamidosalicylate. Calcium Aminacyl B-PAS. Benzoylpas Calcium.
See: Benzapas, Pow., Tab. (Novartis).

calcium benzoyl-p-aminosalicylate.
See: Benzoylpas calcium.

calcium benzoylpas.
See: Benzoylpas calcium.

calcium bis-dioctyl sulfosuccinate.
See: Dioctyl calcium.

calcium carbimide. Calcium cyanamide. Sulfosuccinate.
See: Alka-Mints (Bayer Corp).
Amitone, Tab. (Menley & James).
Antacid Tablets (Zenith Goldline).
Chooz (Schering Plough).
Dicarbosil, Tab. (SmithKline Beecham Pharmaceuticals).
Equilet (Mission Pharmacal).
Extra Strength Antacid (Various Mfr.).
Maalox Antacid (Rhone-Poulenc Rorer).
Mallamint, Tab. (Roberts Pharm).
Mylanta (J & J Merck Consumer Pharm).
Tums (SmithKline Beecham Pharmaceuticals).

•**calcium carbonate.** U.S.P. 23. Formerly calcium carbonate, precipitated.
Use: Antacid.
See: Extra Strength Alkets Antacid, Chew. Tab. (Roberts Pharm).
Tums 500, Chew. Tab. (SmithKline Beecham).

calcium carbonate. (Various Mfr.) Precipitated chalk; carbonic acid, calcium salt (1:1).
Use: Antacid.

calcium carbonate.
Use: Hyperphosphatemia. [Orphan drug]
See: R&D Calcium Carbonate/600 (R&D).

calcium carbonate. (Various Mfr.) 500 mg/Tab. 100s, 120s, UD 100s; 600 mg/Tab. 60s, 72s, 150s, UD 100s; 650 mg/Tab. 100s, 1000s. *otc.*
Use: Antacid, calcium supplement.

calcium carbonate. (Roxane) **Tab.:** 1250 mg. Bot. 100s, UD 100s. **Susp.:** 1250 mg/5 ml. Bot. 500 ml, UD 5 ml. *otc.*
Use: Antacid, calcium supplement.

calcium carbonate, aromatic. (Eli Lilly) Calcium carbonate 10 gr/Tab. Bot. 100s, 1000s. *otc.*
Use: Antacid.

calcium carbonate w/combinations.
See: Accelerase, Cap. (Organon Teknika).
Alkets, Tab. (Pharmacia & Upjohn).
Camalox, Tab., Susp. (Rhone-Poulenc Rorer).
Ca-Plus, Tab. (Miller).
Co-Gel, Tab. (Arco).
Gas-Ban, Tab. (Roberts Pharm).
Lactocal, Tab. (Laser).
Natabec, Prep. (Parke-Davis).
Titralac, Liq., Tab. (3M).

Calcium Carbonate 600mg + Vitamin D. (Major) Ca 600 mg, D 125 IU. Tab. Bot. 60s. *otc.*
Use: Mineral, vitamin supplement.

calcium caseinate.
See: Casec, Pow. (Bristol-Myers).

calcium channel blockers.
Use: Angina pectoris, vasospastic and unstable angina.
See: Adalat, Cap. (Bayer Corp).
Calan, Inj., Tab. (Searle).
Calan SR, SR Cap. (Searle).
Cardene, Cap. (Syntex).
Cardene SR, SR Cap. (Syntex).
Cardene IV, Inj. (DuPont Merck Pharmaceuticals).
Cardizem, Tab. (Hoechst Marion Roussel).
Diltiazem HCl, ER Cap. (Various Mfr.).
DynaCirc, Cap. (Novartis).
Isoptin, Inj., Tab. (Knoll Pharmaceuticals).
Isoptin SR, SR Cap. (Knoll Pharmaceuticals).
Nimotop, Cap. (Bayer Corp).
Plendil, SR Tab. (Merck).
Procardia, Cap. (Pfizer).
Vascor, Tab. (Ortho McNeil).
Verapamil HCl, Inj., Tab. (Various Mfr.).

Calcium Chel 330. (Novartis).
Use: Antidote, heavy metals.
See: Calcium Trisodium Pentetate.

•**calcium chloride.** U.S.P. 23.
Use: Electrolyte, calcium replenisher.

•**calcium chloride Ca 45.** USAN.
Use: Radiopharmaceutical.

•**calcium chloride Ca 47.** USAN.
Use: Radiopharmaceutical.

calcium chloride injection. (Pharmacia & Upjohn) 1 g Amp. 10 ml, 25s. (Torigian) 1 g Amp. 10 ml 12s, 25s, 100s. (Trent) 10% Amp. 10 ml (Bayer Corp) 13.6 mEq./10 ml Vial.
Use: Antihypocalcemic.

•**calcium citrate.** U.S.P. 23.
Use: Mineral supplement.

calcium cyclamate. Calcium cyclohexanesulfamate.

calcium cyclobarbital.
Use: Central depressant.

calcium cyclohexanesulfamate.
See: Calcium Cyclamate.

Calcium 600 + D. (NBTY) Calcium 600 mg, vitamin D 125 IU. Film coat. Tab. Bot. 60s. *otc.*
Use: Mineral, vitamin supplement.

calcium dl-pantothenate. Calcium Pantothenate, Racemic, U.S.P. 23.

calcium dioctyl sulfosuccinate. Docusate Calcium, U.S.P. 23.
See: Surfak (Hoechst Marion Roussel).

calcium disodium edathamil.
See: Edetate Calcium Disodium, U.S.P. 23.

calcium disodium edetate. (KAL-see-uhm die-SO-dee-uhm ed-deh-TATE) Edetate Calcium Disodium, U.S.P. 23.
Use: Antidote for acute and chronic lead poisoning, lead encephalopathy.
See: Calcium Disodium Versenate (3M).

calcium disodium versenate. (3M) Calcium Disodium Edetate U.S.P. Inj.: 200 mg/ml. Amp 5 ml. *Rx.*
Use: IV or IM for lead poisoning and lead encephalopathy.

calcium edetate sodium.
See: calcium disodium edetate.

calcium EDTA.
See: Calcium Disodium Versenate, Amp. (3M).

calcium glubionate syrup. (KAL-see-uhm glue-BYE-oh-nate) U.S.P. 23.
Use: Calcium replenisher.
See: Neo-Calglucon (Novartis).

•**calcium gluceptate.** (KAL-see-uhm GLUE-sep-tate) U.S.P. 23.
Use: Calcium replenisher.
See: Calcium Gluceptate (Abbott Laboratories).
Calcium Gluceptate (I.M.S.).
Calcium Gluceptate (Eli Lilly).

•**calcium gluceptate.** (Various Mfr.) 1.1 g (5 ml) contains 90 mg (4.5 mEq) calcium. Inj.: 1.1 g/5 ml. Amp. 5 ml. Vial 50 ml.
Use: Calcium electrolyte replacement.

calcium glucoheptonate. (Various Mfr.) Cal. D-glucoheptonate O. *otc.*
Use: Nutritional supplement.

•**calcium gluconate.** U.S.P. 23.
Use: Calcium replenisher.

calcium gluconate gel 2.5%. (LTR Pharm)
Use: Topical treatment of hydrogen fluoride burns. [Orphan drug]
See: H-F Gel (Paddock).

calcium glycerophosphate. Neurosin. (Various Mfr.).

•**calcium hydroxide.** U.S.P. 23.
Use: Astringent; pharmaceutic necessity for calamine lotion.

calcium hydroxide powder. (Eli Lilly) Powder 4 oz/Bot.
Use: Lime water.

calcium hypophosphite. (N.Y. Quinine & Chem. Works).

calcium iodide.
W/Codeine phosphate.
See: Calcidrine Syr. (Abbott Laboratories).
W/Chloral hydrate, ephedrine HCl.
See: Iophen, Syr. (Marsh Labs).

calcium iodized.
See: Cal-Lime-1, Tab. (Scrip).
W/Calcium creosotate.
See: Niocrese, Tab. (Noyes).
W/Ipecac, hyoscyamus extract, licorice extract.
See: Kaldifane, Tab. (Noyes).

calcium iodobehenate. Calioben. (Various Mfr.).

calcium ipodate. Ipodate Calcium, U.S.P. 23.
See: Oragrafin Calcium, Granules (Bristol-Myers Squibb).

calcium kinate gluconate. Kinate is hexahydrotetrahydroxybenzoate. Calcium Quinate.

•**calcium lactate.** U.S.P. 23.
Use: Calcium replenisher.
W/Calcium glycerophosphate.
See: Calphosan, Amp., Vial (Carlton).
W/Calcium glycerophosphate, phenol, sodium Cl solution.
See: Calpholac, Vial (Century Pharm).
Calphosan, Inj. (Zeneca).
W/Niacinamide, folic acid, ferrous gluconate, vitamins.
See: Pergrava No. 2, Cap. (Arcum).
W/Phenobarbital, extract hyoscyamus, terpin hydrate, guaifenesin.
W/Theobromine sodium salicylate, phenobarbital.
See: Theolaphen, Tab. (Zeneca).
W/Zinc sulfate.

See: Zinc-220, Cap. (Alto Pharmaceuticals).

•**calcium lactobionate.** U.S.P. 23.
Use: Mineral supplement.

calcium lactophosphate. Lactic acid hydrogen phosphate calcium salt.

calcium leucovorin. Leucovorin Calcium, U.S.P. 23. Inj. Tab. Powder for Oral. Powder for Inj. *Rx.*
Use: For overdosage of folic acid antagonists; megalobastic anemias.
See: Leucovorin Calcium (ESI Lederle Generics).
Wellcovorin (GlaxoWellcome).

•**calcium levulinate.** (KAL-see-uhm LEV-you-lih-nate) U.S.P. 23.
Use: Calcium replenisher.

Calcium Magnesium Chelated. (NBTY) Ca 500 mg, Mg 250 mg/Tab. Bot. 50s, 100s. *otc.*
Use: Mineral supplement.

Calcium Magnesium Zinc. (NBTY) Ca 333 mg, Mg 133 mg, Zn 8.3 mg/Tab. Bot. 100. *otc.*
Use: Mineral supplement.

calcium novobiocin. Calcium salt of an antibacterial substance produced by *Streptomyces niveus.*
Use: Anti-infective.

calcium orotate.
See: Calora, Tab. (Miller).

calcium oxytetracycline. Oxytetracycline Calcium, N.F. XIV.

•**calcium pantothenate.** (KAL-see-uhm pan-toe-THEH-nate) U.S.P. 23.
Use: Pantothenic acid (B_5) deficiency, coenzyme A precursor, vitamin (enzyme co-factor).
See: Calcium Pantothenate (Freeda Vitamins).
Calcium Pantothenate (Fibertone).

W/Ascorbic acid, niacinamide, vitamins B_1, B_2, B_6, B_{12}, A, D, E.
See: Tota-Vi-Caps Gelatin Capsule, Cap. (Zeneca).

W/Calcium carbonate.
See: Ilomel, Pow. (Warren-Teed).

W/Calcium carbonate, ferrous fumarate, niacinamide.
See: Prenatag, Tab. (Solvay).

W/Danthron.
See: Modane, Tab., Liq. (Warren-Teed).
Parlax, Tab. (Parmed).

W/Docusate sodium.
See: Pantyl, Tab. (McGregor).

W/Docusate sodium, acetphenolisatin.
See: Android-Plus, Tab. (Zeneca).
Peri-Pantyl, Tab. (McGregor).

W/Methoscopolamine nitrate, mephobarbital.
See: Ilocalm, Tabs. (Warren-Teed).

W/Niacinamide and vitamins.
See: Allbee C-800, Prods. (Robins).
Allbee T, Cap. (Robins).
Allbee with C, Cap. (Robins).
Ferrovite, Tab. (Laser).
Fumatinic, Tab. (Laser).
Maintenance Vitamin Formula, Tab. (Burgin-Arden).
Mulvidren, Tab. (Zeneca).
OB-Tabs, Tab. (Laser).
Probec, Tab. (Zeneca).
Probec-T, Tab. (Zeneca).
Stuart Hematinic, Tab. (Zeneca).
Stuart Therapeutic Multivitamin, Tab. (Zeneca).

W/Niacinamide, vitamins B_1, B_2, B_6.
See: Noviplex Capsules, Cap. (Zeneca).

W/Vitamins B_1, B_2, B_6, B_{12}, niacinamide, choline Cl, inositol, dl-methionine, testosterone, estrone, procaine.
See: Gerihorm, Inj. (Burgin-Arden).

W/Vitamin complex, ferrous fumarate, folic acid, calcium lactate, niacinamide.
See: Vitanate, Tab. (Century Pharm).

W/Vitamins A, D, B_1, B_2, C, niacinamide, calcium phosphorus, iron, B_6, B_{12}, E, magnesium, manganese, potassium, zinc, choline bitartrate, inositol.
See: Geriatric Vitamin Formula, Tab. (Burgin-Arden).

W/Vitamins A, E, C, zinc sulfate, magnesium sulfate, niacinamide, B_1, B_2, manganese Cl, B_6, folic acid, B_{12}.
See: Vicon Forte, Cap. (GlaxoWellcome).

W/Vitamin C, niacin, zinc sulfate, vitamins E, B_1, B_2, B_6, B_{12}.
See: Z-Bec, Tab. (Robins).

W/Vitamin complex, iron.
See: Vita-iron, Tab. (Century Pharm).

W/Vitamins, minerals, niacinamide.
See: Arcum-VM, Cap. (Arcum).
Capre, Tab. (Hoechst Marion Roussel).
Orovimin, Tab. (Solvay).
Os-Cal Forte, Tab. (Hoechst Marion Roussel).
Os-Vim, Tab. (Hoechst Marion Roussel).
Stuartinic, Tab. (Zeneca).
Theramin, Tab. (Arcum).
Theron, Tab. (Zeneca).
Uplex, Cap. (Arcum).

W/Vitamins, minerals, methyl testosterone, ethinyl estradiol, niacinamide.
See: Geritag, Cap. (Solvay).

W/Vitamin C, niacinamide, zinc sulfate, magnesium sulfate, vitamins B_1, B_2, B_6.

See: Vicon-C, Cap. (GlaxoWellcome).
W/Zinc sulfate, niacinamide, magnesium sulfate, manganese sulfate, vitamin complex.
See: Vicon Plus, Cap. (Glaxo-Wellcome).

•**calcium pantothenate, racemic.** U.S.P. 23.
Use: Vitamin B (enzyme cofactor).
See: Pantholin (Eli Lilly).

•**calcium phosphate, dibasic.** U.S.P. 23.
Use: Calcium replenisher, pharmaceutic aid (tablet base).
See: Dicalcium Phosphate.
Diostate D, Tab. (Pharmacia & Upjohn).

calcium phosphate, monocalcium.
See: Dicalcium Phosphate.

•**calcium phosphate, tribasic.** N.F. 18.
Use: Calcium replenisher.
See: Posture (Wyeth Ayerst).

calcium-phosphorus-free.
See: Fosfree, Tab. (Mission Pharmacal).

•**calcium polycarbophil.** (KAL-see-uhm PAHL-ee-CAR-boe-fill) U.S.P. 23.
Use: Laxative.
See: Equalactin, Chew. Tab. (Numark).
Fibercon, Tab. (ESI Lederle Generics).
Konsyl Fiber, Tab. (Konsyl Pharm).

calcium polysulfide.
Use: Wet dressing, soak.
See: Vlemasque, Cream. (Dormik).
Vleminckx, Soln. (Ulmer).

calcium propionate.
See: Propionate-caprylate mixtures.

calcium quinate.
See: Calcium Kinate Gluconate.

•**calcium saccharate.** U.S.P. 23.
Use: Pharmaceutic aid, sweetener (stabilizer).

calcium saccharin. Saccharin Calcium, U.S.P. 23.
Use: Pharmaceutic aid, sweetener.

calcium salicylate, theobromine.

calcium salts of sennosides A & B.
Use: Laxative.
See: Gentle Nature, Tab. (Novartis).
Nytilax, Tab. (Mentholatum).

•**calcium silicate.** N.F. 18.
Use: Pharmaceutic aid (tablet excipient).

•**calcium stearate.** N.F. 18.
Use: Pharmaceutic aid (tablet and capsule lubricant).

calcium succinate.
W/Aspirin.
See: Ber-Ex, Tab. (Dolcin).
Dolcin, Tab. (Dolcin).

•**calcium sulfate.** N.F. 18.
Use: Pharmaceutic aid (tablet and capsule diluent).

calcium thiosulfate.
Use: Wet dressing, soak.
See: Vlemasque Cream (Dermik Laboratories).
Vleminckx, Soln. (Ulmer).

calcium trisodium pentetate. (KAL-see-uhm try-SO-dee-uhm PEN-teh-tate)
Use: Antidote, heavy metals.
See: Calcium Chel 330 (Novartis).

•**calcium undecylenate.** U.S.P. 23.
Use: Antifungal.

calcium undecylenate. 10% calcium undecylenate Pow.
Use: Antifungal, topical.
See: Caldesene, Pow. (Novartis).
Cruex Squeeze Pow. (Novartis).

calcium with vitamin D tablets.
Use: Mineral, vitamin supplement.

Calcium with Vitamin D. (Schein Pharmaceutical) Calcium 600 mg, vitamin D 125 IU Bot. 60s. *otc.*
Use: Mineral, vitamin supplement.

Caldecort Spray. (Novartis) Hydrocortisone 0.5%. Aerosol can 1.5 oz. *otc.*
Use: Corticosteroid, topical.

Calderol. (Organon Teknika) Calcifediol 20 mcg or 50 mcg/Tab. Bot. 60s. *Rx.*
Use: Antihypocalcemia.

•**caldiamide sodium.** (KAL-DIE-ah-MIDE) USAN.
Use: Pharmaceutic aid.

Cal-D-Mint. (Enzyme Process) Calcium 800 mg, magnesium 150 mg, iron 18 mg, iodine 0.1 mg, copper 2 mg, vitamin D 200 IU/2 Tab. Bot. 100s, 250s. *otc.*
Use: Mineral, vitamin supplement.

Cal-D-Phos. (Archer-Taylor) Dicalcium phosphate 4.5 gr, calcium gluconate 3 gr, vitamin D/Tab. Bot. 1000s. *otc.*
Use: Mineral, vitamin supplement.

Cal-Guard. (Rugby) Calcium carbonate 50 mg. Softgel Cap. Bot. 60s. *otc.*
Use: Mineral supplement.

Calicylic Creme. (Gordon Laboratories) Salicylic acid 10%, mineral oil, cetyl alcohol, propylene glycol, white wax, sodium lauryl sulfate, oleic acid, methyl and propyl parabens, triethanolamine. 60 g. *otc.*
Use: Keratolytic.

Cal-Im. (Standex) Calcium glycerophosphate 1%, calcium levulinate 1.5%. Vial 30 ml. *Rx.*
Use: Mineral supplement.

Calinate-FA. (Solvay) Calcium 250 mg, vitamins A 4000 IU, D 400 IU, B_1 3 mg, B_2 3 mg, B_6 5 mg, B_{12} 1 mcg, folic acid 1 mg, C 50 mg, B_3 (niacinamide) 20 mg, B_5 (d-panthenol 1 mg), iron 60 mg, iodine 0.02 mg, manganese 0.2 mg, magnesium 0.2 mg, zinc 0.1 mg, copper 0.15 mg/Tab. Bot. 100s. *Rx.*
Use: Mineral, vitamin supplement.

calioben.
See: Calcium Iodobehenate.

Calivite. (Apco) Calcium carbonate 885 mg, ferrous sulfate 199 mg, vitamins A 3600 IU, D 400 IU, C 75 mg, B_1 1.5 mg, B_2 1.95 mg, B_6 0.75 mg, nicotinic acid 15 mg, B_{12} activity 0.025 mcg, choline 1500 mcg, inositol 2500 mcg, pantothenic acid 75 mcg, folic acid 25 mcg, p-aminobenzoic acid 12 mcg, potassium 10 mg, magnesium 1 mg, zinc 0.075 mg, manganese 0.02 mg, copper 0.01 mg, cobalt 0.02 mcg/Tab. Bot. 100s. *otc.*
Use: Mineral, vitamin supplement.

Cal-Lime-1. (Scrip) Calcium iodized 1 gr/Tab. Bot. 1000s.

Calmol 4. (Mentholatum) **Supp.:** Cocoa butter 80%, zinc oxide 10%, parabens. Box 12s, 24s. *otc.*
Use: Anorectal preparation.

Calmosin. (Spanner) Calcium gluconate, strontium bromide. Amp. 10 ml. 100s.

Cal-Nor. (Vortech) Calcium glycerophosphate 100 mg, calcium levulinate 150 mg/10 ml. Inj. Vial 100 ml. *Rx.*
Use: Mineral supplement.

Calocarb Tablets. (Pal-Pak) Calcium carbonate 648 mg/Tab. w/cinnamon flavor. Bot. 1000s. *otc.*
Use: Antacid.

calomel. Mercurous Cl.
Use: Cathartic.

Calotabs. Reformulated. (Calotabs) Docusate sodium 100 mg, casanthranol 30 mg/Tab. Box 10s. *otc.*
Use: Laxative.

caloxidine (iodized calcium).
See: Calcium Iodized.

Calphosan. (Glenwood) Calcium glycerophosphate 50 mg, calcium lactate 50 mg/10 ml sodium Cl solution. Contains calcium 0.08 mEq/ml. Inj. Amp. 10 ml, Vial 60 ml. *Rx.*
Use: Mineral supplement.

Calphron. (Nephro-Tech) Calcium acetate 667 mg/Tab. Bot. 200s. *otc.*
Use: Mineral supplement.

Cal-Plus. (Roberts Pharm) Calcium carbonate 1500 mg/Tab. Bot. 100s. *otc.*
Use: Mineral supplement.

Calsan. (Burgin-Arden) Calcium glycerophosphate 10 mg, calcium levulinate 15 mg, chlorobutanol 0.5%/ml. Inj. Vial 100 ml. *Rx.*
Use: Calcium supplement.

Cal Sup Instant 1000. (3M Personal Care Products) Elemental calcium 1000 mg, vitamins D 400 IU, C 60 mg. Pow. Packet 12s. *otc.*
Use: Mineral, vitamin supplement.

Cal Sup 600 Plus. (3M Personal Care Products) Elemental calcium 600 mg, vitamins D 200 IU, C 30 mg/Tab. Bot. 60s. *otc.*
Use: Mineral, vitamin supplement.

•**calteridol calcium.** (KAL-TER-ih-dahl KAL-see-uhm) USAN.
Use: Pharmaceutic aid.

Caltrate 600. (ESI Lederle Generics) Calcium carbonate 1.5 g (calcium 600 mg). Bot. 60s, 120s. *otc.*
Use: Mineral supplement.

Caltrate 600 + D. (ESI Lederle Generics) D 200 IU, Ca 600 mg. Sugar free. Tab. Bot. 60s. *otc.*
Use: Mineral, vitamin supplement.

Caltrate 600 + Iron. (ESI Lederle Generics) Calcium carbonate 600 mg, iron 18 mg, vitamin D 125 IU/Tab. Bot. 60s. *otc.*
Use: Mineral, vitamin supplement.

Caltrate Jr. (ESI Lederle Generics) Calcium carbonate 750 mg (300 mg calcium)/Chew. Tab. Bot. 60s. *otc.*
Use: Mineral supplement.

Caltrate Plus. (ESI Lederle Generics) D 200 IU, Ca 600 mg, Zn 7.5 mg, Mg, Cu, Mn, B. Sugar free. Tab. Bot. 60s. *otc.*
Use: Mineral, vitamin supplement.

Caltro. (Geneva Pharm) Elemental calcium 250 mg, vitamin D 125 IU/Tab. Bot. 100s, 1000s. *otc.*
Use: Mineral, vitamin supplement.

•**calusterone.** USAN.
Use: Antineoplastic.

Cama Arthritis Pain Reliever. (Novartis) Aspirin 500 mg, magnesium oxide 150 mg, aluminum hydroxide 125 mg, methylparaben. Tab. Bot. 100s. *otc.*
Use: Analgesic, antacid.

Cam-Ap-Es. (Camall) Hydrochlorothiazide 15 mg, reserpine 0.1 mg, hydralazine HCl 25 mg/Tab. Bot. 100s. *Rx.*
Use: Antihypertensive.

•**cambendazole.** (kam-BEND-ah-zole) USAN.
Use: Anthelmintic.

Camellia Lotion. (O'Leary) Moisturizer

lotion for face, hands and body. For normal to oily skin. Bot. 4 oz. *otc.*
Use: Emollient.

Cameo Oil. (Medco Lab) Mineral oil, isopropyl myristate, lanolin oil, PEG-8-Dioleate. Plastic Bot. 8 oz, 16 oz, 32 oz. *otc.*
Use: Emollient.

•**camiglibose.** (kah-mih-GLIE-bose) USAN.
Use: Antidiabetic (Glucohydrolase inhibitor).

Camouflage Crayon. (O'Leary) Coverup for minor skin discolorations, under eye concealer, lipstick fixer. Available in 6 shades. Crayon 0.05 oz. *otc.*
Use: Skin coverup.

Campho-Phenique. (Sanofi Winthrop) Camphor 10.8%, phenol 4.7%. **Liq.:** 22.5 ml, 45 ml, 120 ml. **Gel:** 6.9 g, 15 g. *otc.*
Use: Analgesic, antiseptic, local.

Campho-Phenique Antibiotic Plus Pain Reliever. (Sanofi Winthrop) Bacitracin 500 units, neomycin 3.5 mg, polymyxin B 5000 units/g, lidocaine 40 mg. Oint.: Tube 5 g. *otc.*
Use: Anti-infective, topical.

•**camphor.** U.S.P. 23.
Use: Topical antipruritic; anti-infective; pharmaceutic necessity for camphorated phenol, paregoric and flexible collodion, antitussive, expectorant, local counterirritant, nasal decongestant.
See: Vicks Inhaler (Procter & Gamble).
Vicks Regular and Wild Cherry Medicated Cough Drops (Procter & Gamble).
Vicks Medi-Trating Throat Lozenges (Procter & Gamble).
Vicks Sinex, Nasal Spray (Procter & Gamble).
Vicks Vaporub, Oint. (Procter & Gamble).
Vicks Vaposteam, Liq. (Procter & Gamble).
Vicks Va-Tro-Nol, Nose Drops (Procter & Gamble).

camphor, monobromated.

camphorated, parachlorophenol.
Use: Anti-infective (dental).

camphoric acid.

camphoric acid ester. Ester of p-Tolylmethylcarbinal as Diethanolamine Salt.

Camptosar. (Pharmacia & Upjohn) Irinotecan HCl 20 mg/ml, sorbitol/Inj. Vial. 5 ml. *Rx.*
Use: Antineoplastic.

•**candesartan.** (Kan-deh-SAHR-tan) USAN.
Use: Antagonist, angiotensin II receptor, antihypertensive.

•**candesartan cilexetil.** (kan-deh-SAHR-tan sigh-LEX-eh-till)
Use: Antagonist, angiotension II receptor, antihypertensive.

•**candicidin.** (KAN-dih-SIDE-in) U.S.P. 23. An antifungal antibiotic derived from *Strep. griseus.*
Use: Antifungal.
See: Candeptin, Vaginal Tab., Oint. (Julius Schmid).
Vanobid, Oint., Vaginal Tab. (Merrell Dow).

candida albicans skin test antigen.
Use: Diagnostic aid.
See: Candin, Inj. (Allermed, ALK Laboratories).

candida test. (SmithKline Diagnostics) Culture test for candida. 4s.
Use: Diagnostic aid.

Candin. (Allermed, ALK Laboratories) Candida albicans skin test antigen prepared from the culture filtrate and cells of two strains of *Candida albicans.* Vial 1 ml. *Rx.*
Use: Evaluation of cell-mediated immunity; diagnostic aid.

•**candoxatril.** (kan-DOXE-at-trill) USAN.
Use: Antihypertensive.

•**candoxatrilat.** (kan-DOXE-at-trill-at) USAN.
Use: Antihypertensive.

Candycon. (Allison) Chlorprophenpyridamine maleate 2 mg, phenylephrine HCl 5 mg/Tab. Bot. 50s. *otc.*
Use: Antihistamine, decongestant.

cannabinoids. Antiemetic/Antivertigo agent.
See: Dronabinol.

cannabis. Antiemetic, antivertigo.
See: Dronabinol.

Canopar. (GlaxoWellcome).

•**canrenoate potassium.** (kan-REN-oh-ate) USAN.
Use: Aldosterone antagonist.

•**canrenone.** (kan-REN-ohn) USAN.
Use: Aldosterone antagonist.

cantharidin.
Use: Keratolytic.

Cantil. (Hoechst Marion Roussel) Mepenzolate bromide 25 mg/Tab. Bot. 100s. *Rx.*
Use: Anticholinergic, antispasmodic.

Ca-Orotate. (Miller) Calcium (as calcium orotate) 50 mg/Tab. Bot. 100s. *otc.*
Use: Mineral supplement.

C-A-P. (Eastman Kodak) Cellulose acetate phthalate.

Capahist-DMH. (Freeport) Chlorpheniramine maleate 8 mg, phenylpropanolamine HCl 50 mg, atropine sulfate 1/180 gr, dextromethorphan HBr 20 mg/T.R. Cap. *Rx.*
Use: Anticholinergic, antihistamine, antispasmodic, antitussive, decongestant.

Capastat Sulfate. (Dura Pharm) Capreomycin sulfate 1 g/5 ml. Vial 5 ml. *Rx.*
Use: Antituberculous.

•**capecitabine.** (cap-eh-SITE-ah-bean) USAN.
Use: Antineoplastic.
See: Xeloda, Tab. (Roche).

Capital with Codeine. (Carnrick Labs) **Susp.:** Acetaminophen 120 mg, codeine phosphate 12 mg/5 ml. Bot. 473 ml. *c-v.* **Tab.:** Codeine phosphate 30 mg, acetaminophen 325 mg, Tab. scored. Bot. 100s. *c-III.*
Use: Analgesic combination, narcotic.

Capitrol Cream Shampoo. (Westwood Squibb) Tube 85 g. *Rx.*
Use: Antiseborrheic.

Ca-Plus-Protein. (Miller) Calcium (as contained in a calcium-protein complex made with specially isolated soy protein) 280 mg/Tab. Bot. 100s. *otc.*
Use: Mineral supplement.

Capnitro. (Freeport) Nitroglycerin 6.5 mg/TR Cap. Bot. 100s. *Rx.*
Use: Antianginal agent.

•**capobenate sodium.** (CAP-oh-BEN-ate) USAN.
Use: Cardiovascular agent (antiarrhythmic).

•**capobenic acid.** (CAP-oh-BEN-ik) USAN.
Use: Cardiovascular agent (antiarrhythmic).

Capoten. (Bristol-Myers Squibb) Captopril 12.5 mg, 25 mg, 50 mg or 100 mg, lactose. Tab. Bot 100s, 1000s (except 100 mg), UD 100s. *Rx.*
Use: Antihypertensive.

Capozide. (Bristol-Myers Squibb) Captopril/hydrochlorothiazide 25/15 mg, 25/25 mg, 50/15 mg or 50/25 mg/Tab. Bot. 100s. *Rx.*
Use: Antihypertensive.

•**capreomycin sulfate, sterile.** (CAP-ree-oh-MY-sin) U.S.P. 23. An antibiotic derived from *Streptomyces capreolus.* Caprocin.
Use: Anti-infective (tuberculostatic).
See: Capastat Sulfate, Amp. (Eli Lilly).

caprochlorone.

•**capromab pendetide.** (CAP-row-mab PEN-deh-TIDE) USAN.
Use: Monoclonal antibody.
See: Prostascint (Cytogen).

caprylate-propionate mixtures.

caprylate, salts.
See: Sodium Caprylate.
Zinc Caprylate.

caprylate sodium, injection. (Ingram) Amp. 33%, 1 ml Pkg. 12s, 25s, 100s.
Use: Antifungal.
See: Sodium Caprylate Preps.

•**capsaicin.** (kap-SAY-uh-sin) U.S.P. 23.
Use: Analgesic-topical; antineuralgic, specific pain syndromes, topical.
See: Capsin, Lot. (Feming).
Capzasin-P, Cream (Thompson Medical).
Dolorac, Cream (GenDerm).
No Pain-HP, Roll-on (Young Again Products).
Pain Doctor, Cream (Fougera).
Pain-X, Gel (BF Ascher).
R-Gel (Healthline Labs).
Zostrix Cream (GenDerm).

•**capsicum.** (CAP-sih-kum) U.S.P. 23.
Use: Carminative, counterirritant (external), stomachic.

•**capsicum oleoresin.** U.S.P. 23.
Use: Carminative; counterirritant (external); stomachic.

Capsin. (Fleming) Capsaicin 0.025% or 0.075%, benzyl alcohol, propylene glycol, denatured alcohol. Lot. Bot. 59 ml. *otc.*
Use: Analgesic-topical.

capsules, empty gelatin. (Eli Lilly) Lilly markets clear empty gelatin capsules in sizes 000,00,0,1,2,3,4,5.

•**captamine hydrochloride.** (CAP-tameen) USAN.
Use: Depigmentor.

captodiame hydrochloride.

•**captopril.** (KAP-toe-prill) U.S.P. 23.
Use: Antihypertensive, enzyme inhibitor (angiotensin-converting).
See: Capoten, Tab. (Bristol-Myers Squibb).

captopril. (Various Mfr.) Captopril 12.5 mg, 25 mg. Tab. Bot. 100s, 500s, 1000s, 5000s, UD 100s. 50 mg. Tab. 100s, 1000s, 5000s. 100 mg. Tab. 100s, 500s. *Rx.*
Use: Antihypertensive, enzyme inhibitor (angiotensin-converting).

•**capuride.** (CAP-you-ride) USAN.
Use: Hypnotic, sedative.

Capzasin-P. (Thompson Medical) Cap-

saicin 0.025%, benzyl and cetyl alcohol. Cream. 42.5 g. *otc.*
Use: Analgesic, topical.

Caquin. (Forest Pharmaceutical) Hydrocortisone 1%, iodochlorhydroxyquin 3%, hydrophilic base. Cream. Tube 20 g. *otc, Rx.*
Use: Corticosteroid, topical.

•**caracemide.** (car-ASS-eh-MIDE) USAN.
Use: Antineoplastic.

Carafate. (Hoechst Marion Roussel) **Tab.:** Sucralfate 1 g. Bot. 100s, 120s, 500s, UD 100s. **Susp.:** Sucralfate 1 g/10 ml. Bot. 420 ml. *Rx.*
Use: Antiulcerative.

•**caramel.** N.F. 18.
Use: Pharmaceutic aid (color).

caramiphen edisylate.
W/Phenylpropanolamine.
See: Tuss-Ornade, Prods. (SmithKline Beecham Pharmaceuticals).

caramiphen ethanedisulfonate.
W/Phenylephrine HCl, phenindamine tartrate.
See: Dondril, Tab. (Whitehall Robins).

caramiphen hydrochloride.
Use: Proposed antiparkinson.

caraway. N.F. XVI.
Use: Flavoring.

•**carbachol.** (CAR-bah-kole) U.S.P. 23.
Use: Parasympathomimetic, cholinergic (ophthalmic).
See: Carbastat, Soln. (Ciba Vision).
Miostat Intraocular, Soln. (Alcon Laboratories).
Murocarb, Soln. (Muro).
W/Methylcellulose.
See: Carbuptic, Soln. (Optopic).
Isopto Carbachol, Soln. (Alcon Laboratories).

carbacrylamine resins.
Use: Cation-exchange resin.

•**carbadox.** (CAR-bah-dox) USAN.
Use: Anti-infective.

carbamate.
See: Valmid, Tab. (Eli Lilly).

•**carbamazepine.** (KAR-bam-AZE-uh-peen) U.S.P. 23.
Use: Analgesic, anticonvulsant.
See: Atretol, Tab. (Athena Neurosciences).
Carbamazepine (Rugby).
Carbatrol, ER Cap. (Athena Neurosciences).
Epitol, Tab. (Teva USA).
Tegretol, Tab. (Novartis).

carbamazepine. (KAR-bam-AZE-uh-peen) (Various Mfr.) **Chew. Tab.:** 100 mg. Bot. 25s, 100s, UD 100s. **Tab.:** 200 mg. Bot. 25s, 100s, 1000s, UD 100s, 300s. *Rx.*
Use: Treatment of epilepsy and trigeminal neuralgia.

carbamide. (Various Mfr.) Urea. Cream, Lot.
Use: Emollient.
See: Aquacare (Allergan).
Carmol 20 (Syntex).
Elaqua XX (Zeneca).
Nutraplus (Galderma).
Rea-Lo (Whorton).
Ultra Mide Moisturizer (Baker/Cummins).
Ureacin-20 (Pedinol).
Ureacin-40 (Pedinol).

carbamide compounds.
See: Acetylcarbromal (Various Mfr.).
Bromisovalum (Various Mfr.).
Bromural, Tab. (Knoll Pharmaceuticals).
Carbrital, Elix., Kap. (Parke-Davis).
Carbromal (Various Mfr.).

•**carbamide peroxide.** (CAR-bah-mide per-ox-ide) U.S.P. 23. Urea compound w/hydrogen peroxide (1:1).
Use: Anti-infective-topical (dental); anti-inflammatory; analgesic.
See: Gly-Oxide (Hoechst Marion Roussel).
Orajel Brace-aid Rinse (Del Pharmaceuticals).
Orajel Perioseptic, Liq. (Del Pharmaceuticals).
Proxigel (Schwarz Pharma).

carbamide peroxide 6.5% in glycerin.
Use: Otic.
See: Murine Ear Drops (Abbott Laboratories).
Murine Ear Wax Removal System (Abbott Laboratories).

carbamylcholine chloride.
See: Carbachol.

carbamylmethylcholine chloride.
See: Urecholine, Tab., Inj. (Merck).

•**carbantel lauryl sulfate.** (CAR-ban-tell LAH-ruhl) USAN.
Use: Anthelmintic.

carbapenem.
See: Imipenem-Cilastatin.

carbarsone. U.S.P. 21. Caps., U.S.P. 21. (Various Mfr.) N-carbamoylarsanilic acid. Amabevan, ameban, amibiarson, arsambide, fenarsone, leucarsone, aminarsone, amebarsone. p-Ureidobenzenearsonic acid.
Use: Acute and chronic amebiasis and trichomoniasis.

•**carbaspirin calcium.** USAN.
Use: Analgesic.

Carbastat. (Ciba Vision Ophthalmics) Carbachol 0.1%, sodium Cl 0.064%, potassium Cl 0.075%, calcium Cl dihydrate 0.048%, magnesium Cl hexahydrate 0.03%, sodium acetate trihydrate 0.39%, sodium citrate dihydrate 0.17%. Soln. Vial 1.5 ml. *Rx.*
Use: Antiglaucoma.

Carbatrol. (Athena Neurosciences) Carbamazepine 200 mg, 300 mg, lactose, talc. ER Cap. Bot. 120s. *Rx.*
Use: Anticonvulsant.

•**carbazeran.** (CAR-BAY-zeh-ran) USAN.
Use: Cardiovascular agent.

•**carbenicillin disodium, sterile.** (CAR-ben-ih-SILL-in die-SO-dee-uhm) U.S.P. 23.
Use: Anti-infective.
See: Geopen, Vial (Roerig).
Pyopen, Inj. (SmithKline Beecham Pharmaceuticals).

•**carbenicillin indanyl sodium.** (car-BEN-ih-SILL-in IN-duh-nil) U.S.P. 23.
Use: Anti-infective.
See: Geocillin, Tab. (Roerig).

•**carbenicillin phenyl sodium.** (CAR-ben-ih-SILL-in FEN-ill) USAN.
Use: Anti-infective.

•**carbenicillin potassium.** (CAR-ben-ih-SILL-in) USAN.
Use: Anti-infective.

•**carbenoxolone sodium.** (CAR-ben-ox-ah-lone) USAN.
Use: Corticosteroid, topical.

carbetapentane citrate.
Use: Antitussive.
W/Codeine phosphate, chlorpheniramine maleate, guaifenesin.
See: Tussar-2, Syr. (Rhone-Poulenc Rorer).
Tussar SF, Liq. (Rhone-Poulenc Rorer).

carbethoxysyringoyl methylreserpate.

carbethyl salicylate.
See: Sal-Ethyl Carbonate, Tab. (Parke-Davis).

•**carbetimer.** (car-BEH-tih-MER) USAN.
Use: Antineoplastic.

Carbex. (Dupont Pharma) Selegiline HCl 5 mg, lactose/Tab. Bot. 60s. *Rx.*
Use: Used in combination with levodopa/carbidopa for treatment of Parkinson's disease.

•**carbidopa.** (CAR-bih-doe-puh) U.S.P. 23.
Use: Decarboxylase inhibitor.
See: Lodosyn, Tab. (Merck).
W/Levodopa.
See: Sinemet, Tab. (DuPont Pharma).

carbidopa and levodopa tablets.
Use: Antiparkinsonian.
See: Sinemet, Tab. (DuPont Pharma).

carbidopa & levodopa. (Various) Carbidopa 10 mg, levodopa 100 mg; carbidopa 25 mg, levodopa 100 mg; carbidopa 25 mg, levodopa 250 mg. Tab. Bot. 100s, 500s, 1000s. *Rx.*
Use: Antiparkinsonian.

carbimazole.

Carbinoxamine Compound Drops. (Rosemont) Pseudoephedrine HCl 25 mg, carbinoxamine maleate 2 mg, dextromethorphan HBr 4 mg. Grape flavor. Drop. Bot. 30 ml. *Rx.*
Use: Antihistamine, antitussive, decongestant.

Carbinoxamine Compound Syrup. (Rosemont) Pseudoephedrine HCl 60 mg, dextromethorphan HBr 15 mg, carbinoxamine maleate 4 mg. Grape flavor. Syr. Bot. 120 ml, pt, gal. *Rx.*
Use: Antihistamine, antitussive, decongestant.

carbinoxamine drops. (Morton Grove) Carbinoxamine maleate 2 mg, pseudoephedrine HCl 25 mg/ml, sorbitol, parabens, alcohol free, raspberry, fruit flavors. Drops. Bot. 30 ml w/calibrated dropper. *Rx.*
Use: Antihistamine, decongestant.

carbinoxamine maleate and pseudophedrine HCl.
See: Biohist-LA, TR Tab. (Wakefield).
Carbinoxamine Preps. (Morton Grove).

carbinoxamine maleate w/combinations.
See: Sildec-DM, Ped. Drops (Silarx).

Carbinoxamine Syrup. (Morton Grove) Carbinoxamine maleate 4 mg, pseudoephedrine HCl 60 mg/5 ml, sorbitol, parabens, alcohol free, raspberry, fruit flavors. Syr. Bot. 118 ml, 237 ml, 473 ml. *Rx.*
Use: Antihistamine, decongestant.

•**carbiphene hydrochloride.** (CAR-bih-FEEN) USAN.
Use: Analgesic.

Carbiset Tablets. (Nutripharm) Pseudoephedrine 60 mg, carbinoxamine maleate 4 mg/Tab. Bot. 100s, 500s. *Rx.*
Use: Antihistamine, decongestant.

Carbiset-TR. (Nutripharm) Pseudoephedrine HCl 120 mg, carbinoxamine maleate 8 mg/Tab. Bot. 100s. *Rx.*
Use: Antihistamine, decongestant.

Carbocaine. (Cook-Waite) Mepivacaine HCl 3%. Inj. Dental cartridge 1.8 ml. *Rx.*

Use: Anesthetic, local.

Carbocaine. (Sanofi Winthrop) Mepivacaine HCl. **1%:** Vial 30 ml, 50 ml. **1.5%:** Vial 30 ml. **2%:** Vial 20 ml, 50 ml. *Rx.*
Use: Anesthetic, local.

Carbocaine-Neo-Cobefrin. (Cook-Waite) Mepivacaine HCl 2% with levonorefrin 1:20,000. Inj. Dental cartridge 1.8 ml. *Rx.*
Use: Anesthetic, local.

•**carbocloral.** (CAR-boe-KLOR-uhl) USAN.
Use: Hypnotic, sedative.
See: Chloralurethane.
Prodorm (Parke-Davis).

•**carbocysteine.** (car-boe-SIS-teen) USAN.
Use: Mucolytic.

Carbodec. (Rugby) Pseudoephedrine HCl 60 mg, carbinoxamine maleate 4 mg/5 ml. Syr. Bot. 473 ml. *Rx.*
Use: Antihistamine, decongestant.

Carbodec DM Products. (Rugby) **Syr.:** Pseudoephedrine HCl 60 mg, carbinoxamine maleate 4 mg, dextromethorphan HBr 15 mg, alcohol < 0.6%/5 ml. Bot. 30 ml, 120 ml, pt, gal. **Drops (Pediatric Pharmaceuticals):** Pseudoephedrine HCl 25 mg, carbinoxamine maleate 2 mg, dextromethorphan HBr 4 mg, alcohol 0.6%/ml. Bot. 30 ml. *Rx.*
Use: Antihistamine, antitussive, decongestant.

Carbodec Tablets. (Rugby) Pseudoephedrine HCl 60 mg, carbinoxamine maleate 4 mg/Tab. Bot. 100s. *Rx.*
Use: Antihistamine, decongestant.

Carbodec TR. (Rugby) Pseudoephedrine HCl 120 mg, carbinoxamine maleate 8 mg/Tab. Bot. 100s. *Rx.*
Use: Antihistamine, decongestant.

carbol-fuchsin paint. Original fuchsin formula known as Castellani's Paint. Basic Fuchsin 0.3%, phenol 4.5%, resorcinol 10%, acetone 5%, alcohol 10%. Bot. 30 ml, 120 ml, 480 ml.
Use: Antifungal, topical.
See: Carfusin, Soln. (Rhone-Poulenc Rorer).
Castellani's Paint (Various Mfr.).

•**carbol-fuchsin, topical solution.** (CAR-buhl-FOOK-sin) U.S.P. 23.
Use: Antifungal.

carbomer. (CAR-boe-mer) N.F. 18. A polymer of acrylic acid, crosslinked with a polyfunctional agent.
Use: Pharmaceutic aid (emulsifying, suspending agent).
See: Carbopol 934 P (Goodrich).

•**carbomer 910.** (CAR-boe-mer 910) N.F. 18.
Use: Pharmaceutic aid, (emulsifying, suspending agent).

•**carbomer 934.** (CAR-boe-mer 934) N.F. 18.
Use: Pharmaceutic aid (emulsifying, suspending agent).

•**carbomer 934p.** (CAR-boe-mer 934) *Formerly carpolene* N.F. 18.
Use: Pharmaceutic aid (emulsifying, suspending, viscosity, thickening agent).

•**carbomer 940.** (CAR-boe-mer 940) N.F. 18.
Use: Pharmaceutic aid (emulsifying, suspending agent).

•**carbomer 941.** (CAR-boe-mer 941) N.F. 18.
Use: Pharmaceutic aid (emulsifying, suspending agent).

•**carbomer 1342.** (CAR-boe-mer 1342) N.F. 18.
Use: Pharmaceutic aid (emulsifying, suspending agent).

carbomycin. An antibiotic from *Streptomyces halstedii.*
Use: Anti-infective.

•**carbon dioxide.** U.S.P. 23.
Use: Inhalation, respiratory.
See: Ceo-Two, Supp. (Beutlich).

•**carbon monoxide c 11.** (CAR-bahn moe-NOX-ide C11) U.S.P. 23.
Use: Diagnostic aid (blood volume determination), radiopharmaceutical.

carbonic acid, dilithium salt. Lithium Carbonate, U.S.P. 23.

carbonic acid, disodium salt. Sodium Carbonate, N.F. 18.

carbonic acid, monosodium salt. Sodium Bicarbonate, U.S.P. 23.

carbonic anhydrase inhibitors.
See: Acetazolamide, Tab. (Various Mfr.).
AK-ZOL, Tab. (Akorn).
Daranide, Tab. (Merck).
Dazamide, Tab. (Major).
Diamox, Tab., Sequel, Vial (ESI Lederle Generics).
Neptazane, Tab. (ESI Lederle Generics).

Carbonis Detergens, Liquor.
See: Coal Tar Solution.

carbonyl diamide.
See: Chap Cream (Ar-Ex).

carbon tetrachloride. N.F. XVII. Benzinoform. (Various Mfr.).
Use: Pharmaceutic aid (solvent).

•**carboplatin.** (car-boe-PLATT-in) U.S.P. 23.
Use: Antineoplastic.
See: Paraplatin Pow. for Inj. (Bristol-Myers Oncology).

•**carboprost.** (CAR-boe-prahst) USAN.
Use: Oxytocic.

•**carboprost methyl.** (CAR-boe-prahst METH-ill) USAN.
Use: Oxytocic

•**carboprost tromethamine.** (CAR-boe-prahst troe-METH-ah-meen) U.S.P. 23.
Use: Oxytocic.
See: Prostin, Amp. (Pharmacia & Upjohn).

Carboptic. (Optopics) Carbachol 3%. Soln. Bot. 15 ml. *Rx.*
Use: Ophthalmic.

carbose d.
See: Carboxymethylcellulose sodium, Prep.

carbovir. (GlaxoWellcome)
Use: Antiviral, HIV. [Orphan drug]

carbowax. 300, 400, 1540, 4000. Polyethylene glycol 300, 400, 1540, 4000.

•**carboxymethylcellulose calcium.** N.F. 18.
Use: Pharmaceutic aid (tablet disintegrant).

carboxymethylcellulose salt of dextroamphetamine. Carboxyphen.
See: Bontril Timed Tab. (Carnrick Labs).

•**carboxymethylcellulose sodium.** (car-BOX-ee-meth-ill-SELL-you-lohs) U.S.P. 23.
Use: Pharmaceutic aid (suspending agent, tablet excipient), viscosity-increasing; cathartic.
W/Acetphenolisatin, docusate sodium.
See: Scrip-Lax, Tab. (Scrip).
W/Alginic acid, sodium bicarbonate.
See: Pretts, Tabs. (Hoechst Marion Roussel).
W/Belladonna extract, kaolin, pectin, zinc phenosulfonate.
See: Gelcomul, Liq. (Del Pharmaceuticals).
W/Digitoxin.
See: Foxalin, Cap. (Standex).
W/Docusate sodium.
See: Dialose, Cap. (Zeneca).
W/Docusate sodium, casanthranol.
See: Dialose Plus, Cap. (Zeneca).
Tri-Vac, Cap. (Rhode).
W/Docusate sodium, oxyphenisatin acetate.
See: Dialose Plus, Cap. (Zeneca).
W/Methylcellulose.
See: Ex-Caloric, Wafer (Eastern Research).
W/Testosterone, estrone, sodium Cl.
See: Tostestro, Inj. (Jones Medical Industries).

•**carboxymethylcellulose sodium 12.** N.F. 18.
Use: Pharmaceutic aid (suspending, viscosity-increasing agent).
Use: Mucolytic agent.

carboxyphen.
W/Butabarbital.
See: Bontril, Timed Tab. (Carnrick Labs).

Carbromal. (Various Mfr.) Bromodiethylacetylurea, bromadel, nyctal, planadalin, uradal. *Rx.*
Use: Sedative, hypnotic.
W/Bromisovalum (Bromural).
See: Bro-T's, Tab. (Brothers).

carbutamide.
Use: Hypoglycemic.

•**carbuterol hydrochloride.** (car-BYOO-ter-ole) USAN.
Use: Bronchodilator.

cardamon. Oil, seed, Cpd. Tincture.
Use: Flavoring.

Cardec DM Drops. (Various Mfr.) Carbinoxamine maleate 2 mg, pseudoephedrine HCl 25 mg, dextromethorphan HBr 4 mg, alcohol < 0.6%/ml. Drop. Bot. 30 ml. *Rx.*
Use: Antihistamine, antitussive, decongestant.

Cardec DM Pediatric Syrup. (Schein Pharmaceutical) Pseudoephedrine HCl 60 mg, dextromethorphan HBr 15 mg, carbinoxamine maleate 4 mg, < 0.6% alcohol. Bot. pt. *Rx.*
Use: Antihistamine, antitussive, decongestant.

Cardec DM Syrup. (Various Mfr.) Carbinoxamine maleate 4 mg, pseudoephedrine HCl 60 mg, dextromethorphan HBr 15 mg, alcohol > 0.6%/5 ml. Bot. 30 ml, 120 ml, pt, gal. *Rx.*
Use: Antihistamine, antitussive, decongestant.

Cardec-S. (Alphalma USPD) Pseudoephedrine HCl 60 mg, carbinoxamine maleate 4 mg/5 ml. Syr. Bot. 473 ml. *Rx.*
Use: Antihistamine, decongestant.

Cardene. (Syntex) Nicardipine 20 mg or 30 mg/Cap. Bot. 100s, 500s, UD 100s. *Rx.*
Use: Calcium channel blocker.

Cardene IV. (Wyeth Ayerst) Nicardipine HCl 2.5 ml, sorbitol 48 mg/ml. Inj. 10 ml amps. *Rx.*
Use: Calcium channel blocker.

Cardene SR. (Syntex) Nicardipine HCl

30 mg, 45 mg, 60 mg/Cap. SR Bot. 60s, 200s, UD 100s. *Rx.*
Use: Calcium channel blocker.

Cardenz. (Miller) Vitamins C 25 mg, E 5 mg, inositol 30 mg, p-aminobenzoic acid 9 mg, A 2000 IU, B_6 1.5 mg, B_{12} 1 mcg, D 100 IU, niacinamide 20 mg, magnesium 23 mg, iodine 0.05 mg, potassium 8 mg/Tab. Bot. 100s. *otc.*
Use: Mineral, vitamin supplement.

cardiamid.
See: Nikethamide. (Various Mfr.).

cardiazol.
See: Metrazol, Preps. (Knoll Pharmaceuticals).

Cardilate. (GlaxoWellcome) Erythrityl tetranitrate 10 mg/Tab. Bot. 100s.
Use: Antianginal.

Cardio-Green (CG). (Becton Dickinson) Indocyanine Green 25 mg or 50 mg. Inj. Amps 10 ml (2s).
Use: Diagnostic aid.

Cardio-Green Disposable Unit. (Becton Dickinson) Vial Cardio-Green, ampule aqueous solvent and calibrated syringe. 10 mg.
Use: Diagnostic aid.

Cardi-Omega 3. (Thompson Medical) EPA 180 mg, DHA 120 mg, cholesterol 5 mg, less than 2% RDA of vitamins A, B_1, B_2, B_3, C, D, Fe, Ca/Cap. Bot. 60s. *otc.*
Use: Mineral, vitamin supplement.

cardioplegic solution.
Use: During open heart surgery.
See: Plegisol, Soln. (Abbott Laboratories).

Cardioquin Tablets. (Purdue Frederick) Quinidine polygalacturonate 275 mg equivalent to quinidine sulfate 200 mg/Tab. Bot. 100s, 500s. *Rx.*
Use: Antiarrhythmic.

Cardiotrol-CK. (Roche Laboratories) Lyophilized human serum containing three CK isoenzymes from human tissue source. 10 × 2 ml.
Use: Diagnostic aid, quality control.

Cardiotrol-LD. (Roche Laboratories) Lyophilized human serum containing all LD isoenzymes from human tissue source. 10 × 1 ml.
Use: Diagnostic aid, quality control.

Cardizem. (Hoechst Marion Roussel) Diltiazem HCl **30 mg/Tab:** Bot. 100s, 500s, UD 100s. **60 mg/Tab:** Bot. 90s, 100s, 500s, UD 100s. **90 mg/Tab:** Bot 90s, 100s, UD 100s. **120 mg/Tab:** Bot. 100s and UD 100s. *Rx.*
Use: Calcium channel blocker.

Cardizem CD. (Hoechst Marion Roussel) Diltiazem HCl 120 mg, 180 mg, 240 mg, 300 mg/Ext. Rel. Cap. Bot. 30s, 90s, 5000s and UD 100s. *Rx.*
Use: Calcium channel blocker.

Cardizem Injection. (Hoechst Marion Roussel) **25 mg (5 mg/ml)/Inj:** Diltiazem HCl, 3.75 mg citric acid, 3.25 mg sodium citrate dihydrate and 357 mg sorbitol solution. 5 ml vials. **50 mg (5 mg/ml)/Inj:** Diltiazem HCl, 7.5 mg citric acid, 6.5 mg sodium citrate dihydrate and 714 mg sorbitol solution. 10 ml vials. *Rx.*
Use: Calcium channel blocker.

Cardizem SR. (Hoechst Marion Roussel) Diltiazem HCl 60 mg, 90 mg or 120 mg/S.R. Cap. Bot. 100s, UD 100s. *Rx.*
Use: Calcium channel blocker.

Cardophyllin.
See: Aminophylline. (Various Mfr.).

Cardoxin. (Vita Elixir) Digoxin 0.25 mg/Tab. *Rx.*
Use: Cardiovascular agent.

Cardura. (Roerig) Doxazosin mesylate 1 mg, 2 mg, 4 mg, 8 mg/Tab. Bot. 100s, UD 100s. *Rx.*
Use: Antihypertensive.

carena.
See: Aminophylline (Various Mfr.).

•**carfentanil citrate.** (car-FEN-tah-NILL SIH-trate) USAN.
Use: Analgesic, narcotic.

Cargentos.
See: Silver Protein, Mild.

•**carisoprodol.** (car-eye-so-PRO-dole) U.S.P. 23.
Use: Muscle relaxant.
See: Rela, Tab. (Schering Plough). Soma, Tab. (Wallace Laboratories).

carisoprodol. (Various Mfr.) 350 mg. Tab. Bot. 30s, 60s, 100, 500s, 1000s, UD 100s.
Use: Muscle relaxant.

carisoprodol and aspirin tablets.
Use: Analgesic, muscle relaxant.
See: Soma Compound Tab. (Wallace Laboratories).

carisoprodol, aspirin, and codeine phosphate tablets.
Use: Analgesic, muscle relaxant.
See: Soma Compound w/Codeine Tab. (Wallace Laboratories).

Carisoprodol Compound. (Various Mfr.) Carisoprodol 200 mg, aspirin 325 mg/Tab. Bot. 15s, 30s, 40s, 100s, 500s, 1000s. *Rx.*
Use: Analgesic, muscle relaxant.

Cari-Tab. (Jones Medical Industries) Fluoride 0.5 mg, vitamins A 2000 IU, D 200 IU, C 75 mg/Softab. Bot. 100s. *Rx.*
Use: Vitamin supplement, dental caries agent.

•**carmantadine.** (car-MAN-tah-deen) USAN.
Use: Antiparkinsonian.

Carmol 10. (Doak Dermatologics) Urea (carbamide) 10% in hypoallergenic water-washable lotion base. Bot. 6 fl oz. *otc.*
Use: Emollient.

Carmol 20. (Doak Dermatologics) Urea (carbamide) 20% in hypoallergenic vanishing cream base. Tube 3 oz, Jar lb. *otc.*
Use: Emollient.

Carmol HC Cream 1%. (Doak Dermatologics) Micronized hydrocortisone acetate 1%, urea 10% in water-washable base. Tube 1 oz, Jar 4 oz. *Rx.*
Use: Corticosteroid, topical.

•**carmustine (BCNU).** (CAR-muss-teen) USAN.
Use: Antineoplastic.
See: BiCNU, Inj. (Bristol-Myers Oncology).
Gliadel, wafer (Rhone-Poulenc Rorer).

Carnation Follow-Up. (Carnation) Protein (from non-fat milk) 18 g, carbohydrate (from lactose and corn syrup) 89.2 g, fat 27.7 g, vitamins A, D, E, K, C, B_1, B_2, B_3, B_6, B_{12}, B_5, biotin, choline, Ca, P, Cl, Mg, I, Mn, Cu, Zn, Fe 13 mg, inositol, cholesterol 11.4 mg, taurine, sodium 264 mg, potassium 913 mg. Pow. 360 g Con. 390 ml. *otc.*
Use: Nutritional supplement.

Carnation Good-Start. (Carnation) Protein 16 g, carbohydrate 74.4 g, fat 34.5 g, vitamins A, D, E, K, B_1, B_2, B_3, B_5, B_6, B_{12}, C, biotin, choline, inositol, cholesterol 68 mg, taurine, Ca, P, Mg, Fe 10 mg, Zn, Mn, Cu, I, Cl, sodium 162 mg, potassium 663 mg. Pow 360 g Con. 390 ml. *otc.*
Use: Nutritional supplement.

Carnation Instant Breakfast. (Carnation) Non-fat instant breakfast containing 280 K calories w/15 g protein and 8 oz whole milk. Pkt. 35 g, Ctn. 6s. Six flavors. *otc.*
Use: Nutritional supplement.

•**carnidazole.** (car-NIH-dah-zole) USAN. Methyl-nitro-imidazole.
Use: Antiparasitic, antiprotozoal.

Carnitor. (Sigma-Tau Pharmaceuticals) Levocarnitine. **Liq.:** 100 mg/ml. Bot. 10 ml. **Tab.:** 330 mg. Bot. 90s. **Inj.:** 1 g/5 ml. Single-dose amps 5 ml. *Rx.*
Use: Vitamin supplement.

•**caroxazone.** (car-OX-ah-zone) USAN.
Use: Antidepressant.

•**carphenazine maleate.** (car-FEN-azz-een) USAN. U.S.P XXII
Use: Antipsychotic.

•**carprofen.** (car-PRO-fen) USAN.
Use: Analgesic, NSAID.
See: Rimadyl. (Roche Laboratories).

•**carrageenan.** (ka-rah-GEE-nan) N.F. 18.
Use: Pharmaceutic aid (suspending, viscosity-increasing agent).

Carrisyn. (Carrington Labs) Phase I AIDS, ARC. *Rx.*
Use: Antiviral, immunomodulator.

•**carsatrin succinate.** (car-SAT-rin) USAN.
Use: Cardiovascular agent.

•**cartazolate.** (car-TAZZ-oh-late) USAN.
Use: Antidepressant.

•**carteolol hydrochloride.** (CAR-tee-oh-lahl) U.S.P. 23.
Use: Antiadrenergic (β-receptor).
See: Ocupress, Ophth. Soln. (Otuska America).

Carter's Little Pills. (Carter Products) Bisacodyl 5 mg/Pill. Pills 30s, 85s. *otc.*
Use: Laxative.

Cartrol. (Abbott Laboratories) Carteolol 2.5 mg or 5 mg/Tab. Bot. 100s. *Rx.*
Use: Beta-adrenergic blocker.

Cartucho Cook with Ravocaine. (Sanofi Winthrop) Ravocaine, novocaine, levophed or neo-cobefrin. *Rx.*
Use: Anesthetic.

•**carubicin hydrochloride.** (kah-ROO-bih-sin) USAN. *Formerly carminomycin hydrochloride*
Use: Antineoplastic.

•**carumonam sodium.** (kah-roo-MOE-nam) USAN.
Use: Anti-infective.

•**carvedilol.** (CAR-veh-DILL-ole) USAN.
Use: Antianginal, antihypertensive.
See: Coreg, Tab. (SmithKline Beecham).

Car-Vit. (Mericon) Ascorbic acid 60 mg, vitamins A acetate 4000 IU, D-2 400 IU, ferrous fumarate 90 mg (elemental iron 30 mg), oyster shell 600 mg (calcium 230 mg)/Cap. Bot. 90s, 1000s. *otc.*
Use: Mineral, vitamin supplement.

•**carvotroline hydrochloride.** (car-VAH-trah-leen) USAN.
Use: Antipsychotic.

•**carzelesin.** (car-ZELL-eh-sin) USAN.
Use: Antineoplastic (site-selective DNA binding).

carzenide.
Use: Carbonic anhydrase inhibitor.

casa-dicole. (Halsey) Docusate sodium 100 mg, casanthrol 30 mg/Cap. Bot. 100s. *otc.*
Use: Laxative.

•**casanthranol.** (kass-AN-thrah-nole) U.S.P. 23. A purified mixture of the anthranol glycosides derived from *Cascara sagrada.*
Use: Laxative.
See: Black Draught, Prods. (Chattem Consumer Products).
W/Docusate sodium.
See: Bu-Lax-Plus, Cap. (Ulmer).
Calotabs, Tab. (Calotabs).
Comfolax-Plus, Cap. (Rhone-Poulenc Rorer).
Comfolax-Plus, Cap. (Searle).
Comfula-Plus (Searle).
Constiban, Cap. (Quality Formulations).
Diolax, Cap. (Century Pharm).
Dio-Soft (Standex).
Disulans, Cap. (Noyes).
Easy-Lax Plus, Cap. (Walgreens).
Genericace, Cap. (Forest Pharmaceutical).
Neo-Vardin D-S-S-C, Cap. (Scherer).
Nuvac, Cap. (LaCrosse).
Peri-Colace, Cap., Syr. (Bristol-Myers).
W/Docusate sodium, sodium carboxymethylcellulose.
See: Dialose Plus, Cap. (Zeneca).
Tri-Vac, Cap. (Rhode).
W/Mineral oil, irish moss.
See: Neo-Kondremul, Liq. (Medeva).

Cascara. (Eli Lilly) Cascara 150 mg/Tab. Bot. 100s. *otc.*
Use: Laxative.

cascara fluid extract, aromatic.
Use: Laxative.
W/Psyllium husk powder, prune powder.
See: Casyllium, Pow. (Pharmacia & Upjohn).

Cascara Glycosides.
Use: Laxative.

•**cascara sagrada.** (kass-KA-rah sah-GRAH-dah) U.S.P. 23.
Use: Cathartic.
W/Bile salts, papain, phenolphthalein, capsicum oleoresin.
See: Torocol Compound, Tab. (Plessner).
W/Bile salts, phenolphthalein, capsicum oleoresin, peppermint oil.
See: Torocol, Tab. (Plessner).
W/Ox bile (desiccated), phenolphthalein, aloin, podophyllin.
See: Bilgon, Tab. (Solvay).
W/Oxgall, dandelion root, podophyllin, tincture nux vomica.
See: Oxachol, Liq. (Roxane).
W/Pancreatin, pepsin, sodium salicylate.
See: Bocresin, Liq. (Scrip).
W/Phenolphthalein, sodium glycocholate, sodium taurocholate, aloin.
See: Bicholax, Tab. (Zeneca).
Oxiphen, Tab. (PolyMedica).
W/Sodium salicylate, phenolphthalein, chionanthus extract, bile extract, sodium glycocholate, sodium taurocholate.
See: Glycols, Tab. (Jones Medical Industries).

cascara sagrada. (Various Mfr.) 325 mg/Tab. Bot. 100s, 1000s.
Use: Cathartic.

cascara sagrada fluid extract. (Parke-Davis) Alcohol 18%. Bot. pt, gal, UD 5 ml.
Use: Laxative. [Orphan drug]
See: Cas-Evac, Liq. (Parke-Davis).
Bilstan (Standex).

cascara sagrada fluid extract aromatic. Aromatic Cascara Fluid extract. Liq. Alcohol ≈ 18%/5 ml. Bot. 60 ml, 120 ml, pt, gal, UD 5 ml.
Use: Laxative.
W/Psyllium husk powder, prune powder.
See: Casyllium, Granules (Pharmacia & Upjohn).

cascarin.
See: Casanthranol (Various Mfr.).

Casec. (Bristol-Myers) Calcium caseinate (derived from skim milk curd and calcium carbonate). Pow. Can 2.5 oz. *otc.*
Use: Mineral supplement.

Casodex. (Zeneca) Bicalutamide 50 mg, lactose/Tab. In 100s and UD 30s. *Rx.*
Use: Antineoplastic.

CAST. (Biomerica) Color Allergy Screening Test: A visual ELISA test for quantitative determination of Human Immunoglobulin E in serum.
Use: Diagnostic aid.

CAST. (Biomerica) Reagent test for immunoglobulin E in serum. Tube Kit 25s.
Use: Diagnostic aid.

Castellani Paint Modified. (Pedinol) Basic fuchsin, phenol resorcinol, acetone, alcohol. Bot. 30 ml, 120 ml, 480 ml. Also available as colorless solution without basic fuchsin. Bot. 30 ml, 120 ml, 480 ml. *Rx.*
Use: Antifungal, topical.

Castellani's Paint. (Penta) Carbol-fuchsin solution. Fuchsin 0.3%, phenol 4.5%, resorcinol 10%, acetone 1.5%, alcohol 13%. Bot. 1 oz, 4 oz, pt. *Rx.*
Use: Antifungal, topical.

•**castor oil.** (KASS-ter oil) U.S.P. 23.
Use: Laxative, pharmaceutic aid (plasticizer).
See: Neoloid (ESI Lederle Generics).
Purge (Fleming).

castor oil. (KASS-ter oil) Aromatic Caps. Liq. emulsion. Liq. Bot. 60 ml, 120 ml, pt.
Use: Laxative, pharmaceutic aid (plasticizer).

castor oil emulsion.
Use: Cathartic.
See: Emulsoil (Paddock).
Fleet Flavored (C.B. Fleet Co.).

castor oil, hydrogenated.
Use: Laxative.

Cataflam. (Novartis) Diclofenac 50 mg (as potassium), sucrose Tab. Bot. 100s, UD 100s. *Rx.*
Use: Analgesic, NSAID.

Catapres. (Boehringer Ingelheim) Clonidine HCl 0.1 mg, 0.2 mg or 0.3 mg/Tab. Bot. 100s. 0.1 mg, 0.2 mg: Bot. 1000s, UD 100s. *Rx.*
Use: Antihypertensive.

Catapres-TTS. (Boehringer Ingelheim) Clonidine 2.5 mg, 5 mg or 7.5 mg/Transdermal patch. Pkg. 4s, 12s. *Rx.*
Use: Antihypertensive.

Catarase 1:5000. (Ciba Vision Ophthalmics) Chymotrypsin 300 units in a 2-chamber vial with 2 ml sodium Cl. *Rx.*
Use: Ophthalmic enzyme.

Catatrol. (Zeneca) Viloxazine.
Use: Antidepressant.

cathomycin calcium. Calcium novobiocin.
Use: Anti-infective.

cathomycin sodium. Novobiocin sodium.
Use: Anti-infective.

cationic resins.
See: Resins, Sodium-Removing.

Caverject. (Pharmacia & Upjohn) Alprostadil 11.9 mcg (10 mcg/ml) or 23.2 mcg (20 mcg/ml). Lyophilized powd. for inj. In vials with diluent syringes. *Rx.*
Use: Anti-impotence agent.

Cav-X Fluoride Treatment. (Palisades Pharm) Stannous fluoride 0.4% gel. Bot. 121.9 g. *Rx.*
Use: Dental caries agent.

C-Bio. (Barth's) Vitamin C 150 mg, citrus bioflavonoid complex 100 mg, rutin 50 mg/Tab. Bot. 100s, 500s, 1000s. *otc.*
Use: Vitamin supplement.

C-B Time Liquid. (Arco) Vitamins C 300 mg, B_1 15 mg, B_2 10 mg, B_3 100 mg, B_5 20 mg, B_6 5 mg, B_{12} 5 mcg. Liq. Bot. 120 ml. *otc.*
Use: Vitamin supplement.

CCD 1042. (Cocensys)
Use: Treatment of infantile spasms. [Orphan drug]

CC-Galactosidase. Alpha-galactosidase A.
Use: Fabry's disease. [Orphan drug]

CCNU. Lomustine.
Use: Antineoplastic.
See: CeeNu, Tab. (Bristol-Myers Squibb).

C-Crystals. (NBTY) Vitamin C 5,000 mg/tsp. Crystals. Bot. 180 g. *otc.*
Use: Vitamin supplement.

CD4 human truncated 369 AA polypeptide. *Rx.*
Use: Antiviral, HIV.

CD4, recombinant soluble human (rCD4).
Use: Antiviral, HIV. [Orphan drug]

CD-45 monoclonal antibodies.
Use: Prevent graft rejection in organ transplants. [Orphan drug]

CDDP.
Use: Antineoplastic.
See: Cisplatin.

C.D.P. Caps. (Zenith Goldline) Chlordiazepoxide HCl 5 mg, 10 mg or 25 mg/Cap. Bot. 100s, 500s, 1000s. *c-iv.*
Use: Anxiolytic.

Cea. (Abbott Diagnostics) Radioimmunoassay or enzyme immunoassay for quantitative measurement of carcinoembryonic antigen in human serum or plasma. Test kit 100s.
Use: Diagnostic aid.

Cea-Roche. (Roche Laboratories) Radioimmunoassay capable of detecting and measuring plasma levels of CEA in the nanogram range. Sensitivity-0.5 ng./ml of CEA.
Use: Diagnostic aid.

Cea-Roche Test Kit. (Roche Laboratories) Carcinoembryonic antigen, a glycoprotein which is a constituent of the glycocalyx of embryonic entodermal epithelium. Test kit.
Use: Diagnostic aid.

CEA-Scan. (Immunomedics, Mallinckrodt) Arcitumomab 1.25 mg. Reconstitute with Tc 99m sodium pertechnetate in NaCl for Inj. Inj. Single-dose Vial. *Rx.*

Use: For detection of recurrent or metastatic colorectal carcinoma of the liver, extrahepatic abdomen and pelvis; radioimmunoscintigraphy.

Cebid Timecelles. (Roberts Pharm) Ascorbic acid 500 mg/Cap. Bot. 100s. *otc.*
Use: Vitamin supplement.

Ceb Nuggets. (Scott/Cord) Vitamins B_1 15 mg, B_2 15 mg, B_6 5 mg, B_{12} 5 mcg, C 600 mg, niacinamide 100 mg, E 40 IU, calcium pantothenate 20 mg, folic acid 0.1 mg/Nugget. Bot. 60s. *otc.*
Use: Mineral, vitamin supplement.

Cebo-Caps. (Forest Pharmaceutical) Placebo capsules. *otc.*

C & E Capsules. (NBTY) Vitamins C 500 mg, E 400 mg/Cap. Bot. 50s, 100s. *otc.*
Use: Vitamin supplement.

Ceclor. (Eli Lilly) **Pulv.:** Cefaclor 250 mg or 500 mg. Bot. 15s, 30s, 100s, UD 100s. **Oral Susp.:** Cefaclor 125 mg, 187 mg, 250 mg, 375 mg/5 ml. Bot. 50 ml, 75 ml, 100 ml, 150 ml. 375 mg/5 ml.
Use: Anti-infective, cephalosporin.

Ceclor CD. (Eli Lilly) Cefaclor (as monohydrate) 375 mg or 500 mg, mannitol/ ER Tab. Bot. 60s. *Rx.*
Use: Anti-infective.

Cecon Solution. (Abbott Laboratories) Ascorbic acid 10% in propylene glycol. Each drop from enclosed dropper supplies 2.5 mg ascorbic acid; each ml contains 100 mg Bot. w/dropper 50 ml. *otc.*
Use: Vitamin supplement.

Cedax. (Schering Plough) **Cap.:** Ceftibuten 400 mg, parabens/Bot 20s, 100s, UD 40s. **Susp.:** Ceftibuten 90 or 180 mg/5 ml, sucrose/Bot 30, 60, 90, 120 ml. *Rx.*
Use: Anti-infective, cephalosporin.

•**cedefingol.** (seh-deh-FIN-gole) USAN.
Use: Antineoplastic, adjunct; antipsoriatic.

•**cedelizumab.** (sed-eh-LIE-zoo-mab) USAN.
Use: Monoclonal antibody, immunosuppressant.

Ceebevim. (NBTY) Vitamins B_1 15 mg, B_2 10.2 mg, B_3 50 mg, B_5 10 mg, B_6 5 mg, C 300 mg/Cap. Bot. 100s, 300s. *otc.*
Use: Vitamin supplement.

CeeNu. (Bristol-Myers Oncology) Lomustine (CCNU) 10 mg, 40 mg or 100 mg/ Cap. Dose pk. of two cap. each of all three strengths. *Rx.*
Use: Antineoplastic.

Ceepa. (Geneva Pharm) Theophylline 130 mg, ephedrine HCl 24 mg, phenobarbital 8 mg/Tab. Bot. 100s, 1000s. *Rx.*
Use: Bronchodilator, decongestant, hypnotic, sedative.

Ceepryn. Cetylpyridinium Cl. *otc.*
Use: Antiseptic.
See: Cēpacol Lozenges, Soln., Troches (J.B. Williams).

Cee with Bee. (Wesley Pharmacal) Vitamins B_1 15 mg, B_2 10.2 mg, B_3 50 mg, B_5 10 mg, B_6 5 mg, C 300 mg, tartrazine. Bot. 100s, 1000s. *otc.*
Use: Vitamin supplement.

•**cefaclor.** (SEFF-uh-klor) U.S.P. 23.
Use: Anti-infective, cephalosporin.
See: Ceclor Prods. (Eli Lilly).

cefaclor. (Various Mfr.) **Cap.:** 250 mg, 500 mg. Bot. 15s (500 mg), 30s (250 mg), 100s, 500s (250 mg), 1000s (250 mg), UD 100s (500 mg). **Pow. for Oral Susp.:** 125 mg/5 ml, 187 mg/5 ml, 250 mg/5 ml, 375 mg/5 ml, Bot. 50 ml, 75 ml, 100 ml, 150 ml. *Rx.*
Use: Anti-infective

•**cefadroxil.** (SEFF-uh-DROX-ill) U.S.P. 23.
Use: Anti-infective, cephalosporin.
See: Duricef, Cap., Tab., Susp. (Bristol-Myers).

cefadroxil. (Various Mfr.) Cefadroxil **Cap.:** 500 mg/Bot 100s. **Tab.:** 1 g/Bot 24s, 50s, 100s, 500s. *Rx.*
Use: Anti-infective, cephalosporin.

•**cefamandole.** (SEFF-ah-MAN-dole) USAN.
Use: Anti-infective.

•**cefamandole nafate for injection.** (SEFF-uh-MAN-dahl NA-fate) U.S.P. 23.
Use: Anti-infective, cephalosporin.
See: Mandol, Amp. (Eli Lilly).

•**cefamandole sodium for injection.** U.S.P. 23.
Use: Anti-infective, cephalosporin.

Cefanex. (Apothecon) Cephalexin monohydrate 250 mg or 500 mg/Cap. Bot. 100s. *Rx.*
Use: Anti-infective, cephalosporin.

•**cefaparole.** (SEFF-ah-pah-ROLE) USAN.
Use: Anti-infective.

•**cefatrizine.** (SEFF-ah-TRY-zeen) USAN.
Use: Anti-infective, cephalosporin.

•**cefazaflur sodium.** (seff-AZE-ah-flure) USAN.
Use: Anti-infective, cephalosporin.

•**cefazolin.** (seff-AH-zoe-lin) U.S.P. 23.
Use: Anti-infective (systemic), cephalosporin.

•**cefazolin sodium, injection.** (seff-uh-zoe-lin) U.S.P. 23.
Use: Anti-infective (systemic), cephalosporin.
See: Ancef, Vial (SmithKline Beecham Pharmaceuticals).
Kefzol, Amp. (Eli Lilly).

cefazolin sodium. (Apothecon). Cefazolin sodium 250 mg/Vial; 500 mg, 1 g/Vial, piggyback vial; 5 g, 10 g, 20 g,/ bulk pkg.
Use: Anti-infective (systemic), cephalosporin.

•**cefbuperazone.** (SEFF-byoo-PURR-ah-zone) USAN.
Use: Anti-infective, cephalosporin.

•**cefdinir.** (SEFF-dih-ner) USAN.
Use: Anti-infective, cephalosporin.
See: Omnicef, Cap. Oral Susp. (Parke-Davis).

•**cefepime.** (SEFF-eh-pim) USAN.
Use: Anti-infective.

•**cefepime hydrochloride.** (SEFF-eh-pim) USAN.
Use: Anti-infective.
See: Maxipime, Pow. for Inj. (Bristol-Myers Squibb).

•**cefetecol.** (seff-EH-teh-kahl) USAN.
Use: Antibacterial, cephalosporin.

Cefinal II. (Alto Pharmaceuticals) Salicymide 150 mg, acetaminophen 250 mg, doxylamine succinate 25 mg/Tab. Bot. 100s. *otc.*
Use: Analgesic combination.

•**cefixime.** (SEFF-IKS-eem) U.S.P. 23.
Use: Antibacterial, cephalosporin.
See: Suprax (ESI Lederle Generics).

Cefizox. (SmithKline Beecham) Ceftizoxime sodium. **Pow. for Inj.:** 500 mg (single-dose fliptop vials 10 ml); 1 g, 2 g, (vial 20 ml, piggyback vial 100 ml); 10 g (bulk pkg). **Inj.:** 1 g, 2 g. Frozen, premixed, single-dose plastic containers 50 ml. *Rx.*
Use: Anti-infective, cephalosporin.

•**cefmenoxine hydrochloride, sterile.** (SEFF-men-ox-eem) U.S.P. 23.
Use: Anti-infective, cephalosporin.
See: Takeda (Abbott Laboratories).

•**cefmetazole.** (seff-MET-ah-zole) U.S.P. 23.
Use: Anti-infective, cephalosporin.

•**cefmetazole sodium, sterile.** (seff-MET-ah-zole) U.S.P. 23.
Use: Anti-infective, cephalosporin.
See: Zefazone (Pharmacia & Upjohn).

Cefobid. (Roerig) Cefoperazone sodium **Pow. for Inj.:** 1 g or 2 g. Piggyback unit. **Inj.:** 1 g, 2 g. Premixed, frozen, 50 ml plastic container 10 g Pharmacy bulk package. *Rx.*
Use: Anti-infective, cephalosporin.

Cefol Filmtab. (Abbott Laboratories) Vitamins B_1 15 mg, B_2 10 mg, B_6 5 mg, B_{12} 6 mcg, C 750 mg, E 30 mg, B_5 20 mg, B_3 100 mg, folic acid 0.5 mg/Tab. Bot. 100s. *otc.*
Use: Mineral, vitamin supplement.

•**cefonicid monosodium.** (seh-FAHN-ih-SID MAHN-oh-SO-dee-uhm) USAN.
Use: Anti-infective, cephalosporin.

•**cefonicid sodium, sterile.** (seh-FAHN-ih-SID) U.S.P. 23.
Use: Anti-infective, cephalosporin.
See: Monocid, Pow. for Inj. (SmithKline Beecham).

•**cefoperazone sodium.** (SEFF-oh-PUR-uh-zone) U.S.P. 23.
Use: Anti-infective, cephalosporin.
See: Cefobid, Inj. (Roerig).

•**ceforanide for injection.** (seh-FAR-ah-NIDE) U.S.P. 23.
Use: Anti-infective, cephalosporin.

Cefotan. (Zeneca) Cefotetan disodium **Pow. for Inj.:** 1 g, 2 g (*ADD-Vantage* and piggyback vials); 10 g (vial 100 ml). **Inj.:** 1 g/50 ml, 2 g/50 ml, dextrose. Frozen, iso-osmotic, premixed single-dose *Galaxy* containers 50 ml. *Rx.*
Use: Anti-infective, cephalosporin.

•**cefotaxime sodium.** (seff-oh-TAX-eem) U.S.P. 23.
Use: Anti-infective, cephalosporin.
See: Claforan, Inj. (Hoechst Marion Roussel).

•**cefotetan.** (SEFF-oh-tee-tan) U.S.P. 23.
Use: Anti-infective, cephalosporin.

•**cefotetan disodium.** (SEFF-oh-tee-tan die-SO-dee-uhm) U.S.P. 23.
Use: Anti-infective
See: Cefotan (Zeneca).

•**cefotiam hydrochloride sterile.** (SEFF-oh-TIE-am) U.S.P. 23.
Use: Anti-infective, cephalosporin.

•**cefoxitin.** (seff-OX-ih-tin) USAN.
Use: Anti-infective, cephalosporin.
See: Mefoxin, Inj. (Merck).

•**cefoxitin sodium.** (seff-OX-ih-tin) U.S.P. 23.
Use: Anti-infective, cephalosporin.

•**cefpimizole.** (seff-PIH-mih-zole) USAN.
Use: Anti-infective, cephalosporin.

•**cefpimizole sodium.** (seff-PIH-mih-zole) USAN.
Use: Anti-infective, cephalosporin.

See: Mefoxin, Inj., Pow. for Inj. (Merck).

•**cefpiramide.** (SEFF-PIHR-am-ide) U.S.P. 23.
Use: Anti-infective, cephalosporin.

•**cefpiramide sodium.** (SEFF-PIHR-am ide) USAN.
Use: Anti-infective, cephalosporin.

•**cefpirome sulfate.** (SEFF-pihr-ome) USAN.
Use: Anti-infective, cephalosporin.

•**cefpodoxime proxetil.** (SEFF-pode-OX-eem PROX-uh-til) USAN.
Use: Anti-infective, cephalosporin.
See: Vantin Gran. for Susp., Tab. (Pharmacia & Upjohn).

•**cefprozil.** (SEFF-pro-zill) U.S.P. 23.
Use: Anti-infective, cephalosporin.
See: Cefzil Pow. for Susp., Tab. (Bristol Labs.)

•**cefroxadine.** (SEFF-ROX-ah-deen) USAN.
Use: Anti-infective, cephalosporin.

•**cefsulodin sodium.** (SEFF-SULL-oh-din) USAN.
Use: Anti-infective, cephalosporin.

•**ceftazidime.** (seff-TAZE-ih-deem) U.S.P. 23.
Use: Anti-infective, cephalosporin.
See: Ceptaz, Inj. (GlaxoWellcome).
Fortaz, Inj. (GlaxoWellcome).
Tazicef, Inj. (Abbott Laboratories)
Tazidime, Inj. (Eli Lilly).

•**ceftibuten.** (seff-TIE-byoo-ten) USAN.
Use: Anti-infective.
See: Cedax, Cap., Susp. (Schering Plough).

Ceftin. (GlaxoWellcome) Cefuroxime axetil **Tab:** 125 mg, 250 mg or 500 mg/Tab. Bot. 20s, 60s, UD 50s, 100s. *Rx.* **Susp.:** 125 mg/5 ml, 250 mg/5 ml, sucrose/Bot. 50 ml, 100 ml. *Rx.*
Use: Anti-infective, cephalosporin.

•**ceftizoxime sodium.** (SEFF-tih-ZOX-eem) U.S.P. 23.
Use: Anti-infective, cephalosporin.
See: Cefizox, Pow. for Inj. (Fujisawa).

•**ceftriaxone sodium.** (SEFF-TRY-AXE-own) U.S.P. 23.
Use: Anti-infective, cephalosporin.
See: Rocephin, Inj. (Roche Laboratories).

•**cefuroxime.** (SEFF-yur-OX-eem) USAN.
Use: Anti-infective, cephalosporin.
See: Ceftin, Tab. (GlaxoWellcome).

•**cefuroxime axetil.** (SEFF-your-OX-eem ACK-seh-TILL) USAN. U.S.P. 23.
Use: Anti-infective, cephalosporin.
See: Ceftin, Tab. (Allen & Hanburys).

•**cefuroxime pivoxetil.** (SEFF-your-OX-eem pih-VOX-eh-till) USAN.
Use: Anti-infective, cephalosporin.

•**cefuroxime sodium.** U.S.P. 23.
Use: Anti-infective, cephalosporin.
See: Kefurox, Pow. for Inj. (Eli Lilly).
Zinacef, Inj., Pow. for Inj. (GlaxoWellcome).

cefuroxime sodium. (Various) **Pow. for Inj.:** 750, 1.5 g in 10 ml (750 mg only), 20 ml (1.5 g only), 100 ml piggyback vials; 7.5 g/vial pharmacy bulk package. *Rx.*
Use: Anti-infective, cephalosporin.

cefuroxime sodium, sterile.
Use: Anti-infective, cephalosporin.
See: Kefurox, Inj. (Eli Lilly).
Zinacef, Inj. (GlaxoWellcome).

Cefzil. (Bristol-Myers) Cefprozil. **Tab:** 250 mg, 500 mg. Bot. 50s, 100s and UD 100s. **Pow. for Oral Susp.:** 125 mg/5 ml, 250 mg/5 ml. Sucrose, aspartame, phenylalanine 28 mg/5 ml. Bot. 50 ml, 75 ml, 100 ml. *Rx.*
Use: Anti-infective, cephalosporin.

•**celgosivir hydrochloride.** (sell-GO-sih-vihr) USAN.
Use: Antiviral; inhibitor (α-glucoside).

Celestone. (Schering Plough) **Tab.:** Betamethasone 0.6 mg. Bot. 100s, 500s, UD 21s. **Syr.:** Betamethasone 0.6 mg/5 ml, alcohol < 1%. Bot. 120 ml. *Rx.*
Use: Corticosteroid.

Celestone Phosphate Injection. (Schering Plough) Betamethasone sodium phosphate 4 mg/ml equivalent to betamethasone alcohol 3 mg/ml. Vial 5 ml. *Rx.*
Use: Corticosteroid.

Celestone Soluspan. (Schering Plough) Betamethasone sodium phosphate 3 mg, betamethasone acetate 3 mg, dibasic sodium phosphate 7.1 mg, monobasic sodium phosphate 3.4 mg, edetate disodium 0.1 mg, benzalkonium Cl 0.2 mg/ml. Vial 5 ml. *Rx.*
Use: Corticosteroid.

•**celiprolol hydrochloride.** (SEE-lih-PRO-lahl) USAN.
Use: Anti-adrenergic (β-receptor).

Cellaburate. (Eastman Kodak) Cellulose acetate butyrate.
Use: Pharmaceutic aid (plastic filming agent).

Cellase W-100.
W/Alpha-amylase W-100, proteinase W-300, lipase, estrone, testosterone, vitamins, minerals.
See: Geramine, Tab. (Zeneca).

CellCept. (Roche Laboratories) **Cap.:** Mycophenolate mofetil 250 mg. Bot. 100s, 500s, UD 100s. **Tab.:** Mycophenylate mofetil 500 mg, alcohols. Bot. 100s, 500s. *Rx.*
Use: Immunosuppressant.

Cellepacbin. (Arthrins) Vitamins A 1200 IU, B_1 1.5 mg, B_2 1.5 mg, B_6 0.75 mg, niacinamide 7.5 mg, panthenol 3 mg, C 20 mg, B_{12} 2 mcg, E 1 IU/Cap. Bot. 180s. *otc.*
Use: Vitamin supplement.

Cellothyl. (Numark Laboratories) Methylcellulose 0.5 g/Tab. Bot. 100s, 1000s. *otc.*
Use: Laxative.

•**cellulase.** (SELL-you-lace) USAN. A concentrate of cellulose-splitting enzymes derived from *Aspergillus niger* and other sources.
Use: Enzyme (digestive adjunct).
W/Bile salts, mixed conjugated, pancrelipase.
See: Cotazym-B, Tab. (Organon Teknika).
W/Mylase, prolase, calcium carbonate, magnesium glycinate.
See: Zylase, Tab. (Eon Labs Manufacturing).
W/Mylase, prolase, lipase.
See: Ku-Zyme, Cap. (Kremers Urban).
W/Pepsin, glutamic acid, pancreatin, ox bile extract.
See: Kanulase, Tab. (Novartis).
W/Pepsin, pancreatin, dehydrocholic acid.
See: Gastroenterase, Tab. (Wallace Laboratories).

cellulose. (SELL-you-lohs)
W/Hexachlorophene.
See: Zeasorb, Pow. (Stiefel).

•**cellulose acetate.** (SELL-you-lohs) N.F. 18.
Use: Pharmaceutic aid (coating agent), polymer membrane (insoluble).

•**cellulose acetate phthalate.** (SELL-you-lohs) N.F. 18.
Use: Pharmaceutic aid (tablet coating agent).

cellulose, carboxymethyl, sodium salt. (SELL-you-lohs) Carboxymethylcellulose Sodium, U.S.P. 23.

cellulose, hydroxypropyl methyl ether. Hydroxypropyl Methylcellulose, U.S.P. 23.

cellulose methyl ether. (SELL-you-lohs)
See: Methylcellulose, Prep. (Various Mfr.).

•**cellulose microcrystalline.** (SELL-you-lohs) N.F. 18.
Use: Pharmaceutic aid (tablet and capsule diluent).

cellulose, nitrate. Pyroxylin.

•**cellulose, oxidized.** (SELL-you-lohs) U.S.P. 23.
Use: Hemostatic.

•**cellulose, oxidized regenerated.** (SELL-you-lohs) U.S.P. 23.
Use: Hemostatic.

cellulose, powdered. (SELL-you-lohs)
Use: Tablet and capsule diluent.

•**cellulose sodium phosphate.**
Use: Antiurolithic.
See: Calcibind (Mission Pharmacal).

cellulosic acid.
See: Oxidized Cellulose. (Various Mfr.).

cellulolytic.

cellulolytic enzyme.
See: Cellulase (Various Mfr.).
W/Amylolytic, proteolytic enzymes, lipase, phenobarbital, hyoscyamine sulfate, atropine sulfate.
See: Arco-Lipase Plus, Tab. (Arco).
W/Amylolytic enzyme, proteolytic enzyme, lipolytic enzyme, butisol sodium, belladonna.
See: Butibel-zyme, Tab. (Ortho McNeil).
W/Calcium carbonate, glycine, amylolytic and proteolytic enzymes.
See: Co-Gel, Tab. (Arco).
W/Proteolytic enzyme, amylolytic enzyme, lipolytic enzyme.
See: Ku-Zyme, Cap. (Kremers Urban).
Zymme, Cap. (Scrip).
W/Proteolytic, amylolytic, lipolytic enzymes, iron, ox bile.
See: Spaszyme, Tab. (Dooner).

Celluvisc. (Allergan) Carboxymethylcellulose 1%, NaCl, KCl, sodium lactate. Ophthalmic soln. Single use containers 0.3 ml (UD 30s). *otc.*
Use: Artificial tears.

Celontin. (Parke-Davis) Methsuximide 150 mg or 300 mg/Kapseal. Bot. 100s. *Rx.*
Use: Anticonvulsant.

Cel-U-Jec. (Roberts Pharm) Betamethasone sodium phosphate 4 mg (equivalent to betamethasone alcohol 3 mg)/ml. Soln. Inj. Vial 5 ml. *Rx.*
Use: Corticosteroid.

Cenafed. (Century Pharm) **Tab.:** Pseudoephedrine HCl 30 mg or 60 mg. Bot. 100s, 1000s. **Syr.:** Pseudoephedrine HCl 30 mg/5 ml. Bot. 120 ml, pt, gal. *otc.*
Use: Decongestant.

Cenafed Plus. (Century Pharm) Pseudoephedrine HCl 60 mg, triprolidine HCl

2.5 mg/Tab. Bot. 100s. *otc.*
Use: Antihistamine, decongestant.

Cena-K. (Century Pharm) Potassium and Cl 20 mEq/15 ml (10% KCl), saccharin. Bot. pt, gal. *Rx.*
Use: Electrolyte supplement.

Cenalax. (Century Pharm) Bisacodyl. **Tab.:** 5 mg. Bot. 100s, 1000s. **Supp.:** 10 mg. Pkg. 12s, 1000s. *otc.*
Use: Laxative.

Cenolate. (Abbott Hospital Prods) Sodium ascorbate 562.5 mg/ml (equivalent to 500 mg/ml ascorbic acid), sodium hydrosulfate 0.5%. Inj. Amp. 1 ml, 2 ml. *Rx.*
Use: Vitamin supplement.

Centeon Thyroid. (Rhone-Poulenc Rorer) Dessicated animal thyroid glands (active thyroid hormones) T-4 thyroxine, T-3 thyronine 0.25 gr, 0.5 gr, 1 gr, 1.5 gr, 2 gr, 3 gr, 4 gr or 5 gr/Tab. Bot. 100s, 1000s. Handy Hundreds, Carton Strip 100s. *Rx.*
Use: Hormone, thryoid.

Center-Al. (Center Laboratories) Allergenic extracts, alum precipitated 10,000 PNU/ml or 20,000 PNU/ml. Vial 10 ml, 30 ml. *Rx.*
Use: Antiallergic.

Centoxin. (Centocor) Nebacumab.
Use: Antibacterial. [Orphan drug]

Centrafree. (NBTY) Iron 27 mg, vitamins A 5000 IU, D 400 IU, E 30 IU, B_1 2.25 mg, B_2 2.6 mg, B_3 20 mg, B_5 10 mg, B_6 3 mg, B_{12} 9 mcg, C 90 mg, folic acid 0.4 mg, biotin 45 mcg, Ca, Cl, Cr, Cu, I, K, Mg, Mn, Mo, P, Se, Zn/Tab. Bot. 100s. *otc.*
Use: Mineral, vitamin supplement.

central nervous system depressants.
See: Sedatives.

central nervous system stimulants.
See: Amphetamine (Various Mfr.).
D-Amphetamine (Various Mfr.).
Anorexigenic agents.
Caffeine (Various Mfr.).
Coramine, Liq., Inj. (Novartis).
Desoxyephedrine HCl, Tab. (Various Mfr.).
Desoxyn HCl, Tab. Gradumet. (Abbott Laboratories).
Dexedrine, Preps. (SmithKline Beecham Pharmaceuticals).
Methamphetamine HCl (Various Mfr.).
Ritalin HCl, Tab., Inj. (Novartis).

Centrovite Advanced Formula. (Rugby) Fe 18 mg, A 5000 IU, D 400 IU, E 30 IU, B_1 1.5 mg, B_2 1.7 mg, B_3 20 mg, B_5 10 mg, B_6 2 mg, B_{12} 6 mcg, C 60 mg, Fa 0.4 mg, biotin 30 mcg, Ca, Cl, Cr, Cu, I, vitamin K, Mg, Mn, Mo, Ni, P, Se, Si, Sn, V, Zn, K. Tab. Bot. 100s. *otc.*
Use: Miineral, vitamin supplement.

Centrovite Jr. (Rugby) Iron 18 mg, vitamins A 5000 IU, D 400 IU, E 15 IU, B_1 1.5 mg, B_2 1.7 mg, B_3 20 mg, B_5 10 mg, B_6 2 mg, B_{12} 6 mcg, C 60 mg, folic acid 0.4 mg, biotin 45 mcg, Cr, Cu, I, Mg, Mn, Mo, Zn/Chew. Tab. Bot. 60s. *otc.*
Use: Mineral, vitamin supplement.

Centrum. (ESI Lederle Generics) Vitamins A 5000 IU, E 30 IU, C 90 mg, folic acid 400 mcg, B_1 2.25 mg, B_2 2.6 mg, B_6 3 mg, niacinamide 20 mg, B_{12} 9 mcg, D 400 IU, biotin 45 mcg, pantothenic acid 10 mg, calcium 162 mg, phosphorus 125 mg, iodine 150 mcg, iron 27 mg, magnesium 100 mg, potassium 30 mg, manganese 5 mg, chromium 25 mcg, selenium 25 mcg, molybdenum 25 mcg, zinc 15 mg, copper 2 mg, K 25 mcg, Cl 27.2 mg/Tab. *otc.*
Use: Mineral, vitamin supplement.

Centrum, Advanced Formula. (ESI Lederle Generics) Vitamins A 2500 IU, E 30 IU, C 60 mg, B_1 1.5 mg, B_2 1.7 mg, B_3 20 mg, B_5 10 mg, B_6 2 mg, B_{12} 6 mcg, D_2 400 IU, iron 9 mg, biotin 300 mcg per 15 ml. With I, Zn, Mn, Cr, Mo, alcohol. 6.6%. Liq. Bot. 236 ml. *otc.*
Use: Mineral, vitamin supplement.

Centrum Jr. (ESI Lederle Generics) Vitamins A 5000 IU, D 400 IU, E 30 IU, C 60 mg, folic acid 400 mcg, B_1 1.5 mg, B_6 2 mg, B_{12} 6 mcg, riboflavin 1.7 mg, niacinamide 20 mg, iron 18 mg, magnesium 25 mg, copper 2 mg, zinc 10 mg, biotin 45 mcg, panthothenic acid 10 mg, molybdenum 20 mcg, chromium 20 mcg, iodine 150 mcg, manganese 1 mg/Chew. Tab. Bot. 60s. *otc.*
Use: Mineral, vitamin supplement.

Centrum Jr. + Extra C. (ESI Lederle Generics) Vitamins A 5000 IU D 400 IU, E 30 IU, C 300 mg, folic acid 400 mcg, biotin 45 mcg, B_1 1.5 mg, B_5 10 mg, B_2 1.7 mg, B_3 20 mg, B_6 2 mg, B_{12} 6 mcg, K, iron 18 mg, Mg, I, Cu, P, calcium 108 mg, zinc 15 mg, Mn, Mo, Cr, biotin 45 mcg, sugar, lactose/Chew. Tab. Bot. 60s. *otc.*
Use: Mineral, vitamin supplement.

Centrum Jr. + Extra Calcium. (ESI Lederle Generics) Calcium 160 mg, iron 18 mg, vitamins A 5000 IU, D 400 IU, E 30 mg, B_1 1.5 mg, B_2 1.7 mg, B_3 20 mg, B_5 10 mg, B_6 2 mg, B_{12} 6 mcg, C 60 mg, folic acid 400 mcg, Cr, Cu, I, Mn, Mg, Mo, P, Zn 15 mg, vitamin K,

biotin 45 mcg, sugar/Chew. Tab. Bot. 60s. *otc.*
Use: Mineral, vitamin supplement.

Centrum Jr. + Iron. (ESI Lederle Generics) Iron 18 mg, vitamins A 5000 IU, D 400 IU, E 30 IU, B_1 1.5 mg, B_2 1.7 mg, B_3 20 mg, B_5 10 mg, B_6 2 mg, B_{12} 6 mcg, C 60 mg, folic acid 0.4 mg, Ca, Cr, Cu, I, Mg, Mn, Mo, P, zinc 15 mg, biotin 45 mcg, vitamin K/Chew. Tab. Bot. 60s. *otc.*
Use: Mineral, vitamin supplement.

Centrum Silver. (ESI Lederle Generics) Tab.: Vitamin A 5000 IU, D 400 IU, E 45 IU, B_1 1.5 mg, B_2 1.7 mg, B_3 20 mg, B_5 10 mg, B_6 3 mg, B_{12} 25 mcg, C 60 mg, iron 4 mg, folic acid 0.4 mg, Ca 200 mg, Zn 15 mg, biotin 30 mcg, vitamin K, Cu, I, Mg, P, Cl, Cr, Mn, Mo, Ni, Se, Si, V. Bot. 60s, 100s, 180s, *otc.*
Use: Mineral, vitamin supplement.

Centrum Silver Gel-Tabs. (ESI Lederle Generics) Vitamins A 6000 IU, D 400 IU, E 45 IU, B_1 1.5 mg, B_2 1.7 mg, B_3 20 mg, B_5 10 mg, B_6 3 mg, B_{12} 25 mcg, C 60 mg, K 10 mcg, biotin 30 mcg, folic acid 200 mcg, Fe 9 mg. With Ca 200 mg, Cu, I, Mg, P, Zn, Cl, Cr, Mn, Mo, Ni, K, Se, Si and V. Tab. Bot. 60s. *otc.*
Use: Mineral, vitamin supplement.

Centurion A-Z. (Mission Pharmacal) Fe 27 mg, A 5000 IU, D 400 IU, E 30 IU, B_1 2.25 mg, B_2 2.6 mg, B_3 20 mg, B_5 10 mg, B_6 3 mg, B_{12} 9 mcg, C 90 mg, Fa 0.4 mg, biotin 0.45 mg, Ca, Cl, Cr, Cu, I, K, Mg, Mn, Mo, P, Se, Zn, vitamin K. Tab. Bot. 130s. *otc.*
Use: Vitamin/mineral supplement.

Ceo-Two. (Beutlich) Potassium bitartrate, sodium bicarbonate in polyethylene glycol base/Supp. 10s. *otc.*
Use: Laxative.

Cēpacol. (J.B. Williams) Cetylpyridinium Cl 0.05%, alcohol 14%, tartrazine, saccharin. Liq. Bot. 360 ml, 540 ml, 720 ml, 960 ml. *otc.*
Use: Antiseptic.

Cēpacol Anesthetic Lozenges. (J.B. Williams) Benzocaine 10 mg, cetylpyridinium Cl 0.07%, tartrazine. Pkg. 18s, 24s. *otc.*
Use: Anesthetic, local.

Cēpacol Maximum Strength. (J.B. Williams) Benzocaine 10 mg, menthol, cool mint, cherry flavors. Loz. Pkg. 16s. *otc.*
Use: Mouth and throat product.

Cēpacol Throat Lozenges. (J.B. Williams) Cetylpyridinium Cl 0.07%, benzyl alcohol 0.3%, tartrazine. Pkg. 27s, 40s. *otc.*
Use: Antiseptic.

Cēpastat Cherry Lozenges. (SmithKline Beecham Pharmaceuticals) Phenol 14.5 mg, menthol, sorbitol, saccharin. Sugar free. Box 18s. *otc.*
Use: Anesthetic.

Cēpastat Extra Strength. (SmithKline Beecham Pharmaceuticals) Phenol 29 mg, menthol, sorbitol, eucalyptus oil. Sugar free. Loz. Pkg. 18s. *otc.*
Use: Anesthetic.

•**cephacetrile sodium.** (SEFF-ah-seh-TRILE) USAN. U.S.P.XX.
Use: Anti-infective, cephalosporin.

•**cephalexin.** (SEFF-ah-LEX-in) U.S.P. 23.
Use: Anti-infective, cephalosporin.
See: Biocef, Cap., Pow. (Inter. Ethical Labs).
Keflex, Cap., Susp. (Eli Lilly).

Cephalexin. (Various Mfr.) **Cap.:** 250 mg, 500 mg. Bot. 100s, 250s (500 mg), 500s, 1000s, UD 20s, 100s. **Tab.:** 250 mg, 500 mg, 1 g. Bot. 20s, 100s, 500s. Pkg. 24s (1 g only). **Pow. for Oral Susp.:** 125 mg/5 ml, 250 mg/5 ml. Bot. 100 ml, 200 ml. *Rx.*
Use: Anti-infective, cephalosporin.

•**cephalexin hydrochloride.** (SEFF-ah-LEX-in) U.S.P. 23.
Use: Anti-infective, cephalosporin.
See: Keftab, Tab. (Eli Lilly).

cephalexin monohydrate. (SEFF-ah-LEX-in)
Use: Anti-infective, cephalosporin.
See: Biocef, Cap., Pow.. (Inter. Ethical Labs).
Cefalexin, Cap., Tab., Susp. (Various).
Keflex, Cap., Susp. (Eli Lilly).

cephalin.
W/Lecithin with choline base, lipositol.
See: Alcolec, Cap., Granules (American Lecithin).

•**cephaloglycin.** (SEFF-ah-low-GLIE-sin) USAN. U.S.P. XX.
Use: Anti-infective.

•**cephaloridine.** (SEFF-ah-lor-ih-deen) USAN. U.S.P. XX.
Use: Anti-infective, cephalosporin.

•**cephalothin sodium.** (seff-AY-low-thin) U.S.P. 23.
Use: Anti-infective, cephalosporin.

•**cephapirin benzathine.** U.S.P. 23.
Use: Anti-infective.

•**cephapirin sodium, sterile.** (SEFF-uh-PIE-rin) U.S.P. 23.
Use: Anti-infective, cephalosporin.
See: Cefadyl, Vial (Bristol-Myers Squibb).

cephazolin sodium.
See: Cefazolin.

•**cephradine.** (SEFF-ruh-deen) U.S.P. 23.
Use: Anti-infective, cephalosporin.
See: Velosef, Cap., Inj., Susp. (Bristol-Myers Squibb).

cephradine. (Various Mfr.) **Cap.:** 250 mg, 500 mg. Bot. 24s, 40s, 100s, 500s, UD 100s. **Pow. for Oral Susp.:** 125 mg/5 ml, 250 mg/5 ml when reconstituted. Bot. 100 ml, 200 ml. *Rx.*
Use: Anti-infective, cephalosporin.

Cephulac. (Hoechst Marion Roussel) Lactulose syrup 10 g/15 ml (less than galactose 2.2 g, lactose 1.2 g, other sugars 1.2 g). Bot. 473 ml, 1890 ml, UD 15 ml, 30 ml. Box 100s. *Rx.*
Use: Laxative.

Ceptaz. (GlaxoWellcome) Ceftazidime pentahydrate with L-arginine 1 g and 2 g. Infusion packs 1 g, 2 g. Pharmacy bulk packages 10 g. *Rx.*
Use: Anti-infective, cephalosporin.

ceramide trihexosidase/alpha-galactosidase a. (Genzyme)
Use: Fabry's disease. [Orphan drug]

Cerapon. Triethanolamine Polypeptide Oleate-Condensate. (Purdue Frederick).
See: Cerumenex, Drops (Purdue Frederick).

Cerebyx. (Parke-Davis) Fosphenytoin 150 mg (100 mg phenytoin sodium) in 2 ml vials and 750 mg (500 mg phenytoin sodium) in 10 ml vials. *Rx.*
Use: Treatment of certain types of seizures.

Ceredase. (Genzyme) Alglucerase. 10 U/ml or 80 U/ml. Inj. Bot. 50 U with 5 ml fill volume (IOU). 400 U with 5 ml fill volume (800). *Rx.*
Use: Enzyme replacement for Gaucher's disease.

cerelose.
See: Glucose (Various Mfr.).

Ceretex. (Enzyme Process) Iron 15 mg, vitamins B_{12} 10 mcg, B_1 2 mg, B_6 1 mg, niacinamide 1 mg, pantothenic acid 0.15 mg, B_2 2 mg, iodine 15 mg/2 ml. Bot. 60 ml, 8 oz. *otc.*
Use: Mineral, vitamin supplement.

Cerezyme. (Genzyme) Imiglucerase 212 units (equiv. to a withdrawal dose of 200 units). Pow. for Inj. Vials. *Rx.*
Use: Treatment for Gaucher's disease.

•**cerivastatin sodium.** (seh-RIHV-ah-stat-in) USAN.
Use: Antihyperlipidemic; inhibitor.
See: Baycol, Tab. (Bayer).

•**ceronapril.** (seh-ROW-nap-rill) USAN.
Use: Antihypertensive.

Cerose. (Wyeth Ayerst) Dextromethorphan HBr 15 mg, chlorpheniramine maleate 4 mg, phenylephrine HCl 10 mg/5 ml, alcohol 2.4%, saccharin. Sugar free. Liq. Bot. 120 ml, 480 ml. *otc.*
Use: Antihistamine, antitussive, decongestant.

Cerovite. (Rugby) Iron 18 mg, vitamins A 5000 IU, D 400 IU, E 30 IU, B_1 1.5 mg, B_2 1.7 mg, B_3 20 mg, B_5 10 mg, B_6 2 mg, B_{12} 6 mcg, C 60 mg, folic acid 0.4 mg, Ca, Cl, Cr, Cu, I, Mg, Mn, Mo, Ni, P, Se, Si, SN, V, biotin 30 mcg, vitamin K, Zn 15 mg/Tab. Bot. 130s. *otc.*
Use: Mineral, vitamin supplement.

Cerovite Advanced Formula. (Rugby) Iron 18 mg, A 5000 IU, D 400 IU, E 30 IU, B_1 1.5 mg, B_2 1.7 mg, B_3 20 mg, B_5 10 mg, B_6 2 mg, B_{12} 6 mcg, C 60 mg, folic acid 0.4 mg, biotin 30 mcg, Ca, P, I, Mg, Cu, Mn, K, Cl, Cr, Mo, Se, Ni, Si, Sn, V, vitamin K, Zn 15 mg/Tab. Bot. 130s, 200s. *otc.*
Use: Iron with vitamin supplement.

Cerovite Jr. (Rugby) Iron 18 mg, vitamins A 5000 IU, D 400 IU, E 15 IU, B_1 1.5 mg, B_2 1.7 mg, B_3 20 mg, B_5 10 mg, B_6 2 mg, B_{12} 6 mcg, C 60 mg, folic acid 0.4 mg, Cu, I, Mg, Zn, Mn, Mo, biotin 45 mcg, Cr, sugar/Tab. Bot. 60s. *otc.*
Use: Mineral, viatmin supplement.

Cerovite Senior. (Rugby) Vitamins A 6000 IU, D 400 IU, E 45 IU, B_1 1.5 mg, B_2 1.7 mg, B_3 20 mg, B_5 10 mg, B_6 3 mg, B_{12} 25 mcg, C 60 mg, iron 9 mg, folic acid 0.2 mg, Ca 200 mg, Zn 15 mg, biotin 30 mcg, Cu, I, Mg, P, Cl, Cr, Mn, Mo, Ni, Se, Si, V, vitamin K. Tab. Bot. 60s. *otc.*
Use: Mineral, viatmin supplement.

Certagen. (Zenith Goldline) Iron 18 mg, A 5000 IU, D 400 IU, E 30 IU, B_1 1.5 mg, B_2 1.7 mg, B_3 20 mg, B_5 10 mg, B_6 2 mg, B_{12} 6 mcg, C 60 mg, folic acid 0.4 mg, biotin 30 mcg, Ca, P, I, Mg, Cu, Mn, K, Cl, Cr, Mo, Se, Ni, Si, Sn, V, vitamin K, Zn 15 mg/Tab. Bot. 130s, 1000s. *otc.*
Use: Mineral, vitamin supplement.

Certagen Liquid. (Zenith Goldline) Vitamins A 2500 IU, B_1 1.5 mg, B_2 1.7 mg, B_3 20 mg, B_5 10 mg, B_6 2 mg, B_{12} 6 mcg, C 60 mg, D_3 400 IU, E 30 IU, biotin 300 mcg, iron 9 mg, Zn 3 mg, Cr, I, Mn, Mo/15 ml. Alcohol 6.6%. Liq. Bot. 237 ml. *otc.*

Use: Mineral, vitamin supplement.

Certagen Senior. (Zenith Goldline) Vitamin A 6000 IU, B_1 1.5 mg, B_2 1.7 mg, B_6 3 mg, B_{12} 25 mcg, C 60 mg, D 400 IU, E 45 IU, vitamin K, biotin 30 mcg, folic acid 200 mcg, B_3 20 mg, B_5 10 mg, Ca 80 mg, Cl, Cr, Cu, I, Fe 3 mg, Mg, Mn, Mo, Ni, P, K, Se, Si, V, Zn 15 mg/Tab. Bot. 60s. *otc.*
Use: Mineral, vitamin supplement.

Certa-Vite. (Major) Vitamin A 5000 IU, D 400 IU, E 30 IU, K_1, C 60 mg, B_1 1.5 mg, B_2 1.7 mg, B_3 20 mg, B_6 2 mg, B_{12} 6 mcg, B_5 10 mg, folic acid 0.4 mg, biotin 30 mcg, iron 18 mg, Ca, P, I, Mg, Cu, Zn, Mn, K, Cl, Cr, Mo, Se, Ni, Si, V, B. Tab. Bot. 130s, 300s. *otc.*
Use: Mineral, vitamin supplement.

Certa-Vite Golden. (Major) Vitamin A 6000 IU, D 400 IU, E 45 IU, B_1 1.5 mg, B_2 1.7 mg, B_3 20 mg, B_5 10 mg, B_6 3 mg, B_{12} 25 mcg, C 60 mg, vitamin K, calcium 200 mg, zinc 15 mg, biotin 30 mcg, Cl, Cr, Cu, I, K, Mg, Mn, Mo, Ni, P, Se, Si, V. Tab. Bot. 60s. *otc.*
Use: Mineral, vitamin supplement.

cervical ripening agent.
See: Cervidil, Insert. (Forest Pharmaceutical).
Prepidil, Gel. (Pharmacia & Upjohn).

Cervidil. (Forest Pharmaceutical) Dinoprostone 10 mg/Insert. 1 each. *Rx.*
Use: Cervical ripening.

•**ceruletide.** (seh-ROO-leh-tide) USAN.
Use: Stimulant (gastric secretory).

•**ceruletide diethylamine.** (seh-ROO-leh-tide die-ETH-ill-ah-meen) USAN.
Use: Stimulant (gastric secretory).

Cerumenex Drops. (Purdue Frederick) Triethanolamine polypeptide oleate-condensate 10%, chlorobutanol in propylene glycol 0.5%. Liq. Dropper bot. 6 ml, 12 ml. *Rx.*
Use: Otic.

cervical ripening agents.
See: Prepidil (Pharmacia & Upjohn).

Cervidil. (Forest Pharmaceutical) Dinoprostone 10 mg. Insert. 1s. *Rx.*
Use: Cervical ripening.

Ces. (ICN Pharmaceuticals) Conjugated estrogens 0.625 mg, 1.25 mg or 2.5 mg/Tab. *Rx.*
Use: Estrogen.

•**cesium chloride Cs 131.** (SEE-zee-uhm KLOR-ide) USAN.
Use: Radiopharmaceutical agent.

Ceta. (C & M Pharmacal) Soap Free. Propylene glycol, hydroxyethylcellulose, cetyl and cetearyl alcohols, sodium lauryl sulfate, parabens. Liq. Bot. 240 ml. *otc.*
Use: Dermatologic cleanser.

Ceta-Plus. (Seatrace) Hydrocodone bitartrate 5 mg, acetaminophen 500 mg/Cap. Bot. 100s. *c-III.*
Use: Analgesic combination, narcotic.

•**cetaben sodium.** (SEE-tah-ben) USAN.
Use: Antihyperlipoproteinemic.

Cetacaine. (Cetylite Industries) Benzocaine 14%, butyl aminobenzoate 2%, tetracaine HCl 2%, benzalkonium Cl 0.5%, cetyl dimethyl ethyl ammonium bromide 0.005%. **Aerosol Spray:** 56 g. **Liq.:** 56 g. **Oint.:** Jar 37 g, flavored. **Hosp. Gel:** 29 g. *Rx.*
Use: Anesthetic, local.

Cetacort. (Galderma) Hydrocortisone in concentrations of 0.25%, 0.5%, 1% w/ cetyl alcohol, propylene glycol, stearyl alcohol, sodium lauryl sulfate, butylparaben, methylparaben, propylparaben, purified water. Bot. 120 ml (0.25% only), 60 ml (0.5%, 1%). *Rx.*
Use: Corticosteroid, topical.

cetalkonium. (SEET-al-KOE-nee-uhm) F.D.A. Benzylhexadecyldimethylammonium ion.

•**cetalkonium chloride.** (SEET-al-KOE-nee-uhm) USAN.
Use: Anti-infective, topical.
W/Phenylephrine, pyrilamine maleate, thimerosal.
See: Anti-B Mist (DePree).

Cetamide. (Alcon Laboratories) Sulfacetamide sodium 10%. Sterile ophthalmic oint. Tube 3.5 g. *Rx.*
Use: Anti-infective, ophthalmic.

•**cetamolol hydrochloride.** (SEET-AM-oh-lahl) USAN.
Use: Anti-adrenergic (β-receptor).

Cetaphil. (Galderma) Cetyl alcohol, stearyl alcohol, propylene glycol (cream only), sodium lauryl sulfate, methylparaben, propylparaben, butylparaben, purified water. Cream, Lot. Bot. 480 g (cream), 120 ml, 240 ml, 480 ml (lotion). *otc.*
Use: Dermatologic cleanser.

Cetapred. (Alcon Laboratories) Sulfacetamide sodium 10%, prednisolone acetate 0.25%. Ophth. Oint. Tube 3.5 g. *Rx.*
Use: Anti-infective, ophthalmic.

Cetazol. (Professional Pharmacal) Acetazolamide 250 mg/Tab. Bot. 100s. *Rx.*
Use: Anticonvulsant, diuretic.

•**cetiedil citrate.** (see-TIE-eh-DILL SIH-trate) USAN.

Use: Vasodilator (peripheral).

•**cetirizine hydrochloride.** (seh-TIH-rih-zeen) USAN.
Use: Antihistamine.
See: Zyrtec, Syr., Tab. (Pfizer).

•**cetocycline hydrochloride.** (SEE-toe-SIGH-kleen) USAN. *Formerly cetotetrine HCl*
Use: Anti-infective.

•**cetophenicol.** (see-toe-FEN-ih-kole) USAN.
Use: Antibacterial.

•**cetostearyl alcohol.** N.F. 18.
Use: Pharmaceutic aid (emulsifying agent).

•**cetraxate hydrochloride.** (seh-TRAX-ate) USAN.
Use: Antiulcerative (gastrointestinal).

•**cetyl alcohol.** (SEE-till) N.F. 18.
Use: Pharmaceutic aid (emulsifying and stiffening agent).

Cetylcide Solution. (Cetylite Industries) Cetyldimethylethyl ammonium bromide 6.5%, benzalkonium Cl 6.5%, isopropyl alcohol 13%. Inert ingredients 74%, including sodium nitrite. Bot. 16 oz, 32 oz.
Use: Disinfectant.

cetyldimethyl benzyl ammonium chloride.
W/Benzocaine, ascorbic acid.
See: Locane, Troches (Solvay).
W/Phenylephrine HCl, pyrilamine maleate.
See: Dalihist, Nasal Spray (Dalin).

•**cetyl esters wax.** N.F. 18. *Formerly synthetic spermaceti*
Use: Pharmaceutic aid (stiffening agent).

•**cetylpyridinium chloride.** (SEE-till-pihr-ih-DIH-nee-uhm) U.S.P. 23.
Use: Anti-infective (topical), pharmaceutic aid (preservative).
See: Bactalin (LaCrosse).
W/Benzocaine.
See: Axon Throat Loz. (McKesson).
Cēpacol, Throat Loz., (J.B. Williams).
Coirex, Preps. (Solvay).
Oradex-C, Troches (Del Pharmaceuticals).
Semets, Troches (SmithKline Beecham Pharmaceuticals).
Spec-T Sore Throat Loz. (Bristol-Myers Squibb).
Vicks Medi-Trating Throat Lozenges (Procter & Gamble).
W/Benzocaine.
See: Cēpacol Antiseptic Lozenges (J.B. Williams).
W/Benzocaine, menthol, camphor, eucalyptus oil.
See: Vicks Medi-Trating Throat Lozenges (Procter & Gamble).
W/d-Methorphan HBr, phenyltoloxamine dihydrogen citrate, sodium citrate.
See: Exo-Kol, Cough Syrup, Spray, Tab. (Inwood).
W/Phenylephrine HCl, methapyrilene HCl, menthol, eucalyptol, camphor, methyl salicylate.
See: Vicks Sinex Nasal Spray (Procter & Gamble).
W/Phenylpropanolamine HCl, benzocaine, terpin hydrate.
See: S.A.C. Throat Lozenges (Towne).

cetyltrimethyl ammonium bromide. (Bio Labs) Cetrimide B.P., Cetavlon, CTAB.
Use: Antiseptic.
W/Lidocaine, hexachlorophene.
See: Aerosept, Aerosol (Dalin).

Cevalin. (Eli Lilly) Ascorbic acid 100 mg or 500 mg/ml. Inj. Amp. 10 ml (100 mg), 1 ml (500 mg). *Rx.*
Use: Vitamin supplement.

Cevi-Bid. (Roberts Pharm) Ascorbic acid 500 mg/TR Caps. Bot. 30s, 100s, 500s. *otc.*
Use: Vitamin supplement.

Cevi-Fer. (Roberts Pharm) Ascorbic acid 300 mg, ferrous fumarate 20 mg, folic acid 1 mg/TR Cap. Bot. 30s, 100s. *Rx.*
Use: Mineral, vitamin supplement.

•**cevimeline hydrochloride.** (seh-vih-MEH-leen) USAN.
Use: Treatment of Alzheimer's disease, adjunct.

Ce-Vi-Sol. (Bristol-Myers) Ascorbic acid 35 mg/0.6 ml, alcohol 5%. Bot. w/dropper 50 ml. *otc.*
Use: Vitamin supplement.

cevitamic acid.
See: Ascorbic acid.

cevitan.
See: Ascorbic acid.

Cewin Tablets. (Sanofi Winthrop) Ascorbic acid. *otc.*
Use: Vitamin supplement.

ceylon gelatin.
See: Agar.

Cezin. (Forest Pharmaceutical) Vitamins B_1 20 mg, B_2 10 mg, B_3 100 mg, B_5 20 mg, B_6 5 mg, C 300 mg, magnesium sulfate 70 mg, zinc sulfate 80 mg. Cap. Bot. 100s. *otc.*
Use: Vitamin supplement.

Cezin-S. (Forest Pharmaceutical) Vitamins A 10,000 IU, D 50 IU, E 50 IU, B_1 10 mg, B_2 5 mg, B_3 50 mg, B_5 10 mg, B_6 2 mg, C 200 mg, folic acid 0.5 mg,

zinc 18 mg, Mg, Mn/Cap. Bot. 100s. *Rx.*
Use: Vitamin supplement.

C Factors "1000" Plus. (Solgar) Vitamins C with rosehips 1000 mg, citrus bioflavonoids 250 mg, rutin 50 mg, hesperidin complex 25 mg. Tab. Bot. 50s, 100s, 250s. *otc.*
Use: Vitamin supplement. *otc.*

C.G. (Sigma-Tau Pharmaceuticals) Chorionic gonadotropin (lyophilized) 10,000 units, mannitol 100 mg, supplied with diluent. Univial 10 ml. *Rx.*
Use: Hormone, chorionic gonadotropin.

CG Disposable Unit.
See: Cardio Green, Vial (Becton Dickinson).

CG Ria. (Abbott Diagnostics) Radioimmunoassay for the quantitative measurement of total circulating serum cholylglycine.
Use: Diagnostic aid.

Chap Cream. (Ar-Ex) Carbonyl diamide. Tube 1.5 oz, 3.25 oz. Jar 4 oz, 9 oz, 18 oz. *otc.*
Use: Emollient.

Chapoline Cream Lotion. (Wade) Glycerine, boric acid, chlorobutanol 0.5%, alcohol 10%. Bot. 4 oz, pt, gal. *otc.*
Use: Emollient.

Chapstick Medicated Lip Balm. (Robins) **Jar:** Petrolatum 60%, camphor 1%, menthol 0.6%, phenol 0.5%, microcrystalline wax, mineral oil, cocoa butter, lanolin, paraffin wax, parabens 7 g. **Squeezable tube:** Petrolatum 67%, camphor 1%, menthol 0.6%, phenol 0.5%, microcrystalline wax, mineral oil, cocoa butter, lanolin, parabens 10 g. **Stick:** Petrolatum 41%, camphor 1%, menthol 0.6%, phenol 0.5%, paraffin wax, mineral oil, cocoa butter, 2-octyl dodecanol, arachydil propionate, polyphenyl methylsiloxane 556, white wax, oleyl alcohol, isopropyl lanolate, carnauba wax, isopropyl myristate, lanolin, cetyl alcohol, parabens 4.2 g. *otc.*
Use: Mouth and throat preparation.

Chapstick Sunblock 15. (Robins) Padimate O 0.7%, oxybenzone 3%. Stick 4.25 g. *otc.*
Use: Lip protectant.

Chapstick Sunblock 15 Petroleum Jelly Plus. (Robins) White petrolatum 89%, padimate O 7%, oxybenzone 3%, aloe, lanolin. Stick 10 g. *otc.*
Use: Lip protectant.

CharcoAid. (Requa) Activated charcoal 15 g/120 ml, 30 g/150 ml, sorbitol/ Susp. Bot. *otc.*
Use: Antidote.

CharcoAid 2000. (Requa) Activated charcoal 15 g/120 ml, 50 g/240 ml with and without sorbitol/Liq. 15 g/240 ml. Granules. Bot. *otc.*
Use: Antidote.

charcoal. (CHAR-kole) (Various Mfr.) Cap., Tab. *otc.*
Use: Antiflatulent.
See: Charcoal (Paddock).
Charcoal (Rugby).

•**charcoal, activated.** (CHAR-kole) U.S.P. 23.
Use: Antidote (general purpose), pharmaceutic aid (adsorbant).
See: Actidose-Aqua, Liq. (Paddock).
CharcoAid, Susp. (Requa).
Charcoal Plus, EC Tab. (Kramer).
Liqui-Char, Liq. (Jones Medical Industries).

W/Nux vomica, bismuth subgallate, pepsin, berberis, diastase, pancreatin, hydrastis, papain.
See: Charcocaps, Cap. (Requa).
Charcotabs, Tab. (Requa).

Charcoal Plus. (Kramer) Activated charcoal 250 mg, sugar. EC Tab. Bot. 120s. *otc.*
Use: Antiflatulent.

charcoal and simethicone. Antiflatulent.
See: Charcoal Plus (Kramer).
Flatulex (Dayton).

CharcoCaps. (Requa) Activated charcoal 260 mg/Cap. Bot. 36s. *otc.*
Use: Antiflatulent.

Chardonna-2. (Kremers Urban) Belladonna extract 15 mg, phenobarbital 15 mg/Tab. Bot. 100s. *Rx.*
Use: Anticholinergic, antispasmodic, hypnotic, sedative.

Charo Scatter-Paks. (Requa) Activated charcoal 5 g/Packet.
Use: Odor absorbant.

Chaz Scalp Treatment Dandruff Shampoo. (Revlon) Zinc pyrithione 1% in liquid shampoo. *otc.*
Use: Antiseborrheic.

Chealamide Injection. (Vortech) Disodium edetate 150 mg/ml. Vial 20 ml. *Rx.*
Use: Chelating agent.

Checkmate. (Oral-B Laboratories) Acidulated phosphate fluoride 1.23%. Bot. 2 oz, 16 oz. *Rx.*
Use: Dental caries agent.

Chek-Stix Urinalysis Control Strips. (Bayer Corp) Bot. 25s.
Use: Diagnostic aid.

chelafrin.
See: Epinephrine.

Chelated Calcium Magnesium. (NBTY) Calcium^{++} 500 mg, magnesium 250 mg/Tab. Protein coated. Bot. 50s. *otc.*
Use: Mineral supplement.

chelated calcium magnesium zinc. (NBTY) Calcium^{++} 333 mg, magnesium 133 mg, zinc 8.3 mg/Tab. Bot. 100s. *otc.*
Use: Mineral supplement.

Chelated Magnesium. (Freeda Vitamins) Magnesium amino acids chelate 500 mg (magnesium 100 mg)/Tab. Bot. 100s, 250s, 500s. *otc.*
Use: Vitamin supplement.

Chelated Manganese. (Freeda Vitamins) Manganese 20 mg or 50 mg/Tab. Bot. 100s, 250s, 500s. *otc.*
Use: Mineral supplement.

chelating agent.
See: BAL, Amp. (Becton Dickinson).
Calcium Disodium Versenate, Amp., Tab. (3M).
Desferal, Amp. (Novartis).
Endrate Disodium, Amp. (Abbott Laboratories).
Magora, Tab. (Miller).

chelen.
See: Ethyl Chloride.

Chemet. (Sanofi Winthrop) Succimer 100 mg. Cap. Bot. 100s. *Rx.*
Use: Chelating agent.

Chemipen. Potassium phenethicillin.
Use: Anti-infective, penicillin.

Chemovag Supps. (Forest Pharmaceutical) Sulfisoxazole 0.5 g/Supp. Bot. 12s w/applicators. *Rx.*
Use: Anti-infective, sulfonamide.

Chemozine. (Tennessee Pharmaceutic) Sulfadiazine, 0.167 g, sulfamerazine 0.167 g, sulfamethazine 0.167 g/Tab. Bot. 100s, 1000s. Susp. Bot. pt, gal. *Rx.*
Use: Anti-infective, sulfonamide.

Chemstrip 6. (Boehringer Mannheim) Broad range test for glucose, protein, pH, blood, ketones and leukocytes. Bot. strip 100s.
Use: Diagnostic aid.

Chemstrip 7. (Boehringer Mannheim) Broad range test for glucose, protein, pH, blood, ketones, bilirubin and leukocytes. Bot. strip 100s.
Use: Diagnostic aid.

Chemstrip 8. (Boehringer Mannheim) Broad range urine test for glucose, protein, pH, blood, ketones, bilirubin, urobilinogen and leukocytes. Bot. Strip 100s.
Use: Diagnostic aid.

Chemstrip 9. (Boehringer Mannheim) Broad range test for glucose, protein, pH, blood, ketones, bilirubin, urobilinogen, nitrite and leukocytes in urine. Bot. strip 100s.
Use: Diagnostic aid.

Chemstrip 10 SG. (Boehringer Mannheim) Broad range test for glucose, protein, pH, blood, ketones, bilirubin, urobilinogen, nitrite and leukocytes in urine. Bot. Strip 100s.
Use: Diagnostic aid.

Chemstrip 4 the OB. (Boehringer Mannheim) Broad range test for glucose, protein, blood and leukocytes in urine. Bot. Strip 100s.
Use: Diagnostic aid.

Chemstrip bG. (Boehringer Mannheim) Reagent strips for testing blood sugar. Bot. Strip 50s.
Use: Diagnostic aid.

Chemstrip 2 GP. (Boehringer Mannheim) Broad range test for glucose and protein. Bot. strip 100s.
Use: Diagnostic aid.

Chemstrip-K. (Boehringer Mannheim) Reagent papers for ketones in urine. Bot. paper 25s, 100s.
Use: Diagnostic aid.

Chemstrip 2 LN. (Boehringer Mannheim) Broad range test for nitrite and leukocytes. Bot. strip 100s.
Use: Diagnostic aid.

Chemstrip Micral. (Boehringer Mannheim) In vitro reagent strips to detect albumin in urine. In 5s, 30s.
Use: Diagnostic aid.

Chemstrip Mineral. (Boehringer Mannheim) In vitro reagent strips used to detect albumin in urine. Strips. 5s, 30s.
Use: In vitro diagnostic aid.

Chemstrip uG. (Boehringer Mannheim) Reagent strips for glucose in urine. Bot. Strip 100s.
Use: Diagnostic aid.

Chemstrip uGK. (Boehringer Mannheim) Broad range test for glucose and ketones. Bot. strip 50s, 100s.
Use: Diagnostic aid.

Chenatal. (Miller) Calcium 580 mg, magnesium 200 mg, vitamins C 100 mg, folic acid 0.4 mg, A 5000 IU, D 400 IU, B_1 3 mg, B_2 3 mg, B_6 5 mg, B_{12} 9 mcg, niacinamide 30 mg, pantothenic acid 5 mg, tocopherols (mixed) 10 mg, iron 20 mg, copper 1 mg, manganese 2 mg, potassium 10 mg, zinc 25 mg, iodine 0.1 mg/2 Tabs. Bot. 100s. *otc.*

Use: Mineral, vitamin supplement.

Chenix. (Solvay) Chenodil.
Use: Anticholelithogenic. [Orphan drug]

chenodeoxycholic acid.
Use: Urolithic.
See: Chenodiol.

•**chenodiol.** (KEEN-oh-DIE-ahl) USAN.
Formerly chenic acid
Use: Anticholelithogenic. [Orphan drug]
See: Chex (Solvay).

Cheracol. (Roberts Pharm) Codeine phosphate 10 mg, guaifenesin 100 mg/5 ml, alcohol 4.75%. Bot. 2 oz, 4 oz, pt. *c-v.*
Use: Antitussive, expectorant.

Cheracol D. (Roberts Pharm) Dextromethorphan HBr 10 mg, guaifenesin 100 mg/5 ml, alcohol 4.75%. Bot. 2 oz, 4 oz, 6 oz. *otc.*
Use: Antitussive, expectorant.

Cheracol Nasal. (Roberts Pharm) Oxymetazoline HCl 0.05%, phenylmercuric acetate 0.02 mg/ml, benzalkonium chloride, glycine, sorbitol. Soln. Spray 30 ml. *otc.*
Use: Decongestant.

Cheracol Plus. (Roberts Pharm) Phenylpropanolamine HCl 8.3 mg, dextromethorphan HBr 6.7 mg, chlorpheniramine maleate 1.3 mg/5 ml. Bot. 4 oz. *otc.*
Use: Antihistamine, antitussive, decongestant.

Cheracol Sore Throat. (Roberts Pharm) Phenol 1.4%, saccharin, sorbitol, alcohol 12.5%. Spray Bot. 180 ml. *otc.*
Use: Mouth and throat product.

Cheratussin Cough Syrup. (Towne) Dextromethorphan HBr 45 mg, ammonium Cl 575 mg, citrate sodium 280 mg/Fl oz. Bot. 4 oz. *otc.*
Use: Antitussive, expectorant.

Chero-Trisulfa-V. (Vita Elixir) Sulfadiazine 0.166 g, sulfacetamide 0.166 g, sulfamerazine 0.166 g, sodium citrate 0.5 g/5 ml. Susp. Bot. pt.
Use: Anti-infective, sulfonamide.

cherry juice. N.F. XVI.
Use: Flavoring.

cherry syrup.
Use: Pharmaceutic aid (Vehicle).

Chestamine. (Leeds) Chlorpheniramine maleate 8 mg or 12 mg/Cap. Bot. 50s. *Rx.*
Use: Antihistamine.

Chest Throat Lozenges. (Lane) Eucalyptol, anise, horehound, tolu balsam, benzoin tincture, sugar, corn syrup. Pkg. 30s. *otc.*
Use: Antiseptic.

Chewable C. (Health for Life Brands) Vitamin C 100 mg, 250 mg, 300 mg and 500 mg/Tab. Bot. 100s. *otc.*
Use: Vitamin supplement.

Chewable Multivitamins w/Fluoride. (Moore) Tab.: Fluoride 1 mg, vitamins A 2500 IU, D 400 IU, E 15 IU, B_1 1.05 mg, B_2 1.2 mg, B_3 13.5 mg, B_6 1.05 mg, B_{12} 4.5 mcg, C 60 mg, folic acid 0.3 mg, sucrose/ Bot. 100s. *Rx.*
Use: Mineral, vitamin supplement; dental caries agent.

Chew-Vims. (Barth's) Vitamins A 5000 IU, D 400 IU, B_1 3 mg, B_2 6 mg, niacin 1.71 mg, C 100 mg, B_{12} 5 mcg, E 5 IU/Tab. Bot. 30s, 90s, 180s, 360s. *otc.*
Use: Vitamin supplement.

Chew-Vi-Tab. (Halsey) Vitamins A 2500 IU, D 400 IU, E 15 IU, C 60 mg, folic acid 0.3 mg, B_1 1.05 mg, B_2 1.2 mg, niacin 13.5 mg, B_6 1.05 mg, B_{12} 4.5 mcg/Tab. Bot. 100s. *otc.*
Use: Vitamin supplement.

Chew-Vi-Tab with Iron. (Halsey) Vitamins A 5000 IU, C 60 mg, E 15 IU, folic acid 0.4 mg, B_1 1.5 mg, B_2 1.7 mg, niacin 20 mg, B_6 2 mg, B_{12} 6 mcg, D 400 IU, iron 18 mg/Tab. Bot. 100s. *otc.*
Use: Mineral, vitamin supplement.

Chibroxin. (Merck) Norfloxacin 3 mg/ml. Soln. Drop. Bot. 5 ml Ocumeters. *Rx.*
Use: Anti-infective, ophthalmic.

chicken pox vaccine.
See: Varivax (Merck).

Chiggerex. (Scherer) Benzocaine 0.02%, camphor, menthol, peppermint oil, olive oil, clove oils, pegosperse, methylparaben, distilled water. Oint. Jar 50 g. *otc.*
Use: Anesthetic, counterirritant.

Chigger-Tox. (Scherer) Benzocaine 2.1%, benzyl benzoate 21.4%, soft soap, isopropyl alcohol. Liq. Bot. 30 ml. *otc.*
Use: Anesthetic, topical.

Children's Advil. (Wyeth Ayerst) Ibuprofen 100 mg/5 ml. Susp. Bot. 119 ml, 473 ml. *Rx.*
Use: Analgesic, NSAID.

Children's Allerest. (Novartis) Phenylpropanolamine HCl 9.4 mg, chlorpheniramine maleate 1 mg. Chew. Tab. Bot. 24s. *otc.*
Use: Antihistamine, decongestant.

Children's Cēpacol. (J.B. Williams) Acetaminophen 160 mg/5 ml, pseudoephedrine HCl 15 mg/5 ml, benzoic acid, sorbitol, glycerin, grape, cherry flavors. Liq. Bot. 118 ml. *otc.*
Use: Decongestant.

Children's Dramamine. (Pharmacia & Upjohn) Dimenhydrinate 12.5 mg/5 ml, alcohol 5%, sucrose/Bot. 120 ml. *otc.*
Use: Antiemetic, antivertigo.

Children's Dynafed Jr. (BDI) Acetaminophen 80 mg, fruit flavor. Chew. Tab. Bot. 36s. *otc.*
Use: Analgesic.

Children's Feverall. (Upsher-Smith Labs) Acetaminophen 120 mg or 325 mg/Supp. Pkg. 6s. *otc.*
Use: Analgesic.

Children's Formula Cough Syrup. (Pharmakon Labs) Guaifenesin 50 mg, dextromethorphan HBr 5 mg, sucrose, corn syrup. Alcohol free. Grape flavor. Syr. Bot. 118 ml, 236 ml. *otc.*
Use: Antitussive, expectorant.

Children's Hold 4-Hour Cough Suppressant & Decongestant. (Beecham Products) Dextromethorphan HBr 3.75 mg, phenylpropanolamine HCl 6.25 mg/Loz. Pkg. 10s. *otc.*
Use: Antitussive, decongestant.

Children's Kaopectate. (Pharmacia & Upjohn) Attapulgite 600 mg. Liq. Bot. 180 ml. *otc.*
Use: Antidiarrheal.

Children's Mapap. (Major) Acetaminophen 160 mg/5ml, alcohol free/Elixir. Bot. 120 ml. *otc.*
Use: Analgesic.

Children's Motrin. (Ortho McNeil) Ibuprofen 100 mg/5 ml, alcohol free/Susp. Bot. 120 ml, 480 ml. *otc, Rx.*
Use: Analgesic, NSAID.

Children's No Aspirin Elixir. (Walgreens) Acetaminophen 80 mg/2.5 ml. Non-alcoholic. Bot. 4 oz. *otc.*
Use: Analgesic.

Children's No-Aspirin Tablets. (Walgreens) Acetaminophen 80 mg/Tab. Bot. 30s. *otc.*
Use: Analgesic.

Children's Nyquil. (Procter & Gamble) Pseudoephedrine HCl 10 mg, chlorpheniramine maleate 0.6 mg, dextromethorphan HBr 5 mg/5 ml. Bot. 120 ml, 240 ml. *otc.*
Use: Antihistamine, antitussive, decongestant.

Children's Nyquil Nightime Head Cold, Allergy Formula. (Procter & Gamble) Pseudoephedrine HCl 10 mg, chlorpheniramine maleate 0.67 mg/5 ml. Alcohol free. Sorbitol, sucrose. Grape flavor. Liq. Bot. 120 ml. *otc.*
Use: Antihistamine, decongestant.

Children's Silapap. (Silarx) Acetaminophen 80 mg/2.5 ml, sugar free, alcohol free/Liq. Bot. 237 ml. *otc.*
Use: Analgesic.

Children's Silfedrine. (Silarx) Pseudoephedrine HCl 30 mg/5 ml. Liq. Bot. 118 ml. *otc.*
Use: Decongestant, nasal.

Children's Sunkist Multivitamins Complete. (Novartis) Iron 18 mg, vitamin A 5000 IU, D_3 400 IU, E 30 IU, B_1 1.5 mg, B_2 1.7 mg, B_3 20 mg, B_5 10 mg, B_6 2 mg, B_{12} 6 mcg, C 60 mg, folic acid 0.4 mg, Ca, Cu, I, K, Mg, Mn, P, zinc 10 mg, biotin 40 mcg, vitamin K, sorbitol, aspartame, phenylalanine, tartrazine/Chew. Tab. Bot. 60s. *otc.*
Use: Mineral, vitamin supplement.

Children's Sunkist Multivitamins + Extra C. (Novartis) Vitamin A 2500 IU, E 15 IU, D_3 400 IU, B_1 1.05 mg, B_2 1.2 mg, B_3 13.5 mg, B_6 1.05 mg, B_{12} 4.5 mcg, C 250 mg, folic acid 0.3 mg, vitamin K_1 5 mcg, sorbitol, aspartame, phenylalanine, tartrazine. Chew. Tab. Bot. 60s. *otc.*
Use: Mineral, vitamin supplement.

Children's Sunkist Multivitamins + Iron. (Novartis) Iron 15 mg, vitamin A 2500 IU, E 15 IU, D_3 400 IU, B_1 1.05 mg, B_2 1.2 mg, B_3 13.5 mg, B_6 1.05 mg, B_{12} 4.5 mcg, C 60 mg, folic acid 0.3 mg, vitamin K_1 5 mcg, sorbitol, aspartame, phenylalanine, tartrazine. Chew. Tab. Bot. 60s. *otc.*
Use: Mineral, vitamin supplement.

Children's Tylenol Cold Tablets. (McNeil Consumer Products) Pseudoephedrine HCl 7.5 mg, chlorpheniramine maleate 0.5 mg, acetaminophen 80 mg, aspartame, sucrose, phenylalanine 4 mg. Chewable. Grape flavor. Tab. Bot. 24s. *otc.*
Use: Analgesic, antihistamine, decongestant.

Children's Tylenol Cold Liquid. (McNeil Consumer Products) Pseudoephedrine HCl 15 mg, chlorpheniramine maleate 1 mg, acetaminophen 160 mg, sorbitol, sucrose. Alcohol free. Grape flavor. Liq. Bot. 120 ml. *otc.*
Use: Analgesic, antihistamine, decongestant.

Children's Tylenol Cold Multi Symptom Plus Cough. (McNeil Consumer Products) Acetaminophen 160 mg, dextromethorphan HBr 5 mg, chlorpheniramine maleate 1 mg, pseudoephedrine HCl 15 mg/5 ml. Liq. Bot. 120 ml. *otc.*
Use: Antihistamine, antitussive, decongestant.

Children's Tylenol Cold Plus Cough. (Ortho McNeil) Acetaminophen 80 mg, pseudoephedrine HCl 7.5 mg, dextromethorphan HBr 2.5 mg, chlorpheniramine maleate 0.5 mg/Chew. Tab. Pkg. 24s. *otc.*
Use: Analgesic, antihistamine, antitussive, decongestant.

Children's Tylenol Elixir. (McNeil Consumer Products) Acetaminophen 160 mg/5 ml. Elix. Bot. 60 ml, 120 ml. *otc.*
Use: Analgesic.

Children's Ty-Tabs. (Major) Acetaminophen 80 mg. Tab. Bot. 100s, 1000s. *otc.*
Use: Analgesic.

chimeric A2 (human-murine) IgG monoclonal anti-TNF antibody (CA2). (Centocor).
Use: Crohn's disease. [Orphan drug]

chimeric M-t412 (human-murine) igg monoclonal anti-CD4.
Use: Multiple sclerosis. [Orphan drug]

chimeric (murine variable, human constant) Mab (C2B8) to CD20. (Idec Pharm)
Use: Treatment of non-Hodgkin's B-cell lymphoma. [Orphan drug]

chinese gelatin.
See: Agar.

chinese isinglass.
Use: Amebicide.

chiniofon.
Use: Amebicide.

Chinosol. (Vernon) 8-Hydroxyquinoline sulfate 7.5 gr/Tab. Vial 6s. Trit. Tab. (3/5 gr) Bot. 50s. Vial 110s. Pow. 1 oz.
Use: Antiseptic.

chlamydia trachomatis test.
Use: Diagnostic aid.
See: MicroTrak (Syva).

Chlamydiazyme. (Abbott Diagnostics) Enzyme immunoassay for detection of *Chlamydia trachomatis* from urethral or urogenital swabs. Test kit 100s.
Use: Diagnostic aid.

Chlo-Amine. (Bayer Corp) Chlorpheniramine maleate 2 mg/Chew. Tab. Box 24x4 mg Tab. Packages. *otc.*
Use: Antihistamine.

chlophedianol. (KLOE-fee-DIE-ah-nole) F.D.A.

•**chlophedianol hydrochloride.** (KLOE-fee-DIE-ah-nole) USAN.
Use: Antitussive.

Chloracol 0.5%. (Horizon) Chloramphenicol 5 mg/ml with chlorobutanol, hydroxypropyl methylcellulose. Dropper bot. 7.5 ml. *Rx.*
Use: Anti-infective, ophthalmic.

Chlorafed. (Roberts Pharm) Chlorpheniramine maleate 2 mg, pseudoephedrine HCl 30 mg/5 ml, alcohol, dye, sugar and corn free. Liq. Bot. 120 ml, 480 ml. *otc.*
Use: Antihistamine, decongestant.

Chlorafed H.S. Timecelles. (Roberts Pharm) Chlorpheniramine maleate 4 mg, pseudoephedrine HCl 60 mg/SR Cap. Bot. 100s. *Rx.*
Use: Antihistamine, decongestant.

Chlorafed Timecelles. (Roberts Pharm) Chlorpheniramine maleate 8 mg, pseudoephedrine HCl 120 mg/SA timecelles. Bot. 100s. *Rx.*
Use: Antihistamine, decongestant.

Chlorahist. (Evron) Chlorpheniramine maleate **4 mg/Tab.:** Bot. 100s, 1000s. **8 mg or 12 mg/Cap.:** Bot. 250s, 1000s. **Syr. 2 mg/4 ml.:** Bot. qt. *otc, Rx.*
Use: Antihistamine.

•**chloral betaine.** (KLOR-uhl BEE-taheen) USAN. N.F. XIV.
Use: Hypnotic, sedative.

chloralformamide.

•**chloral hydrate.** (KLOR-uhl HIGH-drate) U.S.P. 23.
Use: Sedative, hypnotic.
See: Aquachloral Supprettes, Supp. (PolyMedica).
Noctec, Cap., Syr. (Bristol-Myers Squibb).
Generic Products:
Quality Generics (7.5 gr) Bot. 100s.
G.F. Harvey-Cap. (3 gr) Bot. 100s; (7.5 gr) Bot. 100s.
Lederle-Cap. (500 mg) 100s.
Pacific Pharm. Corp. Cap. (7.5 gr) Bot. 100s, 1000s.
Parke, Davis-Cap. (500 mg) Bot. 100s, UD 100s.
Stayner-Cap. (250 mg or 500 mg) Bot. 100s, (500 mg) Bot. 1000s, Crystals Bot. 1 lb. and 5 lbs.
West-Ward-Cap. (3 gr, 7.5 gr) Bot. 100s.

chloral hydrate betaine (1:1) compound. Chloral Betaine.

chloralpyrine dichloralpyrine.
See: Dichloralantipyrine.

chloralurethane. Name used for Carbochloral.

Chloraman. (Rasman) Chlorpheniramine maleate 12 mg/Tab. Bot. 100s, 500s, 1000s. *Rx.*
Use: Antihistamine.

•**chlorambucil.** (klor-AM-byoo-sill) U.S.P. 23.

Use: Antineoplastic.
See: Leukeran, Tab. (GlaxoWellcome).

Chloramine-T. Sodium paratoluenesulfan chloramide, chloramine, chlorozone.
Lilly-Tab. (0.3 g), Bot. 100s, 1000s.
Robinson, Pow., 1 oz.
Use: Antiseptic, deodorant.
See: Chlorazene (Badger).

chloramphenicol. (KLOR-am-FEN-ih-kahl) (Various Mfr.) **Soln.:** 5 mg/ml Bot. 7.5 ml, 15 ml; **Oint.:** 10 mg/g Tube 3.5 g; **Cap.:** 250 mg Bot. 100s.
Use: Anti-infective, antirickettsial.

•**chloramphenicol.** (KLOR-am-FEN-ih-kole) U.S.P. 23.
Use: Anti-infective, antirickettsial.
See: AK-Chlor, Preps. (Akorn).
Chloromycetin, Preps. (Parke-Davis)
Chloroptic Ophth. Oint. (Allergan).
Chloroptic S.O.P. Ophth. Oint. (Allergan).
Econochlor, Soln., Oint. (Alcon Laboratories).
Mychel, Cap. (Houba).
Ophthochlor, Soln. (Parke-Davis).
W/Polymixin B.
Use: Treatment of superficial ocular infections involving the conjunctiva and/or cornea caused by susceptible organisms.
See: Chloromyxin Ophthalmic Oint. (Parke-Davis).
W/Polymyxin B, Hydrocortisone.
See: Ophthocort, Oint. (Parke-Davis).

chloramphenicol and hydrocortisone acetate for ophthalmic suspension.
Use: Anti-infective, anti-inflammatory.
See: Chloromycetin, Prods. (Parke-Davis).

chloramphenicol and polymyxin b sulfate ophthalmic ointment.
Use: Anti-infective.

chloramphenicol, hydrocortisone acetate and polymyxin b sulfate, ophthalmic ointment.
Use: Anti-infective, anti-inflammatory.
See: Chloromycetin, Prods. (Parke-Davis).

•**chloramphenicol palmitate.** U.S.P. 23.
Use: Anti-infective, antirickettsial.
See: Chloromycetin Palmitate, Oral Susp. (Parke-Davis).

•**chloramphenicol pantothenate complex.** (KLOR-am-FEN-ih-kahl PAN-toe-THEH-nate) USAN.
Use: Anti-infective, antirickettsial.

chloramphenicol and prednisolone ophthalmic ointment.
Use: Anti-infective, steroid combination.
See: Chloromycetin, Prods. (Parke-Davis).

•**chloramphenicol sodium succinate, sterile.** U.S.P. 23.
Use: Anti-infective, antirickettsial.
See: Chloromycetin Succinate, Inj., (Parke-Davis).
Mychel-S, IV. (Houba).

chloramphenicol sodium succinate. (Various Mfr.) 100 mg/ml. Inj. Vial. 1 g in 15 ml.
Use: Anti-infective, antirickettsial.

chloranil.

Chloraseptic Children's Lozenges. (Procter & Gamble) Benzocaine 5 mg/Loz. Pkg. 18s. *otc.*
Use: Anesthetic, local.

Chloraseptic Liquid. (Procter & Gamble) Total phenol 1.4% as phenol and sodium phenolate, saccharin. Menthol and cherry flavors. Bot. 180 ml, 360 ml (mouthwash/gargle); 45 ml, 240 ml, 360 ml (throat spray). *otc.*
Use: Anesthetic, antiseptic, local.

Chloraseptic Lozenge. (Procter & Gamble) Total phenol 32.5 mg/lozenge as phenol and sodium phenolate. Menthol and cherry flavors. Pkg. 18s, 36s. *otc.*
Use: Anesthetic, antiseptic.

chlorazanil hydrochloride.

Chlorazene. (Badger) Chloramine-T, sodium p-toluene-sulfonchloramide.
Pow.: UD Pkg. 20 g, 38 g, 50 g, 88 g, 200 g, 240 g, 320 g, Bot. 1 lb, 5 lb.
Aromatic Pow. (5%): Bot. 1 lb, 5 lb.
Tab. (0.3 g): Bot. 20s, 100s, 1000s, 5000s. *otc.*
Use: Antiseptic, deodorant.

chlorazepate dipotassium.
Use: Anxiolytic anticonvulsant.
See: Clorazepate dipotassium.

chlorazepate monopotassium.
See: Clorazepate monopotassium.

Chlorazine Tabs. (Major) Prochlorperazine 5 mg or 10 mg/Tab. Bot. 100s.
Use: Antiemetic, antipsychotic, antivertigo.

chlorazone.
See: Chloramine-T.

Chlor Benzo Mor, A and D Ointment. (Wade) Vitamins A and D fortified, chlorobutanol 3%, benzocaine 2%, benzyl alcohol 3%, actamer 1%, in lanolin and petrolatum base. Tube 1 oz, Jar 1 oz, lb. *otc.*
Use: Anesthetic, antiseptic, local.

Chlor Benzo Mor Spray. (Wade) Vitamin A and D fortified, chlorobutanol

3%, benzocaine 2%, benzyl alcohol 3%, and actamer 1%, in lanolin and mineral oil base. Bot. 2 oz, 11 oz. *otc.*
Use: Antiseptic, anesthetic, local.

chlorbutanol.
See: Chlorobutanol, N.F. 18.

chlorbutol.
See: Chlorobutanol, N.F. 18.

chlorcyclizine hydrochloride. N.F. XVI.
Use: Antihistamine.
W/Hydrocortisone acetate.
See: Mantadil, Cream (Glaxo-Wellcome).
W/Pseudoephedrine HCl.
See: Fedrazil, Tab. (GlaxoWellcome).

•**chlordantoin.** (CLOR-dan-toe-in) USAN.
Use: Antifungal.

•**chlordiazepoxide.** (klor-DIE-aze-ee-POX-side) U.S.P. 23.
Use: Anxiolytic.
See: A-poxide, Cap. (Abbott Laboratories).
Brigen-G, Tab. (Grafton).
Libritabs, Tab. (Roche Laboratories).
W/Amitriptyline.
See: Limbitrol, Tab. (Roche Laboratories).

chlordiazepoxide and amitriptyline HCl tablets. (klor-DIE-aze-ee-POX-ide and am-ee-TRIP-tih-leen)
Use: Anxiolytic.
See: Limbitrol, Tab. (Roche Laboratories).

•**chlordiazepoxide hydrochloride.** (klor-DIE-aze-ee-POX-ide) U.S.P. 23.
Use: Hypnotic, sedative.
See: A-poxide, Cap. (Abbott Laboratories).
Chlordiazachel, Cap. (Houba).
Librium, Cap., Inj. (Roche Laboratories).
Screen, Cap. (Foy).
Zetran, Cap. (Roberts Pharm).
W/Clidinium bromide.
See: Librax, Cap. (Roche Laboratories).

chlordiazepoxide w/clindinium bromide. (Various Mfr.) Clindinium 2.5 mg, chlordiazepoxide HCl 5 mg/Cap. Bot. 30s, 100s, 500s, 1000s, UD 100s. *c-iv.*
Use: Gastrointestinal, anticholinergic.

chlordiazepoxide and clindinium bromide. (Chelsea Labs) Clindinium bromide 2.5 mg, chlordiazepoxide HCl 5 mg/Cap. Bot. 100s, 500s, 1000s. *Rx. Formerly Clindex (Rugby).*
Use: Anticholinergic, antispasmodic.

Chlordrine S.R. (Rugby) Pseudoephedrine HCl 120 mg, chlorpheniramine maleate 8 mg/Cap. Bot. 100s. *Rx.*
Use: Antihistamine, decongestant.

Chloren 4. (Wren) Chlorpheniramine maleate 4 mg/Tab. Bot. 100s, 1000s. *otc.*
Use: Antihistamine.

Chloren 8 T.D. (Wren) Chlorpheniramine maleate 8 mg/Tab. Bot. 100s, 1000s. *otc.*
Use: Antihistamine.

Chloren 12 T.D. (Wren) Chlorpheniramine maleate 12 mg/Tab. Bot. 100s, 1000s. *otc, Rx.*
Use: Antihistamine.

Chloresium. (Rystan) **Oint.:** Chlorophyllin copper complex 0.5% in hydrophilic base. Tube 1 oz, 4 oz, Jar lb. **Soln.:** Chlorophyllin copper complex 0.2% in isotonic saline soln. Bot. 60 ml, 240 ml, qt. *otc.*
Use: Deodorant, healing agent.

Chloresium Tablets. (Rystan) Chlorophyllin copper complex 14 mg/Tab. Bot. 100s, 1000s. *otc.*
Use: Deodorant, oral.

Chloresium Tooth Paste. (Rystan) Chlorophyllin copper complex. Tube 3.25 oz. *otc.*
Use: Deodorant, oral.

chlorethyl.
See: Ethyl Chloride.

chlorguanide hydrochloride.
See: Chloroguanide HCl (Various Mfr.).

chlorhexadol.

chlorhexidine. (klor-HEX-ih-deen) F.D.A. *otc.*
Use: Antiseptic.
See: BactoShield, Foam, Soln. (Steris Laboratories).
BactoShield 2, Soln. (Steris Laboratories).
Hibiclens. (Zeneca).

•**chlorhexidine gluconate.** (klor-HEX-ih-deen GLUE-koe-nate) USAN.
Use: Antimicrobial.
See: BactoShield, Foam, Soln. (Steris Laboratories).
BactoShield 2, Soln. (Steris Laboratories).
Hibiclens, Liq. (Zeneca).
Hibistat, Liq. (Zeneca).
Peridex (Procter & Gamble).

chlorhexidine gluconate mouthrinse.
Use: Amelioration of oral mucositis associated with cytoreductive therapy for conditioning patients for bone marrow transplantation. [Orphan drug]
See: Peridex (Procter & Gamble).
PerioGard, Oral Rinse (Colgate Oral).

•**chlorhexidine hydrochloride.** (klor-

HEX-ih-deen) USAN.
Use: Anti-infective, topical.

•**chlorhexidine phosphanilate.** (klor-HEX-ih-deen FOSS-fah-nih-LATE) USAN.
Use: Anti-infective.

chlorhydroxyquinolin.
See: Quinolor Compound, Oint. (Bristol-Myers Squibb).

chlorinated and iodized peanut oil. Chloriodized Oil.

•**chlorindanol.** (klor-IN-dah-nahl) USAN.
Use: Antiseptic, spermaticide.

chlorine compound, antiseptic. Antiseptics, Chlorine.

chloriodized oil. Chlorinated and iodized peanut oil.

chlorisondamine chloride.

•**chlormadinone acetate.** (klor-MAD-ih-nohn) USAN. NF XIII.
Use: Hormone, progestin.

Chlor Mal w/Sal + APAP S.C. (Global Source) Chlorpheniramine maleate 2 mg, acetaminophen 150 mg, salicylamide 175 mg/Tab. Bot. 1000s. *otc.*
Use: Analgesic, antihistamine.

chlormerodrin. Mercloran. *Rx.*
Use: Diuretic.

•**chlormerodrin hg 197.** USAN. U.S.P. XX.
Use: Diagnostic aid (renal function determination), radiopharmaceutical.

•**chlormerodrin hg 203.** USAN. U.S.P. XX.
Use: Diagnostic aid (renal function determination), radiopharmaceutical.

chlormezanone. Chlormethazanone. *Rx.*
Use: Anxiolytic.
See: Trancopal, Cap. (Sanofi Winthrop).

Chlor-Niramine Allergy Tabs. (Whiteworth Towne) Chlorpheniramine maleate 4 mg/Tab. Bot. 24s, 100s. *otc.*
Use: Antihistamine.

chloroazodin. Alpha, alpha, Azobis-(chloroformamidine).

•**chlorobutanol.** (Klor-oh-BYOO-tah-nole) N.F. 18.
Use: Anesthetic, antiseptic, hypnotic; pharmaceutic aid (antimicrobial).
See: Cerumenex, Drops (Purdue-Frederick).
Pre-Sert (Allergan).
W/Atropine sulfate, chlorpheniramine maleate, phenylpropanolamine HCl.
See: Decongestant, Inj. (Century Pharm).
W/Calcium glycerophosphate, calcium levulinate.
See: Cal San, Inj. (Burgin-Arden).
W/Cetyltrimethylammonium Br, methapyrilene HCl, phenylephrine HCl, hydrocortisone.
See: T-Spray, Liq. (Saron).
W/Diphenhydramine HCl.
See: Ardeben, Inj. (Burgin-Arden).
W/Ephedrine HCl, sodium Cl.
See: Efedron HCl, Nasal Jelly (Hart).
W/Estradiol cypionate, testosterone cypionate.
See: Depo-Testadiol, Vial (Pharmacia & Upjohn).
Depotestogen, Vial (Hyrex).
W/Glycerin, anhydrous.
See: Ophthalgan, Liq. (Wyeth Ayerst).
W/Liquifilm.
See: Liquifilm Tears (Allergan).
W/Methylcellulose.
See: Lacril (Allergan).
W/Myristyl-gamma-picolinium Cl.
See: Wet Tone, Soln. (3M).
W/Nonionic lanolin derivative.
See: Lacri-Lube, Ophthalmic Ointment (Allergan).
W/Polyethylene glycol, polyoxyl 40 stearate.
See: Blink-N-Clean (Allergan).
W/Sodium Cl.
See: Ocean, Liq. (Fleming).
W/Tannic acid, isopropyl alcohol.
See: Outgro, Soln. (Whitehall Robins).
W/Vitamins B_1, B_2, B_6, niacinamide, calcium pantothenate, benzyl alcohol.

•**chlorocresol.** (KLOR-oh-KREE-sole) N.F. 18.
Use: Antiseptic, disinfectant.

chloroethane.
See: Ethyl Chloride. anticholinergic, antispasmodic.

Chlorofair. (Pharmafair) **Soln.:** Chloramphenicol 5 mg/ml. Bot. 7.5 ml **Oint.:** Chloramphenicol 10 mg/g in white petrolatum base with mineral oil, polysorbate 60. Tube 3.5 g. *Rx.*
Use: Anti-infective, ophthalmic.

chloroguanide hydrochloride. (Various Mfr.) (Proguanil HCl) *Rx.*
Use: Antimalarial.

Chlorohist-LA. (Roberts Pharm) Xylometazoline HCl 0.1%. Soln. Spray 15 ml. *otc.*
Use: Decongestant.

chloro-iodohydroxyquinoline.
See: Clioquinol, U.S.P. 23.

chloromethapyrilene citrate.
See: Chlorothen Citrate.

Chloromycetin. (Monarch) Chloramphenicol. **Ophth. Oint.:** (1%) in base of petrolatum, polyethylene. Tube 3.5 g. **Inj.:** 100 mg/ml (as sodium succinate)

when reconstituted. In 1 g in 15 ml vials. **Ophth. Soln.:** (25 mg) Bot. w/dropper 15 ml (dry). Soln. Plastic dropper Bot. 15 ml. **Oral:** 150 mg/5 ml (palmitate), alcohol, sucrose, sodium benzoate 0.5%. Custard flavor. Bot. 60 ml. **Otic Drops:** (0.5%) 5 mg/ml w/propylene glycol. Bot. 15 ml. *Rx.*
Use: Anti-infective.

Chloromycetin/Hydrocortisone. (Parke-Davis) Hydrocortisone acetate 0.5% (2.5% as powder), chloramphenicol 0.25% (1.25% as powder). Pow. Bot. with dropper 5 ml. *Rx.*
Use: Anti-infective, ophthalmic.

Chloromycetin Sodium Succinate I.V. (Monarch) Chloramphenicol sodium succinate dried powder which when reconstituted contains chloromycetin 100 mg/ml. Steri-vial 1 g, 10s. *Rx.*
Use: Anti-infective.

chlorophenothane.
Use: Pediculicide.

chlorophyll. (Freeda Vitamins) Chlorophyll 20 mg, sugar free/Tab. Bot. 100s, 250s, 500s. *otc.*
Use: Deodorant, oral.

Chlorophyll "A" Ointment.
See: Chloresium Oint. (Rystan).

Chlorophyll "A" Solution. (Chlorophyllin).
See: Chloresium Soln. (Rystan).

chlorophyll derivatives, systemic.
See: chlorophyll (Freeda Vitamins).
Derifil (Rystan).
Chloresium (Rystan).

chlorophyll derivatives, topical.
See: Chloresium (Rystan).

chlorophyll tablets. *otc.*
See: Derifil, Tab. (Rystan).
Nullo, Tab. (Depree).

chlorophyll, water-soluble. (Various Mfr.) Chlorophyllin.
See: Chloresium Prep. (Rystan).
Derifil, Pow. (Rystan).

chlorophyllin. (KLOR-oh-FILL-in)
Use: Deodorant, healing agent.

•**chlorophyllin copper complex.** (KLOR-oh-FILL-in KAHP-uhr) USAN.
Use: Deodorant.
See: Nullo, Tab. (Chattem Consumer Products).
PALS, Tab. (Palisades Pharm).

•**chlorophyllin copper complex sodium.** U.S.P. 23.

•**chloroprocaine hydrochloride.** (Klor-oh-PRO-cane) U.S.P. 23.
Use: Anesthetic, local.
See: Nesacaine, Inj. (Astra).
Nesacaine-MPF, Inj. (Astra).

Chloroptic. (Allergan) Chloramphenicol 0.5%. **Soln.:** Dropper bot. 2.5 ml, 7.5 ml. *Rx.*
Use: Anti-infective, ophthalmic.

Chloroptic S.O.P. (Allergan) Chloramphenicol 10 mg/g. Oint. Tube 3.5 g. *Rx.*
Use: Anti-infective, ophthalmic.

•**chloroquine.** (KLOR-oh-kwin) U.S.P. 23.
Use: Antiamebic, antimalarial.
See: Aralen HCl Prods. (Sanofi Winthrop).

•**chloroquine hydrochloride injection.** U.S.P. 23.
Use: Antiamebic, antimalarial.
See: Aralen HCl (Sanofi Winthrop).

•**chloroquine phosphate.** U.S.P. 23.
Use: Antiamebic, antimalarial, lupus erythematosus agent.
See: Aralen Phosphate, Tab. (Sanofi Winthrop).

chlorothen.
Use: Antihistamine.

chlorothen citrate. (Whittier) Tab., Bot. 100s.
Use: Antihistamine.
W/Pyrilamine, thenylpyramine.
See: Derma-Pax, Liq. (Recsei).

chlorothenylpyramine. Chlorothen, Prep.

Chlorotheophyllinate w/Benadryl.
See: Dramamine, Prep. (Searle).

•**chlorothiazide.** U.S.P. 23.
Use: Diuretic.
See: Diuril, Tab., Susp. (Merck).
W/Methyldopa.
See: Aldoclor, Tab. (Merck).
W/Reserpine. Tab.: Chlorothiazide 250 mg or 500 mg, reserpine 0.125 mg. Bot. 100s.
See: Diupres, Tab. (Merck).
Use: Diuretic.

•**chlorothiazide sodium for injection.** U.S.P. 23.
Use: Antihypertensive, diuretic.
See: Sodium Diuril, Vial (Merck).

chlorothymol. 6-Chlorothymol.
Use: Anti-infective

•**chlorotrianisene.** (klor-oh-try-AN-ih-seen) U.S.P. 23.
Use: Estrogen.

chlorotrianisene capsules.
Use: Estrogen. [/NAME]
See: Placidyl, Cap. (Abbott Laboratories).

•**chloroxine.** (KLOR-ox-een) USAN.
Use: Antiseborrheic.

•**chloroxylenol.** (KLOR-oh-ZIE-len-ole) U.S.P. 23.
Use: Antibacterial.
W/Benzocaine, menthol, lanolin.
See: Unburn, Spray, Cream, Lot. (Leeming-Pacquin).
W/Hexachlorophene.
See: Desitin, Preps. (Leeming-Pacquin).
W/Hydrocortisone, pramoxine.
See: Otomar-HC, Otic Soln. (Marnel).
W/Methyl salicylate, menthol, camphor, thymol, eucalyptus oil, isopropyl alcohol.
See: Gordobalm, Balm (Gordon Laboratories).
W/Pramoxine HCl, hydrocortisone.
See: Oti-Med, Drops. (Hyrex Pharmaceuticals).
Tri-Otic, Drops (Pharmics).
Zoto-HC, Otic Drops (Horizon).

Chlorpazine. (Major) Prochlorperazine maleate 5 mg, 10 mg or 25 mg/Tab. Bot. 100s, UD 100s (5 mg, 10 mg only). *Rx.*
Use: Antipsychotic.

Chlorphed Injection. (Roberts Pharm) Brompheniramine maleate 10 mg/ml. Vial 10 ml. *Rx.*
Use: Antihistamine.

Chlorphed-LA. (Roberts Pharm) Oxymetazoline 0.05%. Soln. Spray 15 ml. *otc.*
Use: Decongestant.

Chlorphedrine SR. (Zenith Goldline) Chlorpheniramine maleate 8 mg, pseudoephedrine HCl 120 mg/Cap. Bot. 100s. *Rx.*
Use: Antihistamine, decongestant.

chlorphenesin. (KLOR-fen-ss-sin) F.D.A.

•**chlorphenesin carbamate.** (KLOR-fenee-sin CAR-bah-mate) USAN.
Use: Muscle relaxant.
See: Maolate, Tab. (Pharmacia & Upjohn).

•**chlorpheniramine maleate.** (klor-fen-IHR-ah-meen) U.S.P. 23.
Use: Antihistamine.
See: Alermine, Tab. (Solvay).
Aller-Chlor, Syr., Tab. (Rugby).
Allergy, Tab. (Major).
Chestamine, Cap. (Leeds).
Chlo-Amine, Tab. (Bayer Corp).
Chloraman, Tab. (Rasman).
Chloren, Preps. (Wren).
Chlor-4, Tab. (Mills).
Chlor-Niramine, Tab. (Whiteworth Towne).
Chlorophen, Vial (Medical Chem.).
Chlor-pen, Tab., Vial (American Chemical & Drug).
Chlor-Span, Cap. (Burlington).
Chlortab, Tab., Cap., Inj. (Vortech).
Chlor-Trimeton Maleate, Preps. (Schering Plough).
Cosea, Preps. (Center Laboratories).
Efidac 24 Chlorpheniramine, ER Tab. (Novartis).
Histacon, Tab., Syr. (Marsh Labs).
Histaspan, Cap. (Rhone-Poulenc Rorer).
Histex, Cap. (Roberts Pharm).
Nasahist (Keene Pharmaceuticals).
Polaramine, Tab., Syr. (Schering Plough).
Pedia Care Allergy Formula, Liq. (Ortho-McNeil)
Pyranistan, Tab. (Standex).
Teldrin, Spansule (SmithKline Beecham Pharmaceuticals).

chlorpheniramine maleate. (Various Mfr.) **Tab.:** Chlorpheniramine maleate 4 mg. Bot. 100s, 1000s. *otc.* **Inj.:** 10 mg/ml, benzyl alcohol 1.5%. Multidose vial. *Rx.*
Use: Antihistamine.

chlorpheniramine maleate w/combinations.
See: Al-Ay, Preps. (Jones Medical Industries).
Alka-Seltzer Plus, Tab. (Bayer Corp).
Allerdec, Cap. (Towne).
Allerest, Prods. (Novartis).
Alumadrine, Tab. (Fleming).
A.R.M., Tab. (SmithKline Beecham Pharmaceuticals).
Atuss DM, Syr. (Atley).
Atussin-D.M. Expectorant, Liq. (Federal).
B.M.E., Liq. (Brothers).
Bobid, Cap. (Boyd).
Breacol Cough Medication, Liq. (Bayer Corp).
Brolade, Cap. (Brothers).
Bur-Tuss Expectorant (Burlington).
Cenahist, Cap. (Century Pharm).
Cenaid, Tab. (Century Pharm).
Centuss, Tab. (Century Pharm).
Chlorpel, Cap. (Santa).
Chlor-Trimeton, Preps. (Schering Plough).
Codimal, Tab. (Schwarz Pharma).
Col-Decon, Tab. (Quality Formulations).
Colrex Compound, Preps. (Solvay).
Comtrex, Tab., Cap., Liq. (Bristol-Myers).
Conalsyn Croncap, Cap. (Cenci).
Contac, Cap. (SmithKline Beecham Pharmaceuticals).
Cophene No. 2, Cap. (Dunhall Pharmaceuticals).

Cophene-S, Syr. (Dunhall Pharmaceuticals).
Coricidin, Preps. (Schering Plough).
Corilin, Liq. (Schering Plough).
Corizahist, Preps. (Mason).
Coryban-D, Cap. (Pfizer).
Co-Tylenol, Preps. (Ortho McNeil).
D.A. II, Tab. (Dura).
Dallergy, Tab., Cap., Syr. (Laser).
Deconamine, Tab., Cap., Syr. (Berlex).
Dehist, Cap. (Forest Pharmaceutical).
Demazin, Tab., Syr. (Schering Plough).
Derma-Pax, Lot. (Recsei).
Dezest, Cap. (Geneva Pharm).
Donatussin, Liq., Syr. (Laser).
Dristan, Preps. (Whitehall Robins).
Drucon, Elix. (Standard Drug).
Efricon Expectorant (Lannett).
Extendryl, Tab., Cap., Syr. (Fleming).
F.C.A.H., Cap. (Scherer).
Fedahist, Prods. (Donner).
Fitacol (Standex).
Histabid, Cap. (GlaxoWellcome).
Histacon, Tab., Syr. (Marsh Labs).
Histapco, Tab. (Apco).
Histaspan-D, Cap. (Rhone-Poulenc Rorer).
Histaspan Plus, Cap. (Rhone-Poulenc Rorer).
Hista-Vadrin, Tab., Cap., Syr. (Scherer).
Histine Prods. (Freeport).
Histine PV, Syr. (Ethex).
Histogesic, Tab. (Century Pharm).
Hycomine Compound, Tab. (DuPont Merck Pharmaceuticals).
Infantuss, Liq. (Scott/Cord).
Iodal HD, Liq. (Iomed).
Iotussin HC, Syr. (Iomed).
Koryza, Tab. (Forest Pharmaceutical).
Kronofed-A, Cap. (Ferndale Laboratories).
Mapap CF, Tab. (Major).
Marhist (Marlop Pharm).
Neo-Pyranistan, Tab. (Standex).
Nilcol, Tab., Elix. (Parke-Davis).
Nolamine, Tab. (Carnrick Labs).
Novafed A, Cap., Liq. (Hoechst Marion Roussel).
Novahistine, Preps. (Hoechst Marion Roussel).
Partuss, Liq. (Parmed).
Partuss T.D., Tab. (Parmed).
Phenahist, Preps. (T.E. Williams).
Phenchlor, Prods. (Freeport).
Polytuss-DM, Liq. (Rhode).
Pyma, Cap., Vial (Forest Pharmaceutical).
Pyristan, Cap., Elix. (Arcum).
Pyranistan (Standex).
Quelidrine, Syr. (Abbott Laboratories).
Rentuss, Cap., Syr. (Wren).
Rhinex D M, Tab., Syr. (Teva USA).
Ryna, Liq. (Wallace Laboratories).
Ryna-tussadine, Tab., Liq. (Wallace Laboratories).
Salphenyl, Cap. (Roberts Pharm).
Scotcof, Liq. (Scott/Cord).
Scotnord (Scott/Cord).
Scotuss Liq. (Scott/Cord).
Shertus, Liq. (Sheryl).
Sialco, Tab. (Foy).
Sinarest, Tab. (Novartis).
Sine-Off, Prods. (SmithKline Beecham Pharmaceuticals).
Sino-Compound, Tab. (Bio-Factor).
Sinovan Timed, Cap. (Drug Ind.).
Sinucol, Cap., Vial (Tennessee Pharmaceutic).
Sinulin, Tab. (Carnrick Labs).
Sinutab Extra Strength, Cap. (Warner Lambert).
Spantuss, Tab., Liq. (Arco).
Statomin Maleate CC, Tab. (Jones Medical Industries).
Sudafed Plus, Tab., Syr. (Glaxo-Wellcome).
Symptrol, Cap. (Saron).
T.A.C., Cap. (Towne).
Tonecol, Tab., Syr. (A.V.P.).
Triaminininic, Prods. (Novartis).
Triaminicin Chewables (Novartis).
Turbilixir, Liq. (Burlington).
Turbispan Leisurecaps, Cap. (Burlington).
Tusquelin, Syr. (Circle).
Tussar, Prods. (Rhone-Poulenc Rorer).
Unituss HC, Syr. (URL).

d-chlorpheniramine maleate.
See: Polaramine Expectorant, Tab., Syr. (Schering Plough).

chlorpheniramine maleate w/pseudoephedrine hydrochloride. (Eon Labs Manufacturing) Pseudoephedrine HCl 120 mg, chlorpheniramine maleate 8 mg/Cap. Bot. 100s, 250s, 1000s. *otc.*
Use: Antihistamine, decongestant.

•**chlorpheniramine polistirex.** (klor-fen-IHR-ah-meen pahl-ee-STIE-rex) USAN.
Use: Antihistamine.

chlorpheniramine resin w/combinations.
See: Omni-Tuss, Liq. (Medeva).

chlorpheniramine tannate.
W/Carbetapentane tannate, ephedrine tannate, phenylephrine tannate.
See: Rynatuss Tab., Susp. (Wallace Laboratories).

W/Phenylephrine tannate, pyrilamine tannate.
See: Rynatan, Tab., Susp. (Wallace Laboratories).
W/Pseudoephedrine tannate.
See: Tanafed, Susp. (Horizon).

•**chlorphentermine hydrochloride.** (klor-FEN-ter-meen) USAN.
Use: Anorexic.

chlorphthalidone.
See: Chlorthalidone.

Chlor-Pro 10. (Schein Pharmaceutical) Chlorpheniramine maleate 10 mg/ml, benzyl alcohol. Inj. Vial 30 ml. *Rx.*
Use: Antihistamine.

•**chlorpromazine.** (klor-PRO-muh-zeen) U.S.P. 23.
Use: Antiemetic, antipsychotic.
See: Chloractil.
Largactil.

•**chlorpromazine hydrochloride.** U.S.P. 23.
Use: Antiemetic, antipsychotic.
See: Chlorzine, Inj. (Roberts Pharm).
Promachlor, Tab. (Geneva Pharm).
Promapar, Tab. (Parke-Davis).
Promaz, Inj. (Keene Pharmaceuticals).
Sonazine, Tab. (Solvay).
Terpium, Tab. (Scrip).
Thorazine, Tab., Cap., Liq., Syr., Supp., Amp. (SmithKline Beecham Pharmaceuticals).

chlorpromazine HCl tablets. (Various Mfr.) Chlorpromazine HCl 10 mg, 25 mg, 50 mg, 100 mg, 200 mg. Tab. Bot. 100s, 1000s, UD 100s. *Rx.*
Use: Antipsychotic.

chlorpromazine HCl injection. (Various Mfr.) Chlorpromazine HCl 25 mg/ml. Inj. Amp. 1 ml, 2 ml. Vial 10 ml. *Rx.*
Use: Antipsychotic.

chlorpromazine hydrochloride intensol oral solution. (Roxane) Chlorpromazine HCl concentrated oral soln. **30 mg/ml:** Bot. 120 ml. **100 mg/ml:** Bot. 60 ml, 240 ml. *Rx.*
Use: Antiemetic, antipsychotic.

•**chlorpropamide.** (klor-PRO-puh-mide) U.S.P. 23.
Use: Antidiabetic.
See: Diabinese, Tab. (Pfizer).

chlorprophenpyridamine maleate.
See: Chlorpheniramine Maleate, U.S.P. 23.

chlorquinaldol. U.S.P. 23. 5,7-Dichloro-8-hydroxyquinal-dine.

chlorquinol. A mixture of the chlorinated products of 8-hydroxyquinoline containing about 65% of 5,7-dichloro-8-hydroxyquinoline. Quixalin.

Chlor-Rest. (Rugby) Phenylpropanolamine HCl 18.7 mg, chlorpheniramine maleate 2 mg/Tab. Bot. 100s. *otc.*
Use: Decongestant, antihistamine.

chlor-span. (Burlington) Chlorpheniramine maleate 8 mg/S.R. Cap. Bot. 60s. *otc.*
Use: Antihistamine.

chlortetracycline and sulfamethazine bisulfates soluble powder.
Use: Anti-infective.

•**chlortetracycline bisulfate.** (klor-the-trah-SIGH-kleen) U.S.P. 23.
Use: Anti-infective; antiprotozoal.

•**chlortetracycline hydrochloride.** U.S.P. 23.
Use: Anti-infective; antiprotozoal.
See: Aureomycin, Oint. (Storz/Lederle)

•**chlorthalidone.** (klor-THAL-ih-dohn) U.S.P. 23.
Use: Antihypertensive, diuretic.
See: Hygroton, Tab. (Rhone-Poulenc Rorer).
Thalitone, Tab. (Horus Therapeutics).
W/Reserpine.
See: Demi-Regroton, Tab. (Rhone-Poulenc Rorer).
Regroton, Tab. (Rhone-Poulenc Rorer).

chlorthalidone. (Various). Tab.: 25, 50, or 100 mg. Bot. 100s (25 mg); 100s, 250s, 1000s, (50 mg); 100s, 500s, 1000s (100 mg). *Rx.*
Use: Diuretic, antihypertensive.

Chlor-Trimeton Allergy 4 Hour. (Schering Plough) **Tab.:** Chlorpheniramine maleate 4 mg, lactose. Bot. 48s. **Syr.:** Chlorpheniramine maleate 2 mg/5ml, parabens, cherry flavor. Bot. 118 ml. *otc.*
Use: Antihistamine.

Chlor-Trimeton Allergy 8 Hour. (Schering Plough) Chlorpheniramine maleate 8 mg, parabens, lactose, sugar. TR Tab. Bot. 24s. *otc.*
Use: Antihistamine.

Chlor-Trimeton Allergy 12 Hour. (Schering Plough) Chlorpheniramine maleate 12 mg, parabens, lactose, sugar. TR Tab. Pgk. 15s. *otc.*
Use: Antihistamine.

Chlor-Trimeton Allergy Sinus. (Schering Plough) Phenylpropanolamine HCl 12.5 mg, chlorpheniramine maleate 2 mg, acetaminophen 500 mg/Capl. Box 24s. *otc.*
Use: Analgesic, antihistamine, decongestant.

Chlor-Trimeton w/Combinations. (Schering Plough) Chlorpheniramine maleate.
W/Acetaminophen.
See: Coricidin, Tab. (Schering Plough).
W/Acetaminophen, phenylpropanolamine.
See: Coricidin "D", Prods. (Schering Plough).
W/Phenylephrine HCl.
See: Demazin, Prods. (Schering Plough).
W/Pseudoephedrine sulfate.
See: Chlor-Trimeton Decongestant Tab. (Schering Plough).
Chlor-Trimeton 12 Hour Allergy (Schering Plough).
W/Salicylamide, phenacetin, caffeine, vitamin C.
See: Coriforte, Cap. (Schering Plough).
W/Sodium salicylate, amino acetic acid.
See: Corilin, Liq. (Schering Plough).

Chlor-Trimeton 4 Hour Relief Tablets. (Schering Plough) Chlorpheniramine maleate 4 mg, pseudoephedrine sulfate 60 mg/Tab. Box 24s, 48s. *otc.*
Use: Antihistamine, decongestant.

Chlor-Trimeton 12 Hour Allergy. (Schering Plough) Chlorpheniramine maleate 8 mg, pseudoephedrine sulfate 120 mg/SR Tab. Box 24s, 48s. UD 96s. *otc.*
Use: Antihistamine, decongestant.

Chlor-Trimeton 12 Hour Relief Tablets. (Schering Plough) Chlorpheniramine 8 mg, pseudoephedrine sulfate 120 mg/Tab. Box 12s. Bot. 36s. *otc.*
Use: Antihistamine, decongestant.

Chlorzide. (Foy) Hydrochlorothiazide 50 mg/Tab. Bot. 1000s. *Rx.*
Use: Diuretic.

•**chlorzoxazone.** (klor-ZOX-uh-zone) U.S.P. 23.
Use: Muscle relaxant.
See: Paraflex, Tab. (Ortho McNeil).
Parafon Forte DSC, Capl. (Ortho McNeil).
Remular-S (Inter. Ethical).
W/Acetaminophen.
See: Blanex, Cap. (Edwards Pharmaceuticals).

chlorzoxazone. (Various Mfr.) 250 mg, 500 mg/Tab. Bot. 100s, 500s (500 mg only), 1000s.
Use: Muscle relaxant.

chlorzoxazone and acetaminophen capsules.
Use: Analgesic, muscle relaxant.

chlorzoxazone and acetaminophen tablets.
Use: Analgesic, muscle relaxant.

Choice 10. (Whiteworth Towne) Potassium Cl 10% soln., unflavored. Bot. gal. *Rx.*
Use: Electrolyte supplement.

Choice 20. (Whiteworth Towne) Potassium Cl 20% soln., unflavored. Bot. gal. *Rx.*
Use: Electrolyte supplement.

Choice dm. (Mead Johnson Nutritionals) Protein 10.6 g, fat 12 g, carbohydrate 25 g, vitamins A, D, E, K, C, FA, B_1, B_2, B_3, B_5, B_6, B_{12}, biotin, Ca, P, I, Fe, Mg, Cu, Zn, Mn, Cl, Na, Se, Cr, Mo, sucrose,, 250 calories/240 ml. Lactose free/Liq. 240 ml. *otc.*
Use: Nutritional supplement, enteral.

Cholac. (Alra Laboratories) Lactulose 10 g/15 ml. Bot. 240 ml, pt, UD 30 ml. *Rx.*
Use: Laxative.

cholacrylamine resin. An anion exchange resin consisting of a water soluble polymer having a molecular weight equivalent between 350 and 360 in which aliphatic quaternary amine groups are attached to an acrylic backbone by ester linkages.

cholalic acid.
See: Cholic Acid.

Cholan-DH. (Medeva) Dehydrocholic acid 250 mg/Tab. Bot. 100s.
Use: Laxative.

cholanic acid. Dehydrodesoxycholic acid.

Cholebrine. (Mallinckrodt) Iocetamic acid (62% iodine) 750 mg/Tab. Bot. 100s, 150s.
Use: Radiopaque agent.

•**cholecalciferol.** (kole-eh-kal-SIH-fer-ole) U.S.P. 23. *Formerly 7-Dehydrocholesterol, activated.*
Use: Vitamin D_3 (antirachitic).
See: Decavitamin Cap., Tab.
Delta-D, Tab. (Freeda).

cholecystography agents.
See: Bilopaque, Cap. (Sanofi Winthrop).
Iodized Oil (Various Mfr.).
Iophendylate Inj.
Pantopaque, Amp. (Lafayette Pharm).
Telepaque, Tab. (Sanofi Winthrop).

Choledyl SA. (Parke-Davis) Oxtriphylline 400 mg or 600 mg/Tab. Bot. 100s, UD 100s. *Rx.*
Use: Bronchodilator.

•**cholera vaccine.** U.S.P. 23.
Use: Immunization.

cholera vaccine. (Wyeth Ayerst) 8 units each of Ogawa and Inaba strains per ml. Vial, 1.5 ml, 20 ml.
Use: Immunization.

choleretic. Bile salts.
See: Bile Preps. and Forms.
Dehydrocholic Acid.
Desoxycholic Acid.
Tocamphyl, Tab. (Various Mfr.).

cholesterin.
See: Cholesterol.

•**cholesterol.** N.F. 18.
Use: Pharmaceutic aid (emulsifying agent).

cholesterol reagent strips. (Bayer Corp) A quantitative strip test for cholesterol in serum. Seralyzer reagent strips. Bot. 25s.
Use: Diagnostic aid.

cholestyramine. (koe-less-TIE-ruh-meen) An antihyperlipidemic agent used to lower cholesterol. Consists of anhydrous cholestyramine 4 g/dose.
See: Cholybar, Bar (Parke-Davis).
Questran, Pow. (Bristol Labs.).
Questran Light, Pow. (Bristol Labs.).

cholestyramine. (koe-less-TIE-ruh-meen) U.S.P. 23.
Use: Ion-exchange resin (bile salts), antihyperlipoproteinemic.

cholestyramine powder. (Zenith Goldline) 4 g (as anhydrous resin), phenylalanine 14.1 mg/5.5 g powder, aspartame/Pow. Packets. 42 and 60 single dose 5.5 g Packets. *Rx.*
Use: Bile acid sequestrant.

•**cholestyramine resin.** (koe-less-TEER-uh-meen) U.S.P. 23.
Use: Antihyperlipidemic, ion-exchange resin (bile salts).
See: Questran, Pow. (Bristol-Myers Squibb).

cholic acid.

Cholidase. (Freeda Vitamins) Choline 450 mg, inositol 150 mg, vitamins B_6 2.5 mg, B_{12} 5 mcg, E 7.5 mg/Tab. Bot. 100s, 250s, 500s. *otc.*
Use: Lipid, vitamin supplement.

choline. (Various Mfr.) Choline. Tab.: **250 mg:** Bot. 100s, 250s, 500s, 1000s. **500 mg:** Bot. 100s. **650 mg:** Bot. 90s, 100s, 250s, 500s. *otc.*
Use: Lipotropic.

choline bitartrate.
W/Bile extract, pancreatic substance, dl-methionine.
See: Licoplex, Tab. (Mills).
W/Methionine, inositol, desiccated liver, vitamin B_{12}.
See: Limvic, Tab. (Briar).
W/Mucopolysaccharide, epinephrine neutralizing factor, pancreatic lipotropic fraction, dl-methionine, inositol, bile extract.
See: Lipo-K, Cap. (Marcen).
W/d-Pantothenyl alcohol.
See: Ilopan-Choline, Tab. (Pharmacia & Upjohn).
W/Safflower oil, whole liver, soybean, lecithin, inositol, methionine, natural tocopherols, vitamins B_6, B_{12}, panthenol.
See: Nutricol, Cap., Vial (Nutrition Control).

choline chloride. (Various Mfr.).
Use: Liver supplement. [Orphan drug]
W/Inositol, methionine, vitamin B_{12}.
See: Lychol-B, Inj. (Burgin-Arden).
W/Methionine, vitamins, niacinamide, panthenol.
See: Minoplex, Vial (Savage).
W/Panthenol, inositol, vitamins, minerals, estrone, testosterone.
See: Geramine, Inj. (Zeneca).
W/Panthenol, inositol, vitamins, minerals, estrone, testosterone, polydigestase.
See: Geramine, Tab. (Zeneca).
W/Vitamin B_1, niacinamide, B_2, B_6, calcium pantothenate, cyanocobalamin, B_{12}, inositol, dl-methionine, testosterone, estrone, procaine.
See: Gerihorm, Inj. (Burgin-Arden).

choline chloride, carbamate. Carbachol, U.S.P. 23.

choline chloride succinate.
See: Succinylcholine Chloride, U.S.P. 23.

choline citrate, tricholine citrate.
W/Inositol, methionine, vitamin B_{12}.
See: Cholimeth Tab. (Schwarz Pharma).

choline dihydrogen citrate. 2-Hydroxyethyl trimethylammonium citrate-U.S. vitamin 0.5 g. Bot. 100s, 500s.
Use: Lipotropic.
See: Cholinate, Liq. (Cenci).

choline magnesium trisalicylate. (Sidmak) 500 mg, 750 mg or 1000 mg. Tab. Bot. 100s, 500s. *Rx.*
Use: Analgesic.
See: Trilisate, Tab. (Purdue Frederick).

cholinergic agents.
(Parasympathomimetic Agents).
See: Mecholyl Cl, Inj. (Baker Norton).
Mestinon, Tab., Syr., Amp. (Roche Laboratories).
Mytelase, Cap. (Sanofi Winthrop).
Pilocarpine Nitrate (Various Mfr.).
Prostigin Bromide, Tab. (Roche Laboratories).
Prostigin Methylsulfate, Inj. (Roche Laboratories).
Tensilon, Inj. (Roche Laboratories).
Urecholine, Inj., Tab. (Merck).

cholinergic blocking agents.
See: Parasympatholytic agents.

•**choline salicylate.** USAN.
Use: Analgesic.

cholinesterase inhibitors. Agents that inhibit the enzyme cholinesterase and enhance the effects of endogenous acetylcholine.
Use: Glaucoma therapy.
See: Eserine Sulfate, Oint., (Various, eg, Harber, Iolab, Pharmaderm).
Isopto Eserine, Soln., (Alcon Laboratories).
Eserine Salicylate, Soln., (Alcon Laboratories).
Use: Muscle stimulants.
See: Prostigin, Tab., (Roche Laboratories).
Neostigine Methylsulfate, Inj., (Various Mfr.).
Prostigin, Inj., (Roche Laboratories).

choline theophyllinate.
See: Oxtriphylline.

Cholinoid. (Zenith Goldline) Choline 111 mg, inositol 111 mg, vitamins B_1 0.33 mg, B_2 0.33 mg, B_3 3.33 mg, B_5 1.7 mg, B_6 0.33 mg, B_{12} 1.7 mcg, C 100 mg, lemon bioflavonoid complex 100 mg/Cap. Bot. 100s. *otc.*
Use: Lipid, vitamin supplement.

Chol Meth in B. (Esco) Choline bitartrate 235 mg, inositol 112 mg, methionine 70 mg, betaine anhydrous 50 mg, vitamins B_{12} 6 mcg, B_1 6 mg, B_6 3 mg, niacin 10 mg/Cap. Bot. 500s, 1000s. *otc.*
Use: Vitamin supplement.

Cholografin Meglumine. (Bristol-Myers Squibb) Iodipamide meglumine **10.3%** (iodine 5.1%)/100 ml, Vial 100 ml. **52%** (26% iodine)/20 ml, Vial 20 ml.
Use: Radiopaque agent.

Cholografin Sodium.

Choloxin. (Knoll Pharmaceuticals) Sodium dextrothyroxine 1 mg/Tab. Bot. 100s. *Rx.*
Use: Antihyperlipidemic.

cholylglycine.
See: CG RIA, Kit (Abbott Laboratories).

chondodendron tomentosum.
See: Curare.

Chondroitinase. (Storz Ophthalmics).
Use: Surgical aid, ophthalmic. [Orphan Drug]

chondrotin sulfate and sodium hyaluronate. A surgical aid in anterior segent procedures including cataract extraction and intraocular lens implantation. *Rx.*
See: Viscoat, Soln., (Cilco).

chondrus. Irish Moss.
W/Petrolatum, Liq.
See: Kondremul, Liq. (Medeva).

Chooz. (Schering Plough) Calcium carbonate 500 mg/Gum tab. Pkg. 16s. *otc.*
Use: Antacid.

Chorex 5. (Hyrex) Chorionic gonadotropin 5000 units, mannitol, benzyl alcohol 0.9%/Vial 10 ml. *Rx.*
Use: Hormone, chorionic gonadotropin.

Chorex 10. (Hyrex) Chorionic gonadotropin 10,000 units. Mannitol, benzyl alcohol 0.9%/Vial 10 ml. *Rx.*
Use: Hormone, chorionic gonadotropin.

chorionic gonadotropin. 5000 units/ Vial w/diluent 10 ml, 10,000 units/Vial w/ diluent 10 ml, 20,000 units/vial w/diluent 10 ml (Various) mannitol, benzyl alcohol 0.9%/10 ml. Vial.
Use: Prepubertal cryptorchidism or induction of ovulation and pregnancy in anovulatory women.
See: Antuitrin-S (Parke-Davis).
A.P.L., Inj. (Wyeth Ayerst).
C-G-10, Vial (Scrip).
Chorex 5, Vial (Hyrex).
Chorex 10, Vial (Hyrex).
Choron 10, Vial (Forest Pharmaceutical).
Gonadex (Continental Dist.).
Gonic, Vial (Hauck).
Khorion (Hickam).
Neovital-Diluent, Inj. (Taylor Pharmaceuticals).
Pregnyl, Vial (Orgamon).
Profasi, Vial (Serono Labs).

Choron 10. (Forest Pharmaceutical) Chorionic gonadotropin 10,000 units/ vial with diluent 10 ml, mannitol, benzyl alcohol 0.9%/Inj. Vial 10 ml. *Rx.*
Use: Hormone, chorionic gonadotropin.

Chromagen. (Savage) **Cap.:** Ferrous fumarate 66 mg, vitamins C 250 mg, B_{12} activity 10 mcg, desiccated stomach substances 100 mg/soft gelatin cap. Bot. 100s, 500s. *Rx.*
Use: Mineral, vitamin supplement.

Chromagen FA. (Savage Labs) Fe 66 mg, vitamin C 250 mg, folic acid 1 mg, B_{12} 10 mcg. Cap. UD 100s. *Rx.*
Use: Mineral, vitamin supplement.

Chromagen Forte. (Savage Labs) Fe 151 mg, vitamin C 60 mg, folic acid 1 mg, B_{12} 10 mcg. Cap. UD 100s. *Rx.*
Use: Mineral, vitamin supplement.

Chroma-Pak. (SoloPak) Chromium **4 mcg/ml:** Vial 10 ml, 30 ml. **20 mcg/ml:** Vial 5 ml. *Rx.*

Use: Nutritional supplement, parenteral.
chromargyre.
See: Merbromin (Various Mfr.).
chromated. Solution (Cr^{51}).
See: Chromitope sodium (Bristol-Myers Squibb).
Chromelin Complexion Blender. (Summers) Dihydroxyacetone 5%, alcohol 50%. Bot. oz. *otc.*
Use: Hyperpigmenting.
chromic acid, disodium salt. Sodium Chromate Cr^{51} Inj., U.S.P. 23.
•**chromic chloride.** U.S.P. 23.
Use: Supplement (trace mineral).
See: Chrometrace, Inj. (Centeon).
•**chromic chloride Cr^{51}.** USAN.
Use: Radiopharmaceutical.
See: Chromitope Cl (Bristol-Myers Squibb).
•**chromic phosphate Cr^{51}.** USAN.
Use: Radiopharmaceutical.
•**chromic phosphate P^{32} suspension.** U.S.P. 23.
Use: Radiopharmaceutical.
Chromitope Sodium. (Bristol-Myers Squibb) Chromate Cr^{51}, Sodium for Inj. 0.25 mCi.
Use: Radiopharmaceutical.
chromium. A trace metal used in IV nutritional therapy that helps maintain normal glucose metabolism and peripheral nerve function.
See: Chromium, Inj. (Various Mfr.).
Chromic Chloride, Inj. (Various Mfr.).
Chromium Chloride, Inj. (Various Mfr.).
Chroma-Pak, Inj. (Solopak).
Chromium Trace Metal Additive, Inj. (IMS, Ltd.).
Concentrated Chromic Chloride, Inj. (American Regent).
•**chromonar hydrochloride.** (KROE-moe-nahr) USAN.
Use: Coronary vasodilator.
Chronulac. (Hoechst Marion Roussel) Lactulose 10 g/15 ml (< 2.2 g galactose, 1.2 g lactose, 1.2 g other sugars). Bot. 473 ml, 1890 ml, UD 15 ml, 30 ml. Box 100s. *Rx.*
Use: Laxative.
chrysazin.
See: Danthron, N.F. 18.
Chur-Hist. (Churchill) Chlorpheniramine 4 mg/Kaptab. Bot. 100s.
Use: Antihistamine.
Chymex. (Pharmacia & Upjohn) Bentiromide 500 mg/7.5 ml w/propylene glycol 40%. Screening test for pancreatic exocrine insufficiency.
Use: Diagnostic aid.
Chymodiactin. (Smith & Nephew United) 4 nKat units, 1.4 mg sodium L-cysteinate HCl with diluent. Pow. for Inj. Vial 2 ml. *Rx.*
Use: Proteolytic enzyme.
•**chymopapain.** (KIE-moe-pap-ANE) USAN.
Use: Proteolytic enzyme.
•**chymotrypsin.** (kye-moe-TRIP-sin) U.S.P. 23.
Use: Proteolytic enzyme.
See: Catarase, Soln. (Ciba Vision Ophthalmics).
W/Trypsin.
See: Orenzyme, Tab. (Hoechst Marion Roussel).
W/Trypsin, neomycin palmitate.
See: Biozyme, Oint. (Centeon).
Cibacalcin. (Novartis) Calcitonin-human for injection.
Use: Paget's disease. [Orphan drug]
C.I. Basic Violet 3. Gentian Violet, U.S.P. 23.
Ciba Vision Cleaner. (Ciba Vision Ophthalmics) Cocoamphocarboxyglycinate, sodium lauryl sulfate, sorbic acid 0.1%, hexylene glycol, EDTA 0.2%. Soln. 5 ml or 15 ml. *otc.*
Use: Contact lens care.
Ciba Vision Saline. (Ciba Vision Ophthalmics) Buffered, isotonic with NaCl, boric acid. Soln. Bot. 90 ml, 240 ml, 360 ml. *otc.*
Use: Contact lens care, rinsing, storage.
cibenzoline. (SIGH-BEN-zoe-leen)
See: Cifenline Succinate. USAN.
•**ciclafrine hydrochloride.** (SICK-lah-freen) USAN.
Use: Antihypotensive.
•**ciclazindol.** (sigh-CLAY-zin-dole) USAN.
Use: Antidepressant.
•**cicletanine.** (sick-LET-ah-neen) USAN.
Use: Antihypertensive.
•**ciclopirox.** (sigh-kloe-PEER-ox) USAN.
Use: Antifungal.
•**ciclopirox olamine.** (sigh-kloe-PEER-ox OLE-ah-meen) U.S.P. 23.
Use: Antifungal.
See: Loprox, Cream (Hoechst Marion Roussel).
•**cicloprofen.** (SICK-low-pro-fen) USAN.
Use: Anti-inflammatory.
•**cicloprolol hydrochloride.** (SIGH-kloe-PRO-lahl) USAN.
Use: Anti-adrenergic (β receptor).
Cidex. (Johnson & Johnson Consumer Products) Activated dialdehyde soln.

Bot. qt, gal, 2.5 gal.
Use: Disinfectant, sterlizing.

Cidex-7. (Johnson & Johnson Consumer Products) Glutaraldehyde 2% and vial of activator with aqueous potassium salt as buffer and sodium nitrite as a corrosive inhibitor. Soln. Bot. qt, 1 gal, 5 gal.
Use: Disinfectant, sterilizing.

Cidex Plus. (Johnson & Johnson Consumer Products) 3.2% glutaraldehyde. Soln. Gal.
Use: Disinfectant, sterilizing.

C.I. Direct Blue 53 Tetrasodium Salt. Evans Blue, U.S.P. 23. *Rx.*

•**cidofovir.** (sigh-DAH-fah-vihr) USAN
Use: Antiviral.
See: Vistide (Gilead Sciences).

•**cidoxepin hydrochoride.** (sih-DOX-eh-PIN) USAN.
Use: Antidepressant.

•**cifenline.** (sigh-FEN-leen) USAN. *Formerly cibenzoline.*
Use: Cardiovascular (antiarrhythmic).

•**cifenline succinate.** (sigh-FEN-leen) USAN.
Use: Cardiovascular agent (antiarrhythmic).

•**ciglitazone.** (sigh-GLIE-tah-ZONE) USAN.
Use: Antidiabetic.

cignolin.
See: Anthralin (Various Mfr.).

•**ciladopa hydrochloride.** (SIGH-lah-doe-pah) USAN.
Use: Antiparkinsonian, dopaminergic.

cilastatin-imipenem. A formulation of imipenem, a thienamycin antibiotic, and cilastatin sodium, the inhibitor of the renal dipeptidase, dehydropeptidase-1.
Use: Anti-infective.
See: Primaxin I.V., Pow. (Merck).
Primaxin I.M., Pow. (Merck).

•**cilastatin sodium.** (SIGH-lah-STAT-in) U.S.P. 23.
Use: Enzyme inhibitor.
W/Imipenem.
See: Primaxin, Inj. (Merck).

•**cilazapril.** (sile-AZE-ah-PRILL) USAN.
Use: Antihypertensive.

•**cilexetil.** (sigh-LEX-eh-till) USAN.
Use: Anti-infective.

Cilfomide Tablets. (Sanofi Winthrop) Inositol hexanicotinate. *Rx.*
Use: Hypolipidimic, peripheral vasodilator.

ciliary neutrotrophic factor (recombinant human). (Regeneron Pharm)
Use: Treatment of motor neuron disease. [Orphan drug]

Cillium. (Whiteworth Towne) Psyllium seed husk pow. 4.94 g, 14 calories/rounded tsp. Bot. 420 g, 630 g. *otc.*
Use: Laxative.

•**cilmostim.** (SILL-moe-stim) USAN. *Formerly rhM-CSF, M-CSF, CSF-1.*
Use: Hematopoietic (macrophage colony-stimulating factor).

•**cilobamine mesylate.** (SIGH-low-BAM-een) USAN. *Formerly clobamine mesylate.*
Use: Antidepressant.

•**cilofungin.** (SIGH-low-FUN-jin) USAN.
Use: Antifungal.

•**cilostazol.** (sill-OH-stah-zole) USAN.
Use: Antithrombotic; platelet inhibitor; vasodilator.

Ciloxan. (Alcon Laboratories) Ciprofloxacin HCl 3.5 mg (equivalent to 3 mg base)/ml. Soln., Drop-Tainer dispensers. 2.5 ml, 5 ml. *Rx.*
Use: Anti-infective.

•**cimaterol.** (sigh-MAH-teh-role) USAN.
Use: Repartitioning agent.

•**cimetidine.** (sigh-MET-ih-deen) U.S.P. 23.
Use: H_2 histamine antagonist.
See: Tagamet, Tab., Inj. (SmithKline Beecham Pharmaceuticals).

cimetidine. (Various Mfr.) 200 mg, 300 mg, 400 mg, 800 mg/Tab. Bot. 30s, 50s, 100s, 500s, 1000s.
Use: Histamine H_2 receptor antagonist.

•**cimetidine hydrochloride.** (sigh-MET-ih-deen) USAN.
Use: Histamine H_2-receptor antagonist

cimetidine hydrochloride. (sigh-MET-ih-deen) (Endo Labs) Cimetidine HCl 150 mg, phenol 5 mg/ml. Inj. In 2 ml vials and 8 ml multiple dose vials. *Rx.*
Use: Histamine H_2 antagonist.

cimetidine. (Endo) Cimetidine 150 mg, phenol 5 mg/ml. Inj. Vial 2 ml. Multidose vial 8 ml. *Rx.*
Use: Histamine H_2 receptor antagonist.

cimetidine oral solution. (sigh-MET-ih-deen) (Alpharma USPD) 300 mg (as HCl)/5 ml. Bot. 240 ml, 470 ml. *Rx.*
Use: Histamine H_2 antagonist.

Cinacort Span. (Foy) Triamcinolone acetonide 40 mg/ml. Vial 5 ml. *Rx.*
Use: Corticosteroid.

•**cinalukast.** (sin-ah-LOO-kast) USAN.
Use: Antiasthmatic (leukotriene antagonist).

•**cinanserin hydrochloride.** (sin-AN-ser-in) USAN.
Use: Serotonin inhibitor.

cinchona bark. (Various Mfr.).
Use: Antimalarial, tonic.
W/Anhydrous quinine, cinchonidine, cinchonine, quinidine, quinine.
See: Totaquine, Pow. (Various Mfr.).
W/Iron oxide, nux vomica, vitamin B_1, alcohol.
See: Briatonic, Liq. (Briar).

cinchonidine sulfate.

cinchonine salts. (Various Mfr.).
Use: Quinine dihydrochloride.

cinchophen.
Use: Analgesic.

•**cinepazet maleate.** (SIN-eh-PAZZ-ett) USAN.
Use: Antianginal.

•**cinflumide.** (SIN-flew-mide) USAN.
Use: Muscle relaxant.

•**cingestol.** (sin-JESS-tole) USAN.
Use: Hormone, progestin.

cinnamaldehyde. N.F. IX.

•**cinnamedrine.** (sin-am-ED-reen) USAN.
Use: Muscle relaxant.
See: Midol, Tab. (Bayer Corp).

cinnamic aldehyde. Name previously used for Cinnamaldehyde.

cinnamon. N.F. XVI.
Use: Flavoring.

cinnamon oil. N.F. XVI. (Various Mfr.).
Use: Pharmaceutic aid.

cinnamyl ephedrine hydrochloride.
W/Acetaminophen, homatropine methylbromide.
See: Periodic, Cap. (Towne).

•**cinnarizine.** (sin-NAHR-ih-zeen) USAN.
Use: Antihistamine.

cinnopentazone. INN for Cintazone.

Cinobac. (Oclassen) Cinoxacin **250 mg/Cap.:** Bot. 40s. **500 mg/Cap.:** Bot. 50s. *Rx.*
Use: Anti-infective, urinary.

•**cinoxate.** (sin-OX-ate) U.S.P. 23.
Use: Ultraviolet screen.
W/Methyl anthranilate.
See: Maxafil Cream (Rydelle).

•**cinperene.** (SIN-peh-reen) USAN.
Use: Antipsychotic.

Cin-Quin. (Solvay) Quinidine sulfate. (Contains 83% anhydrous quinidine alkaloid.) **Tab.:** 100 mg, 200 mg or 300 mg. Bot. 100s, 1000s, UD 100s. **Cap.:** 200 mg. Bot. 100s. 300 mg. Bot. 100s, 1000s, UD 100s. *Rx.*
Use: Antiarrhythmic.

•**cinromide.** (SIN-row-mide) USAN.
Use: Anticonvulsant.

•**cintazone.** (SIN-tah-zone) USAN.
Use: Anti-inflammatory.

•**cintriamide.** (sin-TRY-ah-mid) USAN.
Use: Antipsychotic.

•**cioteronel.** (SIGH-oh-TEH-row-nell) USAN.
Use: Dermatologic, acne; androgenic alopecia and keloid (antiandrogen).

•**cipamfylline.** (sigh-PAM-fih-lin) USAN.
Use: Antiviral.

Cipralan. (Roche Laboratories) Cifenline succinate, formerly cibenzoline. *Rx.*
Use: Antiarrhythmic.

•**ciprefadol succinate.** (sih-PREH-fah-dahl) USAN.
Use: Analgesic.

Cipro. (Bayer Corp) Ciprofloxacin HCl 100 mg, 250 mg, 500 mg or 750 mg/Tab. Bot. 50s (750 mg only), 100s (except 750 mg), UD 100s, 100 mg in *Cipro Cystitis Packs* 6s. *Rx.*
Use: Anti-infective, fluoroquinolone.

Cipro HC Otic. (Bayer) Ciprofloxacin 2 mg, hydrocortisone 10 mg/ml, benzyl alcohol. Susp. Bot. 10 ml. *Rx.*
Use: Otic preparation.

Cipro I.V.. (Bayer Corp) Ciprofloxacin 200 mg and 400 mg (with lactic acid): Inj. Vial: 20 ml (1%), 40 ml (1%). Flex Bot.: 100 ml (in 5% dextrose) and 200 ml (in 5% dextrose). *Rx.*
Use: Anti-infective, fluoroquinolone.

•**ciprocinonide.** (sih-PRO-SIN-oh-nide) USAN.
Use: Adrenocortical steroid.

•**ciprofibrate.** (sip-ROW-FIE-brate) USAN.
Use: Antihyperlipoproteinemic.

•**ciprofloxacin.** (sip-ROW-FLOX-ah-sin) U.S.P. 23.
Use: Anti-infective.

•**ciprofloxacin hydrochloride.** (sip-ROW-FLOX-ah-sin) U.S.P. 23.
Use: Anti-infective.
See: Ciloxan, Soln. (Alcon Laboratories).
Cipro Preps. (Bayer Corp).

•**ciprostene calcium.** (sigh-PRAHS-teen) USAN.
Use: Platelet aggregation inhibitor.

•**ciramadol.** (sihr-AM-ah-dole) USAN.
Use: Analgesic.

•**ciramadol hydrochloride.** (sihr-AM-ah-dole) USAN.
Use: Analgesic.

Cirbed. (Boyd) Papaverine HCl 150 mg/Cap. Bot. 100s. *Rx.*
Use: Antispasmodic.

Circavite-T. (Circle) Iron 12 mg, vitamins A 10,000 IU, D 400 IU, E 15 mg, B_1 10.3 mg, B_2 10 mg, B_3 100 mg, B_5 18.4 mg,

B_6 4.1 mg, B_{12} 5 mcg, C 200 mg, Cu, I, Mg, Mn, zinc 1.5 mg. Bot. 100s. *otc.*
Use: Mineral, vitamin supplement.

•**cirolemycin.** (sih-ROW-leh-MY-sin) USAN.
Use: Anti-infective, antineoplastic.

•**cisapride.** (SIS-uh-PRIDE) USAN.
Use: Gastrointestinal, stimulant (peristaltic).
See: Propulsid, Tab. (Janssen).

•**cisatracurium besylate.** (sis-ah-trah-CURE-ee-uhm BESS-ih-late) USAN.
Use: Nondepolarizing neuromuscular blocking agent; muscle relaxant.
See: Nimbex, Inj. (GlaxoWellcome).

•**cisconazole.** (SIS-KOE-nah-zahl) USAN.
Use: Antifungal.

•**cisplatin.** (SIS-plat-in) U.S.P. 23. *Formerly cis-* Platinum II.
Use: Antineoplastic.
See: Platinol, Inj. (Bristol-Myers Squibb).

cis-retinoic acid. (13-cis-Retinoic Acid). *Rx.*
Use: Antiacne.
See: Isotretinoin.
Accutane (Roche Laboratories).

9-cis retinoic acid. (Allergan)
Use: Promyelocytic leukemia treatment; prevention of retinal detachment due to proliferative vitreoretinopathy. [Orphan drug]

citanest hydrochloride. (Astra) **Plain:** Prilocaine HCl 4%/1.8 ml dental cartridge. *Rx.*
Use: Anesthetic, local.

Citanest Hydrochloride Forte. (Astra) Prilocaine HCl 4% with epinephrine 1: 200,000. Contains sodium metabisulfite. Dental cartridge 1.8 ml. Inj. *Rx.*
Use: Anesthetic, local.

•**citenamide.** (sigh-TEN-ah-MIDE) USAN.
Use: Anticonvulsant.

Cithal Capsules. (Table Rock) Watermelon seed extract 2 gr, theobromine 4 gr, phenobarbital 0.25 gr/Cap. Bot. 100s, 500s. *Rx.*
Use: Antihypertensive.

•**citicoline sodium.** (SIGH-tih koe-leen) USAN.
Use: Post-stroke and post-head trauma treatment.

Citracal. (Mission Pharmacal) Calcium citrate 950 mg/Tab. Bot. 100s. *otc.*
Use: Calcium supplement.

Citracal 1500 + D. (Mission Pharmacal) Calcium citrate 1500 mg, vitamin D 200 IU/Tab. Bot. 60s. *otc.*
Use: Mineral, vitamin supplement.

Citracal Liquitab. (Mission Pharmacal) Calcium citrate 2376 mg/Effervescent tab. Box. 30s. *otc.*
Use: Mineral supplement.

Citra Forte. (Boyle) Hydrocodone bitartrate 5 mg, ascorbic acid 30 mg, pheniramine maleate 2.5 mg, pyrilamine maleate 3.33 mg, potassium citrate 150 mg/5 ml. Bot. pt, gal. *c-III.*
Use: Antihistamine, antitussive, vitamin supplement.

Citramin-500. (Thurston) Vitamin C 500 mg, rose hips, acerola with mixed bioflavonoids/Loz. Bot. 100s, 250s, 1000s. *otc.*
Use: Mineral, vitamin supplement.

Citranox. (Alconox)
Use: Liquid acid detergent for manual and ultrasonic washers.

Citra pH. (ValMed) Sodium citrate dihydrate 450 mg/30 ml. Soln. 30 ml. *otc.*
Use: Antacid.

Citrasan B. (Sandia) Lemon bioflavonoid complex 300 mg, vitamins C 300 mg, B_1 30 mg, B_2 10 mg, B_6 5 mg, B_{12} 4 mcg, calcium pantothenate 10 mg, niacinamide 50 mg/Tab. Bot. 100s, 1000s. *otc.*
Use: Mineral, vitamin supplement.

Citrasan K-250. (Sandia) Vitamins C 250 mg, K 1 mg, lemon bioflavonoid 250 mg/Tab. Bot. 100s, 1000s. *otc.*
Use: Vitamin supplement.

Citrasan K Liquid. (Sandia) Vitamins C 125 mg, K 0.66 mg, lemon bioflavonoid complex 125 mg/5 ml. Bot. pt, gal. *otc.*
Use: Vitamin supplement.

citrate acid.
See: Bicitra Soln. (Baker Norton).

citrate and citric acid solution.
Use: Alkalinizer.
See: Polycitra (Baker Norton).
Polycitra-LC (Baker Norton).
Polycitra-K (Baker Norton).
Oracit (Carolina Medical Products).
Bicitra (Baker Norton).

Citrate of Magnesia. (Various Mfr.) Magnesium citrate. Soln. Bot. 300 ml. *otc.*
Use: Laxative.

citrated normal human plasma.
See: Plasma, Normal Human.

Citresco-K. (Esco) Vitamins C 100 mg, K 0.7 mg, citrus bioflavonoid complex 100 mg/Cap. Bot. 100s, 500s, 1000s. *otc.*
Use: Vitamin supplement.

•**citric acid.** U.S.P. 23.
Use: Component of anticoagulant solu-

tions and drug products.

citric acid and d-gluconic acid irrigant.
Use: Irrigant, genitourinary. [Orphan drug]
See: Renacidin (Guardian Laboratories).

citric acid, glucono-delta-lactone and magnesium carbonate.
Use: Renal and bladder calculi of the apatite or struvite variety. [Orphan drug]

citric acid, magnesium oxide, and sodium carbonate irrigation.
Use: Irrigant, ophthalmic.

citrin.
See: Vitamin P.

Citrin Capsules. (Table Rock) Watermelon seed extract 4 gr/Cap. Bot. 100s, 500s. *Rx.*
Use: Antihypertensive.

Citrocarbonate. (Pharmacia & Upjohn) Sodium bicarbonate 0.78 g, sodium citrate anhydrous 1.82 g/3.9 g. Bot. 4 oz, 8 oz. *otc.*
Use: Antacid.

Citrocarbonate Effervescent Granules. (Roberts Pharm) Sodium bicarbonate 780 mg, sodium citrate anhydrous 1820 mg, sodium 700.6 mg/5 ml. Bot. 150 g. *otc.*
Use: Analgesic, antacid.

Citro Cee, Super. (Marlyn) Bioflavonoids 500 mg, rutin 50 mg, vitamin C 500 mg, rose hips powder 500 mg/Tab. Bot. 50s, 100s. *otc.*
Use: Vitamin supplement.

Citro-Flav 200. (Zenith Goldline) Citrus bioflavonoid compound 200 mg/Cap. Bot. 100s, 1000s. *otc.*
Use: Vitamin supplement.

Citroleum Sunburn Creme. (Citroleum) Bot. 4 oz.

Citrolith. (Beach Pharmaceuticals) Potassium citrate 50 mg, sodium citrate 950 mg/Tab. Bot. 100s, 500s. *Rx.*
Use: Alkalinizer, urinary.

Citroma. (Century Pharm) Magnesium citrate. Oral soln. Bot. 10 oz. *otc.*
Use: Laxative.

Citroma Low Sodium. (National Magnesia) Magnesium citrate. Oral soln w/lemon or cherry flavor in sugar-free vehicle. Bot. 10 oz. *otc.*
Use: Laxative.

Citrotein. (Novartis) Sucrose, pasteurized egg white solids, amino acids, maltodextrin, citric acid, natural and artificial flavors, mono and diglycerides, partially hydrogenated soybean oil, 0.66 cal/ml, protein 40.7 g, carbohydrate 120.7 g, fat 1.55 g, sodium 698 mg, potassium 698 mg/L. Tartrazine (orange flavor only). Pow. 1.57 oz/packet, Can 14.16 oz. Orange, grape and punch flavors. *otc.*
Use: Nutritional supplement, enteral.

citrovorum factor. Leucovorin Calcium, U.S.P. 23.
See: Leucovorin Calcium (ESI Lederle Generics) Folinic Acid.

Citrucel. (SmithKline Beecham Pharmaceuticals) Methylcellulose 2 g/heaping tbsp. dose w/citric acid. Bot. 16 oz, 30 oz. *otc.*
Use: Laxative.

Citrucel Sugar Free. (SmithKline Beecham Pharmaceuticals) Methylcellulose 2 g, aspartame, phenylalanine 52 mg. Pow. Can. 479 g. *otc.*
Use: Laxative.

citrus bioflavonoid compound.
See: Bioflavonoid Compounds (Various Mfr.).
C.V.P., Syr. (Rhone-Poulenc Rorer).
Vitamin P.
W/Ascorbic acid, phenyltoloxamine dihydrogen citrate, salicylamide, acetyl p-aminophenol, caffeine, racemic amphetamine sulfate.
See: Euphenex, Tab. (Westerfield).

Citrus-flav C 500. (Fibertone) Citrus bioflavonoids complex 200 mg, vitamin C 200 mg, hesperidin complex 40 mg, acerola 50 mg, rutin 10 mg, in citrus base of orange and lemon powder, grapefruit concentrate powder and citrus pectin. Tabs. Bot. 100s, 250s. *otc.*
Use: Nutritional supplement.

C-Ject. (Lincoln) Ascorbic acid 2000 mg, sodium bisulfite 0.1%, disodium sequestrene 0.01%/10 ml. Amp. 10 ml, "Score-Break" Box 25s. *Rx.*
Use: Nutritional supplement.

C-Ject with B. (Lincoln) When mixed with 10 ml of diluent, each vial contains: Vitamins C 2000 mg, B_1 50 mg, B_2 5 mg, B_6 10 mg, nicotinamide 100 mg, methylparaben 0.89 mg, propylparaben 0.22 mg, sodium bisulfite 10 mg, disodium sequestrene 1 mg. Box of 6 lyophilized plugs and 6 10 ml vials of Sterile Diluent. *Rx.*
Use: Nutritional supplement.

CKA Canker Aid. (Pannett Prod.) Benzocaine, aluminum hydrate, magnesium trisilicate, sodium acid carbonate. Pow. *otc.*
Use: Cancer, coldsores.

CK(CPK) Reagent Strips. (Bayer Corp) Seralyzer reagent strips for creatinine phosphokinase in serum or plasma. Bot. 25s.
Use: Diagnostic aid.

•**cladribine.** (KLAD-rih-BEAN) USAN.
Use: Antineoplastic. [Orphan drug]
See: Leustatin (Ortho Biotech).

Claforan. (Hoechst Marion Roussel) Cefotaxime sodium **Pow. for Inj.:** 500 mg/Vial Pkg. 10s. 1 g, 2 g Vial. Pkg. 10s, 25s, 50s. Infusion bot. 10s, *ADD-Vantage* system vials 25s. 10g. Bot. **Inj.:** 1 g, 2 g. Premixed, frozen. 50 ml Pkg. 12s. *Rx.*
Use: Anti-infective, cephalosporin.

•**clamoxyquin hydrochloride.** (KLAM-OX-ee-kwin) USAN.
Use: Amebicide.

Claritin-12.
See: Vitamin B_{12}.

•**clarithromycin.** (kluh-RITH-row-MY-sin) U.S.P. 23.
Use: Anti-infective.
See: Biaxin, Tab; Gran. for Oral Susp. (Abbott).

clarithromycin. A semi-synthetic macrolide antibiotic. *Rx.*
Use: Anti-infective, antiulcerative, erythromycin.
See: Biaxin Tabs., Gran. for Oral Susp. (Abbott Laboratories).

Claritin. (Schering Plough) Loratadine 10 mg, lactose/Tab. Bot. 100s, 500s, unit-of-use 14s, 30s and UD 100s. Loratadine 1 mg/ml. Syr. Bot. 16 oz. Loratadine 10 mg, mannitol/Reditabs. Unit-of-use 30s. *Rx.*
Use: Antihistamine.

Claritin-D. (Schering Plough) Loratadine 5 mg, pseudoephedrine sulfate 120 mg. Tab, SR Tab. Bot. 30s, 100s, unit-of-use 10s, 30s, UD 100s. *Rx.*
Use: Antihistamine, decongestant.

Claritin-D 24-Hour. (Schering Plough) Loratadine 10 mg, pseudoephedrine sulfate 240 mg/ER Tab. Bot. 100s, UD 100s. *Rx.*
Use: Antihistamine, decongestant.

•**clavulanate potassium.** (CLAV-you-lah-nate) U.S.P. 23.
Use: Inhibitor (β-lactamase).

clavulanate potassium, sterile. (CLAV-you-lah-nate)
Use: Inhibitor (β-lactamase).

clavulanate potassium and ticarcillin.
Use: Anti-infective, pencillin.
See: Timentin, Pow. for Inj. (SmithKline Beecham Pharmaceuticals).
Timentin, Soln. (SmithKline Beecham Pharmaceuticals).

clavulanic acid/amoxicillin.
Use: Anti-infective, penicillin.
See: Augmentin Tab. (SmithKline Beecham Pharmaceuticals).

clavulanic acid/ticarcillin.
Use: Anti-infective, penicillin.
See: Timentin Pow. for Inj. (SmithKline Beecham Pharmaceuticals).

•**clazolam.** (CLAY-zoe-lam) USAN.
Use: Anxiolytic.

•**clazolimine.** (clay-ZOLE-ih-meen) USAN.
Use: Diuretic.

Clean-N-Soak. (Allergan) Cleaning agent with phenylmercuric nitrate 0.004%. Bot. 120 ml. *otc.*
Use: Contact lens care.

Clearasil 10%. (Proter & Gamble) Benzoyl peroxide 10%. Bot. oz. *otc.*
Use: Dermatologic, acne.

Clearasil Adult Care Cream. (Procter & Gamble) Sulfur, resorcinol, alcohol 10%, parabens. Cream. Tube. 17 g. *otc.*
Use: Dermatologic, acne.

Clearasil Adult Care Medicated Blemish Stick. (Procter & Gamble) Sulfur 8%, resorcinol 1%, bentonite 4%, laureth-4, titanium dioxide. Stick ⅛ oz. *otc.*
Use: Dermatologic, acne.

Clearasil Antibacterial Soap. (Procter & Gamble) Triclosan 0.75%, 92 g. *otc.*
Use: Dermatologic, acne.

Clearasil Clearstick, Maximum Strength. (Procter & Gamble) Salicylic acid 2%, alcohol 39%, menthol, EDTA. Liq. 35 ml. *otc.*
Use: Dermatologic, acne.

Clearasil Clearstick, Regular Strength. (Procter & Gamble) Salicylic acid 1.25%, alcohol 39%, aloe vera gel, menthol, EDTA. Liq. 35 ml. *otc.*
Use: Dermatologic, acne.

Clearasil Clearstick for Sensitive Skin, Maximum Strength. (Procter & Gamble) Salicylic acid 2%, alcohol 39%, aloe vera gel, menthol, EDTA. Liq. 35 ml. *otc.*
Use: Dermatologic, acne.

Clearasil Daily Face Wash. (Procter & Gamble) Triclosan 0.3%, glycerin, aloe vera gel, EDTA. Liq. Bot. 135 ml. *otc.*
Use: Dermatologic, acne.

Clearasil Double Clear. (Procter & Gamble) **Pads, maximum strength:** Salicylic acid 2%, alcohol 40%, witch hazel distillate, menthol, Jar 32s. **Pads,**

regular strength: Salicylic acid 1.25%, alcohol 40%, witch hazel distillate, menthol. Jar 32s. *otc.*
Use: Dermatologic, acne.

Clearasil Double Textured Pads. (Procter & Gamble) **Pads, regular strength:** Salicylic acid 2%, alcohol 40%, glycerin, aloe vera gel, EDTA. In 32s, 40s. **Pads, maximum strength:** Salicylic acid 2%, alcohol 40%, menthol, aloe vera gel, EDTA. In 32s, 40s. *otc.*
Use: Dermatologic, acne.

Clearasil Maximum Strength Cream. (Procter & Gamble) Benzoyl peroxide 10%, parabens in tinted or vanishing base. Tube 18 g, 28 g. *otc.*
Use: Dermatologic, acne.

Clearasil Maximum Strength Lotion. (Procter & Gamble) Benzoyl peroxide 10%, cetyl alcohol, parabens in vanishing base. Bot. 29 ml. *otc.*
Use: Dermatologic, acne.

Clearasil Medicated Deep Cleanser. (Procter & Gamble) Salicylic acid 0.5%, alcohol 42%, menthol, EDTA, aloe vera gel, hydrogenated castor oil. Liq. Bot. 229 ml. *otc.*
Use: Dermatologic, acne.

Clear Away. (Schering Plough) Salicyclic acid 40%. Disc Pck. 18s. *otc.*
Use: Dermatologic, acne.

Clear Away Plantar. (Schering Plough) Salicyclic acid 40%. Disc (for feet) Pck. 24s. *otc.*
Use: Dermatologic, acne.

Clearblue Easy. (Whitehall Robins) Dip stick for in-home pregnancy test. Kit 1, 2s.
Use: Diagnostic aid.

Clearblue Pregnancy Test. (VLI) Dip stick for pregnancy test. Kit 2s.
Use: Diagnostic aid.

Clearex Acne Cream. (Health for Life Brands) Allantoin, sulfur, resorcinol, d-panthenol, isopropanol. Tube 1.5 oz. *otc.*
Use: Dermatologic, acne.

Clear Eyes ACR Eye Drops. (Ross Laboratories) Naphazoline HCl 0.012%. Bot. 15 ml, 30 ml. *otc.*
Use: Mydriatic, vasoconstrictor.

Clear Eyes Eye Drops. (Ross Laboratories) Naphazoline HCl 0.012%. Bot. 15 ml, 30 ml. *otc.*
Use: Mydriatic vasoconstrictor.

Clearly Cala-Gel. (Tec Labs) Diphenhydramine HCl, zinc acetate, menthol, EDTA. Gel In 180 g. *otc.*
Use: Antipruritic, topical.

Clearplan. (VLI) Ovulation prediction test. Box 10s.
Use: Diagnostic aid.

Clear Total Lice Elimination System. (Care Technologies) **Shampoo:** Pyrethrum extract 0.3%, piperonyl butoxide 3%. 2 ml, 4 ml. **Lice egg remover:** Enzymes including oxidoreductase, tranferase, lyase, hydrolase, isomerase, ligase and hydroxyethyl cellulose, sodium benzoate. *otc.*
Use: Pediculicide.

Clear Tussin 30. (Zenith Goldline) Dextromethorphan HBr 15 mg, guaifenesin 100 mg/5 ml, alcohol, dye, sugar free/Liq. Bot. 118 ml. *otc.*
Use: Decongestant, expectorant.

•**clebopride.** (KLEH-boe-PRIDE) USAN.
Use: Antiemetic.

•**clemastine.** (KLEM-ass-teen) USAN.
Use: Antihistamine.
See: Tavist, Tab., Syr. (Novartis).

•**clemastine fumarate.** (KLEM-ass-teen) U.S.P. 23.
Use: Antihistamine.
See: Tavist, Tab., Syr. (Novartis)

clemastine fumarate. (Various Mfr.) Clemastine fumarate 0.5 mg/5 ml Syr. Bot. 118 ml, 480 ml. 1.34 mg, 2.68 mg/Tab. Bot. 100s; 500s, 1000s (2.68 mg only). *Rx. otc.*
Use: Antihistamine.

clemastine fumarate w/combinations.
See: Antihist-D, Tab. (Zenith Goldline)

clemizole hydrochloride.

Clens. (Alcon Laboratories) Cleansing agent with benzalkonium Cl 0.02%, EDTA 0.1%. Soln. Bot. 60 ml. *otc.*
Use: Contact lens care.

•**clentiazem maleate.** (klen-TIE-ah-zem) USAN.
Use: Antianginal, antihypertensive, antagonist (calcium channel).

Cleocin Hydrochloride. (Pharmacia & Upjohn) Clindamycin HCl 75 mg, 150 mg or 300 mg/Cap. Tartrazine. Bot. 100s. (75 mg); 16s, 100s, UD 100s (150 mg, 300 mg). *Rx.*
Use: Anti-infective.

Cleocin Pediatric. (Pharmacia & Upjohn) Clindamycin palmitate HCl equivalent to clindamycin 75 mg/5 ml when reconstituted as directed. Bot. 100 ml. *Rx.*
Use: Anti-infective.

Cleocin Phosphate. (Pharmacia & Upjohn) Clindamycin phosphate equivalent to clindamycin 150 mg/ml. **300 mg:** Vial 2 ml w/disodium edetate 1 mg,

benzyl alcohol 18.9 mg. Pack 25s, 100s. **600 mg:** Vial 4 ml w/disodium edetate 2 mg, benzyl alcohol 37.8 mg. Pack 25s, 100s. **900 mg:** Vial 6 ml. Pack 25s, 100s. **9000 mg:** Bulk Vial 60 ml. Pack 5s. *Rx.*
Use: Anti-infective.

Cleocin T. (Pharmacia & Upjohn) Clindamycin phosphate 10 mg/ml. Topical soln., gel, lot. Bot. 30 ml, 60 ml, pt. (topical soln.). Bot. 7.5 g, 30 g (gel). Lot. Bot. 60 ml (lotion). *Rx.*
Use: Anti-infective.

Cleocin Vaginal. (Pharmacia & Upjohn) Clindamycin phosphate 2%, mineral oil, benzyl alcohol, propylene glycol, polysorbate 60, sorbitan, monostearate. Cream. Tube with 7 disposable applicators 40 g. *Rx.*
Use: Anti-infective, vaginal.

Clerz Drops for Hard Lenses. (Ciba Vision Ophthalmics) Hypertonic solution with hydroxyethylcellulose, sorbic acid, poloxamer 407, EDTA 0.1%, thimerosal 0.001%. Soln. Bot. 25 ml. *otc.*
Use: Contact lens care.

Clerz Drops for Soft Lenses. (Ciba Vision Ophthalmics) Hypertonic solution with hydroxyethylcellulose, sodium borate, poloxamer 407, sorbic acid, thimerosal 0.001%, EDTA 0.1%. Soln. Bot. 25 ml. *otc.*
Use: Contact lens care.

Clerz 2 for Hard Lenses. (Ciba Vision Ophthalmics) Isotonic solution with hydroxyethylcellulose, poloxamer 407, sodium Cl, potassium Cl, sodium borate, boric acid, sorbic acid, EDTA. Soln. Bot. 5 ml, 15 ml, 30 ml. *otc.*
Use: Contact lens care.

Clerz 2 for Soft Lenses. (Ciba Vision Ophthalmics) Isotonic solution with sodium Cl, potassium Cl, hydroxyethylcellulose, poloxamer 407, sodium borate, boric acid, sorbic acid, EDTA. Soln. Bot. 5 ml (2s), 15 ml, 30. *otc.*
Use: Contact lens care.

•**clidinium bromide.** (KLIH-dih-nee-uhm BROE-mide) U.S.P. 23.
Use: Anticholinergic.
See: Quarzan, Cap. (Roche Laboratories).

W/Chlordiazepoxide.
See: Librax, Cap. (Roche Laboratories).

Climara. (Berlex) Estradiol 3.9 mg or 7.8 mg/Transdermal Patch. In 4s. *Rx.*
Use: Estrogen.

•**clinafloxacin hydrochloride.** (klin-ah-FLOX-ah-sin) USAN.
Use: Anti-infective.

Clinda-Derm. (Paddock) Clindamycin phosphate 10 mg/ml, isopropyl alcohol 51.5%, propylene glycol. Soln. Bot. 60 ml. *Rx.*
Use: Dermatologic, acne.

•**clindamycin.** (KLIN-dah-MY-sin) USAN.
Use: Anti-infective, dermatologic, acne. Oral as antibiotic. Vaginal as anti-infective. AIDS associated pneumonia [Orphan drug]
See: Cleocin T (Pharmacia & Upjohn).
Cleocin (Pharmacia & Upjohn).
Cleocin Vaginal Cream (Pharmacia & Upjohn).
Clindets, Pledgets (Stiefel).

•**clindamycin hydrochloride.** (KLIN-dah-MY-sin) U.S.P. 23.
Use: Anti-infective.
See: Cleocin HCl A.D.T., Cap. (Pharmacia & Upjohn).

•**clindamycin palmitate hydrochloride.** (KLIN-dah-MY-sin PAL-mih-tate) U.S.P. 23.
Use: Anti-infective.
See: Cleocin Pediatric (Pharmacia & Upjohn).
Cleocin T, Liq. (Pharmacia & Upjohn).

•**clindamycin phosphate.** (KLIN-dah-MY-sin) U.S.P. 23.
Use: Anti-infective.
See: Cleocin phosphate, Inj. (Pharmacia & Upjohn).
Clinda-Derm, Soln. (Paddock).

clindamycin phosphate. (KLIN-dah-MY-sin) (Various Mfr.) Clindamycin phosphate 10 mg/ml. Topical Soln., gel, lotion. Bot. 30 ml, 60 ml (Topical Soln.). Tube 30 g (gel). Bot. 60 ml (lot.). *Rx.*
Use: Dermatologic, acne.

Clindets. (Stiefel) Clindamycin 190 (10 mg/ml). Pledgets. 60s. *Rx.*
Use: Anti-infective.

Clindex. (Rugby)
See: Chlordiazepoxide and clindinium bromide (Chelsea Labs).

Clinistix Reagent Strips. (Bayer Corp) Glucose oxidase, peroxidase and orthotolidine. Diagnostic test for glucose in urine. Bot. 50s.
Use: Diagnostic aid.

Clinitest. (Bayer Corp) 2-drop and 5-drop combination packages w/color charts for both 2-drop and 5-drop use. Reagent tablets containing copper sulfate, sodium hydroxide, heat-producing agents. Patient's plastic set; Tab. refills. **Box:** 100s, 500s, sealed in foil. **Child-resistant bot.:** 36s, 100s.
Use: Diagnostic aid.

Clinocaine Hydrochloride.
See: Procaine HCl.

Clinoril. (Merck) Sulindac 150 mg or 200 mg/Tab. Bot. 100s, UD 100s. Unit-of-use 60s, 100s. *Rx.*
Use: Analgesic, NSAID.

Clinoxide Capsules. (Geneva Pharm) Clidinium 2.5 mg, chlordiazepoxide HCl, 5 mg. Cap. Bot. 100s, 500s. *c-iv.*
Use: Gastrointestinal, anticholinergic.

•**clioquinol.** (Klye-oh-KWIN-ole) U.S.P. 23. *Formerly Iodochlorhydroxyquin.*
Use: Antiamebic, anti-infective, topical.
See: HCV Cream (Saron).
Quin III, Cream (Teva USA).
Quinoform, Oint., Cream, Lot. (C & M Pharmacal).
Vioform, Prep. (Novartis).
W/Aluminum acetate solution, hydrocortisone.
See: Hydrelt, Cream, Oint. (Zeneca).
Hysone, Cream (Roberts Pharm).
W/Hydrocortisone acetate, lidocaine.
See: Lidaform-HC, Creme, Lot. (Bayer Corp).
W/Hydrocortisone, lidocaine.
See: Bafil Lotion (Scruggs).
HIL-20 Lotion (Solvay).
W/Hydrocortisone, chlorobutanol.
See: Hc-Form, Jelly (Recsei).
W/Hydrocortisone, coal tar extract.
See: Racet LCD, Cream (Teva USA).
W/Hydrocortisone and pramoxine HCl.
See: Dermarex Cream (Hyrex).
Sherform-HC, Oint. (Sheryl).
Stera-Form Creme (Merz).
V-Cort, Cream (Scrip).
W/Methylcellulose, aluminum hydroxide, atropine sulfate, hyoscine HBr, hyoscyamine sulfate.
See: Enterex, Tab. (Person & Covey).
W/Nystatin.
See: Nystaform, Oint. (Bayer Corp).

clioquinol and hydrocortisone cream.
Use: Antifungal.
See: Bafil, Cream (Skruggs).
Caquin Cream (Forest Pharmaceutical).
Coidocort Cream (Coast).
Domeform-HC, Cream (Bayer Corp).
Hi-Form Cream (Blaine).
Hydrelt, Cream (Zeneca).
Hysone, Cream (Roberts Pharm).
Ido-Cortistan Oint. (Standex).
Iodocort, Cream (Ulmer).
Iohydro, Cream (Freeport).
Maso-Form, Cream (Mason).
Mity-Quin Cream (Solvay).
Racet, Cream (Teva USA).
Racet Forte, Cream (Teva USA).
Vioform-Hydrocortisone, Cream, Oint., Lot. (Novartis).
Vio-Hydrocort, Cream, Oint. (Quality Formulations).

clioquinol and hydrocortisone ointment.
Use: Antifungal.
See: Hysone, Cream (Roberts Pharm).
Vioform-Hydrocortisone, Cream, Oint., Lot. (Novartis).
Vio-Hydrocort, Cream, Oint. (Quality Formulations).

•**clioxanide.** (klie-OX-ah-nide) USAN.
Use: Anthelmintic.

Clipoxide. (Schein Pharmaceutical) Clidinium bromide 2.5 mg, chlordiazepoxide HCl 5 mg/Cap. Bot. 100s, 500s. *c-v.*
Use: Anticholinergic, antispasmodic.

•**cliprofen.** (klih-PRO-fen) USAN.
Use: Anti-inflammatory.

clobamine mesylate. (KLOE-bah-meen) Name previously used. See cilobamine mesylate.
Use: Antidepressant.

•**clobazam.** (KLOE-bazz-am) USAN.
Use: Anxiolytic.

clobenztropine.

•**clobetasol propionate.** (kloe-BEE-tah-sahl PRO-ee-oh-nate) U.S.P. 23.
Use: Anti-inflammatory.
See: Cormax, Oint. (Oclassen).
Temovate, Cream, Oint., Scalp application (Glaxo Dermatology).

clobetasol propionate. (Various Mfr.) **Cream:** 0.05%. Tube 15 g, 30 g, 45 g. **Ointment:** 0.05%, white petrolatum. 15 g, 30 g, 45 g.
Use: Corticosteroid, topical.

•**clobetasone butyrate.** (kloe-BEE-tih-sone BYOO-tah-rate) USAN.
Use: Corticosteroid, anti-inflammatory.

•**clocortolone acetate.** (kloe-CORE-toe-lone) USAN.
Use: Corticosteroid, topical.

•**clocortolone pivalate.** (kloe-CORE-toe-lone PIH-vah-late) U.S.P. 23.
Use: Corticosteroid, topical.

Clocream. (Pharmacia & Upjohn) Vitamins A and D in vanishing base. Tube oz. *otc.*
Use: Emollient.

•**clodanolene.** (Kloe-DAN-oh-leen) USAN.
Use: Muscle relaxant.

•**clodazon hydrochloride.** (KLOE-dah-zone) USAN.
Use: Antidepressant.

Cloderm. (Hermal) Clocortolone pivalate cream 0.1%. Tube 15 g, 45 g. *Rx.*

Use: Corticosteroid, topical.

•**clodronic acid.** (kloe-DRAHN-ik acid) USAN.
Use: Calcium regulator.

•**clofazimine.** (kloe-FAZZ-ih-meen) U.S.P. 23.
Use: Anti-infective (tuberculostatic, leprostatic). [Orphan drug]
See: Lamprene, Cap. (Novartis).

•**clofibrate.** (kloe-FIH-brate) U.S.P. 23.
Use: Antihyperlipidemic.
See: Atromid S, Cap. (Wyeth Ayerst).

•**clofilium phosphate.** (KLOE-FILL-ee-uhm) USAN.
Use: Cardiovascular agent (antiarrhythmic).

•**cloflucarban.** (KLOE-flew-CAR-ban) USAN.
Use: Antiseptic, disinfectant.

•**clogestone acetate.** (kloe-JESS-tone ASS-eh-tate) USAN. Under study.
Use: Hormone, progestin.

•**clomacran phosphate.** (KLOE-mah-KRAN) USAN. Under study.
Use: Antipsychotic.

•**clomegestone acetate.** (KLOE-meh-JESS-tone) USAN. Under study.
Use: Hormone, progestin.

•**clometherone.** (kloe-METH-ehr-OHN) USAN.
Use: Antiestrogen.

Clomid. (Hoechst Marion Roussel) Clomiphene citrate 50 mg/Tab. Carton 30s. *Rx.*
Use: Ovulation inducer.

•**clominorex.** (kloe-MEE-no-rex) USAN.
Use: Anorexic.

•**clomiphene citrate.** (KLOE-mih-feen SIH-trate) U.S.P. 23.
Use: Antiestrogen.
See: Clomid, Tab. (Hoechst Marion Roussel).
Milophene, Tab. (Milex).
Serophene, Tab. (Serono Labs).

clomiphene citrate. (Various Mfr.) 50 mg/Tab. Pkg. 10s, 30s. *Rx.*
Use: Ovulation inducer.

•**clomipramine hydrochloride.** (kloe-MIH-pruh-meen) USAN.
Use: Antidepressant.
See: Anafranil (Novartis).

clomipramine hydrochloride. (kloe-MIH-pruh-meen) (Apothecon) Clomipramine HCl 25 mg, 50 mg, 75 mg. Cap. Bot. 100s, 1000s. *Rx.*
Use: Antidepressant.

Clomycin. (Roberts Pharm) Bacitracin 500 U, neomycin sulfate equivalent to 3.5 mg neomycin base, polymyxin B sulfate 5000 U, lidocaine 40 mg, yellow petrolatum, anhydrous, lanolin, light mineral oil/g. Oint. Tube 30 g. *otc.*
Use: Anti-infective, topical.

•**clonazepam.** (kloe-NAY-ze-pam) U.S.P. 23.
Use: Anticonvulsant.
See: Klonopin, Tab. (Roche Laboratories).

clonazepam. 0.5 mg, 1 mg, 2 mg/Tab. Bot. 100s. *c-iv.*
Use: Anticonvulsant.

•**clonidine.** (KLOE-nih-DEEN) USAN.
Use: Antihypertensive.
See: Catapres (Boehringer Ingelheim).

•**clonidine hydrochloride.** (KLOE-nih-DEEN) U.S.P. 23.
Use: Antihypertensive. Epidural use for pain in cancer patients [Orphan drug]
See: Catapres, Tab. (Boehringer Ingelheim).
Duraclon, Inj. (Fujisawa).

clonidine hydrochloride and chlorthalidone tablets. (Various Mfr.) Clonidine HCl 0.1 mg, 0.2 mg or 0.3 mg, chlorthalidone 15 mg/Tab. Bot. 100s, 500s, 1000s.
Use: Antihypertensive; diuretic.
See: Combipres, Tab. (Boehringer Ingelheim).

•**clonitrate.** (KLOE-nye-trate) USAN.
Use: Coronary vasodilator.

•**clonixeril.** (kloe-NIX-ehr-ill) USAN.
Use: Analgesic.

•**clonixin.** (kloe-NIX-in) USAN.
Use: Analgesic.

•**clopamide.** (kloe-PAM-id) USAN.
Use: Antihypertensive, diuretic.
See: Aquex, Tab. (Lannett).

•**clopenthixol.** (KLOE-pen-THIX-ole) USAN.
Use: Antipsychotic.

•**cloperidone hydrochloride.** (KLOE-per-ih-dohn) USAN.
Use: Hypnotic, sedative.

clophedianol hydrochloride.
See: Acutuss, Tab., Expect. (Roxane).

clophenoxate hydrochloride.
Use: Cerebral stimulant.

•**clopidogrel bisulfate.** (kloe-PIH-doe-grell bye-SULL-fate)
Use: Platelet inhibitor.
See: Plavix, Tab. (Sanofi Winthrop).

•**clopimozide.** (KLOE-PIM-oh-zide) USAN.
Use: Antipsychotic.

•**clopipazan mesylate.** (KLOE-pip-ah-ZAN) USAN.
Use: Antipsychotic.

•**clopirac.** (KLOE-pih-rack) USAN.
Use: Anti-inflammatory.

•**cloprednol.** (kloe-PRED-nahl) USAN.
Use: Corticosteroid, topical.

•**cloprostenol sodium.** (kloe-PROSTE-een-ole) USAN.
Use: Prostaglandin.

•**clorazepate dipotassium.** (klor-AZE-eh-PATE DIE-poe-TASS-ee-uhm) U.S.P. 23.
Use: Anxiolytic, anticonvulsant.
See: Tranxene, Prods. (Abbott Laboratories).

clorazepate dipotassium. (Various Mfr.) 3.75 mg, 7.5 mg, 15 mg/Tab. Bot. 30s, 100s, 500s. *c-IV.*
Use: Anxiolytic, anticonvulsant.

•**clorazepate monopotassium.** (clor-AZE-eh-PATE MAHN-oh-poe-TASS-ee-uhm) USAN.
Use: Anxiolytic.

•**clorethate.** (klahr-ETH-ate) USAN.
Use: Hypnotic, sedative.

•**clorexolone.** (KLOR-ex-oh-LONE) USAN.
Use: Diuretic.
See: Nefrolan.

Clorfed II. (Stewart-Jackson) Chlorpheniramine 4 mg, pseudoephedrine 60 mg/Tab. Bot. 100s. *otc.*
Use: Antihistamine, decongestant.

Clorfed Capsules. (Stewart-Jackson) Chlorpheniramine 8 mg, pseudoephedrine 120 mg/Cap. Bot. 100s. *otc, Rx.*
Use: Antihistamine, decongestant.

Clorfed Expectorant. (Stewart-Jackson) Pseudoephedrine 30 mg, guaifensen 100 mg, codeine 10 mg. Bot. pt. *c-v.*
Use: Antitussive, decongestant, expectorant.

•**cloroperone hydrochloride.** (KLOR-oh-PURR-ohn) USAN.
Use: Antipsychotic.

•**clorophene.** (KLOR-oh-feen) USAN.
Use: Disinfectant.

Clorpactin WCS-90. (Guardian Laboratories) Sodium oxychlorosene. Bot. 2 g, 5s.
Use: Antiseptic.

•**clorprenaline hydrochloride.** (klor-PREN-ah-leen) USAN.
Use: Bronchodilator.

•**clorsulon.** (KLOR-sull-ahn) U.S.P. 23.
Use: Antiparasitic, fasciolicide.

•**clortermine hydrochloride.** (klor-TER-meen) USAN.
Use: Anorexic.

•**closantel.** (KLOSE-an-tell) USAN.
Use: Anthelmintic.

•**closiramine aceturate.** (kloe-SIH-rah-meen ah-SEE-tur-ate) USAN.
Use: Antihistamine.

clostridial collagenase.
Use: Dupuytren's disease. [Orphan drug]

•**clothiapine.** (KLOE-THIGH-ah-peen) USAN.
Use: Antipsychotic.

•**clothixamide maleate.** (kloe-THIX-ah-mid) USAN.
Use: Antipsychotic.

•**cloticasone propionate.** (kloe-TICK-ah-SONE PRO-pee-oh-nate) USAN.
Use: Anti-inflammatory.

•**clotrimazole.** (kloe-TRIM-uh-zole) U.S.P. 23.
Use: Antifungal.
See: FemCare, Vaginal Tab., Cream. (Schering Plough).
Fungoid, Cream, Soln. (Pedinol).
Gyne-Lotrimin, Cream, Vaginal Tab. (Schering Plough).
Gyne-Lotrimin Combination Pack. (Schering Plough).
Lotrimin, Cream, Soln. (Schering Plough).
Mycelex, Cream, Soln., Tab. (Bayer Corp).
Mycelex-7, Vaginal Cream, Tab. (Bayer Corp).
Mycelex-7 Combination Pack (Bayer Corp).
Mycelex-G, Vaginal Supp. (Bayer Corp).

clotrimazole. (Various Mfr.) **Vaginal Tab.:** 100 mg, in 7s with applicator. **Vaginal cream:** 1% Tube 45 g with applicator.
Use: Antifungal, candida infections.

clotrimazole. (NMC Labs) Clotrimazole 1%, benzyl alcohol. Vaginal cream. In 45 g with 7 disposable applicators. *otc.*
Use: Antifungal, vaginal.

clotrimazole. (Taro Pharm) Clotrimazole 1% in a vanishing cream base, benzyl alcohol 1%, cetostearyl alcohol. Cream. Tube 15 g, 30 g, 45 g, 2 × 45 g. *otc.*
Use: Antifungal, topical.

clotrimazole and betamethasone dipropionate cream.
Use: Antifungal, anti-inflammatory.

clotrimidazole. (Fujisawa)
Use: Sickle cell disease. [Orphan Drug]

clove oil.
Use: Pharmaceutic aid (flavor).

Cloverine. (Medtech) White salve. Tin oz. *otc.*

Use: Dermatologic, counterirritant.

Clovocain. (Vita Elixir) Benzocaine, oil of cloves. *otc.*
Use: Anesthetic, local.

•**cloxacillin benzathine.** (KLOX-ah-SILL-in BENZ-ah-theen) U.S.P. 23.
Use: Anti-infective.

•**cloxacillin sodium.** (KLOX-ah-SILL-in) U.S.P. 23.
Use: Anti-infective.
See: Cloxapen, Cap. (SmithKline Beecham Pharmaceuticals).
Tegopen, Granules (Bristol-Myers Squibb).

Cloxapen. (SmithKline Beecham Pharmaceuticals) Cloxacillin sodium 250 mg or 500 mg/Cap. Bot. 100s. *Rx.*
Use: Anti-infective, penicillin.

•**cloxyquin.** (KLOX-ee-kwin) USAN.
Use: Anti-infective.

•**clozapine.** (KLOE-zuh-PEEN) USAN.
Use: Antipsychotic.
See: Clozaril (Novartis).

Clozaril. (Novartis) Clozapine 25 mg or 100 mg/Tab. Bot. 100s, 500s, 1000s, 4000s, 5000s. UD 100s, total daily dose packages of 150 mg, 200 mg, 250 mg, 300 mg, 400 mg, 500 mg, 600 mg/day. *Rx.*
Use: Antipsychotic.

Clysodrast. (Rhone-Poulenc Rorer) Tannic acid, 2.5 g, bisacodyl 1.5 mg per packet. Pow. Box 25s, 50s. *Rx.*
Use: Laxative.

C-Max. (Bio-Tech) Vitamin C 1000 mg, magnesium 40 mg, zinc 5 mg, potassium 10 mg, manganese 1 mg, pectin 10 mg in a base of rose hips. Tabs. Bot. 100s. *otc.*
Use: Mineral, vitamin supplement.

C.M.C. Cellulose Gum.
See: Carboxymethylcellulose Sodium, Preps.

CMV. (Wampole Laboratories) Cytomegalovirus antibody test system for the qualitative and semi-quantitative detection of CMV antibody in human serum. Test 100s.
Use: Diagnostic aid.

CMV-IGIV.
Use: Immunization.
See: Cytogam, Vial (Med Immune).
Cytomegalovirus Immune Globulin Intravenous, (Human).
Soln. (Massachusetts Public Health Biologic Laboratories)

Coadvil. (Whitehall Robins) Ibuprofen 200 mg, pseudoephedrine HCl 30 mg/Tab. Bot. 100s. *otc.*
Use: Analgesic, decongestant.

coagulation factor ix.
Use: Antihemophilic. [Orphan drug]
See: Mononine (Armour Pharm).

coagulation factor ix (human).
Use: Antihemophilic. [Orphan drug]
See: AlphaNine (Alpha Therapeutic).

coagulation factor ix (recombinant).
Use: Antihemophilic. [Orphan Drug]
See: BeneFix (Genetics Institute).

coagulants.
See: Hemostatics.

•**coal tar.** U.S.P. 23.
Use: Topical antieczematic; antipsoriatic.
See: Balnetar, Liq. (Westwood Squibb).
Creamy Tar, Shampoo (C&M Pharmacal).
Estar, Gel (Westwood Squibb).
L.C.D. Compound, Oint., Soln. (Almay).
Polytar Bath, Liq. (Stiefel).
Protar Protein, Shampoo (Dermol Pharmaceuticals).
Tarbonis, Cream (Schwarz Pharma).
Zetar, Preps. (Dermik Laboratories).

W/Allantoin, hydrocortisone.
See: Alphosyl-HC, Lot., Cream (Schwarz Pharma).

W/Hydrocortisone.
See: Doak Oil Forte, Liq. (Doak Dermatologics).
Tarcortin, Cream (Schwarz Pharma).

W/Iodoquinol, hydrocortisone.
See: Ze Tar-Quin, Cream (Dermik Laboratories).

W/Zinc oxide.
See: Tarpaste, Paste (Doak Dermatologics).

coal tar, distillate.
Use: Dermatologic, topical.
See: Lavatar, Liq. (Doak Dermatologics).
Syntar, Cream (Zeneca).

W/Sulfur, salicylic acid.
See: Pragatar, Oint. (Menley & James).

coal tar extract.
Use: Dermatologic, topical.
See: Pentrax Gold, Shampoo (Gen Derm).

W/Allantoin, hexachlorophene.
See: Sebical Cream (Schwarz Pharma).

W/Allantoin, hexachlorophene, glycerin, lanolin.
See: Pso-Rite, Cream (DePree).

W/Allantoin, salicylic acid, perhydrosqualine.
See: Skaylos Cream (Ambix Laboratories).
Skaylos Lotion (Ambix Laboratories).

W/Salicylic acid, resorcinol, benzoic acid.
See: Mazon Cream (SmithKline Beecham Pharmaceuticals).

coal tar paste.
Use: Dermatologic, topical.
W/Zinc paste.
See: Tarpaste, Paste (Doak Dermatologics).

coal tar topical solution. Liquor Carbonis Detergens. L.C.D.
Use: Anti-eczematic, topical.
See: Advanced Formula Tegrin, Shampoo (Block Drug).
Balnetar, Liq. (Westwood Squibb).
Creamy Tar, Shampoo (C&M Pharmacal).
Estar, Gel (Westwood Squibb).
High Potency Tar (C&M Pharmacal).
L.C.D. Compound Oint., Soln. (Almay).
MG217 Medicated, Shampoo, Cond. (Triton Consumer Products).
Psorigel, Gel (Galderma).
PsoriNail, Liq. (Summers).
Wright's Soln. (E. Fougera).
Zetar, Emulsion, Shampoo (Dermik Laboratories).
W/Allantoin, psorilan, myristate.
See: Iocon, Shampoo (Galderma).
Psorelief, Cream (Quality Formulations).
W/Hydrocortisone, iodoquinol.
See: Cor-Tar-Quin, Cream, Lot. (Bayer Corp).
W/Hydrocortisone alcohol, clioquinololine, diperodon HCl, vitamins A, D.
See: Pentarcort, Cream (Dalin).
W/Robane (perhydrosqualene).
See: Skaylos Shampoo (Ambix Laboratories).
W/Salicylic acid.
See: Epidol, Soln. (Spirt).
Ionil T, Shampoo (Galderma).
W/Salicylic acid, sulfur, protein.
See: Vanseb-T Tar Shampoo (Allergan).

Co-Apap. (Various Mfr.) Pseudoephedrine HCl 30 mg, chlorpheniramine maleate 2 mg, dextromethorphan HBr 15 mg, acetaminophen 325 mg/Tab. Bot. 24s, 50s, 1000s. *otc.*
Use: Analgesic, antihistamine, antitussive, decongestant.

cobalamine concentrate. U.S.P. 21.
Use: Hematopoietic vitamin.
See: Vitamin B_{12} (Various Mfr.).

cobalt chloride.
W/Ferrous gluconate, vitamin B_{12}, duodenum whole desiccated.
See: Bitrinsic-E, Cap. (Zeneca).

cobalt gluconate.
W/Ferrous gluconate, vitamin B_{12} activity, desiccated stomach substance, folic acid.
See: Chromagen, Cap., Inj. (Savage).

cobalt-labeled vitamin B_{12}.
See: Rubratope-57 (Bristol-Myers Squibb).

cobalt standards for vitamin B_{12}.
See: Cobatope-57, and Cobatope-60 (Bristol-Myers Squibb).

•**cobaltous chloride Co 57.** (koe-BALL-tuss) USAN.
Use: Radiopharmaceutical.

•**cobaltous chloride Co 60.** USAN.
Use: Radiopharmaceutical.

cobatope-57. (Bristol-Myers Squibb) Cobaltous Cl Co 57.

cobex 1000. (Standex) Vitamin B_{12} 1000 mcg/10 ml. Vial 30 ml. *Rx.*
Use: Vitamin supplement.

Co-Bile. (Western Research) Hog bile 64.8 mg, pancreas substance 64.8 mg, papain-pepsin complex 97.2 mg, diatase malt 16.2 mg, papain 48.6 mg, pepsin 48.6 mg/Tab. Bot. 1000s. *otc, Rx.*
Use: Digestive enzyme.

•**cocaine.** (koe-CANE) U.S.P. 23.
Use: Anesthetic, local.

•**cocaine hydrochloride.** U.S.P. 23.
Use: Anesthetic, local.

cocaine HCl. Top. Soln.: Cocaine HCl 4%, 10%/Bot. 10 ml, UD 4 ml. (Various). **Pow.:** 5 g, 25 g. (Mallinckrodt). *c-II.*
Use: Mucosal anesthetic.

cocaine viscous. (Various) Cocaine viscous 4%, 10%/Soln. Top. Bot. 10 ml, UD 4 ml. *c-II.*
Use: Anesthetic, local.

•**coccidioidin.** (cox-id-ee-OY-din) U.S.P. 23.
Use: Diagnostic aid (dermal reactive indicator).
See: BioCox, Vial (Iatric).
Spherulin (ALK Laboratories).

cocculin.
See: Picrotoxin, Inj. (Various Mfr.).

Cocilan Syrup. (Health for Life Brands) Euphorbia, wild lettuce, cocillana, squill, senega, cascarin (bitterless). Bot. gal. Available w/codeine. Bot. gal.

cocillana.
W/Euphorbia pilulifera, squill, antimony potassium tartrate, senega.
See: Cylana Syr. (Jones Medical Industries). [

cocoa. N.F. XVI.
Use: Pharmaceutic aid (flavor; flavored vehicle).

•**cocoa butter.** N.F. 18.
Use: Pharmaceutic aid (suppository base).

Codamine Pediatric Syrup. (Alphalma USPD) Hydrocodone bitartrate 2.5 mg, phenylpropanolamine HCl 12.5 mg. Bot. pt. *c-III.*
Use: Antitussive, decongestant.

Codamine Syrup. (Zenith Goldline) Hydrocodone bitartrate 5 mg, phenylpropanolamine HCl 25 mg/5 ml. Bot. pt, gal. *c-III.*
Use: Antitussive, decongestant.

Codanol Ointment. (A.P.C.) Vitamins A, D, hexachlorophene, zinc oxide. Tube 1.5 oz, 4 oz, Jar lb. *otc.*
Use: Dermatologic, counterirritant.

Codap. (Solvay) Codeine phosphate 32 mg, acetaminophen 325 mg/Tab. Bot. 250s. *c-III.*
Use: Analgesic combination.

Codegest Expectorant. (Great Southern) Guaifenesin 100 mg, phenylpropanolamine HCl 12.5 mg, codeine phosphate 10 mg. Alcohol, dye free. Liq. Bot. pt, gal. *c-v.*
Use: Antitussive, decongestant, expectorant.

Codehist DH Elixir. (Geneva Pharm) Pseudoephedrine 30 mg, chlorpheniramine maleate 2 mg, codeine phosphate 10 mg, alcohol 5.7%. Bot. 120 ml, 480 ml. *c-v.*
Use: Antihistamine, antitussive, decongestant.

•**codeine.** (KOE-deen) U.S.P. 23.
Use: Analgesic, narcotic; antitussive.

codeine combinations.
See: Actifed-C, Expectorant, Syr. (GlaxoWellcome).
Anexsia w/Codeine, Tab. (SmithKline Beecham Pharmaceuticals).
APAP w/Codeine, Tab. (Schwarz Pharma).
A.P.C. w/Codeine, Tab. (Various Mfr.).
Ascriptin W/Codeine No. 2, Tab. (Rhone-Poulenc Rorer).
Ascriptin W/Codeine No. 3, Tab. (Rhone-Poulenc Rorer).
Buff-A-Compound, Tab. (Merz).
Calcidrine Syr. (Abbott Laboratories).
Capital w/Codeine, Susp. (Carnrick Labs).
Cheracol, Syr. (Pharmacia & Upjohn).
Chlor-Trimeton Expectorant (Schering Plough).
Codasa I and II, Cap. (Stayner).
Colrex Compound, Cap., Elix. (Solvay).
Cosanyl Cough Syrup (Health Care Ind.).
Cycofed Pediatric, Syr. (Cypress)
Deconsal Pediatric, Syr. (Adams).
Drucon w/Codeine, Liq. (Standard Drug).
Empirin No. 1, No. 2, No. 3, No. 4, Tab. (GlaxoWellcome).
Fiorinal w/Codeine, Cap. (Novartis).
G-3, Cap. (Roberts Pharm).
Golacol, Syr. (Arcum).
Guaifenesin DAC, Liq. (Cypress).
Novahistine, Expectorant (Hoechst Marion Roussel).
Nucofed, Liq. (Beecham).
Partuss AC (Parmed).
Pediacof, Syr. (Sanofi Winthrop).
Phenaphen #2, #3, #4, Cap. (Robins).
Phenaphen-650, Cap. (Robins).
Phenergan Expectorant w/Codeine, Troches (Wyeth Ayerst).
Proval No. 3, Tab. (Solvay).
Prunicodeine, Syr. (Eli Lilly).
Robitussin A-C, DAC (Robins).
Tolu-Sed, Elix. (Scherer).
Tussar-2, Syr. (Rhone-Poulenc Rorer).
Tussar SF, Liq. (Rhone-Poulenc Rorer).
Tussi-Organidin, Prods. (Wallace Laboratories).
Tylenol w/Codeine No. 1, No. 2, No. 3, No. 4 Tab. (Ortho McNeil).
Tylenol w/Codeine, Elix. (Ortho McNeil).
Vasotus, Liq. (Sheryl).

codeine methylbromide. Eucodin.
Use: Antitussive.

•**codeine phosphate.** (KOE-deen FOSS-fate) U.S.P. 23.
Use: Analgesic, narcotic; antitussive.

codeine phosphate. (Various Mfr.) Pow. Bot. ⅛ oz, 0.25 oz, 0.5 oz, 1 oz.
Use: Analgesic, narcotic; antitussive.

codeine phosphate and guaifenesin. (Zenith Goldline) Codeine phospate 10 mg, guaifenesin 300 mg/Tab. Bot. 100s. *c-III.*
Use: Expectorant, narcotic antitussive.

•**codeine polistirex.** (KOE-deen pahl-ee-STIE-rex) USAN.
Use: Antitussive.

codeine resin complex combinations.
See: Omni-Tuss, Liq. (Medeva).

•**codeine sulfate.** (KOE-deen) U.S.P. 23.
Use: Analgesic, antitussive, narcotic.

codelcortone.
See: Prednisolone.

Codiclear DH Syrup. (Schwarz Pharma) Hydrocodone bitartrate 5 mg, guaifenesin 100 mg/5 ml. Bot. 4 oz, pt. *c-III.*
Use: Antitussive, expectorant.

Codimal. (Schwarz Pharma) Chlorpheniramine maleate 2 mg, pseudoephedrine HCl 30 mg, acetaminophen 325 mg/ Cap. or Tab. Bot. 24s, 100s, 1000s. *otc.*
Use: Analgesic, antihistamine, decongestant.

Codimal DH Syrup. (Schwarz Pharma) Hydrocodone bitartrate 1.66 mg, phenylephrine HCl 5 mg, pyrilamine maleate 8.33 mg/5 ml. Bot. 4 oz, pt, gal. *c-III.*
Use: Antihistamine, antitussive, decongestant.

Codimal DM. (Schwarz Pharma) Dextromethorphan HBr 10 mg, phenylephrine HCl 5 mg, pyrilamine maleate 8.33 mg/ 5 ml, alcohol 4%, saccharin, sorbitol. Sugar free. Bot. 4 oz, pt, gal. *otc.*
Use: Antitussive, antihistamine, decongestant.

Codimal-L.A. (Schwarz Pharma) Chlorpheniramine maleate 8 mg, pseudoephedrine HCl 120 mg/SR Cap. Bot. 100s, 1000s. *Rx.*
Use: Antihistamine, decongestant.

Codimal-L.A. Half Capsules. (Schwarz Pharma) Pseudoephedrine HCl 60 mg, chlorpheniramine maleate 4 mg, sucrose. Cap. Bot. 100s. *Rx.*
Use: Antihistamine, decongestant.

Codimal PH Syrup. (Schwarz Pharma) Codeine phosphate 10 mg, phenylephrine HCl 5 mg, pyrilamine maleate 8.33 mg/5 ml. Bot. 4 oz, pt, gal. *c-v.*
Use: Antihistamine, antitussive, decongestant.

Codimal Tablets. (Schwarz Pharma) Chlorpheniramine maleate 2 mg, pseudoephedrine HCl 30 mg, acetaminophen 325 mg/Tab. Bot. 24s, 100s, 1000s.
Use: Analgesic, antihistamine, decongestant.

•**cod liver oil.** U.S.P. 23. Emulsion.
Use: Vitamin A and D therapy.
See: Cod Liver Oil Concentrate Cap. (Schering Plough).

W/Anesthesin, zinc oxide, hydroxyquinoline.
See: Medicone Dressing. (Medicone).

W/Benzocaine.
See: Morusan, Oint. (SmithKline Beecham Pharmaceuticals).

W/Creosote.
(Bryant) Cod liver oil 9 min, creosote 1 min/Cap. Bot. 100s.

W/Malt extract.
(GlaxoWellcome) Vitamins A 6450 IU, D 645 IU. Bot. 10 fl oz, 20 fl oz.

W/Methylbenzethonium Cl.
See: Benephen, Prods. (Halsted).

W/Viosterol.
(Abbott Laboratories) Vitamins A 2800 IU, D 255 IU/g. Bot. 12 fl oz.
(Bristol-Myers Squibb) Vitamins A 2000 IU, D 440 IU/g. Bot. 4 fl oz, 12 fl oz.

W/Zinc oxide.
See: Desitin, Preps. (Pfizer).

cod liver oil concentrate. (Schering Plough) Concentrate of cod liver oil with vitamins A and D added. **Cap.:** Bot. 40s, 100s. **Tab.:** Bot. 100s, 240s. Also W/Vitamin C. Bot. 100s. *otc.*
Use: Vitamin supplement.

cod liver oil ointment. *otc.*
See: Moruguent, Oint. (SmithKline Beecham Pharmaceuticals).

codorphone hydrochloride. (KOE-dahr-fone) Name previously used.
Use: Analgesic.
See: Conorphone HCl.

•**codoxime.** (CODE-ox-eem) USAN.
Use: Antitussive.

codoxy. (Halsey) Oxycodone HCl 4.5 mg, oxycodone terephthalate 0.38 mg, aspirin 325 mg/Tab. Bot. 100s.
Use: Analgesic combination.

Cogentin. (Merck) Benztropine Mesylate **Tab.:** 0.5 mg Bot. 100s; 1 mg Bot. 100s, UD 100s; 2 mg Bot. 100s, 1000s, UD 100s. **Inj.:** Benztropine mesylate 1 mg/ ml w/sodium Cl 9 mg and water for injection q.s. to 1 ml Amp. 2 ml, Box 6s. *Rx.*
Use: Antiparkinsonian.

Co-Gesic. (Schwarz Pharma) Hydrocodone bitartrate 5 mg, acetaminophen 500 mg/Tab. Bot. 100s, 500s. *c-III.*
Use: Analgesic combination.

Cognex. (Parke-Davis) Tacrine HCl 10 mg, 20 mg, 30 mg, 40 mg/Cap. Bot. 120s, UD 100s. *Rx.*
Use: Psychotherapeutic.

Co-Hep-Tral. (Davis & Sly) Folic acid 10 mg, vitamin B_{12} 100 mcg, liver injection q.s./ml. Vial 10 ml. *Rx.*
Use: Mineral, vitamin supplement.

Co-Hist. (Roberts Pharm) Pseudoephedrine HCl 30 mg, chlorpheniramine 2 mg, acetaminophen 325 mg/Tab. Bot. 500s, 1000s. *otc.*
Use: Analgesic, antihistamine, decongestant.

Colabid Tabs. (Major) Probenecid 500 mg, colchicine 0.5 mg/Tab. Bot. 100s, 1000s. *Rx.*
Use: Antigout.

Colace. (Bristol-Myers) Docusate sodium. **Cap.:** 50 mg or 100 mg. Bot. 30s, 60s, 250s, 1000s, UD 100s. **Syr.:** 60 mg/15 ml with alcohol < 1%. Bot. 240 ml, 480 ml. **Liq.:** 150 mg/15 ml. Bot. 30 ml, 480 ml with calibrated droppers. *otc.*
Use: Laxative.

Colagyn. (Smith & Nephew United) Zinc sulfocarbolate, potassium, oxyquinoline sulfate, lactic acid, boric acid. Jelly. Tube w/applicator and refill 6 oz. Douche Pow. 3 oz, 7 oz, 14 oz. *otc.*

Colana Syrup. (Hance) Euphorbia pilulifera tincture 8 ml, wild lettuce syrup 8 ml, cocillana tincture 2.5 ml, squill compound syrup 1.5 ml, cascara 0.25 g, menthol 4.8 mg/fl oz. Bot. 4 fl oz, gal. Also w/Dionin 15 mg/fl oz. Bot. gal.

Co-Lav. (Copley) Polyethylene glycol 3350 60 g, sodium chloride 1.46 g, potassium chloride 0.745 g, sodium bicarbonate 1.68 g, sodium sulfate 5.68 g per L/Pow. for Soln. Jug 4 L. *Rx.*
Use: Bowel evacuant.

Colax. (Rugby) Docusate sodium 100 mg, phenolphthalein 65 mg/Tab. Bot. 30s. *otc.*
Use: Laxative.

•**colchicine.** (KOHL-chih-seen) U.S.P. 23.
Use: Gout suppressant. Treat multiple sclerosis [Orphan drug]
W/Benemid.
See: Colbenemid, Tab. (Merck).
W/Methyl salicylate. (Parke-Davis) Colchicine gr, methyl salicylate 3 min/Cap. Bot. 100s, 500s, 1000s.
Use: Orally, gout therapy.
W/Probenecid.
See: Benn-C, Tab. (Scrip).
Colbenemid, Tab. (Merck).
Col-Probenecid, Tab. (Various Mfr.).
W/Sodium salicylate, calcium carbonate, dried aluminum hydroxide gel, phenobarbital.
See: Apcogesic, Tabs. (Apco).
W/Sodium salicylate, potassium iodide.
See: Bricolide, Tab. (Briar).

colchicine. (Various Mfr.) Colchicine 0.5 mg, 0.6 mg. Tab. Bot. 100s. *Rx.*
Use: Gout suppressant. Treat multiple sclerosis [Orphan drug].

colchicine salicylate.
W/Phenobarbital, sodium p-aminobenzoate, vitamin B_1, aspirin.
See: Doloral, Tab. (Alamed).

Cold & Allergy Elixir. (Zenith Goldline) Phenylpropanolamine HCl 12.5 mg, brompheniramine maleate 2 mg/5 ml. Liq. Bot. 118 ml, 237 ml, 473 ml, gal. *otc.*
Use: Antihistamine, decongestant.

cold cream. U.S.P. 21.
Use: Emollient; water in oil emulsion ointment base.

Cold-Gest Cold Capsules. (Major) Chlorpheniramine maleate 8 mg, pseudoephedrine HCl 75 mg/Cap. Pkg. 10s, 20s. *otc.*
Use: Antihistamine, decongestant.

Coldloc. (Fleming) Phenylpropanolamine HCl 20 mg, phenylephrine 5 mg, guaifenesin 100 mg/5 ml, sorbitol. Alcohol, sugar, dye free. Elixir. Bot. Pt. *Rx.*
Use: Decongestant, expectorant.

Coldloc-LA. (Fleming) Phenylpropanolamine HCl 75 mg, guaifenesin 600 mg/SR Cap. Bot. 50s, 100s. *Rx.*
Use: Decongestant, expectorant.

Coldonyl. (Dover Pharmaceuticals) Acetaminophen, phenylephrine HCl/Tab. Sugar, lactose and salt free. UD Box 500s. *otc.*
Use: Analgesic, decongestant.

Coldran. (Halsey) Phenylephrine HCl 5 mg, chlorpheniramine maleate 2 mg, salicylamide 1.5 gr, acetaminophen 0.5 gr, caffeine/Tab. Bot. 30s. *otc.*
Use: Analgesic, antihistamine, decongestant.

Cold Relief. (Rugby) Phenylpropanolamine HCl 12.5 mg, chlorpheniramine maleate 2 mg, dextromethorphan HBr 10 mg, acetaminophen 325 mg/Tab. Bot. 50s. *otc.*
Use: Analgesic, antihistamine, antitussive, decongestant.

Coldrine. (Roberts Pharm) Acetaminophen 325 mg, pseudoephedrine HCl 30 mg, sodium metabisulfite/Tab. Bot. 1000s, 500s (packets), 4-dose boxes. *otc.*
Use: Analgesic, decongestant.

Cold Sore Lotion. (Purepac) Camphor, benzoin, aluminum Cl. Bot. 0.5 oz.
Use: Cold sores, fever blisters.

Cold Symptoms Relief. (Major) Pseudoephedrine HCl 30 mg, chlorpheniramine maleate 2 mg, dextromethorphan HBr 10 mg, acetaminophen 325 mg/Tab. Bot. 50s. *otc.*
Use: Analgesic, antihistamine, antitussive, decongestant.

Cold Tablets. (Walgreens) Phenylephrine HCl 5 mg, chlorpheniramine

maleate 2 mg, acetaminophen 325 mg/ Tab. Bot. 50s. *otc.*
Use: Analgesic, antihistamine, decongestant.

Cold Tablets Multiple Symptom. (Walgreens) Acetaminophen 500 mg, pseudoephedrine HCl 30 mg, chlorpheniramine maleate 2 mg, dextromethorphan HBr 10 mg/Tab. Bot. 50s. *otc.*
Use: Analgesic, antihistamine, antitussive, decongestant.

•**colesevelam hydrochloride.** (koe-leh-SEH-veh-lam)
Use: Antihyperlipidemic.

Colestid. (Pharmacia & Upjohn) Colestipol HCl. **Unflavored:** Bot. 300 g, 500 g. Pkt. 5 g. **Flavored:** Bot. 450 g. Pkt. 7.5 g (5 g colestipol HCl). *Rx.*
Use: Antihyperlipidemic.

Colestid Tablets. (Pharmacia & Upjohn) Colestipol HCl 1 g/Tab. 120s and 250s. *Rx.*
Use: Antihyperlipidemic.

•**colestipol hydrochloride.** (koe-LESS-tih-pole) U.S.P. 23.
Use: Antihyperlipidemic.
See: Colestid (Pharmacia & Upjohn).

•**colestolone.** (koe-LESS-toe-LONE) USAN.
Use: Hypolipidemic.

Col-Evac. (Forest Pharmaceutical) Potassium bitartrate, bicarbonate of soda and a blended base of polyethylene glycols. Supp. 2s, 12s.

Colfed-A Capsules. (Parmed) Pseudoephedrine HCl 120 mg, chlorpheniramine maleate 8 mg. Bot 100s. *Rx.*
Use: Antihistamine, decongestant.

•**colforsin.** (kole-FAR-sin) USAN.
Use: Antiglaucoma agent.

•**colfosceril palmitate.** (kahl-FOSE-uhr-ILL PAL-mih-TATE) USAN.
Use: Pulmonary surfactant, antiatelectic; prevention/treatment of hyaline membrane disease. [Orphan drug]
See: Exosurf (GlaxoWellcome).

colfosceril palmitate, cetyl alcohol, tyloxapol.
Use: Hyaline membrane disease; adult respiratory distress syndrome. [Orphan drug]
See: Exosurf Neonatal for Intrathecal Suspension (GlaxoWellcome).

colimycin sodium methanesulfonate. (Parke-Davis).
See: Colistimethate Sodium.

colimycin sulfate. (Parke-Davis).
See: Coly-Mycin, Preps. (Parke-Davis).

•**colistimethate sodium, sterile.** (koe-LISS-tih-METH-ate) U.S.P. 23.
Use: Anti-infective.
See: Coly-Mycin-M, Injectable (Parke-Davis).

colistin base.
W/Neomycin base, hydrocortisone acetate, thonzonium bromide, polysorbate 80, acetic acid, sodium acetate.
See: Coly-Mycin Otic W/Neomycin and Hydrocortisone, Liq. (Parke-Davis).
Cortisporin-TC, Otic Susp. (Monarch).

colistin methanesulfonate.
See: Colistimethate Sodium.

colistin and neomycin sulfates and hydrocortisone acetate otic suspension.
Use: Anti-infective, anti-inflammatory.

Co-Liver. (Standex) Folic acid 1 mg, vitamin B_{12} 100 mcg, liver 10 mcg/ml. Vial 10 ml. *Rx.*
Use: Mineral, vitamin supplement.

Colladerm. (C & M Pharmacal) Purified water, glycerin, soluble collagen, hydrolysed elastin, allantoin, ethylhydroxycellulose, sorbic, octoxynol-9. Bot. 2.3 oz. *otc.*
Use: Emollient.

collagenase.
See: Santyl (Knoll Pharmaceuticals).

collagenase abc ointment. (Advance Biofactures) Collagenase 250 units/g in white petrolatum. 25 g, 50 g. *otc.*
Use: Enzyme, topical.

collagen implant. (Lacrimedics) In 0.2 mm, 0.3 mm, 0.4 mm, 0.5 mm. 0.6 mm. Box 12s. *Rx.*
Use: Collagen implant, ophthalmic.

collagen implant.
See: Zyderm I. (Collagen).
Zyderm II. (Collagen).

collagenase (lyophilized) for injection.
Use: Peyronie's disease. [Orphan drug]
See: Plaquase (Advance Biofactures).

•**collodion.** (kah-LOW-dee-uhm) U.S.P. 23.
Use: Topical protectant.

colloidal aluminum hydroxide.
See: Aluminum Hydroxide Gel, U.S.P. 23.

colloidal gold.
See: Aureotope (Bristol-Myers Squibb).

collodial oatmeal.
Use: Emollient.
See: Aveeno, Preps. (Rydelle).
Actibath, Effer. Tab (Jergens).

colloidal silver iodide.
See: Neo-Silvol, Soln. (Parke-Davis).

Colloral. (AutoImmune) Purified type II collagen.
Use: Juvenile rheumatoid arthritis. [Orphan drug]

Collyrium for Fresh Eyes. (Wyeth Ayerst) Boric acid, sodium borate, benzalkonium Cl. Bot. 120 ml. *otc.*
Use: Irrigant, ophthalmic.

Collyrium Fresh Eye Drops. (Wyeth Ayerst) Tetrahydrozoline HCl 0.05%. Drop. Bot. 15 ml. *otc.*
Use: Mydriatic, vasoconstrictor.

ColoCare. (Helena Labs) In-home fecal test. Kit. 3s.
Use: Diagnostic aid.

Coloctyl. (Eon Labs Manufacturing) Docusate sodium 100 mg/Cap. Bot. 100s, 1000s, UD 1000s. *otc.*
Use: Laxative.

Cologel. (Eli Lilly) Methylcellulose 450 mg/5 ml, alcohol 5%, saccharin. Bot. 16 fl oz. *otc.*
Use: Laxative.

colony stimulating factor.
Use: Adjunct during antineoplastic therapy.
See: Leukine (Immunex)
Neupogen (Amgen).

color allergy screening test.
See: CAST (Biomerica).

Color Ovulation Test. (Biomerica) Monoclonal antibody-based enzyme immunoassay test for hLH in urine. Kit. 9-day test kit.
Use: Diagnostic aid, ovulation.

Coloscreen. (Helena Labs) Occult blood screening test. Kit 12s, 25s, 50s. 3 tests per kit.
Use: Diagnostic aid.

Coloscreen/VPI. (Helena Labs) Occult blood screening test. Box 100s, 1000s.
Use: Diagnostic aid.

Colovage. (Dyna Pharm) Powder for reconstitution to produce 1 gal soln. Containing sodium Cl 5.53 g, potassium Cl 2.82 g, sodium bicarbonate 6.36 g, sodium sulfate anhydrous 21.5 g, polyethylene glycol 3350. Pkg. 1s. *Rx.*
Use: Laxative.

Col-Probenecid. (Various Mfr.) Probenecid 500 mg, colchicine 0.5 mg/Tab. Bot. 100s. *Rx.*
Use: Antigout.

Coltab Children's. (Roberts Pharm) Phenylephrine HCl 2.5 mg, chlorpheniramine maleate 1 mg/Chew. tab. Bot. 30s. *otc.*
Use: Antihistamine, decongestant.

•**colterol mesylate.** (KOLE-ter-ole) USAN.
Use: Bronchodilator.

Coly-Mycin M Parenteral. (Monarch) Colistimethate sodium equivalent 150 mg colistin base per vial. *Rx.*
Use: Anti-infective.

Coly-Mycin S Otic Drops w/ Neomycin and Hydrocortisone. (Parke-Davis) Colistin base as the sulfate 3 mg, neomycin base as the sulfate 3.3 mg, hydrocortisone acetate 10 mg, thonzonium bromide 0.5 mg/ml, polysorbate 80, acetic acid, sodium acetate, thimerosal. Dropper bot. 5 ml, 10 ml. *Rx.*
Use: Anti-infective.

CoLyte. (Schwarz Pharma) **2L:** PEG (Polyethylene glycol-electrolyte solution) 3350 120 g, sodium sulfate 11.36 g, sodium bicarbonate 3.36 g, sodium Cl 2.92 g, potassium Cl 1.49 g. **1 gal:** PEG 3350 227.1 g, sodium sulfate 21.5 g, sodium bicarbonate 6.36 g, sodium Cl 5.53 g, potassium Cl 2.82 g. **6 L:** PEG 3350 360 g, sodium sulfate 34.08 g, sodium bicarbonate 10.08 g, sodium Cl 8.76 g, potassium Cl 4.47 g. Pack 5. Bot. 2 L, gal, 4L, 6L. *Rx.*
Use: Bowel evacuant.

Combichole. (Trout) Dehydrocholic acid 2 gr, desoxycholic acid 1 gr/Tab. Bot. 100s, 1000s. *Rx.*
Use: Hydrocholeretic.

Combipres Tablets. (Boehringer Ingelheim) **0.1 mg:** Clonidine HCl 0.1 mg, chlorthalidone 15 mg/Tab. Bot. 100s, 1000s. **0.2 mg:** Clonidine HCl 0.2 mg, chlorthalidone 15 mg/Tab. Bot. 100s, 1000s. **0.3 mg:** Clonidine HCl 0.3 mg, chlorthalidone 15 mg/Tab. Bot. 100s. *Rx.*
Use: Antihypertensive.

Combistix. (Bayer Corp) Urine test for glucose, protein and pH. In 100s.
Use: Diagnostic aid.

Combistix Reagent Strips. (Bayer Corp) Protein test-tetrabromphenol blue, citrate buffer, protein-absorbing agent; glucose test area-glucose oxidase, orthotolidin and a catalyst; pH test area methyl red and bromthymol blue. Box, strips, 100s.
Use: Diagnostic aid.

Combivent. (Boehringer Ingelheim) Per actuation - ipratropium bromide 18 mg, albuterol sulfate 103 mcg (90 mcg base)/Aerosol Can 14.7 g (200 inhalations). *Rx.*
Use: Secondary treatment of chronic obstructive pulmonary disease (COPD).

Combivir. (GlaxoWellcome) Lamivudine 150 mg, zidovudine 300 mg. Tab. Bot. 60s. *Rx.*
Use: HIV infection.

ComfortCare GP Wetting & Soaking. (PHB Wesley Jessen) Buffered, isotonic. Chlorhexidine gluconate 0.005%, EDTA 0.02%, octylphenoxy (oxyethylene) ethanol, povidone, polyvinyl alcohol, propylene glycol, hydroxyethylcellulose, NaCl. Soln. Bot. 120 ml or 240 ml. *otc.*
Use: Contact lens care.

Comfort Drops. (PHB Wesley Jessen) Isotonic solution containing naphazoline 0.03%, benzalkonium Cl 0.005%, edetate disodium 0.02%. Bot. 15 ml. *otc.*
Use: Contact lens care.

Comfort Eye Drops. (PHB Wesley Jessen) Naphazoline HCl 0.03%. Bot. 15 ml. *otc.*
Use: Decongestant, ophthalmic.

Comfort Gel Liquid. (Walgreens) Aluminum hydroxide compressed gel 200 mg, magnesium hydroxide 200 mg, simethicone 20 mg/5 ml. Bot. 12 oz. *otc.*
Use: Antacid, antiflatulent.

Comfort Gel Tablets. (Walgreens) Magnesium hydroxide 85 mg, simethicone 25 mg, aluminum hydroxide-magnesium carbonate codried gel 282 mg/Tab. Bot. 100s. *otc.*
Use: Antacid, antiflatulent.

Comfort Tears. (PHB Wesley Jessen) Hydroxyethyl cellulose, benzalkonium Cl 0.005%, edetate disodium 0.02%. Bot. 15 ml. *otc.*
Use: Contact lens care.

Comhist L.A. Capsules. (Roberts Pharm) Phenylephrine HCl 20 mg, chlorpheniramine maleate 4 mg, phenyltoloxamine citrate 50 mg/Cap. Bot. 100s. *Rx.*
Use: Antihistamine, decongestant.

Comhist Tablets. (Roberts Pharm) Phenylephrine HCl 10 mg, chlorpheniramine maleate 2 mg, phenyltoloxamine citrate 25 mg/Tab. Bot. 100s. *Rx.*
Use: Antihistamine, decongestant.

Compal. (Solvay) Dihydrocodeine 16 mg, acetaminophen 356.4 mg, caffeine 30 mg/Cap. Bot. 100s. *c-III.*
Use: Analgesic combination.

Compat Nutrition Enteral Delivery System. (Novartis) Top fill feeding containers 600 ml, 1400 ml. Gravity delivery set. Pump delivery set. Compat enteral feeding pump.
Use: Nutritional supplement.

Compazine. (SmithKline Beecham Pharmaceuticals) Prochlorperazine as the maleate. **Tab.:** 5 mg, 10 mg Bot. 100s. **Inj.:** Edisylate salt 5 mg/ml. Amp. 2 ml, vial 10 ml, disposable syringe 2 ml. **SR Spansule:** Maleate salt 10 mg, 15 mg. Bot. 50s. **Supp.:** 2.5 mg, 5 mg or 25 mg. Box 12s. **Syr.:** Edisylate salt 5 mg/5 ml. Bot. 120 ml. *Rx.*
Use: Antiemetic, antipsychotic.

Compete. (Mission Pharmacal) Iron 27 mg, vitamins A 5000 IU, D 400 IU, E 45 IU, B_1 2 mg, B_2 2.6 mg, B_3 30 mg, B_6 20.6 mg, B_{12} 9 mcg, C 90 mg, folic acid 0.4 mg, Zn 22.5/Tab. Bot. 100s. *otc.*
Use: Mineral, vitamin supplement.

Compleat B Meat Base Formula. (Novartis) Beef, nonfat milk, hydrolyzed cereal solids, maltodextrin, pureed fruits and vegetables, corn oil, mono and diglycerides. Bot. 250 ml, Can 250 ml. *otc.*
Use: Nutritional supplement, eternal.

Compleat Modified Formula Meat Base. (Novartis) Hydrolyzed cereal solids, calcium caseinate, pureed fruits and vegetables, corn oil, beef puree, mono and diglycerides. Can 250 ml. *otc.*
Use: Enteral nutritional supplement.

Compleat Regular Formula. (Novartis) Deionized water, beef puree, hydrolyzed cereal solids, green bean puree, pea puree, nonfat milk, corn oil, maltodextrin, peach puree, orange juice, mono and diglycerides, carrageenan, vitamins, minerals. Bot. 250 ml, Can 250 ml. *otc.*
Use: Nutritional supplement, eternal.

Complete. (Mission Pharmacal) Vitamins A 5000 IU, D 400 IU, E 45 IU, C 90 mg, B_1 2.25 mg, folic acid 0.4 mg, B_2 2.6 mg, B_3 30 mg, B_6 25 mg, B_{12} 9 mcg, ferrous gluconate 233 mg, zinc 22.5 mg/Tab. Bot. 100s, 1000s. *otc.*
Use: Mineral, vitamin supplement.

Complete. (Allergan) Buffered, isotonic. Sodium Cl, polyhexamethylene biguanide 0.0001%, tromethamine, tyloxapol, EDTA. Soln. Bot. 15 ml. *otc.*
Use: Contact lens care.

Complete All-In-One. (Allergan) Buffered, isotonic. Sodium Cl, polyhexamethylone biguanide, EDTA. Soln. Bot. 60, 120, 360 ml. *otc.*
Use: Contact lens care.

Complete Weekly Enzymatic Cleaner. (Allergan) Effervescing, buffering and tableting agents. Sublitisin A. Tab. Pkg. 8s. *otc.*

Use: Contact lens care.

Completone Elixir Fort. (Sanofi Winthrop) Ferrous gluconate.
Use: Mineral supplement.

Complex 15 Cream. (Baker/Cummins) Jar 4 oz. *otc.*
Use: Emollient.

Complex 15 Lotion. (Baker/Cummins) Bot. 8 oz. *otc.*
Use: Emollient.

Complex Zinc Carbonates.
See: Zinc (Pharmaceuticals Labs).

Comply Liquid. (Sherwood Medical) Sodium caseinate, calcium caseinate, hydrolyzed cornstarch, sucrose, corn oil, soy lecithin, vitamins A, B_1, B_2, B_3, B_5, B_6, B_{12}, C, D, E, K, folic acid, biotin, choline, Ca, Cl, Cu, Fe, I, Mg, Mn, P, Zn. Can 250 ml, Bot. 200 ml. *otc.*
Use: Nutritional supplement, eternal.

compound 42.
See: Warfarin (Various Mfr.).

compound b.
See: Corticosterone (Various Mfr.).

compound cb3025.
See: Alkeran, Tab. (GlaxoWellcome).

compound e. (McGaw).
See: Cortisone Acetate. (Various Mfr.).

compound f.
See: Hydrocortisone (Various Mfr.).

compound q.
Use: Antiviral.

compound s.
Use: Antiviral.
See: Retrovir (GlaxoWellcome). Zidovudine.

Compound W. (Whitehall Robins) Salicylic acid 17% w/w in flexible collodion vehicle w/ether 63.5%. Bot. 0.31 oz. *otc.*
Use: Keratolytic.

Compoz. (Medtech) **Tab.:** Diphenhydramine HCl 50 mg Pkg. 12s, 24s. **Cap.:** Diphenhydramine HCl 25 mg Pkg. 16s. *otc.*
Use: Sleep aid.

comprecin.
See: Penetrex (Warner Lambert).

Comtrex. (Bristol-Myers) Acetaminophen 325 mg, pseudoephedrine HCl 30 mg, chlorpheniramine maleate 2 mg, dextromethorphan HBr 10 mg/Tab. Bot. 24s, 50s. *otc.*
Use: Analgesic, antihistamine, antitussive, decongestant.

Comtrex Allergy-Sinus. (Bristol-Myers) Pseudoephedrine HCl 30 mg, chlorpheniramine maleate 2 mg, acetaminophen 500 mg/Tab. or Capl. Bot. 24s, 50s. *otc.*
Use: Analgesic, antihistamine, decongestant.

Comtrex Caplets. (Bristol-Myers) Acetaminophen 325 mg, pseudoephedrine HCl 30 mg, chlorpheniramine maleate 2 mg, dextromethorphan HBr 10 mg/ Capl. Bot. 24s, 50s. *otc.*
Use: Analgesic, antihistamine, antitussive, decongestant.

Comtrex Cough Formula. (Bristol-Myers) Pseudoephedrine HCl 15 mg, dextromethorphan 7.5 mg, guaifenesin 50 mg, acetaminophen 125 mg/5 ml, alcohol 20%. Bot. 120 ml, 240 ml. *otc.*
Use: Analgesic, antitussive, decongestant, expectorant.

Comtrex Day-Night. (Bristol-Myers) **Night:** Pseudoephedrine HCl 30 mg, chlorpheniramine maleate 2 mg, dextromethorphan HBr 10 mg, acetaminophen 325 mg/Tab. Pkg. 6s. **Day:** Pseudoephedrine HCl 30 mg, dextromethrophan HBr 10 mg, acetaminophen 500 mg/Tab. Pkg. 18s. *otc.*
Use: Antihistamine, antitussive, decongestant,.

Comtrex Liquid. (Bristol-Myers) Pseudoephedrine HCl 10 mg, dextromethorphan HBr 3.3 mg, chlorpheniramine maleate 0.67 mg, acetaminophen 108.3 mg, alcohol 20%, sucrose. Bot. 180 ml. *otc.*
Use: Antihistamine, antitussive, decongestant.

Comtrex Liquid Multi-Symptom Cold Reliever. (Bristol-Myers) Acetaminophen 650 mg, phenylpropanolamine HCl 25 mg, chlorpheniramine maleate 4 mg, dextromethorphan HBr 20 mg/30 ml, alcohol 20%. Bot. 6 oz, 10 oz. *otc.*
Use: Analgesic, antihistamine, antitussive, decongestant.

Comtrex Liqui-Gels. (Bristol-Myers) Acetaminophen 325 mg, phenylpropanolamine HCl 12.5 mg, chlorpheniramine maleate 2 mg, dextromethorphan HBr 10 mg/Tab. Blister pkg. 24s, 50s. *otc.*
Use: Analgesic, antihistamine, antitussive, decongestant.

Comtrex, Maximum Strength. (Bristol-Myers) Phenylpropanolamine HCl 12.5 mg, dextromethorphan HBr 15 mg, chlorpheniramine maleate 2 mg, acetaminophen 500 mg. Cap. 24s, 50s. *otc.*
Use: Antihistamine, antitussive, decongestant.

Comtrex Maximum Strength Multi-Symptom Cold & Flu Relief. (Bristol-Myers) Phenylpropanolamine HCl 12.5

mg, chlorpheniramine maleate 2 mg, dextromethorphan HBr 15 mg, acetaminophen 500 mg/Capl. or Tab. Pkg. 24s. *otc.*
Use: Analgesic, antihistamine, antitussive, decongestant.

Comtrex Maximum Strength Non-Drowsy. (Bristol-Myers) Pseudoephedrine HCl 30 mg, dextromethorphan HBr 15 mg, acetaminophen 500 mg/Capl. Pkg. 24s. *otc.*
Use: Analgesic, antitussive, decongestant.

Comvax. (Merck) *Haemophilus influenzae* type b and hepatitis b vaccines, combined 7.5 mcg Hib polysaccharide and 5 mcg hepatitis B surface antigen per 0.5 ml. Single-dose vial. *Rx.*
Use: Vaccine.

Conceive Ovulation Predictor. (Quidel) In vitro diagnostic test for luteinizing hormone in urine.
Use: Diagnostic aid, pregnancy.

Concentraid. (Ferring Pharmaceuticals) Desmopressin acetate 0.1 mg/ml (0.1 mg equals 400 IU arginine vasopressin). Soln. Disposable intranasal pipettes containing 20 mcg/2 ml. *Rx.*
Use: Hormone.

Concentrated Cleaner. (Bausch & Lomb) Anionic sulfate surfactant with friction-enhancing agents and sodium chlorine. Soln. Bot. 30 ml. *otc.*
Use: Contact lens care.

Concentrated Milk of Magnesia-Cascara. (Roxane) Magnesium hydroxide 2.34 g, aromatic cascara fluid extract U.S.P. 5 ml, alcohol 7%/Susp. UD 15 ml. *otc.*
Use: Laxative.

Concentrated Multiple Trace Element. (American Regent) Zinc (as sulfate) 5 mg, copper (as sulfate) 1 mg, manganese (as sulfate) 0.5 mg, chromium (as chloride) 10 mcg. Vial. 10 ml. *Rx.*
Use: Trace element supplement.

concentrated oleovitamin a & d.
See: Oleovitamin A & D, Concentrated, Cap. (Various Mfr.).

Concentrated Phillips' Milk of Magnesia. (Roxane) Magnesium hydroxide 800 mg/5 ml, sorbitol and sugar. Strawberry and orange vanilla creme flavors. Liq. 8 fl. oz. *otc.*
Use: Antacid, laxative.

Concentrin Caps. (Parke-Davis) Dextromethorphan HBr 15 mg, pseudoephedrine HCl 30 mg, guaifenesin 100 mg/ Cap. Bot. 12s. *otc.*
Use: Antitussive, decongestant, expectorant.

Conceptrol Contraceptive Inserts. (Advanced Care Products) Nonoxynol-9 150 mg. Supp. 10s. *otc.*
Use: Contraceptive, spermicide.

Conceptrol Disposable Contraceptive. (Advanced Care Products) Nonoxynol-9 4%. Vaginal gel. Tube. 2.7 g (6s, 10s). *otc.*
Use: Contraceptive, spermicide.

Condol Suspension. (Sanofi Winthrop) Dipyrone, chlormezanone. *Rx.*
Use: Analgesic, muscle relaxant.

Condol Tablets. (Sanofi Winthrop) Dipyrone, chlormezanone. *Rx.*
Use: Analgesic, muscle relaxant.

Condrin-LA. (Roberts Pharm) Phenylpropanolamine HCl 75 mg, chlorpheniramine maleate 12 mg. Bot. 1000s. *otc.*
Use: Antihistamine, decongestant.

condylox. (Oclassen) Podofilox 0.5%, alcohol 95%. Soln. Bot. 3.5 ml. *Rx.*
Use: Keratolytic.

Conest. (Grafton) Conjugated estrogens 0.625 mg, 1.25 mg or 2.5 mg/Tab. Bot. 100s, 1000s. *Rx.*
Use: Estrogen.

Conex-DA. (Forest Pharmaceutical) Phenylpropanolamine HCl 37.5 mg, chlorpheniramine maleate 4 mg/Tab. Bot. 100s, 1000s. *otc.*
Use: Antihistamine, decongestant.

Conex Plus. (Forest Pharmaceutical) Phenylpropanolamine HCl 25 mg, chlorpheniramine maleate 4 mg, acetaminophen 325 mg/Tab. Bot. 1000s. *otc.*
Use: Analgesic, antihistamine, decongestant.

Confide. (Direct Access Diagnostics) Reagent kit for HIV blood tests. Kit contains materials to draw a blood sample, a test card and a protective mailer for 1 test. *otc.*
Use: Diagnostic aid.

Confident. (Block Drug) Carboxymethylcellulose gum, ethylene oxide polymer, petrolatum/mineral oil base. Tube 0.7 oz, 1.4 oz, 2.4 oz. *otc.*
Use: Denture adhesive.

Congess. (Fleming) **Sr.:** Guaifenesin 250 mg, pseudoephedrine HCl 120 mg/SR Cap. **Jr.:** Guaifenesin 125 mg, pseudoephedrine HCl 60 mg/TR Cap. Bot. 100s, 1000s. *otc, Rx.*
Use: Decongestant, expectorant.

Congess Jr. (Fleming) Pseudoephedrine HCl 60 mg, guaifenesin 125 mg/Cap. Bot. 100s, 1000s. *Rx.*
Use: Decongestant, expectorant.

Congess Sr. (Fleming) Pseudoephed-

rine HCl 120 mg, guaifenesin 250 mg/Cap. Bot. 100s, 1000s. *Rx.*
Use: Decongestant, expectorant.

Congestac. (Menley & James) Pseudoephedrine HCl 60 mg, guaifenesin 400 mg/Tab. Bot. 24s. *otc.*
Use: Decongestant, expectorant.

Congestant D. (Rugby) Phenylpropanolamine HCl 12.5 mg, chlorpheniramine maleate 2 mg, acetaminophen 325 mg, sucrose. Tab. Bot. 100s, 1000s. *otc.*
Use: Antihistamine, decongestant.

congo red. Injection.
Use: Hemostatic in hemorrhagic disorders.

conjugated estrogens.
See: Estrogens, Conjugated (Various Mfr.).
Use: Estrogen.

Conjunctamide. (Horizon) Prednisolone acetate 0.5%, sodium sulfacetamide 10%, hydroxypropyl methylcellulose, polysorbate 80, sodium thiosulfate, benzalkonium Cl 0.01%. Susp. Dropper bot. 5 ml, 15 ml. *Rx.*
Use: Anti-infective, corticosteroid, ophthalmic.

•**conorphone hydrochloride.** (KOE-nahr-fone) USAN. *Formerly Codorphone.*
Use: Analgesic.

Conray. (Mallinckrodt) Iothalamate meglumine 60% (28.2% iodine), EDTA. Inj. Vial 20 ml, 30 ml, 50 ml, 100 ml, 150 ml. *Rx.*
Use: Radiopaque agent.

Conray-30. (Mallinckrodt) Iothalamate meglumine 30% (14.1% iodine), EDTA. Inj. Vial 300 ml. *Rx.*
Use: Radiopaque agent.

Conray-43. (Mallinckrodt) Iothalamate meglumine 43% (20.2% iodine), EDTA. Inj. Vial 50 ml, 100 ml, 250 ml. *Rx.*
Use: Radiopaque agent.

Conray-325. (Mallinckrodt) Iothalamate sodium 54.3% (32.5% iodine), EDTA. Inj. Vial 30 ml, 50 ml. *Rx.*
Use: Radiopaque agent.

Conray-400. (Mallinckrodt) Iothalamate sodium 66.8% (40% iodine), EDTA. Inj. Vial 25 ml, 50 ml. *Rx.*
Use: Radiopaque agent.

Consin Compound Salve. (Wisconsin Pharm) Carbolic acid ointment. Jar 2 oz, lb. *otc.*
Use: Minor skin irritations.

Constilac. (Alra Laboratories) Lactulose syrup 10 g/15 ml. Bot. 8 oz, 16 oz, UD 30 ml. *Rx.*
Use: Laxative.

Constonate 60. Docusate sodium 100 mg, 250 mg/Cap. Bot. 100s, 1000s. *otc.*
Use: Laxative.

Constulose. (Alphalma USPD) Lactulose 10 g, galactose < 2.2 g, lactose 1.2 g, other sugars ≤ 1.2 g/15 ml. Syr. Bot. 237 ml, 946 ml. *Rx.*
Use: Analgesic, laxative.

Contac-12 Hour Capsules. (SmithKline Beecham Pharmaceuticals) Phenylpropanolamine HCl 75 mg, chlorpheniramine maleate 8 mg/CA Cap. Pkg. 10s, 20s. *otc.*
Use: Antihistamine, decongestant.

Contac Cough & Chest Cold Liquid. (SmithKline Beecham Pharmaceuticals) Pseudoephedrine HCl 15 mg, dextromethorpan HBr 5 mg, guaifenesin 50 mg, acetaminophen 125 mg, alcohol 10%, saccharin, sorbitol. Liq. Bot. 4 fl. oz. *otc.*
Use: Analgesic, antitussive, decongestant, expectorant,.

Contac Cough and Sore Throat Formula. (SmithKline Beecham Pharmaceuticals) Dextromethorphan HBr 5 mg, acetaminophen 125 mg, alcohol 10%. Bot. 120 ml. *otc.*
Use: Analgesic, antitussive.

Contac Day & Night Allergy/Sinus Caplets. (SmithKline Beecham Pharmaceuticals) **Day:** Pseudoephedrine HCl 60 mg, acetaminophen 650 mg/Capl. **Night:** Pseudoephedrine HCl 60 mg, diphenhydramine HCl 50 mg, acetaminophen 650 mg/Capl. Pkg. 20 (15 day; 5 night). *otc.*
Use: Analgesic, antihistamine, decongestant.

Contac Day & Night Cold & Flu Caplets. (SmithKline Beecham Pharmaceuticals) **Night:** Pseudoephedrine HCl 60 mg, diphenhydramine HCl 50 mg, acetaminophen 650 mg/Cap. Pkg. 5s. **Day:** Pseudoephedrine HCl 60 mg, dextromethorphan HRr 30 mg, acetaminophen 650 mg/Cap. Pkg. 15s. *otc.*
Use: Analgesic, antihistamine, antitussive, decongestant.

Contac Jr. (SmithKline Beecham Pharmaceuticals) Pseudoephedrine HCl 15 mg, acetaminophen 160 mg, dextromethorphan HBr 5 mg, saccharin, sorbitol/5 ml. Bot. 4 oz. *otc.*
Use: Analgesic, antitussive, decongestant.

Contac Maximum Strength 12-Hour Caplets. (SmithKline Beecham Pharmaceuticals) Phenylpropanolamine HCl

75 mg, chlorpheniramine maleate 12 mg/Capl. Pkg. 10, 20s. *otc.*
Use: Antihistamine, decongestant.

Contac Nighttime Cold. (SmithKline Beecham Pharmaceuticals) Acetaminophen 167 mg, dextromethorphan HBr 5 mg, pseudoephedrine HCl 10 mg, doxylamine succinate 1.25 mg/5 ml, alcohol 25%. Bot. 177 ml. *otc.*
Use: Analgesic, antihistamine, antitussive, decongestant.

Contac Non-Drowsy Formula Sinus. (SmithKline Beecham Pharmaceuticals) Pseudoephedrine HCl 30 mg, acetaminophen 500 mg/Capl. or Tab. Pkg. 24s. *otc.*
Use: Analgesic, decongestant.

Contac Severe Cold Formula. (SmithKline Beecham Pharmaceuticals) Phenylpropanolamine HCl 12.5 mg, acetaminophen 500 mg, chlorpheniramine maleate 2 mg, dextromethorphan HBr 15 mg/Capl. Pkg. 10s, 20s. *otc.*
Use: Analgesic, antihistamine, antitussive, decongestant.

Contac Severe Cold & Flu Nighttime Liquid. (SmithKline Beecham Pharmaceuticals) Pseudoephedrine HCl 10 mg, chlorpheniramine maleate 0.67 mg, dextromethorphan HBr 5 mg, acetaminophen 167 mg, alcohol 18.5%, saccharin, sorbitol, glucose. Liq. Bot. 180 ml. *otc.*
Use: Antihistamine, antitussive, decongestant.

contact lens products, soft. (Hydrogel). *otc.*
Use: Contact lens care, rising, storage.
See: Allergan Hydrocare Preserved Saline (Allergan).
Boil n Soak (Alcon Laboratories).
Lensrins (Allergan).
Opti-Soft (Alcon Laboratories).
ReNu Saline (Bausch & Lomb).
Saline Solution, Sterile Preserved (Bausch & Lomb).
Murine Preserved All-Purpose Saline Solution (Ross Laboratories).
Sensitive Eyes Plus (Bausch & Lomb).
Sensitive Eyes Saline (Bausch & Lomb).
Soft Mate Saline for Sensitive Eyes (PHB Wesley Jessen).
Allergan Sorbi-Care Saline (Allergan).
Sterile Saline (Bausch & Lomb).
Blairex Sterile Saline (Blairex Labs).
Hypo-Clear (Bausch & Lomb).
Lens Plus Preservative Free (Allergan).
Ciba Vision Saline (Ciba Vision Ophthalmics).
Hypo-Clear (Bausch & Lomb).
Unisol (Wesley-Jessen).
Unisol 4 (Wesley-Jessen).
Soft Mate Saline Preservative-Free (PHB Wesley Jessen).
Use: Salt tablets for normal saline.
See: Soft Rinse 135 (Professional Supplies).
Amcon 250 (Amcon Laboratories).
Easy Eyes (Eaton Medicals).
Marlin Salt System II (Marlin).
Soft Rinse 250 (Professional Supplies).
Use: Surfactant cleaning solutions.
See: Ciba Vision Cleaner (Ciba Vision Ophthalmics).
Daily Cleaner (Bausch & Lomb).
Preflex for Sensitive Eyes (Alcon Laboratories).
DURAcare II (Blairex Labs).
LC-65 (Allergan).
Lens Clear (Allergan).
Lens Plus Daily Cleaner (Allergan).
Mira Flow Extra Strength (Ciba Vision Ophthalmics).
Murine Contact Lens Cleaner (Ross Laboratories).
Opti-Clean II (Alcon Laboratories).
Pliagel (Wesley-Jessen).
Sensitive Eyes Saline/Cleaning Solution (Bausch & Lomb).
Sof/Pro-Clean (Sherman).
Sof/Pro-Clean (s.a.) (Sherman).
Soft Mate Hands Off Daily Cleaner (PHB Wesley Jessen).
Soft Mate Protein Remover (PHB Wesley Jessen).
Soft Mate Daily Cleaning for Sensitive Eyes (PHB Wesley Jessen).
Use: Enzymatic cleaners.
See: Allergan Enzymatic (Allergan).
Extenzyme Protein Cleaner (Allergan).
Opti-zyme Enzymatic Cleaner (Alcon Laboratories).
ReNu Effervescent Enzymatic Cleaner (Bausch & Lomb).
ReNu Thermal Enzymatic Cleaner (Bausch & Lomb).
Ultrazyme Enzymatic Cleaner (Allergan).
Use: Re-wetting solutions.
See: Adapettes for Sensitive Eyes (Alcon Laboratories).
Clerz Drops (Wesley-Jessen).
Clerz 2 (Wesley-Jessen).
Comfort Tears (PHB Wesley Jessen).
Lens Drops (Ciba Vision Ophthalmics).

Lens Fresh (Allergan).
Lens Lubricant (Bausch & Lomb).
Lens Plus Rewetting Drops (Allergan).
Lens-Wet (Allergan).
Murine Sterile Lubricating and Rewetting Drops (Ross Laboratories).
Opti-Tears (Alcon Laboratories).
Sensitive Eye Drops (Bausch & Lomb).
Soft Mate Comfort Drops (PHB Wesley Jessen).
Soft Mate Lens Drops (PHB Wesley Jessen).
Sterile Lens Lubricant (Blairex Labs).
Use: Disinfectant.
See: Allergan Hydrocare Cleaning and Disinfecting (Allergan).
Aosept (Ciba Vision Ophthalmics).
Disinfecting Solution (Bausch & Lomb).
Flex-Care (Alcon Laboratories).
Lens Plus Oxysept System (Allergan).
Lensept (Ciba Vision Ophthalmics).
MiraSept System (Wesley-Jessen).
Opti-Free (Alcon Laboratories).
Pure Sept (Ross Laboratories).
Quik-Sept System (Bausch & Lomb).
ReNu Multi-Action (Bausch & Lomb).
Soft Mate (PHB Wesley Jessen).
Soft Mate Consept (PHB Wesley Jessen).

ConTE-PAK-4. (SoloPak) Zinc 5 mg, copper 1 mg, manganese 0.5 mg, chromium 10 mcg/ml. Soln. Vial 1 ml, 10 ml. *Rx.*
Use: Nutritional supplement, parenteral.

contraceptives.
See: Oral Contraceptives (Various Mfr.).
Foams, Vaginal.
See: Delfen, Vaginal Foam (Ortho McNeil).
Emko, Vaginal Foam (Schering Plough).
Intrauterine System.
See: Progestasert, (Alza).
Jellies & Creams, Vaginal.
See: Colagyn, Jel (Smith & Nephew United).
Colagyn, Jel (Smith & Nephew United).
Conceptrol, Cream, Gel (Ortho McNeil).
Gynol II, Gel (Ortho McNeil).
Immolin, Cream-Jel (Schmid).
Koromex-A, Jelly (Holland-Rantos).
Koromex, Cream or Jelly (Holland-Rantos).
Ortho-Creme (Ortho McNeil).
Ortho-Gynol, Jelly (Ortho McNeil).
Miscellaneous.
See: Norplant (Wyeth Ayerst).
VCF, Film (Apothecus).
Suppositories, Vaginal.
See: Intercept, Inserts (Ortho McNeil).
Lorophyn, Supp., Jelly (Eaton Medical Corp).

Contrin. (Geneva Pharm) Iron (from ferrous fumarate) 110 mg, B_{12} 15 mcg, IFC (intrinisic factor as concentrate or from stomach preparations) 240 mg, C 75 mg, folic acid 0.5 mg/Cap. Bot. 100s. *Rx.*
Use: Mineral, vitamin supplement.

Control. (Thompson Medical) Phenylpropanolamine HCl 75 mg/TR Cap. Bot. 14s, 28s, 56s. *otc.*
Use: Dietary aid.

Contuss Liquid. (Parmed) Phenylpropanolamine HCl 20 mg, phenylephrine HCl 5 mg, guaifenesin 100 mg, alcohol 5%, saccharin, sorbitol, sucrose. Liq. Bot. 16 fl. oz. *Rx.*
Use: Decongestant, expectorant.
Use: Digestive enzymes.

Converspaz. (B.F. Ascher) Cellulase 5 mg, protease 10 mg, amylase 30 mg, lipase 13 mg, l-hyoscamine sulfate 0.0625 mg/Cap. Bot. 100s. *Rx.*
Use: Decongestant, expectorant.

Cool-Mint Listerine. (Warner Lambert) Thymol, eucalyptol, methyl salicylate, menthol, alcohol 21.6%. Liq. Bot. 90 ml, 180 ml, 360 ml, 540 ml, 720 ml, 960 ml. *otc.*
Use: Mouthwash.

Coopervision Balanced Salt Solution. (Ciba Vision Ophthalmics) Sterile intraocular irrigation soln. Bot. 15 ml, 500 ml.
Use: Irrigant, ophthalmic.

Copavin Pulvules. (Eli Lilly) Codeine sulfate 15 mg, papaverine HCl 15 mg/Cap. Bot. 100s. *c-v.*
Use: Antitussive.

Copaxone. (Teva) Glatiramer acetate, mannitol 40 mg/Vial, 2 ml. 32s. *Rx.*
Use: Multiple sclerosis agent.

COPE. (Mentholatum) Aspirin 421 mg, magnesium hydroxide 50 mg, aluminum hydroxide 25 mg, caffeine 32 mg/Tab. Bot. 36s, 60s. *otc.*
Use: Analgesic, antacid.

Cophene #2. (Dunhall Pharmaceuticals) Chlorpheniramine maleate 12 mg, pseudoephedrine HCl 120 mg/Time Cap. Bot. 100s, 500s. *Rx.*
Use: Antihistamine, decongestant.

Cophene Injectable. (Dunhall Pharmaceuticals) Atropine sulfate 0.2 mg,

phenylpropanolamine HCl 12.5 mg, chlorpheniramine maleate 5 mg/ml. Pkg. 10 ml. *Rx.*
Use: Anticholinergic, antihistamine, antispasmodic, decongestant.

Cophene-PL. (Dunhall Pharmaceuticals) Phenylephrine HCl 20 mg, phenylpropanolamine HCl 20 mg, chlorpheniramine maleate 5 mg/5 ml. Bot. 16 oz. *otc, Rx.*
Use: Antihistamine, decongestant.

Cophene-S. (Dunhall Pharmaceuticals) Dihydrocodone bitartrate 3 mg, phenylephrine HCl 20 mg, phenylpropanolamine HCl 20 mg, chlorpheniramine maleate 5 mg/5 ml. Bot. pt. *c-III.*
Use: Antihistamine, antitussive, decongestant.

Cophene-X. (Dunhall Pharmaceuticals) Carbetapentane citrate 20 mg, phenylephrine HCl 10 mg, phenylpropanolamine HCl 10 mg, chlorpheniramine maleate 2.5 mg, potassium guaiacolsulfonate 45 mg/Cap. Bot. 100s. *Rx.*
Use: Antihistamine, antitussive, decongestant, expectorant.

Cophene-XP Syrup. (Dunhall Pharmaceuticals) Carbetapentane citrate 20 mg, phenylephrine HCl 10 mg, phenylpropanolamine HCl 20 mg, chlorpheniramine maleate 2.5 mg, potassium guaiacolsulfonate 45 mg/5 ml. Bot. pt. *Rx.*
Use: Antihistamine, antitussive, decongestant, expectorant.

copolymer 1, (cop 1).
Use: Treat multiple sclerosis. [Orphan drug]

copper. (Abbott Laboratories) Copper 0.4 mg/ml (as 0.85 mg cupric Cl.) Inj. Vial 10 ml, 30 ml. *Rx.*
Use: Nutritional supplement, parenteral.

•**copper gluconate.** U.S.P. 23.
Use: Supplement (trace mineral).

copperhead bite therapy.
See: Antivenin, (crotalidae) Polyvalent Inj. (Wyeth Ayerst).

Copperin. (Vernon) Iron ammonium citrate, copper (6 gr). "A" adult dose, "B" children dose. Bot. 30s, 100s, 500s.
Use: Mineral supplement.

Coppertone. (Schering Plough) A series of sun-care products marketed under the Coppertone name including Waterproof Lotions SPF 4, 6, 8, 15 and 25. Bot. 4 fl oz, 8 fl oz. Oil SPF 2: Bot. 4 fl oz, 8 fl oz; Lite Formula Oil SPF 2: Bot. 4 fl oz; Lite Lotion SPF 4: Bot. 4 fl oz; Dark Tanning Body Mousse SPF 4: Tube 4 oz; Suntanning Gel SPF 4: Tube 3 oz; Noskote SPF 8: Tube 0.44 oz, Jar 1 oz; Noskote SPF-15: Jar 1 oz. Contain one or more of the following ingredients: Padimate O, oxybenzone, homosalate, ethylhexyl p-methocinnamate. *otc.*
Use: Sunscreen.

Coppertone Dark Tanning Spray. (Schering Plough) Padimate O in spray base (SPF 2). Bot. 8 fl oz. *otc.*
Use: Sunscreen.

Coppertone Face. (Schering Plough) A series of sunscreen lotions with SPF 2, 4, 6 and 15 in a non-greasy base with Padimate O, oxybenzone (SPF 15 only). *otc.*
Use: Sunscreen.

Coppertone Kids Sunblock. (Schering Plough) **SPF 15:** Ethylhexyl p-methoxycinnamate, oxybenzone, 2-ethylhexyl salicylate, homosalate. Lot. Bot. 120 ml, 240 ml. **SPF 30:** Octocrylene, ethylhexyl p-methoxycinnamate, oxybenzone, 2-ethylhexyl salicylate. Lot. Bot. 120 ml, 240 ml. *otc.*
Use: Sunscreen.

Coppertone Lipkote. (Schering Plough) Ethylhexyl p-methoxycinnamate, oxybenzone. SPF 15. Stick 4.5 g. *otc.*
Use: Sunscreen.

Coppertone Moisturizing Sunblock. (Schering Plough) **SPF 45:** Ethylhexyl p-methoxycinnamate, 2-ethylhexyl salicylate, octocrylene, oxybenzone. Lot. Bot. 120 ml, 300 ml. **SPF 30, 25:** Ethylhexyl p-methoxycinnamate, oxybenzone, 2-ethylhexyl salicylate, homosalate. Lot. Bot. SPF 30: 120 ml, 240 ml; SPF 25: 120 ml. **SPF 15:** Ethylhexyl p-methoxycinnamate, oxybenzone. Lot. Bot. 120 ml, 240 ml, 300 ml. *otc.*
Use: Sunscreen.

Coppertone Moisturizing Sunscreen. (Schering Plough) Ethylhexyl p-methoxycinnamate, oxybenzone, benzyl alcohol, vitamin E, aloe. PABA free. SPF 6, 8. Waterproof. Lot. Bot. 120 ml, 240 ml. *otc.*
Use: Sunscreen.

Coppertone Moisturizing Suntan. (Schering Plough) **SPF 4:** ethylhexyl p-methoxycinnamate, oxybenzone, benzyl alcohol, vitamin E, aloe. PABA free. Waterproof. Lot. Bot. 120 ml, 240 ml. **SPF 2:** homosalate, vitamin E, aloe. PABA free. Waterproof. Oil. Bot. 120 ml. *otc.*
Use: Sunscreen.

Coppertone Noskote. (Schering Plough) Homosalate 8%, oxybenzone 3%. (SPF 8) Oint. Jar 13.2 g, 30 g. *otc.*

Use: Sunscreen.

Coppertone SPF-25 Sunblock Lotion. (Schering Plough) Ethylhexyl p-methoxycinnamate, oxybenzone, Padimate O in lotion base (SPF-25). Bot. 4 fl oz. *otc.*
Use: Sunscreen.

Coppertone Sport. (Schering Plough) Ethylhexyl p-methoxycinnamate, oxybenzone. SPF 4, 8, 15, 30. Lot. Bot. 120 ml. *otc.*
Use: Sunscreen.

Coppertone Tan Magnifier Suntan. (Schering Plough). **SPF 2:** Triethanolamine salicylate. Oil Bot. 120 ml. **SPF 4: Lotion:** Ethylhexyl p-methoxycinnamate. Bot. 120 ml. **Gel:** 2-phenylbenzimidazole-5-sulfonic acid. Tube 120 g. *otc.*
Use: Sunscreen

copper trace metal additive. (IMS, Ltd.) Copper 1 mg. Inj. Vial 10 ml. *Rx.*
Use: Copper supplement.

•**copper undecylenate.** USAN.

W/Sodium propionate, sodium caprylate, propionic acid, undecylenic acid, salicylic acid.

Co-Pyronil 2. (Eli Lilly) Chlorpheniramine maleate 4 mg, pseudoephedrine HCl 60 mg/Pulvule. Bot. 100s. *otc.*
Use: Antihistamine, decongestant.

Corab. (Abbott Diagnostics) Radioimmunoassay for detection of antibody to hepatitis B core antigen. Test kit 100s.
Use: Diagnostic aid.

Corab-M. (Abbott Diagnostics) Radioimmunoassay for the qualitative determination of specific Ig antibody to hepatitis B virus core antigen (Anti-HBc Ig) in human serum or plasma and may be used as an aid in the diagnosis of acute or recent hepatitis B infection.
Use: Diagnostic aid.

Corace Injection. (Forest Pharmaceutical) Cortisone acetate 50 mg/ml. Vial 10 ml. *Rx.*
Use: Corticosteroid, topical.

Coracin. (Roberts Pharm) Hydrocortisone acetate 1%, neomycin sulfate 0.5%, bacitracin zinc 400 units, polymyxin B sulfate 10,000 units/g in white petrolatum and mineral oil base. Oint. Tube 3.5 g. *Rx.*
Use: Anti-infective, corticosteroid, ophthalmic.

Coral. (Young Dental) Fluoride ion 1.23%, 0.1 molar phosphate. Jar 250 g, Coral II: 180 disposable cup units/carton. *Rx.*
Use: Fluoride, dental.

Coral/Plus. (Young Dental) Free fluoride ion 2.2%, recrystallized kaolinite. Tube 250 g. *Rx.*

coral snake (North American) antivenin.
See: Antivenin (Micrurus fulvius). (Wyeth Ayerst).

Corane Capsules. (Forest Pharmaceutical) Pyrilamine maleate 25 mg, pheniramine maleate 10 mg, phenylpropanolamine HCl 25 mg, phenylephrine HCl 10 mg/Cap. Bot. 100s, 500s, 1000s. *otc.*
Use: Antihistamine, decongestant.

Corbicin-125. (Arthrins) Vitamin C 125 mg/Cap. Bot. 100s. *otc.*
Use: Vitamin supplement.

Cordarone. (Wyeth Ayerst) **Tab.:** Amiodarone HCl 200 mg, lactose. Bot. 60s, UD 100s. **Inj.:** Amiodarone 50 mg/ml, benzyl alcohol 20.2 mg/ml. Amps. 3 ml. *Rx.*
Use: Antiarrhythmic.

Cordran. (Eli Lilly) Flurandrenolide 0.025%, 0.05% in emulsified petrolatum base/g. **0.025%:** Tube 30 g, 60 g, Jar 225 g. **0.05%:** Tube 15 g, 30 g, 60 g, Jar 225 g. *Rx.*
Use: Corticosteroid, topical.

Cordran Lotion. (Eli Lilly) Flurandrenolide 0.05%, cetyl alcohol, benzyl alcohol, stearic acid, glyceryl monostearate, polyoxyl 40 stearate, glycerin, mineral oil, menthol, purified water. Squeeze bot. 15 ml, 60 ml. *Rx.*
Use: Corticosteroid, topical.

Cordran-N Cream & Ointment. (Eli Lilly) Flurandrenolide 0.5 mg, neomycin sulfate 5 mg/g. Tube 15 g, 30 g, 60 g. *Rx.*
Use: Corticosteroid, topical.

Cordran SP. (Eli Lilly) Flurandrenolide 0.025%, 0.05% in emulsified base w/ cetyl alcohol, stearic acid, polyoxyl 40 stearate, mineral oil, propylene glycol, sodium citrate, citric acid, purified water. **0.025%:** Tube 30 g, 60 g, Jar 225 g. **0.05%:** Tube 15 g, 30 g, 60 g, Jar 225 g. *Rx.*
Use: Corticosteroid, topical.

Cordran Tape. (Eli Lilly) Flurandrenolide 4 mcg/sq. cm. Roll 7.5 cm × 60 cm, 7.5 cm 200 cm. *Rx.*
Use: Corticosteroid, topical.

Cordrol. (Vita Elixir) Prednisolone 5 mg, 10 mg or 20 mg/Tab. Bot. 100s. *Rx.*
Use: Corticosteroid.

Coreg. (SmithKline Beecham) Carvedilol

3.125 mg, 6.25 mg, 12.5 mg, 25 mg. lactose, sucrose. Tab. Bot. 100s *Rx.*
Use: Antihypertensive.

Coreg Powder. (Block Drug) Denture adhesive containing polyethyleneoxide polymer w/peppermint oil, karaya gum. Pkg.: pocket 0.7 oz; medium 1.15 oz; economy 3.55 oz. *otc.*
Use: Denture adhesive.

Corgard. (Bristol-Myers Squibb) Nadolol 20 mg, 40 mg, 80 mg, 120 mg or 160 mg/Tab. Bot 100s, 1000s, UD 100s. *Rx.*
Use: Beta-adrenergic blocker.

•**coriander oil.** N.F. XVI.
Use: Pharmaceutic aid (flavor).

Coricidin. (Schering Plough) Chlorpheniramine maleate 2 mg, acetaminophen 325 mg/Tab. Bot. 100s. *otc.*
Use: Analgesic, antihistamine.

Coricidin "D" Tablets. (Schering Plough) Chlorpheniramine maleate 2 mg, acetaminophen 325 mg, phenylpropanolamine HCl 12.5 mg/Tab. Bot. 12s, 24s, 48s, 100s. *otc.*
Use: Analgesic, antihistamine, decongestant,

Coricidin Demilets. (Schering Plough) Phenylpropanolamine HCl 6.25 mg, chlorpheniramine maleate 1 mg, acetaminophen 80 mg, saccharin, lactose. Tab. Bot. 24s, 36s. *otc.*
Use: Analgesic, antihistamine, decongestant.

Coricidin Extra Strength Sinus Headache Tablets. (Schering Plough) Acetaminophen 500 mg, phenylpropanolamine HCl 12.5 mg, chlorpheniramine maleate 2 mg/Tab. Box 24s. *otc.*
Use: Analgesic, antihistamine, decongestant.

Coricidin Maximum Strength Sinus Headache. (Schering Plough) Phenylpropanolamine HCl 12.5 mg, chlorpheniramine maleate 2 mg, acetaminophen 500 mg/Tab. Box 24s. *otc.*
Use: Analgesic, antihistamine, decongestant.

Corilin Infant Liquid. (Schering Plough) Chlorpheniramine maleate 0.75 mg, sodium salicylate 80 mg/ml, alcohol < 1%. Bot. 30 ml. *otc.*
Use: Analgesic, antihistamine.

Corlopam. (Neurex) Fenoldopam mesylate 10 mg/ml, sodium metabisulfite. Inj. single-dose amp. 5 ml. *Rx.*
Use: Antihypertensive.

Cormax. (Oclassen) Clobetasol propionate 0.05%, white petrolatum, sorbitan sesquioleate/Oint. Tube. 15 g and 45 g. *Rx.*
Use: Corticosteroid, topical.

Cormed.
See: Nikethamide (Various Mfr.).

•**cormethasone acetate.** (core-METH-ahsone) USAN.
Use: Anti-inflammatory, topical.

Corn Huskers Lotion. (Warner Lambert) Glycerin 6.7%, SD alcohol, algin, TEA-oleoyl sarcosinate, guar gum, methylparaben, calcium sulfate, calcium Cl, TEA-fumarate, TEA-borate. Bot. 4 oz, 7 oz. *otc.*
Use: Emollient.

•**corn oil.** N.F. 18.
Use: Pharmaceutic aid (solvent, oleaginous vehicle).
See: G. B. Prep Emulsion (Gray).
Lipomul-Oral, Liq. (Pharmacia & Upjohn).

Corns-O-Poppin. (Ries-Hamly) Salicylic acid 6.5%, benzoic acid 12%. *otc.*
Use: Cardiovascular agent.

Corotrope. (Sanofi Winthrop) Milrinone for IV use. *Rx.*
Use: Cardiovascular agent.

corpus luteum, extract (water soluble).
See: Progesterone, Preps. (Various Mfr.).

Corque. (Geneva Pharm) Hydrocortisone 1%, iodochlorhydroxyquin 3%. Cream. Tube 20 g. *Rx.*
Use: Corticosteroid, topical.

Correctol. (Schering Plough) Bisacodyl 5 mg, talc, lactose, sugar. Tab. Bot. 60s. *otc.*
Use: Laxative.

Correctol Extra Gentle. (Schering Plough) Docusate sodium 100 mg. Softgel Cap. Bot. 30s. *otc.*
Use: Laxative.

Cortaid Intensive Therapy. (Pharmacia & Upjohn) Hydrocortisone 1%, alcohols, parabens. Tube 56 g. *otc.*
Use: Corticosteroid, topical.

Cortaid, Maximum Strength. (Pharmacia & Upjohn) **Cream:** Hydrocortisone in parabens 1%, cetyl and stearyl alcohols, glycerin and white petrolatum. Tube 15 g, 30 g. *otc.*
Use: Corticosteroids, topical.

Cortaid Maximum Strength Spray. (Pharmacia & Upjohn) Hydrocortisone 1%, alcohol 55%, glycerin, methylparaben. Pump spray. Bot. 45 ml. *otc.*
Use: Corticosteroid, topical.

Cortan. (Halsey) Prednisone 5 mg/Tab. Bot. 1000s. *Rx.*
Use: Corticosteroid.

Cortane D.C. Expectorant. (Standex)

Brompheniramine maleate 2 mg, guaifenesin 100 mg, phenylephrine HCl 5 mg, phenylpropanolamine HCl 5 mg, codeine phosphate 10 mg, alcohol 3.5%/5 ml. Bot. pt. *c-v.*
Use: Antihistamine, antitussive, decongestant, expectorant.

Cortane Expectorant. (Standex) Brompheniramine maleate 2 mg, guaifenesin 100 mg, phenylephrine 5 mg, phenylpropanolamine HCl 5 mg, alcohol 3.5%/5 ml. Bot. pt. *otc.*
Use: Antihistamine, decongestant, expectorant.

Cortapp Elixir. (Standex) Brompheniramine maleate 5 mg, phenylephrine HCl 5 mg, phenylpropanolamine HCl 5 mg, alcohol 2.3%/5 ml. Bot. pt. *otc.*
Use: Antihistamine, decongestant.

Cortatrigen Ear Suspension. (Zenith Goldline) Hydrocortisone 1%, neomycin sulfate 5 mg, polymyxin B sulfate 10,000 units/ml. Bot. 10 ml. *Rx.*
Use: Anti-infective, corticosteroid, otic.

Cortatrigen Modified Ear Drops. (Zenith Goldline) Bot. 10 ml. *Rx.*
Use: Anti-infective; corticosteroid, otic.

Cort-Dome. (Bayer Corp) Hydrocortisone alcohol. **Cream:** 0.25%: 1 oz, 4 oz; 0.5%: 1 oz; 1%: 1 oz. **Lot.:** 0.25%: 4 oz; 0.5%: 4 oz; 1%: 1 oz. *Rx.*
Use: Corticosteroid, topical.

Cort-Dome High Potency. (Bayer Corp) Hydrocortisone acetate 25 mg in a monoglyceride base. *Rx.*
Use: Corticosteroid, topical.

Cortef Acetate Ointment. (Pharmacia & Upjohn) Hydrocortisone acetate 10 mg/g, lanolin (anhydrous), white petrolatum, mineral oil. Tube 20 g (10 mg/g). *Rx.*
Use: Corticosteroid, topical.

Cortef Feminine Itch Cream. (Pharmacia & Upjohn) Hydrocortisone acetate equivalent to hydrocortisone 5 mg/g. Tube 0.5 oz. *Rx.*
Use: Corticosteroid, topical.

Cortef Oral Suspension. (Pharmacia & Upjohn) Hydrocortisone 10 mg/5 ml (as 13.4 mg hydrocortisone cypionate). Oral susp. Bot. 4 oz. *Rx.*
Use: Corticosteroid.

Cortef Tablets. (Pharmacia & Upjohn) Hydrocortisone. **5 mg/Tab.:** Bot. 50s; **10 mg or 20 mg/Tab.:** Bot. 100s. *Rx.*
Use: Corticosteroid.

Cortenema. (Solvay) Hydrocortisone 100 mg in aqueous solution w/carboxypolymethylene, polysorbate 80, methylparaben 0.18%/60 ml. Bot. w/applicator. UD 1s. *Rx.*
Use: Corticosteroid, topical.

cortenil.
See: Desoxycorticosterone Acetate, Preps. (Various Mfr.).

cortical hormone products.
See: Adrenal Cortex Extract (Various Mfr.).
Aristocort, Preps. (ESI Lederle Generics).
Corticotropin, Preps. (Various Mfr.).
Hydrocortisone, Preps. (Various Mfr.).
Cortisone Acetate, Preps. (Various Mfr.).
Decadron LA, Inj. (Merck).
Decadron, Tab., Elix., Inj. (Merck).
Desoxycorticosterone Acetate, Preps. (Various Mfr.).
Dexamethasone, Tab. (Various Mfr.).
Fludrocortisone (Various Mfr.).
Hydeltrasol, Inj. (Merck).
Hydrocortone Acetate, Inj. (Merck).
Hydrocortone Phosphate, Inj. (Merck & Co.).
Kenacort, Prep. (Bristol-Myers Squibb).
Lipo-Adrenal Cortex, Inj. (Pharmacia & Upjohn).
Medrol, Preps. (Pharmacia & Upjohn).
Methylprednisolone, Tab. (Various Mfr.).
Prednisolone, Tab. (Various Mfr.).
Prednisone, Tab. (Various Mfr.).
Triamcinolone, Tab. (Various Mfr.).

Cortic Ear Drops. (Everett Laboratories) Hydrocortisone 10 mg, pramoxine HCl 10 mg, chloroxylenol 1 mg/ml, propylene glycol diacetate 3%/Drops. Bot. 10 ml. *Rx.*
Use: Otic.

•**corticorelin ovine triflutate.** (core-tih-kah-REH-lin OH-vine TRY-flew-TATE) USAN.
Use: Hormone (corticotropin-releasing); diagnostic aid (adrenocortical insufficiency, Cushing's syndrome. [Orphan drug]
See: Acthrel (Ferring).

corticosteroid/mydriatic combo, ophthalmics. Prednisolone acetate 0.25%, atropine sulfate 1%. *Rx.*
Use: Treatment of anterior uveitis.
See: Mydrapred, Susp. (Alcon Laboratories).

corticotropin highly purified.
See: H. P. Acthar Gel. Vial. (Centeon).

•**corticotropin injection.** (core-tih-koe-TROE-pin) U.S.P. 23. ACTH, Adrenocorticotropic hormone or adrenocortico-

trop(h)in or corticotropin.
Use: Adrenocorticotropic hormone; corticosteroid, topical; diagnostic aid (adrenocortical insufficiency).
See: ACTH.
Acthar (Centeon).
Cortrophin Gel, Vial, Amp. (Organon Teknika).

•**corticotropin, repository, injection.** (core-tih-koe-TROE-pin) U.S.P. 23.
Use: Hormone (adrenocorticotropic); corticosteroid, topical; diagnostic aid (adrenocortical insufficiency).
See: Acthar Gel Vial (Centeon).
ACTH Gel Purified (Various Mfr.).
Cortrophin Gel Amp., Vial (Organon Teknika).
H.P. Acthar Gel, Vial (Centeon).

Cortifoam. (Schwarz Pharma) Hydrocortisone acetate 10% in an aerosol foam w/propylene glycol, emulsifying wax, steareth 10, cetyl alcohol, methylparaben, propylparaben, trolamine, water, inert propellants. Container 20 g w/rectal applicator for 14 applicatorfuls. *Rx.*
Use: Corticosteroid, topical.

cortisol.
See: Hydrocortisone, U.S.P. 23.
Note: Cortisol was the official published name for hydrocortisone in U.S.P. 23. The name was changed back to Hydrocortisone, U.S.P. in Supplement 1 to the U.S.P. 23.

cortisol cyclopentylpropionate.
See: Cortef Fluid, Susp., Tab. (Pharmacia & Upjohn).

•**cortisone acetate.** (CORE-tih-sone) U.S.P. 23.
Use: Corticosteroid, topical.
See: Cortistan (Standex).
Cortone Acetate, Inj. (Merck).

cortisone acetate. (Kendall's Compound E, Pharmacia & Upjohn) 5 mg, 10 mg, 25 mg/Tab. Bot. 50s, 100s, 500s.
Use: Adrenocortical steroid (anti-inflammatory).

Cortisporin Cream. (GlaxoWellcome) Polymyxin B sulfate 10,000 units, neomycin sulfate 5 mg, hydrocortisone acetate 5 mg/g, methylparaben 0.25%. Tube 7.5 g. *Rx.*
Use: Anti-infective, corticosteroid, topical.

Cortisporin Ointment. (GlaxoWellcome) Polymyxin B sulfate 5000 units, bacitracin zinc 400 units, neomycin sulfate 5 mg, hydrocortisone (1%) 10 mg/g in petrolatum base. Tube 30 g. *Rx.*
Use: Anti-infective, corticosteroid, topical.

Cortisporin Ophthalmic Ointment. (GlaxoWellcome) Polymyxin B sulfate 10,000 units, bacitracin 400 units, neomycin sulfate 0.35%, hydrocortisone 0.1%. Tube 3.5 g. *Rx.*
Use: Anti-infective, corticosteroid, ophthalmic.

Cortisporin Ophthalmic Suspension. (GlaxoWellcome) Polymyxin B sulfate 10,000 units, neomycin sulfate 0.35%, hydrocortisone 1%. Dropper bot. 7.5 ml Sterile. *Rx.*
Use: Anti-infective, corticosteroid, ophthalmic.

Cortisporin Otic Solution Sterile. (GlaxoWellcome) Polymyxin B sulfate 10,000 units, neomycin sulfate 5 mg, hydrocortisone 10 mg/ml, glycerin, propylene glycol, vitamin K metabisulfite 0.1%. Dropper bot. 10 ml Sterile. *Rx.*
Use: Anti-infective, corticosteroid, otic.

Cortisporin Otic Suspension. (GlaxoWellcome) Polymyxin B sulfate 10,000 units, neomycin sulfate 5 mg, hydrocortisone free alcohol 10 mg/ml, cetyl alcohol, propylene glycol, polysorbate 80, thimerosal. Dropper bot. 10 ml Sterile. *Rx.*
Use: Anti-infective, corticosteroid, otic.

Cortisporin-TC. (Monarch) Colistin sulfate 3 mg, neomycin 3.3 mg, hydrocortisone acetate 10 mg, thonzonium bromide 0.5 mg, polysorbate 80, acetic acid, sodium acetate. Otic Susp. Bot. 10 ml w/ dropper. *Rx.*
Use: Otic preparation.

Cortistan. (Standex) Cortisone 25 mg/10 ml. *Rx.*
Use: Corticosteroid.

•**cortivazol.** (core-TIH-vah-zole) USAN.
Use: Corticosteroid, topical.

Cortizone-5. (Thompson Medical) Hydrocortisone 0.5%, glycerin, mineral oil, white petrolatum. Tube 30 g. *otc.*
Use: Corticosteroid, topical.

Cortizone-S, Maximum Strength. (Thompson Medical) Hydrocortisone 0.5%. Tube. *otc.*
Use: Corticosteroid, topical.

•**cortodoxone.** (CORE-toe-dox-OHN) USAN.
Use: Anti-inflammatory.

Cortogen Acetate. Cortisone acetate.

Cortone Acetate. (Merck) Cortisone acetate 50 mg/ml. Inj. Vial 10 ml. *Rx.*
Use: Corticosteroid.

Cortril Topical Ointment 1%. (Pfizer) Hydrocortisone 1%, cetyl and stearyl alcohol, propylene glycol, sodium lauryl

sulfate, petrolatum, cholesterol, mineral oil, methyl and propyl parabens in ointment base. Tube 0.5 oz.
Use: Corticosteroid, topical.

Cortrosyn Injection. (Organon Teknika) Cosyntropin 0.25 mg, mannitol 10 mg, lyophilized powder/ml. Vial. Pkg. w/1 ml amp. diluent. Box 10s. Vial. *Rx.*
Use: Corticosteroid.

Corubeen. (Spanner) Vitamin B_{12} crystalline 1000 mcg/ml. Vial 10 ml. *Rx.*
Use: Vitamin supplement.

Corvert. (Pharmacia & Upjohn) Ibutilide fumerate 0.1 mg/ml/Soln. Vial. 10 ml. *Rx.*
Use: Antiarrhythmatic.

Coryza Brengle. (Roberts Pharm) Pseudoephedrine HCl 30 mg, acetaminophen 200 mg/Cap. Bot. 1000s. *otc.*
Use: Analgesic, decongestant.

Corzide. (Bristol-Myers) Nadolol 40 mg, bendroflumethiazide 5 mg/Tab or Nadolol 80 mg, bendroflumethiazide 5 mg/Tab. Bot. 100s. *Rx.*
Use: Antihypertensive.

Corzyme. (Abbott Diagnostics) Enzyme immunoassay for detection of antibody to hepatitis B core antigen in serum or plasma. Test kit 100s.
Use: Diagnostic aid.

Corzyme-M. (Abbott Diagnostics) Enzyme immunoassay for the detection of Ig antibody to hepatitis B core antigen. (Anti-HBc Ig) In human serum or plasma. Test kit 100s.
Use: Diagnostic aid.

Cosmegen. (Merck) Actinomycin D (dactinomycin) 0.5 mg (lyophilized powder)/3 ml. *Rx.*
Use: Antineoplastic.

Cosmoline.
See: Petrolatum.

Cosulid. (Novartis) Sulfachloropyridazine.

•**cosyntropin.** (koe-sin-TROE-pin) USAN.
Use: Hormone (adrenocorticotropic).
See: Cortrosyn, Vial (Organon Teknika).

Cotaphylline Tabs. (Major) Oxtriphylline 100 mg or 200 mg/Tab. Bot. 100s, 500s. *Rx.*
Use: Bronchodilator.

cotarnine chloride. Cotarnine hydrochloride.

cotarnine hydrochloride.
See: Cotarnine Chloride.

Cotazym. (Organon Teknika) Pancrelipase, lipase 8000 units, protease 30,000 units, amylase 30,000 units, calcium carbonate 25 mg/Cap. Bot. 100s, 500s. *Rx.*
Use: Digestive enzymes.

Cotazym-S. (Organon Teknika) Pancrelipase spheres, lipase 5,000 units, protease 20,000 units, amylase 20,000 units/Cap. Bot. 100s, 500s. *Rx.*
Use: Digestive enzyme.

•**cotinine fumarate.** (koe-TIH-neen) USAN.
Use: Antidepressant, psychomotor stimulant.

Cotolate Tabs. (Major) Benztropine 1 mg or 2 mg/Tab. Bot. 100s, 1000s. *Rx.*
Use: Antiparkinsonian.

Cotrim. (Teva USA) Sulfamethoxazole 400 mg, trimethoprim 80 mg/Tab. Bot. 100s, 500s. *Rx.*
Use: Anti-infective.

Cotrim D.S. (Teva USA) Sulfamethoxazole 800 mg, trimethoprim 160 mg/Tab. Bot. 100s, 500s. *Rx.*
Use: Anti-infective.

Cotrim Pediatric. (Teva USA) Sulfamethoxazole 200 mg, trimethoprim 40 mg/5 ml. Bot. 473 ml. *Rx.*
Use: Anti-infective.

•**cotton, purified.** U.S.P. 23.
Use: Surgical aid.

•**cottonseed oil.** N.F. 18.
Use: Pharmaceutic aid, solvent, oleaginous vehicle.

Co-Tuss V Liquid. (Rugby) Hydrocodone bitartrate 5 mg, guaifenesin 100 mg. Bot. 480 ml. *c-III.*
Use: Antitussive, expectorant.

Cotylenol Chewable Cold Tablet. (McNeil Consumer Products) Acetaminophen 80 mg, phenylpropanolamine HCl 3.125 mg, chlorpheniramine maleate 0.5 mg/Tab. Bot. 24s. *otc.*
Use: Analgesic, antihistamine, decongestant.

Cotylenol Children's Chewable Cold Tablet. (McNeil Consumer Products) Acetaminophen 80 mg, chlorpheniramine maleate 0.5 mg, pseudoephedrine HCl 7.5 mg/Tab. Bot. 24s. *otc.*
Use: Analgesic, antihistamine, decongestant.

Cotylenol Children's Liquid Cold Formula. (McNeil Consumer Products) Acetaminophen 160 mg, chlorpheniramine maleate 1 mg, pseudoephedrine HCl 15 mg, sorbitol/5 ml. Bot. 4 oz. *otc.*
Use: Analgesic, antihistamine, decongestant.

Cotylenol Cold Formula. (McNeil Consumer Products) Chlorpheniramine maleate 2 mg, dextromethorphan HBr

15 mg, pseudoephedrine HCl 30 mg, acetaminophen 325 mg/Tab. or Capl. **Tab.:** Box 24s, Bot. 50s, 100s. **Capl.:** Bot. 24s, 50s. *otc.*
Use: Analgesic, antihistamine, antitussive, decongestant.

Cotylenol Liquid Cold Formula. (McNeil Consumer Products) Acetaminophen 650 mg, chlorpheniramine maleate 4 mg, pseudoephedrine HCl 60 mg, dextromethorphan HCl 30 mg/30 ml, alcohol 7.5%, sorbitol. Bot. 5 oz. *otc.*
Use: Analgesic, antihistamine, antitussive, decongestant.

Cough Formula Comtrex. (Bristol-Myers) Pseudoephedrine HCl 15 mg, dextromethorphan HBr 7.5 mg, guaifenesin, saccharin, sucrose. Liq. Bot. 120 ml, 240 ml. *otc.*
Use: Antitussive, expectorant.

Cough Syrup. (Zenith Goldline) Phenylephrine HCl 5 mg, dextromethorphan HBr 10 mg, guaifenesin 100 mg, alcohol free. Bot. 120 ml. *otc.*
Use: Antitussive, decongestant, expectorant.

Cough-X. (B.F. Ascher) Dextromethorphan 5 mg, benzocaine 2 mg, dye free/Loz. Pkg. 9s. *otc.*
Use: Anesthetic, antitussive.

Coumadin. (DuPont) Warfarin sodium crystalline. **Tab.:** 1 mg, 2 mg, 2.5 mg, 4 mg, 5 mg, 7.5 mg or 10 mg. Bot. 100s, 1000s, UD 100s. **Powd. for Inj., lyophilized:** Warfarin sodium 2 mg, sodium phosphate 4.98 mg, dibasic,, heptahydrate, sodium phosphate 0.194 mg, monobasic, monohydrate, NaCl 0.1 mg, mannitol 38 mg/ml when reconstituted. Vial. 5 mg. *Rx.*
Use: Anticoagulant.

coumarin.
Use: Anticoagulant; treat renal cell carcinoma. [Orphan Drug]
See: Oncostate. (Praevomed GmBH).

coumarin and indandione derivatives.
Use: Anticoagulant.
See: Coumadin, Tab. (DuPont Merck Pharmaceuticals).
Warfarin Sodium, Tab. (Various Mfr.).
Panwarfin, Tab. (Abbott Laboratories).
Sofarin, Tab. (Teva USA).
Miradon, Tab. (Schering Plough).

•**coumermycin.** (KOO-mer-MY-sin) USAN.
Use: Anti-infective.

•**coumermycin sodium.** (KOO-mer-MY-sin) USAN.
Use: Anti-infective.

Counterpain Rub. (Squibb Diagnostic) Methyl salicylate, eugenol, menthol. Oint. Tube 1 oz. *otc.*
Use: Analgesic, topical.

Covangesic. (Wallace Laboratories) Phenylpropanolamine HCl 12.5 mg, phenylephrine HCl 7.5 mg, chlorpheniramine maleate 2 mg, pyrilamine maleate 12.5 mg, acetaminophen 275 mg, tartrazine/Tab. Bot. 24s. *otc.*
Use: Analgesic, antihistamine, decongestant.

Covera-HS. (Searle) Verapamil HCl 180 or 240 mg/ER Tab. Bot. 30s, 100s, UD 100s. *Rx.*
Use: Calcium channel blocker.

Covermark. (O'Leary) Neutral cream, hypoallergenic, opaque, greaseless. Jars 1 oz, 3 oz, available in eleven shades. *otc.*
Use: Conceals birthmarks and skin discolorations.

Covermark Stick. (O'Leary) For normal to oily skin, available in 7 shades. *otc.*
Use: Conceals birthmarks and skin discolorations.

Co-Xan Syrup. (Schwarz Pharma) Theophylline anhydrous 150 mg, ephedrine HCl 25 mg, guaifenesin 100 mg, codeine phosphate 15 mg, alcohol 10%/15 ml. Bot. 1 pt. *Rx.*
Use: Antitussive, bronchodilator, decongestant, expectorant.

Cozaar. (Merck) Losartan potassium 25 mg, 50 mg, lactose. Tab. Bot. 30s (50 mg only), 90s, 100s, UD 100s. *Rx.*
Use: Antihypertensive.

CPA TR. (Schein Pharmaceutical) Phenylpropanolamine HCl 75 mg, chlorpheniramine maleate 12 mg/Cap. Bot. 100s, 1000s. *otc.*
Use: Antihistamine, decongestant.

Cplex. (Arcum) Vitamins B_1 10 mg, B_2 10 mg, B_6 5 mg, B_{12} 10 mcg, niacinamide 100 mg, calcium pantothenate 25 mg, C 150 mg, liver 50 mg, dried yeast 50 mg/Cap. Bot. 100s, 1000s. *otc.*
Use: Mineral, vitamin supplement.

C.P.M. Tablets. (Zenith Goldline) Chlorpheniramine 4 mg/Tab. Bot. 1000s. *otc.*
Use: Antihistamine.

c-reactive protein test.
See: LA test-CRP kit. (Fischer).

Cream Camellia. (O'Leary) Jar 2 oz. *otc.*
Use: Emollient.

Creamy Tar. (C & M Pharmacal) Coal tar topical solution 6.65%, crude coal tar 0.67%. Shampoo. Bot. 240 ml. *otc.*
Use: Antiseborrheic.

•**creatinine.** N.F. 18.
Use: Bulking agent for freeze drying.

creatinine reagent strips. (Bayer Corp) Seralyzer reagent strips. A quantitative strip test for creatinine in serum or plasma. Bot. 25s.
Use: Diagnostic aid.

Cremagol. (Cremagol) Emulsion of liquid petrolatum, agar agar, acacia, glycerin. Bot. 14 oz.
W/cascara 11 gr/oz, Bot. 14 oz.
W/phenolphthalein 2 gr/oz, Bot. 14 oz. *otc.*
Use: Laxative.

Creomulsion Cough Medicine. (Creomulsion) Beechwood creosote, cascara, ipecac, menthol, white pine, wild cherry w/alcohol. For adults. Bot. 4 fl oz, 8 fl oz. *otc.*
Use: Cough preparation.

Creomulsion for Children. (Creomulsion) Beechwood creosote, cascara, ipecac, menthol, white pine, wild cherry w/alcohol. For children. Bot. 4 fl oz, 8 fl oz. *otc.*
Use: Cough preparation.

Creon. (Solvay) Lipase 8000 units, amylase 30,000 units, protease 13,000 units, pancreatin 300 mg/Cap. Bot. 100s, 250s. *Rx.*
Use: Digestive enzyme.

Creon 10. (Solvay) Lipase 10,000 USP units, amylase 33,200 USP units, protease 37,500 USP units. DR Cap. Bot. 100s, 250s. *Rx.*
Use: Digestive enzyme.

Creon 20. (Solvay) Lipase 20,000 USP units, amylase 66,400 USP units, protease 75,000 USP units. DR Cap. Bot. 100s, 250s. *Rx.*
Use: Digestive enzyme.

Creon 25. (Solvay) Lipase 25,000 units, amylase 74,700 units, protease 62,500 units, pancreatin 300 mg. Cap. Bot. 100s. *Rx.*
Use: Digestive enzyme.

creosote. Wood creosote, creosote, beechwood creosote.
W/Ipecac, menthol, licorice, white pine, wild cherry, cascara, vitamin C.
See: Creozets, Loz. (Creomulsion).

Creo-Terpin. (Lee) Dextromethorphan HBr 10 mg/15 ml, tartrazine, alcohol 25%, terpin hydrate, creosote, saccharin, corn syrup. Liq. Bot. 120 ml. *otc.*
Use: Antitussive.

Crescormon. (Pharmacia & Upjohn) Somatotropin 4 IU/Vial. IM administration. *Rx.*
Use: Hormone, growth.
Note: Crescormon will be available only for patients who qualify for treatment. Apply to Kabi Group Inc. for approval.

•**cresol.** (KREE-sole) N.F. 18.
Use: Antiseptic, disinfectant.

cresol preparations.
Use: Antiseptic, disinfectant.
See: Cresol, Soln. (Various Mfr.).
Cresylone, Liq. (Parke-Davis).
Saponated Cresol Soln.

m-cresyl-acetate.
See: Cresylate, Liq. (Recsei).

Cresylate. (Recsei) M-cresyl-acetate 25%, isopropanol 25%, chlorobutanol 1%, benzyl alcohol 1%, castor oil 5%, propylene glycol/15 ml. Bot. 15 ml, pt. *Rx.*
Use: Otic.

cresylic acid. Same as Cresol.

•**crilvastatin.** (krill-vah-STAT-in) USAN.
Use: Antihyperlipidemic.

Crinone 8%. (Wyeth Labs) Progesterone 8% (90 mg). Mineral oil, glycerin. Gel. Single-use, one piece 1.125 g applicators. *Rx.*
Use: Assisted reproductive technology treatment.

•**crisnatol mesylate.** (KRISS-nah-tole) USAN.
Use: Antineoplastic.

Criticare HN. (Bristol-Myers Squibb) High nitrogen elemental diet. Protein 14%, fat 4.3%, carbohydrate 81.5%. Bot. 8 oz. *otc.*
Use: Nutritional supplement, enteral.

Crixivan. (Merck) Indinavir sulfate 200 mg, 400 mg, lactose/Cap. Bot. 270s and 360s (200 mg only), 180s (400 mg only). *Rx.*
Use: Antiviral.

Croferrin. (Forest Pharmaceutical) Iron peptonate 50 mg, liver injection 2.5 mcg, vitamin B_{12} 12.5 mcg, lidocaine HCl 1%, phenol 0.5%, sodium citrate 0.125%, sodium bisulfite 0.009%/ml. Vial 10 ml, 30 ml. *Rx.*
Use: Mineral, vitamin supplement.

•**crofilcon A.** (kroe-FILL-kahn A) USAN.
Use: Contact lens material (hydrophilic).

Crolom. (Bausch & Lomb) Cromolyn sodium 4%. Soln. Bot. 2.5 ml, 10 ml w/ controlled drop tip. *Rx.*
Use: Antiallergic, ophthalmic.

Cro-Man-Zin. (Freeda Vitamins) Cr 200 mcg, Mn 5 mg, Zn 25 mg, kosher, sugar free/Tab. Bot. 100s, 250s. *otc.*

Use: Electrolyte, mineral supplement.

•**cromitrile sodium.** (KROE-mih-TRILE) USAN.
Use: Antiasthmatic.

cromolyn sodium.
Use: Mastocytosis. [Orphan drug]
See: Gastrocrom (Fisons).

•**cromolyn sodium.** (KROE-moe-lin) U.S.P. 23.
Use: Antiasthmatic, prophylactic.
See: Gastrocrom (Fisons).
Intal (Medeva).
Nasalcrom (Medeva).
Opticrom (Medeva).

cromolyn sodium. (Dey Labs) **Inhalation:** 20 mg/2 ml. In unit-dose vials. **Soln. for nebulization:** 20 mg/Vial. 2 ml. *Rx.*
Use: Antiasthmatic, prophylactic.

cromolyn sodium 4% ophthalmic solution.
Use: Antiallergic, ophthalmic. [Orphan drug]
See: Crolom, Ophth. Soln. (Bausch & Lomb)

Cronetal.
See: Disulfiram.

•**croscarmellose sodium.** (KRAHS-CAR-mell-ose) N.F. 18. *Formerly Crosslinked Carboxymethylcellulose Sodium and Modified Cellulose Gum.*
Use: Pharmaceutic aid (tablet disintegrant).

•**crospovidone.** N.F. 18.
Use: Pharmaceutic aid (tablet excipient).

Cross Aspirin. (Cross) Aspirin 325 mg/Tab. Sugar, salt and lactose free. Bot. 100s, 1000s. *otc.*
Use: Analgesic.

Crotab. (Therapeutic Antibodies) *Rx.*
See: Antivenin, Polyvalent Crotalic (Ovine) Fab.

Crotalidae Antivenin Polyvalent. (Wyeth Ayerst) 1 vial of lyophilized serum, 1 vial of bacteriostatic water 10 ml, USP, 1 vial normal horse serum. Inj. Vials combination Pkg. *Rx.*
Use: Antivenin.

crotaline antivenin, polyvalent. Antivenin Crotalidae Polyvalent, U.S.P. 23. North and South American Antisnakebite serum. *Rx.*
Use: Immunizing agent.

•**crotamiton.** (kroe-TAM-ih-tuhn) U.S.P. 23.
Use: Scabicide.
See: Eurax, Cream, Lot. (Novartis).
Component of Eurax (Westwood-Squibb).

CRPA, CRPA Latex Test. (Laboratory Diagnostics) Rapid latex agglutination test for the qualitative determination of C reactive protein. CRPA, 1 ml–CRP Positest Control, 0.5 ml CRPA Latex Test Kit.
Use: Diagnostic aid.

Cruex Cream. (Novartis Self-Medication) Total undecylenate 20% as undecylenic acid and zinc undecylenate. Tube 0.5 oz. *otc.*
Use: Antifungal, topical.

Cruex Spray Powder. (Novartis) Undecylenic acid 2% and zinc undecylenate 20%. Aerosol can 1.8 oz, 3.5 oz, 5.5 oz. *otc.*
Use: Antifungal, topical.

Cruex Squeeze Powder. (Novartis) Calcium undecylenate 10%. Plastic squeeze bot. 1.5 oz. *otc.*
Use: Antifungal, topical.

Cryptolin. (Hoechst Marion Roussel) Gonadorelin in nasal spray. *Rx.*
Use: Cryptorchism treatment.

cryptosporidium hyperimmune bovine colostrum IgG concentrate. (Immu-Cell)
Use: Treat diarrhea in AIDS patients. [Orphan drug]

cryptosporidium parvum bovine immunoglobulin concentrate.
Use: Treat infection of GI tract in immunocompromised patients. [Orphan drug]

crystalline trypsin. Highly purified preparation of enzyme as derived from mammalian pancreas glands.

crystal violet.
See: Methylrosaniline Chloride, U.S.P.

Crystamine. (Dunhall Pharmaceuticals) Cyanocobalamin 100 mcg or 1000 mcg/ml, benzyl alcohol. Vial 10 ml, 30 ml. *Rx.*
Use: Vitamin supplement.

Crysti 1000. (Roberts Pharm) Cyanocobalamine crystalline 1000 mcg/ml. Inj. Vial 10 ml, 30 ml. *Rx.*
Use: Vitamin B_{12}.

Crysti-Liver. (Roberts Pharm) Liver injection (equivalent to B_{12} 10 mcg), crystalline B_{12} 100 mcg, folic acid 0.4 mg. Vial 10 ml. *Rx.*
Use: Mineral, vitamin supplement.

Crystodigin. (Eli Lilly) Digitoxin 0.05 mg and 0.1 mg/Tab. Bot. 100s. *Rx.*
Use: Cardiovascular agent.

C Speridin. (Marlyn) Hesperidin 100 mg, lemon bioflavonoids 100 mg, vitamin C 500 mg/SR Tab. Bot. 100s. *otc.*

Use: Vitamin supplement.

CTab.
See: Cetyl Trimethyl Ammonium Bromide.

C/T/S. (Hoechst Marion Roussel) Clindamycin phosphate 10 mg/ml. Top. Soln. 30 ml, 60 ml. *Rx.*
Use: Dermatologic, acne.

C-Tussin. (Century Pharm) Codeine phosphate 10 mg, pseudoephedrine HCl 30 mg, guaifenesin 100 mg/5 ml, alcohol 7.5%. Bot. 120 ml, gal. *c-v.*
Use: Antitussive, decongestant, expectorant.

Culminal. (Culminal) Benzocaine 3% in water miscible cream base. Tube oz. *otc.*
Use: Anesthetic, local.

Culturette 10 Minute Group A Step ID. (Hoechst Marion Roussel) Latex slide agglutination test for group A streptococcal antigen on throat swabs. Kit 55 determinations.
Use: Diagnostic aid.

•**cupric acetate Cu 64.** (koo-prik ASS-eh-tate) USAN.
Use: Radioactive agent.

•**cupric chloride.** U.S.P. 23.
Use: Supplement (trace mineral).
See: Coppertrace, Inj. (Centeon).

•**cupric sulfate.** U.S.P. 23.
Use: Antidote to phosphorus.
W/Zinc sulfate, camphor.
See: Dalibour, Pow. (Doak Dermatologics).

Cuprid. (Merck) Trientine HCl 250 mg/Cap. Bot. 100s. *Rx.*
Use: Chelating agent.

Cuprimine. (Merck) Penicillamine 125 mg or 250 mg/Cap. Bot. 100s. *Rx.*
Use: Chelating agent.

•**cuprimyxin.** (KUH-prih-mix-in) USAN.
Use: Antifungal.

Cupri-Pak. (SoloPak) Copper **0.4 mg/ml:** Vial 10 ml, 30 ml. **2 mg/ml:** Vial 5 ml. *Rx.*
Use: Nutritional supplement, parenteral.

curare.
Use: Muscle relaxant.
See: d-Tubocurarine Salts (Various Mfr.).

curare antagonist.
See: Neostigine Methylsulfate Inj. (Various Mfr.).
Tensilon, Amp. (Roche Laboratories).

Curel. (Bausch & Lomb) Glycerin, petrolatum, dimethicone, parabens. Lot. 180, 300, 390 ml. Cream 90 g. *otc. Rx.*
Use: Emollient.

Curosurf. (Dey Labs) Pulmonary Surfactant Replacement.
Use: Respiratory distress syndrome. [Orphan drug]

curral.
See: Diallyl Barbituric Acid, Tab. (Various Mfr.).

Curretab. (Solvay) Medroxyprogesterone acetate 10 mg/Tab. Bot. 50s. *Rx.*
Use: Hormone, progestin.

Cutar Bath Oil. (Summers) Liquor carbonis detergens 7.5% in liquid petrolatum, isopropyl myristate, acetylated lanolin, lanolin alcohols extract. Bot. 180 ml. *otc.*
Use: Emollient.

Cutemol Emollient Cream. (Summers) Allantoin 0.2%, liquid petrolatum, acetylated lanolin, lanolin alcohols extract, isopropyl myristate, water. Jar 2 oz. *otc.*
Use: Emollient.

Cuticura Medicated Shampoo. (DEP) Sodium lauryl sulfate, sodium stearate, salicylic acid, protein, sulfur. Tube 3 oz. *otc.*
Use: Antidandruff.

Cuticura Medicated Soap. (DEP) Triclocarban 1%, petrolatum, sodium tallowate, sodium cocoate, glycerin, mineral oil, sodium Cl, tetrasodium EDTA, sodium bicarbonate, magnesium silicate, iron oxides. Bar 3.5 oz, 5.5 oz. *otc.*
Use: Anti-infective, topical.

Cutivate. (GlaxoWellcome) Fluticasone propionate. **Cream:** 0.05%. Jar 15,30,60 g. **Oint.:** 0.005%. Jar 15, 30, 60 g. *Rx.*
Use: Corticosteroid, topical.

Cutter Insect Repellent. (Bayer Corp) N,N-Diethyl-meta-toluamide 28.5%, other isomers 1.5%. Vial 1 oz; Foam, Can 2 oz; Spray 7 oz, 14 oz aerosol can; Assortment Pack; First Aid Kits, Trial Pack, 6s; Marine Pack 3s; Camp Pack 4s; Pocket Pack, Travel Pack.
Use: Insect repellent.

CY 1503. (Cytel)
Use: Anti-thromboembolic. [Orphan drug]

CY 1899. (Cytel)
Use: Antiviral, hepatitis B. [Orphan drug]

Cyanide Antidote Package. (Eli Lilly) 2 Amp. (300 mg/10 ml) sodium nitrite; 2 Amp. (12.5 g/50 ml), sodium thiosulfate; 12 aspirols amyl nitrite (0.3 ml), syringes, stomach tube, tourniquet/Pkg. Check exact dosage before administration. *Rx.*

Use: Antidote, cyanide poisoning.

Cyanocob. (Paddock) Vitamin B_{12} 1000 mcg/ml. Bot. 1000 ml, Vial 10 ml. *Rx.*
Use: Vitamin supplement.

•**cyanocobalamin.** (sigh-an-oh-koe-BAL-uh-min) U.S.P. 23. *Formerly Vitamin B_{12}.*
Use: Vitamin (hematopoietic).
See: Redisol, Inj., Tab. (Merck).
Nascobal, Intranasal Gel (Schwarz Pharma).

•**cyanocobalamin Co 57.** (sigh-an-oh-koe-BAL-uh-min) U.S.P. 23.
Use: Diagnostic aid (pernicious anemia); radioactive agent.

•**cyanocobalamin Co 60.** (sigh-an-oh-koe-BAL-uh-min) USAN. U.S.P. XXII.
Use: Diagnostic aid (pernicious anemia), radioactive agent.

cyanocobalamin crystalline. *otc, Rx.*
Use: Vitamin B_{12} supplement.
See: Vitamin B_{12}, Inj., Tab. (Various Mfr.).
Cobex, Inj. (Taylor Pharmaceuticals).
Crystamine, Inj. (Dunhall Pharmaceuticals).
Berubigen, Inj. (Pharmacia & Upjohn).
Betalin 12, Inj. (Eli Lilly).
Crysti-12, Inj. (Roberts Pharm).
Crysti 1000, Inj. (Roberts Pharm).
Cyanoject, Inj. (Merz).
Cyomin, Inj. (Forest Pharmaceutical).
Kaybovite-1000, Inj. (Kay).
Redisol, Inj. (Merck).
Rubesol-1000, Inj. (Schwarz Pharma).
Sytobex, Inj. (Park-Davis).

Cyanoject. (Merz) Vitamin B_{12} 1000 mcg/ml, benzyl alcohol. Vial 10 ml, 30 ml. *Rx.*
Use: Vitamin supplement.

Cyanover. (Research Supplies) Cyanocobalamin 100 mcg, liver injection 10 mcg, folic acid 10 mg/ml. Lyo-layer vial 10 ml with vial of diluent 10 ml. *Rx.*
Use: Mineral, vitamin supplement.

•**cyclacillin.** (SIGH-klah-SILL-in) U.S.P. 23.
Use: Anti-infective.

cyclamate sodium. Cyclohexanesulfamate dihydrate salt.

•**cyclamic acid.** (sigh-KLAM-ik) USAN.
Use: Sweetener (non-nutritive).

cyclandelate. (Various Mfr.) Cyclandelate 200 mg, 400 mg. Cap. Bot. 60s, 100s, 500s, 1000s, UD 100s. *Rx.*
Use: Peripheral vasodilator.

•**cyclazocine.** (SIGH-CLAY-zoe-seen) USAN. Under study.
Use: Analgesic.

•**cyclindole.** (sigh-KLIN-dole) USAN.
Use: Antidepressant.

Cyclinex-1. (Ross Laboratories) Protein 7.5 g (from carnitine, cystine, histidine, isoleucine, leucine, lysine, methionine, phenylalanine, taurine, threonine, tryptophan, tyrosine, valine), fat 27 g (from palm oil, hydrogenated coconut oil, soy oil), carbohydrate 52 g (from hydrolyzed corn starch), linoleic acid 2000 mg, Fe 10 mg, Na 215 mg, K 760 mg, Ca, vitamins A, B_1, B_2, B_3, B_5, B_6, B_{12}, C, D, E, K, biotin, choline, folic acid, inositol, Cl, Cu, I, Mg, Mn, P, Se, Zn and 515 Cal per 100 g. Nonessential amino acid free. Pow. Can 350 g. *otc.*
Use: Nutritional supplement.

Cyclinex-2. (Ross Laboratories) Protein 15 g (from carnitine, cystine, histidine, isoleucine, leucine, lysine, methionine, phenylalanine, taurine, threonine, tryptophan, tyrosine, valine), fat 20.7 g (from palm oil, hydrogenated coconut oil, soy oil), carbohydrate 40 g (from hydrolyzed cornstarch), Fe 17 mg, Na 1175 mg, K 1830 mg, Ca, vitamins A, B_1, B_2, B_3, B_5, B_6, B_{12}, C, D, E, K, biotin, choline, folic acid, inositol, Cl, Cu, I, Mg, Mn, P, Se, Zn and 480 Cal per 100 g. Nonessential amino acid free. Pow. Can 325 g. *otc.*
Use: Nutritional supplement.

•**cycliramine maleate.** (SIGH-klih-rah-meen) USAN.
Use: Antihistamine.

•**cyclizine.** (SIGH-klih-zeen) U.S.P. 23.
Use: Antihistamine.
See: Marzine (hydrochloride).

•**cyclizine hydrochloride.** U.S.P. 23.
Use: Antiemetic.
See: Marezine HCl and lactate, Preps. (GlaxoWellcome).
W/Ergotamine tartrate, caffeine.
See: Migral, Tab. (GlaxoWellcome).

•**cyclizine lactate injection.** U.S.P. 23.
Use: Antihistamine, antinauseant.

cyclobarbital.
Use: Central depressant.

cyclobarbital calcium.
Use: Hypnotic, sedative.

•**cyclobendazole.** (SIGH-kloe-BEN-dah-zole) USAN.
Use: Anthelmintic.

•**cyclobenzaprine hydrochloride.** (SIGH-kloe-BEN-zuh-preen) U.S.P. 23.
Use: Muscle relaxant.
See: Flexeril, Tab. (Merck).
Use: Muscle relaxant.

cyclobenzaprine hydrochloride. (Vari-

ous Mfr.) 10 mg/Tab. Bot. 30s, 100s, 1000s.
Use: Muscle relaxant.

Cyclocort Cream. (ESI Lederle Generics) Amcinonide 0.1% in Aquatain hydrophilic base. Tubes 15 g, 30 g, 60 g. *Rx.*
Use: Corticosteroid, topical.

Cyclocort Ointment. (ESI Lederle Generics) Amcinonide 0.1% in ointment base. Tube 15 g, 30 g, 60 g. *Rx.*
Use: Corticosteroid, topical.

cyclocumarol.
Use: Anticoagulant.

•**cyclofilcon a.** (SIGH-kloe-FILL-kahn A) USAN.
Use: Contact lens material (hydrophilic).

Cyclogen. (Schwarz Pharma) Dicyclomine HCl 10 mg, sodium Cl 0.9%, chlorobutanol hydrate 0.5%. Vial 10 ml, Box 12s. *Rx.*
Use: Antispasmodic.

•**cycloguanil pamoate.** (SIGH-kloe-GWAHN-ill PAM-oh-ate) USAN.
Use: Antimalarial.

Cyclogyl. (Alcon Laboratories) Cyclopentolate HCl Soln. 0.5%, 1% or 2%. Droptainer 2 ml, 5 ml, 15 ml. *Rx.*
Use: Cycloplegic, mydriatic.

•**cycloheximide.** (sigh-KLOE-HEX-ih-mid) USAN.
Use: Antipsoriatic.

•**cyclomethicone.** (sigh-kloe-METH-ih-cone) N.F. 18.
Use: Pharmaceutic aid (wetting agent).

cyclomethycaine and methapyrilene.
Use: Anesthetic, local.
See: Surfadil Cream, Lot. (Eli Lilly).

cyclomethycaine sulfate. U.S.P. XXI.
Use: Anesthetic, local.
See: Surfacaine, Prep. (Eli Lilly).
W/Methapyrilene.
See: Surfadil, Cream, Lot. (Eli Lilly).

cyclomethycaine and thenylpyramine.
See: Surfadil Cream, Lot. (Eli Lilly).

Cyclomydril. (Alcon Laboratories) Phenylephrine HCl 1%, cyclopentolate HCl 0.2%. Droptainer 2 ml, 5 ml. *Rx.*
Use: Mydriatic.

Cyclonil. (Seatrace) Dicyclomine HCl 10 mg/ml. Vial 10 ml. *Rx.*
Use: Anticholinergic, antispasmodic.

Cyclopar. (Parke-Davis) Tetracycline HCl 250 mg or 500 mg/Cap. **250 mg:** Bot. 100s, 1000s. **500 mg:** Bot. 100s, UD 100s. *Rx.*
Use: Anti-infective, tetracycline.

cyclopentamine hydrochloride. U.S.P. XXI.
Use: Adrenergic (vasoconstrictor).
See: Clopane Hydrochloride, Nasal Soln. (Eli Lilly).
W/Aludrine.
See: Aerolone Compound, Soln. (Eli Lilly).
W/Chlorpheniramine.
See: Hista-Clopane, Pulvule (Eli Lilly).

cyclopentenyl-allyl-barbituric acid.
See: Cyclopal.

8 cyclopentyl 1,3-dipropylxanthine. (SciClone Pharm).
Use: Cystic fibrosis. [Orphan drug]

•**cyclopenthiazide.** (SIHG-kloe-pen-THIGH-ah-zide) USAN.
Use: Antihypertensive, diuretic.
See: Navidrex.

•**cyclopentolate hydrochloride.** (sigh-kloe-PEN-toe-tate) U.S.P. 23.
Use: Anticholinergic (ophthalmic).
See: AK-Pentolate, Soln. (Akorn).
Cyclogyl, Soln. (Alcon Laboratories).
W/Phenylephrine HCl.
See: Cyclomydril, Soln. (Alcon Laboratories).

cyclopentolate hydrochloride. (Various Mfr.) 1% Soln. Bot. 2 ml, 15 ml.
Use: Anticholinergic (ophthalmic).

cyclopentylpropionate.
See: Depo-Testosterone, Vial (Pharmacia & Upjohn).

•**cyclophenazine hydrochloride.** (SIGH-kloe-FEH-nazz-een) USAN.
Use: Antipsychotic.

•**cyclophosphamide.** (sigh-kloe-FOSS-fuh-mide) U.S.P. 23.
Use: Antineoplastic, immunosuppressant.
See: Cytoxan, Pow. for Inj. Tab., Vial (Mead Johnson Oncology).
Neosar, Pow. for Inj. (Pharmacia & Upjohn).

•**cyclopropane.** (sigh-kloe-PRO-pane) U.S.P. 23.
Use: Anesthetic, general.

•**cycloserine.** (sigh-kloe-SER-een) U.S.P. 23.
Use: Anti-infective (tuberculostatic).
See: Seromycin, Cap. (Eli Lilly).

l-cycloserine.
Use: Treat Gaucher's disease. [Orphan drug].

cyclosporin a.
Use: Immunosuppressant.
See: Cyclosporine, U.S.P. 23.

•**cyclosporine.** (SIGH-kloe-spore-EEN) U.S.P. 23. *Formerly Cyclosporin A*
Use: Immunosuppressant.
See: Sandimmune, Preps. (Novartis).

Neoral, Cap., Oral Soln. (Novartis).

cyclosporine ophthalmic. (SIGH-kloe-spore-EEN)
Use: Severe keratoconjunctivitis sicca; graft rejection following keratoplasty. [Orphan drug]
See: Optimmune.

cyclosporine 2% ophthalmic ointment. (Allergan)
Use: Treatment of graft rejection after keratoplasty and corneal melting syndromes. [Orphan Drug]

•**cyclothiazide.** (SIGH-kloe-thigh-AZZ-ide) USAN. U.S.P. XXII.
Use: Antihypertensive, diuretic.

Cycofed Pediatric. (Cypress) Codeine phosphate 10 mg, pseudoephedrine HCl 30 mg, guaifenesin 100 mg, alcohol 6%/Syr. Bot. 1 pt. *c-v.*
Use: Antitussive, expectorant.

Cycrin. (ESI Lederle Generics) Medroxyprogesterone acetate 2.5 mg, 5 mg, 10 mg, lactose. Tab. Bot. 100s, 1000s. *Rx.*
Use: Hormone, progestin.

Cydonol Massage Lotion. (Gordon Laboratories) Isopropyl alcohol 14%, methyl salicylate, benzalkonium Cl. Bot. 4 oz, gal. *otc.*
Use: Counterirritant.

•**cyheptamide.** (sigh-HEP-tah-mid) USAN.
Use: Anticonvulsant.

Cyklokapron. (Pharmacia & Upjohn) **Tab.:** Tranexamic acid 500 mg. Bot. 100s. **Inj.:** 100 mg/ml. Amp. 10 ml. *Rx.*
Use: Hemostatic.

Cylert Chewable Tablets. (Abbott Laboratories) Pemoline 37.5 mg/Tab. Bot. 100s. *c-IV.*
Use: Psychotherapeutic.

Cylert Tablets. (Abbott Laboratories) Pemoline 18.75, 37.5 or 75 mg/Tab. Bot. 100s. *c-IV.*
Use: Psychotherapeutic.

Cylex Sugar Free. (Pharmakon Labs) Benzocaine 15 mg, cetylpyridinium Cl 5 mg, sorbitol. Loz. Pkg. 12s. *otc.*
Use: Antiseptic; analgesic, topical.

Cylex Throat. (Pharmakon Labs) Benzocaine 15 mg, cetylpyridinium Cl 5 mg, sorbitol. Loz. Pkg. 12s. *otc.*
Use: Antiseptic; analgesic, topical.

Cynobal. (Arcum) Cyanocobalamin 100 mcg or 1000 mcg/ml. Inj. **100 mcg:** Vial 30 ml. **1000/mcg/ml.:** Inj. Vial 10 ml, 30 ml. *Rx.*
Use: Vitamin supplement.

Cyomin. (Forest Pharmaceutical) Cyanocobalamin 1000 mcg/ml. Vial 10 ml, 30 ml. *Rx.*
Use: Vitamin supplement.

•**cypenamine hydrochloride.** (sigh-PEN-ah-meen) USAN.
Use: Antidepressant.

•**cyprazepam.** (sigh-PRAY-zeh-pam) USAN.
Use: Hypnotic, sedative.

•**cyproheptadine hydrochloride.** (sip-row-HEP-tuh-deen) U.S.P. 23.
Use: Antihistamine, antipruritic.
See: Periactin, Tab., Syr. (Merck).

cyproheptadine hydrochloride. (sip-row-HEP-tuh-deen) (Various Mfr.) **Tab.:** Cyproheptadine HCl 4 mg. Bot. 100s, 250s, 500s, 1000s. **Syr.:** 2 mg/5 ml, alcohol. Bot. 118 ml, pt., gal. *Rx.*
Use: Antihistamine.

•**cyprolidol hydrochloride.** (sigh-PRO-lih-dahl) USAN.
Use: Antidepressant.

•**cyproterone acetate.** (sigh-PRO-ter-ohn) USAN.
Use: Antiandrogen.

•**cyproximide.** (sigh-PROX-ih-MIDE) USAN.
Use: Antidepressant, antipsychotic.

cyren a.
See: Diethylstilbestrol Prep. (Various Mfr.).

cyrimine hydrochloride.
See: Pagitane HCl, Tab. (Eli Lilly).

Cyronine. (Major) Liothyronine sodium 25 mcg/Tab. Bot. 100s. *Rx.*
Use: Hormone, thyroid.

Cystadane. (Orphan Medical) Betaine anhydrous 1 g/1.7 ml/Pow. Bot. 180 g. *Rx.*
Use: Treatment of homocystinuria.
See: Optimmune.

Cystagon. (Mylan) Cysteamine bitartrate 50 mg, 150 mg/Cap. Bot. 100s, 500s. *Rx.*
Use: Urinary tract agent.

Cystamin.
See: Methenamine, Tab. (Various Mfr.).

Cystamine. (Tennessee Pharmaceutic) Methenamine 2 gr, phenyl salicylate 0.5 gr, phenazopyridine HCl 10 mg, benzoic acid 1/8 gr, hyoscyamine sulfate gr, atropine sulfate gr/SC Tab. Bot. 100s, 1000s. *Rx.*
Use: Anti-infective, urinary.

•**cysteamine.** (sis-TEE-ah-MEEN) USAN.
Use: Antiurolithic (cystine calculi), nephropathic cystinosis. [Orphan Drug]
See: Cystagen.

•**cysteamine hydrochloride.** (sis-TEE-ah-MEEN) USAN.
Use: Antiurolithic (cystine calculi) treatment of nephropathic cystinosis.
See: Cystagon.

•**cysteine hydrochloride.** (SIS-teh-een) U.S.P. 23.
Use: Amino acid for replacement therapy, treatment of photosensitivity in erythropoietic protoporphyria. [Orphan Drug]
See: Cysteine HCl (Abbott Laboratories).

Cystex. (Numark Laboratories) Methenamine 162 mg, sodium salicylate 162.5 mg, benzoic acid 32 mg/Tab. Bot. 40s, 100s. *otc.*
Use: Anti-infective, urinary.

cystic fibrosis gene therapy. (Genzyme)
Use: Cystic fibrosis. [Orphan Drug]

cystic fibrosis transmembrane conductance regulator gene. (Genetic Therapy, Genzyme)
Use: Cystic fibrosis. [Orphan Drug]

cystic fibrosis TR gene therapy (recombinant adenovirus). (Gerac)
Use: Cystic fibrosis. [Orphan Drug]
See: AdGVCFTR.10 (GenVec).

•**cystine.** (SIS-TEEN) USAN.
Use: Amino acid replacement therapy, an additive for infants on TPN.

Cysto. (Freeport) Methenamine 40.8 mg, methylene blue 5.4 mg, phenyl salicylate 18.1 mg, atropine sulfate 0.03 mg, hyoscyamine 0.03 mg, benzoic acid 4.5 mg/Tab. Bot. 1000s. *Rx.*
Use: Anti-infective, urinary.

Cysto-Conray. (Mallinckrodt) Iothalamate meglumine 43% (iodine 20.2%) with EDTA. Soln. Vial 50 ml, 100 ml. Bot. 250 ml.
Use: Radiopaque agent.

Cysto-Conray II. (Mallinckrodt) Iothalamate meglumine 17.2% (iodine 8.1%) with EDTA. Soln. Bot. 250 ml, 500 ml.
Use: Radiopaque agent.

Cystografin. (Bristol-Myers Squibb) Meglumine diatrizoate 30% (bound iodine 14%), EDTA 0.04%. Bot. 100 ml, 300 ml.
Use: Radiopaque agent.

Cystografin Dilute. (Bristol-Myers Squibb) Diatrizoate meglumine 18% (organically-bound iodine 85 mg)/ml. Vial 300 ml, 500 ml.
Use: Radiopaque agent.

Cystospaz. (Polymedica) l-Hyoscyamine 0.15 mg/Tab. Bot. 100s. *Rx.*
Use: Anticholinergic, antispasmodic.

Cystospaz-M. (Polymedica) Hyoscyamine sulfate 375 mcg/Cap. Bot. 100s. *Rx.*
Use: Anticholinergic, antispasmodic.

Cytadren. (Novartis) Aminoglutethimide 250 mg/Tab. Bot. 100s. *Rx.*
Use: Adrenal steroid inhibitor; treatment of Cushing's syndrome.

•**cytarabine.** (SIGH-tar-ah-bean) U.S.P. 23.
Use: Antineoplastic, antiviral.
See: Cytosar, Inj. (Pharmacia & Upjohn).

cytarabine. (Various Mfr.) 100 mg, 500 mg/Pow. for Inj. Vials.
Use: Antineoplastic, antiviral.

cytarabine, depofoam encapsulated.
Use: Neoplastic meningitis. [Orphan Drug]

•**cytarabine hydrochloride.** (SITE-ah-rah-been HIGH-droe-KLOR-ide) USAN. *Formerly Cytosine Arabinoside Hydrochloride*
Use: Antiviral management of acute leukemias.
See: Cytosar-U, Vial (Pharmacia & Upjohn).

CytoGam. (MedImmune) Cytomegalovirus immune globulin IV (human) 2500 mg ±500 mg/Inj. Solvent/detergent treated. Vial 2.5 g. *Formerly called cytomegalovirus immune globulin (human) IV. Rx.*
Use: Antiviral, cytomegalovirus.

cytomegalovirus immune globulin (human).
Use: Antiviral, cytomegalovirus. [Orphan drug]
See: CytoGam, Vial (MedImmune).

cytomegalovirus immune globulin (human) iv. Now named CytoGam (MedImmune).
Use: CMV pneumonia in bone marrow transplants. [Orphan Drug]
See: CytoGam, Inj., (MedImmune).

cytomegalovirus immune globulin IV (human). (Miles)
Use: With ganciclovir sodium for the treatment of CMV pneumonia in bone marrow transplant patients. [Orphan drug]

Cytomel. (SmithKline Beecham Pharmaceuticals) Liothyronine sodium 5 mcg, 25 mcg or 50 mcg/Tab. Bot. 100s. 25 mcg: Bot. 100s. *Rx.*
Use: Hormone, thyroid.

Cytosar-U. (Pharmacia & Upjohn) Cytarabine 20 mg/ml in powder, 50

mg/ml reconstituted. Vial 100 mg, 500 mg. *Rx.*
Use: Antineoplastic.

cytosine arabinoside hydrochloride. Cytarabine HCl.
See: Cytosar-U (Pharmacia & Upjohn).

Cytosol. (Cytosol Ophthalmics) Calcium chloride 48 mg, magnesium chloride 30 mg, potassium chloride 75 mg, sodium acetate 390 mg, sodium chloride 640 mg, sodium citrate 170 mg/100 ml. Soln. Bot. 200 ml, 500 ml. *Rx.*
Use: Irrigant.

Cytotec. (Searle) Misoprostol 200 mcg/Tab. Bot. 100s, UD 100s. *Rx.*
Use: Prostaglandins.

Cytovene. (Roche Laboratories) Ganciclovir (as sodium) . **Cap.:** 250 mg/Tab. Bot. 180s. **Inj.:** 500 mg/Pow. Vial. 10 ml. *Rx.*
Use: Antiviral.

Cytox. (MPL) Cyanocobalamin 500 mcg, vitamins B_6 20 mg, B_1 100 mg, benzyl alcohol 2% in isotonic solution of sodium Cl/ml. Inj. Vial 10 ml. *Rx.*
Use: Vitamin supplement.

Cytoxan Lyophilized. (Mead Johnson Oncology) Cyclophosphamide. 100 mg, mannitol 75 mg. Pow. for Inj. Vial 100 mg, 200 mg, 500 mg, 1 g, 2 g. *Rx.*
Use: Antineoplastic.

Cytoxan Powder. (Bristol-Myers Oncology/Immunology) Cyclophosphamide powder 100 mg, 200 mg, 500 mg, 1 g or 2 g/Vial. *Rx.*
Use: Antineoplastic.

Cytoxan Tablets. (Mead Johnson Oncology) Cyclophosphamide 25 mg, 50 mg/Tab. Bot. 100s, 1000s (50 mg only). *Rx.*
Use: Antineoplastic.

Cytra-2. (Cypress) Sodium citrate dihydrate 500 mg, citric acid monohydrate 334 mg/5 ml/Soln. Bot. 16 oz. *Rx.*
Use: Alkalinizer, systemic.

Cytra-3. (Cypress) Potassium citrate monohydrate 550 mg, sodium citrate dihydrate 500 mg, citric acid monohydrate 334 mg/5 ml/Syr. Bot. 480 ml. *Rx.*
Use: Alkalinizer, sysemic.

Cytra-K. (Cypress) Potassium citrate monohydrate 1100 mg, citric acid monohydrate 334 mg/5 ml/Soln. Bot. 473 ml. *Rx.*
Use: Alkalinizer, systemic.

Cytra-LC. (Cypress) Potassium citrate monohydrate 550 mg, sodium citrate dihydrate 500 mg, citric acid monohydrate 334 mg/5 ml/Soln. Bot. 473 ml. *Rx.*
Use: Alkalinizer, systemic.

D

D-2. One of the D vitamins.
See: Ergocalciferol.

D-3. One of the D vitamins.
See: Cholecalciferol.

daa.
See: Dihydroxy Aluminum Aminoacetate.

DAB_{389} IL-2. (Seragen)
Use: Cutaneous T-cell lymphoma. [Orphan drug]

•**dacarbazine.** (da-CAR-buh-zeen) U.S.P. 23.
Use: Antineoplastic.
See: Dtic-Dome, Inj. (Bayer Corp).

D.A. Chew Tabs. (Dura Pharm) Phenylephrine HCl 10 mg, chlorpheniramine 2 mg, methscopolamine nitrate 1.25 mg/Tab. Bot. 100s. *Rx.*
Use: Anticholinergic, antihistamine, decongestant.

D.A. II. (Dura Pharm) Chlorpheniramine maleate 4 mg, phenylephrine HCl 10 mg, methscopolamine nitrate 1.25 mg/Tab. Bot. 100s. *Rx.*
Use: Anticholinergic, antihistamine, decongestant.

•**dacliximab.** (dak-LICK-sih-mab) USAN.
Use: Monoclonal antibody (immunosuppressant).
See: Zenapax, Inj. (Hoffmann-LaRoche).
See: Daclizumab

Daclizumab. USAN.
Use: Immunosuppressant.
See: Zenapax (Hoffman-LaRoche).

Dacodyl. (Major) **Tab.:** Bisacodyl 5 mg/Tab. Bot. 100s, 250s, 1000s. UD 100s. **Supp.:** Bisacodyl 10 mg. Box 12s, 100s. *otc.*
Use: Laxative.

Dacriose. (Ciba Vision Ophthalmics) Sodium Cl, potassium Cl, sodium hydroxide, sodium phosphate, benzalkonium Cl 0.01%, edetate disodium. Bot. 15 ml, 120 ml. *otc.*
Use: Irrigant, ophthalmic.

•**dactinomycin.** (DAK-tih-no-MY-sin) U.S.P. 23.
Use: Antineoplastic.
See: Cosmegen, Vial (Merck).

Daily Cleaner. (Bausch & Lomb) Isotonic solution with sodium Cl, sodium phosphate, tyloxapol, hydroxyethylcellulose, polyvinyl alcohol with thimerosal 0.004%, EDTA 0.2%. Soln. Bot. 45 ml. *otc.*
Use: Contact lens care.

Daily Conditioning Treatment. (Blistex) Padimate O 7.5%, oxybenzone 3.5%, petrolatum. Stick 11.4 g. SPF 15. *otc.*
Use: Lip protectant.

Daily Vitamins Liquid. (Rugby) Vitamins A 2500 IU, D 400 IU, E 15 IU, C 60 mg, B_1 1.2 mg, B_2 1.2 mg, B_6 1.05 mg, B_{12} 4.5 mcg, niacinamide 13.5 mg/5 ml. Bot. 273 ml, 473 ml. *otc.*
Use: Vitamin supplement.

Daily Vitamins Tablets. (Kirkman Sales) Vitamins A 5000 IU, D 400 IU, C 50 mg, B_1 3 mg, B_2 2.5 mg, B_6 1 mg, B_{12} 1 mcg, niacinamide 20 mg, d-calcium pantothenate 1 mg/Tab. Bot. 100s. *otc.*
Use: Vitamin supplement.

Daily Vitamins w/Iron. (Kirkman Sales) Vitamins A 5000 IU, D 400 IU, B_1 2 mg, B_2 2.5 mg, B_6 1 mg, B_{12} 1 mcg, niacinamide 20 mg, d-calcium pantothenate 1 mg, iron 18 mg/Tab. Bot. 100s. *otc.*
Use: Vitamin supplement.

Daily-Vite w/Iron & Minerals. (Rugby) Iron 18 mg, vitamins A 5000 IU, D 400 IU, E 30 mg, B_1 1.5 mg, B_2 1.7 mg, B_3 20 mg, B_5 10 mg, B_6 2 mg, B_{12} 6 mcg, C 60 mg, folic acid 0.4 mg, Ca, Cl, Cr, Cu, I, K, Mg, Mn, Mo, P, Se, zinc 15 mg, biotin, vitamin K/Tab. Bot. 100s. *otc.*
Use: Mineral, vitamin supplement.

Dairy Ease. (Sanofi Winthrop) Lactase 3300 FCC units, mannitol. Tab. Bot. 60s. *otc.*
Use: Digestive enzyme.

Daisy 2 Pregnancy Test. (Advanced Care Products) Home pregnancy test. Test kit 2s.
Use: Diagnostic aid.

Dakin's Solution.
See: Sodium Hypochlorite Solution Diluted.

Dakin's Solution-Full Strength. (Century Pharm) Sodium hypochlorite 0.5%. Soln. Bot. pt, gal. *otc.*
Use: Anti-infective, topical.

Dakin's Solution-Half Strength. (Century Pharm) Sodium hypochlorite 0.25%. Soln. Bot. pt. *otc.*
Use: Anti-infective, topical.

Dalalone. (Forest Pharmaceutical) Dexamethasone sodium phosphate 4 mg/ml, methyl and propyl parabens, sodium bisulfite. Vial 5 ml. *Rx.*
Use: Corticosteroid.

Dalalone D.P. (Forest Pharmaceutical) Dexamethasone acetate 16 mg/ml, polysorbate 80, carboxymethylcellulose, sodium bisulfite, EDTA, benzyl alco-

hol. Vial 1 ml, 5 ml. *Rx.*
Use: Corticosteroid.

Dalalone L.A. (Forest Pharmaceutical) Dexamethasone 8 mg/ml, polysorbate 80, carboxymethylcellulose, sodium bisulfite, EDTA, benzyl alcohol. Vial 5 ml. *Rx.*
Use: Corticosteroid.

d-ala-peptide t.
Use: Antiviral.
See: Peptide T (Carl Biotech/National Institute of Mental Health).

•**daledalin tosylate.** (dah-LEH-dah-lin TAH-sill-ate) USAN.
Use: Antidepressant.

•**dalfopristin.** (dal-FOE-priss-tin) USAN.
Use: Anti-infective.

Dalgan. (Wyeth Ayerst) Dezocine 5 mg, 10 mg or 15 mg/ml. **5 mg/ml:** Vial (SD) 1 ml. **10 mg/ml:** Vial (SD) 1 ml, Vial (MD) 10 ml, syringes (prefilled) 1 ml. **15 mg/ml:** Vial (SD) 1 ml, syringes (prefilled) 1 ml. *Rx.*
Use: Analgesic, narcotic.

Dallergy. (Laser) Chlorpheniramine maleate 8 mg, phenylephrine HCl 20 mg, methscopolamine nitrate 2.5 mg/ER Capl. Bot. 100s. *Rx.*
Use: Anticholinergic, antihistamine, decongestant.

Dallergy-D Syrup. (Laser) Chlorpheniramine maleate 2 mg, phenylephrine HCl 5 mg/5 ml. Bot. 118 ml. *otc.*
Use: Antihistamine, decongestant.

Dallergy-Jr. Capsules. (Laser) Brompheniramine maleate 6 mg, pseudoephedrine HCl 60 mg/Cap. Bot. 100s. *Rx.*
Use: Antihistamine, decongestant.

Dallergy Syrup. (Laser) Chlorpheniramine maleate 2 mg, phenylephrine HCl 10 mg, methscopolamine nitrate 0.625 mg/5 ml. Bot. 473 ml. *Rx.*
Use: Anticholinergic, antihistamine, antispasmodic, decongestant.

Dallergy Tablets. (Laser) Chlorpheniramine maleate 4 mg, phenylephrine HCl 10 mg, methscopolamine nitrate 1.25 mg/Tab. Bot. 100s. *Rx.*
Use: Anticholinergic, antihistamine, antispasmodic, decongestant.

Dalmane. (Roche) Flurazepam HCl 15 mg or 30 mg/Cap. Bot. 100s, 500s, Prescription Pak 300s. RNP (Reverse Numbered Packages) 4 rolls × 25 cap. or 4 cards × 25 cap. UD 100s. *c-IV.*
Use: Hypnotic, sedative.

•**dalteparin sodium.** (dal-TEH-puh-rin) USAN.
Use: Anticoagulant, antithrombotic.
See: Fragmin, Soln. (Pharmacia & Upjohn).

•**daltroban.** (DAL-troe-ban) USAN.
Use: Platelet aggregation inhibitor, immunosuppressant.

•**dalvastatin.** (DAL-vah-STAT-in) USAN.
Use: Antihyperlipidemic.

Damacet-P. (Mason) Hydrocodone bitartrate 5 mg, acetaminophen 500 mg/Tab. Bot. 100s, 500s. *c-III.*
Use: Analgesic combination, narcotic.

Damason-P. (Mason) Hydrocodone bitartrate 5 mg, aspirin 500 mg/Tab. Bot. 100s, 500s, 1000s. *c-III.*
Use: Analgesic combination, narcotic.

Dambose.
See: Inositol, Tabs.

•**danaparoid sodium.** (dan-AHP-ah-royd) USAN.
Use: Antithrombotic.
See: Orgaran, Inj. (Organon).

Danatrol Capsules. (Sanofi Winthrop) Danazol. *Rx.*
Use: Gonadotropin inhibitor.

•**danazol.** (DAN-uh-ZOLE) U.S.P. 23.
Use: Anterior pituitary suppressant.
See: Danocrine, Cap. (Sanofi Winthrop) Chronogyn (Sterling Winthrop).

danazol. (Various Mfr.) Danazol 200 mg/Cap. Bot. 50s, 60s, 100s, 500s.
Use: Anterior pituitary suppressant.

Dandruff Shampoo. (Walgreen) Zinc pyrithione 2 g/100 ml. Bot. 11 oz. Tube 7 oz. *otc.*
Use: Antiseborrheic.

•**daniplestim.** (dan-ih-PLEH-stim) USAN.
Use: Antineutroenic, hematopoietic stimulant, treatment of chemotherapy-induced bone marrow suppression.

Danocrine. (Sanofi Winthrop) Danazol 50 mg, 100 mg or 200 mg/Cap. Bot. 100s. *Rx.*
Use: Gonadotropin inhibitor.

Danogar Tablets. (Sanofi Winthrop) Danazol. *Rx.*
Use: Gonadotropin inhibitor.

Danol Capsules. (Sanofi Winthrop) Danazol. *Rx.*
Use: Gonadotropin inhibitor.

Dantrium. (Procter & Gamble) Dantrolene sodium. **25 mg/Cap.:** Bot. 100s, 500s, UD 100s; **50 mg/Cap.:** Bot. 100s; **100 mg/Cap.:** Bot. 100s, UD 100s. *Rx.*
Use: Muscle relaxant.

Dantrium IV. (Procter & Gamble) Dantrolene sodium 20 mg/Vial. Vial 70 ml. *Rx.*
Use: Muscle relaxant.

•**dantrolene.** (dan-troe-LEEN) USAN.
Use: Muscle relaxant.

•**dantrolene sodium.** (dan-troe-LEEN) USAN.
Use: Muscle relaxant.
See: Dantrium, Cap., I.V. (Procter & Gamble).

Dapa Extra Strength Tablets. (Ferndale Laboratories) Acetaminophen 500 mg/ Cap. Bot. 50s, 100s, 1000s, UD 100s. *otc.*
Use: Analgesic.

Dapa Tablets. (Ferndale Laboratories) Acetaminophen 324 mg/Tab. Bot. 100s, 1000s, UD 100s. *otc.*
Use: Analgesic.

Dapco. (Schlicksup) Salicylamide 300 mg, butabarbital 15 mg/Tab. Bot. 100s, 1000s. *c-III.*
Use: Analgesic, hypnotic, sedative.

•**dapiprazole hydrochloride.** (DAP-ih-PRAY-zole) USAN.
Use: Alpha-adrenergic blocker, antiglaucoma agent, neuroleptic, psychotherapeutic agent.
See: Rēv-Eyes, Pow. (Storz/Lederle).

•**dapoxetine hydrochloride.** (dap-OX-eh-teen) USAN.
Use: Antidepressant.

•**dapsone.** (DAP-sone) U.S.P. 23. *Formerly Diaminodiphenylsulfone.*
Use: Anti-infective (leprostatic), dermitis herpetiformis suppressant, prevention/treatment of *Pneumocystis carinii* pneumonia. [Orphan drug]
See: Dapsone (Jacobus Pharm).

Dapsone. (Jacobus Pharm) 25 mg or 100 mg/Tab. Bot. 100s.
Use: Anti-infective (leprostatic), dermitis herpetiformis suppressant, prevention/treatment of *Pneumocystis carinii* pneumonia. [Orphan drug]

•**daptomycin.** (DAP-toe-MY-sin) USAN.
Use: Anti-infective.

Daragen. (Galderma) Collagen polypeptide, benzalkonium Cl in a mild amphoteric base. Shampoo. Bot. 8 oz. *otc.*
Use: Dermatologic.

Dara Soapless Shampoo. (Galderma) Purified water, potassium coco hydrolyzed protein, sulfated castor oil, pentasodium triphosphate, sodium benzoate, sodium lauryl sulfate, fragrance. Shampoo. Bot. 8 oz, 16 oz. *otc.*
Use: Dermatologic, scalp.

Daranide. (Merck) Dichlorphenamide 50 mg/Tab. Bot. 100s. *Rx.*
Use: Antiglaucoma agent.

Daraprim. (GlaxoWellcome) Pyrimethamine 25 mg/Tab. Bot. 100s. *Rx.*
Use: Antimalarial.

Darco G-60. (Zeneca) Activated carbon from lignite.
Use: Purifier.

•**darglitazone sodium.** (dahr-GLIH-tah-zone) USAN.
Use: Oral hypoglycemic.

•**darodipine.** (DA-row-dih-PEEN) USAN.
Use: Antihypertensive, bronchodilator, vasodilator.

Darvocet-N 100. (Eli Lilly) Propoxyphene napsylate 100 mg, acetaminophen 650 mg/Tab. Bot. 100s (Rx Pak) 500s, UD 100s, 500s, RN 500s. *c-IV.*
Use: Analgesic combination, narcotic.

Darvon. (Eli Lilly) Propoxyphene HCl 65 mg/Pulv. Bot. 100s. Rx Pak 500s; Blister pkg. 10 × 10s; UD 20 rolls 25s. *c-IV.*
Use: Analgesic combination, narcotic.

Darvon Compound-65. (Eli Lilly) Propoxyphene HCl 65 mg, aspirin 389 mg, caffeine 32.4 mg/Pulv. Bot. 100s (Rx Pak) 500s. *c-IV.*
Use: Analgesic combination, narcotic.

Darvon-N. (Eli Lilly) Propoxyphene napsylate. **Tab.:** 100 mg. Bot. 100s (Rx Pak), 500s; Blister pkg. 10 × 10s; Rx Pak 20 × 50s. *c-IV.*
Use: Analgesic, narcotic.

Da-Sed Tablet. (Sheryl) Butabarbital 0.5 gr/Tab. Bot. 100s. *c-III.*
Use: Hypnotic, sedative.

Dasin. (SmithKline Beecham Pharmaceuticals) Ipecac 3 mg, acetylsalicylic acid 130 mg, camphor 15 mg, caffeine 8 mg, atropine sulfate 0.13 mg/ Cap. Bot. 100s, 500s. *Rx.*
Use: Analgesic, anticholinergic, antispasmodic.

Daturine Hydrobromide.
See: Hyoscyamine Salts (Various Mfr.)

•**daunorubicin hydrochloride.** (DAW-no-RUE-bih-sin) U.S.P. 23.
Use: Antineoplastic.
See: DaunoXome (NeXstar), Cerubidine, Inj. (Bedford Labs).

daunorubicin citrate liposome. (DAW-no-RUE-bih-sin)
Use: Treatment of advanced HIV-associated Kaposi's sarcoma. [Orphan drug]
See: DaunoXome (NeXstar).

DaunoXome. (NeXstar) Daunorubicin citrate liposomal 2 mg/ml (equivalent to 50 mg daunorubicin base). Inj. Vials. 1, 4, 10 unit packs. *Rx.*
Use: Treatment of advanced HIV-asso-

ciated Kaposi's sarcoma.

Davitamon K.
See: Menadione Inj., Tab. (Various Mfr.)

Davosil. (Colgate Oral) Silicon carbide in glycerin base. Jar 8 oz, 10 oz. *otc.*
Use: Agent for oral hygiene.

Dayalets. (Abbott Laboratories) Vitamins B_1 1.5 mg, B_2 1.7 mg, A 5000 IU, C 60 mg, D 400 IU, niacinamide 20 mg, B_6 2 mg, B_{12} 6 mcg, E 30 IU, folic acid 0.4 mg/Filmtab. Bot. 100s. *otc.*
Use: Vitamin supplement.

Dayalets + Iron. (Abbott Laboratories) Vitamins B_1 1.5 mg, B_2 1.7 mg, niacinamide 20 mg, B_6 2 mg, C 60 mg, A 5000 IU, D 400 IU, E 30 IU, B_{12} 6 mcg, iron 18 mg, folic acid 0.4 mg/Filmtab. Bot. 100s. *otc.*
Use: Mineral, vitamin supplement.

Day Caps. (Towne) Vitamins A 5500 IU, D 400 IU, B_1 3 mg, B_2 3 mg, B_6 0.5 mg, B_{12} 4 mcg, C 50 mg, calcium pantothenate 5 mg, niacinamide 20 mg/Cap. Bot. 120s, 300s.
Use: Vitamin supplement.

Day Cap Tabs-M. (Towne) Vitamins A 5500 IU, D 400 IU, B_1 3 mg, B_2 3 mg, B_6 0.5 mg, B_{12} 4 mcg, C 50 mg, niacinamide 20 mg, calcium pantothenate 5 mg, l-Lysine HCl 15 mg, iron 10 mg, zinc 1.5 mg, manganese 1 mg, iodine 0.1 mg, copper 1 mg, potassium 5 mg, magnesium 6 mg/Cap. or Tab. Bot. 100s, 250s.
Use: Mineral, vitamin supplement.

Daycare. (Procter & Gamble) Pseudoephedrine HCl 10 mg, dextromethorphan HBr 3.3 mg, guaifenesin 33.3 mg, acetaminophen 108 mg, alcohol 10% and saccharin. Expectorant Liq. Bot. 180 ml, 300 ml. *otc.*
Use: Analgesic, antitussive, decongestant, expectorant.

Day-Night Comtrex. (Bristol-Myers) Pseudoephedrine HCl 30 mg, chlorpheniramine maleate 2 mg, dextromethorphan HBr 10 mg, acetaminophen 325 mg/Tab. Pkg. 6s. *otc.*
Use: Analgesic, antihistamine, antitussive, decongestant.

Daypro. (Searle) Oxaprozin 600 mg/capl. Bot. 100s, 500s, UD 100s. *Rx.*
Use: Analgesic, NSAID.

Day Tab. (Towne) Vitamins A 5000 IU, D 400 IU, B_1 15 mg, B_2 10 mg, C 600 mg, niacinamide 20 mg, B_6 5 mg, folic acid 400 mcg, pantothenic acid 10 mg, zinc 15 mg, copper 2 mg, B_{12} 5 mcg/Tab. Bot. 100s, 200s. *otc.*
Use: Mineral, vitamin supplement.

Day Tab Essential. (Towne) Vitamins A 5000 IU, D 400 IU, E 15 IU, C 60 mg, folic acid 0.4 mg, B_1 1.5 mg, B_2 1.7 mg, niacin 20 mg, B_6 2 mg, B_{12} 6 mcg/Tab. Bot. 200s. *otc.*
Use: Vitamin supplement.

Day Tabs, New. (Towne) Vitamins A 5000 IU, E 15 IU, D 400 IU, C 60 mg, folic acid 0.4 mg, B_1 1.5 mg, B_2 1.7 mg, niacin 20 mg, B_6 20 mg, B_{12} 6 mcg/Tab. Bot 100s, 250s. *otc.*
Use: Vitamin supplement.

Day Tab Plus Iron. (Towne) Iron 18 mg, vitamins A 5000 IU, D 400 IU, B_1 1.5 mg, B_2 1.7 mg, niacinamide 20 mg, C 60 mg, B_6 2 mg, pantothenic acid 10 mg, B_{12} 6 mcg, folic acid 0.1 mg/Tab. Bot. 100s. *otc.*
Use: Mineral, vitamin supplement.

Day Tabs Plus Iron, New. (Towne) Vitamins A 5000 IU, E 15 IU, D 400 IU, C 60 mg, folic acid 0.4 mg, B_1 1.5 mg, B_2 1.7 mg, niacin 20 mg, B_6 20 mg, B_{12} 6 mcg, iron 18 mcg/Tab. Bot. 250s. *otc.*
Use: Mineral, vitamin supplement.

Day Tab Stress Complex. (Towne) Vitamins A 5000 IU, C 600 mg, B_1 15 mg, B_2 10 mg, niacin 100 mg, D 400 IU, E 30 IU, B_6 5 mg, folic acid 400 mcg, B_{12} 6 mcg, pantothenic acid 20 mg, iron 18 mg, zinc 15 mg, copper 2 mg/Tab. Bot. 60s. *otc.*
Use: Mineral, vitamin supplement.

Day Tab with Iron. (Towne) Vitamins A 5000 IU, D 400 IU, E 15 IU, C 60 mg, folic acid 1.5 mg, B_1 15 mg, B_2 1.7 mg, niacin 20 mg, B_6 2 mg, B_{12} 6 mcg, iron 18 mg/Tab. Bot. 200s. *Rx.*
Use: Mineral, vitamin supplement.

Dayto-Anase. (Dayton) Bromelains 50,000 IU (protease activity). Tab. Bot. 60s. *otc.*
Use: Enzyme.

Dayto Himbin. (Dayton) Yohimbine 5.4 mg/Tab. Bot. 60s. *Rx.*
Use: Alpha-adrenergic blocker.

Dayto Sulf. (Dayton) Sulfathiazole 3.42%, sulfacetamide 2.86%, sulfabenzamide 3.7%, urea 0.64%. Cream. Tube 78 g with 8 disposable applicators. *Rx.*
Use: Anti-infective, vaginal.

•**dazadrol maleate.** (DAY-zah-drole) USAN.
Use: Antidepressant.

Dazamide Tabs. (Major) Acetazolamide 250 mg/Tab. Bot. 100s, 250s, 1000s, UD 100s. *Rx.*
Use: Diuretic.

•**dazepinil hydrochloride.** (dahz-EH-pih-NILL) USAN.
Use: Antidepressant.

•**dazmegrel.** (DAZE-meh-grell) USAN.
Use: Inhibitor (thromboxane synthetase).

•**dazopride fumarate.** (DAY-zoe-PRIDE) USAN.
Use: Peristaltic stimulant.

•**dazoxiben hydrochloride.** (DAZE-OX-ih-ben) USAN.
Use: Antithrombotic.

DB Electrode Paste. (Day-Baldwin) Tube 5%.

Dbed. Dibenzylethylenediamine dipenicillin G.
Use: Anti-infective, penicillin.
See: Benzathine penicillin G, Susp.

DCA.
See: Desoxycorticosterone acetate preps. (Various Mfr.)

DCF. Pentostatin (2'-deoxycoformycin). *Rx.*
Use: Anti-infective.
See: Nipent, Pow. (Parke-Davis).

DCP. (Towne) Calcium 180 mg, phosphorus 105 mg, vitamins D 66.7 IU/Tab. Bot. 100s. *otc.*
Use: Mineral, vitamin supplement.

DC Softgels. (Zenith Goldline) Docusate calcium 240 mg/Cap. Bot. 100s, 500s. *otc.*
Use: Laxative.

DC 240. (Zenith Goldline) Docusate calcium 240 mg/Cap. Bot. 100s, 500s. *otc.*
Use: Laxative.

DDAVP Injection. (Rorer). Desmopressin acetate 4 mcg, chlorobutanol 5 mg/ml. Amp. 1 ml. Vials. 10 ml. 15 mcg/ml, sodium chloride 9 mg/ml. Amp. 1 ml, 2 ml. *Rx.*
Use: Antidiuretic.

DDAVP Nasal. (Rhone-Poulenc Rorer) **Soln:** 0.1 mg/ml (0.1 mg equivalent to 400 IU arginine vasopressin). **Spray Pump:** Sodium chloride 7.5 mg. Bot. 5 ml w/ spray pump (50 doses of 10 mcg). *Rx.*
Use: Antidiuretic.

DDAVP Spray. (Rorer) Desmopressin acetate 0.1 mg, chlorobutanol 5 mg/ml. Bot. 5 ml. Vial 2.5 ml w/applicator tubes for nasal administration. *Rx.*
Use: Antidiuretic.

DDAVP Tablets. (Rhone-Poulenc Rorer) Desmopressin acetate 0.1 or 0.2 mg/Tab. Bot 100s. *Rx.*
Use: Antidiuretic.

ddC. Dideoxycytidine.
Use: Antiviral.
See: HIVID (Roche).

ddI. Didanosine.
Use: Antiviral.
See: Videx, Tab., Pow. (Bristol-Myers Squibb).

D-Diol. (Burgin-Arden) Testosterone cypionate 50 mg, estradiol cypionate 2 mg/ml. Vial 10 ml. *Rx.*
Use: Androgen, estrogen combination.

DDS.
See: Dapsone Tab., U.S.P. 23.

DDT.
See: Chlorophenothane.

Deacetyllanatoside C.
See: Deslanoside, U.S.P. 23.

deadly nightshade leaf.
See: Belladonna Leaf, U.S.P. 23.

1-deamino-8-d-arginine vasopressin. Desmopressin acetate.
Use: Hormone.
See: Concentraid, Soln. (Ferring Labs.).
DDAVP, Inj., Soln. (Rhone-Poulenc Rorer).

deba.
See: Barbital (Various Mfr.)

Debrisan. (Johnson & Johnson Consumer Products) Dextranomer. **Beads:** Spherical hydrophilic 0.1-0.3 mm diameter. Bot. 25 g, 60 g, 120 g. Pk. 7 × 4 g, 14 × 14 g. U.S. distributor Johnson & Johnson Consumer Products. **Paste:** 10 g. Foil packets 6s. *otc.*
Use: Dermatologic, wound therapy.

•**debrisoquin sulfate.** (deb-RICE-oh-kwin) USAN.
Use: Antihypertensive.

Debrox. (Hoechst Marion Roussel) Carbamide peroxide 6.5% in anhydrous glycerol. Plastic squeeze bot. 0.5 oz, 1 oz. *otc.*
Use: Otic.

Decabid. (Eli Lilly) Indecainide HCl 50 mg, 75 mg or 100 mg/SR tab. Bot. 100s, UD 100s. [Approved but not marketed].
Use: Antiarrhythmic.

Deca-Bon. (Barrows) Vitamins A 3000 IU, D 400 IU, C 60 mg, B_1 1 mg, B_2 1.2 mg, niacinamide 8 mg, B_6 1 mg, panthenol 3 mg, B_{12} 1 mcg, biotin 30 mcg/0.6 ml. Drops Bot. 50 ml. *otc.*
Use: Vitamin supplement.

Decaderm. (Merck) Dexamethasone 0.1% w/isopropyl myristate gel, wood alcohols, refined lanolin alcohol, microcrystalline wax, anhydrous citric acid, anhydrous sodium phosphate dibasic. Tube 30 g. *Rx.*

Use: Corticosteroid.

Decadron. (Paddock) Dexamethasone sodium phosphate 4 mg/ml. Vial 5 ml. *Rx.*
Use: Corticosteroid.

Decadron. (Merck) Dexamethasone. **Tab.:** 0.5 mg: Bot. 100s, UD 100s; 0.75 mg: 100s, UD 100s; 4 mg: Bot. 50s, UD 100s. **Elix.:** 0.5 mg/5 ml, benzoic acid 0.1%, alcohol 5% Bot. w/dropper 100 ml, Bot. w/out dropper 237 ml. *Rx.*
Use: Corticosteroid.
W/Neomycin sulfate.
See: NeoDecadron, Ophth. Soln., Ophth. Oint., Topical, Cream (Merck).

Decadron Phosphate. (Merck) Dexamethasone sodium phosphate equivalent in various forms: **Ophth. Soln.:** 0.1%. Ocumeter dispenser 5 ml. *Rx.* **Ophth. Oint.:** 0.05%. Tube 3.5 g. *Rx.* **Cream:** 0.1% w/stearyl alcohol, cetyl alcohol, mineral oil, polyoxyl 40 stearate, sorbitol solution, methyl polysilicone emulsion, creatinine, purified water, sodium citrate, disodium edetate, sodium hydroxide to adjust pH, methylparaben 0.15%, sorbic acid 0.1%. Tube 15 g, 30 g.
Use: Corticosteroid, ophthalmic.

Decadron Phosphate Injection. (Merck) Dexamethasone sodium phosphate 4 mg or 24 mg/ml, creatinine 8 mg, sodium citrate 10 mg, disodium edetate 0.5 mg (24 mg/ml only), sodium hydroxide to adjust pH, sodium bisulfite 1 mg, methylparaben 1.5 mg, propylparaben 0.2 mg/ml. **4 mg/ml:** Vial 1 ml, 5 ml, 25 ml. **24 mg/ml** (for I.V. use only): Vial 5 ml, 10 ml. *Rx.*
Use: Corticosteroid.

Deca-Durabolin. (Organon) Nandrolone decanoate injection w/benzyl alcohol 10%. **50 mg/ml:** Multidose vial 2 ml. **100 mg/ml:** Multidose vial 2 ml, syringe 1 ml. **200 mg/ml:** Multidose vial 1 ml, syringe 1 ml. *c-III.*
Use: Anabolic steroid.

Deca-Durabolin Rediject Syringes. (Organon) Nandrolone decanoate 50 mg, 100 mg or 200 mg/ml. Syringe 1 ml Box 25s. *c-III.*
Use: Anabolic steroid.

Decagen. (Zenith Goldline) Iron 18 mg, vitamins A 5000 IU, D 400 IU, E 30 IU, B_1 1.7 mg, B_2 2 mg, B_3 20 mg, B_5 10 mg, B_6 3 mg, B_{12} 6 mcg, C 60 mg, folic acid 0.4 mg, Ca, Cl, Cr, Cu, B, I, K, Mg, Mn, Mo, Ni, P, Se, Si, Sn, V, Zn 15 mg, vitamin K, biotin 30 mcg/Tab. Bot. 130s. *otc.*
Use: Mineral, vitamin supplement.

Decaject. (Mayrand) Dexamethasone sodium phosphate 4 mg/ml. Vial 5 ml, 10 ml. *Rx.*
Use: Corticosteroid.

Decaject-L.A. (Mayrand) Dexamethasone acetate 8 mg/ml suspension, polysorbate 80, carboxymethylcellulose, sodium bisulfite, EDTA, benzyl alcohol. Inj. vial 5 ml. *Rx.*
Use: Corticosteroid.

Decalix. (Pharmed) Dexamethasone 0.5 mg/5 ml. Bot. 100 ml. *Rx.*
Use: Corticosteroid.

Decameth. (Foy) Dexamethasone sodium phosphate injection 4 mg/5 cc vial. *Rx.*
Use: Corticosteroid.

Decameth L.A. (Foy) Dexamethasone sodium phosphate injection 8 mg/ml. Vial/5 ml. *Rx.*
Use: Corticosteroid.

Decameth Tablets. (Foy) Dexamethasone 0.75 mg/Tab. Bot. 1000s. *Rx.*
Use: Corticosteroid.

Decapryn. (Hoechst Marion Roussel) Doxylamine succinate 12.5 mg/Tab. Bot. 100s. *otc.*
Use: Antihistamine.
W/Pyridoxine HCl.
See: Bendectin, Tab. (Hoechst Marion Roussel).

Decasone Injection. (Forest Pharmaceutical) Dexamethasone sodium phosphate equivalent to dexamethasone phosphate 4 mg/ml. Vial 5 ml. *Rx.*
Use: Corticosteroid.

decavitamin. U.S.P. XXI. Vitamins A 4000 IU, D 400 IU, C 70 mg, calcium pantothenate 10 mg, B_{12} 5 mcg, folic acid 100 mcg, nicotinamide 20 mg, B_6 2 mg, B_2 2 mg, B_1 2 mg/Cap. or Tab. *otc.*
Use: Vitamin supplement.

Decholin. (Bayer Corp) Dehydrocholic acid 250 mg/Tab. Bot. 100s, 500s. *otc.*
Use: Hydrocholeretic.

Decicain. Tetracaine HCl.

•**decitabine.** (deh-SIGH-tah-BEAN) USAN.
Use: Antineoplastic.

declaben. (DEH-klah-BEN) (previously used name) see lodelaben.
Use: Antiarthritic, emphysema therapy adjunct.

Declomycin Hydrochloride. (ESI Lederle Generics) Demeclocycline HCl. **Cap.:** 150 mg. Bot. 100s. **Tab.:** 150 mg. Bot. 100s; 300 mg. Bot. 48s. *Rx.*

Use: Anti-infective, tetracycline.

Decofed. (Various Mfr.) Pseudoephedrine HCl 30 mg/5 ml. Syr. Bot. 120 ml, 240 ml, pt, gal. *otc.*
Use: Decongestant.

Decohist Capsules. (Towne) Chlorpheniramine maleate 1 mg, phenylpropanolamine HCl 12.5 mg, salicylamide 180 mg, caffeine 15 mg/Cap. Bot. 18s. *otc.*
Use: Analgesic, antihistamine, decongestant.

Decohistine DH Liquid. (Morton Grove) Pseudoephedrine HCl 30 mg, chlorpheniramine maleate 2 mg, codeine phosphate 10 mg, alcohol. Liq. Bot. 120 ml, pt and gal. *c-v.*
Use: Antihistamine, antitussive, decongestant.

Decohistine Elixir. (Rosemont) Phenylephrine HCl 5 mg, chlorpheniramine maleate 2 mg, alcohol 5%. Elix. Bot. 120 ml, pt. and gal. *otc.*
Use: Antihistamine, decongestant.

Deconade. (H.L. Moore) Phenylpropanolamine HCl 75 mg, chlorpheniramine maleate 12 mg/Cap. Bot. 100s, 1000s. *otc.*
Use: Antihistamine, decongestant.

Deconamine CX Liquid. (Bradley) Hydrocodone bitartrate 5 mg, pseudoephedrine HCl 60 mg, guaifenesin 200 mg/5 ml. Bot. 480 ml. *Rx.*
Use: Antitussive, expectorant.

Deconamine CX Tablets. (Bradley) Hydrocodone bitartrate 5 mg, pseudoephedrine HCl 30 mg, guaifenesin 300 mg/Tab. Bot. 100s. *Rx.*
Use: Antitussive, expectorant.

Deconamine SR Capsules. (Bradley) Chlorpheniramine maleate 8 mg, d-pseudoephedrine HCl 120 mg/Cap. Bot. 100s, 500s. *Rx.*
Use: Antihistamine, decongestant.

Deconamine Syrup. (Bradley) Chlorpheniramine maleate 2 mg, d-pseudoephedrine HCl 30 mg/5 ml, sorbitol. Bot. 473 ml. *Rx.*
Use: Antihistamine, decongestant.

Deconamine Tablets. (Bradley) Chlorpheniramine maleate 4 mg, d-pseudoephedrine HCl 60 mg/Tab. Bot. 100s. *Rx.*
Use: Antihistamine, decongestant.

Decongestabs. (Various Mfr.) Phenylpropanolamine HCl 40 mg, phenylephrine HCl 10 mg, chlorpheniramine maleate 5 mg, phenyltoloxamine citrate 15 mg/Tab. Bot. 100s, 1000s. *Rx.*
Use: Antihistamine, decongestant.

Decongestant Expectorant Liquid. (Schein) Pseudoephedrine HCl 30 mg, codeine phosphate 10 mg, guaifenesin 100 mg, alcohol 7.5%. Bot. 480 ml. *c-v.*
Use: Antitussive, decongestant, expectorant.

Decongestant Formula Mediquell. (Parke-Davis) Dextromethorphan HBr 30 mg, pseudoephedrine HCl 60 mg/Square.
Use: Antitussive, decongestant.

Decongestant Tablets, Extended Release. (Various Mfr.) Phenylpropanolamine HCl 40 mg, phenylephrine HCl 10 mg, chlorpheniramine maleate 5 mg, phenyltoloxamine citrate 15 mg/Tab. Bot. 50s, 100s, 1000s. *Rx.*
Use: Antihistamine, decongestant.

Deconhist L.A. (Zenith Goldline) Phenylephrine HCl 25 mg, phenylpropanolamine HCl 50 mg, chlorpheniramine maleate 8 mg, hyoscyamine sulfate 0.19 mg, atropine sulfate 0.04 mg, scopolamine hydrobromide 0.01 mg/SR Tab. Bot. 100s, 250s, 500s, 1000s. *Rx.*
Use: Anticholinergic, antihistamine, decongestant.

Deconomed. (Iomed Labs) Chlorpheniramine maleate 8 mg, pseudoephedrine HCl 120 mg/Cap. Bot. 100s, 500s. *Rx.*
Use: Antihistamine, decongestant.

Deconsal II Capsules. (Adams Labs) Pseudoephedrine 60 mg, guaifenesin 600 mg/Cap. Bot. 100s. *Rx.*
Use: Decongestant, expectorant.

•**dectaflur.** (DECK-tah-flure) USAN.
Use: Dental caries agent.

Decubitex. (I.C.P) **Oint.:** Biebrich scarlet red sulfonated 0.1%, balsam Peru, castor oil, zinc oxide, starch, sodium propionate, parabens. Jar 15 g, 60 g, 120 g, lb. **Pow.:** Biebrich scarlet red sulfonated 0.1%, starch, zinc oxide, sodium propionate, parabens. Bot. 30 g, UD 1 g. *otc.*
Use: Antipruritic; dermatologic, wound therapy; emollient.

Decylenes. (Rugby) Undecylenic acid, zinc undecylenate. Oint. Tube 30 g, lb. *otc.*
Use: Antifungal, topical.

Deep-Down Pain Relief Rub. (SmithKline Beecham Pharmaceuticals) Methyl salicylate 15%, menthol 5%, camphor 0.5%. Tube 1.25 oz, 3 oz. *otc.*
Use: Analgesic, topical.

Deep Strength Musterole. (Schering Plough) Methyl salicylate 30%, menthol 3%, methyl nicotinate 0.5%. Tube 1.25 oz, 3 oz. *otc.*
Use: Analgesic, topical.

Defen-LA. (Horizon) Pseudoephedrine HCl 60 mg, guaifenesin 600 mg/SR Tab. Bot. 100s. *Rx.*
Use: Decongestant, expectorant.

•**deferoxamine.** (DEE-fer-OX-ah-meen) USAN.
Use: Chelating agent (iron).

•**deferoxamine hydrochloride.** (DEE-fer-OX-ah-meen) USAN.
Use: Chelating agent for iron.

•**deferoxamine mesylate.** (DEE-fer-OX-ah-meen) U.S.P. 23.
Use: Iron depleter, antidote to iron poisoning, chelating agent.
See: Desferal Mesylate, Pow. for Inj. (Novartis).

defibrotide. (Crinos International)
Use: Thrombotic thrombocytopenic purpura. [Orphan drug]

Deficol. (Vangard) Bisacodyl 5 mg/Tab. Bot. 100s, 1000s. *otc.*
Use: Laxative.

•**deflazacort.** (deh-FLAZE-ah-cart) USAN.
Use: Anti-inflammatory.

d4T.
Use: Antiviral.
See: Stavudine (B-M Squibb).

Degas. (Invamed) Simethicone 80 mg, sucrose, mannitol. Tab. Chewable. Bot. 100s. *otc.*
Use: Antiflatulent.

Degest 2. (Akorn) Naphazoline HCl 0.012%. Bot. 15 ml. *otc.*
Use: Decongestant, ophthalmic.

dehydrex. (Holles Labs)
Use: Recurrent corneal erosion. [Orphan drug]

dehydrocholate sodium inj.. U.S.P. XXI.
Use: Relief of liver congestion, diagnosis of cardiac failure.
See: Decholin Sodium, Inj. (Bayer Corp).

7-dehydrocholesterol, activated. (Various Mfr.) Vitamin D-3.
Use: Vitamin supplement.

•**dehydrocholic acid.** (dee-HIGH-droe-KOLE-ik) U.S.P. 23.
Use: Orally, hydrocholeretic and choleretic.
See: Atrocholin,Tab. (GlaxoWellcome).
Cholan-DH, Tab. (Medeva).
Decholin (Bayer Corp).
Dilabil (Sterling Winthrop).
Ketocholanic acid.
Neocholan, Tab. (Hoechst Marion Roussel).
Procholon (Bristol-Myers Squibb).
W/Amylolytic and proteolytic enzymes, desoxycholic acid.
See: Bilezyme, Tab. (Roberts Pharm).
W/Bile, homatropine methylbromide, pepsin.
See: Biloric, Caps. (Arcum).
W/Bile, homatropine methylbromide, phenobarbital.
See: Bilamide, Tab. (Norgine).
W/Bile extract, pepsin, pancreatin.
See: Progestive, Tab. (NCP).
W/Desoxycholic acid.
See: Combichole, Tab. (F. Trout).
Ketosox, Tab. (B.F. Ascher).
W/Docusate sodium.
See: Dubbalax-B, Cap. (Redford).
Dubbalax-N, Cap. (Redford).
Neolax, Tab. (Schwarz Pharma).
W/Docusate sodium, phenolphthalein.
See: Bolax, Cap. (Boyd).
Sarolax (Saron).
Tripalax, Cap. (Redford).
W/Homatropine methylbromide.
See: Cholan V, Tab. (Medeva).
Dranochol, Tab. (Marin).
W/Homatropine methylbromide, sodium pentobarbital.
See: Homachol, Tab. (Teva USA).
W/Methscopolamine, ox bile, amobarbital.
See: Hydrochol Plus, Tab. (Zeneca)
W/Ox bile, homatropine methylbromide, phenobarbital.
See: Bilamide, Tab. (Norgine).
W/Pancreatin, pepsin, ox bile, belladonna extract.
See: Ro-Bile, Tab. (Solvay).
W/Pepsin, pancreatin, ox bile extract, papain.
See: Canz, Tab. (Cole).
W/Pepsin, pancreatin enzyme concentrate, cellulase.
See: Gastroenterase, Tab (Wallace).
W/Phenobarbital, homatropine methylbromide.
See: Cholan-HMB, Tab. (Medeva).
W/Phenobarbital, homatropine methylbromide, gerilase, geriprotase, desoxycholic acid.
See: Bilezyme Plus, Tabs. (Roberts Pharm).
W/Phenolphthalein, docusate sodium.
See: Sarolax, Cap. (Saron).

dehydrocholin.
Use: Hydrocholeretic.
See: Dehydrocholic acid.

dehydroepiandrosterone. (Genelabs)
Use: Treatment of systemic lupus ery-

thematosus (SLE). [Orphan drug].

dehydroeiandrosterone sulfate sodium. (Pharmadigm)
Use: Treatment of serious burns, accelerate re-epithelialization of donor sites in autologous skin grafting. [Orphan Drug]

dehydrodesoxycholic acid.
See: Cholanic acid.

Dekasol. (Seatrace) Dexamethasone phosphate 4 mg/ml. Vial 5 ml, 10 ml. *Rx.*
Use: Corticosteroid.

Dekasol L.A. (Seatrace) Dexamethasone acetate 8 mg/ml. Vial 5 ml. *Rx.*
Use: Corticosteroid.

De-Koff. (Whiteworth Towne) Terpin hydrate w/dextromethorphan. Elix. Bot. 4 oz. *otc.*
Use: Antitussive, expectorant.

Delacort Lotion. (Mericon) Hydrocortisone 0.5%. Bot. 4 oz. *otc.*
Use: Corticosteroid, topical.

•**delapril hydrochloride.** (DELL-ah-prill) USAN.
Use: Antihypertensive, angiotensin-converting enzyme inhibitor.

Del Aqua-5. (Del-Ray) Benzoyl peroxide 5%. Tube 42.5 g. *Rx.*
Use: Dermatologic, acne.

Del Aqua-10. (Del-Ray) Benzoyl peroxide 10%. 42.5 g. *Rx.*
Use: Dermatologic, acne.

Delaquin Lotion. (Schlicksup) Hydrocortisone 0.5%, iodoquin 3%. Bot. 3 oz. *Rx.*
Use: Antifungal, corticosteroid.

Delatest. (Dunhall Pharmaceuticals) Testosterone enanthate 100 mg/ml, chlorobutanol in sesame oil. Amp. 10 ml. *c-III.*
Use: Androgen.

Delatestadiol. (Dunhall Pharmaceuticals) Testosterone enanthate 90 mg, estradiol valerate 4 mg/ml, chlorobutanol in sesame oil. Amp. 10 ml. *Rx.*
Use: Androgen, estrogen combination.

Delatestryl. (Bio-Technology General) Testosterone enanthate 200 mg/ml in sesame oil, chlorobutanol 0.5%. Vial 5 ml. *c-III.*
Use: Androgen.

•**delavirdine mesylate.** USAN.
Use: Antiviral.
See: Rescriptor, Tab. (Pharmacia & Upjohn).

Delcid. (SmithKline Beecham Pharmaceuticals) Aluminum hydroxide 600 mg, magnesium hydroxide 665 mg/5 ml, alcohol 0.3%, saccharin. Bot. 8 oz. *otc.*
Use: Antacid.

Del-Clens. (Del-Ray) Soapless cleanser. Bot. 8 oz. *otc.*
Use: Dermatologic, cleanser.

Delcort. (Lee Pharm) Hydrocortisone 0.5% or 1%. Cream. Pack. 1 g, 20 g, 1 lb. (1% only). *otc.*
Use: Corticosteroid, topical.

Delco-Lax. (Delco) Bisacodyl 5 mg/Tab. Bot. 1000s. *otc.*
Use: Laxative.

Delcozine. (Delco) Phendimetrazine tartrate 70 mg/Tab. Bot. 1000s, 5000s. *c-III.*
Use: Anorexiant.

•**delequamine hydrochloride.** (deh-LEH-kwah-meen) USAN.
Use: Anti-impotence agent.

Delestrec. Estradiol 17-undecanoate. *Rx.*
Use: Estrogen.

Delestrogen. (Bristol-Myers) Estradiol valerate **10 mg/ml:** In sesame oil, chlorobutanol 0.5%. Vial 5 ml. **20 mg/ml:** In castor oil, benzyl benzoate 20%, benzyl alcohol 2%. Vial 5 ml or 1 ml unimatic single dose syringe. **40 mg/ml:** In castor oil, benzyl benzoate 40%, benzyl alcohol 2%. Vial 5 ml. *Rx.*
Use: Estrogen.

Delfen Contraceptive Foam. (Advanced Care Products) Nonoxynol-9 12.5% in an oil-in-water emulsion at pH 4.5 to 5.0. Starter can with applicator 20 g. Refill 20 g, 42 g. *otc.*
Use: Contraceptive, spermicide.

delinal. Propenzolate HCl.

•**delmadinone acetate.** (del-MAD-ih-nohn ASS-eh-tate) USAN.
Use: Antiandrogen; antiestrogen; hormone, progestin.
See: Delmate (Syntex).

Del-Mycin. (Del-Ray) Erythromycin 2%, ethyl alcohol 66%. Topical soln. Bot. 60 ml. *Rx.*
Use: Dermatologic, acne.

Del-Stat. (Del-Ray) Abradent cleaner. Jar 2 oz. *otc.*
Use: Dermatologic, acne.

Delsym Cough Suppressant Liquid. (McNeil Prods) Dextromethorphan HBr 30 mg/5 ml. Bot. 3 oz. *otc.*
Use: Antitussive.

delta-1-cortisone.
Use: Corticosteroid.
See: Deltasone, Tab. (Pharmacia & Upjohn).

delta-1-hydrocortisone.
Use: Corticosteroid.

See: Prednisolone (Various Mfr.)

Delta-Cortef. (Pharmacia & Upjohn) Prednisolone 5 mg/Tab. Bot. 100s, 500s. *Rx.*
Use: Corticosteroid.

Deltacortone. Prednisone.
Use: Corticosteroid.

Delta-Cortril. Prednisolone.
Use: Corticosteroid.

Delta-D. (Freeda Vitamins) Vitamin D_3 400 IU/Tab. Bot. 250s, 500s. *otc.*
Use: Vitamin supplement.

•**deltafilcon a.** (DELL-tah-FILL-kahn A) USAN.
Use: Contact lens material, hydrophilic.

•**deltafilcon b.** (DELL-tah-FILL-kahn B) USAN.
Use: Contact lens material (hydrophilic).
See: Amsof (Lombart).
Amsof-Thin (Lombart).

Deltasone. (Pharmacia & Upjohn) Prednisone. **2.5 mg:** Tab. Bot. 100s. **5 mg:** Tab. Bot. 100s, 500s, UD 100s, Dosepak 21s. **10 mg, 20 mg:** Tab. Bot. 100s, 500s, UD 100s. **50 mg:** Tab. Bot. 100s, UD 100s. *Rx.*
Use: Corticosteroid.

Delta-Tritex. (Dermol) Triamcinolone acetonide. **Cream:** 0.1% Tube 30 and 80 g. **Oint.:** 0.1% Tube 30 g. *Rx.*
Use: Corticosteroid, topical.

Del-Trac. (Del-Ray) Acne lotion. Bot. 2 oz. *otc.*
Use: Dermatologic, acne.

Deltastab.
Use: Corticosteroid.
See: Prednisolone (Various Mfr.)

•**deltibant.** (DELL-tih-bant) USAN.
Use: Antagonist (bradykinin).

Del-Vi-A. (Del-Ray) Vitamin A 50,000 IU/Cap. Bot. 100s. *Rx.*
Use: Vitamin supplement.

Delysid. Lysergic acid diethylamide.
Use: Potent psychotogenic.

Demadex. (Boehringer Mannheim) **Tab.:** Torsemide 5 mg, 10 mg, 20 mg, 100 mg. Bot. UD 100s. **Inj.:** Torsemide 10 mg/ml. Amps. 2 ml or 5 ml. *Rx.*
Use: Diuretics.

Demazin. (Schering Plough) **Syr.:** Chlorpheniramine maleate 2 mg, phenylpropanolamine HCl 12.5 mg/5 ml, alcohol 7.5%, menthol. Bot. 118 ml. **Tab.:** Chlorpheniramine maleate 4 mg, phenylpropanolamine HCl 25 mg. Box 24s. Bot. 100s. *otc.*
Use: Antihistamine, decongestant.

•**demecarium bromide.** (deh-meh-CARE-ee-uhm BROE-mide) U.S.P. 23.
Use: Cholinergic, (ophthalmic).
See: Humorsol, Soln. (Merck).

•**demeclocycline.** (DEH-meh-kloe-SIGH-kleen) U.S.P. 23. *Formerly Demethylchlortetracycline.*
Use: Anti-infective.
See: Declomycin Prods. (ESI Lederle Generics).
Ledermycin Prods. (ESI Lederle Generics).

•**demeclocycline hydrochloride.** (DEH-meh-kloe-SIGH-kleen) U.S.P. 23.
Use: Anti-infective.
See: Declomycin HCl, Preps. (ESI Lederle Generics).

demeclocycline hydrochloride and nystatin tablets.
Use: Anti-infective.
See: Declostatin, Tab. (ESI Lederle Generics).

•**demecycline.** (DEH-meh-SIGH-kleen) USAN.
Use: Anti-infective.

Demerol Hydrochloride. (Sanofi Winthrop) Meperidine HCl. **Syr.:** 50 mg/5 ml, saccharin. Bot. 16 fl oz. **Inj.:** Detecto-Seal, Carpuject, Sterile Cartridge-Needle Unit. **2.5%** (25 mg/ml), **5%** (50 mg/ml), **7.5%** (75 mg/ml), **10%** (100 mg/ml), Box 10s. **Uni-Amp 5%:** 0.5 ml (25 mg)/Amp., 1 ml (50 mg)/Amp., 1.5 ml (75 mg)/Amp., 2 ml (100 mg)/Amp. Box 25s; **10%:** 1 ml (100 mg)/Amp. Box 25s. **Uni-Nest 5%:** 0.5 ml (25 mg)/Amp., 1 ml (50 mg)/Amp., 1.5 ml (75 mg)/Amp., 2 ml (100 mg)/Amp. Box 25s; **10%:** 1 ml/Amp. Box 25s. **Vial: 5%** multiple-dose vial/30 ml Box 1s. **Tab.:** 50 mg or 100 mg. Bot. 100s, 500s. *c-II.*
Use: Analgesic, narcotic.

demethylchlortetracycline hydrochloride.
Use: Anti-infective, tetracycline.
See: Demeclocycline HCl, U.S.P. 23.

Demi-Regroton. (Rhone-Poulenc Rorer) Chlorthalidone 25 mg, reserpine 0.125 mg/Tab. Bot. 100s. *Rx.*
Use: Antihypertensive, diuretic.

•**demoxepam.** (dem-OX-eh-pam) USAN.
Use: Anxiolytic.

Demser. (Merck) Metyrosine 250 mg/Cap. Bot. 100s. *Rx.*
Use: Antihypertensive.

Demulen 1/35-21. (Searle) Ethynodiol diacetate 1 mg, ethinyl estradiol 35 mcg/Tab. Compack disp. 21s, 6 × 21, 2421. Refill 21s, 1221. *Rx.*
Use: Contraceptive.

Demulen 1/35-28. (Searle) Ethynodiol di-

acetate 1 mg, ethinyl estradiol 35 mcg/ Tab. Compack 28s: 21 active tabs, 7 placebo tabs. Compack 6 × 28, 2428. Refill 28s, 1228. *Rx.*
Use: Contraceptive.

Demulen 1/50-21. (Searle) Ethynodiol diacetate 1 mg, ethinyl estradiol 50 mcg/ Tab. Compack Disp. 21s, 6 × 21, 2421. Refill 21s, 1221. *Rx.*
Use: Contraceptive.

Demulen 1/50-28. (Searle) Ethynodiol diacetate 1 mg, ethinyl estradiol 50 mcg/ Tab. Compack 28s: 21 active tabs, 7 placebo tabs. Compack Disp. of 28, 6 × 28, 2428. Refill 28s, 1228. *Rx.*
Use: Contraceptive.

Denalan Denture Cleanser. (Whitehall Robins) Sodium percarbonate 30%. Bot. 7 oz., 13 oz. *otc.*
Use: Agent for oral hygiene.

•**denatonium benzoate.** (DEE-nah-TOE-nee-uhm BEN-zoh-ate) N.F. 18.
Use: Pharmaceutic aid (flavor, alcohol denaturant).
See: Bitrex.

Denavir. (SmithKline Beecham) Penciclovir 10 mg/g Cream. Tube 2 g. *Rx.*
Use: Cold sores.

Dencorub. (Last) Methyl salicylate 20%, menthol 0.75%, camphor 1%, eucalyptus oil 0.5%. Tube 1.25 oz, 2.75 oz. *otc.*
Use: Analgesic, topical.

Dencorub Analgesic Liquid. (Last) Oleoresin capsicum suspension in aqueous vehicle. Bot. 6 oz. *otc.*
Use: Analgesic, topical.

•**denofungin.** (DEE-no-FUN-jin) USAN.
Use: Antifungal, antibacterial.

Denorex. (Whitehall Robins) Coal tar solution 9%, menthol 1.5%. Shampoo Bot. 4 oz, 8 oz. *otc.*
Use: Antiseborrheic.

Denorex, Extra Strength. (Whitehall Robins) Coal tar solution 12.5%, menthol 1.5%, alcohol 10.4%. Shampoo. Bot. 120, 240, 360 ml. *otc.*
Use: Antiseborrheic.

Denorex Mountain Fresh. (Whitehall Robins) Coal tar solution 9%, menthol 1.5%. Bot. 4 oz, 8 oz. *otc.*
Use: Antiseborrheic.

Denorex with Conditioners. (Whitehall Robins) Coal tar solution 9%, menthol 1.5%. Bot 4 oz, 8 oz. *otc.*
Use: Antiseborrheic.

Denquel. (Procter & Gamble) Potassium nitrate 5%, calcium carbonate, glycerin, flavors. Tube 1.6 oz, 3 oz, 4.5 oz. *otc.*
Use: Dentrifice.

Dental Caries Preventive. (Colgate Oral) Fluoride ion 1.2%, alumina abrasive. 2 g Box 200s, Jar 9 oz. *Rx.*
Use: Dental caries agent.

Dentipatch. (Noven) Lidocaine 23 mg or 46.1 mg/2 cm^2 patch, aspartame/Patch. Box 50s, 100s. *Rx.*
Use: Anesthetic, local.

Dentrol. (Block Drug) Carboxymethylcellulose, polyethelyne oxide homopolymer, peppermint and spearmint in mineral oil base. Bot. 0.9 oz, 1.8 oz. *otc.*
Use: Denture adhesive.

Dent's Dental Poultice. (C.S. Dent) Glycerin, mineral oil, polyoxyethylene sorbitan monooleate. Bot. 0.125 oz, 0.25 oz. *otc.*
Use: Dental poultice.

Dent's Ear Wax Drops. (C.S. Dent) Glycerin, mineral oil, polyoxyethylene sorbitan monooleate. Bot. 0.125 oz, 0.25 oz. *otc.*
Use: Otic.

Dent's Extra Strength Toothache Gum. (C.S. Dent) Benzocaine. Box. 1 g. *otc.*
Use: Anesthetic, local.

Dent's Lotion-Jel. (C.S. Dent) Benzocaine in special base. Tube 0-2 oz. *otc.*
Use: Anesthetic, local.

Dent's Maximum Strength Toothache Drops. (C.S. Dent) Benzocaine, alcohol 74%, chlorobutanol anhydrous 0.09%. Liq. 3.7 ml. *otc.*
Use: Anesthetic, local.

Dent's Toothache Drops Treatment. (C.S. Dent) Alcohol 60%, chlorobutanol anhydrous (chloroform derivative) 0.09%, propylene glycol, eugenol. Bot. 0.125 oz. *otc.*
Use: Anesthetic, local.

Dent's Toothache Gum. (C.S. Dent) Benzocaine, eugenol, petrolatum in base of cotton and wax. Box 0.035 oz. *otc.*
Use: Anesthetic, local.

Denture Orajel. (Del Pharmaceuticals) Benzocaine 10%, saccharin. Gel. Tube. 9.45 g. *otc.*
Use: Anesthetic, local.

Dent-Zel-Ite. (Last) **Oral Mucosal Analgesic:** Benzocaine 5%, alcohol, glycerin. Bot. 1/16 oz. **Temporary Dental Filling:** Sandarac gum, alcohol. Bot. oz. **Toothache Drops:** Eugenol 85% in alcohol. Bot. oz. *otc.*
Use: Anesthetic, local.

denyl sodium.

Use: Anticonvulsant.
See: Diphenylhydantoin Sodium, Cap. (Various Mfr.)

deodorizers, systemic. Chlorophyll derivatives (chlorophyllin). *otc.*
Use: **Oral:** Control of fecal and urinary odors in colostomy, ileostomy or incontinence. **Topical:** Reduce pain and inflammation (wounds, burns, surface ulcers, skin irritation).
See: Chlorophyll, Tab. (Freeda Vitamins).
Derifil, Tab. (Rystan).
Chloresium, Tab., Soln., Oint. (Rystan).

deoxyadenosine, 2-chloro-2'. (St. Jude Children's Hospital)
Use: Antineoplastic. [Orphan drug]

deoxycholic acid.
See: Desoxycholic Acid, Tab. (Various Mfr.)

2'deoxycoformycin. Pentostatin.
Use: Antibiotic, antineoplastic.
See: Nipent, Pow. (Parke-Davis).

deoxycytidine (5-AZA-2'). (Pharmachemie U.S.A.)
Use: Antineoplastic. [Orphan drug]

deoxynojirmycin. (Searle) Butyl-DNJ. *Rx.*
Use: Antiviral.

Depacon. (Abbott Laboratories) Valproic acid 5 ml (as valproic sodium)/Inj. Vial 10s. *Rx.*
Use: Anticonvulsant.

Depade. (Mallinckrodt) Naltrexone HCl 50 mg/Tab. Bot. 50s. *Rx.*
Use: Antidote.

Depakene. (Abbott Laboratories) Valproic acid. **Cap.:** 250 mg. Bot. 100s, UD 100s. **Syr.:** 250 mg/5 ml, sorbitol. Bot. 480 ml. *Rx.*
Use: Anticonvulsant.

Depakote. (Abbott Laboratories) Divalproex sodium 125 mg, 250 mg or 500 mg/Delayed Release Tab and 125 mg/sprinkle cap. **DR Tab.:** Bot. 100s, 500s, UD 100s. **Sprinkle Cap.:** Bot. 100s, UD 100s. *Rx.*
Use: Anticonvulsant.

DepAndro 100. (Forest Pharmaceutical) Testosterone cypionate in cottonseed oil 100 mg/ml, benzyl alcohol. Vial 10 ml. *c-III.*
Use: Androgen.

DepAndro 200. (Forest Pharmaceutical) Testosterone cypionate in cottonseed oil 200 mg/ml, benzyl benzoate, benzyl alcohol. Vial 10 ml. *c-III.*
Use: Androgen.

DepAndrogyn. (Forest Pharmaceutical) Testosterone cypionate 50 mg, estradiol cypionate 2 mg/ml. Vial 10 ml. *Rx.*
Use: Androgen, estrogen combination.

Depa-Syrup. (Alra Laboratories) Valproic acid syrup 250 mg/5 ml. Bot. 4 oz, 16 oz. *Rx.*
Use: Anticonvulsant.

Depen Tablets. (Wallace) Penicillamine 250 mg/Tab. Bot. 100s. *Rx.*
Use: Chelating agent.

depepsen. Amylosulfate sodium.
Use: Digestive aid.

depGynogen. (Forest Pharmaceutical) Estradiol cypionate in cottonseed oil 5 mg/ml, cottonseed oil, chlorobutanol. Vial 10 ml. *Rx.*
Use: Estrogen.

depMedalone 40. (Forest Pharmaceutical) Methylprednisolone acetate in aqueous suspension 40 mg/ml, polyethylene glycol, myristyl-gamma-picolinium Cl. Vial 5 ml. *Rx.*
Use: Corticosteroid.

depMedalone 80. (Forest Pharmaceutical) Methylprednisolone acetate 80 mg/ml, polyethylene glycol, myristyl-gamma-picolinium Cl. Vial 5 ml. *Rx.*
Use: Corticosteroid.

Depoestra. (Tennessee Pharmaceutic) Estradiol cypionate 5 mg/ml. Vial 10 ml. *Rx.*
Use: Estrogen.

Depo-Estradiol. (Pharmacia & Upjohn) Estradiol cypionate 1 mg or 5 mg/ml, chlorobutanol anhydrous 5.4 mg/ml, cottonseed oil. **1 mg/ml:** Vial 10 ml. **5 mg/ml:** Vial 5 ml. *Rx.*
Use: Estrogen.

Depofoam encapsulated cytarabine. (Depo Tech).
Use: Neoplastic meningitis. [Orphan drug]

DepoGen. (Hyrex) Estradiol cypionate 5 mg/ml, cottonseed oil, chlorobutanol. Vial 10 ml. *Rx.*
Use: Estrogen.

Depoject. (Mayrand) Methylprednisolone acetate 40 mg or 80 mg/ml suspension with polyethylene glycol and myristyl-gamma-picolinium Cl. Inj. Vial 5 ml. *Rx.*
Use: Corticosteroid.

Depo-Medrol. (Pharmacia & Upjohn) Methylprednisolone acetate, 20 mg/Inj. Vial. 5 ml, 10 ml. Methylprednisolone acetate, 40 mg/Inj. Vial. 5 ml, 10 ml. Methylprednisolone acetate 80 mg/Inj. Vial. 1 ml, 5 ml. *Rx.*
Use: Corticosteroid.

Deponit. (Schwarz Pharma Kremers Urban) Nitroglycerin transdermal delivery system containing 16 mg or 32 mg. Box 30s, 100s. *Rx.*
Use: Antianginal, vasodilator.

Depopred-40. (Hyrex) Methylprednisolone acetate suspension 40 mg/ml, polyethylene glycol, myristyl-gamma-picolinum Cl. Vial 5 ml, 10 ml. *Rx.*
Use: Corticosteroid.

Depopred-80. (Hyrex) Methylprednisolone acetate 80 mg/Inj. Vial. 5 ml. *Rx.*
Use: Corticosteroid.

Depo-Provera. (Pharmacia & Upjohn) Medroxyprogesterone acetate 400 mg/ml. Suspended in polyethylene glycol 3350 20.3 mg, sodium sulfate (anhydrous) 11 mg, myristyl-gamma-picolinium Cl 1.69 mg/ml. Vial 2.5 ml, 10 ml, 1 ml U-Ject. *Rx.*
Use: Hormone, progestin.

Depo-Provera Contraceptive Injection. (Pharmacia & Upjohn) Medroxyprogesterone acetate 150 mg/ml, with PEG-3350 28.9 mg, polysorbate 80 2.41 mg, sodium Cl 8.68 mg, methylparaben 1.37 mg, propylparaben 0.15 mg/Inj. Vial. 1 ml. *Rx.*
Use: Contraceptive.

Depotest. (Hyrex) Testosterone cypionate. **100 mg:** With cottonseed oil, benzyl alcohol. **200 mg:** With cottonseed oil, benzyl benzoate, benzyl alcohol. Vial 10 ml. *c-III.*
Use: Androgen.

Depo-Testadiol. (Roberts Pharm) Testosterone cypionate 50 mg, estradiol cypionate 2 mg/ml. Vial 10 ml. *Rx.*
Use: Androgen, estrogen combination.

Depotestogen. (Hyrex) Testosterone cypionate 50 mg, estradiol cypionate 2 mg/ml. Vial 10 ml. *Rx.*
Use: Androgen, estrogen combination.

Depo-Testosterone. (Pharmacia & Upjohn) Testosterone cypionate. **100 mg/ml:** In benzyl alcohol 9.45 mg, cottonseed oil 736 mg/ml. Vial 1 ml, 10 ml. **200 mg/ml:** In benzyl benzoate 0.2 ml, benzyl alcohol 9.45 mg, cottonseed oil 560 mg/ml. Vial 1 ml, 10 ml. *c-III.*
Use: Androgen.

deprenyl. Selegiline HCl.
See: Eldepryl (Somerset).

Deproist Expectorant/Codeine. (Geneva Pharm) Pseudoephedrine HCl 30 mg, codeine phosphate 10 mg, guaifenesin 100 mg/5 ml. Bot. 120 ml, 480 ml. *c-v.*
Use: Antitussive, decongestant, expectorant.

•**deprostil.** (deh-PRAHST-ill) USAN.
Use: Antisecretory, gastric.

Dep-Test. (Sig) Testosterone cypionate 100 mg/ml. Vial 10 ml. *c-III.*
Use: Androgen.

Dequasine. (Miller) L-lysine 20 mg, l-cysteine 100 mg, dl-methionine 50 mg, vitamin C 200 mg, iron 5 mg, Cu, I, Mg, Mn, Zn. Tab. Bot. 100s. *otc.*
Use: Mineral, vitamin supplement.

Derifil. (Rystan) Chlorophyllin copper complex 100 mg/Tab. Bot. 30s, 100s, 1000s. *otc.*
Use: Deodorant, oral.

Dermabase. (Paddock) Mineral oil, petrolatum, cetostearyl alcohol, propylene glycol, sodium lauryl sulfate, isopropyl palmitate, imidazolidinyl urea, methyl and propylparabens. Cream. Jar 1 lb. *otc.*
Use: Emollient.

Dermacoat Aerosol Spray. (Century Pharm) Benzocaine 4.5%. Bot. 7 oz. *otc.*
Use: Anesthetic, local.

Dermacort Cream. (Solvay) Hydrocortisone 0.5% or 1% in a water soluble cream of stearyl alcohol, cetyl alcohol, isopropyl palmitate, citric acid, polyoxyethylene 40 stearate, sodium phosphate, propylene glycol, water, benzyl alcohol, buffered to pH 5.0. 0.5% in 30 g, 1% in 1 lb. *Rx.*
Use: Corticosteroid, topical.

Dermacort Lotion. (Solvay) Hydrocortisone 1% in lotion base, buffered to pH 5.0. Paraben free. Bot. 120 ml. *Rx.*
Use: Corticosteroid, topical.

Derma-Cover. (Scrip) Sulfur, salicylic acid, hyamine 10x, isopropyl alcohol 22%, in powder film forming base. Bot. 2 oz. *otc.*
Use: Keratolytic.

DermaFlex. (Zila) Lidocaine 2.5%, alcohol 79%. Gel. Tube 15 g. *otc.*
Use: Anesthetic, local.

Derma-Guard. (Greer Laboratories) Protective adhesive pow. Can w/sifter top, 4 oz. Spray top Bot. 4 oz, pkg. 1 lb. Rings. Pkg. 5s, 10s. *otc.*
Use: Dermatologic, protectant.

Dermal-Rub Balm. (Roberts Pharm) Menthol racemic 7%, camphor 1%, methyl salicylate 1%, cajuput oil 1%. Cream. Jar 1 oz, 1 lb. *otc.*
Use: Analgesic, topical.

Dermamycin. (Pfeiffer) **Cream:** Diphenhydramine HCl 2% in a base of parabens, polyethylene glycol monostearate

and propylene glycol. 28.35 g. **Spray:** Diphenhydramine HCl 2 %, menthol 1%, alcohol, methylparaben. Bot. 60 ml. *otc.*
Use: Antihistamine, topical.

Dermaneed. (Hanlon) Zirconium oxide 4.5%, calamine 6%, zinc oxide 4%, actamer 0.1% in bland lotionized base. Bot. 4 oz. *otc.*
Use: Antipruritic, topical.

Derma-Pax. (Recsei) Methapyrilene HCl 0.22%, chlorothenylpyramine maleate 0.06%, pyrilamine maleate 0.22%, benzyl alcohol 1%, chlorobutanol 1%, isopropyl alcohol 40%. Liq. 4 oz, pt. *otc.*
Use: Antihistamine, topical; antipruritic, topical.

Derma-Pax HC. (Recsei) Hydrocortisone 0.5%, pyrilamine maleate 0.2%, pheniramine maleate 0.2%, chlorpheniramine 0.06%, benzyl alcohol 1%. Liq. Bot. 60 ml, 120 ml, 480 ml.
Use: Antihistamine, topical; corticosteroid, topical.

Dermarest. (Del Pharmaceuticals) Diphenhydramine HCl 2%, resorcinol 2%, aloe vera gel, benzalkonium chloride, EDTA, menthol, methylparaben, propylene glycol. Gel Tube 29.25 g, 56.25 g. *otc.*
Use: Antihistamine, topical.

Dermarest Dricort. (Del Pharmaceuticals) Hydrocortisone 1%, white petrolatum cream. Bot. 14 g. *otc.*
Use: Corticosteroid, topical.

Dermarest Plus. (Del Pharmaceuticals) **Gel:** Diphenhydramine HCl 2%, menthol 1%, aloe vera gel, benzalkonium chloride, isopropyl alcohol, methylparaben; propylene glycol. Tube 15 g, 30 g. **Spray:** Diphenhydramine HCl 2%, menthol 1%, aloe vera gel, benzalkonium chloride, methylparaben propylene glycol, SDA 40 alcohol, EDTA. Bot. 60 ml. *otc.*
Use: Antihistamine, topical.

Dermasept Antifungal. (PharmaKon) Tannic acid 6.098%, zinc Cl 5.081%, benzocaine 2.032%, methylbenzethonium HCl, tolnaftate 1.017%, undecylenic acid 5.081%, ethanol 38B 58.539%, phenol, benzyl alcohol, benzoic acid, coal tar, camphor, menthol. Liq. Bot. 30 ml. *otc.*
Use: Antifungal, topical.

Dermasil. (Chesebrough-Ponds) Glycerin and dimethicone in a base containing cyclomethicone, sunflower seed oil, petrolatum, borage seed oil, lecithin, vitamin E acetate, vitamin A palmitate, vitamin D_3, corn oil, EDTA, methylparaben. Lot. Bot. 120 ml, 240 ml. *otc.*
Use: Emollient.

Derma-Smoothe/FS Oil. (Hill) Fluocinolone acetonide 0.01%. Oil. Bot. 4 oz. *Rx.*
Use: Antipsoriatic; antiseborrheic, topical.

Derma-Smoothe Oil. (Hill) Refined peanut oil, mineral oil in lipophilic base. *otc.*
Use: Antipruritic; dermatologic, protectant.

Derma Soap. (Ferndale Laboratories) Dowicil 0.1%. 4 oz w/dispenser. *otc.*
Use: Antiseptic.

Derma-Soft. (Vogarell) Medicated cream. Salicylic acid, castor oil, triethanolamine. Tube ¾ oz. *otc.*
Use: Keratolytic.

Derma-Sone 1%. (Hill) Hydrocortisone 1%, pramoxine HCl 1%, cetyl alcohol, glyceryl monosterate, isopropyl myristate, potassium sorbate, furcelleran. *otc, Rx.*
Use: Anesthetic; corticosteroid, local.

Dermasorcin. (Lamond) Resorcin 2%, sulfur 5%. Bot. 1 oz, 2 oz, 4 oz, 8 oz, pt, 32 oz, 0.5 gal. *otc.*
Use: Dermatologic, acne; antiseborrheic, topical.

Dermastringe. (Lamond) Bot. 4 oz, 6 oz, 8 oz, pt, 32 oz, gal. *otc.*
Use: Dermatologic, cleanser.

Dermasul. (Lamond) Sulfur 5%. Bot. 1 oz, 2 oz, 4 oz, 8 oz, pt, 32 oz, 0.5 gal, gal. *otc.*
Use: Dermatologic, acne; antiseborrheic, topical.

Dermathyn. (Davis & Sly) Benzyl alcohol 3%, benzocaine 3.5%, butyl-p-aminobenzoate 1%, phenylmercuric borate. Tube 1 oz. *otc.*
Use: Anesthetic, local.

Dermatic Base. (Whorton) Compounding cream base. Bot. 16 oz.
Use: Pharmaceutical aid, emollient base.

Dermatol.
See: Bismuth subgallate, Preps. (Various Mfr.)

Dermatop. (Hoechst Marion Roussel) Prednicarbate 0.1%, white petrolatum, lanolin alcohols, mineral oil, cetostearyl alcohol, EDTA, lactic acid. Cream 15 g, 60 g. *Rx.*
Use: Corticosteroid, topical.

Derma Viva. (Rugby) Mineral oil, glyceryl stearate, laureth-4, lanolin oil, PEG-100 stearate, PEG-40 stearate,

PEG-4 dilaurate, trolamine, diocetyl sodium sulfosuccinate, parabens. Lot. Bot. 237 ml. *otc.*
Use: Emollient.

Dermed. (Holloway) Vitamins A and D with hydrogenated vegetable oil. Cream. Tube 60 g, 120 g. *otc.*
Use: Emollient.

Dermeze. (Premo) Thenylpyramine HCl 2%, benzocaine 2%, tyrothricin 0.25 mg/g. Massage Lot. Bot. 5¾ oz. *otc.*
Use: Anesthetic, antihistamine, anti-infective.

Dermolate Anti-Itch. (Schering Plough) Hydrocortisone 0.5% petrolatum, mineral oil, chlorocresol. Cream Tube 15 g, 30 g. *otc.*
Use: Corticosteroid, topical.

Dermol HC. (Dermol) **Cream:** Hydrocortisone 1% or 2.5%. Tube 30 g. **Oint.:** Hydrocortisone 1%. Tube 30 g. *Rx.*
Use: Anorectal preparation.

Dermolin. (Roberts Pharm) Menthol racemic, methyl salicylate, camphor, mustard oil, isopropyl alcohol 8%. Bot. 3 oz, pt, gal. *otc.*
Use: Liniment.

Dermoplast. (Whitehall-Robins) **Spray:** Benzocaine 20%, menthol, methylparaben, aloe, lanolin. Bot. 82.5 ml. **Lot.:** Benzocaine 8%, menthol, aloe, glycerin, parabens, lanolin. Bot. 90 ml. *otc.*
Use: Anesthetic, local.

Dermovan. (Galderma) Glyceryl stearate, spermaceti, mineral oil, glycerin, cetyl alcohol, butylparaben, methylparaben, propylparaben, purified water. Vanishing-type base, Jar 1 lb. *otc.*
Use: Dermatologic, protectant.

Dermtex HC. (Pfeiffer) Hydrocortisone 0.5% in a glycerin base. Tube 15 g. *otc.*
Use: Corticosteroid, topical.

Dermuspray. (Warner-Chilcott) Trypsin 0.1 mg, Balsam Peru 72.5 mg, castor oil 650 mg/0.82 ml. Aer. Bot. 120 g. *Rx.*
Use: Enzyme, topical.

DES.
See: Diethylstilbestrol.

desacchromin. A nonprotein bacterial colloidal dispersion of polysaccharide.

•**desciclovir.** (DESS-sigh-kloe-veer) USAN.
Use: Antiviral.

•**descinolone acetonide.** (DESS-SIN-ole-ohn ah-SEE-toe-nide) USAN.
Use: Corticosteroid, topical.

Desenex. (Novartis) **Cream:** Total 25% (Undecylenic acid, zinc undecylenate) lanolin, parabens, white petrolatum. Tube 15 g. **Oint.:** Total 25% (Undecylenic acid, zinc undecylenate) lanolin, parabens, white petrolatum. Tube 14 g. **Pow.:** Total 25% (Undecylenic acid, zinc undecylenate), talc. 45 g. **Liq.:** Undecylenic acid 10%, isopropyl alcohol 47.1%. Pump spray bot. 1.5 oz. **Spray Pow.:** Total 25% (Undecylenic acid, zinc undecylenate), menthol, talc. Aerosol can 81 g. **Penetrating Foam:** Undecylenic acid 10%, isopropyl alcohol 29.2%. Can 45 g. *otc.*
Use: Antifungal, topical.

Desenex Antifungal, Maximum. (Novartis) Miconazole nitrate 2% Pow. Tube 14 g. *otc.*
Use: Antifungal, topical.

Desenex Foot & Sneaker Spray. (Novartis) Aluminum chlorhydrex w/alcohol 89.3%. Aerosol can 2.7 oz. *otc.*
Use: Foot deodorant, antiperspirant.

Desenex Maximum Strength. (Medeva) Total undecylenate 25%, lanolin, parabens, white petrolatum. Oint. Tube 15 g. *otc.*
Use: Antifungal, topical.

De Serpa. (de Leon) Reserpine 0.25 mg or 0.5 mg/Tab. Bot. 100s, 500s, 1000s (0.25 mg only).
Use: Antihypertensive.

Desert Pure Calcium. (Cal-White Mineral Co.) Calcium (from calcium carbonate) 500 mg, vitamin D 125 IU. Tab. Bot. 200s. *otc.*
Use: Mineral, vitamin supplement.

Desferal. (Novartis) Deferoxamine mesylate 500 mg/5 ml. Amp. 4s. *Rx.*
Use: Antidote.

•**desflurane.** (dess-FLEW-rane) U.S.P. 23.
Use: Anesthetic.
See: Suprane (Ohmeda).

•**desipramine hydrochloride.** (dess-IPP-ruh-meen) U.S.P. 23.
Use: Antidepressant.
See: Norpramin, Tab. (Hoechst Marion Roussel).
Pertofrane, Cap. (Rhone-Poulenc Rorer).

•**desirudin.** (deh-SIHR-uh-din) USAN.
Use: Anticoagulant.

Desitin. (Pfizer) **Pow.:** Talc. Can 3 oz, 7 oz, 10 oz. **Oint.:** Cod liver oil, zinc oxide 40%, talc, petrolatum, lanolin. Tube 1 oz, 2 oz, 4 oz, 8 oz, Jar 1 lb. *otc.*
Use: Astringent, skin protectant.

Desitin Creamy. (Pfizer) Zinc oxide 10%, mineral oil, white petrolatum, parabens. Oint. Tube 57 g . *otc.*

Use: Antifungal, topical.

Desitin Powder with Zinc Oxide. (Pfizer) Cornstarch 88.2%, zinc oxide 10%. Pow. 28 g, 397 g. *otc.*
Use: Diaper rash preparation.

•**deslanoside.** (dess-LAN-oh-side) U.S.P. 23.
Use: Cardiovascular agent.
See: Cedilanid-D (Sandoz Consumer).

•**deslorelin.** (DESS-low-REH-lin) USAN.
Use: Gonadotropin inhibitor. [Orphan drug], LHRH agonist.
See: Somagard [as acetate] (Roberts Pharm).

Desma. (Tablicaps) Diethylstilbestrol 25 mg/Tab. Patient dispenser 10s. *Rx.*
Use: Estrogen.

•**desmopressin acetate.** (DESS-moe-PRESS-in) USAN.
Use: Treatment of diabetes insipidus, mild hemophilia A, and von Willebrand's disease [Orphan drug], antidiuretic.
See: Stimate (Centeon).
DDAVP, Liq. (Rhone-Poulenc Rorer).

desmopressin acetate. (Rhone-Poulenc Rorer).
Use: Treatment of mild hemophilia A and von Willebrand's disease. [Orphan drug]

desmopressin acetate. (Various Mfr.) Desmopressin acetate 4 mcg/ml. Inj. 1 ml, 10 ml. *Rx.*
Use: Treatment of diabetes insipidus.

Desogen. (Organon) Desogestrel 0.15 mg, ethinyl estradiol 0.03 mg/Tab. Pck. 28s. *Rx.*
Use: Contraceptive.

•**desogestrel.** (DESS-oh-JESS-trell) USAN.
Use: Hormone, progestin.
W/ Ethinyl estradiol.
See: Desogen, Tab. (Organon).
Ortho-Cept, Tab. (Ortho).

•**desonide.** (DESS-oh-nide)
Use: Anti-inflammatory.
See: Tridesilon, Cream (Bayer Corp).

desonide. (Various Mfr.) Desonide 0.05%. Oint. Cream 15 g, 60 g. *Rx.*
Use: Anti-inflammatory; corticosteroid, topical.

desonide cream. (Galderma) Desonide 0.05% in cream base. Tube 15 g, 60 g. *Rx.*
Use: Corticosteroid, topical.

DesOwen. (Galderma) Desonide 0.05%. Cream. Tube 15 g, 60 g. *Rx.*
Use: Corticosteroid, topical.

•**desoximetasone.** (dess-OX-ee-MET-ah-sone) U.S.P. 23.
Use: Anti-inflammatory; corticosteroid, topical.
See: Topicort (Hoechst Marion Roussel).

•**desoxycorticosterone acetate.** (dess-OX-ee-core-tih-koe-STURR-ohn ASS-eh-tate) U.S.P. 23.
Use: Adrenocortical steroid (salt-regulating).

•**desoxycorticosterone pivalate.** U.S.P. 23.
Use: Adrenocortical steroid (salt-regulating).

desoxycorticosterone pivalate injectable suspension.
Use: Adrenocortical steroid (salt-regulating).

desoxycorticosterone trimethylacetate. U.S.P. XVI.
Use: Adrenocortical steroid (salt-regulating).

desoxyephedrine hydrochloride. (Various Mfr.) *c-II.*
Use: CNS stimulant.
See: Methamphetamine HCl, Prep.

Desoxyn. (Abbott Laboratories) Methamphetamine HCl. **Tab.:** 5 mg. Bot. 100s. **Gradumets:** 5 mg. Bot. 100s; 10 mg. Bot. 100s; 15 mg. Bot. 100s. *c-II.*
Use: CNS stimulant.

desoxy norephedrine.
Use: CNS stimulant.
See: Amphetamine HCl, Preps. (Various Mfr.)

desoxyribonuclease.
W/Fibrinolysin.
Use: Enzyme, topical.
See: Elase, prep. (Parke-Davis).

Desquam-E 2, 5, & 10. (Westwood Squibb) Benzoyl peroxide 5% or 10%. Gel. Tube 42.5 g. *Rx.*
Use: Dermatologic, acne.

Desquam-X 5% or 10% Gel. (Westwood Squibb) Benzoyl peroxide 5% or 10%, water base with EDTA. Tube 42.5 ml; 85 g (5% only). *Rx.*
Use: Dermatologic, acne.

Desquam-X 5% or 10% Wash. (Westwood Squibb) Benzoyl peroxide 5% or 10%, EDTA. Bot. 150 ml. *Rx.*
Use: Dermatologic, acne.

D-Est. (Burgin-Arden) Estradiol cypionate 5 mg/ml. Vial 10 ml. *Rx.*
Use: Estrogen.

de-Stat. (Sherman) Surfactant cleaner, benzalkonium Cl 0.01%, EDTA 0.25%. Soln. Bot. 118 ml. *otc.*
Use: Contact lens care.

de-Stat 3. (Sherman) Octylphenoxy poly-

ethoxyethanol, benzyl alcohol 0.1%, EDTA 0.5%, lauryl sulfate salt of imidazoline. Soln. Bot. 118 ml. *otc.*
Use: Contact lens care.

de-Stat 4. (Sherman) Benzyl alcohol 0.3%, EDTA 0.5%, lauryl sulfate, salt of imidazole, octylphenoxypolyethoxyethanol. Thimerosol free. Soln. Bot. 118 ml. *otc.*
Use: Contact lens care.

Desyrel. (Bristol-Myers) Trazodone HCl 50 mg or 100 mg. **50 mg:** Bot. 100s, 1000s, UD 100s. **100 mg:** Bot. 500s. *Rx.*
Use: Antidepressant.

Desyrel Dividose. (Bristol-Myers) Trazodone HCl 150 mg or 300 mg/Dividose tab. Dividose design breakable into fragments for dosing convenience. Bot. 100s, 500s (150 mg). *Rx.*
Use: Antidepressant.

Detachol. (Ferndale Laboratories) Bland, nonirritating liquid for removing adhesive tape. Pkg. 4 oz.
Use: Adhesive remover.

De Tal. (de Leon) Phenobarbital 0.25 gr, hyoscyamine sulfate 0.1037 mg, atropine sulfate 0.0194 mg, hyoscine HBr 0.0065 mg/Tab. or 5 ml. **Tab.:** Bot. 100s. **Elix.:** With alcohol 20%. Bot. pt. *Rx.*
Use: Anticholinergic, antispasmodic, hypnotic, sedative.

Detane. (Del Pharmaceuticals) Benzocaine 7.5%. Tube 0.5 oz. *otc.*
Use: Anesthetic, local.

•**deterenol hydrochloride.** (dee-TEER-eh-nahl) USAN.
Use: Adrenergic, ophthalmic.

detergents. surface-active.
See: pHisoDerm, Liq. (Sanofi Winthrop).
pHisoHex, Liq. (Sanofi Winthrop).
Zephiran, Prods. (Sanofi Winthrop).

detigon hydrochloride.
See: Chlophedianol HCl (Various Mfr.)

•**detirelix acetate.** (DEH-tih-RELL-ix) USAN.
Use: Antagonist (LHRH).

•**detomidine hydrochloride.** (deh-TOE-mih-deen HIGH-droe-KLOR-ide) USAN.
Use: Hypnotic, sedative.

Detrol. (Pharmacia & Upjohn) Tolerodine tartrate 1 mg, 2 mg /Tab. Bot. 60s, 500s. UD 140s. *Rx.*
Use: Urinary tract product.

Detussin. (Various Mfr.) Phenylpropanolamine HCl 75 mg and caramiphen edisylate 40 mg/TR Cap. Bot. 100s, 500s, 1000s. *otc.*
Use: Antitussive, decongestant.

Detussin Expectorant Liquid. (Various Mfr.) Pseudoephedrine HCl 60 mg, hydrocodone bitartrate 5 mg, guaifenesin 200 mg, alcohol. Liq. Bot. 480 ml. *c-III.*
Use: Antitussive, decongestant, expectorant.

Detussin Liquid. (Various Mfr.) Pseudoephedrine HCl 60 mg, hydrocodone bitartrate 5 mg. Liq. Bot. Pt, Gal. *c-III.*
Use: Antitussive, decongestant.

•**deuterium oxide.** (doo-TEER-ee-uhm) USAN.
Use: Radiopharmaceutical.

•**devazepide.** (dev-AZE-eh-PIDE) USAN.
Use: Antagonist (cholecystokinin); antispasmodic, gastrointestinal.

Devrom. (Parthenon). Bismuth subgallate 200 mg, lactose, sugar/chew. tab. Bot. 100s. *otc.*
Use: Deodorant, systemic.

Dex 4 Glucose. (Can-Am Care) Glucose. Tab. Bot. 10s, 50s. *otc.*
Use: Hyperglycemic.

Dexacidin Ointment. (Ciba Vision Ophthalmics) Neomycin sulfate 0.35%, dexamethasone 0.1% polymyxin B sulfate 10,000 units. Tube 3.5 g. *Rx.*
Use: Anti-infective; corticosteroid, ophthalmic.

Dexacidin Ophthalmic Suspension. (Ciba Vision Ophthalmics) Neomycin 0.35%, polymyxin B sulfate 10,000 units, dexamethasone 1%. Bot. 5 ml. *Rx.*
Use: Anti-infective; corticosteroid, ophthalmic.

Dexacort Phosphate in Turbinaire. (Adams Labs) Dexamethasone sodium phosphate 0.1 mg equivalent to dexamethasone 0.084 mg w/fluorochlorohydrocarbons as propellants and alcohol 2%. Aerosol w/nasal applicator. Container 170 sprays; refill package without nasal applicator.
Use: Nasal corticosteroid.

Dexacort Phosphate Respihaler. (Adams Labs) Dexamethasone sodium phosphate equivalent to 0.1 mg dexamethasone phosphate (approximately 0.084 mg dexamethasone) w/fluorochlorohydrocarbons as propellants, alcohol 2%. Aerosol for oral inhalation, 170 sprays in 12.6 g pressurized container.
Use: Bronchodilator.

Dex-a-Diet Caffeine Free. (Columbia) Phenylpropanolamine HCl 75 mg/Cap. or Capl. Pkg. 3s, 6s, 20s, 40s.
Use: Dietary aid.

Dex-a-Diet Original Formula. (Columbia) Phenylpropanolamine HCl 75 mg, ascorbic acid 200 mg/Cap. Pkg. 3s, 6s, 10s, 24s, 48s.
Use: Dietary aid.

Dexafed. (Mallard) Phenylephrine HCl 5 mg, dextromethorphan HBr 10 mg, guaifenesin 100 mg/5 ml. Syr. Bot. 120 ml. *otc.*
Use: Antitussive, decongestant, expectorant.

Dexameth. (Major) **Tab.:** Dexamethasone 0.25 mg, 0.5 mg, 0.75 mg, 1.5 mg or 4 mg. Bot. 100s (0.25 mg, 0.5 mg, 1.5 mg); Bot. 100s, 1000s, Unipak 12s (0.75 mg); Bot. 50s, 100s (4 mg). **Elix.:** 0.5 mg/5 ml, alcohol 5%. Bot. 100 ml, 240 ml. *Rx.*
Use: Corticosteroid.

•**dexamethasone.** (DEX-uh-METH-uh-sone) U.S.P. 23.
Use: Adrenal corticosteroid (anti-inflammatory); corticosteroid, topical.
See: Aeroseb-Dex, Aerosol (Allergan).
Decaderm in Estergel (Merck).
Decadron, Tab., Elix. (Merck).
Decameth, Inj. (Foy).
Decameth L.A., Inj. (Foy).
Dexaport, Tab. (Freeport).
Dexone TM, Tab. (Solvay).
Dezone, Tab. (Solvay).
Hexadrol, Tab., Elix., Cream (Organon).
Maxidex Ophth. Liq. (Alcon Laboratories).
W/Neomycin sulfate.
See: NeoDecadron, Prep. (Merck)
NeoDecaspray, Aerosol (Merck).
W/Neomycin sulfate, polymyxin B sulfate.
See: Maxitrol Ophth. Susp., Oint. (Alcon Laboratories).

dexamethasone. (Steris) 0.1%. Susp. Bot. 5 ml. *Rx.*
Use: Corticosteroid, ophthalmic.

•**dexamethasone acefurate.** (DEX-ah-METH-ah-sone ASS-eh-fer-ate) USAN.
Use: Anti-inflammatory, topical steroid.

•**dexamethasone acetate.** (DEX-ah-METH-ah-sone) U.S.P. 23.
Use: Adrenocortical steroid (anti-inflammatory).
See: Dalalone (Forest Pharmaceutical).
Decadronal (Merck)
Dexone LA, Ind. (Kay).

•**dexamethasone dipropionate.** (DEX-ah-METH-ah-sone die-PRO-pee-oh-nate) USAN.
Use: Anti-inflammatory, steroid.

Dexamethasone Intensol Oral Solution. (Roxane) Dexamethasone 1 mg/ml concentrated oral soln. Bot. 30 ml w/calibrated dropper. *Rx.*
Use: Corticosteroid.

dexamethasone ophthalmic. (Various Mfr.) Dexamethasone 0.1%. Susp. Bot. 5 ml. *Rx.*
Use: Corticosteroid.

•**dexamethasone sodium phosphate.** (DEX-ah-METH-ah-sone) U.S.P. 23.
Use: Adrenocortical steroid (anti-inflammatory); corticosteroid, topical.
See: AK-Dex, Soln., Oint. (Akorn).
Dalalone (Forest Pharmaceutical).
Decadron Phosphate, Preps. (Merck).
Decaject, Vial (Mayrand).
Decameth, Inj. (Foy).
Dexone, Inj. (Keene, Hauck).
Dezone, Inj. (Solvay).
Hexadrol Phosphate, Inj. (Organon).
Maxidex, Oint. (Alcon Laboratories).
Savacort D, Inj. (Savage).
Solurex, Inj. (Hyrex).
W/Lidocaine (Xylocaine).
W/Neomycin sulfate.
See: NeoDecadron, Prods. (Merck).
W/Neomycin and polymixin B sulfates.
See: Dexacidin, Prods. (Ciba Vision Ophthalmics).

dexamethasone sodium phosphate. (Various Mfr.) **Soln.:** 0.1%. Bot. 5 ml; **Oint.:** 0.05%. Tube 3.5 g.
Use: Adrenocortical steroid (anti-inflammatory); corticosteroid, topical.

•**dexamisole.** (DEX-AM-ih-sole) USAN.
Use: Antidepressant.

dexamphetamine.
See: Dextroamphetamine (Various Mfr.)

Dexaphen-S.A. Tablets. (Major) Pseudoephedrine sulfate 120 mg, dexbrompheniramine maleate 6 mg. In 100s, 500s. *Rx.*
Use: Antihistamine, decongestant.

Dexaport. (Freeport) Dexamethasone 0.75 mg/Tab. Bot. 1000s. *Rx.*
Use: Corticosteroid.

Dexasone. (Various Mfr.) Dexamethasone sodium phosphate 4 mg/ml, methyl and propyl parabens, sodium bisulfite. Vial 5 ml, 10 ml, 30 ml. *Rx.*
Use: Corticosteroid.

Dexasone Injection. (Roberts Pharm) Dexamethasone sodium phosphate 4 mg/ml. Vial 5 ml, 30 ml. *Rx.*
Use: Corticosteroid.

Dexasone L.A. Injection. (Roberts Pharm) Dexamethasone acetate 8 mg/ml. Vial 5 ml. *Rx.*
Use: Corticosteroid.

Dexasporin Ointment. (Bausch & Lomb) Dexamethasone 0.1%, neomycin sulfate equivalent to 0.35% neomycin base and 10,000 units polymyxin B sulfate. Ophth. Oint. Tube 3.5 g. *Rx.*
Use: Steroid; anti-infective, ophthalmic.

Dexasporin Suspension. (Various Mfr.) Dexamethasone 0.1%, neomycin sulfate equivalent to 0.35%, neomycin base and 10,000 units polymyxin B sulfate/ml, hydroxypropyl methylcellulose, polysorbate 20, benzalkonium chloride. Drops. Bot. 5 ml. *Rx.*
Use: Anti-infective; corticosteroid, ophthalmic.

Dexatrim-15. (Thompson) Phenylpropanolamine HCl 75 mg/TR Cap. Bot. 20s, 40s. *otc.*
Use: Dietary aid.

Dexatrim-15 w/Vitamin C. (Thompson) Phenylpropanolamine HCl 75 mg, vitamin C 180 mg/TR Cap. Bot. 20s. *otc.*
Use: Dietary aid.

Dexatrim Maximum Strength. (Thompson) Phenylpropanolamine HCl 75 mg/Tab. ER Bot. 20s. *otc.*
Use: Dietary aid.

•**dexbrompheniramine maleate.** (dex-brome-fen-EER-ah-meen MAL-ee-ate) U.S.P. 23.
Use: Antihistamine.
W/Pseudoephedrine sulfate.
See: Disophrol Chronotab, Tab. (Schering Plough).
Drixoral S.A., Tab. (Schering Plough).

•**dexchlorpheniramine maleate.** U.S.P. 23.
Use: Antihistamine.
See: Polaramine, Repetabs Tab., Tab., Syr. (Schering Plough).
W/Pseudoephedrine sulfate, guaifenesin, alcohol.
See: Polaramine Expectorant (Schering Plough).

dexchlorpheniramine maleate. (Various Mfr.) Dexchlorpheniramine maleate 4 mg, 6 mg/TR Tab. Bot. 100s. *Rx.*
Use: Antihistamine.

•**dexclamol hydrochloride.** (DEX-clay-mahl) USAN.
Use: Hypnotic, sedative.

Dexedrine. (SmithKline Beecham Pharmaceuticals) Dextroamphetamine sulfate. **Tab.:** 5 mg Bot. 100s, 1000s. **Spansule:** 5 mg Bot. 50s; 10 mg, 15 mg Bot. 50s, 500s. *c-II.*
Use: CNS stimulant.

•**dexetimide.** (dex-ETT-ih-mid) USAN.
Use: Anticholinergic, antiparkinsonian.

DexFerrum. (American Regent) Elemental iron 50 mg/ml (as dextran)/Inj. Vial. 2 ml (single dose). *Rx.*
Use: Hematinic.

Dex4 Glucose. (Can-Am-Care) Glucose, lemon, orange, raspberry, grape flavors. Chew. Tab. 10s, 50s. *otc.*
Use: Glucose-elevating agent.

•**dexibuprofen.** (dex-EYE-byoo-PRO-fen) USAN.
Use: Analgesic; anti-inflammatory.

•**dexibuprofen lysine.** (dex-EYE-byoo-PRO-fen LIE-seen) USAN.
Use: Analgesic (cyclooxygenase inhibitor), anti-inflammatory.

•**deximafen.** (dex-IH-mah-fen) USAN.
Use: Antidepressant.

•**dexivacaine.** (dex-IH-vah-CANE) USAN.
Use: Anesthetic.

•**dexmedetomidine.** (DEX-meh-dih-TOE-mih-deen) USAN.
Use: Anxiolytic.

Dexone. (Solvay) Dexamethasone 0.5 mg, 0.75 mg, 1.5 mg or 4 mg/Tab. Bot. 100s, UD 100s. Box 1s, 10s, 150s. *Rx.*
Use: Corticosteroid.

Dexone. (Roberts Pharm) Dexamethasone sodium phosphate 4 mg/ml. Amp. 5 ml. *Rx.*
Use: Corticosteroid.

Dexone. (Solvay) Dexamethasone sodium phosphate 4 mg/ml, methyl and propyl parabens, sodium bisulfite. Vial 5 ml, 10 ml. *Rx.*
Use: Corticosteroid.

Dexone LA. (Keene Pharmaceuticals) Dexamethasone acetate suspension equivalent to dexamethasone 8 mg, polysorbate 80, carboxymethylcellulose, sodium bisulfite, EDTA, benzyl alcohol. Vial 5 ml. *Rx.*
Use: Corticosteroid.

•**dexormaplatin.** (DEX-ore-mah-PLAT-in) USAN.
Use: Antineoplastic.

•**dexoxadrol hydrochloride.** (dex-OX-ah-drole) USAN.
Use: Antidepressant; stimulant (central); analgesic.

•**dexpanthenol.** (DEX-PAN-theh-nahl) U.S.P. 23.
Use: Treatment of paralytic ileus and postoperative distention, cholinergic.
See: Ilopan, Inj. (Pharmacia & Upjohn).
Panthoderm (Rhone-Poulenc Rorer).

dexpanthenol/choline bitartrate.
See: Ilopan-choline (Pharmacia & Upjohn).

•**dexpemedolac.** (dex-peh-MED-oh-lack) USAN.
Use: Analgesic.

•**dexpropanolol hydrochloride.** (DEX-pro-PRAN-oh-lole) USAN.
Use: Antiadrenergic (β-receptor); cardiovascular agent (antiarrhythmic).

•**dexrazoxane.** (dex-ray-ZOX-ane) USAN.
Use: Cardioprotectant. [Orphan drug]
See: Zinecard, Pow. for Inj., (Pharmacia & Upjohn).

•**dexsotalol hydrochloride.** (DEX-ah-tah-lahl) USAN
Use: Cardiovascular agent (antiarrhythmic).

dextran 1.
See: Promit (Pharmacia & Upjohn).

dextran 6%. (Abbott Laboratories). *Rx.*
See: Dextran 75, I.V. (Abbott Laboratories).

•**dextran 40.** (DEX-tran 40) USAN. Polysaccharide (m.w. 40,000) produced by the action of *Leuconostoc mesenteroidesо*n sucrose.
Use: Blood flow adjuvant, plasma volume extender.
See: Gentran 40 (Baxter Healthcare).
Rheomacrodex (Medisan)
10% LMD, Inj. (Abbott Laboratories).

dextran 40. (McGaw) Dextran 40 10% with 0.9% sodium chloride or in 5% dextrose. Inj. 500 ml. *Rx.*
Use: Plasma expander.

dextran 45, 75. Polysaccharide (m.w. 45,000, 75,000) produced by the action of Leuconostoc mesenteroides on saccharose. Rheotran (45). *Rx.*
Use: Blood volume expander.

•**dextran 70.** (DEX-tran 70) USAN. Polysaccharide (m.w.70,000) produced by the action of *Levconostoc mesenteroides* on sucrose.
Use: Plasma volume extender.
See: Aquasite (Ciba Vision Ophthalmics).
Dextran 70, Inj. (McGaw).
Gentran 70, Inj. (Baxter).
Hyskon (Kabi Pharmacia & Upjohn).
Macrodex (Medisan).

dextran 70. (DEX-tran 70) (McGaw) Dextran 70 6% in 0.9% sodium chloride. Inj. 500 ml. *Rx.*
Use: Plasma expander.

•**dextran 75.** (DEX-tran 75) USAN Polysaccharide (m.w. 75,000) produced by the action of *Leuconostoc mesenteroides* on sucrose.
Use: Plasma volume extender.
See: Dextran 75, Inj. (Abbott Laboratories).
Macrodex, Inj. (Medisan).

dextran 75. (Abbott Laboratories) Dextran 75 6% in 0.9% sodium chloride or 5% dextrose. Inj. 500 ml. *Rx.*
Use: Plasma expander.

dextran adjunct. *Rx.*
Use: Plasma expander.
See: Promit, Inj. (Pharmacia & Upjohn).

dextran and deferoxamine.
Use: Acute iron poisoning. [Orphan drug]
See: Bio-Rescue (Biomedical Frontiers).

dextran sulfate, inhaled aerosolized.
Use: Antiviral. [Orphan drug]
See: Uendex (Ueno Fine Chem Industry Ltd.)

dextran sulfate sodium. (Ueno Fine Chemicals)
Use: AIDS drug. [Orphan drug]

•**dextrates.** (DEX-traytz) N.F. 18. Mixture of sugars (approximately 92% dextrose monohydrate and 8% higher saccharides; dextrose equivalent is 95% to 97%) resulting from the controlled enzymatic hydrolysis of starch.
Use: Pharmaceutic aid (tablet binder, diluent).

•**dextrin.** N.F. 18.
Use: Pharmaceutic aid (suspending, viscosity-increasing agent; tablet binder; tablet, capsule diluent).

•**dextroamphetamine.** (DEX-troe-am-FET-ah-meen) USAN.
Use: Stimulant (central).

dextroamphetamine with amphetamine as resin complex.
See: Biphetamine 12.5, 20, Cap. (Medeva).

dextroamphetamine phosphate. Monobasic d-a-methylphenethlyamine phosphate. (+)-α-Methylphenethylamine phosphate.
Use: CNS stimulant.
See: d-Amphetamine phosphate combinations.

dextroamphetamine saccharate.
See: Adderall, Tab. (Richwood).

•**dextroamphetamine sulfate.** (DEX-troe-am-FET-uh-meen) U.S.P. 23.
Use: CNS stimulant.
See: Adderall. Tab. (Richwood) .Dexampex, Cap., Tab. (Teva USA).
Dexedrine, Preps. (SmithKline Beecham Pharmaceuticals).
Dextrostat, Tab. (Richwood).

Diphylets, Granucaps (Solvay).
Tidex Tab. (Allison).

dextroamphetamine sulfate w/combinations.
Use: CNS stimulant.
See: Adderall, Tab. (Richwood).
Amphodex, Cap. (Jamieson-McKames).
Delcobese (Delco).
Min-Gera, Tab. (Scrip).
Trimex, Trimex #2, Cap. (Mills).

Dextro-Check Normal Control. (Bayer Corp) Clear liquid containing measured amount of glucose 0.10% w/v.
Use: Glucometer calibration aid.

Dextro-Chek Calibrators. (Bayer Corp) Clear liquid soln. containing measured amounts of glucose. Low calibrator contains 0.05% w/v glucose. High calibrator contains 0.30% w/v glucose.
Use: Glucometer calibration aid.

Dextro-Chlorpheniramine Maleate.
Use: Antihistamine.
See: Polaramine, Repetab, Tab., Expect., Syr. (Schering Plough).

•**dextromethorphan.** (DEX-troe-meth-OR-fan) U.S.P. 23.
Use: Cough suppressant, antitussive.

•**dextromethorphan hydrobromide.** (DEX-troe-meth-OR-fan HIGH-droe-BROE-mide) U.S.P. 23.
Use: Antitussive.
See: Benylin, Preps. (Parke-Davis).
Creo-Terpin, Liq. (Lee).
Delsym, Liq. (Medeva).
Mediquell, Tab. (Warner Lambert).
Silphen DM, Syr. (Silarx).
St. Joseph Cough Syr. (Schering Plough).
Sucrets 4-Hour Cough, Loz. (SmithKline Beecham).
Symptom 1, Liq. (Parke-Davis).
Tus-F, Liq. (Orbit).

W/Benzocaine, menthol, peppermint oil.
See: Vicks Formula 44 Cough Control Discs, Loz. (Procter & Gamble).

dextromethorphan hydrobromide w/ benzocaine.
Use: Nonnarcotic antitussives.
See: Cough-X, Loz. (Archer).
Spec-T, Loz. (Apothecon).
Vicks Cough Silencers, Loz. (Procter & Gamble).
Vicks Formula 44 Cough Control Discs, Loz. (Procter & Gamble).

dextromethorphan hydrobromide w/ combinations.
See: Ambenyl-D, Liq. (Hoechst Marion Roussel).
Anatuss DM, Syr., Tab. (Mayrand).
Anti-Tuss D.M., Liq. (Century Pharm).
Anti-Tussive, Tab. (Canright).
Atuss DM, Syr. (Atley).
Bayer Prods. (Bayer Corp).
Benylin Multi-Symptom, Liq. (Glaxo Wellcome).
Breacol Cough Medication, Liq. (Bayer Corp).
Capahist-DMH, Cap. (Freeport).
Centuss, MLT, Tab. (Century Pharm).
Cerose-DM, Liq. (Wyeth Ayerst).
Cheracol-D, Cough Syr. (Upjohn).
Cheratussin, Cough Syr. (Towne).
Chexit, Tab. (Sandoz Consumer).
Children's Hold 4-Hour Cough Suppressant & Decongestant, Loz. (SmithKline Beecham Pharmaceuticals).
Codimal DM, Liq. (Schwarz Pharma).
Colrex, Syr. (Solvay).
Comtrex, Cap., Liq. Tab. (Bristol-Myers).
Congespirin Cough Syrup (Bristol-Myers).
Contac Jr., Liq. (SmithKline Beecham Pharmaceuticals).
Coricidin Children's Cough Syrup (Schering Plough).
Diabetic Tussin, Liq. (Roberts Pharm).
Dimacol, Cap. (Robins).
Donatussin, Syr. (Laser).
Dorcol Ped. Cough Syr. (Sandoz Consumer).
Dristan Cough Formula, Syr. (Whitehall Robins).
End-A-Koff, Jr. Syr. (Quality Generics).
Fenesin DM, Tab. (Dura).
Formula 44 Prods. (Procter & Gamble).
Halls Mentho-Lyptus Decongestant Cough Formula, Liq. (Warner Lambert).
Histalet, DM, Syr. (Reid Provident).
Infantuss, Liq. (Scott/Cord).
Iobid DM, SR Tab. (Iomed).
Iohist DM, Syr. (Iomed).
Liqui-Histine DM, Syr. (Liquipharm).
Mapap CF, Tab. (Major).
Maximum Strength Tylenol Flu, Tab. (McNeil-CPC).
Monafed DM, TR Tab. (Monarch).
Muco-Fen-DM, TR Tab. (Wakefield Pharm).
Niltuss, Syr. (Minn. Pharm)
Nyquil, Liq. (Procter & Gamble).
Orthoxicol, Syr. (Pharmacia & Upjohn).
Partuss, Liq. (Parmed).
Pediacon DX Preps. (Zenith Goldline).

Phenadex, Preps. (Barre National).
Phenergan, Pediatric, Liq. (Wyeth Ayerst).
Polytuss-DM, Liq. (Rhode).
Profen II DM, TR Tab. (Wakefield).
Rentuss, Tab., Syr. (Wren).
Rentuss, Tab. (Wren).
Respa-DM, SR Tab. (Respa)
Robitussin-DM, Syr., Loz. (Robins).
Robitussin Cold & Cough, Preps. (Robins).
Robitussin-CF (Robins).
Rondec DM, Drops, Syr. (Ross).
Scotcof Liq. (Scott/Cord).
Scotuss, Pediatric Cough Syr. (Scott/Cord).
Scot-Tussin Senior Clear, Liq. (Scot-Tussin Pharm).
Shertus, Liq. (Sheryl).
Sildec-DM, Ped. Drops. (Silarx).
Siltapp with Dextromethorphan HBr Cold & Cough, Elix. (Silarx).
Siltussin Preps. (Silarx).
Sorbase Cough Syr. (Fort David).
Spec-T Sore Throat-Cough Suppressant Loz. (Squibb).
Sudafed Cough Syr. (Glaxo-Wellcome).
Synacol CF, Tab. (Roberts).
Synatuss-One, Liq. (Freeport).
Thor, Cough Syr. (Towne).
Tolu-Sed DM, Liq. (Scherer).
Tonecol, Syr., Tab. (A.V.P.).
Triaminic, Preps. (Sandoz Consumer).
Triaminicol, Syr. (Sandoz, Consumer).
Trind-DM, Syr. (Bristol-Myers).
Tusibron-DM, Liq. (Kenwood/Bradley).
Tussi-Organidin DM NR, Liq. (Wallace).
Tussi-Organidin DM-S NR, Liq. (Wallace).
Tusquelin, Syr. (Circle).
Tussagesic, Tab., Susp. (Sandoz, Consumer).
Tylenol, Preps. (McNeil).
Unproco, Cap. (Solvay).
Vicks Cough Prods. (Procter & Gamble).
Vicks Daycare, Liq. (Procter & Gamble).
Vicks Formula 44 Prods. (Procter & Gamble).
Vicks Nyquil, Liq. (Procter & Gamble).
Wal-Tussin DM, Syr. (Walgreen).

•**dextromethorphan polistirex.** (DEX-troe-meth-OR-fan pahl-ee-STIE-rex) USAN.
Use: Antitussive.

dextromoramide tartrate.
Use: Analgesic, narcotic.

dextro-pantothenyl alcohol.
See: Panthenol (Various Mfr.)
Ilopan (Pharmacia & Upjohn).

dextropropoxyphene hydrochloride. *c-IV.*
Use: Analgesic.
See: Propoxyphene HCl, Cap. (Various Mfr.)

•**dextrorphan hydrochloride.** (DEX-trore-fan) USAN.
Use: Treatment of cerebral ischemia, vasospastic therapy adjunct.

•**dextrose.** (DEX-trose) U.S.P. 23.
Use: Fluid and nutrient replenisher.
W/Calcium ascorbate and benzyl alcohol injection
See: Calscorbate, Amp. (Cole).
W/Psyllium mucilloid.
See: V-lax, Pow. (Century Pharm).

5% Dextrose and Electrolyte No. 48. (Baxter) Dextrose 50 g, calories 180/L with Na^+ 25 mEq, K^+ 20 mEq, Mg^{++} 3 mEq, Cl^- 24 mEq, phosphate 3 mEq, acetate 23 mEq with osmolarity 348 mOsm/L. Soln. Bot. 250 ml, 500 ml, 1000 ml. *Rx.*
Use: Nutritional supplement, parenteral.

5% Dextrose and Electrolyte No. 75. (Baxter) Dextrose 50 g, calories 180/L with Na^+ 40 mEq, K^+ 35 mEq, Cl^- 48 mEq, phosphate 15 mEq and lactate 20 mEq with osmolarity 402 mOsm/L. Soln. Bot. 250 ml, 500 ml, 1000 ml. *Rx.*
Use: Nutritional supplement, parenteral.

dextrose-alcohol injection. *Rx.*
Use: Nutritional supplement, parenteral.
See: 5% alcohol and 5% dextrose in water (Abbott, Baxter, Kendall McGaw)

dextrose-electrolyte solution. *Rx.*
Dextrose 2.5% w/0.45% sodium chloride (Various Mfr.) Soln. 250, 500, 1000 ml.
Dextrose 5% w/0.11% sodium chloride (Kendal McGaw). Soln. 500, 1000 ml.
Dextrose 5% w/0.2% sodium chloride (Various Mfr.) Soln. 250, 500, 1000 ml.
Dextrose 5% w/0.33% sodium chloride (Various Mfr.) Soln. 250, 500, 1000 ml.
Dextrose 5% w/0.45% sodium chloride (Various Mfr.) Soln. 250, 500, 1000 ml.
Dextrose 5% w/0.9% sodium chloride (Various Mfr.) Soln. 250, 500, 1000 ml.

Dextrose 10% w/0.45% sodium chloride (McGaw). Soln. 1000 ml.
Dextrose 10% w/0.9% sodium chloride (Various Mfr.) Soln. 500, 1000 ml.
Potassium chloride 0.075% in D-5-W (Baxter). Soln. 1000 ml.
Potassium chloride 0.15% in D-5-W (Various Mfr.) Soln. 1000 ml.
Potassium chloride 0.224% in D-5-W (Various Mfr.) Soln. 1000 ml.
Potassium chloride 0.3% in D-5-W (Various Mfr.) Soln. 500, 1000 ml.
0.075% potassium chloride in 5% dextrose and 0.2% sodium chloride (Various Mfr.) Soln. 1000 ml.
0.15% potassium chloride in 5% dextrose and 0.2% sodium chloride (Various Mfr.) Soln. 250, 500, 1000 ml.
0.224% potassium chloride in 5% dextrose and 0.2% sodium chloride (Various Mfr.) Soln. 1000 ml.
0.3% potassium chloride in 5% dextrose and 0.2% sodium chloride (Various Mfr.) Soln. 1000 ml.
0.15% potassium chloride in 5% dextrose and 0.33% sodium chloride (Baxter). Soln. 500, 1000 ml.
0.224% potassium chloride in 5% dextrose and 0.33% sodium chloride (Baxter). Soln. 1000 ml.
0.3% potassium chloride in 5% dextrose and 0.33% sodium chloride (Various Mfr.) Soln. 1000 ml.
0.075% potassium chloride in 5% dextrose and 0.45% sodium chloride (Various Mfr.) Soln. 1000 ml.
0.15% potassium chloride in 5% dextrose and 0.45% sodium chloride (Various Mfr.) Soln. 500, 1000 ml.
0.224% potassium chloride in 5% dextrose and 0.45% sodium chloride (Various Mfr.) Soln. 1000 ml.
0.3% potassium chloride in 5% dextrose and 0.45% sodium chloride (Various Mfr.) Soln. 1000 ml.
0.15% potassium chloride in 5% dextrose and 0.9% sodium chloride (Baxter). Soln. 1000 ml.
0.3% potassium chloride in 5% dextrose and 0.9% sodium chloride (Baxter). Soln. 1000 ml.
Isolyte G with 5% dextrose (McGaw) 70 mEq NH_4+. Soln. 1000 ml.
Isolyte G with 10% dextrose (McGaw) 70 mEq NH_4+. Soln. 1000 ml.
5% dextrose and electrolyte #75 (Baxter). Soln. 250, 500, 1000 ml.
Ionosol T and 5% dextrose (Abbott Laboratories). Soln. 250, 500, 1000 ml.
Isolyte M and 5% dextrose (McGaw). Soln. 1000 ml.
Dextrose 5% in Ringer's (Various Mfr.) Soln. 500, 1000 ml.
Dextrose 2.5% in half-strength lactated Ringer's (Various Mfr.) Soln. 250, 500, 1000 ml.
Dextrose 5% in lactated Ringer's (Various Mfr.) Soln. 250, 500, 1000 ml.
5% dextrose and electrolyte #48 (Baxter). Soln. 250, 500, 1000 ml.
Ionosol MB and 5% dextrose (Abbott Laboratories). Soln. 250, 500, 1000 ml.
Ionosol B and 5% dextrose (Abbott Laboratories). Soln. 500, 1000.
Isolyte H with 5% dextrose (McGaw). Soln. 1000 ml.
Normosol-M and 5% dextrose (Abbott Laboratories). Soln. 500, 1000.
Plasma-Lyte 56 and 5% dextrose (Baxter). Soln. 500, 1000.
Isolyte P with 5% dextrose (McGaw). Soln. 250, 500, 1000.
Isolyte S with 5% dextrose (McGaw). 23 mEq gluconate. Soln. 1000 ml.
Normosol-R and 5% dextrose (Abbott Laboratories). 23 mEq gluconate. Soln. 500, 1000 ml.
Plasma-Lyte 148 and 5% dextrose (Baxter). 23 mEq gluconate. Soln. 500, 1000 ml.
Ionosol MB and 10% dextrose (Abbott Laboratories). Soln. 500 ml.
10% dextrose with electrolytes (Abbott Laboratories). Soln. 21 mEq gluconate. Soln. 500 ml in 1000 ml partial fill container.
10% dextrose and electrolyte no. 48 injection (Baxter). Soln. 250 ml.
Isolyte R with 5% dextrose (McGaw). Soln. 1000 ml.
Plasma-Lyte M and 5% dextrose (Baxter). Soln. 500, 1000 ml.
Plasma-Lyte R and 5% dextrose (Baxter). Soln. 1000 ml.
Isolyte E with 5% dextrose (McGaw). 8 mEq citrate. Soln. 1000 ml.
Use: Nutritional supplement, parenteral.

•**dextrose excipient.** N.F. 18.
Use: Pharmaceutic aid (tablet excipient).

50% Dextrose/Electrolyte Pattern A. (McGaw) Dextrose 500 g/L, calories 1700 cal/L, Na^+ 84 mEq, K^+ 40 mEq, Ca^{++} 10 mEq, Mg^{++} 16 mEq, Cl^- 115 mEq, osmolarity 2,800 mOsm/L, sulfate 16 mEq, gluconate 13 mEq. Soln. 500 ml in 1000 ml partial fill container. *Rx.*

Use: Nutritional supplement, parenteral.

50% Dextrose/Electrolyte Pattern B. (McGaw) Dextrose 500 g/L, calories 1700 cal/L, Na^+ 32 mEq, Ca^{++} 9 mEq, Mg^{++} 16 mEq, Cl^- 32 mEq, osmolarity 2,615 mOsm/L, sulfate 16 mEq, gluconate 4.2 mEq. Soln. 500 ml in 1000 ml partial fill container. *Rx.*
Use: Nutritional supplement, parenteral.

50% Dextrose/Electrolyte Pattern N. (McGaw) Dextrose 500 g/L, calories 1,700 cal/L, Na^+ 90 mEq, K^+ 80 mEq, Mg^{++} 16 mEq, Cl^- 150 mEq, phosphate 28 mEq, osmolarity 2,875 mOsm/L, sulfate 16 mEq. 500 ml in 1000 ml partial fill container. *Rx.*
Use: Nutritional supplement, parenteral.

dextrose large volume parenterals. (Abbott Hospital Prods). *Rx.*
Dextrose 2 0.5% in Water-1000 ml.
Dextrose 2 0.5% in 0.5 Sterile Lactose Ringer's or in 0.5 Sterile Saline-1000 ml.
Dextrose 5% in Water-150 ml, 250 ml, 500 ml, 1000 ml in Abbo-Vac glass or LifeCare flexible plastic container; partial-fill glass: 50 in 200 ml, 50 in 300 ml, 100 in 300 ml, 400 in 500 ml; partial-fill plastic: 50 in 150 ml, 100 in 150 ml.
Dextrose 5% in Lactose Ringer's-250 ml, 500 ml, 1000 ml glass; 500 ml, 1000 ml plastic container.
Dextrose 5% in Ringer's-500 ml, 1000 ml.
Dextrose 5% in Saline 0.9% or in 0.25, 0.33 or 0.5 Sterile Saline-250, 500, 1000 ml glass or plastic container.
Dextrose 10% in Water-250 ml, 500 ml, 1000 ml containers.
Dextrose 20% in Water-500 ml.
Dextrose 50% in Water-500 ml. Dextrose 20%, 30%, 40%, 50%, 60%, 70% Injections, U.S.P. in partial-fill container, 500 ml in 1000 ml.
Dextrose Injection 50%. Bot. 1000 ml.
Dextrose 50% and Injection w/Electrolytes in partial-fill container, 500 ml in 1000 ml.
Dextrose Injection 70%. Bot. 1000 ml.
Use: Nutritional supplement, parenteral.

dextrose small volume parenterals. (Abbott Hospital Prods) **Dextrose 5%:** 50 ml, 100 ml pressurized pintop vial. **Dextrose 10%:** 5 ml amp.; **Dextrose 25%:** 10 ml syringe. **Dextrose 50%:** 50 ml Abboject syringe (18 g × 1.5″), 50 ml Fliptop vial. **Dextrose 70%:** 70 ml pressurized pintop vial. *Rx.*
Use: Nutritional supplement, parenteral.

dextrose-sodium chloride injection. (Abbott Laboratories) 10% Dextrose and 0.225% Sodium Cl. Inj. Single dose container 500 ml.
Use: Nutritional supplement, parenteral.

Dextrostat. (Richwood) Dextroamphetamine sulfate 5 mg, sucrose, lactose, tartrazine/Tab. Bot. 100s. *c-II.*
Use: CNS Stimulant.

Dextrostix. (Bayer Corp) A cellulose strip containing glucose oxidase and indicator system. Box 10s.
Use: Diagnostic aid, glucose.

•**dextrothyroxine sodium.** (dex-troe-thigh-ROX-een) USAN. U.S.P. XXI.
Use: Anticholesteremic, antihyperlipidemic.

Dexule. (Health for Life Brands) Vitamins A 1333 IU, D 133 IU, B_1 0.33 mg, B_2 0.4 mg, C 10 mg, niacinamide 3.3 mg, iron 3.3 mg, calcium 29 mg, phosphorous 15 mg, methylcellulose 100 mg, benzocaine 3 mg/Cap. Bot. 21s, 90s. *otc.*
Use: Mineral, vitamin supplement.

Dexyl. (Pinex) Dextromethorphan HBr 15 mg, vitamin C 20 mg/Tab. Box 20s. *otc.*
Use: Antitussive, vitamin supplement.

Dey-Dose Epinephrine. (Dey Labs) Racemic epinephrine (as HCl) equal to 2.25% epinephrine base, chlorobutanol, sodium metabisulfite. Soln. for nebulization. Vial 0.25 ml. *otc.*
Use: Bronchodilator.

Dey-Dose Isoetharine Hydrochloride. (Dey Labs) Isoetharine HCl 1% with glycerin, sodium metabisulfite and parabens. Soln. for nebulization. Vial 0.25 ml, 0.5 ml. *Rx.*
Use: Bronchodilator.

Dey-Dose Isoproterenol Hydrochloride. (Dey Labs) Isoproterenol HCl 0.5% (1:200). Soln. for nebulization. Vial 0.5 ml. *Rx.*
Use: Bronchodilator.

Dey-Dose Metaproterenol Sulfate. (Dey Labs) Metaproterenol sulfate 0.5%. Inhaler 0.3 ml. *Rx.*
Use: Bronchodilator.

Dey-Lute. (Dey Labs) Isoetharine HCl with sodium metabisulfite, glycerin. Soln. **0.08%:** UD 3 ml; **0.1%:** UD 5 ml; **0.17%:** UD 3 ml; **0.25%:** UD 2 ml. *Rx.*
Use: Bronchodilator.

Dey-Lute Metaproterenol Sulfate. (Dey Labs) Metaproterenol sulfate 0.6%. Soln. for inhalation 2.5 ml. *Rx.*

Use: Bronchodilator.

Dey Pak Sodium Chloride Solution 3%. (Dey Labs) Sodium chloride 3%. Soln. Vial 10 ml, 15 ml single-use. 50s.
Use: To induce sputum production for specimen collection.

Dey-Pak Sodium Chloride Solution 10%. (Dey Labs) Sodium chloride 10%. Soln. Vial 10 ml, 15 ml single-use. 50s.
Use: To induce sputum production for specimen collection.

•dezaguanine. (DEH-zah-GWAHN-een) USAN.
Use: Antineoplastic.

•dezaguanine mesylate. (DEE-zah-GWAHN-een MEH-sih-late) USAN.
Use: Antineoplastic.

Dezest. (Armenpharm, Ltd.) Atropine sulfate, phenylpropanolamine HCl, chlorpheniramine maleate. Bot. 100s.
Use: Anticholinergic, antihistamine, antispasmodic, decongestant.

•dezinamide. (deh-ZIN-ah-mide) USAN.
Use: Anticonvulsant.

•dezocine. (DESS-oh-seen) USAN.
Use: Analgesic.
See: Dalgan (Wyeth Ayerst).

D-Film. (Ciba Vision Ophthalmics) Poloxamer 407, EDTA 0.25%, benzalkonium Cl 0.025%. Gel Tube 25 g. *otc.*
Use: Contact lens care.

DFMO. Eflornithine HCl. *Rx.*
Use: Anti-infective.
See: Ornidyl, Inj. (Hoechst Marion Roussel).

DFP. Disopropyl fluorophosphate (Various Mfr.)

d-Glucose. Dextrose. *Rx.*
Use: Nutritional supplement, parenteral.
See: D-2½-W, Soln. (Various Mfr.)
D-5-W, Soln. (Various Mfr.)
D-7.7-W, Soln. (McGaw).
D-10-W, Soln. (Various Mfr.)
D-20-W, Soln. (Various Mfr.)
D-25-W, Soln. (Various Mfr.)
D-30-W, Soln. (Various Mfr.)
D-38-W, Soln. (McGaw).
D-38.5-W, Soln. (Abbott Laboratories).
D-40-W, Soln. (Various Mfr.)
D-50-W, Soln. (Various Mfr.)
D-60-W, Soln. (Various Mfr.)
D-70-W, Soln. (Various Mfr.)

DHC Plus. (Purdue Frederick) Dihydrocodeine bitartrate 16 mg, acetaminophen 356.4 mg, caffeine 30 mg. Cap. Bot. 100s. *c-III.*
Use: Analgesic combination, narcotic.

DHEA. (Elan Corp) EL10. *Rx.*
Use: Antiviral, immunomodulator.

D.H.E. 45. (Sandoz) Dihydroergotamine mesylate 1 mg/ml, methanesulfonic acid, alcohol 6.1%, glycerin 15%. Inj. in 1 ml amps. *Rx.*
Use: Antimigraine.

DHPG. Ganciclovir sodium. *Rx.*
Use: Antiviral.
See: Cytovene, Pow. (Syntex).
BW B759U (GlaxoWellcome).

DHS Conditioning Rinse. (Person & Covey) Conditioning ingredients. Bot. 8 oz. *otc.*
Use: Dermatologic, hair.

DHS Shampoo. (Person & Covey) Blend of cleansing surfactants and emulsifiers. Plastic bot. w/dispenser 8 oz, 16 oz. *otc.*
Use: Dermatologic, hair and scalp.

DHS Tar Gel Shampoo. (Person & Covey) Coal Tar, U.S.P. 0.5% Bot. 8 oz. *otc.*
Use: Antipsoriatic, antiseborrheic.

DHS Tar Shampoo. (Person & Covey) Coal tar 0.5% in DHS shampoo. Bot. 4 oz, 8 oz, 16 oz. *otc.*
Use: Antipsoriatic, antiseborrheic.

DHS Zinc Shampoo. (Person & Covey) Zinc pyrithione 2% in DHS shampoo. Bot. 6 oz, 12 oz. *otc.*
Use: Antiseborrheic.

DHT. (Roxane) Dihydrotachysterol. **Tab.:** 0.125 mg, 0.2 mg or 0.4 mg/Tab. Bot. 50s, UD 100s (0.125 mg). 100s, UD 100s (0.2 mg). 50s (0.4 mg). **Intensol:** Dihydrotachysterol 0.2 mg/ml, alcohol 20%. Bot. 30 ml w/dropper. *Rx.*
Use: Antihypocalcemic.

DiaBeta Tablets. (Hoechst Marion Roussel) Glyburide. **1.25 mg:** Bot. 50s. **2.5 mg:** Bot. 60s, 100s, 500s, UD 100s. **5 mg:** Bot. 30s, 60s, 90s, 100s, 500s, 1000s, UD 1000s. *Rx.*
Use: Antidiabetic.

Diabetes CF. (Scot-Tussin) Sugarfree. Syr. Bot. 120 ml. *otc.*
Use: Antitussive, expectorant.

Diabetic Tussin. (Roberts Pharm) Dextromethorphan HBr 10 mg, guaifenesin 100 mg, phenylephedrine 5 mg/5 ml. Liq. Bot. 120 ml. *otc.*
Use: Antitussive, decongestant, expectorant.

Diabetic Tussin DM. (Roberts Pharm) Dextromethorphan HBr 10 mg, guaifenesin 100 mg, saccharin, methylparaben, menthol, alcohol & dye free. Liq. Bot. 118 ml. *otc.*
Use: Antitussive, expectorant.

Diabetic Tussin EX. (Health Care Products) Guaifenesin 100 mg/5 ml, saccharin, menthol, methylparaben. Liq. Bot. 118 ml. *otc.*
Use: Expectorant.

Diabinese. (Pfizer Laboratories) Chlorpropamide. **100 mg/Tab.:** Bot. 100s, UD 100s; **250 mg/Tab.:** Bot. 100s, 1000s. *Rx.*
Use: Antidiabetic.

diacetic acid test.
See: Acetest, Tab. (Bayer Corp).

Diaceto w/Codeine. (Archer-Taylor) Codeine 0.25 gr, 0.5 gr/Tab. or Cap. Bot. 500s, 1000s. *c-II.*
Use: Analgesic, narcotic.

Diaceto w/Gelsemium. (Archer-Taylor) Phenobarbital 0.5 gr, gelsemium 3 min./Tab. Bot. 1000s. *c-IV.*
Use: Hypnotic, sedative.

•**diacetolol hydrochloride.** (DIE-ah-SEET-oh-lahl HIGH-droe-KLOR-ide) USAN.
Use: Antiadrenergic (β-receptor).

diacetrizoate, sodium.
See: Diatrizoate (Various Mfr.)

•**diacetylated monoglycerides.** N.F. 18.
Use: Pharmaceutic aid (plasticizer).

diacetylcholine chloride. Succinylcholine Cl.
See: Anectine Chloride, Inj., Pow. (Burroughs-Wellcome).

diacetyl-dihydroxydiphenylisatin.
See: Oxyphenisatin acetate (Various Mfr.)

diacetyldioxyphenylisatin.
See: Oxyphenisatin acetate (Various Mfr.)

diacetylmorphine salts. Heroin. Illegal in U.S.A. by Federal statute because of its addiction potential.

Di-Ademil.
See: Hydroflumethiazide, Tab. (Various Mfr.)

diagniol.
See: Sodium Acetrizoate.

diagnostic agents.
See: Acholest, Kit (E. Fougera).
allergic extracts.
Aplisol (Parke-Davis).
Aplitest (Parke-Davis).
BioCox (Iatric).
Candida Skin Test Antigen (Allermed, ALK).
Candin (Allermed, ALK).
Cardio-Green, Vial (Becton Dickinson).
Cardiografin, Vial (Squibb).
Cea-Roche, Kit (Roche).
Cholografin, Prep. (Squibb).
Coccidioidin, Vial (ALK, Iatric).
Dextrostix, Strip (Bayer Corp).
Dey-Pak Sodium Chloride (Dey Labs).
Evans Blue Dye, Inj. (New World Trading Corp).
EZ Detect Strep-A Test (Biomerica).
Fertility Tape (Weston Labs.).
First Choice (Polymer Technology Int.).
Fluorescein Sodium Ophth. Soln. (Various Mfr.)
Fluor-I-Strip (Wyeth Ayerst).
Fluor-I-Strip A.T. (Wyeth Ayerst).
Fluress, Ophth. Soln. (Pilkington Barnes Hind).
Glucola, Soln. (Bayer Corp).
Hema-Combistix Strips (Bayer Corp).
Hemastix Strips (Bayer Corp).
Histalog, Amp. (Eli Lilly).
Histolyn-CYL (ALK).
Histoplasmin, Vial (Parke-Davis).
Hymenoptera venoms.
Indigo Carmine (Various Mfr.)
HIVAB HIV-1/HIV-2 (rDNA) EIA (Abbot).
Immunex CRP (Wampole).
Mannitol Soln., Inj. (Merck).
Mono-Latex (Wampole).
Mono-Plus (Wampole).
MSTA (Pasteur Merieux Connaught).
Multitest-CMI (Pasteur Merieux Connaught).
Mumps skin test antigen (Pasteur Merieux Connaught).
Persantine IV (DuPont Merck Pharmaceuticals).
Pharmalgen (ALK).
Phenolsulfonphthalein (Various Mfr.)
Phentolamine Methanesulfonate, Inj. (Various Mfr.)
Prepen (Schwartz Pharma).
Regitine, Amp., Tab. (Novartis).
Rheumanosticon Slide Test (Organon).
Rheumatex (Wampole).
Rheumaton (Wampole).
Spherulin (ALK).
SureCell Chlamydia Test (Kodak).
SureCell Herpes (HSV) Test (Kodak).
SureCell Strep A Test (Kodak).
Sodium Dehydrocholate, Inj. (Various Mfr.).
Tes-Tape (Eli Lilly).
Tine Test (Wyeth Ayerst).
True Test (GlaxoWellcome).
Tubersol (Pasteur Merieux Connaught).
Venomil (Bayer Corp.).
See: Cholecystography Agents.
Kidney Function Agents.

Liver Function Agents.
Urography Agents.

diagnostic agents for urine.
See: Acetest, Tab. (Bayer Corp).
Albustix, Strip (Bayer Corp).
Biotel Diabetes (Biotel).
Biotel Kidney (Biotel).
Biotel U.T.I. (Biotel).
Bumintest, Tab. (Bayer Corp).
Chemstrip Micral, Strips (Boehringer Mannheim).
Clinistix, Strip (Bayer Corp).
Clinitest, Tab. (Bayer Corp).
Fortel Midstream (Biomerica).
Fortel Plus (Biomerica).
Hema-Combistix, Strip (Bayer Corp).
HCG-nostick (Organon Teknika).
Hemastix, Strip (Bayer Corp).
Hematest, Tab. (Bayer Corp).
Ictotest, Tab. (Bayer Corp).
Ketostix, Strip (Bayer Corp).
Pheniplate, Preps. (Bayer Corp).
Phenistix, Strip (Bayer Corp).
SureCell hCG-Urine Test (Kodak).
Uristix, Strip (Bayer Corp).
Wampole One-Step hCG (Wampole).

diallybarbituric acid. Allobarbital, Allobarbitone, Curral.

diallylamicol. Diallyl-diethylaminoethyl phenol di HCl.

diallylnortoxiferine.
See: Alloferin (Roche).

dialminate. Mixture of magnesium carbonate and (alminate) dihydroxyaluminum glycinate.
W/Aspirin.
See: Bufferin, Preps. (Bristol-Myers).

Dialose. (Merck) Docusate sodium 100 mg., lactose, sugar. Tab. Bot. 36s. *otc.*
Use: Laxative.

Dialose Plus. (Merck) **Cap.:** Docusate sodium 100 mg, yellow phenolphthalein 65 mg/Cap. Bot. 36s, 100s, 500s. **Tab.:** Docusate sodium 100 mg, yellow phenolphthalein 65 mg, sugar/Tab. Bot 100s. *otc.*
Use: Laxative.

Dialyte Pattern LM w/1.5% Dextrose. (Gambro) Dextrose 15 g/L, Na^+ 131, Ca^{++} 3.5, Mg^{++} 0.5, Cl^- 94 and lactate 40 with osmolarity 345 mOsm/L. Soln. Bot. 1000 ml, 2000 ml, 4000 ml. *Rx.*
Use: Peritoneal dialysis solution.

Dialyte Pattern LM w/2.5% Dextrose. (Gambro) Dextrose 25 g/L, Na^+ 131.5, Ca^{++} 3.5, Mg^{++} 0.5, Cl^- 94 and lactate 40 with osmolarity 395 mOsm/L. Soln. Bot. 1000 ml, 2000 ml, 4000 ml. *Rx.*
Use: Peritoneal dialysis solution.

Dialyte Pattern LM w/4.25% Dextrose. (Gambro) Dextrose 42.5 g/L, Na^+ 131.5, Ca^{++} 3.5, Mg^{++} 0.5, Cl^- 94 and lactate 40 with osmolarity 485 mOsm/L. Soln. Bot. 1000 ml, 2000 ml, 4000 ml. *Rx.*
Use: Peritoneal dialysis solution.

diamethine.
See: Dimethyl tubocurarine (Various Mfr.)

diaminedipenicillin g.
See: Benzethacil (Various Mfr.)

di-amino acetate complex w/calcium aluminum carbonate. Cap. IU.
See: Ancid Tab., Susp. (Sheryl).

diaminodiphenylsulfone. Dapsone, U.S.P. 23.
Use: Antimalarial.

diaminopropyl tetramethylene.
See: Spermine.

3,4-diaminopyridine. (Jacobus Pharm)
Use: Lambert-Eaton myasthenic syndrome. [Orphan drug]

•**diamocaine cyclamate.** (die-AM-oh-CANE SIH-klah-mate) USAN.
Use: Anesthetic, local.

Diamox. (ESI Lederle Generics) Acetazolamide. **Tab.:** 125 mg Bot. 100s. 250 mg Bot. 100s, 1000s, UD 10 × 10s. **Inj. Vial:** Sterile sodium salt 500 mg (sodium hydroxide to adjust pH). *Rx.*
Use: Anticonvulsant, diuretic.

Diamox Sequels. (ESI Lederle Generics) Acetazolamide 500 mg/Cap. Bot. 30s, 100s. *Rx.*
Use: Anticonvulsant, diuretic.

diamthazole dihydrochloride. Asterol.

Dianeal w/1.5% Dextrose. (Baxter) Dextrose 15 g/L, Na^+ 141, Ca^{++} 3.5, Mg^{++} 1.5, Cl^- 101, lactate 45 with osmolarity 364 mOsm/L. Soln. Bot. 1000 ml, 2000 ml. *Rx.*
Use: Peritoneal dialysis solution.

Dianeal 137 w/1.5% Dextrose. (Baxter) Dextrose 15 g/L, Na^+ 132, Ca^{++} 3.5, Mg^{++} 1.5, Cl102, lactate 35 with osmolarity 347 mOsm/L. Soln. Bot. 2000 ml. *Rx.*
Use: Peritoneal dialysis solution.

Dianeal w/4.25% Dextrose. (Baxter) Dextrose 42.5 g/L, Na^+ 141, Ca^{++} 3.5, Mg^{++} 1.5, Cl^- 101, lactate 45 with osmolarity 503 mOsm/L. Soln. Bot. 2000 ml. *Rx.*
Use: Peritoneal dialysis solution.

Dianeal 137 w/4.25% Dextrose. (Baxter) Dextrose 42.5 g/L, Na^+ 132, Ca^{++} 3.5, Mg^{++} 1.5, Cl^- 102, lactate 35 with osmolarity 486 mOsm/L. Soln. Bot. 2000 ml. *Rx.*

Use: Peritoneal dialysis solution.

dianeal PD-2 peritoneal dialysis soln with 1.1% amino acid.
Use: Nutritional supplement for dialysis patients. [Orphan drug]
See: Nutrineal Peritoneal Dialysis Solution with 1.1% Amino Acid (Baxter Healthcare).

•**diapamide.** (die-APP-am-ide) USAN.
Use: Antihypertensive, diuretic.

Diapantin. (Janssen) Isopropamide bromide. *Rx.*
Use: Anticholinergic.

Diaparene. (Bayer Corp) Methylbenzethonium Cl. Pow. Bot. 4 oz, 9 oz, 12.5 oz, 14 oz.
Use: Disinfectant, surface active agent.

Diaparene Medicated. (Reckitt & Coleman) Methylbenzethonium Cl with white petrolatum 0.1%, glycerin, mineral oil, stearyl alcohol. Cream. Tube 30, 60, 120 g. *otc.*
Use: Antimicrobial, topical.

Diaparene Ointment. (Bayer Corp) Methylbenzethonium Cl 0.1% w/petrolatum, glycerin. Tube 1 oz, 2 oz, 4 oz. *otc.*
Use: Antimicrobial, topical.

Diaparene Peri-Anal Cream. (Bayer Corp) Methylbenzethonium Cl 1:1000, zinc oxide, starch, cod liver oil, white petrolatum, lanolin, calcium caseinate. Cream Tube 1 oz, 2 oz, 4 oz. *otc.*
Use: Antimicrobial, astringent.

Diaper Guard. (Del Pharmaceuticals) Dimethicone 1%, white petrolatum 66%, cocoa butter, parabens, vitamins A, D_3, E, zinc oxide. Oint. Tube 49.6 g, 99.2 g. *otc.*
Use: Diaper rash preparation.

Diaper Rash. (Various Mfr.) Zinc oxide, cod liver oil, lanolin, methylparaben, petrolatum, talc. Oint. Tube 113 g. *otc.*
Use: Diaper rash preparation.

diaphenylsulfone. Dapsone, U.S.P. 23.
Use: Leprostatic.

Diapid. (Sandoz,) Lypressin synthetic lysine-8-vasopressin. Equiv. to 50 U.S.P. units posterior pituitary/ml (0.185 mg/ml). Nasal spray. Bot. 8 ml. *Rx.*
Use: Pituitary hormone.

Di-Ap-Trol. (Foy) Phendimetrazine tartrate 35 mg/Tab. Bot. 100s, 1000s. *c-III.*
Use: Anorexiant.

Diarrest. (Dover Pharmaceuticals) Calcium carbonate, pectin/Tab. Sugar, lactose and salt free. UD box 500s. *otc.*
Use: Antidiarrheal.

diarrhea therapy.
See: Antidiarrheal.

Diaserp Tabs. (Major) Chlorothiazide 250 mg or 500 mg/Tab. w/reserpine. Bot. 100s. *Rx.*
Use: Antihypertensive.

Diasorb. (Columbia) Activated nonfibrous attapulgite. **Liq.:** 750 mg per 5 ml. Bot. 120 ml. **Tab.:** 750 mg. Pkg. 24s. *otc.*
Use: Antidiarrheal.

Diasporal Cream. (Doak Dermatologics) Formerly Sulfur Salicyl Diasporal. Sulfur 3%, salicylic acid 2%, isopropyl alcohol in diasporal base. Cream Jar 3¾ oz. *otc.*
Use: Antiseptic, topical.

Diastase.
See: Aspergillus oryzae enzyme.

Diastat. (Atheria) Diazapam. **Pediatric:** 2.5 mg, 5 mg, 10 mg. **Adult:**10 mg, 15 mg, 20 mg. Rectal gel. Twin pack. Includes lubricating jelly, plastic applicator with flexible, molded tip in two lengths. *c-iv.*
Use: Anticonvulsant.

Diastix Reagent Strips. (Bayer Corp) Broad range test for glucose in urine. Containing glucose oxidase, peroxidase, potassium iodide/w blue background dye. Tab. Pkg. 50s, 100s.
Use: Diagnostic aid.

diatrizoate.

•**diatrizoate meglumine.** (die-ah-TRIH-zoe-ate meh-GLUE-meen) U.S.P. 23.
Use: Diagnostic aid (radiopaque medium).
See: Angiovist 282, Inj. (Berlex).
Cardiografin, Vial (Squibb).
Cystografin, Inj. (Squibb).
Gastrografin, Liq. (Squibb).
Hypaque-Cysto, Liq. (Sanofi Winthrop).
Hypaque Meglumine (Sanofi Winthrop).
Renografin, Inj. (Squibb).
Reno-M-DIP, Inj. (Squibb).
Reno-M-30, Inj. (Squibb).
Reno-M-60, Inj. (Squibb).
Urovist, Prods. (Berlex).

W/Iodipamide methylglucamine.
See: Sinografin, Vial (Squibb).

W/Sodium Diatrizoate.
See: Renovist, Inj. (Squibb).

diatrizoate meglumine and diatrizoate sodium injection.
Use: Diagnostic aid (radiopaque medium).
See: Angiovist 292, Inj. (Berlex).
Angiovist 370, Inj. (Berlex).
Gastrovist, Soln. (Berlex).

Hypaque-M Prods. (Sanofi Winthrop).

diatrizoate meglumine and diatrizoate sodium solution.
Use: Diagnostic aid (radiopaque medium).
See: Gastrografin Soln. (Squibb).
Renografin-60, Soln. (Squibb).
Renografin-76, Soln. (Squibb).
Renovist, Soln. (Squibb).

diatrizoate meglumine 52.7% and iodipamide meglumine 25.8% (38% iodine).
Use: Diagnostic aid (radiopaque agent).
See: Sinografin, Inj. (Bracco Diagnostics).

diatrizoate methylglucamine.
Use: Diagnostic aid (radiopaque medium).
See: Diatrizoate Meglumine, U.S.P. 23.

diatrizoate methylglucamine sodium.
Use: Diagnostic aid (radiopaque medium).

•**diatrizoate sodium.** U.S.P. 23.
Use: Diagnostic aid (radiopaque medium).
See: Hypaque Prods. (Sanofi Winthrop).
Urovist Sodium, Inj. (Berlex).
W/Meglumine diatrizoate.
See: Gastrografin, Liq. (Squibb).
Renografin-60, -76, Vial (Squibb).
Renovist II, Vial (Squibb).
W/Methylglucamine diatrizoate, sodium citrate, disodium ethylenediamine tetraacetate dihydrate, methylparaben, propylparaben.
See: Renovist, Vial (Squibb).

diatrizoate sodium 41.66% (24.9% iodine).
Use: Diagnostic aid (radiopaque agent).
See: Hypaque sodium, Soln. (Sanofi Winthrop).

diatrizoate sodium (59.87% iodine).
Use: Diagnostic aid (radiopaque agent).
See: Hypaque Sodium, Soln. (Sanofi Winthrop).

•**diatrizoate sodium I-125.** USAN.
Use: Radiopharmaceutical.

•**diatrizoate sodium I-131.** USAN.
Use: Radiopharmaceutical.

•**diatrizoic acid.** (DIE-at-rih-ZOE-ik) U.S.P. 23.
Use: Diagnostic aid (radiopaque medium).
See: Amidotrizoic Acid.
Hypaque sodium salt.

•**diaveridine.** (DIE-ah-ver-ih-deen) USAN.
Use: Anti-infective.

•**diazepam.** (DIE-aze-uh-pam) U.S.P. 23.
Use: Agent for control of emotional disturbances, anxiolytic, hypnotic, sedative.
See: Diastat, Rectal Gel. (Athena).
Diazepam Intensol, Soln. (Roxane).
Dizac, Inj. (Ohmeda).
Valium, Tab. (Roche).

diazepam. (Various Mfr.) **Tab.:** 2 mg, 5 mg, 10 mg. Bot. 100s, 500s, 1000s; 5 mg or 10 mg. Bot. 100s, 500s, 1000s; **Inj.:** 5 mg/ml Amps 2 ml; vial 1, 2, 10 ml; syringe 1, 2 ml; cartridge 1, 2 ml. **Oral Soln.** (Roxane): 1 mg/1 ml orange, spice, wintergreen flavor. In 500 ml, UD 5 ml, 10 ml. **Concentrated Oral Soln.** (Roxane): 5 mg/ml In 30 ml w/dropper. *c-iv.*
Use: Agent for control of emotional disturbances, anxiolytic, hypnotic, sedative.

Diazepam Intensol. (Roxane) Diazepam 5 mg/ml. Oral Soln. In 30 ml with dropper. *c-iv.*
Use: Anxiolytic.

diazepam viscous rectal solution. (Athena)
Use: To treat acute repetitive seizures. [Orphan drug]

•**diaziquone.** (DIE-azz-ih-kwone) USAN.
Use: Antineoplastic.

diazomycins a, b, & c. Antibiotic obtained from *Streptomyces ambofaciens.* Under study.

•**diazoxide.** (DIE-aze-OX-ide) U.S.P. 23.
Use: Antihypertensive.
See: Proglycem Capsules (Medical Market Specialists).
Proglycem Suspension (Medical Market Specialists).

diazoxide, parenteral. (DIE-aze-OX-ide)
Use: Antihypertensive.
See: Diazoxide Injection USP, Inj. (Various Mfr.)
Hyperstat IV, Inj. (Schering Plough).

dibasic calcium phosphate dihydrate.
Use: Replenisher (calcium); pharmaceutic aid (tablet base).
See: D.C.P. 340, Tab. (Parke-Davis).
Diostate D, Tab. (Pharmacia & Upjohn).

Dibatrol. (Lexis) Chlorpropamide 100 mg or 250 mg/Tab. Bot. 100s, 1000s. *Rx.*
Use: Antidiabetic.

dibencil.
See: Benzathine Penicillin G. (Various Mfr.)

Dibent. (Roberts Pharm) Dicyclomine 10 mg/ml with chlorobutanol. Inj. Vial 10 ml. *Rx.*

Use: Gastrointestinal, anticholinergic.

•**dibenzepin hydrochloride.** (die-BEN-zeh-pin) USAN.
Use: Antidepressant.

•**dibenzothiophene.** (die-BEN-zoe-THIGH-oh-feen) USAN.
Use: Keratolytic.

Dibenzyline. (SmithKline Beecham Pharmaceuticals) Phenoxybenzamine HCl 10 mg/Cap. Bot. 100s. *Rx.*
Use: Antihypertensive.

dibromodulcitol. (Biopharmaceutics)
Use: Antineoplastic. [Orphan drug]

•**dibromsalan.** (die-BROME-sah-lan) USAN.
Use: Antimicrobial, disinfectant.

•**dibucaine.** (DIE-byoo-cane) U.S.P. 23.
Use: Local anesthetic.
See: D-Caine, Oint. (Century Pharm).
Dulzit, Cream (Del Pharmaceuticals).
Nupercainal, Oint., Cream, Supp. (Novartis).
Nupercainal Heavy, Soln. (Novartis).
W/Dextrose.
See: Nupercaine Heavy Soln. (Novartis).
W/Sodium bisulfite.
See: Nupercainal, Cream, Oint. (Novartis).
W/Zinc oxide, bismuth subgallate, acetone sodium bisulfite.
See: Nupercainal, Oint., Supp. (Novartis).

•**dibucaine hydrochloride.** U.S.P. 23.
Use: Anesthetic, local.
See: Nupercaine HCl, soln., (Novartis).
W/Antipyrine, hydrocortisone, polymyxin B sulfate, neomycin sulfate.
See: Otocort, Liq. (Teva USA).
W/Colistin sodium methanesulfonate, citric acid, sodium citrate.
See: Coly-Mycin M, Injectable (Warner-Chilcott).

dibutoline sulfate. Ethyl(2-hydroxyethyl)-dimethylammonium sulfate (2:1) bis(dibutyl-carbamate).
Use: Anticholinergic, antispasmodic.

•**dibutyl sebacate.** N.F. 18.
Use: Pharmaceutic aid (plasticizer).

Dical Captabs. (Rugby) Calcium 116 mg, vitamin D 133 IU, phosphorus 90 mg. Bot. 1000s. *otc.*
Use: Mineral, vitamin supplement.

dicalcium phosphate. (Various Mfr.) Dibasic calcium phosphate, monocalcium phosphate. **Cap.:** 7.5 gr or 10 gr. **Tab.:** 7.5 gr, 10 gr or 15 gr. **Wafer:** 15 gr. *otc.*
Use: Mineral supplement.
W/Calcium gluconate and Vitamin D. (Various Mfr.) Cap., Tab., Wafer.
See: CalciCaps, Tab. (Nion).
W/Iron and Vitamin D. (Various Mfr.) Lilly–Pulv., Bot. 100s.
W/Vitamin D. (Squibb) Calcium 85 mg, phosphorous 60 mg, vitamin D 41 IU.

Dical-D. (Abbott Laboratories) Calcium 117 mg, vitamin D 133 IU, phosphorus 90 mg. Tab. Bot. 100s, 500s. *otc.*
Use: Mineral, vitamin supplement.

Dical-D with Vitamin C. (Abbott Laboratories) Dibasic calcium phosphate containing calcium 116.7 mg, phosphorus 90 mg, vitamin D 133 IU, ascorbic acid 15 mg/Cap. Bot. 100s.
Use: Mineral, vitamin supplement.

Dical-Dee. (Alphalma USPD) Vitamins D 350 IU, dibasic calcium phosphate 4.5 gr, calcium gluconate 3 gr/Cap. Bot. 100s, 1000s. *otc.*
Use: Mineral, vitamin supplement.

Dicaldel. (Faraday) Dibasic calcium phosphate 300 mg, calcium gluconate 200 mg, vitamin D 33 IU/Cap. Bot. 100s, 250s, 500s, 1000s. *otc.*
Use: Mineral, vitamin supplement.

Dical-D Wafers. (Abbott Laboratories) Dibasic calcium phosphate containing calcium 232 mg, phosphorus 180 mg, vitamin D 200 IU/Wafer. Box 51s. *otc.*
Use: Mineral, vitamin supplement.

Dicaltabs. (Faraday) Dibasic calcium phosphate 108 mg, calcium gluconate 140 mg, vitamin D 35 IU/Tab. Bot. 100s, 250s, 1000s. *otc.*
Use: Mineral, vitamin supplement.

Dicarbosil. (BIRA) Calcium carbonate 500 mg/Chew. Tab. Roll 12s. *otc.*
Use: Antacid.

Di-Cet. (Sanford & Son) Methylbenzethonium Cl 24.4 g, sodium carbonate monohydrate 48.8 g, sodium nitrite 24.4 g, trisodium ethylenediamine tetra-acetate monohydrate 2.4 g. Pow. Pkg. 2.4 g, Box 24s.
Use: Disinfectant.

dichloralantipyrine. Dichloralphenazone. Chloralpyrine. A complex of 2 mol. chloral hydrate with 1 mol. antipyrine. Sominat.
W/Isometheptene mucate, acetaminophen.
See: Midrin, Cap. (Schwarz Pharma).

•**dichloralphenazone.** (die-klor-al-FEN-ah-zone) U.S.P. 23.
Use: Hypnotic, sedative.

Dichloramine T. (Various Mfr.) (1% to 5% in chlorinated paraffin). P-Toluenesulfone-dichloramine.

Use: Antiseptic.

dichloren.
See: Mechlorethamine HCl, Sterile Inj. (Various Mfr.)

dichlorisone acetate.

dichlormethazanone.

dichloroacetate sodium.
Use: Lactic acidosis; hypercholesterolemia. [Orphan drug]

dichloroacetic acid. *Rx.*
Use: Cauterizing agent.
See: Bichloracetic Acid, Liq. (Glenwood).

•**dichlorodifluoromethane.** (die-KLOR-oh-die-flure-oh-METH-ane) N.F. 18.
Use: Pharmaceutic aid (aerosol propellant).

dichlorodiphenyl trichloroethane.
See: Chlorophenothane (Various Mfr.)

dichlorophenarsine hydrochloride. (Chlorarsen, Clorarsen, Fontarsol, Halarsol).

dichlorophene. Related to hexachlorophene.
W/Undecylenic acid.
See: Onychomycetin, Liq. (Gordon Laboratories).
W/Undecylenic acid, salicylicacid, hexachlorophene.
See: Podiaspray, aerosol pow. (Dalin).

•**dichlorotetrafluoroethane.** (die-KLOR-oh-teh-trah-flur-oh-ETH-ane) N.F. 18.
Use: Pharmaceutic aid (aerosol propellant).

•**dichlorphenamide.** (die-klor-FEN-ah-mide) U.S.P. 23.
Use: Carbonic anhydrase inhibitor.

dichlorphenamide. *Rx.*
Use: Antiglaucoma.

•**dichlorvos.** (DIE-klor-vahs) USAN.
Use: Anthelmintic.
See: Atgard (Fermenta).
Equigard (Fermenta).
Task (Fermenta).

•**dicirenone.** (die-sigh-REN-ohn) USAN.
Use: Hypotensive, aldosterone antagonist.

Dickey's Old Reliable Eye Wash. (Dickey Drug) Berberine sulfate, boric acid, propyl parasept, methyl parasept. Plastic dropper bot. 8 ml, 12 ml, 1 oz. *otc.*
Use: Counterirritant, ophthalmic.

•**diclofenac potassium.** (die-KLOE-fen-ak) USAN.
Use: Analgesic, NSAID.
See: Cataflam, Tab. (Novartis).

•**diclofenac sodium.** (die-KLOE-fen-ak) U.S.P. 23.
Use: Analgesic, NSAID.
See: Voltaren (Novartis).
Voltaren Ophthalmic (Ciba Vision Ophthalmic).

diclofenac sodium. (Various Mfr.) 25 mg, 50 mg or 75 mg/DR Tab. Bot. 60s, 100s, 1000s, UD 100s. *Rx.*
Use: Analgesic, NSAID.

diclofenac sodium and misoprostol.
Use: Arthritis treatment.
See: Arthrotec, Tab. (Searle).

Dicloxacil. (Zenith Goldline) Dicloxacillin sodium 250 mg or 500 mg/Cap. Bot. 100s. *Rx.*
Use: Anti-infective, penicillin.

•**dicloxacillin.** (DIE-klox-uh-SILL-in) USAN.
Use: Anti-infective.
See: Dynapen, Cap., Susp. (Bristol-Myers Squibb).
Pathocil, Cap., Susp. (Wyeth Ayerst).

•**dicloxacillin sodium.** (DIE-klox-uh-SILL-in) U.S.P. 23.
Use: Anti-infective.
See: Dycill, Cap. (SmithKline Beecham Pharmaceuticals).
Dynapen, Cap., Soln. (Bristol-Myers Squibb).

Dicole. (Halsey) Docusate sodium 100 mg/Cap. Bot. 100s. *otc.*
Use: Laxative.

dicophane.
Use: Pediculicide.
See: Chlorophenothane (Various Mfr.), DDT.

dicoumarin.
Use: Anticoagulant.
See: Dicumarol, Preps. (Various Mfr.)

dicoumarol.
Use: Anticoagulant.
See: Dicumarol, U.S.P. 23.

•**dicumarol.** (die-KUME-ah-rahl) USAN. U.S.P. XXII. *Formerly Bishydroxycoumarin.*
Use: Anticoagulant.

dicumarol. (Abbott Laboratories) 25 mg/Tab. Bot. 100s, 1000s.
Use: Anticoagulant.

•**dicyclomine hydrochloride.** (die-SIGH-kloe-meen) U.S.P. 23.
Use: Anticholinergic, antispasmodic.
See: Antispas, Inj. (Keene Pharmaceuticals).
Bentyl, Amp. Syringe, Cap., Tab., Syr. (Hoechst Marion Roussel).
Dysaps, Tab., Liq., Inj. (Savage).
Nospaz, Vial (Solvay).
Stannitol (Standex).
W/Aluminum hydroxide, magnesium

hydroxide, methylcellulose.
See: Triactin Liq., Tab. (Procter & Gamble).
W/Phenobarbital.
See: Bentyl with Phenobarbital, Prods. (Hoechst Marion Roussel).

Dicynene. (Baxter) *Rx.*
Use: Hemostatic.
See: Ethamsylate.

dicysteine.
See: Cystine, Pow. (Various Mfr.)

•**didanosine.** (die-DAN-oh-SEEN) USAN.
Use: Antiviral.
See: Videx, Tab., Pow. (Bristol-Myers Squibb).

didehydrodideoxythymidine.
Use: Antiviral.
See: Stavudine (B-M Squibb).

Di-Delamine Gel. (Del Pharm) Tripelennamine HCl 0.5%, diphenhydramine HCl 1%, benzalkonium Cl 0.12% in clear gel. Tube 1.25 oz. *otc.*
Use: Antipruritic, topical.

Di-Delamine Spray. (Del Pharm) Tripelennamine HCl 0.5%, diphenhydramine HCl 1%, benzalkonium Cl 0.12%. Spray pump 4 oz. *otc.*
Use: Antipruritic, topical.

dideoxycytidine. (Roche). *Rx.*
Use: Antiviral.
See: HIVID.

2,3 dideoxycytidine. (Roche; NCI; Bristol-Myers). *Rx.*
Use: Antiviral (AIDS).

dideoxyinisine.
Use: Antiviral.
See: Videx, Tab., Pow. (Bristol-Myers Squibb).

Didrex. (Pharmacia & Upjohn) Benzphetamine HCl. **25 mg/Tab.:** Bot. 100s; **50 mg/Tab.:** Bot. 100s, 500s. *c-III.*
Use: Anorexiant.

Didronel. (Procter & Gamble) Etidronate disodium 200 mg or 400 mg/Tab. Bot. 60s. *Rx.*
Use: Antihypercalcemia.

Didronel IV. (MGI Pharma) Etidronate disodium 300 mg/6 ml amp. Amp. 6 ml. *Rx.*
Use: Antihypercalcemla.

•**dienestrol.** (die-en-ESS-trole) U.S.P. 23.
Use: Estrogen therapy, atrophic vaginitis.
See: D V, Cream (Hoechst Marion Roussel).
D V, Supp. (Hoechst Marion Roussel).
Ortho Dienestrol Cream (Ortho).
W/Sulfanilamide, aminacrine HCl, allantoin.
See: AVC/Dienestrol Cream, Supp. (Hoechst Marion Roussel).

dienestrol. (Ortho) 0.01%. Tube 78 g w/ applicator.
Use: Estrogen.

Diet-Aid, Maximum Strength. (Columbia) Phenylpropanolamine HCl 75 mg/ Cap. Pkg. 20s. *otc.*
Use: Dietary aid.

Diet-Aid Plus Vitamin C, Maximum Strength. (Columbia) Phenylpropanolamine HCl 75 mg, vitamin C 180 mg/ Cap. Pkg. 20s. *otc.*
Use: Dietary aid.

diet aids, nonprescription.
Use: Dietary aid.
See: Appedrine, Tab. (Thompson).
Dex-A-Diet Plus Vitamin C, Cap. (Columbia).
Diet Ayds, Candy (DEP Corp).
Dieutrim T.D., Cap. (Legere).
Extra Strength Grapefruit Diet Plan w/ Diadax, Cap. (Columbia).
Grapefruit Diet Plan w/Diadax, Cap., Tab. (Columbia).
Maximum Strength Dexatrim Plus Vitamin C, Cap. (Thompson).
Slim-Mint, Gum (Thompson).

•**diethanolamine.** N.F. 18.
Use: Pharmaceutic acid (alkalizing agent).

diethanolamine.
See: Diolamine.

diethazine hydrochloride. 10-(β-Diethylaminoethyl)-pheno-thiazine HCl. Diparcol.
Use: Parkinsonism.

diethoxin. Intracaine HCl.

•**diethyl phthalate.** N.F. 18.
Use: Pharmaceutic aid (plasticizer).

diethyldithiocarbamate.
Use: Trial drug for AIDS. [Orphan drug]
See: Imuthiol (Connaught).

diethylenediamine citrate. Piperazine Citrate, Piperazine Hexahydrate.
See: Antepar, Syr., Tab., Wafer (Glaxo-Wellcome).

diethylmalonylurea.
See: Barbital, Tab. (Various Mfr.)

•**diethylcarbamazine citrate.** (die- ETH-ill-car-BAM-ah-zeen SIH-trate) U.S.P. 23.
Use: Anthelmintic.
See: Nemacide (Fermenta).

•**diethylpropion hydrochloride.** (die-ETH-uhl-PRO-pee-ahn) U.S.P. 23.
Use: Anorexic.
See: D.E.P.-75
Tenuate, Tab. (Hoechst Marion Roussel).

Tepanil, Tab. (3M).
Tepanil Ten-Tab, Tab. (3M).

diethylpropion. (Various Mfr.) **Tab.:** Diethylpropion 25 mg. Bot. 100s, 500s, 1000s. **SR Tab.:** Diethylpropion 75 mg. Bot. 100s, 250s, 500s, 1000s. *c-iv.*
Use: Anorexiant.

•**diethylstilbestrol diphosphate.** (die-ETH-uhl-still-BESS-trahl die-FOSS-fate) U.S.P. 23.
Use: Estrogen.
See: Stilphostrol, Inj., Tab. (Bayer Corp).

diethylstilbestrol dipropionate. (Various Mfr.) Amp. in oil, 0.5 mg, 1 mg or 5 mg/ml. Tab. 0.5 mg, 1 mg or 5 mg.
Use: Estrogen.

•**diethyltoluamide.** (die-ETH-ill-toe-LOO-ah-mide) U.S.P. 23.
Use: Repellent (arthropod).
See: RV Pellent, Oint. (Zeneca)

n, n-diethylvanillamide.
See: Ethamivan, Inj. (Various Mfr.)

Diet-Tuss. (Health for Life Brands) Dextromethor- phan 30 mg, thenylpyramine HCl, pyrilamine maleate 80 mg, sodium salicylate 200 mg, sodium citrate 600 mg, ammonium Cl 100 mg/fl oz. Sugar free. Bot. 4 oz. *otc.*
Use: Analgesic, antihistamine, antitussive, expectorant.

Dieutrim T.D. (Legere) Phenylpropanolamine 75 mg, benzocaine 9 mg, sodium carboxymethylcellulose 75 mg/SR Cap. Bot. 100s, 1000s. *otc.*
Use: Dietary aid.

•**difenoximide hydrochloride.** (DIE-fen-OX-ih-mid) USAN.
Use: Antiperistaltic.

•**difenoxin.** (DIE-fen-OX-in) USAN.
Use: Antidiarrheal, antiperistaltic.
W/Atropine sulfate.
See: Motofen (Schwarz Pharma).

Differin. (Galderma) Adapalene 0.1%, propylene glycol, EDTA, methylparaben/Gel. Tube. 15 g, 45 g. *Rx.*
Use: Dermatologic, acne.

•**diflorasone diacetate.** (die-FLORE-ah-sone die-ASS-eh-tate) U.S.P. 23.
Use: Anti-inflammatory, topical; antipruritic.
See: Florone, Cream, Oint. (Pharmacia & Upjohn).
Maxiflor, Cream, Oint. (Allergan).
Psorcon, Cream, Oint. (Dermik Laboratories).

•**difloxacin hydrochloride.** (die-FLOX-ah-SIN) USAN.
Use: Anti-infective (DNA gyrase inhibitor).

•**difluanine hydrochloride.** (die-FLEW-an-EEN) USAN.
Use: CNS stimulant.

Diflucan. (Roerig) Fluconazole. **Tab.:** 50 mg. Bot. 30s, 100 mg or 200 mg. Bot. 30s, UD 100s; 150 mg. 1s. **Inj.:** 2 mg/ml Vial with sodium chloride 9 mg/ml or *Viaflex Plus* 100 ml, 200 ml. **Pow. for Oral Susp.:** 10 mg/ml in 350 mg or 40 mg/ml in 1400 mg. *Rx.*
Use: Antifungal.

•**diflucortolone.** (die-flew-CORE-toe-lone) USAN.
Use: Corticosteroid, topical.

•**diflucortolone pivalate.** USAN.
Use: Corticosteroid, topical.

•**diflumidone sodium.** (die-FLEW-mih-DOHN) USAN.
Use: Anti-inflammatory.

•**diflunisal.** (die-FLOO-nih-sal) U.S.P. 23.
Use: Analgesic, NSAID.
See: Dolobid, Tab. (Merck).

diflunisal. (Various Mfr.) Diflunisal 250 mg or 500 mg/Tab. Pkg. UD 60s, 100s, 500s. *Rx.*
Use: Analgesic, NSAID.

•**difluprednate.** (DIE-flew-PRED-nate) USAN.
Use: Anti-inflammatory.

•**diftalone.** (DIFF-tah-lone) USAN.
Use: Anti-inflammatory, analgesic.

•**digalloyl trioleate.** USAN.

Di-Gel, Advanced. (Schering Plough) Magnesium hydroxide 128 mg, calcium carbonate 280 mg, simethicone 20 mg/Tab. Bot. 30s, 60s, 90s. *otc.*
Use: Antacid, antiflatulent.

Di-Gel Liquid. (Schering Plough) Aluminum hydroxide (equivalent to dried gel) 200 mg, magnesium hydroxide 200 mg, simethicone 20 mg/5 ml, saccharin, sorbitol. Bot. 180 ml, 360 ml. *otc.*
Use: Antacid, antiflatulent.

Digepepsin. (Kenwood/Bradley) Pepsin 250 mg, pancreatin 300 mg, bile salts 150 mg/Tab. Bot. 60s. *Rx.*
Use: Digestive enzyme.

Digestamic. (Lexis) Pancrelipase 300 mg, pepsin 100 mg/Tab. Bot. 50s. *otc, Rx.*
Use: Digestive aid.

Digestamic Liquid. (Lexis) Belladonna leaf fluid extract 0.64 min./5 ml. Bot. 8 oz. *otc, Rx.*
Use: Anticholinergic, antispasmodic.

Digestant. (Canright) Pancreatin 5.25 gr, ox bile extract 2 gr, pepsin 5 gr, betaine HCl 1 gr/Tab. Bot. 100s, 1000s. *otc, Rx.*

Use: Digestive aid.

Digestive Compound. (Thurston) Betaine HCl 3.25 gr, pepsin 1 gr, papain 2 gr, mycozyme 2 gr, ox bile 2 gr/2 Tab. Bot. 100s, 500s. *otc, Rx.*
Use: Digestive aid.

digestive enzymes.
See: Cotazym Capsules (Organon).
Cotazym-S Capsules (Organon).
Creon Capsules (Solvay).
Dizymes Tablets (Recsei Labs.).
Festal II Tablets (Hoechst Marion Roussel).
Hi-Vegi-Lip Tablets (Freeda Vitamins).
Ilozyme Tablets (Pharmacia & Upjohn).
Ku-Zyme HP Capsules (Kremers Urban).
Pancrease Capsules (McNeil Pharm)
Pancreatin Enseals Tablets (Eli Lilly).
Pancreatin Tablets (Eli Lilly).
Viokase Pow., Tab. (Robins).

digestive products, miscellaneous.
Use: Digestive enzyme supplement.
See: Ku-Zyme, Cap. (Kremers Urban).
Arco-Lase, Tabs. (Arco).
Converzyme, Cap. (B.F. Ascher).
Digestozyme, Tab. (Various Mfr.)
Nu'Leven, Tab. (Teva USA).
Enzobile Improved (Roberts Pharm).
Sto-Zyme (Misemer).

Digestozyme Tabs. (Zenith Goldline) Pancreatin, pepsin, bile salts. Bot. 1000s. *Rx.*
Use: Digestive aid.

Digibind. (GlaxoWellcome) Digoxin Immune Fab (ovine) fragments 38 mg, sorbitol 75 mg/Vial. Box 1s. *Rx.*
Use: Antidote.

Digidote. (Boehringer Mannheim)
Use: Antidote. [Orphan drug].

•**digitalis.** (dih-jih-TAL-iss) U.S.P. 23.
Use: Cardiovascular agent.
See: Acylanid, Tab. (Sandoz).
Cedilanid, Tab. (Sandoz).
Cedilanid-D, Amp. (Sandoz).
Crystodigin, Tab. Amp., Vial (Eli Lilly).
Deslanoside, Inj. (Various Mfr.)
Digiglusin, Tab. (Eli Lilly).
Digitaline Nativelle, Soln., Tab., Elix. (Savage).
Digitoxin, Preps. (Various Mfr.)
Digoxin, Preps. (Various Mfr.)
Gitaligin, Tab. (Schering).
Gitalin, Tab. (Various Mfr.)
Lanatoside C, Inj., Tab. (Various Mfr.)
Lanoxin, Tab., Inj., Elix. (GlaxoWellcome).

digitalis leaf, powdered.
Use: Cardiovascular agent.
See: Pil-Digis, Pill (Key Pharm).

digitalis tincture.
Use: Cardiovascular agent.

•**digitoxin.** (dih-jih-TOX-in) U.S.P. 23.
Use: Cardiovascular agent.
See: Crystodigin, Tab. (Eli Lilly).

digitoxin. (Various Mfr.) **Amp.:** (0.2 mg/ml) 1 ml, **Cap. in oil:** 0.1 mg or 0.2 mg. **Tab.:** 0.1 mg, 0.2 mg.
Use: Cardiovascular agent.

digitoxin, acetyl.
Use: Cardiovascular agent.
See: Acylanid, Tab. (Sandoz).

α-digitoxin monoacetate.
Use: Cardiovascular agent.
See: Acetyldigitoxin, Tab. (Various Mfr.)

•**digoxin.** (dih-JOX-in) U.S.P. 23.
Use: Cardiovascular agent.
See: Lanoxicaps (GlaxoWellcome).
Lanoxin, Preps. (GlaxoWellcome).
Masoxin, Tab. (Mason).

digoxin. (Roxane) Digoxin 0.05 mg/ml, alcohol 10%. Bot 60 ml, UD 2.5 ml, UD 5 ml. *Rx.*
Use: Cardiovascular agent.

digoxin antibody.
See: Digibind (GlaxoWellcome).

Digoxin Elixir. (Roxane) 0.05 mg/ml. Liq. Bot. 60 ml, UD 2.5 ml, 5 ml. *Rx.*
Use: Cardiovascular agent.

digoxin i-125 imusay. (Abbott Diagnostics) Digoxin diagnostic kit for the quantitative determination of serum digoxin. 100s, 300s.
Use: Diagnostic aid.

digoxin immune fab (ovine) fragments.
Use: Antidote. [Orphan drug]
See: Digibind, Pow. for Inj. (GlaxoWellcome).
Digidote (Boehringer Mannheim).

Digoxin Riabead. (Abbott Diagnostics) Solid-phase radioimmunoassay for quantitative measurement of serum digoxin. Test kit 100s, 300s.
Use: Diagnostic aid.

dihematoporphyrin ethers.
Use: Photodynamic therapy of transitional cell carcinoma in situ of urinary bladder or primary or recurrent obstructing esophageal carcinoma. [Orphan drug]
See: Photofrin (QLT Phototherapeutics).

•**dihexyverine hydrochloride.** (die-HEX-ih-ver-een) USAN.
Use: Anticholinergic.

Dihistine DH. (Zenith Goldline) Pseudoephedrine HCl 30 mg, chlorpheniramine maleate 2 mg, codeine phos-

phate 10 mg. Elix. Bot. 4 oz, pt, gal. *c-v.*
Use: Antihistamine, antitussive, decongestant.

Dihistine Elixir. (Various Mfr.) Phenylephrine HCl 5 mg, chlorpheniramine maleate 2 mg/5 ml. Bot. pt, gal. *otc.*
Use: Antihistamine, decongestant.

Dihistine Expectorant. (Zenith Goldline) Pseudoephedrine HCl 30 mg, codeine phosphate 10 mg, guaifenesin 100 mg, alcohol 7.5%. Bot. 4 oz, pt, gal. *c-v.*
Use: Antitussive, decongestant, expectorant.

dihydan soluble.
See: Phenytoin Sodium (Various Mfr.)

dihydrocodeine. Paracodin. Drocode.
Use: Analgesic, antitussive.

•**dihydrocodeine bitartrate.** (die-high-droe-KOE-deen bye-TAR-trate) U.S.P. 23.
Use: Analgesic.
See: Hydrocodone Bitartrate, U.S.P. 23.
W/Caffeine, phenacetin, aspirin.
See: Drocogesic #3, Tab. (Rand).
Duradyne DHC, Liq. (Forest Pharmaceutical).
W/Caffeine, aspirin.
See: Synalgos-DC, Cap. (Wyeth Ayerst).
W/Caffeine, acetaminophen.
See: DHC Plus, Cap. (Purdue Frederick).

dihydrocodeinone resin complex.
W/Phenyltoloxamine resin complex.
See: Tussionex, Preps. (Medeva).

dihydro-diethylstilbestrol.
See: Hexestrol, Tab., Vial (Various Mfr.)

dihydroergocornine. Ergot alkaline component of hydergine.
See: Circanol, Tab. (3M).
Deapril-ST, Tab. (Bristol-Myers).

dihydroergocristine. Ergot alkaloid component of hydergine.
See: Circanol, Tab. (3M).
Deapril-ST, Tab. (Bristol-Myers).

dihydroergocryptine. Ergot alkaloid component of hydergine.
See: Circanol, Tab. (3M).
Deapril-ST, Tab. (Bristol-Myers).

dihydroergotamine. (D.H.E. 45) (Sandoz) Dihydroergotamine mesylate. Amp. *Rx.*
Use: Agent for migraine, antiadrenergic.

•**dihydroergotamine mesylate.** (DIE-high-droe-err-GOT-uh-meen) U.S.P. 23. Dihydroergotamine methanesulfonate.
Use: Antiadrenergic, antimigraine.
See: DHE 45, Amp. (Sandoz). *Rx.*
W/Scopolamine HBr, phenobarbital sodium, barbital sodium, Sandoptal.
See: Plexonal, Tab. (Sandoz).

dihydroergotoxine. Ergoloid mesylate. *Rx.*
Use: Psychotherapeutic agent.
See: Gerimal, Tab. (Rugby).
Hydergine, Tab. (Sandoz).
Ergoloid Mesylates, Tab. (Various Mfr.)
Ergoloid Mesylates, Tab. (Various Mfr.)
Hydergine, Tab. (Sandoz).
Niloric, Tab. (B.F. Ascher).
Hydergine LC, Cap. (Sandoz).
Hydergine, Liq. (Sandoz).

5,6-dihydro-5-azacytidine. (Ilex Oncology)
Use: Antineoplastic. [Orphan Drug]

dihydrofollicular hormone.
See: Estradiol (Various Mfr.)

dihydrofolliculine.
See: Estradiol (Various Mfr.)

dihydrohydroxycodeinone. Oxycodone. (Ducodal, Eukodal, Eucodal). *c-II.*
Use: Analgesic, narcotic.

dihydrohydroxycodeinone hydrochloride or bitartrate. Oxycodone HCl or Bitartrate.
W/Combinations.
See: Cophene-S, Syr. (Dunhall Pharmaceuticals).
Corizahist-D, Syr. (Mason).
Damason-P, Tab. (Mason).
Percobarb, Cap. (DuPont Merck Pharmaceuticals).
Percodan, Tab. (DuPont Merck Pharmaceuticals).
Triaprin-DC, Cap. (Dunhall Pharmaceuticals).

dihydromorphinone hydrochloride.
See: Dilaudid, Preps. (Knoll Pharmaceuticals).

•**dihydrostreptomycin sulfate.** (die-HIGH-droe-strep-toe-MY-sin) U.S.P. 23.
Use: Anti-infective.

dihydrotachysterol. (die-HIGH-droe-tack-ISS-ter-ole) (Roxane) 0.2 mg/Tab. Bot. 100s, UD 100s.
Use: Antihypocalcemic.
See: Hytakerol, Cap. (Sanofi Winthrop).

dihydrotachysterol. (Roxane) 0.2 mg/Tab. Bot. 100s, UD 100s.
Use: Antihypocalcemic.

dihydrotestosterone.
Use: AIDS [Orphan drug].
See: Androgel-DHT. (Unimed).

dihydrotheelin.

See: Estradiol (Various Mfr.)

dihydroxyacetone.
See: Chromelin, Liq. (Summers).
QT, Liq. (Schering Plough).
Sudden Tan, Liq. (Schering Plough).

•**dihydroxyaluminum aminoacetate.** (die-high-DROX-ee-ah-LOO-min-uhm ah-MEE-no-ASS-eh-tate) U.S.P. 23.
Use: Antacid.
W/Methscopolamine bromide, sodium lauryl sulfate, magnesium hydroxide.
See: Alu-Scop, Cap., Susp. (Westerfield).
W/Phenobarbital and atropine methyl nitrate.
See: Harvatrate A, Tab. (O'Neal).
W/Salicylsalicylic acid, aspirin.
See: Salsprin, Tab. (Seatrace).

•**dihydroxyaluminum sodium carbonate.** U.S.P. 23.
Use: Antacid.
See: Rolaids (Parke-Davis).

dihydroxycholecalciferol.
See: Rocaltrol. (Roche).

24,25 dihydroxycholecalciferol. (Lemmon/Tag)
Use: Uremic osteodystrophy. [Orphan drug]

dihydroxyestrin.
See: Estradiol (Various Mfr.)

dihydroxyfluorane. Fluorescein.

dihydroxyphenylisatin.
See: Oxyphenisatin (Various Mfr.)

dihydroxyphenyloxindol.
See: Oxyphenisatin (Various Mfr.)

dihydroxypropyl Theophylline. Dyphylline.
See: Neothylline, Tab., Elix., Inj. (Teva USA).

dihydroxy(stearato)aluminum. Aluminum Monostearate, N.F. 18.

diiodohydroxyquin.
Use: Amebicide.
See: Iodoquinol, U.S.P. 23.

diiodohydroxyquinoline.
See: Iodoquinol, U.S.P. 23.

diisopromine hydrochloride. (Lab. for Pharmaceutical Development, Inc.).
See: Desquam-X (Westwood Squibb).

diisopropyl phosphorofluoridate.
See: Isofluorophate, U.S.P. 23.
Floropryl, Oint. (Merck).

diisopropyl sebacate.
Use: Moisturizing agent.
See: Delavan, Cream (Bayer Corp).

Dilacor XR. (Rhone-Poulenc Rorer) Diltiazem HCl 120 mg, 180 mg, or 240 mg/Cap. SR 100s, UD 100s. *Rx.*
Use: Calcium channel blocker.

dilaminate. Mixture of magnesium carbide and dihydroxy aluminum glycinate. *otc.*
Use: Antacid.

Dilantin. (Parke-Davis) Phenytoin. **30' Susp.:** 30 mg/5 ml. Bot. 8 oz, UD 5 ml. **125 Susp.:** 125 mg/5 ml. Bot. 8 oz, UD 5 ml. **Infatab:** 50 mg/Tab. Bot. 100s, UD 100s. *Rx.*
Use: Anticonvulsant.

Dilantin Sodium. (Parke-Davis) Extended phenytoin sodium. **Kapseal:** 30 mg, 100 mg. Bot. 100s, 1000s, UD 100s. **Amp.:** (w/propylene glycol 40%, alcohol 10%, sodium hydroxide) 100 mg/2 ml. UD 10s; 250 mg/5 ml. Amp. 10s, UD 10s. *Rx.*
Use: Anticonvulsant.

Dilantin Sodium w/Phenobarbital Kapseal. (Parke-Davis) Phenytoin sodium 100 mg, phenobarbital 16 mg or 32 mg/Cap. Bot. 100s, 1000s, UD 100s (32 mg only). *Rx.*
Use: Anticonvulsant, hypnotic, sedative.

Dilantin-30 Pediatric. (Parke-Davis) Phenytoin 30 mg/5 ml, alcohol 0.6%. Susp. Bot. 240 ml, 5 ml. *Rx.*
Use: Anticonvulsant.

Dilatrate-SR. (Schwarz Pharma) Isosorbide dinitrate 40 mg/SR Cap. Bot. 60s, 100s. *Rx.*
Use: Antianginal.

Dilaudid. (Knoll Pharmaceuticals) Hydromorphone HCl. **Amp.** (w/sodium citrate 0.2%, citric acid soln. 0.2%): 1 mg, 2 mg or 4 mg/ml. Box 10s. 2 mg. Box 25s. **Multiple Dose Vial:** 2 mg/ml. Bot. 20 ml. **Tab.:** 2 mg Bot. 100s, 500s. Strip pack 4 × 25s. 4 mg 100s, 500s. Strip pack 4 × 25s. 8 mg. Bot. 100s. **Pow:** Vial, 15 gr Multiple dose vial 10 ml, 20 ml. 2 mg/ml. **Rectal Supp.:** (in cocoa butter base, w/colloidal silica 1%): 3 mg/Supp. Box 6s. *c-II.*
Use: Analgesic, narcotic.
W/Guaifenesin.
See: Dilaudid Cough Syrup. (Knoll Pharmaceuticals).

Dilaudid Cough Syrup. (Knoll Pharmaceuticals) Hydromorphone HCl 1 mg, guaifenesin 100 mg/ 5ml. Alcohol 5%. Bot. pt. *c-II.*
Use: Analgesic, narcotic; expectorant.

Dilaudid-5. (Knoll Pharmaceuticals) Hydromorphone HCl 5 mg/5 ml. Liq. Bot. Pt. *c-II.*
Use: Analgesic, narcotic.

Dilaudid HP Ampule. (Knoll Pharmaceuticals) Hydromorphone 10 mg/ml. Box

10s; 50 mg/5 ml. Box 1s. *c-II*.
Use: Analgesic, narcotic.

Dilaudid-HP Injection. (Knoll Pharmaceuticals) Hydromorphone HCl 250 mg (10 mg/ml when reconstituted). Vial 1 ml, 5 ml, 50 ml, 250 mg (lyophilized) single-dose. *c-II*.
Use: Analgesic, narcotic.

•**dilevalol hydrochloride.** (DIE-LEV-ah-lole) USAN.
Use: Antihypertensive, antiadrenergic (β-receptor).

dilithium carbonate. Lithium Carbonate, U.S.P. 23.
Use: Antipsychotic.

Dilocaine. (Hauck) Lidocaine HCl 1% or 2%. Bot. 50 ml. *Rx.*
Use: Anesthetic, local.

Dilor. (Savage) Dyphylline. **Tab.:** 200 mg. Bot. 100s, 1000s, UD 100s. **Elix.:** 160 mg/15 ml. Bot. pt. *Rx.*
Use: Bronchodilator.

Dilor 400. (Savage) Dyphylline 400 mg. Bot. 100s, 1000s, UD 100s. *Rx.*
Use: Bronchodilator.

Dilor G Liquid. (Savage) Dyphylline 300 mg, guaifenesin 300 mg/15 ml. Bot. pt, gal. *Rx.*
Use: Bronchodilator, expectorant.

Dilor G Tablets. (Savage) Dyphylline 200 mg, guaifenesin 200 mg/Tab. Bot. 100s, 1000s, UD 100s. *Rx.*
Use: Bronchodilator, expectorant.

diloxaride furoate.
Use: Anti-infective.

•**diltiazem hydrochloride.** (dill-TIE-uh-zem) U.S.P. 23.
Use: Vasodilator (coronary).

diltiazem hydrochloride extended-release capsules. (Various Mfr.) Diltiazem HCl 60 mg, 90 mg or 120 mg. Bot. 100s. *Rx.*
Use: Calcium channel blocker.
See: Tiazac, ER CAP. (Forest Pharm).

diltiazem hydrochloride tablets. (Various Mfr.) Diltiazem HCl 30 mg, 60 mg, 90 mg or 120 mg. Bot. 100s, 500s, 1000s and unit of issue 30s, 60s, 90s, 120s. *Rx.*
Use: Calcium channel blocker.

diltiazem injection. (Bedford Labs) Diltiazem 5 mg/ml, 71.4 mg/ml sorbitol solution. Vial 5 ml, 10 ml. *Rx.*
Use: Calcium channel blocker.

•**diltiazem malate.** (dill-TIE-ah-zem MAL-ate) USAN.
Use: Calcium channel blocker, antihypertensive.

Dimacol. (Robins) Pseudoephedrine HCl 30 mg, dextromethorphan HBr 10 mg, guaifenesin 100 mg/Cap. or 5 ml. **Cap.** Bot. 100s, 500s, Pre-Pack 12s, 24s. **Liq.** (w/alcohol 4.75%) Bot. pt. *otc.*
Use: Antitussive, decongestant, expectorant.

Dimaphen Elixir. (Major) Phenylpropanolamine HCl 12.5 mg, brompheniramine maleate 2 mg, 237 ml. *otc.*
Use: Antihistamine, decongestant.

Dimaphen Release. (Major) Phenylpropanolamine HCl 75 mg, brompheniramine maleate 12 mg/Tab. Bot. 12s. *otc.*
Use: Antihistamine, decongestant.

Dimaphen Tablets. (Major) Phenylpropanolamine HCl 25 mg, brompheniramine maleate 4 mg. Tab. Bot. 24s. *otc.*
Use: Antihistamine, decongestant.

•**dimefadane.** (DIE-meh-fah-dane) USAN.
Use: Analgesic.

•**dimefilcon a.** (DIE-meh-FILL-kahn A) USAN.
Use: Contact lens material (hydrophilic).

•**dimefline hydrochloride.** (DIE-meh-fleen) USAN.
Use: Respiratory.

•**dimefocon a.** (DIE-meh-FOE-kahn A) USAN.
Use: Contact lens material (hydrophobic).

Dimenest. (Forest Pharmaceutical) Dimenhydrinate 50 mg/ml. Vial 10 ml. *Rx.*
Use: Antiemetic, antivertigo.

•**dimenhydrinate.** (die-men-HIGH-drih-nate) U.S.P. 23.
Use: Antiemetic, antihistamine.
See: Dimenest, Inj. (Forest Pharmaceutical)
Dimentabs, Tab. (Jones Medical Industries).
Dramamine, Preps. (Pharmacia & Upjohn).
Dramocen, Inj. (Schwarz Pharma).
Dymenate, Inj. (Keene Pharmaceuticals).
Eldadryl, Preps. (Zeneca)
Eldodram, Tab. (Zeneca)
Hydrate, Vial (Hyrex).
Signate, Inj. (Sig).
Trav-Arex, Cap. (Quality Generics).
Traveltabs, Tab. (Geneva Pharm)
Vertab, Cap. (UAD).

Dimentabs. (Jones Medical Industries) Dimenhydrinate 50 mg/Tab. Bot. 100s. *otc.*
Use: Antiemetic, antivertigo.

•**dimepranol acedoben.** (DIE-MEH-prah-

nahl ah-SEE-doe-BEN) USAN.
Use: Immunomodulator.

•**dimercaprol.** (die-mer-CAP-role) U.S.P. 23. *Formerly BAL.*
Use: Antidote to gold, arsenic and mercury poisoning; metal complexing agent.
See: BAL in oil, Inj. (Becton Dickinson).

Dimetane-DC Cough Syrup. (Robins) Brompheniramine maleate 2 mg, phenylpropanolamine HCl 12.5 mg, codeine phosphate 10 mg/5 ml w/alcohol 0.95%. Bot. pt, gal. *c-v.*
Use: Antihistamine, antitussive, decongestant.

Dimetane Decongestant Caplets. (Robins) Brompheniramine maleate 4 mg, phenylephrine HCl 10 mg/Capl. Bot. 24s, 48s. *otc.*
Use: Antihistamine, decongestant.

Dimetane Decongestant Elixir. (Robins) Brompheniramine maleate 2 mg, phenylephrine HCl 5 mg/5 ml, alcohol 2.3%. Bot. 120 ml. *otc.*
Use: Antihistamine, decongestant.

Dimetane-DX Cough Syrup. (Robins) Pseudoephedrine HCl 30 mg, brompheniramine maleate 2 mg, dextromethorphan HBr 10 mg, alcohol 0.95%, saccharin, sorbitol. Bot. pt. *Rx.*
Use: Antihistamine, antitussive, decongestant.

Dimetapp Allergy. (AH Robins) Brompheniramine maleate 4 mg, sorbitol/ Liqui-gels. 24s. *otc.*
Use: Antihistamine.

Dimetapp Cold & Allergy. (Robins) Brompheniramine maleate 1 mg, phenylpropanolamine HCl 6.25 mg, aspartame, phenylalanine 8 mg, sorbitol. Tab. Chew. Bot. 24s. *otc.*
Use: Antihistamine, decongestant.

Dimetapp Cold & Flu Caplet. (Robins) Phenylpropanolamine HCl 12.5 mg, brompheniramine maleate 2 mg, acetaminophen 500 mg/Capl. Bot. 24s, 48s. *otc.*
Use: Analgesic, antihistamine, decongestant.

Dimetapp DM Elixir. (Robins) Phenylpropanolamine HCl 12.5 mg, brompheniramine maleate 2 mg, dextro- methorphan HBr 10 mg, 2.3% alcohol, saccharin, sorbitol. Elix. Bot. 120 ml, 240 ml. *otc.*
Use: Antihistamine, antitussive, decongestant.

Dimetapp Elixir. (Robins) Brompheniramine maleate 2 mg, phenylpropanolamine HCl 12.5 mg/5 ml. Bot. 120 ml, 240 ml, 360 ml, 473 ml, gal, UD 5 ml. *otc.*
Use: Antihistamine, decongestant.

Dimetapp Extentabs. (Robins) Brompheniramine maleate 12 mg, phenylpropanolamine HCl 75 mg/Tab. Bot. 100s, 500s, UD 100s. Blister pack 12s, 24s, 48s. *otc.*
Use: Antihistamine, decongestant.

Dimetapp 4-Hour Liqui-Gels. (Robins) Brompheniramine maleate 4 mg, phenylpropanolamine HCl 25 mg, sorbitol. Cap. Pck. 12s. *otc.*
Use: Antihistamine, decongestant.

Dimetapp Sinus. (Robins) Pseudoephedrine HCl 30 mg, ibuprofen 200 mg/Cap. Bot. 20s, 40s. *otc.*
Use: Analgesic, decongestant.

Dimetapp Tablets. (Robins) Brompheniramine maleate 4 mg, phenylpropanolamine HCl 25 mg/Tab. Blisterpak 24s. *otc.*
Use: Antihistamine, decongestant.

•**dimethadione.** (DIE-meth-ah-DIE-ohn) USAN.
Use: Anticonvulsant.

dimethazan.

•**dimethicone.** (DIE-meth-ih-cone) N.F. 18.
Use: Prosthetic aid (soft tissue), component of barrier creams, lubricant and hydrophobing agent.
See: Covicone, Cream (Abbott Laboratories).
Silicone, Oint. (Various Mfr.)

•**dimethicone 350.** (DIE-meth-ih-cone 350) USAN.
Use: Prosthetic aid for soft tissue.

•**dimethindene maleate.** (DIE-METH-in-deen) USAN. U.S.P. XX.
Use: Antihistamine.

•**dimethisoquin hydrochloride.** (die-meh-THIGH-so-kwin) USAN.

•**dimethisterone.** (DIE-meth-ISS-ter-ohn) USAN. N.F. XIV.
Use: Hormone, progestin.

dimetholizine phosphate.

dimethoxyphenyl penicillin sodium.
Use: Anti-infective.
See: Methicillin sodium (Various Mfr.)

dimethpyridene maleate. Dimethindene Maleate, U.S.P. 23.
See: Dimethindene Maleate, U.S.P. 23.

dimethylaminophenazone.
See: Aminopyrine (Various Mfr.)

dimethylamino pyrazine sulfate.
See: Ampyzine Sulfate.

dimethylcarbamate. of 3-Hydroxy-1-Methylpyridinium Bromide.
See: Mestinon, Tab. (Roche).

dimethylhexestrol dipropionate. Promethestrol Dipropionate.
See: Meprane Dipropionate, Tab. (Schwarz Pharma).

dimethyl polysiloxane.
See: Dimethicone (Various Mfr.)
W/Benzocaine, bismuth subcarbonate, carbamide, hexachlorophene, phenylephrine HCl, pyrilamine maleate, zinc oxide.
W/Hexachlorophene, zinc oxide, pyrilamine maleate, tetracaine HCl, methyl salicylate, zirconium oxide.

•**dimethyl sulfoxide.** (die-METH-uhl sull-FOX-ide) U.S.P. 23.
Use: Anti-inflammatory, topical.
See: Rimso-50 (Research Ind.).

dimethyl sulfoxide. (Pharma 21)
Use: Increased intracranial pressure. [Orphan Drug]

dimethyl-tubocurarine iodide.
Use: Muscle relaxant.
See: Metocurine Iodide, U.S.P. 23.

dimethylurethimine.
See: Meturedepa (Centeon).

•**dimoxamine hydrochloride.** (die-MOX-AH-meen) USAN.
Use: Memory adjuvant.

Dimycor. (Standard Drug) Pentaerythritol tetranitrate 10 mg, phenobarbital 15 mg/Tab. Bot. 1000s. *Rx.*
Use: Antianginal, hypnotic, sedative.

Dinacrin. (Sanofi Winthrop) Isonicotinic acid, hydrazide. *Rx.*
Use: Antituberculous.

Dinate. (Blaine) Dimenhydrinate 50 mg/ml. Vial 10 ml. *Rx.*
Use: Antiemetic, antivertigo.

•**dinoprost.** (DIE-no-proste) USAN.
Use: Oxytocic; prostaglandin.

•**dinoprost tromethamine.** (DIE-no-proste troe-METH-ah-meen) U.S.P. 23.
Use: Oxytocic, prostaglandin.

•**dinoprostone.** (DIE-no-PROSTE-ohn) USAN.
Use: Abortifacient, agent for cervical ripening, oxytocic, prostaglandin.
See: Cervidil, Insert (Forest Pharmaceutical).
Prepidil, Gel (Pharmacia & Upjohn).
Prostin E_2, Supp. (Pharmacia & Upjohn).

Diocto. (Purepac) Docusate sodium 100 mg or 200 mg/Cap. Bot. 100s. *otc.*
Use: Laxative.

Diocto C. (Various Mfr.) Docusate sodium 60 mg, casanthranol 30 mg/15 ml. Syr. Bot. 240 ml, pt, gal. *otc.*
Use: Laxative.

Diocto-K. (Rugby) Docusate potassium 100 mg/Cap. Bot. 100s, 1000s. *otc.*
Use: Laxative.

Diocto-K Plus. (Rugby) Docusate sodium 100 mg, casanthranol 30 mg. Cap. Bot. 100s, 1000s. *otc.*
Use: Laxative.

Dioctolose. (Zenith Goldline) Docusate potassium 100 mg/Cap. Bot. 100s, 1000s.
Use: Laxative.

Dioctolose Plus Capsules. (Zenith Goldline) Docusate 100 mg, casanthranol 30 mg/Cap. Bot. 100s, 1000s. *otc.*
Use: Laxative.

dioctyl calcium sulfosuccinate. (die-OCK-till SULL-foe-SUCK-sih-nate) Docusate Calcium.
Use: Laxative.

dioctyl potassium sulfosuccinate. *otc.*
W/Glycerin, potassium oleate and stearate.
See: Rectalad, Liq. (Wallace).

dioctyl sodium sulfosuccinate.
See: Docusate Sodium, U.S.P. 23.
Use: Non-laxative fecal softener.

diodone injection.
See: Iodopyracet injection.

Dioeze. (Century Pharm) Dioctyl sodium sulfosuccinate 250 mg/Cap. Bot. 100s, 1000s. *otc.*
Use: Laxative.

•**diohippuric acid I 125.** USAN.
Use: Radiopharmaceutical.

•**diohippuric acid I 131.** USAN.
Use: Radiopharmaceutical.

Dio-Hist. (Health for Life Brands) Dextromethorphan 30 mg, thenylpyramine HCl 80 mg, phenylephrine HCl 20 mg, potassium tartrate 1/24 gr/oz. Bot. 4 oz. *otc.*
Use: Antihistamine.

D-Diol. (Burgin-Arden) Testosterone cypionate 50 mg, estradiol cypionate 2 mg/ml. Vial 10 ml. *Rx.*
Use: Androgen, estrogen combination.

diolamine. Diethanolamine.

diolostene.
See: Methandriol.

Dionex. (Henry Schein) Docusate sodium 100 mg or 250 mg/Cap. Bot. 100s, 250s, 1000s. *otc.*
Use: Laxative.

dionin. Ethylmorphine HCl.
Use: Orally; cough depressant, ocular lymphagogue.

Dionosil Oily. (GlaxoWellcome) Propyliodone 60% in peanut oil. Inj. Vial 20 ml.
Use: Radiopaque agent.

diophyllin.
See: Aminophylline, Preps. (Various Mfr.)

diopterin. Pteroylglutamic acid, PDGA, Pteroyl-alpha-glutamylglutamic acid.
Use: Antineoplastic.

Diorapin. (Standex) Estrogenic conjugate 0.625 mg, methyltestosterone 5 mg/Tab. Bot. 100s. Estrone 2 mg, testosterone 25 mg/ml. Inj. Vial 10 ml. *Rx.*
Use: Androgen, estrogen combination.

Diosate D. (Towne) Docusate sodium. Cap. 100 mg or 250 mg/Tab. Bot. 100s. *otc.*
Use: Laxative.

Diosmin. Buchu resin obtained from lvs. of barosma serratifolia and alliedrutaceae.

Dio-Soft. (Standex) Docusate sodium 100 mg, casanthranol 30 mg/Cap. Bot. 100s. *otc.*
Use: Laxative.

Diostate D. (Pharmacia & Upjohn) Vitamin D 400 IU, calcium 343 mg, phosphorus 265 mg/3 Tab. Bot. 100s. *otc.*
Use: Mineral, vitamin supplement.

•**diotyrosine I 125.** (die-oh-TIE-row-seen) USAN.
Use: Radiopharmaceutical.

•**diotyrosine I 131.** USAN.
Use: Radiopharmaceutical.

Diovan. (Novartis) Valsartan 80 mg, 160 mg/Cap. Bot. 100s, 4000s, UD blister 100s. *Rx.*
Use: Antihypertensive.

Diovocylin. (Novartis)
See: Estradiol, Preps. (Various Mfr.)

•**dioxadrol hydrochloride.** (die-OX-ah-drole) USAN.
Use: Antidepressant.

dioxindol. Diacetylhydroxyphenylisatin.

dioxyanthranol.
See: Anthralin, N.F. (Various Mfr.)

dioxyanthraquinone.
See: Danthron, U.S.P. 23.

•**dioxybenzone.** (die-ox-ee-BEN-zone) U.S.P. 23.
Use: Ultraviolet screen.
W/Oxybenzone, benzophene.
See: Solbar, Lot. (Person & Covey).

dipalmitoylphosphatidylcholine. Colfosceril palmitate.
Use: Synthetic lung surfactant.
See: Exosurf Neonatal, Pow. (GlaxoWellcome).

dipalmitoylphosphatidylcholine/phosphatidylglycerol.
Use: Neonatal respiratory distress syndrome. [Orphan drug]
See: ALEC (Forum Products).

diparcol hydrochloride. Diethazine.

Dipegyl.
See: Nicotinamide, Preps. (Various Mfr.)

dipenicillin g.
See: Benzethacil.

Dipentum. (Pharmacia & Upjohn) Osalazine sodium 250 mg/Cap. Bot. 100s, 500s. *Rx.*
Use: Gastrointestinal.

diperodon hydrochloride.
Use: Anesthetic.
See: Diothane Oint. (Hoechst Marion Roussel).
Proctodon, Cream (Solvay).
W/Bacitracin, neomycin sulfate, polymyxin.
See: Epimycin A, Oint. (Delta).
W/Benzalkonium Cl, ichthammol, thymol, camphor, juniper tar.
See: Boro Oint. (Scrip).
W/Furacin (nitrofurazone).
See: Furacin E Urethral Inserts (Eaton Medical).
Furacin H.C. Urethral Inserts (Eaton Medical).
W/Furacin (nitrofurazone) and Microfur (nituroxime).
See: Furacin Otic, Drops. (Eaton Medical).
W/Hydrocortisone, polymyxin B sulfate, neomycin.
See: My Cort Otic #1, Ear Drops (Scrip).
W/Hydroxyquinoline Benzoate.
See: Diothane, Oint. (Hoechst Marion Roussel).
W/Methapyrilene HCl, pyrilamine maleate, allantoin, benzocaine, menthol.
See: Antihistamine Cream (Towne).
W/Thimerosal, isopropyl alcohol.
See: Earobex, Ear Drops (Roberts Pharm).

diphenadione.
Use: Anticoagulant.
See: Dipaxin, Tab. (Pharmacia & Upjohn).

Diphen AF. (Morton Grove) Diphenhydramine HCl 6.25 mg/5 ml, saccharine, sugar, cherry flavor. Liq. Bot. 237 ml. *otc.*
Use: Antihistamine.

diphenatil.
See: Diphemanil methylsulfate.

Diphenatol. (Rugby) Diphenoxylate HCl 2.5 mg, atropine sulfate 0.025 mg. Tab. Bot. 100s, 500s, 1000s.

Use: Antidiarrheal.

Diphen Cough. (Rosemont) Diphenhydramine HCl 12.5 mg/5 ml., alcohol 5.1%, methol, sucrose, parabens. Syr. Bot. 118 ml. *otc.*
Use: Antitussive.

Diphendydramine 50. (Moore) Diphenhydramine HCl 50 mg, lactose, bisulfites/cap. Bot. 100s, 1000s. *otc.*
Use: Antihistamine.

Diphenhist. (Rugby) Diphenhydramine HCl. **Captabs, cap. softgels:** 25 mg lactose, parabens (soft gels) Bot. 100s. Soln. 12.5 mg/5 ml, saccharin, sucrose. Bot. 118 ml. *otc.*
Use: Antihistamine.

•**diphenhydramine citrate.** (die-fen-HIGH-druh-meen SIH-trate) U.S.P. 23.
Use: Antihistamine.

diphenhydramine and pseudoephedrine capsules.
Use: Antihistamine, decongestant.

diphenhydramine citrate.
Use: Antihistamine.

diphenhydramine hydrochloride. (die-fen-HIGH-druh-meen) (Various Mfr.) Diphenhydramine HCl. **Cap. Softgels:** 25 mg. 30s, 100s, 1000s. **Cap.:** 50 mg. Bot. 100s, 1000s. **Syrup:**12.5 mg/5 ml, alcohol. Bot. 118 ml. **Inj.** 50 mg/ml. Single-dose Amp. 1 ml, Multidose vial 10 ml. *otc, Rx.*
Use: Antihistamine.

•**diphenhydramine hydrochloride.** (die-fen-HIGH-druh-meen) U.S.P. 23.
Use: Antihistamine.
See: AllerMax, Preps. (Pfeiffer).
Banophen, Preps. (Major).
Bax, Cap., Elix., Expectorant (McKesson).
Benadryl Hydrochloride, Preps. (Parke-Davis).
Benahist, Preps. (Keene Pharmaceuticals).
Benylin Cough Syrup (Warner Lambert).
Clearly Cala-gel (Tec Labs).
Diphen, Preps. (Morton Grove).
Diphen-Ex, Syr. (Quality Generics).
Diphendrydramine 50, Cap. (Moore).
Diphenhist, Preps. (Rugby).
Diphenhydramine HCl (Weeks & Leo).
Fenylhist, Cap. (Roberts Pharm).
Genahist, Liq (Zenith Goldline).
Histine Prods. (Freeport).
Hyrexin, Inj. (Hyrex).
Mouthkote P/R, Oint., Spray (Parnell).
Nighttime Sleep Aid, Tab. (Rugby).
Scot-Tussin Allergy DM, Liq. (Scot-Tussin Pharmacal).
Siladryl, Elix. (Silarx).
Silphen DM, Syr. (Silarx).
Span-Lanin, Cap. (Scrip).
Snooze Fast, Tab. (BDI).
40 Winks, Cap. (Roberts Pharm).
Tusstat, Expectorant (Century Pharm).
W/Acetaminophen.
See: Excedrin PM, Preps. (Bristol-Myers Squibb).
Legatrin PM, Capl. (Columbia).
Midol PM, Capl. (Sterling Health).
W/Ammonium Cl, menthol.
See: Eldadryl Expectorant, Liq. (Zeneca)
Fenylex, Expectorant (Roberts Pharm).
Tusstat Expectorant (Century Pharm).
W/Antihistamines.
See: Symptrol, Syr., Cap., Inj. (Saron).
W/Benzethonium Cl.
See: Bendylate, Inj. (Solvay).
W/Chlorobutanol.
See: Ardeben, Inj. (Burgin-Arden).
W/Pheniramine maleate pyrilamine maleate, phenylephrine HCl, phenylpropanolamine HCl.
See: Symptrol, Syr. (Saron).
W/Zinc oxide.
See: Ziradryl, Lot. (Parke-Davis).

diphenhydramine w/combinations.
Benadryl Itch, Preps. (Glaxo-Wellcome).
Dermaycin, Cream, Spray (Pfeiffer).
Dermarest, Gel (Del).
Dermarest Plus, Gel, Spray (Del).

•**diphenidol hydrochloride.** (die-FEN-ih-dahl) USAN.
Use: Antiemetic.

•**diphenidol pamoate.** (die-FEN-ih-dahl) USAN.
Use: Antiemetic.

diphenmethanil methylsulfate.
See: Diphemanil Methylsulfate (Various Mfr.)

•**diphenoxylate hydrochloride.** (die-fen-OX-ih-late) U.S.P. 23.
Use: Antiperistaltic to treat diarrhea.
W/Atropine.
See: Diaction, Tab. (Knoll Pharmaceuticals)
Lomotil, Tab., Liq. (Searle).

diphenoxylate hydrochloride and atropine sulfate. (die-fen-OX-ih-late and AT-troe-peen)
Use: Antiperistaltic.

diphenylhydroxycarbinol. Benzhydrol HCl.

diphenylhydantoin. Phenytoin, U.S.P. 23.
Use: Anticonvulsant.

diphenylhydantoin sodium. Phenytoin Sodium, U.S.P. 23.
Use: Anticonvulsant.

diphenylisatin.
See: Oxyphenisatin (Various Mfr.)

diphosphonic acid.
See: Etidronic acid.

diphosphopyridine (dpn).
Use: Antialcoholic. Under study.

diphosphothiamin. Cocarboxylase.
See: Coenzyme-B, Cap., and Inj. (Inwood).

diphoxazide.

diphtheria, acellular pertussis, tetanus vaccine. (diff-THEER-ee-uh, ay-SELL-you-luhr per-TUSS-iss, TET-ah-nus)
Use: Immunization.
See: Acel-Imune (Wyeth Lederle).
Infanrix (SKB).
Tripedia (Pasteur Merieux Connaught).

•**diphtheria antitoxin.** (diff-THEER-ee-uh) U.S.P. 23.
Use: Passive immunizing agent.

diphtheria antitoxin. (Pasteur Merieux Connaught) 20,000 units, tricresol 4%/vial. (Biocine-Sclavo) 20,000 units, m-cresol 0.3%/vial. (not < 500 units/ml).
Use: I.M. slow I.V. infusion; protection/treatment of diphtheria; immunization.

diphtheria equine antitoxin. *Rx.*
Use: Prophylaxis and treatment of diphtheria.

diphtheria & tetanus toxoids. (diff-THEER-ee-uh & TET-ah-nus)
Use: Immunization.

diphtheria & tetanus toxoids & acellular pertussis vaccine.
See: Acel-Imune, Vial (Wyeth Lederle).
Infanrix, Vial (SmithKline Beecham Pharmaceuticals).
Tripedia, Vial (Pasteur-Merieux-Connaught).

diphtheria & tetanus toxoids, aluminum phosphate adsorbed. (Wyeth Lederle) Tubex 0.5 ml. Vial 5 ml. Pkg. 10s. Available in pediatric and adult strengths. 10 Lf units diphtheria and 5 Lf units tetanus per 0.5 ml dose. 1.5 Lf units diphtheria, 5 Lf units tetanus per 0.5 ml dose. *Rx.*
Use: Immunization.

diphtheria & tetanus toxoids.
Pediatric: (Pasteur-Merieux-Connaught) 6.6 Lf units diphtheria and 5 Lf units tetanus/0.5 ml dose. Vial 5 ml.
(Wyeth Lederle) 12.5 Lf units diphtheria, 5 Lf units tetanus per 0.5 ml dose. Vial 5 ml.
(Massachusetts Public Health Biologic Labs) 7.5 Lf units diphtheria and 7.5 Lf units tetanus/0.5 ml dose. Vial, multidose. *Rx.*
Adult:
(Pasteur-Merieux-Connaught) 2 Lf units diphtheria and 5 Lf units tetanus/0.5 ml dose. Vial 5 ml, 30 ml.
(Wyeth Lederle) 2 Lf units diphtheria and 5 Lf units tetanus per 0.5 ml dose. Vial 5 ml, disp. syringe 0.5 ml, vial 5 ml.
(Massachusetts Public Health Biologic Labs) 2 Lf units diphtheria and 2 Lf units tetanus/0.5 ml dose. Vial, multidose. *Rx.*
Use: Immunization.

diphtheria & tetanus toxoids & whole-cell pertussis vaccine. (diff-THEER-ee-uh & TET-ah-nus & per-TUSS-iss)
(Pasteur-Merieux-Connaught) 6.5 Lf units diphtheria, 5 Lf units tetanus, 4 Lf units pertussis/0.5 ml dose. Vial 2.5 ml, 5 ml, 7.5 ml.
(Massachusetts Public Health Biologic Labs) 10 Lf units diphtheria, 5.5 Lf units tetanus and 4 units pertussis/0.5 ml dose. Vial 5 ml.
Use: Prevention against diphtheria, tetanus and pertussis; immunization.
See: DTwP (Michigan Dept. of Public Health/SmithKline Beecham Pharmaceuticals).
Tri-immunol, Vial (Wyeth Lederle).

diptheria & tetanus toxoids & acellular pertussis vaccine. (U-Line)
Use: Prevention against diphtheria, tetanus, and pertussis; immunizing agent.
See: Acel-Imune, Vial (Wyeth Lederle).
Infanrix, Vial (SKB).
TriHIBit, Kit (Pasteur Merieux Connaught).
Tripedia, Vial (Pasteur Merieux Connaught).

diphtheria & tetanus toxoids & pertussis vaccine adsorbed. (Wyeth Lederle) Vaccine Vial 7.5 ml. *Rx.*
Use: Immunization.

diphtheria & tetanus toxoids & pertussis vaccine combined, aluminum phosphate-adsorbed.
Use: Immunization.
See: Tri-Immunol, Vial (Wyeth Lederle).

•**diphtheria toxin for Schick Test.** (diff-

THEER-ee-uh). U.S.P. 23. *Formerly Diphtheria Toxin, Diagnostic.*
Use: Diagnostic aid (dermal reactivity indicator).

•**diphtheria toxoid.** (diff-THEER-ee-uh) U.S.P. 23.
Use: Immunization (active).

•**diphtheria toxoid adsorbed.** (diff-THEER-ee-uh) U.S.P. 23.
Use: Immunization (active).

diphylline.
See: Diazma, Vial (Pharmex).

Dipimol. (Everett Laboratories) Dipyridamole 25 mg, 50 mg or 75 mg/Tab. Bot. 100s, 500s, 1000s.
Use: Antianginal.

dipivalyl epinephrine.
See: Propine (Allergan).

•**dipivefrin.** (die-PIHV-eh-FRIN) USAN. *Formerly Dipivalyl Epinephrine.*
Use: Adrenergic, ophthalmic.

•**dipivefrin hydrochloride.** (die-PIHV-eh-FRIN) U.S.P. 23.
Use: Antiglaucoma agent.
See: Propine, Soln. (Allergan).

dipivefrin hydrochloride. (Various Mfr.) 0.1% Soln. 5 ml, 10 ml, 15 ml. *Rx.*
Use: Antiglaucoma agent.

Dipyridamole. (Foy) Dipyridamole 25 mg/Tab. Bot. 1000s. *Rx.*
Use: Antianginal.

Diprivan. (Zeneca) Propofol 10 mg/ml. Inj. Amp. 20 ml, 50 ml or 100 ml infusion vials. *Rx.*
Use: Anesthetic, general.

Diprolene AF Cream. (Schering Plough) Betamethasone dipropionate cream equivalent to 0.05% betamethasone. 15 g, 45 g. *Rx.*
Use: Corticosteroid, topical.

Diprolene Cream 0.05%. (Schering Plough) Betamethasone dipropionate 0.05% in cream base. Tube 15 g. *Rx.*
Use: Anti-inflammatory; antipruritic, topical.

Diprolene Ointment 0.05%. (Schering Plough) Betamethasone dipropionate 0.05%, in ointment base. Tube 15 g, 45 g. *Rx.*
Use: Anti-inflammatory; antipruritic, topical.

dipropylacetic acid.
See: Valproic Acid.

Diprosone Aerosol 0.1%. (Schering Plough) Betamethasone dipropionate 6.4 mg (equiv. to 5 mg betamethasone) in vehicle of mineral oil, caprylic-capric triglyceride w/isopropyl alcohol 10%, inert hydrocarbon propellants. (propane and isobutane). Can 85 g. *Rx.*
Use: Corticosteroid, topical.

Diprosone Cream 0.05%. (Schering Plough) Betamethasone dipropionate 0.64 mg (equiv. to 0.5 mg betamethasone) w/mineral oil, white petrolatum, polyethylene glycol 1000 monocetyl ether, cetostearyl alcohol, phosphoric acid, monobasic sodium phosphate with 4-chloro-m-cresol as preservative. Tube 15 g, 45 g. *Rx.*
Use: Corticosteroid, topical.

Diprosone Lotion 0.05%. (Schering Plough) Betamethasone dipropionate 0.64 mg (equivalent to 0.5 mg betamethasone) w/isopropyl alcohol (46.8%), purified water. Bot. 20 ml, 60 ml. *Rx.*
Use: Corticosteroid, topical.

Diprosone Ointment 0.05%. (Schering Plough) Betamethasone dipropionate 0.64 mg (equivalent to 0.5 mg betamethasone) in white petrolatum and mineral oil base. Tube 15 g, 45 g.
Use: Corticosteroid, topical.

•**dipyridamole.** (DIE-pih-RID-uh-mole) U.S.P. 23.
Use: Coronary vasodilator.
See: Persantine, Tab. (Boehringer Ingelheim).
Persantine IV (DuPont Merck Pharmaceuticals).

dipyridamole. (DIE-pih-RID-uh-mole) (Various Mfr.) **25 mg/Tab.:** Bot. 90s, 100s, 500s, 1000s, 5000s, UD 100s. **50 mg, 75 mg/Tab.:** Bot. 100s, 500s, 1000s, UD 100s.
Use: Coronary vasodilator.
See: Persantine (Boehringer Ingelheim).

•**dipyrithione.** (DIE-pihr-ih-THIGH-ohn) USAN.
Use: Antifungal, anti-infective.

•**dipyrone.** (DIE-pie-rone) USAN. *Formerly Methampyrone.*
Use: Analgesic, antipyretic.
See: Novaldin (Sterling Winthrop).

•**dirithromycin.** (die-RITH-row-MY-sin) USAN.
Use: Anti-infective.
See: Dynabac, Tab. (Bock Pharmacal).

disaccharide tripeptide glycerol dipalmitoyl.
Use: Antineoplastic. [Orphan drug]
See: ImmTher (Immuno Therapeutics).

Disalcid. (3M) Salsalate. **Tab.:** 500 mg or 750 mg. Bot. 100s, 500s, UD 100s. **Cap.:** 500 mg. Bot. 100s. *Rx.*
Use: Analgesic.

Discase. (Omnis Surgical) Chymopapain 5 units/2 ml. Vial 5 ml. *Rx.*
Use: Intradiscal injection for herniated lumbar intervertebral discs.

Disinfecting Solution. (Bausch & Lomb) Sodium Cl, sodium borate, boric acid, chlorhexidine 0.005%, EDTA 0.1%, thimerosal 0.001%. Bot. 355 ml. *otc.*
Use: Contact lens care.

•**disiquonium chloride.** (die-SIH-CONE-ee-uhm) USAN.
Use: Antiseptic.

Dismiss Douche. (Schering Plough) Sodium Cl, sodium citrate, citric acid, cetaryl octoate, ceteareth-27, fragrance. Pow. for dilution. Pkg. 2s.
Use: Vaginal agent.

Disobrom. (Geneva Pharm) Pseudoephedrine sulfate 120 mg, dexbrompheniramine maleate 6 mg Tab. Bot 100s, 1000s. *Rx.*
Use: Antihistamine, decongestant.

•**disobutamide.** (DIE-so-BYOO-tam-ide) USAN.
Use: Cardiovascular agent (antiarrhythmic).

disodium carbonate. Sodium Carbonate, N.F. 18.

disodium chromate. Sodium Chromate Cr 51 Injection, U.S.P. 23.

disodium chromoglycate.
See: Intal (Medeva).
Nasalcrom (Medeva).

disodium clodronate. (Discovery Experimental & Development)
Use: Antihypercalcemic. [Orphan drug]

disodium clodronate tetrahydrate.
Use: Increased bone resorption due to malignancy. [Orphan drug]
See: Bonefos (Leiras Pharm).

disodium edathamil.
See: Edathamil Disodium (Various Mfr.)

disodium edetate. Disodium ethylenediaminetetra acetate.
See: Edetate Disodium, U.S.P. 23.

disodium phosphate.
See: Sodium Phosphate, U.S.P. 23.

disodium phosphate heptahydrate. Sodium Phosphate, U.S.P. 23.

disodium thiosulfate pentahydrate. Sodium Thiosulfate, U.S.P. 23.

di-sodium versenate.
See: Edathamil Disodium (Various Mfr.)

•**disofenin.** (DIE-so-FEN-in) USAN.
Use: Diagnostic aid (carrier agent).

Disophrol. (Schering Plough) Pseudoephedrine sulfate 60 mg, dexbrompheniramine maleate 2 mg. Tab. Bot. 100s. *otc.*
Use: Antihistamine, decongestant.

Disophrol Chronotabs. (Schering-Plough) Dexbrompheniramine maleate 6 mg, pseudoephedrine sulfate 120 mg/SA Tab. Bot. 100s. *otc.*
Use: Antihistamine, decongestant.

•**disopyramide.** (DIE-so-PIR-uh-mide) USAN.
Use: Cardiovascular agent (antiarrhythmic).

•**disopyramide phosphate.** (DIE-so-PIHR-ah-mid) U.S.P. 23.
Use: Cardiovascular agent, antiarrhythmic.
See: Norpace (Searle).

disopyramide phosphate extended-release capsules. (DIE-so-PIHR-ah-mid)
Use: Cardiovascular agent, antiarrhythmic.

Disotate. (Steris) Edetate disodium 150 mg/ml. Vial 20 ml. *Rx.*
Use: Antihypercalcemic.

•**disoxaril.** (die-SOX-ar-ILL) USAN.
Use: Antiviral.

Di-Spaz. (Vortech) Dicyclomine HCl. **Cap.:** 10 mg. Bot. 1000s. **Inj.:** 10 mg. Vial 10 ml. *Rx.*
Use: Gastrointestinal, anticholinergic.

Dispos-a-Med. (Parke-Davis) Isoetharine HCl 0.5% or 1%. Can of prefilled sterile tubes 0.5 ml, 50s. *Rx.*
Use: Bronchodilator.

distaquaine.
See: Penicillin V.

distigmine bromide. Hexamarium bromide.

•**disulfiram.** (die-SULL-fih-ram) U.S.P. 23.
Use: Alcohol deterrent.
See: Antabuse, Tab. (Wyeth Ayerst).

disulfonamide.
See: Dia-Mer-Sulfonamides (Various Mfr.)

Dital. (UAD) Phendimetrazine tartrate 105 mg/SR Cap. Bot. 100s. *c-III.*
Use: Anorexiant.

Ditate D.S. (Savage) Testosterone enanthate 360 mg, estradiol valerate 16 mg, benzyl alcohol 2% in sesame oil. Syringe 2 ml Box 10s. Vial 2 ml. *Rx.*
Use: Androgen, estrogen combination.

•**ditekiren.** (DIE-teh-KIE-ren) USAN.
Use: Antihypertensive.

dithranol.
See: Anthralin, U.S.P. 23. (Various Mfr.)

D.I.T.I. Creme. (Dunhall Pharmaceuticals) Iodoquinol 100 mg, sulfanilamide 500 mg, diethylstilbestrol 0.1 mg/g Jar. 4 oz. *Rx.*

Use: Anti-infective, vaginal.

D.I.T.I.-2 Creme. (Dunhall Pharmaceuticals) Sulfanilamide 15%, aminacrine HCl 0.2%, allantoin 2%. Tube 142 g. *Rx.*
Use: Anti-infective, vaginal.

Ditropan. (Alza) Oxybutynin Cl 5 mg, lactose/Tab. Bot. 100s, 1000s, UD 100s. *Rx.*
Use: Urinary tract agent.

Ditropan Syrup. (Alza) Oxybutynin Cl. 5 mg/5 ml sorbitol, sucrose, methylparaben. Syr. Bot. 473 ml. *Rx.*
Use: Genitourinary.

Diucardin. (Wyeth Ayerst) Hydroflumethiazide 50 mg/Tab. Bot. 100s. *Rx.*
Use: Antihypertensive, diuretic.

Diulo. (Searle) Metolazone. 2.5 mg, 5 mg or 10 mg/Tab. Bot. 100s. *Rx.*
Use: Antihypertensive, diuretic.

Diurese. (American Urologicals) Trichlormethiazide 4 mg/Tab. Bot. 100s, 1000s. *Rx.*
Use: Diuretic.

diuretic combinations.
See: Moduretic, Tab. (Merck).
Spironolactone w/Hydrochlorothiazide, Tab. (Various Mfr.)
Alazide, Tab. (Major).
Aldactazide, Tab. (Searle).
Dyazide, Cap. (SKB).
Maxzide, Tab. (ESI Lederle Generics).
Maxzide-25 MG, Tab. (ESI Lederle Generics).
Spironazide, Tab. (Schein).
Spirozide, Tab. (Rugby).
Triamterene w/Hydrochlorthiazide, Cap. (Various Mfr.)
Triamterene w/Hydrochlorothiazide, Tab. (Various Mfr.)

diuretics, loop.
See: Bumex, Inj., Tab. (Roche).
Edecrin, Tab. (Merck).
Edecrin Sodium, Inj. (Merck).
Fumide, Tab. (Everett Laboratories).
Furomide M.D., Inj. (Hyrex).
Furosemide, Inj., Tab. (Various Mfr.)
Furosemide, Oral Soln. (Roxane).
Lasix, Inj., Oral Soln., Tab. (Hoechst Marion Roussel).
Luramide, Tab. (Major).

diuretics, osmotic.
See: Glyrol, Soln. (Ciba Vision Ophthalmics).
Ismotic, Soln. (Alcon Laboratories).
Mannitol, Inj. (Various Mfr.)
Osmitrol, Inj. (Baxter).
Osmoglyn, Soln. (Alcon Laboratories).
Ureaphil, Inj. (Abbott Laboratories).

diuretics, potassium-sparing.
See: Alatone, Tab. (Major).
Aldactone, Tab. (Searle).
Amiloride HCl, Tab. (Various Mfr.)
Dyrenium, Cap. (SmithKline Beecham Pharmaceuticals).
Midamor, Tab. (Merck).
Spironolactone, Tab. (Various Mfr.)

diuretics, thiazides.
See: Anhydron, Tab. (Eli Lilly).
Aquatag, Tab. (Solvay).
Aquatensen, Tab. (Wallace).
Chlorothiazide, Tab. (Various Mfr.)
Chlorthalidone, Tab. (Various Mfr.)
Diachlor, Tab. (Major).
Diaqua, Tab. (Roberts Pharm).
Diucardin, Tab. (Wyeth Ayerst).
Diulo, Tab. (Searle).
Diurese, Tab. (American Urologicals).
Diurigen, Tab. (Zenith Goldline).
Diuril, Oral Susp., Tab. (Merck).
Diuril Sodium, Inj. (Merck).
Enduron, Tab. (Abbott Laboratories).
Esidrix, Tab. (Novartis).
Ethon, Tab. (Major).
Exna, Tab. (Robins).
Hydrex, Tab. (Trimen).
Hydrochlorothiazide, Tab. (Various Mfr.)
Hydrochlorothiazide, Oral Soln. (Roxane).
HydroDIURIL, Tab. (Merck).
Hydroflumethiazide, Tab. (Various Mfr.)
Hydromal, Tab. (Roberts Pharm).
Hydromox, Tab. (ESI Lederle Generics).
Hydro-T, Tab. (Major).
Hydro-Z-50, Tab. (Mayrand).
Hydrozide-50, Tab. (T.E. Williams).
Hygroton, Tab. (Rhone-Poulenc Rorer).
Hylidone, Tab. (Major).
Lozol, Tab. (Rhone-Poulenc Rorer).
Metahydrin, Tab. (Hoechst Marion Roussel).
Methyclothiazide, Tab. (Various Mfr.)
Mictrin, Tab. (Econo Med Pharmaceuticals).
Mykrox (Medeva).
Naqua, Tab. (Schering Plough).
Naturetin, Tab. (Bristol-Myers).
Niazide, Tab. (Major).
Oretic, Tab. (Abbott Laboratories).
Proaqua, Tab. (Solvay).
Renese, Tab. (Pfizer).
Saluron, Tab. (Bristol-Myers).
Thalitone, Tab. (Boehringer Ingelheim).
Thiuretic, Tab. (Warner-Chilcott).
Trichlormethiazide, Tab. (Various Mfr.)

Zaroxolyn, Tab. (Medeva).

Diuretic Tablets. (Faraday) Buchu leaves 150 mg, uva ursi leaves 150 mg, juniper berries 120 mg, bone meal, parsley, asparagus/Tab. Bot. 100s. *Rx.*
Use: Diuretic.

Diurigen Tablets. (Zenith Goldline) Chlorothiazide 500 mg/Tab Bot. 100s, 1000s. *Rx.*
Use: Diuretic.

Diurigen w/Reserpine 250 Tablets. (Zenith Goldline). Chlorothiazide 250 mg, reserpine 0.125 mg. Tab. Bot. 100s, 1000s. *Rx.*
Use: Antihypertensive combination.

Diurigen w/Reserpine 500 Tablets. (Zenith Goldline). Chlorothiazide 500 mg, reserpine 0.125 mg. Tab. Bot. 100s, 1000s. *Rx.*
Use: Antihypertensive combination.

Diuril. (Merck) Chlorothiazide, U.S.P. **Tab.:** 250 mg Bot. 100s, 1000s; 500 mg Bot. 100s, 1000s, UD 100s. **Oral Susp.:** 250 mg/5 ml w/methylparaben 0.12%, propylparaben 0.02%, benzoic acid 0.1%, alcohol 0.5%. Bot. 237 ml. *Rx.*
Use: Antihypertensive, diuretic.
W/Methyldopa.
See: Aldoclor, Tab. (Merck).
W/Reserpine.
See: Diupres, Tab. (Merck).

Diuril Sodium Intravenous. (Merck) Chlorothiazide sodium equivalent to 0.5 g chlorothiazide w/mannitol 0.25 g sodium hydroxide, thimerosal 0.4 mg. Vial 20 ml. *Rx.*
Use: Antihypertensive, diuretic.

Diutensen-R. (Wallace) Methyclothiazide 2.5 mg, reserpine 0.1 mg/Tab. Bot. 100s, 500s, 5000s. *Rx.*
Use: Antihypertensive combination.

•**divalproex sodium.** (die-VAL-pro-ex) USAN.
Use: Anticonvulsant.
See: Depakote (Abbott Laboratories).

divinyl oxide. Vinyl ether, divinyl ether.
Use: Inhalation anesthetic.

Dizac. (Ohmeda) Diazepam 5 mg/ml, preservative free. Inj. Vial 3 ml. *c-IV.*
Use: Anxiolytic, anticonvulsant, muscle relaxant.

Dizmiss. (Jones Medical Industries) Meclizine HCl 25 mg/Tab. Bot. 100s, 1000s. *otc.*
Use: Antiemetic, antivertigo.

•**dizocilpine maleate.** (die-ZOE-sill-PEEN) USAN.
Use: Neuroprotective.

dl-desoxyephedrine hydrochloride.
See: dl-Methamphetamine HCl.

dl-methamphetamine hydrochloride. dl-Desoxyephedrine HCl.
See: Oxydess, Tab. (Vortech).
W/Pyrilamine maleate, phenyltoloxamine dihydrogen citrate, didesoxyephedrine HCl, codeine phosphate, ammonium Cl, potassium guaiacolsulfonate, chloroform, phenylpropanolamine tartar emetic.
See: Meditussin-X Liquid (Roberts Pharm).

dl-norephedrine hydrochloride.
See: Phenylpropanolamine Hydrochloride (Various Mfr.)

DM Cough. (Rosemont) Dextromethorphan HBr 10 mg/5 ml, alcohol 5%. Syr. Bot. 120 ml, pt, gal. *otc.*
Use: Antitussive.

DMCT. (ESI Lederle Generics) Demethylchlortetracycline. *Rx.*
Use: Anti-infective, tetracycline.
See: Declomycin HCl, Preps. (ESI Lederle Generics).

d-methorphan hydrobromide.
See: Dextromethorphan HBr (Various Mfr.).

d-methylphenylamine sulfate.
See: Dextroamphetamine Sulfate, U.S.P. 23. (Various Mfr.).

DML Dermatological Moisturizing Lotion. (Person & Covey) Purified water, petrolatum, glycerin, methyl glucose sesquisterate, dimethicone, methyl gluceth-20 sesquisterate, benzyl alcohol, volatile silicone, glyceryl stearate, stearic acid, palmitic acid, cetyl alcohol, xanthan gum, magnesium aluminum silicate carbomer 941, sodium hydroxide. Bot. 8 oz. *otc.*
Use: Emollient.

DML Facial Moisturizer. (Person & Covey) Octyl methoxycinnamate 8%, oxybenzone 4%, benzyl alcohol, petrolatum, EDTA. SPF 15. Cream 45 g. *otc.*
Use: Sunscreen.

DML Forte. (Person & Covey) Petrolatum, PPG-2 myristyl ether propionate, glyceryl stearate, glycerin, stearic acid, d-panthenol, DEA-cetyl phosphate, simethicone, PVP eicosene copolymer, benzyl alcohol, cetyl alcohol, silica, disodium EDTA, BHA, magnesium aluminum silicate, sodium carbomer 1342. Tube 113 g. *otc.*
Use: Emollient.

dmp 777. (DuPont Merck)
Use: Cystic fibrosis. [Orphan drug].

DMSO.
See: Dimethyl sulfoxide.
n-DNA.

DNR.
See: Cerubidine (Wyeth Ayerst).

Doak Tar Distillate. (Doak Dermatologics) Coal tar distillate 40%. Liq. Bot. 59 ml. *otc.*
Use: Antiseborrheic.

Doak Tar Lotion. (Doak Dermatologics) Tar distillate 5%. Bot. 118 ml. *otc.*
Use: Antiseborrheic.

Doak Tar Oil. (Doak Dermatologics) Tar distillate 2%. Liq. Bot. 237 ml. *otc.*
Use: Antiseborrheic.

Doak Tar Oil Forte. (Doak Dermatologics) Tar distillate 5%. Bot. 4 oz.
Use: Antiseborrheic.

Doak Tar Shampoo. (Doak Dermatologics) Tar distillate 3% in shampoo base. Bot. 237 ml. *otc.*
Use: Antiseborrheic.

Doak Tersaseptic. (Doak Dermatologics) Liquid cleanser, pH 6.8. Bot. 4 oz, pt, gal. *otc.*
Use: Detergent.

Doan's Backache Spray. (DEP Corp) Methyl salicylate 15%, menthol 8.4%, methyl nicotinate 0.6%. Aerosol can 4 oz. *otc.*
Use: Analgesic, topical.

Doan's PM, Extra Strength.
See: Extra Strength Doan's PM, Capl. (Ciba).

Doan's Pills. (DEP Corp) Magnesium salicylate 325 mg/Tab. Ctn. 24s, 48s. *otc.*
Use: Analgesic.

•**dobutamine for injection.** (doe-BYOOT-ah-meen) U.S.P. 23
Use: Cardiovascular agent.

•**dobutamine hydrochloride.** (doe-BYOOT-ah-meen) U.S.P. 23.
Use: Cardiovascular agent.
See: Dobutrex, Inj. (Eli Lilly).

dobutamine hydrochloride. (Various Mfr.) 12.5 mg/ml. May contain sulfites. Inj. Vial 20 ml.
Use: Cardiovascular agent.

•**dobutamine lactobionate.** (doe-BYOOT-ah-meen) USAN.
Use: Cardiovascular agent.

•**dobutamine tartrate.** (doe-BYOOT-ah-meen) USAN.
Use: Cardiovascular agent.

Dobutrex Solution. (Eli Lilly) Dobutamine HCl 250 mg. Inj. Vial 20 ml. *Rx.*
Use: Cardiovascular agent.

•**docebenone.** (dah-SEH-beh-nohn) USAN.
Use: Inhibitor (5-lipoxygenase).
See: Antiallergic, antiasthmatic.

•**docetaxel.** (doe-seh-TAX-ehl) USAN.
Use: Antineoplastic.
See: Taxotere (Rhone-Poulenc Rorer).

•**doconazole.** (doe-KOE-nah-zole) USAN.
Use: Antifungal.

Doctar. (Savage) Coal tar 0.5%, conditioner. Shampoo. Bot. 100 ml. *otc.*
Use: Antiseborrheic.

Doctase. (Purepac) Docusate sodium 100 mg, casanthranol 30 mg/Cap. Bot. 100s. *otc.*
Use: Laxative.

Doctyl. (Health for Life Brands) Docusate sodium 100 mg/Tab. Bot. 40s, 100s, 1000s. *otc.*
Use: Laxative.

Doctylax. (Health for Life Brands) Docusate sodium 100 mg, acetophenolisatin 2 mg, prune conc. ¾ mg/Tab. Bot. 40s, 100s, 1000s. *otc.*
Use: Laxative.

Docucal-P Softgels. (Parmed) Docusate (as calcium) 60 mg, phenolphthalein 65 mg/Cap. Bot. 100s, 1000s. *otc.*
Use: Laxative.

•**docusate calcium.** (DOCK-you-sate) U.S.P. 23. *Formerly Dioctyl Calcium Sulfosuccinate.*
Use: Laxative, stool softener.
See: Surfak, Cap. (Hoechst Marion Roussel).
Doxidan, Cap. (Hoechst Marion Roussel).
Danthron, Tab. (Zenith Goldline).

docusate with casanthranol. (DOCK-you-sate) (Various Mfr.) Docusate (as sodium) 100 mg, casanthranol 30 mg/Cap. Bot. 100s, 1000s, UD 100s. *otc.*
Use: Laxative, stool softener.

•**docusate potassium.** U.S.P. 23.
Use: Laxative, stool softener.
See: Dialose, Cap. (Stuart).
Dialose Plus, Cap. (Stuart).
Kasof, Cap. (Stuart).

•**docusate sodium.** (DOCK-you-sate) U.S.P. 23. *Formerly Dioctyl Sodium Sulfosuccinate.*
Use: Pharmaceutical aid (surfactant), stool softener.
See: Colace, Cap., Liq., Syr. (Bristol-Myers).
Coloctyl, Cap. (Eon Labs Manufacturing).
Comfolax, Cap. (Searle).
Correctol Extra Gentle, Cap. (Schering Plough).

Dialose Preps. (Merck).
Diomedicone, Tab (Medicone).
Diosate Caps. (Towne).
Doss, Super Doss, Tab. (Ferndale Laboratories).
Doxinate, Cap., Liq. (Hoechst Marion Roussel).
DSS (Parke-Davis).
Duosol, Cap. (Kirkman Sales).
Dynoctol, Cap. (Solvay).
Easy-Lax, Cap. (Walgreen).
Konsto, Cap. (Freeport).
Laxatab, Tab. (Freeport).
Liqui-Doss, Liq. (Ferndale Laboratories).
Modane Soft, Cap. (Pharmacia & Upjohn).
Peri-Doss, Cap. (Ferndale Laboratories).
Phillips Laxative, Gelcaps (Sterling Health).
Regul-Aid, Syr. (Quality Generics).
Regutol, Tab. (Schering Plough).
Silace, Syr. (Silarx).
Silace-C, Syr. (Silarx).
Stulex, Tab. (Jones Medical Industries).
Surfak, Cap. (Hoechst Marion Roussel).

W/Ascorbic acid, ferrous fumarate.
See: Hemaspan Cap. (Bock Pharmacal).

W/Betaine HCl, zinc, manganese, molybdenum.
See: Hemaferrin (Western Research).

W/Bisacodyl.
See: Laxadan, Supp. (Teva USA).

W/Brewer's yeast.
See: Doss or Super Doss, Tab. (Ferndale Laboratories).

W/Casanthranol.
See: Calotabs, Tab. (Calotabs).
Constiban (Quality Generics).
Diolax, Cap. (Century Pharm).
Dio-Soft (Standex). (Drug).
Easy-Lax Plus, Cap. (Walgreen).
Genericace, Cap. (Forest Pharmaceutical)
Neo-Vadrin D-D-S, Cap. (Scherer).
Nuvac, Cap. (LaCrosse).
Peri-Colace, Cap., Syr. (Bristol-Myers).

W/Casanthranol, sodium carboxymethylcellulose.
See: Dialose Plus, Cap. (Stuart).
Tri-Vac, Cap. (Rhode).

W/Dehydrocholic acid.
See: Dubbalax-B, Cap. (Redford).
Dubbalax-N, Cap. (Redford).
Neolax, Tab. (Schwarz Pharma).

W/D-calcium pantothenate and acetphenolisatin.
See: Peri-Pantyl, Tab. (McGregor).

W/Ferrous fumarate, Vitamin C.
See: Hemaspan, Cap. (Bock Pharmacal).
Recoup, Tab. (ESI Lederle Generics).

W/Ferrous fumarate, vitamins.
See: Bevitone, Tab. (Teva USA).

W/Ferrous fumarate, betaine HCl, desiccated liver, vitamins, minerals.
See: Hemaferrin, Tab. (Western Research).

W/Glycerin.
See: Rectalad Enema, Liq. (Wampole).

W/Isobornyl thiocyanoacetate.
See: Barc, Cream, Liq. (Del Pharm)

W/Petrolatum.
See: Milkinol, Liq., Emulsion (Kremers Urban).

W/Phenolphthalein.
See: Correctol, Tab. (Schering Plough).
Ex-Lax Prods. (Sandoz Consumer).
Feen-A-Mint, Pills (Schering Plough).

W/Phenolphthalein, dehydrocholic acid.
See: Bolax, Cap. (Boyd).
Sarolax, Cap. (Saron).
Tripalax, Cap. (Redford).

W/Polyoxyethylene nonyl phenol, sodium edetate, and 9-aminoacridine HCl.
See: Vagisec Plus Supp. (Schmid).

W/Senna concentrate.
See: Gentlax S, Tab. (Blair Laboratories).
Sarolax (Saron).
Senokap-DDS, Cap. (Purdue Frederick).
Senokot S, Tab. (Purdue Frederick).

W/Sodium propionate, propionic acid, salicylic acid.
See: Prosal, Liq. (Gordon Laboratories).

W/Vitamin-mineral combination.
See: Geriplex-FS, Kapseal (Parke-Davis).
Materna 1.60, Tab. (ESI Lederle Generics).

doderlein bacilli.
See: Redoderlein, Vial (Forest Pharmaceutical)

•**dofetilide.** (doe-FEH-till-ide) USAN.
Use: Cardiovascular agent (antiarrhythmic).

Dofus. (Miller) Freeze dried *Lactobacillus acidophilus* minimum of 100,000,000 organisms/Cap. w/*Lactobacillus bifidus* organisms added. Bot. 60s. *otc.*
Use: Nutritional supplement, antidiarrheal.

DOK. (Major) Docusate sodium. **Caps.:** 250 mg. Bot. 100s, 1000s. **Liq.:** 150 mg/15 ml. Bot. pt. **Syrup:** 60 mg/15 ml. Bot. pt, gal. *otc.*

Use: Laxative, stool softener.

DOK-250. (Major) Docusate sodium 250 mg. Cap. Bot. 100s. *otc.*
Use: Laxative, stool softener.

Doktors Spray. (Scherer) Phenylephrine HCl 0.25%, chlorobutanol, sodium bisulfite, benzalkonium chloride. Soln. Bot. 30 ml. *otc.*
Use: Decongestant.

Dolacet. (Roberts Pharm) Hydrocodone bitartrate 5 mg, acetaminophen 500 mg/Cap. Bot. 100s. *c-III.*
Use: Analgesic combination, narcotic.

Dolamide Tabs. (Major) Chlorpropamide 100 mg or 250 mg/Tab. Bot. 100s, 500s, 1000s. *Rx.*
Use: Antidiabetic.

Dolamin. (Harvey) Ammonium sulfate 0.75% with sodium Cl, benzyl alcohol. Amp. 10 ml. In 12s, 25s, 100s. *Rx.*
Use: Antineuralgic.

dolantin.
See: Meperidine HCl, U.S.P. 23.

•**dolasetron mesylate.** (dahl-AH-set-rahn) USAN.
Use: Antiemetic, antimigraine.
See: Anzemet Tab., Inj. (Hoechst Marion Roussel).

Dolcin. (Dolcin) Aspirin 3.7 gr, calcium succinate 2.8 gr/Tab. Bot. 100s, 200s. *otc.*
Use: Analgesic.

Doldram. (Dram) Salicylamide 7.5 gr/Tab. Bot. 100s.
Use: Analgesic.

Dolene AP-65. (ESI Lederle Generics) Propoxyphene HCl 65 mg, acetaminophen 650 mg/Tab. Bot. 100s, 500s. *c-IV.*
Use: Analgesic combination, narcotic.

Dolene Compound-65. (ESI Lederle Generics) Propoxyphene HCl 65 mg, aspirin 389 mg, caffeine 32.4 mg/Cap. Bot. 100s, 500s. *c-IV.*
Use: Analgesic combination, narcotic.

Dolene Plain. (ESI Lederle Generics) Propoxyphene HCl 65 mg/Cap. Bot. 100s, 500s. *c-IV.*
Use: Analgesic, narcotic.

Dolobid. (Merck) Diflunisal 250 mg or 500 mg/Tab. Unit-of-use 60s, UD 100s. *Rx.*
Use: Analgesic.

Dolomite. (NBTY) Magnesium 78 mg, calcium 130 mg/Tab. Bot. 100s, 250s. *otc.*
Use: Mineral supplement.

Dolomite. (Halsey) Calcium 426 mg, magnesium 246 mg/3 Tab. w/guar and acacia gum. Bot. 250s. *otc.*
Use: Mineral supplement.

Dolomite Plus Capsules. (Barth's) Magnesium 37 mg, calcium 187 mg, phosphorous 50 mg, iodine 0.25 mg/Cap. Bot. 100s, 500s, 1000s. *otc.*
Use: Mineral supplement.

Dolomite Tablets. (Faraday) Calcium 150 mg, magnesium 90 mg/Tab. Bot. 250s. *otc.*
Use: Mineral supplement.

dolonil. (Parke-Davis)
See: Pyridium Plus, Tab. (Parke-Davis).

Dolophine Hydrochloride. (Eli Lilly) Methadone HCl. **Amp.:** (10 mg/ml; sodium Cl 0.9%) 1 ml 12s, 100s. **Vial:** (10 mg/ml) 20 ml (sodium Cl 0.9%, chlorobutanol 0.5%). 1s, 25s. **Tab.:** 5 mg, Bot. 100s. 10 mg, Bot. 100s. *c-II.*
Use: Analgesic, narcotic.

Dolopirona Tablets. (Sanofi Winthrop) Dipyrone with chlormezanone. *Rx.*
Use: Analgesic, anxiolytic, muscle relaxant.

Dolorac. (GenDerm) Capsaicin 0.25%, benzyl alcohol, cetyl alcohol/Cream. Tube 28 g. *otc.*
Use: Analgesic, topical.

Doloral. (Progressive Enterprises) Colchicine salicylate 0.1 mg, phenobarbital 8 mg, sodium p-amino-benzoate 15 mg, vitamins B_1 25 mg, aspirin 325 mg/Tab. Bot. 100s, 1000s. *Rx.*
Use: Antiarthritic, antigout.

dolosal.
See: Meperidine HCl.

Dolsed. (American Urologicals) Methenamine 40.8 mg, phenylsalicylate 18.1 mg, atropine sulfate 0.03 mg, hyoscyamine 0.03 mg, benzoic acid 4.5 mg, methylene blue 5.4 mg. Tab. Bot. 100s, 1000s. *Rx.*
Use: Anti-infective, urinary.

dolvanol.
Use: Analgesic, narcotic.
See: Meperidine HCl.

•**domazoline fumarate.** (DOME-AZE-oh-leen) USAN.
Use: Anticholinergic.

Domeboro. (Bayer Corp) Aluminum sulfate and calcium acetate when added to water gives therapeutic effect of Burow's. One pkg. or Tab./pt. water approximately equivalent to 1:40 dilution. **Pkg.:** 2.2 g, 12s, 100s. **Effervescent Tab.:** Box 12s, 100s, 1000s. *otc.*
Use: Anti-inflammatory, topical.

Domeboro Otic. (Bayer Corp) Acetic acid 2% (in aluminum acetate solution).

Soln. Bot. 60 ml with dropper. *Rx.*
Use: Otic.

Dome-Paste Bandage. (Bayer Corp) Zinc oxide, calamine and gelatin bandage. Pkg. 4"×10 yd. and 3"×10 yd. impregnated gauze bandage. *otc.*
Use: Dermatologic, wound therapy.

domestrol.
See: Diethylstilbestrol, Preps. (Various Mfr.)

D.O.M.F.
Use: Antimicrobial.
See: Merbromin (Mercurochrome) (City Chem.).

•**domiodol.** (dome-EYE-oh-DOLE) USAN.
Use: Mucolytic.

•**domiphen bromide.** (DOE-mih-fen) USAN.
Use: Antiseptic; anti-infective, topical.
See: Bradosol.
Domibrom.

Domol Bath and Shower Oil. (Bayer Corp) D_1-isopropyl sebacate, isopropyl myristate with mineral oil. Bot. 240 ml. *otc.*
Use: Emollient.

•**domperidone.** (dome-PEH-rih-dohn) USAN.
Use: Antiemetic.
See: Motilium (Janssen).

Donatussin DC Syrup. (Laser) Hydrocodone bitartrate 2.5 mg, phenylephrine HCl 7.5 mg, guaifenesin 50 mg/5 ml. Bot. 120 ml, 480 ml. *c-III.*
Use: Antitussive, decongestant, expectorant.

Donatussin Pediatric Drops. (Laser) Guaifenesin 20 mg, chlorpheniramine maleate 1 mg, phenylephrine HCl 2 mg/ml. Drop. Bot. 30 ml. *Rx.*
Use: Antihistamine, decongestant, expectorant.

Donatussin Syrup. (Laser) Phenylephrine 10 mg, chlorpheniramine maleate 2 mg, dextromethorphan HBr 7.5 mg, guaifenesin 100 mg. Bot. pt, gal. *Rx.*
Use: Antihistamine, antitussive, decongestant, expectorant.

Dondril. (Whitehall Robins) Dextromethorphan HBr 10 mg, phenylephrine HCl 5 mg, chlorpheniramine maleate 1 mg/Tab. Bot. 24s. *otc.*
Use: Antihistamine, antitussive, decongestant.

donepezil HCl. (Eisai/Pfizer)
Use: Treatment of mild to moderate dementia of the Alzheimer's type.
See: Aricept, Tab. (Eisai/Pfizer).

•**donetidine.** (doe-NEH-tih-DEEN) USAN.
Use: Antiulcerative.

Donna. (Arcum) Menthol, thymol, eucalyptol, exsiccated alum, boric acid. 4 oz, 14 oz. *Rx.*
Use: Vaginal agent.

Donnagel. (Wyeth Ayerst) Attapulgite 600 mg. Chew. Tab. Pkg. 18s; Liq. Bot. 120 ml, 240 ml. *otc.*
Use: Antidiarrheal.

Donnamar. (H.L. Moore) Atropine sulfate 0.0194 mg, scopolamine HBr 0.0065 mg, hyoscyamine HBr or SO_4 0.1037 mg, phenobarbital 16.2 mg/5 ml, alcohol 23%. Elix. Bot. 120 ml, pt, gal. *Rx.*
Use: Anticholinergic, antispasmodic.

Donnamar. (Marnel) Hyoscyamine sulfate 0.125 mg. Tab. Bot. 100s. *Rx.*
Use: Anticholinergic, antispasmodic.

Donnaphen Elixir. (Health for Life Brands) Phenobarbital 16.2 mg, hyoscyamine sulfate 0.1037 mg, atropine sulfate 0.0194 mg, hyoscine HBr 0.0065 mg/5 ml. Bot. pt, gal. *Rx.*
Use: Anticholinergic, antispasmodic.

Donna-Sed Elixir. (Vortech) Atropine sulfate 0.0194 mg, scopolamine HBr 0.0065, hyoscyamine HBr or SO_4 0.1037 mg, phenobarbital 16.2 mg, alcohol 23%. Liq. Bot. 118 ml, gal. *Rx.*
Use: Gastrointestinal, anticholinergic.

Donnatal. (Robins) Hyoscyamine sulfate 0.1037 mg, atropine sulfate 0.0194 mg, scopolamine HBr 0.0065 mg, phenobarbital 16.2 mg. **Cap. & Tab.:** Bot. 100s, 1000s. **Elix.:** w/alcohol 23%. Bot. 4 oz, pt, gal, Dis-Co pack 5 ml, 100s. *Rx.*
Use: Anticholinergic, antispasmodic, sedative.

Donnatal Dis-Co UD Pack. (Robins) Hyoscyamine sulfate 0.1037 mg, atropine sulfate 0.0194 mg, hyoscine HBr 0.0065 mg, phenobarbital 16.2 mg (0.25 gr)/Tab. or 5 ml. **Tab.:** UD 100s. **Elix.:** UD (5 ml) 25s. *Rx.*
Use: Anticholinergic, antispasmodic, sedative.

Donnatal Elixir. (Robins) Atropine sulfate 0.0194 mg, scopolamine HBr 0.0065 mg, hyoscyamine HBr or sulfate 0.1037 mg, phenobarbital 16.2 mg, alcohol 23%, glucose, saccharin/5 ml. Bot. 120 ml, pt., gal, Dis-Co pack 5 ml. *Rx.*
Use: Gastrointestinal, anticholinergic.

Donnatal Extentabs. (Robins) Hyoscyamine sulfate 0.3111 mg, atropine sulfate 0.0582 mg, scopolamine HBr 0.0195 mg, phenobarbital 48.6 mg (¾

gr)/Tab. Bot. 100s, 500s, Dis-Co pack 100s. *Rx.*
Use: Anticholinergic, antispasmodic, sedative.

Donnatal #2. (Robins) Phenobarbital 32.4 mg (0.5 gr), hyoscyamine sulfate 0.1037 mg, atropine sulfate 0.0194 mg, scopolamine HBr 0.0065 mg/Tab. Bot. 100s, 1000s. *Rx.*
Use: Anticholinergic, antispasmodic, sedative.

Donnazyme. (Robins) Hyoscyamine sulfate 0.0518 mg, atropine sulfate 0.0097 mg, scopolamine HBr 0.0033 mg, phenobarbital 8.1 mg (1/8 gr), pepsin 150 mg/Tab. in outer layer, pancreatin 300 mg, bile salts 150 mg/Tab. in core. Bot. 100s, 500s. *Rx.*
Use: Anticholinergic, antispasmodic, digestive aid.

Don't. (Del Pharm) Sucrose octa acetate 5%, isopropyl alcohol 54%. Bot. 0.45 oz. *otc.*
Use: Nail biting deterrent.

•**dopamantine.** (DOE-pah-MAN-teen) USAN.
Use: Antiparkinsonian.

dopamine. (DOE-pah-meen) (Astra) Dopamine. **Amp.:** 200 mg/5 ml Amp. Box 10s; 400 mg/10 ml Amp. Box 5s. **Additive Syringe:** 200 mg/5 ml Syr. Box 1s; 400 mg/10 ml Syr. Box 1s. *Rx.*
Use: Inotropic agent.

•**dopamine hydrochloride.** (DOE-puh-meen) U.S.P. 23.
Use: Adrenergic.
See: Intropin, Amp. (DuPont Merck Pharmaceuticals).

dopamine hydrochloride and dextrose injection. (DOE-pah-meen)
Use: Adrenergic, emergency treatment of low blood pressure.

Dopar. (Procter & Gamble) Levodopa 100 mg or 250 mg/Cap. Bot. 100s. 500 mg/Cap. Bot. 100s, 1000s. *Rx.*
Use: Antiparkinsonian.

•**dopexamine.** (doe-PEX-ah-MEEN) USAN.
Use: Cardiovascular agent.

•**dopexamine hydrochloride.** (doe-PEX-ah-MEEN) USAN.
Use: Cardiovascular agent.

Dopram. (Robins) Doxapram HCl 20 mg/ml, 0.9% benzyl alcohol. Vial 20 ml. *Rx.*
Use: Respiratory.

Doral. (Wallace) Quazepam 7.5 mg or 15 mg/Tab. Bot. 100s, UD 100s. *c-IV.*
Use: Hypnotic, sedative.

•**dorastine hydrochloride.** (DAHR-ass-teen HIGH-droe-KLOR-ide) USAN.
Use: Antihistamine.

Dorcol Children's Cold Formula. (Sandoz Consumer) Pseudoephedrine HCl 15 mg, chlorpheniramine maleate 1 mg/5 ml. Bot. 120 ml. *otc.*
Use: Antihistamine, decongestant.

Dorcol Children's Cough Syrup. (Sandoz Consumer) Dextromethorphan HBr 5 mg, pseudoephedrine HCl 15 mg, guaifenesin 50 mg/5 ml. Bot. 120 ml, 240 ml. *otc.*
Use: Antitussive, decongestant, expectorant.

Dorcol Children's Decongestant Liquid. (Sandoz Consumer) Pseudoephedrine HCl 15 mg/5 ml. Bot. 4 oz. *otc.*
Use: Decongestant.

Dorcol Fever and Pain Reducer. (Sandoz Consumer) Acetaminophen 160 mg/5 ml. Bot. 4 oz. *otc.*
Use: Analgesic.

•**doretinel.** (DOE-REH-tin-ell) USAN.
Use: Antikeratinizing agent.

Doriglute Tabs DEA. (Major) Glutethimide 0.5 g/Tab. Bot. 100s, 250s, 1000s. *c-II.*
Use: Hypnotic.

Dormeer. (Taylor Pharmaceuticals) Scopolamine aminoxide HBr 0.2 mg/Cap. Bot. 100s, 1000s. *Rx.*
Use: Hypnotic, sedative.

dormethan.
See: Dextromethorphan HBr. (Various Mfr.)

Dormin. (Randob) Diphenhydramine HCl 25 mg, lactose. Cap. Bot. 32s, 72s *otc.*
Use: Sleep aid.

Dormin Sleeping Caplets. (Randob) Diphenhydramine HCl 25 mg/Cap. Bot. 32s. *otc.*
Use: Sleep aid.

dormiral.
See: Phenobarbital, Preps. (Various Mfr.).

dormonal.
See: Barbital, Preps. (Various Mfr.).

Dormutol. (Health for Life Brands) Scopolamine aminoxide HBr 0.2 mg/Cap. Bot. 24s, 60s. *Rx.*
Use: Hypnotic, sedative.

dornase alfa. (DOR-nace AL-fuh)
Use: Cystic fibrosis. [Orphan drug]
See: Pulmozyme, Soln. (Genentech).

Doryx Pellets. (Parke-Davis) Doxycycline hyclate 100 mg/Cap. Bot. 50s. *Rx.*
Use: Anti-infective, tetracycline.

•**dorzolamide hydrochloride.** (dore-ZOLE-lah-mide) USAN.
Use: Carbonic anhydrase inhibitor.
See: TruSopt, Soln. (Merck).

Dosaflex. (Richwood) Senna fruit extract, parabens, sucrose, alcohol 7%. Bot. 237 ml. *otc.*
Use: Laxative.

Dosalax. (Richwood) Extract of senna fruit, parabens, sucrose, alcohol 7%. Syrup. Bot. 237 ml.*Rx.*
Use: Laxative.

DOS Caps. (Zenith Goldline) Dioctyl sodium sulfosuccinate SG 100 mg or 250 mg/Cap. Bot. 100s, 1000s. *otc.*
Use: Laxative.

Doss Syrup. (Rosemont) Docusate sodium 20 mg/5 ml. Bot. pt, gal. *otc.*
Use: Laxative, stool softener.

Dostinex. (Pharmacia & Upjohn) Cabergoline 0.5 mg/Tab. Bot. 8s. *Rx.*
Use: Antihyperprolacinemic.

•**dothiepin hydrochloride.** (DOE-THIGH-eh-pin) USAN.
Use: Antidepressant.
See: Prothiaden.

Dotirol. (Sanofi Winthrop) Ampicillin trihydrate available in Cap, Susp., Inj. (IV, IM.). *Rx.*
Use: Anti-infective, penicillin.

Double-Action Toothache Kit. (C.S. Dent) **Liquid**: benzocaine, alcohol 74%, chlorobutanol anhydrous 0.09%. Bot. 3.7 ml. **Maronox Pain Relief Tablets**: acetaminophen 325 mg/Tab. Box. 8s. *otc.*
Use: Analgesic, topical.

Double Sal Tablets. (Pal-Pak) Sodium salicylate 648 mg/EC Tab. Bot. 1000s. *otc.*
Use: Analgesic.

Double Strength Gaviscon-2. (SmithKline Beecham Pharmaceuticals) Aluminum hydroxide 160 mg, magnesium trisilicate 40 mg, alginic acid, calcium stearate, sodium bicarbonate, sucrose. Tab. Bot. 48s. *otc.*
Use: Antacid.

Dovacet Capsules. (Pal-Pak) Dover's powder 24.3 mg, aspirin 324 mg, caffeine 32.4 mg/Tab. Bot. 1000s.
Use: Analgesic.

Dover's Powder. Ipecac 1 part, opium 1 part, lactose 8 parts.
Use: Analgesic, diaphoretic, sedative.

W/Acetophenetidin, atropine sulfate, aspirin, camphor, caffeine, sodium sulfate, dried.
See: Dovium, Cap. (Hance).

W/Acetophenetidin, camphor, aspirin, caffeine, atropine sulfate.
See: Analgestine, Cap. (Roberts Pharm).

W/Acetophenetidin, sodium citrate, potassium guaiacolsulfonate.
See: Doverlyn, Cap., Tab. (Davis & Sly).

W/A.P.C. camphor monobromated.
See: Coldate, Tab. (Zeneca)

W/Aspirin, phenacetin, camphor monobromated, caffeine.
See: Coldate, Tab. (Zeneca)

W/Atropine sulfate, A.P.C., camphor.
See: Dasin, Cap. (SmithKline Beecham Pharmaceuticals).

Dovonex. (Westwood Squibb) Calcipotreine 0.005% alcohols, EDTA, mineral oil. Oint. Tube 30, 60 or 100 g. Soln. Bot. 50 ml. Cream Tube 30, 60, 100 g. *Rx.*
Use: Dermatologic, antipsoriatic.

Dowicil 200.
See: Derma Soap (Ferndale Laboratories).

Dow-Isoniazid. (Hoechst Marion Roussel) Isoniazid 300 mg/Tab. Bot. 30s. *Rx.*
Use: Antituberculous.

•**doxacurium chloride.** (dox-ah-cure-ee-uhm) USAN.
Use: Neuromuscular blocker.
See: Nuromax (GlaxoWellcome).

Doxamin. (Forest Pharmaceutical) Thiamine HCl 100 mg, vitamin B_6 100 mg/ml. Vial 10 ml. *Rx.*
Use: Vitamin supplement.

Doxapap-N Tabs. (Major) Propoxyphene napsylate 100 mg, acetaminophen 650 mg Bot. 100s, 500s. *c-iv.*
Use: Analgesic combination, narcotic.

Doxaphene Capsules. (Major) Propoxyphene HCl 65 mg/Cap. Bot. 1000s. *c-iv.*
Use: Analgesic, narcotic.

Doxaphene Compound 65 Caps. (Major) Propoxyphene HCl, acetaminophen. Bot. 1000s. *c-iv.*
Use: Analgesic combination, narcotic.

•**doxapram hydrochloride.** (DOX-uh-pram) U.S.P. 23.
Use: Respiratory and CNS stimulant.
See: Dopram, Vial (Robins).

doxapram hydrochloride. (Various Mfr.) 20 mg/ml. Benzyl alcohol. Inj. Vial. 20 ml.
Use: Respiratory and CNS stimulant.

•**doxaprost.** (DOX-ah-proste) USAN.
Use: Bronchodilator.

Doxate. Docusate sodium. *otc.*
Use: Laxative.

•**doxazosin mesylate.** (DOX-uh-ZOE-sin) USAN.
Use: Antihypertensive.
See: Cardura, Tab. (Roerig).

•**doxepin hydrochloride.** (DOX-uh-pin) U.S.P. 23.
Use: Psychotherapeutic agent, antidepressant.
See: Sinequan, Cap. (Roerig).

doxepin hydrochloride. (Various Mfr.) Doxepin HCl 10 mg, 25 mg, 50 mg, 75 mg, 100 mg, 150 mg/Cap. Bot. 100s, 500s, 1000s, UD 100s; 10 mg/ml Oral Conc. Bot. 120 ml. *Rx.*
Use: Anxiolytic.

Doxidan. (Hoechst Marion Roussel) Yellow phenolphthalein 65 mg, docusate calcium 60 mg/Cap. Bot. 30s, 100s, 1000s, UD 100s, Display Pack 10s. *otc.*
Use: Laxative.

Doxil. (Sequus) Doxorubicin HCl 20 mg/10 ml vial. *Rx.*
Use: Antineoplastic.

•**doxofylline.** (DOX-oh-fill-een) USAN.
Use: Bronchodilator.
See: Maxivent (Roberts Pharm).

•**doxorubicin.** (DOX-oh-ROO-bih-sin) USAN.
Use: Antineoplastic.

•**doxorubicin hydrochloride.** (DOX-oh-ROO-bih-sin) U.S.P. 23.
Use: Antineoplastic.
See: Adriamycin, Inj. (Pharmacia & Upjohn).
Rubex, Pow. for Inj. (Bristol-Myers Oncology).

doxorubicin HCl. (Chiron Therapeutics) Doxorubicin HCl. **Pow. for Inj.: 10 mg:** w/lactose 50 mg. **20 mg:** w/lactose 100 mg. **50 mg:** w/lactose 250 mg. **Inj., aqueous:** 2 mg/ml, sodium chloride 0.9%. Vials 5, 10, 25, 100 ml. *Rx.*
Use: Antibiotic.

•**doxpicomine hydrochloride.** (DOX-PIH-koe-meen) USAN. *Formerly Doxpicodin hydrochloride.*
Use: Analgesic.

Doxy 100. (Fujisawa) Doxycycline hyclate for injection. Pow. 100 mg/Vial. *Rx.*
Use: Anti-infective, tetracycline.

Doxy 200. (Fujisawa) Doxycycline hyclate. Pow. 200 mg/Vial. *Rx.*
Use: Anti-infective, tetracycline.

Doxy Caps. (Edwards Pharmaceuticals) Doxycycline hyclate 100 mg/Cap. Bot. 50s. *Rx.*
Use: Anti-infective, tetracycline.

Doxychel Capsules. (Houba Inc.) Doxycycline hyclate 50 mg or 100 mg/Cap. Bot. 50s, 500s, UD 100s. *Rx.*
Use: Anti-infective, tetracycline.

Doxychel Injectable. (Houba Inc.) Doxycycline hyclate 100 mg or 200 mg/Vial. *Rx.*
Use: Anti-infective, tetracycline.

Doxychel Tablets. (Houba Inc.) Doxycycline hyclate 50 mg or 100 mg/Tab. Bot. 50s, 500s. *Rx.*
Use: Anti-infective, tetracycline.

•**doxycycline.** (DOX-ee-SIGH-kleen) U.S.P. 23.
Use: Anti-infective.
See: Monodex, Cap. (Oclassen).
Vibramycin for Oral Susp. (Pfizer Laboratories).
Vibramycin IV. (Roerig).

•**doxycycline calcium oral suspension.** (DOX-ee-SIGH-kleen) U.S.P. 23.
Use: Anti-infective, antiprotozoal.

•**doxycycline fosfatex.** USAN. (DOX-ee-SIGH-kleen foss-FAH-tex)
Use: Anti-infective.

•**doxycycline hyclate.** (DOX-ee-SIGH-kleen HIGH-klate) U.S.P. 23.
Use: Anti-infective.
See: Bio-Tab, Tab. (Inter. Ethical Labs).
Doxy-Caps, Cap. (Edwards Pharmaceuticals).
Vibra-Tabs, Tab. (Pfizer Laboratories).
Vibramycin, Cap., Tab., Vial (Pfizer Laboratories).

•**doxylamine succinate.** U.S.P. 23.
Use: Antihistamine.
See: Decapryn, Prep. (Hoechst Marion Roussel).
Unisom, Tab. (Pfizer).
W/Acetominophen, ephedrine sulfate, dextromethorphan HBr, alcohol.
See: Nyquil, Liq. (Vick).
W/Dextromethorphan HBr, alcohol.
See: Consotuss Antitussive, Syr. (Hoechst Marion Roussel).
W/Dextromethorphan HBr, sodium citrate, alcohol.
See: Vicks Formula 44 Cough Mixture, Syr. (Procter & Gamble).

Doxy-Lemmon Capsules. (Teva USA) Doxycycline hyclate equivalent to 100 mg of doxycycline base/Cap. Bot. 50s, 500s, UD 100s. *Rx.*
Use: Anti-infective, tetracycline.

Doxy-Lemmon Tablets. (Teva USA) Doxycycline hyclate equivalent to 100 mg of doxycycline base/Tab. Bot. 50s, 500s, UD 100s. *Rx.*
Use: Anti-infective, tetracycline.

Doxy-Tabs. (Houba Inc.) Doxycycline hyclate 100 mg/FC Tab. Bot. 50s, 500s. *Rx.*

Use: Anti-infective, tetracycline.

Doxy-Tabs-50. (Houba Inc.) 50 mg/Tab. Bot. 50s. *Rx.*
Use: Anti-infective, tetracycline.

DPPC. Colfosceril palmitate. *Rx.*
Use: Lung surfactant.
See: Exosurf Neonatal (Glaxo-Wellcome).

•**draflazine.** (DRAFF-lah-ZEEN) USAN.
Use: Cardioprotectant.

Dramamine II. (Pharmacia & Upjohn) Meclizine HCl 25 mg, lactose/Tab. 8s. *otc.*
Use: Antiemetic, antivertigo.

Dramamine, Children's. (Pharmacia & Upjohn) Dimenhydrinate 12.5 mg/5 ml, alcohol 5%, sucrose. Liq. Bot. 120 ml. *otc.*
Use: Antiemetic, antivertigo.

Dramamine Liquid. (Pharmacia & Upjohn) Dimenhydrinate 12.5 mg/4 ml Bot. 90 ml, pt. *otc.*
Use: Antiemetic, antivertigo.

Dramamine Tablets. (Pharmacia & Upjohn) Dimenhydrinate 50 mg/Tab. Bot. 36s, 100s, 1000s, Blister pkg. 12s, UD 100s. *otc.*
Use: Antiemetic, antivertigo.

Dramanate. (Pasadena) Dimenhydrinate 50 mg/ml. Inj. Vial 10 ml. *Rx.*
Use: Antiemetic, antivertigo.

dramarin.
See: Dramamine, Preps. (Searle).

dramyl.
See: Dramamine, Preps. (Searle).

Drawing Salve. (Whiteworth Towne) Tube oz. *otc.*
Use: Dermatologic, wound therapy.

Drawing Salve with Triquinodin. (Towne) Tube 2 oz. *otc.*
Use: Dermatologic, wound therapy.

Dr. Berry's Skin Toner. (Last) Hydroquinone 2%. Jar oz. *Rx.*
Use: Dermatologic.

Dr. Caldwell Senna Laxative. (Mentholatum) Senna 7%, alcohol 4.5%. Bot. 130 ml, 360 ml. *otc.*
Use: Laxative.

DRC Peri-Anal Cream. (Xttrium) Lassar's paste 37.5%, anhydrous lanolin, U.S.P. 37.5%, cold cream 25%. Tube 5 oz. *otc.*
Use: Dermatologic protectant, perianal.

Dr. Dermi-Heal. (Quality Formulations) Zinc oxide 25%, allantoin 1%, peruvian balsam, castor oil, white petrolatum. Oint. Tube 75 g. *otc.*
Use: Astringent.

Dr. Drake's Cough Medicine. (Last) Dextromethorphan HBr 10 mg/5 ml Bot. 2 oz. *otc.*
Use: Antitussive.

•**dribendazole.** (dry-BEN-dah-ZOLE) USAN.
Use: Anthelmintic.

Dri-A Caps. (Barth's) Vitamin A 10,000 IU/Cap. Bot. 100s, 500s. *otc.*
Use: Vitamin supplement.

Dri A & D Caps. (Barth's) Vitamins A 10,000 IU, D 400 IU/Cap. Bot. 100s, 500s. *otc.*
Use: Vitamin supplement.

Dri-E. (Barth's) Vitamin E. **100 IU/Cap.:** Bot. 100s, 500s, 1000s. **200 IU/Cap.:** Bot. 100s, 250s, 500s. **400 IU/Cap.:** Bot. 100s, 250s. *otc.*
Use: Vitamin supplement.

Dri/Ear. (Pfeiffer) Boric acid 2.75% in isopropyl alcohol. Soln. Dropper Bot. 30 ml. *otc.*
Use: Otic.

dried aluminum hydroxide gel.
Use: Antacid.
See: Aluminum Hydroxide Gel, dried.

dried yeast.
See: Yeast, dried.

Driminate Tabs. (Major) Dimenhydrinate 50 mg/Tab. Bot. 100s, 1000s. *otc.*
Use: Antiemetic, antivertigo.

•**drinidene.** (DRIH-nih-deen) USAN.
Use: Analgesic.

Drisdol Drops. (Sanofi Winthrop) Ergocalciferol (Vitamin D_2) 8000 IU/ml in propylene glycol. Bot. 60 ml. *otc.*
Use: Refractory rickets, hypophosphatemia, hypoparathyroidism.

Drisdol 50,000 Unit Capsules. (Sanofi Winthrop) Vitamin D_2, 50,000 IU/Cap. Bot. 50s. *Rx.*
Use: Refractory rickets, hypophosphatemia, hypoparathyroidism.

Dristan 12 Hour. (Whitehall Robins) Chlorpheniramine maleate 4 mg, phenylephrine HCl 20 mg/Cap. Bot. 6s, 10s, 15s. *otc.*
Use: Antihistamine, decongestant.

Dristan Allergy. (Whitehall Robins) Pseudoephedrine HCl 60 mg, brompheniramine maleate 4 mg/Cap. Bot. 20s. *otc.*
Use: Antihistamine, decongestant.

Dristan Capsules. (Whitehall Robins) Phenylephrine HCl 5 mg, chlorpheniramine maleate 2 mg, acetaminophen 325 mg/Cap. Bot. 16s, 36s, 75s. *otc.*
Use: Analgesic, antihistamine, decongestant.

Dristan Cold. (Whitehall Robins) Pseudoephedrine HCl 30 mg, acetaminophen 500 mg/Capl. Bot. 20s, 40s. *otc.*
Use: Analgesic, decongestant.

Dristan Cold & Flu. (Whitehall Robins) Acetaminophen 500 mg, pseudoephedrine HCl 60 mg, chlorpheniramine maleate 4 mg, dextromethorphan HBr 20 mg/Pow. Pkts. 6s. *otc.*
Use: Analgesic, antihistamine, antitussive, decongestant.

Dristan Cold Multi-Symptom Formula. (Whitehall Robins) Phenylephrine HCl 5 mg, chlorpheniramine maleate 2 mg, acetaminophen 325 mg/Tab. Bot. 20s, 40s, 75s. *otc.*
Use: Analgesic, antihistamine, decongestant.

Dristan Juice Mix-In. (Whitehall Robins) Acetaminophen 500 mg, pseudoephedrine HCl 60 mg, dextromethorphan 20 mg/Pow. Pkts. 5s. *otc.*
Use: Analgesic, antitussive, decongestant.

Dristan 12-Hr Nasal. (Whitehall Robins) Oxymetazoline HCl 0.05%, benzalkonium Cl 1:5000, thimerosal 0.002%, hydroxypropylmethylcellulose. Spray. Bot. 15 ml, 30 ml. *otc.*
Use: Decongestant, nasal.

Dristan Maximum Strength Caplets. (Whitehall Robins) Pseudoephedrine HCl 30 mg, acetaminophen 500 mg/Capl. Bot. 24s. *otc.*
Use: Analgesic, decongestant.

Dristan Menthol Nasal Mist. (Whitehall Robins) Phenylephrine HCl 0.5%, pheniramine maleate 0.2%. Bot. 0.5 oz, 1 oz. *otc.*
Use: Antihistamine, decongestant.

Dristan Nasal Mist. (Whitehall Robins) Phenylephrine HCl 0.5%, pheniramine maleate 0.2%. Regular: 15 ml, 30 ml. Menthol: 15 ml. *otc.*
Use: Antihistamine, decongestant.

Dristan No Drowsiness Cold. (Whitehall Robins) Pseudoephedrine HCl 30 mg, acetaminophen 500 mg/Cap. Bot. 20s. *otc.*
Use: Analgesic, decongestant.

Dristan Saline Spray. (Whitehall Robins) Sodium chloride. Soln. Bot. 15 ml.
Use: Nasal product.

Dristan Sinus. (Whitehall Robins) Pseudoephedrine HCl 30 mg, ibuprofen 200 mg/Cap. Pkg. 20s. Bot. 24s, 40s. *otc.*
Use: Analgesic, decongestant.

Drithocreme. (Dermik Laboratories) Anthralin 0.1%, 0.25% or 0.5%. Tube 50 g. *Rx.*
Use: Antipsoriatic.

Drithocreme HP 1.0%. (Dermik Laboratories) Anthralin 1%. Tube 50 g. *Rx.*
Use: Antipsoriatic.

Dritho-Scalp. (Dermik Laboratories) Anthralin 0.25% or 0.5%. Tube 50 g. *Rx.*
Use: Antipsoriatic.

Drixomed. (Iomed Labs) Dexbrompheniramine maleate 6 mg, pseudoephedrine sulfate 120 mg/SR Tab. Bot. 100s, 500s. *Rx.*
Use: Antihistamine, decongestant.

Drixoral. (Schering Plough) Dexbrompheniramine maleate 6 mg, pseudoephedrine sulfate 120 mg. SA Tab. Box 10s, 20s, 40s. Bot. 48s, 100s. *otc.*
Use: Antihistamine, decongestant.

Drixoral. (Schering Plough) Pseudoephedrine sulfate 30 mg, brompheniramine maleate 2 mg, sorbitol, sugar. Syrup. Bot. 118 ml. *otc.*
Use: Antihistamine, decongestant.

Drixoral Cold & Allergy. (Schering Plough) Dexbrompheniramine maleate 6 mg, pseudoephedrine sulfate 120 mg/SR Tab. Pkg. 10s. *otc.*
Use: Antihistamine, decongestant.

Drixoral Cold & Flu. (Schering Plough) Pseudoephedrine HCl 60 mg, dexbrompheniramine maleate 3 mg, acetaminophen 500 mg/Tab. Bot. 12s, 24s, 48s. *otc.*
Use: Analgesic, antihistamine, decongestant.

Drixoral Cough & Congestion Liquid Caps. (Schering Plough) Pseudoephedrine HCl 60 mg, dextromethorphan HBr 30 mg/Cap. Pkg. 10s. *otc.*
Use: Antihistamine, decongestant.

Drixoral Cough & Sore Throat Liquid Caps. (Schering Plough) Dextromethorphan HBr 15 mg, acetaminophen 325 mg, sorbitol. Cap. Pkg. 10s. *otc.*
Use: Analgesic, antitussive.

Drixoral Non-Drowsy Formula. (Schering Plough) Pseudoephedrine sulfate 120 mg, sugar. Tab. Pkg. 10s, 20s. *otc.*
Use: Decongestant.

Drixoral Plus. (Schering Plough) Pseudoephedrine sulfate 60 mg, dexbrompheniramine maleate 3 mg, acetaminophen 500 mg/TR Tab. Bot. 12s, 24s. *otc.*
Use: Analgesic, antihistamine, decongestant.

Drixoral Sustained-Action Tablets. (Schering Plough) Pseudoephedrine sulfate 120 mg, dexbrompheniramine maleate 6 mg, sugar, lactose. Tab. Pkg. 10s. Bots. 20s, 40s. *otc.*
Use: Antihistamine, decongestant.

Drize. (Jones Medical Industries) Phenylpropanolamine HCl 75 mg, chlorpheniramine maleate 12 mg/SR Cap. Bot. 100s. *Rx.*
Use: Antihistamine, decongestant.

•**drobuline.** (DROE-byoo-leen) USAN.
Use: Cardiovascular agent (antiarrhythmic).

•**drocinonide.** (droe-SIN-oh-nide) USAN.
Use: Anti-inflammatory.

drocode.
See: Dihydrocodeine.

•**droloxifene.** (drole-OX-ih-feen) USAN.
Use: Antineoplastic.

•**droloxifene citrate.** (drole-OX-ih-feen) USAN.
Use: Antineoplastic.

•**drometrizole.** (DROE-meh-TRY-zole) USAN.
Use: Ultraviolet screen.

•**dromostanolone propionate.** (DRAHM-oh-STAN-oh-lone) USAN. U.S.P. XX.
Use: Antineoplastic.

•**dronabinol.** (droe-NAB-ih-nahl) U.S.P. 23.
Use: Antiemetic. [Orphan drug]
See: Marinol, Gel Cap. (Roxane).

drop chalk. (Various Mfr.) Calcium carbonate, prepared. Prepared chalk.

•**droperidol.** (dro-PER-i-dahl) U.S.P. 23.
Use: Antipsychotic, anxiolytic.
See: Inapsine, Inj. (Janssen).
W/Fentanyl citrate.
Use: Anxiolytic.
See: Innovar, Inj. (Janssen).

•**droprenilamine.** (droe-preh-NILL-ah-meen) USAN.
Use: Vasodilator (coronary).

Drotic Sterile Otic Solution. (B.F. Ascher) Hydrocortisone 10 mg (1%), polymyxin B sulfate 10,000 units, neomycin 5 mg/ml, preservatives. Dropper bot. 10 ml. *Rx.*
Use: Otic.

•**droxacin sodium.** (DROX-ah-sin) USAN.
Use: Anti-infective.

•**droxifilcon a.** (DROX-ih-fill-kahn A) USAN.
Use: Contact lens material (hydrophilic).

•**droxinavir hydrochloride.** (drox-IN-ah-veer HIGH-droe-KLOR-ide) USAN.
Use: Antiviral.

Dr. Scholl's Advanced Pain Relief Corn Removers. (Schering Plough) Salicylic acid 40% in a rubber-based vehicle. Disc. 6s. *otc.*
Use: Keratolytic.

Dr. Scholl's Athlete's Foot. (Schering Plough) **Pow.:** Tolnaftate 1%. Talc. 63 g. **Spray Liq.:** Tolnaftate 1%, alcohol 36%. 113 ml. *otc.*
Use: Antifungal, topical.

Dr. Scholl's Athlete's Foot Cream. (Schering Plough) Tolnaftate 1%. Tube 0.5 oz. *otc.*
Use: Antifungal, topical.

Dr. Scholl's Callus Removers. (Schering Plough) Salicylic acid 40% in a rubber-based vehicle. 6 pads, 4 discs. Extra thick in 4 discs. *otc.*
Use: Keratolytic.

Dr. Scholl's Clear Away. (Schering Plough) Salicylic acid 40% in a rubber-based vehicle. Disc 18s. *otc.*
Use: Keratolytic.

Dr. Scholl's Clear Away One Step. (Schering Plough) Salicylic acid 40% in a rubber-based vehicle. Strip 14s. *otc.*
Use: Keratolytic.

Dr. Scholl's Clear Away Plantar. (Schering Plough) Salicylic acid 40% in a rubber-based vehicle. Disc 24s. *otc.*
Use: Keratolytic.

Dr. Scholl's Corn/Callus Remover. (Schering Plough) Salicylic acid 12.6% in a flexible collodion, alcohol 18%, ether 55%, hydrogenated vegetable oil. Liq. 10 ml with 3 cushions. *otc.*
Use: Keratolytic.

Dr. Scholl's Corn/Callus Salve. (Schering Plough) Salicylic acid 15%. Tube 0.4 oz. *otc.*
Use: Keratolytic.

Dr. Scholl's Corn Remover. (Schering Plough) Salicylic acid 40% in a rubber-based vehicle. Discs: 6s as wraparounds, 9s as ultra thin, small, waterproof, regular, soft and extra-thick. *otc.*
Use: Keratolytic.

Dr. Scholl's Corn Salve. (Schering Plough) Salicylic acid 15%. Jar 0.4 oz. *otc.*
Use: Keratolytic.

Dr. Scholl's Cracked Heel Relief. (Schering Plough) Lidocaine 2%, benzalkonium Cl 0.13%. Cream 5.6 g. *otc.*
Use: Anesthetic, local.

Dr. Scholl's Ingrown Toenail Reliever. (Schering Plough) Sodium sulfide 1%. Bot. 0.33 oz. *otc.*
Use: Foot preparation.

Dr. Scholl's Moisturizing Corn Remover Kit. (Schering Plough) Salicylic acid 40% in a rubber-based vehicle, moisturizing cream, pain relief cushions. Disc 6s. *otc.*
Use: Keratolytic.

Dr. Scholl's One Step Corn Removers. (Schering Plough) Salicylic acid 40% in a rubber-based vehicle. Strips 6s. *otc.*
Use: Keratolytic.

Dr. Scholl's Pro Comfort Jock Itch Spray. (Schering Plough) Tolnaftate 1%. Aerosol can 3.5 oz. *otc.*
Use: Antifungal, topical.

Dr. Scholl's Wart Remover Kit. (Schering Plough) Salicylic acid 17% in a flexible collodion, alcohol 17%, ether 52%. Liq. 10 ml with brush and 6 adhesive pads. *otc.*
Use: Keratolytic.

Dr. Scholl's Zino Pads/with Medicated Disks. (Schering Plough) Salicylic acid 20% or 40%. Protective pads designed for use with and without salicylic acid-impregnated disks. *otc.*
Use: Keratolytic.

Drucon. (Standard Drug) Phenylephrine HCl 5 mg, chlorpheniramine maleate 2 mg, menthol 1 mg, alcohol 5%/5 ml Elix. Bot. pt, gal. *otc.*
Use: Antihistamine, decongestant.

Drucon C R. (Standard Drug) Phenylephrine HCl 25 mg, chlorpheniramine maleate 4 mg/Tab. Bot. 100s. *otc.*
Use: Antihistamine, decongestant.

Drucon with Codeine. (Standard Drug) Codeine phosphate 10 mg, phenylephrine HCl 10 mg, chlorpheniramine maleate 2 mg, menthol 1 mg, alcohol 5%/5 ml. Bot. pt. *c-v.*
Use: Antihistamine, antitussive, decongestant.

Dry Eyes. (Bausch & Lomb) White petrolatum, mineral oil, lanolin. Oint. Tube 3.5 g. *otc.*
Use: Lubricant, ophthalmic.

Dry Eyes Solution. (Bausch & Lomb) Polyvinyl alcohol 1.4%, benzalkonium Cl 0.01%, sodium phosphate, EDTA, NaCl. Bot. 15 ml. *otc.*
Use: Lubricant, ophthalmic.

Dry Eye Therapy. (Bausch & Lomb) Glycerin 0.3%, potassium Cl, sodium Cl, sodium citrate, sodium phosphate, zinc Cl. Drop. Single-use Bot. 0.3 ml (UD 32s). *otc.*
Use: Ophthalmic.

Dryox 2.5, 10. (C & M Pharmacal.) Benzoyl peroxide 2.5%, 5%, 10%, 20%. Gel. Tube. 30 g, 60 g. *otc.*
Use: Dermatologic, acne.

Dryox 20S 5. (C & M Pharm) Benzoyl peroxide 20%, sulfur 10%, methylparaben. Gel. Tube. 30 g, 60 g. *otc.*
Use: Dermatologic, acne.

Dry Skin Creme. (Gordon Laboratories) Cetyl alcohol, lubricating oils in a water soluble base. Jar 2 oz, 1 lb, 5 lb. *otc.*
Use: Emollient.

Drysol. (Person & Covey) Aluminum Cl hexahydrate 20% in 93% SD alcohol 40. Bot. 37.5 ml. *Rx.*
Use: Astringent.

Drysum Shampoo. (Summers) Alcohol 15%, acetone 6%. Plastic bot. 4 oz. *otc.*
Use: Dermatologic, hair.

Drytergent. (C & M Pharmacal.) TEA-dodecylbenzenesulfonate, boric acid, lauramide DEA, propylene glycol, tartrazine, purified water, color, fragrance. Liq. Bot. 240 ml, 480 ml. *otc.*
Use: Dermatologic, acne.

Drytex. (C & M Pharmacal) Salicylic acid 2%, benzalkonium Cl 0.1%, acetone 10%, isopropyl alcohol 40%, tartrazine. Lot. Bot. 240 ml. *otc.*
Use: Dermatologic, acne.

DSMC Plus. (Geneva Pharm) Docusate potassium 100 mg. Cap. Bot. 100s. *otc.*
Use: Laxative.

DSS. (Dioctyl sodium sulfosuccinate) Docusate sodium. *otc.*
Use: Laxative.
See: Regutol, Tab. (Schering Plough).
Colace, Cap. (Bristol-Myers).
Docusate Sodium, Cap. (Various, eg, Geneva, Marsam, Lederle, Major, Purepac, Rugby, Schein, URL).
DOK, Cap. (Major).
DOS, Softgel, Cap. (Zenith Goldline).
D-S-S, Cap. (Warner Chilcott).
Modane Soft, Cap. (Pharmacia & Pharmacia & Upjohn).
Pro-Sof, Cap. (Vangard).
Regulax SS, Cap. (Republic).

D-S-S. (Warner-Chilcott) Docusate sodium 100 mg/Cap. Bot. 100s, 1000s and UD 100s. *otc.*
Use: Laxative, stool softener.

DST. Dihydrostreptomycin.
See: Dihydrostreptomycin, Preps. (Various Mfr.)

D-Test 100. (Burgin-Arden) Testosterone cypionate 100 mg/ml. Vial 10 ml. *c-III.*
Use: Androgen.

D-Test 200. (Burgin-Arden) Testosterone cypionate 200 mg/ml. Vial 10 ml. *c-III.*

Use: Androgen.

DTIC. Dacarbazine. *Rx.*
Use: Antineoplastic.
See: Decarbazine, Inj. (Various Mfr.)
DTIC-Dome, Inj. (Bayer Corp).

DTIC-Dome. (Bayer Corp) Dacarbazine 100 mg or 200 mg/Vial. Vial 10 ml, 20 ml. *Rx.*
Use: Antineoplastic.

DTP. Diphtheria and tetanus toxoids and pertussis vaccine, adsorbed. *Rx.*
Use: Immunization.
See: Acel-Imune, Vial (Wyeth Lederle).
Diphtheria and Tetanus Toxoids and whole-cell Pertussis Vaccine, Inj. (Pasteur-Merieux-Connaught, Massachusetts Public Health Biologic Labs) Infanarix (SKB).
DTwP, Inj. (Michigan Dept of Public Health/SmithKline Beecham Pharmaceuticals).
Tri-Immunol, Vial, Inj. (Wyeth Lederle).
Tripedia, Vial (Pasteur-Merieux-Connaught).

DTwP. (Michigan Dept. of Public Health/SmithKline Beecham Pharmaceuticals) 10 Lf units diphtheria, 5.5 Lf units tetanus and 4 Lf units pertussis/0.5 ml. Vial 5 ml. *Rx.*
Use: Immunization.

Duadacin. (Kenwood/Bradley) Phenylpropanolamine HCl 12.5 mg, chlorpheniramine maleate 2 mg, acetaminophen 325 mg/Cap. Bot. 100s, 1000s. Dispense-A-Pak 1000s. *otc.*
Use: Analgesic, antihistamine, decongestant.

Dual-Wet. (Alcon Lenscare) Polyvinyl alcohol, duasorb water soluble polymetric system, benzalkonium Cl 0.01%, disodium edetate 0.05%. Bot. 2 oz. *otc.*
Use: Contact lens care.

•**duazomycin.** (doo-AZE-oh-MY-sin) USAN. Antibiotic isolated from broth filtrates of *Streptomyces ambofaciens.*
Use: Antineoplastic.

Duazomycin A. Name used for Duazomycin.
Use: Antineoplastic.

Duazomycin B. Name used for Azotomycin.
Use: Antineoplastic.

Duazomycin C. Name used for Ambomycin.
Use: Antineoplastic.

Dulcagen Suppositories. (Zenith Goldline) Bisacodyl 10 mg/Supp. Box 12s, 100s. *otc.*
Use: Laxative.

Dulcagen Tablets. (Zenith Goldline) Bisacodyl 5 mg/Tab. Bot. 100s. *otc.*
Use: Laxative.

Dulcolax. (Novartis Consumer Health) Bisacodyl. **EC Tab.:** 5 mg. Box 10s, 25s, 50s, 100s. Bot. 1000s, UD 100s. **Supp.:** 10 mg. Box 2s, 4s, 8s, 50s, 500s. **Bowel Prep Kit:** 4 tab., 1 supp./Kit. 5s/box. *otc.*
Use: Laxative.

Dull-C. (Freeda Vitamins) Ascorbic acid 4 g/tsp. Pow. Bot. 100 g, 500 g, 1000 g. *otc.*
Use: Vitamin supplement.

•**duloxetine hydrochloride.** (doo-LOX-eh-teen) USAN.
Use: Antidepressant.

Dulphalac. (Solvay) Lactulose 10 g/5 ml. Syr. Bot. 240 ml, 480 ml, 960 ml, UD 30 ml. *Rx.*
Use: Laxative.

Duo. (Norcliff Thayer) Tube 0.5 oz.
Use: Adhesive.

Duocet. (Mason) Hydrocodone bitartrate 5 mg, acetaminophen 500 mg/Tab. Bot. 100s. *c-III.*
Use: Analgesic combination, narcotic.

Duo-Cyp. (Keene Pharmaceuticals) Testosterone cypionate 50 mg, estradiol cypionate 2 mg/ml. Vial 10 ml. *Rx.*
Use: Androgen, estrogen combination.

duodenal substance.
W/Ox bile extract, pancreatin, papain.
See: Digenzyme, Tab. (Burgin-Arden).

duodenum whole, desiccated & defatted.
W/Ferrous gluconate, Vitamin B_{12}, cobalt Cl.
See: Bitrinsic-E, Cap. (Zeneca)

DuoDerm. (ConvaTec) **Sterile dressing:** 10 cm × 10 cm. Pack 5s. 20 cm 20 cm. Pack 3s. **Sterile gran:** Packet 4 g. Pack 5s. *otc.*
Use: Dermatologic, wound therapy.

Duoderm Extra Thin. (ConvaTec) Flexible hydroactive sterile dressings. 4" × 4", 6"×6". Pck. 10s. *otc.*
Use: Dressing, topical.

DuoFilm. (Stiefel) Salicylic acid 16.7%, lactic acid 16.7% in flexible collodion. Bot. 15 ml w/applicator. *otc.*
Use: Keratolytic.

Duo-Flow. (Ciba Vision Ophthalmics) Poloxamer 188, benzalkonium Cl 0.013%, EDTA 0.25%. Soln. Bot. 120 ml. *otc.*
Use: Contact lens care.

Duo-K. (Various Mfr.) Potassium 20 mEq, chloride 3.4 mEq/15 ml (from potas-

sium gluconate and potassium Cl). Bot. pt, gal. *Rx*.
Use: Mineral supplement.

Duolube. (Bausch & Lomb) White petrolatum, mineral oil. Sterile, preservative and lanolin free. Oint. Tube 3.5 g. *otc*.
Use: Lubricant, ophthalmic.

duomycin.
See: Aureomycin, Preps. (ESI Lederle Generics).

•**duoperone fumarate.** (DOO-oh-per-OHN) USAN.
Use: Neuroleptic.

DuoPlant. (Stiefel). Salicylic acid 27%, alcohol 50%, flexible collodion, hydroxypropylcellulose, lactic acid. Liq. Bot. 14 g. *otc*.
Use: Ketatolytic (wart removal).

Duosol. (Kirkman Sales) Docusate sodium 100 mg or 250 mg/Cap. Bot. 100s, 1000s. *otc*.
Use: Laxative.

Duotal. (Health for Life Brands) 1.5 gr: Secobarbital sodium ¾ gr, amobarbital gr/Cap. 3 gr: Secobarbital sodium 1.5 gr, amobarbital 1.5 gr/Cap. Bot. 100s, 500s, 1000s. *c-II*.
Use: Hypnotic, sedative.

duotal.
See: Guaiacol Carbonate (Various Mfr.).

Duo-Trach Kit. (Astra) Lidocaine HCl 4%. Inj. 5 ml disp. syringe with laryngotracheal cannula. *Rx*.
Use: Anesthetic, local.

Duotrate 30. (Jones Medical Industries) Pentaerythritol tetranitrate 30 mg/SR Cap. Bot. 100s. *Rx*.
Use: Antianginal.

Duotrate 45. (Jones Medical Industries) Pentaerythritol tetranitrate 45 mg/SR Cap. Bot. 100s. *Rx*.
Use: Antianginal.

Duovin-S. (Spanner) Estrone 2.5 mg, progesterone 25 mg/ml. Vial 10 ml. *Rx*.
Use: Estrogen, progestin combination.

Duo-WR, No. 1 & No. 2. (Whorton) **No. 1:** Salicylic acid, compound tincture benzoin. **No. 2:** Compound tincture benzoin, formaldehyde. Bot. 0.25 oz. *otc*.
Use: Keratolytic.

Duphalac. (Solvay) Lactulose 10 g/15 ml (< 2.2 g galactose, 1.2 g lactose, 1.2 g or less of other sugars). Syr. Bot. 240 ml, pt, qt, UD 30 ml. *Rx*.
Use: Laxative.

Duplast. (Beiersdorf) Adhesive coated elastic cloth. 8" X 4" Strip. Box 10s. 10" X 5"; Strip. Box 8s, 10s.

Duplex. (C & M Pharmacal) Sodium lauryl sulfate 15%, lauramide DEA. Liq. Bot. 480 ml. *otc*.
Use: Dermatologic, cleanser.

Duplex Shampoo. (C & M Pharmacal) Sodium lauryl sulfate 15%, lauramide DEA, purified water. Bot. pt, gal. *otc*.
Use: Dermatologic.

Duplex T Shampoo. (C & M Pharmacal) Sodium lauryl sulfate, purified water, lauramide DEA, solution of coal tar, alcohol 8.3%. Bot. pt, gal. *otc*.
Use: Antiseborrheic.

duponol.
See: Gardinol-type detergents (Sodium Lauryl Sulfate) (Various Mfr.)

Durabolin. (Organon) Nandrolone phenpropionate 25 mg/ml in sesame oil, benzyl alcohol 5%. Inj. Vial 5 ml. *c-III*.
Use: Anabolic steroid.
See: Deca-Durabolin, Inj. (Organon).

Durabolin. (Organon) Nandrolone phenpropionate 50 mg/ml in sterile sesame oil, benzyl alcohol 10%. Inj. Vial 2 ml. *c-III*.
Use: Anabolic steroid.

DURAcare. (Blairex Labs) Buffered hypertonic salt solution, non-ionic detergents with thimerosal 0.004%, EDTA 0.1%. Soln. Bot. 30 ml. *otc*.
Use: Contact lens care.

DURAcare II. (Blairex Labs) Buffered hypertonic, ethylene and propylene oxide, octylphenoxypolyethoxyethanol, lauryl sulfate salt of imidazoline, sodium bisulfite 0.1%, sorbic acid 0.1%, EDTA 0.25%. Soln. Bot. 30 ml. *otc*.
Use: Contact lens care.

Duraclon. (Fujisawa) Clonidine HCl 100 mcg/ml/Inj. Vials. 10 ml. *Rx*.
Use: Analgesic.

Dura-Estrin. (Roberts Pharm) Estradiol cypionate in oil 5 mg/ml. Inj. Vial 10 ml. *Rx*.
Use: Estrogen.

Duragen. (Roberts Pharm) Estradiol valerate in oil 20 mg or 40 mg/ml. Inj. Vial 10 ml. *Rx*.
Use: Estrogen.

Duragesic. (Janssen) Fentanyl 2.5 mg, 5 mg, 7.5 mg or 10 mg/transdermal patch. Carton 5s. *c-II*.
Use: Analgesic, narcotic.

Dura-Gest. (Dura Pharm) Phenylpropanolamine HCl 45 mg, phenylephrine HCl 5 mg, guaifenesin 200 mg/Cap. Bot. 100s, 500s. *Rx*.
Use: Decongestant, expectorant.

Duralex. (American Urologicals) Pseudo-

ephedrine HCl 120 mg, chlorpheniramine maleate 8 mg/SR Cap. Bot. 100s, 1000s. *Rx.*
Use: Antihistamine, decongestant.

Duralone Injection. (Roberts Pharm) Methylprednisolone acetate 40 mg or 80 mg/ml Susp. for Inj. **40 mg:** Vial 10 ml. **80 mg:** Vial 5 ml. *Rx.*
Use: Corticosteroid.

Duralutin Injection. (Roberts Pharm) Hydroxyprogesterone caproate in oil 250 mg/ml. Vial 5 ml. *Rx.*
Use: Hormone, progesterone.

Dura-Meth. (Foy) Methylprednisolone 40 mg/ml. Vial 5 ml, 10 ml. *Rx.*
Use: Corticosteroid.

Duramist Plus. (Pfeiffer) Oxymetazoline HCl 0.05%. Spray. 15 ml. *otc.*
Use: Decongestant.

Duramorph. (Elkins-Sinn) Morphine sulfate. Inj. 0.5 mg/ml or 1 mg/ml. Amp. 10 ml Box 10s. Preservative free. *c-II.*
Use: Analgesic, narcotic.

Duranest. (Astra) Etidocaine HCl 1.5%, epinephrine 1:200,000, sodium metabisulfite. Dental cartridges 1.8 ml. *Rx.*
Use: Anesthetic, local.

Duranest-MPF. (Astra) Etidocaine. **1%:** w/epinephrine 1:200,000. Vial 30 ml. **1.5%:** w/epinephrine 1:200,000. Amp. 20 ml. *Rx.*
Use: Anesthetic, local.

Durapam. (Major) Flurazepam HCl 15 mg or 30 mg/Cap. Bot. 100s, 500s. *c-IV.*
Use: Hypnotic, sedative.

•**durapatite.** (der-APP-ah-tite) USAN.
Use: Prosthetic aid.
See: Alveograf (Sterling Winthrop). Periograf (Sterling Winthrop).

Duraquin. (Parke-Davis) Quinidine gluconate 330 mg/SR Tab. Bot. 100s, UD 100s. *Rx.*
Use: Cardiovascular agent.

DuraScreen. (Schwarz Pharma) SPF 30. Octyl methoxycinnamate, octyl salicylate, oxybenzone, 2-phenylbenzimidazole-sulfonic acid, titanium dioxide, cetearyl alcohol, diazolidinyl urea, parabens, shea butter. Lot. Bot. 105 ml. *otc.*
Use: Sunscreen.

DuraScreen SPF 15. (Schwarz Pharma) SPF 15. Ethylhexyl p-methoxycinnamate, 2-ethylhexyl salicylate, oxybenzone, parabens, titanium dioxide. Lot. Bot. 105 ml. *otc.*
Use: Sunscreen.

Dura-Tap/PD. (Dura Pharm) Pseudoephedrine HCl 60 mg, chlorpheniramine maleate 4 mg. Cap. Bot. 100s. *Rx.*
Use: Antihistamine, decongestant.

Duratears Naturale. (Alcon Laboratories) White petroleum, anhydrous liquid lanolin, mineral oil. Oint. Tube 3.5 g. *otc.*
Use: Lubricant, ophthalmic.

Duratest-200/Duratest-100. (Roberts Pharm) Testosterone cypionate in oil 100 mg or 200 mg/ml. Inj. Vial 10 ml. *c-III.*
Use: Androgen.

Duratestrin. (Roberts Pharm) Estradiol cypionate 2 mg, testosterone cypionate 50 mg/ml. Vial 10 ml. *Rx.*
Use: Androgen, estrogen combination.

Durathate-200 Injection. (Roberts Pharm) Testosterone enanthate in oil 200 mg/ml. Vial 10 ml. *c-III.*
Use: Androgen.

Duration Mentholated Vapor Spray. (Schering Plough) Oxymetazoline HCl 0.05%, aromatics. Squeeze bot. 15 ml. *otc.*
Use: Decongestant.

Duration Mild Nasal Spray. (Schering Plough) Phenylephrine HCl 0.5%. Bot. 15 ml. *otc.*
Use: Decongestant.

Duration Nasal Spray. (Schering Plough) Oxymetazoline HCl 0.05%. Aqueous soln. Squeeze bot. 15 ml, 30 ml. *otc.*
Use: Nasal decongestant; androgen, estrogen combination.

Duratuss. (Whitby) Pseudoephedrine HCl 120 mg, guaifenesin 600 mg. LA Tab. Bot. 100s. *Rx.*
Use: Decongestant, expectorant.

Duratuss-G. (UCB Pharmaceuticals) 1200 mg guaifenesin (UCB/620)/Tab. Bot. 100s. *Rx.*
Use: Expectorant.

Duratuss HD. (Whitby) Hydrocodone bitartrate 2.5 mg, pseudoephedrine HCl 30 mg, guaifenesin 100 mg, alcohol 5%. Elixir Bot. 473 ml. *c-III.*
Use: Antitussive, decongestant, expectorant.

Dura-Vent. (Dura Pharm) Phenylpropanolamine HCl 75 mg, guaifenesin 600 mg. SR Tab. Bot. 100s. *Rx.*
Use: Decongestant, expectorant.

Dura-Vent/A. (Dura Pharm) Phenylpropanolamine HCl 75 mg, chlorpheniramine maleate 10 mg. SR Cap. Bot. 100s. *Rx.*
Use: Antihistamine, decongestant.

Dura-Vent/DA. (Dura Pharm) Phenylephrine HCl 20 mg, chlorpheniramine maleate 8 mg, methscopolamine nitrate 2.5 mg. SR Tab. Bot. 100s. *Rx.*
Use: Anticholinergic, antihistamine, decongestant.

Durazyme. (Blairex Labs) Nonionic detergent preserved w/thimerosal 0.004%, EDTA 0.1% in sterile buffered hypertonic salt soln. Bot. 30 ml. *otc.*
Use: Contact lens care.

Duricef. (Mead-Johnson) Cefadroxil.
Tab.: 1 g. Bot. 50s, 100s, UD 100s.
Cap.: 500 mg. Bot. 50s, 100s, UD 100s.
Susp.: 125 mg/5 ml, 250 mg/5 ml or 500 mg/5 ml Bot. 50 ml, 75 ml (500 mg/5 ml), 100 ml. *Rx.*
Use: Anti-infective, cephalosporin.

Dusotal. (Harvey) Sodium amobarbital ¾ gr, sodium secobarbital gr/Cap. Bot. 1000s. (3 gr) Bot. 1000s. *c-II.*
Use: Hypnotic, sedative.

•**dusting powder, absorbable.** U.S.P. 23.
Use: Lubricant.

dusting powder, surgical.
See: B-F-I Powder (SmithKline Beecham Pharmaceuticals).

Dutch Drops. Oil of turpentine, sulfurated.

dutch oil. Oil of turpentine, sulfurated.

Duvoid. (Roberts Pharm) Bethanechol Cl 10 mg, 25 mg or 50 mg/Tab. Bot. 100s, UD ctn. 100s. *Rx.*
Use: Genitourinary.

D V Cream. (Hoechst Marion Roussel) Dienestrol 0.01% w/lactose, propylene glycol, stearic acid, diglycol stearate, TEA, benzoic acid, butylated hydroxytoluene, disodium edetate, buffered w/lactic acid to an acid pH. Tube 3 oz, w/applicator. *Rx.*
Use: Estrogen.

D-Vaso-S. (Dunhall Pharmaceuticals) Pentylenetetrazol 50 mg, niacin 50 mg, dimenhydrinate 25 mg, alcohol 18%, sherry wine vehicle. Bot. pt. *Rx.*
Use: Respiratory.

D-10-W. (Various Mfr.) Dextrose in water injection 10% (amps 3 ml); vials 250 ml, 500 ml, 1000 ml; 17 ml fill in 20 ml, 500 ml fill in 1000 ml, 1000 ml fill in 2000 ml vials. *Rx.*
Use: Carbohydrate supplement.

Dwelle. (Dakryon) EDTA 0.09%, sodium chloride, potassium chloride, boric acid, povidone, NPX 0.001%. Drop. Bot. 15 ml. *otc.*
Use: Artificial tears.

d-xylose.
See: Xylo-Pfan. (Pharmacia & Upjohn).

Dyantoin Caps. (Major) Phenytoin sodium 100 mg/Cap. Bot. 100s, 1000s. *Rx.*
Use: Anticonvulsant.

DX 114 Foot Powder. (Amlab) Zinc undecylenate 1%, salicylic acid 1%, benzoic acid 1%, ammonium alum 5%, boric acid 10.5% w/zinc stearate, chlorophyll, talc, kaolin, starch, calcium silicate, oil of wormwood. Cont. 2 oz. *otc.*
Use: Antifungal, topical.

Dyazide. (SmithKline Beecham Pharmaceuticals) Triamterene 37.5 mg, hydrochlorothiazide 25 mg/Cap. Bot. 1000s, UD 100s, Patient Pack 100s. *Rx.*
Use: Antihypertensive, diuretic.

Dycill. (SmithKline Beecham Pharmaceuticals) Dicloxacillin sodium 250 mg or 500 mg/Cap. Bot. 100s. *Rx.*
Use: Anti-infective, penicillin.

Dyclone. (Astra) Dyclonine HCl 0.5% or 1%. Soln. Bot. 30 ml. *Rx.*
Use: Anesthetic, local.

•**dyclonine hydrochloride.** (DIE-kloe-neen) U.S.P. 23.
Use: Anesthetic, topical.
See: Dyclone, Soln. (Astra).
W/Benzethonium chloride
See: Skin Shield, Liq. (Del Pharmaceuticals).
W/Neomycin sulfate, polymyxin B sulfate, hydrocortisone acetate.
See: Neo-polycin HC, Oint. (Hoechst Marion Roussel).

Dycomene. (Hance) Hydrocodone bitartrate ⅙ gr, pyrilamine maleate 1 gr/fl. oz. Bot. 3 oz, gal. *c-III.*
Use: Antitussive, sleep aid.

•**dydrogesterone.** (DIE-droe-JESS-ter-ohn) U.S.P. 23.
Use: Hormone, progestin.

dyes.
See: Antiseptic, Dyes.

Dyflex-200 Tablets. (Econo Med Pharmaceuticals) Dyphylline 200 mg/Tab. Bot. 100s, 1000s. *Rx.*
Use: Bronchodilator.

Dyflex-G Tablets. (Econo Med Pharmaceuticals) Dyphylline 200 mg, guaifenesin 200 mg/Tab. Bot. 100s, 1000s. *Rx.*
Use: Bronchodilator, expectorant.

dylate. Clonitrate.
Use: Coronary vasodilator.

Dyline-G.G. Liquid. (Seatrace) Dyphylline 300 mg, guaifenesin 300 mg/15 ml. Bot. pt, gal. *Rx.*
Use: Bronchodilator, expectorant.

Dyline-GG Tablets. (Seatrace) Dyphylline 200 mg, guaifenesin 200 mg/Tab. Bot. 100s, 1000s. *Rx.*
Use: Bronchodilator, expectorant.

•**dymanthine hydrochloride.** (DIE-man-theen) USAN.
Use: Anthelmintic.

Dymelor. (Eli Lilly) Acetohexamide 250 mg or 500 mg/Tab. Bot. 200s. *Rx.*
Use: Antidiabetic.

Dymenate. (Keene Pharmaceuticals) Dimenhydrinate 50 mg/ml. Vial 10 ml. *Rx.*
Use: Antiemetic, antivertigo.

Dynabac. (Sanofi Winthrop) Dirithromycin 250 mg/Tab. Enteric coated. Bot. 60s. *Rx.*
Use: Anti-infective.

Dynacin. (Medicis Dermatologics) Minocycline HCl 50 mg, 100 mg. Cap. Bot. 100s (50 mg). 50s (100 mg). *Rx.*
Use: Anti-infective, tetracycline.

DynaCirc. (Sandoz Consumer) Isradipine. 2.5 mg or 5 mg/Cap. Bot. 60s, 100s, UD 100s. *Rx.*
Use: Calcium channel blocker.

DynaCirc CR. (Novartis) Isradipine 5 mg, 10 mg/CR Tab. Bot. 30s, 100s. *Rx.*
Use: Calcium channel blocker.

Dynacoryl.
See: Nikethamide, Preps. (Various Mfr.)

Dynafed Asthma Relief. (BDI Pharm) Ephedrine HCl 25 mg, guaifenesin 200 mg/Tab. Bot. 60s. *otc.*
Use: Decongestant, expectorant.

Dynafed Jr., Children's. (BDI).
See: Children's Dynafed Jr., Chew Tab. (BDI).

Dynafed Ex, Extra Strength. (BDI)
See: Extra Strength Dynafed, Tab. (BDI).

Dynafed IB. (BDI) Ibuprofen 200 mg/Tab. 36s. *otc.*
Use: Analgesic.

Dynafed Plus, Maximum Strength. (BDI)
See: Maximum Strength Dynafed Plus, Tab. (BDI).

Dynafed Pseudo. (BDI Pharm) Pseudoephedrine HCl 60 mg/Tab. Bot. 60s. *otc.*
Use: Decongestant.

Dyna-Hex Skin Cleanser. (Western Medical) Chlorhexidine gluconate 4%, isopropyl alcohol 4%. Liq. Bot. 120 ml, 240 ml, 480 ml, 1 gal. *otc.*
Use: Antimicrobial, antiseptic.

Dyna-Hex 2 Skin Cleanser. (Western Medical) Chlorhexidine gluconate 2%, isopropyl alcohol 4%. Liq. Bot. 120 ml, 2409 ml, 480 ml, 1 gal. *otc.*
Use: Anitmicrobial, antiseptic.

dynamine. (Mayo Foundation)
Use: Antispasmodic, Lambert-Eaton myasthenic syndrome, hereditary motor and sensory neuropathy type I (Charcot-Marie-Tooth Disease). [Orphan drug]

Dynapen. (Bristol-Myers Squibb) Sodium dicloxacillin. **Cap.:** 125 mg, 250 mg or 500 mg. Bot. 24s, 50s, 100s. **Susp.:** 62.5 mg/5 ml. Bot. 80 ml, 100 ml, 200 ml. *Rx.*
Use: Anti-infective, penicillin.

Dynaplex. (Alton) Vitamin B complex. Bot. 100s, 1000s. *otc.*
Use: Vitamin supplement.

dynarsan.
See: Acetarsone, Tab.

Dy-O-Derm. (Galderma) Purified water, isopropyl alcohol, acetone, dihydroxyacetone, FD&C; yellow No. 6, FD&C; blue No. 1, FD&C; red No. 33. Bot. 4 oz.
Use: Dermatologic, vitiligo stain.

Dy-Phyl-Lin. (Foy) Dyphylline 250 mg/ml with benzyl alcohol. Inj. Vial 10 ml. *Rx.*
Use: Bronchodilator.

•**dyphylline.** (DIE-fih-lin) U.S.P. 23.
Use: Vasodilator, bronchodilator.
See: Brophylline, Inj., Granucaps (Solvay).
Dilor, Preps. (Savage).
Emfabid TD, Tab. (Saron).
Lardet, Inj. (Standex).
Neothylline, Tab. (Teva USA).
Prophyllin, Oint., Pow. (Rystan).
W/Chlorpheniramine maleate, guaifenesin, dextromethorphan HBr, phenylephrine HCl.
See: Hycoff-A, Syr. (Saron).
W/Guaifenesin.
See: Bronkolate-G, Tab. (Parmed).
Dilor-G, Liq., Tab. (Savage).
Embron, Syr., Cap. (T.E. Williams).
Neothylline GG, Liq. (Teva USA).

Dyphylline GG Elixir. (Various Mfr.) Dyphylline 100 mg, guaifenesin 100 mg/15 ml. Bot. 473 ml. *Rx.*
Use: Bronchodilator.

Dyprotex. (Blistex) Micronized zinc oxide 40%, petrolatum 37.6%, dimethicone 2.5%, cod liver oil, aloe extract, zinc stearate. Pads. Pkgs. 3s (9 applications). *otc.*
Use: Astringent.

Dyrenium. (SmithKline Beecham Pharmaceuticals) Triamterene. **50 mg/Cap.:** Bot. 100s, UD 100s. **100 mg/Cap.:**

Bot. 100s, 1000s, UD 100s. *Rx.*
Use: Diuretic.

Dyretic. (Keene Pharmaceuticals) Furosemide 10 mg/ml. Vial 10 ml. *Rx.*
Use: Diuretic.

Dyrexan-OD. (Trimen) Phendimetrazine tartrate 105 mg/SR Cap. Bot. 100s. *c-III.*
Use: Anorexiant.

Dyspel. (Dover Pharmaceuticals) Acetaminophen, ephedrine sulfate, atropine sulfate. Sugar, lactose and salt free. Tab. UD Box 500s. *Rx.*
Use: Analgesic.

E

Ease. (Neuro Genesis/Matrix) D, L-phenylalanine 500 mg, L-glutamine 15 mg, L-tyrosine 25 mg, L-carnitine 10 mg, L-arginine pyroglutamate 10 mg, L-ornithine/L-aspartate 10 mg, Cr 0.033 mg, Se 0.012 mg, B_1 0.33 mg, B_2 5 mg, B_3 3.3 mg, B_5 0.33 mg, B_6 0.33 mg, B_{12} 1 mcg, E 5 IU, biotin 0.05 mg, FA 0.066 mg, Fe 1 mg, Zn 2.5 mg, Ca 35 mg, I 0.25 mg, Cu 0.33 mg, Mg 25 mg/Cap. Bot. 42s *otc.*
Use: Nutritional supplement.

EACA. (Lederle Consumer Products) Epsilon aminocaproic acid. *Rx.*
Use: Antifibrinolytic.
See: Amicar (Lederle Consumer Products).

Ear Drops. (Weeks & Leo) Carbamide peroxide 6.5% in an anhydrous glycerin base. Bot. oz. *otc.*
Use: Otic.

Ear-Dry. (Scherer) Isopropyl alcohol, boric acid 2.75%. Dropper bot. 30 ml. *otc.*
Use: Otic.

Earex Ear Drops. (Health for Life Brands) Benzocaine 0.15 g, antipyrine 0.7 g/0.5 oz. Bot. 0.5 oz. *Rx.*
Use: Otic.

Ear-Eze. (Hyrex) Hydrocortisone 1%, chloroxylenol 0.1%, pramoxine HCl 1%. Dropper bot. 15 ml. *Rx.*
Use: Anesthetic, local; anti-infective, corticosteroid.

Earocol Ear Drops. (Roberts Pharm) Benzocaine 1.4%, antipyrine 5.4%, glycerin, oxyquinoline sulfate. Soln. Dropper bot. 15 ml. *Rx.*
Use: Otic.

earthnut oil. Peanut Oil.

Easprin. (Parke-Davis) Aspirin 15 gr/EC Tab. Bot. 100s. *Rx.*
Use: Analgesic.

East-A. (Eastwood) Therapeutic lotion. Bot. 16 oz. *otc.*
Use: Emollient.

Easy-Lax. (Walgreens) Docusate sodium 100 mg/Cap. Bot. 60s. *otc.*
Use: Laxative, stool softener.

Easy-Lax Plus. (Walgreens) Docusate sodium 100 mg, casanthranol 30 mg/Cap. Bot. 60s. *otc.*
Use: Laxative, stool softener.

Eazol. (Roberts Pharm) Fructose, dextrose, orthophosphoric acid with controlled hydrogen ion concentration. Bot. 473 ml. *otc.*
Use: Antinauseant.

E-Base. (Barr Laboratories) Erythromycin. **Cap.:** 333 mg. Bot. 100s, 500s, 1000s. **Tab.:** 500 mg. Bot. 100s, 500s. *Rx.*
Use: Anti-infective, erythromycin.

•**ebastine.** (EBB-ass-teen) USAN.
Use: Antihistamine.

EBV-VCA. (Wampole Laboratories) Epstein-Barr virus, viral capsid antigen antibody test. Qualitative and semi-quantitative detection of EBV antibody in human serum. Test 100s.
Use: Diagnostic aid.

EBV-VCA Ig. (Wampole Laboratories) Epstein-Barr virus, viral capsid antigen Ig antibody. Qualitative and semi-qualitative detection of EBV-VCA Ig antibody in human serum. Test 50s.
Use: Diagnostic aid.

•**ecadotril.** (ee-CAD-oh-trill) USAN.
Use: Antihypertensive.

•**ecamsule.** (eh-KAM-sool) USAN.
Use: Sunscreen.

Ecee Plus. (Edwards Pharmaceuticals) Vitamin E 165 mg, ascorbic acid 100 mg, magnesium sulfate 70 mg, zinc sulfate 80 mg/Tab. Bot. 100s. *otc.*
Use: Mineral, vitamin supplement.

•**echothiophate iodide.** (eck-oh-THIGH-oh-fate EYE-oh-dide) U.S.P. 23.
Use: Antiglaucoma agent; cholinergic (ophthalmic).
See: Echodide, Ophth. Soln. (Alcon Laboratories).
Phospholine Iodide, Pow. (Wyeth Ayerst).

•**eclanamine maleate.** (eh-KLAN-ah-MEEN) USAN.
Use: Antidepressant.

•**eclazolast.** (eh-CLAY-zole-AST) USAN.
Use: Antiallergic, inhibitor (mediator release).

Eclipse After Sun. (Novartis) Petrolatum, glycerin, oleth-3 phosphate, carbomer-934, imidazolidinyl urea, benzyl alcohol, cetyl esters wax. Lot. Bot. 180 ml. *otc.*
Use: Emollient.

Eclipse Lip and Face Protectant. (Novartis) Padimate O, oxybenzone. Stick 4.5 g. *otc.*
Use: Lip protectant.

Eclipse Original Sunscreen. (Novartis) Padimate O, glyceryl PABA. Lot. Bot. 120 ml. *otc.*
Use: Sunscreen.

Eclipse Suntan, Partial. (Novartis) Padimate O. Lot. Bot. 120 ml. *otc.*
Use: Sunscreen.

EC-Naprosyn. (Syntex) Naproxen 375 mg or 500 mg/TR Tab. Bot. 100s. *Rx.*
Use: NSAID.

•**econazole.** (ee-CON-uh-zole) USAN.
Use: Antifungal.

•**econazole nitrate.** (ee-CON-uh-zole) U.S.P. 23.
Use: Antifungal.
See: Spectazole (Ortho Pharm).

Econo B & C. (Vangard) Vitamins B_1 15 mg, B_2 10.2 mg, B_3 50 mg, B_5 10 mg, B_6 5 mg, C 300 mg/Capl. Bot. 100s, UD 100s. *otc.*
Use: Vitamin supplement.

Econopred Ophthalmic. (Alcon Laboratories) Prednisolone acetate 0.125% Susp. Drop-Tainer 5 ml, 10 ml. *Rx.*
Use: Corticosteroid, ophthalmic.

Econopred Plus. (Alcon Laboratories) Prednisolone acetate 1%. Susp. Drop-Tainer 5 ml, 10 ml. *Rx.*
Use: Corticosteroid, ophthalmic.

Ecotrin Adult Low Strength. (SmithKline Beecham) Aspirin 81 mg., tartrazine/Tab. ent. ctd. Bot. 36s *otc.*
Use: Analgesic.

Ecotrin Maximum Strength. (SmithKline Beecham) Acetylsalicylic acid 500 mg. **Tab.:** Bot. 60s, 150s. **Cap.:** Bot. 60s. *otc.*
Use: Analgesic.

Ecotrin Regular Strength Tablets. (SmithKline Beecham) Aspirin 325 mg/EC Tab. Bot. 100s, 250s, 1000s. *otc.*
Use: Analgesic.

Ed A-Hist. (Edwards Pharmaceuticals) Phenylephrine HCl 10 mg, chlorpheniramine maleate 4 mg/5 ml, alcohol 5%. Liq. Bot. 473 ml. *Rx.*
Use: Antihistamine, decongestant.

Ed A-Hist Tablets. (Edwards Pharmaceuticals) Chlorpheniramine maleate 8 mg, phenylephrine HCl 20 mg/SR Tab. Bot. 100s. *Rx.*
Use: Antihistamine, decongestant.

edathamil. Edetate ethylenediaminetetraacetic acid.
See: Nullapons (General Aniline).

edathamil calcium-disodium. Calcium disodium ethylenediamine tetraacetate.
See: Calcium Disodium Versenate, Amp. & Tab. (3M).

edathamil disodium. Disodium salt of ethylene diamine tetraacetic acid.
See: Endrate, Amp. (Abbott Laboratories).

•**edatrexate.** (EE-dah-TREX-ate) USAN.
Use: Antineoplastic.

Edecrin. (Merck) Ethacrynic acid 25 mg or 50 mg/Tab. Bot. 100s. *Rx.*
Use: Diuretic.

Edecrin Sodium Intravenous. (Merck) Ethacrynate sodium equivalent to 50 mg ethacrynic acid w/mannitol 62.5 mg, thimerosal 0.1 mg/Vial. Vial 50 ml for reconstitution. *Rx.*
Use: Diuretic.

•**edetate calcium disodium.** (EH-duh-tate) U.S.P. 23. *Formerly Edathamil.*
Use: Chelating agent (metal).
See: Calcium Disodium Versenate, Amp., Tab. (3M).

•**edetate dipotassium.** (EH-deh-tate) USAN.
Use: Pharmaceutic aid (chelating agent).

•**edetate disodium.** (EH-duh-tate) U.S.P. 23.
Use: Chelating agent (metal); pharmaceutic aid (chelating agent).
See: Disotate, Inj. (Steris)
Endrate, Amp. (Abbott Laboratories).

W/Benzalkonium Cl, boric acid, potassium Cl, sodium carbonate anhydrous.
See: Swim-Eye Drops (Savage).

W/Phenylephrine HCl, methapyrilene HCl, benzalkonium Cl, sodium bisulfite.
See: Allerest Nasal Spray (Novartis Pharmaceuticals).

W/Phenylephrine HCl, benzalkonium Cl, sodium bisulfate.
See: Sinarest, Aerosol (Novartis Pharmaceuticals).

W/Potassium Cl, benzalkonium Cl, isotonic boric acid.
See: Dacriose (Smith, Miller & Patch).

W/Prednisolone sodium phosphate, niacinamide, sodium bisulfite, phenol.
See: P.S.P. IV. Inj. (Solvay).

W/Sodium thiosulfate, salicylic acid, isopropyl alcohol, propylene glycol, menthol, colloidal alumina.
See: Tinver Lotion (PBH Wesley Jessen).

edetate disodium. (Various Mfr.) Edetate disodium 150 mg/ml. Vial 20 ml. *Rx.*
Use: Antihypercalcemia, cadiovascular agent.

•**edetate sodium.** (EH-deh-tate) USAN.
Use: Chelating agent.
See: Disodium Versenate (3M).
Vagisec, Liq. (Julius Schmid).

•**edetate trisodium.** (EH-deh-tate) USAN.
Use: Chelating agent.

•**edetic acid.** (ED-eh-tic) N.F. 18.
Use: Pharmaceutic aid (chelating agent).
See: Versene Acid (Dow Chemical).

•**edetol.** (eh-deh-TOLE) USAN.
Use: Pharmaceutic aid (alkalinizing agent).
See: Neutrol TE (BASF).

Edex. (Schwarz Pharma) Alprostadil 5 mcg, 10 mcg, 20 mcg, 40 mcg (after reconstitution), lactose. Single-dose Vial or Kit 5 mcg, 10 mcg, 20 mcg, 40 mcg. *Rx.*
Use: Treatment for impotence.

•**edifolone acetate.** (EH-DIH-fah-LONE) USAN.
Use: Cardiovascular agent (antiarrhythmic).

edithamil.
See: Edathamil.

•**edobacomab.** (eh-dah-BACK-ah-mab) USAN.
Use: Antiendotoxin monoclonal antibody.

•**edoxudine.** (ee-DOX-you-DEEN) USAN.
Use: Antiviral.

•**edrecolomab.** (edd-reh-KOE-lah-mab) USAN.
Use: Monoclonal antibody (antineoplastic adjuvant).

edrofuradene. Name used for Nifurdazil.

•**edrophonium chloride.** (eh-droe-FOE-nee-uhm) U.S.P. 23.
Use: Antidote to curare principles; diagnostic aid, myasthenia gravis.
See: Enlon, Inj. (Ohmeda Pharmaceuticals).
Reversol (Organon Teknika).
Tensilon Chloride, Vial (Roche Laboratories).

edrophonium chloride/atropine sulfate.
See: atropine sulfate/edrophonium chloride.

ED-SPAZ. (Edwards Pharmaceuticals) Hyoscyamine sulfate 0.125 mg/Tab. Bot. 100s. *Rx.*
Use: Anticholinergic, antispasmodic.

EDTA.
See: Edathamil (Various Mfr.).

ED-TIC. (Edwards Pharmaceuticals) Phenylephrine HCl 5 mg, chlorpheniramine maleate 2 mg, hydrocodone bitartrate 1.67 mg/5 ml. Liq. Bot. 473 ml. *c-III.*
Use: Antihistamine, antitussive, decongestant.

Ed Tuss HC. (Edwards Pharmaceuticals) Phenylephrine HCl 10 mg, chlorpheniramine maleate 4 mg, hydrocodone bitartrate 2.5 mg, alcohol 5%/5 ml. Liq. Bot. 480 ml. *c-III.*
Use: Antihistamine, antitussive, decongestant.

E.E.S. 400 Filmtab. (Abbott Laboratories) Erythromycin ethylsuccinate representing 400 mg erythromycin activity/Tab. Pkg. 100s, 500s, UD 100s. *Rx.*
Use: Anti-infective, erythromycin.

E.E.S. Drops. (Abbott Laboratories) Erythromycin ethylsuccinate representing erythromycin activity 100 mg/2.5 ml when reconstituted w/water. Dropper Bot. 50 ml. *Rx.*
Use: Anti-infective, erythromycin.

E.E.S. Granules. (Abbott Laboratories) Erythromycin ethylsuccinate representing erythromycin activity 200 mg/5 ml oral susp. Gran. Bot. 60 ml, 100 ml, 200 ml, UD 5 ml. *Rx.*
Use: Anti-infective, erythromycin.

E.E.S. Liquid-200 & 400. (Abbott Laboratories) Erythromycin ethylsuccinate representing erythromycin activity 200 mg/5 ml. Bot. 100 ml, 480 ml; erythromycin activity 400 mg/5 ml. Bot. 100 ml, 480 ml. *Rx.*
Use: Anti-infective, erythromycin.

Efed-II. (Alto Pharmaceuticals) Ephedrine sulfate 25 mg/Cap. Box 24s. *otc.*
Use: Decongestant.

Efedron Nasal. (Hyrex) Ephedrine HCl 0.6%, chlorobutanol 0.5% w/sodium Cl, menthol and cinnamon oil in a water-soluble jelly base. Tube 20 g. *otc.*
Use: Decongestant.

•**efegatran sulfate.** (EH-feh-GAT-ran) USAN.
Use: Antithrombotic.

E-Ferol Spray. (Forest Pharmaceutical) Alpha tocopherol equivalent to 30 IU Vitamin E/ml. Can 6 oz. *otc.*
Use: Emollient.

E-Ferol Succinate. (Forest Pharmaceutical) d-alpha Tocopherol acid succinate, equivalent to Vitamin E. *otc.* **100 or 400 IU/Cap.:** Bot. 100s, 500s, 1000s. **200 IU/Cap.:** Bot. 50s, 100s, 500s, 1000s. **50 IU/Tab.:** Bot. 100s, 500s, 1000s.
Use: Vitamin supplement.

E-Ferol Vanishing Cream. (Forest Pharmaceutical) Alpha tocopherol. Jar 2 oz. *otc.*
Use: Emollient.

Effectin Tablets. (Sanofi Winthrop) Bitolterol mesylate. *Rx.*
Use: Bronchodilator.

Effective Strength Cough Formula. (Alphalma USPD) Chlorpheniramine maleate 2 mg, dextromethorphan HBr 15 mg, alcohol 10%. Liq. Bot. 240 ml. *otc.*
Use: Antihistamine, antitussive.

Effective Strength Cough w/Decongestant. (Alphalma USPD) Pseudoephedrine HCl 20 mg, dextromethorhan HBr 10 mg, alcohol 10%. Liq. Bot. 240 ml. *otc.*
Use: Antitussive, decongestant.

Effer-K. (Nomax) Potassium 25 mEq. (as bicarbonate and citrate), saccharin. Effervescent tab. Box foil 30s, 250s. *Rx.*
Use: Mineral supplement.

Effexor. (Wyeth Ayerst) Venlafaxine 25 mg, 37.5 mg, 50 mg, 75 mg or 100 mg/Tab. Bot. 100s, Redipak 100s. *Rx.*
Use: Antidepressant.

Effexor XR. (Wyeth-Ayerst) Venlafaxine HCl 37.5 mg, 75 mg, 150 mg/ER Cap. Bot. 100s, UD 100s. *Rx.*
Use: Antidepressant.

Efficol Cough Whip, Suppressant, Decongestant. (Block Drug) Phenylpropanolamine HCl 6.25 mg, dextromethorphan HBr 2.5 mg/5 ml Bot. 8 oz. *otc.*
Use: Antitussive, decongestant.

Efficol Cough Whip, Suppressant, Decongestant, Antihistamine. (Block Drug) Dextromethorphan HBr 2.5 mg, phenylpropanolamine HCl 6.25 mg, chlorpheniramine maleate 1 mg/5 ml Bot. 8 oz. *otc.*
Use: Antihistamine, antitussive, decongestant.

Efidac/24. (Novartis Pharmaceuticals) Pseudoephedrine HCl 240 mg/Tab. Pkg. 6s, 12s. *otc.*
Use: Decongestant.

Efidac 24 Chlorpheniramine. (Novartis Pharmaceuticals) Chlorpheniramine maleate 16 mg/ER Tab. Pkg. 6s, 12s. *otc.*
Use: Antihistamine.

•**eflornithine hydrochloride.** (ee-FLAHR-nih-THEEN) USAN.
Use: Antineoplastic, antiprotozoal. [Orphan drug]
See: Ornidyl (Hoechst Marion Roussel).

EfoDine Ointment. (E. Fougera) Povidone-iodine oint. Foilpac oz, Tube oz. Jar lb. *otc.*

Efudex. (Roche Laboratories) Fluorouracil. **Soln:** Fluorouracil 2% or 5%, w/ propylene glycol, hydroxypropyl cellulose, parabens, disodium edetate. Drop Dispenser 10 ml. **Cream:** Fluorouracil 5%, in vanishing cream base w/white petrolatum, stearyl alcohol, propylene glycol, polysorbate 60, parabens. Tube 25 g. *Rx.*
Use: Antineoplastic.

egraine. A protein binder from oats.

•**egtazic acid.** (egg-TAY-zik) USAN.
Use: Pharmaceutic aid.

EHDP.
See: Etidronate Disodium.

ehrlich 606.
See: Arspheramine (Various Mfr.).

EL 10. (Elan) *Rx.*
Use: Antiviral, immunomodulator.

•**elacridar hydrochloride.** (eh-LACK-rih-dahr) USAN.
Use: Potentiation of chemotherapy in cancer (multidrug resistance inhibitor in cancer); antineoplastic (adjunct).

•**elantrine.** (EL-an-treen) USAN.
Use: Anticholinergic.

Elase. (Parke-Davis) **Pow.:** Fibrinolysin 25 units, desoxyribonuclease 15,000 units, thimerosal 0.1 mg/Vial as lyophilized powder. May be reconstituted with 10 ml of isotonic sodium Cl Soln. **Oint.:** Fibrinolysin 30 units, desoxyribonuclease 20,000 units, thimerosal 0.12 mg/30 g Tube. Fibrinolysin 10 units, desoxyribonuclease 6,666 units/10 g w/ thimerosal 0.04 mg as preservative. Ointment base of liquid petrolatum, polyethylene w/sucrose, sodium Cl. Tube 10 g, 30 g. *Rx.*
Use: Enzyme, topical.

Elase-Chloromycetin Ointment. (Parke-Davis) Fibrinolysin 10 units, desoxyribonuclease 6666 units, chloramphenicol 100 mg. Tube 10 g. Fibrinolysin 30 units, desoxyribonuclease 20,000 units, chloramphenicol 300 mg and thimerosal. In 30 g. *Rx.*
Use: Enzyme, topical.

•**elastofilcon a.** (ee-LASS-toe-FILL-kahn A) USAN.
Use: Contact lens material, hydrophilic.

Elavil. (Zeneca) Amitriptyline HCl. **Tab.: 10 mg:** Bot. 100s, 1000s; **25 mg:** Bot. 100s, 1000s; **50 mg:** Bot. 100s, 1000s; **75 mg, 100 mg:** Bot. 100s; **150 mg:** Bot. 30s, 100s. All strengths in UD 100s. **Inj.:** Vial 10 mg/ml w/dextrose 44 mg, methylparaben 1.5 mg, propylparaben 0.2 mg/ml w/water for injection. q.s. Vial 1 ml, 10 ml. *Rx.*
Use: Antidepressant, tricyclic.

elcatonin. (Innapharma).
Use: Intrathecal treatment of intractable pain. [Orphan drug]

•**eldacimibe.** (ell-DASS-ih-mibe) USAN.
Use: Antiatherosclerotic, antihyperlipidemic.

Eldec Kapseals. (Parke-Davis) Elemental iron 3.3 mg, Vitamins A 1667 IU, E

10 mg, B_1 10 mg, B_2 0.9 mg, B_3 17 mg, B_5 10 mg, B_6 0.7 mg, B_{12} 2 mcg, C 67 mg, folic acid 0.3 mg, calcium iodine/ Cap. Bot. 100s. *otc.*
Use: Mineral, vitamin supplement.

Eldecort. (Zeneca) Hydrocortisone 2.5%, light mineral oil, propylene glycol, allantoin/Cream. Tube 15 g, 30 g. *Rx.*
Use: Corticosteroid, topical.

Eldepryl. (Somerset) Selegiline HCl 5 mg. lactose. Cap. Bot. 60s, 300s. *Rx.*
Use: Antiparkinsonian.

Eldercaps. (Merz) Vitamins A 4000 IU, D 400 IU, E 25 IU, B, 10mg. B_2 5 mg., B_3 25 mg., B_5 10 mg., B_6 2 mg., C 200 mg, folic acid 1 mg , Zn 15.8 mg. Mg, Mn. /Cap. Bot. 100s. *Rx.*
Use: Mineral, vitamin supplement.

Elder's RVP. Red Vet. Petrolatum.
Use: Dermatoses.

Eldertonic. (Merz) Vitamins B_1 0.17 mg, B_2 0.19 mg, B_3 2.22 mg, B_5 1.11 mg, B_6 0.22 mg, B_{12} 0.67 mcg, alcohol 13.5%, Mg, Mn, zinc 1.7 mg/5 ml. Bot. 473 ml. *otc.*
Use: Mineral, vitamin supplement.

Eldisine. (Eli Lilly).
See: Vindesine sulfate.

Eldo-B & C. (Canright) Vitamins C 250 mg, B_1 25 mg, B_2 10 mg, niacinamide 150 mg, B_6 5 mg, d-calcium pantothenate 20 mg/Tab. Bot. 100s, 1000s. *otc.*
Use: Mineral, vitamin supplement.

Eldofe. (Canright) Ferrous fumarate 225 mg/Chew. tab. Bot. 100s, 1000s. *otc.*
Use: Mineral supplement.

Eldofe-C. (Canright) Ferrous fumarate 225 mg, ascorbic acid 50 mg/Tab. Bot. 100s. *otc.*
Use: Mineral, vitamin supplement.

Eldopaque. (ICN Pharmaceuticals) Hydroquinone 2% in a tinted sunblocking cream base. Tube 15 g, 30 g. *otc.*
Use: Dermatologic.

Eldopaque-Forte. (ICN Pharmaceuticals) Hydroquinone 4% in a tinted sunblocking cream base. Tube 15 g, 30 g. *Rx.*
Use: Dermatologic.

Eldoquin. (ICN Pharmaceuticals) Hydroquinone 2% in a vanishing cream base. Tube 15 g, 30 g. *otc.*
Use: Dermatologic.

Eldoquin Forte. (ICN Pharmaceuticals) Hydroquinone 4% in vanishing cream base. Tube 15 g, 30 g. *Rx.*
Use: Dermatologic.

Elecal. (Western Research) Calcium 250 mg, magnesium 15 mg/Tab. Bot. 1000s. *otc.*
Use: Mineral supplement.

Electrolyte #48 Injection. Pediatric maintenance electrolyte solution. Dextrose 5% in electrolyte #48 w/sodium 25 mEq, potassium 20 mEq, magnesium 3 mEq, chloride 22 mEq, lactate 23 mEq, phosphate 3 mEq/L. *Rx.*
Use: Water, caloric, electrolyte supplement.

Electrolyte #75 and 5% Dextrose.
See: 5% Dextrose and Electrolyte #75.

Elegen-G. (Grafton) Amitriptyline 10 mg, 25 mg or 50 mg/Tab. Bot. 100s, 1000s. *Rx.*
Use: Antidepressant, tricyclic.

Elevites. (Barth's) Vitamins A 6000 IU, D 400 IU, B_1 1.5 mg, B_2 3 mg, C 60 mg, B_{12} 10 mcg, niacin 1 mg, E 10 IU, malt diastase 15 mg, iron 15 mg, calcium 381 mg, phosphorus 0.172 mg, citrus bioflavonoid complex 15 mg, rutin 15 mg, nucleic acid 3 mg, red bone marrow 30 mg, peppermint leaves 10 mg, wheat germ 30 mg/Tab. or Cap. Bot. 100s, 500s, 1000s. *Rx.*
Use: Mineral, vitamin supplement.

Elimite. (Allergan) Permethrin 5%. Cream. Tube 60 g. *Rx.*
Use: Scabicide, pediculicide.

Elixicon. (Berlex) Theophylline 100 mg/ 5 ml with methyl and propyl parabens. Susp. Bot. 237 ml. *Rx.*
Use: Bronchodilator.

Elixiral. (Vita Elixir) Phenobarbital 16.2 mg, hyoscyamine sulfate 0.1037 mg, atropine sulfate 0.194 mg, hyoscine HBr 0.0065 mg/5 ml. Liq. pt, gal. *Rx.*
Use: Anticholinergic, antispasmodic, hypnotic, sedative.

Elixophyllin Capsules, Dye-Free. (Forest Pharmaceutical) Anhydrous theophylline 100 mg or 200 mg/Cap. **100 mg:** Bot. 100s; **200 mg:** Bot. 100s, 500s, UD 100s. *Rx.*
Use: Bronchodilator.

Elixophyllin Elixir. (Forest Pharmaceutical) Anhydrous theophylline 80 mg, alcohol 20%/15 ml. Bot. pt, qt, gal. *Rx.*
Use: Bronchodilator.

Elixophyllin GG Liquid. (Forest Pharmaceutical) Theophylline 100 mg, guaifenesin 100 mg/15 ml. Alcohol free. Bot. 237, 480 ml. *Rx.*
Use: Antiasthmatic combination.

Elixophyllin-KI Elixir. (Forest Pharmaceutical) Anhydrous theophylline 80 mg, potassium iodide 130 mg/15 ml. Bot. 237 ml. *Rx.*

Use: Antiasthmatic combination.

Ellesdine. (Janssen) Pipenperone. *Rx.*
Use: Anxiolytic.

Elliot's B Solution. (Orphan Medical)
Use: Acute lymphatic leukemias and acute lymphoblastic lymphomas. [Orphan drug].

•**elm.** U.S.P. 23. Dried inner bark of *Ulmus rubra* Muhlenberg (*Ulmus fulva* Michaux).
Use: Pharmaceutic aid (suspending agent), demulcent.

Elmiron. (Baker Norton) Pentosan polysulfate 100 mg/ Cap. Bot. 100s *Rx.*
Use: Relief of bladder pain associated with interstitial cystitis.

Elocon Cream. (Schering Plough) Mometasone furoate 0.1%, hexylene glycol, phosphoric acid, propylene glycol stearate, stearyl alcohol, ceteareth-20, titanium dioxide, aluminum starch octenyl succinate, white wax, white petrolatum. 15 g, 45 g. *Rx.*
Use: Corticosteroid, topical.

Elocon Lotion. (Schering Plough) Mometasone furoate 0.1%. Bot. 30 ml, 60 ml. *Rx.*
Use: Corticosteroid, topical.

Elocon Ointment. (Schering Plough) Mometasone furoate 0.1%, hexylene glycol, propylene glycol stearate, white wax, white petrolatum. 15 g, 45 g. *Rx.*
Use: Corticosteroid, topical.

Elphemet. (Canright) Phendimetrazine tartrate 35 mg/Tab. Bot. 100s, 1000s. *c-III.*
Use: Anorexiant.

Elprecal. (Canright) Vitamins A 5000 IU, D 400 IU, B_1 3 mg, B_2 2 mg, B_6 0.1 mg, B_{12} 1 mcg, C 50 mg, E 2 IU, calcium pantothenate 2.5 mg, niacinamide 15 mg, inositol 5 mg, choline 5 mg, calcium lactate 500 mg, ferrous sulfate 50 mg, copper 1 mg, manganese 1 mg, magnesium 2 mg, potassium 2 mg, zinc 0.5 mg, sulfur 1 mg/Cap. Bot. 100s. *otc.*
Use: Mineral, vitamin supplement.

•**elsamitrucin.** (els-AM-ih-TRUE-sin) USAN.
Use: Antineoplastic.

Elserpine. (Canright) Reserpine 0.25 mg/ Tab. Bot. 100s, 1000s. *Rx.*
Use: Antihypertensive.

Elspar. (Merck) Asparaginase 10,000 IU, mannitol 80 mg/Inj. Vial 10 ml. *Rx.*
Use: Antineoplastic.

•**elucaine.** (eh-LOO-cane) USAN.
Use: Anticholinergic, gastric.

Eltroxin. (Roberts Pharm) Levothyroxine sodium 0.05 mg, 0.1 mg, 0.15 mg, 0.2 mg, 0.3 mg/Tab. Bot. 100s, 500s. *Rx.*
Use: Hormone, thyroid.

Elvanol. (DuPont Merck Pharmaceuticals) Polyvinyl alcohol.
Use: Pharmaceutical aid.

Emadine. (Alcon) Emedastine difumarate 0.05% (0.5 mg/ml), benzalkonium chloride 0.01%. Ophth. Soln. Dispenser 5 ml. *Rx.*
Use: Antihistamine, ophthalmic.

embechine. Aliphatic chloroethylamine.
Use: Antineoplastic.

Emcodeine Tabs. (Major) Aspirin with codeine as #2, #3 or #4. Bot. 100s, 500s. *c-III.*
Use: Analgesic combination, narcotic.

Emcyt. (Pharmacia & Upjohn) Estramustine phosphate sodium equivalent to 140 mg estramustine phosphate sodium 12.5 mg/Cap. Bot. 100s. *Rx.*
Use: Antineoplastic.

Emdol. (Health for Life Brands) Salicylamide, para-aminobenzoic acid, sodium calcium succinate, vitamin D-1250. Bot. 100s, 1000s. *otc.*
Use: Analgesic combination.

•**emedastine difumarate.** (eh-meh-DASS-teen die-FEW-mah-rate) USAN.
Use: Management of allergic conjunctivitis, antiasthmatic, antiallergic, antihistamine (H_1-receptor).
See: Emadine, Ophth. Soln. (Alcon).

emergency kits.
See: Ana-Kit (Bayer Corp).
AtroPen Auto-Injector (Survival Technology).
Cyanide Antidote Package (Eli Lilly).
Emergent-Ez Kit (Healthfirst Corp).
EpiPen Auto-Injector (Center Labs).
EpiEZPen (Center Labs).
EpiEZPen Jr. (Center Labs).
EpiPen Jr. Auto-Injector (Center Labs).
LidoPen Auto-Injector (Survival Technology).
Poison Antidote Kit (Jones Medical Industries).

Emergent-Ez. (Healthfirst Corp) Adrenalin 2 amp., aminophylline 1 amp., ammonia inhalants (3), amyl nitrite inhalants (2), atropine 2 amp., diazepam (2 amp), epinephrine (2 amp), Benadryl 2 amp., nitroglycerin 1 bottle, Solu-Cortef 1 mix-o-vial, Talwin 1 amp., Tigan 1 amp., Valium 2 amp., Wyamine 2 amp., plastic air way (1), disposable syringes, tracheotomy needle (1) and tourniquet (1)/kit. *Rx.*
Use: Emergency kit.

Emeroid. (Delta) Zinc oxide 5%, diperodon HCl 0.25%, bismuth subcarbonate 0.2%, pyrilamine maleate 0.1%, phenylephrine HCl 0.25%, in a petrolatum base containing cod liver oil. Tube 1.25 oz. *otc.*
Use: Anorectal preparation.

Emersal. (Medco Lab) Ammoniated mercury 5%, salicylic acid 2.5%. Lot. Bot. 120 ml. *Rx.*
Use: Antipsoriatic.

Emerson 1% Sodium Fluoride Dental Gel. (Emerson) Red and plain. Bot. 2 oz. *Rx.*
Use: Dental caries agent.

emetics.
See: Apomorphine HCl. Cupric Sulfate. Ipecac Syr.

•**emetine hydrochloride.** (EM-eh-teen) U S. P. 23.
Use: Antiamebic.

Emetrol. (Pharmacia & Upjohn) Dextrose 1.87 g; fructose 1.87g; phosphoric acid 21.5 mg; methylparaben; lemon, mint, or cherry flavor. Sol. Bot. 118 ml, 236 ml, 473 ml. *otc.*
Use: Antiemetic.

Emgel. (GlaxoWellcome) Erythromycin 2%. Gel. Tube 27 g. *Rx.*
Use: Dermatologic, acne.

EM-GG. (Econo Med Pharmaceuticals) Guaifenesin 100 mg/5 ml. Bot. pt. *otc.*
Use: Expectorant.

•**emilium tosylate.** (EE-MILL-ee-uhm TAH-sill-ate) USAN.
Use: Cardiovascular agent (antiarrhythmic).

Eminase. (Roberts Pharm) Anistreplase 30 units/Pow. for Inj. Vials. *Rx.*
Use: Thrombolytic enzyme.

Emitrip Tabs. (Major) Amitriptyline **10 mg or 25 mg/Tab.:** Bot. 100s, 250s, 1000s, UD 100s. **50 mg/Tab.:** Bot. 100s, 250s, 1000s, UD 100s. **75 mg/Tab.:** Bot. 100s, 250s, UD 100s. **100 mg/ Tab.:** Bot. 100s, 250s, 1000s, UD 100s. **150 mg/Tab.:** Bot. 100s, 250s. *Rx.*
Use: Antidepressant, tricyclic.

Emko Because Contraceptor. (Schering Plough) Nonoxynol-9 (8% concentration). Contraceptor container w/applicator. Tube 10 g. *otc.*
Use: Vaginal contraceptive.

EMLA. (Astra) Lidocaine 2.5%, prilocaine 2.5%/Cream. Tube 5 g, 30 g. *Rx.*
Use: Anesthetic, local.

Emollia-Creme. (Gordon Laboratories) Cetyl alcohol, lubricating oils in water-soluble base. Jar 4 oz, 5 lb. *otc.*
Use: Emollient.

Emollia-Lotion. (Gordon Laboratories) Water-dispersable waxes, lubricating bland oils in a water-soluble lotion base. Bot. 1 oz, 4 oz, gal. *otc.*
Use: Emollient.

Empirin Aspirin Tablets. (Glaxo-Wellcome) Aspirin 325 mg/Tab. Bot. 50s, 100s, 250s. *otc.*
Use: Analgesic.

Empirin w/Codeine. (GlaxoWellcome) Aspirin 325 mg with codeine phosphate 15 mg, 30 mg or 60 mg/Tab. **No. 2:** Codeine phosphate 15 mg. Bot. 100s. **No. 3:** Codeine phosphate 30 mg. Bot. 100s, 500s, 1000s, Dispenserpak 25s. **No. 4:** Codeine phosphate 60 mg. Bot. 100s, 500s, Dispenserpak 25s. *c-III.*
Use: Analgesic combination, narcotic.

Emulave. (Rydelle)
See: Aveenobar Oilated (Rydelle).

Emul-O-Balm. (Medeva) Menthol, camphor, methyl salicylate. Bot. 2 oz, 8 oz, gal.
Use: Analgesic, topical.

Emulsoil. (Paddock) Castor oil 95%. Bot. 60 ml. *otc.*
Use: Laxative.

E-Mycin. (Pharmacia & Upjohn) Erythromycin. 333 mg/EC Tab. Bot. 100s, 500s, UD 100s. *Rx.*
Use: Anti-infective, erythromycin.

•**enadoline hydrochloride.** (en-AHD-ole-en) USAN.
Use: Analgesic. Severe head injury. [Orphan drug]

•**enalapril maleate.** (EH-NAL-uh-prill) U.S.P. 23.
Use: Antihypertensive.
See: Vasotec, Tab. (Merck).
W/ Diltiazem maleate.
See: Teczem, ER Tab. (Hoechst-Marion Roussel).
W/Felodipine.
See: Lexxel, ER Tab. (Astra Merck).
W/Hydrochlorothiazide.
See: Vaseretic, Tab. (Merck).

•**enalaprilat.** (EH-NAL-uh-prill-at) U.S.P. 23.
Use: Antihypertensive.
See: Vasotec Inj(Merck).

•**enalkiren.** (en-al-KIE-ren) USAN.
Use: Antihypertensive.

•**enazadrem phosphate.** (eh-NAZZ-ah-drem FOSS-fate) USAN.
Use: Antipsoriatic; inhibitor (5-lipoxygenase).

encapsulated porcine islet prepara-

tion.
Use: Type 1 diabetes. [Orphan drug]
See: BetaRx (VivoRx).

Encare. (Thompson Medical) Nonoxynol-9 (2.27%). Supp. 12s. *otc.*
Use: Vaginal contraceptive.

•**enciprazine hydrochloride.** (en-SIH-PRAH-zeen) USAN.
Use: Anxiolytic.

•**enclomiphene.** (en-KLOE-mih-FEEN) USAN. *Formerly Ciscolomiphene.*

•**encyprate.** (en-SIGH-prate) USAN.
Use: Antidepressant.

Endafed. (Forest Pharmaceutical) Pseudoephedrine HCl 120 mg, brompheniramine maleate 12 mg/SR Cap. Bot. 100s. *Rx.*
Use: Antihistamine, decongestant.

Endagen-HD. (Jones Medical Industries) Phenylephrine HCl 5 mg, chlorpheniramine maleate 2 mg, hydrocodone bitartrate 1.67 mg. Bot. 473 ml. *c-III.*
Use: Antihistamine, antitussive, decongestant.

Endal. (Forest Pharmaceutical) Phenylephrine HCl 20 mg, guaifenesin 300 mg/TR tab., dye free. Bot. 100s. *Rx.*
Use: Decongestant, expectorant.

Endal Expectorant. (Forest Pharmaceutical) Codeine phosphate 10 mg, phenylpropanolamine HCl 12.5 mg, guaifenesin 100 mg/5 ml w/alcohol 5%. Bot. pt. *c-IV.*
Use: Antitussive, decongestant, expectorant.

Endal-HD. (Forest Pharmaceutical) Phenylephrine HCl 5 mg, chlorpheniramine maleate 2 mg, hydrocodone bitartrate 1.67 mg w/menthol, sucrose. Liq. Bot. 480 ml. *c-III.*
Use: Antihistamine, antitussive, decongestant.

Endal-HD Plus. (Forest Pharmaceutical) Hydrocodone bitartrate 2 mg, phenylephrine HCl 5 mg, chlorpheniramine maleate 2 mg/5 ml. Liq. Bot. 473 ml. *c-III.*
Use: Antihistamine, antitussive, decongestant.

Endecon. (DuPont Merck Pharmaceuticals) Phenylpropanolamine HCl 25 mg, acetaminophen 325 mg/Tab. Bot. 60s. *otc.*
Use: Analgesic, decongestant.

Endep. (Roche Laboratories) Amitriptyline HCl 10 mg, 25 mg, 50 mg, 75 mg, 100 mg or 150 mg/Tab. **10 mg:** Bot. 100s, Tel-E-Dose 100s. **25 mg:** Bot. 100s, 500s, Tel-E-Dose 100s. **50 mg:** Bot. 100s, 500s, Tel-E-Dose 100s. **75 mg:** Bot. 100s, Tel-E-Dose 100s. **100 mg:** Bot. 100s, Tel-E-Dose 100s. **150 mg:** Bot 100s. *Rx.*
Use: Antidepressant, tricyclic.

End Lice. (Thompson Medical) Pyrethrins 0.3%, piperonyl butoxide technical 3%. Liq. Bot. 177 ml. *otc.*
Use: Pediculicide.

endobenziline bromide.
Use: Anticholinergic.

endocaine. Pyrrocaine.
Use: Anesthetic, local.

endojodin.
See: Entodon.

Endolor. (Keene Pharmaceuticals) Butalbital 50 mg, caffeine 40 mg, acetaminophen 325 mg/Cap. Bot. 100s. *Rx.*
Use: Analgesic, hypnotic, sedative.

endomycin. A new antibiotic obtained from cultures of *Streptomyces endus.* Under study.

endophenolphthalein. (Roche Laboratories) Diacetyldioxyphenylisatin-isacenbisatin. *otc.*
Use: Laxative.
See: Diacetylhydroxphenylisatin, Prep. (Various Mfr.)

•**endralazine mesylate.** (en-DRAL-ah-zeen MEH-sih-late) USAN.
Use: Antihypertensive.
See: Migranol (Novartis).

Endrate. (Abbott Hospital Prods) Edetate disodium 150 mg/ml. Amp. 20 ml. *Rx.*
Use: Antihypercalcemic, cardiovascular agent.

•**endrysone.** (EN-drih-sone) USAN.
Use: Anti-inflammatory, topical; ophthalmic.

Enduron. (Abbott Laboratories) Methyclothiazide 5 mg/Tab. Bot. 100s, 1000s, UD 100s. *Rx.*
Use: Diuretic.

Enduronyl. (Abbott Laboratories) Methyclothiazide 5 mg, deserpidine 0.25 mg/Tab. Bot. 100s, 1000s, UD 100s. *Rx.*
Use: Antihypertensive, diuretic.

Enduronyl Forte. (Abbott Laboratories) Methyclothiazide 5 mg, deserpidine 0.5 mg/Tab. Bot. 100s, 1000s. *Rx.*
Use: Antihypertensive, diuretic.

Enebag 2. (Lafayette Pharm) Air contrast barium enema bag. Case 24s.
Use: Radiopaque agent.

Enebag XL. (Lafayette Pharm) Air contrast barium enema bag 3000 ml w/lumen tubing, enema tip and side clamp. Case 24s.

Use: Radiopaque agent.

Enecat. (Lafayette Pharm) Barium sulfate suspension CT colon exam kit. Case 12s.
Use: Radiopaque agent.

Enemark. (Lafayette Pharm) Rectal marker. 85% w/v liquid barium. Case of 12 kits.
Use: Rectal marker during radiation therapy.

Enerjets. (Chilton) Caffeine 65 mg/Loz. pkg. 10s. *otc.*
Use: CNS stimulant.

Eneset 1. (Lafayette Pharm) Barium sulfate suspension 300 ml/air contrast examination kit. Unit-of-use kit. Case 12s.
Use: Radiopaque agent.

Eneset 2. (Lafayette Pharm) Barium sulfate suspension 450 ml/contrast examination kit. Unit-of-use kit. Case 12s.
Use: Radiopaque agent.

Eneset 600. (Lafayette Pharm) Barium sulfate suspension 600 ml/air contrast examination kit. Unit-of-use kit. Case 12s.
Use: Radiopaque agent.

Enfamil. (Bristol-Myers) Vitamins A 2000 IU, D 400 IU, E 20 IU, C 52 mg, B_1 0.5 mg, B_2 1 mg, B_6 0.4 mg, B_{12} 1.5 mcg, niacin 8 mg, calcium 440 mg, phosphorus 300 mg, folic acid 100 mcg, pantothenic acid 3 mg, inositol 30 mg, biotin 15 mcg, K-1 55 mcg, choline 100 mg, iron 1.4 mg, potassium 650 mg, chloride 400 mg, copper 0.6 mg, iodine 65 mcg, sodium 175 mg, magnesium 50 mg, zinc 5 mg, manganese 100 mg/Qt. Concentrated Liq. 13 fl oz, Instant Pow. lb. *otc.*
Use: Nutritional supplement.

Enfamil Human Milk Fortifier. (Bristol-Myers) Whey protein, casein, corn syrup solids, lactose, protein 0.7 g, carbohydrate 2.7 g, fat 0.04 g, calories 14. Pow. Packet 0.95 g, Box 100s. *otc.*
Use: Nutritional supplement.

Enfamil w/Iron. (Bristol-Myers) Iron 12 mg/Qt. Pkg. Con. Liq. 13 fl oz. 24s. Pow. 1 lb. 6s. *otc.*
Use: Nutritional supplement.

Enfamil with Iron Ready to Use. (Bristol-Myers) Ready-to-use Enfamil with Iron infant formula 20 kcal/fl oz. Can 8 fl oz, 6-can pack; 32 fl oz, 6 cans per case. *otc.*
Use: Nutritional supplement.

Enfamil Next Step. (Bristol-Myers) Protein 17.3 g, carbohydrates 74 g, fat 33.3 g/liter, with appropriate vitamins and minerals. **Liq.:** 390 ml concentrate, 1 qt ready-to-use. **Pow.:** 360 g, 720 g. *otc.*
Use: Nutritional supplement.

Enfamil Nursette. (Bristol-Myers) Ready-to-feed Enfamil 20 kcal/fl oz, 4 fl oz, 6 fl oz and 8 fl oz. 4 bottles/sealed carton. W/Iron. Ready to use. Bot. 6 fl oz 4s, 24s. *otc.*
Use: Nutritional supplement.

Enfamil Premature Formula. (Bristol-Myers) Nonfat milk, whey protein concentrate, corn syrup solids, lactose, coconut oil, corn oil, medium chain triglycerides, soy lecithin. Protein 2.8 g, carbohydrate 10.7 g, fat 4.9 g, calories 96. Pow. Nursettes 120 ml. *otc.*
Use: Nutritional supplement.

Enfamil Ready To Use. (Bristol-Myers) Ready-to-use Enfamil infant formula 20 kcal/fl oz. Can 8 fl oz, 6-can pack; 32 fl oz, 6 cans per case. *otc.*
Use: Nutritional supplement.

•**enflurane.** (EN-flew-rane) U.S.P. 23.
Use: Anesthetic, inhalation.
See: Ethrane (Ohmeda).

enflurane. (Abbott Laboratories) Enflurane 125 ml and 250 ml/Inhalation. *Rx.*
Use: Anesthetic, inhalation.

Engerix-B. (SmithKline Beecham) Hepatitis B vaccine (recombinant). **Adult:** 20 mcg hepatitis B surface antigen. Vial 1 ml single-dose; 10 ml multidose vial; 1 ml Disp. Single-Dose Syr. **Pediatric:** 10 mcg/0.5 ml hepatitis B surface antigen Vial dose, 0.5 ml single-dose; 0.5 ml Disp. Single-Dose Syr. *Rx.*
Use: Vaccine.

•**englitazone sodium.** (EN-GLIH-tah-zone) USAN.
Use: Antidiabetic.

•**enilconazole.** (EE-nill-KOE-nah-zole) USAN.
Use: Antifungal.

•**eniluracil.** (en-ill-YOUR-ah-sill) USAN.
Use: Potentiator of antineoplastic activity of fluorouracil (uracil reductase inhibitor); antineoplastic (adjunct).

•**enisoprost.** (en-EYE-so-prahst) USAN.
Use: Antiulcerative.

Enisyl. (Person & Covey) L-Lysine monohydrochloride 334 mg or 500 mg/Tab. Bot. 100s, 250s. *otc.*
Use: Nutritional supplement.

•**enlimomab.** (en-LIE-moe-mab) USAN.
Use: Anti-inflammatory; monoclonal antibody.

Enlon Injection. (Ohmeda Pharmaceuticals) Edrophonium Cl 10 mg/ml, phe-

nol 0.45%, sodium sulfite 0.2%. Vial 15 ml. *Rx.*
Use: Cholinergic muscle stimulant.

Enlon-Plus. (Ohmeda Pharmaceuticals) Edrophonium chloride 10 mg, atropine sulfate 0.14 mg. Inj. Amp. 5 ml, Multi-dose Vial 15 ml. *Rx.*
Use: Muscle stimulant.

•**enloplatin.** (en-LOW-PLAT-in) USAN.
Use: Antineoplastic.

Ennex Ointment. (Ennex) Aloe vera extract 37.5%. **Skin Oint.:** Zinc oxide 12.5%, coal tar 1.5%, alcohol 4.5%. Tube oz. **Hemorrhoidal Oint.:** Tube oz. *otc.*
Use: Anti-inflammatory, astringent, antipruritic.

•**enofelast.** (EE-no-fell-ast) USAN.
Use: Antiasthmatic.

•**enolicam sodium.** (ee-NO-lih-kam) USAN.
Use: Anti-inflammatory, antirheumatic.

Enomine Capsules. (Major) Phenylpropanolamine 45 mg, phenylephrine 5 mg, guaifenesin 200 mg/Cap. Bot. 100s, 500s. *Rx.*
Use: Decongestant, expectorant.

Enovid-E 21. (Searle) Norethynodrel 2.5 mg, mestranol 0.1 mg/Tab. Compack disp. 21s, 6 × 21. Refill 21s, 12 × 21. *Rx.*
Use: Estrogen, progestin combination.

Enovil. (Roberts Pharm) Amtriptyline HCl 10 mg/ml. Vial 10 ml. *Rx.*
Use: Antidepressant.

•**enoxacin.** (en-OX-ah-SIN) USAN.
Use: Anti-infective.
See: Penetrex (Rhone-Poulenc Rorer).

•**enoxaparin sodium.** (ee-NOX-ah-PAR-in) USAN.
Use: Antithrombotic.
See: Lovenox Inj.(Rhone-Poulenc Rorer).

•**enoximone.** (EN-ox-ih-MONE) USAN.
Use: Cardiovascular agent.
See: Perfar (Hoechst Marion Roussel).

•**enpiroline phosphate.** (en-PIHR-oh-LEEN) USAN.
Use: Antimalarial.

•**enprofylline.** (en-PRO-fih-lin) USAN.
Use: Bronchodilator.

•**enpromate.** (EN-pro-mate) USAN.
Use: Antineoplastic.

•**enprostil.** (en-PRAHS-till) USAN.
Use: Antisecretory, antiulcerative.
See: Gardrin (Syntex).

Enrich. (Ross Laboratories) Liquid food with fiber providing complete, balanced nutrition as a full liquid diet, liquid supplement, or tube feeding. One serving provides 5 g dietary fiber. 1100 calories/L. 1530 calories provides 100% US RDA for vitamins and minerals. Can Ready-to-Use 8 fl oz (vanilla, chocolate). *otc.*
Use: Nutritional supplement, enteral.

Ensidon. (Novartis Pharmaceuticals) Opipramol HCl. *Rx.*
Use: Antidepressant.

Ensure. (Ross Laboratories) Liquid food providing 1.06 calories/ml. Can be used as a full liquid diet, liquid supplement or tube feeding. Two quarts (2000 calories) provides 100% US RDA for vitamins and minerals for adults and children over 4 yrs. **Ready-to-Use:** Bot. 8 fl oz (vanilla). Can 8 fl oz (chocolate, black walnut, coffee, strawberry, eggnog, vanilla), 32 fl oz (vanilla, chocolate). **Pow.:** Can 14 oz (400 g) (vanilla). *otc.*
Use: Nutritional supplement.

Ensure HN. (Ross Laboratories) High nitrogen low residue liquid food providing complete, balanced nutrition as tube feeding or oral supplement with 1.06 calories/ml. Provides 100% US RDA for vitamins and minerals for adults and children over 4 yrs. 1400 calories (1321 ml). Ready-to-Use: Can 8 fl oz (vanilla). *otc.*
Use: Nutritional supplement.

Ensure High Protein. (Ross Laboratories) Protein 50.4 g, carbohydrate 129.4 g, fat 25.2 g, < 21 mg cholesterol, Na 1218 mg, K 2100 mg, vitamin A 5250 IU, D 420 IU, E 47.5 IU, K 84 mcg, C 125 mg, folic acid 420 mg, B_1 1.6 mg, B_2 1.8 mg, B_3 21 mg, B_5 10.5 mg, B_6 2.1 mg, B_{12} 6.3 mcg, biotin 315 mcg, Ca 1050 mg, Cl, P, Mg, I, Mn, Cu, Zn 24 mg, Fe 19 mg, Se, Cr, Mo, 945 calories/237 ml. Liq. Bot. 237 ml. *otc.*
Use: Nutritional supplement.

Ensure Osmolite. (Ross Laboratories).
See: Osmolite (Ross Laboratories).

Ensure Plus. (Ross Laboratories) High-calorie liquid food w/caloric density of 1500 calories/L. Six servings (8 oz and 2130 calories each) provides 100% US RDA for vitamins and minerals for adults and children. Ready-to-Use: Bot. 8 fl oz (vanilla). Can 8 fl oz (chocolate, vanilla, eggnog, coffee, strawberry). *otc.*
Use: Nutritional supplement.

Ensure Plus HN. (Ross Laboratories) High-calorie, high-nitrogen liquid food

providing 1.5 calories/ml; 1420 calories provides 100% US RDA for vitamins and minerals for adults and children. Calorie/nitrogen ratio is 150:1. Can 8 fl oz (vanilla). *otc.*
Use: Nutritional supplement.

Ensure Pudding. (Ross Laboratories) Protein 6.8 g (nonfat milk), carbohydrate 34 g (sucrose, modified food starch), fat 9.7 g (partially hydrogenated soybean oil), vitamin A 850 IU, D 68 IU, E 7.7 IU, K 12 mcg, C 15.4 mg, folic acid 68 mcg, B_1 0.25 mg, B_2 0.29 mg, B_6 0.34 mg, B_{12} 1.1 mcg, B_3 3.4 mg, choline, biotin, B_5 1.7 mg, Na 240 mg, K 330 mg, Cl 220 mg, Ca 200 mg, P, Mg, I, Mn, Cu, Zn 3.83 mg, Fe 3.06 mg, 250 calories/can. Pudding. 150 g. *otc.*
Use: Nutritional supplement.

Entab 650. (Merz) Aspirin 650 mg/EC tab. Bot. 100s. *otc.*
Use: Analgesic.

Entero-Test. (HDC) Cap. To identify duodenal parasites; to diagnose and locate upper GI bleeding, pH disorders, achlorhydria and esophageal reflux. Bot. 10s, 25s.
Use: Diagnostic aid.

Entero-Test Pediatric. (HDC) To identify duodenal parasites; to diagnose and locate upper GI bleeding, pH disorders, achlorhydria and esophageal reflux. Cap. Bot. 10s, 25s.
Use: Diagnostic aid.

Enterotube. (Roche Laboratories) Culture-identification method for enterobacteriaceae ACA. Test kit 25s.
Use: Diagnostic aid.

Entertainer's Secret Spray. (KLI Corp) Sodium carboxymethylcellulose, potassium Cl, dibasic sodium phosphate, aloe vera gel, glycerin, parabens. Soln. 60 ml spray. *otc.*
Use: Saliva substitute.

Entex. (Procter & Gamble) Phenylephrine HCl 5 mg, phenylpropanolamine HCl 45 mg, guaifenesin 200 mg/Cap. Bot. 100s, 500s. *Rx.*
Use: Decongestant, expectorant.

Entex LA. (Procter & Gamble) Phenylpropanolamine HCl 75 mg, guaifenesin 400 mg/T.R. Tab. Bot. 100s, 500s. *Rx.*
Use: Decongestant, expectorant.

Entex Liquid. (Procter & Gamble) Phenylephrine HCl 5 mg, phenylpropanolamine HCl 20 mg, guaifenesin 100 mg/5 ml, alcohol 5%. Elix. Bot. 480 ml. *Rx.*
Use: Decongestant, expectorant.

Entex PSE. (Procter & Gamble) Pseudoephedrine 120 mg, guaifenesin 600 mg. Prolonged action. Tab. Bot. 100s. *Rx.*
Use: Decongestant, expectorant.

entodon.

entoidoin.
See: Entodon.

Entolase HP. (Robins) Lipase 8,000 units, protease 50,000 units, amylase 40,000 units/Cap. (enteric coated microbeads). Bot. 100s, 250s. *Rx.*
Use: Digestive enzyme.

Entrition Half Strength. (Biosearch Medical Products) Calcium and sodium caseinates, maltodextrin, corn oil, soy lecithin, mono- and diglycerides, protein 17.5 g, carbohydrate 68 g, fat 17.5 g, sodium 350 mg, potassium 600 mg, calories 0.5/ml, osmolarity 120 mOsm/kg, water, vitamins A, B_1, B_2, B_3, B_5, B_6, B_{12}, C, D, E, K, Ca, P, Mg, I, Fe, Zn, Mn, Cu, Cl, biotin, choline, folic acid. Pouch 1 L. *otc.*
Use: Nutritional supplement.

Entrition HN Entri-Pak. (Biosearch Medical Products). Sodium and calcium caseinates, soy protein isolate, maltodextrin, corn oil, soy lecithin, mono and diglycerides, vitamins A, B_1, B_2, B_3, B_5, B_6, B_{12}, C, D, E, K, folic acid, biotin, choline, Ca, Cl, Cu, Fe, I, Mg, Mn, P, Zn. Pouch 1 L. *otc.*
Use: Nutritional supplement.

Entrobag Set. (Lafayette Pharm) Enteroclysis set. Case 6 sets.
Use: Enteroclysis of the small intestine.

Entrobar. (Lafayette Pharm) Barium sulfate 50% w/v susp. Bot. 500 ml, case 12 bot.
Use: Radiopaque agent.

Entrokit. (Lafayette Pharm) Barium sulfate susp. (Entrobar), methylcellulose (Entrolcel). Case 4 kits.
Use: Radiopaque agent.

Entrolcel. (Lafayette Pharm) Methylcellulose 1.8% w/w concentrate for dilution at time of use. Bot. 500 ml, case 24 Bot.
Use: Diagnostic aid.

•**entsufon sodium.** (ENT-sue-fahn) USAN.
Use: Detergent.

E.N.T. Syrup. (Springbok) Brompheniramine maleate 4 mg, phenylephrine HCl 5 mg, phenylpropanolamine HCl 5 mg/5 ml. Bot. 16 oz. *Rx.*
Use: Antihistamine, decongestant.

Entuss. (Roberts Pharm) **Tab.:** Hydro-

codone bitartrate 5 mg, guaifenesin 300 mg/Tab. Bot. 100s. **Syr.:** 5 mg hydrocodone bitartate, 300 mg potassium guaiacolsulfonate/5 ml. Alcohol free. Bot. 120 ml, 480 ml. *c-III*.
Use: Antitussive, expectorant.

Entuss-D Junior. (Roberts Pharm) Pseudoephedrine HCl 30 mg, hydrocodone bitartrate 2.5 mg, guaifenesin 100 mg w/alcohol 5%, saccharin, sorbitol, sucrose. Liq. Bot.120 ml, pt. *c-III*.
Use: Antitussive, expectorant combination.

Entuss-D Liquid. (Roberts Pharm) Hydrocodone bitartrate 5 mg, pseudoephedrine 30 mg/5 ml. 473 ml. *c-III*.
Use: Antitussive, decongestant.

Entuss-D Tablets. (Roberts Pharm) Pseudoephedrine 30 mg, hydrocodone bitartrate 5 mg, guaifenesin 300 mg/ Tab. Bot. 100s. *c-III*.
Use: Antitussive, decongestant, expectorant.

Enuclene. (Alcon Laboratories) Tyloxapol 0.25%. Soln. Drop-tainer 15 ml. *otc*.
Use: Artificial eye care.

Enulose. (Alphalma USPD) Lactulose 10 g, galactose 2.2 g, lactose 1.2 g, other sugars ≤ 1.2 g. Syr. pt, 2 qt. *Rx*.
Use: Laxative.

•**enviradene.** (en-VIE-rah-DEEN) USAN.
Use: Antiviral.

Enviro-Stress. (Vitaline) Vitamins B_1 50 mg, B_2 50 mg, B_3 100 mg, B_5 50 mg, B_6 50 mg, B_{12} 25 mcg, C 600 mg, E 30 IU, folic acid 0.4 mg, zinc 30 mg, Mg, Se, PABA. SR Tab. Bot. 90s, 1000s. *otc*.
Use: Mineral, vitamin supplement.

•**enviroxime.** (en-VIE-rox-eem) USAN.
Use: Antiviral.

Envisan Treatment Multipack. (Hoechst Marion Roussel) Dextranomer with PEG 3000 and PEG 600. Paste 10 g packets with nylon net and semi-occlusive film. *otc*.
Use: Dermatologic, wound therapy.

Enzest. (Barth's) Seven natural enzymes, calcium carbonate 250 mg/Tab. Bot. 100s, 250s, 500s. *otc*.
Use: Digestive enzymes, antacid.

Enzobile Improved. (Roberts Pharm) Pancreatic enzyme concentrate 100 mg, ox bile extract 100 mg, cellulase 10 mg in inner core and pepsin 150 mg in outer layer. EC tab. Bot. 100s. *otc, Rx*.
Use: Digestive enzymes.

Enzone. (Forest Pharmaceutical) Hydrocortisone acetate 1%, pramoxine HCl 1% in hydrophilic base w/stearic acid, aquaphor, isopropyl palmitate, polyoxyl-40, stearate, triethanolamine lauryl sulfate. Cream. Tube 30 g w/rectal applicator. *Rx*.
Use: Corticosteroid combination.

Enzymatic Cleaner for Extended Wear. (Alcon Laboratories) Highly purified pork pancreatin to dilute in saline solution. Tab. Pkg. 12s. *otc*.
Use: Contact lens care.

Enzyme Formula #E-2. (Barth's) Amylase 30 mg, lipase 25 mg, bile salts 1 gr, wilzyme 10 mg, pepsin 2 gr, pancreatin 0.5 gr, calcium carbonate 4 gr/ Tab. Bot. 100s, 250s. *otc, Rx*.
Use: Digestive aid.

enzymes.
See: Alpha Chymar, Vial (Centeon).
Ananase, Tab. (Rhone-Poulenc Rorer).
Cholinesterase (Various Mfr.).
Chymotrypsin.
Cotazym, Cap. (Organon Teknika).
Creon (Solvay).
Diastase (Various Mfr.).
Dornavac, Vial (Merck).
Fibrinolysin. Hyaluronidase (Various Mfr.).
Neutrapen, Vial (3M).
Pancreatin (Various Mfr.).
Papain (Various Mfr.).
Papase, Tab. (Warner Chilcott).
Penicillinase (Various Mfr.).
Pepsin (Various Mfr.).
Plasmin. Rennin (Various Mfr.).
Taka-Diastase, Prep. (Parke-Davis).
Travase, Oint. (Knoll Pharmaceuticals).
Thrombolysin, I.V. Inj. (Merck).
Varidase, Prep. (Lederle Consumer Products).

EPA Capsules. (NBTY) N-3 fat content (mg) EPA 180 mg, DHA 120 mg, vitamin E 1 IU. Bot. 50s, 100s. *otc*.
Use: Nutritional supplement.

•**eperezolid.** (eh-per-EH-zoe-lid) USAN.
Use: Anti-infective.

•**ephedrine.** (eh-FED-rin) U.S.P. 23.
Use: Adrenergic (bronchodilator).
See: Bofedrol Inhalant (Jones Medical Industries).
Racephedrine HCl (Various Mfr.).
W/Procaine.
See: Ephedrine and Procaine, Rx A', Amp. (Eli Lilly).
W/Pyrilamine maleate, guaifenesin, theophylline.
W/Theophylline, guaifenesin, phenobarbital.

See: Duovent, Tab. (3M).

•**ephedrine hydrochloride.** (eh-FED-rin) U.S.P. 23.
Use: Bronchodilator

ephedrine hydrochloride. (Various Mfr.) Cryst. Box 0.25 oz, 4 oz.
Use: Bronchodilator.

ephedrine hydrochloride w/combinations.
See: Asma-lief, Tab., Susp. (Quality Formulations).
Ceepa, Tab. (Geneva Pharm).
Co-Xan, Elix. (Schwarz Pharma).
Derma Medicone (Medicone).
Derma Medicone HC, Oint. (Medicone).
Dynafed Asthma Relief, Tab. (BDI).
Ectasule, Ectasule Minus, Cap. (Fleming).
Golacal, Syr. (Arcum).
Kie, Tab., Syr. (Laser).
Lardet Expectorant, Tab. (Standex).
Lardet, Tab. (Standex).
Mini Thin Asthma Relief, Tab. (BDI).
Mudrane GG, Tab. (ECR Pharmaceuticals).
Mudrane, Tab. (ECR Pharmaceuticals).
Quadrinal, Tab., Susp. (Knoll Pharmaceuticals).
Quelidrine, Syr. (Abbott Laboratories).
Quibron Plus (Bristol-Myers Squibb).
Tedral-25, Tab. (Parke-Davis).
T-E-P Compound, Tab. (Stanlabs).
Theofenal, Susp., Tab. (Rugby).

ephedrine hydrochloride nasal jelly.
See: Efedron Nasal (Hyrex).

•**ephedrine sulfate.** (eh-FED-rin) U.S.P. 23.
Use: Adrenergic (bronchodilator, nasal decongestant).
See: Ectasule Minus Jr. and Sr., Cap. (Fleming).
Slo-Fedrin, Cap. (Dooner).

ephedrine sulfate. (Various Mfr.) Inj. 50 mg/1mL Amp.
Use: Adrenergic (bronchodilator, nasal decongestant).

ephedrine sulfate w/combinations.
See: B.M.E., Elix. (Brothers).
Bronkaid, Preps. (Sanofi Winthrop).
Bronkolixir, Elix. (Sanofi Winthrop).
Bronkotabs (Sanofi Winthrop).
Ectasule, Cap. (Fleming).
Ectasule Minus, Cap. (Fleming).
Eponal, Prep. (Cenci).
Marax DF, Syr. (Roerig).
Marax, Tab., Syr. (Roerig).
Neogen, Supp. (Premo).
Pazo, Oint., Supp. (Bristol-Myers).
Rectacort, Supp. (Century Pharm).
Va-Tro-Nol, Nose Drops (Procter & Gamble).
Wyanoids, Preps. (Wyeth Ayerst).

ephedrine sulfate and phenobarbital capsules.
Use: Bronchodilator, hypnotic, sedative.

1-ephenamine penicillin g. Compenamine.

Ephenyllin. (CMC) Theophylline 130 mg, ephedrine HCl 24 mg, phenobarbital 8 mg/Tab. Bot. 100s, 500s, 1000s. *Rx.*
Use: Bronchodilator, decongestant, hypnotic, sedative.

Ephrine Nasal Spray. (Walgreens) Phenylephrine HCl 0.5%. Bot. 20 ml. *otc.*
Use: Decongestant.

Epi-C. (Lafayette Pharm) Barium sulfate 150%. Susp. Bot. 450 ml.
Use: Diagnostic aid.

•**epicillin.** (EH-pih-SILL-in) USAN.
Use: Anti-infective.
See: Dexacillin.

epidermal growth factor (human). (Chiron Therapeutics)
Use: Accelerate corneal healing. [Orphan drug]

Epi-Derm Balm. (Pedinol) Methyl salicylate, menthol, propylene glycol, alcohol. Bot. gal. *otc.*
Use: Analgesic, topical.

EpiEZPen Autoinjector. (Center Laboratories) Epinephrine injection 1:2000. Delivers single dose of 0.3 mg. *Rx.*
Use: Emergency kit, anaphylaxis.

EpiEZPen Jr. Autoinjector. (Center Laboratories) Epinephrine injection 1:2000. Delivers single dose of 0.15 mg. *Rx.*
Use: Emergency kit, anaphylaxis.

Epifoam. (Schwarz Pharma) Hydrocortisone acetate 1%, pramoxine HCl 1% in base of propylene glycol, cetyl alcohol, PEG-100 stearate, glyceryl stearate, laureth-23, polyoxyl-40 stearate, methylparaben, propylparaben, trolamine, or hydrochloric acid to adjust pH, purified water, butane, propane inert propellant. Aerosol container 10 g. *Rx.*
Use: Corticosteroid, topical.

Epiform-HC. (Delta) Hydrocortisone 1%, iodohydroxyquin 3% in cream base. Tube 20 g. *Rx.*
Use: Antifungal; corticosteroid, topical.

Epifrin Sterile Ophthalmic Solution. (Allergan) Epinephrine HCl 0.5%, 1% or 2%. Bot. w/dropper 15 ml. *Rx.*

Use: Antiglaucoma.

E-Pilo. (Ciba Vision Ophthalmics) Pilocarpine HCl 1%, 2%, 3%, 4% or 6%, epinephrine bitartrate 1%. Soln. Bot. 10 ml w/dropper-tip plastic vial. *Rx.*
Use: Antiglaucoma.

Epilyt. (Stiefel) Propylene glycol, glycerin, oleic acid, quaternium-26, lactic acid, BHT. Lotion. Bot. 118 ml. *otc.*
Use: Emollient.

•**epimestrol.** (EH-pih-MESS-trole) USAN.
Use: Anterior pituitary activator.

Epinal. (Alcon Laboratories) Epinephrine borate 0.5%, 1%. Dropper Bot. 7.5 ml *Rx.*
Use: Antiglaucoma.

epinephran.
See: Epinephrine, Preps. (Various Mfr.).

•**epinephrine.** (epp-ih-NEFF-rin) U.S.P. 23.
Use: Asthma, hayfever, acute allergic states, cardiac arrest, acute hypersensitivity reactions, adrenergic (vasoconstrictor).
See: Asthma Meter, Aerosol (Rexall).
Asmolin, Vial (Lincoln).
Emergency Ana-Kit (Bayer Corp).
W/Chlorobutanol, sodium bisulfite.
W/Lidocaine HCl.
See: Ardecaine 1%, 2%, Inj. (Burgin-Arden).

epinephrine. (Abbott Laboratories) Epinephrine 0.01 mg/ml/Soln (Pediatric Inj). Box. 5 ml single-dose Abboject Syringe. *otc, Rx.*
Use: Asthma, hayfever, acute allergic states, cardiac arrest, acute hypersensitivity reactions, adrenergic (vasoconstrictor).

•**epinephrine bitartrate.** (epp-ih-NEFF-rim) U.S.P. 23.
Use: Adrenergic, ophthalmic.

epinephrine borate.
Use: Adrenergic, ophthalmic.
See: Epinal Ophth. Soln. (Alcon Laboratories).

epinephrine hydrochloride. (Ciba Vision Ophthalmics) 0.1%. Soln. 1 ml Dropperettes (12s). *Rx.*
Use: Adrenergic, ophthalmic. Emergency kit, anaphylaxis.
See: Adrenalin Cl, Soln. (Parke-Davis).
Ana-Guard Epinephrine, Inj. (Burgin-Arden).
EpiEZPen (Center Labs).
EpiEZPen Jr. (Center Labs).
EpiPen (Center Labs).
EpiPen Jr. (Center Labs).
Epifrin, Ophth. Soln. (Allergan).
Epinal, Ophth. Soln. (Alcon Laboratories).
Sus-Phrine, Amp., Vial (Berlex).
Vaponefrin Solution & Nebulizer, Vial (Medeva).
W/Benzalkonium Cl, sodium Cl, sodium metabisulfite.
See: Glaucon, Soln. (Alcon Laboratories).
W/Pilocarpine HCl.
See: Epicar, Soln. (PBH Wesley Jessen).

epinephrine, racemic.
See: Asthmanefrin Solution (SmithKline Beecham).

epinephrine-related compounds.
See: Sympathomimetic Agents.

•**epinephryl borate ophthalmic solution.** (EPP-ih-NEFF-rill) U.S.P. 23.
Use: Adrenergic.

epinephryl borate ophthalmic solution.
Use: Adrenergic, ophthalmic.
See: Epinal (Alcon Laboratories).
Eppy (PBH Wesley Jessen).

EpiPen Auto-Injector. (Center Laboratories) Epinephrine injection 1:1000. Delivers dose of 0.3 mg. Pkg. 1s, 2s, 2 ml injectors. *Rx.*
Use: Emergency kit.

EpiPen Jr. Auto-Injector. (Center Laboratories) Epinephrine injection 1:2000. Delivers dose of 0.15 mg. Pkg. 1s, 2s, 2 ml injectors. *Rx.*
Use: Emergency kit.

epiphenethicillin.

•**epipropidine.** (EPP-ih-PRO-pih-deen) USAN.
Use: Antineoplastic.

epirenan.
See: Epinephrine (Various Mfr.).

•**epirizole.** (eh-PEER-IH-zole) USAN.
Use: Analgesic, anti-inflammatory.

•**epirubicin hydrochloride.** (EH-pih-ROO-bih-sin) USAN.
Use: Antineoplastic.
See: Pharmorubicin (Pharmacia & Upjohn).

•**epitetracycline hydrochloride.** (epp-ih-TEH-trah-SIGH-kleen HIGH-droe-KLOR-ide) U.S.P. 23.
Use: Anti-infective.

•**epithiazide.** (EH-pih-THIGH-azz-ide) USAN.
Use: Antihypertensive, diuretic.

Epitol. (Teva USA) Carbamazepine 200 mg/Tab. Bot. 100s. *Rx.*
Use: Anticonvulsant.

Epivir. (GlaxoWellcome) Lamivudine 150 mg/Tab. Bot. 60s. Lamivudine 10 mg/ml/Oral soln. Bot. 240 ml. *Rx.*

Use: Treatment of HIV infection.

•**eplerenone.** (eh-PLER-en-ohn) USAN.
Use: Antihypertensive; aldosterone antagonist.

EPO.
See: Epogen (Amgen).
Procrit (Ortho Biotech).

•**epoetin alfa.** (eh-POE-eh-tin) USAN.
Use: Antianemic; hematinic, hematopoietic. [Orphan drug]
See: Epogen (Amgen).
Procrit (Ortho Biotech).

•**epoetin beta.** (eh-POE-eh-tin) USAN.
Use: Hematopoietic, hematinic, antianemic. [Orphan drug]
See: Marogen (Chugai-USA)

Epogen. (Amgen) Epoetin Alfa (Erythropoietin; EPO) 2,000 units, 3,000 units, 4,000 units, 10,000 units. Preservative free w/ 2.5 mg albumin (human) per ml. Vial 1 ml and 10,000 units in 2 ml multidose vials (1% benzyl alcohol). *Rx.*
Use: Hematopoietic.

•**epoprostenol.** (EH-poe-PROSTE-eh-nole) USAN. *Formerly Prostacyclin, PGI_2, Prostagland in I_2, Prostaglandin X, PGX.*
Use: Inhibitor (platelet). Primary pulmonary hypertension.
See: Flolan (GlaxoWellcome) [Orphan drug]

•**epoprostenol sodium.** (EH-poe-PROSTE-eh-nole) USAN.
Use: Inhibitor (platelet).
See: Flolan (GlaxoWellcome).

•**epostane.** (EH-poe-stain) USAN.
Use: Interceptive.

epoxytropine tropate methylbromide.
See: Methscopolamine Bromide (Various Mfr.).

Eppy/N. (PBH Wesley Jessen) Epinephryl borate ophthalmic soln. 0.5%, 1% or 2%. Bot. 7.5 ml. *Rx.*
Use: Antiglaucoma.

•**epristeride.** (eh-PRISS-the-ride) USAN.
Use: Inhibitor (alpha reductase).

Epromate. (Major) Aspirin 325 mg, meprobamate 200 mg Tab. Bot. 100s, 500s. *c-IV.*
Use: Analgesic, anxiolytic.

•**eprosartan.** (eh-pro-SAHR-tan) USAN.
Use: Antihypertensive.

•**eprosartan mesylate.** (eh-pro-SAHR-tan) USAN.
Use: Antihypertensive.

Epsal. (Press) Saturated soln. of epsom salts 80% in ointment form. Jar 0.5 oz, 2 oz. *otc.*
Use: Drawing ointment.

Epsivite 100. (Standex) Vitamin E 100 IU/Cap. Bot. 100s. *otc.*
Use: Vitamin supplement.

Epsivite 200. (Standex) Vitamin E 200 IU/Cap. Bot. 100s. *otc.*
Use: Vitamin supplement.

Epsivite 400. (Standex) Vitamin E 400 IU/Cap. Bot. 100s. *otc.*
Use: Vitamin supplement.

Epsivite Forte. (Standex) Vitamin E 1000 IU/Cap. Bot. 100s. *otc.*
Use: Vitamin supplement.

epsom salt.
See: Magnesium Sulfate.

e.p.t. Stick Test. (Parke-Davis) Reagent in-home kit for urine testing. Pregnancy test. Kit 1s. *otc.*
Use: Diagnostic aid.

eptifibatide.
Use: Acute coronary syndrome.
See: Integrilin, Inj. (Cor Therpeutics).

eptoin.
See: Phenytoin Sodium (Various Mfr.).

Equagesic. (Wyeth Ayerst) Meprobamate 200 mg, aspirin 325 mg/Tab. Bot. 100s, UD 100s. *c-IV.*
Use: Analgesic, anxiolytic.

Equal. (Nutrasweet) Aspartame. **Packet:** 0.035 oz. (1 g). Box 50s, 100s, 200s. **Tab.:** Bot. 100s. *otc.*
Use: Artificial sweetener.

Equalactin. (Numark Laboratories) Polycarbophil 625 mg (as calcium polycarbophil) dextrose, citric acid flavor. Chew. Tab. Bot. 48s. *otc.*
Use: Antidiarrheal or laxative.

Equanil. (Wyeth Ayerst) Meprobamate 200 mg or 400 mg/Tab. **200 mg:** Bot. 100s. **400 mg:** Bot. 100s, 500s, Redipak 25s. *c-IV.*
Use: Anxiolytic.

Equazine M. (Rugby) Aspirin 325 mg, meprobamate 200 mg, tartrazine tab. Bot. 100s, 500s. *c-IV.*
Use: Analgesic, anxiolytic.

•**equilin.** U.S.P. 23.
Use: Estrogen.

Equipertine Capsules. (Sanofi Winthrop) Oxypertine. *Rx.*
Use: Anxiolytic.

Eradacil Capsules. (Sanofi Winthrop) Rosoxacin.
Use: Antigonococcal agent.

Eramycin. (Wesley Pharmacal) Erythromycin FC Tab. Bot. 100s, 500s. *Rx.*
Use: Anti-infective, erythromycin.

•**erbulozole.** (ehr-BYOO-low-zole) USAN.
Use: Radiosensitizer; antineoplastic (adjunct).

Ercaf. (Geneva Pharm) Ergotamine tartrate 1 mg, caffeine 100 mg/Tab. Bot. 100s, 1000s. *Rx.*
Use: Antimigraine.

Ergamisol. (Janssen) Levamisole (base) 50 mg/Tab. Blister pack 36s. *Rx.*
Use: Antineoplastic.

Ergo Caff. (Rugby) Ergotamine tartrate 1 mg, caffeine 100 mg/Tab. Bot. 100s. *Rx.*
Use: Antimigraine.

•**ergocalciferol.** (ehr-go-kal-SIFF-eh-role) U.S.P. 23. *Formerly Oleovitamin D, Synthetic; Calciferol.*
Use: Treatment of refractory rickets; familial hypophosphatemia; hypoparathyroidism, vitamin (antirachitic).
See: Calciferol, Preps. (Schawrz Pharma).,
Drisdol, Liq., Cap. (Sanofi Winthrop).
Vitamin D, Preps. (Various Mfr).

ergocornine. (Various Mfr.) Ergot alkaloid. *Rx.*
Use: Peripheral vascular disorders.

ergocristine. (Various Mfr.) Ergot alkaloid. *Rx.*
Use: Vascular disorders.

ergocryptine. (Various Mfr.) Ergot alkaloid. *Rx.*
Use: Peripheral vascular disorders.

•**ergoloid mesylates.** (err-GO-loyd) U.S.P. 23. *Formerly Dihydroergotoxine Mesylate; Dihydroergotoxine Methanesulfonate; Dihydrogenated Ergot Alkaloids, Hydrogenated Ergot Alkaloids.*
Use: Psychotherapeutic, cognition adjuvant.
See: Hydergine Prods. (Novartis).

ergoloid mesylates.
Use: Psychotherapeutic agent, cognition adjuvant.

Ergomar. (Lotus) Ergotamine tartrate 2 mg, lactose, peppermint oil, saccharin/ Sublingual Tab. Pkg. 20s. *Rx.*
Use: Antimigraine.

ergometrine maleate.
See: Ergonovine (Various Mfr.).

Ergonal. (Vita Elixir) Ergot powder 259.2 mg, aloin 8.1 mg, apiol fluid green 290 mg, oil pennyroyal 28 mg/Cap. Bot. 24s. *Rx.*
Use: Oxytocic.

ergonovine. (Various Mfr.) Ergobasine, erolklinine, ergometrine, ergostetrine, ergotocine. *Rx.*
Use: Oxytocic.
See: Ergonovine Maleate.

•**ergonovine maleate.** (ehr-go-NO-veen MAL-ee-ate) U.S.P. 23.
Use: Oxytocic.
See: Methergine, Ing., Tab. (Novartis).

ergosterol, activated or irradiated.
See: Ergocalciferol, U.S.P. 23.

ergostetrine.
See: Ergonovine (Various Mfr.).

Ergot Alkalside Dihydrogenated.
See: ergoloid mesylates.

•**ergotamine tartrate.** (ehr-GOT-ah-mean TAR-trate) U.S.P. 23.
Use: Analgesic (specific in migraine).
See: Ergomar, Tab. (Lotus).
Gynergen, Amp., Tab. (Novartis).
W/Belladonna alkaloids, acetophenetidin, caffeine.
See: Wigraine, Tab. (Organon Teknika).
W/Belladonna alkaloids, pentobarbital.
See: Cafergot P-B, Supp. (Novartis).
W/Belladonna alkaloids, phenobarbital.
See: Bellergal, Tab. (Novartis).
W/Caffeine.
See: Cafergot, Supp. (Novartis).
W/Caffeine, homatropine methylbromide.
See: Ergotatropin, Tab. (Cole).
W/Cyclizine HCl, caffeine.
See: Migral Tab. (GlaxoWellcome).
W/1-Hyoscyamine sulfate, phenobarbital.
See: Ergkatal, Tab. (Gilbert).

ergotamine tartrate and caffeine suppositories.
Use: Vascular headache; analgesic (specific in migraine).

ergotamine tartrate and caffeine tablets.
Use: Vascular headache; analgesic (specific in migraine).

ergotamine tartrate w/combinations.
See: Folergot-DF, Tab. (Mernel).

ergot, fluid extract. (Various Mfr.) Ergot 1 g/ml Bot. 4 oz, pt.

ergotidine.
See: Histamine (Various Mfr.).

ergotocine.
See: Ergonovine (Various Mfr.).

Ergotrate Maleate. (Bedford Labs) Ergonovine maleate 0.2 mg/ml. Inj. Vial 1 ml. *Rx.*
Use: Oxytocic.

ergot-related products.
See: Cafergot, Supp., Tab. (Novartis).
Cafergot P-B, Tab., Supp. (Novartis).
DHE-45, Amp. (Novartis).
Ergonovine (Various Mfr.).
Ergotamine (Various Mfr.).
Ergotrate (Various Mfr.).
Gynergen, Amp., Tab. (Novartis).
Hydergine, Sub. Tab. (Novartis).
Hydro-Ergot, Tab. (Henry Schein).

Methergine, Amp., Tab. (Novartis).
Wigraine, Supp., Tab. (Organon Teknika).

eriodictin.
See: Vitamin P & Rutin.

eriodictyon. Flext., Aromatic Syrup.
Use: Pharmaceutic aid (flavor).
See: Vitamin P & Rutin.

E-R-O. (Scherer) Propylene glycol, glycerol. Bot. w/dropper tip 15 ml. *otc.*
Use: Otic.

•**ersofermin.** (EER-so-FEER-min) USAN.
Use: Dermatologic, wound therpy.
See: Trofak (Synergen).

Ertine. (Health for Life Brands) Hexachlorophene, benzocaine, cod liver oil, allantoin, boric acid, lanolin. Tube 1.5 oz. *Rx.*
Use: Burn and first aid remedy.

Erwinase. (Porton) Erwinia L-asparaginase.
Use: Acute lymphocytic leukemia. [Orphan drug]

erwina L-asparaginase.
Use: Acute lymphocytic leukemia.
See: Erwinase (Porton).

Eryc. (Warner-Chilcott) Erythromycin enteric coated 250 mg/Tab. Bot. 40s, 100s, 500s, UD 100s. *Rx.*
Use: Anti-infective, erythromycin.

Erycette. (Ortho McNeil) Erythromycin 2%. Pkg. 60 pledgets. *Rx.*
Use: Dermatologic, acne.

EryDerm 2%. (Abbott Laboratories) Erythromycin topical soln. 2%. Bot. 60 ml. *Rx.*
Use: Dermatologic, acne.

Erygel. (Allergan) Erythromycin 2%. Gel Tube 30 g, 60 g, *Erygel 6* in 5 g (6s). *Rx.*
Use: Anti-infective, topical.

Erymax. (Allergan) Erythromycin 2% Soln. 59 ml, 118 ml. *Rx.*
Use: Dermatologic, acne.

Erypar. (Parke-Davis) Erythromycin stearate 250 mg or 500 mg/Filmseal. **250 mg:** Bot. 100s, 500s. **500 mg:** Bot. 100s. *Rx.*
Use: Anti-infective, erythromycin.

EryPed. (Abbott Laboratories) Erythromycin ethylsuccinate granules for oral susp. representing erythromycin activity of 400 mg/5 ml. Bot. 60 ml, 100 ml, 200 ml, UD 5 ml, 100s. *Rx.*
Use: Anti-infective, erythromycin.

Ery-Tab. (Abbott Laboratories) Erythromycin enteric coated 250 mg, 333 mg or 500 mg/Tab. **250 mg:** Bot. 30s, 40s, 100s, 500s, UD 100s. **333 mg:** Bot. 100s, 500s, UD 100s. **500 mg:** Bot. 100s, UD 100s. *Rx.*
Use: Anti-infective, erythromycin.

Erythra-Derm. (Paddock) Erythromycin 2%, alcohol 66%. Soln. Bot. 60 ml. *Rx.*
Use: Dermatologic, acne.

•**erythrityl tetranitrate, diluted.** (eh-RITH-rih-till TEH-trah-NYE-trate) U.S.P. 23. *Formerly Erythrol Tetranitrate.*
Use: Coronary vasodilator.
See: Cardilate (GlaxoWellcome).

erythrityl tetranitrate tablets. (eh-RITH-rih-till TEH-trah-NYE-trate) (Various Mfr.) Erythritol, erythrol tetranitrate, nitroerythrite, tetranitrin, tetranitrol.
Use: Coronary vasodilator.
See: Anginar, Tab. (Pasadena Research Labs.). Cardilate, Tab. (GlaxoWellcome).
W/Phenobarbital.
See: Cardilate-P, Tab. (GlaxoWellcome).

Erythrocin Lactobionate, I.V. (Abbott Hospital Prods) Erythromycin lactobionate. Pow. 500 mg/vial w/benzyl alcohol 90 mg; 1 g/vial w/benzyl alcohol 180 mg. Pkg. Vial 5s. *Rx.*
Use: Anti-infective, erythromycin.

Erythrocin Lactobionate Piggyback. (Abbott Hospital Prods) Erythromycin lactobionate for injection, 500 mg/dispensing vial. 5 mg/ml of erythromycin after reconstitution w/90 mg benzyl alcohol. Pow. Pkg. 5100 ml dispensing vials. *Rx.*
Use: Anti-infective, erythromycin.

•**erythromycin.** (eh-RITH-row-MY-sin) U.S.P. 23.
Use: Anti-infective.
See: AK-Mycin, Oint. (Akorn).
A/T/S, Gel (Hoechst Marion Roussel).
Del-Mycin, Soln. (Del Ray).
Emgel, Gel (GlaxoWellcome).
E-Mycin, Tab. (Pharmacia & Upjohn).
Erymax, Soln. (Allergan).
EryDerm, Soln. (Abbott Laboratories).
Ery-sol, Soln. (Dermol Pharmaceuticals).
Erythrocin, Prep. (Abbott Laboratories).
Erythromycin, Pledgets (Glades).
Erythromycin Base, Filmtab (Abbott Laboratories).
Ilotycin, Prep. (Eli Lilly).
PCE, Tab. (Abbott Laboratories).
Robimycin, Tab. (Robins).
Romycin, Topical Soln. (Roberts Pharm).
RP-Mycin, Tab. (Solvay).

T-Stat, Pads (Westwood Squibb).
Theramycin Z, Soln. (Medicis Dermatologics).

erythromycin. (Pharmacia & Upjohn) Tab. 100 mg. Bot. 100s; 250 mg. Bot. 25s, 100s. (Various Mfr.) 5 mg/g Oint. Tube 3.5 g, 3.75 g, UD 1 g.
Use: Anti-infective.

erythromycin. (Glades) Erythromycin 2%, alcohol 95% / Gel. Tube 30 g, 60 g. *Rx.*
Use: Dermatologic, acne.

•**erythromycin acistrate.** (eh-RITH-row-MY-sin ass-IH-strate) USAN.
Use: Anti-infective.

erythromycin and benzoyl peroxide topical gel. (eh-RITH-row-MY-sin and BEN-zoyl per-OX-ide)
Use: Anti-infective.

erythromycin base filmtab. (Abbott Laboratories) Erythromycin base 250 mg or 500 mg/Tab. **250 mg:** Bot. 100s, 500s, UD 100s. **500 mg:** Bot 100s. *Rx.*
Use: Anti-infective, erythromycin.

•**erythromycin estolate.** (eh-RITh-row-MY-sin ESS-toe-late) U.S.P. 23. *Formerly Erythromycin Propionate Lauryl Sulfate.*
Use: Anti-infective, erythromycin.
See: Ilosone, Preps. (Eli Lilly).

•**erythromycin ethylsuccinate.** (eh-RITH-row-MY-sin ETH-il-SUX-i-nate) U.S.P. 23.
Use: Anti-infective, erythromycin.
See: E.E.S. Prods. (Abbott Laboratories).
E-mycin E, Liq. (Pharmacia & Upjohn).
Pediamycin Prods. (Ross Laboratories).
Pediazole, Liq. (Ross Laboratories).
Wyamycin-E, Liq. (Wyeth Ayerst).

erythromycin ethylsuccinate and sulfisoxazole acetyl for oral suspension. (eh-RITH-row-MY-sin Eth-ill-SUCK-sihnate and sull-fih-SOX-ah-zole ASS-eh-till)
Use: Anti-infective.
See: Pediazole, Susp. (Ross Laboratories).

•**erythromycin gluceptate, sterile.** (eh-RITH-row-MY-sin glue-SEP-tate) U.S.P. 23.
Use: Anti-infective, erythromycin.
See: Ilotycin Gluceptate, Amp. (Eli Lilly).

erythromycin glucoheptonate.
See: Erythromycin Gluceptate, U.S.P. 23. Ilotycin Glucoheptonate, Amp. (Eli Lilly).

•**erythromycin lactobionate for injection.** (eh-RITH-row-MY-sin lack-toe-BYE-oh-nate) U.S.P. 23.
Use: Anti-infective, erythromycin.
See: Erythrocin Lactobionate, Vial (Abbott Laboratories).

erythromycin 2-propionate dodecyl sulfate. Erythromycin Estolate, U.S.P. 23.
Use: Anti-infective, erythromycin.

erythromycin pledgets. (eh-RITH-row-MY-sin)
Use: Anti-infective, erythromycin.

Erythromycin Pledgets. (Glades) Erythromycin 2%, alcohol 68.5%/Pledgets. Bot. 60s. *Rx.*
Use: Anti-infective, erythromycin.

•**erythromycin propionate.** (eh-RITH-row-MY-sin PRO-pee-oh-nate) USAN.
Use: Anti-infective.

erythromycin propionate lauryl sulfate.
Use: Anti-infective, erythromycin.
See: Erythromycin Estolate. Ilosone, Preps. (Eli Lilly).

•**erythromycin salnacedin.** (eh-RITH-row-MY-sin sal-NAH-seh-din) USAN.
Use: Dermatologic, acne.

•**erythromycin stearate.** (eh-RITH-row-MY-sin STEE-ah-rate) U.S.P. 23.
Use: Anti-infective, erythromycin.
See: Erypar Filmseal, Tab. (Parke-Davis).
Wyamycin-S, Tab. (Wyeth Ayerst).

erythromycin sulfate.
Use: Anti-infective, erythromycin.

erythromycin topical. (Various Mfr.) 2% Gel. Tube 30 g, 60 g. 2% Soln. Bot. 60 ml. *Rx.*
Use: Dermatologic, acne.
See: Benzamycin (Dermik Laboratories).
Emgel (GlaxoWellcome).
Erygel (Allergan).

erythropoietin (recombinant human). (Boeing).
Use: Antianemic. [Orphan drug]

erythrosine sodium. U.S.P. XXII.
Use: Diagnostic aid (dental disclosing agent).

Eryzole. (Alra Laboratories) Erythromycin ethylsuccinate 200 mg, acetyl sulfisoxazole 600 mg/5 ml when reconstituted. Gran for Susp. 100 ml, 150 ml, 200 ml. *Rx.*
Use: Anti-infective.

esclabron. Guaithylline.
Use: Antiasthmatic.

Eserdine Forte Tabs. (Major) Methyclo-

thiazide, reserpine 0.5 mg/Tab. Bot. 100s. *Rx.*
Use: Antihypertensive, diuretic.

Eserdine Tabs. (Major) Methyclothiazide, reserpine 0.25 mg/Tab. Bot. 100s, 250s. *Rx.*
Use: Antihypertensive, diurectic.

Eserine. Physostigmine as alkaloid, salicylate or sulfate salt. *Rx.*
Use: Antiglaucoma.

Eserine Salicylate. (Alcon Laboratories) Physostigmine 0.5%. Soln. 2 ml. *Rx.*
Use: Antiglaucoma.

Eserine Sulfate Sterile Ophthalmic Ointment. (Ciba Vision Ophthalmics) Physostigmine sulfate 0.25%. Tube 3.5 g. *Rx.*
Use: Antiglaucoma.

Eserine Sulfate. (Ciba Vision Ophthalmics) Physostigmine sulfate 0.25%. Oint. Tube 3.5 g. *Rx.*
Use: Antiglaucoma.

Esgic Capsules. (Forest Pharmaceutical) Butalbital 50 mg, caffeine 40 mg, acetaminophen 325 mg/Cap. Bot. 100s. *Rx.*
Use: Analgesic, hypnotic, sedative.

Esgic Tablets. (Forest Pharmaceutical) Butalbital 50 mg, caffeine 40 mg, acetaminophen 325 mg/Tab. Bot. 100s, 500s. *Rx.*
Use: Analgesic, hypnotic, sedative.

Esgic-Plus. (Forest Pharmaceutical) Acetaminophen 500 mg, butalbital 50 mg, caffeine 40 mg/Tab. Bot. 100s, 500s. *Rx.*
Use: Analgesic, hypnotic, sedative.

Esidrix. (Novartis Pharmaceuticals) Hydrochlorothiazide 25 mg, 50 mg/Tab. **25 mg:** Bot. 100s, 1000s, UD 100s. **50 mg:** Bot. 100s, 360s, 720s, 1000s, UD 100s. *Rx.*
Use: Antihypertensive, diuretic.
W/Apresoline.
See: Apresoline-Esidrix, Tab. (Novartis Pharmaceuticals).

Esimil. (Novartis Pharmaceuticals) Hydrochlorothiazide 25 mg, guanethidine monosulfate 10 mg/Tab. Bot. 100s. *Rx.*
Use: Antihypertensive, diuretic.

Eskalith. (SmithKline Beecham) Lithium carbonate. **Cap.:** 300 mg. Bot. 100s, 500s; **Tab.:** 300 mg. Bot. 100s. *Rx.*
Use: Antipsychotic.

Eskalith CR. (SmithKline Beecham) Lithium carbonate 450 mg/CR Tab. Bot. 100s. *Rx.*
Use: Antipsychotic.

•**esmolol hydrochloride.** (ESS-moe-lahl) USAN.
Use: Short-acting beta-adrenergic blocker; antiadrenergic (β-receptor)
See: Brevibloc, Inj. (DuPont Merck Pharmaceuticals).

•**esorubicin hydrochloride.** (ESS-oh-ROO-bih-sin) USAN.
Use: Antineoplastic.

Esoterica Dry Skin Treatment Lotion. (SmithKline Beecham) Bot. 13 fl oz. *otc.*
Use: Emollient.

Esoterica Facial. (SmithKline Beecham) Hydroquinone 2%, padimate O 3.3%, oxybenzone 2.5%, sodium bisulfites, parabens, EDTA. Cream, Tube 85 g. *otc.*
Use: Dermatologic.

Esoterica Medicated Fade Cream. (SmithKline Beecham) Hydroquinone 2%, padimate O 3.3%, oxybenzone 2.5%. Cream. Jar 90 g. *otc.*
Use: Dermatologic.

Esoterica Medicated Fade Cream, Facial. (SmithKline Beecham) Hydroquinone 2%, padimate O 3.3%, oxybenzone 2.5% in cream base. Jar 90 g, scented or unscented. *otc.*
Use: Dermatologic.

Esoterica Medicated Fade Cream, Regular. (SmithKline Beecham) Hydroquinone 2%. Cream. Jar 90 g. *otc.*
Use: Dermatologic.

Esoterica Sensitive Skin Formula. (SmithKline Beecham) Hydroquinone 1.5% with mineral oil, sodium bisulfite, parabens, EDTA. Cream. Jar 85 g. *otc.*
Use: Dermatologic.

Espotabs. (Combe) Yellow phenolphthalein 97.2 mg/Tab. Bot. 12s, 30s, 60s. *otc.*
Use: Laxative.

•**esproquin hydrochloride.** (ESS-pro-kwin) USAN.
Use: Adrenergic.

Essential-8. Liquid amino acid protein supplement.
Use: Protein supplement.
See: Vivonex Diets, Liq. (Procter & Gamble).

Estar. (Westwood Squibb) Tar equivalent to 5% coal tar, U.S.P. in a hydro-alcoholic gel w/alcohol 13.8%. Tube 3 oz. *otc.*
Use: Antipsoriatic, antipruritic.

•**estazolam.** (ess-TAZZ-OH-lam) USAN.
Use: Hypnotic, sedative.
See: ProSom (Abbott Laboratories).

estazolam. (Zenith Goldline) Estazolam 1 mg, 2 mg Tab. Bot. 30s, 100s, 500s, 1000s. *Rx.*
Use: Hypnotic, sedative.

Ester-C Plus. (Solgar) Vitamin C 500 mg, citrus bioflavonoid complex 25 mg, acerola 10 mg, rutin 5 mg, rose hips 10 mg, calcium 62 mg/Cap. Bot. 50s. *otc.*
Use: Mineral, vitamin supplement.

Ester-C Plus, Extra Potency. (Solgar) Vitamin C 1000 mg, citrus bioflavonoid complex 200 mg, acerola 25 mg, rutin 25 mg, rose hips 25 mg, calcium 125 mg/Tab. Bot. 30s. *otc.*
Use: Mineral, vitamin supplement.

esterified estrogens.
See: estrogens, esterified.

•**esterifilcon a.** (ess-TER-ih-FILL-kahn A) USAN.
Use: Contact lens material (hydrophilic).

Estilben.
See: Diethylstilbestrol Dipropionate (Various Mfr.).

Estinyl. (Schering Plough) Ethinyl estradiol. **0.02 mg, 0.05 mg/Tab., coated:** Bot. 100s, 250s; **0.5 mg/Tab.:** Bot. 100s. *Rx.*
Use: Estrogen.

estopen.
See: Benzylpenicillin 2-diethylaminoethyl ester HI.

Estrace. (Bristol-Myers) Estradiol micronized 0.5 mg, 1 mg or 2 mg/Tab. Bot. 100s. *Rx.*
Use: Estrogen.

Estrace Vaginal Cream. (Bristol-Myers) Estradiol 0.1 mg/g in a nonliquefying base, EDTA, methylparaben. Tube w/ applicator 42.5 g. *Rx.*
Use: Estrogen.

Estracon. (Freeport) Conjugated estrogens 1.25 mg/Tab. Bot. 1000s. *Rx.*
Use: Estrogen.

Estraderm Transdermal. (Novartis Pharmaceuticals) Estradiol. **0.05:** Each 10 × 10 cm. system contains 4 mg of estradiol for nominal delivery of 0.05 mg estradiol/day. Patient calendar packs of 8 and 24 systems. Ctn 6s. **0.1:** Each 20 × 20 cm. system contains 8 mg estradiol for nominal delivery of 0.1 mg estradiol/day. Patient calendar packs of 8 and 24 systems. Ctn. 6s. *Rx.*
Use: Estrogen.

•**estradiol.** (ESS-truh-DIE-ole) U.S.P. 23. The form now known to be physiologically active is the β form rather than the α.
Use: Estrogen.
See: Aquagen, Vial, Aq. (Remsen).
Estrace, Tab., Vaginal Creme (Bristol-Myers).
Estraderm, Transdermal (Novartis Pharmaceuticals).
Estring, Vaginal ring (Pharmacia & Upjohn).
FemPatch, Transd. Sys. (Parke-Davis)
Femogen, Susp., Tab. (Fellows-Testagar).
Progynon, Pellets (Schering Plough).
W/Estriol, estrone. Hormonin No. 1 and 2, Tab. (Schwarz Pharma).
W/Estrone, estriol.
See: Sanestro, Tab. (Sandia).
W/Estrone, potassium estrone sulfate.
See: Tri-Estrin, Inj. (Keene Pharmaceuticals).
W/Progesterone, testosterone, procaine HCl, procaine base.
See: Horm-Triad, Vial (Bell).
W/Testosterone and chlorobutanol in cottonseed oil.
See: Depo-Testadiol, Vial (Pharmacia & Upjohn).
Transdermal.
Estraderm, Patch (Novartis Pharmaceuticals).
Climara, Patch (Berlex).
Vivelle, Patch (Novartis Pharmaceuticals).

estradiol cyclopentylpropionate. Estradiol 17-beta(3-cyclopentyl)propionate. Estradiol Cypionate, U.S.P. 23.
W/Testosterone cypionate.
See: Depo-Testadiol, Vial (Pharmacia & Upjohn).

•**estradiol cypionate.** (ESS-trah-DIE-ole SIP-ee-oh-nate) U.S.P. 23.
Use: Estrogen.
See: Estradiol cyclopentylpropionate.
Depo-Estradiol Cypionate, Inj. (Pharmacia & Upjohn).
Depogen, Inj. (Hyrex).
D-Est, Inj. (Burgin-Arden).
Estroject-L.A., Vial (Merz).
Hormogen Depot, Inj. (Roberts Pharm).
Span-F, Inj. (Scrip).
W/Testosterone cypionate.
See: D-Diol, Inj. (Burgin-Arden).
Dep-Testestro, Inj. (Zeneca).
Duo-Cyp, Vial (Keene Pharmaceuticals).
Duracrine, Inj. (B.F. Ascher).
Menoject, L.A., Vial (Merz).
T.E. Ionate P.A., Inj. (Solvay).
W/Testosterone cypionate, chlorobutanol.
See: Depo-Testadiol (Pharmacia & Upjohn).

Span F.M., Inj. (Scrip).
T.E. Ionate P.A., Inj. (Solvay).

estradiol cypionate. (Forest Pharmaceutical) Estradiol cypionate 5 mg/ml/ Inj. Vial. 10 ml. *Rx.*
Use: Estrogen.

estradiol dipropionate.
Use: Estrogen.

•**estradiol enanthate.** (ESS-trah-DIE-ole eh-NAN-thate) USAN.
Use: Estrogen.

estradiol, ethinyl.
See: Ethinyl Estradiol.

estradiol monobenzonate.
See: Estradiol Benzoate.

estradiol phosphate.
See: Estradurin, Secule (Wyeth Ayerst).

•**estradiol undecylate.** (ESS-trah-DIE-ole UHN-DEH-sill-ate) USAN.
See: Delestrec.

estradiol vaginal cream. (ESS-trah-DIE-ole)
Use: Estrogen.

•**estradiol valerate.** (ESS-trah-DIE-ole VAL-eh-rate) U.S.P. 23.
Use: Estrogen.
See: Ardefem 10, 20, Inj. (Burgin-Arden).
Deladiol, Inj. (Steris).
Delestrogen, Vial (Bristol-Myers).
Depogen, Inj. (Sigma-Tau Pharmaceuticals).
Dioval, Preps. (Keene Pharmaceuticals).
Duragen, Inj. (Roberts Pharm).
Duratrad, Inj. (B.F. Ascher).
Estate, Inj. (Savage).
Estra-L, Inj. (Taylor Pharmaceuticals).
Gynogen L.A., Inj. (Forest Pharmaceutical).
Span-Est, Inj. (Scrip).
Valergen, Inj. (Hyrex).
W/Benzyl alcohol.
See: Estate, Vial (Savage).
W/Hydroxyprogesterone caproate.
See: Hy-Gestradol, Inj. (Taylor Pharmaceuticals).
Hylutin-Est, Inj. (Hyrex).
W/Testosterone cypionate.
See: Depo-Testadiol, Inj. (Pharmacia & Upjohn).
W/Testosterone enanthate.
See: Ardiol 90/4, 180/8, Inj. (Burgin-Arden).
Deladumone, Vial (Squibb Diagnostic).
Delatestadiol, Vial (Dunhall Pharmaceuticals).
Duoval-P.A., I.M. (Solvay).
Estra-Testrin, Inj. (Taylor Pharmaceuticals).
Span-Est-Test 4, Inj. (Scrip).
Teev, Inj. (Keene Pharmaceuticals).
Tesogen L.A., Inj. (Sigma-Tau Pharmaceuticals).
Valertest, Inj. (Hyrex).
W/Testosterone enanthate, benzyl alcohol, sesame oil.
See: Repose-TE (Paddock).

estradiol valerate. (Various Mfr.) Inj. 10 mg/ml. 20 mg/ml. Vial 10 ml. 40 mg/ ml. Vial 10 ml.
Use: Estrogen.

Estra-L. (Taylor Pharmaceuticals) Estradiol valerate in castor oil. **20 mg/ml:** Vial 10 ml. **40 mg/ml:** Vial 10 ml. *Rx.*
Use: Estrogen.

Estralutin.

•**estramustine.** (ESS-truh-muss-TEEN) USAN.
Use: Antineoplastic.

•**estramustine phosphate sodium.** (Ess-truh-muss-TEEN) USAN.
Use: Antineoplastic.
See: Emcyt, Cap. (Pharmacia & Upjohn).

Estratab. (Solvay) **Tab.:** Esterified estrogens, principally sodium estrone sulfate 0.3 mg, 0.625 mg, 1.25 mg or 2.5 mg/Tab. Bot. 100s, 1000s. *Rx.*
Use: Estrogen.

Estratest. (Solvay) Esterified estrogens 1.25 mg, methyltestosterone 2.5 mg/ Tab. Bot. 100s, 1000s. *Rx.*
Use: Estrogen, androgen combination.

Estratest H.S. (Solvay) Esterified estrogens 0.625 mg, methyltestosterone 1.25 mg/Tab. Bot. 100s. *Rx.*
Use: Estrogen, androgen combination.

•**estrazinol hydrobromide.** (ESS-trazz-ih-nahl) USAN.
Use: Estrogen.

estrin.
See: Estrone.

Estrinex. (Pharmacia & Upjohn)
See: Toremifene.

Estring. (Pharmacia & Upjohn). Estradiol 2 mg/Vaginal ring. Single packs. *Rx.*
Use: Treatment of postmenopausal atrophy of the vagina or lower urinary tract.

•**estriol.** (ESS-tree-ole) U.S.P. 23.
Use: Estrogen.

Estrobene DP.
See: Diethylstilbestrol Dipropionate (Various Mfr.).

Estrofem. (Taylor Pharmaceuticals) Estradiol cypionate 5 mg/ml in oil. Inj. Vial 10 ml.

Use: Estrogen.

•**estrofurate.** (ESS-troe-FYOOR-ate) USAN.
Use: Estrogen.

estrogen-androgen therapy.
See: Androgen-Estrogen Therapy.

estrogenic substances, conjugated. (Water-soluble) A mixture containing the sodium salts of the sulfate esters of the estrogenic substances, principally estrone and equilin that are of the type excreted by pregnant mares. *Rx.*
Cream.
See: Premarin Vaginal Cream (Wyeth Ayerst).
Intravenous.
See: Estroject, Vial (Merz).
Premarin (Wyeth Ayerst).
Tab.
See: Aquagen, Inj. (Remsen).
Ces (Zeneca).
Estroquin, Tab. (Sheryl).
Estrosan, Tab. (Recsei).
Evestrone, Tab. (Delta).
Genisis, Tab. (Organon Teknika).
Menotabs, Tab. (Fleming).
Orapin (Standex).
Prelestrin, Tab. (Taylor Pharmaceuticals).
Premarin, Tab. (Wyeth Ayerst).
Tag-39 H, Tab. (Solvay).
W/Ethinyl estradiol.
See: Demulen, Tab. (Searle).
W/Meprobamate.
See: Milprem, Tab. (Wallace Laboratories).
PMB 200, Tab. (Wyeth Ayerst).
PMB 400, Tab. (Wyeth Ayerst).
W/Methyltestosterone.
See: Estratest, Tab. (Solvay).
Estratest H.S., Tab (Solvay).
Premarin with Methyltestosterone, Tab. (Wyeth Ayerst).

estrogenic substances in aqueous suspension. (Wyeth Ayerst) Sterile estrone suspension 2 mg/ml. Vial 10 ml. *Rx.*
Use: Estrogen.

estrogenic substance aqueous. (Various) Estrogenic substance or estrogens (mainly estrone) 2 mg/ml/Inj. Vial 10 or 30 ml. *Rx.*
Use: Estrogen.

estrogenic substances mixed. May be a crystalline or an amorphous mixture of the naturally occurring estrogens obtained from the urine of pregnant mares.
Aqueous Susp.
See: Gravigen Inj. (Bluco).
Cap.
W/Androgen therapy, vitamins, iron, d-desoxyephedrine HCl.
See: Mediatric, Preps. (Wyeth Ayerst).
W/Methyltestosterone.
See: Premarin w/methyltestosterone, Tab. (Wyeth Ayerst).
W/Testosterone.
See: Andrestraq, Vial (Schwarz Pharma).

•**estrogens, conjugated.** (ESS-truh-janz KAHN-juh-gay-tuhd) U.S.P. 23.
Use: Estrogen.
See: Conest, Tab. (Century Pharm).
Congens, Tab. (Blaine).
Estrocon, Tab. (Savage).
Ganeake, Tab. (Geneva Pharm).
Menotab, Tab. (Fleming).
PMB, Tab. (Wyeth Ayerst).
Premarin, Tab., I.V. (Wyeth Ayerst).
Premarin Vaginal Cream (Wyeth Ayerst).
Premarin with Methyltestosterone, Tab. (Wyeth Ayerst).
Sodestrin and Sodestrin-H, Tab. (Solvay).
Tag-39, Tab. (Solvay).

estrogens equine.
See: Estrogen.
PMB, Tab. (Wyeth Ayerst).
Premarin, Tab., I.V. (Wyeth Ayerst).
Premarin Vaginal Cream (Wyeth Ayerst).
Premarin with Methyltestosterone, Tab. (Wyeth Ayerst).

•**estrogens, esterified.** (ESS-troe-jenz, ess-TER-ih-fide) U.S.P. 23.
Use: Estrogen.
See: Amnestrogen, Tab. (Bristol-Myers Squibb).
Estratab (Solvay).
Evex, Tab. (Syntex).
Menest, Tab. (SmithKline Beecham).
Menogen, Tab. (Breckenridge).
Menogen HS, Tab. (Breckenridge).
Ms-Med, Tab. (Dunhall Pharmaceuticals).

estrogens, esterified & androgens.
Use: Estrogen, androgen supplement.
See: Estratest.

estrogens, natural.
Use: Estrogen.
See: Depogen, Vial (Hyrex).
Estradiol, Preps. (Various Mfr.).
Estrone, Preps. (Various Mfr.).
Estrogenic Substance (Various Mfr.).
PMB, Tab. (Wyeth Ayerst).
Premarin, Tab., I.V. (Wyeth Ayerst).
Premarin Vaginal Cream (Wyeth Ayerst).

Premarin with Methyltestosterone, Tab. (Wyeth Ayerst).

estrogens, synthetic.
See: Dienestrol, Preps. (Various Mfr.).
Diethylstilbestrol, Preps. (Various Mfr.).
Hexestrol, Preps. (Various Mfr.).
Meprane, Tab. (Schwarz Pharma).
TACE, Cap. (Hoechst Marion Roussel).

Estrogestin A. (Harvey) Estrogenic substance 1 mg, progesterone 10 mg/ml in peanut oil. Vial 10 ml. *Rx.*
Use: Estrogen, progestin combination.

Estrogestin C. (Harvey) Estrogenic substance 1 mg, progesterone 12.5 mg/ml in peanut oil. Vial 10 ml. *Rx.*
Use: Estrogen, progestin combination.

•**estrone.** (ESS-trone) U.S.P. 23.
Use: Estrogen.
See: Bestrone Suspension, Inj. (Bluco).
Estrogenic Substances in Aqueous Susp. (Wyeth Ayerst).
Kestrone 5, Inj. (Hyrex).
Foygen, Vial (Foy).
Menagen, Cap. (Parke-Davis).
Menformon (A), Vial (Organon Teknika).
Par-Supp, Vag. Supp. (Parmed).
Propagon-S, Inj. (Spanner).
Theelin, Vial, Aqueous and Oil (Parke-Davis).
W/Hydrocortisone acetate.
See: Estro-V HC, Supp. (PolyMedica).
W/Estradiol, potassium estrone sulfate.
Tri-Orapin (Standex).
W/Estradiol, vitamin B_{12}.
See: Ovulin, Inj. (Sigma-Tau Pharmaceuticals).
W/Estriol, estradiol. Hormonin, Tab. (Schwarz Pharma).
W/Estrogens.
See: Estrogenic Mixtures, Preps. (Various Mfr.).
Estrogenic Substances, Preps. (Various Mfr.).
W/Lactose.
See: Estrovag, Supp. (Fellows-Testagar).
W/Potassium estrone sulfate.
See: Mer-Estrone, Inj. (Keene Pharmaceuticals).
Sodestrin, Inj. (Solvay).
W/Progesterone.
See: Duovin-S, Inj. (Spanner).
W/Testosterone.
See: Andesterone, Vial (Lincoln).
Anestro, Inj. (Roberts Pharm).
Di-Hormone, Susp. (Paddock).
Di-Met Susp. (Organon Teknika).
Diorapin (Standex).
Dl-Steroid, Vial (Kremers Urban).
Estratest, Tab. (Solvay).
W/Testosterone, progesterone.
W/Testosterone, sodium carboxymethylcellulose, sodium Cl.
See: Tostestro, Inj. (Jones Medical Industries).
W/Testosterone, vitamins.
See: Android-G, Vial (ICN Pharmaceuticals).
Geratic Forte, Inj. (Keene Pharmaceuticals).
Geriamic, Tab. (Vortech).
Geritag, Inj., Cap. (Solvay).
W/Testosterone, vitamin and mineral formula, amino acids.
See: Geramine, Tab., Inj. (ICN Pharmaceuticals).
W/Testosterone propionate.

estrone aqueous. (Various Mfr.) Estrone aqueous 2 mg and 5 mg/ml/Inj. Vial 10 ml or 30 ml. *Rx.*
Use: Estrogen.

estrone sulfate, piperazine.
See: Ogen, Tab., Vaginal Cream (Abbott Laboratories).

estrone sulfate, potassium.
See: Estrogen, Vial (Med Chem).
Kaytron, Inj. (Taylor Pharmaceuticals).

•**estropipate.** (ESS-troe-PIH-pate) U.S.P. 23. *Formerly Piperazine Estrone Sulfate.*
Use: Estrogen.
See: Ogen, Tab., Vaginal Cream (Abbott Laboratories).
Ortho-Est (Ortho Pharma).

estropipate. (Various Mfr.) Estropipate 0.625 mg, 1.25 mg and 2.5 mg/Tab. Bot. 50s, 100s. *Rx.*
Use: Estrogen.

Estroquin Tablet. (Sheryl) Purified conjugated estrogens 1.25 mg/Tab. Bot. 100s. *Rx.*
Use: Estrogen.

Estrostep Fe. (Parke-Davis) Norethindrone acetate 1 mg, ethinyl estradiol 20 mcg/Triangular Tab. Norethindrone acetate 1 mg, ethinyl estradiol 30 mcg/ Square Tab. Norethindrone acetate 1 mg, ethinyl estradiol 35 mcg/Round Tab. Ferrous fumarate 75 mg, lactose. Box. 28s. *Rx.*
Use: Contraceptive.

Estrostep 21. (Parke-Davis) Norethindrone acetate 1 mg, ethinyl estradiol 20 mcg/Triangular Tab. Norethindrone acetate 1 mg, ethinyl estradiol 30 mcg/ Square Tab. Norethindrone acetate 1 mg, ethinyl estradiol 35 mcg/Round

Tab. Lactose. Box. 21s. *Rx.*
Use: Contraceptive.

•**etafedrine hydrochloride.** (EH-tah-FED-rin) USAN.
Use: Bronchodilator, adrenergic.
See: Mercodol w/Decapryn, Liq. (Merrell Dow).
Nethamine (Merrell Dow).

•**etafilcon a.** (EH-tah-FILL-kahn A) USAN.
Use: Contact lens material (hydrophilic.)
See: Acuvine (Vistacon).

Etalent. (Roger) Ethaverine HCl 100 mg/Cap. Bot. 50s, 500s. *Rx.*
Use: Vasodilator.

•**etanidazole.** (ETT-ah-NIDE-ah-zole) USAN.
Use: Antineoplastic (hypoxic cell radiosensitizer).

E-Tapp Elixir. (Edwards Pharmaceuticals) Brompheniramine maleate 4 mg, phenylephrine HCl 5 mg, phenylpropanolamine HCl 5 mg/5 ml, alcohol 2.3%. Bot. gal. *otc.*
Use: Antihistamine, decongestant.

•**etarotene.** (ett-AHR-oh-teen) USAN.
Use: Keratolytic.

•**etazolate hydrochloride.** (eh-TAY-zoe-late) USAN.
Use: Antipsychotic.

Eterna 27 Cream. (Revlon) Pregnenolone acetate 0.5% in cream base. *otc.*
Use: Emollient.

•**eterobarb.** (ee-TEER-oh-barb) USAN.
Use: Anticonvulsant.

•**ethacrynate sodium for injection.** (ETH-ah-KRIN-ate) U.S.P. 23.
Use: Diuretic.
See: Edecrin Sodium I.V., Inj. (Merck).

•**ethacrynic acid.** (eth-uh-KRIN-ik) U.S.P. 23.
Use: Diuretic.
See: Edecrin, Tab. (Merck).

•**ethambutol hydrochloride.** (eth-AM-byoo-tahl) U.S.P. 23.
Use: Anti-infective (tuberculostatic).
See: Myambutol HCl (Lederle Consumer Products).

Ethamicort.
See: Hydrocortamate.

•**ethamivan.** (eth-AM-ih-van) USAN. U.S.P. XX.
Use: Stimulant (central and respiratory).

Ethamolin. (Schwarz Pharma) Ethanolamine oleate 5%. Inj. Amp. 2 ml. *Rx.*
Use: Sclerosing agent.

•**ethamsylate.** (ETH-AM-sill-ate) USAN.
Use: Hemostatic.

ethanol. (Various Mfr.) Alcohol, anhydrous. Alcohol, U.S.P. 23.

ethanolamine. Olamine.

•**ethanolamine oleate.** (ETH-ah-nahl-ah-MEEN OH-lee-ate) USAN.
Use: Sclerosing agent. [Orphan drug]
See: Ethamolin (Schwarz Pharma).

ethasulfate sodium. Sodium 2-Ethyl-1-hexanol sulfate.

•**ethchlorvynol.** (eth-klor-VIH-nahl) U.S.P. 23.
Use: Hypnotic, sedative.
See: Placidyl, Cap. (Abbott Laboratories).
Serensil, Prods. (Novartis Pharmaceuticals).

ethenol, homopolymer. Polyvinyl Alcohol, U.S.P. 23.

ethenzamide. o-Ethoxybenzamide.

•**ether.** (EE-ther) U.S.P. 23.
Use: Anesthetic, general; inhalation.

•**ethinyl estradiol.** (ETH-in-ill ess-trah-DIE-ole) U.S.P. 23.
Use: Estrogen.
See: Estinyl, Tab. (Schering Plough).
Feminone, Tab. (Pharmacia & Upjohn).
Lynoral, Tab. (Organon Teknika).
Menolyn, Tab. (Arcum).
Ovogyn, Tab. (Taylor Pharmaceuticals).

ethinyl estradiol. (Bio-Technology)
Use: Turner's syndrome. [Orphan drug]

ethinyl estradiol w/combinations.
See: Ardiatric, Tab. (Burgin-Arden).
Alesse-21, Tab. (Wyeth-Ayerst).
Alesse-28, Tab. (Wyeth-Ayerst).
Brevicon, Tab. (Syntex).
Demulen, Tab. (Searle).
Desogen, Tab. (Organon Teknika).
GenCept, Tab. (Gencon).
Estrostep Fe, Tab. (Parke-Davis).
Estrostep 21, Tab (Parke-Davis).
Halodrin, Tab. (Pharmacia & Upjohn).
Jenest-28, Tab. (Organon Teknika).
Levora 0.15/30-21, Tab. (SCS).
Levora 0.15/30-28. Tab. (SCS).
Loestrin, Tab. (Parke-Davis).
Loestrin 1.5/30, Tab. (Parke-Davis).
Lo/Ovral, Tab. (Wyeth Ayerst).
Modicon 21 and 28, Tab. (Ortho McNeil).
Nelulen, Tab. (Watson Laboratories).
Nordette, Tab. (Wyeth Ayerst).
Norinyl, Prods. (Syntex).
Norlestrin, Tab. (Parke-Davis).
Norlestrin Fe, Tab. (Parke-Davis).
Ortho-Cept, Tab. (Ortho McNeil).
Ortho-Cyclen, Tab. (Ortho McNeil).
Ortho-Novum 1/35, 21 and 28 (Ortho McNeil).

Ortho Tri-Cyclen, Tab. (Ortho McNeil).
Os-Cal-Mone, Tab. (Hoechst Marion Roussel).
Ovcon-35, Tab. (Bristol-Myers).
Ovcon-50, Tab. (Bristol-Myers).
Ovlin, Vial (Zeneca).
Ovral, Tab. (Wyeth Ayerst).
Triphasil, Tab. (Wyeth Ayerst).
Zovia, Tab. (Watson).

ethinyl estradiol and dimethisterone tablets.
Use: Estrogen, progestin combination.

ethinyl estrenol.
See: Lynestrenol (Organon Teknika).

•**ethiodized oil injection.** (eth-EYE-oh-dized) U.S.P. 23.
Use: Diagnostic aid (radiopaque medium).
See: Ethiodol, Inj. (Savage).

•**ethiodized oil I 131.** (eth-EYE-oh-dized OIL I 131) USAN.
Use: Antineoplastic, radiopharmaceutical.

ethiodol. (Savage) Ethiodized oil. Fatty acid Ethyl ester of poppy seed oil, iodine 37%. Inj. Amp. 10 ml, Box 2s.
Use: Diagnostic aid.

Ethiofos. (eh-THIGH-oh-foss)
See: Amifostine.

•**ethionamide.** (eh-THIGH-ohn-ah-mide) U.S.P. 23.
Use: Anti-infective (tuberculostatic).
See: Trecator S.C., Tab. (Wyeth Ayerst).

ethisterone.
See: Anhydrohydroxyprogesterone (Various Mfr.).

Ethmozine. (Roberts Pharm) Moricizine HCl 200 mg, 250 mg or 300 mg/Tab. Bot. 21s, 100s, UD 100s. *Rx.*
Use: Antiarrhythmic.

Ethocaine.
See: Procaine HCl (Various Mfr.).

ethocylorvynol. β-Chlorovinyl ethyl ethynyl carbinol. Ethchlorvynol, U.S.P. 23.

ethodryl.
See: Diethylcarbamazine Citrate.

ethoheptazine citrate.

ethohexadiol. Ethyl hexanediol, 2-ethylhexane-1,3-diol, Rutgers 612. Used in Comp. Dimethyl Phthalate.
Use: Insect repellent.

•**ethonam nitrate.** (ETH-oh-nam NYE-trate) USAN.
Use: Antifungal.

•**ethosuximide.** (ETH-oh-SUX-ih-mide) U.S.P. 23.
Use: Anticonvulsant.
See: Zarontin, Cap., Syr. (Parke-Davis).

ethosuximide. (Copley) Ethosuximide 250 mg/5 ml, saccharin, sucrose, raspberry flavor. Syr. Bot. 483 ml. *Rx.*
Use: Anticonvulsant.

•**ethotoin.** (ETH-oh-toyn) U.S.P. 23.
Use: Anticonvulsant.
See: Peganone (Abbott Laboratories)

ethovan. Ethyl Vanillin.

•**ethoxazene hydrochloride.** (eth-OX-ah-zeen) USAN.
Use: Analgesic.

ethoxzolamide.
Use: Carbonic anhydrase inhibitor.

Ethrane. (Ohmeda Pharmaceuticals) Enflurane. Volatile Liq. Bot. 125 ml, 250 ml. *Rx.*
Use: Anesthetic, general.

•**ethybenztropine.** (ETH-ih-BENZ-troe-peen) USAN.
Use: Anticholinergic.

•**ethyl acetate.** (ETH-ill ASS-eh-tate) N.F. 18.
Use: Pharmaceutic aid, flavoring; solvent.

ethyl aminobenzoate. Anesthesin, anesthrone, benzocaine, parathesin.
Use: Anesthetic, local.
See: Benzocaine (Various Mfr.).

ethyl biscoumacetate.

ethyl bromide. (Various Mfr.) Bromoethane. *Rx.*
Use: Anesthetic, general.

ethyl carbamate.
See: Urethan (Various Mfr.).

•**ethylcellulose.**
Use: Tablet binder, pharamaceutic aid.

ethylcellulose aqueous dispersion.
Use: Tablet binder, pharamaceutic aid.

ethyl chaulmoograte.
Use: Hansen's disease, sarcoidosis.

•**ethyl chloride.** (ETH-ill KLOR-ide) U.S.P. 23.
Use: Anesthetic, topical.
See: Gebauer-Spra-Pak. Stratford-Cook-Spray, 100 g.

ethyl chloride. (Various) Ethyl chloride 100 g chloroethane/Spray. Bot. 105 ml, 120 ml. *Rx.*
Use: Anesthetic, local.

•**ethyl dibunate.** (ETH-ill DIE-byoo-nate) USAN.
Use: Cough suppressant, antitussive.

ethyl diiodobrassidate. Iodobrassid. Lipoiodine.

ethyldimethylammonium bromide.
See: Ambutonium Bromide.

ethylene. (Various Mfr.) Ethene. *Rx.*
Use: Anesthetic, general.

•**ethylenediamine.** (eth-ih-leen-DIE-ah-meen) U.S.P. 23.
Use: Component of aminophylline injection.
ethylenediamine solution. (67% w/v).
Use: Solvent (Aminophylline Inj.).
ethylenediaminetetraacetic acid.
See: Edathamil, EDTA (Various Mfr.).
ethylenediamine tetraacetic acid disodium salt.
See: Endrate Disodium, Amp. (Abbott Laboratories).
•**ethylestrenol.** (ETH-ill-ESS-tree-nahl) USAN.
Use: Anabolic.
ethylhydrocupreine hydrochloride.
Use: Antiseptic.
ethylmorphine hydrochloride.
Use: Narcotic.
ethyl nitrite spirit. Ethyl nitrite. Sweet Spirit of Niter. Spirit of Nitrous Ether.
•**ethyl oleate.** (ETH-ill) N.F. 18.
Use: Pharmaceutic aid (vehicle).
ethyl oxide; ethyl ether.
Use: Solvent.
ethylpapaverine hydrochloride.
See: Ethaverine HCl (Various Mfr.).
•**ethylparaben.** (eth-ill-PAR-ah-ben) N.F. 18.
Use: Pharmaceutic aid (antifungal preservative).
ethylstibamine. Astaril, neostibosan.
Use: Antimony therapy.
ethyl vanillate.
•**ethyl vanillin.** (ETH-ill) N.F. 18.
Use: Pharmaceutic aid (flavor).
•**ethynerone.** (eth-EYE-ner-ohn) USAN.
Use: Hormone, progestin.
•**ethynodiol diacetate.** (eh-THIN-oh-die-ole die-ASS-eh-tate) U.S.P. 23.
Use: Progesterone, progestin.
See: Ovulen, Tab. (Searle).
W/Ethinyl estradiol.
Demulen, Preps. (Searle).
Estrostep Fe, Tab. (Parke-Davis).
Estrostep 21, Tab. (Parke-Davis).
Nelulen, Tab. (Watson Laboratories).
Zovia, Tab. (Watson).
W/Mestranol.
See: Ovulen, Tab. (Searle).
ethynodiol diacetate and ethinyl estradiol tablets.
Use: Contraceptive.
ethynodiol diacetate and mestranol tablets.
Use: Contraceptive.
ethynylestradiol.
See: Ethinyl Estradiol, U.S.P. (Various Mfr.)
Mestranol (Various Mfr.).
ethynylestradiol 3-methyl ether.
See: Enovid, Tab. (Searle).
Ethyol. (Alza/US Bioscience) Pow. for Inj. Lyophilized: 500 mg (anhydrous basis) 500 mg mannitol in 10 ml single-use vials. *Rx.*
Use: Cyto-protective agent.
•**etibendazole.** (eh-tie-BEN-dah-ZOLE) USAN.
Use: Anthelmintic.
Eticylol. (Novartis Pharmaceuticals) Ethinyl estradiol. *Rx.*
Use: Estrogen.
•**etidocaine.** (eh-TIE-doe-cane) USAN.
Use: Anesthetic, local.
See: Duranest, Inj. (Astra).
Duranest-MPF, Inj. (Astra).
•**etidronate disodium.** (eh-TIH-DROE-nate) U.S.P. 23.
Use: Bone resorption inhibitor. Treatment of symptomatic Paget's disease of bone (osteitis deformans). Degenerative metabolic bone disease [Orphan drug]
See: Didronel, Tab. (Procter & Gamble).
•**etidronic acid.** (eh-tih-DRAH-nik) USAN.
Use: Calcium regulator.
•**etifenin.** (EH-tih-FEN-in) USAN.
Use: Diagnostic aid.
•**etintidine hydrochloride.** (ett-IN-tih-DEEN) USAN.
Use: Antiulcerative.
etiocholanedoine. (SuperGen).
Use: Aplastic anemia; Prader-Willi syndrome. [Orphan drug]
•**etocrylene.** (EH-toe-KRIH-leen) USAN.
Use: Ultraviolet screen.
•**etodolac.** (EE-toe-DOE-lak) USAN.
Use: Analgesic, NSAID.
See: Lodine (Wyeth Ayerst).
Lodine XL, ER Tab. (Wyeth-Ayerst).
etodolac. (Zenith Goldline). Etodolac 400 mg, lactose, polyethylene glycol, povidone. Tab. Bot. 100s, 500s, 1000s. *Rx.*
Use: Analgesic.
•**etofenamate.** (EH-toe-FEN-am-ate) USAN.
Use: Analgesic, anti-inflammatory.
•**etoformin hydrochloride.** (EH-toe-FORE-min) USAN.
Use: Antidiabetic
•**etomidate.** (eh-TAHM-ih-date) USAN.
Use: Hypnotic, sedative.
See: Amidate (Abbott Laboratories).
etomide hydrochloride. (ETT-oh-mide) Bandol. Carbiphene HCl.
•**etonogestrel.** (ETT-oh-no-JESS-trell) USAN.

Use: Hormone, progestin.

•**etoperidone hydrochloride.** (EH-toe-PURR-ih-dohn) USAN.
Use: Antidepressant.
See: Vepesid, Inj., Cap. (Bristol-Myers Squibb).

Etopophos. (Bristol-Myers Oncology/Immunology) Etoposide phosphate diethanolate 119.3 mg (100 mg etoposide), dextran 40 300 mg/Pow. for Inj. Vials. Single dose. *Rx.*
Use: Antineoplastic.

•**etoposide.** (EH-toe-POE-side) U.S.P. 23.
Use: Antineoplastic.
See: Etopophos, Pow. for Inj. (Bristol-Myers Oncology/Immunology).
Toposar, Inj. (Pharmacia & Upjohn).
Vepesid, Inj., Cap. (Bristol-Myers Squibb).

etoposide. (EH-toe-POE-side) (Various Mfr.) Etoposide 20 mg/ml, alcohol 30.5%, benzyl alcohol 30 mg, polysorbate 80 80 mg, PEG 300 650 mg, citric acid 2 mg/ml. Inj. Vials 5 ml, 12.5 ml, 25 ml. *Rx.*
Use: Antineoplastic.

•**etoposide phosphate.** (ee-toe-POE-side) USAN.
Use: Antineoplastic.
See: Etopophos, Pow. for Inj. (Bristol-Myers Oncology).

•**etoprine.** (ETT-oh-preen) USAN.
Use: Antineoplastic.

etoquinol sodium. Name used for Actinoquinol sodium.

etoval.
See: Butethal, N.F. (Various Mfr.).

•**etoxadrol hydrochloride.** (eh-TOX-ah-drole) USAN.
Use: Anesthetic.

•**etozolin.** (EAT-oh-zoe-lin) USAN.
Use: Diuretic.

Etrafon (2-10). (Schering Plough) Perphenazine 2 mg, amitriptyline HCl 10 mg/Tab. Bot. 100s, 500s, UD 100s. *Rx.*
Use: Psychotherapeutic combination.

Etrafon (2-25). (Schering Plough) Perphenazine 2 mg, amitriptyline HCl 25 mg/Tab. Bot. 100s, 500s, UD 100s. *Rx.*
Use: Psychotherapeutic combination.

Etrafon-A (4-10). (Schering Plough) Perphenazine 4 mg, amitriptyline HCl 10 mg/Tab. Bot. 100s, UD 100s. *Rx.*
Use: Psychotherapeutic combination.

Etrafon Forte Tablets (4-25). (Schering Plough) Perphenazine 4 mg, amitriptyline HCl 25 mg/Tab. Bot. 100s, 500s, UD 100s. *Rx.*
Use: Psychotherapeutic combination.

•**etretinate.** (eh-TRETT-ih-nate) USAN.
Use: Antipsoriatic.

etrynit. Propatyl nitrate.
Use: Cardiovascular agent.

•**etryptamine acetate.** (ee-TRIP-tah-meen) USAN.
Use: Central stimulant.
See: Monase (Pharmacia & Upjohn).

E.T.S.-2%. (Paddock) Erythromycin topical 2%. Soln. Bot. 60 ml. *Rx.*
Use: Dermatologic, acne.

ettriol trinitrate.
See: Propatyl nitrate.

etybenzatropine. Ethybenztropine.

etynodiol acetate. Ethynodiol Diacetate.

eubasin.
See: Sulfapyridine (Various Mfr.).

eucaine hydrochloride. (Novartis Pharmaceuticals) Menthol 8%, eucalyptus oil, SD 3A alcohol. Gel. Tube 60 g. *otc.*
Use: Liniments.

Eucalyptamint. (Novartis) Menthol 8%, eucalyptus oil, SD 3A alcohol. Gel 6g. *otc.*
Use: Liniment.

Eucalyptamint, Maximum Strength. (Novartis Pharmaceuticals) Menthol 16%, lanolin, eucalyptus oil. Oint. Tube 60 ml. *otc.*
Use: Liniments.

•**eucalyptol.** USAN.
Use: Pharmaceutic aid (flavor); antitussive; decongestant, nasal.
See: Vicks Sinex, Nasal Spray (Procter & Gamble).
Vicks Va-Tro-Nol, Nose Drops (Procter & Gamble).
Vicks Prods. (Procter & Gamble).

eucalyptus oil.
Use: Flavor; antitussive; decongestant, nasal; expectorant; analgesic, topical.
See: Vicks Prods. (Procter & Gamble).
Victors Regular, Cherry Loz. (Procter & Gamble).

•**eucatropine hydrochloride.** (you-CAT-troe-peen) U.S.P. 23.
Use: Pharmaceutical necessity for ophthalmic dosage form; anticholinergic, ophthalmic.

eucatropine hydrochloride. (Glogau) Crystal, Bot. g.
Use: Pharmaceutical necessity for ophthalmic dosage form; anticholinergic, ophthalmic.

Eucerin. (Beiersdorf) Unscented moisturizing formula. **Creme:** Jar 120 g, lb. **Lot.:** Bot. 240 ml, 480 ml. *otc.*
Use: Emollient.

Eucerin Cleansing. (Beiersdorf) Sodium laureth sulfate, cocoamphocarboxyglycinate, cocamidopropyl betaine, cocamide MEA, PEG-7 glyceryl cocoate, PEG-5 lanolate, PEG-120 methyl glucose dioleate, lanolin alcohol, imidazolidinyl urea. Soap free. Lot. Bot. 240 ml. *otc.*
Use: Dermatologic, cleanser.

Eucerin Dry Skin Care Daily Facial. (Beiersdorf) Ethylhexyl p-methoxycinnamate, titanium dioxide, 2-phenylbenzimidazole-5-sulfonic acid, 2-ethylhexyl salicylate, mineral oil, cetearyl alcohol, castor oil, lanolin alcohol, EDTA. SPF 20. Lot. Bot. 120 ml. *otc.*
Use: Sunscreen.

Eucerin Plus. (Beiersdorf) Mineral oil, hydrogenated castor oil, sodium lactate 5%, urea 5%, glycerin, lanolin alcohol. Lot. Bot. 177 ml. *otc.*
Use: Emollient.

eucodal.
See: Oxycodone.

Eucoran.
See: Nikethamide (Various Mfr.).

eucupin dihydrochloride. Isoamylhydrocupreine dihydrochloride.

Eudal-SR. (Forest Pharmaceutical) Pseudoephedrine 120 mg, guaifenesin 400 mg/SR Tab. Bot. 100s. *Rx.*
Use: Decongestant, expectorant.

euflavine.
See: Acriflavine (Various Mfr.).

•**eugenol.** (you-jeh-nole) U.S.P. 23.
Use: Dental analgesic, oral anesthetic.
See: Benzodent, Oint. (Procter & Gamble).

eukadol.
See: Dihydrohydroxycodeinone, Preps. (No Mfr. currently lists).

Eulcin. (Leeds) Methscopolamine bromide 2.5 mg, butabarbital sodium 10 mg, aluminum hydroxide gel, dried, 250 mg, magnesium trisilicate 250 mg/Tab. Bot. 100s. *Rx.*
Use: Antacid, anticholinergic, antispasmodic, hypnotic, sedative.

Eulexin. (Schering Plough) Flutamide 125 mg/Cap. 100s, 500s, UD 100s. *Rx.*
Use: Antineoplastic.

Eumydrin Drops. (Sanofi Winthrop) Atropine methonitrate. *Rx.*
Use: Anticholinergic, antispasmodic.

euneryl.
See: Phenobarbital (Various Mfr.).

Euphorbia Compound. (Sherwood Medical) Euphorbia pilulifera fluidextract 1.5 ml, iobelia tincture 2.2 ml, nitroglycerin spirit 0.29 ml, sodium iodide 1.04 g, sodium bromide 1.04 g, alcohol 24%/30 ml. Bot. pt, gal. *Rx.*
Use: Expectorant, hypnotic, sedative.

euphorbia pilulifera.
W/Cocillana, squill, antimony potassium tartrate, senega.
See: Cylana, Syr. (Jones Medical Industries).
W/Phenyl salicylate and various oils.
See: Rayderm, Oint. (Velvet Pharmacal).

Eupractone. (Baxter) Dimethadione.

•**euprocin hydrochloride.** (YOU-pro-sin) USAN.
Use: Anesthetic, local.
See: Eucupin HCl.

euquinine. Quinine ethyl carbonate.
Use: Antimalarial, antipyretic.

Eurax. Albutoin.

Eurax Cream. (Westwood Squibb) Crotamiton 10% in vanishing-cream base of glyceryl monostearate, anhydrous lanolin, PEG 6-32, glycerin, polysorbate 80, water, benzyl alcohol, mineral oil, white wax, quaternium-15, fragrance. Tube 60 g. *Rx.*
Use: Scabicide, pediculicide.

Eurax Lotion. (Westwood Squibb) Crotamiton 10% in emollient-lotion base of glyceryl monostearate, anhydrous lanolin, PEG 6-32, glycerin, polysorbate 80, water, benzyl alcohol, light mineral oil, carboxymethylcellulose, simethicone, quaternium-15, fragrance. Bot. 60 g, 454 g. *Rx.*
Use: Scabicide, pediculicide.

Evac-Q-Kit. (Pharmacia & Upjohn) Each kit contains: **Evac-Q-Mag:** Magnesium citrate 300 ml, citric acid, potassium citrate. **Evac-Q-Tabs:** 2 tab. phenolphthalein 130 mg/Tab. **Evac-Q-Sert:** 2 supp. containing potassium bitartrate, sodium bicarbonate/supp. in polyethylene glycol base. Patient instruction sheet. *otc.*
Use: Bowel evacuant.

Evac-Q-Kwik. (Pharmacia & Upjohn) Each kit contains: **Evac-Q-Mag:** magnesium citrate 300 ml, citric acid, potassium citrate in cherry-flavored base. **Evac-Q-Tabs:** 2 tab. phenolphthalein 130 mg. **Evac-Q-Kwik Supp.:** bisacodyl 10 mg. *otc.*
Use: Bowel evacuant.

Evac Suppositories. (Burgin-Arden) Sodium bicarbonate, sodium biphosphate, dioctyl sodium sulfosuccinate 50 mg/Supp. *otc.*
Use: Laxative.

Evac Tablets. (Burgin-Arden) Guar gum 300 mg, danthron 50 mg, sodium 100 mg/Tab. *otc.*
Use: Laxative.

Evactol. (Delta) Docusate sodium 100 mg, sodium carboxymethyl cellulose 200 mg/Cap. Pkg. 10s, Bot. 10s, 30s, 100s. *otc.*
Use: Laxative.

Evac-U-Gen. (Walker Corp) Yellow phenolphthalein 97.2 mg w/corn syrup, lactose, saccharin/Chew. Tab. Bot. 35s, 100s. *otc.*
Use: Laxative.

Evac-U-Lax. (Roberts Pharm) Yellow phenolphthalein 80 mg/Chew. tab. Bot. 100s. *otc.*
Use: Laxative.

Evalose. (Copley) Lactulose 10 g/15 ml, galactose < 1.6 g, lactose < 1.2 g, other sugars ≤ 1.2 g/Syrup. Bot. 240 ml, 960 ml. *Rx.*
Use: Laxative.

evans blue. U.S.P. XXII.
Use: Diagnostic aid (blood volume determination).

Evans Blue Dye. (New World Trading Corp) Evans blue dye 5 ml/Inj. *Rx.*
Use: Diagnostic aid.

Everone. (Hyrex) Testosterone enanthate in oil 100 mg or 200 mg/ml. Vial 10 ml. *c-III.*
Use: Androgen.

Evicyl Tablets. (Sanofi Winthrop) Inositol hexanicotinate. *Rx.*
Use: Hypolipidemic, peripheral vasodilator.

Eviron. (Delta) Ferrous fumarate 160 mg, copper 1 mg, ascorbic acid 75 mg/Tab. *otc.*
Use: Mineral, vitamin supplement.

Evista. (Eli Lilly) Raloxifene HCl, lactose/Tab. Bot. 30s, 100s, 2000s. *Rx.*
Use: Osteoporosis prevention.

E-Vital Creme. (Taylor Pharmaceuticals) Vitamins E 100 IU, A 250 IU, D 100 IU, d-panthenol 0.2%, allantoin 0.1%/g. Jar 2 oz, lb. *otc.*
Use: Emollient.

Ewin Ninos Tablets. (Sanofi Winthrop) Aspirin. *otc.*
Use: Analgesic.

Exact. (Advanced Polymer Systems) Benzoyl peroxide 5%, cetyl and steryl alcohol, parabens. Cream Jar 18 g. *otc.*
Use: Dermatologic, acne.

Exact Liquid. (Advanced Polymer Systems) Salicylic acid 2%, propylene glycol, aloe vera gel, disodium EDTA, menthol, parabens, glycerin, diazolidinyl urea. Liq. Bot. 118 ml. *otc.*
Use: Dermatologic, acne.

•**exametazime.** (EX-ah-MET-ah-zeen) USAN.
Use: Diagnostic aid (regional cerebral perfusion imaging).

•**exaprolol hydrochloride.** (EX-ah-PRO-lahl) USAN.
Use: Antiadrenergic (β-receptor).

Ex-Caloric Wafers. (Eastern Research) Carboxymethylcellulose 181 mg, methylcellulose 272 mg/Wafer. Bot. 100s, 500s, 5000s. *otc.*
Use: Dietary aid.

Excedrin Aspirin Free. (Bristol-Myers) Acetaminophen 500 mg, caffeine 65 mg/Cap. Bot. 24s, 50s, 100s. *otc.*
Use: Analgesic combination.

Excedrin Extra Strength. (Bristol-Myers) Acetaminophen 250 mg, aspirin 250 mg, caffeine 65 mg. **Capl.:** Bot. 24s, 50s, 80s. **Tab.:** Bot. 12s, 30s, 60s, 100s, 165s, 225s. *otc.*
Use: Analgesic combination.

Excedrin Extra Strength. (Bristol-Myers Squibb) Acetaminophen 500 mg, caffeine 65 mg, parabens, mineral oil. Geltab 40s. *otc.*
Use: Analgesic combination.

Excedrin P.M.. (Bristol-Myers) Acetaminophen 500 mg, diphenhydramine citrate 38 mg. **Tab.:** Bot. 50s. **Capl.:** Bot. 30s, 50s. **Liquigels:** Diphenhydramine 25 mg. Bot. 20s, 40s. **Liq.:** Acetaminophen 1000 mg, diphenhydramine HCl 50 mg/30 ml, alcohol 10%, sucrose. Bot. 180 ml. **Geltab**: Bot. 50s. *otc.*
Use: Analgesic, sleep aid.

Excedrin Sinus. (Bristol-Myers) Pseudoephedrine HCl 30 mg, acetaminophen 500 mg/Tab. Capl. Bot. 24s. *otc.*
Use: Analgesic, decongestant.

Excita Extra. (Schmid) Nonoxynol 9 8% (Ribbed). Condom. Box 3s, 12s, 36s.. *otc.*
Use: Condom with spermicide.

exemestane. (Pharmacia & Upjohn)
Use: Hormonal therapy of metastatic breast carcinoma. [Orphan drug]

Exgest LA Tablets. (Schwarz Pharma) Phenylpropanolamine HCl 75 mg, guaifenesin 400 mg. Bot. 100s or 500s. *Rx.*
Use: Decongestant, expectorant.

Ex-Histine. (WE Pharma) Phenylephrine 10 mg, chlorpheniramine 2 mg, methscopolamine 1.25 mg/5 ml, root beer

flavor. Syr. Bot. 16 oz. *Rx.*
Use: Antihistamine, decongestant.

Exidine-2 Scrub. (Baxter) Chlorhexidine gluconate 2%, isopropyl alcohol 4%. Soln. Bot. 120 ml. *otc.*
Use: Antiseptic, antimicrobial.

Exidine-4 Scrub. (Baxter) Chlorhexidine glucoante 4%, isopropyl alcohol 4%. Soln. Bot. 120 ml, 240 ml, 480 ml, 887 ml, 1 gal. *otc.*
Use: Antiseptic, antimicrobial.

Exidine Skin Cleanser. (Xttrium) Chlorhexidine gluconate 4%, isopropyl alcohol 4%. Bot. 120 ml, 240 ml, 16 oz, 32 oz, gal. *otc.*
Use: Antiseptic, antimicrobial.

Ex-Lax. (Novartis) Yellow phenolphthalein 90 mg/chocolate Chew. Tab. or unflavored pill. Chocolate Tab. 6s, 18s, 48s, 72s. Unflavored pill 8s, 30s, 60s. *otc.*
Use: Laxative.

Ex-Lax Maximum Relief. (Novartis) Yellow phenolphthalein 135 mg. Tab. Pkg. 24s. *otc.*
Use: Laxative.

Exna. (Robins) Benzthiazide 50 mg/Tab. Bot. 100s. *Rx.*
Use: Diuretic, antihypertensive.

Exocaine Plus. (Del Pharmaceuticals) Methyl salicylate 30%. Jar 4 oz, Tube 1.3 oz. *otc.*
Use: Analgesic, topical.

exol. Di-isobutyl ethoxy ethyl dimethyl benzyl ammonium Cl.

exonic ot. Dioctyl Sodium Sulphosuccinate.
Use: Laxative.

Exosurf Neonatal. (GlaxoWellcome) Colfosceril palmitate; dipalmitoylphosphatidylcholine (DPPC). Lyophilized pow. Vial 10 ml. *Rx.*
Use: Synthetic lung surfactant.

Expectorant DM Cough Syrup. (Weeks & Leo) Dextromethorphan HBr 15 mg, guaifenesin 100 mg/5 ml, alcohol 7.125%. Bot. 6 oz. *otc.*
Use: Antitussive, expectorant.

Expendable Blood Collection Unit ACD. (Baxter) Citric acid 540 mg, sodium citrate 1.49 g, dextrose 1.65 g/ 67.5 ml. *Rx.*
Use: Anticoagulant.

Exten Strone 10. (Schlicksup) Estradiol valerate 10 mg/ml. Vial 10 ml. *Rx.*
Use: Estrogen.

Extendryl Chewable Tablets. (Fleming) Chlorpheniramine maleate 2 mg, phenylephrine HCl 10 mg, methscopolamine nitrate 1.25 mg/Chew. Tab. Bot. 100s, 1000s. *Rx.*
Use: Anticholinergic, antihistamine, antispasmodic, decongestant.

Extendryl Junior. (Fleming) Chlorpheniramine maleate 4 mg, phenylephrine HCl 10 mg, methscopolamine nitrate 1.25 mg/TD Cap. 100s, 1000s. *Rx.*
Use: Anticholinergic, antihistamine, antispasmodic, decongestant.

Extendryl S.R. (Fleming) Chlorpheniramine maleate 8 mg, phenylephrine HCl 20 mg, methscopolamine nitrate 2.5 mg/TD Cap. Bot. 100s, 1000s. *Rx.*
Use: Anticholinergic, antihistamine, antispasmodic, decongestant.

Extendryl Syrup. (Fleming) Chlorpheniramine maleate 2 mg, phenylephrine HCl 10 mg, methscopolamine nitrate 1.25 mg/5 ml. Bot. 473 ml, gal. *Rx.*
Use: Anticholinergic, antihistamine, antispasmodic, decongestant.

Extenzyme Soflens Protein Cleaner. (Allergan) Papain, sodium Cl, sodium carbonate, sodium borate, edetate disodium. Vial w/Tab. 24s. Refill 36s. *otc.*
Use: Contact lens care.

Extra Action Cough. (Rugby) Dextromethorphan HBr 15 mg, guaifenesin 100 mg w/alcohol 1.4%, corn syrup, saccharin. Syr. Bot. 118 ml. *otc.*
Use: Antitussive, expectorant.

Extra Strength Adprin-B. (Pfeiffer) Aspirin with calcium carbonate 500 mg, magnesium carbonate, magnesium oxide/Tab, buffered. *otc.*
Use: Analgesic.

Extra Strength Alka-Seltzer Effervescent. (Bayer Corp) Sodium bicarbonate (heat-treated) 1985 mg, aspirin 500 mg, citric acid 1000 mg, sodium 588 mg/Tab. Bot. 12s and 24s. *otc.*
Use: Antacid.

Extra Strength Alkets Antacid. (Roberts Pharm) Calcium carbonate 750 mg/Tab. Chew. Bot. 96s. *otc.*
Use: Antacid.

Extra Strength Aspirin Capsules. (Walgreens) Aspirin 500 mg/Cap. Bot. 80s. *otc.*
Use: Analgesic.

Extra Strength Bayer Plus. (Bayer Corp) Aspirin buffered with calcium carbonate, magnesium carbonate, magnesium oxide 500 mg/Capl. Bot. 30s, 60s. *otc.*
Use: Analgesic.

Extra Strength Bayer Enteric 500 Aspirin. (Bayer Corp) Aspirin 500 mg. Tab.

Enteric coated. Bot. 60s. *otc.*
Use: Analgesic.

Extra Strength Doan's PM. (Novartis Pharmaceuticals) Magnesium salicylate 500 mg, diphenhydramine HCl 25 mg/Capl. Pkg. 20s. *otc.*
Use: Sleep aid.

Extra Strength Dynafed Ex. (BDI) Acetaminophen 500 mg, fruit favor. Tab. Bot. 36s. *otc.*
Use: Analgesic.

Extra Strength Excedrin Capsules and Tablets. (Bristol-Myers) Acetaminophen 250 mg, aspirin 250 mg, caffeine 65 mg. Cap. Bot. 24s, 50s, 80s. Tab. Bot. 30s, 60s, 100s, 165s, 225s, Pkg. 12s. *otc.*
Use: Analgesic combination.

Extra Strength 5 mg Biotin Forte. (Vitaline) Vitamins B_1 10 mg, B_2 10 mg, B_3 40 mg, B_5 10 mg, B_6 25 mg, B_{12} 10 mcg, C 100 mg, biotin 5 mg, FA 800 mcg/Tab. Bot. 60s, 1000s. *otc.*
Use: Mineral, vitamin supplement.

Extra Strength Gas-X. (Novartis) Simethicone 125 mg/Tab. Pkg. 18s. *otc.*
Use: Antiflatulent.

Extra Strength Tylenol PM. (McNeil Consumer Products) Diphenhydramine 25 mg, acetaminophen 500 mg/**Tab.:** 24s, 50s; **Capl.:** 24s, 50s; **Gelcap:** 20s, 40s. *otc.*
Use: Sleep aid.

Extra Strength Vicks Cough Drops. (Procter & Gamble) Menthol 8.4 mg (menthol flavor) or menthol 10 mg (cherry and honey lemon flavors), corn syrup, sucrose/Loz. Pkg. 9s, 30s. *otc.*
Use: Mouth and throat preparation.

Extreme Cold Formula. (Major) Pseudoephedrine HCl 30 mg, chlorpheniramine maleate 1 mg, dextromethorphan HBr 15 mg, acetaminophen 500 mg/Cap. Bot. 10s. *otc.*
Use: Analgesic, antihistamine, antitussive, decongestant.

Eye Drops. (Bausch & Lomb) Tetrahydrozoline HCl 0.05%. Drop. Bot. 15 ml. *otc.*
Use: Ophthalmic vasoconstrictor, mydriatic.

Eye Face and Body Wash Station. (Lavoptik) Sodium Cl 0.49 g, sodium biphosphate 0.4 g, sodium phosphate 0.45 g/100 ml, benzalkonium Cl 0.005%. Bot. 32 oz.
Use: Emergency wash.

Eye Irrigating Solution. (Rugby) Sodium Cl, sodium phosphate mono- and dibasic, benzalkonium Cl, EDTA. Soln. Bot. 118 ml. *otc.*
Use: Irrigant, ophthalmic.

Eye Irrigating Wash. (Roberts Pharm) Boric acid, potassium Cl, sodium carbonate anhydrous, EDTA 0.01%, benzalkonium Cl. Soln. Bot. 120 ml. *otc.*
Use: Irrigant, ophthalmic.

Eye-Lube-A. (Optopics) Glycerin 0.25%, EDTA, NaCl, benzalkonium chloride. Soln. Bot. 15 ml. *otc.*
Use: Lubricant, opthalmic.

Eye Mo. (Sanofi Winthrop) Boric acid, benzalkonium Cl, phenylephrine HCl, zinc sulfate. *otc.*
Use: Astringent, ophthalmic.

Eye Scrub. (Ciba Vision Ophthalmics) PEG-200 glyceryl monotallawate, disodium laureth sulfosuccinate, cocoamidopropylamineoxide, PEG-78 glyceryl monococoate, benzyl alcohol, EDTA/Soln. Bot. 240 ml. *otc.*
Use: Cleanser, opthalmic.

Eye-Sed Ophthalmic Solution. (Scherer) Zinc sulfate 0.25%. Bot. 15 ml. *otc.*
Use: Astringent, ophthalmic.

Eyesine. (Akorn) Tetrahydrozoline HCl 0.05%. Drops. Bot. 15 ml. *otc.*
Use: Mydriatic, vasoconstrictor.

Eye-Stream. (Alcon Laboratories) Sodium Cl 0.64%, potassium Cl 0.075%, magnesium Cl hexahydrate 0.03%, calcium Cl dihydrate 0.048%, sodium acetate trihydrate 0.39%, sodium citrate dihydrate 0.17%, benzalkonium Cl 0.013%. Bot. 30 ml, 118 ml. *otc.*
Use: Irrigant, ophthalmic.

Eye Wash. (Bausch & Lomb) Boric acid, potassium Cl, EDTA, sodium carbonate, benzalkonium Cl 0.01%. Soln. Bot. 118 ml. *otc.*
Use: Irrigant, ophthalmic.

Eye Wash. (Zenith Goldline) Boric acid, potassium Cl, EDTA, anhydrous sodium carbonate, benzalkonium Cl 0.1%. Soln. Bot. 118 ml. *otc.*
Use: Irrigant, opthalmic.

Eye Wash. (Lavoptik) Sodium Cl 0.49%, sodium biphosphate 0.4%, sodium phosphate 0.45%, benzalkonium Cl 0.005%. Soln. Bot. 180 ml with eye cup. *otc.*
Use: Irrigant, opthalmic.

EZ-Detect. (Biomerica) Occult blood screening test. Kit 3s.
Use: Diagnostic aid.

EZ Detect Strep-A Test. (Biomerica) Coated stick test for detection of group

A streptococci taken directly from a throat swab.
Use: Diagnostic aid.

Eze Pain. (Halsey) Acetaminophen 2.5 gr, salicylamide, caffeine/Cap. Bot. 21s. *otc.*
Use: Analgesic combination.

Ezide. (Econo Med Pharmaceuticals) Hydrochlorothiazide 50 mg/Tab. Bot. 100s, 1000s. *Rx.*
Use: Diuretic.

Ezol. (Stewart-Jackson) Butalbital 50 mg, caffeine 40 mg, acetaminophen 325 mg. Bot. 100s. *Rx.*
Use: Analgesic, hypnotic, sedative.

Ezol #3. (Stewart-Jackson) Acetaminophen 650 mg, codeine 30 mg. Bot. 100s. *c-III.*
Use: Analgesic combination, narcotic.

F

Fabrase.
Use: Fabry's disease. [Orphan drug]

Faces Only Moisturizing Sunblock by Coppertone. (Schering Plough) Ethylhexyl p-methoxycinnamate, oxybenzone. SPF 15. Lot. Bot. 55.5 ml. *otc.*
Use: Sunscreen.

Fact Home Pregnancy Test. (Advanced Care Products) Accurate test for pregnancy in 45 minutes, for use as early as 3 days after a missed period. 1 Test kit 1s.
Use: Diagnostic aid.

factor VIIa recombinant, DNA orgin. (Novo-Nordisk)
Use: Antihemophilic, von Willebrand's disease. [Orphan drug]

factor VIII.
See: Antihemophilic factor.

•**factor IX complex,** (FAK-tuhr-[IX] KAHM-plex) U.S.P. 23.
Use: Hemostatic.
See: Alpha Nine SD. (Alpha Therapeutics).
Konyne 80. (Bayer Corp)
Mononine. (Centeon)
Profilnine SD (Alpha Therapeutics).
Proplex T. (Baxter).

factor IX, coagulation.
See: Coagulation factor ix.

factor XIII (plasma-derived).
Use: Congenital Factor XIII deficiency. [Orphan drug]
See: Fibrogammin P (Behringwerke Aktiengesellschaft, AG).

Fact Plus. (Advanced Care Products) Reagent in-home kit for urine testing. Pregnancy test. Kit 1s, 2s.
Use: Diagnostic aid.

Factrel. (Wyeth Ayerst) Gonadorelin HCl 100 mcg or 500 mcg/Vial w/Amp. of 2 ml sterile diluent. *Rx.*
Use: Diagnostic aid.

•**fadrozole hydrochloride.** (FAHD-rah-ZOLE) USAN.
Use: Antineoplastic.

Falgos Tablets. (Sanofi Winthrop) Acetylsalicylic acid. *otc.*
Use: Analgesic.

•**famciclovir.** (fam-SIGH-kloe-veer) USAN.
Use: Antiviral.
See: Famvir, Tab. (SmithKline Beecham Pharmaceuticals).

Falmonox. (Sanofi Winthrop) Teclozan. Susp., Tab. *Rx.*
Use: Amebicide.

•**famotidine,** (fah-MOE-tih-den) U.S.P. 23.
Use: Antiulcerative.
See: Pepcid, Tab., Susp., Inj. (Merck).
Pepcid RPD, Tab. (Merck).

•**famotine hydrochloride.** (FAM-oh-teen) USAN.
Use: Antiviral.

•**fampridine.** (FAHM-prih-DEEN) USAN.
Use: Symptomatic treatment of multiple sclerosis.
See: Neurelan (Elan).

Famvir. (SmithKline Beecham Pharmaceuticals) Famciclovir 125 mg, lactose/Tab. Bot 30s, UD 100s. Famciclovir 250 mg, lactose/Tab. Bot. 30s. Famciclovir 500 mg, lactose/Tab. Bot. 30s, UD 50s. *Rx.*
Use: Management of acute herpes zoster (shingles).

•**fananserin.** (fan-AN-ser-in) USAN.
Use: Antipsychotic, antischizophrenic (dual dopamine D_4 and serotonin 5-HT_2 receptor antagonist).

•**fanetizole mesylate.** (fan-EH-tih-zole) USAN.
Use: Immunoregulator.

Fansidar. (Roberts Pharm) Sulfadoxine 500 mg, pyrimethamine 25 mg/Tab. Box 25s. *Rx.*
Use: Antimalarial.

•**fantridone hydrochloride.** (FAN-trih-dohn) USAN.
Use: Antidepressant.

Faramals. (Faraday) Vitamins A 10,000 IU, D 2000 IU, B_1 6 mg, B_2 4 mg, B_6 0.5 mg, folic acid 0.1 mg, C 100 mg, calcium pantothenate 5 mg, niacinamide 30 mg, E 5 IU, B_{12} 3 mcg/Tab. Bot. 100s, 250s, 500s, 1000s. *otc.*
Use: Mineral, vitamin supplement.

Faramals-M. (Faraday) Faramals plus calcium 103 mg, cobalt 0.1 mg, copper 1 mg, iodine 0.15 mg, iron 10 mg, magnesium 6 mg, molybdenum 0.2 mg, phosphorus 80 mg, potassium 5 mg, zinc 1.2 mg/Tab. Bot. 100s, 250s, 500s, 1000s. *otc.*
Use: Mineral, vitamin supplement.

Faramins. (Faraday) Vitamins B_1 20 mg, B_2 6 mg, C 40 mg, niacinamide 20 mg, calcium pantothenate 3 mg, B_6 0.5 mg, powdered whole dried liver 125 mg, dried debittered yeast 125 mg, choline dihydrogen citrate 20 mg, inositol 20 mg, dl-methionine 20 mg, folic acid 0.1 mg, B_{12} 10 mcg, ferrous gluconate 30 mg, dicalcium phosphate 250 mg, copper sulfate 5 mg, magnesium sulfate 10 mg, manganese sulfate 5 mg, cobalt sulfate 0.2 mg, potassium Cl 2 mg,

potassium iodide 0.15 mg/Tab. Bot. 100s, 250s, 500s, 1000s. *otc.*
Use: Mineral, vitamin supplement.

Faratol. (Faraday) Vitamins A 12,500 IU, D 1000 IU, B_1 20 mg, B_2 6 mg, B_6 0.5 mg, B_{12} 15 mcg, folic acid 0.1 mg, niacinamide 10 mg, calcium pantothenate 3 mg, C 60 mg, E 5 IU, choline dihydrogen citrate 20 mg, inositol 20 mg, dl-methionine 20 mg, whole dried liver 100 mg, dried debittered yeast 100 mg, dicalcium phosphate 200 mg, ferrous gluconate 30 mg, potassium iodide 0.2 mg, magnesium sulfate 7.2 mg, copper sulfate 5 mg, manganese sulfate 3.4 mg, cobalt sulfate 0.2 mg, potassium Cl 1.3 mg, zinc sulfate 2 mg, molybdenum 0.2 mg in a base of alfalfa/Tab. Bot. 100s, 250s, 500s, 1000s. *otc.*
Use: Mineral, vitamin supplement.

Farbee with Vitamin C. (Major) Vitamins B_1 15 mg, B_2 10.2 mg, B_3 50 mg, B_5 10 mg, B_5 5 mg, C 300 mg/Capl. Bot. 100s, 130s, 1000. *otc.*
Use: Vitamin supplement.

Farbital Compound Capsules. (Major) Butalbital, caffeine, aspirin. Bot. 100s. *c-III.*
Use: Analgesic, hypnotic, sedative.

Farbital Compound with Codeine #3. (Major) Butalbital, caffeine, aspirin, codeine 30 mg. Bot. 1000s. *c-III.*
Use: Analgesic, hypnotic, sedative.

Farbital Tabs. (Major) Butalbital. Bot. 100s. *c-III.*
Use: Hypnotic, sedative.

Fareston. (Schering) Toremifene citrate 60 mg, lactose. Tab. Bot. 30s, 100s. *Rx.*
Use: Antiestrogen agent.

farnoquinone.

Fastin. (SmithKline Beecham Pharmaceuticals) Phentermine HCl 30 mg/Cap. Bot. 100s, 450s. Pack 150s. (5 × 30s). *c-IV.*
Use: Anorexiant.

fat emulsion, intravenous.
See: Liposyn 10% (Abbott Laboratories).
Liposyn 20% (Abbott Laboratories).
Travamulsion 10% (Baxter).
Travamulsion 20% (Baxter).
Intralipid 10% (Pharmacia & Upjohn).
Intralipid 20% (Pharmacia & Upjohn).
Soyacal 10% (Alpha Therapeutics).
Soyacal 20% (Alpha Therapeutics).
Liposyn II 10% (Abbott Laboratories).
Liposyn II 20% (Abbott Laboratories).

•**fat, hard.** N. F. 18.
Use: Pharmaceutic aid (suppository base).

Father John's Medicine Plus. (Oakhurst) Phenylephrine HCl 2.5 mg, chlorpheniramine maleate 1 mg, dextromethorphan HBr 7.5 mg, guaifenesin 30 mg, ammonium Cl 100 mg, sodium citrate/5 ml. Bot. 120 ml, 240 ml. *otc.*
Use: Antihistamine, antitussive, decongestant, expectorant.

Fattibase. (Paddock) Preblended fatty acid suppository base composed of triglycerides of coconut oil and palm kernel oil. Jar 1 lb, 5 lb.
Use: Pharmaceutical aid, suppository base.

fazadinium bromide.
Use: Neuromuscular blocking agent.

•**fazarabine.** (fah-ZAY-rah-BEAN) USAN.
Use: Antineoplastic.

F.C.A.H. Capsules. (Scherer) Chlorpheniramine maleate 4 mg, acetaminophen 162 mg, salicylamide 162 mg/Cap. Bot. 100s, 500s. *otc.*
Use: Analgesic, antihistamine.

Fe_{50}. (UCB Pharma) Ferrous sulfate. 160 mg (iron 50 mg), PEG. ER Capl. UD 100s. *otc.*
Use: Mineral supplement.

Feberin. (Arcum) Ferrous gluconate 3 gr, vitamins C 25 mg, B_1 2 mg, B_6 1 mg, B_2 1 mg, niacinamide 5 mg/Tab. Bot. 100s, 1000s. *otc.*
Use: Mineral, vitamin supplement.

febrile antigens. (Laboratory Diagnostics) Group O antigens (somatic) are dyed blue and group H antigens (flagellars) are dyed red for clear identification for detection of bacterial agglutinins, bacterial infections. Vial 5 ml.
Use: Diagnostic aid.

Febrinol. (Eon Labs Manufacturing) Acetaminophen 325 mg/Tab. Bot. 100s, 1000s. *otc.*
Use: Analgesic.

Fe-Brone. (Forest Pharmaceutical) Vitamins B_{12} 1 IU, folic acid 1 mg, ferrous sulfate exsiccated (powdered) 200 mg, ferrous sulfate exsiccated (timed) 200 mg, C acid 100 mg, B_6 0.5 mg, B_1 2 mg, B_2 1 mg, copper 0.9 mg, zinc 0.5 mg, manganese 0.3 mg/Cap. Bot. 30s, 100s, 1000s. *Rx.*
Use: Mineral, vitamin supplement.

Fedahist Expectorant. (Schwarz Pharma) Guaifenesin 200 mg, pseudoephedrine HCl 20 mg/5 ml, sorbitol, alcohol free. *otc.*
Use: Antihistamine, decongestant.

Fedahist Gyrocaps. (Schwarz Pharma) Pseudoephedrine HCl 65 mg, chlor-

pheniramine maleate 10 mg/SR Cap. Bot. 100s. *Rx.*
Use: Antihistamine, decongestant.

Fedahist Timecaps. (Schwarz Pharma) Pseudoephedrine HCl 120 mg, chlorpheniramine maleate 8 mg/SR Cap. Bot. 100s. *Rx.*
Use: Antihistamine, decongestant.

Fedahist Tablets. (Schwarz Pharma) Pseudoephedrine HCl 60 mg, chlorpheniramine maleate 4 mg, sorbitol (alcohol and sugar free)/Tab. Bot. 100s. *Rx.*
Use: Antihistamine, decongestant.

Feen-a-Mint Dual Formula. (Schering Plough) Docusate sodium 100 mg, yellow phenolphthalein 65 mg/Tab. Box 15s, 30s, 60s. *otc.*
Use: Laxative.

Feen-a-Mint Gum. (Schering Plough) Yellow phenolphthalein 97.2 mg/Chewing gum Tab. Box 5s, 16s, 40s. *otc.*
Use: Laxative.

Feen-a-Mint. (Schering Plough) Yellow phenolphthalein 97.2 mg/Chewable mint tab. Box 20s. *otc.*
Use: Laxative.

Feen-a-Mint Pills. (Schering Plough) Docusate sodium 100 mg, yellow phenolphthalein 65 mg/Tab. Box 15s, 30s, 60s. *otc.*
Use: Laxative.

Feen-a-Mint Tablets. (Schering Plough) Bisacodyl 5 mg, talc, lactose, sugar. Tab. 10s. *otc.*
Use: Laxative.

Fe_{50}. (UCB Pharam) Fe 160 mg (as dried ferrous sulfate equivalent to 50 mg elemental iron), PEG. Capl. Bot. 100s. *otc.*
Use: Mineral supplement.

Feg-I. (Western Research) Ferrous gluconate 300 mg/Tab. Handicount 28s (36 bags of 28 tab.). *otc.*
Use: Mineral supplement.

Feiba VH Immuno. (Immuno-U.S.) Freeze-dried anti-inhibitor coagulant complex. Heparin free. Vapor heated. Inj. Vial with diluent and needle.
Use: Antihemophilic.

•**felbamate.** (FELL-buh-MATE) USAN.
Use: Antiepileptic; treatment of Lennox-Gastaut Syndrome. [Orphan drug]
See: Felbatol (Wallace Laboratories).

Felbatol. (Wallace Laboratories) Felbamate 400 mg or 600 mg, lactose/Tab., Felbamate, 600 mg/5 ml, sorbitol, parabens, saccharin/Susp. **Tab.:** Bot. 100s and UD 100s. **Susp.:** Bot. 240 ml and 960 ml. *Rx.*
Use: Antiepileptic. It has been recommended that use of this drug be discontinued if aplastic anemia or hepatic failure occurs unless, in the judgement of the physician, continued therapy is warranted. For further information contact Wallace Labs at 800-526-3840.
Lennox-Gastaut Syndrome. [Orphan drug]

•**felbinac.** (FELL-bih-nak) USAN.
Use: Anti-inflammatory.

Feldene. (Pfizer) Piroxicam 10 mg or 20 mg/Cap. **10 mg:** Bot 100s. **20 mg:** Bot. 100s, 500s, UD 100s. *Rx.*
Use: Analgesic, NSAID.

Fellobolic Injection. (Forest Pharmaceutical) Methandriol dipropionate 50 mg/ml. Vial 10 ml. *Rx.*

•**felodipine.** (feh-LOW-dih-peen) USAN.
Use: Vasodilator.
See: Plendil, Tab. (Merck).

feldopine and enalapril maleate.
Use: Antihypertensive.
See: Lexxel, ER Tab. (Astra Merck).

•**felvizumab.** (fell-VYE-zoo-mab) USAN.
Use: Antiviral (systemic); monoclonal antibody.

•**felypressin.** (fell-ih-PRESS-in) USAN.
Use: Vasoconstrictor.

Femagene. (Tennessee Pharmaceutic) Boric acid, sodium borate, lactic acid, menthol, methylbenzethonium Cl, parachlorometaxylenol, lactose, surface-active agents. Pow. 6 oz. *otc.*
Use: Feminine hygiene.

Femara. (Novartis) Letrozole 2.5 mg, lactose/Tab. Bot. 30s. *Rx.*
Use: Breast cancer treatment.

Femazole Tabs. (Major) Metronidazole 250 mg or 500 mg/Tab. **250 mg:** Bot. 100s, 250s, 500s. **500 mg:** Bot. 50s, 100s. *Rx.*
Use: Anti-infective.

Femcal. (Freeda Vitamins). Calcium carbonate 250 mg, vitamin D_3 100 IU, B_1 100 mg, Mg, Mn, Si, kosher, sugar free/Tab. Bot. 100s and 250s. *otc.*
Use: Electrolyte, mineral supplement.

Femcaps. (Buffington) Acetaminophen, caffeine, ephedrine sulfate, atropine sulfate/Tab. Sugar, lactose and salt free Dispens-a-Kit 500s, Aidpaks 100s. *Rx.*
Use: Analgesic, anticholinergic, antispasmodic, bronchodilator.

Femcet. (Russ Pharmaceuticals) Acetaminophen 325 mg, butalbital 50 mg, caffeine 40 mg/Cap. Bot. 100s. *Rx.*
Use: Analgesic, hypnotic, sedative.

femergin.
See: Ergotamine Tartrate (Various Mfr.)

Femidyn.
See: Estrone (Various Mfr.)

Femilax. (G & W Laboratories) Docusate sodium 100 mg, phenolphthalein 65 mg/Tab. Bot. 30s, 60s, 90s. *otc.*
Use: Laxative.

Feminique Disposable Douche. (Schmid) Sodium benzoate, sorbic acid, lactic acid, octoxynol-9. Twin-pack Bot. 120 ml. *otc.*
Use: Douche.

Feminique Disposable Douche. (Schmid) Vinegar and water. Soln. Twin-packs. Bot. 180 ml. *otc.*
Use: Douche.

Feminone. (Pharmacia & Upjohn) Ethinyl estradiol 0.05 mg/Tab. Bot. 100s. *Rx.*
Use: Estrogen.

Femiron. (Menley & James) Ferrous fumarate 63 mg (iron 20 mg)/Tab. Bot. 40s, 120s. *otc.*
Use: Mineral supplement.

Femiron Multi-Vitamins and Iron. (Menley & James) Iron 20 mg, vitamins A 5000 IU, D 400 IU, B_1 1.5 mg, riboflavin 1.7 mg, B_3 20 mg, C 60 mg, B_6 2 mg, B_{12} 6 mcg, B_5 10 mg, folic acid 0.4 mg, E 15 mg/Tab. Bot. 35s, 60s, 90s. *otc.*
Use: Mineral, vitamin supplement.

Femizol-M. (Lake Consumer Products) Miconazole nitrate 2%/Vaginal cream. Tube, with applicator. 45 g. *otc.*
Use: Antifungal, vaginal.

Fem-1. (BDI) Acetaminophen 500 mg, pamabrom 25 mg/Tab. Bot. 30s. *otc.*
Use: Analgesic.

Femotrone. (Bluco) Progesterone in oil 50 mg/ml. Vial 10 ml. *Rx.*
Use: Hormone, progestin.

FemPatch. (Parke-Davis) Estradiol 10.3 mg (0.025 mg/day)/Patch. Box. 4s. *Rx.*
Use: Estrogen.

Femstat 3. (Procter-Syntex) Butoconazole nitrate 2%, parabens, cetyl alcohol, mineral oil, steryl alcohol/Cream. Three 5 g prefilled applicators and 20 g with applicators. *otc.*
Use: Antifungal, vaginal.

Femizol-M. (Lake Consumer Products) Miconazole nitrate 2%, mineral oil. Vag. Cream. Tube 45 g with applicator. *otc.*
Use: Vaginal preparation.

•**fenalamide.** (fen-AL-am-IDE) USAN.
Use: Muscle relaxant.

fenamisal. Phenyl aminosalicylate.

•**fenamole.** (FEN-ah-mole) USAN.
Use: Anti-inflammatory.

Fenaprin Tablets. (Sanofi Winthrop) Aspirin, chlormezanone. *Rx.*
Use: Analgesic, anxiolytic.

Fenarol. (Sanofi Winthrop) Chlormezanone 100 mg or 200 mg/Tab. Bot. 100s.
Use: Anxiolytic.

fenarsone.
See: Carbarsone (Various Mfr.)

•**fenbendazole.** (FEN-BEND-ah-zole) USAN.
Use: Anthelmintic.
See: Panacure (Hoechst-Roussel)

•**fenbufen.** (FEN-byoo-fen) USAN.
Use: Anti-inflammatory.
See: Cinopal (ESI Lederle Generics)

•**fencibutirol.** (fen-sih-BYOO-tih-role). USAN.
Use: Choleretic.

•**fenclofenac.** (FEN-kloe-fen-ACK) USAN.
Use: Anti-inflammatory.

•**fenclonine.** (fen-KLOE-neen) USAN. Under study by Pfizer.
Use: Serotonin inhibitor.

•**fenclorac.** (FEN-kloe-rack) USAN.
Use: Anti-inflammatory.

Fend. (Mine Safety Appliances).
- **A-2**– Water soluble cream which forms a physical barrier to water insoluble irritants. Tube 3 oz, Jar lb.
- **E-2**– This cream combines the functions of the water soluble Fend A-2 and water insoluble Fend I-2 creams. Tube 3 oz, Jar lb.
- **I-2**– Water insoluble cream which forms a physical barrier to water soluble irritants. Tube 3 oz, Jar lb.
- **S-2**– A silicone cream which forms a barrier against a combination of water soluble and water insoluble irritants. Tube 3 oz, Jar lb.
- **X**– Industrial cold cream which rubs well into the skin and serves as a skin conditioner. Tube 3 oz, Jar lb.

Use: Skin protectant.

Fendol. (Buffington) Salicylamide, caffeine, acetaminophen, phenylephrine HCl/Tab. Sugar, lactose and salt free. Dispens-A-Kit 500s. Bot. 100s. *otc.*
Use: Analgesic combination.

•**fendosal.** (FEN-doe-sal) USAN.
Use: Anti-inflammatory.

Fenesin. (Dura Pharm) Guaifenesin 600 mg/SR Tab. Bot. 100s, 600s. *Rx.*
Use: Expectorant.

Fenesin DM. (Dura Pharm) Dextrometh-

orphan HBr 30 mg, guaifenesin 600 mg/ Tab. Bot. 100s. *Rx.*
Use: Antitussive, expectorant.

•**fenestrel.** (feh-NESS-trell) USAN. Under study.
Use: Estrogen.

•**fenethylline hydrochloride.** (FEN-ETH-ill-in) USAN.
Use: Stimulant (central).

•**fengabine.** (FEN-GAH-bean) USAN.
Use: Mood regulator.

•**fenimide.** (FEN-ih-mid) USAN.
Use: Anxiolytic, antipsychotic.

•**fenisorex.** (fen-EYE-so-rex) USAN.
[use]Use:Anorexigenic, anorexic.

•**fenmetozole hydrochloride.** (FEN-MET-oh-zole) USAN.
Use: Antidepressant, antagonist (to narcotics).

•**fenmetramide.** (fen-MEH-trah-mide) USAN.
Use: Antidepressant.

fennel oil.
Use: Pharmaceutic aid (flavor).

•**fenobam.** (FEN-oh-bam) USAN.
Use: Hypnotic, sedative.

•**fenoctimine sulfate.** (fen-OCK-tih-MEEN) USAN.
Use: Gastric antisecretory.

fenofibrate.
Use: Antihyperlipidemic.
See: Lipidil, Cap. (Fournier).

•**fenoldopam mesylate.** (feh-NAHL-doe-pam) USAN.
Use: Antihypertensive, dopamine agonist.
See: Corlopam, Inj. (Neurex).

•**fenoprofen.** (FEN-oh-PRO-fen) USAN.
Use: Anti-inflammatory, analgesic.

•**fenoprofen calcium,** (FEN-oh-PRO-fen) U.S.P. 23.
Use: Anti-inflammatory, analgesic.
See: Nalfon, Cap., Tab. (Eli Lilly).

•**fenoterol.** (FEN-oh-TER-ahl) USAN.
Use: Bronchodilator.

•**fenpipalone.** (FEN-PIP-ah-lone) USAN.
Use: Anti-inflammatory.

•**fenprinast hydrochloride.** (fen-PRIH-nast) USAN.
Use: Bronchodilator (antiallergic).

•**fenprostalene.** (FEN-PRAHST-ah-leen) USAN.
Use: Luteolysin.

•**fenquizone.** (FEN-kwih-zone) USAN.
Use: Diuretic.

•**fenretinide.** (fen-RET-ih-nide) USAN.
Use: Antineoplastic.

•**fenspiride hydrochloride.** (fen-SPIH-rid) USAN.
Use: Bronchodilator, antiadrenergic (α-receptor).

fentanyl.
Use: Analgesic, narcotic.
See: Duragesic, Transdermal (Janssen).

•**fentanyl citrate,** (FEN-tuh-nill) U.S.P. 23.
Use: Analgesic, narcotic.
See: Sublimaze, Inj. (Janssen).
Oralet (Abbott Laboratories).

fentanyl citrate. (Various Mfr.) 0.05 mg/ ml. Inj. Amp. 2 ml, 5 ml, 10 ml, 20 ml. Vial. 30 ml, 50 ml.
Use: Analgesic, narcotic.

Fentanyl Citrate & Droperidol. (Astra) Fentanyl 0.05 mg, droperidol 2.5 mg/ ml. Inj. Amp and Vial 2 ml, 5 ml. *c-II.*
Use: Anesthetic, general.
See: Innovar, Inj. (Janssen).

Fentanyl Oralet. (Abbott Laboratories) Fentanyl 200 mcg, 300 mcg, 400 mg sucrose, liquid glucose/2 oz. 25s. *c-II.*
Use: Anesthetic, general.

Fentanyl Transdermal System. (FEN-tuh-nill) *c-II.*
See: Duragesic-25 (Janssen).
Duragesic-50 (Janssen).
Duragesic-75 (Janssen).
Duragesic-100 (Janssen).

•**fentiazac.** (fen-TIE-azz-ACK) USAN.
Use: Anti-inflammatory.

•**fenticlor.** (FEN-tih-Klor) USAN.
Use: Antifungal; antiseptic, topical.

•**fenticonazole nitrate.** (FEN-tih-KOE-nah-zole) USAN.
Use: Antifungal.

Fenton Elixir. (Sanofi Winthrop) Ferrous gluconate. *otc.*
Use: Mineral supplement.

Fenylhist. (Roberts Pharm) Diphenhydramine HCl 25 mg or 50 mg/Cap. Bot. 1000s. *otc.*
Use: Antihistamine.

fenyramidol hydrochloride. Phenyramidol HCl.

•**fenyripol hydrochloride.** (FEH-nee-rih-pahl) USAN.
Use: Muscle relaxant.

Feocyte. (Dunhall Pharmaceuticals) Iron 110 mg, vitamins C 100 mg, B_6 2 mg, B_{12} 50 mcg, copper sulfate, folic acid 0.8 mg, desiccated liver 15 mg/Prolonged Action Tab. Bot. 100s. *Rx.*
Use: Mineral, vitamin supplement.

Feocyte Injectable. (Dunhall Pharmaceuticals) Peptonized iron 15 mg, vitamin B_{12} 200 mcg, liver injection N.F. beef 10 units, sodium citrate 10 mg, benzyl alcohol 2%/ml. Vial 10 ml. *Rx.*

Use: Mineral, vitamin supplement.

Feosol Caplets. (SmithKline Beecham) Carbonyl iron 50 mg, lactose, sorbitol, PEG. Capl. Bot. 60s. *otc.*
Use: Mineral supplement.

Feosol Elixir. (SmithKline Beecham Pharmaceuticals) Ferrous sulfate (44 mg iron) 220 mg/5 ml, alcohol 5%. Bot. 16 oz. *otc.*
Use: Mineral supplement.

Feosol Tablets. (SmithKline Beecham Pharmaceuticals) Ferrous sulfate, exsiccated 200 mg (65 mg iron), glucose/ Tab. Bot. 100s. *otc.*
Use: Mineral supplement.

Feostat. (Forest Pharmaceutical) **Tab.:** Ferrous fumarate 100 mg (33 mg iron)/ Chew. tab. Bot. 100s, UD 100s. **Drops:** Ferrous fumarate 45 mg (15 mg iron)/0.6 ml, methylparaben 0.2%. Bot. 60 ml. **Susp.:** Ferrous fumarate 100 mg (iron 33 mg)/5 ml, methylparaben 0.2%. Bot. 240 ml. *otc.*
Use: Mineral supplement.

Feostat Suspension. (Forest Pharmaceutical) Ferrous fumarate 100 mg (33 mg iron)/5 ml. Bot. 240 ml. *otc.*
Use: Mineral supplement.

FE-Plus Protein. (Miller) Iron (as an iron-protein complex) 50 mg/Tab. Bot. 100s. *otc.*
Use: Mineral supplement.

Feratab. (Upsher-Smith Labs) Ferrous sulfate 187 mg (60 mg iron)/Tab. Bot. UD 100s. *otc.*
Use: Mineral supplement.

Ferate-C. (Pal-Pak) Ferrous fumarate 150 mg, ascorbic acid 200 mg, docusate sodium 25 mg/Tab. Bot. 100s, 1000s. *otc.*
Use: Mineral, vitamin supplement; stool softener.

Fer-gen-sol Drops. (Zenith Goldline) Ferrous sulfate 75 mg/0.6 ml (iron 15 mg/0.6 ml), alcohol 0.2%, sodium bisulfite, sorbitol, sugar. Drops. Bot. 50 ml. *otc.*
Use: Mineral supplement.

Fergon. (Bayer) Ferrous gluconate 240 mg (iron 27 mg), sucrose. Tab. Bot. 100s. *otc.*
Use: Mineral supplement.

Feridex I.V. (Berlex) Iron 11.2 mg, mannitol 61.3 mg/ml, dextran 5.6 to 9.1 mg/ ml/Inj. Vial. 5 ml. *Rx.*
Use: Radiopaque agent.

Fer-In-Sol. (Bristol-Myers) **Drops:** Elemental iron 15 mg/0.6 ml, alcohol 0.02%, sodium bisulfite, sorbitol, sugar. Droppter Bot. 50 ml. **Syr.:** 18 mg/5 ml. Alcohol 5%. Bot. 480 ml. *otc.*
Use: Mineral supplement.

Fer-Iron. (Rugby) Ferrous sulfate 75 mg (iron 15 mg)/0.6 ml, alcohol 0.2%, sodium bisulfite, sorbitol, sugar. Dropper Bot. 50 ml. *otc.*
Use: Mineral supplement.

Ferocyl. (Arco) Ferrous fumarate 150 mg (iron 50 mg), docusate sodium 100 mg/ TR Cap. Bot. 100s. *otc.*
Use: Mineral supplement, stool softener.

Fero-Folic 500. (Abbott Laboratories) Ferrous sulfate controlled-release (equivalent to 105 mg iron), vitamin C 500 mg, folic acid 0.8 mg/Filmtab. Bot. 100s, 500s. *Rx.*
Use: Mineral, vitamin supplement.

Fero-Grad 500. (Abbott Laboratories) Sodium ascorbate 500 mg, ferrous sulfate equivalent to 105 mg iron/TR Tab. Bot. 30s. *otc.*
Use: Mineral supplement.

Ferolix. (Century Pharm) Ferrous sulfate 5 gr, alcohol 5%/10 ml Elix. Bot. 8 oz, pt, gal. *otc.*
Use: Mineral supplement.

Ferosan Forte. (Sandia) Ferrous fumarate 300 mg, liver-stomach concentrate 150 mg, vitamin B_{12} w/intrinsic factor concentrate 7.5 mcg, intrinsic factor concentrate 150 mg, B_{12} 7.5 mcg, ascorbic acid 75 mg, folic acid 1 mg, sorbitol 50 mg/Tab. Bot. 100s. *Rx.*
Use: Mineral, vitamin supplement.

Ferosan Syrup. (Sandia) Ferrous fumarate 91.2 mg, B_1 10 mg, B_6 3 mg, B_{12} 25 mcg/5 ml 16 oz, gal. *otc.*
Use: Mineral, vitamin supplement.

Ferospace. (Hudson) Ferrous sulfate 250 mg (iron 50 mg)/TR Cap. Bot. 100s. *otc.*
Use: Mineral supplement.

Ferotrinsic. (Rugby) Iron 110 mg (from ferrous fumarate), vitamins B_{12} 15 mcg, C 75 mg, intrinsic factor (as concentrate or from stomach preparations) 240 mg, folic acid 0.5 mg/Cap. 100s, 500s, 1000s. *Rx.*
Use: Mineral, vitamin supplement.

Feroweet. (Barth's) Vitamins B_1 6 mg, B_2 12 mg, niacin 4 mg, iron 30 mg, B_{12} 10 mcg, B_6 95 mcg, pantothenic acid 50 mcg/3 Cap. Bot. 100s, 500s, 1000s. *otc.*
Use: Mineral, vitamin supplement.

Ferracomp. (Roberts Pharm) Liver 2 mcg, vitamins B_{12} 15 mcg, B_1 10 mg, B_2 5 mg, B_6 1 mg, calcium pantothenate

1 mg, niacinamide 10 mg, iron 31.3 mg/ml. Vial 30 ml. *otc.*
Use: Mineral, vitamin supplement.

Ferralet Plus. (Mission Pharmacal) Ferrous gluconate equivalent to 46 mg iron, C 400 mg, folic acid 0.8 mg, vitamin B_{12} 25 mcg/Tab. Bot. 60s. *otc.*
Use: Mineral, vitamin supplement.

Ferrets. (Pharmics) Ferrous fumarate 325 mg, iron 106 mg/Tab. Bot. 100s. *otc.*
Use: Mineral supplement.

ferric ammonium citrate. Ammonium iron (Fe^{+++}) citrate.
Use: Mineral supplement.

ferric ammonium sulfate. (Various Mfr.)
Use: Astringent.

ferric ammonium tartrate. (Various Mfr.)
Use: Mineral supplement.

ferric cacodylate. (Various Mfr.)
Use: Leukemias, hematinic.

ferric chloride. (Various Mfr.)
Use: Astringent.

•**ferric chloride Fe 59.** (FER-ik KLOR-ide) USAN.
Use: Radiopharmaceutical.

ferric citrochloride tincture. Iron (3+) chloride citrate.
Use: Hematinic.

•**ferric fructose.** (FER-ik FRUKE-tose) USAN.
Use: Hematinic.

ferric glycerophosphate. Glycerol phosphate iron (3+) salt.
Use: Pharmaceutic necessity.

ferric hypophosphite. Iron (3+) phosphinate.
Use: Pharmaceutic necessity.

•**ferriclate calcium sodium.** (fer-ih-KLATE) USAN.
Use: Hematinic.

•**ferric oxide,** (FER-ik) N.F. 18.
Use: Pharmaceutic aid (color).

ferric oxide, yellow.
Use: Pharmaceutic aid (color).

ferric "peptonate". (Various Mfr.)
See: Iron Peptonized.

ferric pyrophosphate, soluble. Iron (3+) citrate pyrophosphate.

ferric quinine citrate, "green". (Various Mfr.)
Use: Mineral supplement.

ferric subsulfate solution. (Various Mfr.)
Use: Local use on the skin.

•**ferristene.** (FER-ih-steen) USAN.
Use: Diagnostic aid (paramagnetic).

Ferrizyme. (Abbott Diagnostics) Enzyme immunoassay for qualitative determination of ferritin in human serum or plasma. Test kit 100s.
Use: Diagnostic aid, paramagnetic.

ferrocholate.
See: Ferrocholinate.

ferrocholinate. Ferrocholate. Ferrocholine. A chelate prepared by reacting equimolar quantities of freshly precipitated ferric hydroxide with choline dihydrogen citrate.
Use: Mineral supplement.
See: Chel-Iron, Preps. (Kinney).

ferrocholine.
See: Ferrocholinate.
Kelex, Tabseal. (Nutrition).

Ferro-Cyte. (Spanner) Iron peptonate 20 mg, liver injection (20 mg/ml) 0.25 ml, vitamins B_1 22 mg, B_2 0.5 mg, B_6 2.5 mg, B_{12} 30 mcg, niacinamide 25 mg, panthenol 1 mg/ml. Inj. Multiple dose vial 10 ml. *Rx.*
Use: Mineral, vitamin supplement.

Ferro-Docusate TR. (Parmed) Ferrous fumarate 150 mg (iron 50 mg), docusate sodium 100 mg/TR Cap. Bot. 100s. *otc.*
Use: Mineral supplement, stool softener.

Ferro-Dok TR. (Major) Ferrous fumarate 150 mg (iron 50 mg), docusate sodium 100 mg/TR Cap. Bot. 100s. *otc.*
Use: Mineral supplement, stool softener.

Ferrodyl Chewable Tablets. (Arcum) Ferrous fumarate 320 mg, vitamin C 200 mg/Tab. Bot. 100s, 1000s. *otc.*
Use: Mineral, vitamin supplement.

Ferromar. (Marnel) Ferrous fumarate 201.5 mg (iron 65 mg), vitamin C 200 mg/SR Capl. Bot. 100s. *otc.*
Use: Mineral supplement.

Ferroneed. (Hanlon) Ferrous gluconate 300 mg, ascorbic acid 60 mg/Cap. Bot. 100s. *otc.*
Use: Mineral, vitamin supplement.

Ferroneed T-Caps. (Hanlon) Ferrous fumarate 250 mg, thiamine HCl 5 mg, ascorbic acid 50 mg/TD Cap. Bot. 100s. *otc.*
Use: Mineral, vitamin supplement.

Ferronex. (Taylor Pharmaceuticals) Iron from ferrous gluconate 2.9 mg, Vitamins B_{12} equivalent 1 mcg, B_2 0.75 mg, B_3 50 mg, B_5 1.25 mg, B_{12} 15 mcg, procaine 2%/ml. Inj. Vial 30 ml. *Rx.*
Use: Mineral, vitamin supplement.

Ferro-Sequels. (Selfcare, Inc.) Ferrous fumarate equivalent to iron 50 mg, docusate sodium, lactose. TR Tab. Bot. 30s, 90s. *otc.*

Use: Mineral supplement.

Ferrospan Capsules. (Imperial Lab) Ferrous fumarate 200 mg, ascorbic acid 100 mg/Tab. Bot. 100s, 1000s. *otc.*
Use: Mineral, vitamin supplement.

Ferrosyn Injection. (Standex) Cyanocobalamin 30 mcg, liver 2 mcg, ferrous gluconate 100 mg, riboflavin 1.5 mg, panthenol 2.5 mg, niacinamide 100 mg, procaine 2%. Vial 30 ml. *Rx.*
Use: Mineral, vitamin supplement.

Ferrosyn S.C. (Standex) Iron 60 mg, vitamin B_{12} 5 mcg, magnesium 0.6 mg, copper 0.3 mg, manganese 0.1 mg, potassium 0.5 mg, zinc 0.15 mg/Tab. Bot. 100s, 1000s. *otc.*
Use: Mineral, vitamin supplement.

Ferrosyn See Tabs. (Standex) Iron 34 mg, ascorbic acid 60 mg/Tab. Bot. 100s, 1000s. *otc.*
Use: Mineral, vitamin supplement.

Ferrosyn Tab. (Standex) Iron 60 mg, vitamin B_{12} 5 mcg, magnesium 0.6 mg, copper 0.3 mg, manganese 0.1 mg, potassium 0.5 mg, zinc 0.15 mg/Tab. Bot. 100s. *otc.*
Use: Mineral, vitamin supplement.

ferrous bromide. (FER-uhs) (Various Mfr.)
Use: In chorea & tuberculous cervical adenitis.

ferrous carbonate mass. Vallet's mass. (Various Mfr.)
Use: Mineral supplement.

ferrous carbonate, saccharated. (Various Mfr.)
Use: Mineral supplement.

•**ferrous citrate Fe 59,** (FER-uhs SIH-trate) USAN.
Use: Radiopharmaceutical.

•**ferrous fumarate,** (FER-uhs FEW-mah-rate) U.S.P. 23.
Use: Hematinic.
See: Children, Susp. (Fleming).
Eldofe, Tab. (Canright).
El-Ped-Ron, Liq. (Zeneca).
Farbegen, Cap. (Hickam).
Feco-T, Cap. (Blaine).
Femiron, Tab. (Menley & James).
Feostat, Preps. (Forest Pharm).
Ferretts, Tab. (Pharmics).
Fumasorb, Tab. (Hoechst Marion Roussel).
Fumerin, Tab. (Laser).
Hemocyte, Tab. (US Pharm).
Ircon, Tab. (Key Pharm).
Laud-Iron, Tab., Susp. (Amfre-Grant).
Maniron, Meltab. (Jones Medical Industries).
Nephro-Fer, Tab. (R & D Labs).
W/Ascorbic Acid.
See: C-Ron, Preps. (Solvay).
Cytoferin, Tab. (Wyeth Ayerst).
Eldofe-C, Tab. (Canright).
Ferancee, Tab. (J & J Merck Consumer Pharm).
Ferancee-HP, Tab. (Zeneca).
Ferrodyl Chewable Tab. (Arcum).
Ferromar, SR Cap. (Marnel).
Min-Hema Chewable, Tab. (Scrip).
W/Ascorbic acid and folic acid.
See: Fer-Regules, Cap. (Quality Formulations).
Ferro-Docusate T.R., Cap. (Parmed)
Ferro Dok TR, Cap. (Major)
Ferro-DSS S.R., Cap. (Geneva Pharm)
Ferro-Sequels, Cap. (ESI Lederle Generics).
W/Norethindrone, mestranol.
See: Ortho Novum Fe-28, Fe-28, 1 mg Fe-28, Tab. (Ortho McNeil).
W/Vitamins and minerals.
See: Stuart Formula, Tab. (Zeneca).
Stuart Prenatal, Tab. (Zeneca).
Stuartnatal 1 + 1, Tab. (Zeneca).
Theron, Tab. (Zeneca).
Vitanate, Tab. (Century Pharm).

ferrous fumarate. (Mission) Ferrous fumarate 200 mg (iron 66 mg), sugar/Tab. Bot. 100s. Ferrous fumarate 300 mg (iron 106 mg) Tab. Bot. 100s. *otc.*
Use: Mineral supplement.

ferrous fumarate and docusate sodium extended-release tablets.
Use: Mineral supplement.

•**ferrous gluconate,** (FER-uhs)U.S.P. 23.
Use: Hematinic.
See: Fergon Prods. (Sanofi Winthrop).
W/Ascorbic acid, desiccated liver, vitamin B complex.
See: I.L.X. w/B_{12}, Tab. (Kenwood Labs).
Stuart Hematinic, Liq. (Zeneca).
W/Polyoxyethylene glucitan monolaurate.
See: Simron, Cap. (Hoechst Marion Roussel).

ferrous gluconate. (Various Mfr.) Ferrous gluconate 325 mg (iron 36 mg). Tab. Bot. 100s, 1000s. *otc.*
Use: Mineral supplement.

ferrous iodide. (Various Mfr.)
Use: In chronic tuberculosis.

ferrous iodide syrup. (Various Mfr.)
Use: In chronic tuberculosis.

ferrous lactate. (Various Mfr.)
Use: Mineral supplement.

•**ferrous sulfate.** (FER-uhs SULL-fate) U.S.P. 23.
Use: Hematinic.
See: Feosol, Spansule, Tab., Elix.

(SmithKline Beecham Pharmaceuticals).
Fe^{50}, Capl. (UCB Pharma).
Fer-gen-sol, Drops (Zenith Goldline).
Fer-Iron, Drops (Rugby).
Fer-In-Sol, Syr. Drops (Mead Johnson).
Fero-Gradumet, Tab. (Abbott Laboratories).
Ferolix, Elix. (Century Pharm).
Ferrous Sulfate Filmseals, Tab. (Parke-Davis).
Fesotyme SR, Cap. (Zeneca).
Irospan, Cap., Tab. (Fielding).
Mol-Iron, Prods. (Schering Plough).

W/Ascorbic acid.
See: Fero-Grad-500, Tab. (Abbott Laboratories).
Mol-Iron W/Vitamin C, Chronosules (Schering Plough).

W/Ascorbic acid, folic acid.
See: Fero-Folic-500, Tab. (Abbott Laboratories).

W/Cyanocobalamin, ascorbic acid, folic acid.
See: Intrin, Cap. (Merit).

W/Folic acid.
See: Folvron, Cap. (ESI Lederle Generics).

W/Maalox.
See: Fermalox, Tab. (Rhone-Poulenc Rorer).

ferrous sulfate. (Various) Ferrous sulfate. **Tab.:** 324 mg (iron 65 mg) UD 100s; 325 mg (iron 65 mg) Bot. 100s. **Elix.:** 220 mg/5 ml (iron 44 mg/5 ml) Bot. 473 ml. **Drops:** 75 mg/0.6 ml (iron 15 mg/0.6 ml) Bot. 50 ml. *otc.*
Use: Mineral supplement.

•**ferrous sulfate, dried,** (FER-uhs SULL-fate) U.S.P. 23.
Use: Antianemic.
See: Fer-In-Sol (Bristol-Myers Squibb Nutritionals).
Feosol (SmithKline Beecham).
Ferrous Sulfate (Various).
Ferra-TD (Zenith Goldline).
Slow Fe (Novartis Pharmaceuticals).

ferrous sulfate exsiccated.
Use: Mineral supplement.
See: Fe$_{50}$, ER Capl. (UCB Pharma).
Feosol, Tab. (SmithKline Beecham).
Feratab, Tab. (Upsher-Smith).
Slow FE, SR Tab. (Novartis).

•**ferrous sulfate Fe 59.** (FER0uhs SULL-fate) USAN.
Use: Radiopharmaceutical.

ferrous sulfate. (Zenith Goldline) Ferrous sulfate 325 mg (elemental iron 65 mg)/Tab. Bot. 100s. *otc.*
Use: Mineral supplement.

Ferrous Sulfate Filmseals. (Parke-Davis) Ferrous sulfate 5 gr/DR Tab. Bot. 1000s, UD 100s. *otc.*
Use: Iron supplement.

Fertility Tape. (Weston Labs.) Regular, extrasensitive, less-sensitive. W/Fertility Testor, cervical glucose test. Pkg. test 60s.
Use: Diagnostic aid.

Fertinex. (Serono Labs) Urofollitropin 75 IU/Pow. for Inj. Amp. 1, 10, 100 ml amps with diluent. Urofollitropin 150 IU/Pow. for Inj. Ampules. Single with diluent. Lactose 10 mg. *Rx.*
Use: Ovulation inducer.

•**ferucarbotran.** (fur-you-CAR-boe-tran) USAN.
Use: Diagnostic aid (superparamagnetic).

•**ferumoxides.** (feh-roo-MOX-ides) USAN.
Use: Diagnostic aid (paramagnetic).
See: Ferides (Advanced Magnetics)

•**ferumoxsil.** (feh-roo-MOX-sill) USAN.
Use: Diagnostic aid (paramagnetic).
See: Gastromark (Advanced Magnetics).

•**ferumoxtran-10.** (fur-you-MOX-tran 10)
Use: Diagnostic aid (superparamagnetic).

Ferusal. (Eon Labs Manufacturing) Ferrous sulfate 325 mg/Tab. *otc.*
Use: Mineral supplement.

Festalan. (Hoechst Marion Roussel) Lipase 6000 units, amylase 30,000 units, protease 20,000 units, atropine methylnitrate 1 mg/EC Tab. Bot. 100s, 1000s. *Rx.*
Use: Digestive enzyme.

Fetinic. (Roberts Pharm) Iron 3.6 mg, vitamins B_{12} equivalent 2 mcg, B_1 10 mg, B_2 0.5 mg, B_3 10 mg, B_5 1 mg, B_6 1 mg, B_{12} 15 mcg, chlorobutanol 0.5%, benzyl alcohol 2%/ml. Vial 30 ml. *Rx.*
Use: Mineral, vitamin supplement.

Fetinic-MW. (Roberts Pharm) Iron 66 mg (from ferrous fumarate), vitamins B_{12} 5 mcg, C 60 mg/SR Cap. Bot. 100s. *otc.*
Use: Mineral, vitamin supplement.

•**fetoxylate hydrochloride.** (fee-TOX-ih-LATE) USAN.
Use: Muscle relaxant.

Feverall Children's. (Upsher-Smith Labs) Acetaminophen 120 mg/Supp. Pkg. 6s. *otc.*
Use: Analgesic.

Feverall, Infants'. (Upsher-Smith Labs) Acetaminophen 80 mg. Supp. Pkg. 6s. *otc.*

Use: Analgesic.

Feverall, Junior Strength. (Upsher-Smith Labs) Acetaminophen 325 mg/Supp. Pkg. 6s. *otc.*
Use: Analgesic.

Feverall Sprinkle. (Upsher-Smith Labs) Acetaminophen 80 mg or 160 mg/Cap. Bot. 20s. *otc.*
Use: Analgesic.

•**fexofenadine hydrochloride.** (fex-oh-FEN-ah-deen) USAN.
Use: Antihistamine.
See: Allegra, Tab. (Hoechst Marion Roussel).
Allegra-D, ER Tab. (Hoechst-Marion Roussel).

•**fezolamine fumarate.** (feh-ZOLE-ah-MEEN) USAN.
Use: Antidepressant.

fgn-1. (Cell Pathways)
Use: Treatment of adenomatous polyposis coli. [Orphan drug]

•**fiacitabine.** (fih-AH-sit-ah-BEEN) USAN.
Use: Antiviral.

•**fialuridine.** (fie-al-YOUR-ih-deen) USAN.
Use: Antiviral.

fiau. (Oclassen)
Use: Antiviral, hepatitis B. [Orphan drug]

Fiberall. (Novartis Consumer Health) Calcium carbophil 1250 mg (equiv. to 1000 mg polycarbophil). Chew. Tab. Lemon-flavor. Pkg. 18s. *otc.*
Use: Laxative.

Fiberall Natural Flavor. (Novartis Self-Medication) **Pow.:** Psyllium hydrophilic mucilloid 3.4 g, wheat bran, sodium < 10 mg, potassium 60 mg, calories 6/5.9 g, saccharin. Can 150 g, 300 g, 450 g. **Wafer:** Psyllium hydrophilic mucilloid 3.4 g, wheat bran, oats, sucrose. Box 14s. *otc.*
Use: Laxative.

Fiberall Orange Flavor. (Novartis Consumer Health) Psyllium hydrophilic mucilloid 3.4 g, wheat bran, sodium < 10 mg, potassium 60 mg, calories 6/5.9 g Pow. Can 150 g, 300 g, 450 g. *otc.*
Use: Laxative.

FiberCon. (ESI Lederle Generics) Calcium polycarbophil 500 mg/Tab. Bot. 36s, 60s. *otc.*
Use: Laxative.

Fiber Guard. (Wyeth Ayerst) All natural high fiber supplement 530 mg/Tab. Bot. 100s, 200s. *otc.*
Use: Fiber supplement.

Fiberlan. (Elan) Protein 50 g, fat 40 g, carbohydrates 160 g, Na 920 mg, K 1.56 g, fiber 14 g/per L. With vitamins A, C, B, B_2, B_3, D, E, B_5, B_6, B_{12}, K, Ca, Fe, folic acid, P, I, Mg, Zn, Cu, biotin, Mn, choline, Cl, Se, Cr, Mo. Liq. Bot. 237 ml. *otc.*
Use: Nutritional supplement.

Fiber-Lax. (Rugby) Calcium polycarbophil 625 mg (equiv. to 500 mg polycarbophil)/Tab. Bot. 60s. *otc.*
Use: Laxative.

Fibermed High-Fiber Snacks. (Purdue Frederick) One serving (15 snacks) contains 5 g dietary fiber. Box 8 oz. Packs of 24 × 1.3 oz. *otc.*
Use: Fiber supplement.

Fibermed High-Fiber Supplement. (Purdue Frederick) Each supplement contains 5 g dietary fiber. Box 14s. Institutional pack, Box 144s of two supplements. *otc.*
Use: Fiber supplement.

FiberNorm. (G & W Laboratories) Calcium polycarbophil 625 mg/Tab. Bot. 60s. *otc.*
Use: Laxative.

Fiber Rich. (Columbia) Phenylpropanolamine HCl 75 mg/Tab. Bot. 24s. *otc.*
Use: Dietary aid.

Fibre Trim Tablets. (Schering Plough) Grain and citrus fruit concentrated dietary fiber. Bot. 100s, 250s. *otc.*
Use: Dietary aid.

Fibre Trim w/Calcium Tablets. (Schering Plough) Grain and citrus fruit concentrated dietary fiber w/calcium. Bot. 90s, 225s. *otc.*
Use: Dietary aid.

fibrin hydrolysate.
See: Aminosol, Soln. (Abbott Laboratories).

•**fibrinogen I 125.** (FIE-BRIN-oh-jen I 125) USAN.
Use: Diagnostic aid (vascular patency); radiopharmaceutical.

fibrinogen (human). (Alpha Therapeutics) Partially purified fibrinogen prepared by fractionation from normal human plasma.
Use: Coagulant (clotting factor). [Orphan drug]

fibrinolysin (human) with desoxyribonuclease. Plasmin. An enzyme prepared by activating a human blood plasma fraction with streptokinase. *Rx.*
Use: Enzyme, topical.
See: Elase, Oint., Pow. (Parke-Davis).

fibrinolysis inhibitor.
See: Amicar Syr., Tab., Vial (ESI Lederle Generics).

Fibrogammin P. (Behringwerke Aktiengesellschaft AG)
Use: Congenital Factor XIII deficiency. [Orphan drug]

fibronectin (human plasma derived). (Melville Biologics)
Use: Treatment of nonhealing corneal ulcers or epithelial defects. [Orphan drug]

•**filaminast.** (fih-LAM-in-ast) USAN.
Use: Antiasthmatic (selective phosphodiesterase IV inhibitor).

Filaxis. (Amlab) Vitamins A 25,000 IU, D 1250 IU, C 150 mg, E 5 IU, B_1 12 mg, B_2 5 mg, B_6 0.5 mg, B_{12} 5 mcg, calcium pantothenate 5 mg, niacinamide 100 mg, iron 15 mg, iodine 0.15 mg, magnesium 10 mg, potassium 5 mg, calcium 75 mg, phosphorous 60 mg/Tab. Bot. 30s, 100s. Available w/B_{12}. Bot. 30s, 60s, 100s. *otc.*
Use: Mineral, vitamin supplement.

•**filgrastim.** (fill-GRAH-stim) USAN.
Use: Biological response modifier, antineoplastic adjunct, antineutropenic, hematopoietic stimulant. [Orphan drug]
See: Neupogen (Amgen).

•**filipin.** (FIH-lih-pin) USAN.
Use: Antifungal.

Finac. (C & M Pharmacal) Salicylic acid 2%, isopropyl alcohol 22.5%, propylene glycol, acetone in lotion base. Bot. 60 ml. *otc.*
Use: Dermatologic, acne.

•**finasteride.** (fih-NASS-teer-ide) USAN.
Use: Benign prostatic hypertrophy therapy, antineoplastic, antineutropenic, inhibitor (alpha-reductase).
See: Propecia, Tab. (Merck).
Proscar, Tab. (Merck).

Fiogesic. (Novartis) Phenylpropanolamine HCl 25 mg, pyrilamine maleate 12.5 mg, pheniramine maleate 12.5 mg, calcium carbaspirin 382 mg (equiv. to 300 mg ASA)/Tab. Bot. 100s. *otc.*
Use: Analgesic, antihistamine, decongestant.

Fioricet. (Novartis) Acetaminophen 325 mg, butalbital 50 mg, caffeine 40 mg/Tab. Bot. 100s, 500s, UD 100s. *Rx.*
Use: Analgesic, hypnotic, sedative.

Fioricet Codeine. (Novartis) Codeine phosphate 30 mg, acetaminophen 325 mg, caffeine 40 mg, butalbital 50 mg/Cap. Bot. 100s, Control pak 25s. *c-III.*
Use: Analgesic combination, narcotic.

Fiorinal. (Novartis) Butalbital (Sandoptal) 50 mg, caffeine 40 mg, aspirin 325 mg/Tab. or Cap. **Tab.:** Lactose Bot. 100s, 1000s. UD 100s. **Cap.:** Benzyl alcohol, parabens. Bot. 100s, 500s, UD 25s. *c-III.*
Use: Analgesic, hypnotic, sedative.

Fiorinal w/Codeine No. 3 Capsules. (Novartis) Butalbital 50 mg, caffeine 40 mg, aspirin 325 mg, codeine phosphate 30 mg/Cap. Bot. 100s. Control Pak 25s. *c-III.*
Use: Analgesic combination, hypnotic, sedative.

Fiorpap. (Geneva) Butalbital 50 mg, acetaminophen 325 mg, caffeine 40 mg/Tab. Bot 100s, 500s. *Rx.*
Use: Analgesic.

Fiortal. (Geneva) Aspirin 325 mg, caffeine 40 mg, butalbital 50 mg, benzyl alcohol, parabens. Cap. Bot. 100s. *c-III.*
Use: Analgesic.

fire ant venom, allergenic extract, imported.
Use: Dermatologic aid-skin test, immunotherapy. [Orphan drug]

Firmdent. (Moyco) Formerly Moy. Karaya gum 94.6%, sodium borate 5.36% Pkg. 3 oz. *otc.*
Use: Denture adhesive.

First Aid Cream. (Johnson & Johnson Consumer Products) Cetyl alcohol, glyceryl stearate, isopropyl palmitate, stearyl alcohol, synthetic beeswax. Tube 0.8 oz, 1.5 oz, 2.5 oz. *otc.*
Use: Antiseptic; dermatologic, protectant.

First Aid Cream. (Walgreens) Benzocaine 3%, allantoin 0.2%, benzyl alcohol 4%, phenol 0.25%. Tube 1.5 oz. *otc.*
Use: Anesthetic, antiseptic.

First Choice. (Polymer Technology International) 50s.
Use: Diagnostic aid.

First Response Ovulation Predictor. (Tambrands) Monoclonal antibody-based enzyme immunoassay test for hLH in urine. Test kit 1s. *otc.*
Use: Diagnostic aid.

First Response Pregnancy Test. (Tambrands) Reagent in-home kit for urine testing. Test kit 1s.
Use: Diagnostic aid.

fish oil concentrate, natural. Natural fish oil concentrate containing EPA (Eicosanoic acid) and DHA (Docosahexaenoic acid).
Use: Nutritional supplement.
See: Comega, Cap. (Upsher-Smith Labs).

Fitacol. (Standex) Atropine sulfate 0.2 mg, phenylpropanolamine 12.5 mg, chlorpheniramine maleate 0.5 mg, chlorobutanol 0.5 mg, water q.s./ml. Bot. pt. *Rx.*
Use: Anticholinergic, antihistamine, antispasmodic, decongestant.

Fitacol Stankaps. (Standex) Belladonna alkaloidal salts 0.16 mg (atropine sulfate 0.024 mg, scopolamine HBr 0.014 mg, hyoscyamine sulfate 0.122 mg), phenylpropanolamine HCl 50 mg, chlorpheniramine maleate 1 mg, pheniramine maleate 12.5 mg/Cap. Bot. 100s. *Rx.*
Use: Anticholinergic, antihistamine, antispasmodic, decongestant.

5-FC.
See: Flucytosine.

5-FU.
See: Fluorouracil.

523 Tablets. (Enzyme Process) Pancreatin 200 mg 4x/Tab. Tryspin, chymotrypsin, amylase, lipase enzymes from pancreatin, raw beef pancreas. Bot. 100s, 250s.
Use: Digestive enzyme.

Fixodent. (Procter & Gamble) Calcium sodium poly (vinyl methyl ether-maleate), carboxymethylcellulose sodium in a petrolatum base. Tube 0.75 oz, 1.5 oz, 2.5 oz. *otc.*
Use: Denture adhesive.

FK506.
See: Prograf (Fujisawa).

FK-565.
Use: Immunomodulator.

Flagyl Capsules. (Searle) Metronidazole 375 mg/Cap. Bot. 50s, 100s, UD 100s. *Rx.*
Use: Anti-infective.

Flagyl I.V. (Searle) Metronidazole HCl sterile lyophilized powder in single-dose vials equivalent to 500 mg metronidazole. Carton 10s. *Rx.*
Use: Anti-infective.

Flagyl I.V. RTU. (Searle) Metronidazole ready-to-use, premixed, 500 mg/100 ml Soln. Vial (glass), Box 6s; Container, (plastic), Box 24s. *Rx.*
Use: Anti-infective.

Flagyl Tablets. (Searle) Metronidazole 250 mg or 500 mg/Tab. **250 mg:** Bot. 50s, 100s, 250s, 1000s, 2500s, UD 100s; **500 mg:** Bot. 50s, 100s, 500s, UD 100s. *Rx.*
Use: Anti-infective.

Flagyl 375. (Searle) Metronidazole 375 mg/Cap. Bot. 50s, UD 100s. *Rx.*
Use: Anti-infective.

Flanders Buttocks Ointment. (Flanders) Zinc oxide, castor oil, balsam peru, boric acid in an emollient base. 60 g. *otc.*
Use: Dermatologic, counterirritant.

Flarex. (Alcon Laboratories) Fluorometholone acetate 0.1%. Susp. Bot. 2.5 ml, 5 ml, 10 ml Drop-Tainers. *Rx.*
Use: Corticosteroid, ophthalmic.

Flatulence Tablets. (Pal-Pak) Nux vomica 16.2 mg, cascara sagrada extract 64.8 mg, ginger 48.6 mg, capsicum 16.2 mg/Tab. w/asafetida. *otc.*
Use: Antiflatulent, laxative.

Flatulex. (Dayton) **Tab.:** Simethicone 80 mg, activated charcoal 250 mg/Tab. Bot. 100s. **Drops:** Simethicone 40 mg/ 0.6 ml. Bot. 30 ml with calibrated dropper. *otc.*
Use: Antiflatulent.

Flatus. (Foy) Nux vomica extract 0.25 gr, cascara extract 1 gr, ginger ¾ gr, capsicum gr/Tab. w/asfetida qs. Bot. 1000s. *otc.*
Use: Antiflatulent, laxative.

Flav-A-D. (Kirkman Sales) Vitamins A 5000 IU, D 1000 IU, C 100 mg/Tab. Bot. 100s, 1000s. Also w/fluoride. Bot. 100s, 1000s. *otc, Rx.*
Use: Vitamin supplement.

flavine.
See: Acriflavine Hydrochloride (Various Mfr.)

Flavinoid-C. (Barth's) **Tab.:** Vitamin C 150 mg, hesperidin complex 10 mg, citrus bioflavonoid 50 mg, rutin 20 mg/ Tab. Bot. 100s, 500s, 1000s. **Liq.:** Vitamin C 100 mg, bioflavonoid complex 100 mg/5 ml. Bot. 4 oz. *otc.*
Use: Vitamin supplement.

•**flavodilol maleate.** (FLAY-voe-DILL-ole) USAN.
Use: Antihypertensive.

flavolutan.
See: Progesterone (Various Mfr.)

flavonoid compounds.
See: Bio-Flavonoid Compounds; Vitamin P.

Flavons-500. (Freeda Vitamins) Citrus bioflavonoids complex 500 mg, hesperidin complex/Tab. Bot. 100s, 250s, 500s. *otc.*
Use: Vitamin supplement.

Flavorcee. (NBTY) Ascorbic acid 100 mg or 250 mg/Chew. Tab. **100 mg:** Bot. 100s; **250 mg:** Bot. 250s. *otc.*
Use: Vitamin supplement.

flavored diluent. (Roxane) Flavored vehicle for the immediate administration

of crushed tablet or capsule product. Bot. 500 ml, UD 15 ml × 100.
Use: Flavored vehicle.

•**flavoxate hydrochloride.** (flay-VOKES-ate) USAN.
Use: Antispasmodic, urinary; muscle relaxant.
See: Urispas, Tab. (SmithKline Beecham Pharmaceuticals).

flavurol. Merbromin.
Use: Antiseptic.

•**flazalone.** (FLAY-zah-lone) USAN.
Use: Anti-inflammatory.

•**flecainide acetate,** (fleh-CANE-ide) U.S.P. 23.
Use: Cardiovascular agent.
See: Tambocor (3M Pharm)

Fleet Babylax. (C.B. Fleet) Glycerin 4 ml in disposable pre-lubricated rectal applicator. Liq. pkg. 6s. *otc.*
Use: Laxative.

Fleet Bagenema. (C.B. Fleet) Castile soap or Fleets bisacodyl prep. *otc.*
Use: Laxative.

Fleet Bisacodyl Prep Packets. (C.B. Fleet) Bisacodyl 10 mg/10 ml packet. 36 packets/box. *otc.*
Use: Laxative.

Fleet Enema. (C.B. Fleet) Sodium biphosphate 19 g, sodium phosphate 7 g/118 ml. Bot. w/rectal tube 4.5 oz. Pediatric size 67.5 ml, 135 ml. *otc.*
Use: Laxative.

Fleet Flavored Castor Oil Emulsion. (C.B. Fleet) 1 oz delivers 30 ml castor oil. Bot. 1.5 oz, 3 oz. *otc.*
Use: Laxative.

Fleet Glycerin Suppositories. (C.B. Fleet) Adult: Jar 12s, 24s, 50s. Child Size: Jar 12s. *otc.*
Use: Laxative.

Fleet Laxative. (C.B. Fleet) Bisacodyl. **EC Tab.:** 5 mg/Tab. Bot. 24s. **Supp.:** 10 mg. Box 4s. *otc.*
Use: Laxative.

Fleet Medicated Wipes. (C.B. Fleet) Hamamelis water 50%, alcohol 7%, glycerin 10%, benzalkonium Cl, methylparaben. Rectal pads. 100s. *otc.*
Use: Perianal hygiene.

Fleet Mineral Oil Enema. (C.B. Fleet) Mineral oil 4.5 fl oz in an unbreakable vinyl squeeze bottle. *otc.*
Use: Laxative.

Fleet Pain Relief. (C.B. Fleet) Pramoxine HCl 1%, glycerin 12%. Pads. 100s. *otc.*
Use: Anorectal preparation.

Fleet Phospho-Soda. (C.B. Fleet) Sodium phosphate 18 g, sodium biphosphate 48 g/100 ml (96.4 mEq sodium/20 ml). Bot. 45 ml, 90 ml, 240 ml. *otc.*
Use: Laxative.

Fleet Prep Kits. (C.B. Fleet) A series of different laxative kits for use prior to barium enema, bowel surgery, proctoscopy, colonoscopy, etc. w/complete patient instruction form:
Prep Kit #1: Fleet Phospho-Soda 45 ml, Fleet Bisacodyl Tablets 45 mg, Fleet Bisacodyl Suppository 110 mg. *otc.*
Prep Kit #2: Fleet Phospho-Soda 45 ml, Fleet Bisacodyl Tablets 45 mg, 1 Fleet Bagenema set for large volume enema, including optional Castile Soap Packet. 20 ml. *otc.*
Prep Kit #3: Fleet Phospho-Soda 45 ml, Fleet Bisacodyl Tablets 45 mg, Fleet Bisacodyl Enema 130 ml. 10 mg. *otc.*
Prep Kit #4: Fleet Flavored Castor Oil Emulsion 45 ml, Fleet Bisacodyl Tablets 45 mg, Fleet Bisacodyl Suppository 110 mg. *otc.*
Prep Kit #5: Fleet Flavored Castor Oil Emulsion 45 ml, Fleet Bisacodyl Tablets 45 mg, 1 Fleet Bagenema set for large volume enema, including optional Castile Soap Packet. 20 ml. *otc.*
Prep Kit #6: Fleet Flavored Castor Oil Emulsion 45 ml, Fleet Bisacodyl Tablets 45 mg, Fleet Bisacodyl Enema 130 ml. 10 mg. *otc.*
Use: Laxative.

•**fleroxacin.** (fler-OX-ah-SIN) USAN.
Use: Anti-infective.
See: Megalone (Roche Laboratories).

•**flestolol sulfate.** (FLESS-toe-lahl) USAN.
Use: Antiadrenergic (β-receptor).

•**fletazepam.** (FLET-AZE-eh-pam) USAN.
Use: Muscle relaxant.

Fletcher's Castoria for Children. (Mentholatum) Senna 6.5%, alcohol 3.5%. Liq. Bot. 75 ml, 150 ml. *otc.*
Use: Laxative.

Flexall 454. (Chattem Consumer Products) Menthol 7%, alcohol, allantoin, aloe vera gel, boric acid, carbomer 940, diazolidinyl urea, eucalyptus oil, glycerin, iodine, parabens, methyl salicylate, peppermint oil, polysorbate 60, potassium iodide, propylene glycol, thyme oil, triethanolamine. Gel Tube. 240 g. *otc.*
Use: Analgesic, topical.

Flexall 454, Maximum Strength. (Chat-

tem Consumer Products) Menthol 16%, aloe vera gel, eucalyptus oil, methysalicylate, SD alcohol 38-B, thyme oil. Gel 90 mg. *otc.*
Use: Analgesic, topical.

Flex Anti-Dandruff Shampoo. (Revlon) Zinc pyrithione 1% in liquid shampoo. *otc.*
Use: Antiseborrheic.

Flex Anti-Dandruff Styling Mousse. (Revlon) Zinc pyrithione 0.1%. Aerosol foam. *otc.*
Use: Antiseborrheic.

Flexaphen. (Trimen) Chlorzoxazone 250 mg, acetaminophen 300 mg/Cap. Bot 100s. *Rx.*
Use: Muscle relaxant.

Flex-Care Especially for Sensitive Eyes. (Alcon Laboratories) EDTA 0.1%, chlorhexidine gluconate 0.005%, sodium Cl, sodium borate, boric acid. Soln. Bot. 118 ml, 237 ml, 355 ml, 360 ml. *otc.*
Use: Contact lens care.

Flexeril. (Merck) Cyclobenzaprine HCl 10 mg/Tab. Bot. 100s, UD 100s. *Rx.*
Use: Muscle relaxant.

flexible hydroactive dressings/granules.
See: Intra Site (Smith & Nephew United).
Shur-Clens (SmithKline Beecham Pharmaceuticals).
DuoDerm (ConvaTec)
Sorbsan (Dow Hickam).

Flexoject. (Merz) Orphenadrine citrate 30 mg/ml. Inj. Vial 10 ml, amps 2 ml. *Rx.*
Use: Muscle relaxant.

Flexon. (Keene Pharmaceuticals) Orphenadrine citrate 30 mg/ml. Inj. Vial 10 ml. *Rx.*
Use: Muscle relaxant.

Flexsol. (Alcon Lenscare) Sterile, buffered, isotonic aqueous soln. of sodium Cl, sodium borate, boric acid, adsorbobase. Bot. 6 oz. *otc.*
Use: Contact lens care.

Flintstones Children's Tablets. (Bayer Corp) Vitamin A 2500 IU, E 15 mg, C 60 mg, folic acid 0.3 mg, B_1 1.05 mg, B_2 1.2 mg, B_3 13.5 mg, B_6 1.05 mg, B_{12} 4.5 mcg, D 400 IU/Chew. Tab. Bot. 60s, 100s. *otc.*
Use: Vitamin supplement.

Flintstones Complete. (Bayer Corp) Elemental iron 18 mg, vitamins A 5000 IU, D 400 IU, E 30 mg, B_1 1.5 mg, B_2 1.7 mg, B_3 20 mg, B_5 10 mg, B_6 2 mg, B_{12} 6 mcg, C 60 mg, folic acid 0.4 mg, biotin 40 mcg, Ca, Cu, I, Mg, P, zinc 15 mg/Chew. Tab. Bot. 60s, 120s. *otc.*
Use: Mineral, vitamin supplement.

Flintstones Plus Calcium. (Bayer Corp) Vitamin A 2500 IU, D IU 400, E 15 IU, C 60 mg, folic acid 0.3 mg, B_1 1.05 mg, B_2 1.2 mg, B_3 13.5 mg, B_6 1.05 mg, B_{12} 4.5 mcg, Ca 200 mg/Tab. Chewable. Bot. 60s. *otc.*
Use: Mineral, vitamin supplement.

Flintstones Plus Extra C Children's. (Bayer Corp) Vitamins A 2500 IU, D 400 IU, E 15 mg, C 250 mg, folic acid 0.3 mg, B_1 1.05 mg, B_2 1.2 mg, niacin 13.5 mg, B_6 1.05 mg, B_{12} 4.5 mcg/Tab. Bot. 60s, 100s. *otc.*
Use: Vitamin supplement.

Flintstones Plus Iron Multivitamins. (Bayer Corp) Vitamins A 2500 IU, E 15 mg, C 60 mg, folic acid 0.3 mg, B_1 1.05 mg, B_2 1.2 mg, niacin 13.5 mg, B_6 1.05 mg, B_{12} 4.5 mcg, D 400 IU, iron 15 mg/Chew. Tab. Bot. 60s, 100s. *otc.*
Use: Mineral, vitamin supplement.

Flo-Coat. (Lafayette Pharm) Barium sulfate 100%. Susp. Bot. 1850 ml.
Use: Radiopaque agent.

•**floctafenine.** (FLOCK-tah-FEN-een) USAN.
Use: Analgesic.

Flolan. (GlaxoWellcome) Epoprostenol sodium 0.5 or 1.5 mg, mannitol, NaCl/Vial. Pow. for Inj. 17 ml. *Rx.*
Use: Antihypertensive.

Flomax. (Boehringer Ingelheim) Tamsulosin HCl 0.4 mg/Cap. Bot. 100s, 1000s. *Rx.*
Use: Benign prostatic hyperplasia treatment.

Flonase. (GlaxoWellcome) Fluticasone proprionate 50 mcg/actuation. Bot. 16 g (120 actuations). *Rx.*
Use: Corticosteroid, nasal.

Flor-D Chewable Tab. (Derm Pharm) Fluoride 1 mg, vitamins A 4000 IU, D 400 IU, C 75 mg, B_1 1.5 mg, B_2 1.8 mg, niacinamide 15 mg, B_6 1 mg, B_{12} 3 mcg, calcium pantothenate 10 mg/Tab. Bot. 100s. *Rx.*
Use: Mineral, vitamin supplement.

Flor-D Drops. (Derm Pharm) Fluoride 0.5 mg, vitamins A 3000 IU, D 400 IU, C 60 mg, B_1 1 mg, B_2 1.2 mg, niacinamide 8 mg/0.6 ml. Bot. 60 ml. *Rx.*
Use: Mineral, vitamin supplement.

•**flordipine.** (FLORE-dih-peen) USAN.
Use: Antihypertensive.

Florical. (Mericon) Sodium fluoride 8.3

mg, calcium carbonate 364 mg (equivalent to 145.6 mg calcium)/Cap. Bot. 100s, 500s. *otc.*
Use: Mineral supplement.

Florida Foam. (Hill) Benzalkonium Cl, aluminum subacetate, boric acid 2%. Bot. 8 oz. *otc.*
Use: Soap substitute, antiseborrheic, antifungal, dermatologic-acne.

Florida Sunburn Relief. (Pharmacel) Benzyl alcohol 3%, phenol 0.4%, camphor 0.2%, menthol 0.15%. Lot. Bot. 60 ml. *otc.*
Use: Sunburn relief.

Florinef Acetate Tablets. (Apothecon) Fludrocortisone acetate, 0.1 mg/Tab. Bot. 100s. *Rx.*
Use: Corticosteroid.

Florone Cream. (Dermik Laboratories) Diflorasone diacetate 0.5 mg/g (0.05%) w/stearic acid, sorbitan mono-oleate, polysorbate 60, sorbic acid, citric acid, propylene glycol, purified water. Tube 15 g, 30 g, 60 g. *Rx.*
Use: Corticosteroid, topical.

Florone E. (Dermik Laboratories) Diflorasone diacetate 0.5 mg. Tube 15 g, 30 g, 60 g. *Rx.*
Use: Corticosteroid, topical.

Florone Ointment. (Dermik Laboratories) Diflorasone diacetate 0.5 mg/g (0.05%) W/polyoxypropylene 15-stearyl ether, stearic acid, lanolin alcohol and white petrolatum. Tube 15 g, 30 g, 60 g. *Rx.*
Use: Corticosteroid, topical.

Floropryl. (Merck) Isoflurophate 0.025% in sterile ophthalmic ointment in polyethylene-mineral oil gel. Tube 3.5 g. *Rx.*
Use: Agent for glaucoma.

Florvite Chewable Tablets. (Everett Laboratories) Vitamins, fluoride 0.5 mg/Chew. tab. Bot 100s. *Rx.*
Use: Dental caries agent.

Florvite Half Strength. (Everett Laboratories) Elemental fluoride 0.5 mg, vitamins A 2500 IU, D 400 IU, E 15 mg, B_1 1.05 mg, B_2 1.2 mg, B_3 13.5 mg, B_6 1.05 mg, B_{12} 4.5 mcg, C 60 mg, folic acid 0.3 mg/Chew. Tab. Bot. 100s. *Rx.*
Use: Mineral, vitamin supplement; dental caries agent.

Florvite + Iron Drops. (Everett Laboratories) Elemental fluorine. **0.25 mg:** Vitamins A 1500 IU, D 400 IU, E 5 mg, B_1 0.5 mg, B_2 0.6 mg, B_3 8 mg, B_6 0.4 mg, C 35 mg, iron 10 mg/ml. **0.5 mg:** Vitamins A 1500 IU, D 400 IU, E 5 mg, B_1 0.5 mg, B_2 0.6 mg, B_3 8 mg, B_6 0.4 mg, C 35 mg, iron 10 mg/ml/Liq. Bot. 50 ml. *Rx.*
Use: Mineral, vitamin supplement; dental caries agent.

Florvite + Iron Chewable. (Everett Laboratories) Fluoride 1 mg, iron 12 mg, vitamins A 2500 IU, D 400 IU, E 15 mg, B_1 1.05 mg, B_2 1.2 mg, B_3 13.5 mg, B_6 1.05 mg, B_{12} 4.5 mcg, C 60 mg, folic acid 0.3 mg, Cu, Zn 10 mg, sucrose/Chew. tab. Bot. 100s. *Rx.*
Use: Mineral, vitamin supplement; dental caries agent.

Florvite Pediatric Drops. (Everett Laboratories) Elemental fluorine. **0.25 mg/ml:** vitamins A 1500 IU, D 400 IU, E 5 mg, B_1 0.5 mg, B_2 0.6 mg, B_3 8 mg, B_6 0.4 mg, B_{12} 2 mcg, C 35 mg/ml. **0.5 mg/ml:** vitamins A 1500 IU, D 400 IU, E 5 mg, B_1 0.5 mg, B_2 0.6 mg, B_3 8 mg, B_6 0.4 mg, B_{12} 2 mcg, C 35 mg, iron 10 mg/ml Bot. 50 ml. *Rx.*
Use: Mineral, vitamin supplement; dental caries agent.

Florvite Tablets. (Everett Laboratories) Fluoride 1 mg, vitamins A 2500 IU, D 400 IU, E 15 mg, B_1 1.05 mg, B_2 1.2 mg, B_3 13.5 mg, B_6 1.05 mg, B_{12} 4.5 mcg, C 60 mg, folic acid 0.3 mg/Chew. tab. Bot. 100s, 1000s. *Rx.*
Use: Mineral, vitamin supplement; dental caries agent.

Florvite Drops. (Everett Laboratories) Fluoride 0.25 mg or 0.5 mg, A 1500 IU, D 400 IU, E 5 IU, B_1 0.5 mg, B_2 0.6 mg, B_3 8 mg, B_6 0.4 mg, B_{12} 2 mcg, C 35 mg/Drop. Bot. 50 ml. *Rx.*
Use: Mineral, vitamin supplement; dental caries agent.

•**flosequinan.** (flow-SEH-kwih-NAHN) USAN.
Use: Antihypertensive (vasodilator).
See: Manoplax (Knoll Pharmaceuticals).

Flovent. (GlaxoWellcome) Fluticasone propionate 44 mcg/Actuation/Aerosol spray. Canister. 7.9 g (60 actuations) and 13 g (120 actuations). Fluticasone propionate 110 mcg/actuation/Aerosol spray. Canister 13 g (120 actuations). Fluticasone propionate 220 mcg/actuation/Aerosol spray. Canister. 13 g (120 actuations). *Rx.*
Use: Antiallergic.

•**floxacillin.** (FLOX-ah-SILL-in) USAN.
Use: Anti-infective.

Floxin. (Ortho McNeil) **Tab.:** Ofloxacin, 200 mg, 300 mg or 400 mg. Bot. 50s, 100s. **Inj.:** 200 mg flexible container; 400 mg Vial 10 ml, 20 ml; Bot. 100 ml; flexible container. *Rx.*
Use: Anti-infective, fluoroquinolone.

Floxin Otic Solution. (Daiichi) Ofloxacin 3 mg/ml, benzalkonium chloride, sodium chloride, sodium hydroxide. Otic Soln. 5 ml. *Rx.*
Use: Anti-infective, otic.

•**floxuridine,** (flox-YUR-ih-deen) U.S.P. 23.
Use: Antiviral, antineoplastic.
See: FUDR, Vial (Roberts Pharm).

•**fluazacort.** (flew-AZE-ah-kort) USAN.
Use: Anti-inflammatory.

•**flubanilate hydrochloride.** (flew-BAN-ill-ate) USAN.
Use: Antidepressant; CNS stimulant.

•**flubendazole.** (FLEW-BEN-dah-zole) USAN.
Use: Antiprotozoal.

flucarbril.
Use: Muscle relaxant, analgesic.

•**flucindole.** (flew-SIN-dole) USAN.
Use: Antipsychotic.

•**flucloronide.** (flew-KLOR-oh-nide) USAN.
Use: Corticosteroid, topical.

Flu, Cold & Cough Medicine. (Major) Pseudoephedrine HCl 60 mg, chlorpheniramine 4 mg, dextromethorphan HBr 20 mg, acetaminophen 500 mg. Pow. Pck. 6s. *otc.*
Use: Analgesic, antihistamine, antitussive, decongestant.

•**fluconazole.** (flew-KOE-nuh-sole) USAN.
Use: Antifungal.
See: Diflucan (Roerig).

•**flucrylate.** (FLEW-krih-late) USAN.
Use: Surgical aid (tissue adhesive).

•**flucytosine,** (flew-SITE-oh-seen) U.S.P. 23.
Use: Antifungal.
See: Ancobon, Cap. (Roberts Pharm).

•**fludalanine.** (flew-DAL-AH-neen) USAN.
Use: Anti-infective.

Fludara. (Berlex) Fludarabine 50 mg. Pow. for recon. Vial. 6 ml. *Rx.*
Use: Antineoplastic.

•**fludarabine phosphate.** (flew-DAR-uh-BEAN) USAN.
Use: Antineoplastic. [Orphan drug]
See: Fludara, Pow. (Berlex).

•**fludazonium chloride.** (FLEW-dazz-OH-nee-uhm) USAN.
Use: Anti-infective, topical.

•**fludeoxyglucose F 18 injection,** (FLEW-dee-OX-ee-GLUE-kose F 18) U.S.P. 23.
Use: Diagnostic aid (brain disorders, thyroid disorders, liver disorders, cardiac disease and neoplastic disease); radiopharmaceutical.

•**fludorex.** (FLEW-doe-rex) USAN.
Use: Anorexic, antiemetic.

•**fludrocortisone acetate,** (flew-droe-CORE-tih-sone) U.S.P. 23.
Use: Adrenocortical steroid (salt-regulating).
See: Florinef Acetate, Tab. (Apothecon).

•**flufenamic acid.** (FLEW-fen-AM-ik) USAN.
Use: Anti-inflammatory.

•**flufenisal.** (flew-FEN-ih-sal) USAN.
Use: Analgesic.

Fluidex. (Columbia) Natural botanical ingredients. Tab. Bot. 36s, 72s.
Use: Diuretic.

Flu-Imune. (Wyeth Lederle) Influenza virus vaccine. Vial 5 ml (10 doses). (Purified surface antigen). *Rx.*
Use: Immunization.

fluitran. Trichlormethiazide.

Flumadine. (Forest Pharmaceutical) **Tab.:** Rimantadine HCl 100 mg. Bot. 20s, 100s, 500s, 1000s. **Syr.:** Rimantadine HCl 50 mg/5ml. Bot. 60 ml, 240 ml, 480 ml. *Rx.*
Use: Antiviral.

•**flumazenil.** (flew-MAZ-ah-nil) USAN.
Use: Antagonist (to benzodiazepine).
See: Mazicon (Roberts Pharm).
Romazicon, Inj. (Roberts Pharm).

flumecinol.
Use: Hyperbilirubinemia in newborns. [Orphan drug]
See: Zixoryn (Farmacon).

•**flumequine.** (FLEW-meh-kwin) USAN.
Use: Anti-infective.

•**flumeridone.** (FLEW-MER-ih-dohn) USAN.
Use: Antiemetic.

•**flumethasone.** (FLEW-meth-ah-zone) USAN.
Use: Corticosteroid, topical.
See: Locorten [21-pivalate] (Novartis Pharmaceuticals).

•**flumethasone pivalate,** (FLEW-meth-ah-zone PIH-vah-late) U.S.P. 23.
Use: Corticosteroid, topical.

flumethiazide.
Use: Diuretic.
See: Rautrax, Tab. (Bristol-Myers Squibb).

•**flumetramide.** (flew-MEH-trah-mide) USAN.
Use: Muscle relaxant.

•**flumezapine.** (FLEW-MEZZ-ah-peen) USAN.
Use: Antipsychotic, neuroleptic.

•**fluminorex.** (flew-MEE-no-rex) USAN.
Use: Anorexic.

•**flumizole.** (FLEW-mih-zole) USAN.
Use: Anti-inflammatory.

•**flumoxonide.** (flew-MOX-OH-nide) USAN.
Use: Adrenocortical steroid.

flunarizine.
Use: Alternating hemiplegia. [Orphan drug]
See: Sibelium (Janssen).

•**flunarizine hydrochloride.** (flew-NAR-ih-zeen) USAN.
Use: Vasodilator.

•**flunidazole.** (FLEW-nih-dah-ZOLE) USAN.
Use: Antiprotozoal.

•**flunisolide,** (flew-NIH-sole-ide) U.S.P. 23.
Use: Corticosteroid, topical.
See: AeroBid, Aer. (Forest Pharm).
Nasarel, Sol. Spray (Roche).

•**flunisolide acetate.** (flew-NIH-sole-ide) USAN.
Use: Anti-inflammatory.

•**flunitrazepam.** (flew-NYE-TRAY-zeh-pam) USAN.
Use: Hynoptic, sedative.

•**flunixin.** (flew-NIX-in) USAN.
Use: Analgesic, anti-inflammatory.

•**flunixin meglumine.** (flew-NIX-in meh-GLUE-meen) U.S.P. 23.
Use: Analgesic, anti-inflammatory.

Fluocet. (NMC Labs) Fluocinolone acetonide cream 0.025% or 0.01%. Tube 15 g, 60 g. *Rx.*
Use: Corticosteroid, topical.

fluocinolide. (flew-oh-SIN-oh-lide)
See: Fluocinonide.

•**fluocinolone acetonide,** (flew-oh-SIN-oh-lone ah-SEE-toe-nide) U.S.P. 23.
Use: Corticosteroid, topical.
See: Fluonid, Cream, Oint., Soln. (Allergan).
Synalar, Cream, Oint., Soln. (Syntex).
W/Neomycin sulfate.
See: Neo-Synalar (Syntex).

•**fluocinonide,** (FLEW-oh-SIN-oh-nide) U.S.P. 23. *Formerly Fluocinolide.*
Use: Corticosteroid, topical.
See: Lidex, Cream, Oint., Soln. (Syntex).
Lidex-E, Cream (Syntex).
Metosyn.

fluocinonide. (E. Fougera) 0.05%. Tube 15 g, 60 g.
Use: Corticosteroid, topical.

fluocinonide topical solution. (E. Fougera) 0.05%. Soln. Bot. 60 ml.
Use: Corticosteroid, topical.

•**fluocortin butyl.** (FLEW-oh-CORE-tin BYOO-tuhl) USAN.
Use: Anti-inflammatory.

•**fluocortolone.** (FLEW-oh-CORE-toe-lone) USAN.
Use: Corticosteroid, topical.

•**fluocortolone caproate.** (FLEW-oh-CORE-toe-lone) USAN.
Use: Corticosteroid, topical.

Fluogen. (Parke-Davis) Influenza virus vaccine, trivalent–Immunizing antigen, ether extracted. Vial 5 ml, UD syringe 0.5 ml. The 5 ml vial contains sufficient product to deliver ten 0.5 ml doses. *Rx.*
Use: Immunization.

Fluonex. (Zeneca) Fluocinonide 0.05%. Cream. Tube. 15 g, 30 g. *Rx.*
Use: Corticosteroid, topical.

Fluonid. (Allergan) Fluocinolone Acetonide. **Soln.:** 0.01%. Bot. 20 ml, 60 ml. *Rx.*
Use: Corticosteroid, topical.

Fluoracaine. (Akorn) Proparacaine HCl 0.5%, fluorescein sodium 0.25%. Dropper Bot. 5 ml. *Rx.*
Use: Anesthetic, local; ophthalmic.

•**fluorescein.** (FLURE-eh-seen) U.S.P. 23.
Use: Diagnostic aid (corneal trauma indicator).
See: Fluorescite (Alcon Laboratories).

•**fluorescein sodium,** U.S.P. 23. *Formerly Fluorescein, soluble.*
Use: Diagnostic aid (corneal trauma indicator).
See: AK-Fluor, Amp., Vial (Akorn).
Fluor-I-Strip. (Wyeth Ayerst).
Fluorets, Strips (Akorn).
Ful-Glo, Strips (PBH Wesley Jessen).
Funduscein, Amp. (Ciba Vision Ophthalmics).
Plak-Lite Soln. (Internat. Pharm).

fluorescein sodium. (Various Mfr.) 2% Ophth. Soln. Bot. 1 ml, 2 ml, 15 ml.
Use: Diagnostic aid (corneal trauma indicator).

fluorescein sodium i.v.
See: Fluorescite, Amp. (Alcon Laboratories).

Fluorescein Sodium 2% Solution. (Alcon Laboratories) Drop-Tainer 15 ml, Steri-Unit 2 ml 12s.
Use: Diagnostic aid, ophthalmic.

Fluorescein Sodium 2%. (Ciba Vision Ophthalmics) A sterile aqueous solution containing fluorescein sodium 2%. Dropperette 1 ml, Box 12s.
Use: Diagnostic aid, ophthalmic.

Fluorescein Sodium w/Proparacaine

Hydrochloride. (Taylor Pharmaceuticals) Proparacaine HCl 0.5%, fluorescein sodium 0.25%. Ophthalmic soln. Bot. 5 ml. *Rx.*
Use: Anesthetic, local; diagnostic aid, ophthalmic.

Fluorescein Sodium/Sodium Hyaluronate.
See: Sodium Hyaluronate and Fluorescein Sodium Healon Yellow (Pharmacia & Upjohn).

Fluorescite. (Alcon Laboratories) Fluorescein as sodium salt. Inj. Soln. **10%:** Amp. 5 ml with syringes; **25%:** Amp 2 ml. *Rx.*
Use: Diagnostic aid, ophthalmic.

Fluoresoft. (Various Mfr.) Fluorexon 0.35%. Soln. Pipette 0.5 ml, Box 12s. *otc.*
Use: Diagnostic aid, ophthalmic.

Fluorets. (Akorn) Fluorescein sodium 1 mg. Strip. Box 100s. *otc.*
Use: Diagnostic aid, ophthalmic.

fluorexon.
See: Fluoresoft (Holles).

fluoride. (Kirkman Sales) Fluoride 1 mg (sodium fluoride 2.21 mg). Tab. Bot. 1000s. *Rx.*
Use: Dental caries agent.

Fluoride Loz. (Kirkman Sales) Fluoride 1 mg (sodium fluoride 2.21 mg). Loz. Bot. 1000s. *Rx.*
Use: Dental caries agent.

fluoride sodium.
See: Dentafluor Chewable, Tab. (Western Pharm).
Fluoride Loz. (Kirkman).
Fluoride, Tab. (Kirkman).
Karidium, Top. Soln., Tab. (Young Dental).
Karigel, Gel (Young Dental).
Luride, Drops, Gel (Colgate-Hoyt).
Luride Lozi-Tabs, Chew. Tab. (Colgate-Hoyt).

fluoride therapy.
See: Adeflor Preps. (Pharmacia & Upjohn).
Cari-Tab, Softab Tab. (Zeneca).
Coral Prods. (Young Dental).
Fluorineed, Chew. Tab. (Hanlon).
Fluorinse, Liq. (Pacemaker).
Fluora, Loz. (Kirkman Sales).
Gal-Kam, Preps. (Scherer).
Luride Preps. (Colgate Oral).
Mulvidren-F, Softab Tab. (Zeneca).
Point Two, Rinse (Colgate Oral).
Poly-Vi-Flor, Drops, Tab. (Bristol-Myers).
Soluvite-F, Drops (Pharmics).
Tri-Vi-Flor, Drops, Tab. (Bristol-Myers).

Fluorigard. (Colgate Oral) Fluoride 0.02% (from sodium fluoride 0.05%), alcohol 6%, tartrazine. Bot. 180 ml, 300 ml, 480 ml. *Rx.*
Use: Dental caries agent.

Fluori-Methane Spray. (Gebauer) Dichlorodifluoromethane 15%, trichloromonofluoromethane 85%. Bot. 4 oz. *Rx.*
Use: "Painful motion" syndromes.

Fluorineed. (Hanlon) Fluoride 1 mg/Chew. Tab. Bot. 100s, 1000s. *Rx.*
Use: Dental caries agent.

Fluorinse. (Oral-B Laboratories) Fluoride 0.09% from sodium fluoride 0.2%. Bot. 480 ml. *Rx.*
Use: Dental caries agent.

Fluorinse. (Pacemaker) Fluoride mouthwash. Pack. Fluoride ion level 0.05% or 0.2%. UD Bot. 32 oz. Concentrate 1 oz, 4 oz, gal. *Rx.*
Use: Dental caries agent.

Fluor-I-Strip. (Wyeth Ayerst) Fluorescein sodium 9 mg/ophthalmic strip. Box. 300s. *Rx.*
Use: Diagnostic aid, ophthalmic.

Fluor-I-Strip-A.T. (Wyeth Ayerst) Fluorescein sodium 1 mg/ophthalmic strip. Box 300s. *Rx.*
Use: Diagnostic aid, ophthalmic.

Fluoritab. (Fluoritab) Sodium fluoride 2.2 mg equivalent to 1 mg of fluorine (as fluoride ion) w/inert organic filler 75.8 mg/Tab. Bot. 100s; Liq. dropper bot. (fluorine 0.25 mg from 0.55 mg sodium fluoride/Drop) 19 ml. *Rx.*
Use: Dental caries agent.

5-fluorocytosine.
See: Ancobon, Cap. (Roberts Pharm).

•**fluorodopa F 18 injection.** (FLEW-roe-DOE-pah) U.S.P. 23.
Use: Diagnostic aid (brain imaging), radiopharmaceutical.

fluorogestone acetate.
Use: Hormone, progestin.

fluorohydrocortisone acetate. 9-α-Fluorohydrocortisone.
See: Fludrocortisone Acetate (Various Mfr.)

•**fluorometholone,** (flure-oh-METH-oh-lone) U.S.P. 23.
Use: Corticosteroid, topical.
See: Fluor-Op, Susp. (Ciba Vision Ophthalmics).
FML, Liquifilm, Ophth. Susp., Oint. (Allergan).
Oxylone, Cream Ophth. Susp. (Pharmacia & Upjohn).
W/Neomycin sulfate.
See: Neo-Oxylone, Oint. (Pharmacia & Upjohn).

•**fluorometholone acetate.** (flure-oh-METH-oh-LONE) USAN.
Use: Corticosteroid, topical; anti-inflammatory.

Fluor-Op. (Ciba Vision Ophthalmics) Fluorometholone 0.1%. Susp. Bot. 5 ml, 10 ml, 15 ml. *Rx.*
Use: Corticosteroid, ophthalmic.

fluorophene.
Use: Antiseptic.

Fluoroplex Topical. (Allergan) **Soln.:** Fluorouracil 1% in a propylene glycol base. Plastic bot. w/dropper 30 ml. **Cream:** Fluorouracil 1% in emulsion base w/benzyl alcohol 0.5%, emulsifying wax, mineral oil, isopropyl myristate, sodium hydroxide, purified water. Tube 30 g. *Rx.*
Use: Topical treatment of multiple actinic (solar) keratoses.

fluoroquinolones.
Use: Anti-infective.
See: Ciloxan (Alcon Laboratories).
Cipro (Bayer Corp).
Cipro I.V. (Bayer Corp).
Floxin (Ortho McNeil).
Maxaquin (Searle).
Noroxin (Merck).
Penetrex (Rhone-Poulenc Rorer).

•**fluorosalan.** (FLEW-oh-row-SAH-lan) USAN.
Use: Antiseptic, disinfectant.

fluorothyl. Bis (2, 2, 2-trifluoroethyl) ether.
See: Flurothyl.

•**fluorouracil,** (FLURE-oh-YUR-uh-sill) U.S.P. 23.
Use: Antineoplastic. [Orphan drug]
See: Adrucil, Inj. (Pharmacia & Upjohn).
Efudex, Soln., Cream (Roberts Pharm).
Fluoroplex, Soln., Cream (Allergan).

fluorouracil. (Roberts Pharm) Amp. 10 ml, 500 mg. Box 10s.
Use: Antineoplastic. [Orphan drug.]

Fluothane. (Wyeth Ayerst) Halothane. Bot. 125 ml, 250 ml. *Rx.*
Use: Anesthetic, general.

•**fluotracen hydrochloride.** (FLEW-oh-TRAY-sen) USAN.
Use: Antipsychotic, antidepressant.

•**fluoxetine.** (flew-OX-eh-teen) USAN.
Use: Antidepressant.
See: Prozac, Pulv., Liq. (Eli Lilly).

•**fluoxetine hydrochloride.** (flew-OX-eh-teen) USAN.
Use: Antidepressant.
See: Prozac (Eli Lilly).

Flu-Oxinate. (Taylor Pharmaceuticals) Benoxinate HCl 0.4%, fluorescein sodium 0.25%. Ophthalmic Soln. Bot. 5 ml. *Rx.*
Use: Local anesthetic, diagnostic aid, ophthalmic.

•**fluoxymesterone,** (flew-ox-ee-MESS-teh-rone) U.S.P. 23.
Use: Androgen.
See: Android-F, Tab. (Zeneca).
Halotestin, Tab. (Pharmacia & Upjohn).
Ora-Testryl, Tab. (Squibb Diagnostic).
W/Ethinyl estradiol.
See: Halodrin, Tab. (Pharmacia & Upjohn).

fluoxymestrone. (Various) 10 mg/Tab. Bot. 100s *c-III.*
Use: Androgen.

•**fluparoxan hydrochloride.** (flew-pah-ROX-an) USAN
Use: Antidepressant.

•**fluperamide.** (flew-purr-ah-mide) USAN.
Use: Antiperistaltic.

•**fluperolone acetate.** (FLEW-per-oh-lone) USAN.
Use: Corticosteroid, topical.

•**fluphenazine decanoate,** (flew-FEN-uh-zeen) U.S.P. 23.
Use: Antipsychotic.
See: Prolixin Decanoate Soln. (Apothecon).

•**fluphenazine enanthate,** (flew-FEN-uh-zeen)U.S.P. 23.
Use: Antipsychotic, anxiolytic.
See: Prolixin Enanthate Prods. (Apothecon).

•**fluphenazine hydrochloride,** (flew-FEN-uh-zeen) U.S.P. 23.
Use: Antipsychotic, anxiolytic.
See: Permitil, Preps. (Schering Plough).
Prolixin, Preps (Apothecon).

fluphenazine HCl concentrate. (Copley) Fluphenazine HCl 5 mg/ml. Conc. Bot. 120 ml. *Rx.*
Use: Antipsychotic.

fluphenazine HCl injection. (Quad) Fluphenazine HCl 2.5 mg/ml. Inj. Vial 10 ml. *Rx.*
Use: Antipsychotic.

fluphenazine HCl tablet. (Various Mfr.) Fluphenazine HCl 1 mg, 2.5 mg, 5 mg, 10 mg/Tab. Bot. 50s, 100s, 500s, 1000s, UD 100s. *Rx.*
Use: Antipsychotic.

•**flupirtine maleate.** (flew-PIHR-teen) USAN.
Use: Analgesic.

•**fluprednisolone.** (FLEW-pred-NIH-so-lone) USAN.

Use: Corticosteroid, topical.

•**fluprednisolone valerate.** (FLEW-pred-NIH-so-lone VAL-eh-rate) USAN.
Use: Corticosteroid, topical.

•**fluproquazone.** (FLEW-PRO-kwah-zone) USAN.
Use: Analgesic.

•**fluprostenol sodium.** (flew-PROSTE-een-ole) USAN.
Use: Prostaglandin.
See: Equimate (Bayer Corp).

•**fluquazone.** (FLEW-kwah-zone) USAN.
Use: Anti-inflammatory.

•**fluradoline hydrochloride.** (FLURE-ade-OLE-een) USAN.
Use: Analgesic.

Flura-Drops. (Kirkman Sales) Fluoride. **Drops:** 0.25 mg (from 0.55 mg sodium fluoride). Bot. 30 ml. **Rinse:** 0.02% (from 0.05% sodium fluoride). Bot. 480 ml. *Rx.*
Use: Dental caries agent.

Flura-Loz. (Kirkman Sales) Sodium fluoride 2.2 mg providing 1 mg fluoride/ Loz. Bot. 100s, 1000s. *Rx.*
Use: Dental caries agent.

•**flurandrenolide,** (FLURE-an-DREEN-oh-lide) U.S.P. 23. *Formerly Flurandrenolone.*
Use: Corticosteroid, topical.
See: Cordran, Preps. (Eli Lilly).

flurandrenolone. (FLURE-an-DREE-nahl-ohn)
Use: Corticosteroid, topical.

Flura-Tablets. (Kirkman Sales) Sodium fluoride 2.21 mg, equivalent to 1 mg fluoride ion/Tab. Bot. 100s, 1000s. *Rx.*
Use: Dental caries agent.

Flurate. (Bausch & Lomb) Benoxinate HCl 0.4%, fluorescein sodium 0.25%, chlorobutanol 1%, povidone/Soln. Bot. 5 ml. *Rx.*
Use: Diagnostic aid, ophthalmic.

•**flurazepam hydrochloride,** (flure-AZE-uh-pam) U.S.P. 23.
Use: Anticonvulsant, hypnotic, muscle relaxant, sedative.
See: Dalmane, Cap. (Roberts Pharm).

•**flurbiprofen,** (FLURE-bih-PRO-fen) U.S.P. 23.
Use: Analgesic, anti-inflammatory.
See: Ansaid (Pharmacia & Upjohn).

flurbiprofen. (FLURE-bih-PRO-fen) (Various Mfr.) Flurbiprofen 50 mg or 100 mg. Tab. 100s, 500s. *Rx.*
Use: Analgesic, NSAID.
See: Ansaid (Pharmacia & Upjohn).

•**flurbiprofen sodium,** (FLURE-bih-PRO-fen) U.S.P. 23.
Use: Analgesic, NSAID; prostaglandin synthesis inhibitor.
See: Ocufen, Drops (Allergan).

flurbiprofen sodium ophthalmic. (FLURE-bih-PRO-fen) (Various) Flurbiprofen sodium 0.03%, polyvinyl alcohol 1.4%, thimerosal 0.005%, EDTA/ Soln. Bot. 2.5 ml *Rx.*
Use: Analgesic, NSAID.

Fluress. (PBH Wesley Jessen) Fluorescein sodium 0.25%. Bot. 5 ml. *Rx.*
Use: Anesthetic, diagnostic aid.

•**fluretofen.** (flure-EH-TOE-fen) USAN.
Use: Anti-inflammatory, antithrombotic.

flurfamide. (FLURE-fah-MIDE)
Use: Enzyme inhibitor.

•**flurocitabine.** (FLEW-row-SIGH-tah-bean) USAN.
Use: Antineoplastic.

Fluro-Ethyl. (Gebauer) Ethyl Cl 25%, dichlorotetrafluoroethane 75%/Spray. Can 270 g. *Rx.*
Use: Anesthetic-topical.

•**flurofamide.** (FLEW-row-fah-MIDE) USAN. *Formerly Flurfamide.*
Use: Enzyme inhibitor (urease).

•**flurogestone acetate.** (FLEW-row-JEST-ohn) USAN.
Use: Hormone, progestin.

Flurosyn. (Rugby) **Cream:** Fluocinolone acetonide 0.01% or 0.025%. Tube 15 g, 60 g, 425 g. **Oint:** Fluocinolone acetonide 0.025% in a white petrolatum base. Tube 15 g, 60 g. *Rx.*
Use: Corticosteroid, topical.

•**flurothyl.** (FLURE-oh-thill) USAN.
Use: Stimulant (central).

•**fluroxene.** (flure-OX-een) USAN. N.F. XIV.
Use: General inhalation anesthetic.

FluShield. (Wyeth Ayerst) Influenza virus vaccine, trivalent - Immunizing antigen, ether extracted. Vial 5 ml, 0.5 ml. Tubex. *Rx.*
Use: Immunization.

•**fluspiperone.** (FLEW-spih-per-OHN) USAN.
Use: Antipsychotic.

•**fluspirilene.** (flew-SPIRE-ih-leen) USAN.
Use: Antipsychotic, anxiolytic.
See: Imap (Ortho McNeil).

•**flutamide,** (FLEW-tuh-mide) U.S.P. 23.
Use: Antiandrogen.
See: Eulexin Cap. (Schering Plough).

•**fluticasone propionate.** (flew-TICK-ah-SONE PRO-pee-oh-nate) USAN.
Use: Anti-inflammatory.
See: Cutivate (GlaxoWellcome).
Flonase, spray. (Allen & Hanburys).

Flovent, Aer. Spray (GlaxoWellcome).

Flutra. Trichlormethiazide.
Use: Diuretic.

•**flutroline.** (FLEW-troe-LEEN) USAN.
Use: Antipsychotic.

•**fluvastatin sodium.** (FLEW-vah-STAT-in) USAN.
Use: Antihyperlipidemic inhibitor (HMG-CoA reductase).
See: Lescol, Cap. (Novartis).

Fluvirin. (Adams) Influenza virus vaccine. Vial 5 ml, 0.5 ml pre-filled syringes. *Rx.*
Use: Immunization.

•**fluvoxamine maleate.** (flew-VOX-ah-meen) USAN.
Use: Antidepressant; antiobsessional agent.
See: Luvox, Tab. (Solvay).

•**fluzinamide.** (flew-ZIN-ah-mide) USAN.
Use: Anticonvulsant.

Fluzone. (Pasteur Merieux Connaught) Influenza virus vaccine, thimerosal 0.01%. Vial 5 ml, 25 ml, syringes 0.5 ml (Whole virus); vial 5 ml, 5 yr. 5 ml (Split-virus). *Rx.*
Use: Immunization.

FML Forte. (Allergan) Fluorometholone 0.25%. Susp. Bot. 2 ml, 5 ml, 10 ml, 15 ml. *Rx.*
Use: Corticosteroid, ophthalmic.

FML Liquifilm. (Allergan) Fluorometholone 0.1%. Bot. 1 ml, 5 ml, 10 ml, 15 ml. *Rx.*
Use: Corticosteroid, ophthalmic.

FML-S. (Allergan) Fluorometholone 0.1%, sulfacetomide sodium 10%. Susp. Dropper Bot. 5 ml, 10 ml. *Rx.*
Use: Corticosteroid, ophthalmic.

FML S.O.P. (Allergan) Fluorometholone 0.1% Oint. Tube 3.5 g. *Rx.*
Use: Corticosteroid, ophthalmic.

Foamicon. (Invamed) Aluminum hydroxide 80 mg, magnesium trisilicate 20 mg, alginic acid, calcium stearate, compressible sugar, sodium bicarbonate, sucrose. Chew. Tab. Bot. 100s. *otc.*
Use: Antacid.

•**focofilcon a.** (FOE-koe-FILL-kahn A) USAN.
Use: Contact lens material (hydrophilic).

Foille. (Blistex) Benzocaine 2%, benzyl alcohol 4% in a bland vegetable oil base. Oint. Tube 30 g. *otc.*
Use: Anesthetic, local.

Foillecort. (Blistex) Hydrocortisone acetate 0.5%. Cream. Tube 3.5 g. *otc.*
Use: Corticosteroid, topical.

Foille Medicated First Aid. (Blistex) **Aerosol:** Benzocaine 5% with chloroxylenol 0.1% in a bland vegetable oil base with benzyl alcohol. Spray 92 g. **Oint.:** Benzocaine 5%, chloroxylenol 0.1% in a bland vegetable oil base. Tube 30 g. **Lot.:** Benzocaine 5%, chloroxylenol 0.1% in a bland vegetable oil base with benzyl alcohol 30 ml. **Oint:** Benzocaine 5%, chloroxylenol, benzyl alcohol, EDTA, corn oil. 3.5 g, 28 g. **Spray:** Benzocaine 5%, chloroxylenol, benzyl alcohol, corn oil. 92 ml. *otc.*
Use: Anesthetic, local.

Foille Plus. (Blistex) **Cream:** Benzocaine 5%, benzyl alcohol 4% in a nonstaining washable base. Tube 3.5 g. **Soln.:** Benzocaine 5%, benzyl alcohol, alcohol 77.8%. Aerosol spray 105 g. **Spray:** Benzocaine 5%, chloroxylenol, alcohol. 105 ml. *otc.*
Use: Anesthetic, local.

Folabee. (Vortech) Liver inj. B_{12} equivalent to 10 mcg, crystalline B_{12} 100 mcg, folic acid 0.4 mg. Inj. Vial 10 ml. *Rx.*
Use: Anemia.

folacin.
See: Folic acid.

folacine.
See: Folic acid. (Various Mfr.)

folate, sodium.
See: Folvite, Soln. (ESI Lederle Generics).

Folergot-DF. (Marnel) Phenobarbital 40 mg, ergotamine tartrate 0.6 mg, levorotatory alkaloids of belladonna 0.2 mg, dye-free. Tab. Bot. 100s. *Rx.*
Use: Anticholinergic, gastrointestinal.

Folex PFS Injection. (Pharmacia & Upjohn) Methotrexate sodium 25 mg/ml. Preservative free. Inj. Vial. 2 ml, 4 ml, 8 ml. *Rx.*
Use: Antineoplastic.

•**folic acid,** (FOLE-ik) U.S.P. 23.
Use: Anemia; vitamin (hematopoietic).
See: Folvite, Tab., Soln. (ESI Lederle Generics).

folic acid. (Various Mfr.) Tab. **0.4 mg:** Bot. 100s. **0.8 mg:** Bot. 100s. **1 mg:** Bot. 30s, 100s, 1000s, UD 100s. *Rx.*
Use: Vitamin supplement.

folic acid. (Fujisawa) 5 mg/ml w/ benzyl alcohol 1.5%, EDTA. Inj. Vials 10 ml. *Rx.*
Use: Vitamin supplement.

folic acid antagonists.
See: Methotrexate Inj., Tab. (ESI Lederle Generics).

folic acid salts.

See: Folvite, Tab., Soln. (ESI Lederle Generics).

folinic acid. Leucovorin Calcium, U.S.P. 23. (Various Mfr.)

Fol-Li-Bee. (Foy) Liver inj. equivalent to cyanocobalamin 10 mcg, folic acid 1 mg, cyanocobalamin 100 mcg/ml, phenol 0.5% pH adjusted w/sodium hydroxide and/or HCl. Vial 10 ml multidose, Monovials. *Rx.*
Use: Anemia.

follicle stimulating hormone, human. Menotropins, Pergonal.

follicormon.
See: Estradiol Benzoate. (Various Mfr.).

follicular hormones.
See: Estrone (Various Mfr.).

folliculin.
See: Estrone (Various Mfr.).

Follistim. (Organon) FSH activity 75 IU (as follitropin beta), sucrose. Inj. Vial 1s, 5s with diluent. *Rx.*
Use: Ovulation inducer.

follitropin alpha.
See: Gonal-F, Inj. (Serono)

follitropin beta.
See: Follistim, Inj. (Organon).

Foltrin. (Eon Labs Manufacturing) Liver and stomach concentrate 240 mg, B_{12} 15 mcg, iron 110 mg, C 75 mg, folic acid 0.5 mg/Cap. Bot. 100s, 1000s. *Rx.*
Use: Mineral, vitamin supplement.

•**fomepizole.** (foe-MEH-pih-ZOLE) USAN.
Use: Antidote (alcohol dehydrogenase inhibitor).
See: Antizol (Orphan Medical).

•**fomivirsen sodium.** (foe-MIH-vihr-sen) USAN.
Use: Antiviral (CMV retinitis).

fonatol.
See: Diethylstilbestrol (Various Mfr.).

•**fonazine mesylate.** (FAH-nazz-een) USAN
Use: Serotonin inhibitor.

fontarsol.
See: Dichlorophenarsine Hydrochloride.

Foralicon Plus Elixir. (Forbes) Vitamins B_{12} 16.7 mcg, B_6 4 mg, iron 200 mg (equivalent to elemental iron 24 mg), niacinamide 40 mg, folic acid 0.8 mg, sorbitol soln. q.s./15 ml. Bot. 8 oz, 16 oz. *Rx.*
Use: Mineral, vitamin supplement.

Forane. (Ohmeda Pharmaceuticals) Isoflurane. Gas. Volume 100 ml. *Rx.*
Use: Anesthetic, general.

•**forasartan.** (far-ah-SAHR-tan) USAN.
Use: Antihypertensive.

Fordustin. (Sween) Cornstarch based powder with deodorizing action. Bot. 3 oz, 8 oz. *otc.*
Use: Powder, topical.

Formadon Solution. (Gordon Laboratories) Formalin solution 3.7% to 4% (10% of U.S.P. strength) in an aqueous perfumed base. Bot. 1 oz, 4 oz, 0.5 gal, gal.
Use: Bromhidrosis, hyperhidrosis agent.

•**formaldehyde solution,** (for-MAL-deh-hide) U.S.P. 23.
Use: For poison ivy, fungus infections of the skin, hyperhidrosis and as an astringent, disinfectant.

formalin.
See: Formaldehyde Solution (Various Mfr.).

Formalyde-10. (Pedinol) Formaldehyde 10%, FDA-40 alcohol. Spray Bot. 60 ml. *Rx.*
Use: Bromhidrosis, hyperhidrosis agent.

Forma-Ray Solution. (Gordon Laboratories) Formalin 7.4% to 8% (20% of USP strength) in aqueous, scented, tinted solution. Bot. 1.5 oz, 4 oz. *otc.*
Use: Drying.

formic acid.
W/Silicic acid.
See: Nyloxin, Inj. (Becton Dickinson).

•**formocortal.** (FORE-moe-CORE-tal) USAN.
Use: Corticosteroid, topical.

Formula 44 Cough Control Discs. (Procter & Gamble).
See: Vicks Formula 44 Cough Discs (Procter & Gamble).

Formula 44 Cough Mixture. (Procter & Gamble) Chlorpheniramine maleate 2 mg, dextromethorphan HBr 15 mg, alcohol 10%/5 ml. Liq. Bot. 120 ml, 240 ml. *otc.*
Use: Antihistamine, antitussive.

Formula 44D Decongestant Cough Mixture. (Procter & Gamble) Pseudoephedrine HCl 20 mg, dextromethorphan HBr 10 mg, guaifenesin 67 mg, alcohol 10%/5 ml. Liq. Bot. 120 ml, 240 ml. *otc.*
Use: Antitussive, decongestant, expectorant.

Formula 44M Cough and Cold. (Procter & Gamble) Pseudoephedrine HCl 15 mg, dextromethorphan HBr 7.5 mg, chlorpheniramine maleate 1 mg, acetaminophen 125 mg/5 ml, alcohol 20%, saccharin, sucrose. Liq. Bot. 120 ml, 240 ml. *otc.*
Use: Analgesic, antihistamine, antitus-

sive, decongestant.

Formula No. 81. (Fellows) Liver (beef) for inj. 1 mcg, ferrous gluconate 100 mg, niacinamide 100 mg, B_2 1.5 mg, panthenol 2.5 mg, B_{12} 3 mcg, procaine HCl 25 mg/2 ml. Vial 30 ml. *otc.*
Use: Mineral, vitamin supplement.

Formula 405. (Doak Dermatologics) Sodium tallowate, sodium cocoate, Doak Additive A, PPF- 20 methyl glucose ether, titanium dioxide, trochbrocarbanilide, pentasodium pentatate, EDTA. Bar 100 g. *otc.*
Use: Dermatologic, cleanser.

Formula 1207. (Thurston) Iodine, liver fraction No. 2, caseinates/Tab. Bot. 100s, 250s. *otc.*
Use: Mineral supplement.

Formula B. (Major) Vitamins B_1 15 mg, B_2 15 mg, B_3 100 mg, B_5 18 mg, B_6 4 mg, B_{12} 5 mcg, C 500 mg, folic acid 0.5 mg/Tab. Bot 250 g. *Rx.*
Use: Vitamin supplement.

Formula B Plus. (Major) Iron 27 mg, A 5000 IU, E 30 IU, B_1 20 mg, B_2 20 mg, B_3 100 mg, B_5 25 mg, B_6 25 mg, B_{12} 50 mcg, C 500 mg, folic acid 0.8 mg, biotin 0.15 mg, Cr, Cu, Mg, Mn, Zn/Tab. Bot 100s, 500s. *Rx.*
Use: Mineral, vitamin supplement.

Formula VM-2000 Tablets. (Solgar) Iron 5 mg, A 12,500 IU, D 200 IU, E 100 IU, B_1 50 mg, B_2 50 mg, B_3 50 mg, B_5 50 mg, B_6 50 mg, B_{12} 50 mcg, C 150 mg, folic acid 0.2 mg, B, Ca, Cr, Cu, I, K, Mg, Mn, Mo, Se, Zn 7.5 mg, betaine, biotin 50 mcg, choline, bioflavonoids, amino acids, hesperidin, inositol, l-glutethione, PABA, rutin/Tab. Bot. 30s, 60s, 90s, 180s. *otc.*
Use: Mineral, vitamin supplement.

formyl tetrahydropteroylglutamic acid. Leucovorin Calcium, U.S.P. 23.

Forta Drink Powder. (Ross Laboratories) Whey protein concentrate, sucrose, vitamins A, B_1, B_2, B_3, B_5, B_6, B_{12}, C, D, E, folic acid, biotin, Ca, Cu, Fe, I, Mg, Mn, P, Zn. Can. 482 g. *otc.*
Use: Nutritional supplement.

Forta-Flora. (Barth's) Whey-lactose 90%, pectin. **Pow.** Jar lb. **Wafer:** Bot. 100s.

Forta Instant Cereal. (Ross Laboratories) Lactose-free oat or bran cereal provides 6.25 g dietary fiber/serving. Can 1 lb 1 oz. *otc.*
Use: Nutritional supplement.

Forta Instant Pudding. (Ross Laboratories) Lactose-free in pudding base. Can 1 lb 12 oz. Vanilla, chocolate, butterscotch flavors. *otc.*
Use: Nutritional supplement.

Forta Pudding Mix. (Ross Laboratories) Milk protein isolate, sucrose, hydrolyzed cornstarch, modified tapioca starch, partially hydrogenated soybean oil, vitamins A, B_1, B_2, B_3, B_5, B_6, B_{12}, C, D, E, folic acid, biotin, Ca, Fe, P, I, Mg, Zn, Cu, Mn, tartrazine. Can 794 g. *otc.*
Use: Nutritional supplement.

Forta Shake Powder. (Ross Laboratories) Nonfat dry milk, sucrose, vitamins A, B_1, B_2, B_3, B_5, B_6, B_{12}, C, D, E, folic acid, biotin, Ca, Cu, Fe, I, Mg, Mn, P, Zn, tartrazine. Can lb, pkt. 1.4 oz. Can 1 lb 2.7 oz, pkt. 1.6 oz. *otc.*
Use: Nutritional supplement.

Forta Soup Mix. (Ross Laboratories) Milk protein isolate, sodium and calcium caseinate, hydrolyzed cornstarch, modified tapioca starch, powdered shortening (partially hydrogenated coconut oil), vitamins A, B_1, B_2, B_3, B_5, B_6, B_{12}, C, D, E, folic acid, biotin, Ca, Cu, Fe, I, Mg, Mn, P, Zn. Chicken flavor. Can. 454 g. *otc.*
Use: Nutritional supplement.

Fortaz. (GlaxoWellcome) Ceftazidime powder for parenteral administration 500 mg, 1 g, 2 g, or 6 g Vial. **Pow.: 500 mg:** Vial. **1 g:** Vial, Infusion Pack. **2 g:** Vial, Infusion Pack. **6 g:** Pharmacy Bulk Pkg. **Inj.:** 1 g, 2 g Vial 50 ml, premixed, frozen. *Rx.*
Use: Anti-infective, cephalosporin.

Forte L.I.V. (Foy) Cyanocobalamin 15 mcg liver injection equivalent to vitamin B_{12} activity 1 mcg, ferrous gluconate 50 mg, B_2 0.75 mg, panthenol 1.25 mg, niacinamide 50 mg, citric acid 8.2 mg, sodium citrate 118 mg/ml, procaine HCl 2%. Bot. 30 ml. *otc.*
Use: Mineral, vitamin supplement.

Fortel Midstream. (Biomerica) Reagent in-home urine test for pregnancy. 1 test stick per kit.
Use: Diagnostic aid, pregnancy.

Fortel Ovulation. (Biomerica) Monoclonal antibody-based home test to predict ovulation. Kit 1s.
Use: Diagnostic aid.

Fortel Plus. (Biomerica) Reagent in-home urine pregnancy test. Kit contains urine collection cup, dropper, test device.
Use: Diagnostic aid, pregnancy.

Fortovase. (Roche) Saquinavir 200 mg/Cap. Bot. 180s. *Rx.*
Use: Antiviral.

Fortral. (Sanofi Winthrop) Pentazocine as solution and tablets. *c-iv.*
Use: Analgesic, narcotic.

Fortramin. (Thurston) Vitamins E 200 IU, A 6000 IU, D 600 IU, B_1 4.5 mg, B_2 4.5 mg, B_6 4.5 mg, B_{12} 5 mcg, C 2.75 mg, rutin 8 mg, hesperidin complex 10 mg, lemon bioflavonoids 15 mg, d-calcium pantothenate 50 mg, para-aminobenzoic acid 7.5 mg, biotin 10 mg, folic acid 24 mcg, niacinamide 20 mg, desiccated liver 25 mg, iron 3 mg, calcium 75 mg, phosphorous 34 mg, manganese 10 mg, copper 0.5 mg, zinc 0.5 mg, iodine 0.375 mg, potassium 500 mg, magnesium 5 mg/Tab. Bot. 100s, 250s. *otc.*
Use: Mineral, vitamin supplement.

40 Winks. (Roberts Pharm) Diphenhydramine HCl 50 mg/Cap. Bot. 30s. *otc.*
Use: Sleep aid.

Fosamax. (Merck) Alendronate sodium 5 mg, 10 mg or 40 mg, lactose/Tab. Bot. 100s, UD 30s, UD 100s. *Rx.*
Use: Bone resorption inhibitor.

•**fosarilate.** (FOSS-ah-RILL-ate) USAN.
Use: Antiviral.

•**fosazepam.** (foss-AZZ-eh-pam) USAN.
Use: Hypnotic, sedative.

•**foscarnet sodium.** (foss-CAR-net) USAN.
Use: Antiviral.
See: Foscavir, Inj. (Astra).

Foscavir. (Astra) Foscarnet sodium 24 mg/ml. Inj. Bot. 250 ml, 500 ml. *Rx.*
Use: Anti-infective, antiviral.

•**fosfomycin.** (foss-foe-MY-sin) USAN.
Use: Anti-infective.
See: Monurol (Zambon).

•**fosfomycin tromethamine.** (foss-foe-MY-sin troe-METH-ah-meen) USAN.
Use: Anti-infective.
See: Monurol, Granules (Forest Pharmaceutical).

•**fosfonet sodium.** (FOSS-foe-net) USAN.
Use: Antiviral.

Fosfree. (Mission Pharmacal) Iron 14.5 mg, A 1500 IU, D 150 IU, B_1 4.5 mg, B_2 2 mg, 10.5 mg, B_5 1 mg, B_6 2.5 mg, B_{12} 2 mcg, C 50 mg, Ca 175.5 mg, sugar/Tab. Bot. 120s. *otc.*
Use: Mineral, vitamin supplement.

fosinopril. (FAH-sen-oh-PRIL)
Use: Angiotensin-converting enzyme inhibitor, antihypertensive.
See: Monopril (Bristol-Myers).

•**fosinopril sodium.** (FAH-sen-oh-PRIL) USAN.
Use: Antihypertensive, enzyme inhibitor (angiotensin-converting).
See: Monopril, Tab. (Bristol-Myers Squibb).

•**fosinoprilat.** (fah-SIN-oh-prill-at) USAN.
Use: Antihypertensive.

•**fosphenytoin sodium.** (FOSS-FEN-ih-toe-in) USAN.
Use: Anticonvulsant.
See: Cerebyx, Inj. (Parke-Davis).

•**fosquidone.** (FOSS-kwih-dohn) USAN.
Use: Antineoplastic.

•**fostedil.** (FOSS-teh-dill) USAN.
Use: Vasodilator (calcium channel blocker).

Fostex. (Bristol-Myers) Benzoyl peroxide 10%, EDTA, urea. Bar. 106 g. *otc.*
Use: Dermatologic, acne.

Fostex Acne Cleansing Cream. (Westwood Squibb) Salicylic acid 2%, EDTA, stearyl alcohol. Cream. 118 g. *otc.*
Use: Dermatologic, acne.

Fostex Acne Medication Cleansing Bar. (Westwood Squibb) Salicyclic acid 2%, EDTA. Bar. 106 g. *otc.*
Use: Dermatologic, acne.

Fostex 10% BPO. (Westwood Squibb) Benzoyl peroxide 10%, EDTA. Gel 42.5 g. *otc.*
Use: Dermatologic, acne.

Fostex 10% Wash. (Bristol-Myers) Benzoyl peroxide 10% with water base. Liq. Bot. 150 ml. *otc.*
Use: Dermatologic, acne.

•**fostriecin sodium.** (FOSS-try-eh-SIN) USAN.
Use: Antineoplastic.

Fostril. (Westwood Squibb) Sulfur, zinc oxide, parabens, EDTA. Lot. Tube 28 ml. *otc.*
Use: Dermatologic, acne.

Fototar Cream. (Zeneca) Coal tar 1.6% (from 2% coal tar extract) in emollient moisturizing cream base. Tube 90 g, 480 g. *otc.*
Use: Dermatologic.

4-Way Cold Tablets. (Bristol-Myers) Aspirin 324 mg, phenylpropanolamine HCl 12.5 mg, chlorpheniramine maleate 2 mg/Tab. Bot. 36s, 60s, Card 15s. *otc.*
Use: Analgesic, antihistamine, decongestant.

4 Hair Softgel. (Marlyn) Iron 2.5 mg, A 1250 IU, E 10 IU, B_3 5mg, B_5 2.5 mg, B_6 1.5 mg, B_{12} 44 mcg, C 25 mg, folic acid 33.3 mg, biotin 250 mcg, I, Mg, Cu, Zn 7.5 mg, choline bitartrate, inositol, Mn, Methionine, PABA, B_1, L-cysteine, tyrosine, Si/Cap. Bot 60s. *otc.*
Use: Mineral, vitamin supplement.

4 Nails Softgel. (Marlyn) Ca 167 mg, iron 3 mg , A 833 IU, D 67, E 10 mg, B_1 3.3 mg, B_2 1.7 mg, B_3 8.3 mg, B_5 8.3 mg, B_6 8.3 mg, B_{12} 8.3 mg, C 10 mg, folic acid 33.3 mg, biotin 8.3 mcg, P, I, Mg, Cu, Zn 3.3 mg, Cr, Mn, methionine, inositol, choline bitartrate, Se, PABA, protein isolate, gelatin, lecithin, unsaturated fatty acid, predigested protein L-cysteine, B mucopolysaccharides, silicon amino acid chelate, S/Cap. Bot. 60s. *otc.*
Use: Mineral, vitamin supplement.

4-Way Fast Acting Nasal Spray. (Bristol-Myers) Phenylephrine HCl 0.5%, naphazoline HCl 0.05%, pyrilamine maleate 0.2%, buffered isotonic aqueous soln., thimerosal. Atomizer 15 ml, 30 ml. *otc.*
Use: Antihistamine, decongestant.

4-Way Long Acting Nasal Spray. (Bristol-Myers) Oxymetazoline HCl 0.05% in isotonic buffered soln. Spray Bot. 15 ml. *otc.*
Use: Decongestant.

Fowler's Solution. Potassium Arsenite Solution (Various Mfr.).

Foxalin. (Standex) Digitoxin 0.1 mg, sodium carboxymethylcellulose/Cap. Bot. 100s. *Rx.*
Use: Cardiovascular agent.

foxglove.
See: Digitalis (Various Mfr.).

Foygen Aqueous. (Foy) Estrogenic substance or estrogens 2 mg/ml with sodium carboxymethylcellulose, povidone, benzyl alcohol, methyl and propyl parabens. Inj. Vial 10 ml. *Rx.*
Use: Estrogen.

Foyplex Injection. (Foy) Sterile injectable soln. of nine water-soluble vitamins. Packaged as 2 separate solutions for extemporaneous combination. *Rx.*
Use: Nutritional supplement, parenteral.

Fragmin. (Pharmacia & Upjohn) Dalteparin sodium 16 mg/0.2 ml, 32 mg/0.2 ml, preservative free. Soln. Bot. 10s. *Rx.*
Use: Anticoagulant.

FreAmine III. (McGaw) Amino acid 8.5% or 10%. Bot. 500 ml, 1000 ml. *Rx.*
Use: Nutritional supplement, parenteral.

FreAmine III 3% w/Electrolytes. (McGaw) Amino acid 3% with electrolytes. Bot. 1000 ml. *Rx.*
Use: Nutritional supplement, parenteral.

FreAmine III 8.5% w/Electrolytes. (McGaw) Sodium 60 mEq/L, potassium 60 mEq/L, magnesium 10 mEq/L, Cl 60 mEq/L, phosphate 40 mEq/L, acetate 125 mEq/L. Soln. Bot. 500 ml, 1000 ml. *Rx.*
Use: Nutritional supplement, parenteral.

FreAmine HBC 6.9%. (American McGaw) High branched 6.9% amino acid formulation for hypercatabolic patients. Bot. 1000 ml. *Rx.*
Use: Nutritional supplement, parenteral.

Free & Clear. (Pharmaceutical Specialties) Ammonium laureth sulfate, disodium cocamide MEA sulfosuccinate, cocamidopropyl hydroxysultaine, cocamide DEA, PEG-120 methyl glucose dioleate, EDTA, potassium sorbate, citric acid. Shampoo. Bot. 240 ml. *otc.*
Use: Dermatologic, cleanser.

Freedavite. (Freeda Vitamins) Iron 10 mg (from ferrous fumarate), vitamins A 5000 IU, D 400 IU, E 3 IU, B_1 5 mg, B_2 3 mg, B_3 25 mg, B_5 5 mg, B_6 2 mg, B_{12} 2 mcg, C 60 mg, choline, inositol, potassium iodide, Ca, Cu, K, Mg, Mn, Se, Zn 0.2 mg. Bot. 100s, 250s. *otc.*
Use: Mineral, vitamin supplement.

Freedox. (Pharmacia & Upjohn) Tirilazad.
Use: A 21 aminosteroid antioxidant.

•**frentizole.** (FREN-tih-zole) USAN.
Use: Immunoregulator.

FreshBurst Listerine. (Warner Lambert) Thymol 0.064%, eucalyptol 0.092%, methyl salicylate 0.06%, menthol 0.042%, alcohol 21.6%. Rinse. Bot. 250 ml. *otc.*
Use: Mouthwash.

Fresh n' Feminine. (Walgreens) Benzethonium Cl 0.2% Bot. 8 oz. *otc.*
Use: Vaginal agent.

•**fructose.** (Various Mfr.) Soln. 10%. Bot. 1000 ml.
Use: Nutritional supplement.
See: Frutabs, Tab. (Pfanstiehl).

•**fructose,** U.S.P. 23.
Use: Nutritional supplement.

fructose and sodium chloride injection.
Use: Electrolyte, fluid, nutrient replacement.

Fruity Chews. (Zenith Goldline) Vitamins A 2500 IU, D 400 IU, E 15 mg, B_1 1.05 mg, B_2 1.2 mg, B_3 13.5 mg, B_6 1.05 mg, B_{12} 4.5 mcg, C (as sodium ascorbate and ascorbic acid) 60 mg, folic acid 0.3 mg/Chew. Tab. Bot. 100s. *otc.*
Use: Mineral, vitamin supplement.

Fruity Chews w/Iron. (Zenith Goldline) Elemental iron 12 mg, vitamins A 2500 IU, D 400 IU, E 15 mg, B_1 1.05 mg, B_2 1.2 mg, B_3 13.5 mg, B_6 1.05 mg, B_{12}

4.5 mcg, C (as sodium ascorbate and ascorbic acid) 60 mg, folic acid 0.3 mg, zinc 8 mg/Chew. Tab. Bot. 100s. *otc.*
Use: Mineral, vitamin supplement.

frusemide.
See: Lasix.

Frutabs. (Pfanstiehl) Fructose 2 g. Tab. Bot. 100s.
Use: Carbohydrate supplement.

FTA-ABS. (Wampole Laboratories) Fluorescent treponemal antibody-absorbed test in vitro for confirming a positive reagin test for syphillis. Test 100s.
Use: Diagnostic aid.

AFT-ABS/DS. (Wampole Laboratories) Fluorescent treponemal antibody-absorbed test in vitro for confirming a positive reagin test for syphilis. Test 100s.
Use: Diagnostic aid.

•**fuchsin, basic,** (FYOO-sin) U.S.P. 23.
Use: Anti-infective, topical.

FUDR. (Roberts Pharm) Floxuridine 500 mg sterile pow. for inj. Vial 5 ml. *Rx.*
Use: Antineoplastic.

Ful-Glo. (PBH Wesley Jessen) Fluorescein sodium 0.6 mg/Strip. Box 300s. *otc.*
Use: Diagnostic aid, ophthalmic.

Fuller. (Birchwood) Pkg. 1 shield.
Use: Anorectal preparation.

Fulvicin P/G. (Schering Plough) Griseofulvin ultramicrosize 125 mg, 165 mg, 250 mg or 330 mg/Tab. Bot. 100s. *Rx.*
Use: Antifungal.

Fulvicin U/F. (Schering Plough) Griseofulvin microsize 250 mg or 500 mg/Tab. Bot. 60s, 250s. *Rx.*
Use: Antifungal.

•**fumaric acid,** (fyoo-MAR-ik) N.F. 18.
Use: Acidifier.

Fumatinic Capsules. (Laser) Iron 90 mg (from ferrous fumarate), vitamins C 100 mg, B_{12} 15 mcg, folic acid 1 mg/SR Cap. Bot. 100s. *Rx.*
Use: Mineral, vitamin supplement.

Fumeron. (Eon Labs Manufacturing) Ferrous fumarate 330 mg, vitamin B_1 5 mg/TR Cap. *otc.*
Use: Mineral, vitamin supplement.

•**fumoxicillin.** (fyoo-MOX-ih-SILL-in) USAN.
Use: Antibacterial.

Funduscein. (Ciba Vision Ophthalmics) Fluorescein sodium. Inj. **10%:** Amp. 5 ml. **25%:** Amp. 3 ml. *Rx.*
Use: Diagnostic aid, ophthalmic.

Fungacetin Ointment. (Blair Laboratories) Triacetin (glyceryl triacetate) 25% in a water-miscible ointment base. Tube 30 g. *Rx.*
Use: Antifungal, topical.

Fungatin. (Major) Tolnaftate 1%. Cream Tube 15 g. *otc.*
Use: Antifungal, topical.

fungicides.
See: Aftate, Prods. (Schering Plough).
Amphotericin B (Fujisawa).
Ancobon (Roberts Pharm).
Arcum, Preps. (Arcum).
Asterol.
Basic Fuchsin (Various Mfr.).
Desenex, Prods. (Novartis Pharmaceuticals).
Dichlorophene.
Diflucan (Roerig).
Fungizone Intravenous (Bristol-Myers Squibb).
Fulvicin P/G (Schering Plough).
Fulvicin U/F (Schering Plough).
Grifulvin V (Advanced Care Products).
Grisactin, Prods. (Wyeth Ayerst).
Griseofulvin Ultramicrosize (Various Mfr.).
Gris-PEG (Allergan).
Miconazole Nitrate (Various Mfr.).
Monistat I.V. (Janssen).
Mycostatin (Apothecon).
Nifuroxime (Various Mfr.).
Nilstat (ESI Lederle Generics).
Nitrofurfuryl Methyl Ether (Various Mfr.).
Nizoral (Janssen).
Nystatin (Various Mfr.).
Phenylmercuric Preps. (Various Mfr.).
Sporanox, Cap. (Janssen).
Undecylenic Acid (Various Mfr.).

•**fungimycin.** (FUN-jih-MY-sin) USAN.
Use: Antifungal.

Fungi-Nail. (Kramer) Resorcinol 1%, salicyclic acid 2%, parachlorometaxylenol 2%, benzocaine 0.5%, acetic acid 2.5%, propylene glycol, hydroxypropyl methylcellulose, alcohol 0.5%. Bot. 30 ml. *otc.*
Use: Antifungal, topical.

Fungizone. (Bristol-Myers Squibb) Amphotericin B 3%, thimerosal, titanium dioxide. **Lot.:** Plastic bot. 30 ml. **Cream, Oint:** Tube 20 g. **Oral Susp.:** Amphotericin B 100 mg/ml, alcohol ≤ 0.55%, parabens, sodium metabisulfite/Bot. 24 ml w/dropper. *Rx.*
Use: Antifungal, topical.

Fungizone Intravenous. (Bristol-Myers Squibb) Amphotericin B 50 mg, as desoxycholate. Pow for Inj. Vial. *Rx.*
Use: Antifungal.

Fungizone for Laboratory Use in Tissue Culture. (Bristol-Myers Squibb) Amphotericin B 50 mg, sodium desoxy-

cholate 41 mg/Vial 20 ml.
Use: Diagnostic aid.

Fungoid AF. (Pedinol) Undecylenic acid 25%/Soln. Bot. 30 ml. *otc.*
Use: Antifungal, topical.

Fungoid Creme. (Pedinol) Clotrimazole 1%, benzyl alcohol. Tube 45 g. *Rx.*
Use: Antifungal,topical.

Fungoid-HC Creme. (Pedinol) Miconazole nitrate 2%, hydrocortisone 1%. In 56.7 g, 1 g dual packets. *Rx.*
Use: Antifungal, topical.

Fungoid Solution. (Pedinol) Clotrimazole 10 mg in polyethylene glycol 400. Bot. 30 ml. *Rx.*
Use: Anti-infective, topical.

Fungoid Tincture. (Pedinol) Miconazole nitrate 2%, alcohol. Soln. Bot. with brush applicator 7.39 ml, 29.57 ml. *otc.*
Use: Antifungal, topical.

Furacin Soluble Dressing. (Roberts Pharm) Nitrofurazone 0.2%, polyethylene glycol base. Oint. (soluble) Jar 454 g, Tube 28 g, 56 g. *Rx.*
Use: Burn therapy.

Furacin Topical Cream. (Roberts Pharm) Nitrofurazone 0.2% in a water miscible cream, cetyl alcohol, mineral oil, parabens. Tube 28 g. *Rx.*
Use: Burn therapy.

Furacin Topical Solution. (Roberts Pharm) Nitrofurazone 0.2%. Bot. 480 ml. *Rx.*
Use: Burn therapy.

Furadantin Oral Suspension. (Procter & Gamble) Nitrofurantoin 5 mg/ml. Bot. 60 ml, 470 ml. *Rx.*
Use: Anti-infective, urinary.

furalazine hydrochloride.
Use: Antimicrobial compound.

furaltadone.

Furanite Tabs. (Major) Nitrofurantoin 50 mg or 100 mg/Tab. Bot. 100s.
Use: Anti-infective, urinary. *Rx.*

•**furaprofen.** (FYOOR-ah-PRO-fen) USAN. *Formerly Enprofen*
Use: Anti-inflammatory.

•**furazolidone,** (fyoor-ah-ZOE-lih-dohn) U.S.P. 23.
Use: Anti-infective, topical; antiprotozoal (Trichomonas, topical).
See: Furoxone Tab., Susp. (Procter & Gamble).

•**furazolium chloride.** (FYOOR-ah-zoe-lee-uhm). USAN.
Use: Anti-infective.

•**furazolium tartrate.** (FYOOR-ah-ZOE-lee-uhm) USAN.
Use: Anti-infective.

furazosin hydrochloride. (FYOOR-ah-zoe-sin) Under study.
Use: Antihypertensive.

•**furegrelate sodium.** (fyoor-eh-GRELL-ate) USAN.
Use: Inhibitor (thromboxane synthetase).

furethidine.

•**furobufen.** (FER-oh-BYOO-fen) USAN.
Use: Anti-inflammatory.

•**furodazole.** (fyoor-OH-dah-zole) USAN.
Use: Anthelmintic.

Furonatal FA. (Lexis) Vitamins A 8000 IU, D 400 IU, E 30 IU, C 60 mg, folic acid 1 mg, B_1 2 mg, B_2 2.8 mg, B_6 2.5 mg, B_{12} 8 mcg, niacinamide 20 mg, iron 65 mg, calcium 125 mg/Tab. Bot. 100s, 1000s. *Rx.*
Use: Mineral, vitamin supplement.

•**furosemide,** (fyu-ROH-se-mide) U.S.P. 23.
Use: Diuretic.
See: Fumide, Tab. (Everett Laboratories).
Furomide, Vial (Hyrex).
Lasix, Tab., Inj., Soln. (Hoechst Marion Roussel).

furosemide. (Roxane) Furosemide. **10 mg/ml:** Soln. Dropper bot. 60 ml. **40 mg/5 ml:** Soln. Bot. 5 ml, 10 ml, 500 ml. *Rx.*
Use: Diuretic.

furosemide. (Various Mfr.) **Tab.: 20 mg or 80 mg:** Bot. 100s, 500s, 1000s, UD 100s; **40 mg:** Bot. 60s, 100s, 500s, 1000s, UD 100s. **Oral Soln.:** 10 mg/ml Bot. 60 ml, 120 ml. **Inj.:** 10 mg/ml Vial 10 ml; single dose vial 2 ml, 10 ml; partial fill single dose vial 4 ml. *Rx.*
Use: Diuretic.

Furoxone. (Procter & Gamble) Furazolidone. **Tab.:** 100 mg. Bot. 20s, 100s. **Liq.:** 50 mg/15 ml. Bot. 60 ml, 473 ml. *Rx.*
Use: Anti-infective.

•**fursalan.** (FYOOR-sal-an) USAN. Under study.
Use: Disinfectant.

•**fusidate sodium.** (FEW-sih-DATE) USAN.
Use: Anti-infective.
See: Fucidine (Bristol-Myers Squibb).

•**fusidic acid.** (few-SIH-dik) USAN.
Use: Anti-infective.

G

G-4.
See: Dichlorophene.

G-11. (Givaudan) Hexachlorophene Pow. for mfg.
See: Hexachlorophene, U.S.P. 23.

•**gabapentin.** (GAB-uh-PEN-tin) USAN.
Use: Anticonvulsant; amyotrophic lateral sclerosis agent. [Orphan drug]
See: Neurontin, Cap. (Warner Lambert).

gabbromicina. Aminosidine.
Use: Anti-infective. [Orphan drug]

Gabitril. (Abbott) Tiagabine HCl 4 mg, 12 mg, 16 mg, 20 mg lactose/Tab. Bot. 100s, 500s, Abbo-Pac 100s. *Rx.*
Use: Partial seizure treatment.

Gacid Tab. (Arcum) Magnesium trisilicate 500 mg, aluminum hydroxide 250 mg/Tab. Bot. 100s, 1000s. *otc.*
Use: Antacid.

•**gadobenate dimeglumine.** (gad-oh-BEN-ate die-meh-GLUE-meen) USAN.
Use: Diagnostic aid (paramagnetic), brain tumors, spine disorders.

•**gadodiamide.** (GAD-oh-DIE-ah-mide) USAN.
Use: Diagnostic aid (paramagnetic); brain and spine disorders.
See: Omniscan, Vial (Sanofi Winthrop).

gadodiamide/caltiamide.
Use: Radiopaque agent.
See: Omniscan (Sanofi Winthrop).

•**gadopentetate dimeglumine injection.** (GAD-oh-PEN-teh-tate die-meh-GLUE-meen) U.S.P. 23.
Use: Radiopaque agent; diagnostic aid.
See: Magnevist (Berlex).

•**gadoteridol.** (GAD-oh-TER-ih-dahl) USAN.
Use: Diagnostic aid (paramagnetic).
See: ProHance, Inj. (Bracco Diagnostics).

•**gadoversetamide.** (gad-oh-ver-SET-ah-mide) USAN.
Use: Diagnostic aid (paramagnetic; brain and spine disorders).

•**gadoxanum.** (gad-oh-ZAN-uhm) USAN.
Use: Diagnostic aid.

•**gadozelite.** (gad-oh-ZEH-lite) USAN.
Use: Diagnostic aid.

Galardin. (Glycomed) Matrix Metalloproteinase inhibitor.
Use: Corneal ulcers. [Orphan drug].

•**galdansetron hydrochloride.** (gahl-DAN-seh-trahn) USAN.
Use: Antiemetic.

•**gallamine triethiodide.** (GAL-ah-meen try-eth-EYE-oh-dide) U.S.P. 23.
Use: Neuromuscular blocker.

•**gallium citrate Ga 67 injection.** (GAL-ee-uhm SIH-trate) U.S.P. 23.
Use: Diagnostic aid (radiopaque medium); radiopharmaceutical.

•**gallium nitrate.** (GAL-ee-uhm NYE-trate) USAN.
Use: Calcium regulator; antihypercalcemic. [Orphan drug]
See: Ganite, Inj. (Fujisawa).

gallochrome.
See: Merbromin (Various Mfr.).

gallotannic acid.
See: Tannic Acid, Preps. (Various Mfr.).

gallstone solubilizing agents.
See: Actigall, Cap. (Novartis).
Chenix, Tab. (Solvay).
Moctanin. (Ethitek Pharmaceuticals).

Galzin. (Lemmon) Zinc acetate.
Use: Wilson's disease. [Orphan drug]

Gamazole Tabs. (Major) Sulfamethoxazole 500 mg/Tab. Bot. 100s, 500s, 1000s. *Rx.*
Use: Anti-infective, sulfonamide.

•**gamfexine.** (gam-FEX-ine) USAN.
Use: Antidepressant.

Gamimune N 5%. (Bayer Corp) Immune globulin IV (human) 5%. Inj. in maltose 10% 500 mg, 2.5 g, 5 g, 10 g. *Rx.*
Use: Immunization.

Gamimune N 10%. (Bayer Corp) Immune globulin IV (human) 10%. Inj. 5 g, 10 g, 20 g. Vial 50 ml, 100 ml, 200 ml. *Rx.*
Use: Immunization.

Gammagard S/D. (Baxter) Immune globulin IV (human) 2.5 g, 5 g or 10 g/Bot. Freeze-dried, solvent/detergent treated w/ sterile water for injection. 500 mg. *Rx.*
Use: Immunization.

gamma benzene hexachloride.
See: lindane.

gamma globulin.
See: Immune Globulin Intramuscular.
Immune Globulin Intravenous.

gamma-hydroxybutyrate. (Biocraft, Orphan Medical)
Use: Narcolepsy. [Orphan drug]

gamma interferon. 1-b.
See: Actimmune (Genentech).

gammalinolenic acid.
Use: Juvenile rheumatoid arthritis. [Orphan drug]

Gammar-P I.V. (Centeon) Immune globulin (human). Sucrose 5%, albumin 3% (1 g or 5 g). In 1 g single-dose vial

with 20 ml sterile water for inj.; 2.5 g single-dose vial with 50 ml sterile water for inj.; 5 g single-dose vial with 100 ml sterile water for inj.; 5 g pharmacy bulk pack, 10 g. *Rx.*
Use: Immunization.

Gamulin Rh. (Centeon) Rho (D) Immune globulin (Human). Vial, syringe 1 dose. *Rx.*
Use: Immunization, Rh.

ganaxolone. (CoCensys)
Use: Infantile spasms. [Orphan drug]

•**ganciclovir.** (gan-SIGH-kloe-VIHR) USAN.
Use: Antiviral.
See: Cytovene, Cap., Pow for Inj., (Roche Laboratories).

ganciclovir intravitreal free implant.
Use: Cytomegalovirus retinitis. [Orphan drug]
See: Vitrasert, Implant (Chiron Vision).

•**ganciclovir sodium.** (gah-SIGH-kloe-VIHR) USAN.
Use: Antiviral.
See: Cytovene (Roche Laboratories).

G & W products. (G & W Laboratories) G & W markets the following products under the G & W Laboratories brand name:
Aminophylline Rectal Supp., 250 mg, 500 mg.
Aspirin Rectal Supp., 125 mg, 300 mg, 600 mg.
Bisacodyl Supp., 10 mg.
Glycerin Supp., Adult and Infant Sizes.
Hemorrhoidal Rectal Ointment.
Hemorrhoidal Rectal Supp., Formula C-116 and Formula C-119.
Hemorrhoidal Rectal Supp. w/Hydrocortisone Acetate 10 mg or 25 mg/Supp.
Vaginal Sulfa Cream.

Ganeake. (Geneva Pharm) Conjugated Estrogens, 0.625 mg, 1.25 mg or 2.5 mg/Tab. Bot. 100s, 1000s. *Rx.*
Use: Estrogen.

ganglionic blocking agents.
See: Arfonad, Amp. (Roche Laboratories).
Dibenzyline HCl, Cap. (SmithKline Beecham Pharmaceuticals).
Hexamethonium Cl and Bromide (Various Mfr.).
Hydergine, Amp., Tab. (Novartis).
Inversine, Tab. (Merck).
Priscoline HCl, Tab., Vial (Novartis).
Regitine, Amp., Tab. (Novartis).

gangliosides as sodium salts.
Use: Retinitis pigmentosa.
See: Cronassial (FIDIA Pharm).

•**ganirelix acetate.** (gah-nih-RELL-ix ASS-eh-tate) USAN.
Use: Gonad-stimulating principle.

Ganite. (Fujisawa). Gallium nitrate. 25 mg/ml. Vial. 20 ml. *Rx.*
Use: Antihypercalcemic.

Gantanol. (Roche Laboratories) Sulfamethoxazole. **Tab.:** 500mg/Tab. Bot. 100s, Tel-E-Dose 100s. *Rx.*
Use: Anti-infective, sulfonamide.

Gantanol DS. (Roche Laboratories) Sulfamethoxazole 1 g/Tab. Bot. 100s. *Rx.*
Use: Anti-infective, sulfonamide.

Gantrisin Injectable. (Roche Laboratories) Sulfisoxazole diolamine 4 mg/ml. *Rx.*
W/sodium metabisulfite 2 mg. Pkg. 10s.
Use: Anti-infective, sulfonamide.

Gantrisin, Lipo. (Roche Laboratories) Acetyl Sulfisoxazole. *Rx.*
Use: Anti-infective, sulfonamide.
See: Lipo Gantrisin, Susp. (Roche Laboratories).

Garamycin. (Schering Plough) **Cream:** Gentamicin sulfate 1.7 mg (equivalent to gentamicin base 1 mg). Methylparaben 1 mg, butylparaben 4 mg as preservatives, stearic acid, propylene glycol monostearate, isopropyl myristate, propylene glycol, polysorbate 40, sorbitol soln., water/g. Tube 15 g. **Oint.:** Gentamicin sulfate 1.7 mg (equivalent to gentamicin base 1 mg), methylparaben 0.5 mg, propylparaben 0.1 mg in petrolatum base/g. Tube 15 g. *Rx.*
Use: Anti-infective, topical.

Garamycin I.V. Piggyback. (Schering Plough) Gentamicin sulfate equivalent to 1 mg gentamicin base, 8.9 mg sodium Cl, (no preservatives). Inj. Bot. 60 ml (60 mg), 80 ml (80 mg). *Rx.*
Use: Anti-infective, aminoglycoside.

Garamycin Ophthalmic Ointment-Sterile. (Schering Plough) Gentamicin sulfate 3 mg/g. Tube 3.5 g. *Rx.*
Use: Anti-infective, ophthalmic.

Garamycin Ophthalmic Solution, Sterile. (Schering Plough) Gentamicin sulfate 3 mg/ml. Dropper Bot. 5 ml. *Rx.*
Use: Anti-infective, ophthalmic.

gardenal.
See: Phenobarbital. (Various Mfr.).

gardinol type detergents. Aurinol, Cyclopon, Dreft, Drene, Duponol, Lissapol, Maprofix, Modinal, Orvus, Sandopan, Sadipan.
Use: Detergent.

gardol. Sodium Lauryl Sarcosinate.

Garfield. (Menley & James) Vitamin A 2500 IU, D 400 IU, E 15 IU, C 60 mg, folic acid 0.3 mg, Vitamin B_1 1.05 mg, B_2 1.2 mg, B_3 13.5 mg, B_6 1.05 mg, B_{12} 4.5 mcg, sucrose, lactose. Chew. Tab. Bot. 60s. *otc.*
Use: Vitamin supplement.

Garfield Complete w/ Minerals. (Menley & James) Vitamin A 5000 IU, D 400 IU, E 30 IU, C 60 mg, folic acid 0.4 mg, B_1 1.5 mg, B_2 1.7 mg, B_3 20 mg, B_6 2 mg, B_{12} 6 mcg, biotin 40 mcg, B_5 10 mg, iron 18 mg, Ca, Cu, P, I, Mg, zinc 15 mg, aspartame, phenylalanine, sorbital/Chew. Tab. Bot. 60s. *otc.*
Use: Mineral, vitamin supplement.

Garfield Plus Extra C. (Menley & James) Vitamin A 2500 IU, D 400 IU, E 15 IU, C 250 mg, folic acid 0.3 mg, B_1 1.05 mg, B_2 1.2 mg, B_3 13.5 mg, B_6 1.05 mg, B_{12} 4.5 mcg, sucrose, lactose/Chew. Tab. Bot. 60s. *otc.*
Use: Vitamin supplement.

Garfield Plus Iron. (Menley & James) Vitamin A 2500 IU, D 400 IU, E 15 IU, C 60 mg, folic acid 0.3 mg, B_1 1.05 mg, B_2 1.2 mg, B_3 13.5 mg, B_6 1.05 mg, B_{12} 4.5 mcg, iron 15 mcg, sucrose, lactose. Chew. Tab. Bot. 60s. *otc.*
Use: Mineral, vitamin supplement.

Garfields Tea. (Last) Senna leaf powder 68.3%. Bot. 2 oz. *otc.*
Use: Laxative.

Garitabs. (Halsey) Iron 50 mg, vitamins B_1 5 mg, B_2 5 mg, C 75 mg, niacinamide 30 mg, B_5 2 mg, B_6 0.5 mg, B_{12} 3 mcg Bot. 1000s. *otc.*
Use: Mineral, vitamin supplement.

Gari-Tonic Hematinic. (Halsey) Vitamins B_1 5 mg, niacinamide 100 mg, B_2 5 mg, pantothenic acid 4 mg, B_6 1 mg, B_{12} 6 mcg, choline bitartrate 100 mg, iron 100 mg/30 ml Bot. 16 oz. *otc.*
Use: Mineral, vitamin supplement.

garlic. Allium.
Use: Antispasmodic.
See: Allimin, Tab. (Mosso).

garlic capsules. (Miller) Garlic 166 mg/Cap. Bot. 100s. *otc.*
Use: Antispasmodic.

garlic concentrate.
W/Parsley Concentrate.
See: Allimin, Tab. (Mosso).

garlic oil.
See: Natural Garlic Oil, Cap. (Spirt).

garlic oil capsules. (Kirkman Sales) Bot. 100s. *otc.*

Gas Ban. (Roberts Pharm) Calcium carbonate 300 mg, simethicone 40 mg/Tab. Bot. UD 8s, 1000s. *otc.*
Use: Antacid.

Gas Ban DS. (Roberts Pharm) Aluminum hydroxide 400 mg, magnesium hydroxide 400 mg, simethicone 40 mg/5 ml. Liq. Bot. 150 ml. *otc.*
Use: Antacid.

Gas Permeable Daily Cleaner. (PHB Wesley Jessen) Potassium sorbate 0.13%, EDTA 2%, ethoxylated polyoxypropylene glycol, tris (hydroxymethyl) amino methane, hydroxymethylcellulose. Thimerosal free. Sol. Bot. 30 ml. *otc.*
Use: Contact lens care.

Gas Permeable Lens Starter System. (PHB Wesley Jessen) Daily cleanser, Bot. 3 ml, Wetting and soaking soln., Bot. 60 ml, Hydra-Mat II spin cleansing unit. Kit. *otc.*
Use: Contact lens care.

Gas Permeable Wetting & Soaking Solution. (PHB Wesley Jessen) Sterile aqueous, isotonic soln. of low viscosity, buffered to physiological pH. Bot. 60 ml, 120 ml. *otc.*
Use: Contact lens care.

gastric acidifiers.
See: Acidulin, Pulv. (Eli Lilly)
Glutamic Acid HCl (Various Mfr.).

Gastroccult. (SmithKline Diagnostics) Occult blood screening test. In 40s.
Use: Diagnostic aid.

Gastrocrom. (Medeva) Cromolyn sodium 100 mg/Cap. Bot. 100s. *Rx.*
Use: Antiallergic.
See: Cromolyn Sodium.

Gastrografin. (Bristol-Myers Squibb) Diatrizoate methyl-glucamine 66%, sodium diatrizoate 10%. Soln. Bot. 120 ml.
Use: Radiopaque agent.

gastrointestinal tests.
See: Entero-test, Cap. (HDC)
Entero-Test, Ped. Cap. (HDC).
Gastro-Test (HDC).

Gastrosed. (Roberts Pharm) Hyoscyamine sulfate. **Soln.:** 0.125 mg/ml. Dropper Bot. 5 ml. Alcohol free. **Tab.:** 0.125 mg. Bot. 100s. *Rx.*
Use: Anticholinergic, antispasmodic.

Gastro-Test. (HDC) To determine stomach pH and to diagnose and locate gastric bleeding. Test 25s.
Use: Diagnostic aid.

Gas-X. (Novartis) Simethicone 80 mg/Chew. Tab. Pkg. 12s, 30s. *otc.*
Use: Antiflatulent.

Gas-X, Extra Strength. (Novartis) Si-

methicone 125 mg, sorbitol/Chew. Tab. Box 30s, 100s. *otc.*
Use: Antiflatulent.

•**gauze, absorbent.** U.S.P. 23.
Use: Surgical aid.

•**gauze, petrolatum.** U.S.P. 23.
Use: Surgical aid.

Gaviscon. (SmithKline Beecham Pharmaceuticals) Aluminum hydroxide 80 mg, magnesium trisilicate 20 mg, alginic acid, sodium bicarbonate, sucrose, calcium stearate. Chew. Tab. Bot. 30s, 100s. *otc.*
Use: Antacid.

Gaviscon-2, Double Strength Tablets. (SmithKline Beecham Pharmaceuticals) Aluminum hydroxide 160 mg, magnesium trisilicate 40 mg, alginic acid, sodium bicarbonate, sucrose, Chew. Tab. Bot. 48s. *otc.*
Use: Antacid.

Gaviscon Extra Strength Relief Formula Liquid. (SmithKline Beecham Pharmaceuticals) Aluminum hydroxide 254 mg, magnesium carbonate 237.5 mg, parabens, EDTA, saccharin, sorbitol, simethicone, sodium alginate/5 ml. Bot. 355 ml. *otc.*
Use: Antacid.

Gaviscon Extra Strength Relief Formula Tablets. (SmithKline Beecham Pharmaceuticals) Aluminum hydroxide 160 mg, magnesium carbonate 105 mg, alginic acid, sodium bicarbonate, sucrose, calcium stearate. Chew. Tab. Bot. 30s, 100s. *otc.*
Use: Antacid.

Gaviscon Liquid. (SmithKline Beecham Pharmaceuticals) Aluminum hydroxide 31.7 mg, magnesium carbonate 119.3 mg/5 ml Bot. 177 ml, 355 ml. *otc.*
Use: Antacid.

GBA.
See: Gamma hydroxybutyrate.

G.B.H. Lotion. (Century Pharm) Gamma benzene hexachloride 1%. Bot. 2 oz, pt, gal.
Use: Scabicide, pediculicide.

G.B.S. (Forest Pharmaceutical) Dehydrocholic acid 125 mg, phenobarbital 8 mg, homatropine methylbromide 2.5 mg/Tab. 100s, 1000s. *Rx.*
Use: Hydrocholeretic.

G-CSF.
See: Neupogen (Amgen).

Gebauer's 114. (Gebauer) Dichlorotetrafluoroethane 100%. Can 8 oz.
Use: Anesthetic, local.

Gee-Gee. (Jones Medical Industries) Guaifenesin 200 mg/Tab. Bot. 1000s. *otc.*
Use: Expectorant.

Geladine. (Barth's) Gelatin, protein, vitamin D/Cap. Bot. 100s, 500s. *otc.*

Gelamal. (Halsey) Magnesium-aluminum hydroxide gel. Bot. 12 oz. *otc.*
Use: Antacid.

•**gelatin.** N.F. 18.
Use: Pharmaceutic aid (encapsulating, suspending agent, tablet binder, tablet coating agent).

•**gelatin film, absorbable.** U.S.P. 23.
Use: Local hemostatic.
See: Gelfilm (Pharmacia & Upjohn).

gelatin film, sterile.
See: Neupogen (Amgen).

gelatin powder, sterile.
See: Gelfoam Powder (Pharmacia & Upjohn).

gelatin sponge.
See: Gelfilm (Pharmacia & Upjohn).

•**gelatin sponge, absorbable.** U.S.P. 23.
Use: Hemostatic, local.
See: Gelfoam, Paks (Pharmacia & Upjohn).

gelatin, zinc.
See: Zinc gelatin. (Various Mfr.).

Gel-Clean. (PHB Wesley Jessen) Gel formulated with nonionic surfactant. Tube 30 g. *otc.*
Use: Contact lens care.

Gelfilm. (Pharmacia & Upjohn) Sterile, absorbable gelatin film. Envelope 1s. 100 mm × 125 mm. Also available as Ophth. Sterile 25 × 50 mm. Box 6s. *Rx.*
Use: Hemostatic, topical.

Gelfoam. (Pharmacia & Upjohn) **Sterile Sponges:**
Size 12-3 mm. 20 × 60 mm (12 sq. cm) × 3 mm. *Rx.*
Box 4 sponges in individual envelopes. *Rx.*
Size 12-7 mm. 20 × 60 mm (12 sq. cm.) × 7 mm.
Box 12 sponges in individual envelopes, jar 4 sponges. *Rx.*
Size 50-10 mm. 62.5 × 80 mm (50 sq. cm.) × 10 mm. Box 4 sponges in individual envelopes. *Rx.*
Size 100-10 mm. 80 × 125 mm (100 sq. cm.) × 10 mm. *Rx.*
Box 6 sponges in individual envelopes. *Rx.*
Size 200-10 mm. 80 × 250 mm (200 sq. cm.) × 10 mm.
Box 6 sponges in individual envelopes. *Rx.*

Compressed Size 100. (intended primarily for application in the dry state). 80 × 125 mm. Boxes of 6 sponges in individual envelopes. *Rx.*
Packs: Packs size 2 cm. (Designed particularly for nasal packing). 2 × 40 cm. Single jar. (Packing cavities). *Rx.*
Size 6 cm. 6 × 40 cm. Box 6 sponges in individual envelopes. *Rx.*
Use: Hemostatic, topical.

Gelfoam Dental Pack. (Pharmacia & Upjohn) Size 4, 20 mm × 20 mm × 7 mm. Jar 15 sponges. *Rx.*
Use: Hemostatic, topical.

Gelfoam Powder. (Pharmacia & Upjohn) Sterile Jar 1 g. *Rx.*
Use: Hemostatic, topical.

Gelfoam Prostatectomy Cones. (Pharmacia & Upjohn) Prostatectomy cones (for use with Foley catheter). 13 cm, 18 cm in diameter. Box 6s. *Rx.*
Use: Hemostatic.

Gel Jet Gelatin Capsules. (Kirkman Sales) Bot. 100s, 250s.

Gel Kam. (Scherer) Fluoride 0.1% (stannous fluoride 0.4%). Cinnamon flavor. Gel. Bot. w/applicator tip 69 g, 105 g, 129 g. *Rx.*
Use: Dental caries agent.

Gelocast. (Beiersdorf) Unna's Boot medicated bandage: Semi-rigid cast impregnated with zinc oxide mixtures. Box 4 inches × 10 yd, 3 inches × 10 yd.
Use: Unna's cast dressing.

Gelpirin. Acetaminophen 125 mg, aspirin 240 mg, caffeine 32 mg. Tab. Bot. 100s, 1000s. *otc.*
Use: Analgesic combination.

Gelpirin-CCF. (Alra Laboratories) Acetaminophen 325 mg, guaifenesin 25 mg, chlorpheniramine maleate 1 mg, phenylpropanolamine HCl 12.5 mg/Tab. Bot. 50s. *otc.*
Use: Analgesic, decongestant, expectorant.

gelsemium. (Various Mfr.) Pkg. oz.
Use: Neuralgia.
W/APC.
See: APC Combinations.

gelsemium w/combinations.
See: Briacel, Tab. (Briar).
Bricor, Tab. (Briar).
Cystitol, Tab. (Briar).
Ricor, Tab. (Vortech).
UB, Tab. (Scrip).
Urisan-P, Tab. (Sandia).
U-Tract, Tab. (Jones Medical Industries).

gelsolin, recombinant human. (Biogen)
Use: Cystic fibrosis. [Orphan drug]

Gel-Tin. (Young Dental) Fluoride 0.1% (from stannous flouride 0.4%) Gel Bot. 57 g, 623 g. *Rx.*
Use: Dental caries agent.

•**gemcadiol.** (JEM-kah-DIE-ole) USAN.
Use: Antihyperlipoproteinemic.

•**gemcitabine.** (JEM-sit-ah-BEAN) USAN.
Use: Antineoplastic.

•**gemcitabine hydrochloride.** (JEM-sit-ah-BEAN) USAN.
Use: Antineoplastic.
See: Gemzar (Eli Lilly).

•**gemeprost.** (JEH-meh-PRAHST) USAN.
Use: Prostaglandin.

•**gemfibrozil.** (gem-FIE-broe-ZILL) U.S.P. 23.
Use: Antihyperlipidemic.
See: Lopid, Cap. (Parke-Davis).

gemfibrozil, (Various Mfr.) 300 mg/Cap., Bot. 100s, 500s, 1000s. 600 mg/Tab., Bot. 60s, 100s, 500s, 1000s.
Use: Antihyperlipidemic.

Gemzar. (Eli Lilly) Gemcitabine HCl 20 mg/ml/Pow for Inj. Vials 10 and 50 ml. *Rx.*
Use: Antineoplastic.

Genac Tablets. (Zenith Goldline) Triprolidine HCl 2.5 mg, pseudoephedrine HCl 60 mg/Tab. Bot. 24s, 100s. *otc.*
Use: Antihistamine, decongestant.

Genacol Tablets. (Zenith Goldline) Pseudoephedrine HCl 30 mg, chlorpheniramine maleate 2 mg, dextromethorphan HBr 10 mg, acetaminophen 325 mg/Tab. Bot. 50s. *otc.*
Use: Analgesic, antihistamine, antitussive, decongestant.

Genagesic Tabs. (Zenith Goldline) Propoxyphene HCl 165 mg, acetaminophen 650 mg/Tab. Bot. 100s, 500s. *c-IV.*
Use: Analgesic combination, narcotic.

Genahist. (Zenith Goldline) Diphenhydramine HCl 12.5 mg/5 ml, alcohol 14%. Liq. Bot. 120 ml. *otc.*
Use: Antihistamine.

Genahist Liquid. (Zenith Goldline) Diphenhydramine 12.5 mg/5 ml. Elix. 120 ml. *otc.*
Use: Antihistamine.

Genallerate Tablets. (Zenith Goldline) Chlorpheniramine maleate 4 mg, lactose/Tab. Bot. 24s. *otc.*
Use: Antihistamine.

Genamin Cold Syrup. (Zenith Goldline) Phenylpropanolamine HCl 6.25 mg, chlorpheniramine maleate 1 mg. Alcohol free. In 118 ml. *otc.*

Use: Antihistamine, decongestant.

Genamin Expectorant. (Zenith Goldline) Phenylpropanolamine 12.5 mg, guaifenesin 100 mg, alcohol 5%. In 120 ml. *otc.*
Use: Decongestant, expectorant.

Genapap, Children's Chewable Tabs. (Zenith Goldline) Acetaminophen 80 mg/Tab. Bot. 30s. *otc.*
Use: Analgesic.

Genapap, Children's Elixir. (Zenith Goldline) Acetaminophen 160 mg/5 ml. Cherry flavor. Bot. 120 ml. *otc.*
Use: Analgesic.

Genapap, Infants' Drops. (Zenith Goldline) Acetaminophen 100 mg/ml, alcohol 7%. Soln. Dropper bot. 15 ml. *otc.*
Use: Analgesic.

Genapap Tablets. (Zenith Goldline) Acetaminophen 325 mg/Tab. Bot. 100s. *otc.*
Use: Analgesic.

Genapax. (Key Pharm) Gentian violet 5 mg/tampon. Box 12s.
Use: Antifungal, vaginal.

Genaphed Tablets. (Zenith Goldline) Pseudoephedrine HCl 30 mg/Tab. Bot. 24s, 100s. *otc.*
Use: Decongestant.

Genasal. (Zenith Goldline) Oxymetazoline 0.05%. Soln. 15 ml, 30 ml. *otc.*
Use: Decongestant.

Genasoft Capsules. (Zenith Goldline) Docusate sodium 100 mg/Cap. Bot. 60s. *otc.*
Use: Laxative, stool softener.

Genasoft Plus Capsules. (Zenith Goldline) Docusate sodium 100 mg, casanthranol 30 mg/Cap. Bot. 60s. *otc.*
Use: Laxative, stool softener.

Genaspor Antifungal Cream. (Zenith Goldline) Tolnaftate 1%. Bot. 15 g. *otc.*
Use: Antifungal, topical.

Genasyme Tablets. (Zenith Goldline) Simethicone 80 mg/Tab. Bot. 100s. *otc.*
Use: Antiflatulent.

Genatap Elixir. (Zenith Goldline) Brompheniramine maleate 2 mg, phenylpropanolamine HCl 12.5 mg/5 ml. Bot. 118 ml. *otc.*
Use: Antihistamine, decongestant.

Genaton. (Zenith Goldline) Aluminum hydroxide 80 mg, magnesium trisilicate 20 mg, alginic acid, sodium bicarbonate, sodium 18.4 mg, sucrose, sugar. Chew. Tab. Bot. 100s. *otc.*
Use: Antacid.

Genaton, Extra Strength Tablets. (Zenith Goldline) Aluminum hydroxide 160 mg, magnesium carbonate 105 mg, alginic acid, sodium bicarbonate, sodium 29.9 mg, sucrose, calcium stearate. Chew. Tab. Bot. 100s. *otc.*
Use: Antacid.

Genaton Liquid. (Zenith Goldline) Aluminum hydroxide 31.7 mg, magnesium carbonate 137.3 mg, sodium alginate, sodium 13 mg, EDTA, saccharin, sorbitol/5 ml. Bot. 355 ml. *otc.*
Use: Antacid.

genatropine hydrochloride. (jen-AT-row-peen) Atropine-N-oxide HCl. Aminoxytropine Tropate HCl.
See: X-tro, Cap. (Xttrium).

Genatuss DM Syrup. (Zenith Goldline) Dextromethorphan HBr 10 mg, guaifenesin 100 mg. Bot. 120 ml. *otc.*
Use: Antitussive, expectorant.

Genatuss Syrup. (Zenith Goldline) Guaifenesin 100 mg/5 ml, alcohol 3.5%. Bot. 120 ml. *otc.*
Use: Expectorant.

Gen-bee with C. (Zenith Goldline) Vitamins B_1 15 mg, B_2 10.2 mg, B_3 50 mg, B_5 10 mg, B_6 5 mg, C 300 mg/Cap. Bot. 130s, 1000s. *otc.*
Use: Vitamin supplement.

Gencalc 600 Tablets. (Zenith Goldline) Calcium 600 mg (from calcium carbonate 1.5 g)/Tab. Bot. 60s. *otc.*
Use: Mineral supplement.

Gencept. (Gencon) **0.5/35:** Norethindrone 0.5 mg, ethinyl estradiol, 35 mcg/Tab (with 7 inert tabs) Pkgs 21s and 28s; **1/35:** norethindrone 1 mg, ethinyl estradiol 35 mcg/Tab (with 7 inert tabs) Pkgs 21s and 28s; **10/11:** norethindrone 0.5 mg and 1 mg, ethinyl estradiol 35 mcg/Tab (with 7 inert tabs). Pkg 21s and 28s. *Rx.*
Use: Contraceptive.

Gencold Capsules. (Zenith Goldline) Phenylpropanolamine HCl 75 mg, chlorpheniramine maleate 8 mg/SR Tab. Pkg. 10s. *otc.*
Use: Antihistamine, decongestant.

Gendecon. (Zenith Goldline) Phenylephrine HCl 5 mg, chlorpheniramine maleate 2 mg, acetaminophen 325 mg/Tab. Bot. 50s. *otc.*
Use: Analgesic, antihistamine, decongestant.

Genebs Extra Strength Caplets. (Zenith Goldline) Acetaminophen 500 mg/Cap. Bot. 100s, 1000s. *otc.*
Use: Analgesic.

Genebs Extra Strength Tablets. (Zenith Goldline) Acetaminophen 500 mg/Tab.

Bot. 100s, 1000s. *otc.*
Use: Analgesic.

Genebs Tablets. (Zenith Goldline) Acetaminophen 325 mg/Tab. Bot. 100s, 1000s. *otc.*
Use: Analgesic.

Generet-500. (Zenith Goldline) Iron 105 mg, Vitamins B_1 6 mg, B_2 6 mg, B_3 30 mg, B_5 10 mg, B_6 5 mg, B_{12} 25 mcg, C (as sodium ascorbate) 500 mg. TR Tab. Bot. 60s. *otc.*
Use: Mineral, vitamin supplement.

Generix-T. (Zenith Goldline) Iron 15 mg, vitamins A 10,000 IU, D 400 IU, E 5.5 mg, B_1 15 mg, B_2 10 mg, B_3 100 mg, B_5 10 mg, B_6 2 mg, B_{12} 7.5 mcg, C 150 mg, Cu, I, Mg, Mn, zinc 1.5 mg/Tab. Bot. 100s. *otc.*
Use: Mineral, vitamin supplement.

GenESA. (Gensia Automedics) Arbutamine HCl 0.05 mg/ml. Inj. Syringe 20 mg (containing 1 mg arbutamine). *Rx.*
Use: Diagnostic aid.

Genex Caps. (Zenith Goldline) Phenylpropanolamine HCl 18 mg, acetaminophen 325 mg/Cap. Bot. 100s, 1000s. *otc.*
Use: Analgesic, decongestant.

Geneye. (Zenith Goldline) Tetrahydrozoline HCl 0.05%. Drop. Bot. 15 ml. *otc.*
Use: Mydriatic, vasoconstrictor.

Geneye Extra. (Zenith Goldline) Tetrahydrozoline HCl 0.05%, PEG 400 1%, benzalkonium Cl, EDTA/Drops. 15 ml. *otc.*
Use: Ophthalmic vasoconstrictor.

genital herpes treatment.
See: Acyclovir.
Zovirax Cap., Oint. (GlaxoWellcome).

Genite. (Zenith Goldline) Pseudoephedrine HCl 10 mg, doxylamine succinate 1.25 mg, dextromethorphan HBr 5 mg, acetaminophen 167 mg, alcohol 25%/5 ml. Bot. 177 ml. *otc.*
Use: Analgesic, antihistamine, antitussive, decongestant.

genitourinary irrigants.
See: Acetic acid for irrigation (Various Mfr.).
Glycine (Aminoacetic Acid) For Irrigation (Various Mfr.).
Neosporin G.U. Irrigant, Soln. (Burroughs-Wellcome).
Renacidin, Pow., Soln. (Guardian Laboratories).
Resectisol, Soln. (McGaw).
Sorbitol (Various Mfr.).
Sorbitol-Mannitol (Abbott Laboratories).
Sodium Chloride for Irrigation (Various Mfr.).
Sterile Water for Irrigation (Various Mfr.).
Suby's Solution G (Various Mfr.).

Gen-K Powder. (Zenith Goldline) Potassium Cl. Pow. 20 mEq/packet. Box 30s. *Rx.*
Use: Electrolyte supplement.

Gen-K Tabs. (Zenith Goldline) Effervescent potassium. Bot. 30s. *Rx.*
Use: Electrolyte supplement.

Genna Tablets. (Zenith Goldline) Senna concentrate 217 mg/Tab. Bot. 100s, 1000s. *otc.*
Use: Laxative.

Gennin Tablets. (Zenith Goldline) Buffered aspirin 5 gr. Bot. 100s. *otc.*
Use: Analgesic.

genophyllin.
See: Aminophylline (Various Mfr.).

Genoptic Liquifilm Sterile Ophthalmic Solution. (Allergan) Gentamicin sulfate 3 mg/ml. Bot. 1 ml, 5 ml. *Rx.*
Use: Anti-infective, ophthalmic.

Genoptic S.O.P. Sterile Ophthalmic Ointment. (Allergan) Gentamicin sulfate 3 mg/g. Oint. Tube 3.5 g. *Rx.*
Use: Anti-infective, ophthalmic.

Genora 0.5/35 Tablets. (Rugby) Norethindrone 0.5 mg, ethinyl estradiol 0.035 mg/Tab. Pkg. 21s; 28s (7 inert tab.) *Rx.*
Use: Contraceptive.

Genora 1/35-21 Tablets. (Rugby) Norethindrone 1 mg, ethinyl estradiol 0.035 mg/Tab. Pkg. 126s (6-pak). *Rx.*
Use: Contraceptive.

Genora 1/35-28 Tablets. (Rugby) Norethindrone 1 mg, ethinylestradiol 0.035 mg/Tab., 7 inert tab. Pkg. 168s (6-pak). *Rx.*
Use: Contraceptive.

Genora 1/50-21 Tablets. (Rugby) Norethindrone 1 mg, mestranol 0.05 mg/Tab. Pkg. 126s (6-pak). *Rx.*
Use: Contraceptive.

Genora 1/50-28 Tablets. (Rugby) Norethindrone 1 mg, mestranol 0.05 mg/Tab., 7 inert tab. Pkg. 168s (6-pak). *Rx.*
Use: Contraceptive.

Genotropin. (Pharmacia & Upjohn) Somatropin 1.5 mg (≈4 IU/ml), preservative free. In 1.5 mg Intra-Mix two-chamber cartridge with pressure-release needle. 5s. Somatropin 5.8 mg (≈15 IU/ml). In 5.8 Intra-Mix two-chamber cartridge with pressure-release needle. 1s, 5s. Pow. for Inj. *Rx.*
Use: Hormone.

Genprep Ointment. (Zenith Goldline)

Live yeast cell derivative supplying 2000 units skin respiratory factor/oz of ointment w/shark liver oil 3%, phenylmercuric nitrate 1:10,000. Tube 2 oz. *otc.*
Use: Anorectal preparation.

Genpril. (Zenith Goldline) Ibuprofen 200 mg. Tab. 50s, 100s. *otc.*
Use: Analgesic, NSAID.

Genprin. (Zenith Goldline) Aspirin 325 mg. Tab. 100s. *otc.*
Use: Analgesic.

gensalate sodium. Sodium gentisate. (Sodium salt of 2,5-dihydroxybenzoic acid).
Use: Analgesic.

Gensan Tablets. (Zenith Goldline) Aspirin 400 mg, caffeine 32 mg/Tab. Bot. 100s. *otc.*
Use: Analgesic combination.

Gentacidin Ophthalmic Ointment. (Ciba Vision Ophthalmics) Gentamicin 3 mg/g. Oint. Tube 3.5 g. *Rx.*
Use: Anti-infective, ophthalmic.

Gentacidin Ophthalmic Solution. (Ciba Vision Ophthalmics) Gentamicin sulfate 3 mg/ml. Soln. Bot. 5 ml. *Rx.*
Use: Anti-infective, ophthalmic.

Gentafair. (Bausch & Lomb) **Oint.:** Gentamicin 3 mg/g with liquid lanolin, white petrolatum, mineral oil, parabens. Tube 3.75 g, 15 g. **Soln.:** Gentamicin 3 mg/ml, polyoxyl 40 stearate, polyethylene glycol. Dropper bot. 5 ml, 15 ml. *Rx.*
Use: Anti-infective, ophthalmic.

Gentak. (Akorn) **Oint.:** Gentamicin 3 mg/g. Tube 3.5 g. **Soln.:** Gentamicin 3 mg/ml. Bot. 5 ml, 15 ml. *Rx.*
Use: Anti-infective, ophthalmic.

gentamicin impregnated PMMA beads on surgical wire.
Use: Chronic osteomyelitis. [Orphan drug]

gentamicin liposome injection.
Use: Mycobacterium avium-intracellulare infection. [Orphan drug]

•**gentamicin sulfate.** (JEN-tuh-MY-sin) U.S.P. 23.
Use: Anti-infective.
See: Genoptic Inj. (Allergan).
Gentacidin, Preps. (Ciba Vision Ophthalmics).
Gentak, Preps. (Akorn).

gentamicin sulfate. (Schering Plough) Produced by *Micromonospora purpurea.* (Various Mfr.) **Ophthalmic Oint.:** 3 mg/g Tube 3.5 g; **Ophthalmic Soln.:** 3 mg/ml Bot. 5 ml, 15 ml. **Inj.:** 40 mg/ml. Vial 2 ml, 20 ml. Cartridge-needle units 1.5 ml, 2 ml. **Ped. Inj.:** 10 mg/ml. Vial 2 ml. *Rx.*
Use: Anti-infective.

gentamicin and prednisolone acetate ophthalmic suspension.
Use: Anti-infective, anti-inflammatory.

•**gentian violet.** (JEN-shun) U.S.P. 23. *Formerly Methylrosaniline Chloride.*
Use: Anti-infective, topical.

gentian violet. (JEN-shun) (Various Mfr.) Gentian violet 1%, 2%. Soln. Bot. 30 ml. *otc.*
Use: Anti-infective, topical.

gentisate sodium.

•**gentisic acid ethanolamide,** N.F. 18.
Use: Pharmaceutic aid, complexing agent.

Gentlax. (Blair Laboratories) Standardized senna concentrate 326 mg, malt extract, sucrose/Gran. 180 g. *otc.*
Use: Laxative.

Gentlax S Tablets. (Blair Laboratories) Standardized senna concentrate 187 mg, docusate sodium 50 mg. Tab. Bot. 30s, 60s. *otc.*
Use: Laxative.

Gentle Nature Natural Vegetable Laxative. (Novartis) Sennosides A and B as calcium salts. 20 mg/Tab. Box 16s, 32s. *otc.*
Use: Laxative.

Gentle Shampoo. (Ulmer) Bot. 4 oz, gal. *otc.*
Use: Dermatologic, hair.

Gentran 40. (Baxter) Dextran 40 10% w/ sodium Cl 0.9% or Dextran 40 10% w/ dextrose 5%. Inj. Plastic Bot. 500 ml. *Rx.*
Use: Plasma expander.

Gentran 70. (Baxter) Dextran 70 6% w/ sodium Cl 0.9%. Inj. Plastic Bot. 500 ml. *Rx.*
Use: Plasma expander.

Gentran 75. (Baxter) Dextran 75 6% in sodium Cl 0.9%. Inj. Bot. 500 ml. *Rx.*
Use: Plasma expander.

Gentrasul. (Bausch & Lomb) Gentamicin 3 mg. **Oint.:** 3.5 g. **Soln.:** Dropper bot. 5 ml. *Rx.*
Use: Anti-infective, ophthalmic.

Gentz Rectal Wipes. (Roxane) Pramoxine HCl 1%, alcloxa 0.2%, witch hazel 50%, propylene glycol 10%. Box 100s, 120s (individually wrapped disposable wipes). *otc.*
Use: Anorectal preparation.

Genuine Bayer Aspirin. (Bayer Corp) Aspirin 325 mg/FC Tab. Bot. 12s, 24s,

50s, 200s, 300s. *otc.*
Use: Analgesic.

Gen-Xene. (Alra Laboratories) Clorazepate dipotassium 3.75 mg, 7.5 mg or 15 mg/Tab. Bot. 30s, 100s, 500s, UD 100s. *c-IV.*
Use: Anticonvulsant, anxiolytic.

Geocillin. (Roerig) Carbenicillin indanyl sodium 382 mg/Tab. Bot. 100s, UD 100s. *Rx.*
Use: Anti-infective, penicillin.

Geopen. (Roerig) Carbenicillin disodium. Inj. **Vial:** 1 g, 2 g, 5 g. Pkg. 10s. **Piggyback Vial:** 2 g, 5 g, 10 g. **Bulk Pharmacy Pack:** 30 g. *Rx.*
Use: Anti-infective, penicillin.

•**gepirone hydrochloride.** (jeh-PIE-rone) USAN.
Use: Anxiolytic.

Gera Plus. (Towne) Iron 50 mg, vitamins B_1 5 mg, B_2 5 mg, C 75 mg, niacinamide 30 mg, calcium pantothenate 2 mg, B_6 0.5 mg, B_{12} 3 mcg/Tab. Bot. 100s. *otc.*
Use: Mineral, vitamin supplement.

Geravim. (Major) Vitamins B_1 0.83 mg, B_2 0.42 mg, B_3 8.3 mg, B_5 1.67 mg, B_6 0.17 mg, B_{12} 0.17 mg, I, Fe 2.5 mg, Zn 0.3 mg, choline, Mn, alcohol 18%. Liq. Bot. pt., gal. *otc.*
Use: Mineral, vitamin supplement.

Geravite Elixir. (Roberts Pharm) Elix.: Vitamins B_1 0.3 mg, B_2 0.4 mg, B_3 33.3 mg, B_{12} 3.3 mcg, L-lysine, alcohol 15%, parabens, sorbitol, sucrose. Bot. 480 ml. *otc.*
Use: Mineral, vitamin supplement.

Gerber Baby Formula Low Iron Formula. (Bristol-Myers) Protein (from non-fat milk) 14.7 g, carbohydrate (from lactose) 71.3 g, fat (from palm olein, soy, coconut and high oleic sunflower oils) 36 g, linoleic acid 5.9 g, vitamins A, D, E, K, C, B_1, B_2, B_3, B_5, B_6, B_{12}, folic acid, biotin, choline, inositol, Ca, P, Mg, Fe 3.4 mg, Zn, Mn, Cu, I, Na 220 mg, K 720 mg, Cl, taurine, calories per L 666.7. **Ready to use liq.:** Bot. 943 ml. **Concentrated liq.:** Bot. 433 ml. **Pow.:** Can 457 g and 914 g. *otc.*
Use: Nutritional supplement.

Gerber Baby Formula with Iron. (Bristol-Myers) Protein (from non-fat milk) 14.7 g, carbohydrate (from lactose) 71.3 g, fat (from palm olein, soy, coconut and high oleic sunflower oils) 36 g, with linoleic acid 5.9 g, vitamins A, D, E, K, C, B_1, B_2, B_6, B_{12}, B_3, folic acid, B_5, biotin, choline, inositol, Ca, P, Mg, Fe 12 mg, Zn, Mn, Cu, I, Na 220 mg, K 720 mg, Cl, taurine, calories per L 666.7./concentrated Liq. Bot. 943 ml. *otc.*
Use: Nutritional supplement.

Geref. (Serono Labs) Sermorelin acetate 50 mcg (lyophilized). Pow. for Inj. Amp. 2 ml w/sodium Cl. 0.9%.
Use: Diagnostic aid.

Geri-All-D. (Barth's) Vitamins A 10,000 IU, D 400 IU, B_1 7 mg, B_2 14 mg, C 200 mg, niacin 4.17 mg, B_{12} 25 mcg, E 50 IU, B_6 0.35 mg, pantothenic acid 0.63 mg, trace minerals and other factors. 2 Cap. Bot. 1 mo., 3 mo. and 6 mo. supply of Geri-All regular and Geri-All-D. *otc.*
Use: Mineral, vitamin supplement.

geriatric supplements w/multivitamins/minerals.
See: Geravite, Elix. (Roberts Pharm).
Gerimed, Tab. (Fielding).
Geriplex FS, Caps. (Parke-Davis).
Hep-Forte, Cap. (Marlyn).
Megadose, Tab. (Arco).
Mega VM-80, Tab. (NBTY).
Optivite P.M.T., Tab. (Optimox).
Strovite Plus, Tab. (Everett Laboratories).
Ultra-Freeda, Tab. (Freeda Vitamins)
Ultra-Freeda Iron Free, Tab. (Freeda Vitamins).
Vigortol, Liq. (Rugby).
Viminate, Elix. (Various Mfr).
Vita-Plus G Softgels (Scot-Tussin Pharmacal).

Geriatroplex. (Morton) Cyanocobalamin 30 mcg, liver inj. 0.1 ml vitamins B_{12} activity 2 mcg, ferrous gluconate 50 mg, B_2 1.5 mg, calcium pantothenate 2.5 mg, niacinamide 100 mg, citric acid 16.4 mg, sodium citrate 23.6 mg/2 ml. Vial 30 ml. *otc.*
Use: Mineral, vitamin supplement.

Geri-Derm. (Barth's) Vitamins A 400,000 IU, D 40,000 IU, E 200 IU, panthenol 800 mg/4 oz. Jar 4 oz. *otc.*
Use: Skin supplement.

Geridium Tablets. (Zenith Goldline) Phenazopyridine HCl 100 mg or 200 mg/Tab. Bot. 100s, 1000s. *Rx.*
Use: Analgesic; anti-infective, urinary.

Gerifort Plus. (A.P.C.) Vitamins A 10,000 IU, B_1 5 mg, B_2 6 mg, B_6 2 mg, C 75 mg, D-2 1000 IU, niacinamide 60 mg, iron 10 mg, calcium 115 mg, phosphorous 83 mg, iodine 0.1 mg, calcium pantothenate 10 mg, d-alpha tocopheryl acid succinate 3 IU, cobalamin concentrate 3 mcg, choline bitartrate 70 mg, inositol 35 mg, biotin 15 mcg, Zn 0.2 mg, magnesium 2 mg, manganese

0.5 mg, potassium 0.15 mg/Amcap. Bot. 100s. *otc.*
Use: Mineral, vitamin supplement.

Gerilets. (Abbott Laboratories) Vitamins A 5000 IU, D 400 IU, E 45 IU, C 90 mg (from sodium ascorbate), folic acid 0.4 mg, B_1 2.25 mg, B_2 2.6 mg, niacin 30 mg, B_6 3 mg, B_{12} 9 mcg, biotin 0.45 mg, pantothenic acid 15 mg, iron 27 mg (from ferrous sulfate)/Tab. Bot. 100s. *otc.*
Use: Mineral, vitamin supplement.

Gerimal. (Rugby) Ergoloid mesylates 0.5 mg or 1 mg/**Sublingual Tab.:** Bot. 100s, 500s, 1000s; 1 mg/**Oral Tab.:** Bot. 100s, 500s, 1000s. *Rx.*
Use: Psychotherapeutic agent.

Gerimed. (Fielding) Vitamins A 5000 IU, D 400 IU, E 30 mg, B_1 3 mg, B_2 3 mg, B_3 25 mg, B_6 2 mg, B_{12} 6 mcg, C 120 mg, calcium 370 mg, zinc 15 mg, Mg, P/Tab. Bot. 60s. *otc.*
Use: Mineral, vitamin supplement.

Gerineed. (Hanlon) Vitamins A 5000 IU, B_1 20 mg, B_2 5 mg, niacinamide 20 mg, B_6 0.5 mg, calcium pantothenate 5 mg, B_{12} 5 mcg, rutin 25 mg, C 50 mg, E 10 IU, choline 50 mg, inositol 50 mg, calcium lactate 1.64 mg, iron sulfate 10 mg, copper 1 mg, iodine 0.5 mg, manganese 1 mg, magnesium sulfate 1 mg, potassium sulfate 5 mg, zinc sulfate 0.5 mg/Cap. Bot. 100s. *otc.*
Use: Mineral, vitamin supplement.

Geriot. (Zenith Goldline) Iron 50 mg (from ferrous sulfate), A 6000 IU, D 400 IU, E 30 IU, B_1 1.5 mg, B_2 1.7 mg, B_3 20 mg, B_5 10 mg, B_6 2 mg, B_{12} 6 mcg, C 60 mg, folic acid 0.4 mg, biotin 45 mcg, Ca, Cl, Cr, Cu, I, K, Mg, Mn, Mo, Ni, P, Se, Si, Sn, V, Zn, vitamin K/Tab. Bot. 100s. *otc.*
Use: Mineral, vitamin supplement.

Geri-Plus. (Health for Life Brands) Vitamins A 12,500 IU, D 1200 IU, B_1 15 mg, B_2 10 mg, C 75 mg, niacinamide 30 mg, calcium pantothenate 2 mg, B_6 0.5 mg, E 5 IU, Brewer's yeast 10 mg, B_{12} 15 mcg, iron 11.58 mg, desiccated liver 15 mg, choline bitartrate 30 mg, inositol 30 mg, calcium 59 mg, phosphorous 45 mg, zinc 0.68 mg, francium dicalcium phosphate 200 mg, Mn, enzymatic factors, amino acids/Cap. Bot. 50s, 100s, 1000s. *otc.*
Use: Mineral, vitamin supplement.

Geri-Plus Elixir. (Health for Life Brands) Vitamins B_1 25 mg, B_2 10 mg, B_6 1 mg, niacinamide 100 mg, calcium pantothenate 5 mg, B_{12} 20 mcg, iron ammonium citrate 100 mg, choline 200 mg, inositol 100 mg, magnesium Cl 2 mg, manganese citrate 2 mg, zinc acetate 2 mg, amino acids/fl oz. Bot. pt. *otc.*
Use: Mineral, vitamin supplement.

Geritol Complete Tablets. (SmithKline Beecham Pharmaceuticals) Vitamins A 6000 IU, E 30 IU, C 60 mg, folic acid 400 mcg, B_1 1.5 mg, B_2 1.7 mg, B_3 20 mg, B_6 2 mg, B_{12} 6 mcg, D 400 IU, K, biotin 45 mcg, B_5 10 mg, iron 18 mg, Ca, Cl, Cr, Cu, I, K, Mg, Mn, Mo, Ni, P, Se, Si, Sn, V, Zn, vitamin K /Tab. Bot. 14s, 40s, 100s, 180s. *otc.*
Use: Mineral, vitamin supplement.

Geritol Extended Caplets. (SmithKline Beecham) Capl.: Iron 10 mg, vitamins A 3333 IU, D 200 IU, E 15 IU, B_1 1.2 mg, B_2 1.4 mg, B_3 15 mg, B_6 2 mg, B_{12} 2 mg, C 60 mg, folic acid 0.2 mg, vitamin K, Ca, I, Mg, Se, Zn 15 mg. Bot. 40s, 100s. *otc.*
Use: Mineral, vitamin supplement.

Geritol Tonic Liquid. (SmithKline Beecham Pharmaceuticals) Iron 18 mg, Vitamins B_1 2.5 mg, B_2 2.5 mg, B_3 50 mg, B_5 2 mg, B_6 0.5 mg, methionine 25 mg, choline bitartrate 50 mg/15 ml. Alcohol 12%. Bot. 120 ml, 360 ml. *otc.*
Use: Mineral, vitamin supplement.

Gerivite. (Zenith Goldline) Liq.: Vitamins B_1 0.8 mg, B_2 0.4 mg, B_3 8.3 mg, B_5 1.7 mg, B_6 0.2 mg, B_{12} 0.2 mcg, iron 0.3 mg, Zn 0.3 mg, choline, I Mg, Mn, alcohol 18%, methylparaben, sorbitol. Bot. 473 ml. *otc.*
Use: Mineral, vitamin supplement.

Gerivites. (Rugby) Iron (from ferrous sulfate) 50 mg, A 5000 IU, D 400 IU, E 30 IU, B_1 1.5 mg, B_2 1.7 mg, B_3 20 mg, B_5 10 mg, B_6 2 mg, B_{12} 300 mcg, C 60 mg, folic acid 400 mg, Ca, Cl, Cr, Cu, I, K, Mg, Mn, Mo, Ni, Se, Si, P, Zn 15 mg/Tab. 40s. *otc.*
Use: Mineral, vitamin supplement.

Gerix Elixir. (Abbott Laboratories) Vitamins B_1 6 mg, B_2 6 mg, niacin 100 mg, iron 15 mg, B_6 1.6 mg, cyanocobalamin 6 mcg, alcohol 20%/30 ml. Bot. 480 ml. *otc.*
Use: Mineral, vitamin supplement.

germanin. (CDC) *Rx.*
Use: Anti-infective.
See: Suramin sodium (Naphuride sodium).

Germicin. (CMC) Benzalkonium Cl 50%. Bot. pt., gal. *otc.*
Use: Antiseptic, antimicrobial.

Ger-O-Foam. (Roberts Pharm) Methylsalicylate 30%, benzocaine 3%, vola-

tile oils. Aerosol can 4 oz. *otc.*
Use: Analgesic, anesthetic.

Geroton Forte. (Kenwood/Bradley) Vitamin B_1 1.7 mg, B_2 1.9 mg, B_3 2.22 mg, B_5 1.11 mg, B_6 0.22 mg, B_{12} 0.67 mcg, Zn 1.7 mg, Mg, Mn, alcohol 13%. Liq. Bot. 473 ml. *otc.*
Use: Mineral, vitamin supplement.

Gerterol Depo. (Fellows) Medroxyprogesterone acetate 50 mg or 100 mg/ml. Vial 5 ml. *Rx.*
Use: Hormone, progestin.

Gesic. (Lexalabs) Aspirin 226.8 mg, caffeine 32.4 mg, codeine 32.4 mg/Tab. Bot. 100s. *c-III.*
Use: Analgesic combination, narcotic.

•**gestaclone.** (JEST-ah-klone) USAN.
Use: Hormone, progestin.

•**gestodene.** (JEST-oh-deen) USAN.
Use: Hormone, progestin.

Gestoneed. (Hanlon) Calcium lactate 1069 mg, vitamins C 100 mg, nicotinic acid 18 mg, B_2 2.4 mg, B_1 1.8 mg, B_6 9 mg, D 500 IU, A 6000 IU/Cap. Bot. 100s. *otc.*
Use: Mineral, vitamin supplement.

•**gestonorone caproate.** (jess-TOE-nore-ohn CAP-row-ate) USAN.
Use: Hormone, progestin.

•**gestrinone.** (JESS-trih-nohn) USAN.
Use: Hormone, progestin.

Gets-It. (Oakhurst) Salicyclic acid, zinc Cl, collodion in ether ≈ 35%, alcohol ≈ 28%. Liq. Bot. 12 ml. *otc.*
Use: Keratolytic.

•**gevotroline hydrochloride.** (jeh-VOE-troe-LEEN) USAN.
Use: Antipsychotic.

Gevrabon. (ESI Lederle Generics) Vitamins B_1 0.83 mg, B_2 0.42 mg, B_3 8.3 mg, B_5 1.67 mg, B_6 0.17 mg, B_{12} 0.17 mcg, Fe 2.5 mg, choline, I, Mg, Mn, Zn 0.3 mg, alcohol 18%. Liq. Bot. 480 ml. *otc.*
Use: Mineral, vitamin supplement.

Gevral. (ESI Lederle Generics) Vitamins A 5000 IU, B_1 1.5 mg, B_2 1.7 mg, B_6 2 mg, B_{12} 6 mcg, folic acid 0.4 mg, C 60 mg, E 30 mg, B_3 20 mg, Ca, P, iron 18 mg, Mg, I, lactose, parabens, sucrose/Tab. Bot. 100s. *otc.*
Use: Mineral, vitamin supplement.

Gevral Protein. (ESI Lederle Generics) Calcium caseinate, sucrose, protein 15.6 g, carbohydrate 7.05 g, fat 0.52 g, sodium 50 mg, potassium 13 mg, calories 95.3/26 g. Pow. Can. 8 oz, 5 lb. *otc.*
Use: Nutritional supplement.

GG-Cen Capsules. (Schwarz Pharma) Guaifenesin 200 mg/Cap. Bot. 24s, 100s. *otc.*
Use: Expectorant.

GI stimulants.
See: Clopra, Tab. (Quantum).
Maxolon, Tab. (SmithKline Beecham Pharmaceuticals).
Metoclopramide, Tab. (Various Mfr.).
Metoclopramide HCl, Inj. (Quad).
Octamide, Tab. (Pharmacia & Upjohn).
Reclomide, Tab. (Major).
Reglan, Inj., Syr., Tab. (Robins).

GL-2 Skin Adherent. (Gordon Laboratories) Ready to use. Bot. pt, qt, gal. *otc.*

GL-7 Skin Adherent. (Gordon Laboratories) Plastic material which may be used full strength or diluted with 3 to 10 parts 99% isopropyl alcohol, acetone or naphtha. Pkg. pt, qt, gal. *otc.*

Glandosane. (Kenwood Labs) Sodium carboxymethylcellulose 0.51 g, sorbitol 1.52 g, sodium Cl 0.043 g, potassium Cl 0.061 g, calcium Cl 0.007 g, magnesium Cl 0.003 g, dipotassium hydrogen phosphate 0.017 g/50 ml. Soln. Spray Bot. 50 ml. *otc.*
Use: Saliva substitute.

glandubolin.
See: Estrone (Various Mfr.).

•**glatiramer acetate.** (glah-TEER-ah-mer ASS-eh-tate) USAN.
Use: Multiple sclerosis; immunomulator.
See: Copaxone (Lemmon).

glauber's salt.
See: Sodium Sulfate (Various Mfr.).

Glaucon Solution. (Alcon Laboratories) Epinephrine HCl 1% or 2%. Drop-Tainers. 10 ml. *Rx.*
Use: Antiglaucoma.

GlaucTabs. (Akorn) Methazolamide 25 mg, 50 mg. Tab. Bot. 100s. *Rx.*
Use: Diuretic.

•**glaze, pharmaceutical,** N.F. 18.
Use: Pharmaceutic aid (tablet coating agent).

•**glemanserin.** (gleh-MAN-ser-in) USAN.
Use: Anxiolytic.

Gliadel. (Rhone-Poulenc Rorer) Carmustine (BCNU) 7.7 mg. Wafer. Single dose treatment box with 8 individually pouched wafers. *Rx.*
Use: Alkylating agent.

•**gliamilide.** (glie-AM-ih-lide) USAN.
Use: Antidiabetic.

glibenclamide.
See: Glyburide.

•**glibornuride.** (glie-BORN-you-ride) USAN.
Use: Oral hypoglycemic agent; antidiabetic.

•**glicetanile sodium.** (glie-SET-AH-nile) USAN. *Formerly Glydanile Sodium.*
Use: Antidiabetic.

•**gliflumide.** (GLIH-flew-mide) USAN.
Use: Antidiabetic.

glim.
See: Gardinol Type Detergents (Various Mfr.).

•**glimepiride.** (GLIE-meh-pie-ride) USAN.
Use: Hypoglycemic.
See: Amaryl, Tab. (Hoechst Marion Roussel).

•**glipizide,** (GLIP-ih-zide) U.S.P. 23.
Use: Antidiabetic.
See: Glucotrol, Tab. (Pratt).

glipizide. (GLIP-ih-zide) (Various Mfr.) 5 or 10 mg/Tab. 100s, 500s, UD 100s. *Rx.*
Use: Antidiabetic.

globulin, cytomegalovirus immune.
See: CytoGam, Vial (MedImmune).

globulin, gamma.
See: Immune Globulin Intramuscular.
Immune Globulin Intravenous.

globulin, hepatitis b immune.
See: BayHep B (Bayer Corp).
H-BIG, Vial (Abbott Laboratories).

•**globulin, immune.** (GLAH-byoo-lin) U.S.P. 23. *Formerly Globulin, Immune Human Serum.*
Use: IM, measles prophylactic and polio; immunization.
See: Gammar-IM (Centeon).

globulin, immune, IV.
Use: Immunodeficiency; immune thrombocytopinea purpura; Kawasaki syndrome.
See: Gamimune-N (Bayer Corp).
Gammagard S/D (Hyland).
Gammar-P IV (Centeon).
Iveegam (Immuno).
Polygam S/D (American Red Cross).
Sandoglobulin (Novartis).
Venoglobulin-I (Alpha Therapeutics).
Venoglubulin-S (Alpha Therapeutics).

globulin, rabies immune.
Use: Immunization.
See: Bayrab (Bayer Corp).
Imogam Rabies (Pasteur Merieux Connaught).

globulin, rho(d) immune.
Use: Prevention of Rh isoimmunization; immune thrombocytopenic purpura.
See: BayRhoD (Centeon).
Gamulin Rh (Centeon).
Mini-Gamulin Rh (Centeon).
MICRhoGAM (Ortho McNeil).
RhoGAM (Ortho McNeil).
WinRho SD (Univax Biologics).

•**globulin serum, anti-human.** U.S.P. 23.

globulin, tetanus immune.
Use: Immunization.
See: Baytet (Bayer Corp).

globulin, vaccinia immune.
Use: Immunization.

globulin, varicella-zoster immune.
Use: Immunization.
See: varicella-zoster immune globulin (VZIG) (Massachusetts Public Health Biologic Laboratories).

•**gloximonam.** (GLOX-ih-MOE-nam) USAN.
Use: Anti-infective.

glubionate calcium.
See: Neo-Calglucon, Syrup (Novartis).

•**glucagon.** (GLUE-kuh-gahn) U.S.P. 23.
Use: Emergency treatment of hypoglycemia; antidiabetic.

glucagon. (Eli Lilly) 1 unit/ml w/diluent. 10 units w/10 ml diluent. Glucagon HCl 1 mg or 10 mg w/diluent; soln. contains lactose, glycerin 1.6% w/phenol 0.2% as a preservative. Vial.
Use: Hypoglycemic shock; antidiabetic.

Glucagon Emergency Kit. (Eli Lilly) Glucagon 1 mg or 10 mg, lactose w/diluent. Inj. 1 ml, 10 ml. *Rx.*

Glucamide. (Teva USA) Chlorpropamide 100 mg or 250 mg/Tab. Bot. 100s, 250s, 500s, 1000s, UD 100s. *Rx.*
Use: Antidiabetic.

•**gluceptate sodium.** (GLUE-sep-tate) USAN.
Use: Pharmaceutic aid.

Glucerna Liquid. (Ross Laboratories) Protein 41 g (amino acids), carbohydrate 93 g (hydrolyzed cornstarch, fructose, soy fiber), fat 55 g (high oleic safflower oil, soy oil, soy lecithin), sodium 917 mg (40 mEq), potassium 1542 mg (40 mEq), vitamins A, B_1, B_2, B_3, B_5, B_6, B_{12}, C, D, E, K, folic acid, Cl, Ca, P, Mg, I, Mn, Cu, Zn, Fe, Se, Cr, Mo, biotin, choline. Liq. Can 240 ml, Cont. 1L. Ready-to-use. *otc.*
Use: Nutritional supplement.

d-glucitol(d-Sorbitol)/Homatropine methylbromide.
See: ProBilagol, Liq. (Purdue Frederick).

glucocerebrosidase-beta-glucosidase.
Use: Treatment of Gaucher's disease.
See: Ceredase, Inj. (Genzyme).

glucocerebrosidase (PEG).
See: PEG-glucocerebrosidase.

glucocerebrosidase, recombinant retroviral vector. (Genetic Therapy)
Use: Treatment for Gaucher's disease. [Orphan drug]

glucocorticoids.
See: Cortical Hormone Products.

Glucolet Automatic Lancing Device. (Bayer Corp) To obtain sample for blood glucose testing. Automatic spring loaded lancing device.
Use: Diagnostic aid.

Glucolet Endcaps. (Bayer Corp) To obtain sample for blood glucose testing. Controls depth of lancet penetration. Regular or super puncture.
Use: Diagnostic aid.

Glucometer II Blood Glucose Meter. (Bayer Corp) Electronic meter for blood glucose testing. *otc.*
Use: Diagnostic aid.

d-gluconic acid, calcium salt. Calcium Gluconate.

gluconic acid salts.
See: Calcium Gluconate.
Ferrous Gluconate.
Magnesium Gluconate.
Potassium Gluconate.

•**gluconolactone.** (glue-koe-no-LACK-tone) U.S.P. 23.
Use: Chelating agent.

Glucophage. (Bristol-Myers Squibb) Metformin HCl 500 mg or 850 mg/Tab. Bot. 100s. *Rx.*
Use: Antidiabetic.

•**glucosamine.** (glue-KOSE-ah-meen) USAN.
Use: Pharmaceutic aid.
W/Nystatin, oxytetracycline.
W/Tetracycline HCl, nystatin.
W/Tetracycline.
See: Tetracyn, Cap., Syr. (Roerig).
W/Oxytetracycline.
See: Terramycin, Prep (Pfizer).

glucose.
See: Glutose, Gel. (Paddock).
Insta-Glucose, Gel. (ICN Pharmaceuticals).
Pal-A-Dex, Pow. (Baker Norton).

Glucose-40 Ophthalmic Ointment. (Ciba Vision Ophthalmics) Liquid glucose 40% in white petrolatum, anhydrous lanolin with parabens. Tube 3.5 g. *Rx.*
Use: Hyperosmolar preparation.

glucose elevating agents.
See: B-D Glucose, Chew. Tab. (Becton Dickinson).
Insta-Glucose, Gel. (ICN Pharmaceuticals).
Glucagon, Pow. for Inj. (Eli Lilly).
Glutose, Gel. (Paddock).
Insta-Glucose, Gel. (ICN Pharmaceuticals).
Insulin Reaction, Gel. (Sherwood Medical).
Proglycem, Cap., Oral. Susp. (Medical Market).

glucose enzymatic test strip.
Use: Diagnostic aid (in vitro, reducing sugars in urine).

glucose (hk) reagent strips. Reagent strip test for detection of glucose in serum or plasma. Bot. 50s.
Use: Diagnostic aid.

Glucose & Ketone Urine Test. (Major) Reagent test for glucose and ketones in urine. Bot. 100s.
Use: Diagnostic aid.

•**glucose, liquid.** (GLUE-kose) N.F. 18.
Use: As a 5% to 50% solution as nutrient; for acute hepatitis and dehydration; to increase blood volume; pharmaceutic aid (tablet binder, tablet coating agent).

d-glucose, monohydrate. Dextrose.

glucose oxidase. W/peroxidase, potassium iodide.
See: Diastix, Vial, Tab. (Bayer Corp).

glucose polymers.
See: Polycose, Pow., Liq. (Ross Laboratories).

Glucose Reagent Strips. (Bayer Corp) A quantitative strip test for glucose in serum or plasma. Seralyzer reagent strips. Bot. 50s.
Use: Diagnostic aid.

glucose test.
See: Combistix (Bayer Corp).
First Choice, Strips (Polymer Technology Int.).
Glucose Reagent Strips (Bayer Corp).

glucose tolerance test preparation.
See: Glucola (Bayer Corp).

Glucostix Reagent Strips. (Bayer Corp) Cellulose strip containing glucose oxidase and indicator system. Bot. 50s, 100s, UD 25s. *otc.*
Use: Diagnostic aid.

glucosulfone sodium, inj..
See: Sodium Glucosulfone Injection.

Gluco System Lancets. (Bayer Corp) Disposable lancets for use in Miles Diagnostic Autolet or Glucolet.
Use: Diagnostic aid.

Glucotrol. (Roerig) Glipizide 5 mg or 10 mg, lactose/Tab. Bot. 100s, 500s, UD 100s. *Rx.*

Use: Antidiabetic.

Glucotrol XL. (Pfizer) Glipizide 5 mg or 10 mg. ER Tab. Bot. 100s, 500s. *Rx.*
Use: Antidiabetic.

Glucovite. (Pal-Pak) Ferrous gluconate 260 mg, vitamins B_1 1 mg, B_2 0.5 mg, C 10 mg/Tab. Bot. 1000s, 5000s. *otc.*
Use: Mineral, vitamin supplement.

glucurolactone. Gamma lactone of glucofuranuronic acid.
See: Preltron-Oral, Tab. (Taylor Pharmaceuticals).

glucuronate sodium.
See: Preltron, Inj. (Taylor Pharmaceuticals).

Glu-K. (Western Research) Potassium gluconate 486 mg/Tab. Bot. 1000s. *otc.*
Use: Electrolyte supplement.

gluside.
See: Saccharin (Various Mfr.).

glutamate sodium.
W/Niacin, vitamins, minerals.
See: L-Glutavite, Cap. (Rydelle).

•**glutamic acid.** USAN.
Use: Nutritional supplement.
See: Glutamic Acid Tablets (Various Mfr.).
Glutamic Acid Powder (J.R. Carlson).

Glutamic Acid Tablets. (Various Mfr.) 500 mg. In 100s, 500s. *otc.*
Use: Nutritional supplement.

Glutamic Acid Powder. (J.R. Carlson) Bot. 100 g. *otc.*
Use: Nutritional supplement.

glutamic acid hydrochloride. Acidogen, aciglumin, glutasin. *otc.*
Use: Gastric acidifier.

glutamic acid salts.
See: Calcium Glutamate (Various Mfr.).

glutamine. (Nutritional Restart)
Use: Treatment of short bowel syndrome. [Orphan drug]

•**glutaral concentrate.** (GLUE-tah-ral) U.S.P. 23.
Use: Disinfectant.
See: Cidex (Surgikos).

glutaraldehyde.
Use: Sterilizing, disinfecting agent.
See: Cidex (J&J Medical).
Cidex-7 (J&J Medical).
Cidex Plus (J&J Medical).

Glutarex-1. (Ross Laboratories) Protein 15 g, fat 23.9 g, carbohydrates 46.3 g, linoleic acid 1800 mg, Fe 9 mg, Na 190 mg, K 675 mg, Ca, vitamins A, B_1, B_2, B_3, B_5, B_6, B_{12}, C, D, E, K, biotin, choline, folic acid, inositol, Cl, Cu, I, Mg, Mn, P, Se, Zn and 480 Cal per 100 g. Lysine and tryptophan free. Pow. Can 350 g. *otc.*
Use: Nutritional supplement.

Glutarex-2. (Ross Laboratories) Protein 30 g, fat 15.5 g, carbohydrates 30 g, Fe 13 mg, Na 880 mg, K 1370 mg, Ca, vitamins A, B_1, B_2, B_3, B_5, B_6, B_{12}, C, D, E, K, biotin, choline, folic acid, inositol, Cl, Cu, I, Mg, Mn, P, Se, Zn and 410 Cal per 100 g. Lysine and tryptophan free. Pow. Can 325 g. *otc.*
Use: Nutritional supplement.

l-glutathione.
Use: Treatment of AIDS-associated cachexia. [Orphan drug]
See: Cachexon (Telluride Pharm).

•**glutethimide.** (glue-TETH-ih-mide) U.S.P. 23.
Use: Hypnotic, sedative.

Glutofac. (Kenwood/Bradley) Capl.: Vitamins A 500 IU, E 30 IU, B_1 15 mg, B_2 10 mg, B_3 50 mg, B_5 20 mg, B_6 50 mg, C 300 mg, Zn 5 mg, Ca, Cr, Cu, Fe, K, Mg, Mn, P, Se/Tab. Bot. 90s. *otc.*
Use: Mineral, vitamin supplement.

Glutol. (Paddock) Dextrose 100 g/180 ml. Bot. 180 ml.
Use: Diagnostic aid.

Glutose. (Paddock) Liquid glucose (40% dextrose). Concentrated glucose for insulin reactions. Gel. Bot. 60 g. *otc.*
Use: Hyperglycemic.

Glyate. (Geneva Pharm) Guaifenesin 100 mg/5 ml, alcohol 3.5%. Syr. Bot. 118 ml, 480 ml. *otc.*
Use: Expectorant.

•**glyburide.** (glie-BYOO-ride) U.S.P. 23.
Use: Antidiabetic.
See: DiaBeta (Hoechst Marion Roussel).
Glynase, Tab. (Pharmacia & Upjohn).
Micronase, Tab. (Pharmacia & Upjohn).

glyburide. (Various Mfr.) **1.25 mg:** Tab. Bot. 50s, 100s. **2.5 & 5 mg:** Tab. Bot. 100s, 500s, 1000s, UD 100s.
Use: Antidiabetic.

glyburide, micronized. (Copley) Micronized glyburide 1.5 mg, 3 mg. Tab. Bot. 100s, 500s (only 3 mg), 1000s (only 3 mg), UD 100s. *Rx.*
Use: Antidiabetic.

glycarnine iron.
See: Ferronord, Tab. (Rydelle).

Glycate Chewables. (Forest Pharmaceutical) Glycine 150 mg, calcium carbonate 300 mg/Tab. Bot. 1000s. *otc.*
Use: Antacid.

•**glycerin.** (GLIH-suh-rin) U.S.P. 23.
Use: Pharmaceutic aid (humectant, solvent).

See: Corn Huskers Lot. (Warner Lambert).
Ophthalgan Ophthalmic, Soln. (Wyeth Ayerst).
Osmoglyn (Alcon Laboratories).
W/ Dimethicone.
See: Dermasil, Lot. (Chesebrough-Ponds).
W/Urea.
See: Kerid Ear Drops (Blair Laboratories).

glycerin. (Various Mfr.) Various concentrations from 10% to > 95% for use as sterile allergen-extract diluents.

glycerin suppositories. (Various Mfr.) Glycerin, sodium stearate. *otc.*
Use: Roctal evacuant, cathartic.

glycerol.
See: Glycerin.

•**glycerol, iodinated.** (GLIH-ser-ole EYE-oh-dih-nay-tehd) USAN.
Use: Expectorant.

•**glyceryl behenate,** N.F. 18.
Use: Pharmaceutic aid (tablet/capsule lubricant).

glyceryl guaiacolate.
Use: Expectorant.
See: Guaifenesin, U.S.P. 23.

glyceryl guaiacolate carbamate. Methocarbamol.
See: Robaxin, Tab., Inj. (Robins).
Robaxin 750, Tab. (Robins).

glyceryl guaiacolether.
See: Guaifenesin.

•**glyceryl monostearate.** N.F. 18.
Use: Pharmaceutic aid (emulsifying agent).

Glyceryl-T. (Rugby) Theophylline 150 mg, guaifenesin 90 mg/Cap. Bot. 100s. *Rx.*
Use: Bronchodilator, expectorant.

Glyceryl-T Liquid. (Rugby) Theophylline 150 mg, guaifenesin 90 mg/15 ml. Liq. Bot. 480 ml. *Rx.*
Use: Bronchodilator, expectorant.

glyceryl triacetate.
See: Triacetin.

glyceryl triacetin. (Various Mfr.) Triacetin.
See: Enzactin, Aerosal, Pow., Cream (Wyeth Ayerst).
Fungacetin, Oint, Liq. (Blair Labs.).

glyceryl trierucate.
Use: Adrenoleukodystrophy. [Orphan drug]

glyceryl trinitrate ointment.
See: Nitrol, Oint. (Kremers Urban).

glyceryl trinitrate tablets.
See: Nitroglycerin (Various Mfr.)
Nitroglyn, Tab. (Key Corp).

glyceryl trioleate.
Use: Adrenoleuko-dystrophy. [Orphan drug]

Glycets-Antacid Tablets. (Weeks & Leo) Calcium carbonate 350 mg, simethicone 25 mg/Chew. Tab. Bot. 100s. *otc.*
Use: Antacid, antiflatulent.

glycinato dihydroxyaluminum hydrate.
See: Dihydroxyaluminum Aminoacetate, U.S.P. 23.

•**glycine.** (GLIE-seen) U.S.P. 23. *Formerly Aminoacetic Acid.*
Use: Myasthenia gravis treatment, irrigating solution.
W/Aluminum hydroxide-magnesium carbonate coprecipitated gel.
See: Glycogel, Tab., Susp. (Schwarz Pharma).
W/Calcium Carbonate.
See: Antacid No. 6, Tab. (Jones Medical Industries).
Glycate Chewables, Tab. (O'Neal).
P.H. Tab. (Scrip).
Titralac, Liq., Tab. (3M).
W/Calcium carbonate, amylolytic, proteolytic cellulolytic enzymes.
See: Co-gel, Tab. (Arco).
W/Chlor-Trimeton, sodium salicylate.
See: Corilin, Liq. (Schering Plough).
W/Glutamic acid, alanine.
See: Prostall, Cap. (Metabolic Prods.).
W/Magnesium trisilicate, calcium carbonate.
See: P.H. Tab., Chewable, Mix (Scrip).

glycine, aluminum salt.
See: Dihydroxyaluminum Aminoacetate, U.S.P. 23.

glycine hydrochloride. (Various Mfr.)
Use: Gastric acidifier.

glycobiarsol. U.S.P. XXI. Bismuthyl-N-Glycolylarsanilate, Chemo Puro, Pow. for Mfr. (Hydrogen N-glycoloylarsanilato) oxobismuth.
Use: Amebiasis, Trichomonas vaginalis, Monilia albicans.

glycocoll. Glycine.
See: Aminoacetic Acid (Various Mfr.).

glycocyamine. Guanidoacetic acid.

Glycofed Tablets. (Pal-Pak) Pseudoephedrine 30 mg, guaifenesin 100 mg. Bot. 1000s. *otc.*
Use: Decongestant, expectorant.

•**glycol distearate.** (GLIE-kole dih-STEE-ah-rate) USAN.
Use: Pharmaceutic aid (thickening agent).

glycol monosalicylate.
W/Oil of mustard, camphor, menthol, methyl salicylate.

See: Musterole, Oint., Cream (Schering Plough).

glycophenylate bromide.
See: Mepenzolate Methylbromide.

•**glycopyrrolate.** (glie-koe-PIE-row-late) U.S.P. 23.
Use: Anticholinergic.
See: Robinul, Tab., Inj. (Robins).
Robinul Forte, Tab. (Robins).

Glycotuss. (Pal-Pak) Guaifenesin 100 mg/Tab. Bot. 100s, 1000s. *otc.*
Use: Expectorant.

Glycotuss-dM. (Pal-Pak) Guaifenesin 100 mg, dextromethorphan HBr 10 mg/Tab. Bot. 100s, 1000s. *otc.*
Use: Antitussive, expectorant.

glycyrrhiza. Pure extract, Fluidextract. Licorice root.
Use: Flavoring agent.

glycyrrhiza extract, pure.
Use: Flavoring agent.

glycyrrhiza fluidextract.
Use: Flavoring agent.
W/Camphorated opium tincture, tartar emetic, glycerin.
See: Brown Mixture. (Jones Medical Industries).
W/Pepsin-papain complex, pancreas, malt diastase, charcoal, ox bile.
See: Pepsocoll, Tab. (Western Research Labs.).

glydanile sodium. (GLIE-dah-neel SO-dee-uhm)
Use: Antidiabetic.

•**glyhexamide.** (glie-HEX-ah-mid) USAN.
Use: Antidiabetic.

Glylorin. (Cellegy Pharmaceuticals) Monolaurin.
Use: Congenital primary ichthyosis. [Orphan drug]

•**glymidine sodium.** (GLIE-mih-deen) USAN.
Use: Oral hypoglycemic agent; antidiabetic.

glymol.
See: Petrolatum Liquid (Various Mfr.)

Glynase PresTab. (Pharmacia & Upjohn) Glyburide (micronized) **1.5 mg:** Tab. Bot. 100s, UD 100s. **3 mg:** Tab. Bot. 100s, 500s, 1000s, UD 100s. **6 mg:** Tab. Bot. 100s, 500s. *Rx.*
Use: Antidiabetic.

•**glyoctamide.** (glie-OCKT-am-id) USAN.
Use: Hypoglycemic agent; antidiabetic.

Gly-Oxide. (SmithKline Beecham Consumer Healthcare) Carbamide peroxide 10% in flavored anhydrous glycerol. Liq. Bot. 15 ml, 60 ml. *otc.*
Use: Mouth and throat preparation.

glyoxyldiureide.
See: Allantoin (Various Mfr.).

•**glyparamide.** (glie-PAR-am-ide) USAN.
Use: Oral hypoglycemic agent; antidiabetic.

Glypressin. (Ferring Pharmaceuticals) Terlipressin.
Use: Bleeding esophageal varicies. [Orphan drug]

Glyset. (Bayer Corp) Miglitol 25 mg, 50 mg, 100 mg/Tab. Bot. 100s, 1000s (except 25 mg), UD 100. *Rx.*
Use: Antidiabetic.

Glytuss. (Merz) Guaifenesin 200 mg/Tab. Bot. 100s. *otc.*
Use: Expectorant.

GM-CSF. Granulocyte macrophage colony stimulating factor.
See: Leukine (Immunex).

G-myticin Creme and Ointment. (Pedinol) Gentamicin sulfate equivalent to gentamicin base 1 mg. Tube 15 g. *Rx.*
Use: Anti-infective, topical.

gododiamide.
Use: Diagnostic aid.

Go-Evac. (Copley) Polyethylene glycol 3350 59 g, sodium sulfate 5.685 g, sodium bicarbonate 1.685 g, sodium chloride 1.465 g, potassium chloride 0.743 g/L. Pow. for soln. Jug 4 L. *Rx.*
Use: Bowel evacuants.

Golacol. (Arcum) Codeine sulfate 30 mg, papaverine HCl 30 mg, emetine HCl 2 mg, ephedrine HCl 15 mg, q.s./30 ml. Alcohol 6.25%. Syr. Bot. 4 oz, 16 oz, gal. Orange flavor. *c-III.*
Use: Antitussive, bronchodilator.

Gold Alka-Seltzer Effervescent. (Bayer Corp) Sodium bicarbonate (heat treated) 958 mg, citric acid 832 mg, potassium bicarbonate 312 mg/Tab. 20s, 36s. *otc.*
Use: Antacid.

•**gold Au^{198}.** USAN. U.S.P. XX.
Use: Antineoplastic, diagnostic aid (liver imaging), radiopharmaceutical.
See: Radio Gold (Au^{198}).

gold Au 198 injection.
Use: Antineoplastic; diagnostic for liver scanning.

gold compounds.
See: Gold Sodium Thiosulfate (Various Mfr.).
Ridaura, Cap. (SmithKline Beecham Pharmaceuticals).
Solganal, Vial (Schering Plough).

Gold Seal Calcium 600. (Walgreens) Calcium 1200 mg/Tab. Bot. 60s. *otc.*
Use: Mineral supplement.

Gold Seal Calcium 600 with Vitamin D. (Walgreens) Calcium 1200 mg, vitamin D/Tab. Bot. 60s. *otc.*
Use: Mineral supplement.

Gold Seal Chewable Vitamin C. (Walgreens) Ascorbic acid 250 mg or 500 mg/Tab. Bot. 100s. *otc.*
Use: Vitamin supplement.

Gold Seal Ferrous Gluconate. (Walgreens) Iron 37 mg/Tab. Bot. 100s. *otc.*
Use: Mineral supplement.

Gold Seal Ferrous Sulfate Tablets. (Walgreens) Ferrous sulfate 325 mg/Tab. Bot. 100s, 1000s. *otc.*
Use: Mineral supplement.

Gold Seal Time Release Ferrous Sulfate. (Walgreens) Iron 50 mg/Tab. Bot. 100s. *otc.*
Use: Mineral supplement.

•**gold sodium thiomalate.** (gold SO-dee-uhm thigh-oh-MAL-ate) U.S.P. 23.
Use: Antirheumatic.
See: Aurolate, Inj. (Taylor Pharmaceuticals).
Myochrysine, Amp. (Merck).

gold sodium thiosulfate. Sterile, Auricidine, Aurocidin, Aurolin, Auropin, Aurosan, Novacrysin, Solfocrisol and Thiochrysine.
Use: Antirheumatic.

gold thioglucose.
See: Aurothioglucose, U.S.P. 23.

Golden-West Compound. (Golden-West) Gentian root, licorice root, cascara sagrada, damiana leaves, senna leaves, psyllium seed, buchu leaves, crude pepsin. Box 1.5 oz. *otc.*
Use: Laxative.

Goldicide Concentrate. (Pedinol) Bot. (Conc.) oz. Ctn. 10s.
Use: Distinfectant.

GoLYTELY. (Braintree Laboratories) Pow. for oral soln. after reconstitution containing PEG-3350 236 g, sodium sulfate 22.74 g, sodium bicarbonate 6.74 g, sodium Cl 5.86 g, potassium Cl 2.97 g when made up to 4 L. Disposable container 4800 ml. *Rx.*
Use: Bowel evacuant.

gonacrine.
See: Acriflavine (Various Mfr.).

•**gonadorelin acetate.** (go-NAD-oh-RELL-in) USAN. *Formerly Luteinizing Hormone-releasing Factor Diacetate Tetrahydrate.*
Use: Gonad-stimulating principle. [Orphan drug]
See: Cryptolin Prods. (Hoechst Marion Roussel).
Lutrepulse. (Ferring Labs).

•**gonadorelin hydrochloride.** (go-NAD-oh-RELL-in) USAN. *Formerly Luteinizing Hormone-releasing Factor Dihydrochloride.*
Use: Gonad-stimulating principle.

gonadotropic substance.
See: Gonadotropin Chorionic.

gonadotropins.
See: Pergonal, Pow. for Inj. (Serono Labs).

•**gonadotropin, chorionic.** (go-NAD-oh-TROE-pin, core-ee-AHN-ik) U.S.P. 23.
Use: Gonad-stimulating principle. In the female: Chronic cystic mastitis, functional sterility, dysmenorrhea, premenstrual tension, threatened abortion. In the male: Cryptorchidism, hypogenitalism, dwarfism, impotency, enuresis.
See: Android HCG, Inj. (Zeneca).
Antuitrin "S", Vial (Parke-Davis).
A.P.L., Secules (Wyeth Ayerst).
Corgonject, Vial (Merz).
Follutein Pow. (Bristol-Myers Squibb).
Libigen, Vial (Savage).
Pregnyl, Amp. (Organon Teknika).
W/Vitamin B_1, glutamic acid, procaine HCl.
See: Glukor, Vial (Zeneca).

gonadotropin, pituitary ant. lobe. Extracted from anterior lobe of equine pituitaries (not pregnant mare urine) (rat unit = 1 Fevold-Hisaw unit).

gonadotropin releasing hormone analog.
See: Lupron, Inj. Susp. (TAP Pharm)
Zoladex, Implant (Zeneca)

gonadotropin releasing hormones.
See: Lutrepulse, Pow. for Inj. (Ortho McNeil).
Supprelin, Inj. (Ortho McNeil).
Synarel, Soln. (Syntex).

gonadotropin serum. Pregnant mare's serum.

Gonak. (Akorn) Hydroxypropyl methylcellulose 2.5%. Soln. Bot. 15 ml. *otc.*
Use: Ophthalmic.

Gonal-F. (Serono) Follitropin alfa 75 IU, 150 IU, sucrose 30 mg. Inj. Amp. 1s, 10s. 100s, with diluent. *Rx.*
Use: Ovulation induction.

Gonic. (Roberts Pharm) Chorionic gonadotropin 10,000 units w/diluent/vial. Pow. for inj. Vial 10 ml. *Rx.*
Use: Hormone, chorionic gonadotropin.

gonioscopic hydroxypropyl methylcellulose.
See: Goniosol Lacrivial, Soln. (Smith, Miller & Patch).

Gonioscopic Solution. (Alcon Laboratories) Hydroxyethyl cellulose. Drop-Tainer 15 ml. *Rx.*
Use: Ophthalmic.

Goniosol. (Ciba Vision Ophthalmics) Gonioscopic hydroxypropyl methylcellulose 2.5%. Bot. 15 ml. *otc.*
Use: Ophthalmic.

Gonodecten Test Kit. (United States Packaging) Tube test for urethral discharge from males, for detection of *Neisseria gonorrhoeae.* Test kit 10s, 25s.
Use: Diagnostic aid.

gonorrhea tests.
See: Biocult-GC (Orion Diagnostica).
Gonodecten Test Kit (United States Packaging).
Gonozyme Diagnostic Kit (Abbott Laboratories).
Isocult for Neisseria gonorrhoeae (SmithKline Diagnostics).
MicroTrak Neisseria gonorrhoeae Culture Test (Syva).

Gonozyme. (Abbott Diagnostics) Enzyme immunoassay for detection of *Neisseria gonorrhoeae* in urogenital swab specimens. Test kit 100s.
Use: Diagnostic aid.

Good Samaritan Ointment. (Good Samaritan) Tube 1.25 oz. *otc.*
Use: Counterirritant.

Goody's Headache Powders. (Goody) Aspirin 520 mg, acetaminophen 260 mg, caffeine 32.5 mg/dose. Pow. Pkg. 2s, 6s, 24s, 50s. *otc.*
Use: Analgesic.

Gordobalm. (Gordon Laboratories) Chloroxylenol, methyl salicylate, menthol, camphor, thymol, eucalyptus oil, isopropyl alcohol 16%, fast-drying gum base. Bot. 4 oz, gal. *otc.*
Use: Analgesic, topical.

Gordochom. (Gordon Laboratories) Undecylenic acid 25%, chloroxylenol 3%, penetrating oil base. Liq. Bot. 15 ml, 30 ml w/applicator. *otc.*
Use: Antifungal, topical.

Gordofilm. (Gordon Laboratories) Salicylic acid 16.7%, lactic acid 16.7% in flexible colloidan. Bot. 15 ml. *otc.*
Use: Keratolytic.

Gordogesic Cream. (Gordon Laboratories) Methyl salicylate 10% in absorption base. Jar 2.5 oz, 1 lb. *otc.*
Use: Analgesic, topical.

Gordomatic Crystals. (Gordon Laboratories) Sodium borate, sodium bicarbonate, sodium Cl, thymol, menthol, eucalyptus oil. Jar 8 oz, 7 lb. *otc.*
Use: Counterirritant.

Gordomatic Lotion. (Gordon Laboratories) Menthol, camphor, propylene glycol, isopropyl alcohol. Bot. 1 oz, 4 oz, gal. *otc.*
Use: Counterirritant.

Gordomatic Powder. (Gordon Laboratories) Menthol, thymol camphor, eucalyptus oil, salicylic acid, alum bentonite, talc. Shaker can 3.5 oz. Can 1 lb, 5 lb. *otc.*
Use: Counterirritant.

Gordon's Urea. (Gordon Laboratories) Urea 40% in petrolatum base. Jar oz. *Rx.*
Use: Emollient.

Gordophene. (Gordon Laboratories) Neutral coconut oil soap 15%, glycerin with Septi-Chlor (trichlorohydroxy diphenyl ether) broad spectrum antimicrobial and bacteriostatic agent. Bot. 4 oz, gal.
Use: Dermatologic, cleanser.

Gordo-Vite A Creme. (Gordon Laboratories) Vitamin A 100,000 IU/oz. in water soluble base. Jar 0.5 oz, 2.5 oz, 4 oz, lb, 5 lb. *otc.*
Use: Emollient.

Gordo-Vite A Lotion. (Gordon Laboratories) Vitamin A 100,000 IU/oz. Plastic bot. 4 oz, gal. *otc.*
Use: Emollient.

Gordo-Vite E Creme. (Gordon Laboratories) Vitamin E 1500 IU/oz in water soluble base. Jar 2.5 oz, lb. *otc.*
Use: Emollient.

Gormel Cream. (Gordon Laboratories) Urea 20% in emollient base. Jar 0.5 oz, 2.5 oz, 4 oz, 1 lb, 5 lb. *otc.*
Use: Emollient.

•**goserelin.** (GO-suh-REH-lin) USAN.
Use: LHRH agonist.
See: Zoladex, Implant (Zeneca).

goserelin acetate. (GO-suh-REH-lin ASS-uh-TATE)
Use: Gonadotropin-releasing hormone analog.
See: Zoladex, Implant (Zeneca).

gossypol.
Use: Antineoplastic. [Orphan drug]

gotamine. (Vita Elixir) Ergotamine tartrate 1 mg, caffeine 100 mg/Tab. *Rx.*
Use: Antimigraine.

gout, agents for.
See: Allopurinol, Tab. (Various Mfr.).
Anturane, Tab., Cap. (Novartis).
Benemid, Tab. (Merck).
ColBenemid, Tab. (Merck).

Colchicine, Inj. (Eli Lilly).
Colchicine, Tab. (Various Mfr.).
Col-Probenecid, Tab. (Various Mfr.).
Proben-C, Tab. (Various Mfr.).
Probenecid, Tab. (Various Mfr.).
Probenecid w/Colchicine, Tab. (Various Mfr.).
Sulfinpyrazone, Tab., Cap. (Various Mfr.).
Zyloprim, Tab. (GlaxoWellcome).

•**govafilcon a.** (GO-vaff-ILL-kahn A) USAN.
Use: Contact lens material (hydrophilic).

gp 100 adenoviral gene therapy. (Genzyme).
Use: Antineoplastic. [Orphan drug]

GP-500. (Marnel) Pseudoephedrine HCl 120 mg, guaifenesin 500 mg. Tab. Bot. 100s. *Rx.*
Use: Decongestant, expectorant.

•**gramicidin.** (gram-ih-SIH-din) U.S.P. 23.
Use: Anti-infective.
W/Neomycin.
See: Spectrocin Oint. (Bristol-Myers Squibb).
W/Neomycin sulfate, polymyxin B sulfate, thimerosal.
See: Neo-Polycin Ophthalmic Soln. (Merrell Dow).
W/Neomycin sulfate, polymyxin B sulfate, benzocaine.
See: Tricidin, Oint. (Amlab).
W/Neomycin, triamcinolone, nystatin.
See: Mycolog Cream, Oint. (Bristol-Myers Squibb).
W/Polymyxin B sulfate, neomycin sulfate.
See: AK-Spore Ophth. Soln. (Akorn).
Neosporin, Ophthalmic Soln. (GlaxoWellcome).
Neosporin-G Cream (GlaxoWellcome).
Ocutricin Ophth. Soln. (Bausch & Lomb).
W/Polymyxin B sulfate, neomycin sulfate, hydrocortisone acetate.
See: Cortisporin, Cream (GlaxoWellcome).

•**granisetron.** (gran-IH-SEH-trahn) USAN.
Use: Antiemetic.
See: Kytril, Inj. (SmithKline Beecham Pharmaceuticals).

•**granisetron hydrochloride.** (gran-IH-SEH-trahn) USAN.
Use: Antiemetic.
See: Kytril Injection (SmithKline Beecham).

Granulderm. (Copley) Trypsin 0.1 mg, balsam Peru 72.5 mg, castor oil 650 mg/0.82 ml. Aerosol Spray 113.4 g. *Rx.*
Use: Enzyme, topical.

Granulex. (Hickam) Trypsin 0.1 mg, balsam Peru 72.5 mg, castor oil 650 mg w/ emulsifier/0.82 ml. Spray can 2 oz, 4 oz. *Rx.*
Use: Dermatologic, wound therapy.

granulocyte colony stimulating factor.
See: Neupogen (Amgen).

granulocyte macrophage-colony stimulating factor.
See: Leukine (Immunex).

gratus strophanthin. Ouabain.

Gravineed. (Hanlon) Vitamins C 100 mg, E 10 IU, B_1 3 mg, B_2 2 mg, B_6 10 mg, B_{12} 5 mcg, A 4000 IU, D 400 IU, niacin 10 mg, folic acid 0.1 mg, iron fumarate 40 mg, calcium 67 mg/Cap. Bot. 100s. *otc.*
Use: Mineral, vitamin supplement.

Green mint. (Block Drug) Urea, glycine, polysorbate 60, sorbitol, alcohol 12.2%, peppermint oil, menthol, chlorophyllin-copper complex. Bot. 7 oz, 12 oz. *otc.*
Use: Mouth and throat preparation.

green soap.
Use: Detergent.

•**grepafloxacin hydrochloride.** (grep-ah-FLOX-ah-sin) USAN.
Use: Antibacterial.

Grifulvin V. (Advanced Care Products) Griseofulvin microsize. **Tab:** 250 mg. Bot. 100s; 500 mg. Bot. 100s, 500s. **Susp:** 125 mg/5 ml. Bot. 120 ml. *Rx.*
Use: Antifungal.

Grisactin Ultra. (Wyeth Ayerst) Griseofulvin ultramicrosize 125 mg, 250 mg or 330 mg/Tab. Bot. 100s. *Rx.*
Use: Antifungal.

•**griseofulvin.** (griss-ee-oh-FULL-vin) U.S.P. 23.
Use: Antifungal.
See: Fulvicin P/G, Tab. (Schering Plough).
Fulvicin-U/F, Tab. (Schering Plough).
Grifulvin V, Tab., Susp. (Ortho McNeil).
Grisactin, Cap., Tab. (Wyeth Ayerst).
Grisactin Ultra, Tab. (Wyeth Ayerst).

griseofulvin. (Various Mfr.) 165 mg or 330 mg. Tab. Bot. 100s.
Use: Antifungal.

griseofulvin microcrystalline.
Use: Antifungal.
See: Fulvicin U/F, Tab. (Schering Plough).
Grifulvin V, Tab., Susp. (Ortho McNeil).
Grisactin, Cap., Tab. (Wyeth Ayerst).

griseofulvin, ultramicrosize. (Various Mfr.) Griseofulvin ultramicrosize 165

mg and 330 mg/Tab. Bot. 100s.
Use: Antifungal.
See: Fulvicin P/G, Tab. (Schering Plough).
Grisactin Ultra, Tab. (Wyeth Ayerst)
Gris-PEG, Tab. (Allergan).

Gris-PEG Tablets. (Allergan) Griseofulvin ultramicrosize 125 mg or 250 mg/Tab. **125 mg:** Bot. 100s. **250 mg:** Bot. 100s, 500s. *Rx.*
Use: Antifungal.

group b streptococcus immune globulin. (North American Biologicals)
Use: Anti-infective. [Orphan drug]

growth hormone. Extract of human pituitaries containing predominantly growth hormone.
See: Crescormon.

growth hormone releasing factor. (ICN Pharm)
Use: Long-term treatment of growth failure. [Orphan drug]

g-strophanthin. Ouabain.

guaiacol carbonate. (Various Mfr.) (Duotal).
Use: Expectorant.

guaiacol glyceryl ether.
See: Guaifenesin.

guaiacol potassium sulfonate.
See: Bronchial, Syr. (DePree).
W/Ammonium Cl, sodium citrate, benzyl alcohol, carbinoxamine maleate.
See: Clistin Expectorant, Syr. (Ortho McNeil).
W/Dextromethorphan HBr.
Bronchial DM, Syr. (DePree).
W/Pheniramine maleate, pyrilamine maleate, codeine phosphate.
See: Tritussin, Syr. (Towne). *Rx.*

guaianesin.
See: Guaifenesin.
Use: Expectorant.

•**guaiapate.** (GWIE-ah-pate) USAN.
Use: Antitussive.

Guaifed Capsules. (Muro) Guaifenesin 250 mg, pseudoephedrine HCl 120 mg/TR Cap. Bot. 100s, 500s. *Rx.*
Use: Decongestant, expectorant.

Guaifed-PD Capsules. (Muro) Pseudoephedrine HCl 60 mg, guaifenesin 300 mg/TR Cap. Bot. 100s, 500s. *Rx.*
Use: Decongestant, expectorant.

Guaifed Syrup. (Muro) Pseudoephedrine HCl 30 mg, guaifenesin 200 mg. Bot. 118 ml, 473 ml. *Rx.*
Use: Decongestant, expectorant.

•**guaifenesin.** (GWHY-fen-ah-sin) U.S.P. 23. *Formerly Glyceryl Guaiacolate.*
Synonyms:
Glyceryl Guaiacolate.
Glyceryl Guaiacol Ether.
Guaianesin.
Guaifylline.
Guayanesin.
Use: Expectorant.
See: Anti-tuss, Liq. (Century Pharm).
Consin-GG, Syr. (Wisconsin Pharm).
Diabetic Tussin Ex, Liq. (Health Care Products).
Dilyn, Liq., Tab. (Zeneca).
Duratuss-G, Tab. (UCB Pharma).
2/G, Liq. (Merrell Dow).
G-100, Syr. (Sanofi Winthrop).
GG-Cen, Syr. (Schwarz Pharma).
Glycotuss, Tab., Syr. (Pal-Pak).
Glytuss, Tab. (Merz).
G-Tussin, Syr. (Quality Formulations).
Guaifenex LA, ER Tab. (Ethex).
Humibid L.A., Tab. (Adams Labs).
Hytuss, Tab., Cap. (Hyrex).
Liquibid, SR Tab. (Ion).
Monafed, SR Tab. (Monarch Pharmaceuticals).
Muco-Fen-La, TR Tab. (Wakefield).
Organidin NR, Tab. Liq. (Wallace).
Pheunomist, SR Tab. (ECR Pharm).
Respa-GF, SR Tab. (Respa).
Siltussin, Syr. (Silarx).
Touro EX, SR Cap. (Dartmouth Pharm).
Tusibron, Liq. (Kenwood/Bradley).
Robitussin, Syr. (Robins).
Wal-Tussin, Syr. (Walgreens).
W/Combinations.
See: Actifed C Expectorant, Liq. (Glaxo-Wellcome).
Actol Exp., Syr., Tab. (SmithKline Beecham Pharmaceuticals).
Airet G.G., Cap., Elix. (Baylor Labs).
Ambenyl-D, Liq. (Hoechst Marion Roussel).
Anatuss DM, Syr., Tab. (Merz).
Anti-tuss D.M., Liq. (Century Pharm).
Antitussive Guaiacolate, Syr. (Med Chem).
Asbron G, Tab., Elix. (Novartis).
Aspirin-Free Bayer Select Head & Chest Cold, Capl. (Bayer).
Atuss-Ex, Syr. (Atley).
Atuss G, Syr. (Atley).
Benylin Multi-Symptom, Liq. (Glaxo-Wellcome).
Brexin, Cap., Liq. (Savage).
Bri-stan, Liq. (Briar).
Broncholate, Cap., Elix. (Sanofi Winthrop).
Bronchovent, Tab. (Mills).
Bronkaid Dual Action, Capl. (Sterling Health).
Brontex, Tab. Liq. (Procter & Gamble).

Bronkolate-G, Tab. (Parmed).
Bronkolixir, Elix. (Sanofi Winthrop).
Bronkotabs, Tab. (Sanofi Winthrop).
Bro-Tane, Expectorant (Scrip).
Bur-Tuss Expectorant (Burlington).
Cerylin, Liq. (Rugby).
Cheracol-D, Syr. (Pharmacia & Upjohn).
Chlor-Trimeton, Expectorant (Schering Plough).
Clear Tussin 30, Liq. (Zenith Goldline).
Codeine Phosphate and Guaifenesin, Tab. (Zenith Goldline).
Coldloc, Elix. (Fleming).
Coldloc-LA, SR Capl. (Fleming).
Colrex, Expectorant (Solvay).
Conar-A, Susp., Tab. (SmithKline Beecham Pharmaceuticals).
Conar Expectorant, Liq. (SmithKline Beecham Pharmaceuticals).
Congestac, Tab. (SmithKline Beecham Pharmaceuticals).
Consin-DM, Syr. (Wisconsin Pharm).
Coricidin Children's Cough Syr. (Schering Plough).
Cortane D.C., Exp. (Standex).
Cycofed Pediatric, Syr. (Cypress).
Deconamine CX, Tab., Liq. (Bradley).
Deconsal Pediatric, Syr. (Adams).
Defen-LA, SR Tab. (Horizon).
Dextro-Tuss GG, Liq. (Ulmer).
Diabetes CF, Syr. (Scot-Tissin).
Diabetic Tussin, Liq. (Roberts Pharm).
Diabetic Tussin DM, Liq. (Roberts Pharm).
Dilaudid, Syr. (Knoll Pharmaceuticals).
Dilor-G, Tab., Liq. (Savage).
Dilyn, Liq. (Zeneca).
Dimacol, Cap. (Robins).
Dimetane Expectorant, Liq. (Robins).
Dimetane Expectorant-DC, Liq. (Robins).
DM Plus, Liq. (West-Ward).
Donatussin, Syr. (Laser).
Duovent, Tab. (3M).
Dynafed Asthma Relief, Tab. (BDI).
Emfaseem, Liq., Tab. (Saron).
Entex, Cap., Liq. (Procter & Gamble).
Fenesin DM, Tab. (Dura).
Formula 44D Decongestant Cough Mixture, Syr. (Procter & Gamble).
G-100/DM, Syr. (Sanofi Winthrop).
G-Bron Elix. (Laser).
2G/DM, Liq. (Merrell Dow).
Glycotuss-DM, Tab. (Pal-Pak).
Guanifenex, Liq. (Ethex).
Guaifenex, PPA 75, ER Tab. (Ethex).
Guaifenex PSE 60, ER Tab. (Ethex).
Guaifenex PSE 120, ER Tab. (Ethex).
Guaifenex Rx, DM Tab. (Ethex).
Guaifenex RX, ER Tab. (Ethex).
Guaitex, Cap. Liq. (Rugby).
Guiatex LA, Tab. (Rugby).
Guaitex PSE, Tab. (Rugby).
Guiavent PD, Cap. (Ethex).
Guai-Vent/PSE, SR Tab. (Dura).
Guiatussin w/Codeine, Liq. (Rugby).
Guistrey Fortis, Tab. (Jones Medical Industries).
Histussinol, Syr. (Sanofi Winthrop).
Hycoff-A, Syr. (Saron).
Hycotuss Expectorant, Liq. (DuPont Merck Pharmaceuticals).
Hycoclear Tuss, Syr. (Ethex).
Hydrocodone GF, Syr. (Morton Grove).
Hylate, Tab., Syr. (Hyrex).
Iobid DM, SR Tab (Iomed).
Iosol II, ER Tab. (Iomed).
Isoclor Expectorant (DuPont Merck Pharmaceuticals).
Lardet Expectorant, Tab. (Standex).
Liquibid-D, SR Tab. (ION).
Med-RX, DM, CR Tab. (Iomed).
Med-RX, CR Tab. (Iomed).
Mini Thin Asthma Relief. Tab. (BDI).
Monafed DM, ER Tab. (Monarch Pharmaceuticals).
Muco-Fen-DM, TR Tab. (Wakefield Pharm).
Mudrane GG, Tab., Elix. (ECR Pharmaceuticals).
Nasabid, PA Cap. (Jones Medical).
Nasabid SR, LA Tab. (Jones Medical).
Nasatab LA, LA Tab. (ECR Pharmaceuticals).
Neospect, Tab. (Teva USA).
Novahistine Cough Formula, Liq. (Merrell Dow).
Novahistine DMX, Liq. (Merrell Dow).
Novahistine, Expectorant (Merrell Dow).
Norel, Cap. (US Pharmaceutical).
Panaphyllin, Susp. (Panamerican).
Panmist JR, LA Tab. (Pan Am Labs).
Partuss-A, Tab. (Parmed).
Partuss AC (Parmed).
Pediacon DX Children's, Syr. (Zenith Goldline).
Pediacon DX Pediatric, Drops. (Zenith Goldline).
Pediacon EX, Drops (Zenith Goldline).
Phenatuss, Liq. (Dalin).
Phenylfenesin LA, EA Tab. (Zenith Goldline).
PMP, Expectorant, Syr. (Schlicksup).
Polaramine Expectorant (Schering Plough).
Poly-Histine Expectorant (Sanofi Winthrop).

Polytuss-DM, Liq. (Rhode).
Profen LA, TR Tab. (Wakefield).
Profen II DM, TR Tab. (Wakefield).
Profen II, TR Tab. (Wakefield).
P.R. Syrup, Liq. (Fleming).
Quibron, Cap., Liq. (Bristol-Myers Squibb).
Quibron-300, Cap. (Bristol-Myers Squibb).
Quibron Plus, Cap., Elix. (Bristol-Myers Squibb).
Rentuss, Cap., Syr. (Wren).
Respa-DM, SR Tab. (Respa).
Respa-1st, SR Tab. (Respa).
Rhinex DM (Teva USA).
Robitussin AC, CF, DAC, DM, PE (Robins).
Robitussin-DM Cough Calmers, Loz. (Robins).
Robitussin Cold & Cough, Cap. Liquigels (Robins).
Robitussin Severe Congestion, Cap., LiquiGels (Robins).
Rondec-DM, Syr. (Ross Laboratories).
Rymed, Prods. (Edwards Pharmaceuticals).
Santussin, Cap. (Sandia).
Scotcof, Liq. (Scott/Cord).
Scot-Tussin Senior Clear, Liq. (Scot-Tussin Pharm).
Silaminic Expectorant, Liq. (Silarx).
Sildicon-E, Ped. Drops (Silarx).
Sil-Tex, Liq. (Silarx).
Siltussin-CF, Liq. (Roberts Pharm).
Siltussin DM, Syr. (Silarx)
Sinutab Non-Drying, Liquicaps (GlaxoWellcome).
Slo-Phyllin GG, Cap., Syr. (Dooner).
Sorbase Cough Syr. (Fort David).
Sorbase II Cough Syr. (Fort David).
Spen-Histine Expectorant (Rugby).
Sudafed Cough Syr. (Glaxo-Wellcome).
Sudal 60/500, TR Tab. (Atley Pharm).
Sudal 120/600, SR Tab. (Atley Pharm).
Synacol CF, Tab. (Roberts).
Syn-Rx, CR Tab. (Adams).
Tolu-Sed, Liq. (Scherer).
Tolu-Sed DM, Liq. (Scherer).
Touro LA, LA Capl. (Dartmouth).
Triaminic Expectorant (Novartis).
Trihista-Phen, Liq. (Recsei).
Tri-Histin Expectorant (Recsei).
Tri-Mine, Expectorant (Rugby).
Trind-DM, Liq. (Bristol-Myers).
Trind, Liq. (Bristol-Myers).
Tusibron-DM, Liq. (Kenwood/Bradley).
Tussafed, Expectorant (Calvital).
Tussar-2, Syr. (Rhone-Poulenc Rorer).
Tussar SF, Liq. (Rhone-Poulenc Rorer).
Tussend, Liq. (Merrell Dow).
Tussi-Organidin DM NR, Liq. (Wallace).
Tussi-Organidin DM-S, Liq. (Wallace).
Tussi-Organidin NR, Liq. (Wallace).
Tussi-Organidin-S NR, Liq. (Wallace).
Verequad, Tab., Susp. (Knoll Pharmaceuticals).
Vicks Cough Syr. (Procter & Gamble).
Vicks Formula 44D Decongestant Cough Mixture, Syr. (Procter & Gamble).
Vicks 44E, Liq. (Procter & Gamble).
Wal-Tussin DM, Syr. (Walgreens).

guaifenesin and codeine phosphate syrup.
Use: Antitussive, expectorant.

Guaifenesin DAC. (Cypress) Codeine phosphate 10 mg, pseudoephedrine HCl 30 mg, guaifenesin 100 mg, alcohol 1.9%, saccharin, sorbitol. Liq. Bot. 480 ml. *otc.*
Use: Antitussive, decongestant, expectorant.

guaifenesin/phenylpropanolamine hydrochloride.
See: Phenylpropanolamine hydrochloride & guaifenesin tablets.

guaifenesin & pseudoephedrine hydrochloride & codeine phosphate syrup. (Schein Pharmaceutical) Pseudoephedrine HCl 30 mg, codeine phosphate 10 mg, guaifenesin 100 mg, alcohol 1.4 %. Bot. 473 ml. *c-v.*
Use: Antitussive, decongestant, expectorant.
See: Guaifenesin DAC, Liq. (Cypress).

Guaifenex. (Ethex) Guaifenesin 100 mg, phenylpropanolamine HCl 20 mg, phenylephrine HCl 5 mg, parabens, sorbitol/5 ml. Liq. Bot. 118 ml, 473 ml. *Rx.*
Use: Decongestant, expectorant.

Guaifenex DM. (Ethex) Guaifenesin 600 mg, dextromethorphan HBr 30 mg/ER Tab. Bot. 100s, 500s, 1000s. *Rx.*
Use: Antitussive, expectorant.

Guaifenex LA. (Ethex) Guaifenesin 600 mg, lactose/ER Tab. Bot. 100s. *Rx.*
Use: Expectorant.

Guaifenex PPA 75. (Ethex) Guaifenesin 600 mg, phenylpropanolamine HCl 75 mg, lactose/ER Tab. Bot. 100s. *Rx.*
Use: Decongestant, expectorant.

Guaifenex PSE 120. (Ethex) Guaifenesin 600 mg, pseudoephedrine HCl 120

mg/ER Tab. Bot. 100s. *Rx.*
Use: Decongestant, expectorant.

Guaifenex PSE 60. (Ethex) Guaifenesin 600 mg, pseudoephedrine HCl 60 mg, lactose/ER Tab. Bot. 100s. *Rx.*
Use: Decongestant, expectorant.

Guaifenex Rx. (Ethex) **AM:** Guaifenesin 600 mg, pseudoephedrine HCl 60 mg. **PM:** Guaifenesin 600 mg, dextromethorphan 30 mg. ER Tab. 28s. *Rx.*
Use: Decongestant, expectorant.

Guaifenex Rx DM. (Ethex) Guaifenesin 600 mg, pseudoephedrine HCl 60 mg/ Tab. 28s. *Rx.*
Use: Decongestant, expectorant.

Guaimax-D. (Schwarz Pharma) Pseudoephedrine HCl 120 mg, guaifenesin 600 mg. ER Tab. Bot. 100s. *Rx.*
Use: Decongestant, expectorant.

Guaipax Tablets. (Vitarine) Phenylpropanolamine HCl 75 mg, guaifenesin 400 mg/Tab. Bot. 100s, 500s, 1000s. *Rx.*
Use: Decongestant, expectorant.

Guaiphotol. (Foy) Iodine 1/30 gr, calcium cresoate 4 gr/Tab. Bot. 1000s. *Rx.*
Use: Expectorant.

Guaitab Tablets. (Muro) Pseudoephedrine HCl 60 mg, guaifenesin 400 mg, lactose/Tab. Bot. 100s. *otc.*
Use: Decongestant, expectorant.

•**guaithylline.** (GWIE-thill-in) USAN.
Use: Bronchodilator, expectorant.

Guaivent. (Ethex) Guaifenesin 600 mg, pseudoephedrine HCl 120 mg, parabens, EDTA, sucrose. Cap. Bot. 100s, 500s. *Rx.*
Use: Decongestant, expectorant.

Guaivent PD. (Ethex) Guaifenesin 600 mg, pseudoephedrine HCl 60 mg, parabens, EDTA, sucrose. Cap. Bot. 100s, 500s. *Rx.*
Use: Decongestant, expectorant.

Guai-Vent/PSE. (Dura Pharm) Pseudoephedrine HCl 120 mg, guaifenesin 600 mg/SR Tab. Bot. 100s. *Rx.*
Use: Expectorant.

guamide.
See: Sulfaguanidine (Various Mfr.).

•**guanabenz.** (GWAHN-uh-benz) USAN.
Use: Antihypertensive.
See: Wytensin, Tab. (Wyeth Ayerst).

•**guanabenz acetate.** (GWAHN-uh-benz) U.S.P. 23.
Use: Antihypertensive.

guanabenz acetate. (Various Mfr.) 4 mg or 8 mg/Tab. Bot. 30s, 100s, 500s.
Use: Antihypertensive.

•**guanacline sulfate.** (GWAHN-ah-kleen) USAN.
Use: Antihypertensive.

•**guanadrel sulfate.** (GWAHN-uh-drell) U.S.P. 23.
Use: Antihypertensive.
See: Hylorel, Tab. (Medeva).

•**guancydine.** (GWAHN-sigh-deen) USAN.
Use: Antihypertensive.

•**guanethidine monosulfate.** (gwahn-ETH-ih-deen MAH-no-SULL-fate) U.S.P. 23.
Use: Antihypertensive. Reflex sympathetic dystrophy and causalgia [Orphan drug]
See: Ismelin (Novartis).
W/Hydrochlorothiazide.
See: Esimil, Tab. (Novartis).

•**guanethidine sulfate.** (gwahn-ETH-ih-deen) USAN. U.S.P. XXI.
Use: Antihypertensive.
See: Ismelin, Tab. (Novartis).
W/Hydrochlorothiazide.
See: Esimil, Tab. (Novartis).

•**guanfacine hydrochloride.** (GWAHN-fay-seen) U.S.P. 23.
Use: Antihypertensive.
See: Tenex, Tab. (Robins).

guanidine hydrochloride. (Key Pharm) Guanidine HCl 125 mg/Tab. Bot. 100s. *Rx.*
Use: Muscle stimulant.

guanisoquin. (GWAN-eye-so-KWIN)
Use: Antihypertensive.

•**guanisoquin sulfate.** (GWAHN-eye-so-kwin) USAN.
Use: Antihypertensive.

•**guanoclor sulfate.** (GWAHN-oh-klahr) USAN.
Use: Antihypertensive.

•**guanoctine hydrochloride.** (GWAHN-ock-teen) USAN.
Use: Antihypertensive.

•**guanoxabenz.** (gwahn-OX-ah-benz) USAN.
Use: Antihypertensive.

•**guanoxan sulfate.** (GWAHN-ox-an) USAN.
Use: Antihypertensive.

•**guanoxyfen sulfate.** (GWAHN-OX-eh-fen) USAN.
Use: Antihypertensive, antidepressant.

Guardal. (Morton) Vitamins A 10,000 IU, B_1 20 mg, B_2 8 mg, C 50 mg, niacinamide 10 mg, calcium d-pantothenate 5 mg, iron 10 mg, dried whole liver 100 mg, yeast 100 mg, choline bitartrate 30 mg, B_6 0.5 mg, B_{12} 8 mcg, mixed tocopherols 5 mg, dicalcium phosphate anhydrous 150 mg, magnesium sulfate

dried 7.2 mg, sodium 1 mg, potassium Cl 1.3 mg/Tab. Bot. 100s. *otc.*
Use: Mineral, vitamin supplement.

Guardex. (Archer-Taylor) Tube 4 oz, 1 lb, 4.5 lb. *otc.*
Use: Emollient.

•**guar gum.** N.F. 18.
Use: Pharmaceutic aid (tablet binder; tablet disintegrant).
W/Danthron, docusate sodium.
See: Guarsol, Tab. (Western Research).
W/Standardized senna concentrate.
See: Gentlax B, Granules, Tab. (Blair Laboratories).

guayanesin.
Use: Expectorant.
See: Guaifenesin (Various Mfr.).

GuiaCough CF Liquid. (Schein Pharmaceutical) Phenylpropanolamine HCl 12.5 mg, dextromethorphan HBr 10 mg, guaifenesin 100 mg. Bot. 118 ml. *otc.*
Use: Antitussive, decongestant, expectorant.

GuiaCough PE Liquid. (Schein Pharmaceutical) Pseudoephedrine HCl 30 mg, guaifenesin 100 mg, alcohol 1.4%. Bot. 118 ml. *otc.*
Use: Decongestant, expectorant.

Guiamid Expectorant. (Vangard) Guaifenesin 100 mg/5 ml, alcohol 3.5%. Bot. pt, gal. *otc.*
Use: Expectorant.

Guiaphed Elixir. (Various Mfr.) Theophylline 45 mg, ephedrine sulfate 36 mg, guaifenesin 150 mg, phenobarbital 12 mg, alcohol 19%/15 ml Liq. Bot. 480 ml. *Rx.*
Use: Antiasthmatic combination.

Guaitex. (Rugby) **Cap.:** Phenylephrine HCl 5 mg, phenylpropanolamine HCl, guaifenesin 200 mg. **Liq.:** Phenylephrine HCl 5 mg, phenylpropanolamine 20 mg, quaifenesin 100 mg. *Rx.*
Use: Antitussive, expectorant.

Guiatex PSE. (Rugby) Pseudophedrine HCl, guaifenesin 500 mg/Tab. Bot. 100s. *Rx.*
Use: Decongestant, expectorant.

Guiatex LA. (Rugby) Phenylpropanolamine HCl 75 mg, guaifenesin 400 mg/Tab. Bot. 100s, 1000s. *Rx.*
Use: Antitussive, expectorant.

Guiatuss AC Syrup. (Various Mfr.) Codeine phosphate 10 mg, guaifenesin 100 mg, alcohol 3.5%/5 ml. Syr. Bot. 120 ml, pt, gal. *c-v.*
Use: Antitussive, expectorant.

Guiatuss CF Syrup. (Alphalma USPD) Phenylpropanolamine HCl 12.5 mg, dextromethorphan HBr 10 mg, guaifenesin 100 mg/Syr. Bot. 120 ml. *otc.*
Use: Antitussive, expectorant.

Guiatuss DAC Liquid. (Various Mfr.) Pseudoephedrine HCl 30 mg, codeine phosphate 10 mg, guaifenesin 100 mg, alcohol. Liq. Bot. 120 ml, 480 ml. *c-v.*
Use: Antitussive, decongestant, expectorant.

Guiatuss-DM Liquid. (Various Mfr.) Dextromethorphan HBr 10 mg, guaifenesin 100 mg. Bot. 120 ml, 240 ml, pt, gal. *otc.*
Use: Antitussive, expectorant.

Guiatuss Syrup. (Various Mfr.) Guaifenesin 100 mg/5 ml. Syr. Bot. 120 ml, 240 ml, pt, gal. *otc.*
Use: Expectorant.

Guiatuss PE. (Alphalma USPD) Pseudoephedrine HCl 30 mg, guaifenesin 100 mg, alcohol 1.4%. Liq. Bot. In 120 ml. *otc.*
Use: Decongestant, expectorant.

Guiatussin/Codeine Expectorant. (Rugby) Codeine phosphate 10 mg, guaifenesin 100 mg/5 ml, alcohol 3.5%. Syr. Bot. 120 ml, pt, gal. *c-v.*
Use: Antitussive, expectorant.

Guiatussin/Dextromethorphan. (Rugby) Dextromethorphan HBr 15 mg, guaifenesin 100 mg, alcohol 1.4%. Liq. Bot. 480 ml. *otc.*
Use: Antitussive, expectorant.

Guaivent. (Ethex) Guaifenesin 250 mg, pseudoephedrine HCl 120 mg, 100s, 500s. *Rx.*
Use: Expectorant.

Guaivent PD. (Ethex) Guaifenesin 300 mg, pseudoephedrine HCl 60 mg, parabens, sucrose. 100s, 500s. *Rx.*
Use: Expectorant.

Guistrey Fortis. (Jones Medical Industries) Guaifenesin 100 mg, phenylephrine HCl 10 mg, chlorpheniramine maleate 1 mg/Tab. Bot. 1000s. *otc.*
Use: Antihistamine, decongestant, expectorant.

Gulfasin Tabs. (Major) Sulfisoxazole 500 mg/Tab. Bot. 100s, 250s, 1000s.
Use: Anti-infective, sulfonamide.

guncotton, soluble. Pyroxylin.

gusperimus.
Use: Acute renal graft-rejection episodes.
See: Spanidin (Bristol-Myers Squibb).

•**gusperimus trihydrochloride.** (guss-PURR-ih-muss try-HIGH-droe-KLOR-ide) USAN.
Use: Immunosuppressant.

Gustalac. (Roberts Pharm) Calcium carbonate 300 mg, defatted skim milk pow. 200 mg/Tab. Bot. 100s, 250s, 1000s. *otc.*
Use: Antacid, calcium supplement.

Gustase. (Roberts Pharm) Gerilase (standard amylolytic enzyme) 30 g, geriprotase (standard proteolytic enzyme) 6 mg, gericellulase (standard cellulolytic enzyme) 2 mg/Tab. Bot. 42s, 100s, 500s. *otc.*
Use: Digestive aid.

Gustase Plus. (Roberts Pharm) Phenobarbital 8 mg, homatropine methylbromide 2.5 mg, gerilase 30 mg, geriprotase 6 mg, gericellulase 2 mg/Tab. Bot. 42s, 100s, 500s. *Rx.*
Use: Anticholinergic, antispasmodic, digestive aid, hypnotic, sedative.

•**gutta percha,** U.S.P. 23.
Use: Dental restoration agent.

G-vitamin.
See: Riboflavin (Various Mfr.).

G-well Shampoo. (Zenith Goldline) Lindane 1%. Bot. 2 oz, pt, gal. *Rx.*
Use: Pediculicide.

Gynecort 10, Extra Strength. (Combe) Hydrocortisone acetate 1%, parabens, zinc pyrithione. Cream. Tube 15 g. *otc.*
Use: Corticosteroid, topical.

Gyne-Lotrimin Combination Pack. (Schering Plough) **Vaginal Tab.:** Clotrimazole 100 mg. Pkg. 7s; **Topical Cream:** Clotrimazole 1%. Tube 7 g. *otc.*
Use: Antifungal, vaginal.

Gyne-Lotrimin Vaginal Cream 1%. (Schering Plough) Clotrimazole ≈ 5 g/applicatorful. Tube 45 g, 45 g twinpacks w/applicator. *otc.*
Use: Antifungal, vaginal.

Gyne-Lotrimin Vaginal Tablets. (Schering Plough) Clotrimazole 100 mg/Tab. Box 7 Tab. w/applicator, Box 6s. *otc.*
Use: Antifungal, vaginal.

gynergon.
See: Estradiol (Various Mfr.)

Gyne-Sulf. (G & W Laboratories) Sulfathiazole 3.42%, sulfacetamide 2.86%, sulfabenzamide 3.7%, urea 0.64%. Cream. Tube with applicator 82.5 g. *Rx.*
Use: Anti-infective, vaginal.

Gynogen L.A. 10. (Forest Pharmaceutical) Estradiol valerate in sesame oil 10 mg/ml. Vial 10 ml. *Rx.*
Use: Estrogen.

Gynogen L.A. 20. (Forest Pharmaceutical) Estradiol valerate in castor oil 20 mg/ml. Vial 10 ml. *Rx.*
Use: Estrogen.

Gynogen L.A. 40. (Forest Pharmaceutical) Estradiol valerate in castor oil 40 mg/ml. Inj. Vial 10 ml. *Rx.*
Use: Estrogen.

Gynol II Contraceptive. (Advanced Care Products) Nonoxynol-9 in 2% concentration. Starter 75 g tube w/applicator. Refill 75 g, 114 g/Tube. *otc.*
Use: Contraceptive.

Gynol II Extra Strength Contraceptive. (Advanced Care Products) Nonoxynol-9 3%. Jelly. 75 g, 114 g. *otc.*
Use: Contraceptive, spermicide.

Gyno-Petraryl. (Janssen) Econazole nitrate. *Rx.*
Use: Antifungal, vaginal.

Gynovite Plus. (Optimox) Vitamins A 833 IU, D 67 IU, E 67 mg (as d-alpha tocopheryl acid succinate), B_1 1.7 mg, B_2 1.7 mg, B_3 3.3 mg, B_5 1.7 mg, B_6 3.3 mg, B_{12} 21 mcg, C 30 mg, calcium 83 mg, iron 3 mg, folic acid 0.07 mg, boron, betaine, biotin, Cr, Cu, hesperidin, I, inositol, Mg, Mn, PABA, pancreatin, rutin, Se, Zinc 2.5 mg. Tab. Bot. 100s. *otc.*
Use: Mineral, vitamin supplement.

H

Habitrol. (Novartis Pharmaceuticals) Nicotine transdermal system. Dose absorbed in 24 hours, 21 mg, 14 mg, 7; total nicotine content (respectively) 52.5 mg, 35 mg, 17.5. Patch. Box 30 systems. *Rx.*
Use: Smoking deterrent.

haemophilus b conjugate vaccine.
Use: Vaccine, bacterial.
See: ActHIB, Pow. For Inj. (Connaught).
HibTITER, Inj. (Wyeth Ayerst).
OmniHIB, Pow. for Inj. (SmithKline Beecham Pharmaceuticals)
Pedvax HIB, Pow. (Merck).
ProHIBIT, Inj. (Pasteur Merieux Connaught).
W/DTP vaccine.
See: ActHIB/DTP, Set of DTwP vial plus Hib Pow. for Inj. (Pasteur Merieux Connaught).
Tetramune, vial (Wyeth Ayerst).

haemophilus influenzae type b and hepatitis vaccines, combined.
See: Comvax (Merck).

Hair Booster Vitamin. (NBTY) Vitamin B_3 35 mg, B_5 100 mg, B_{12} 6 mcg, folic acid 0.4 mg, zinc 15 mg, Cu, iron 18 mg, I, Mn, choline bitatrate, inositol, PABA, protein/Tab. Bot. 60s. *otc.*
Use: Mineral, vitamin supplement.

•**halazepam.** (hal-AZE-uh-pam) USAN. U.S.P. XXII.
Use: Hypnotic, sedative.

•**halazone.** (HAL-ah-zone) U.S.P. 23.
Use: Disinfectant.

•**halcinonide.** (hal-SIN-oh-nide) U.S.P. 23.
Use: Corticosteroid, topical; anti-inflammatory.
See: Halog Cream, Oint., Soln. (Westwood Squibb).

Halcion. (Pharmacia & Upjohn) Triazolam 0.125 mg or 0.25 mg/Tab. **0.125 mg:** Bot. 100s, Visipak 100s. (4 × 25s). **0.25 mg:** Bot. 100s, UD 100s, Visipak 100s. (4 × 25s). *c-IV.*
Use: Hypnotic, sedative.

Haldol. (Ortho McNeil) Haloperidol. **Tab.:** 0.5 mg, 1 mg, 2 mg, 5 mg or 10 mg. 20 mg/Tab. Bot. 100s. **Conc. Soln.:** 2 mg/ml. Bot. 15 ml, 120 ml. **Inj.:** 5mg/ml, parabens. Amp. 1ml. Vial 10 ml. *Rx.*
Use: Antipsychotic.

Haldol Decanoate 50. (Ortho McNeil) Haloperidol 50 (70.5 mg decanoate), sesame oil, benzyl alcohol 1.2%. Amp. 1 ml. Vial 5 ml. *Rx.*
Use: Antipsychotic.

Haldol Decanoate 100. (Ortho McNeil) Haloperidol 100 mg/ml (141.04 mg decanoate), sesame oil, benzyl alcohol 1.2%. Amp. 1 ml. Vial 5 ml. *Rx.*
Use: Antipsychotic.

Haldrone. (Eli Lilly) Paramethasone acetate 1 mg or 2 mg/Tab. Bot. 100s. *Rx.*
Use: Corticosteroid.

Halenol Children's. (Halsey) Acetaminophen 160 mg/5 ml. Elix. Bot. 120 ml, 240 ml, pt, gal. *otc.*
Use: Analgesic.

Halercol. (Roberts Pharm) Vitamins A 5000 IU, D 400 IU, E 1.36 mg, B_1 1.5 mg, B_2 2 mg, B_3 20 mg, B_5 1 mg, B_6 0.1 mg, B_{12} 1 mcg, C 37.5 mg/Cap. Bot. 100s. *otc.*
Use: Vitamin supplement.

Haley's M-O. (Bayer Corp) Mineral oil 25%, milk of magnesia in emulsion base. Flavored or regular. Bot. 240 ml, 480 ml, 960 ml. *otc.*
Use: Laxative.

Halfan. (SmithKline Beecham Pharmaceuticals) 250 mg/Tab. Bot. 60s. *Rx.*
Use: Antimalarial. [Orphan drug]

Halfort-T. (Halsey) Vitamins C 300 mg, B_1 15 mg, B_2 10 mg, niacin 100 mg, B_6 5 mg, B_{12} 4 mcg, pantothenic acid 20 mg/Tab. Bot. 100s. *otc.*
Use: Vitamin supplement.

Halfprin 81. (Kramer) Aspirin 81 mg. EC Tab. Bot. 90s. *otc.*
Use: Analgesic.

Half Strength Entrition Entri-Pak. (Biosearch Medical Products) Protein 17.5 g (Na and Ca caseinates), carbohydrate 68 g (maltodextrin), fat 17.5 g (corn oil, soy lecithin, mono- and diglycerides), sodium 350 mg, potassium 600 mg, m Osm/120 kg H_20, calories 0.5/ml, vitamins A, B_1, B_2, B_3, B_5, B_6, B_{12}, C, D, E, K, P, Ca, Mg, I, Fe, Zn, Mn, Cu, Cl, biotin, choline, folic acid. Liq. Pouch 1 L. *otc.*
Use: Nutritional supplement.

Half Strength Florvite with Iron. (Everett Laboratories) Flouride 0.5 mg, Vitamins A 2500 IU, D 400 IU, E 15 IU, B_1 1.05 mg, B_2 1.2 mg, B_3 13.5 mg, B_6 1.05 mg, B_{12} 4.5 mcg, C 60 mg, folic acid 0.3 mg, Cu, iron 12 mg, Zn 10 mg, sucrose/Tab. Bot. 100s. *Rx.*
Use: Mineral, vitamin supplement; dental caries agent.

Half Strength Introlan. (Elan) Protein 22.5 g, fat 18 g, carbohydrates 70 g, Na 345 mg, K 585 mg/L. Vitamins A, C, B_1, B_2, B_3, D, E, B_6, B_{12}, B_5, K, Ca, Fe, folic acid, P, I, Mg, Zn, Cu, biotin, Mn,

choline, Cl, Se, Cr, Mo. Liq. In 1000 ml New Pak closed systems with and without color check. *otc.*
Use: Nutritional supplement.

Hali-Best. (Barth's) Vitamins A 10,000 IU, D 400 IU/Cap. Bot. 100s, 500s. *otc.*
Use: Vitamin supplement.

halibut liver oil.
Use: Vitamin supplement.

haliver oil.
See: Halibut Liver Oil (Various Mfr.).

Hall's Mentho-Lyptus Decongestant Liquid. (Warner Lambert) Dextromethorphan HBr 15 mg, phenylpropanolamine HCl 37.5 mg, menthol 14 mg, eucalyptus oil 12.7 mg/10 ml, alcohol 22%. Bot. 90 ml. *otc.*
Use: Antitussive, decongestant.

Hall's Mentho-Lyptus Cough Lozenges. (Warner Lambert) Menthol and eucalyptus oil in varying amounts and flavors. Stick-Pack 9s. Bag 30s. *otc.*
Use: Mouth and throat preparation.

Hall's-Plus Maximum Strength. (Warner Lambert) Menthol 10 mg, corn syrup, sugar. Cherry, honey-lemon and regular flavors. Tab. Pkg. 10s, 25s. *otc.*
Use: Mouth and throat preparation.

Hall's Mentho-Lyptus Sugar Free. (Warner Lambert) Menthol 5 mg or 6 mg, eucalyptus oil 2.8 mg/Tab. Pkg. 25s. *otc.*
Use: Mouth and throat preparation.

Hall's Zinc Defense. (Warner-Lambert) Zinc acetate 5 mg, sugar, cherry or peppermint flavor. Loz. 24s. *otc.*
Use: Mineral supplement.

•**halobetasol propionate.** (hal-oh-BEH-tah-sahl PRO-pee-oh-nate) USAN.
Use: Anti-inflammatory; corticosteroid, topical.
See: Ultravate (Westwood Squibb).

•**halofantrine hydrochloride.** (HAY-low-FAN-trin) USAN.
Use: Antimalarial. [Orphan drug]
See: Halfan, Tab. (SmithKline Beecham Pharmaceuticals).

Halofed. (Halsey) **Tab.:** Pseudoephedrine HCl 30 mg or 60 mg. Bot. 100s, 1000s. **Syr.:** Pseudoephedrine HCl 30 mg/5 ml. Bot. 120 ml, 240 ml, pt, gal. *otc.*
Use: Decongestant.

•**halofenate.** (HAY-low-FEN-ate) USAN.
Use: Antihyperlipoproteinemic, uricosuric.
See: Livipas (Merck).

•**halofuginone hydrobromide.** (HAY-low-FOO-jin-ohn HIGH-droe-BROE-mide) USAN.
Use: Antiprotozoal.

Halog Cream. (Westwood Squibb) Halcinonide 0.025% or 0.1%, in specially formulated cream base consisting of glyceryl monostearate, cetyl alcohol, myristyl stearate, isopropyl palmitate, polysorbate 60, propylene glycol, purified water. **0.1%:** Tube 15 g, 30 g, 60 g, Jar 240 g. **0.025%:** Tube 15 g, 60 g. *Rx.*
Use: Corticosteroid-topical.

Halog-E Cream. (Westwood Squibb) Halcinonide 0.1% in hydrophilic vanishing cream base consisting of propylene glycol dimethicone 350, castor oil, cetearyl alcohol, ceteareth-20, propylene glycol stearate, white petrolatum, water. Tube 15 g, 30 g, 60 g. *Rx.*
Use: Corticosteroid-topical.

Halog Ointment. (Westwood Squibb) Halcinonide 0.1%, in Plastibase (plasicized hydrocarbon gel), PEG 400, PEG 6000 distearate, PEG 300, PEG 1540, butylated hydroxy toluene. Tube 15 g, 30 g, 60 g, Jar 240 g. *Rx.*
Use: Corticosteroid-topical.

Halog Solution. (Westwood Squibb) Halcinonide 0.1%, edetate disodium, PEG 300, purified water, butylated hydroxy toluene as preservative. Bot. 20 ml, 60 ml. *Rx.*
Use: Corticosteroid-topical.

•**halopemide.** (hay-LOW-PEH-mid) USAN.
Use: Antipsychotic.

•**haloperidol.** (HAY-low-PURR-ih-dahl) U.S.P. 23.
Use: Antipsychotic, tranquilizer; antidyskinetic (in Gilles de la Tourette's disease).
See: Haldol, Preps. (Ortho McNeil).

haloperidol. (Various Mfr.) Haloperidol. **Tab.:** 0.5 mg, 1 mg, 2 mg, 5 mg, 10 mg, 20 mg/Tab. Bot. 100s, 500s (except 20 mg), 1000s (except 20 mg), 1000s. **Conc.:** 2 mg/ml. Bot. 15 ml, 120 ml, UD 100s 5 ml and 10 ml. **Inj.:** 5 mg/ml. Amp. 1 ml, Syr. 1 ml, Vial 1 ml, 2 ml, 2.5 ml, 10 ml. *Rx.*
Use: Antipsychotic.

•**haloperidol decanoate.** (HAY-low-PURR-ih-dahl deh-KAN-oh-ate) USAN.
Use: Antipsychotic.

•**halopredone acetate.** (HAY-low-PREH-dohn) USAN.
Use: Anti-inflammatory, topical.

•**haloprogesterone.** (HAL-oh-pro-jeh-STEE-rone) USAN.

Use: Hormone-progestin.

•**haloprogin,** (hal-oh-PRO-jin) U.S.P. 23.
Use: Antimicrobic, topical; anti-infective.
See: Halotex, Cream, Soln. (Westwood Squibb).

Halotestin. (Pharmacia & Upjohn) Fluoxymesterone 2 mg, 5 mg or 10 mg. Tartrazine, lactose, sucrose. **2 mg:** Bot. 100s; **5 mg:** Bot. 100s; **10 mg:** Bot. 30s, 100s. *c-III.*
Use: Androgen.
W/Ethinyl estradiol.
See: Halodrin, Tab. (Pharmacia & Upjohn).

Halotex Cream. (Westwood Squibb) Haloprogin 1% in water dispersible base composed of PEG-400, PEG-4000, diethyl sebacate, polyvinylpyrrolidone. Tube 15 g, 30 g. *Rx.*
Use: Antifungal-topical.

Halotex Solution. (Westwood Squibb) Haloprogin 1% in a clear colorless vehicle of diethyl sebacate w/alcohol 75%. Bot. 10 ml, 30 ml. *Rx.*
Use: Antifungal-topical.

•**halothane.** (HAL-oh-thane) U.S.P. 23.
Use: General anesthetic, inhalation.
See: Fluothane, Liq. (Wyeth Ayerst).
Halothane, 250 ml Liq. (Abbott Laboratories).

Halotussin. (Halsey) Guaifenesin 100 mg/5 ml. Bot. 4 oz, 8 oz, pt, gal. *otc.*
Use: Expectorant.

Halotussin-DM. (Halsey) Dextromethorphan HBr 10 mg, guaifenesin 100 mg. In 120 ml, 240 ml, pt, gal. *otc.*
Use: Antitussive, expectorant.

Halotussin-DM Sugar-Free Liquid. (Halsey) Dextromethorphan HBr 10 mg, guaifenesin 100 mg. In 120 ml, 240 ml, 480 ml, gal. *otc.*
Use: Antitussive, expectorant.

•**halquinols.** (HAL-kwin-oles) USAN.
Use: Anti-infective, topical; antimicrobial.
See: Quinolor (Bristol-Myers Squibb).

Haltran Tablets. (Roberts Pharm) Ibuprofen 200 mg/ Tab. Bot. 30s, 50s. Blister pkg. 12s. *otc.*
Use: Analgesic, NSAID.

HAMA. Hydroxy-aluminum magnesium aminoacetate.

hamamelis water.
See: Succus Cineraria Maritima, Soln. (Walker Pharm).
Witch hazel (Various Mfr.).
Tucks Preps., (GlaxoWellcome).

•**hamycin.** (HAY-MY-sin) USAN.
Use: Antifungal.

Hang-Over-Cure. (Silvers) Calcium carbonate, glycine, thiamine HCl, pyridoxine HCl, aspirin. Cont. Tab. 6 g. *otc.*
Use: Antacid, analgesic combination.

Haniform. (Hanlon) Vitamins A 25,000 IU, D 1000 IU, B_1 10 mg, B_2 5 mg, C 150 mg, niacinamide 150 mg/Cap. Bot. 100s. *otc.*
Use: Vitamin supplement.

Haniplex. (Hanlon) Vitamins B_1 20 mg, B_2 10 mg, B_6 1 mg, calcium pantothenate 10 mg, B_{12} 5 mcg, niacin 20 mg, liver concentrate 50 mg, C 150 mg/ Cap. Bot. 100s. *otc.*
Use: Mineral, vitamin supplement.

Harbolin. (Arcum) Hydralazine HCl 25 mg, hydrochlorothiazide 15 mg, reserpine 0.1 mg/Tab. Bot. 100s, 1000s. *Rx.*
Use: Antihypertensive combination.

hard fat.
Use: Pharmaceutic necessity.

hartshorn. Ammonium Carbonate.

Haugase. (Madland) Trypsin, chymotrypsin. Bot. 50s, 250s.
Use: Enzyme preparation.

Havab. (Abbott Diagnostics) Radioimmunoassay or enzyme immunoassay for detection of antibody to hepatitis A virus. Test kit 100s.
Use: Diagnostic aid.

Havab EIA. (Abbott Diagnostics) Enzyme immunoassay for the detection of antibody to hepatitis A virus.
Use: Diagnostic aid.

Havab-M. (Abbott Diagnostics) Radioimmunoassay for the detection of specific Ig antibody to hepatitis A virus. Test kit 100s.
Use: Diagnostic aid.

Havab-M EIA. (Abbott Diagnostics) Enzyme immunoassay for the detection of Ig antibody to hepatitis A virus.
Use: Diagnostic aid.

Havrix. (SmithKline Beecham Pharmaceuticals) Hepatitis A vaccine. **Adult:** 1440 ELU units/ml. Single-dose vial, prefilled syringe. **Pediatric:** 720 ELU/ 0.5 ml. Single-dose vial, prefilled syringe. *Rx.*
Use: Immunization.

Hawaiian Tropic Aloe Paba Sunscreen. (Tanning Research) Padimate 0, oxybenzone. Cream Bot. 120 g. *otc.*
Use: Sunscreen.

Hawaiian Tropic Baby Faces. (Tanning Research) SPF 20. Octyl methoxycinnamate, octocrylene, benzophenone-3,

menthyl anthranilate, PABA free, waterproof. Gel Tube 120 g. *otc.*
Use: Sunscreen.

Hawaiian Tropic Baby Faces Sunblock. (Tanning Research) Octyl methoxycinnamate, benzophenone-3, octyl salicylate, titanium dioxide, octocrylene, PABA free, waterproof. **SPF 35:** Lot. Bot. 60 ml, 120 ml, 300 ml. **SPF 50:** Lot. Bot. 120 ml. *otc.*
Use: Sunscreen.

Hawaiian Tropic Cool Aloe with I.C.E. (Tanning Research) Lidocaine, menthol, aloe, SD alcohol 40, diazolidinyl urea, EDTA, vitamins A and E, tartrazine. Gel. Jar 360 g. *otc.*
Use: Emollient.

Hawaiian Tropic Dark Tanning. (Tanning Research) **Gel:** Phenylbenzimidazole sulfonic acid. SPF 2. Bot. 240 ml. **Oil:** 2-ethylhexyl methoxycinnamate, octyl dimethyl PABA, waterproof. Bot. 240 ml. *otc.*
Use: Sunscreen.

Hawaiian Tropic Dark Tanning with Sunscreen. (Tanning Research) **Oil:** Ethylhexyl p-methoxycinnamate, octyl dimethyl PABA. Waterproof. SPF 4. Bot. 240 ml. **Gel:** Phenylbenzimidazole, sulfonic acid. PABA free. SPF 4. Tube 240 g. *otc.*
Use: Sunscreen.

Hawaiian Tropic Just for Kids Sunblock. (Tanning Research) **SPF 30:** Homosalate, octyl methoxycinnamate, benzophenone-3, menthyl anthranilate, octyl salicylate. PABA free. Waterproof. Lot. Bot. 88.7 ml. **SPF 45:** Octyl methoxycinnamate, benzophenone-3, octyl salicylate, octocrylene, titanium dioxide. PABA free. Waterproof. Lot. Bot. 88.7 ml. *otc.*
Use: Sunscreen.

Hawaiian Tropic Lip Balm Sunblock. (Tanning Research) Padimate 0, oxybenzone. Stick 4 g. *otc.*
Use: Sunscreen.

Hawaiian Tropic 8 Plus. (Tanning Research) Octyl methoxycinnamate, benzophenone-3, menthyl anthranilate. PABA free. Waterproof. SPF 8+. Gel 120 g. *otc.*
Use: Sunscreen.

Hawaiian Tropic 10 Plus. (Tanning Research) Octyl methoxycinnamate, benzophenone-3, menthyl anthranilate. PABA free. Waterproof. SPR 10+. Gel 120 g. *otc.*
Use: Sunscreen.

Hawaiian Tropic 15 Plus. (Tanning Research) Octyl methoxycinnamate, octocrylene, benzophenone-3, menthyl anthranilate, PABA free, waterproof. Gel Tube 120 g. *otc.*
Use: Sunscreen.

Hawaiian Tropic 15 Plus Sunblock. (Tanning Research) Menthyl anthranilate, octyl methoxycinnamate, benzophenone-3. PABA free. Waterproof. Lot. Bot. 7.5 ml, 15 ml, 60 ml, 120 ml, 240 ml, 300 ml. *otc.*
Use: Sunscreen.

Hawaiian Tropic 15 Plus Sunblock Lip Balm. (Tanning Research) Padimate O, oxybenzone. SPF 15, waterproof. Stick 4.2 g. *otc.*
Use: Sunscreen.

Hawaiian Tropic 45 Plus Sunblock Lip Balm. (Tanning Research) Octyl methoxycinnamate, benzophenone-3, octyl salicylate, titanium dioxide, menthyl anthranilate. PABA free. Waterproof. SPF 45+. Lip balm 4.2 g. *otc.*
Use: Sunscreen.

Hawaiian Tropic Protective Tanning. (Tanning Research) Titanium dioxide. PABA free. Waterproof. SPF 6. Lot. Bot. 240 ml. *otc.*
Use: Sunscreen.

Hawaiian Tropic Protective Tanning Dry. (Tanning Research) SPF 6. **Oil:** 2-ethylhexyl p-methoxycinnamate, homosalate, menthyl anthranilate. Waterproof. Bot. 180 ml. **Gel:** Phenylbenzimidazole, sulfonic acid, benzophenone-4. Tube 180 g. *otc.*
Use: Sunscreen.

Hawaiian Tropic Self Tanning Sunblock. (Tanning Research) Octyl methoxycinnamate, benzophenone-3, aloe, cetyl alcohol, stearyl alcohol, cocoa butter, parabens, vitamin E. PABA free. SPF 15. Cream 93.75 ml. *otc.*
Use: Sunscreen.

Hawaiian Tropic Sport Sunblock. (Tanning Research) SPF 15, SPF 30. Methoxycinnamate, octocrylene, benzophenone-3, octyl salicylate, titanium dioxide. PABA free. Waterproof. Lot. Bot. 88.7 ml. *otc.*
Use: Sunscreen.

Hawaiian Tropic Sunblock. (Tanning Research) Titanium dioxide, octyl methoxycinnamate, benzophenone-3, octyl salicylate, octocrylene. PABA free. Waterproof. **SPF 30+:** Lot. Bot. 120 ml. **SPF 45+:** Lot. Bot. 120 ml, 300 ml. *otc.*
Use: Sunscreen.

Hawaiian Tropic Swim n Sun. (Tanning Research) Padimate O, oxybenzone. Lot. Bot. 120 ml. *otc.*
Use: Sunscreen.

Hayfebrol Liquid. (Scot-Tussin Pharmacal) Pseudoephedrine HCl 30 mg, chlorpheniramine 2 mg/Syr. Bot. 118 ml. *otc.*
Use: Antihistamine, decongestant.

Hazogel Body and Foot Rub. (Vortech) Witch hazel 70%, isopropanol 20% in a neutralized resin vehicle. Bot. 4 oz. *otc.*
Use: Astringent, antipruritic.

H-BIG Hepatitis B Immune Globulin (Human). (North American Biologicals) Hepatitis B immune globulin (human). Vial 1 ml, 5 ml. Syr. 0.5 ml. *Rx.*
Use: Immunization.

H-BIGIV,. (NABI) Hepatitis B immune globulin IV.
Use: Prophylaxis against hepatitis B virus reinfectioin in liver transplant patients. [Orphan drug]

1% HC. (C & M Pharmacal) Hydrocortisone 1%, petrolatum base. Oint. Tube 15, 20, 30, 60, 120, 240 g, lb. *otc.*
Use: Corticosteroid, topical.

HC Derma-Pax. (Recsei) Hydrocortisone 0.5% in liquid base. Dropper Bot. 2 oz. *otc.*
Use: Corticosteroid, topical.

HCG.
See: Chorionic Gonadotropin.

HCG-Nostick. (Organon Teknika) Sol Particle Immunoassay (SPIA) for detection of hCG in urine. Stick 30s.
Use: Diagnostic aid, pregnancy.

HD 85. (Lafayette Pharm) High density barium suspension 85% w/v. Bot. 4 x 2000 ml.
Use: Radiopaque agent.

HD 200 Plus. (Lafayette Pharm) Barium sulfate 98%. Pow. Bot. 312 g.
Use: Radiopaque agent.

Head & Shoulders Conditioner. (Procter & Gamble) Pyrithione zinc 0.3%. Bot. 4 oz, 11 oz. *otc.*
Use: Antiseborrheic.

Head & Shoulders Dry Scalp. (Procter & Gamble) Pyrithione zinc 1%, regular and conditioning formulas. Shampoo. Bot. 210 ml, 330 ml, 450 ml. *otc.*
Use: Antiseborrehic.

Head & Shoulders Intensive Treatment Dandruff Shampoo. (Procter & Gamble) Selenium sulfide 1%, regular and conditioning forumlas. Shampoo. Bot. 120 ml, 210 ml, 330 ml. *otc.*
Use: Antiseborrehic.

Head & Shoulders Shampoo. (Procter & Gamble) Pyrithione zinc 1%. **Cream:** Tube 51 g, 75 g, 120 g, 210 g. **Lot:** 120 ml, 210 ml, 330 ml, 450 ml. *otc.*
Use: Antiseborrheic.

Healon. (Pharmacia & Upjohn) Sodium hyaluronate 10 mg/ml Inj. Syringe 0.4 ml, 0.55 ml, 0.85 ml, 2 ml. *Rx.*
Use: Surgical aid, ophthalmic.

Healon GV. (Pharmacia & Upjohn) Sodium hyaluronate 14 mg/ml Inj. Syringe 0.55 ml, 0.85 ml. *Rx.*
Use: Surgical aid, ophthalmic.

Healon Yellow. (Pharmacia & Upjohn) Sodium hyaluronate 10 mg, fluorescein sodium 0.005 mg/ml Inj. Syringe 0.55 ml, 0.85 ml.
Use: Surgical and diagnostic aid, ophthalmic.

Healthbreak. (Lemar Labs) Silver acetate 6 mg. Chewing gum. Pack 24s. *otc.*
Use: Smoking deterrent.

Heartburn Antacid. (Walgreens) Aluminum hydroxide dried gel 80 mg, magnesium trisilicate 60 mg/ Tab. Bot. 100s. *otc.*
Use: Antacid.

Heartline. (BDI) Aspirin 81 mg/Tab. Enteric coated Bot. 36s. *otc.*
Use: Anti-inflammatory.

heavy metal poisoning, antidote.
See: BAL., Amp. (Becton Dickinson).
Calcium Disodium Versenate, Amp., Tab. (3M).

Heet Liniment. (Whitehall Robins) Methyl salicylate 15%, camphor 3.6%, oloeoresin capsicum 0.025%, alcohol 70%. Bot. 2⅓ oz, 5 oz. *otc.*
Use: Analgesic-topical.

•**hefilcon a.** (heh-FILL-kahn A) USAN.
Use: Contact lens material (hydrophilic).

•**helfilcon b.** (heh-FILL-kahn B) USAN.
Use: Contact lens material (hydrophilic).

•**helfilcon c.** (heh-FILL-kahn C) USAN.
Use: Contact lens material (hydrophilic).

Helidac. (Procter & Gamble) Bismuth subsalicylate 264.4 mg/Tab. Metronidazole 250 mg/Tab. Tetracycline 500 mg/ Cap. Box. 4s, 8s (bismuth subsalicylate only). *Rx.*
Use: Antiulcerative.

Helistat. (Hoechst Marion Roussel) Absorbable collagen hemostatic sponge. 1"×2" and 3"×4" in 10s, 9"×10" in 5s. *Rx.*

Use: Hemostatic.

•**helium.** (HEE-lee-uhm) U.S.P. 23.
Use: Diluent for gases.

Helixate. (Centeon) Concentrated recombitant hemophilic factor. After reconstitution, also contains glycine 10 to 30 mg, imidazole ≤ 500 mcg/1000 IU, polysorbate 80 ≤ 600 mcg/1000 IU, Calcium Cl 2 to 5 mM, sodium 100 to 130 mEq/L, chloride 100 to 130 mEq/L, albumin (human) 4 to 10 mg/ml. IU 250, 500, 1000. *Rx.*
Use: Antihemophilic.

Hemabate. (Pharmacia & Upjohn) Carboprost tromethamine equivalent to 250 mcg carboprost, tromethamine 83 mcg/ml. Inj. Amp 1 ml. *Rx.*
Use: Abortifacient.

Hema-Chek Slides. (Bayer Corp) Fecal occult blood test containing slide tests, developer and applicators. Pkg. 100s, 300s, 1000s.
Use: Diagnostic aid.

Hema-Combistix Reagent Strips. (Bayer Corp) Four-way strip test for urinary pH, glucose, protein and occult blood. Strip. Bot. 100s.
Use: Diagnostic aid.

Hemaferrin Tablets. (Western Research) Ferrous fumarate 150 mg, desiccated liver 50 mg, docusate sodium 25 mg, betaine HCl 100 mg, folic acid 0.4 mg, vitamins C 50 mg, B_6 2 mg, manganese 2 mg, B_{12} 5 mcg, copper 1 mg, zinc 2 mg, molybdenum 0.4 mg/Tab. 28 Pack 1000s. *otc.*
Use: Mineral, vitamin supplement; stool softener.

Hemafolate. (Canright) Ferrous gluconate 293 mg, liver fraction II 250 mg, gastric substance 100 mg, vitamins C 50 mg, B_{12} 10 mcg/Tab. Bot. 100s, 1000s. *otc.*
Use: Mineral, vitamin supplement.

Hemalive Liquid. (Barth's) Vitamins B_1 3.15 mg, B_2 3.33 mg, niacin 22.5 mg, B_6 0.81 mg, B_{12} 6 mcg, biotin 3.6 mcg, iron 60 mg, choline, inositol, liver fraction No. 1, pantothenic acid/15 ml. Bot. 8 oz, 24 oz. *otc.*
Use: Mineral, vitamin supplement.

Hemalive Tablets. (Barth's) Vitamins B_{12} 25 mcg, iron 75 mg, B_1 2.5 mg, B_2 5 mg, niacin 1.4 mg, C 30 mg, liver 240 mg, B_6, pantothenic acid, aminobenzoic acid, choline, inositol, biotin, Mg, Mn, Cu/3 Tab. Bot. 100s, 500s, 1000s. *otc.*
Use: Mineral, vitamin supplement.

Hemaneed. (Hanlon) Hematinic B_{12}, intrinsic factor, Fe/Cap. Bot. 100s. *otc.*
Use: Mineral, vitamin supplement.

Hemaspan Tablets. (Bock Pharmacal) Iron 110 mg (from ferrous fumarate), ascorbic acid 200 mg, docusate sodium 20 mg/Tab. Bot. 100s, 1000s. *otc.*
Use: Mineral, vitamin supplement; stool softener.

Hemastix Reagent Strips. (Bayer Corp) Cellulose strip, impregnated with a peroxide and orthotolidine for detection of hematuria and hemoglobinuria. Strip Bot. 50s.
Use: Diagnostic aid.

Hematest Reagent Tablets. (Bayer Corp) Reagent Tab. for blood in the feces. Bot. 100s.
Use: Diagnostic aid.

Hematinic. (Canright) Ferrous gluconate 180 mg, desiccated liver 200 mg, vitamins B_{12} 1 mcg, C 25 mg, B_1 3.3 mg, copper gluconate 0.3 mg/Tab. Bot. 100s, 1000s. *otc.*
Use: Mineral, vitamin supplement.

hematinics.
See: Iron Products.
Ferric Compounds.
Ferrous Compounds.
Liver Products.
Vitamin B_{12}.
Vitamin Products.

Hematrin. (Towne) Iron 50 mg, vitamins B_{12} 10 mcg, B_1 10 mg, B_2 10 mg, B_6 2 mg, C 150 mg, copper 2 mg, niacinamide 50 mg, calcium pantothenate 5 mg, desiccated liver 200 mg/Captab. Bot. 60s, 100s. *otc.*
Use: Mineral, vitamin supplement.

heme arginate.
Use: Acute porphyria; myelodysplastic syndromes. [Orphan drug]
See: Normosang (Leiras).

HemeSelect. (SmithKline Diagnostics) Occult blood screening test. Box 40 test kits.
Use: Diagnostic aid, fecal.

Hemex. Hemin and zinc mesoporphyrin.
Use: Acute porphyric syndromes. [Orphan drug]

Hemiacidrin. Citric acid, glucono-delta-lactone, magnesium carbonate.
Use: Genitourinary irrigant.
See: Renacidin, Pow. (Guardian Laboratories).
Renacidin, Soln. (Guardian Laboratories).

Hemex. (Vogarell) Oint. Tube 1.25 oz. Supp. Box 12s.

Use: Anorectal preparation.

hemin.
Use: Acute intermittent porphyria. [Orphan drug]
See: Panhematin, Inj. (Abbott Laboratories).

hemin and zinc mesoporphyrin.
Use: Acute porphyric syndromes. [Orphan drug]
See: Hemex.

hemisine.
See: Epinephrine (Various Mfr.).

Hemoccult SENSA. (SmithKline Diagnostics) Occult blood screening tests.
Use: Diagnostic aid, fecal.

Hemoccult Slides. (SmithKline Diagnostics) Occult blood detection (fecal). In 100s, 1000s and tape dispensers (test 100s).
Use: Diagnostic aid.

Hemoccult II. (SmithKline Diagnostics) Occult blood detection (fecal). In 102s, kit 100s.
Use: Diagnostic aid.

Hemocitrate. (Hemotec Medical) Trisodium citrate concentrate.
Use: Leukapheresis procedures. [Orphan drug]

Hemocyte. (US Pharmaceutical) Ferrous fumarate 324 mg (FE 106 mg)/Tab. Bot. 100s. *otc.*
Use: Mineral supplement.

Hemocyte-F. (US Pharmaceutical) Iron 106 mg (from ferrous fumarate), folic acid 1 mg/Tab. 100s. *Rx.*
Use: Mineral supplement.

Hemocyte Plus. (US Pharmaceutical) Iron 106 mg (from ferrous fumarate), sodium ascorbate 200 mg, vitamins B_1 10 mg, B_2 6 mg, B_6 5 mg, B_{12} 15 mcg, folic acid 1 mg, B_3 30 mg, B_5 10 mg, zinc 18.2 mg, Mg, Mn sulfate, Cu/Tabule. Bot. 100s. *Rx.*
Use: Mineral, vitamin supplement.

Hemocyte Plus Elixir. (US Pharmaceutical) Polysaccharide iron complex 12 mg, vitamin B_3 13.3 mg, B_5 3.3 mg, B_6 1.3 mg, B_{12} 4 mcg, folic acid 0.33 mg, zinc 5 mg, Mn 1.3 mg/15 ml. Bot. 473 ml. *Rx.*
Use: Mineral, vitamin supplement.

Hemofil M. (Baxter) Stable dried preparation of Antihemophilic Factor in concentrated form. Albumin (human) 12.5 mg/ml when reconstituted. Bot. 10 ml, 20 ml, 30 ml with diluent. *Rx.*
Use: Antihemophilic.

Hemofil T. (Baxter) Antihemophilic Factor (Human), method four, dried, heat-treated 225-375 IU/10 ml; 450-650 IU/20 ml; 675-999 IU/30ml; 1000-1600 IU/30 ml. *Rx.*
Use: Antihemophilic.

•**hemoglobin crosfumaril.** (HEE-moe-GLOBE-in CROSS-FEW-mah-ril) USAN.
Use: Red cell substitute; treatment of prefusion deficit disorders.

Hemoglobin Reagent Strips. (Bayer Corp) Seralyzer reagent strips. Bot. 50s. Quantitive strip test for hemoglobin in whole blood.
Use: Diagnostic aid.

Hemopad. (Astra) Fibrous absorbable collagen hemostat. 2.5 cm×5 cm, 5 cm×8 cm, 8 cm×10 cm. *Rx.*
Use: Hemostatic.

hemorheologic agent. Pentoxifylline.
See: Trental, Tab. (Hoechst Marion Roussel).

Hemorid for Women. (Thompson Medical) **Lotion:** Mineral oil, petrolatum, diazolidinyl urea, cetyl alcohol, glycerin, parabens. Bot. 118 ml. **Cream:** white petrolatum 30%, mineral oil 20%, pramoxine HCl 1%, phenylephrine HCl 0.25%, aloe vera gel, parabens, cetyl and stearyl alcohols. In 28.3 g. **Supp:** zinc oxide 11%, phenylephrine HCl 0.25%, hard fat 88.25%, aloe vera. In 12s. *otc.*
Use: Perianal hygiene.

Hemorrhoidal HC. (Various Mfr.) Hydrocortisone acetate 25 mg/Supp. Bot. 12s, 24s, 50s, 100s, UD 12s. *Rx.*
Use: Anorectal preparation.

Hemorrhoidal Ointment. (Zenith Goldline) Live yeast cell derivative supplying skin respiratory factor 2000 units/oz of ointment w/shark liver oil 3%, phenyl mercuric nitrate 1:10,000. *otc.*
Use: Anorectal preparation.

Hemorrhoidal Suppositories. (Zenith Goldline) Bismuth subgallate 2.25%, bismuth resorcin compound 1.75%, benzyl benzoate 1.2%, balsam Peru 1.8%, zinc oxide 11%/Supp. Box 12s. *otc.*
Use: Anorectal preparation.

Hemorrhoidal Uniserts. (Upsher-Smith Labs) Bismuth subgallate 2.25%, bismuth resorcin compound 1.75%, benzyl benzoate 1.2%, balsam Peru 1.8%, zinc oxide 11%/Supp. Carton 12s, 50s. *otc.*
Use: Anorectal preparation.

hemostatics, local.
See: Absorbable Gelatin Sponge (Pharmacia & Upjohn).

Gelfilm (Pharmacia & Upjohn).
Gelfoam, Preps. (Pharmacia & Upjohn).
Helistat (Hoechst Marion Roussel).
Hemotene (Astra).
Oxidized Cellulose.
Thrombin (Various Mfr.).

hemostatic topical. Thrombin.
See: Thrombinar, Pow. (Centeon).
Thrombostat, Pow. (Parke-Davis).

hemostatin.
See: Epinephrine (Various Mfr.).

Hemotene. (Astra) Absorbable collagen hemostat. 1 g. Pkg. 5s. *Rx.*
Use: Hemostatic-topical.

Hemozyme Elixir. (Barrows) Vitamins B_1 5 mg, B_2 5 mg, B_6 1 mg, panthenol 4 mg, niacinamide 100 mg, B_{12} 3 mcg, iron 100 mg, choline bitartrate 100 mg, dl-methionine 100 mg, yeast extract, alcohol 12%/fl oz. Bot. 12 oz. *otc.*
Use: Mineral, vitamin supplement.

Hem-Prep. (G & W Laboratories) Phenylephrine HCl 0.25%, zinc oxide 11%. Supp. Bot. 12s. *otc.*
Use: Anorectal preparation.

Hem-Prep Ointment. (G & W Laboratories) Phenylephrine HCl 0.025%, zinc oxide 11%, white petrolatum. Oint. 42.5 g. *otc.*
Use: Anorectal preparation.

Hemril-HC Uniserts. (Upsher-Smith Labs) Hydrocortisone acetate 25 mg/ Supp. 12s. *Rx.*
Use: Anorectal preparation.

Hemril Uniserts. (Upsher-Smith Labs) Bismuth subgallate 2.25%, bismuth resorcin compound 1.75%, benzyl benzoate 1.2%, balsam Peru 1.8%, zinc oxide 11%/Supp. 12s, 50s. *otc.*
Use: Anorectal preparation.

henbane.
See: Hyoscyamus (Various Mfr.).

Henydin-M. (Arcum) Thyroid desiccated pow. 0.5 gr, vitamins B_1 1 mg, B_2 0.5 mg, B_6 0.5 mg, niacinamide 2.5 mg/Tab. Bot. 100s, 1000s. *Rx.*
Use: Vitamin supplement.

Henydin-R. (Arcum) Thyroid desiccated pow. 1 gr, vitamins B_1 2 mg, B_2 1 mg, B_6 1 mg, niacinamide 5 mg/Tab. Bot. 100s, 1000s. *Rx.*
Use: Vitamin supplement.

Hepandrin. (Bio-Technology) Oxandrolone.
Use: Turner's syndrome; AIDS; growth delay; alcoholic hepatitis; malnutrition. [Orphan drug]

heparin, 2-0-desulfated. (HEP-uh-rin)
Use: Cystic fibrosis. [Orphan drug]
See: Aeropin.

heparin antagonist.
See: Protamine Sulfate (Various Mfr.).

heparin calcium. *Rx.*
Use: Anticoagulant.
See: Calciparine, Inj. (DuPont Merck Pharmaceuticals).

•**heparin calcium,** (HEP-uh-rin KAL-see-uhm) U.S.P. 23.
Use: Anticoagulant.

heparin lock flush solution. (Sanofi Winthrop) **10 USP units/1 ml:** Cartridge 2 ml HEP-PAK containing 1 cartridge heparin lock flush Soln. (1 ml) and 2 cartridges sodium Cl Inj. HEP-PAK-2 containing 1 cartridge heparin lock flush soln. (1 ml) and 1 cartridge sodium Cl Inj. **10 USP units/2 ml:** Cartridge 2 ml. **100 USP units/1 ml:** Cartridge 2 ml HEP-PAK containing 1 cartridge heparin lock flush soln (1 ml) and 2 cartridges sodium Cl Inj. HEP-PAK-2 containing 1 cartridge of heparin lock flush soln (1 ml) and 1 cartridge sodium Cl Inj. **100 USP units/2 ml:** Cartridge 2 ml. *Rx.*
Use: Catheter patency agent.

heparin lock flush solution. (Wyeth Ayerst) Heparin sodium 10 units or 100 units/1 ml vial. Pkg. 50 Tubex 1 ml, 2 ml. *Rx.*
Use: Infusion set patency agent.

•**heparin sodium.** (HEP-uh-rin SO-dee-uhm) U.S.P. 23.
Use: Anticoagulant. Note: Protamine sulfate is antidote.
See: Hepathrom, Amp., Vial (Fellows-Testagar).
Heprinar, Inj. (Centeon).
Lipo-Hepin, Amp., Vial (3M).
Lipo-Hepin/BL, Amp., Vial (3M).
Liquaemin, Vial (Organon Teknika).

W/Vit. B_{12}, folic acid, niacinamide, choline Cl.
See: Heparin-B, Vial (Medical Chem.).

heparin sodium. (Pharmacia & Upjohn) 1000 units/ml. Vial 10 ml, 30 ml 5000 units/ml. Vial 1 ml, 10 ml 10,000 units/ ml. Vial 1 ml, 4 ml (Sanofi Winthrop) 5000 USP units/1 ml. Carpuject 1 ml fill in 2 ml cartridge.
Use: Anticoagulant. Note: Protamine sulfate is antidote.

heparin sodium and 0.45% sodium chloride. (Abbott Laboratories) 12,500, 25,000 units in 250 ml Inj. *Rx.*
Use: Anticoagulant.

heparin sodium and 0.9% sodium chloride. (Baxter) Inj.: 1000 units in 500

ml Viaflex. 2000, 5000 units in 1000 ml Viaflex. *Rx.*
Use: Anticoagulant.

heparin sodium lock flush solution. *Rx.*
Use: Anticoagulant.
See: Heparin Lock Flush, Inj. (Various).
Hep-Lock, Inj. (ESI Lederle Generics).
Hep-Lock U/P, Inj. (ESI Lederle Generics).

HepatAmine. (McGaw) Amino acid 8%. Inj. Bot. 500 ml. *Rx.*
Use: Nutritional supplement, parenteral.

Hepatic-Aid II Instant Drink Powder. (McGaw) Amino acids (high BCAA, low AAA), maltodextrin, sucrose, partially hydrogenated soybean oil, lecithin, mono and diglycerides. In 3 oz packet of 12s. *otc.*
Use: Nutritional supplement.

hepatitis A vaccine, inactivated. (hep-uh-TIGHT-iss) *Rx.*
Use: Immunization.
See: Havrix, Inj. (SmithKline Beecham Pharmaceuticals).
Vaqta, Inj. (Merck).

hepatitis B and haemophilus type b vaccines, combined.
See: Comvax (Merck).

•**hepatitis B immune globulin.** (hep-uh-TIGHT-iss B ih-myoon GLAH-byoo-lin) U.S.P. 23.
Use: Immunization.
See: BayHep B, Vial, Syr. (Bayer Corp).
H-BIG, Vial, syr. (North American Biologicals).

hepatitis B immune globulin IV. (hep-uh-TIGHT-iss)
Use: Prophylaxis against hepatitis B virus reinfection in liver transplant patients. [Orphan drug]
See: H-BIGIV (NABI).

hepatitis B vaccine, recombinant. (hep-uh-TIGHT-iss) *Rx.*
Use: Immunization.
See: Engerix-B (SmithKline Beecham Pharmaceuticals).
Recombivax-HB, Inj. (Merck).

•**hepatitis B virus vaccine inactivated.** (hep-uh-TIGHT-iss B vak-SEEN) U.S.P. 23.
Use: Immunization.

Hepfomin R Injection. (Keene Pharmaceuticals) Liver inj. equivalent to cyanocobalamin 10 mcg, folic acid 0.4 mg, cyanocobalamin 100 mcg. Vial 10 ml. *Rx.*
Use: Nutritional supplement, parenteral.

Hep-Forte. (Marlyn) Vitamins A 1200 IU, E 10 mg, B_1 1 mg, B_2 1 mg, B_3 10 mg, B_5 2 mg, B_6 0.5 mg, B_{12} 1 mcg, C 10 mg, folic acid 0.06 mg, zinc 0.5 mg, choline, inositol, biotin, dl-methionine, desiccated liver, liver concentrate, liver fraction number 2/Cap. Bot. 100s, 300s, 500s. *otc.*
Use: Vitamin, liver supplement.

Hep-Lock. (ESI Lederle Generics) Sterile heparin sodium soln. in saline 10 units or 100 units/ml. Dosette 1 ml, 2 ml, multiple dose vial 10 ml, 30 ml. *Rx.*
Use: Catheter patency agent.

Hep-Lock PF. (ESI Lederle Generics) Preservative-free heparin flush soln. 10 units/ml or 100 units/ml. Vial 1 ml. *Rx.*
Use: Catheter patency agent.

heprofax.
See: Mucoplex (Zeneca).

Heptalac. (Copley) Lactulose 10 g/15 ml, galactose < 1.6 g, lactose < 1.2 g, other sugars ≤ 1.2 g/ Syrup. Bot. 473 ml, 1920 ml. *Rx.*
Use: Laxative.

Herbal Cellulex. (NBTY) Vitamin C 83 mg, K 33 mg, iron 9 mg/Tab. Bot. 90s. *otc.*
Use: Vitamin supplement.

Herbal Laxative. (NBTY) Senna concentrate 125 mg, cascara sagrada 20 mg, buckthorn bark PDR. Tab. Bot. 100s. *otc.*
Use: Laxative.

Hermal Bath Oil. (Hermal) Soybean oil-based bath oil. Bot. 8 oz, 32 oz. *otc.*
Use: Emollient.

Herpecin-L. (Campbell) Allantoin, octylp-(dimethylamino)-benzoate (Padimate O), titanium dioxide, pyridoxine HCl in a balanced, acidic lipid system. Lip balm. Tube 2.5 g. *otc.*
Use: Cold sores.

herpes simplex virus gene. (Genetic Therapy)
Use: Antineoplastic. [Orphan drug]

Herrick Lacrimal Plug. (Lacrimedics) Silicone plug 0.3 mm or 0.5 mm Pkg. 2 plugs. *Rx.*
Use: Punctal plug.

HES. Hetastarch.
Use: Plasma expander.
See: Hespan, Inj. (DuPont Merck Pharmaceuticals).

Hespan Injection. (DuPont Merck Pharmaceuticals) Hetastarch 6 g, sodium Cl 0.9%/100 ml. Bot. 500 ml. *Rx.*
Use: Plasma volume expander.

hesperidin.

Use: Capillary fragility and permeability, hemorrhage.
See: Vitamin P; also Rutin.
W/Combinations.
See: A.C.N., Tab. (Person & Covey).
Ceebec, Tab. (Person & Covey).
Hesper Bitabs, Tab. (Hoechst Marion Roussel).
Nialex, Tab. (Roberts Pharm).
Norimex-Plus, Cap. (Vortech).
Pregent, Tab. (Beutlich).
Vita Cebus, Tab. (Cenci).

Hesperidin w/C. (Various Mfr.).
Use: Vitamin supplement.
See: Min-Hest, Cap. (Scrip).

hesperidin methyl chalcone.
Use: Vitamin P supplement.

•**hetacillin.** (HET-ah-SILL-in) USAN. U.S.P. XXII
Use: Anti-infective.

•**hetacillin potassium.** (HET-ah-SILL-in poe-TASS-ee-uhm) U.S.P. 23.
Use: Anti-infective.

•**hetaflur.** (HEH-tah-flure) USAN.
Use: Dental caries prophylactic.

•**hetastarch.** (HET-uh-starch) USAN.
Use: Plasma volume extender.
See: Hespan, Inj. (DuPont Merck Pharmaceuticals).

•**heteronium bromide.** (HET-er-oh-nee-uhm) USAN.
Use: Anticholinergic.

Hexabamate #1. (Rugby) Tridihexethyl Cl 25 mg, meprobamate 200 mg/Tab. Bot. 100s, 500s. *Rx.*
Use: Anticholinergic combination.

Hexabamate #2. (Rugby) Tridihexethyl Cl 25 mg, meprobamate 400 mg/Tab. Bot. 100s, 500s. *Rx.*
Use: Anticholinergic combination.

Hexa-Betalin. (Eli Lilly) Pyridoxine HCl. Inj. Vial 100 mg/ml. Ctn. 10s, vial 10 ml. *Rx.*
Use: Vitamin supplement.

Hexabrix Solution. (Mallinckrodt Chemical) Ioxaglate meglumine 39.3%, ioxaglate sodium 19.6% (32% iodine). Vial 20 ml, 30 ml, 50 ml, 100 ml fill in bot. 150 ml, 200 ml fill in bot. 250 ml, bot. 150 ml.
Use: Radiopaque agent.

hexachlorcyclohexane.
See: Benzene Hexachloride, Gamma.

•**hexachlorophene,** (hex-ah-KLOR-oh-feen) U.S.P. 23.
Use: Anti-infective, topical; antiseptic; detergent.
See: Derl.
Gamophen, Leaves, Bar (Arbrook).
pHisoHex Prods. (Sanofi Winthrop).
W/Soya protein complex.
See: Soy-Dome Cleanser, Liq. (Bayer Corp).

hexachlorophene cleansing emulsion.
Use: Anti-infective, topical detergent.

hexachlorophene liquid soap, detergent liquid.
See: pHisoHex Liq. Prods. (Sanofi Winthrop).
Use: Anti-infective, topical detergent.

hexacose. Mixture of C-6 alcohols derived from oxidation of tetracosane–$C_{24}H_{50}$.
See: Hexathricin, Aerospra (Lincoln).

hexadecadrol.
See: Dexamethasone.

hexadienol. Hexacose.

Hexadrol. (Organon Teknika) Dexamethasone. **Tab.:** 4 mg. Bot. 100s, UD 100s, Strip 10 X 10s. **Elix.:** 0.5 mg/5 ml, alcohol 5%. Bot. 120 ml. *Rx.*
Use: Corticosteroid.

Hexadrol Phosphate. (Organon Teknika) Dexamethasone sodium phosphate 4 mg/ml, 10 mg/ml or 20 mg/ml, benzyl alcohol. **4 mg/ml:** Vial 1 ml, 5 ml, disposable syringe 1 ml. **10 mg/ml:** Vial 10 ml, disposable syringe 1 ml. **20 mg/ml:** Vial 5 ml, disposable syringe 5 ml. *Rx.*
Use: Corticosteroid.

•**hexafluorenium bromide.** (HEK-sah-flure-EE-nee-uhm) USAN. U.S.P. XXI.
Use: Muscle relaxant, synergist (succinycholine).

hexafluorodiethyl ether. Name used for Flurothyl.

hexahydroxycyclohexane.
See: Inositol, Preps. (Various Mfr.).

hexakose. Mixture of tetracosanes and oxidation products.
See: Hexathricin, Aerospra (Lincoln).
W/Benzethonium Cl, p-chloro-m-xylenol, ethyl p-aminobenzoate and tyrothricin.
See: Hexathricin, Aeropak (Lincoln).

Hexalen. (US Bioscience) Altretamine. *Rx.*
Use: Antineoplastic.

hexamarium bromide.

hexamethonium.
W/Rauwiloid.
See: Rauwiloid w/hexamethonium, Tab. (3M).

hexamethonium chloride. (Various Mfr.) Hexamethylene (bistrimethylammonium) Cl.

hexamethylamine.
See: Hexastat. Hypotensive.

hexamethylenamine.
See: Methenamine (Various Mfr.).

hexamethylenetetramine.
See: Methenamine, U.S.P. 23. Hexamethylenetetramine Mandelate.

hexamethylmelamine. Altretamine.
Use: Antineoplastic.
See: Hexalen.

hexamethylpararosaniline chloride.
See: Bismuth Violet, Soln. (Table Rock).

hexamethylrosaniline chloride.
See: Gentian Violet.

hexamine.
See: Methenamine (Various Mfr.).

hexapradol hydrochloride. a-(1-Aminohexyl) benzhydrol HCl.
Use: CNS stimulant.

Hexate. (Davis & Sly) Atropine sulfate 1/2000 gr, extract of hyoscyamus 0.25 gr, methylene blue gr, methanamine 0.5 gr, benzoic acid 0.5 gr, salol 0.5 gr./Tab. Bot. 1000s. *Rx.*
Use: Anti-infective, urinary.

Hexavitamin Tablets. (Various Mfr.) Vitamins A 5000 IU, B_1 2 mg, B_2 3 mg, C 75 mg, D 400 IU, B_3 20 mg/Tab. or Cap. Bot. 100s, 1000s, UD 100s. *otc.*
Use: Vitamin supplement.
See: Hepicebrin, Tab. (Eli Lilly).

Hexavitamin Tablets. (Forest Pharmaceutical) Vitamin A 1.5 mg, D 10 mcg, C 75 mg, B_1 2 mg, B_2 3 mg, nicotinamide 20 mg/SC Tab. Bot. 1000s. *otc.*
Use: Vitamin supplement.

Hexavitamin SC. (Halsey).
Use: Vitamin supplement.

hexcarbacholine bromide.

•**hexedine.** (HEX-eh-deen) USAN.
Use: Anti-infective.

hexene-ol. Hexacose.

hexenol. Hexacose.

hexitol irrigants.
Use: Irrigant, genitourinary.
See: Resectisol, Soln. (McGaw).
Sorbitol, Soln. (McGaw).
Sorbitol, Soln. (Baxter).
Sorbitol-Mannitol, Soln. (Abbott Laboratories).

hexobarbital, U.S.P. XXI.
W/Dihydrohydroxycodeinone HCl, dihydrohydroxy-codeinone terephthalate, homatropine terephthalate, aspirin, phenacetin, caffeine.
See: Percobarb, Cap. (DuPont).
W/Dihydrohydroxycodeinone terephthalate, dihydrohydroxycodeinone HCl, homatropine terephthalate, aspirin, phenacetin, caffeine.
See: Percobarb-Demi, Cap. (DuPont).

•**hexobendine.** (HEX-oh-BEN-deen) USAN.
Use: Vasodilator.

hexoestrol.
See: Hexestrol (Various Mfr.).

Hexopal. (Bayer Corp) Inositol hexanicotinate. *Rx.*
Use: Hypolipidemic, peripheral vasodilator.

•**hexoprenaline sulfate.** (hex-oh-PREN-ah-leen) USAN.
Use: Bronchodilator; tocolytic.

•**hexylene glycol,** N.F. 18.
Use: Pharmaceutic aid (humectant, solvent).

•**hexylresorcinol,** (hex-ill-reh-SORE-sih-nole) U.S.P. 23.
Use: Anthelmintic (intestinal roundworms and trematodes), throat preparation.
See: Sucrets Sore Throat Loz. (SmithKline Beecham Pharmaceuticals).

H-F Gel. (Paddock) Calcium gluconate gel 2.5%.
Use: Emergency burn treatment. [Orphan drug]

H.H.R. (Geneva Pharm) Hydralazine HCl 25 mg, hydrochlorothiazide 15 mg, reserpine 0.1 mg/Tab. Bot. 100s, 1000s. *Rx.*
Use: Antihypertensive.

Hibiclens. (J & J Merck Consumer Pharm) Chlorhexidine gluconate 4%, isopropyl alcohol 4%, in a non-alkaline base. Bot. 4 oz, 8 oz, 16 oz, 32 oz, gal. Packette 15 ml. *otc.*
Use: Antimicrobial, antiseptic.

Hibiclens Sponge Brush. (J & J Merck Consumer Pharm) Chlorhexidine gluconate impregnated sponge brush. Unit-of-use 22 ml sponge brushes. *otc.*
Use: Antimicrobial, antiseptic.

Hibistat. (J & J Merck Consumer Pharm) Chlorhexidine gluconate 0.5%. **Liq.:** Isopropyl alcohol 70%, emollients. Bot. 4 oz, 8 oz. **Towelettes:** Unit-of-use pocket-size towelette impregnated with 5 ml Hibistat. *otc.*
Use: Antimicrobial, antiseptic.

Hibplex. (Standex) Vitamins B_1 100 mg, B_2 2 mg, B_3 100 mg, panthenol 2 mg/ml. Vial 30 ml. *Rx.*
Use: Vitamin supplement.

HibTITER Vaccine. (Wyeth Ayerst) Purified Haemophilus b saccharide 10 mcg, diphtheria CRM_{197} protein 25 mcg. Inj. 0.5 ml, 2.5 ml, 5 ml vials. *Rx.*
Use: Immunization.

Hi B with C. (Towne) Vitamin C 300 mg,

B_1 15 mg, B_2 10.2 mg, niacin 50 mg, B_6 5 mg, pantothenic acid 10 mg/Cap. Bot. 100s. *Rx.*
Use: Vitamin supplement.

Hi-Cor 1.0. (C & M Pharmacal) Hydrocortisone 1% in a nonionic, ester-free, salt-free, paraben-free washable base. Tube 30 g, Jar 60 g, lb. *Rx.*
Use: Corticosteroid, topical.

Hi-Cor 2.5. (C & M Pharmacal) Hydrocortisone 2.5% in a nonionic, esterfree, saltfree, parabenfree washable base. Tube 30 g. Jar 60 g. *Rx.*
Use: Corticosteroid, topical.

hiestrone.
See: Estrone (Various Mfr.).

High B12. (Barth's) Vitamin B_{12}, desiccated liver. Cap. Bot. 100s, 500s. *otc.*
Use: Vitamin supplement.

High Potency Cold Cap. (Weeks & Leo) Salicylamide 325 mg, chlorpheniramine maleate 4 mg, dextromethorphan HBr 15 mg, caffeine 16.2 mg/Tab. Bot. 18s. *otc.*
Use: Analgesic, antihistamine, antitussive.

High Potency N-Vites. (Nion) Vitamins B_1 15 mg, B_2 10 mg, B_3 100 mg, B_5 20 mg, B_{12} 10 mcg, C 500 mg/Tab. Bot. 100s. *otc.*
Use: Vitamin supplement.

High Potency Pain Relievers. (Weeks & Leo) Acetaminophen 300 mg, salicylamide 300 mg/Cap. Bot. 20s, 40s. *otc.*
Use: Analgesic.

High Potency Tar. (C & M Pharmacal) Coal tar topical solution 25%. Shampoo, gel. Bot. 240 ml. *otc.*
Use: Antiseborrheic.

High Potency Vitamins and Minerals. (Burgin-Arden) Vitamins A 25,000 IU, D 400 IU, B_1 10 mg, B_2 5 mg, C 150 mg, niacinamide 100 mg, calcium 103 mg, phosphorous 80 mg, iron 10 mg, B_6 1 mg, B_{12} 5 mcg, magnesium 5.5 mg, manganese 1 mg, potassium 5 mg, zinc 1.4 mg/Tab. Bot. 100s. *otc.*
Use: Mineral, vitamin supplement.

Hill-Shade Lotion. (Hill) Para-aminobenzoic acid, alcohol 65%. SPF 22. *otc.*
Use: Sunscreen.

Hi-Po-Vites Tablets. (Hudson) Iron 6 mg, vitamins A 10,000 IU, D 400 IU, E 13 mg, B_1 25 mg, B_2 25 mg, B_3 50 mg, B_5 12.5 mg, B_6 15 mg, B_{12} 50 mcg, C 150 mg, folic acid 0.4 mg, Ca, Cr, Cu, I, K, Mg, Mn, Mo, P, Se, Zn 5 mg, biotin 1 mg, bioflavonoids, bone meal, PABA, choline bitartrate, betaine, inositol, lecithin, desiccated liver, rutin/Tab. Bot. 100s. *otc.*
Use: Mineral, vitamin supplement.

•**hioxifilcon a.** (high-ock-sih-FILL-kahn A) USAN.
Use: Contact lens material (hydrophilic).

hippramine.
See: Methenamine hippurate.

hipputope. (Bristol-Myers Squibb) Radioiodinated sodium iodohippurate (^{131}I) Inj. Bot. 1 m Ci, 2 m Ci.
Use: Diagnostic aid.

Hipotest. (Marlop Pharm) Ca 53.5 mg, iron 50 mg, vitamins A 10,000 IU, D 400 IU, E 2.5 mg, B_1 25 mg, B_2 25 mg, B_3 50 mg, B_5 13 mg, B_6 15 mg, B_{12} 50 mcg, C 150 mg, choline, betaine, PABA, rutin, bioflavonoids, biotin 1 mg, dessicated liver, bone meal, Cu, Mg, Mn, Zn 2.2 mg, I, P, lecithin/Tab. Bot. 100s. *otc.*
Use: Mineral, vitamin supplement.

Hiprex. (Hoechst Marion Roussel) Methenamine hippurate 1 g/Tab. Bot. 100s. *Rx.*
Use: Anti-infective, urinary.

Hismanal. (Janssen) Astemizole 10 mg, lactose, povidone. Tab. 30s, 100s. *Rx.*
Use: Antihistamine.

Histacon. (Marsh Labs) Chlorpheniramine maleate 12 mg, ephedrine HCl 15 mg/SR Tab. Bot. 100s, 1000s. *otc.*
Use: Antihistamine, decongestant.

Histacon Syrup. (Marsh Labs) Chlorpheniramine maleate 3 mg, ephedrine HCl 4 mg/5 ml, alcohol 5%. Bot. pt.
Use: Antihistamine, decongestant.

Histagesic D.M. (Jones Medical Industries) Phenylpropanolamine HCl 25 mg, chlorpheniramine maleate 4 mg, dextromethorphan HBr 10 mg, acetaminophen 324 mg/Tab. Bot. 100s, 1000s. *otc.*
Use: Analgesic, antihistamine, antitussive, decongestant.

Histagesic Modified. (Jones Medical Industries) Acetaminophen 324 mg, phenylephrine HCl 10 mg, chlorpheniramine maleate 4 mg/Tab. *otc.*
Use: Analgesic, antihistamine, decongestant.

Histagesic Modified Tablets. (Jones Medical Industries) Phenylephrine HCl 10 mg, chlorpheniramine maleate 4 mg, acetaminophen 324 mg/Tab. Bot. 1000s. *otc.*
Use: Analgesic, antihistamine, decongestant.

Histalet. (Solvay) **Syr.:** Pseudoephedrine HCl 45 mg, chlorpheniramine maleate 3 mg/5 ml. Bot. 473 ml. *Rx.*
Use: Antihistamine, decongestant.

Histalet Forte. (Major). Phenylpropanolamine HCl 50 mg, phenylephrine HCl 10 mg, chlorpheniramine maleate 4 mg, pyrilamine maleate 25 mg, lactose, sugar. Tab. Bot. 100s, 250s. *Rx.*
Use: Antihistamine, decongestant.

Histalet X. (Solvay) **Syr.:** Pseudoephedrine HCl 45 mg, guaifenesin 200 mg/5 ml, alcohol 15%. Bot. 480 ml. **Tab.:** Pseudoephedrine HCl 120 mg, guaifenesin 400 mg/Tab. Bot. 100s. *Rx.*
Use: Decongestant, expectorant.

Histamic Capsules. (Lexis) Phenylpropanolamine HCl 50 mg, phenylephrine HCl 25 mg, phenyltoloxamine citrate 30 mg, chlorpheniramine maleate 12 mg/SR Cap. Bot. 100s, 1000s. *otc.*
Use: Antihistamine, decongestant.

Histamic Tablets. (Lexis) Phenylpropanolamine HCl 40 mg, phenylephrine HCl 10 mg, phenyltoloxamine citrate 15 mg, chlorpheniramine maleate 5 mg/Tab. Bot. 100s, 1000s. *otc.*
Use: Antihistamine, decongestant.

Histamine.
Use: Diagnostic aid.

•**histamine dihydrochloride,** (HISS-tah-meen die-HIGH-droe-KLOR-ide) U.S.P. 23.
W/Methyl nicotinate, oleoresincapicum, glycomonosalicylate.
Use: Analgesic, topical.
W/Menthol, thymol, methyl salicylate.
See: Imahist Unction (Gordon Laboratories).

histamine H_2 antagonists.
See: Axid Pulvules, Cap. (Eli Lilly).
Cimetidine HCl, Inj. (Endo Labs).
Pepcid, Tab., Pow. (Merck).
Pepcid IV, Inj. (Merck).
Tagamet, Tab., Liq., Inj. (SmithKline Beecham Pharmaceuticals).
Zantac, Tab. Syr. Inj. (Glaxo and Roche).

Histapco. (Apco) Chlorpheniramine maleate 4 mg, ipecac and opium pow. 0.25 gr, (contains opium 0.025 gr), camphor monobromated ⅛ gr, salicylamide 2 gr, phenacetin 1.5 gr, caffeine alkaloid gr, atropine sulfate gr/Tab. *Rx.*
Use: Analgesic, anticholinergic, antihistamine combination.

Histatab Plus. (Century Pharm) Chlorpheniramine maleate 2 mg, phenylephrine HCl 5 mg/Tab. Bot. 100s. *otc.*
Use: Antihistamine, decongestant.

Histatime Forte. (Major) Phenylpropanolamine HCl 50 mg, phenylephrine HCl 10 mg, chlorpheniramine maleate 4 mg, pyrilamine maleate 25 mg/Cap. Bot. 100s. *Rx.*
Use: Antihistamine, decongestant.

Histatrol. (Center Laboratories) 2.75 mg/ml histamine phosphate, equivalent ot 1 ml/ml histamine base, in 50% glycerin w/v, 5 ml vial; available in a Multitest dosage form or dropper bottle; 0.275 mg/ml histamine phosphate, equivalent to 0.1 mg/ml histamine base, 5 ml vial.
Use: Diagnostic aid, skin test control.

Hista-Vadrin Syrup. (Scherer) Phenylpropanolamine HCl 20 mg, chlorpheniramine maleate 2 mg, phenylephrine HCl 2.5 mg, alcohol 2%/5 ml. Bot. pt. *Rx.*
Use: Antihistamine, decongestant.

Hista-Vadrin Tablets. (Scherer) Phenylpropanolamine HCl 40 mg, chlorpheniramine maleate 6 mg, phenylephrine HCl 5 mg/Tab. Bot. 100s. *Rx.*
Use: Antihistamine, decongestant.

Hista-Vadrin T.D. Capsules. (Scherer) Phenylpropanolamine HCl 50 mg, chlorpheniramine maleate 4 mg, belladonna alkaloids 0.2 mg/Cap. Bot. 50s, 250s. *otc.*
Use: Antihistamine, decongestant combination.

Histerone Injection. (Roberts Pharm) Testosterone aqueous susp. 50 mg or 100 mg/ml. Vial 10 ml. *c-III.*
Use: Androgen.

•**histidine.** (HISS-tih-deen) U.S.P. 23.
Use: Amino acid.

histidine monohydrochloride.
Use: I.M., peptic and jejunal ulcers.

Histine-1. (Freeport) Diphenhydramine HCl 10 mg, alcohol 12% to 14%/4 ml. Bot. 4 oz. *otc.*
Use: Antihistamine with anticholinergic, antitussive, antiemetic and sedative effects.

Histine-2. (Freeport) Diphenhydramine HCl 12.5 mg/5 ml w/alcohol 5%. Bot. 4 oz. *otc.*
Use: Antihistamine with anticholinergic, antitussive, antiemetic and sedative effects.

Histine-4. (Freeport) Chlorpheniramine maleate 4 mg/Tab. Bot. 1000s. *otc.*
Use: Antihistamine.

Histine-8. (Freeport) Chlorpheniramine maleate 8 mg/TR Tab. Bot. 1000s. *otc.*
Use: Antihistamine.

Histine-12. (Freeport) Chlorpheniramine

maleate 12 mg/TR Tab. Bot. 1000s. *otc.*
Use: Antihistamine.

Histine-25. (Freeport) Diphenhydramine HCl 25 mg/Cap. Bot. 1000s. *otc.*
Use: Antihistamine with anticholinergic, antitussive, antiemetic and sedative effects.

Histine-50. (Freeport) Diphenhydramine HCl 50 mg/Cap. Bot. 1000s. *otc.*
Use: Antihistamine with anticholinergic, antitussive, antiemetic and sedative effects.

Histine DM Syrup. (Ethex) Phenylpropanolamine HCl 12.5 mg, brompheniramine maleate 2 mg, dextromethorphan HBr 10 mg, parabens, saccharin. Bot. 120 ml or 480 ml. *Rx.*
Use: Antihistamine, antitussive, decongestant.

Histinex HC. (Ethex) Hydrocodone bitartrate 2.5 mg, phenylephrine HCl 5 mg, chlorpheniramine maleate 2 mg/5 ml. Syrup. Alcohol and sugar free. Bot. 473 ml. *c-III.*
Use: Antitussive, decongestant, antihistamine.

Histinex PV. (Ethex) Hydrocodone bitartrate 2.5 mg, pseudoephedrine HCl 30 mg, chlorpheniramine maleate 2 mg, parabens, saccharin, sorbitol/5ml. Syrup. Alcohol and sugar free. Bot. 120 ml, 480 ml. *c-III.*
Use: Antihistamine, antitussive, decongestant.

Histolyn-CYL. (ALK Laboratories) Histoplasmin sterile filtrate from yeast cells of *Histoplasma capsulatum.* Vial 1.3 ml. *Rx.*
Use: Diagnostic aid, skin test.

•**histoplasmin.** (hiss-toe-PLAZZ-min) U.S.P. 23. (Parke-Davis) An aqueous solution containing standardized sterile culture filtrate of *Histoplasma capsulatum* grown on liquid synthetic medium.
Use: Diagnostic aid (dermal reactivity indicator).
See: Histolyn-CYL, Inj. (ALK Labs).
Histoplasmin, diluted (Parke-Davis)

histoplasmin, diluted. (Parke-Davis) 1:100 w/v. Standardized sterile filtrate from cultures of *Histoplasma capsulatum,* 0.5% phenol, polysorbate 80. 1 ml/Inj. *Rx.*
Use: Diagnostic aid.

Histosal. (Ferndale Laboratories) Pyrilamine maleate 12.5 mg, phenylpropanolamine HCl 20 mg, acetaminophen 324 mg, caffeine 30 mg/Tab. Bot. 100s. *otc.*
Use: Analgesic, antihistamine, decongestant.

•**histrelin.** (hiss-TRELL-in) USAN.
Use: LHRH agonist. Treatment of porphyria [Orphan drug]
See: Supprelin, Inj. (Ortho McNeil).

histrelin acetate.
Use: Central procotious puberty. [Orphan drug]
See: Supprelin, Inj. (Roberts Pharm).

Histussin D. (Bock Pharmacal) Hydrocodone bitartrate 5 mg, pseudoephedrine HCl 60 mg/5 ml/Liq. Bot. 480 ml. *c-III.*
Use: Antitussive, decongestant.

Histussin HC Syrup. (Sanofi Winthrop) Phenylephrine HCl 5 mg, chlorpheniramine maleate 2 mg, hydrocodone bitartrate 2.5 mg. In 480 ml. *c-III.*
Use: Analgesic, antihistamine, decongestant, narcotic.

Hitone. (Lafayette Pharm) Barium sulfate suspension 125% w/v. Bot. 2000 ml. Case 4s.
Use: Radiopaque agent.

Hi-Tor. (Barth's) Vitamins B_{12} 15 mcg, niacin 1.5 mg, B_1 6 mg, B_2 12 mg, B_6 54 mcg, pantothenic acid 150 mcg, choline 3.75 mg, inositol 5.25 mg/Tab. Bot. 100s, 500s, 1000s. *otc.*
Use: Vitamin supplement.

Hi-Tor 900. (Barth's) Vitamins B_1 13.5 mg, B_2 5.2 mg, niacin 15 mg, B_6 0.6 mg, pantothenic acid 1.2 mg, biotin, B_{12} 2.5 mcg, iron 0.9 mg, protein 7.5 g, inositol 50 mg, choline 40 mg, aminobenzoic acid 0.15 to 2.4 mg/15 g. Bot. 1 lb, 3 lb. *otc.*
Use: Mineral, vitamin supplement.

HIVAB HIV-1/HIV-2 (rDNA) EIA. (Abbott Laboratories) Enzyme immunoassay for qualitative detection of antibodies to human immunodeficiency viruses Type 1 or Type 2 in human serum or plasma. Test kits 100s, 1000s, 5000s.
Use: Diagnostic aid.

Hi-Vegi-Lip Tablets. (Freeda Vitamins) Pancreatin 2400 mg, lipase 12,000 units, protease 60,000 units, amylase 60,000 units/Tab. Bot. 100s, 250s. *otc.*
Use: Digestive aid.

Hivid. (Roche Laboratories) Zalcitamine 0.375 mg or 0.75 mg/Tab. Bot. 100s. *Rx.*
Use: Antiviral (Phase II/III AIDS).

Hivig. (NABI) Human immunodeficiency virus immune globulin.
Use: Antiviral, HIV. [Orphan drug]

Hiwolfia. (Jones Medical Industries) Rauwolfia 25 mg, 50 mg or 100 mg/Tab. Bot. 100s, 1000s.

Use: Antihypertensive.

HMG-CoA Reductase Inhibitors. *Rx.*
Use: Antihyperlipidemic.
See: Lescol, Cap. (Novartis).
Mevacor, Tab. (Merck).
Pravachol, Tab. (Bristol-Myers Squibb).
Zocor, Tab. (Merck).

HMM.
See: Hexamethylmelamine.

HMS Liquifilm. (Allergan) Medrysone 1%. Ophth. Susp. Bot. 5 ml, 10 ml. *Rx.*
Use: Anti-inflammatory, ophthalmic.

HN_2. Mechlorethamine HCl.
Use: Antineoplastic.
See: Mustargen, Pow. (Merck).

H_2 OEX. (Fellows) Benzthiazide 50 mg/Tab. Bot. 100s, 1000s. *Rx.*
Use: Diuretic.

Hold. (SmithKline Beecham Pharmaceuticals) Dextromethorphan HBr 5 mg/Loz. Plastic tube 10 Loz. *otc.*
Use: Antitussive.

Hold DM. (Menley & James) Dextromethorphan HBr 5 mg, corn syrup, sucrose. Loz. Pkg. 10s. *otc.*
Use: Antitussive.

Hold Lozenges (Children's Formula). (SmithKline Beecham Pharmaceuticals) Phenylpropanolamine HCl 6.25 mg, dextromethorphan HBr 3.75 mg/Loz. Roll 10s. *otc.*
Use: Antitussive, decongestant.

holocaine hydrochloride. (Various Mfr.) Phenacaine HCl.
Use: Anesthetic, local.

homarylamine hydrochloride. N-Methyl-3,4-methylenedioxyphenethylamine HCl.

•**homatropine hydrobromide,** (hoe-MAT-troe-peen HIGH-droe-BROE-mide) U.S.P. 23.
Use: Anticholinergic, ophthalmic; mydriatic, cycloplegic.
See: Homatropine HBr, Soln. (Ciba Vision Ophthalmics).
Isopto Homatropine, Soln. (Alcon Laboratories).
Murocoll, Liq. (Muro).

homatropine hydrobromide. (Various Mfr.) 5% Soln. Bot. 1 ml, 2 ml, 5 ml. *Rx.*
Use: Mydriatic, cycloplegic.

homatropine hydrochloride.
Use: Anticholinergic, topical; mydriatic, cycloplegic.

•**homatropine methylbromide,** U.S.P. 23.
Use: Anticholinergic.

homatropine methylbromide w/combinations.
Use: Anticholinergic.
See: Dranochol, Tab. (Marin).
Homapin, Tab. (Mission Pharmacal).
Hycodan, Tab., Pow., Syr. (DuPont).
Panitol H.M.B., Tab. (Wesley Pharmacal).
Spasmatol, Tab. (Pharmed).
Tapuline, Tab. (Wesley Pharmacal).

homatropine methylbromide and phenobarbital combinations.
Use: Anticholinergic.
See: Gustase-Plus, Tab. (Roberts Pharm).

Hominex-1. (Ross Laboratories) Protein 15 g, fat 23.9 g, carbohydrate 46.3 g, linoleic acid 1800 mg, Fe 9 mg, Na 190 mg, K 675 mg, Ca, vitamins A, B_1, B_2, B_3, B_5, B_6, B_{12}, C, D, E, K, biotin, choline, folic acid, inositol, Cl, Cu, I, Mg, Mn, P, Se, Zn and 480 Cal per 100 g. Methionine free. Pow. Can 350 g. *otc.*
Use: Nutritional supplement.

Hominex-2. (Ross Laboratories) Protein 30 g, fat 15.5 g, carbohydrate 30 g, Fe 13 mg, Na 880 mg, K 1370 mg, Ca, vitamins A, B_1, B_2, B_3, B_5, B_6, B_{12}, C, D, E, K, biotin, choline, folic acid, inositol, Cl, Cu, I, Mg, Mn, P, Se, Zn and 410 Cal per 100 g. Methionine free. Pow. Can 325 g. *otc.*
Use: Nutritional supplement.

Homogene-S. (Spanner) Testosterone 25 mg, 50 mg or 100 mg/ml. Vial 10 ml. *c-III.*
Use: Androgen.

•**homosalate.** (hoe-moe-SAL-ate) USAN. *Formerly Homomenthyl Salicylate.*
Use: Ultraviolet screen.
W/Combinations.
See: Coppertone, Prods. (Schering Plough).

honey bee venom.
See: Albay (Bayer Corp).
Pharmalgen (ALK Laboratories).
Venomil (Bayer Corp).

•**hoquizil hydrochloride.** (HOE-kwih-zill) USAN.
Use: Bronchodilator.

hormofollin.
See: Estrone (Various Mfr.).

hornet venom.
See: Albay (Bayer Corp).
Pharmalgen (ALK Laboratories).
Venomil (Bayer Corp).

Hospital Foam Cleaner. (Health & Medical Techniques) 0-phenylphenol 0.1%, 4-chloro-2-cyclopentyl-phenol 0.08%, lauric diethanolamide 0.2%, triethanolamine dodecylbenzenesulfonate 0.3%.

Aerosol spray 19 oz.
Use: Antimicrobial, disinfectant.

Hospital Lotion. (Paddock) Diisobutylcresoxyethoxy-ethyl dimethyl benzyl ammonium Cl, menthol, lanolin, mineral and vegetable oils. Bot. 4 oz, 8 oz, gal. *otc.*
Use: Emollient.

12-Hour Antihistamine Nasal Decongestant. (United Research Laboratories) Pseudoephedrine sulfate 120 mg, dexbrompheniramine maleate 6 mg, sugar, sucrose. Tab. Pkg. 10s. *otc.*
Use: Antihistamine, decongestant.

12-Hour Cold. (Hudson) Phenylpropanolamine HCl 75 mg, chlorpheniramine maleate 4 mg/Cap. Pkg. 10s. *otc.*
Use: Antihistamine, decongestant.

HPA-23. (antimoniotungstate) An experimental compound developed at the Pasteur Institute in Paris to stop or slow the reproduction of the Acquired Immune Deficiency Syndrome (AIDS) virus, at least temporarily.

H.P. Acthar Gel. (Centeon) Repository corticotropin injection highly purified 40 U.S.P. units/1 ml. Vial 1 ml, 5 ml; 80 U.S.P. units/1 ml. Vial 1 ml, 5 ml. *Rx.*
Use: Corticosteroid.

H-R Lubricating Jelly. (Wallace Laboratories) Hydroxypropyl methycellulose, parabens. Jelly 150 g. *otc.*
Use: Lubricant.

HRC-Tylaprin Elixir. (Cenci) Acetaminophen 120 mg, alcohol 7%/5 ml. Bot. 2 oz, 4 oz. *otc.*
Use: Analgesic.

H.S. Need. (Hanlon) Chloral hydrate 3¾ gr, 7.5 gr/Cap. Bot. 100s. *Rx.*
Use: Sedative.

HSV-1. (Wampole Laboratories) Herpes simplex virus type I test system. For the qualitative and semi-quantitative detection of HSV-1 antibody in human serum. Test 100s.
Use: Diagnostic aid.

HSV-2. (Wampole Laboratories) Herpes simplex virus type II antibody test. For the qualitative and semi-quantitative detection of HSV-2 antibody in human serum. Test 100s.
Use: Diagnostic aid.

H.T. Factorate. (Centeon) Antihemophilic factor (human) dried, heat treated for I.V. administration only. Single-dose vial w/diluent and needles. *Rx.*
Use: Antihemophilic.

H.T. Factorate Generation II. (Centeon) Antihemophilic factor (human) dried, heat treated for I.V. administration only. Single dose vial w/diluent and needles. *Rx.*
Use: Antihemophilic.

HTSH EIA. (Abbott Diagnostics) Enzyme immunoassay for the quantitative determination of human thyroid stimulating hormone (HTSH) in human serum or plasma.
Use: Diagnostic aid.

HTSH RIAbead. (Abbott Diagnostics) Immunoradiometric assay for the quantitative measurement of human thyroid stimulating hormone (HTSH) in serum.
Use: Diagnostic aid.

H-Tuss-D. (Cypress) Hydrocodone bitartrate 5 mg, pseudoephedrine HCl 60 mg/5 ml, Liq. Bot. 473 ml. *Rx.*
Use: Expectorant.

Hulk Hogan Multi-Vitamins Plus Extra C. (S.G. Labs) Vitamins A 2500 IU, E 15 IU, D_3 400 IU, B_1 1.05 mg, B_2 1.2 mg, B_3 13.5 mg, B_6 1.05 mg, B_{12} 4.5 mcg, C 300 mg, folic acid 300 mcg, sucrose. Tab. chew. Bot. 60s. *otc.*
Use: Mineral, vitamin supplement.

Humalog. (Eli Lilly) Insulin lispro 100 units/ml. Inj. Vial, 10 ml. Cartridge 1.5 ml. *Rx.*
Use: Antidiabetic.

human acid alphaglucosidase. (Pharmain BV)
Use: Glycogne storage disease type II. [Orphan drug]

human antihemophilic factor.
See: Antihemophilic.

human growth hormone. (Nutritional Restart)
Use: With glutamine in the treatment of short bowel syndrome. [Orphan drug]

human growth hormone function test.
See: R-Gene 10, Inj. (Pharmacia & Upjohn).

human immunodeficiency virus immune globulin.
Use: Antiviral-HIV. [Orphan drug]

human insulin. Insulin Human, U.S.P. 23.
Use: Hypoglycemic.
See: Humulin Prods. (Eli Lilly).

humanized anti-tac.
Use: Immunosuppressant. [Orphan drug]
See: Zenapax (Hoffman-La Roche).

human serum albumin.
See: Albumotope (Bristol-Myers Squibb).

human thyroid stimulating hormone (THS).

Use: Diagnostic aid. [Orphan drug]
See: Thyrogen (Genzyme).

human t-lymphotropic virus type III gp 160 antigens.
Use: AIDS. [Orphan drug]
See: Vaxsyn HIV-1.

Humate-P. (Centeon). Pasteurized, purified lyophilized concentrate of antihemophilic factor (human). Inj. single dose vial. *Rx.*
Use: Antihemophilic.

Humatin Capsules. (Monarch) Paromomycin sulfate 250 mg/Cap. Bot. 16s. *Rx.*
Use: Amebicide.

Humatrope. (Eli Lilly) Somatropin 5 mg (≈15 IU/vial), sucrose, mannitol 25 mg, glycine 5 mg, m-cresol 0.3%, glycerin 1.7%, water for injection. Pow. For Inj. (lyophilized). *Rx.*
Use: Hormone, growth.

Humegon. (Organon Teknika) Follicle-stimulating hormone activity 75 IU or 150 IU, lutienizing hormone activity 75 IU or 150 IU. Powd. for Inj. Vial 2 ml NaCl. *Rx.*
Use: Gonadotropin.

Humibid DM. (Adams Labs) Dextromethorphan HBr 30 mg, guaifenesin 600 mg/ Tab. Bot. 100s. *Rx.*
Use: Antitussive, expectorant.

Humibid L.A. (Adams Labs) Guaifenesin 600 mg/SR Tab. Bot. 100s. *Rx.*
Use: Expectorant.

Humibid Sprinkle. (Adams Labs) Dextromethorphan HBr 15 mg, guaifenesin 300 mg/SR Cap. Bot. 100s. *Rx.*
Use: Antitussive, expectorant.

HuMist. (Scherer) Sodium Cl 0.65%, chlorobutanol 0.35%. Soln. Bot. 45 ml. *Rx.*
Use: Decongestant combination.

Humorsol. (Merck) Demecarium bromide 0.125% or 0.25% ophthalmic soln. 5 ml Ocumeter. *Rx.*
Use: Antiglaucoma agent.

Humulin 50/50. (Eli Lilly) Isophane insulin suspension (50%) and insulin injection (50%), 100 units human insulin (rDNA)/ml Inj. Vial 10 ml. *otc.*
Use: Antidiabetic.

Humulin 70/30. (Eli Lilly) Isophane insulin suspension (70%) and insulin injection (30%), 100 units/ml human insulin (rDNA) Inj. Bot. 10 ml. *otc.*
Use: Antidiabetic.

Humulin L. (Eli Lilly) Lente human insulin (recombinant DNA origin) 100 units/ ml. Inj. Bot. 10 ml. Cartridge 1.5 ml. *otc.*
Use: Antidiabetic.

Humulin N. (Eli Lilly) NPH human insulin (recombinant DNA origin) 100 units/ ml. Bot. 10 ml. Cartridge 1.5 ml. *otc.*
Use: Antidiabetic.

Humulin U Ultralente. (Eli Lilly) Ultralente human insulin (recombinant DNA origin) 100 units/ml. Inj. Bot. 10 ml. *otc.*
Use: Antidiabetic.

Hurricaine. (Beutlich) Benzocaine 20%. Liq.: 0.25 ml, 3.75 ml, 30 ml. Gel: 3.75 ml, 30 g. Spray: 60 ml. *otc.*
Use: Anesthetic, topical.

Hurricaine Topical Anesthetic Spray Kit. (Beutlich) Benzocaine 20%. Kit: Aerosol 60 g plus 200 disposable extension tubes. *otc.*
Use: Anesthetic, topical.

HVS 1 & 2. (Chemi-Tech Laboratories) Benzalkonium Cl in a specially formulated base. Soln. Bot. 15 ml. *otc.*
Use: Cold sores, fever blisters, herpes virus.

Hyacide. (Niltig) Benzethonium Cl 0.1%, sodium nitrite 0.55%. Soln. Bot. oz. *otc.*
Use: Antiseptic.

Hyalex. (Miller) Magnesium salicylate 260 mg, magnesium p-aminobenzoate 163 mg, vitamins A 1500 IU, C 30 mg, D 100 IU, E 3 IU, B_{12} 2 mcg, pantothenic acid 5 mg, zinc 0.7 mg/Tab. Bot. 100s. *otc.*
Use: Mineral, vitamin supplement.

Hyalgen. (Sanofi Winthrop) Sodium hyaluronate 20 mg/2 ml. *Rx.*
Use: Antiarthritic.

hyalidase.
See: Hyaluronidase (Various Mfr.).

•**hyaluronidase injection.** (high-uhl-yur-AHN-ih-dase) U.S.P. 23. Hyalidase, Hydase Enzymes which depolymerize hyaluronic acid. Hyalase, Rondase.
Use: Hypodermoclyses, promotion of diffusion, spreading agent.
See: Alidase, Vial (Searle).
Wydase, Vial (Wyeth Ayerst).

hyamagnate. Hydroxy-Aluminum-Magnesium-Aminoacetate, Sodium-free.

Hybec Forte. (Amlab) Vitamins B_1 100 mg, B_2 20 mg, B_6 2.5 mg, niacinamide 25 mg, C 200 mg, B_{12} 10 mcg, calcium pantothenate 5 mg, iron 10 mg, choline bitartrate 24 mg, inositol 10 mg, biotin 5 mcg, liver 50 mg, yeast 100 mg/ Tab. Bot. 30s, 100s. *otc.*
Use: Mineral, vitamin supplement.

Hybolin Decanoate. (Hyrex) Nandrolone decanoate 50 mg or 100 mg/ml in oil. Vial 2 ml. *c-III.*

Use: Anabolic steroid.

Hybolin Improved. (Hyrex) Nandrolone phenpropionate 25 mg or 50 mg/ml in oil. Vial 2 ml. *c-III.*
Use: Anabolic steroid.

Hycamtin. (SmithKline Beecham Pharmaceuticals) Topotecan HCl 4 mg (free base), mannitol 48 mg/Pow. for Inj. vial. single dose. *Rx.*
Use: Antineoplastic.

•**hycanthone.** (HIGH-kan-thone) USAN.
Use: Antischistosomal.

Hyclorite. Sodium Hypochlorite soln., U.S.P. 23.

HycoClear Tuss. (Ethex) Hydrocodone bitartrate 5 mg, guaifenesin 100 mg/5 ml. Syrup. Alcohol, dye, sugar free. Bot. 118 ml, 473 ml. *c-III.*
Use: Antitussive, expectorant.

Hycodan. (DuPont Merck Pharmaceuticals) Hydrocodone bitartrate 5 mg, homatropine methylbromide 1.5 mg/5 ml or Tab. **Syr.:** Bot. 473 ml. **Tab.:** Bot. 100s, 500s. *c-III.*
Use: Antitussive combination.

Hycomine Compound Tablets. (DuPont Merck Pharmaceuticals) Hydrocodone bitartrate 5 mg, chlorpheniramine maleate 2 mg, phenylephrine HCl 10 mg, acetaminophen 250 mg, caffeine (anhydrous) 30 mg/Tab. Bot. 100s, 500s. *c-III.*
Use: Analgesic, antihistamine, antitussive, decongestant.

Hycomine Pediatric Syrup. (DuPont Merck Pharmaceuticals) Hydrocodone bitartrate 2.5 mg, phenylpropanolamine HCl 12.5 mg/5 ml. Bot. 480 ml. *c-III.*
Use: Antitussive, decongestant.

Hycomine Syrup. (DuPont Merck Pharmaceuticals) Hydrocodone bitartrate 5 mg, phenylpropanolamine HCl 25 mg/5 ml. Syr. Bot. pt, gal. *c-III.*
Use: Antitussive, decongestant.

Hycort Cream. (Everett Laboratories) Hydrocortisone 1% in a cream base. Tube oz. *Rx.*
Use: Corticosteroid, topical.

Hycort Ointment. (Everett Laboratories) Hydrocortisone 1% in ointment base. Tube oz. *Rx.*
Use: Corticosteroid, topical.

Hycortole. (Teva USA) Hydrocortisone. **Cream:** 0.5%: 5 g, 20 g; 1%: 5 g, 20 g, 4 oz; 2.5%: Tube 5 g, 20 g; **Oint.:** 1% or 2.5%. Tube 5 g, 20 g.
Use: Corticosteroid, topical.

Hycotuss Expectorant. (DuPont Merck Pharmaceuticals) Hydrocodone bitartrate 5 mg, guaifenesin 100 mg, alcohol 10%(v/v)/5 ml. Bot. 480 ml. *c-III.*
Use: Antitussive, expectorant.

hydantoin derivatives.
Use: Anticonvulsant.
See: Dilantin, Preps. (Parke-Davis).
Diphenylhydantoin Sodium, U.S.P.
Ethotoin.
Mesantoin, Tab. (Novartis).
Phenantoin.

hydase.
Use: Hypodermoclyses, promotion of diffusion.
See: Hyaluronidase (Various Mfr.).

Hydeltrasol Injection. (Merck) Prednisolone sodium phosphate 20 mg/ml w/ niacinamide 25 mg, sodium hydroxide to adjust pH, disodium edetate 0.5 mg, sodium bisulfite 1 mg, phenol 5 mg, water for injection q.s. 1 ml. Vial 2 ml, 5 ml. *Rx.*
Use: Corticosteroid.

Hydergine LC Liquid Capsules. (Novartis) Ergoloid mesylates 1 mg/Cap. Bot. 100s, 500s. SandoPak 100s, 500s. *Rx.*
Use: Psychotherapeutic agent.

Hydergine Liquid. (Novartis) Equal parts of dihydroergocornine, dihydroergocristine, dihydroergocryptine. (Ergoloid Mesylates). 1 mg/ml. Bot. 100 ml w/ dropper. *Rx.*
Use: Psychotherapeutic agent.

Hydergine, Oral. (Novartis) Equal parts of dihydroergocornine, dihydroergocristine, dihydroergocryptine (Ergoloid Mesylates). 1 mg/Tab. Bot. 100s, 500s. SandoPak (UD) 100s, 500s. *Rx.*
Use: Psychotherapeutic agent.

Hydergine, Sublingual. (Novartis) Equal parts of dihydroergocornine, dihydroergocristine, dihydroergocryptine (Ergoloid Mesylates). 0.5 mg or 1 mg/Tab. Bot. 100s, 1000s, SandoPak (UD) 100s. *Rx.*
Use: Psychotherapeutic agent.

Hydoril. (Cenci) Hydrochlorthiazide 25 mg or 50 mg/Tab. Bot. 100s, 1000s. *Rx.*
Use: Diuretic.

hydrabamine phenoxymethyl penicillin.
See: Penicillin V Hydrabamine.

hydracrylic acid beta lactone.
See: Propiolactone.

hydralazine. (Solopak) Hydralazine HCl 20 mg/ml Inj. Vial 1 ml. *Rx.*
Use: Antihypertensive.

•**hydralazine hydrochloride.** (high-DRAL-uh-zeen) U.S.P. 23.

Use: Antihypertensive.
See: Apresoline, Amp., Tab. (Novartis Pharmaceuticals).
Dralzine, Tab. (Teva USA).
W/Hydrochlorothiazide.
See: Apresazide, Cap. (Novartis Pharmaceuticals).
Apresoline-Esidrix, Tab. (Novartis Pharmaceuticals).
Hydralazide, Tab. (Zenith Goldline).
Hydroserpine Plus, Tab. (Zenith Goldline).
W/Reserpine.
See: Dralserp, Tab. (Teva USA).
Serpasil-Apresoline, Tab. (Novartis Pharmaceuticals).
W/Reserpine, hydrochlorothiazide (Esidrix).
See: Harbolin, Tab. (Arcum).
Ser-Ap-Es, Tab. (Novartis Pharmaceuticals).
Unipres, Tab. (Solvay).

hydralazine hydrochloride. (Various Mfr.) **10 mg, 25 mg, 50 mg:** Tab. Bot. 100s, 1000s, UD 100s; **100 mg:** Tab. Bot. 100s, 1000s.
Use: Antihypertensive.

•**hydralazine polistirex.** (high-DRAL-ah-zeen pahl-ee-STIE-rex) USAN.
Use: Antihypertensive.

Hydra Mag Tablets. (Pal-Pak) Aluminum hydroxide gel, dried, 195 mg, magnesium trisilicate 195 mg, kaolin 162 mg/Tab. Bot. 1000s. *otc.*
Use: Antacid.

Hydrap-ES. (Parmed) Hydrochlorothiazide 15 mg, reserpine 0.1 mg, hydralazine HCl 25 mg/Tab. Bot. 100s, 500s, 1000s. *Rx.*
Use: Antihypertensive.

Hydraserp. (Geneva Pharm) Hydrochlorothiazide 25 mg or 50 mg, reserpine 0.1 mg/Tab. Bot. 100s, 1000s. *Rx.*
Use: Antihypertensive combination.

hydrastine hydrochloride. (Penick) Pow. Bot. oz.
Use: Hemostatic.

Hydrate. (Hyrex) Dimenhydrinate 50 mg/ml w/propylene glycol 50%, benzyl alcohol 5%. Amp. 1 ml. Box 25s, 100s; Vial 10 ml. *Rx.*
Use: Antiemetic, antihistamine, antivertigo.

Hydrazide Capsules. (Zenith Goldline) **25/25:** Hydrochlorothiazide 25 mg, hydralazine 25 mg/Cap. **50/50:** Hydrochlorothiazide 50 mg, hydralazine 50 mg/Cap. Bot. 100s. *Rx.*
Use: Antihypertensive.

Hydra-Zide Capsules. (Par Pharm) Hydralazine HCl 50 mg, hydrochlorothiazide 50 mg/Cap. Bot. 100s, 500s, 1000s. *Rx.*
Use: Antihypertensive.

hydrazone.
Use: Pulmonary tuberculosis.
See: Rimactane, Cap. (Novartis Pharmaceuticals).

Hydrea. (Bristol-Myers Squibb) Hydroxyurea. 500 mg, lactose/Cap. Bot. 100s. *Rx.*
Use: Antineoplastic.

hydriodic acid. (Various Mfr.).
Use: Expectorant.

hydriodic acid therapy.
See: Aminoacetic Acid HI.

Hydrisinol Creme and Lotion. (Pedinol) Sulfonated hydrogenated castor oil. **Cream:** Spout Cap Jar 4 oz, lb. **Lot.:** Bot. 8 oz. *otc.*
Use: Emollient.

Hydro-12. (Table Rock) Crystalline hydroxocobalamin 1000 mcg/ml Pkg. 10 ml. *Rx.*
Use: Vitamin supplement.

Hydro-Ban Capsules. (Whiteworth Towne) Juniper oil 10 mg, uva ursi 50 mg, buchu extract 50 mg, parsley piert extract 50 mg, iron 6 mg/Cap. Bot. 42s. *otc.*
Use: Diuretic.

Hydrocare Cleaning and Disinfecting. (Allergan) Tris(2-hydroxyethyl) tallow ammonium Cl, thimerosal 0.002%, bis(2-hydroxyethyl) tallow ammonium Cl, sodium bicarbonate, sodium phosphates, hydrochloric acid, propylene glycol, polysorbate 80, polyhema. Soln. Bot. 240 ml, 360 ml. *otc.*
Use: Contact lens care, disinfective.

Hydrocare Preserved Saline. (Allergan) Isotonic, buffered, NaCl, sodium hexametaphosphate, boric acid, sodium borate, EDTA 0.01%, thimerosal 0.001%. Soln. Bot. 240 ml, 360 ml. *otc.*
Use: Contact lens care-rinsing/storage solution.

Hydrocet. (Carnrick Labs) Hydrocodone bitartrate 5 mg, acetaminophen 500 mg/Cap. Bot. 100s. *c-III.*
Use: Narcotic analgesic combination.

hydrochlorate. Same as Hydrochloride.

•**hydrochloric acid,** N.F 18.
Use: Well diluted, achlorhydria; pharmaceutic aid (acidifying agent).

hydrochloric acid. (Various Mfr.) Muriatic Acid, Absolute 38%. Diluted 10%.

hydrochloric acid therapy.

Use: Well diluted, achlorhydria; pharmaceutic aid (acidifying agent).
Use: Gastric acidifier.
See: Betaine HCl (Various Mfr.).
Glutamic Acid HCl (Various Mfr.).
Glycine HCl (Various Mfr.).

Hydrochloroserpine. (Freeport) Hydralazine HCl 25 mg, hydrochlorthiazide 15 mg, reserpine 0.1 mg/Tab. Bot. 1000s.
Use: Antihypertensive combination.

•**hydrochlorothiazide,** (high-droe-klor-oh-THIGH-uh-zide) U.S.P. 23.
Use: Diuretic.
See: Chlorzide, Tab. (Foy).
Delco-Retic, Tab. (Delco).
Diu-Scrip, Cap. (Scrip).
Esidrix, Tab. (Novartis Pharmaceuticals).
Hydromal, Tab. (Roberts Pharm).
HydroDiuril, Tab. (Merck).
Hydrozide-50, Tab. (Merz).
Microzide, Cap. (Watson).
Oretic, Tab. (Abbott Laboratories).
Thiuretic, Tab. (Parke-Davis).
Zide, Tab. (Solvay).
W/Deserpidine.
See: Oreticyl, Tab. (Abbott Laboratories).
W/Enalapril.
See: Vaseretic, Tab. (Merck).
W/Guanethidine monosulfate.
See: Esimil, Tab. (Novartis Pharmaceuticals).
W/Hydralazine HCl.
See: Apresazide, Cap. (Novartis Pharmaceuticals).
Apresoline-Esidrix, Tab. (Novartis Pharmaceuticals).
Hydralazide, Tab. (Zenith Goldline).
W/Labetalol.
W/Lisinopril.
See: Prinzide, Tab. (Merck).
Zestoretic, Tab. (Zeneca).
W/Methyldopa.
See: Aldoril, Tab. (Merck).
W/Moexipril.
See: Uniretic, Tab. (Schwarz Pharma).
W/Propranolol.
See: Inderide, Tab. (Wyeth Ayerst).
W/Reserpine.
See: Aquapres-R, Tab. (Castal).
Hydropres, Tab. (Merck).
Hydroserp, Tab. (Zenith Goldline).
Hydroserpine, Tab. (Geneva Pharm).
Hydrotensin-50, Tab. (Merz).
Hyperserp, Tab. (Zeneca).
Mallopress, Tab. (Roberts Pharm).
Serpasil-Esidrix, Tab. (Novartis Pharmaceuticals).
W/Reserpine, Hydralazine HCl.
See: Harbolin, Tab. (Arcum).
Hydroserpine Plus, Tab. (Zenith Goldline).
Ser-Ap-Es, Tab. (Novartis Pharmaceuticals).
Unipres, Tab. (Solvay).
W/Spironolactone.
See: Aldactazide, Tab. (Searle).
W/Timolol maleate.
See: Timolide, Tab. (Merck).
W/Triamterene.
See: Dyazide, Cap. (SmithKline Beecham Pharmaceuticals).

hydrochlorothiazide/amiloride.
See: Amiloride hydrochloride and hydrochlorthiazide tablets.

hydrochlorothiazide w/combinations.
See: Hyzaar, Tab. (Merck).

hydrochlorothiazide/hydralazine. (Various Mfr.) Hydrochlorothiazide 25 mg, hydralazine HCl 25 mg/Cap, or hydrochlorothiazide 50 mg, hydralazine HCl 50 mg/Cap. Bot. 100s, 500s, 1000s. *Rx.*
Use: Antihypertensive.

hydrochlorothiazide/reserpine. (Various Mfr.)
See: Reserpine and hydrochlorothiazide.

hydrocholeretics.
See: Bile Salts (Various Mfr.).
Dehydrocholic Acid (Various Mfr.).
Desoxycholic Acid (Various Mfr.).
Ox Bile Extract (Various Mfr.).

hydrocholeretic combinations.
See: G.B.S., Tab. (Forest Pharmaceutical).

Hydrocil Instant. (Solvay) Blond psyllium coating containing psyllium 3.5 g/3.7 g dose. Tan granular, instant mix, sugar-free, low sodium, low potassium powder. UD packets. 3.7 g in 30s, 500s, Jar 250 g. *otc.*
Use: Laxative.

Hydro Cobex. (Taylor Pharmaceuticals) Hydroxocobalamin 1000 mcg/Vial 30 ml. *Rx.*
Use: Vitamin B_{12} supplement.

hydrocodone w/acetaminophen. (HIGH-droe-KOE-dohn with ass-eet-ah-MEE-no-fen) (Pharmics) Hydrocodone bitartrate 7.5 mg, acetaminophen 500 mg. Tab. Bot. 100s, 500s. *c-III.*
Use: Analgesic combination, narcotic.
See:
Alor 5/500, Tab. (Atley).
Anexsia 10/660, Tab. (Mallinckrodt).
Lortab, Preps. (UCB Pharma).
Vicodin, Tab. (Knoll Pharmaceuticals).

•**hydrocodone bitartrate,** (HIGH-droe-KOE-dohn by-TAR-TRATE) U.S.P. 23. Dihydrocodeinone bitartrate.
Use: Antitussive.
W/Combinations.
See: Atuss-EX, Syr. (URL).
Atuss G, Syr. (Atley).
Atuss HD, Liq. (Atley).
Deconamine CX, Tab. (Bradley).
Histinex HC, Syr. (Ethex).
Histinex PV, Syr. (Ethex).
Histussin D, Liq. (Bock).
H-Tuss-D, Liq. (Cypress).
Hycoclear Tuss, Syr. (Ethex).
Hydrocet, Cap. (Carnrick Labs).
Hydrocodone/APAP, Tab. (Pharmics).
Hydrocodone CP, Liq. (Morton Grove).
Hydrocodone GF, Liq. (Morton Grove).
Hydrocodone HD, Liq. (Morton Grove).
Hydrocodone PA, Liq. (Morton Grove).
Iodal HD, Liq. (Iomed).
Panacet 5/500, Tab. (ECR Pharmaceuticals).
Panasal 5/500, Tab. (ECR Pharmaceuticals).
Pancof-HC, Liq. (Pan Am Labs).
Protuss-D, Liq. (Horizon).
Tussend, Syr. (Monarch).
Tyrodone, Liq. (Major).
Unituss HC, Syr. (URL).
Vetuss HC, Syr. (Cypress).

hydrocodone bitartrate & acetaminophen capsules. (Various) Hydrocodone bitartrate 5 mg, acetaminophen 500 mg/Cap. Bot. 100s, 500s. *c-III.*
Use: Analgesic combination.

hydrocodone bitartrate & acetaminophen caplets. (Various Mfr.) Hydrocodone bitartrate 7.5 mg, acetaminophen 650 mg. 100s, 500s. *c-III.*
Use: Analgesic combination, narcotic.

hydrocodone bitartrate & acetaminophen tablets. (Watson Laboratories) Hydrocodone bitartrate 5 mg, acetaminophen 500 mg/Tab. Bot. 100s, 500s. (King Pharm) Hydrocodone bitartrate 7.5 mg, acetaminophen 650 mg/capl. Bot. 100s, 500s. *c-III.*
Use: Analgesic combination-narcotic.

hydrocodone bitartrate & phenylpropanolamine hydrochloride pediatric syrup. (Rosemont) Phenylpropanolamine HCl 12.5 mg, hydrocodone bitartrate 2.5 mg/Syr. Bot. 118 ml, pt, gal. *c-III.*
Use: Antitussive combination.

hydrocodone comp. syrup. (Various Mfr.) Hydrocodone bitartrate 5 mg, homatropine methylbromide 1.5 mg. Bot. 473 ml, gal. *c-III.*
Use: Antitussive.

Hydrocodone CP. (Morton Grove) Hydrocodone bitartrate 2.5 mg, phenylephrine 5 mg, chlorpheniramine maleate 2 mg/5 ml/Liq. Bot. 473 ml. *c-III.*
Use: Antitussive.

Hydrocodone GF Syrup. (Morton Grove) Hydrocodone bitartrate 5 mg, guaifenesin 100 mg/5 ml/Syrup. Bot. 473 ml. *c-III.*
Use: Antitussive, expectorant.

Hydrocodone HD. (Morton Grove) Hydrocodone bitartrate 1.67 mg, phenylephrine HCl 5 mg, chlorpheniramine maleate 2 mg/5 ml/Liq. Bot. 473 ml. *c-III.*
Use: Antitussive, expectorant.

Hydrocodone PA Syrup. (Morton Grove) Hydrocodone bitartrate 5 mg, phenylpropanolamine HCl 25 mg/5 ml/Syrup. Bot. 473 ml. *c-III.*
Use: Antitussive, decongestant.

Hydrocodone PA Pediatric Syrup. (Morton Grove) Hydrocodone bitartrate 2.5 mg, phenylpropanolamine HCl 12.5 mg/5 ml/Syrup. Bot. 473 ml. *c-III.*
Use: Antitussive, decongestant.

•**hydrocodone polistirex.** (high-droe-KOE-dohn pahl-ee-STIE-rex) USAN.
Use: Antitussive.

hydrocodone resin complex.
Use: Antitussive.
W/Phenyltoloxamine resin complex.
See: Tussionex, Prods. (Medeva).

hydrocortamate hydrochloride. 17-Hydroxycorticoster-one-21-diethylaminoaceate HCl.
Use: Anti-inflammatory, topical.

•**hydrocortisone,** (HIGH-droe-CORE-tihsone) U.S.P. 23.
Use: Anti-inflammatory, topical; corticosteroid, topical.
See: Acticort Lotion 100. (Baker Norton).
Aeroseb-HC, Aerosol (Allergan).
Alphaderm, Cream (Procter & Gamble).
Caldecort Spray (Novartis Pharmaceuticals).
Cetacort, Lot. (Galderma).
Cortaid Intensive Therapy, Cream (Pharmacia & Upjohn).
Cort-Dome, Cream, Lot., Supp. (Bayer Corp).
Cortef, Tab., Cream, Oint. (Pharmacia & Upjohn).

Cortenema, Enema (Solvay).
Cortril, Oint. (Pfizer).
Delacort, Lot. (Mericon).
Dermacort, Cream, Lot. (Solvay).
Dermol HC, Cream, Oint. (Dermol Pharmaceuticals).
Dermolate, Prods. (Schering Plough).
Ecosone, Cream (Star).
Eldecort, Cream (Zeneca).
HC Derma-Pax, Liq. (Recsei).
HI-COR-1.0, Cream, (C & M Pharmacal).
HI-COR-2.5, Cream (C & M Pharmacal).
Hycort, Cream, Oint. (Everett Laboratories).
Hycortole,Cream, Oint. (Premo).
Hydrocortone, Tab. (Merck).
Hytone, Cream, Oint., Lot. (Dermik Laboratories).
KeriCort-10, Cream (Bristol-Myers Squibb).
Lexocort, Pow., Lot. (Lexington).
Lipo-Adrenal Cortex, Vial (Pharmacia & Upjohn).
Maso-Cort, Lot. (Mason).
Microcort, Lot. (Alto Pharm).
My Cort, Cream (Scrip).
Optef, Soln. (Pharmacia & Upjohn).
Proctocort, Oint. (Solvay).
Scalpicin, Liq. (Combe).
Signef, Supp. (Forest Pharmaceutical).
Synacort, Cream (Syntex).
T/Scalp, Liq. (Neutrogena).
Tarcortin, Cream (Schwarz Pharma).
Texacort 25, 50, Lot. (Rydelle).

hydrocortisone. (Pharmacia & Upjohn). Micronized nonsterile powder for prescription compounding.
Use: Anti-inflammatory, topical; corticosteroid, topical.

hydrocortisone w/combinations.
See: Achromycin W/Hydrocortisone, Oint., Ophth. Oint. (ESI Lederle Generics).
Acrisan w/Hydrocortisone, Liq. (Recsei).
Bafil, Cream. (Scruggs).
Barseb HC, Scalp Lot. (PBH Wesley Jessen).
Barseb Thera-spray, Aerosol (PBH Wesley Jessen).
Bro-Parin, Otic Susp. (3M).
Calmurid HC, Cream (Pharmacia & Upjohn).
Carmol HC, Cream (Ingram).
Coidocort, Cream (Coast).
Cor-Tar-Quin, Cream, Lot. (Bayer Corp).
Cortef, Preps. (Pharmacia & Upjohn).
Cortin, Cream (C & M Pharmacal).
Cortisporin, Prep. (GlaxoWellcome).
Derma-Cover-HC, Liq., Oint. (Scrip).
Dermarex, Cream (Hyrex-Key).
Dicort, Cream, Supp. (Hickam).
Doak Oil Forte, Liq. (Doak Dermatologics).
Drotic No. 2, Drops (B.F. Ascher).
Fostril HC, Lot. (Westwood Squibb).
HC-Form, Jelly (Recsei).
HC-Jel, Jelly (Recsei).
Heb-Cort., Cream, Lot. (PBH Wesley Jessen).
Heb-Cort MC, Lot. (PBH Wesley Jessen).
Heb-Cort. V, Cream, Lot. (PBH Wesley Jessen).
Hi-Cort N Cream (Blaine).
Hill-Cortac, Cream, Lot. (Hill).
Hysone, Oint. (Roberts Pharm).
Kleer, Spray (Scrip).
Loroxide-HC, Lot. (Dermik Laboratories).
Maso-Form, Cream (Mason).
Mity-quin, Cream (Solvay).
Myci-Cort, Liq., Spray (Misemer).
My-Cort, Drops, Lot., Oint., Spray (Scrip).
Neocort, Oint. (H.V.P.).
Neo-Cort Dome, Cream, Lot., Drops (Bayer Corp).
Neo Cort Top, Oint. (Standex).
Neo-Domeform-HC, Cream, Lot., Susp. (Bayer Corp).
Nutracort, Cream, Gel, Lot. (Galderma).
1 + 1 Creme, 1 + 1-F Creme (Dunhall Pharmaceuticals).
Ophthel, Liq. (Zeneca).
Ophthocort, Oint. (Parke Davis).
Orlex HC Otic (Baylor).
Oto, Drops (Solvay).
Otobiotic, Soln. (Schering Plough).
Otocalm-H Ear Drops (Parmed).
Otostan H.C. (Standex).
Pyocidin-Otic, Soln. (Berlex).
Racet Forte, Cream (Teva USA).
Racet LCD, Cream (Teva USA).
Rectal Medicone-HC (Medicone).
Sherform-HC, Creme (Sheryl).
Stera-Form, Creme (Merz).
Steramine Otic, Drops (Merz).
Syntar HC Cream, Oint. (Zeneca).
Tarcortin, Cream (Schwarz Pharma).
Tenda HC, Cream (Dermik Laboratories).
Terra-Cortril, Preps. (Pfipharmecs).
Vanoxide-HC, Lot. (Dermik Laboratories).
V-Cort, Cream (Scrip).
Vioform-Hydrocortisone, Preps. (Nov-

artis Pharmaceuticals).
Vio-Hydrocort, Oint., Cream (Quality Formulations).
Vytone, Cream, (Dermik Laboratories).

•**hydrocortisone acetate,** U.S.P. 23.
Use: Glucocorticoid.
See: Anucort-HC, Supp. (G & W Laboratories).
Anuprep HC, Supp. (Great Southern).
Anusol-HC, Supp. (Parke-Davis).
Caldecort, Cream (Novartis Pharmaceuticals).
Caldecort Light, Cream (Novartis Pharmaceuticals).
Cortef Acetate, Ophth. Oint., Inj. (Pharmacia & Upjohn).
Cortifoam, Aerosol (Schwarz Pharma).
Cortiprel, Cream (Taylor Pharmaceuticals).
Cortril Acetate, Aqueous Susp., Oint. (Pfipharmecs).
Ferncort, Lot. (Ferndale Laboratories).
Fernisone Inj., Vial (Ferndale Laboratories).
Gynecort, Oint. (Combe).
Hemril-HC Uniserts, Supp. (Upsher-Smith Labs).
Hydro-Can (Paddock).
Hydrocort, Vial (Dunhall Pharmaceuticals).
Hydrocortone Acetate, Inj. (Merck).
Hydrosone, Inj. (Sigma-Tau Pharmaceuticals).
Maximum Strength Corticaine, Cream (UCB Pharmaceuticals).
Maximum Strength Dermarest Dricort Creme (Del Pharmaceuticals).
My-Cort, Lot. (Scrip).
Pramosone Cream, Lot. (Ferndale Laboratories).
Span-Ster, Inj. (Scrip).
Tucks-HC (Parke-Davis).

hydrocortisone acetate. (Pharmacia & Upjohn) Micronized non-sterile powder for prescription compounding.
Use: Anti-inflammatory, topical; corticosteroid, topical.

hydrocortisone acetate w/combinations.
See: Anusol-HC, Cream, Supp. (Parke-Davis).
Biotic-Opth W/HC, Oint. (Scrip).
Biotres HC, Cream (Schwarz Pharma).
Carmol HC, Cream (Ingram).
Chloromycetin-Hydrocortisone Ophth. Susp. (Parke-Davis).
Coly-Mycin-S Otic, Soln. (Warner Chilcott).
Cor-Oticin, Liq. (Maurry).
Cortaid, Cream, Lot., Oint. (Pharmacia & Upjohn).
Cortef Acetate, Inj., Oint., Susp. (Pharmacia & Upjohn).
Corticaine Cream (GlaxoWellcome).
Cortisporin-TC, Otic Susp. (Monarch).
Derma Medicone-HC, Oint. (Medicone).
Dicort, Supp. (Hickam).
Doctient HC, Supp. (Suppositoria).
Epifoam, Aerosol (Schwarz Pharma).
Estro-V HC, Supp. (PolyMedica).
Eye-Cort, Soln. (Roberts Pharm).
Furacin-HC Otic (Eaton Medical).
Furacin HC Urethral Inserts (Eaton Medical).
Furacort Cream (Eaton Medical).
Komed HC, Lot. (PBH Wesley Jessen).
Lida-Mantle HC, Cream (Bayer Corp).
Mantadil, Cream (GlaxoWellcome).
Neo-Cortef, Preps. (Pharmacia & Upjohn).
Neo-Hytone Cream (Dermik Laboratories).
Neopolycin-HC, Oint., Ophth. Oint. (Hoechst Marion Roussel).
Ophthocort, Oint. (Parke-Davis).
Otomar-HC, Otic Soln. (Marnel).
Proctofoam-HC, Aerosol (Schwarz Pharma).
Pyracort, Liq. (Teva USA).
Racet Forte, Cream (Teva USA).
Rectacort, Supp. (Century Pharm).
Rectal Medicone-HC, Supp. (Medicone).
Wyanoids HC, Supp. (Wyeth Ayerst).

hydrocortisone and acetic acid otic solution.
Use: Anti-inflammatory, otic.

•**hydrocortisone buteprate.** (HIGH-droe-CORE-tih-sone BYOO-teh-prate) USAN.
Use: Anti-inflammatory; corticosteroid, topical.
See: Pandel, Cream (Savage).

•**hydrocortisone butyrate.** (HIGH-droe-CORE-tih-sone BYOO-tih-rate) U.S.P. 23.
Use: Corticosteroid, topical.
See: Locoid, Soln. (Ferndale Laboratories).

hydrocortisone cypionate. U.S.P. XXII. Oral Susp., U.S.P. XXII. Hydrocortisone Cypionate.
Use: Corticosteroid, topical.

hydrocortisone diethylaminoacetate hcl.
See: Hydrocortamate.

hydrocortisone dypropionate.
See: Cortef, Fluid (Pharmacia & Upjohn).

•**hydrocortisone hemisuccinate.** (HIGH-droe-CORE-tih-sone hem-ih-SUCK-sih-nate) U.S.P. 23.
Use: Adrenocortical steroid.

hydrocortisone I.V.
See: A-Hydro Cort, Vial (Abbott Laboratories).
Solu-Cortef, Vial (Pharmacia & Upjohn).

hydrocortisone/iodochlorhydroxyquin. (Various Mfr.) **Cream:** Hydrocortisone 0.5% or 3%, iodochlorhydroxyquin 3%. 15 g, 30 g, 480 g. **Oint.:** Hydrocortisone 1%, iodochlorhydroxyquin 3%. 20 g, 30 g. *otc, Rx.*
Use: Corticosteroid, topical.

hydrocortisone-neomycin. (Various Mfr.) Hydrocortisone 1%, neomycin sulfate 0.5%. Oint. 20 g. *otc, Rx.*
Use: Corticosteroid, topical.

hydrocortisone phosphate.
See: Hydrocortone Phosphate, Inj. (Merck).

•**hydrocortisone sodium phosphate.** (HIGH-droe-CORE-tih-sone) U.S.P. 23.
Use: Adrenocortical steroid (anti-inflammatory); corticosteroid, topical.

•**hydrocortisone sodium succinate.** (HIGH-droe-CORE-tih-sone) U.S.P. 23.
Use: Adrenocortical steroid (anti-inflammatory); corticosteroid, topical.
See: A-hydroCort, Vial (Abbott Laboratories).
Solu-Cortef, Vial (Pharmacia & Upjohn).

•**hydrocortisone valerate.** (HIGH-droe-CORE-tih-sone VAL-eh-rate) U.S.P. 23.
Use: Corticosteroid, topical.
See: Westcort Cream, Oint. (Westwood Squibb).

Hydrocortone Acetate Saline Suspension. (Merck) Hydrocortisone acetate 25 mg or 50 mg/ml, sodium Cl 9 mg, polysorbate 80 4 mg, sodium carboxymethylcellulose 5 mg/ml, benzyl alcohol 9 mg q.s. water for injection to 1 ml. Vial 5 ml. *Rx.*
Use: Corticosteroid.

Hydrocortone Phosphate Injection. (Merck) Hydrocortisone sodium phosphate equivalent to hydrocortisone 50 mg/ml, creatinine 8 mg, sodium citrate 10 mg/ml, sodium hydroxide to adjust pH, sodium bisulfite 3.2 mg, methylparaben 1.5 mg, propylparaben 0.2 mg, water for injection q.s./ml. Vial 2 ml multiple dose, 10 ml multiple dose. Disposable syringe 2 ml single dose. *Rx.*
Use: Corticosteroid.

Hydrocortone Tablets. (Merck) Hydrocortisone 10 mg or 20 mg/Tab. Bot. 100s. *Rx.*
Use: Corticosteroid.

Hydrocream Base. (Paddock) Petrolatum, mineral oil, woolwax alcohol, imidazolidinyl urea, methyl propylparabens. Cream. Jar lb.
Use: Emollient.

Hydro-Crysti 12. (Roberts Pharm) Hydroxocobalamin, crystalline (vitamin B_{12}) 1000 mcg/ml Inj. Vial 30 ml. *Rx.*
Use: Vitamin B supplement.

HydroDIURIL. (Merck) Hydrochlorothiazide **25 mg/Tab.:** Bot. 100s, 1000s, UD 100s; **50 mg/Tab.:** Bot. 100s, 1000s, UD 100s. *Rx.*
Use: Diuretic.

Hydro-D Tablets. (Halsey) Hydrochlorothiazide. 25 mg or 50 mg/Tab. Bot. 1000s. *Rx.*
Use: Diuretic.

Hydro-Ergot. (Henry Schein) Hydrogenated ergot alkaloids 0.5 mg or 1 mg/Tab. Bot. 100s. *Rx.*
Use: Psychotherapeutic agent.

•**hydrofilcon a.** (HIGH-droe-FILL-kahn A) USAN.
Use: Contact lens material (hydrophilic).

•**hydroflumethiazide.** (HIGH-droe-flew-meth-EYE-ah-zide) U.S.P. 23.
Use: Antihypertensive, diuretic.
See: Diucardin, Tab. (Wyeth Ayerst).
Saluron, Tab. (Bristol-Myers Squibb).
W/Reserpine.
See: Salutensin, Tab. (Bristol-Myers Squibb).
Salutensin-Demi, Tab. (Bristol-Myers Squibb).

hydrogen dioxide.
See: Hydrogen Peroxide.

hydrogen iodide.
Use: Expectorant.
See: Hydriodic acid.

•**hydrogen peroxide concentrate.** (HIGH-droe-jen per-OX-ide) U.S.P. 23.
Use: Anti-infective, topical.

hydrogen peroxide solution 30%. Perhydrol, hydrogen pioxide. Bot. 0.25 lb, 0.5 lb, 1 lb.
Use: Dentistry, preparing the 3% solution.

hydrogen peroxide topical solution.

(Various Mfr.) (3%). 4 oz, 8 oz, pt.
Use: Anti-infective, topical.

Hydrogesic. (Edwards Pharmaceuticals) Hydrocodone bitartrate 5 mg, acetaminophen 500 mg/Cap. Bot. 100s. *c-III.*
Use: Analgesic combination, narcotic.

Hydroloid-G Sublingual. (Major) Ergoloid mesylates. **0.5 mg/Tab.:** Bot. 100s, 250s, 500s, UD 100s. **1 mg/Tab.:** Bot. 100s, 250s, 1000s, UD 100s. *Rx.*
Use: Psychotherapeutic agent.

Hydroloid-G Tabs. (Major) Ergoloid mesylates 1 mg/Tab. Bot. 100s, 250s, 1000s, UD 100s. *Rx.*
Use: Psychotherapeutic agent.

Hydromal. (Roberts Pharm) Hydrochlorothiazide 50 mg/Tab. Bot. 1000s. *Rx.*
Use: Diuretic.

Hydromet. (Alphalma USPD) Hydrocodone bitartrate 5 mg, homatropine MBr 1.5 mg/Syr. Bot. 473 ml, gal. *c-III.*
Use: Antitussive.

hydromorphone. (HIGH-droe-MORE-phone) *c-II.*
Use: Analgesic, narcotic.

•**hydromorphone hydrochloride.** (HIGH-droe-MORE-phone) U.S.P. 23. *Formerly Dihydromorphinone Hydrochloride.*
Use: Analgesic, narcotic.
See: Dilaudid Prods. (Knoll Pharmaceuticals).
W/sodium citrate, antimony potassium tartrate and chloroform. Inj.
See: Dilocor, Liq. (Table Rock).

hydromorphone sulfate.
Use: Analgesic, narcotic.

Hydromox. (ESI Lederle Generics) Quinethazone 50 mg/Tab. Bot. 100s, 500s. *Rx.*
Use: Diuretic.

Hydromox-R. (ESI Lederle Generics) Quinethazone 50 mg, reserpine 0.125 mg/Tab. Bot. 100s, 500s. *Rx.*
Use: Antihypertensive combination.

Hydropane. (Halsey) Hydrocodone bitartrate 5 mg, homatropine methylbromide 1.5 mg. Pt, gal. *c-III.*
Use: Antitussive combination.

Hydropel. (C & M Pharmacal) Silicone 30%, hydrophobic starch derivative 10%, petrolatum. Jar. 2 oz, lb. *otc.*
Use: Emollient.

Hydrophed Tablets. (Rugby) Theophylline 130 mg, ephedrine sulfate 25 mg, hydroxyzine HCl 10 mg/Tab. Bot. 100s, 1000s. *Rx.*
Use: Antiasthmatic combination.

Hydrophen Pediatric Syrup. (Rugby) Phenylpropanolamine HCl 12.5 mg, hydrocodone bitartrate 2.5 mg/5 ml. Bot. 480 ml. *c-III.*
Use: Antitussive, decongestant.

Hydrophen Syrup. (Rugby) Phenylpropanolamine HCl 25 mg, hydrocodone bitartrate 5 mg/5 ml. Bot. pt, gal. *c-III.*
Use: Antitussive, decongestant.

hydrophilic ointment. Stearyl alcohol, white petrolatum, propylene glycol, sodium lauryl sulfate, water. Jar lb. (E. Fougera).
Use: Pharmaceutic aid, ointment base.

hydrophilic ointment base. Oil in water emulsion bases. (Emerson) 1 lb.
Use: Pharmaceutic aid, ointment base.
See: Aquaphilic Ointment (Medco Research)
Cetaphil, Cream, Lot. (Texas Pharmacal).
Dermovan, Cream (Texas Pharmacal).
Lanaphilic Ointment (Medco Research).
Polysorb, Oint. (Savage).
Unibase, Oint. (Parke-Davis).

Hydropine. (Rugby) Hydroflumethiazide 25 mg, reserpine 0.125 mg/Tab. Bot. 100s. *Rx.*
Use: Antihypertensive combination.

Hydropine H.P. Tablets. (Rugby) Hydroflumethiazide 50 mg, reserpine 0.125 mg/Tab. Bot. 100s, 500s, 1000s. *Rx.*
Use: Antihypertensive combination.

Hydropres-50. (Merck) Hydrochlorothiazide 50 mg, reserpine 0.125 mg/Tab. Bot. 100s, 1000s. *Rx.*
Use: Antihypertensive combination.

•**hydroquinone.** (high-DROE-KWIN-ohn) U.S.P. 23.
Use: Depigmentor.
See: Artra Skin Tone Cream (Schering Plough).
Black and White Bleaching Cream (Schering Schering Plough).
Derma-Blanch, Cream (Chattem Consumer Products).
Eldopaque Cream, Oint. (Zeneca).
Eldopaque Forte Cream, Oint. (Zeneca).
Eldoquin, Cream, Lot. (Zeneca).
Esoterica Medicated Cream Prods. (SmithKline Beecham Pharmaceuticals).
Melpaque HP, Cream (Stratus).
Melquin HP, Cream (Stratus).
Nuquin HP, Cream, Gel (Stratus).

hydroquinone. (Glades) Hydroquinone 3%, SD Alcohol 45%, propylene glycol, isopropyl alcohol 4%/Soln. 30 ml

with applicator. Hydroquinone 4%, padimate 0.5%, dioxybenzone 3%, EDTA, sodium metabisulfite, hydroalcoholic base.
Use: Depigmentor.

hydroquinone monobenzyl ether.
See: Benoquin, Oint., Lot. (Zeneca).

Hydrosal. (Hydrosal Co.) Aluminum acetate 5%. **Susp.:** Bot. 16 oz, gal. **Oint.:** 54 g, 113.4 g, Jar 54 g, 454 g. *otc.*
Use: Astringent.

Hydro-Serp. (Zenith Goldline) Hydrochlorothiazide 25 mg or 50 mg, reserpine 0.125 mg or 0.1 mg/Tab. Bot. 100s, 1000s. *Rx.*
Use: Antihypertensive combination.

Hydroserpine #1. (Various Mfr.) Hydrochlorothiazide 25 mg, reserpine. Bot. 100s, 1000s. *Rx.*
Use: Antihypertensive combination.

Hydroserpine #2. (Various Mfr.) Hydrochlorothiazide 50 mg, reserpine. Bot. 100s, 250s, 400s, 1000s. *Rx.*
Use: Antihypertensive combination.

Hydrosine 25 Tablets. (Major) Hydrochlorothiazide 25 mg, reserpine 0.125 mg/Tab. Bot. 100s. Tartrazine. *Rx.*
Use: Antihypertensive combination.

Hydrosine 50 Tablets. (Major) Hydrochlorothiazide 50 mg, reserpine 0.125 mg/Tab. Bot. 100s. *Rx.*
Use: Antihypertensive combination.

Hydrosone. (Sigma-Tau Pharmaceuticals) Hydrocortisone acetate 25 mg or 50 mg, lactose/ml. Vial 5 ml. *Rx.*
Use: Corticosteroid.

Hydrotensin-50. (Merz) Hydrochlorothiazide 50 mg, reserpine 0.125 mg/Tab. Bot. 100s, 1000s. *Rx.*
Use: Antihypertensive combination.

Hydro-T Tabs. (Major) Hydrochlorothiazide. **25 mg/Tab:** Bot. 100s, 1000s, UD 100s; **50 mg/Tab:** Bot. 100s, 1000s, UD 100s; **100 mg/Tab:** Bot. 100s, 250s, 1000s, UD 100s. *Rx.*
Use: Diuretic.

hydroxindasol hydrochloride.

•**hydroxocobalamin.** (high-DROX-oh-koe-BAL-ah-meen) U.S.P. 23.
Use: Treatment of megaloblastic anemia, vitamin (hematopoietic).
See: AlphaRedisol, Inj. (Merck).
Alpha-Ruvite, Vial (Savage).
Cobavite L.A., Vial (Teva USA).
Droxomin, Inj. (Solvay).
Hydrobexan, Vial (Keene Pharmaceuticals).
Rubesol-L.A. 1000, Inj. (Schwarz Pharma).
Span-12, Inj. (Scrip).
Sytobex-H, Vial (Parke-Davis).

hydroxocobalamin, crystalline. (Various Mfr.) 1000 mcg/ml Inj. 30 ml. *Rx.*
Use: Vitamin supplement.
See: Hydroxocobalamin (Various).
Alphamin (Vortech).
AlphaRedisol (Merck).
Codroxomin (Forest Pharmaceutical).
Hybalamin (Roberts Pharm).
Hydrobexan (Keene Pharmaceuticals).
Hydro Cobex (Taylor Pharmaceuticals).
Hydro-Crysti (Roberts Pharm).
LA-12 (Hyrex).

hydroxocobalamin/sodium thiosulfate.
Use: Antidote, cyanide. [Orphan drug]

•**hydroxyamphetamine hydrobromide.** (high-DROX-ee-am-FET-uh-meen HIGH-droe-BROE-mide) U.S.P. 23.
Use: Adrenergic (ophthalmic); mydriatic.
See: Paredrine (Pharmics).

2-hydroxybenzamide.
See: Salicylamide.

hydroxy bis(acetato)aluminum. Aluminum Subacetate Topical Soln.

hydroxybis (salicylato) aluminum diacetate.
See: Aluminum aspirin.

hydroxybutyrate, sodium/gamma.
See: sodium gamma-hydroxybutyrate acid.

hydroxycholecalciferol. (D_3).
Use: Antihypocalcemia.
See: Calcifediol.

•**hydroxychloroquine sulfate.** (high-drox-ee-KLOR-oh-kwin) U.S.P. 23.
Use: Antimalarial, lupus erythematosus suppressant.

hydroxychloroquine sulfate. (Copley) 200 mg/Tab. Bot. 100s, 500s.
Use: Antimalarial, lupus erythematosus suppressant.

hydroxydione sodium.

•**hydroxyethyl cellulose.** (high-drox-ee-ETH-ill SELL-you-lohs) N.F. 18.
Use: Pharmaceutic aid (suspending, viscosity-increasing agent).
See: Gonioscopic, Soln. (Alcon Laboratories).

hydroxyethyl starch. (HES).
Use: Plasma volume expander.
See: Hespan, Inj. (DuPont Merck Pharmaceuticals).

hydroxyisoindolin. Under study.
Use: Antihypertensive.

hydroxymagnesium aluminate.

Use: Antacid.
See: Magaldrate.

hydroxymycin. An antibiotic substance obtained from cultures of *Streptomyces paucisporogenes.*

•**hydroxyphenamate.** (high-DROX-ee-FEN-ah-mate) USAN.
Use: Anxiolytic.

•**hydroxyprogesterone caproate.** (high-DROX-ee-pro-JESS-ter-ohn CAP-ROW-ate) U.S.P. 23.
Use: Hormone, progestin.
See: Delalutin, Vial (Bristol-Myers Squibb).
Duralutin, Inj. (Roberts Pharm).
Gesterol L.A. 250, Inj. (Forest Pharmaceutical).
Hy-Gestrone, Vial (Taylor Pharmaceuticals).
Hylutin, Inj. (Hyrex).
Hyprogest 250, Inj. (Keene Pharmaceuticals).
W/Estradiol valerate.
See: Hy-Gestradol, Inj. (Taylor Pharmaceuticals).
Hylutin-Est., Inj. (Hyrex).

hydroxyprogesterone caproate. (Various Mfr.) **125 mg/ml:** Inj. Vial 10 ml; **250 mg/ml:** Inj. Vial 5 ml. *Rx.*
Use: Hormone, progestin.

•**hydroxypropyl cellulose.** (high-drox-ee-PRO-pill SELL-you-lohs) N.F. 18.
Use: Topical protectant; pharmaceutical aid, emulsifying tablet coating agent.

•**hydroxypropyl methylcellulose.** U.S.P. 23.
Use: Pharmaceutic aid (suspending, viscosity-increasing agent; tablet excipient).
See: Anestacon (Alcon Laboratories).
Econopred, Susp. (Alcon Laboratories).
Occucoat, Soln. (Storz Ophthalmics).
W/benzalkonium Cl.
See: Gonak, Soln. (Akorn).
Goniosol (Ciba Vision Ophthalmics).
Isopto Tears (Alcon Laboratories).
Ultra Tears, Soln. (Alcon Laboratories).

•**hydroxypropyl methylcellulose phthalate.** N.F. 18.
Use: Pharmaceutic aid (coating agent).

hydroxypropyl methylcellulose phthalate 200731.
Use: Pharmaceutic aid (coating agent).

hydroxypropyl methylcellulose phthalate 220824.
Use: Pharmaceutic aid (coating agent).

hydroxystearin sulfate. Sulfonate hydrogenated castor oil.

L-5 Hydroxytryptophan (L-5HTP). (Bolar)
Use: Postanoxic intention myoclonus. [Orphan drug]

•**hydroxyurea.** (high-DROX-ee-you-REE-uh) U.S.P. 23.
Use: Antineoplastic. Sickle cell disease. [Orphan drug]
See: Hydrea, Cap. (Bristol-Myers Squibb).

hydroxyurea. (Roxane) Hydroxyurea 500 mg, lactose. Cap. Bot. 100s, UD 100s. *Rx.*
Use: Antineoplastic.

•**hydroxyzine hydrochloride.** (high-DROX-ih-zeen) U.S.P. 23.
Use: Anxiolytic, antihistamine.
See: Atarax, Syr., Tab. (Roerig).
Vistaril Isoject. (Roerig).
Vistaril, Cap., Susp. (Pfizer).
W/Ephedrine sulf., theophylline.
See: Marax DF, Syr. (Roerig).
Marax Tab. (Roerig).
Theo-Drox, Tab. (Quality Formulations).
W/Pentaerythritol tetranitrate.
See: Cartrax 10, 20, Tab. (Roerig).

hydroxyzine hydrochloride. (Various Mfr.). **Tab.:** 10 mg, 25 mg. Bot. 20s, 30s, 50s, 100s, 250s, 500s, 1000s, UD 32s, 100s. 50 mg. Bot. 30s, 100s. **Syr.:** 10 mg/5 ml. Bot. 16 ml, 120 ml, 473 ml, UD 5 ml, 12.5 ml, 25 ml. **Inj.:** 25 mg/ml. Syr. 2 ml. Vial 1 ml, 10 ml; 50 mg/ml. Amp. 2 ml; Syr. 1 ml, 2 ml; Vial 1 ml, 2 ml, 10 ml. *Rx.*
Use: Antihistamine, anxiolytic.

•**hydroxyzine pamoate.** U.S.P. 23.
Use: Tranquilizer (minor), antihistamine.
See: Hy-Pam 25 Cap. (Teva USA).
Vistaril, Cap., Susp. (Pfizer).

hydroxyzine pamoate. (Various). Hydroxyzine pamoate 25 mg, 50 mg. Bot. 12s, 20s, 100s, 500s, 100s, UD 32s, 100s. 100 mg. Bot. 100s, 500s, 1000s, UD 100s. *Rx.*
Use: Antihistamine, anxiolytic.

Hydro-Z-50 Tablets. (Merz) Hydrochlorothiazide 50 mg/Tab. Bot. 100s, 1000s. *Rx.*
Use: Diuretic.

Hy-Flow Solution. (Ciba Vision Ophthalmics) Polyvinyl alcohol with hydroxyethylcellulose, benzalkonium Cl, EDTA. Bot. 60 ml. *otc.*
Use: Contact lens care.

Hy-Gestrone. (Taylor Pharmaceuticals) Hydroxyprogesterone caproate. **125 mg/ml.:** Vial 10 ml. **250 mg/ml.:** Vial 5 ml. *Rx.*

Use: Hormone, progestin.

Hygienic Cleansing. (Rugby) Witch hazel 50%, glycerin, benzalkonium Cl, methylparaben. Pads. 100s. *otc.*
Use: Anorectal preparation.

Hygienic Powder.
See: Bo-Car-Al, Pow. (SmithKline Beecham Pharmaceuticals).

Hygroton. (Rhone-Poulenc Rorer) Chlorthalidone 25 mg or 50 mg/Tab. Lactose (25, 50 mg). Bot. 100s. *Rx.*
Use: Diuretic.

Hylidone Tabs. (Major) Chlorthalidone. **25 mg or 50 mg/Tab:** Bot. 100s, 250s, 1000s, UD 100s. **100 mg/Tab:** Bot. 100s, 250s, 500s, 1000s. *Rx.*
Use: Diuretic.

Hyliver Plus. (Hyrex) Folic acid 0.4 mg, liver 10 mcg, vitamin B_{12} 100 mcg/ml. Vial 10 ml with phenol. *Rx.*
Use: Vitamin supplement.

Hylorel Tablets. (Medeva) Guanadrel sulfate 10 mg or 25 mg/Tab. Bot. 100s. *Rx.*
Use: Antihypertensive.

Hylutin Injectable. (Hyrex) Hydroxyprogesterone caproate in oil 125 mg/ml, 250 mg/ml. Castor oil with benzyl benzoate and benzyl alcohol. Vial 5 ml (250 mg), 10 ml (125 mg). *Rx.*
Use: Hormone, progestin.

•**hymecromone.** (HIGH-meh-KROE-mone) USAN.
Use: Choleretic.

hymenoptera venom/venom protein. Purified venoms of honeybee, wasp, white faced hornet, yellow hornet, yellow jacket and mixed vespids (both hornets and yellow jackets). *Rx.*
Use: Allergenic extract.
See: Albay (Miles).
Phamalgen (ALK).
Venomil (Bayer Corp).

HY-N.B.P. Ointment. (Jones Medical Industries) Bacitracin zinc 400 units, neomycin sulfate 5 mg, polymixin B sulfate 10,000 units/g. Tube ⅛ oz. *Rx.*
Use: Anti-infective, topical.

hyoscine hydrobromide. Scopolamine HBr, U.S.P. 23.
Use: Antispasmodic.

hyoscine-hyoscyamine-atropine.
Use: Anticholinergic.
See: Atropine w/hyoscyamine w/hyoscine.

•**hyoscyamine.** (high-oh-SIGH-ah-meen) U.S.P. 23.
Use: Anticholinergic.
See: Bellafoline, Amp., Tab. (Novartis).
Cysto-Spaz, Tab. (PolyMedica).

hyoscyamine-atropine-hyoscine.
Use: Anticholinergic.
See: Atropine w/hyoscyamine w/hyoscine.

•**hyoscyamine hydrobromide.** U.S.P. 23.
Use: Anticholinergic.
W/Physostigmine salicylate.

hyoscyamine hydrochloride. (Various Mfr.).

hyoscyamine maleate.
See: Bellafoline, Amp., Tab. (Novartis).

hyoscyamine salts.
Use: Anticholinergic.
W/Atropine salts.
See: Atropine W/Hyoscyamine.

•**hyoscyamine sulfate.** U.S.P. 23.
Use: Anticholinergic.
See: Anaspaz, Tab. (B.F. Ascher).
A-Spas SK, Tab. Subl. (Hyrex).
Cystospaz-M, Cap. (PolyMedica).
Donnamar, Tab. (Marnel).
ED-SPAZ, Tab. (Edwards Pharmaceuticals).
Gastrosed, Drops, Tab. (Roberts Pharm).
Levbid, ER Tab. (Schwarz Pharma).
Levsin/SL, Sublingual Tab. (Schwarz Pharma).
W/Atropine sulfate, hyoscine HBr, phenobarbital.
See: DeTal, Elix., Tab. (DeLeon).
Donnatal, Prods. (Robins).
Hyonal C.T., Tab. (Paddock).
Maso-Donna, Elix., Tab. (Mason).
Peece, Tab. (Scrip).
Sedamine, Tab. (Dunhall Pharmaceuticals).
Spasaid, Cap. (Century Pharm).
Spasquid, Elix. (Geneva Pharm).
W/Atropine sulfate, hyoscine HBr, phenobarbital, pepsin, pancreatin, bile salts.
See: Donnazyme, Tab. (Robins).
W/Atropine sulfate. Scopolamine HCl, phenobarbital.
See: Ultabs, Tab. (Burlington).
W/Belladonna Alkaloids.
See: Belladonna Prods.
W/Butabarbital.
See: Cystospaz-SR, Cap. (PolyMedica).
W/Methenamine, atropine sulfate, methylene blue, salol, benzoic acid, gelsemium.
W/Phenobarbital, simethicone, atropine sulfate, scopolamine HBr.
See: Kinesed, Tab. (Zeneca).

hyoscyamine sulfate. (Various Mfr.) 0.375 mg/ER Cap. 100s. *Rx.*
Use: Anticholinergic.

hyoscyamine sulfate. (Zenith Goldline) 0.125 mg/ml, alcohol 5%/Soln. Bot. with dropper. 15 ml. *Rx.*
Use: Anticholinergic.

hyoscyamus extract.
W/A.P.C.
See: Valacet Junior, Tab. (Pal-Pak).
W/A.P.C., gelsemium extract.
See: Valacet, Tab. (Pal-Pak).

hyoscyamus products and phenobarbital combinations.
Use: Anticholinergic, sedative.
See: Anaspaz PB, Tab. (Taylor Pharmaceuticals).
Donnatal, Preps. (Robins).
Elixiral, Elix. (Vita Elixir).
Floramine, Tab. (Teva USA).
Kinesed, Tab. (Zeneca).
Neoquess, Tab. (O'Neal).
Nevrotose, Cap. (Pal-Pak).

Hyosophen Elixir. (Rugby) Atropine sulfate 0.0194 mg, scopolamine HBr 0.0065 mg, hyoscyamine HBr or sulfate 0.1037 mg, phenobarbital 16.2 mg, alcohol 23%, sugar, sorbitol. 120 ml, pt, gal. *Rx.*
Use: Gastrointestinal, anticholinergic.

Hyosophen Tablets. (Rugby). Atropine sulfate 0.0194 mg, scopolamine HBr 0.0065 mg, hyoscyamine HBr or SO_4 0.1037 mg, phenobarbital 16.2 mg. In 1000s. *Rx.*
Use: Anticholinergic combination.

Hypaque 76. (Sanofi Winthrop) Diatrizoate meglumine 66%, diatrizoate sodium 10%, iodine 37%, EDTA. Vial 30 ml, 50 ml, 100 ml.
Use: Radiopaque agent.

Hypaque-Cysto. (Sanofi Winthrop) Diatrizoate meglumine 30% soln., iodine 14.1%. 250 ml in 500 ml dilution bottle. Pediatric: 100 ml in 300 ml dilution bottle.
Use: Radiopaque agent.

Hypaque-M 75%. (Sanofi Winthrop) Diatrizoate meglumine 50%, diatrizoate sodium 25%, iodine 38.5%, EDTA. Vial 20 ml, 50 ml.
Use: Radiopaque agent.

Hypaque-M 90%. (Sanofi Winthrop) Diatrizoate meglumine 60%, diatrizoate sodium 30%, EDTA. Vial 50 ml.
Use: Radiopaque agent.

Hypaque Meglumine 30%. (Sanofi Winthrop) Diatrizoate meglumine 30%, iodine 14.1%. Bot. 100 ml, 300 ml w/ and w/o I.V. infusion set.
Use: Radiopaque agent.

Hypaque Meglumine 60%. (Sanofi Winthrop) Diatrizoate meglumine 60%, iodine 28%, EDTA. Vial 20 ml, 30 ml, 50 ml, 100 ml.
Use: Radiopaque agent.

Hypaque Oral. (Sanofi Winthrop) **Pow.:** Diatrizoate sodium oral pow. containing iodine 600 mg/g. Can 250 g, Bot. 10 g. **Liq.:** Soln. 41.66%. Bot. 120 ml.
Use: Radiopaque agent.

Hypaque Sodium 20%. (Sanofi Winthrop) Diatrizoate sodium 20%, iodine 12%, EDTA. Vial 100 ml.
Use: Radiopaque agent.

Hypaque Sodium 25%. (Sanofi Winthrop) Diatrizoate sodium 25%, iodine 15%. Bot. 300 ml, w/ and w/out I.V. infusion set.
Use: Radiopaque agent.

Hypaque Sodium 50%. (Sanofi Winthrop) Diatrizoate sodium 50%, iodine 30%. **Vial:** 20 ml, 30 ml, 50 ml. **Dilution Bottle:** 200 ml with EDTA.
Use: Radiopaque agent.

Hyperab.
See: Bayrab, Vial. (Bayer Corp).

HyperHep.
See: BayHep B, Vial. (Bayer Corp).

hypericin. (VIMRxyn Pharm/NIH) *Rx.*
Use: Antiviral.

hyperlipidemia, agents for.
See: Atromid-S (Wyeth Ayerst).
Choloxin (Knoll Pharmaceuticals).
Cholybar (Parke-Davis).
Clofibrate (Various).
Colestid (Pharmacia & Upjohn).
Lescol (Novartis).
Lopid (Parke-Davis).
Lorelco (Hoechst Marion Roussel).
Mevacor (Merck).
Pravachol (Bristol-Myers Squibb).
Questran (Bristol-Myers).
Questran Light (Bristol-Myers).
Zocor (Merck).

Hyperlyte. (American McGaw) Sodium 25 mEq, potassium 40.5 mEq, calcium 5 mEq, magnesium 8 mEq, chloride 33.5 mEq, acetate 40.6 mEq, gluconate 5 mEq, 6050 mOsm/L. Inj. Vial 25 ml fill in 50 ml. *Rx.*
Use: Nutritional supplement, parenteral.

Hyperlyte CR. (American McGaw) Sodium 25 mEq, potassium 20 mEq, calcium 5 mEq, magnesium 5 mEq, chloride 30 mEq, acetate 30 mEq, 5500 mOsm/L. Inj. Super-vial 150 ml, 250 ml fill. *Rx.*
Use: Nutritional supplement, parenteral.

Hyperlyte R. (American McGaw) Sodium 25 mEq, potassium 20 mEq, calcium 5 mEq, magnesium 5 mEq, chlor-

ide 30 mEq, acetate 25 mEq, 4200 mOsm/L. Inj. Vial 25 ml fill in 50 ml. *Rx.*
Use: Nutritional supplement, parenteral.

Hypermune RSV. (MedImmune) Respiratory syncytial virus immune globulin, human.
Use: Respiratory syncytial virus treatment. [Orphan drug]

Hyperopto 5%. (Professional Pharmacal) Sodium Cl 5%. Oint. Tube 3.5 g. *otc.*
Use: Ophthalmic.

Hyperopto Ointment. (Professional Pharmacal) Sodium HCl 50 mg, D.I. water 150 mg, anhydrous lanolin 150 mg, liquid petrolatum 50 mg, white petrolatum 599 mg, methylparaben 7 mg, propylparaben 3 mg/g. Tube 3.5 g. *otc.*
Use: Ophthalmic.

hyperosmolar agents.
Use: Laxative.
See: Glycerin, USP (Various).
Sani-Supp, Supp. (G & W Laboratories).
Fleet Babylax, Liq. (C.B. Fleet).

Hyperstat IV Injection. (Schering Plough) Diazoxide 15 mg/ml. Amp. 20 ml. *Rx.*
Use: Antihypertensive.

hypertension diagnosis.
See: Regitine, Amp., Tab. (Novartis Pharmaceuticals).

hypertensive emergency drugs.
See: Arfonad, Inj. (Roche Laboratories).
Diazoxide Injection (Quad).
Hyperstat IV, Inj. (Schering Plough).
Nitropress, Inj. (Abbott Laboratories).

Hyper-Tet.
See: Baytet, Vial. (Bayer Corp).

Hy-Phen Tablets. (B.F. Ascher) Hydrocodone bitartrate 5 mg, acetaminophen 500 mg. Bot. 100s. *c-III.*
Use: Analgesic, antitussive.

Hyphylline. Dyphylline. *Rx.*
See: Neothylline, Elix., Amp., Tab. (Teva USA).

hypnogene.
See: Barbital (Various Mfr.).

Hypnomidate. (Janssen) Etomidate. *Rx.*
Use: Anesthetic, general.

hypnotics.
See: Sedatives.

"hypo".
See: Sodium Thiosulfate (Various Mfr.).

Hypo-Bee. (Towne) Vitamins B_1 50 mg, B_2 20 mg, B_6 5 mg, B_{12} 15 mcg, niacinamide 25 mg, calcium pantothenate 5 mg, C 300 mg, E 200 IU, iron 10 mg/Tab. Bot. 30s, 100s. *otc.*
Use: Mineral, vitamin supplement.

hypochlorite preps.
See: Antiformin.
Dakin's Soln.
Hyclorite.

Hypoclear. (Bausch & Lomb) Isotonic soln. with sodium Cl 0.9%. Aerosol soln. 240 ml, 300 ml. *otc.*
Use: Contact lens care.

hypoglycemic agents.
See: Chlorpropamide.
Diabeta, Tab. (Hoechst Marion Roussel).
Diabinese, Tab. (Pfizer).
Dymelor, Tab. (Eli Lilly).
Glucotrol, Tab. (Roerig).
Glynase, Tab. (Pharmacia & Upjohn).
Micronase, Tab. (Pharmacia & Upjohn).
Orinase, Tab., Vial (Pharmacia & Upjohn).
Phenformin HCl.
Tolbutamide.
Tolinase, Tab. (Pharmacia & Upjohn).

α-**hypophamine.** Oxytocin.

•**hypophosphorous acid.** (high-poe-FOSS-for-uhs) N.F. 18.
Use: Pharmaceutic aid (antioxidant).

HypoTears Ophthalmic Liquid. (Ciba Vision Ophthalmics) Polyvinyl alcohol 1%, PEG-400, dextrose 1%, benzalkonium Cl 0.01%, EDTA. Bot. 15 ml, 30 ml. *otc.*
Use: Lubricant, ophthalmic.

HypoTears Ophthalmic Ointment. (Ciba Vision Ophthalmics) White petrolatum, light mineral oil. Tube 3.5 g. *otc.*
Use: Lubricant, ophthalmic.

HypoTears PF. (Ciba Vision Ophthalmics) Polyvinyl alcohol 1%, PEG 400, dextrose and EDTA. Soln. In 0.6 ml. *otc.*
Use: Artificial tears.

hypotensive agents.
See: Hypertension Therapy.

HypRh$_O$-D.
See: BayRh$_O$ D, Vial. (Bayer Corp).

HypRh$_O$-D Mini-Dose. (Bayer Corp) RH$_O$ (D) Immune Globulin Micro-Dose. Each package contains a single dose syringe. *Rx.*
Use: Immunization.

Hyrexin-50. (Hyrex) Diphenhydramine HCl 50 mg/ml, benzethonium chloride. Vial 10 ml. Amp. 1 ml. *Rx.*
Use: Antihistamine.

Hyscorbic Plus Tablets. (Sanofi Win-

throp) Vitamins E 45 IU, C 600 mg, folic acid 400 mcg, B_1 20 mg, B_2 10 mg, niacinamide 100 mg, B_6 10 mg, B_{12} 25 mcg, pantothenic acid 25 mg, copper 3 mg, zinc 23.9 mg/Tab. Bot. 60s. *otc.*
Use: Mineral, vitamin supplement.

Hyserp. (Freeport) Reserpine alkaloid 0.25 mg/Tab. Bot. 1000s. *Rx.*
Use: Antihypertensive.

Hyskon. (Pharmacia & Upjohn) Dextran 70 32% in 10% w/v dextrose. Bot. 100 ml, 250 ml. *Rx.*
Use: Diagnostic aid. For distending the uterine cavity and in irrigating and visualizing its surfaces.

Hysone. (Roberts Pharm) Clioquinol 30 mg, hydrocortisone 10 mg/g. Cream. Tube. 20 g. *otc.*
Use: Antifungal; corticosteroid, topical.

hysteroscopy fluid.
Use: Diagnostic aid.
See: Hyskon (Pharmacia & Upjohn).

Hytakerol. (Sanofi Winthrop) Dihydrotachysterol. **Cap.:** 0.125 mg. Bot. 50s. **Soln.:** 0.25 mg/ml in oil. Bot. 15 ml. *Rx.*
Use: Treatment of tetany and hypoparathyroidism.

Hytinic. (Hyrex) Polysaccharide-iron complex **Cap.:** 150 mg. Bot. 50s, 500s. **Elix.:** 100 mg/5 ml, alcohol 10%. Bot. 240 ml. *otc.*
Use: MIneral supplement.

Hytinic Injection. (Hyrex) Ferrous gluconate 3 mg, liver equivalent to vitamins B_{12} 1 mcg, vitamins B_2 0.75 mg, B_3 50 mg, B_5 1.25 mg, B_{12} equivalent 15 mcg. Vial 30 ml. *Rx.*
Use: Mineral, vitamin supplement.

Hytone Cream. (Dermik Laboratories) Hydrocortisone in cream base. **1%:** 1 oz. Jar 4 oz. **2.5%:** Tube 1 oz, 2 oz. *otc, Rx.*
Use: Corticosteroid, topical.

Hytone Lotion 1%. (Dermik Laboratories) Hydrocortisone 1% (10 mg/ml). Bot. 120 ml. *Rx.*
Use: Corticosteroid, topical.

Hytone Lotion 2.5%. (Dermik Laboratories) Hydrocortisone 2 1/2% (25 mg/ml) in lotion base. Bot. 60 ml. *Rx.*
Use: Corticosteroid, topical.

Hytone Ointment. (Dermik Laboratories) Hydrocortisone in ointment base, mineral oil, white petrolatum. **1%:** Tube 28.3 g, 113.4 g. **2.5%:** Tube 28.3 g. *Rx.*
Use: Corticosteroid, topical.

Hytone Spray. (Dermik Laboratories) Hydrocortisone 1%. 45 ml. *Rx.*
Use: Corticosteroid, topical.

Hytrin. (Abbott Laboratories) Terazosin HCl 1 mg, 2 mg, 5 mg, 10 mg, parabens. Cap. Bot. 100s, UD 100s. *Rx.*
Use: Antihypertensive.

Hytuss Tablets. (Hyrex) Guaifenesin 100 mg/Tab. Bot. 100s, 1000s. *otc.*
Use: Expectorant.

Hytuss 2X. (Hyrex) Guaifenesin 200 mg/Cap. Bot. 100s, 1000s. *otc.*
Use: Expectorant.

Hyzaar. (Merck) Losartan potassium 50 mg, hydrochlorothiazide 12.5 mg, potassium 4.24 mg, lactose/Tab. Bot. 30s, 90s, 100s, UD 100s. *Rx.*
Use: Antihypertensive.

Hyzine-50. (Hyrex) Hydroxyzine HCl 50 mg as HCl/ml. Vial 10 ml. *Rx.*
Use: Anxiolytic.

I

•**ibafloxacin.** (ih-BAH-FLOX-ah-sin) USAN.
Use: Anti-infective.

ibenzmethyzin. Name used for Procarbazine Hydrochloride.

Iberet. (Abbott Laboratories) Ferrous sulfate 105 mg, ascorbic acid 150 mg, vitamins B_{12} 25 mcg, B_1 6 mg, B_2 6 mg, niacinamide 30 mg, B_5 10 mg, B_6 5 mg/ CR Filmtab. Bot. 60s. *Rx.*
Use: Mineral, vitamin supplement.

Iberet-500. (Abbott Laboratories) Ascorbic acid 500 mg, ferrous sulfate 105 mg, vitamins B_1 6 mg, B_2 6 mg, B_3 30 mg, B_5 10 mg, B_6 5 mg, B_{12} 25 mcg/ CR Filmtab. Bot. 60s, 100s, Abbo-Pac 100s. *Rx.*
Use: Mineral, vitamin supplement.

Iberet-500 Liquid. (Abbott Laboratories) Ferrous sulfate 78.75 mg, vitamins B_1 4.5 mg, B_2 4.5 mg, B_3 22.5 mg, B_5 7.5 mg, B_6 3.75 mg, B_{12} 18.75 mcg, C 375 mg, sorbitol, parabens/5 ml. Bot. 240 ml. *Rx.*
Use: Mineral, vitamin supplement.

Iberet-Folic-500 Filmtab. (Abbott Laboratories) Ferrous sulfate 105 mg, vitamin C 500 mg, B_3 30 mg, B_5 10 mg, B_1 6 mg, B_2 6 mg, B_6 5 mg, B_{12} 25 mcg, folic acid 0.8 mg/CR Filmtab. Bot. 60s. *Rx.*
Use: Mineral, vitamin supplement.

Iberet Liquid. (Abbott Laboratories) Ferrous sulfate 78.75 mg, vitamins C 112.5 mg, B_{12} 18.75 mcg, B_1 4.5 mg, B_2 4.5 mg, B_3 22.5 mg, B_5 7.5 mg, B_6 3.75 mg/ 15 ml. Bot. 240 ml. *Rx.*
Use: Mineral, vitamin supplement.

•**ibopamine.** (EYE-BOE-pah-meen) USAN.
Use: Dopaminergic (peripheral).

IBU. (Knoll Pharmaceuticals) Ibuprofen 400, 600 or 800 mg/Tab. 100s, 500s. *Rx.*
Use: Analgesic, NSAID.

•**ibufenac.** (eye-BYOO-feh-nak) USAN.
Use: Antirheumatic (anti-inflammatory, analgesic, antipyretic).
See: Dytransin.

Ibuprin. (Thompson Medical) Ibuprofen 200 mg/Tab. Bot. 50s, 100s. *otc.*
Use: Analgesic, NSAID.

•**ibuprofen,** (eye-BYOO-pro-fen) U.S.P. 23.
Use: Anti-inflammatory, analgesic.
See: Advil, Tab. (Whitehall Robins).
Children's Advil, Susp. (Wyeth Ayerst).
Dynafed IB, Tab. (BDI).
Genpril, Tab. (Zenith Goldline).
Haltran, Tab. (Pharmacia & Upjohn).
IBU, Tab. (Knoll Pharmaceuticals).
Ibuprin, Tab. (Thompson Med).
Junior Strength Advil, Tab. (Whitehall Robins).
Junior Strength Motrin, Tab. (Ortho McNeil).
Menadol, Tab. (Rugby).
Midol IB, Tab. (Bayer Corp).
Motrin, Tab., Drops, Chew. Tab., Susp. (Pharmacia & Upjohn).
Motrin IB, Tab. (Pharmacia & Upjohn).
Nuprin, Tab. (Bristol-Myers Squibb).
Pediatric Advil Drops, Oral Susp. (Whitehall-Robins).
Rufen, Tab. (Knoll Pharmaceuticals).
Saleto, Tab. (Roberts Pharm).
Salprofen (Farmacon).

ibuprofen. (Various Mfr.) 200, 300, 400, 600, 800 mg/Tab. 12s, 15s, 21s, 30s, 40s, 50s, 60s, 100s, 360s, 500s, UD 100s. *otc. Rx.*
Use: Analgesic, NSAID.

•**ibuprofen aluminum.** (eye-BYOO-profen) USAN.
Use: Anti-inflammatory.

•**ibuprofen piconol.** (eye-BYOO-pro-fen PIK-oh-nahl) USAN.
Use: Topical anti-inflammatory.

ibuprofen suspension. (Various Mfr.) 100 mg/5 ml. UD 50s. *Rx.*
Use: Analgesic, NSAID.

•**ibutilide fumarate.** (ih-BYOO-tih-lide FEW-muh-rate) USAN.
Use: Cardiac depressant (antiarrhythmic).
See: Corvert, Soln. (Pharmacia & Upjohn).

ICAPS Plus. (Ciba Vision Ophthalmics) Vitamin A 6000 IU, C 200 mg, E 60 IU, B_2 20 mg, Zn 14.25 mg, Cu, Se, Mn/ Tab. Sugar free. Bot. 60s, 120s. *otc.*
Use: Mineral, vitamin supplement.

ICAPS Time Release. (Ciba Vision Ophthalmics) Vitamin A 7000 IU, C 200 mg, E 100 IU, B_2 20 mg, Zn 14.25 mg, Cu, Se/Tab. Sugar free. Bot. 60s, 120s. *otc.*
Use: Mineral, vitamin supplement.

•**icatibant acetate.** (eye-CAT-ih-bant ASS-eh-tate) USAN.
Use: Bradykinin antagonist.

Ice Mint. (Westwood Squibb) Stearic acid, synthetic cocoa butter, lanolin oil, camphor, menthol, beeswax, mineral oil, sodium borate, aromatic oils, emulsifiers, water. Jar 4 oz. *otc.*
Use: Emollient, counterirritant.

I-Chlor 0.5%. (Americal) Chloramphenicol 5 mg/ml. Bot. 7.5 ml, 15 ml. *Rx.*
Use: Anti-infective, ophthalmic.

•**ichthammol,** (ICK-thah-mole) U.S.P. 23.
Use: Topical anti-infective.
W/Aluminum hydroxide, phenol, zinc oxide, camphor, eucalyptol.
See: Almophen, Oint. (Jones Medical Industries).
W/Benzocaine, resin cerate, carbolic acid, thymol, camphor, juniper tar, hexachlorophene.
See: Boil-Ease Anesthetic Drawing Salve (Del Pharmaceuticals).
W/Hydrocortisone acetate, benzocaine, oxyquinoline sulfate, ephedrine HCl.
See: Derma Medicone-HC (Medicone).
W/Naftalan, calamine, amber pet.
See: Naftalan, Oint. (Paddock).

ichthammol. (Eli Lilly). 10%, 20% Oint.

ichthammol. (NMC Labs) Ichthammol 10% or 20% in a lanolin-petrolatum base. Oint. Tube 28.4 g. *otc.*
Use: Antiseptic.

ichthynate.
See: Ichthammol.

•**icopezil maleate.** (eye-KOE-peh-zill MAL-ee-ate) USAN.
Use: Alzheimer's disease treatment (cognition enhancer), cognition adjuvant, acetylcholinesterase inhibitor.

•**icotidine.** (eye-KOE-tih-DEEN) USAN.
Use: Antagonist (to histamine H_2 and H_1 receptors).

•**ictasol.** (IK-tah-sahl) USAN.
Use: Disinfectant.

Ictotest Reagent Tablets. (Bayer Corp) Reagent Tab. For urinary bilirubin. Bot. 100s.
Use: Diagnostic aid.

Icy Hot Balm. (Procter & Gamble) Methyl salicylate 29%, menthol 7.6%. Jar 3.5 oz, 7 oz. *otc.*
Use: Analgesic, topical.

Icy Hot Cream. (Procter & Gamble) Methyl salicylate 30%, menthol 10%. Tube 0.25 oz, 1.25 oz, 3 oz. *otc.*
Use: Analgesic, topical.

Icy Hot, Extra Strength. (Procter & Gamble) Methyl salicylate 30%, menthol 10%, ceresin, cyclomethicone, hydrogenated castor oil, PEG-150 distearate, propylene glycol, stearic acid, stearyl alcohol. Stick 52.5 g. *otc.*
Use: Liniment.

Icy Hot Stick. (Procter & Gamble) Methyl salicylate 15%, menthol 8%. Stick 1.75 oz. *otc.*
Use: Analgesic, topical.

I.D.A. Capsules. (Zenith Goldline) Isometheptene mucate 65 mg, dichloralphenazone 100 mg, acetaminophen 324 mg/Cap. Bot. 100s. *Rx.*
Use: Analgesic.

Idamycin. (Pharmacia & Upjohn) Idarubicin HCl. Lactose 50 mg/5 mg. Lactose 100 mg/10 mg. Lactose 200 mg/20 mg Pow. for Inj. *Rx.*
Use: Anti-infective.

Idamycin PFS. (Pharmacia & Upjohn) Idarubicin HCl 1 mg/ml Inj. Vial. 5, 10 and 20s. *Rx.*
Use: Anti-infective (anthracycline).

•**idarubicin hydrochloride,** (eye-DUH-RUE-bih-sin) U.S.P. 23.
Use: Antineoplastic. [Orphan drug]
See: Idamycin, Pow. for Inj. (Pharmacia & Upjohn).

•**idoxifene.** (ih-dox-ih-feen) USAN.
Use: Antineoplastic, hormone replacement therapy (estrogen receptor antagonist), osteoporosis treatment and prevention.

I-Drops. (Americal) Tetrahydrozoline HCl 0.5%. Ophthalmic soln. Bot. 0.5 oz
Use: Mydriatic, vasoconstrictor.

IDU. Idoxuridine. *Rx.*
Use: Antiviral, ophthalmic.
See: Herplex Liquifilm, Soln. (Allergan).
Stoxil, Soln. (SmithKline Beecham Pharmaceuticals).
Stoxil, Oint. (SmithKline Beecham Pharmaceuticals).

Ifen. (Everett Laboratories) Ibuprofen 400 mg or 600 mg/Tab. Bot. 100s, 500s. *Rx.*
Use: Analgesic.

•**ifetroban.** (ih-FEH-troe-ban) USAN.
Use: Antithrombotic.

•**ifetroban sodium.** (ih-FEH-troe-ban) USAN.
Use: Antithrombotic.

Ifex. (Bristol-Myers) Ifosfamide 1 g or 3 g. Pow. for Inj. Vial single dose. *Rx.*
Use: Antineoplastic.

•**ifosfamide,** (eye-FOSS-fuh-MIDE) U.S.P. 23.
Use: Antineoplastic.
See: Ifex, Pow. for Inj. (Mead Johnson Oncology).

ifosfamide, sterile. (eye-FOSS-fah-MIDE)
Use: Antineoplastic.

I-Gent. (Americal) Gentamicin sulfate 3 mg/ml. Ophthalmic soln. Bot. 5 ml. *Rx.*
Use: Anti-infective, ophthalmic.

Igepal Co-430. (General Aniline & Film) Non-oxynol 4. *otc.*
Use: Contraceptive, spermicide.

Igepal Co-730. (General Aniline & Film) Non-oxynol 15. *otc.*
Use: Contraceptive, spermicide.

Igepal Co-880. (General Aniline & Film) Non-oxynol 30. *otc.*
Use: Contraceptive, spermicide.

igG monoclonal anti-CD4.
See: Chimeric m-t412 (human-murine) igG monoclonal anti-cd4

IGIV. (Various Mfr.) Immune globulin IV. *Rx.*
Use: Immunomodulator (Phase II/III pediatric HIV), immunization.
See: Gamimune N, Inj. (Bayer Corp).
Gammagard S/D, Pow. (Baxter).
Gammar-P IV, Pow. (Centeon).
Iveegam, Pow. (Immuno)
Polygam S/D (American Red Cross).
Sandoglobulin, Pow. (Novartis).
Venoglobulin-I, Pow. (Alpha Therapeutics).
Venoglobulin-S (Alpha Therapeutics).

I-Homatrine 5%. (Americal) Homatropine hydrobromide 5%. Ophthalmic soln. Bot. 5 ml. *Rx.*
Use: Cycloplegic, mydriatic.

IL-2. (Various Mfr.) Interleukin-2. *Rx.*
Use: Immunomodulator.
See: Proleukin (Chiron).

•**ilepcimide.** (eye-LEPP-sih-mide) USAN. *Formerly antiepilepsirine.*
Use: Anticonvulsant.

Iletin I. (Eli Lilly) Regular and modified insulin products from beef and pork. *otc.*
Regular: 100 units/ml. Bot. 10 ml.
Lente: 100 units/ml. Bot. 10 ml.
NPH: 100 units/ml. Bot. 10 ml.
Use: Antidiabetic.

Iletin II. (Eli Lilly) Special insulin products prepared from purified beef or purified pork. *otc.*
Regular: 100 units/ml. Bot. 10 ml.
Lente: 100 units/ml. Bot. 10 ml.
NPH: 100 units/ml. Bot. 10 ml.
Use: Antidiabetic.

Iletin II Concentrated. (Eli Lilly) Purified pork regular insulin 500 units/ml. Vial 20 ml. *Rx.*
Use: Antidiabetic.

•**ilmofosine.** (ill-MOE-fose-een) USAN.
Use: Antineoplastic.

•**ilonidap.** (ile-OHN-ih-dap) USAN.
Use: Anti-inflammatory.

Ilopan. (Pharmacia & Upjohn) Dexpanthenol 250 mg/ml. Amp. 2 ml, Disp. Syringe 2 ml. *Rx.*
Use: Gastrointestinal stimulant.

Ilopan-Choline. (Pharmacia & Upjohn) Ilopan 50 mg, choline bitartrate 25 mg/Tab. Bot. 100s, 500s. *Rx.*
Use: Gastrointestinal stimulant.

•**iloperidone.** (ill-oh-PURR-ih-dohn) USAN.
Use: Antipsychotic.

iloprost infusion solution. (Berlex) Raynaud's phenomenon secondary to systemic sclerosis. [Orphan drug]

Ilosone. (Eli Lilly) Erythromycin estolate. **Cap.:** (Erythromycin base) 250 mg/Pulv. Bot. 24s, 100s, UD 100s, Blister pkg. 10 × 10s. **Liq.:** 125 mg or 250 mg/5 ml. Bot. 100 ml, 16 fl oz. **Tab.:** Bot. 50s. **Susp.:** 125 mg or 250 mg/5 ml. Bot. 10 ml. *Rx.*
Use: Anti-infective, erythromycin.

Ilosone Chewable. (Eli Lilly) Erythromycin estolate 125 mg or 250 mg/Tab. Bot. 50s. *Rx.*
Use: Anti-infective, erythromycin.

Ilotycin Gluceptate I.V. (Eli Lilly) Erythromycin gluceptate. Vial. I.V. 1 g, vial 30 ml. Box 1s. *Rx.*
Use: Anti-infective, erythromycin.

Ilotycin Ophthalmic Ointment. (Eli Lilly) Erythromycin 5 mg/g. Tube 3.5 g. *Rx.*
Use: Anti-infective, ophthalmic.

Ilozyme. (Pharmacia & Upjohn) Pancrelipase equivalent to lipase 11,000 units, protease 30,000 units, amylase 30,000 units/Tab. Bot. 250s. *Rx.*
Use: Digestive enzymes.

I-Lube. (Americal) Petrolatum ophthalmic ointment. Tube 0.125 oz.
Use: Lubricant, ophthalmic.

I.L.X. B12 Elixir. (Kenwood/Bradley) Liver fraction 98 mg, iron 102 mg, vitamins B_1 5 mg, B_2 2 mg, B_3 10 mg, B_{12} 10 mcg/15 ml. Bot. 240 ml. *otc.*
Use: Mineral, vitamin supplement.

I.L.X. B12 Tablets and Caplets. (Kenwood/Bradley) Iron 37.5 mg, vitamins C 120 mg, B_{12} 12 mcg, desiccated liver 130 mg, B_1 2 mg, B_2 2 mg, B_3 20 mg/Tab. Bot. 100s. *otc.*
Use: Mineral, vitamin supplement.

I-L-X Elixir. (Kenwood/Bradley) Iron 70 mg, liver concentrate 98 mg, vitamins B_1 5 mg, B_2 2 mg, B_3 10 mg/15 ml. Bot. 240 ml. *otc.*
Use: Mineral, vitamin supplement.

•**imafen hydrochloride.** (IH-mah-fen) USAN.
Use: Antidepressant.

•**imazodan hydrochloride.** (ih-MAY-zoe-DAN) USAN.
Use: Cardiovascular agent.

•**imciromab pentetate.** (im-SIHR-ah-mab PEN-teh-tate) USAN.

Use: Monoclonal antibody (antimyosin). [Orphan drug]
See: Myoscint (Centocor).

Imdur. (Key Pharm) Isosorbide mononitrate 30 mg, 60 mg, 120 mg. ER Tab. Bot. 30s, 100s, UD 100s. *Rx.*
Use: Antianginal.

Imenol. (Sigma-Tau Pharmaceuticals) Guaiacol 0.1 g, eucalyptol 0.08 g, iodoform 0.02 g, camphor 0.05 g/ml. Vial 30 ml. *Rx.*
Use: Expectorant.

l-methorphinan levorphanol.
See: Levo-Dromoran, Amp., Tab., Vial (Roche Laboratories).

Imferon. (Fisons) An iron-dextran complex containing iron 50 mg/ml. Amp. 2 ml. Box 10s. Vial (w/phenol 0.5%) 10 ml. Box 2s. *Rx.*
Use: Mineral supplement.

imexon. (Amplimed)
Use: Multiple myeloma. [Orphan drug]

imidazole carboxamide. *Rx.*
Use: Antineoplastic.
See: Dacarbazine, Inj. (Various Mfr.).
DTIC-Dome, Inj. (Bayer Corp).

•**imidecyl iodine.** (IH-mih-DEH-sill EYE-uh-dine) USAN.
Use: Anti-infective, topical.

•**imidocarb hydrochloride.** (ih-MIH-doe-KARB) USAN.
Use: Antiprotozoal (Babesia).

•**imidoline hydrochloride.** (im-ID-oh-leen) USAN.
Use: Anxiolytic, antipsychotic.

•**imidurea,** (ih-mid-your-EE-ah) N.F. 18.
Use: Antimicrobial.

•**imiglucerase.** (ih-mih-GLUE-ser-ACE) USAN.
Use: Enzyme replenisher, treatment for Gaucher's disease (glucocerebrosidase). [Orphan drug]
See: Cerezyme (Genzyme).

•**imiloxan hydrochloride.** (ih-mill-OX-ahn) USAN.
Use: Antidepressant.

imipemide. (ih-MIH-peh-MIDE)
Use: Anti-infective.
See: Imipenem, U.S.P 23.

•**imipenem,** (ih-mih-PEN-em) U.S.P. 23.
Formerly imipemide.
Use: Anti-infective.
W/Cilastatin for Injection.
See: Primaxin, Inj (Merck).

•**imipramine hydrochloride,** (im-IPP-ruh-meen) U.S.P. 23.
Use: Antidepressant.
See: Janimine, Tab. (Abbott Laboratories).
Presamine, Tab. (Rhone-Poulenc Rorer).
Tofranil, Tab., Amp. (Novartis).
W.D.D., Tab. (Solvay).

imipramine pamoate. *Rx.*
Use: Antidepressant.
See: Tofranil-PM, Cap. (Novartis).

•**imiquimod.** (ih-mih-KWIH-mahd) USAN.
Use: Immunomodulator.
See: Aldara Cream (3M Pharmaceuticals).

Imitrex Injection. (GlaxoWellcome) Sumatriptan succinate. 12 mg/ml, sodium chloride 7 mg/ml. Inj. Unit-of-use syringes: 0.5 ml in 2 ml; Single-dose vial: 6 mg; SELFdose system kit: 2 unit-of-use syringes, 1 SELFdose unit. *Rx.*
Use: Antimigraine.

Imtrex Nasal Spray. (GlaxoWellcome) Sumatriptan 5 mg, 20 mg. Nasal spray devices 100 mcL. 6s. *Rx.*
Use: Antimigraine.

Imitrex Tablets. (GlaxoWellcome) Sumatriptan succinate 25 mg or 50 mg, lactose/Tab. Pkg. 9s. *Rx.*
Use: Antimigraine.

ImmTher. (Immuno Therapeutics) Disaccharide tripeptide glycerol dipalmitoyl.
Use: Antineoplastic. [Orphan drug]

Immun-Aid. (McGaw) A custard flavored liquid containing 18.5 g protein, 60 g carbohydrate, 11 g fat per liter sodium 290 mg, potassium 530 mg. 1 calorie/ml. With appropriate vitamins and minerals. Pow. Packets 123 g. 24s. *otc.*
Use: Nutritional supplement, enteral.

immune globulin. (ih-MYOON GLAH-byoo-lin) Immune Serum Globulin Human. Gamma-globulin fraction of normal human plasma. Vial 10 ml. Tubex 1 ml, 2 ml w/thimerosal 1:10,000. *Rx.*
Use: Modification of active measles, prophylaxis of hepatitis A; treatment of immune deficiencies; prevention of infection associated with bone marrow transplantation (BMT); decrease frequency of certain pediatric HIV-related infections and conjunctive therapy for Kawasaki syndrome.
See: Gamimune N (Bayer Corp).
Gammagard S/D (Baxter).
Gammar-P IV (Centeon).
Iveegam (Immuno).
Polygam S/D (American Red Cross).
Sandoglobulin (Novartis).
Venoglobulin-I (Alpha Therapeutics).
Venoglobulin-S (Alpha Therapeutics).

immune globulin, cytomegalovirus.
See: CytoGam, Vial (MedImmune).

immune globulin, hepatitis B.
See: BayHep B, Vial, Syr. (Bayer Corp).
H-BIG, Vial, Syr. (North American Biologicals).

immune globulin IM.
Use: Immunization.
See: Gammar-IM (Centeon).

•**immune globulin intravenous pentetate.** (ih-MYOON GLAH-byoo-lin intrah-VEE-nuhs PEN-teh-tate) USAN.
Use: Diagnostic aid.

immune globulin IV.
Use: Immunization. [Orphan drug]
See: Gamimune N, Inj. (Bayer Corp).
Gammagard, Pow. (Baxter).
Gammar-P IV, Pow. (Centeon).
Iveegam, Pow. (Immuno).
Polygam S/D (American Red Cross).
Sandoglobulin, Pow. (American Red Cross, Novartis).
Venoglobulin-I, Pow. (Alpha Therapeutics).
Venoglobulin-S (Alpha Therapeutics).

immune globulin, rabies.
Use: Immunization.
See: Bayrab (Bayer Corp).
Imogam Rabies (Pasteur Merieux Connaught).

immune globulin, Rh_o(D).
See: Gamulin Rh (Centeon).
BayRho D (Bayer Corp).
MICRhoGAM (Ortho Diagnostics).
Mini-Gamulin Rh (Centeon).
RhoGAM (Ortho Diagnostics).
WinRho SD (Univax Biologics).

immune globulin, tetanus.
Use: Immunization.
See: Bay Tet (Bayer Corp).

immune globulin, vaccinia.
Use: Immunization.

immune globulin, varicella-zoster.
Use: Immunization.

immune serums.
See: Cytomegalovirus Immune Globulin Intravenous (Human) (Massachusetts Public Health Biologic Laboratories).
Hepatitis b immune globulin.
Immune globulin IM.
Immune globulin IV.
Immune Serum Globulin (Human).
Rabies immune globulin.
Rho(D) immune globulin.
Tetanus immune globulin.
Vaccina immune globulin.
Varicella-zoster immune globulin.

immune serum (animal).
See: Antivenins
Botulism Antitoxin, Vial (Connaught).
Diphtheria Antitoxin.

Immunex C-RP. (Wampole Laboratories) Two-minute latex agglutination slide test for the qualitative detection of C-Reactive protein in serum. Kit 100s.
Use: Diagnostic aid.

Immuno. Immune globulin IV (human).
Use: Immunosuppressant. [Orphan drug]

Immuno-C. (Biomune Systems) Bovine Whey Protein Concentrate.
Use: Cryptosporidiosis treatment. [Orphan drug]

immunosuppressive drugs.
See: Atgam (Pharmacia & Upjohn).
Imuran (GlaxoWellcome).
Neoral (Novartis).
Orthoclone OKT3, Inj. (Ortho McNeil).
Prograf (Fujisawa).
Sandimmune, Cap., Oral Soln. or IV Soln. (Novartis).
Zenapax (Hoffman-LaRoche).

Immunorex. (Antigen Laboratories) Allergenic extracts, various. Vial. *Rx.*
Use: Allergen desensitization.

Immuraid. (Immunomedics) Technetium Tc-99M murine monoclonal antibody to hCG and human AFP.
Use: Diagnostic aid.[Orphan drug]

Immurait. (Immunomedics) Iodine I^{131} murine monoclonal antibody IgG2a to B cell.
Use: Antineoplastic.

Imodium A-D Liquid. (Ortho McNeil) Loperamide 1 mg/5 ml, alcohol 5.25%. *otc.*
Use: Antidiarrheal.

Imodium Capsules. (Janssen) Loperamide 2 mg/Cap. Bot. 100s, 500s, UD 100s. *Rx.*
Use: Antidiarrheal.

Imogam Rabies Immune Globulin. (Pasteur Merieux Connaught) Rabies immune globulin (human) 150 IU/ml. Vials 2 ml, 10 ml. *Rx.*
Use: Immunization, rabies.

Imovax Rabies I.D. (Connaught) Rabies vaccine 0.25 IU/0.1 ml for I.D. administration for pre-exposure treatment only. Wistar rabies virus strain PM-1503-3M grown in human diploid cell culture. Powd. Inj. in single dose syringe w/1 vial diluent. *Rx.*
Use: Immunization, rabies.

Imovax Rabies Vaccine. (Connaught) Merieux rabies vaccine, Wistar rabies virus strain PM-1503-3M grown in human diploid cell cultures. Rabies Vaccine ≥ 2.5 IU/ml. Powd. Inj. In single dose vial with disposable needle and

syring containing diluent and disposable needle for administration. *Rx.*
Use: Immunization, rabies.

Impact. (Health for Life Brands) Belladonna alkaloids 0.16 mg, phenylpropanolamine HCl 50 mg, chlorpheniramine maleate 1 mg, pheniramine maleate 12.5 mg/Cap. Pack 12s, 24s. Vial 15s, 30s, Bot. 1000s. *Rx.*
Use: Anticholinergic, antihistamine, antispasmodic, decongestant.

imported fire ant venom, allergenic extract. (ALK Labs)
Use: Allergy testing. [Orphan drug]

Impromen. (Janssen) Bromperidol decanoate. *Rx.*
Use: Antipsychotic.

Impromen Decanoate. (Janssen) Bromperidol decanoate. *Rx.*
Use: Antipsychotic.

•**impromidine hydrochloride.** (im-PRAH-mid-deen) USAN.
Use: Diagnostic aid (gastric secretion indicator).

Improved Congestant Tablets. (Rugby) Chlorpheniramine maleate 2 mg, acetaminophen 325 mg/Tab. Bot. 100s, 1000s. *otc.*
Use: Antihistamine, analgesic.

Imreg-1. (Imreg) *Rx.*
Use: Immunomodulator.

Imreg-2. (Imreg)
Use: Immunomodulator.

Imuran. (GlaxoWellcome) **Tab.:** Azathioprine 50 mg/Tab. Bot. 100s, UD 100s. **Inj.:** Azathioprine 100 mg/20 ml. Vial. *Rx.*
Use: Immunosuppressant.

Imuthiol. (Connaught) Diethyldithiocarbamate. *Rx.*
Use: Immunomodulator.

Imuvert. (Cell Technology) Serratia marcescens extract (polyribosomes).
Use: Primary brain malignancies. [Orphan drug]

Inapsine. (Janssen) Droperidol 2.5 mg/ml. Amp. 2 ml, 5 ml, 10 ml. Box 10s. Multi-dose Vial w/methylparaben 1.8 mg, propylparaben 0.2 mg, lactic acid/10 ml. Box 10s. *Rx.*
Use: Anesthetic, general.
W/Fentanyl citrate.
See: Innovar, Inj. (Janssen).

•**indacrinone.** (IN-dah-KRIH-nohn) USAN.
Use: Antihypertensive, diuretic.

indalone.
See: Butopyronoxyl (Various Mfr.).

indandione derivative. *Rx.*
Use: Anticoagulant.
See: Anisindione (Various Mfr.).

•**indapamide,** (IN-DAP-uh-mide) U.S.P. 23.
Use: Antihypertensive, diuretic.
See: Lozol, Tab. (Rhone-Poulenc Rorer).

indapamide. (IN-DAP-uh-mide) (Various Mfr.) Indapamide 2.5 mg, lactose/Tab. Bot. 100s, 1000s. *Rx.*
Use: Antihypertensive, diuretic.

•**indecainide hydrochloride.** (in-deh-CANE-ide) USAN.
Use: Cardiovascular agent.
See: Decabid (Eli Lilly).

•**indeloxazine hydrochloride.** (in-DELL-OX-ah-zeen) USAN.
Use: Antidepressant.

Inderal Injection. (Wyeth Ayerst) Propranolol HCl 1 mg/ml. Amp. 1 ml. Box 10s. *Rx.*
Use: Beta-adrenergic blocker.

Inderal LA. (Wyeth Ayerst) Propranolol HCl 60 mg, 80 mg, 120 mg or 160 mg/SR Cap. Bot. 100s, 1000s, UD 100s. *Rx.*
Use: Beta-adrenergic blocker.

Inderal Tablets. (Wyeth Ayerst) Propranolol HCl 10 mg, 20 mg, 40 mg, 60 mg or 80 mg/Tab. Bot. 100s, 1000s, UD 100s. *Rx.*
Use: Beta-adrenergic blocker.

Inderide. (Wyeth Ayerst) Propranolol HCl 40 mg, hydrochlorothiazide 25 mg/Tab. Bot. 100s, 1000s, UD 100s. Propranolol HCl 80 mg, hydrochlorothiazide 25 mg/Tab. Bot. 100s. *Rx.*
Use: Antihypertensive combination.

Inderide LA Capsules. (Wyeth Ayerst) Propranolol HCl/hydrochlorothiazide Long Acting Caps: 80 mg/50 mg, 120 mg/50 mg or 160 mg/50 mg. Bot. 100s. *Rx.*
Use: Antihypertensive combination.

indian gum.
See: Karaya Gum.

indigo carmine. (Becton Dickinson) Sodium indigotindisulfonate 8 mg/ml. Amp. 5 ml. Box 10s, 100s.
Use: Diagnostic aid.
See: Sodium indigotindisulfonate.

indigo carmine solution. (Becton Dickinson) Indigotindisulfonate sodium inj. (0.8% aqueous soln. sodium salt of indigotindisulfonic acid) 40 mg/5 ml. Amp. 5 ml, 10s.
Use: Diagnostic aid.

•**indigotindisulfonate sodium,** (IN-dih-go-tin-die SULL-foe-nate) U.S.P. 23. Indigo Carmine.

Use: Diagnostic aid (cystoscopy).
See: Sodium Indigotindisulfonate.

•**indinavir.** USAN.
Use: Antiviral (HIV-protease inhibitor).

•**indinavir sulfate.** (in-DIN-ah-veer) USAN.
Use: Antiviral.
See: Crixivan, Cap. (Merck).

•**indium chlorides In 113m.** (IN-dee-uhm) USAN. U.S.P. XX.
Use: Radiopharmaceutical.

•**indium In 111 chloride solution,** U.S.P. 23.
Use: Radiopharmaceutical.

indium In 111 murine monoclonal antibody fab to myosin.
Use: Diagnostic aid in myocarditis. [Orphan drug]
See: Myoscint (Centocor).

•**indium In 111 oxyquinoline solution,** (IN-dee-uhm OX-ee-KWIN-oh-lin) U.S.P. 23.
Use: Radiopharmaceutical, diagnostic aid.

•**indium In 111 pentetate injection,** (IN-dee-uhm In 111 PEN-teh-tate) U.S.P. 23.
Use: Diagnostic aid (radionuclide cisternography), radiopharmaceutical.

•**indium In 111 pentetreotide,** (IN-dee-uhm In 111 pen-teh-TREE-oh-tide) U.S.P. 23.
Use: Diagnostic aid, radiopharmaceutical.

•**indium In 111 satumomab pendetide.** (IN-dee-uhm sat-YOU-mah-mab PEN-deh-TIDE) USAN.
Use: Radiodiagnostic monoclonal antibody (ovarian and colorectal carcinoma), radiopharmaceutical.

Indochron E-R. (Inwood) Indomethacin 75 mg. SR Cap. Bot. 60s, 100s. *Rx.*
Use: Analgesic, NSAID.

Indocin. (Merck) Indomethacin. **Cap.:** 25 mg. Bot. 100s, 1000s, UD 100s. Unit-of-use 100s; 50 mg. Bot. 100s, UD 100s. **Supp.:** 50 mg. Pkg. 30s. **Oral Susp.:** 25 mg/5 ml, alcohol 1%, sorbitol 0.1%. Bot. 237 ml. *Rx.*
Use: Analgesic, NSAID.

Indocin I.V. (Merck) Indomethacin sodium trihydrate equivalent to 1 mg indomethacin/Vial. Vial single dose. *Rx.*
Use: Arterial patency agent.

Indocin SR. (Merck) Indomethacin 75 mg/SR Cap. Unit-of-Use 30s, 60s.
Use: Analgesic, NSAID.

•**indocyanine green,** (in-doe-SIGH-ah-neen green) U.S.P. 23.
Use: Diagnostic aid (cardiac output determination, hepatic function determination).
See: Cardio-Green, Inj. (Beckton-Dickinson).

Indogesic. (Century Pharm) Acetaminophen 32.5 mg, butalbital 50 mg/Tab. Bot. 100s, 1000s. *Rx.*
Use: Analgesic, hypnotic, sedative.

Indoklon. Hexafluorodiethyl ether. Flurothyl. Bis-(2,2,2-trifluorethyl)ether. *Rx.*
Use: Shock inducing agent (convulsant).

•**indolapril hydrochloride.** (in-DAHL-ah-PRILL) USAN.
Use: Antihypertensive.

Indo-Lemmon. (Teva USA) Indomethacin 25 mg or 50 mg/Cap. Bot. 100s, 500s, 1000s. *Rx.*
Use: Analgesic, NSAID.

•**indolidan.** (in-DOE-lih-DAN) USAN.
Use: Cardiovascular agent.

Indometh Caps. (Major) Indomethacin 25 mg or 50 mg/Tab. **25 mg:** Bot. 100s, 1000s. **50 mg:** Bot. 100s, 500s. *Rx.*
Use: Analgesic, NSAID.

•**indomethacin,** (in-doe-METH-ah-sin) U.S.P. 23.
Use: Anti-inflammatory, analgesic.
See: Indochron E-R, Cap. (Inwood).
Indocin, Cap., S.R. Cap., I.V., Oral Susp., Supp. (Merck).
Indo-Lemmon, Cap. (Teva USA).

indomethacin. (Various Mfr.) **Cap.: 25 mg:** 60s, 100s, 500s, 1000s, UD 100s; **50 mg:** 23s, 72s, 100s, 250s, 500s, UD 100s; **SR Cap.:** 75 mg. Bot. 60s, 100s.
Use: Anti-inflammatory.

indomethacin. (Roxane) Indomethacin 25 mg/5ml. Oral susp. Bot. 500 ml. *Rx.*
Use: Analgesic, NSAID.

•**indomethacin sodium,** (in-doe-METH-ah-sin) U.S.P. 23.
Use: Anti-inflammatory, analgesic.

indomethacin sodium trihydrate. *Rx.*
Use: Arterial patency agent.
See: Indocin I.V., Pow. (Merck).

•**indoprofen.** (in-doe-PRO-fen) USAN.
Use: Analgesic, anti-inflammatory.

•**indoramin.** (in-DAHR-ah-min) USAN.
Use: Antihypertensive.

•**indoramin hydrochloride.** (in-DAHR-ah-min) USAN.
Use: Antihypertensive.

•**indorenate hydrochloride.** (in-DAHR-en-ATE) USAN.

Use: Antihypertensive.

•**indoxole.** (IN-dox-OLE) USAN.
Use: Antipyretic, anti-inflammatory.

•**indriline hydrochloride.** (IN-drih-leen) USAN.
Use: Stimulant (central).

I-Neocort. (American) Neomycin sulfate 5 mg, hydrocortisone acetate 15 mg/5 ml. Ophthalmic susp. Bot. 5 ml. *Rx.*
Use: Anti-infective, corticosteroid.

I-Neospor. (American) Polymixin B sulfate, gramicidin, neomycin sulfate ophthalmic soln. Bot. 10 ml. *Rx.*
Use: Anti-infective, ophthalmic.

Infalyte Oral Solution. (Bristol-Myers Squibb) Electrolyte mixture with 30 g/L rice syrup solids containing 4.2 calories/fl. oz. In 1 liter. *otc.*
Use: Nutritional supplement.

Infanrix. (SmithKline Beecham Pharmaceuticals) Diphtheria toxoid 25 Lf units, tetanus toxoid 10 Lf units, acellular pertussis vaccine (pertussis toxin 25 mcg, filamentous hemagglutinin 25 mcg, pertactin 8 mcg) and aluminum ≤ 0.625 mg/0.5 ml. With 2-phenoxyethanol 5 mg/ml. Vial 0.5 ml. *Rx.*
Use: Immunization.

infant foods.
Use: Nutritional supplement.
See: Enfamil (Bristol-Myers).
Enfamil Human Milk Fortifier (Bristol-Myers).
Enfamil Premature 20 Formula (Bristol-Myers).
RCF Liquid (Ross Laboratories).
Similac (Ross Laboratories).
Similac PM 60/40 Liquid (Ross Laboratories).

infant foods, hypoallergenic.
Use: Nutritional supplement.
See: Alimentation (Ross Laboratories).
Isomil (Ross Laboratories).
Isomil SF (Ross Laboratories).
I-Soyalac (Mt. Vernon Foods).
Nutramigen (Bristol-Myers).
Pregestimil Powder (Bristol-Myers).
ProSobee (Bristol-Myers).
Soyalac (Mt. Vernon Foods).

Infant's Feverall. (Upsher-Smith Labs) Acetaminophen 80 mg/Supp. 6s. *otc.*
Use: Analgesic.

Infants' No-Aspirin Drops. (Walgreens) Acetaminophen 80 mg/0.8 ml. Nonalcoholic. Bot. 15 ml. *otc.*
Use: Analgesic.

Infants' Silapap. (Silarx) Acetaminophen 80 mg/0.8 ml. Drops. Bot. 15 ml. Alcohol free. *otc.*
Use: Analgesic, antipyretic.

Infarub Cream. (Whitehall Robins) Methyl salicylate 35%, menthol 10% in vanishing cream base. Tube 1.25 oz, 3.5 oz. *otc.*
Use: Analgesic, topical.

Infasurf. (ONY) Surface active extract of saline lavage of bovine lungs.
Use: Prevent or treat respiratory failure due to pulmonary surfactant deficiency in preterm infants. [Orphan drug]

Infatuss. (Scott/Cord) Dextromethorphan HBr 7.2 mg, chlorpheniramine maleate 1.1 mg, phenylpropanolamine HCl 4.8 mg, ammonium Cl 50 mg/5 ml. Bot. 4 oz, pt, gal. *otc.*
Use: Antihistamine, antitussive, decongestant, expectorant.

Infectrol Ointment. (Bausch & Lomb) Dexamethasone 0.1%, neomycin sulfate equivalent to 0.35% neomycin base and 10,000 units polymyxin B sulfate/g. White petrolatum, lanolin, mineral oil, parabens. Oint. Tube 3.5, 3.75 g. *Rx.*
Use: Anti-infective, corticosteroid, topical.

Infectrol Suspension. (Bausch & Lomb) Dexamethasone 0.1%, neomycin sulfate equivalent to 0.35% neomycin base and 10,000 units polymyxin B sulfate/ml. Hydroxypropyl methylcellulose, polysorbate 20, benzalkonium chloride. Drop. Bot. 5 ml. *Rx.*
Use: Anti-infective, corticosteroid, ophthalmic.

InFeD. (Schein Pharmaceutical) Iron 50/ml (as dextran), sodium chloride 0.9%. Inj. Vial 2 ml. *Rx.*
Use: Mineral supplement.

Infergen. (Amgen) Interferon alfacon-1 9 mcg, 15 mcg, preservative free. Single-dose Vial 0.3 ml. Pack 6s. *Rx.*
Use: Antiviral.

Inflamase Forte. (Ciba Vision Ophthalmics) Prednisolone sodium phosphate 1%. Bot. 5 ml, 10 ml, 15 ml. *Rx.*
Use: Corticoisteroid, ophthalmic.

Inflamase Mild. (Ciba Vision Ophthalmics) Prednisolone sodium phosphate 0.125%. Bot. 3 ml, 5 ml, 10 ml. *Rx.*
Use: Corticosteroid, ophthalmic.

•**influenza virus vaccine,** (in-flew-EN-zuh) U.S.P. 23.
Use: Immunization.
See: Flu-Shield, Inj. (Wyeth Ayerst).
Fluvirin, Inj. (Evans Medical).
Fluzone, Inj. (Connaught).

InfraRUB. (Whitehall Robins) Methyl

salicylate 35%, menthol 10%. Cream. Jar 37.5, 90 g. *otc.*
Use: Analgesic, topical.

Infumorph 200. (ESI Lederle Generics) Morphine sulfate 10 mg/ml/Inj. Ampuls 20 ml. Preservative free. *c-II.*
Use: Analgesic, narcotic.

Infumorph 500. (ESI Lederle Generics) Morphine sulfate 25 mg/ml/Inj. Ampuls 20 ml. Preservative free. *c-II.*
Use: Analgesic, narcotic.

Ingadine Tabs. (Major) Guanethidine sulfate 10 mg or 25 mg/Tab. Bot. 100s, 1000s. *Rx.*
Use: Antihypertensive.

INH. (Novartis) Isoniazid 300 mg/Tab. *Rx.*
Use: Antituberculous.
See: Rimactane/INH, Dual Pack (Novartis).

Inhal-Aid. (Key Pharm)
Use: Respiratory drug delivery system.

Inhibace. (Roche/Glaxo Wellcome) Cilazapril. *Rx.*
Use: Antihypertensive.

Innerclean Herbal Laxative. (Last) Senna leaf powder, psyllium seed, buckthorne, anise seed, fennel seed. Bot. 1 oz, 2 oz. *otc.*
Use: Laxative.

Innertabs. (Last) Senna leaf powder and psyllium seed tablets. Bot. 80s, 200s. *otc.*
Use: Laxative.

InnoGel Plus. (Hogil Pharm) Pyrethrins 0.3%, piperonyl butoxide technical 3%. Gel. Kits contain 3 pre-dosed gel paks and a comb. *otc.*
Use: Pediculicide.

Innovar Injection. (Janssen) Fentanyl citrate 0.05 mg, droperidol 2.5 mg/ml. Amp. 2 ml, 5 ml. Box of 10s. *c-II.*
Use: Analgesic, narcotic; anesthetic, general.

Inocor Lactate. (Sanofi Winthrop) Amrinone lactate (base equivalent) 5 mg/ml, sodium metabisulfite 0.25 mg/Inj. Amp. 20 ml. Box 5s. *Rx.*
Use: Inotropic.

•**inocoterone acetate.** (ih-NO-koe-ter-ohn) USAN.
Use: Dermatologic, acne.

in-111 murine mab. (2B8-MX-DTPA).
Use: B-cell non-Hodgkin's lymphoma. [Orphan drug]

inophylline.
See: Aminophylline (Various Mfr.).

inosine pranobex. Isoprinosine.
Use: Antiviral. [Orphan drug]
See: Isoprinosine (Newport).

Inosiplex. (Newport Pharmaceuticals) Isoprinosine. *Rx.*
Use: Antiviral.

inosit.
See: Inositol (Various Mfr.).

inositol. 1,2,3,5/4,6-Cyclohexanehexol. Commercial solvents (Bios 1,Hexahydroxycyclohexane, Inosit, Dambose).
Use: Lipotropic.
W/Choline bitartrate, vitamins, minerals.
W/Methionine, choline bitartrate, liver desiccated, vitamin B_{12}.
See: Limvic, Tab. (Briar).
W/Panthenol, choline Cl, vitamins, minerals, estrone, testosterone.
See: Geramine, Inj. (ICN Pharmaceuticals).
W/Panthenol, choline Cl, vitamins, minerals, estrone, testosterone, polydigestase.
See: Geramine, Tab. (ICN Pharmaceuticals).

•**inositol niacinate.** (in-OH-sih-tole NIE-ah-sin-ate) USAN. Myo-Inositol hexanicotinate. Meso-inositol hexanicotinate, hexanicotinate. Meso-inositol hexanicotinate. Hexopal; Mesonex.
Use: Vasodilator.

inositol nicotinate.
See: Inositol Niacinate.

Inotropin. (Faulding USA) Dopamine 40 mg/ml, sodium metabisulfite 1%/Inj. In 5 ml. *Rx.*
Use: Vasoconstrictor.

Inspirease. (Key Pharm). *Rx.*
Use: Respiratory drug delivery system.

Insta-Char. (Kerr) **Regular:** Aqueous suspension activated charcoal 50 g/8 oz. **Pediatric:** Aqueous suspension activated charcoal 15 g/4 oz. *otc.*
Use: Antidote.

Insta-Glucose. (ICN Pharmaceuticals) Undiluted USP glucose. UD tube containing liquid glucose 31 g. *otc.*
Use: Hyperglycemic.

Inst-E-Vite. (Barth's) Vitamin E 100 IU or 200 IU/Cap. **100 IU:** Bot 100s, 500s, 1000s. **200 IU:** Bot. 100s, 250s, 500s. *otc.*
Use: Vitamin supplement.

Insulatard NPH Human. (Nordisk-USA) Human insulin isophane suspension 100 IU/ml. *otc.*
Use: Antidiabetic.

•**insulin,** (IN-suh-lin) U.S.P. 23.
Use: Antidiabetic.
See: Humulin Prods. (Eli Lilly).
Iletin Prods. (Eli Lilly).
Insulin Prods. (Bristol-Myers Squibb).

Novolin Prod. (Novo Nordisk).
Velosulin Human BR, Inj. (Novo Nordisk).

insulin. (IN-suh-lin) (Nordisk) Insulatard NPH Mixtard Velosulin. *otc.*
Use: Antidiabetic.

•**insulin, dalanated.** USAN.
Use: Antidiabetic.

•**insulin human,** (IN-suh-lin) U.S.P. 23.
Use: Antidiabetic.
See: Humulin (Eli Lilly).

•**insulin human, isophane, suspension,** U.S.P. 23.
Use: Antidiabetic.

•**insulin human zinc suspension,** (IN-suh-lin) U.S.P. 23.
Use: Antidiabetic.

•**insulin human zinc, extended, suspension,** (IN-suh-lin) U.S.P. 23.
Use: Antidiabetic.

•**insulin, isophane, suspension,** U.S.P. 23.
Use: Antidiabetic.
See: NPH (Novo Nordisk).

•**insulin I-125.** (IN-suh-lin) USAN.
Use: Radiopharmaceutical.

•**insulin I-131.** (IN-suh-lin) USAN.
Use: Radiopharmaceutical.

insulin-like growth factor-1.
Use: Amyotrophic lateral sclerosis. [Orphan drug]
See: Myotrophin (Cephalon).

•**insulin lispro.** (IN-suh-lin LICE-pro) USAN.
Use: Antidiabetic.
See: Humalog, Tab. (Bayer Corp).

•**insulin, neutral.** (IN-suh-lin) USAN.
Use: Antidiabetic.

insulin novo rapitard. Biphasic Insulin.

insulin, protamine zinc suspension, (IN-suh-lin PRO-tah-meen zingk) U.S.P. XXII. 40 or 100 units/ml. Vials 10 ml.
Use: Antidiabetic.

insulin, regular.
Use: Antidiabetic.
See: Regular Iletin I (Beef and Pork), Inj. (Eli Lilly).
Regular Insulin (Pork), Inj. (Novo Nordisk).
Pork Regular Iletin II (Pork), Inj. (Eli Lilly).
Regular Purified Pork Insulin, Inj. (Novo Nordisk).
Velosulin (Pork), Inj. (Novo Nordisk).
Humulin R, Inj. (Eli Lilly).
Humulin BR, Inj. (Eli Lilly).
Novolin R, Inj. (Novo Nordisk).
Velosulin, Inj. (Novo Nordisk).
Novolin R PenFill, Cartridges (Novo Nordisk).

insulin, regular concentrate.
Use: Antidiabetic.
See: Semilente Iletin I (Beef or Pork), Inj. (Eli Lilly).
Semilente Insulin (Beef), Inj. (Novo Nordisk).

insulin suspension, isophane.
Use: Antidiabetic.
See: Humulin 50/50, Inj. (Eli Lilly).
Humulin 70/30, Inj. (Eli Lilly).
Mixtard, Inj. (Novo Nordisk).
Novolin 70/30, Inj. (Novo Nordisk).
Novolin 70/30 PenFill, Cartridge (Novo Nordisk).

insulin suspension, lente.
Use: Antidiabetic.
See: Lente Insulin, Cial (Novo Nordisk).
Lente L, Vial (Novo Nordisk).
Novolin L, Vial (Novo Nordisk).
Lente Iletin I (Beef and Pork), Inj. (Eli Lilly).
Lente Insulin (Beef), Inj. (Novo Nordisk).
Lente Iletin II (Pork), Inj. (Eli Lilly).
Lente Iletin II (Beef), Inj. (Eli Lilly).
Lente Purified Pork Insulin, Inj. (Novo Nordisk).
Humulin L, Inj. (Eli Lilly).
Novolin L, Inj. (Novo Nordisk).

insulin suspension, NPH.
Use: Antidiabetic.
See: NPH Iletin I (Beef and Pork), Inj. (Eli Lilly).
NPH Insulin (Beef), Inj. (Novo Nordisk).
Beef NPH Iletin II, Inj. (Eli Lilly).
NPH-N Purified (Pork), Inj. (Novo Nordisk).
Pork NPH Iletin II, Inj. (Eli Lilly).
Insulatard NPH (Pork), Inj. (Novo Nordisk).
Humulin N, Inj. (Eli Lilly).
Insulatard NPH, Inj. (Novo Nordisk).
Novolin N, Inj. (Novo Nordisk).
Novolin N PenFill, Cartridge (Novo Nordisk).

insulin suspension, PZI. *otc.*
Use: Antiadiabetic.
See: Humulin U Ultralente, Inj. (Eli Lilly).

insulin suspension semilente. *otc.*
Use: Antidiabetic.
See: Semilente Iletin I (Beef or Pork), Inj. (Eli Lilly).
Semilente Insulin (Beef), Inj. (Novo Nordisk).

insulin suspension, ultralente. *otc.*
Use: Antidiabetic.
See: Ultralente Insulin (Beef), Inj. (Novo Nordisk).

Humulin U Ultralente, Inj. (Eli Lilly).

•**insulin zinc suspension,** (IN-suh-lin) U.S.P. 23.
Use: Antidiabetic.
See: Humulin L, Bot. (Eli Lilly).
Lente Insulin, Vial (Eli Lilly).
Lente Insulin, Vial (Novo Nordisk).
Lente L, Vial (Novo Nordisk).
Novolin L, Vial (Novo Nordisk).

•**insulin zinc, suspension, extended,** (IN-suh-lin) U.S.P. 23.
Use: Antidiabetic.
See: Humulin U Ultralente, Bot. (Eli Lilly).
Ultralente U, Vial (Novo Nordisk).

•**insulin zinc, prompt, suspension,** (IN-suh-lin) U.S.P. 23.
Use: Antidiabetic.

Intal Inhaler. (Fisons) Cromolyn sodium inhalation aerosol 800 mcg/actuation. Canister 8.1 g, 14.2 g. *Rx.*
Use: Respiratory.

Intal Nebulizer Solution. (Fisons) Cromolyn sodium 20 mg in 2 ml distilled water for use with a power operated nebulizer unit. Box 60s, 120s, Amp. 2 ml. *Rx.*
Use: Respiratory.

Integrilin. (Cor Therapeutics) Eptifibatide 2 mg/ml, sodium hydroxide. Vial 10 ml. *Rx.*
Use: Acute coronary syndrome treatment.

Integrin Caps. (Sanofi Winthrop) Oxypertine. *Rx.*
Use: Anxiolytic.

Intensol. (Roxane) A system of concentrated solutions of drugs w/calibrated dropper:
Chlorpromazine HCl 30 mg or 100 mg/ml.
Dexamethasone 1 mg/ml.
Dihydrotachysterol 0.2 mg/ml.
Hydrochlorothiazide 100 mg/ml.
Prednisone 5 mg/ml.
Thioridazine HCl 30 mg or 100 mg/ml.

interferon. (IN-ter-FEER-ahn) A family of naturally occurring, small protein molecules with molecular weights of approximately 15,000 to 21,000 daltons. They are formed by the interaction of animal cells with viruses capable of conferring on animal cells resistance to virus infection. Three major classes of interferons have been identified: alpha, beta, and gamma. Interferon was first derived from human white blood cells and originally used in Finland.
Use: Antineoplastic, antiviral. Treatment of breast cancer lymphoma, multiple melanoma and malignant melanoma.
See: Actimmune (Genentech).
Alferon-N (Purdue Frederick).
Avonex (Biogen).
Betaseron (Berlex).
Intron-A, Inj. (Schering Plough).
Roferon-A (Roche Laboratories).

interferon alfacon-1.
See: Infergen (Amgen).

•**interferon alfa-2a.** (IN-ter-FEER-ahn AL-fuh-2a) USAN.
Use: Antineoplastic, antiviral; biological response modifier. [Orphan drug]
See: Roferon-A (Roche Laboratories).

•**interferon alfa-2b.** (IN-ter-FEER-ahn AL-fuh-2b) USAN.
Use: Antineoplastic, antiviral; biological response modifier. [Orphan drug]
See: Intron-A (Schering Plough).

•**interferon alfa-n1.** (IN-ter-FEER-ahn AL-fuh-nl) USAN.
Use: Antineoplastic, antiviral, biological response modifier. [Orphan drug]
See: Wellferon (GlaxoWellcome).

interferon, beta. (IN-ter-FEER-ahn BAY-tuh) *Rx.*
Use: Immunomodulator, treatment of multiple sclerosis.
See: Avonex (Biogen).
Betaseron (Berlex).

•**interferon beta-1a.** (in-ter-FEER-ohn BAY-tah-1a) USAN
Use: Antineoplastic, biological response modifier, immunomodulator, antineoblast. [Orphan drug]
See: Avonex (Berlex).

•**interferon beta-1b.** (IN-ter-FEER-ahn BAY-tah-1b) USAN.
Use: Immunomodulator.
See: Betaseron (Berlex).

interferon beta (recombinant).
Use: Immune therapy.
See: Antril (Amgen). [Orphan drug]
See: Avonex (Biogen).
Rebif (Biogen).
r-IFN-beta (Serono).

•**interferon gamma-1b.** (IN-ter-FEER-ahn GAM-uh-1b). USAN.
Use: Antineoplastic, antiviral, immunoregulator, biological response modifier. [Orphan drug]
See: Actimmune (Genentech).

interleukin-1 receptor antagonist, human recombinant.
Use: Juvenile rheumatoid arthritis, graft-v-host disease in transplant patients. [Orphan drug]
See: Antril (Amgen).

interleukin-2.
Use: Immunomodulator, antineoplastic. [Orphan drug]
See: Proleukin (Chiron).
Teceleukin (Hoffman-LaRoche).

interleukin-2, recombinant liposome encapsulated.
Use: Antineoplastic. [Orphan drug]

interleukin-2 PEG. (Cetus). *Rx.*
Use: Immunomodulator.

interleukin-3, recombinant human. (Novartis).
Use: Immunomodulator. [Orphan drug]

interleukin-11.
See: Opelvekrin, Neumega (Genetics Institute).

Intralipid 10% I.V. Fat Emulsion. (Pharmacia & Upjohn) IV fat emulsion containing soybean oil 10%, egg yolk phospholipids 1.2%, glycerin 2.25% and water for injection. I.V. Flask 50 ml, 100 ml, 250 ml, 500 ml. *Rx.*
Use: Nutritional supplement, parenteral.

Intralipid 20% I.V. Fat Emulsion. (Pharmacia & Upjohn) IV fat emulsion containing soybean oil 20%, egg yolk phospholipids 1.2%, glycerin 2.25% and water for injection. I.V. Flask 50 ml, 100 ml, 250 ml, 500 ml. *Rx.*
Use: Nutritional supplement, parenteral.

intranasal steroids.
See: Beconase AQ Nasal (Allen & Hanburys).
Beconase Inhalation (Allen & Hanburys).
Decadron Phosphate Turbinaire (Merck).
Flonase (Allen & Hanburys).
Nasalide (Syntex).
Nasacort (Rhone-Poulenc Rorer).
Vancenase Nasal Inhaler (Schering Plough).
Rhinocort (Astra).
Vancenase AQ Nasal (Schering Plough).

IntraSite. (Smith & Nephew United) Graft T starch copolymer 2%, water 8%, propylene glycol 20%. Sterile amorphous interactive hydrogel dressing. 25 g. *Rx.*
Use: Dermatologic, wound therapy.

intrauterine progesterone system. *Rx.*
Use: Contraceptive.
See: Progestasert (Alza).

intraval sodium.
See: Pentothal Sodium, Preps. (Abbott Laboratories).

•**intrazole.** (IN-trah-zole) USAN. 1-(p-Chlorobenzoyl)-3-(1H-tetrazol-5-ylmethyl) indole.
Use: Anti-inflammatory.

•**intriptyline hydrochloride.** (in-TRIP-tih-leen) USAN.
Use: Antidepressant.

Introlite. (Ross Laboratories) Protein 22.2 g, carbohydrate 70.5 g, fat 18.4 g, sodium 930 mg, potassium 1570 mg/L with 200 mOsm/kg water, with appropriate vitamins and minerals, 0.53 Cal/ml. Liq. *otc.*
Use: Nutritional supplement.

Intron A for Injection. (Schering Plough) Interferon alfa-2b (recombinant). **Pow. for Inj.:** 3 million/1 ml vial diluent; 5 million IU/1 ml vial diluent or syringe; 10 million IU/2 ml vial diluent, 10 million IU/1 ml syringe diluent; 18 million IU/3.8 ml vial diluent/Multidose vial; 25 million IU/5 ml vial diluent/Multidose vial; 50 million IU/1 ml vial diluent/Multidose vial. **Soln:** 3 million IU/0.5 ml Vial, Pack-3 (6 vials, 6 syringes); 5 million IU/0.5 ml Vial, Pak-5 (6 vials, 6 syringes); 10 million IU/1 ml Vial, Pak-10 (6 vials, 6 syringes); 18 million IU/Multi-dose Vial (22.8 million IU/3.8 ml); 25 million IU/Multidose Vial (32 million IU/3.2 ml). *Rx.*
Use: Antineoplastic.

Intropaque Liquid. (Lafayette Pharm) Barium sulfate 60% w/v suspension. Bot. gal. Case 4 Bot.
Use: Radiopaque agent.

Intropin 200 mg. (DuPont Merck Pharmaceuticals) Dopamine HCl 40 mg/ml, sodium bisulfite 1% as an antioxidant. Vial 5 ml. Box 20s; Amp. 5 ml. Box 20s; Prefilled additive Syr. 5 ml. Box 5s. *Rx.*
Use: Vasoconstrictor.

Intropin 400 mg. (DuPont Merck Pharmaceuticals) Dopamine HCl 80 mg/ml, sodium bisulfite 1% as an antioxidant. Vial 5 ml. Box 20s.; Prefilled additive Syringe 5 ml. Box 5s. *Rx.*
Use: Vasoconstrictor.

Intropin 800 mg. (DuPont Merck Pharmaceuticals) Dopamine HCl 160 mg/ml, sodium bisulfite 1% as an antioxidant. Vial 5 ml. Box 20s.; Prefilled additive syringe 5 ml. Box 5s. *Rx.*
Use: Vasoconstrictor.

inulin. (DuPont Merck Pharmaceuticals) Purified inulin 5 g/50 ml sodium Cl 0.9%, sodium hydroxide to adjust pH. Amp. 50 ml.
Use: Diagnostic aid.

•**inulin,** (IN-you-lin) U.S.P. 23.
Use: Diagnostic aid (renal function determination).

invert sugar. (Abbott Laboratories) 10% soln. Bot. 1000 ml. *otc, Rx.*
Use: Nutritional supplement, parenteral.
See: Travert, Soln. (Baxter).

invert sugar-electrolyte solutions. *Rx.*
Use: Nutritional supplement, parenteral.
See: Ionosol G and 10% Invert Sugar (Abbott Laboratories).
Multiple Electrolyte 2 w/5% Invert Sugar (McGaw).
5% Travert and Electrolyte No. 2 (Baxter).
Ionosol B and 10% Invert Sugar (Abbott Laboratories).
10% Travert and Electrolyte No. 2 (Baxter).
Multiple Electrolyte 2 w/10% Invert Sugar (McGaw).
Ionosol D and 10% Invert Sugar (Abbott Laboratories).

invert sugar injection.
Use: Fluid, nutrient replacement.

Invirase. (Roche Laboratories) Saquinavir mesylate 200 mg, lactose/Cap. 270s. *Rx.*
Use: Antiviral.

•**iobenguane I 123 injection,** (EYE-oh-BEN-gwane) U.S.P. 23.
Use: Radiopharmaceutical.

•**iobenguane I 131.** (EYE-oh-BEN-gwane) USAN.
Use: Diagnostic aid, radiopharmaceutical.

•**iobenguane sulfate I 123.** (EYE-oh-BEN-gwane) USAN.
Use: Diagnostic aid, radioactive, adrenomedullary disorders and neuroendocrine tumors); radiopharmaceutical.

•**iobenguane sulfate I 131.** (EYE-oh-BEN-gwane) USAN.
Use: Diagnostic aid, radiopharmaceutical.

•**iobenzamic acid.** (EYE-oh-ben-ZAM-ik) USAN.
Use: Diagnostic aid (radiopaque medium, cholecystographic).

Iobid DM. (Iomed Labs) Dextromethorphan HBr 30 mg, guaifenesin 600 mg/SR Tab. Bot. 100s, 500s. *Rx.*
Use: Antitussive, expectorant.

•**iocanlidic acid I 123.** (eye-oh-kan-LIH-dik) USAN.
Use: Diagnostic aid (radioactive, cardiac disease) for assessment of viable myocardium.

Iocare Balanced Salt Solution. (Ciba Vision Ophthalmics) Sodium Cl 0.64%, potassium Cl 0.075%, magnesium Cl 0.03%, calcium Cl 0.048%, sodium acetate 0.39%, sodium citrate 0.17%, sodium hydroxide or hydrochloric acid. Soln. Bot. 15 ml. *Rx.*
Use: Irrigant, ophthalmic.

•**iocarmate meglumine.** (EYE-oh-CAR-mate meh-GLUE-meen) USAN.
Use: Diagnostic aid (radiopaque medium).

•**iocarmic acid.** (EYE-oh-CAR-mik) USAN.
Use: Diagnostic aid (radiopaque medium).

•**iocetamic acid,** (eye-oh-seh-TAM-ik) U.S.P. 23.
Use: Diagnostic aid (radiopaque medium).

i-octadecanol.
See: Stearyl Alcohol, N.F. 18.

Iodal HD. (Iomed Labs) Hydrocodone bitartrate 1.67 mg, phenylephrine HCl 2 mg, chlorpheniramine maleate 2 mg/5 ml. Liq. Bot. 473 ml. *c-III.*
Use: Antihistamine, antitussive, decongestant.

•**iodamide.** (EYE-oh-dah-mide) USAN.
Use: Diagnostic aid (radiopaque medium).

•**iodamide meglumine.** (EYE-oh-dah-MIDE meh-GLUE-meen) USAN.
Use: Diagnostic aid (radiopaque medium).
W/Combinations:
See: Renovue-65, Vial (Bristol-Myers Squibb).
Renovue-Dip, Vial (Bristol-Myers Squibb).

Iodex. (KM Lee) Iodine 4.7% in petrolatum ointment base. Jar 1 oz, 14 oz. *otc.*
Use: Antimicrobial, antiseptic.

Iodex w/Methyl Salicylate. (KM Lee) Iodine 4.7%, methyl salicylate 4.8% in petrolatum ointment base. *otc.*
Use: Antiseptic, analgesic, topical.

iodinated I-125 albumin injection.
Use: Diagnostic aid (blood volume determination), radiopharmaceutical.
See: albumin, iodinated I 125.

iodinated I-131 albumin aggregated injection.
Use: Radiopharmaceutical.
See: albumin, aggregated iodinated I 131 serum.

iodinated I-131 albumin injection.
Use: Diagnostic aid (blood volume determination and intrathecal imaging), radiopharmaceutical.
See: albumin, iodinated I-131.

iodinated glycerol and codeine phosphate liquid. (Various Mfr.) Codeine phosphate 10 mg, iodinated glycerol 30 mg/Liq. Bot. pt and gal. *c-v.*
Use: Antitussive, expectorant, narcotic.

iodinated glycerol/theophylline.
See: Iophylline (Various Mfr.).

iodinated human serum albumin.
See: Albumotope (Bristol-Myers Squibb).

•**iodine,** (EYE-uh-dine) U.S.P. 23.
Use: Anti-infective, topical; source of iodine.
See: Kelp, Tab. (Quality Formulations).

iodine cacodylate, colloidal. Cacodyne Iodine.

iodine 131: capsules diagnostic - capsules therapeutic - solution therapeutic oral.
See: Iodotope (Bristol-Myers Squibb).

iodine combination.
See: Calcidrine, Syr. (Abbott Laboratories).

iodine I^{123} murine monoclonal antibody to alpha-fetoprotein. (Immunomedics)
Use: Diagnostic aid. [Orphan drug]

iodine I^{123} murine monoclonal antibody to hCG. (Immunomedics)
Use: Diagnostic aid. [Orphan drug]

iodine I^{131} 6b-iodomethyl-19-norcholesterol.
Use: Diagnostic aid. [Orphan drug]

iodine I^{131} metaiodobenzylguanidine sulfate.
Use: Diagnostic aid. [Orphan drug]

iodine I^{131} murine monoclonal antibody to alpha-fetoprotein. (Immunomedics)
Use: Antineoplastic. [Orphan drug]

iodine I^{131} murine monoclonal antibody to hCG. (Immunomedics)
Use: Antineoplastic. [Orphan drug]

iodine I^{131} murine monoclonal antibody IgG2a to B cell.
Use: Antineoplastic. [Orphan drug]
See: Immurait (Immunomedics).

iodine-iodophor.
See: Betadine, Preps. (Purdue Frederick).
Isodine, Preps. (Blair Laboratories).

iodine povidone.
See: Efodine, Oint. (E. Fougera).
Iodophor.
Mallsol, Liq. (Roberts Pharm).

iodine products, anti-infective.
See: Anayodin.
Betadine, Preps. (Purdue Frederick).
Chiniofon.
Diodoquin, Tab. (Searle).
Diiodo-Hydroxyquinoline (Various Mfr.).
Isodine, Preps. (Blair Laboratories).
Prepodyne, Soln., Scrub (West).
Quinoxyl.
Surgidine, Liq. (Continental Consumer Products).
Vioform, Preps. (Novartis).

iodine products, diagnostic.
See: Chloriodized Oil (Various Mfr.).
Ethyl Iodophenylundecylate (Various Mfr.).
Iodized Oil.
Iodoalphionic Acid (Various Mfr.).
Iodobrassid.
Iodohippurate Sodium (Various Mfr.).
Iodopanoic Acid (Various Mfr.).
Iodophthalein Sodium (Various Mfr.).
Iodopyracet, Preps. (Various Mfr.).
Lipiodol Lafay, Amp., Vial (Savage).
Optiray 350, Inj. (Mallinckrodt Medical).
Methiodal Sodium (Various Mfr.).
Pantopaque, Amp. (Lafayette Pharm).
Sodium Acetrizoate (Various Mfr.).
Sodium Iodomethamate (Various Mfr.).
Telepaque, Tab. (Sanofi Winthrop).

iodine products, nutritional.
See: Calcium Iodobehenate (Various Mfr.).
Entodon.
Hydriodic Acid (Various Mfr.).
Iodobrassid (Various Mfr.).
Potassium Iodide (Various Mfr.).

iodine ration, (Barth's) Iodine (from kelp) 0.15 mg, trace minerals/Tab. Bot. 90s, 180s, 360s. *otc.*
Use: Mineral supplement.

iodine ration. (Nion) Iodine (from kelp) 0.15 mg/3 Tab. Bot. 175s, 500s. *otc.*
Use: Mineral supplement.

iodide, sodium, I-123 capsules. (EYE-uh-dine SO-dee-uhm)
Use: Diagnostic aid (thyroid function determination).

iodide, sodium, I-123 tablets.
Use: Diagnostic aid (thyroid function determination).

iodide, sodium, I-125 capsules.
Use: Diagnostic aid (thyroid function determination), radiopharmaceutical.

iodide, sodium, I-125 solution.
Use: Diagnostic aid (thyroid function determination), radiopharmaceutical.

iodide, sodium, I-131 capsules.
Use: Antineoplastic, diagnostic aid (thyroid function determination), radiopharmaceutical.

See: Iodotope, Cap. (Bracco Diagnostics).

iodide, sodium, I-131 solution.
Use: Antineoplastic, diagnostic aid (thyroid function determination), radiopharmaceutical.
See: Iodotope, Oral Soln. (Bracco Diagnostics).

iodine soluble.
See: Burnham Soluble Iodine, Soln. (Burnham).

iodine surface active complex.
See: Ioprep, Soln. (Arbrook).

iodine tincture, strong.
Use: Anti-infective, topical.

•**iodipamide,** (eye-oh-DIH-pa-mide) U.S.P. 23.
Use: Pharmaceutic necessity for Iodipamide Meglumine Injection.

•**iodipamide meglumine injection,** U.S.P. 23.
Use: Diagnostic aid (radiopaque medium).

iodipamide methylglucamine. Also sodium salt inj.
W/Diatrizoate methylglucamine.
See: Sinografin, Vial (Bristol-Myers Squibb).

•**iodipamide sodium I 131.** USAN.
Use: Radiopharmaceutical.

iodipamide sodium injection.
See: Cholografin Sodium, Soln. (Various Mfr.).

•**iodixanol.** (EYE-oh-DIX-an-ole) USAN
Use: Diagnostic aid (radiopaque medium).
See: Visipaque, Inj. (Nycomed).

iodized oil. A vegetable oil containing not less than 38% and not more than 42% of organically combined iodine.
Use: Diagnostic aid.
See: Lipiodol Lafay, Amp., Vial (Savage).

iodized poppy-seed oil.
See: Lipiodol Lafay, Amp., Vial (Savage).

iodoalphionic acid. Biliselectan dikol, pheniodol.

•**iodoantipyrine I 131.** USAN.
Use: Radiopharmaceutical.

iodobehenate calcium. Calcium iododocosanoate.
Use: Antigoitrogenic.

iodobrassid. Ethyl Diiodobrassidate. Lipoiodine.

•**iodocetylic acid I 123.** (eye-OH-doe-SEE-till-ik) USAN.
Use: Diagnostic aid, radiopharmaceutical.

•**iodocholesterol I 131.** (EYE-oh-DOE-koe-LESS-teh-role) USAN.
Use: Radiopharmaceutical.

iodochlorhydroxyquin. Clioquinol, U.S.P. 23.

Iodo Cream. (Day-Baldwin) Clioquinol 3%. Tube 1 oz, Jar 1 lb. *otc.*
Use: Antifungal, topical.

Iodo H-C. (Day-Baldwin) Clioquinol 3%, hydrocortisone 1%. **Oint.:** Tube 20 g, Jar 1 lb. **Cream:** Tube 20 g, Jar 1 lb. *Rx.*
Use: Antifungal, corticosteroid.

•**iodohippurate sodium I 123 injection,** (EYE-oh-doe-HIP-you-rate) U.S.P. 23.
Use: Radiopharmaceutical, diagnostic aid (renal function determination).

•**iodohippurate sodium I 125.** (EYE-oh-doe HIP-you-rate) USAN.
Use: Radiopharmaceutical.
See: Hipputope I 125 (Bristol-Myers Squibb).

•**iodohippurate, sodium I 131 injection,** (EYE-oh-doe-HIP-you-rate) U.S.P. 23.
Use: Diagnostic aid (renal function determination), radiopharmaceutical.
See: Hipputope (Bristol-Myers Squibb).

iodo-hippuric acid.
See: Hipputope (Bristol-Myers Squibb).

iodol. 2,3,4,5-Tetraiodopyrrole.

Iodo Ointment. (Day-Baldwin) Clioquinol 3%. Tube oz, Jar lb. *Rx.*
Use: Antifungal, topical.

Iodo-Pak. (SoloPak) Iodine 100 mcg/ml. Inj. Vial 10 ml. *Rx.*
Use: Nutritional supplement, parenteral.

iodopanoic acid.
Use: Diagnostic aid (radiopaque medium).

Iodopen. (Fujisawa) Sodium iodide 118 mcg/ml. Vial 3 ml, 10 ml. *Rx.*
Use: Nutritional supplement, parenteral.

iodophene. Iodophthalein.

iodophene sodium.
See: Iodophthalein Sodium (Various Mfr.).

iodophor.
See: Betadine, Preps. (Purdue Frederick).
Isodine, Preps. (Blair Laboratories).

iodophthalein sodium. Tetraiodophenolphthalein Sodium, Tetraiodophthalein Sodium, Tetiothalein Sodium (Antinosin, Cholepulvis, Cholumbrin, Foriod, Iodophene, Iodorayoral, Nosophene Sodium, Opacin, Photobiline, Piliophen, Radiotetrane).
Use: Radiopaque agent.

iodopropylidene glycerol.
See: Organidin, Elix., Tab., Soln. (Wampole Laboratories).

•**iodopyracet I 125.** USAN.
Use: Radiopharmaceutical.

•**iodopyracet I 131.** USAN.
Use: Radiopharmaceutical.
See: Diodrast (R)-131.

iodopyracet inj. (Diatrast, Diodone, Iopyracil, Neo-Methiodal, NeoSkiodan).
Use: Radiopaque medium.

iodopyracet compound. Diodrast.

iodopyracet concentrated. Diodrast.

iodopyrine. Antipyrine iodide.
Use: Iodides, analgesic.

•**iodoquinol,** (EYE-oh-doe-KWIH-nole) U.S.P. 23. *Formerly Diiodohydroxyquin.*
Use: Antiamebic.
See: Floraquin (Searle).
Sebaquin, Shampoo (Summers Labs).
W/9-Aminoacridine HCl.
See: Vagitric, Cream (ICN Pharmaceuticals).
Yodoxin, Tab., Pow. (Glenwood).
W/Hydrocortisone alcohol.
See: Vytone, Cream (Dermik Laboratories).
W/Hydrocortisone, coal tar solution.
See: Cor-Tar-Quin, Cream, Lot. (Bayer Corp).
W/Stilbestrol, sulfadiazine, tartaric acid, boric acid, etc.
See: Gynben, Vag. Insert, Cream (I. C. N).
Gynben Insufflate, Pow. (I. C. N).
W/Surfactants.
See: Lycinate, Supp. (Hoechst Marion Roussel).
W/Sulfanilamide, diethylstilbestrol.
See: Amide V/S, Vaginal Insert. (Scrip).
D.I.T.I. Creme (Dunhall Pharmaceuticals).

Iodotope (Diagnostic). (Bristol-Myers Squibb) Sodium iodide I-131 for oral use. 7, 14, 28, 70, 106 units Ci/Vial of 5, 10, 15, 20 Cap.
Use: Diagnostic aid.

Iodotope (Therapeutic). (Bracco Diagnostics) Sodium iodide I-131. 1 to 50 mCi Cap. Sodium iodide I-151 7.05 m Ci/ml. Vial 7, 14, 28, 70, 106 mCi, EDTA 1 mg/solution. *Rx.*
Use: Antithyroid agent.

•**iodoxamate meglumine.** (EYE-oh-DOX-ah-mate meh-GLUE-meen) USAN.
Use: Diagnostic aid (radiopaque medium).

•**iodoxamic acid.** (EYE-oh-dox-AM-ik) USAN.
Use: Diagnositc aid (radiopaque medium).

iodoxyl.
See: Sodium Iodomethamate (Various Mfr.).

Iofed. (Iomed Labs) Brompheniramine maleate 12 mg, pseudoephedrine HCl 120 mg/ER Cap. Bot. 100s. *Rx.*
Use: Antihistamine, decongestant.

Iofed PD. (Iomed Labs) Brompheniramine maleate 6 mg, pseudoephedrine HCl 60 mg/ER Cap. Bot. 100s. *Rx.*
Use: Antihistamine, decongestant.

•**iofetamine hydrochloride I 123.** (EYE-oh-FET-ah-meen) USAN.
Use: Diagnostic aid, radiopharmaceutical.

•**ioglicic acid.** (eye-oh-GLIH-sick) USAN.
Use: Diagnostic aid (radiopaque medium).

•**ioglucol.** (EYE-oh-GLUE-kahl) USAN.
Use: Diagnostic aid (radiopaque medium).

•**ioglucomide.** (EYE-oh-GLUE-koe-mide) USAN.
Use: Diagnostic aid (radiopaque medium).

•**ioglycamic acid.** (EYE-oh-glie-KAM-ik) USAN.
Use: Diagnostic aid (radiopaque medium, cholecystographic).

•**iogulamide.** (EYE-oh-GULL-ah-mide) USAN.
Use: Diagnostic aid (radiopaque medium).

•**iohexol.** (EYE-oh-HEX-ole) U.S.P. 23.
Use: Diagnostic aid (radiopaque medium).

Iohist D. (Iomed Labs) Phenylopropanolamine HCl 25 mg, phenyltoloxamine citrate 4 mg, pyrilamine maleate 4 mg, pheniramine maleate 4 mg, alcohol 4 %/ 5 ml. Pt. *Rx.*
Use: Antihistamine, decongestant.

Iohist DM. (Iomed Labs) Dextromethorphan HBr 10 mg, phenylpropanolamine HCl 12.5 mg, brompheniramine maleate 2 mg/5 ml. Syrup. Alcohol and sugar free. Bot. pt. *Rx.*
Use: Antihistamine, antitussive, decongestant.

Iohydro Cream. (Freeport) Hydrocortisone 1%, clioquinol 3%, pramoxine HCl 0.5%/0.5 oz. Tube 0.5 oz. [use]Use:Anesthetic, antifungal, corticosteroid, topical.

•**iomeprol.** (EYE-oh-MEH-prole) USAN
Use: Diagnostic aid (radiopaque medium).

•**iomethin I 125.** (EYE-oh-METH-in) USAN.

Use: Diagnostic aid (neoplasm); radiopharmaceutical.

•**iomethin I 131.** (EYE-o-METH-in) USAN.
Use: Diagnostic aid (neoplasm); radiopharmaceutical.

•**iometopane I 123.** (eye-oh-meh-TOE-pane) USAN.
Use: Diagnostic aid.

Ionamin. (Medeva) Phentermine. Resin base 15 mg and 30 mg, lactose/Cap. Bot. 100s, 400s. *c-IV.*
Use: Anorexiant.

Ionax Astringent Cleanser. (Galderma) Isopropyl alcohol 48%, acetone, salicylic acid. Bot. 240 ml. *otc.*
Use: Dermatologic, acne.

Ionax Foam. (Galderma) Benzalkonium Cl, propylene glycol. Aerosol can 150 ml. *otc.*
Use: Dermatologic, acne.

Ionax Scrub. (Galderma) SD Alcohol 40, benzalkonium Cl. Tube 60 g, 120 g. *otc.*
Use: Dermatologic, acne.

ionaze.
See: Propazolamide.

I-131 radiolabeled b1 monoclonal antibody. (Coulter)
Use: Treatment for non-Hodgkin's B-cell lymphoma. [Orphan drug]

ion-exchange resins.
See: Polyamine Methylene Resin.
Resins, Sodium Removing.

Ionil Plus Shampoo. (Galderma) Salicylic acid 2%, water, sodium laureth sulfate, lauramide dea, quaternium-22, talloweth-60 myristyl glycol, laureth-23, tea lauryl sulfate, glycol disterate, laureth-4, tea-abietoyl hydrolyzed collagen, DMDM hydantoin, tetrasodium EDTA, sodium hydroxide, fragrance, FD&C; blue No. 1. Bot. 4 oz, 8 oz. *otc.*
Use: Antiseborrheic.

Ionil Rinse. (Galderma) Conditioners with benzalkonium Cl in water base. Bot. 16 oz. *otc.*
Use: Dermatologic, hair.

Ionil Shampoo. (Galderma) Salicylic acid, benzalkonium Cl, alcohol 12%, polyoxyethylene ethers. Plastic bot. w/ dispenser cap 4 oz, 8 oz, 16 oz, 32 oz. *otc.*
Use: Antiseborrheic.

Ionil T. (Galderma) A nonionic/cationic foaming shampoo w/coal tar, salicylic acid, benzalkonium Cl, alcohol 12%, polyoxyethylene ethers. Plastic bot. 4 oz, 8 oz, 16 oz, 32 oz. *otc.*
Use: Antiseborrheic.

Ionil-T Plus Shampoo. (Galderma) Owentar II (equivalent to 2% coal tar), water, sodium laureth sulfate, lauramide dea, quaternium-22, laureth-23, talloweth-60 myristyl glycol, tea lauryl sulfate, glycol distearate, laureth-4, tea abietoyl hydrolyzed collagen, DMDM hydantoin, disodium EDTA, fragrance, FD&C; blue No.1, FD&C; yellow No. 70. Bot. 4 oz, 8 oz. *otc.*
Use: Antiseborrheic.

Ionosol D-CM. (Abbott Hospital Prods) Sodium Cl 516 mg, potassium Cl 89.4 mg, calcium Cl anhydrous 27.8 mg, magnesium Cl anhydrous 14.2 mg, sodium lactate 560 mg/100 ml. Bot. 1000 ml. *Rx.*
Use: Nutritional supplement, parenteral.

•**iopamidol,** (EYE-oh-PAM-ih-dahl) U.S.P. 23.
Use: Diagnostic aid (radiopaque medium).
See: Isovue-300, Inj. (Bristol-Myers Squibb).
Isovue-370, Inj. (Bristol-Myers Squibb).
Isovue-M 200, Inj. (Bristol-Myers Squibb).
Isovue-M 300, Inj. (Bristol-Myers Squibb).

•**iopanoic acid,** (eye-oh-pan-OH-ik) U.S.P. 23.
Use: Diagnostic aid (radiopaque medium).
See: Telepaque, Tab. (Sanofi Winthrop).

•**iopentol.** (EYE-oh-PEN-tole) USAN.
Use: Diagnostic aid (radiopaque medium).

Iophen. (Various Mfr.) 30 mg/Tab., 100s. 60 mg/5 ml/Elixer, 120 and 480 ml. 50 mg/ml/Soln., 30 ml. *Rx.*
Use: Expectorant.

•**iophendylate,** (eye-oh-FEN-dih-late) U.S.P. 23. Benzenedecanoic acid, iodo-t-methyl-, ethyl ester.
Use: Diagnostic aid (radiopaque medium).

iophendylate injection. Ethiodan, Myodil. Ethyl Iodophenylundecylate.
Use: Diagnostic aid (radiopaque medium).
See: Pantopaque, Amp. (LaFayette Pharm).

iophenoxic acid. (EYE-oh-pro-SEH-mik Acid) Tab.

Iophylline. (Various Mfr.) Theophylline 120 mg, iodinated glycerol 30 mg/15 ml. Elixir. Bot. 480 ml. *Rx.*
Use: Antiasthmatic combination.

Iopidine. (Alcon Laboratories) Apraclonidine 0.5% or 1%, benzalkonium Cl

0.01%. Dispenser Bot. 0.25 ml (1%), Drop-Tainer 5 ml (0.5%). *Rx.*
Use: Antiglaucoma agent.

iopodate sodium.
See: Ipodate Sodium.

Ioprep. (Johnson & Johnson) Nonylphenoxypolyethylenoxy (4) ethanol and nonylphenoxypolyethyleneoxy (15) ethanol iodine complex 5.5%, nonylphenoxypolyethyleneoxy (30) ethanol 10%. Solution provides 1% available iodine. Plastic bot. gal.
Use: Antiseptic.

•**ioprocemic acid.** (EYE-oh-pro-SEH-mik acid) USAN.
Use: Diagnostic aid (radiopaque medium).

•**iopromide.** (eye-oh-PRO-mide) USAN.
Use: Diagnostic aid (radiopaque medium).
See: Ultravist, Inj. (Berlex).

•**iopronic acid.** (eye-oh-PRO-nik acid) USAN.
Use: Diagnostic aid (radiopaque medium, cholecystographic).

•**iopydol.** (eye-oh-PIE-dahl) USAN.
Use: Diagnostic aid (radiopaque medium, bronchographic).

•**iopydone.** (eye-oh-PIE-dohn) USAN.
Use: Diagnostic aid (radiopaque medium, bronchographic).

Iosal II. (Iomed Labs) Pseudoephedrine HCl 60 mg, guaifenesin 600 mg/Tab. ER. 100s. *Rx.*
Use: Expectorant.

•**iosefamic acid.** (EYE-oh-seh-FAM-ik) USAN.
Use: Diagnostic aid; radiopaque medium.

•**ioseric acid.** (eye-oh-SEH-rik) USAN.
Use: Diagnostic aid (radiopaque medium).

Iosopan. (Zenith Goldline) Magaldrate 540 mg/5 ml. Liq. Bot. 355 ml. *otc.*
Use: Antacid.

Iosopan Plus. (Zenith Goldline) Magaldrate 540 mg, simethicone 40 mg/5 ml. Liq. Bot. 355 ml. *otc.*
Use: Antacid.

•**iosulamide meglumine.** (eye-oh-SULL-ah-mide meh-GLUE-meen) USAN.
Use: Diagnostic aid (radiopaque medium).

•**iosumetic acid.** (eye-oh-sue-MEH-tick) USAN.
Use: Diagnostic aid (radiopaque medium).

•**iotasul.** (EYE-oh-tah-sull) USAN.
Use: Diagnostic aid (radiopaque medium).

•**iotetric acid.** (eye-oh-TEH-trick) USAN.
Use: Diagnostic aid (radiopaque medium).

iothalamate meglumide and iothalmate sodium injection.
Use: Diagnostic aid (radiopaque medium).

•**iothalamate meglumine injection,** (eye-oh-THAL-am-ate meh-GLUE-meen) U.S.P. 23.
Use: Diagnostic aid (radiopaque medium).

•**iothalamate sodium injection,** (eye-oh-THAL-am-ate) U.S.P. 23.
Use: Diagnostic aid (radiopaque medium).

•**iothalamate sodium I 125 injection,** (eye-oh-THAL-am-ate) U.S.P. 23.
Use: Radiopharmaceutical.

•**iothalamate sodium I 131,** (eye-oh-THAL-am-ate) USAN.
Use: Radiopharmaceutical.

•**iothalamic acid,** (eye-oh-THAL-am-ik) U.S.P. 23
Use: Diagnostic aid (radiopaque medium).

iothiouracil sodium. Sodium salt of 5-iodo-2-thiouracil.

•**iotrolan.** (EYE-oh-TRAHL-an) USAN.
Formerly Iotrol.
Use: Diagnostic aid, (radiopaque medium).

•**iotroxic acid.** (EYE-oh-TRAHK-sick) USAN.
Use: Diagnostic aid (radiopaque medium).

Iotussin HC. (Iomed Labs) Hydrocodone bitartrate 2.5 mg, phenylephrine HCl 5 mg, chlorpheniramine maleate 2 mg/5 ml. Alcohol and sugar free. Syr. Bot. 473 ml. *c-III.*
Use: Antihistamine, antitussive, decongestant.

•**iotyrosine I 131.** USAN.
Use: Radiopharmaceutical.

•**ioversol.** (EYE-oh-ver-SAHL) U.S.P. 23.
Use: Diagnostic aid (radiopaque medium).
See: Optiray 350, Inj. (Mallinckrodt Medical).

•**ioxaglate meglumine.** (eye-ox-AGG-late meh-GLUE-meen) USAN.
Use: Diagnostic aid (radiopaque medium).
See: Hexabrix, Inj. (Wallace Laboratories).

ioxaglate meglumine/ioxaglate sodium.
Use: Radiopaque agent.

See: Hexabrix (Mallinckrodt).

•**ioxaglate sodium.** (eye-ox-AGG-late) USAN.
Use: Diagnostic aid (radiopaque medium).

•**ioxaglic acid,** (eye-ox-AGG-lick) U.S.P. 23.
Use: Diagnostic aid (radiopaque medium).

•**ioxilan.** (eye-OX-ee-lan) USAN
Use: Diagnostic aid.

•**ioxotrizoic acid.** (eye-OX-oh-TRY-zoe-ik) USAN.
Use: Diagnostic aid (radiopaque medium).

•**ipazilide fumarate.** (ih-PAZZ-ih-LIDE) USAN
Use: Cardiovascular agent.

•**ipecac,** (IPP-uh-kak) U.S.P. 23.
Use: Emetic.
W/Combinations.
See: Balmial Cough Syrup, Syr. (Clapp).
Creozets, Loz. (Creomulsion Co.).
Derfort, Cap. (Cole).
Ipsatol/DM, Cough Syr. (Key Pharm).
Ipsatol, Syr. (Key Pharm).
Mallergan, Liq. (Roberts Pharm)
Polyectin, Liq. (T.E. Williams).
Rubacac, Tab. (Scrip).
Spenlaxo, Tab. (Rugby).
Terpium, Tab. (Scrip).

ipecac. (Various Mfr.) 1.5% to 1.75% alcohol/Syrup. 15, 30 ml. *otc.*
Use: Antidote.

ipecac. (Various Mfr.) 2% alcohol/Syrup. 15, 30 ml. *Rx.*
Use: Antidote.

•**ipexidine mesylate.** (eye-PEX-ih-DEEN) USAN.
Use: Dental caries agent.

I-Pilopine. (Akorn) Pilocarpine HCl 1%. Ophthalmic soln. Bot. 15 ml. *Rx.*
Use: Antiglaucoma agent.

•**ipodate calcium,** (EYE-poe-date) U.S.P. 23.
Use: Diagnostic aid (radiopaque medium).
See: Oragrafin calcium, Granules (Bristol-Myers Squibb).

•**ipodate sodium,** U.S.P. 23.
Use: Diagnostic aid (radiopaque medium).
See: Bilivist, Cap. (Berlex).
Oragrafin sodium, Cap., Vial (Bristol-Myers Squibb).

IPOL. (Pasteur Merieux Connaught) Suspension of 3 types of poliovirus (Types 1, 2 and 3) grown in monkey kidney cell cultures. Inj. Single-dose syringe 0.5 ml. *Rx.*
Use: Immunization.

Ipran. (Major) Propranolol HCl 10 mg, 20 mg, 40 mg, 60 mg, 80 mg, 90 mg/Tab. **10 mg, 20 mg, 40 mg:** Bot. 100s, 250s, 1000s, UD 100s; **60 mg:** Bot. 100s, 500s; **80 mg:** Bot. 100s, 500s, 1000s, UD 100s; **90 mg:** Bot. 100s, 500s. *Rx.*
Use: Beta-adrenergic blocker.

•**ipratropium bromide.** (IH-pruh-TROE-pee-uhm) USAN.
Use: Bronchodilator.
See: Atrovent, Aerosol (Boehringer Ingelheim).

ipratropium bromide. (Dey Labs) Ipratropium bromide 0.02% (500 mcg/vial/Soln. for Inhalation. Vials. 25 and 60 unit dose (2.5 ml each). *Rx.*
Use: Anticholinergic.

ipratropium bromide/albuterol sulfate. (Boehringer Ingelheim)
Use: Secondary treatment of chronic obstructive pulmonary disease (COPD).
See: Combivent, Inhalation aerosol. (Boehringer Ingelheim).

I-Pred. (Akorn) Prednisolone sodium phosphate 0.5% or 1%. Ophthalmic soln. Bot. 5 ml. *Rx.*
Use: Corticosteroid, ophthalmic.

I-Prednicet. (Akorn) Prednisolone acetate 1%. Ophthalmic soln. Bot. 5 ml, 10 ml. *Rx.*
Use: Corticosteroid, ophthalmic.

•**iprindole.** (IH-prin-dole) USAN.
Use: Antidepressant.

•**iprofenin.** (IH-pro-FEN-in) USAN.
Use: Diagnostic aid (hepatic funtion determination).

•**ipronidazole.** (ih-pro-NIH-dah-zole) USAN.
Use: Antiprotozoal (*Histomonas*).

•**iproplatin.** (IH-pro-PLAT-in) USAN.
Use: Antineoplastic.

iproveratril. Name used for verapamil.

•**iproxamine hydrochloride.** (IH-PROX-ah-meen) USAN.
Use: Vasodilator.

•**ipsapirone hydrochloride.** (ipp-sah-PIE-rone) USAN.
Use: Anxiolytic.

Ipsatol Cough Formula Liquid for Children and Adults. (Kenwood Labs) Guaifenesin 100 mg, dextromethorphan HBr 10 mg, phenylpropanolamine HCl 9 mg/5 ml. Bot. 118 ml. *otc.*
Use: Antitussive, decongestant, expectorant.

IPV.
Use: Immunization.
See: IPOL (Connaught).
Polio Virus Vaccine, Inactivated.

•**irbesartan.** (ihr-beh-SAHR-tan) USAN.
Use: Antihypertensive (angiotensin II receptor antagonist).
See: Avapro, Tab. (Sanogi Winthrop).

Ircon. (Kenwood) Ferrous fumarate 200 mg/Tab. Bot. 100s. *otc.*
Use: Mineral supplement.

Ircon-FA. (Kenwood Labs) Ferrous fumarate 82 mg, folic acid 0.8 mg/Tab. Bot. 100s. *otc.*
Use: Mineral supplement.

Irgasan CF3. Cloflucarban.
Use: Antiseptic, topical.

•**iridium Ir 192.** (ih-RID-ee-uhm) USAN.
Use: Radioactive agent.
See: Iriditope (Bristol-Myers Squibb).

Irigate Eye Wash. (Optopics) Sodium Cl, sodium phosphate mono- and dibasic, benzalkonium Cl, EDTA. Soln. Bot. 118 ml. *otc.*
Use: Irrigant, ophthalmic.

•**irinotecan hydrochloride.** (eye-rih-no-TEE-can) USAN.
Use: Antineoplastic (DNA topoisomerase I inhibitor).
See: Camptosar, Inj. (Pharmacia & Upjohn).

irisin. A polysaccharide found in several species of iris.

irocaine.
See: Procaine HCl (Various Mfr.).

Irodex. (Keene Pharmaceuticals) Iron dextran complex 50 mg/ml. Vial 10 ml. *Rx.*
Use: Mineral supplement.

Iromin-G. (Mission Pharmacal) Ferrous gluconate 260 mg (iron 30 mg), vitamins B_{12} (crystalline on resin) 2 mcg, C 100 mg, A acetate 4000 IU, D 400 IU, B_1 5 mg, B_2 2 mg, B_6 20.6 mg, B_3 10 mg, B_5 1 mg, folic acid 0.8 mg, Ca/Tab. Bot. 100s. *otc.*
Use: Mineral, vitamin supplement.

iron (2+) fumarate. Ferrous Fumarate, U.S.P. 23.

iron (2+) gluconate.
See: Ferrous Gluconate, U.S.P. 23.

iron bile salts.
See: Bilron, Pulvules (Eli Lilly).

iron carbonate complex.
See: Polyferose.

iron choline citrate complex.
See: Chel-Iron, Tab. (Kinney).
Kelex, Tabseals (Nutrition Control).

•**iron dextran injection,** (iron DEX-tran) U.S.P. 23.
Use: Hematinic.
See: Dexferrum, Inj. (American Regent).
Ferrodex, Inj. (Keene Pharmaceuticals).
Hydextran, Inj. (Hyrex).
Imferon, Amp., Vial (Merrell Dow).
InFeD, Inj. (Schein).

Iron-Folic 500. (Major) Ferrous sulfate 105 mg, B_1 6 mg, B_2 6mg, B_3 30 mg, B_5 10 mg, B_{12} 25 mcg, C 500 mg, folic acid 0.8 mg/Tab. Bot. 100s, 500s. *otc.*
Use: Mineral, vitamin supplement.

iron/liver combinations, injection.
See: Rogenic (Forest Pharmaceutical).
Hemocyte (US Pharmaceutical).
Hytinic (Hyrex).
Licoplex DS (Keene Pharmaceuticals).
Hemocyte-V (US Pharmaceutical).
Liver-Iron B Complex w/Vitamin B_{12} (Akorn).

iron/liver combination, oral.
See: Arcotinic, Tab. (Arco).
Feocyte, Tab. (Dunhill).
Rogenic, Tab. (Forest Pharmaceutical).
I-L-X B_{12}, Tab. (Kenwood Labs).
Livitamin, Cap. (SmithKline Beecham Pharmaceuticals).
Liquid Geritonic (Roberts Pharm).
I-L-X B_{12} Elixir (Kenwood Labs).
I-L-X Elixir (Kenwood Labs).
Arcotinic Liquid (Arco).
Livitamin Liquid (SmithKline Beecham Pharmaceuticals).

iron oxide mixture with zinc oxide.
Calamine, U.S.P. 23.

iron peptonized.
See: Saferon, Tab. (ICN Pharmaceuticals).

iron products, injection.
See: InFeD (Schein Pharmaceutical).

iron protein complex.

•**iron sorbitex injection,** (SORE-bih-tex) U.S.P. 23.
Use: Hematinic.
See: Jectofer, Amp. (Astra).

iron sulfate. W/Maalox.
See: Fermalox, Tab. (Rhone-Poulenc Rorer).

iron with vitamin B_{12} and IFC.
See: Pronemia Hematinic Capsules (ESI Lederle Generics).
Contrin Capsules (Geneva Pharm).
Ferotrinsic Capsules (Rugby).
Livitrinsic-f Capsules (Zenith Goldline).

Trinsicon Capsules (UCB Pharmaceuticals).
Fergon Plus Caplets (Sanofi Winthrop).
TriHEMIC 600 Tablets (ESI Lederle Generics).
Heptuna Plues Capsules (Roerig).
Livitamin w/Intrinsic Factor Capsules (Savage).
Chromagen Capsules (Savage).

Ironco-B. (Pal-Pak) Ferrous sulfate 120.4 mg, manganese sulfate 21.6 mg, dicalcium phosphate 129.6 mg, vitamins B_1 1 mg, B_2 1 mg, niacin 6 mg, D 100 IU/Tab. Bot. 100s, 1000s. *otc.*
Use: Mineral, vitamin supplement.

Irospan. (Fielding) Ferrous sulfate 65 mg, vitamin C 150 mg/Cap. Bot. 60s. Tab. Bot. 100s. *otc.*
Use: Mineral, vitamin supplement.

irradiated ergosterol.
See: Calciferol.

Irrigate Eye Wash. (Optopics) Sodium Cl, mono- and dibasic sodium phosphate, benzalkonium Cl, EDTA. Bot. 118 ml. *otc.*
Use: Irrigant, ophthalmic.

irrigating solutions, physiological.
Use: Irrigant.
See: 0.45% Sodium Chloride Irrigation (Abbott Laboratories).
0.9% Sodium Chloride Irrigation (Abbott Laboratories).
Tis-U-Sol (Baxter).
Lactated Ringer's Irrigation (Abbott Laboratories).
Physiolyte (American McGaw).
PhysioSol (Abbott Laboratories).

irrigating solutions, urinary.
Use: Irrigant.
See: Neosporin G.U. Irrigant (Glaxo-Wellcome).
Renacidin (Guardian Laboratories).
Resectisol (McGaw).
Sorbitol-Mannitol (Abbott Laboratories).
Acetic Acid (Various Mfr.).
Glycine (Aminoacetic acid) (Various Mfr.).
Sodium Chloride (Various Mfr.).
Sterile Water (Various Mfr.).

•**irtemazole.** (ihr-TEH-mah-zole) USAN.
Use: Uricosuric.

isacen.
See: Oxyphenisatin, Preps. (Various Mfr.).

•**isamoxole.** (eye-SAH-MOX-ole) USAN.
Use: Antiasthmatic.

iscador. (Hiscia).
Use: Antiviral.

•**isepamicin.** (eye-SEP-ah-MY-sin) USAN.
Use: Antibacterial (aminoglycoside).

ISG. Immune globulin intramuscular. *Rx.*
Use: Immunization.
See: Gammar-IM, Inj. (Centeon).

Ismelin. (Novartis) Guanethidine monosulfate 10 mg or 25 mg/Tab. Bot. 100s. *Rx.*
Use: Antihypertensive.

ISMO. (Wyeth Ayerst) Isosorbide mononitrate 20 mg/Tab. Bot. 100s, UD 100s. *Rx.*
Use: Antianginal.

Ismotic. (Alcon Surgical) Isosorbide solution. W/sodium 4.6 mEq, potassium 0.9 mEq/220 ml, alcohol, saccharin, sorbitol. In 220 ml. *Rx.*
Use: Diuretic.

iso-alcoholic elixir.
Use: Vehicle.

isoamylhydrocupreine dihydrochloride.
See: Eucupin Dihydrochloride.

isoamyl nitrate.
See: Amyl Nitrite, U.S.P. 23.

isoamyne.
See: Amphetamine (Various Mfr.).

Iso-B. (Tyson and Associates) B_1 25 mg, B_2 25 mg, B_3 75 mg, B_5 125 mg, B_6 50 mg, B_{12} 100 mcg, FA 0.2 mg, pyridoxal 5 phosphate 2.5 mg, PABA 50 mg, inositol 50 mg, choline bitartrate 125 mg, biotin 100 mcg/Cap. Bot. 120s. *otc.*
Use: Mineral, vitamin supplement.

isobornyl thiocyanoacetate, technical.
Use: Pediculicide.
See: Barc, Liq. (Del Pharmaceuticals).
W/Anhydrous soap.
W/Docusate sodium and related terpenes.
See: Barc, Cream (Del Pharmaceuticals).

isobucaine hydrochloride, U.S.P. XXI.
Use: Anesthetic, local.

isobucaine hydrochloride & epinephrine injection, U.S.P. XXI.
Use: Anesthetic, local.

•**Isobutamben.** (EYE-so-BYOO-tam-ben) USAN.
Use: Anesthetic, local.

•**isobutane,** (eye-so-BYOO-tane) N.F. 18.
Use: Aerosol propellant.

isobutylallylbarbituric acid.
W/Aspirin, phenacetin, caffeine.
See: Buff-A-Comp, Tab., Cap. (Merz).
Fiorinal, Tab., Cap. (Novartis).
Palgesic, Tab., Cap. (Pan Amer.).
Tenstan, Tab. (Standex).
W/Codeine phosphate.

See: Fiorinal w/codeine, Cap. (Novartis).

isobutyl p-aminobenzoate.
See: Isobutamben, U.S.A.N.

isobutyramide. (Vertex)
Use: Sickle cell disease, beta-thalassemia. [Orphan drug]

isobutyramide oral solution. (Alpha Ther)
Use: Sickle call disease, beta-thalassemia. [Orphan drug]

isocaine. Isobutamben, USAN.

Isocaine Hydrochloride. (Novocol Chemical) Mepivacaine HCl 3%: 1.8 ml (dental cartridge). 2%: w/levonordefrin 1:20,000, sodium bisulfite. 1.8 ml (dental cartridge). *Rx.*
Use: Anesthetic, local.
See: Isocaine HCl, Inj. (Novocol Chemical).

Isocal. (Bristol-Myers) Lactose-free isotonic liquid containing as a percentage of the calories protein 13% as caseinate and soy protein; fat 37% as soy oil and medium chain triglycerides; carbohydrate 50% as corn syrup solids w/vitamins and minerals for the tube fed patient. Bot. 8 fl oz, 12 fl oz, 32 fl oz. *otc.*
Use: Nutritional supplement.

Isocal HCN. (Bristol-Myers) High calorie, nitrogen nutritionally complete food. Protein 15%, fat 45%, carbohydrate 40%. Can 8 fl oz. *otc.*
Use: Nutritional supplement.

Isocal HN. (Bristol-Myers) ≈ 1 Kcal/ml with protein 44 g, fat 45 g, carbohydrates 124 g/L. In 237 ml. *otc.*
Use: Nutritional supplement.

•**isocarboxazid,** (eye-so-car-BOX-ah-zid) U.S.P. 23.
Use: Antidepressant.
See: Marplan (Roche Laboratories).

Isocet. (Rugby) Acetaminophen 325 mg, caffeine 40 mg, butalbital 50 mg/Tab. Bot. 100s. *Rx.*
Use: Analgesic combination.

Isoclor Expectorant. (Fisons) Codeine phosphate 10 mg, pseudoephedrine HCl 30 mg, guaifenesin 100 mg/5 ml, alcohol 5%. Bot. pt. *c-v.*
Use: Antitussive, decongestant, expectorant.

isococaine. Pseudococaine.

Isocom. (Nutripharm) Isometheptene mucate 65 mg, dichloralphenazone 100 mg, acetaminophen 325 mg/Cap. Bot. 50s, 100s, 250s. *Rx.*
Use: Antimigraine.

•**isoconazole.** (EYE-so-CONE-ah-zole) USAN.
Use: Anti-infective, antifungal.

Isocult Test for Bacteriuria. (SmithKline Diagnostics)
Use: Diagnostic aid.

Isocult Test for Candida. (SmithKline Diagnostics)
Use: Diagnostic aid.

Isocult Test for Neisseria Gonorrhoeae. (SmithKline Diagnostics)
Use: Diagnostic aid.

Isocult Test for N Gonorrhoeae and Candida. (SmithKline Diagnostics)
Use: Diagnostic aid.

Isocult Test for Pseudomonas Aeruginosa. (SmithKline Diagnostics)
Use: Diagnostic aid.

Isocult Test for Staphylococcus Aureus. (SmithKline Diagnostics)
Use: Diagnostic aid.

Isocult Test for Throat Streptococci. (SmithKline Diagnostics)
Use: Diagnostic aid.

Isocult Test for Trichomonas Vaginalis. (SmithKline Diagnostics)
Use: Diagnostic aid.

Isocult Test for T Vaginalis/Candida. (SmithKline Diagnostics)
Use: Diagnostic aid.

Iso D. (Dunhall Pharmaceuticals) Isosorbide dinitrate. **Cap.:** 40 mg. Bot. 100s, 1000s. **Tab.:** 5 mg (sublingual). Bot. 100s. *Rx.*
Use: Antianginal.

isoephedrine hydrochloride. d-Isoephedrine HCl.
See: Pseudoephedrine HCl.
W/Chlorpheniramine maleate.
See: Isoclor, Tab., Expectorant Timesule, Liq. (Arnar-Stone).
W/Chlorprophenpyridamine maleate.
See: Isoclor, Tab. (Arnar-Stone).
W/Theophylline sodium glycinate, guaifenesin.
See: Iso-Tabs 60 Tab. (Solvay).

d-isoephedrine sulfate.
See: Pseudoephedrine Sulfate.

•**isoetharine.** (EYE-so-ETH-uh-reen) USAN.
Use: Bronchodilator.

•**isoetharine hydrochloride,** (EYE-so-ETH-uh-reen) U.S.P. 23.
Use: Bronchodilator.
See: Bronkosol, Soln. (Sanofi Winthrop).

isoetharine inhalation solution.
Use: Bronchodilator.

•**isoetharine mesylate,** (EYE-so-ETH-uh-reen) U.S.P. 23.
Use: Bronchodilator.
See: Bronkometer, Aerosol (Sanofi Winthrop).

•**isoflupredone acetate.** (eye-so-FLEW-PREH-dohn) USAN.
Use: Anti-inflammatory.

•**isoflurane,** (EYE-so-FLEW-rane) U.S.P. 23.
Use: Anesthetic, general.

•**isoflurophate,** (eye-so-FLURE-oh-fate) U.S.P. 23.
Use: Cholinergic, ophthalmic.
See: Floropryl, Oint. (Merck).

iso-iodeikon.
See: Phentetiothalein Sodium (No Mfr. currently lists).

Isoject. (Roerig) A purified, sterile, disposable injection system.
Permapen (benzathine pencillin G) aqueous soln. 1,200,000 units/2 ml. 10s.
Terramycin (oxytetracycline) intramuscular soln. 250 mg/2 ml. 10s.
Use: Injection system.

I-Sol Solution. (Dey Labs) Sodium Cl 0.64%, potassium Cl 0.075%, calcium Cl 0.048%, magnesium Cl 0.03%, sodium acetate 0.39%, sodium citrate 0.17%, sodium hydroxide or hydrochloric acid. Soln. Bot. 20 ml, 200 ml. *otc.*
Use: Irrigant, ophthalmic.

Isolan. (Elan) Protein 40 g, fat 36 g, carbohydrates 144 g, Na 690 g, K 1.17 g/L, with appropriate vitamins and minerals. Lactose free. Liq. In 237 ml Tetra Pak containers and 1000 ml New Pak closed systems with and without Color Check. *otc.*
Use: Nutritional supplement.

Isolate Compound Elixir. (Various Mfr.) Theophylline 45 mg, ephedrine sulfate 12 mg, isoproterenol HCl 2.5 mg, potassium iodide 150 mg, phenobarbital 6 mg/15 ml, alcohol 19%. Elix. Bot. pt, gal. *Rx.*
Use: Antiasthmatic combination.

•**isoleucine,** (EYE-so-LOO-seen) U.S.P. 23.
Use: Amino acid.

isoleucine. (EYE-so-LOO-seen) (Pfaltz & Bauer) Pow. 10 g.
Use: Amino acid.

Isolyte G with Dextrose. (American McGaw) Sodium 65 mEq, potassium 17 mEq, chloride 150 mEq, NH_4 70 mEq, dextrose 50 g, 170 Cal, 555 mOsm/L. Bot. 1000 ml. *Rx.*
Use: Nutritional supplement, parenteral.

Isolyte H/5% Dextrose. (American McGaw) Sodium 70 mEq, potassium 13 mEq, magnesium 3 mEq, chloride 40 mEq, acetate 16 mEq, dextrose 50 g, 170 Cal, 370 mOsm/L. Inj. Soln. 1000 ml. *Rx.*
Use: Nutritional supplement, parenteral.

Isolyte M/5% Dextrose. (American McGaw) Sodium 38 mEq, potassium 35 mEq, chloride 44 mEq, phosphate 15 mEq, acetate 20 mEq, dextrose 50 g, 175 Cal, 405 mOsm/L. Inj. Soln. 1000 ml. *Rx.*
Use: Nutritional supplement, parenteral.

Isolyte P/5% Dextrose. (American McGaw) Sodium 25 mEq, potassium 19 mEq, magnesium 3 mEq, chloride 23 mEq, phosphate 3 mEq, acetate 23 mEq, dextrose 50 g, 175 Cal, 350 mOsm/L. Inj. Soln. 250 ml, 500 ml, 1000 ml. *Rx.*
Use: Nutritional supplement, parenteral.

Isolyte R/5% Dextrose. (American McGaw) Sodium 41 mEq, potassium 16 mEq, calcium 5 mEq, magnesium 3 mEq, chloride 40 mEq, acetate 24 mEq, dextrose 50 g, 175 Cal, 380 mOsm/L. Inj. Soln. 1000 ml. *Rx.*
Use: Nutritional supplement, parenteral.

Isolyte S H 7.4. (American McGaw) Sodium 140 mEq, potassium 5 mEq, magnesium 3 mEq, chloride 98 mEq, acetate 27 mEq, gluconate 23 mEq, 295 mOsm/L. Inj. Soln. 500 ml, 1000 ml. *Rx.*
Use: Nutritional supplement, parenteral.

Isolyte S/5% Dextrose. (American McGaw) Sodium 140 mEq, potassium 5 mEq, magnesium 3 mEq, chloride 98 mEq, acetate 27 mEq, gluconate 23 mEq, dextrose 50 g, 185 Cal, 550 mOsm/L. Inj. Soln. 1000 ml. *Rx.*
Use: Nutritional supplement, parenteral.

•**isomazole hydrochloride.** (eye-SO-mah-ZOLE) USAN.
Use: Cardiovascular agent.

Isomeprobamate.
See: Carisoprodol (Various Mfr.).

•**isomerol.** (EYE-so-MER-ole) USAN. *Formerly Parahydrecin.*
Use: Antiseptic.

isometheptane mucate/dichloralphenazone/acetaminophen. (eye-so-meth-EPP-teen MYOO-kate, die-klor-uhl-FEN-uh-zone and ASS-et-ah-MEE-noe-fen)

isometheptene/dichloralphenazone/acetaminophen.

Use: Antimigraine.
See: Isometheptene/Dichloralphenazone/Acetaminophen, Cap. (Various Mfr.).
Isocam, Cap. (Nutripharm).
Midchlor, Cap. (Schein Pharmaceutical).
Midrin, Cap. (Carnrick Labs).
Migratine, Cap. (Major).

•**isometheptene mucate,** (eye-so-meth-EPP-teen MYOO-kate) U.S.P. 23.
See: Midrin, Cap. (Carnick).

Isomil. (Ross Laboratories) Soy protein isolate infant formula containing 20 calories/fl oz. **Pow.:** Can 14 oz. **Concentrated Liq.:** Can 13 fl oz. **Ready-to-feed:** Can 32 fl oz. **Nursing Bottles:** Hospital use. Bot. 8 fl oz. *otc.*
Use: Nutritional supplement.

Isomil DF. (Ross Laboratories) Protein 17.9 g, carbohydrates 67.3 g, fat 36.7 g, Fe 12 mg, Na 293 mg, K 720 mg, with appropriate vitamins and minerals. 676 cal/L. Lactose free. Liq. 960 ml prediluted, ready-to-use cans. *otc.*
Use: Nutritional supplement.

Isomil SF. (Ross Laboratories) Low osmolar sucrose-free soy protein isolate infant formula containing 20 calories/fl oz. **Concentrated Liq.:** Can 13 fl oz. **Ready-to-feed:** Can 32 fl oz. **Nursing Bottles:** Hospital use. Bot. 8 fl oz. *otc.*
Use: Nutritional supplement, enteral.

Isomune-CK. (Roche Laboratories) Rapid immunochemical separation method of the heart specific CK-MB isoenzyme for quantitation when used with an appropriate CK substrate reagent. Test kit 100s, 250s.
Use: Diagnostic aid.

Isomune-LD. (Roche Laboratories) Rapid immunochemical separation method of the heart specific LD-1 isoenzyme for quantitation when used with an appropriate LD substrate reagent. Test kit 40s, 100s.
Use: Diagnostic aid.

•**isomylamine hydrochloride.** (EYE-so-MILL-ah-meen) USAN.
Use: Muscle relaxant.

isomyn.
See: Amphetamine (Various Mfr.).

Isonate Sublingual. (Major) Isosorbide 2.5 mg or 5 mg/Sublingual Tab. Bot. 100s, 1000s, UD 100s. *Rx.*
Use: Antianginal.

Isonate Tablets. (Major) Isosorbide 5 mg, 10 mg, 20 mg or 30 mg/Tab. **5 mg or 10 mg:** Bot. 100s, 1000s, UD 100s. **20 mg or 30 mg:** Bot. 100s, 1000s. *Rx.*
Use: Antianginal.

Isonate TD-Caps. (Major) Isosorbide 40 mg/TD Cap. Bot. 100s, 1000s. *Rx.*
Use: Antianginal.

Isonate T.R. Tabs. (Major) Isosorbide 40 mg/TD Tab. Bot. 100s, 1000s. *Rx.*
Use: Antianginal.

isoniazid. (eye-so-NYE-uh-zid) (Carolina Medical Products) Isoniazid 50 mg/5 ml. Syr. Bot. pt. *Rx.*
Use: Antituberculous.

•**isoniazid,** (eye-so-NYE-uh-zid) U.S.P. 23.
Use: Anti-infective (tuberculostatic).
See: Dow-Isoniazid, Tab. (Merrell Dow).
INH, Tab. (Novartis).
Laniazid, Syr. (Lannett).
Niconyl, Tab. (Parke-Davis).
Nydrazid, Inj. (Squibb Diagnostic).
Nydrazid, Tab. (Marsam Pharmaceuticals).
Triniad, Tab. (Kasar).
Uniad, Tab. (Kasar).
W/Calcium paraminosalicylate.
See: Calpas-INH, Tab. (American Chem. & Drug).
W/Calcium p-aminosalicylate, vitamin B_6.
See: Calpas Isoxine, Tab. (American Chem. & Drug).
Calpas-INAH-6, Tab. (American Chem. & Drug).
W/Pyridoxine HCl. (vitamin B_6).
See: Niadox, Tab. (PBH Wesley Jessen).
Teebaconin w/B_6 (Consoln. Mid.).
Triniad Plus 30, Tab. (Kasar).
Uniad-Plus, Tab. (Kasar).
W/Pyridoxine HCl, sodium aminosalicylate.
See: Pasna, Tri-Pack 300, Granules (PBH Wesley Jessen).
W/Rifampin.
See: Rifater, Tab. (Hoechst Marion Roussel).
Rimactane/INH DuoPack (Novartis).
W/Sodium aminosalicylate, pyridoxine.
See: Pasna Tri-Pack, Granules (PBH Wesley Jessen).

isoniazid. (Various Mfr.) 50 mg/Tab. Bot. 100s, 500, 1000s.
Use: Anti-infective (tuberculostatic).

isonicotinic acid hydrazide.
See: Isoniazid, U.S.P. 23. (Various Mfr.).

isonicotinyl hydrazide.
See: Isoniazid, U.S.P. 23. (Various Mfr.).

isonipecaine hydrochloride.
See: Meperidine Hydrochloride, U.S.P. 23. (Various Mfr.).

isopentaquine.
Use: Antimalarial.

isophane insulin suspension.
Use: Hypoglycemic agent.
See: Humulin, Vial (Eli Lilly).
insulin, isophane.
Novolin, Vial (Novo Nordisk).
NPH Insulin, Vial (Novo Nordisk).
NPH Iletin, Vial (Eli Lilly).

isophane insulin suspension/insulin injection.
Use: Antidiabetic.
See: Humulin 50/50 (Eli Lilly).
Humulin 70/30 (Eli Lilly).
Novolin 70/30 (Novo Nordisk).
Novolin 70/30 Penfill (Novo Nordisk).

isopregnenone.
See: Duphaston, Tab. (Roxane).
Dydrogesterone.

Isoprinosine. (Newport Pharmaceuticals) Inosine pranobex.
Use: Antiviral, immunomodulator.

•**isopropamide iodide,** (eye-so-PRO-pah-mide EYE-oh-dide) U.S.P. 23.
Use: Anticholinergic.
See: Darbid, Tab. (SmithKline Beecham Pharmaceuticals).
W/Prochlorperazine maleate.
See: Iso-Perazine, Cap. (Teva USA).

isoprophenamine hydrochloride. Name used for Clorprenaline HCl.

isopropicillin potassium.
Use: Anti-infective.

•**isopropyl alcohol,** (eye-so-PRO-pill AL-koe-hahl) U.S.P. 23.
Use: Topical anti-infective; pharmaceutic aid (solvent).

isopropyl alcohol, azeotropic.

isopropyl alcohol spray. (Morton) Isopropyl alcohol w/propellant. Aerosol Can 6 oz. *otc.*
Use: Anti-infective.

isopropylarterenol hydrochloride.
Use: Asthma, vasoconstrictor and allergic states.

isopropylarterenol sulfate.
See: Isoproterenol Sulfate.

•**isopropyl myristate,** N.F. 18.
Use: Pharmaceutic aid (emollient).

iso-noradrenaline.
See: Isoproterenol.

isopropyl-noradrenaline hydrochloride.
See: Isoproterenol HCl, U.S.P. 23.

•**isopropyl palmitate,** N.F. 18.
Use: Pharmaceutic aid (oleaginous vehicle).

isopropyl phenazone. 4-Isopropyl antipyrine. Larodon.

isopropyl rubbing alcohol.
Use: Rubefacient, solvent.

isoproterenol. (eye-so-pro-TER-uh-nahl)
See: Norisidrine (Abbott Laboratories).
W/Butabarbital, theophylline, ephedrine HCl.
See: Medihaler-Iso, Vial (3M).

•**isoproterenol hydrochloride,** (eye-so-pro-TER-uh-nahl) U.S.P. 23.
Use: Bronchodilator, vasoconstrictor.
See: Isuprel HCl, Prods. (Sanofi Winthrop).
Norisodrine, Aerotrol, Syr. (Abbott Laboratories).
Proternol, Tab. (Key Pharm).
Vapo-Iso, Soln. (Fisons).
W/Aminophylline, ephedrine sulfate, phenobarbital.
See: Asminorel, Tab. (Solvay).
W/Clopane (clopentamine) HCl, propylene glycol, ascorbic acid.
See: Aerolone Compound, Soln. (Eli Lilly).
W/Phenobarbital sodium, ephedrine sulfate, theophylline hydrous.
See: Iso-asminyl, Tab. (Cole).

isoproterenol inhalation solution.
Use: Bronchodilator.

•**isoproterenol sulfate,** (eye-so-pro-TER-uh-nahl) U.S.P. 23.
Use: Bronchodilator.
See: Medihaler-Iso, Vial (3M).
W/Calcium iodide (anhydrous), alcohol.
See: Norisodrine, Syr. (Abbott Laboratories).

Isoptin. (Knoll Pharmaceuticals) Verapamil HCl 5 mg/2 ml. Inj. 2 ml and 4 ml amps, vials and disp. syringes. *Rx.*
Use: Calcium channel blocker.

Isoptin SR Tablets. (Knoll Pharmaceuticals) Verapamil HCl **120 mg, 180 mg/SR Tab.:** Bot. 100s, 500s, UD 100s. **240 mg/SR Tab.:** Bot. 100s, 500s, UD 100s. *Rx.*
Use: Calcium channel blocker.

Isoptin Tablets. (Knoll Pharmaceuticals) Verapamil HCl Tab. Bot. 100s, 500s, 1000s, UD 100s. *Rx.*
Use: Calcium channel blocker.

Isopto Alkaline. (Alcon Laboratories) Hydroxypropyl methylcellulose 1%, benzalkonium Cl 0.01%. Sterile ophthalmic soln. Dropper bot. 15 ml. *otc.*
Use: Artificial tears.

Isopto Atropine. (Alcon Laboratories) Atropine sulfate 0.5% or 1%. **0.5%:** Drop-Tainer 5 ml. **1%:** Drop-Tainer 5 ml, 15 ml. *Rx.*
Use: Cycloplegic, mydriatic.

Isopto Carbachol. (Alcon Laboratories) Carbachol U.S.P. 0.75%, 1.5%, 2.25% or 3%, in a sterile buffered solution of methylcellulose 1%. **2.25%:** Drop-Tainer 15 ml. **0.75%, 1.5% or 3%:** Drop-Tainer 15 ml, 30 ml. *Rx.*
Use: Antiglaucoma agent.

Isopto Carpine. (Alcon Laboratories) Pilocarpine HCl 0.5%, 1%, 2%, 4%, 5%, 6%, or 8%. Soln. Bot. 15 ml, 30 ml (except 5%). *Rx.*
Use: Antiglaucoma agent.

Isopto Cetamide. (Alcon Laboratories) Sodium sulfacetamide 15%. Soln. Drop-Tainer 5 ml, 15 ml. *Rx.*
Use: Anti-infective, ophthalmic.

Isopto Cetapred. (Alcon Laboratories) Sulfacetamide sodium 10%, prednisolone 0.25%. Susp. Drop-Tainer 5 ml, 15 ml. *Rx.*
Use: Anti-infective, corticosteroid, ophthalmic.

Isopto Frin. (Alcon Laboratories) Phenylephrine HCl 0.12% in a methylcellulose soln. Drop-Tainer 15 ml. *Rx.*
Use: Mydriatic, vasoconstrictor.

Isopto Homatropine. (Alcon Laboratories) Homatropine HBr 2% or 5%. Soln. Drop-Tainer 5 ml, 15 ml. *Rx.*
Use: Cycloplegic, mydriatic.

Isopto Hyoscine. (Alcon Laboratories) Hyoscine HBr 0.25%. Soln. Drop-Tainer 5 ml, 15 ml. *Rx.*
Use: Cycloplegic, mydriatic.

Isopto Plain. (Alcon Laboratories) Hydroxypropyl methylcellulose 2910 0.5%, benzalkonium Cl 0.01%, sodium Cl, sodium phosphate, sodium citrate. Drop-Tainer 15 ml. *otc.*
Use: Artificial tears.

Isopto Tears. (Alcon Laboratories) Hydroxypropyl methylcellulose 0.5%, benzalkonium Cl 0.01%, sodium Cl, sodium phosphate, sodium citrate. Bot. Drop-Tainer 15 ml, 30 ml. *otc.*
Use: Artificial tears.

Isordil Sublingual. (Wyeth Ayerst) Isosorbide dinitrate 2.5 mg, 5 mg or 10 mg/Tab. **2.5 mg or 5 mg:** Bot. 100s, 500s, Redi-pak 100s. **10 mg:** Bot. 100s. *Rx.*
Use: Antianginal.

Isordil Tembids. (Wyeth Ayerst) Isosorbide dinitrate 40 mg/Tab. or Cap. **SR Tab.:** Bot. 100s, 500s, 1000s. **SR Cap.:** Bot. 100s, 500s. *Rx.*
Use: Antianginal.

Isordil Titradose Tablets. (Wyeth Ayerst) Isosorbide dinitrate 5 mg, 10 mg, 20 mg, 30 mg or 40 mg/Tab. **5 mg.:** Bot. 100s, 500s, 1000s, Redi-pak 100s. **10 mg:** Bot. 100s, 500s, 1000s, Redi-pak 100s. **20 mg:** Bot. 100s, 500s, Redi-pak 100s. **30 mg:** Bot. 100s, 500s. Redi-pak 100s. **40 mg:** Bot. 100s, Redi-pak 100s. *Rx.*
Use: Antianginal.

Isorgen-G. (Grafton) Isosorbide 5 mg or 10 mg/Tab. Bot. 1000s. *Rx.*
Use: Antianginal.

•**isosorbide concentrate.** (EYE-sos-ORE-bide) U.S.P. 23.
Use: Diuretic.

•**isosorbide dinitrate diluted,** (EYE-sos-ORE-bide die-NYE-trate) U.S.P. 23.
Use: Coronary vasodilator.
See: Dilatrate-SR, Cap. (Schwarz Pharma).
Iso-Bid, Cap. (Roberts Pharm).
Iso-D, Tab., Cap. (Dunhall Pharmaceuticals).
Isordil, Tab. (Wyeth Ayerst).
Isordil Tembids Cap., Tab. (Wyeth Ayerst).
Nitromed, Tab. (U.S. Ethicals).
Onset, Tab. (Sanofi Winthrop).
Sorbitrate, Tab. (Zeneca).
Sorquad, Tab. (Solvay).
W/Phenobarbital.
See: Sorbitrate w/Phenobarbital, Tab. (Zeneca).

isosorbide dinitrate. (Various Mfr.) **Sublingual:** 2.5 mg, 5 mg, 10 mg. **2.5 mg:** Bot. 100s, 500s, 1000s, UD 100s. **5 mg:** Bot. 100s, 1000s, UD 100s. **10 mg:** Bot. 100s, 1000s. **Oral:** 5 mg, 10 mg, 20 mg, 30 mg/Tab. 40 mg/SR Tab. **5 mg:** Bot. 100s, 1000s, UD 100s. **10 mg:** Bot. 100s, 500s, 1000s, UD 100s. **20 mg:** Bot. 90s, 100s, 120s, 180s, 240s, 360s, 500s, 1000s, UD 100s. **30 mg:** Bot. 100s, 500s, 1000s, UD 100s. **40 mg:** Bot. 90s, 100s, 250s, 1000s, UD 100s. *Rx.*
Use: Coronary vasodilator.

•**isosorbide mononitrate.** (EYE-sos-ORE-bide MAH-no-NYE-trate) USAN.
Use: Coronary vasodilator.
See: Imdur, ER Tab. (Key Pharm).
ISMO, Tab. (Wyeth Ayerst).
Monoket, Tab. (Schwarz Pharma).

isosorbide oral solution.
Use: Diuretic.

Isosource. (Novartis) Protein (Ca and Na caseinate, soy protein isolate) 43.2 g, carbohydrate (maltodextrin) 1755 g, fat (MCT, canola oil, lecithin) 443.9 g, Na 760 mg, K 1182 mg, mOsm/kg H_2O 390, Cal/ml 1.2, vitamins A, B_1, B_2, B_3,

B_5, B_6, B_{12}, C, D, E, K, FA, biotin, choline, Ca, Cl, Cu, Fe, I, Mg, Mn, P, Zn, Se, Cr, Mo. Liq. Bot. 250 ml, 1000 ml. *otc.*
Use: Nutritional supplement.

Isosource HN. (Novartis) Protein (Ca and Na caseinate, soy protein isolate) 56.1 g, carbohydrate (maltodextrin) 165 g, fat (MCT, canola oil, lecithin) 43.9 g, Na 760 mg, K 1772 mg, mOsm/kg H_2O 390, Cal/ml 1.2, vitamins A, B_1, B_2, B_3, B_5, B_6, B_{12}, C, D, E, K, FA, biotin, choline, Ca, P, I, Fe, Mg, Cu, Zn, Cl, Mn, Se, Cr, Mo. Liq. Bot. 250 ml, 1000 ml. *otc.*
Use: Nutritional supplement.

•**isostearyl alcohol.** (FYE-so-STEE-rill) USAN.
Use: Pharmaceutic aid (emollient, solvent).

•**isosulfan blue.** (EYE-so-SULL-fan) USAN.
Use: Diagnostic aid, lymphangiography.

Isotein HN. (Novartis) Vanilla Flavor. Maltodextrin, delactosed lactalbumin, partially hydrogenated soy oil with BHA, fructose, medium chain triglycerides, artificial flavor, sodium caseinate, mono and diglycerides, sodium Cl, vitamins, minerals. Pow. Packet 2.75 oz. *otc.*
Use: Nutritional supplement.

•**isotiquimide.** (eye-so-TIH-kwih-MIDE) USAN.
Use: Antiulcerative.

•**isotretinoin,** (EYE-so-TREH-tin-NO-in) U.S.P. 23.
Use: Keratolytic.
See: Accutane, Cap. (Roche Laboratories).

•**isotretinoin anisatil.** (eye-so-TRETT-ih-noyn ah-NIH-sah-till) USAN.
Use: Dermatologic, acne.

isovorin. (ESI Lederle Generics) L-Leucovorin.
Use: Antineoplastic. [Orphan drug]

Isovue-128. (Bracco Diagnostics) Iopamidol 26% (12.8% iodine). Inj. Vial 50 ml.
Use: Radiopaque agent.

Isovue-200. (Bracco Diagnostics) Iopamidol 41% (20% iodine). Inj. Vial 50. Bot. 100 ml, 200 ml.
Use: Radiopaque agent.

Isovue-300 Injection. (Bristol-Myers Squibb) Iopamidol 612 mg, tromethamine 1 mg, edetate calcium disodium 0.39 mg/ml. Vial 50 ml, Box 10s. Bot. 100 ml, Box 10s.
Use: Radiopaque agent.

Isovue-370 Injection. (Bristol-Myers Squibb) Iopamidol 755 mg, tromethamine 1 mg, edetate calcium disodium 0.48 mg/ml. Vial 50 ml, Box 10s; Bot. 100 ml, Box 10s; 150 ml, Box 10s; 200 ml, Box 10s.
Use: Radiopaque agent.

Isovue-M 200 Injection. (Bristol-Myers Squibb) Iopamidol 408 mg, tromethamine 1 mg, edetate calcium disodium 0.26 mg/ml. Vial 20 ml, Box 10s.
Use: Radiopaque agent.

Isovue-M 300 Injection. (Bristol-Myers Squibb) Iopamidol 612 mg, tromethamine 1 mg, edetate calcium disodium 0.39 mg/ml. Vial 20 ml, Box 10s.
Use: Radiopaque agent.

•**isoxepac.** (EYE-SOX-eh-pack) USAN.
Use: Anti-inflammatory.

•**isoxicam.** (eye-SOX-ih-kam) USAN.
Use: Anti-inflammatory.

•**isoxsuprine hydrochloride,** (eye-SOX-you-preen) U.S.P. 23.
Use: Vasodilator.
See: Vasodilan, Tab. (Bristol-Myers).

I-Soyalac. (Mt. Vernon Foods) P-soy protein isolate, l-methionine, CHO-sucrose, tapioca dextrin. F-soy oil, soy lecithin. Corn free. Protein 20.2 g, carbohydrate 63.4 g, fat 35.5 g, iron 12 mg, 640 Cal/serving (1 qt). Concentrate 390 ml, ready to use 1 qt. *otc.*
Use: Nutritional supplement.

•**isradipine.** (iss-RAHD-ih-peen) USAN.
Use: Calcium channel blocker; antagonist (calcium channel).
See: DynaCirc (Novartis).

I-Sulfacet. (American) Sulfacetamide sodium 10%, 15% or 30% ophthalmic soln. Bot. 2 ml, 5 ml, 15 ml. *Rx.*
Use: Anti-infective, ophthalmic.

I-Sulfalone Suspension. (American) Sulfacetamide sodium 100 mg, prednisolone acetate 5 mg. Ophthalmic susp. Bot. 5 ml, 15 ml. *Rx.*
Use: Anti-infective, ophthalmic.

Isuprel Inhalation Solution. (Sanofi Winthrop) Isoproterenol HCl inhalation soln. 1:200 or 1:100. Bot. 10 ml, 60 ml. *Rx.*
Use: Bronchodilator.

Isuprel Mistometer. (Sanofi Winthrop) Isoproterenol HCl. Complete nebulizing unit of aerosol soln. containing 10 ml or 15 ml of isoproterenol HCl w/inert propellants, alcohol 33%, ascorbic acid. Measured dose of approximately 131 mcg. Aerosol Unit. Bot. 15 ml, 22.5 ml.

Refill 15 ml, 22.5 ml. *Rx.*
Use: Bronchodilator.

Isuprel Sterile Injection. (Sanofi Winthrop) Isoproterenol HCl 0.2 mg/ml with sodium metabisulfite in 1:5000 solution in 1 and 5 ml amps.; 0.02 mg/ml with sodium metabisulfite in 1:50,000 solution in 10 ml with needle. *Rx.*
Use: Sympathomimetic.

isuprene.
See: Isoproterenol (Various Mfr.).

•**itasetron.** (eye-tah-SEH-trahn) USAN.
Use: Antidepressant; antiemetic; anxiolytic.

•**itazigrel.** (ih-TAY-zih-GRELL) USAN.
Use: Platelet aggregation inhibitor.

Itchaway. (Moyco) Zinc undecylenate 20%, undecylenic acid 2%. Pow. Can 1.5 oz. *otc.*
Use: Antifungal, topical.

Itch-X. (B.F. Ascher) Pramoxine HCl 1%. Gel: Benzyl alcohol, aloe vera gel, diazolidinyl urea, SD alcohol 40, parabens. 35.4 g. Spray: Benzyl alcohol, aloe vera gel, SD alcohol 40. In 60 ml. *otc.*
Use: Anesthetic, local.

itobarbital.
W/Acetaminophen.
See: Panitol, Tab. (Wesley Pharmacal).

•**itraconazole.** (ih-truh-KAHN-uh-zole) USAN.
Use: Antifungal.
See: Sporanox, Cap. (Janssen).

I-Trol. (Akorn) Neomycin sulfate-polymyxin B sulfate-dexamethasone 0.1%. Ophthalmic susp. Bot. 5 ml. *Rx.*
Use: Anti-infective, corticosteroid, ophthalmic.

I-Valex-1. (Ross Laboratories) Protein 15 g, fat 23.9 g, carbohydrates 46.3 g, linoleic acid 1800 mg, Fe 9 mg, Na 190 mg, K 675 mg, with appropriate vitamins and minerals. 480 Cal per 100 g. Leucine free. Pow. Can 350 g. *otc.*
Use: Nutritional supplement.

I-Valex-2. (Ross Laboratories) Protein 30 g, fat 15.5 g, carbohyrates 30 g, Na 880 mg, K 1370 mg, with appropriate vitamins and minerals. 410 Cal per 100 g. Leucine free. Pow. Can 325 g. *otc.*
Use: Nutritional supplement.

Ivarest. (Blistex) Calamine 14%, benzocaine 5%. **Cream:** 60 g. **Lot.:** 120 ml. *otc.*
Use: Dermatologic, poison ivy.

Iveegam. (Immune) Immune globulin 50 mg/ml IgG/Pow. for Inj. in 1000 mg with diluent, double-ended spike and filter needle; and 2500 and 5000 mg with diluent, double-ended spike and infusion set with filter. *Rx.*
Use: Immunization.

•**ivermectin.** (eye-VER-MEK-tin) USAN.
Use: Antiparasitic.
See: Cardomec (Merck).
Equalan (Merck).
Ivomec (Merck).

Ivocort. (Roberts Pharm) Micronized hydrocortisone alcohol 0.5% or 1%. Bot. 4 oz. *otc.*
Use: Corticosteroid, topical.

Ivy-Chex. (Jones Medical Industries) Polyvinyl pyrrolidone-vinyl acetate, benzalkonium Cl 1:1000 in alcohol acetone base. Aerosol can 4 oz. *otc.*
Use: Dermatologic, poison ivy.

Ivy Dry. (Ivy) Tannic acid 10%, isopropyl alcohol 12.5% Liq. 4 oz, Cream 1 oz, Super 6 oz. *otc.*
Use: Poison ivy therapy, topical.

Ivy-Rid. (Roberts Pharm) Polyvinyl pyrrolidone-vinyl acetate, benzalkonium Cl. Spray can 2.75 oz. *otc.*
Use: Poison ivy therapy, topical.

I-Wash. (Akorn) Phosphate buffered saline soln. Bot. 4 oz, 8 oz. *otc.*
Use: Irrigant, ophthalmic.

I-White. (Akorn) Phenylephrine 0.12%, polyvinyl alcohol, hydroxyethyl cellulose. Soln. Bot. 15 ml. *otc.*
Use: Mydriatic, vasoconstrictor.

Izonid tablets. (Major) Isoniazid 300 mg/Tab. Bot. 100s. *Rx.*
Use: Antituberculous.

J

jalovis.
See: Hyaluronidase (Various Mfr.).

Janimine. (Abbott Laboratories) Imipramine HCl 10 mg, 25 mg or 50 mg/Tab. Bot. 100s, 1000s. *Rx.*
Use: Antidepressant.

japan agar.
See: Agar (Various Mfr.).

japan gelatin.
See: Agar (Various Mfr.).

japan isinglass.
See: Agar (Various Mfr.).

japanese encephalitis virus vaccine.
Use: Immunization.
See: JE-VAX.

JE-VAX. (Connaught) Japanese encephalitis virus vaccine 2-3 mcg nitrogen content per ml.. Pow. for Inj. single-dose vial with 1.3 ml diluent; 10-dose vial with 11 ml diluent. *Rx.*
Use: Immunization.

Jenest-28. (Organon Teknika) 7 white tablets norethindrone 0.5 mg, ethinyl estradiol 35 mcg; 14 peach tablets norethindrone 1 mg, ethinyl estradiol 35 mcg; 7 inert tablets. Cyclic dispenser of 28. *Rx.*
Use: Contraceptive.

Jeri-Bath. (Dermik Laboratories) Concentrated moisturizing bath oil. Plastic Bot. 8 oz. *otc.*
Use: Dermatologic.

Jets. (Freeda Vitamins) Lysine 300 mg, vitamins C 25 mg, B_{12} 25 mcg, B_6 5 mg, B_1 10 mg/Chew. tab. Bot. 30s, 250s, 500s. *otc.*
Use: Vitamin supplement.

Jevity Liquid. (Ross Laboratories) Calcium and sodium caseinates, soy fiber, hydrolyzed cornstarch, MCT (fractionated coconut oil) soy oil, corn oil, soy lecithin, vitamins A, B_1, B_2, B_3, B_5, B_6, B_{12}, C, D, E, K, folic acid, biotin, choline, Ca, P, Mg, Fe, Mn, Cu, Zn, I, Cl. In 240 ml. *otc.*
Use: Nutritional supplement.

Jiffy. (Block Drug) Benzocaine, menthol, eugenol in glycerin-water base with SD alcohol 38-B 76%. Bot. 0.125 oz. *otc.*
Use: Anesthetic, local.

J-Liberty. (J Pharmacal) Chlordiazepoxide HCl 5 mg, 10 mg or 25 mg/Cap. *C-IV.*
Use: Anxiolytic.

Johnson's Baby Cream. (Johnson & Johnson Consumer Products) Dimethicone 2%. Jar 4 oz, 6 oz, Tube 2 oz. *otc.*
Use: Dermatologic protectant.

Johnson's Baby Sunblock Cream. (Johnson & Johnson Consumer Products) Octyl methoxycinnamate, octyl salicylate, oxybenzone, titandium dioxide, benzyl alcohol, cetyl alcohol. PABA free. SPF 15. Waterproof. Cream. Bot. 60 Gm. *otc.*
Use: Sunscreen.

Johnson's Baby Sunblock Extra Protection. (Johnson & Johnson Consumer Products) Octyl methoxycinnamate, octyl salicylate, titanium dioxide, oxybenzone, C12-15 alcohols benzoate, cetyl alcohol, EDTA, vitamin E. Lot. Bot. 120 ml. *otc.*
Use: Sunscreen.

Johnson's Baby Sunblock Lotion. (Johnson & Johnson Consumer Products) **SPF 30:** Benzophenone-3, octyl methoxycinnamate, octyl salicylate, titanium dioxide. PABA free. Waterproof. Bot. 120 ml. **SPF 15:** Octyl methoxycinnamate octyl salicylate, oxybenzone, titanium dioxide, benzyl alcohol, cetyl alcohol. PABA free. Waterproof. Bot. 60 Gm. *otc.*
Use: Sunscreen.

Johnson's Medicated Powder. (Johnson & Johnson Consumer Products) Bentonite, kaolin, talc, zinc oxide. Pow. Small, Medium, Large. *otc.*
Use: Diaper rash preparation.

•**josamycin.** (JOE-sah-MYsin) USAN.
Use: Anti-Infective.

Junior Strength Advil. (Whitehall Robins) Ibuprofen 100 mg, sucrose, parabens/Tab. Bot. 24s. *otc.*
Use: Analgesic, NSAID.

Junior-Strength Feverall. (Upsher-Smith Labs) Acetaminophen 120 mg or 325 mg/Supp. Pkg 6s. *otc.*
Use: Analgesic.

Junior Strength Motrin. (Ortho McNeil) Ibuprofen 100 mg, phenylalanine 6 mg, aspartame/Chew. Tab. Bot. 24s. *otc.*
Use: Analgesic, NSAID.

Junior Strength Panadol. (Bayer Corp) Acetaminophen 160 mg. Capl. 30s. *otc.*
Use: Analgesic.

•**juniper tar.** (JOO-nih-per tar) U.S.P. 23.
Use: Local antieczematic, pharmaceutic necessity.

Junyer-All. (Barth's) Vitamins A 6000 IU, D 400 IU, B_1 3 mg, B_2 6 mg, C 120 mg, niacin 1 mg, E 12 IU, B_{12} 10 mcg, calcium 217 mg, phosphorus 97.5 mg, red bone marrow 10 mg, organic iron 15 mg, iodine 0.1 mg, beef peptone 20

mg/2 Cap. Bot. 10 month, 3 month, 6 month supply. *otc.*
Use: Vitamin supplement.

Just Tears. (Blairex Labs) Benzalkonium chloride, EDTA, NaCl, polyvinyl alcohol 1.4%. Soln. Bot. 15 ml. *otc.*
Use: Lubricant, ophthalmic.

juvocaine.
See: Procaine HCl (Various Mfr.)

K

K-1. Phytonadione.
Use: Vitamin K.
See: Mephyton, Tab. (Merck).
Aqua MEPHYTON, Inj. (Merck).
KonaKion, Inj. (For IM use only) (Roche Laboratories).

K-4. Menadiol sodium diphosphate.
Use: Vitamin K.

K+8. (Alra Laboratories) Potassium chloride 8 mEq. ER Tab. Bot. 100s, 500s. *Rx.*
Use: Electrolyte supplement.

K+10. (Alra Laboratories) Potassium Cl 10 mEq/Tab. Bot. 100s, 500s, 1000s. *Rx.*
Use: Electrolyte supplement.

K 34. Hexachlorophene.

K + Care. (Alra Laboratories) Potassium chloride, saccharin. Soln. Pkt. 15, 20, 25 mEq, 30s, 100s. *Rx.*
Use: Electrolyte supplement.

Kabikinase. (Pharmacia & Upjohn) Streptokinase 250,000 IU, 600,000 IU or 750,000 IU or 1,500,000 IU/vial. Pow. for inj. Vial 5 ml, 10 ml. *Rx.*
Use: Thrombolytic.

Kadian. (Zeneca) Morphine sulfate 20 mg, 50 mg and 100 mg, sucrose/SR Cap. Bot. 60s, 100s, 500s (except 100 mg) and UD 100s. *c-II.*
Use: Analgesic, narcotic.

Kaergona.
See: Menadione (Various Mfr.).

Kala. (Freeda Vitamins) Soy-based acidophilus 2 million units/Tab. Bot. 100s, 250s and 500s. *otc.*
Use: Nutritional supplement.

•**kalafungin.** (kal-ah-FUN-jin) USAN.
Use: Antifungal.

Kalory-Plus. (Tyler) Thyroid 3 gr, amphetamine sulfate 15 mg, atropine sulfate 1/180 gr, aloin 0.25 gr, phenobarbital 0.25 gr/TR cap. Bot. 100s, 1000s.
Use: Anorexiant.

Kaltostat. (SmithKline Beecham Pharmaceuticals) Calcium-sodium alginate fiber, 3"×4¾" sterile dressing. In 1s. *otc.*
Use: Dressing, hydroactive.

Kaltostat Forte. (SmithKline Beecham Pharmaceuticals) Calcium-sodium alginate fiber, 4"×4" sterile dressing. In 1s. *otc.*
Use: Dressing, hydroactive.

Kamfolene. (Wade) Camphor, menthol, methyl salicylate, oils turpentine and eucalyptus, carbolic acid 2%, calamine, zinc oxide in lanolin base. Jar 2 oz, lb. *otc.*
Use: Antiseptic.

•**kanamycin sulfate.** (kan-uh-MY-sin) U.S.P. 23.
Use: Anti-infective.
See: Kantrex, Cap., Vial (Bristol-Myers Squibb).
Klebcil, Inj. (SmithKline Beecham Pharmaceuticals).

Kank-A. (Blistex) Benzocaine 5%, cetylpyridinium chloride, castor oil, benzoin compound. Liq. Bot. 3.75 ml. *otc.*
Use: Anesthetic, local.

Kantrex. (Bristol-Myers Squibb) Kanamycin sulfate. **Cap.:** 0.5 g. Bot. 20s, 100s. **Vial:** 0.5 g/2 ml or 1 g/3 ml. **Pediatric Inj.:** 75 mg/2 ml. **Disposable Syringe:** 500 mg/2 ml. *Rx.*
Use: Anti-infective aminoglycoside.

Kaochlor 10% Liquid. (Pharmacia & Upjohn) Potassium and chloride 20 mEq/15 ml (potassium Cl 10%), alcohol 5%, saccharin, FD&C; Yellow No. 5. Bot. pt. *Rx.*
Use: Electrolyte supplement.

Kaochlor-Eff. (Pharmacia & Upjohn) Elemental potassium 20 mEq, chloride 20 mEq/Tab. Supplied by: Potassium Cl 0.6 g, potassium citrate 0.22 g, potassium bicarbonate 1 g, betaine HCl 1.84 g, saccharin 20 mg, artificial fruit flavor, tartrazine (color)/Tab. Sugar free. Carton 60s. *Rx.*
Use: Electrolyte supplement.

Kaochlor S-F 10% Liquid. (Pharmacia & Upjohn) Potassium 20 mEq, chloride 20 mEq/15 ml, saccharin, flavoring, alcohol 5%. Sugar free. Bot. 4 oz, pt. *Rx.*
Use: Electrolyte supplement.

Kaodene Non-Narcotic. (Pfeiffer) Kaolin 3.9 g, pectin 194.4 mg/30 ml, bismuth subsalicylate. Alcohol free. Liq. Bot. 120 ml. *otc.*
Use: Antidiarrheal.

Kaodene with Codeine. (Pfeiffer) Codeine phosphate 32.4 mg, kaolin 3.9 g, pectin 194.4 mg, sodium carboxymethylcellulose, bismuth subsalicylate/30 ml. Susp. Bot. 120 ml.
Use: Antidiarrheal.

•**kaolin.** (KAY-oh-lin) U.S.P. 23.
Use: Adsorbent.
W/Atropine sulfate, phenobarbital.
W/Belladonna, phenobarbital.
See: Bellkata, Tab. (Ferndale Laboratories).
W/Bismuth compound.

See: Kaomine, Pow. (Eli Lilly).
W/Bismuth subgallate.
See: Diastop, Liq. (ICN Pharm).
W/Bismuth subgallate, pectin, zinc phenolsulfonate, opium pow.
See: Diastay, Tab. (ICN Pharm).
W/Bismuth subsalicylate, salol, methyl salicylate, benzocaine, pectin.
W/Cornstarch, camphor, zinc oxide, eucalyptus oil.
See: Mexsana, Pow. (Schering Plough).
W/Furazolidone, pectin.
See: Furoxone, Liq. (Eaton Medical).
W/Hyoscyamine sulfate, sodium benzoate, atropine sulfate, hyoscine HBR, pectin.
See: Donnagel, Susp. (Robins).
W/Neomycin sulfate, pectin.
See: Pecto-Kalin, Liq. (Harvey).
W/Pectin.
See: Kaopectate, Liq. (Pharmacia & Upjohn).
Kapectin, Liq. (Health for Life Brands).
Pecto-Kalin, Susp. (Teva USA).
Pectokay Mixture (Jones Medical Industries).
W/Pectin, belladonna alkaloids.
W/Pectin, bismuth subcarbonate.
See: B-K-P Mixture, Liq. (Sutliff & Case).
W/Pectin, bismuth subcarbonate, belladonna.
See: Kay-Pec, Liq. (Case).
W/Pectin, bismuth subcarbonate, opium pow.
See: KBP/O, Cap. (Cole).
W/Pectin, bismuth subsalicylate.
W/Pectin, bismuth subsalicylate, paregoric, zinc sulfocarbolate.
W/Pectin, hyoscyamine sulfate, atropine sulfate, hyoscine HBr.
See: Kapigam, Liq. (Solvay).
Palsorb Improved, Liq. (Roberts Pharm).
W/Pectin, pow. opium extract.
See: Pecto-Kalin, Susp. (Teva USA).
W/Pectin, opium pow., bismuth subgallate, zinc phenolsulfonate.
See: Cholactabs, Tab. (Roxane).
B.P.P., Tab. (Teva USA).
W/Pectin, paregoric (equivalent).
See: Duosorb, Liq. (Solvay).
Kaoparin, Liq. (McKesson).
Kapectin, Liq. (Health for Life Brands).
Ka-Pek w/Paregoric, Liq. (APC).
Parepectolin, Susp. (Rhone-Poulenc Rorer).
W/Pectin, zinc phenolsulfonate.
See: Pectocel, Susp. (Eli Lilly).
W/Phenobarbital, atropine sulfate, aluminum hydroxide gel.
See: Kao-Lumin, Tab. (Roxane).
W/Salol, zinc sulfocarbolate, aluminum hydroxide, bismuth subsalicylate, pectin.
See: Wescola Antidiarrheal-Stomach Upset (Western Research).

kaolin colloidal.
W/Bismuth subcarbonate.
See: Bisilad, Susp. (Schwarz Pharmaceuticals).
W/Magnesium trisilicate, aluminum hydroxide dried gel.
See: Kamadrox, Tab. (ICN Pharm).
Kathmagel, Tab. (Mason).
W/Pectin, aromatics.
See: Paocin, Susp. (SmithKline Beecham Pharmaceuticals).
W/Pectin, belladonna alkaloids.
See: Kamabel, Liq. (Towne).

kaolin w/pectin. (KAY-oh-lin with PECK-tin) (Various Mfr.) Kaolin 90 g, pectin 2 g/30 ml. Susp. Bot. 180, pt, UD 30 ml. *otc.*
Use: Antidiarrheal combination.

Kaon Cl^{-}10 controlled release tablets. (Pharmacia & Upjohn) Potassium Cl 750 mg/Tab. Bot. 100s, 500s, 1000s. Stat-Pak 100s. *Rx.*
Use: Electrolyte supplement.

Kaon-Cl 20%. (Pharmacia & Upjohn) Potassium and chloride 40 mEq (to potassium Cl 3 g)/15 ml, saccharin, flavoring, alcohol 5%. Bot. pt. *Rx.*
Use: Electrolyte supplement.

Kaon Cl Controlled Release Tablets. (Pharmacia & Upjohn) Potassium Cl 500 mg/Tab., FD&C Yellow No. 5. Bot. 100s, 250s, 1000s. *Rx.*
Use: Electrolyte supplement.

Kaon Elixir. (Pharmacia & Upjohn) Elemental potassium 20 mEq (as potassium gluconate 4.68 g)/15 ml, aromatics, grape and lemon-lime flavors, alcohol 5%, saccharin. Unit pkg. pt, gal. *Rx.*
Use: Electrolyte supplement.

Kaon Tablets. (Pharmacia & Upjohn) Elemental potassium 5 mEq obtained from potassium gluconate 1.17 g/SC Tab. Bot. 100s, 500s. *Rx.*
Use: Electrolyte supplement.

Kaopectate. (Pharmacia & Upjohn) Kaolin 5.85 g, pectin 130 mg/oz. Bot. 8 oz, 12 oz, 16 oz, 1 gal, UD pkg. 3 oz. *otc.*
Use: Antidiarrheal.

Kaopectate, Advanced Formula. (Pharmacia & Upjohn) Attapulgite 750 mg/15 ml, sucrose, methylparaben, alcohol free. Regular and peppermint flavor. Liq. Bot. 354 ml. *otc.*

Use: Antidiarrheal combination.

Kaopectate, Children's. (Pharmacia & Upjohn) Attapulgite 600 mg/15 ml. Bot. 180 ml. *otc.*
Use: Antidiarrheal combination.

Kaopectate, Maximum Strength. (Pharmacia & Upjohn) Attapulgite 750 mg, Capl. Pkg. 12s, 20s. *otc.*
Use: Antidiarrheal combination.

Kaopectate Tablet Formula. (Pharmacia & Upjohn) Attapulgite 750 mg/Tab. Blister pak 12s, 20s. *otc.*
Use: Antidiarrheal.

Kaophen Tablets. (Pal-Pak) Phenobarbital 6.5 mg, belladonna extract 0.1 mg, kaolin 388.8 mg/Tab. Bot. 100s, 1000s.
Use: Antidiarrheal.

Kao-Spen. (Century Pharm) Kaolin 5.2 g, pectin 260 mg/30 ml. Susp. Bot. 120 ml, pt, gal. *otc.*
Use: Antidiarrheal.

Kao-Tin. (Major) Kaolin 5.85 g, pectin 130 mg/30 ml. Susp. Bot. 120 ml, 240 ml, pt, gal. *otc.*
Use: Antidiarrheal.

Kapectin. (Health for Life Brands) Kaolin 90 gr, pectin 2 gr/oz. Bot. gal.
Use: Antidiarrheal.

Kapectolin. (Various Mfr.) Kaolin 90 g, pectin 2 g/30 ml. Susp. Bot. 360 ml. *otc.*
Use: Antidiarrheal.

Ka-Pek. (APC) Kaolin 90 gr, pectin 4.5 gr/fl oz. Bot. 6 oz, gal. *otc.*
Use: Antidiarrheal.

kapilin.
See: Menadione (Various Mfr.).

karaya gum. (Penick) Indian Gum. Sterculia gum,
See: Tri-Costivin (Prof. Lab.).
W/Frangula.
W/Psyllium seed, plantago ovata, brewers yeast.
See: Plantamucin Gran. (ICN Pharm).
W/Cortex rhamni frangulae.
See: Movicol (Norgine).
W/Refined psyllium mucilloid.
See: Hydrocil regular (Solvay).

karaya powder. (Sween) Bot. 3 oz.
Use: Deodorant, ostomy.

Kareon.
See: Menadione (Various Mfr.).

Karidium. (Lorvic) **Tab.:** Sodium fluoride 2.21 mg, sodium Cl 94.49 mg, disintegrant 0.5 mg. Bot. 180s, 1000s. **Liq.:** Sodium fluoride 2.21 mg, sodium Cl 10 mg, purified water q.s./8 drops. Bot. 30 ml, 60 ml. *Rx.*
Use: Dental caries agent.

Karigel. (Lorvic) Fluoride ion 0.5%, pH 5.6. Gel. Bot. 30 ml, 130 ml, 250 ml. *Rx.*
Use: Dental caries agent.

Karigel-N. (Lorvic) Fluoride ion 0.5% in neutral pH gel. Bot. 24 ml, 125 ml. *Rx.*
Use: Dental caries agent.

•**kasal.** (KAY-sal) USAN. Approximately $Na_8Al_2(OH_2(PO_4)_4$ with about 30% of dibasic sodium phosphate; sodium aluminum phosphate, basic.
Use: Food additive.

Kasof. (J & J Merck Consumer Pharm) Docusate potassium 240 mg/Cap. Bot. 30s, 60s. *otc.*
Use: Laxative.

kasugamycin. Under study.
Use: Anti-infective.

Kaviton.
See: Menadione, U.S.P. 23. (Various Mfr.).

Kay Ciel Elixir. (Forest Pharmaceutical) Potassium Cl 1.5 g/15 ml. (20 mEq/15 ml), alcohol 4%. Bot. 120 ml, 473 ml, gal. *Rx.*
Use: Electrolyte supplement.

Kay Ciel Powder. (Forest Pharmaceutical) Potassium chloride 1.5 g/Packette. (20 mEq/Packet), 4% alcohol. Box 30s, 100s, 500s. *Rx.*
Use: Electrolyte supplement.

Kayexalate. (Sanofi Winthrop) Sodium polystyrene sulfonate sodium content ≈100 mg/g. Jar lb. *Rx.*
Use: Potassium removing resin.

K-C. (Century Pharm) Kaolin 5.2 g, pectin 260 mg, bismuth subcarbonate 260 mg/30 ml. Susp. Bot. 120 ml, pt, gal. *otc.*
Use: Antidiarrheal.

K + Care ET. (Alra Laboratories) Potassium bicarbonate 25 mEq/Effervescent tab. Bot. 30s, 100s, 1000s. *Rx.*
Use: Electrolyte supplement.

K-C Liquid. (Century Pharm) Kaolin 5.2 g, pectin 260 mg, bismuth subcarbonate 260 mg/oz. Bot. 4 oz, pt, gal. *otc.*
Use: Antidiarrheal.

K-C Suspension. (Century Pharm) Kaolin 5.2 g, pectin 260 mg, bismuth subcarbonate 260 mg/30 ml. Bot. 120 ml, pt, gal. *otc.*
Use: Antidiarrheal.

KCl-20. (Western Research) Potassium Cl 1.5 g (potassium 20 mEq, chloride 20 mEq)/Packet. Box 30s. *Rx.*
Use: Electrolyte supplement.

K-Dur 10 & 20. (Key Pharm) **10:** Potassium Cl 750 mg (10 mEq)/SR Tab. **20:**

Potassium Cl 1500 mg (20 mEq)/SR Tab. Bot. 100s. *Rx.*
Use: Electrolyte supplement.

KE.
See: Cortisone Acetate (Various Mfr.).

Keelamin. (Mericon) Zinc 20 mg, manganese 5 mg, copper 3 mg/Tab. Bot. 100s. *otc.*
Use: Mineral supplement.

Keflex. (Eli Lilly) **Cap.:** Cephalexin 250 mg, 500 mg/Capl. Bot. 20s, 100s (250 mg only), UD 100s. *Rx.* **Pow. for Oral Susp.:** Cephalexin 125 mg/5 ml, 250 mg/5 ml. 100 ml, 200 ml, UD 100 ml (250 mg/5 ml only).
Use: Anti-infective, cephalosporin.

Keftab. (Eli Lilly) Cephalexin HCl monohydrate 500 mg/Tab. Bot. 100s. *Rx.*
Use: Anti-infective, cephalosporin.

Kefurox. (Eli Lilly) Cefuroxime sodium 750 mg or 1.5 g/Vial. ADD-vantage and Faspak **750 mg:** Vial 10 ml, 100 ml. **1.5 g:** Vial 20 ml, 100 ml. **7.5 g:** Vial. Pharmacy bulk pkg. *Rx.*
Use: Anti-infective, cephalosporin.

Kefzol. (Eli Lilly) Cefazolin sodium. **Pow. for Inj. In Vials:** 500 mg, 1 g. **In 100 ml Bulk Vials:** 10 g, 20 g. **Inj.:** 500 mg, 1g. In 10 ml Redi-vials, Faspacks and ADD-Vantage vials. *Rx.*
Use: Cephalosporin.

Kell E. (Canright) di-α Tocopheryl 100 IU, 200 IU or 400 IU. Bot. 100s. *otc.*
Use: Vitamin supplement.

Kellogg's Tasteless Castor Oil. (SmithKline Beecham Pharmaceuticals) Castor oil 100%. Bot. 2 oz. *otc.*
Use: Laxative.

Kelp. (Arcum) Tab. Bot. 100s, 1000s.

Kelp Plus. (Barth's) Iodine from kelp plus 16 trace minerals/Tab. Bot. 100s, 500s, 1000s.

Kelp Tablets. (Faraday) Iodine from kelp 0.15 mg/Tab. Bot. 100s.

Kemadrin. (GlaxoWellcome) Procyclidine HCl 5 mg/Tab. Bot. 100s. *Rx.*
Use: Antiparkinsonian.

kemithal. Thialbarbital. 5-Allyl-5-cyclohex-2-enyl-2-thiobarbituric acid.

Kenac Cream. (NMC Labs) Triamcinolone acetonide cream 0.025% or 0.1%. Tube 15 g, 60 g, 80 g, Jar 240 g. *Rx.*
Use: Corticosteroid, topical.

Kenac Ointment. (NMC Labs) Triamcinolone acetonide ointment 0.1%. Tube 15 g, 80 g. *Rx.*
Use: Corticosteroid, topical.

Kenaject-40. (Merz) Triamcinolone acetonide 40 mg/ml/Inj. Vial 5 ml. *Rx.*
Use: Corticosteroid.

Kenakion. (Harriett Lane Home of Johns Hopkins Hospital) Vitamin K-1 oxide. *Rx.*
Use: Vitamin K-induced kernicterus.

Kenalog. (Westwood Squibb) Triamcinolone acetonide. **0.1% Cream:** Tube 15 g, 60 g, 80 g, Jar 240 g, in aqueous lotion base w/propylene glycol, cetyl and stearyl alcohols, glyceryl monostearate, sorbitan monopalmitate, polyoxyethylene sorbitan monolaurate, methylparaben, propylparaben, polyethylene glycol monostearate, simethicone, sorbic acid. **0.5% Cream:** Tube 20 g. **0.1% Oint.:** (w/base of polyethylene, mineral oil) Tube 15 g, 60 g, 80 g; Jar 240 g, **0.5% Oint.:** Tube 20 g. **0.1% Lot.:** Bot. 15ml, 60 ml. **Spray:** 6.6 mg/100 g, alcohol 10.3%. Can 23 g, 63 g. *Rx.*
Use: Corticosteroid, topical.

Kenalog 0.025%. (Westwood Squibb) Triamcinolone acetonide. **Cream:** Tube 15 g, 80 g, Jar 240 g. **Lot.:** In aqueous lotion base w/propylene glycol, cetyl and stearyl alcohols, glyceryl monostearate, sorbitan monopalmitate, polyoxyethylene sorbitan monolaurate, methylparaben, propylparaben, polyethylene glycol monostearate, simethicone, sorbic acid, tinted in an isopropyl palmitate vehicle with alcohol (4.7%). Bot. 60 ml. **Oint.:** Plastibase (w/base of polyethylene and mineral oil gel). 15 g, 80 g, 240 g. *Rx.*
Use: Corticosteroid, topical.

Kenalog-H. (Westwood Squibb) Triamcinolone acetonide cream USP 0.1%. Each g of cream provides 1 mg of triamcinolone acetonide in a specially formulated hydrophilic vanishing cream base containing propylene glycol, dimethicone 350, castor oil, cetearyl alcohol and ceteareth-20, propylene glycol stearate, white petrolatum, purified water. Tube 15 g, 60 g. *Rx.*
Use: Corticosteroid, topical.

Kenalog-10 Injection. (Squibb Diagnostic) Sterile triamcinolone acetonide suspension 10 mg/ml, sodium Cl for isotonicity, benzyl alcohol 0.9% (w/v) as a preservative, sodium carboxymethylcellulose 0.75%, polysorbate 80 0.04%. Sodium hydroxide or HCl acid may be present to adjust pH to 5 to 7.5. Nitrogen packed at the time of manufacture. Vial 5 ml. *Rx.*
Use: Corticosteroid.

Kenalog-40 Injection. (Squibb Diagnos-

tic) Sterile triamcinolone acetonide suspension 40 mg/ml, sodium chloride for isotonicity, benzyl alcohol 0.9% (w/v) as a preservative, sodium carboxymethylcellulose 0.75%, polysorbate 80 0.04%. Sodium hydroxide or HCl acid may be present to adjust pH to 5 to 7.5. Nitrogen packed at the time of manufacture. Vial 1 ml, 5 ml, 10 ml. *Rx.*
Use: Corticosteroid.

Kenalog in Orabase. (Apothecon) Triamcinolone acetonide 0.1% in Orabase. Triamcinolone acetonide 1 mg/g. Tube 5 g. *Rx.*
Use: Corticosteroid, topical.

Kendall's "Compound B".
See: Corticosterone (Various Mfr.).

Kendall's "Compound E".
See: Cortisone Acetate (Various Mfr.).

Kendall's "Compound F".
See: 17-Hydroxycorticosterone (Various Mfr.).

Kendall's "Desoxy Compound B".
See: Desoxycorticosterone Acetate (Various Mfr.).

Kenwood Therapeutic Liquid. (Kenwood Labs) Vitamins A 3333 IU, D 133 IU, E 1.5 IU, C 50 mg, B_1 2 mg, B_2 1 mg, B_3 20 mg, B_5 2 mg, B_6 0.33 mg, Ca, K, Mg, Mn, P/Liq. Bot. 240 ml. *otc.*
Use: Mineral, vitamin supplement.

keratolytics.
See: Condylox (Oclassen).

Keri Facial Soap. (Westwood Squibb) Sodium tallowate, sodium cocoate, water, mineral oil, octyl hydroxystearate, fragrance, glycerin, titanium dioxide, PEG-75, lanolin oil, docusate sodium, PEG-4 dilaurate, propylparaben, PEG-40 stearate, glyceryl monostearate, PEG-100 stearate, sodium Cl, BHT, EDTA. Bar 3.25 oz. *otc.*
Use: Dermatologic cleanser.

Keri Light Lotion. (Westwood Squibb) Water, stearyl alcohol, ceteareath-20, cetearyl octaneoate, glycerin, stearyl heptanoate, stearyl alcohol, Carbomer 934, sodium hydroxide, squalane, methylparaben, propylparaben, fragrance. Bot. 6.5 oz, 13 oz. *otc.*
Use: Emollient.

Keri Lotion. (Westwood Squibb) Mineral oil, lanolin oil, water, propylene glycol, glyceryl stearate, PEG-100 stearate, PEG 40 stearate, PEG-4 dilaurate, laureth-4, parabens, docusate sodium, triethanolamine, quaternium 15, carbomer 934, fragrance. Bot. 6.5 oz, 13 oz, 20 oz. *otc.*
Use: Emollient.

Kerlone. (Searle) Betaxolol HCl 10 mg or 25 mg/Tab. Bot. 100s, UD 100s. *Rx.*
Use: Beta-adrenergic blocker.

Kerocaine.
See: Procaine HCl (Various Mfr.).

Kerodex. (Wyeth Ayerst) *otc.*
No. 51: Water-miscible. Tube 4 oz, Jar lb.
No. 71: Water-repellent. Tube 4 oz, Jar lb.
Use: Emollient.

kerohydric. A de-waxed, oil-soluble fraction of lanolin.
Use: Emollient, cleanser.
See: Alpha-Keri, Soap, Spray (Westwood Squibb).
Keri, Cream, Lot. (Westwood Squibb).
W/Docusate sodium, sodium alkyl polyether sulfonate, sodium sulfoacetate, sulfur, salicylic acid, hexachlorophene.
See: Sebulex, Cream, Liq. (Westwood Squibb).

Kerr Insta-Char. (Kerr) **Regular:** Aqueous suspension activated charcoal 50 g/8 oz. **Pediatric:** Aqueous suspension activated charcoal 15 g/4 oz. *otc.*
Use: Antidote.

Kerr Triple Dye. (Kerr) Gentian violet, proflavine hemisulfate, brilliant green in water. Dispensing bot. 15 ml. Single Use Dispos-A-Swab 0.65 ml, Box 10s, Case 10 × 50 Box. *otc.*
Use: Antiseptic.

Kestrone 5. (Hyrex) Estrone 5 mg/ml, sodium carboxymethylcellulose, povidone, benzyl alcohol, parabens/Inj. Vial 10 ml. *Rx.*
Use: Estrogen.

Ketalar. (Monarch) Ketamine HCl, sodium Cl, benzethonium Cl. **10 mg/ml:** Vial 20 ml, 25 ml and 50 ml. Pkg. 10s; **50 mg/ml:** Vial 10 ml. **100 mg/ml:** Vial 5 ml. Pkg. 10s. *Rx.*
Use: Anesthetic, general.

•**ketamine hydrochloride.** (KEET-uh-MEEN) U.S.P. 23.
Use: Anesthetic.
See: Ketaject, Vial (Bristol-Myers Squibb).
Ketalar, Inj. (Parke-Davis).

•**ketanserin.** (KEET-AN-ser-in) USAN.
Use: Serotonin antagonist.

•**ketazocine.** (key-TAY-zoe-seen) USAN.
Use: Analgesic.

•**ketazolam.** (keet-AZE-oh-lam) USAN.
Use: Anxiolytic.

•**kethoxal.** (KEY-thox-al) USAN.
Use: Antiviral.

•**ketipramine fumarate.** (key-TIH-prah-MEEN) USAN.
Use: Antidepressant.

•**ketoconazole.** (KEY-toe-KOE-nuh-zole) U.S.P. 23.
Use: Antifungal.
See: Nizoral, Tab. (Janssen).

Ketodestrin.
See: Estrone (Various Mfr.).

Keto-Diastix Reagent Strips. (Bayer Corp) Dip and read reagent strip test for glucose and ketones in urine. Two test areas: glucose levels from 30 mg to 5000 mg/dL; Ketone test (acetoacetic acid) negative 5 mg, 40 mg, 80 mg, 160 mg/dL. Strip Bot. 50s, 100s.
Use: Diagnostic aid.

ketohexazine. 4, 6-Diethyl-3(2H)-pyridazinono (ESI Lederle Generics).
Use: Hypnotic.

ketohydroxyestratriene.
See: Estrone.

ketohydroxyestrin.
See: Estrone (Various Mfr.).

ketone tests.
Use: Diagnostic aid.
See: Acetest Reagent, Tab. (Bayer Corp).
Chemstrip K, Reagent paper (Boehringer Mannheim).
Ketostix Strips, Reagent Strips (Bayer Corp).

Ketonex-1. (Ross Laboratories) Protein 15 g, fat 23.9 g, carbohydrates 46.3 g, linoleic acid 1800 mg, Fe 9 mg, Na 190 mg, K 675 mg. With appropriate vitamins and minerals. 480 Cal/100 g. Isoleucine, leucine and valine free. Pow. Can 350 g. *otc.*
Use: Nutritional supplement.

Ketonex-2. (Ross Laboratories) Protein 30 g, fat 15.5 g, carbohydrates 30 g, Fe 13 mg, Na 880 mg, K 1370 mg. With appropriate vitamins and minerals. 410 Cal/100 g. Isoleucine, leucine and valine free. Pow. Can 325 g. *otc.*
Use: Nutritional supplement.

•**ketoprofen.** (KEY-to-pro-fen) U.S.P. 23.
Use: Anti-inflammatory.
See: Orudis, Cap. (Wyeth Ayerst).
Oruvail, Cap. (Wyeth Ayerst).

ketoprofen. (Various Mfr.) 25 mg, 50 mg, 75 mg. Cap. Bot. 100s, 500s.
Use: Anti-inflammatory.

•**ketorfanol.** (key-TAR-fan-AHL) USAN.
Use: Analgesic.

•**ketorolac tromethamine.** (KEY-TOR-oh-lak tro-METH-uh-meen) U.S.P. 23.
Use: Analgesic.
See: Toradol (Syntex).

ketorolac tromethamine. (Ethex). 10 mg/Tab. Bot. 100s. *Rx.*
Use: Analgesic.

ketorolac tromethamine.
Use: NSAID, ophthalmic.
See: Acular (Allergan).

Ketostix Reagent Strips. (Bayer Corp) Sodium nitroprusside, sodium phosphate, glycine. Stick test for ketones in urine (measures acetoacetic acid). Bot. 50s, 100s, UD 20s.
Use: Diagnostic aid.

•**ketotifen fumarate.** (KEY-toe-TIE-fen) USAN.
Use: Antiasthmatic.

Key-Plex. (Hyrex) Vitamins B_1 50 mg, B_2 5 mg, B_{12} 1000 mcg, pyridoxine HCl 5 mg, d-panthenol 6 mg, niacinamide 125 mg, ascorbic acid 50 mg/ml. Vial 10 ml. *Rx.*
Use: Nutritional supplement, parenteral.

Key-Pred. (Hyrex) Prednisolone. **25 mg/ml:** Vial 10 ml, 30 ml; **50 mg/ml:** Vial 10 ml. *Rx.*
Use: Corticosteroid.

Key-Pred-SP. (Hyrex) Prednisolone sodium phosphate 20 mg/ml. Vial 10 ml. *Rx.*
Use: Corticosteroid.

K-G Elixir. (Geneva Pharm) Potassium (as potassium gluconate) 20 mEq/15 ml, alcohol 5%. Elix. Bot. pt. *Rx.*
Use: Electrolyte supplement.

kharophen.
See: Acetarsone (Various Mfr.).

khellin.
Use: Coronary vasodilator.

Kiddie Powder. (Gordon Laboratories) Pure fine Italian talc. Can 3.5 oz. *otc.*
Use: Antifungal.

Kiddi-Vites, Improved. (Geneva Pharm) Vitamins A 5000 IU, D 500 IU, B_1 1 mg, B_2 1.5 mg, B_{12} 2 mcg, C 50 mg, B_6 1 mg, pantothenate 2 mg, niacinamide 10 mg/Tab. Bot. 100s, 1000s. *otc.*
Use: Vitamin supplement.

kidney function agents.
See: Biotel Kidney (Biotel).
Indigo Carmine Soln. (Various Mfr.).
Inulin, Amp. (Arnar-Stone).
Iodohippurate, Sodium.
Mannitol Soln., Amp. (Merck).
Methylene Blue (Various Mfr.).
Phenolsulfonphthalein (Various Mfr.).

KIE Syrup. (Laser) Potassium iodide 150 mg, ephedrine HCl 8 mg/5 ml. Syr. Bot. pt, gal. *Rx.*
Use: Decongestant, expectorant.

Kindercal. (Mead Johnson Nutritionals) Protein 13%, carbos 50%, fat 37%, sucrose, vanilla flavor, lactose free. 30 cal/oz. Liq. Cans 8 oz. *otc.*
Use: Nutritional supplement.

kinate. Hexahydrotetra hydroxybenzoate salt, quinic acid salt.

Kinevac. (Bristol-Myers Squibb) Sincalide 5 mcg/vial. For gallbladder, pancreatic secretion and cholecystography.
Use: Diagnostic aid.

Kin White. (Whiteworth Towne) Triamcinolone acetonide. **Cream:** 0.025% or 1%. Tube 15 g, 80 g. **Oint.:** 1%. Tube 15 g, 80 g. *Rx.*
Use: Corticosteroid, topical.

•**kitasamycin.** (kit-ah-sah-MY-sin) USAN. An antibiotic substance obtained from cultures of *Streptomyces kitasatoensis.* Under study.
Use: Anti-infective.

Klaron. (Dermik Laboratories) Sodium sulfacetamide 10%, propylene glycol, polyethylene glycol 400, methylparaben, EDTA/Lot. Bot. 59 ml. *Rx.*
Use: Dermatologic.

Klavikordal. (U.S. Ethicals) Nitroglycerin 2.6 mg/SR Tab. Bot. 100s, 1000s. *Rx.*
Use: Antianginal.

KLB6 Complete. (NBTY) Vitamins A 833.3 IU, E 5 mg (as IU), B_3 3.3 mg, C 10 mg, soya lecithin 200 mg, kelp 25 mg, cider vinegar 40 mg, wheat bran 83.3 mg, D 66.7 IU, FA 0.067 mg, B_1 0.25 mg, B_2 0.28 mg, B_6 8.3 mg, B_{12} 1 mcg, biotin 0.05 mg/Tab. Bot. 100s. *otc.*
Use: Vitamin supplement.

KLB6 Softgels. (NBTY) Vitamin B_6 mcg, soya lecithin 100 mg, kelp 25 mg, cider vinegar 80 mg/Capl. Bot. 100s. *otc.*
Use: Vitamin supplement.

K-Lease. (Pharmacia & Upjohn) Potassium chloride 10 mEq (750 mg). ER Cap. Bot. 100s, 500s, 1000s, 2500s, UD 100s. *Rx.*
Use: Electrolyte supplement.

Kleen-Handz. (American Medical) Ethyl alcohol 62%, aloe vera, purified water. Sol. Bot. 60 ml. *otc.*
Use: Antiseptic.

Kleer Compound. (Scrip) Acetaminophen 300 mg, phenylpropanolamine HCl 35 mg, guaifenesin. Tab. Bot. 100s. *otc.*
Use: Analgesic, decongestant, expectorant.

Kleer Improved. (Scrip) Atropine sulfate 0.2 mg, chlorpheniramine maleate 5 mg/ml. *Rx.*
Use: Anticholinergic, antihistamine.

Klerist-D. (Nutripharm) **Cap. SR:** Pseudoephedrine HCl 120 mg, chlorpheniramine maleate 8 mg. Bot. 100s, 500s. **Tab.:** Pseudoephedrine HCl 60 mg, chlorpheniramine maleate 4 mg. Bot. 24s, 100s. *Rx.*
Use: Antihistamine, decongestant.

Kler-Ro Liquid. (Ulmer) Surgical cleanser and laboratory detergent. Bot. gal.
Use: Antiseptic.

Kler-Ro Powder. (Ulmer) Surgical cleanser and laboratory detergent. Can 2 lb, Bot. 6 lb.
Use: Antiseptic.

KL4-Surfactant. (Acute Therapeutics)
Use: Treatment of acute respiratory distress syndrome. [Orphan drug]

Klonopin. (Roche Laboratories) Clonazepam 0.5 mg, 1 mg or 2 mg, lactose/Tab. 100s. *c-IV.*
Use: Anticonvulsant.

K-Lor. (Abbott Laboratories) Potassium Cl equivalent to potassium 20 mEq and Cl 20 mEq/2.6 g for oral soln. w/ saccharin. Pkg. 30s, 100s. 15 mEq/2 g Pkg. 100s. *Rx.*
Use: Electrolyte supplement.

Klor-Con 8. (Upsher-Smith Labs) Potassium Cl 8 mEq/ER Tab. Bot. 100s, 500s. *Rx.*
Use: Electrolyte supplement.

Klor-Con 10. (Upsher-Smith Labs) Potassium Cl 10 mEq/ER Tab. Bot. 100s, 500s. *Rx.*
Use: Electrolyte supplement.

Klor-Con/25 Powder. (Upsher-Smith Labs) Potassium Cl for oral soln 25 mEq/Pkt. Carton 30s, 100s, 250s. *Rx.*
Use: Electrolyte supplement.

Klor-Con/EF. (Upsher-Smith Labs) Potassium bicarbonate 25 mEq/Tab. Carton 30s, 100s. *Rx.*
Use: Electrolyte supplement.

Klor-Con Powder. (Upsher-Smith Labs) Potassium Cl for oral soln. 20 mEq/ Packet w/saccharin. Packet 1.5 g. Box 30s, 100s. *Rx.*
Use: Electrolyte supplement.

Klorvess Effervescent Granules. (Novartis) Potassium 20 mEq, Cl 20 mEq supplied by potassium Cl 1.125 g, potassium bicarbonate 0.5 g, L-lysine monohydrochloride 0.913 g/Packet. w/ saccharin. Box 30s. *Rx.*
Use: Electrolyte supplement.

Klorvess Effervescent Tablets. (Novartis) Potassium Cl 1.125 g, potassium bi-

carbonate 0.5 g, L-lysine HCl 0.913 g/ Effervescent Tab. Sodium and sugar free. w/saccharin. Pkg. 60s, 1000s. *Rx.*
Use: Electrolyte supplement.

Klorvess Liquid. (Novartis) Potassium Cl 1.5 g (20 mEq)/15 ml, alcohol 0.75%. Bot. pt. *Rx.*
Use: Electrolyte supplement.

Klotrix. (Bristol-Myers) Potassium Cl 10 mEq/SR Tab. Bot. 100s, 1000s, UD 100s. *Rx.*
Use: Electrolyte supplement.

K-Lyte. (Bristol-Myers Squibb) Potassium bicarbonate and citrate 25 mEq, saccharin. Lime and orange flavors. Effervescent Tab. Pkg. 30s, 100s, 250s. *Rx.*
Use: Electrolyte supplement.

K-Lyte/Cl. (Bristol-Myers Squibb) Potassium Cl 25 mEq, saccharin. Citrus and fruit punch flavor. Effervescent Tab. Pkg. 30s, 100s, 250s. Bulk powder 225 g/Can. *Rx.*
Use: Electrolyte supplement.

K-Lyte/Cl 50. (Bristol-Myers Squibb) Potassium Cl 50 mEq, saccharin. Citrus and fruit punch flavors. Pkg. 30s, 100s. *Rx.*
Use: Electrolyte supplement.

K-Lyte DS. (Bristol-Myers Squibb) Potassium bicarbonate and citrate 50 mEq, saccharin. Lime and orange flavor. Effervescent Tab. Pkg. 30s, 100s. *Rx.*
Use: Electrolyte supplement.

K-Norm. (Fisons) Potassium Cl 10 mEq/ CR Cap. Bot. 100s, 500s. *Rx.*
Use: Electrolyte supplement.

Koate HP. (Bayer Corp) A stable dried concentrate of Anti-hemophilic Factor. When reconstituted, contains heparin ≤ 5 U/ml, PEG ≤ 1500 ppm, glycine ≤ 0.05 M glycine, polysorbate 80 ≤ 25 ppm, calcium chloride ≤ 3 mM, aluminum ≤ 1 ppm, histidine ≤ 0.06 M, albumin (human) ≤ 10 mg/ml. Includes Sterile Water for Injection, double-ended transfer needle, filter needle and administration set. Pow. Bot. 250, 500, 1000 and 1500 IU Factor VIII activity (approximate). *Rx.*
Use: Antihemophilic.

Kodonyl Expectorant. (Halsey) Bromodiphenhydramine HCl 3.75 mg, diphenhydramine HCl 8.75 mg, ammonium Cl 80 mg, potassium guaiacolsulfonate 80 mg, menthol 0.5 mg/5 ml. Bot. 16 oz. *otc.*
Use: Antihistamine, expectorant.

Kof-Eze. (Roberts Pharm) Menthol 6 mg. Loz. Pkg. 4s, Bot. 500s. *otc.*
Use: Mouth and throat preparation.

Kogenate. (Bayer Corp) Recombinant antihemophilic factor (Factor VIII). Pow. for inj. Bot. 250 IU, 500 IU, 1000 IU. *Rx.*
Use: Antihemophilic.

Kolephrin Caplets. (Pfeiffer) Pseudoephedrine HCl 30 mg, chlorpheniramine maleate 2 mg, acetaminophen 325 mg/Capl. Bot. 24s, 36s. *otc.*
Use: Analgesic, antihistamine, decongestant.

Kolephrin/DM Caplets. (Pfeiffer) Pseudoephedrine HCl 30 mg, chlorpheniramine maleate 2 mg, dextromethorphan HBr 10 mg, acetaminophen 325 mg/Capl. Bot. 30s. *otc.*
Use: Analgesic, antihistamine, antitussive, decongestant.

Kolephrin GG/DM Expectorant. (Pfeiffer) Dextromethorphan HBr 10 mg, guaifenesin 150 mg/5 ml. Alcohol free. Bot. 120 ml. *otc.*
Use: Antitussive, expectorant.

Kolephrin NN Liquid. (Pfeiffer) Phenylpropanolamine HCl 12.5 mg, pyrilamine maleate 10 mg, dextromethorphan HBr 7.5 mg/5 ml. Alcohol free. Bot. 120 ml. *otc.*
Use: Antihistamine, antitussive, decongestant.

•**kolfocon a.** (KAHL-FOE-kahn A) USAN.
Use: Contact lens material (hydrophobic).

•**kolfocon b.** (KAHL-FOE-kahn B) USAN.
Use: Contact lens material (hydrophobic).

•**kolfocon c.** (KAHL-FOE-kahn C) USAN.
Use: Contact lens material (hydrophobic).

•**kolfocon d.** (KAHL-FOE-kahn D) USAN.
Use: Contact lens material (hydrophobic).

Kolyum Liquid. (Fisons) Potassium ion 20 mEq, chloride ion 3.4 mEq from potassium gluconate 3.9 g, potassium Cl 0.25 g/15 ml or 5 g/15 ml. w/saccharin, sorbitol. **Liq.:** Bot. pt, gal. *Rx.*
Use: Electrolyte supplement.

Kondon's Nasal Jelly. (Kondon) Tube 20 g w/ephedrine alkaloid. Tube 20 g. *otc.*
Use: Decongestant.

Kondremul. (Fisons) Mineral oil 55%, Irish moss. Emulsion Bot. pt. *otc.*
Use: Laxative.

W/Phenolphthalein 2.2 gr/Tbsp. Bot. pt.
W/Cascara 0.66 g/15 ml. Bot. 14 oz.

Konsto. (Freeport) Docusate sodium 100

mg/Cap. Bot. 1000s. *otc.*
Use: Laxative.

Konsyl-D Powder. (Konsyl Pharm) Psyllium hydrophilic mucilloid, dextrose. Canister 325 g, 500 g, Packet 6.5 g, Ctn. 25s. *otc.*
Use: Laxative.

Konsyl Fiber. (Konsyl Pharm) Calcium polycarbophil 625 mg/Tab. Bot. 90s. *otc.*
Use: Laxative.

Konsyl-Orange. (Konsyl Pharm) Psyllium fiber 3.4 g/Tbsp., sucrose, orange flavor. Pow. 12 g, 538 g. *otc.*
Use: Laxative.

Konsyl Powder. (Konsyl Pharm) Psyllium hydrophyllic mucilloid. Canister 300 g, 450 g, Packet 6 g, Ctn. 25s. *otc.*
Use: Laxative

Konyne 80. (Bayer Corp) Dried plasma fraction of coagulation factors II, VII, IX and X. Heparin free. Heat treated. Vial. 10 ml and 20 ml. *Rx.*
Use: Antihemophilic.

Kophane Cough & Cold Formula Liquid. (Pfeiffer) Phenylpropanolamine HCl 12.5 mg, chlorpheniramine maleate 2 mg, dextromethorphan HBr 10 mg. Bot. 120 ml. *otc.*
Use: Antihistamine, antitussive, decongestant.

Koro-Flex. (Holland-Rantos) Improved contouring spring natural latex diaphrag 60 mm-95 mm.
Use: Contraceptive.

Koromex Coil Spring Diaphragm. (Holland-Rantos) Diaphragm made of pure latex rubber, cadmium plated coil spring. Koromex Jelly and Cream/kit. 50 mm-95 mm at graduations of 5 mm.
Use: Contraceptive.

Koromex Combination. (Holland-Rantos) Diaphrag 50 mm-95 mm, Koromex Jelly and Cream/Kit.
Use: Contraceptive.

Koromex Crystal Clear Gel. (Schmid) Nonoxynol-9 2%. Tube 126 g with or without applicator. *otc.*
Use: Contraceptive.

Koromex Jelly. (Schmid) Nonoxynol-9 3%. Vaginal Jelly. 126 g. *otc.*
Use: Contraceptive, spermicide.

Korum. (Geneva Pharm) Acetaminophen 5 gr/Tab. Bot. 1000s. *otc.*
Use: Analgesic.

Kotabarb. (Wesley Pharmacal) Phenobarbital 1/4 gr/Tab. Bot. 1000s. *Rx.*
Use: Hypnotic, sedative.

Kovitonic Liquid. (Freeda Vitamins) Iron 42 mg, vitamins B_1 5 mg, B_6 10 mg, B_{12} 30 mcg, folic acid 0.1 mg, l-lysine 10 mg/15 ml. Liq. Bot. 120 ml, 240 ml. *otc.*
Use: Mineral, vitamin supplement.

K-Pek. (Rugby) Attapulgite 600 mg/15 ml. Susp. Bot. 237 ml, pt, gal. *otc.*
Use: Antidiarrheal.

K-Phos M.F. (Beach Pharmaceuticals) Potassium acid phosphate 155 mg, sodium acid phosphate 350 mg/Tab. Bot. 100s, 500s. *Rx.*
Use: Acidifier, urinary.

K-Phos Neutral. (Beach Pharmaceuticals) Dibasic sodium phosphate 852 mg, potassium acid phosphate 155 mg, sodium acid phosphate 130 mg/Tab. Bot. 100s, 500s. *Rx.*
Use: Mineral supplement.

K-Phos No. 2. (Beach Pharmaceuticals) Potassium acid phosphate 305 mg, sodium acid phosphate, anhydrous 700 mg/Tab. Bot. 100s, 500s. *Rx.*
Use: Acidifier, urinary.

K-Phos Original. (Beach Pharmaceuticals) Potassium acid phosphate 500 mg/Tab. Bot. 100s, 500s. *Rx.*
Use: Urinary acidifier, electrolyte supplement.

K.P.N. (Freeda Vitamins) Vitamins C 333 mg, Fe 11 mg, A 2667 IU, D 133 IU, E 10 mg, B_1 2 mg, B_2 2 mg, B_3 10 mg, B_5 3.3 mg, B_6 0.83 mg, B_{12} 2 mcg, C 33 mg, FA 0.27 mg, I, Cu, Mn, K, Mg, Zn 6.7 mg, bioflavonoids/Tab. Bot. 100s, 250s, 500s. *otc.*
Use: Mineral, vitamin supplement.

K-P Suspension. (Century Pharm) Kaolin 5.2 g, pectin 260 mg/oz. Bot. gal. *otc.*
Use: Antidiarrheal.

Kronofed-A. (Ferndale Laboratories) Pseudoephedrine HCl 120 mg, chlorpheniramine maleate 8 mg/Cap. Bot. 100s, 500s. *Rx.*
Use: Antihistamine, decongestant.

Kronofed-A Jr. (Ferndale Laboratories) Pseudoephedrine HCl 60 mg, chlorpheniramine maleate 4 mg/Cap. Bot. 100s, 500s. *Rx.*
Use: Antihistamine, decongestant.

Kronohist Kronocaps. (Ferndale Laboratories) Chlorpheniramine maleate 4 mg, pyrilamine maleate 25 mg, phenylpropanolamine HCl 50 mg/Cap. Bot. 100s, 1000s. *otc.*
Use: Antihistamine, decongestant.

•**krypton clathrate Kr 85.** (KRIPP-tahn KLATH-rate) USAN.

Use: Radiopharmaceutical.

•**krypton Kr 81m.** (KRIP-tahn Kr 81 m) U.S.P. 23.
Use: Radiopharmaceutical.

K-Tab. (Abbott Laboratories) Potassium Cl (10 mEq) 750 mg/ER Tab. Bot. 100s, 1000s, UD 100s. *Rx.*
Use: Electrolyte supplement.

K.T.V. Tablets. (Knight) Vitamin B_{12}, minerals. Bot. 50s. *otc.*
Use: Mineral, vitamin supplement.

Kudrox Double Strength Suspension. (Schwarz Pharma) Aluminum hydroxide 500 mg, magnesium hydroxide 450 mg, simethicone 40 mg/5 ml. Bot. 355 ml. *otc.*
Use: Antacid.

Kutapressin. (Kremers Urban) Liver derivative complex composed of peptides and amino acids. Inj. Vial 20 ml. *Rx.*
Use: Nutritional supplement.

Kutrase. (Kremers Urban) Amylase 30 mg, protease 6 mg, lipase 25 mg, cellulase 2 mg, l-hyoscyamine sulfate 0.0625 mg, phenyltoloxamine citrate 15 mg/Cap. Bot. 100s, 500s. *Rx.*
Use: Digestive aid.

Ku-Zyme. (Kremers Urban) Amylase 30 mg, protease 6 mg, lipase 75 mg, cellulase 2 mg/Cap. Bot. 100s, 500s. *Rx.*
Use: Digestive aid.

Ku-Zyme HP. (Kremers Urban) Lipase 8000 units, protease 30,000 units, amylase 30,000 units/Cap. Bot. 100s. *Rx.*
Use: Digestive aid.

Kwelcof. (B.F. Ascher) Hydrocodone bitartrate 5 mg, guaifenesin 100 mg/5 ml. Bot. pt, UD 5 ml. Pkg. 10s, 100s. Alcohol, dye, sugar, and corn free. *c-III.*
Use: Antitussive, expectorant.

Kwikderm Cream. (NMC Labs) Tolnaftate 1%. Cream. Tube 15 g. *otc.*
Use: Antifungal, topical.

Kwikderm Solution. (NMC Labs) Tolnaftate 1%. Soln. Bot. 10 ml.
Use: Antifungal, topical.

Kwildane Shampoo. (Major) Gamma benzene hexachloride 1%. Bot. 60 ml, pt, gal.
Use: Pediculicide.

K-Y. (Johnson & Johnson Consumer Products) Glycerin, methylparaben, hydroxyethylcellulose. Sterile or regular. Jelly Tube 12 g, 60 g, 120 g. *otc.*
Use: Lubricant.

Kyodex Reagent Strips. (Kyoto) A disposable plastic reagent strip for determination of glucose in whole blood. Vial 25s.
Use: Diagnostic aid.

Kyotest UG Reagent Strips. (Kyoto) Reagent strips for glucose and ketones in urine.
Use: Diagnostic aid.

Kyotest UGK Reagent Strip. (Kyoto) Disposable reagent strip for measurement of glucose and ketones in the urine. Vial 50s, 100s.
Use: Diagnostic aid.

Kyotest UK Reagent Strips. (Kyoto) Reagent strip for ketones in urine. Vial 50s.
Use: Diagnostic aid.

KY Plus. (Johnson & Johnson Consumer Products) Nonoxynol-9 2%, methylparaben. Non-greasy. 113 g. *otc.*
Use: Lubricant.

Kytril. (SmithKline Beecham Pharmaceuticals) Granisetron HCl. **Inj.:** 1.12 mg/ml. Inj. Single-use vial 1 ml, 4 ml multidose vial (w/benzyl alcohol). **Tab:** 1.12 mg/Tab. Pkg. 20s, unit-of-use 2s. *Rx.*
Use: Antiemetic (cancer therapy).

L

LA-12. (Hyrex) Hydroxocobalamin 1000 mcg/ml. Vial 30 ml. *Rx.*
Use: Vitamin supplement.

•**labetalol hydrochloride.** (la-BET-ul-lahl) U.S.P. 23.
Use: Antihypertensive, antiadrenergic, (α-receptor, β-receptor).
See: Normodyne, Inj., Tab. (Schering Plough).
Trandate Inj., Tab. (GlaxoWellcome).
W/Hydrochlorothiazide.
See: Trandate HCT, Tab. (GlaxoWellcome).
Normodyne, Inj., Tab. (Schering Plough).

Labstix Reagent Strips. (Bayer Corp) Urine screening test. Bot 100s.
Use: Diagnostic aid.

Lac-Hydrin Lotion. (Westwood Squibb) Lactic acid 12% neutralized w/ammonium hydroxide, light mineral oil, cetyl alcohol, parabens. Tube 150 ml, 360 ml. *Rx.*
Use: Emollient.

•**lacidipine.** (lah-SIH-dih-PEEN) USAN.
Use: Antihypertensive.

Laclede Cleaner. (Laclede) Container. 2 lb.
Use: Detergent.

Laclede Disclosing Swab. (Laclede) Swabs 6″. 100s, 500s, 1000s.
Use: Dentrifice.

Laclede Topi-Fluor A.P.F. Topical Cream. (Laclede) Fluoride ion 1.23% (from sodium fluoride) in orthophosphoric acid 0.98%. Jar 50 ml, 500 ml, 1000 ml, 2000 ml. *Rx.*
Use: Dental caries agent.

Lacotein. (Christina) Protein digest 5% w/preservatives. Vial 30 ml (w/iodochin), Vial 30 ml. *Rx.*
Use: Protein supplement.

Lacril. (Allergan) Hydroxypropyl methylcellulose 0.5%, gelatin A 0.01%, chlorobutanol 0.5%, polysorbate 80, dextrose, magnesium Cl, sodium borate, sodium chloride. Soln. Dropper bot. 15 ml. *otc.*
Use: Lubricant, ophthalmic.

Lacri-Lube NP. (Allergan) White petrolatum 55.5%, mineral oil 42.5%, petrolatum/lanolin alcohol 2%. Oint. 0.7 g. *otc.*
Use: Lubricant, ophthalmic.

Lacri-Lube S.O.P. (Allergan) White petrolatum 56.8%, mineral oil 41.5%, lanolin alcohols, chlorobutanol. Tube 3.5 g, 7 g. *otc.*
Use: Lubricant, ophthalmic.

Lacrisert. (Merck) Hydroxypropyl cellulose 5 mg/insert. Pkg. 60s w/applicators. *Rx.*
Use: Artificial tears.

LactAid. (Ortho McNeil) **Liq.:** Beta-D-galactosidase derived from *Kluyveromyces lactis* yeast (1000 Neutral Lactase units/5 drop dosage) in carrier of glycerol 50%, water 30%, inert yeast dry matter 20%. Units of 4, 12, 30 and 75 one-quart dosages at 5 drops/dose. **Tab.:** Beta-D-galactosidase from *Aspergillus oryzae* (3300 FCC lactase units/Tab.) In 12s, 100s. *otc.*
Use: Digestive aid.

lactalbumin hydrolysate.
See: Aminonat.

lactase enzyme.
Use: Digestive aid.
See: LactAid, Capl. Liq. (Ortho McNeil).
Lactogest, Cap. (Thompson Medical).
Lactrase, Cap. (Schwarz Pharma).
Dairy Ease, Tabs. (Sanofi Winthrop).
SureLac, Tab. (Caraco).

lactated ringer's injection.
Use: Electrolyte, fluid replacement; alkalizer, systemic.

•**lactic acid.** (LACK-tick) U.S.P. 23.
Use: Pharmaceutic necessity for sodium lactate injection.
See: Penecare, Cream, Lot. (Reed & Carnrick).
W/Sodium pyrrolidone carboxylate.
See: LactiCare (Stiefel).
Lactinol, Lot. Creme (Pedinol).

LactiCare Lotion. (Stiefel) Lactic acid 5%, sodium pyrrolidone carboxylate 2.5% in an emollient lotion base. Bot. 8 oz, 12 oz, w/pump dispenser. *otc.*
Use: Emollient.

LactiCare-HC Lotion. (Stiefel) Hydrocortisone lotion 1% or 2.5%. **1%:** Bot 4 oz. **2.5%:** Bot. 2 oz. *Rx.*
Use: Corticosteroid, topical.

Lactinex. (Becton Dickinson) *Lactobacillus acidophilus & Lactobacillus bulgaricus* mixed culture. Tab. 250 mg, Bot. 50s. Gran. 1 g pk. Box 12s. *otc.*
Use: Antidiarrheal, nutritional supplement.

Lactinol. (Pedinol) Lactic acid 10%. Lot. Bot. 237 ml. *Rx.*
Use: Emollient.

Lactinol-E Creme. (Pedinol) Lactic acid 10%, Vitamin E 3500 IU/30 g. Cream 56.7 g. *Rx.*
Use: Emollient.

lactobacillus acidophilus. Preparation made from acid-producing bacterium.
Use: Antidiarrheal, nutritional supplement.
See: Bacid (Novartis Pharmaceuticals).
DoFUS (Miller).
More Dophilus (Freeda Vitamins).
Pro-Bionate (Natren).
Superdophilus (Natren).

lactobacillus acidophilus & bulgaricus mixed culture.
See: Lactinex, Tab., Gran. (Becton Dickinson).

lactobacillus acidophilus, viable culture.
See: DoFus, Tab. (Miller).
Lactinex Granules, Tab. (Becton Dickinson).

lactobin. (Roxane)
Use: AIDS-associated diarrhea. [Orphan drug]

Lactocal-F. (Laser) Vitamin A 4000 IU, D 400 IU, E 30 IU, C 100 mg, folic acid 1 mg, B_1 3 mg, B_2 3.4 mg, B_3 20 mg, B_6 5 mg, B_{12} 12 mcg, calcium 200 mg, I, iron 65 mg, Mg, Cu, zinc 15 mg/Tab. Bot. 100s, 1000s. *Rx.*
Use: Mineral, vitamin supplement.

lactoflavin.
See: Riboflavin, U.S.P. 23. (Various Mfr.).

Lactofree. (Bristol-Myers) Protein 14.7 g, carbohydrates 69.3 g, fat 36.7 g, linoleic acid 6 g, Fe 12 mg, Na 200 mg, K 733.3 mg, with appropriate vitamins and minerals. Lactose free. 666.7 cal/L. Pow. Can 400 g. *otc.*
Use: Nutritional supplement, enteral.

lactose. Milk sugar.
Use: Pharmaceutic aid (tablet and capsule diluent).
See: Natur-Aid, Pow. (Scott/Cord).

•**lactose anhydrous.** (LACK-tohs an-HIGH-druss) N.F. 18.
Use: Pharmaceutic aid (tablet and capsule diluent).

•**lactose monohydrate.** N.F. 18.
Use: Pharmaceutic aid (tablet and capsule diluent).

Lactrase. (Rhone-Poulenc Rorer) Standardized enzyme lactase (β-D-galactosidase) 125 mg dispersed in maltodextrins. Cap. Bot. 100s. *otc.*
Use: Nutritional supplement.

Lactrodectus Mactans Antivenin. (Merck) Antivenin 6000 units per vial (with 1:10,000 thimersol), supplied with a 2.5 ml vial of Sterile Water for Injection and a 1 mg vial (with 1:10,000 thimersol) of normal horse serum (1:10 dilution) for sensitivity testing. *Rx.*
Use: Antivenin (Black Widow spider).
See: antivenin (Lactrodectus Mactans).

•**lactulose concentrate.** (LAK-tyoo-lohs) U.S.P. 23.
Use: Laxative, treatment of hepatic coma and chronic constipation.
See: Cephulac, Syr. (Hoechst Marion Roussel).
Chronulac, Liq. (Hoechst Marion Roussel).
Evalose, Syr. (Copley).
Heptalac, Syr. (Copley).

ladakamycin.
Use: Refractory acute myelogenous leukemia (AML) agent.
See: Azacitidine.

Ladogal. (Sanofi Winthrop) Danazol. *Rx.*
Use: Androgen.

Ladogar. (Sanofi Winthrop) Danazol. *Rx.*
Use: Androgen.

Lady Esther. (Menley & James) Mineral oil. Cream. 120 g. *otc.*
Use: Emollient.

L.A.E. 20. (Seatrace) Estradiol valerate 20 mg/ml. Vial 10 ml. *Rx.*
Use: Estrogen.

L.A.E. 40. (Seatrace) Estradiol valerate 40 mg/ml. Vial 10 ml. *Rx.*
Use: Estrogen.

Lamictal. (GlaxoWellcome) Lamotrigine 25 mg, 100 mg, 150 mg or 200 mg/Tab. Bot. 25s (25 mg), 60s (150 mg, 200 mg), 100s (100 mg). *Rx.*
Use: Anticonvulsant.

•**lamifiban.** (la-mih-FIE-ban) USAN.
Use: Antithrombotic, platelet aggregation inhibitor, fibrinogen receptor antagonist.

Lamisil. (Novartis) Terbinafine HCl. 1%. Cream/Tube 15 and 30 g. 250 mg/Tab. Bot. 30s and 100s.
Use: Antifungal.

•**lamivudine.** (la-MIH-view-deen) USAN.
Use: Antiviral; treatment of HIV infection.
See: Epivir, Tab., Oral Soln. (GlaxoWellcome).

lamivudine and zidovudine.
Use: AIDS.
See: Combivir, Tab. (GlaxoWellcome).

•**lamotrigine.** (lah-MOE-trih-JEEN) USAN.
Use: Anticonvulsant; Lennox-Gestaut syndrome. [Orphan drug]
See: Lamictal, Tab. (GlaxoWellcome)

Lampit. (Bayer 2502) Nifurtimox.
Use: Anti-infective.

Lamprene. (Novartis Pharmaceuticals)

Clofazimine 50 mg/Cap. Bot. 100s. *Rx.*
Use: Leprostatic.

Lanabiotic. (Combe) Polymyxin B sulfate 5000 units, neomycin (as sulfate) 3.5 mg, bacitracin 500 units, lidocaine 40 mg/g. Oint. 15 g, 30 g. *otc.*
Use: Anti-infective, anesthetic, local.

Lanacane. (Combe) Spray: Benzocaine 20%, benzethonium Cl, ethanol, aloe extract. 113 ml. Cream: Benzocaine 6%, benzethonium Cl, aloe, parabens, castor oil, glycerin, isopropyl alcohol. 28 g, 56 g. *otc.*
Use: Anesthetic, local.

Lanacort 10. (Combe) Hydrocortisone acetate 1% **Cream.** Tube 15, 30 g. **Oint.** Tube 15 g. *otc.*
Use: Corticosteroid, topical.

Lanacort Cream. (Combe) Hydrocortisone acetate 0.5%. Tube 0.5 oz, 1 oz. *otc.*
Use: Corticosteroid, topical.

Lanaphilic Ointment. (Medco Lab) Sorbitol, isopropyl palmitate, stearyl alcohol, white petrolatum, lanolin oil, sodium lauryl sulfate, propylene glycol, methylparaben, propylparaben. Jar 16 oz. Also available w/urea 10% or 20%. *otc.*
Use: Emollient.

Lanaphilic w/Urea 10%. (Medco Lab) Urea, stearyl alcohol, white petrolatum, isopropyl palmitate, propylene glycol, sorbitol, sodium lauryl sulfate, lactic acid, parabens. Oint. Jar lb. *otc.*
Use: Emollient.

•**lanolin.** (LAN-oh-lin) U.S.P. 23. *Formerly Anhydrous lanolin.*
Use: Pharmaceutic aid (ointment base, absorbant).
See: Kerohydric (Westwood Squibb).
W/Coconut oil, pine oil, castor oil, cholesterols, lecithin and parachlorometaxylenol.
See: Sebacide, Liq. (Paddock).
W/Diiosbutylcresoxyethoxyethyl, dimethyl benzyl ammonium Cl, menthol.
See: Hospital Lot. (Paddock).

•**lanolin alcohols.** N.F. 18.
Use: Pharmaceutic aid (emulsifying agent).

•**lanolin, modified.** U.S.P. 23.
Use: Pharmaceutic aid (ointment base, absorbant).

Lanoline. (GlaxoWellcome) Perfumed emollient. Oint. Tube 1.75 oz. *otc.*
Use: Pharmaceutic aid, ointment base, absorbant, emollient.

Lano-Lo Bath Oil. (Whorton) 8 oz.

Lanolor. (Numark Laboratories) Cream. Jar 8 oz, tube 2 oz. *otc.*
Use: Emollient.

Lanorinal. (Lannett) Aspirin 325 mg, caffeine 40 mg, butalbitaL 50 mg. Cap., Tab. Bot. 100s (Cap. only), 1000s. *c-III.*

•**lanoteplase.** (lan-OH-teh-place) USAN.
Use: Thrombolytic, plasminogen activator.

Lanoxicaps. (GlaxoWellcome) Digoxin 0.05 mg, 0.1 mg, 0.2 mg. Soln. in cap. Bot. 100s. *Rx.*
Use: Cardiovascular agent.

Lanoxin. (GlaxoWellcome) Digoxin. **Tab. 0.125 mg:** Bot. 100s, 1000s, Unit-of-use 30s, UD 100s. **0.25 mg:** Bot. 100s, 1000s, 5000s, UD 100s, Unit-of-use 30s. **Pediatric Elix.:** 0.05 mg/ml, alcohol 10%. Bot. 60 ml. **Inj.:** (w/propylene glycol 40%, alcohol 10%, sodium phosphate 0.3%, anhydrous citric acid 0.08%) Amp. 0.5 mg/2 ml. Amp. 10s, 50s. **Pediatric Inj.:** 0.1 mg/ml. Amp. 1 ml 10s. *Rx.*
Use: Cardiovascular agent.

•**lanreotide acetate.** (lan-REE-oh-tide) USAN.
Use: Antineoplastic.

•**lansoprazole.** (lan-SO-pruh-zole) USAN.
Use: Gastric acid pump inhibitor, antiulcerative, maintenance of healing of erosive esophagitis and gastric ulcers.
See: Prevacid, Cap. (TAP Pharm).

Lanturil. (Sanofi Winthrop) Oxypertine. *Rx.*
Use: Anxiolytic.

lanum. (Various Mfr.) Lanolin. *otc.*
Use: Pharmaceutic aid.

•**lapyrium chloride.** (LAH-pihr-ee-uhm KLOR-ide) USAN.
Use: Pharmaceutic aid (surfactant).

Lardet. (Standex) Phenobarbital 8 mg, theophylline 130 mg, ephedrine HCl 24 mg/Tab. Bot. 100s. *Rx.*
Use: Antiasthmatic combination.

Lardet Expectorant. (Standex) Phenobarbital 8 mg, theophylline 130 mg, ephedrine HCl 24 mg, guaifenesin 100 mg/Tab. Bot. 100s. *Rx.*
Use: Antiasthmatic combination.

Largon. (Wyeth Ayerst) Propiomazine HCl 20 mg/ml w/ sodium formaldehyde sulfoxylate, sodium acetate buffer. Amp. 1 ml, 2 ml. Pkg. 25s, Tubex syringe 1 ml. *Rx.*
Use: Hypnotic, sedative.

Lariam. (Roche Laboratories) Mefloquine HCl 250 mg/Tab. UD 25s. *Rx.*
Use: Antimalarial.

Larodopa Capsules. (Roche Laboratories) Levodopa 100 mg, 250 mg or 500 mg/Cap. **100 mg:** Bot. 100s. **250 mg:** Bot. 100s, 500s. **500 mg:** Bot. 100s, 500s. *Rx.*
Use: Antiparkinsonian.

Larodopa Tablets. (Roche Laboratories) Levodopa 100 mg, 250 mg or 500 mg. **100 mg:** Bot. 100s. **250 mg and 500 mg:** Bot. 100s, 500s. *Rx.*
Use: Antiparkinsonian.

Larotid. (SmithKline Beecham Pharmaceuticals) Amoxicillin. **Cap.: 250 mg:** Bot. 100s, 500s, UD 100s, unit-of-use 18s. **500 mg:** Bot. 50s, 500s. **Oral Susp.:** 125 mg or 250 mg (as trihydrate)/5 ml. Bot. 80 ml, 100 ml, 150 ml. **Pediatric drops:** 50 mg (as trihydrate)/ml. Bot. 15 ml. *Rx.*
Use: Anti-infective, penicillin.

Larynex. (Dover Pharmaceuticals) Benzocaine. Sugar, lactose and salt free. Loz. UD Box 500s. *otc.*
Use: Anesthetic, local.

Lasix. (Hoechst Marion Roussel) Furosemide. **Tab.:** 20 mg or 40 mg/Tab. Bot. 100s, 500s, 1000s, UD 100s; 80 mg/Tab. Bot. 50s, 500s, UD 100s. **Inj.:** 10 mg/ml. 2 ml/Amp. Box 5s, 50s, 4 ml/Amp. Box 5s, 25s; 10 ml/Amp. Box 5s, 25s; Syringe 2 ml, 4 ml, 10 ml. Box 5s. Single Use Vial 2 ml, 4 ml, 10 ml. *Rx.*
Use: Diuretic.

lassar's paste.
See: Zinc Oxide Paste, U.S.P. 23. (Various Mfr.).

•**latanoprost.** (lah-TAN-oh-prahst) USAN.
Use: Antiglaucoma agent.
See: Xalatan, Sol. (Pharmacia & Upjohn).

Latest-CRP Kit. (Fischer) Measures C-reactive protein in serum. Kit 1s.
Use: Diagnostic aid.

•**laureth 4.** (LAH-reth 4) USAN.
Use: Pharmaceutic aid (surfacant).

•**laureth 9.** (LAH-reth 9) USAN.
Use: Pharmaceutical aid (surfactant), emulsifier, spermaticide.

•**laureth 10s.** (LAH-reth 10s) USAN.
Use: Spermaticide.

•**laurocapram.** (LAHR-oh-KAH-pram) USAN.
Use: Pharmaceutic aid (excipient).

lauromacrogol 400. Laureth 9.

•**lauryl isoquinolinium bromide.** (LAH-rill EYE-so-KWIN-oh-lih-nee-uhm) USAN.
Use: Anti-infective.

lauryl sulfoacetate.
See: Lowila, Cake, Liq., Oint. (Westwood Squibb).

Lavacol. (Parke-Davis) Ethyl alcohol 70%. Bot. pt. *otc.*
Use: Anti-infective, topical.

Lavatar. (Doak Dermatologics) Coal tar distillate 25.5% in a bath oil base. Liq. Bot. 4 oz, pt. *otc.*
Use: Antipsoriatic, antipruritic.

lavender oil.
Use: Perfume.

•**lavoltidine succinate.** (lahv-OLE-tih-DEEN) USAN. *Formerly Loxotidine.*
Use: Antiulcerative (histamine H_2-receptor blocker).

Lavoptik Emergency Wash. (Lavoptik) Eye, face, body wash. 32 oz/Emergency station. *otc.*
Use: Emergency wash.

Lavoptik Eye Wash. (Lavoptik) Sodium Cl 0.49%, sodium biphosphate 0.4%, sodium phosphate 0.45%/100 ml w/ benzalkonium Cl 0.005%. Bot. 6 oz. *otc.*
Use: Irrigant, ophthalmic.

Lavoris. (Procter & Gamble) Zinc Cl, glycerin, poloxamer 407, saccharin, polysorbate 80, flavors, clove oil, alcohol, citric acid, water. Bot. 6 oz, 12 oz, 18 oz, 24 oz. *otc.*
Use: Mouthwash.

Laxative Caps. (Weeks & Leo) Docusate sodium 100 mg, casanthranol 30 mg/Cap. Bot. 30s, 60s. *otc.*
Use: Laxative.

laxatives.
See: Agar-Gel (Various Mfr.).
Aloe (Various Mfr.).
Aloin (Various Mfr.).
Bile Salts (Various Mfr.).
Bisacodyl, Tab., Supp. (Various Mfr.).
Bisacodyl Tannex (PBH Wesley Jessen).
Carboxymethylcellulose Sodium (Various Mfr.).
Casanthranol, Cap., Tab. (Various Mfr.).
Cascara Sagrada (Various Mfr.).
Cascara Sagrada Fluidextract, Liq. (Parke-Davis).
Cascara Tab. (Various Mfr.).
Castor Oil (Various Mfr.).
Citrucel (SmithKline Beecham Pharmaceuticals).
Correctol, Tab. (Schering Plough).
Docusate Sodium (Various Mfr.).
Ex-Lax, Tab., Pow. (Ex-Lax. Inc.).
Feen-a-Mint, Gum, Mints (Schering Plough).
Karaya Gum (Penick).
Liquid Petrolatum, Liq. (Various Mfr.).

Magnesia Maga (Various Mfr.).
Maltsupex (Wallace Laboratories).
Methylcellulose (Various Mfr.).
Mucilloid of Psyllium Seed W/Dextrose (Searle).
Mylanta Natural Fiber Supplement (J & J-Merck).
Nature's Remedy (SmithKline Beecham Pharmaceuticals).
Nujol, Liq. (Schering Plough).
Oxyphenisatin Acetate (Various Mfr.).
Petrolatum, Liq. (Various Mfr.).
Petrolatum, Liq., Emulsion (Various Mfr.).
Phenolphthalein (Various Mfr.).
Plantago ovata, Coating (Various Mfr.).
Poloxalkol, Cap., Soln. (Various Mfr.).
Prune Concentrate, Tab., Cap. (Various Mfr.).
Prune Preps. (Various Mfr.).
Psyllium Granules W/Dextrose (Med Chem).
Psyllium Husk Pow. (Pharmacia & Upjohn).
Psyllium Hydrocolloid, Pow. (Zeneca).
Psyllium Hydrophilic Mucilloid (Various Mfr.).
Psyllium Seed, Gel, Gran. (Various Mfr.).
Regutol, Tab. (Schering Plough).
Restore (Inagra).
Senna, Alexandrian, Liq., Tab. (Various Mfr.).
Senna, Cassia angustifolia, Tab. (Brayten).
Senna Conc., Standardized, Gran., Tab., Pow., Supp. (Various Mfr.).
Senna Fruit Extract, Liq. (Various Mfr.).
Sennosides A & B, Tab. (Novartis).
Sodium Biphosphate (Various Mfr.).
Sodium Phosphate (Various Mfr.).
Unifiber (Dow Hickam).

Laxinate 100. (Roberts Pharm) Dioctyl sodium sulfosuccinate 100 mg/Cap. Bot. 100s, 1000s. *otc.*
Use: Laxative.

Lax Pills. (G & W Laboratories) Yellow phenolphthalein 90 mg/Tab. Bot. 30s, 60s. *otc.*
Use: Laxative.

layor carang.
See: Agar (Various Mfr.).

•**lazabemide.** (lazz-AH-bem-ide) USAN.
Use: Antiparkinsonian.

Lazer Creme. (Pedinol) Vitamins E 3500 units, A 100,000 units/oz. Jar 2 oz. *otc.*
Use: Emollient.

Lazer Formalyde Solution. (Pedinol) Formaldehyde 10%, polysorbate 20, hydroxyethyl cellulose. Bot. 3 oz. *Rx.*
Use: Drying.

LazerSporin-C Solution. (Pedinol) Neomycin sulfate 3.5 mg, polymyxin B sulfate 10,000 units, hydrocortisone 1%. Bot. 10 ml. *Rx.*
Use: Anti-infective combination, topical.

l-baclofen.
Use: Antispasmodic. [Orphan drug]

l-bulgaricus. (Antidiarrheal).
See: Bacid (Medeva).
Lactinex B (Becton Dickinson).
More-Dophilus (Freeda Vitamins).

LC-65 Daily Contact Lens Cleaner. (Allergan) Daily cleaning solution for all hard, soft (hydrophilic), rigid gas permeable contact lenses. Bot. 15 ml, 60 ml. *otc.*
Use: Contact lens care.

L-Caine E. (Century Pharm) Lidocaine HCl 1% or 2%, epinephrine 1:100,000/ml. Inj. 20 ml, 50 ml. *Rx.*
Use: Anesthetic, local.

L-Caine Viscous. (Century Pharm) Lidocaine HCl 2% with sodium carboxymethylcellulose. Soln. Bot. 100 ml. *Rx.*
Use: Anesthetic, local.

l-carnitine. Amino acid derivative 250 mg/Cap. Bot. 60s.
Use: Nutritional supplement.
See: Vitacarn.
Carnitor (Sigma-Tau Pharmaceuticals).

L.C.D. (Almay) Alcohol extractions of crude coal tar. Cream, soln. Bot. 4 oz, pt. *otc.*
Use: Antipsoriatic, antipruritic, topical.
See: Coal Tar Topical Soln., U.S.P. 23.

LCR. *Rx.*
Use: Antineoplastic.
See: Vincristine sulfate.

LCx Neisseria gonorrhoeae Assay. (Abbott Laboratories) Reagent kit for the detection of *Neisseria gonorrhoeae* in female endocervical, male urethral and urine swab specimens. Kit. 96s. *Rx.*
Use: Diagnostic aid.

l-cycloserine.
Use: Gaucher's disease. [Orphan drug]

l-cysteine. (Tyson)
Use: Erythropoietic protoporphyria. [Orphan drug]

l-deprenyl.
See: Selegiline HCl.

LDH Reagent Strip. (Bayer Corp) A quantitative strip test for LDH in serum or plasma. Seralyzer reagent strip. Bot. 25s. *Rx.*

Use: Diagnostic aid.

Leber Tabulae. (Paddock) Aloe 0.09 g, extract of rhei 0.03 g, myrrh 0.01 g, frangula 5 mg, galbanum 2 mg, olibanum 3 mg/Tab. Bot. 100s, 500s, 1000s.

Lec-E-Plex. (Barth's) Vitamin E 100 IU, 200 IU or 400 IU/Cap. w/lecithin. Bot. 100s, 500s, 1000s. *otc.*
Use: Vitamin E supplement.

•**lecimibide.** (leh-SIM-ih-bide) USAN.
Use: Antihyperlipidemic.

lecithin. (Various Mfr.) Lecithin. **Cap.:** 520 mg. Bot. 100s, 250s, 1000s; 650 mg. Bot. 90s, 100s, 250s, 500s. **Pow.:** 120 g, kg, lb. *otc.*
Use: Nutritional supplement.

•**lecithin.** (LESS-ih-thin) N.F. 18.
Use: Pharmaceutic aid (emulsifying agent).
W/Choline base, cephalin, lipositol.
See: Alcolec Cap., Gran. (American Lecithin).
W/Coconut oil, pine oil, castor oil, lanolin, cholesterols, parachlorometaxylenol.
See: Sebacide, Liq. (Paddock).
W/Vitamins.
See: Acletin, Cap. (Associated Concentrates).
Lec-E-Plex, Cap. (Barth's).

lecithin. (Arcum) 1200 mg/Cap. Bot. 100s, 1000s; Gran. Bot. 8 oz; Pow. Bot. 4 oz.
Use: Pharmaceutic aid (emulsifying agent).
(Barth's) 8 gr/Cap. Bot. 100s, 500s, 1000s; Gran. Can 8 oz, 16 oz; Pow. Can 10 oz.
(Cavendish) Tab. (0.5 gr) Bot. 500s.
(Quality Formulations) 1200 mg, Cap. 100s.
(De Pree) Cap. Bot. 100s.
(Pfanstiehl) 25 g, 100 g, 500 g/Pkg.

leflunomide.
Use: Organ transplant rejection. [Orphan drug]

Legatrin PM. (Columbia) Acetaminophen 500 mg, diphenhydramine HCl 50 mg/ Capl. Bot. 30s, 50s. *otc.*
Use: Sleep aid.

lemon oil.
Use: Pharmaceutic aid (flavor).

lenetran. Mephenoxalone.
Use: Anxiolytic.

lenicet.
See: Aluminum Acetate, Basic (Various Mfr.).

•**leniquinsin.** (LEN-ih-KWIN-sin) USAN. Under study.
Use: Antihypertensive.

Lenium Medicated Shampoo. (Sanofi Winthrop) Selenium sulfide. *otc.*
Use: Antiseborrheic.

•**lenograstim.** (leh-no-GRAH-stim) USAN.
Use: Antineutropenic, hematopoietic stimulant, immunomodulator (granulocyte colony-stimulating factor).

•**lenperone.** (LEN-per-OHN) USAN.
Use: Antipsychotic.

Lens Clear. (Allergan) Sterile, isotonic solution surfactant cleaner w/sorbic acid 0.1%, edetate disodium 0.2%. Bot. 15 ml. *otc.*
Use: Contact lens care.

Lens Drops. (Ciba Vision Ophthalmics) Sodium chloride, borate buffer, carbamide, poloxamer 407, EDTA 0.2%, sorbic acid 0.15%. Soln. Bot. 15 ml. *otc.*
Use: Contact lens care-rewetting.

Lensept Disinfecting Solution. (Ciba Vision Ophthalmics) Micro-filtered hydrogen peroxide with sodium stannate 3%, sodium nitrate, phosphate buffers. Soln. Bot. 237, 355 ml. *otc.*
Use: Disinfecting solution.

Lensept Rinse and Neutralizer. (Ciba Vision Ophthalmics) Sodium chloride, sodium borate decahydrate, boric acid, bovine catalase, sorbic acid, EDTA. Soln. Bot. 237 ml. System includes lens cup and holder. *otc.*
Use: Contact lens care, rinsing, neutralizing.

Lens Fresh. (Allergan) Sterile, buffered, isotonic aqueous soln. W/hydroxyethyl cellulose, sodium Cl, boric acid, sodium borate, sorbic acid 0.1%, edetate disodium 0.2%. Bot. 0.5 oz. *otc.*
Use: Contact lens care.

Lensine Extra Strength. (Ciba Vision Ophthalmics) Cleaning agent with benzalkonium Cl 0.01%, EDTA 0.1%. Soln. Bot. 45 ml. *otc.*
Use: Contact lens care.

Lens Lubricant. (Bausch & Lomb) Povidone and polyoxyethylene with thimerosal 0.004%, EDTA 0.1% Soln. Bot. 15 ml. *otc.*
Use: Contact lens care, lubricant.

Lens Plus. (Allergan) Isotonic soln. w/ sodium Cl 0.9%. Aerosol 3 oz, 8 oz, 12 oz. Preservative free. *otc.*
Use: Contact lens care.

Lens Plus Daily Cleaner. (Allergan) Buffered solution with cocoamphocarboxyglycinate, sodium lauryl sulfate, hexylene glycol, sodium chloride, sodium phosphate. Preservative free. Soln. Bot. 15 ml or 30 ml. *otc.*

Use: Contact lens care, cleanser.

Lens Plus Oxysept Disinfecting Solution. (Allergan) Hydrogen peroxide with sodium stannate 3%, sodium nitrate and phosphate buffer. Soln. Bot. 240 ml. *otc.*
Use: Contact lens care.

Lens Plus Oxysept 2 Neutralizing. (Allergan) Catalase with buffering agents used to neutralize the Lens Plus Oxysept 1 disinfecting solution in a chemical lens care system. For soft contact lens. Tabs. Box 12s. Bot. 36s. *otc.*
Use: Contact lens care.

Lens Plus Oxysept Rinse and Neutralizer. (Allergan) Isotonic with sodium chloride, mono- and dibasic sodium phosphates, catalytic neutralizing agent, EDTA. Soln. Bot. 15 ml. *otc.*
Use: Contact lens care.

Lens Plus Preservative Free. (Allergan) Isotonic sodium chloride 9%. Soln. Bot. 90, 240, 360 ml. *otc.*
Use: Contact lens care.

Lens Plus Rewetting Drops. (Allergan) Sterile, non-preserved isotonic solution w/sodium Cl, boric acid. 0.35 ml (30s). *otc.*
Use: Contact lens care.

Lens Plus Rewetting Drops. (Allergan) Isotonic solution with sodium chloride and boric acid. Thimerosol and preservative free. Soln. Bot. 0.3 ml (30s). *otc.*
Use: Contact lens care.

Lens Plus Sterile Saline. (Allergan) Sodium Cl, boric acid, nitrogen. Soln. Bot. 90 ml, 240 ml, 360 ml. Aerosol. *otc.*
Use: Contact lens care.

Lensrins. (Allergan) Sterile preserved saline for heat disinfection, rinsing and storage of soft (hydrophilic) contact lenses; rinsing solution for chemical disinfection. Soln. Bot. 8 oz. *otc.*
Use: Contact lens care.

Lens-Wet. (Allergan) Isotonic, buffered soln. of polyvinyl alcohol, thimerosal 0.002%, EDTA 0.01%. Bot. 0.5 fl oz. *otc.*
Use: Contact lens care.

Lente Iletin I. (Eli Lilly) Insulin zinc suspension 100 units/ml. Beef and pork. Inj. Vial. 10 ml. *otc.*
Use: Antidiabetic.

Lente Iletin II. (Eli Lilly) Insulin zinc suspension 100 units/ml. Purified pork. Inj. Bot. 10 ml. *otc.*
Use: Antidiabetic.

lente insulin. Susp. of zinc insulin crystals. *otc.*
See: Iletin Lente, Vial (Eli Lilly).

lente insulin. (Novo Nordisk) Insulin zinc susp. 100 units/ml Beef. Inj. Vial 10 ml. *otc.*
Use: Antidiabetic.

Lente L. (Novo Nordisk) Insulin zinc suspension 100 units/ml. Purified pork. Inj. Vial 10 ml. *otc.*
Use: Antidiabetic.

lentinan. (Lenti-Chemico Pharmaceuticals)
Use: Immunomodulator.

lepirudin.
Use: Heparin-associated thrombocytopenia Type II. [Orphan drug]
See: Refludan (Behring Werke AG).

lepromin. (Louisiana State University) Lepromin, 30 to 40 million acid-fast bacilli per ml. Vial 5 ml, 10 ml, 20 ml, 50 ml.

leprostatics.
Use: Bactericidal.
See: Dapsone, Tab. (Jacobus).
Lamprene, Cap. (Novartis Pharmaceuticals).

leptazol.
See: Pentylenetetrazol.

•**lergotrile.** (LER-go-trill) USAN.
Use: Enzyme inhibitor (prolactin).

•**lergotrile mesylate.** (LER-go-trill) USAN.
Use: Enzyme inhibitor (prolactin).

Lerton Ovules. (Vita Elixir) Caffeine 250 mg/Cap. *otc.*
Use: CNS stimulant.

Lescol. (Novartis) Fluvastatin sodium 20 mg or 40 mg. Cap. Bot. 30s, 100s. *Rx.*
Use: Antihyperlipidemic.

Lesterol. (Dram) Nicotinic acid 500 mg/Tab. Bot. 250s. *otc.*
Use: Antihyperlipidemic.

•**letimide hydrochloride.** (LET-ih-mide) USAN.
Use: Analgesic.

•**letrozole.** (let-ROW-zahl) USAN.
Use: Antineoplastic.
See: Femara, Tab. (Novartis).

letusin. (Eli Lilly).

•**leucine.** (LOO-SEEN) U.S.P. 23.
Use: Amino acid.

leucomax. (Various Mfr.). Leucomax. Granulocyte-Macrophage colony-stimulating factor (Recombinant). Molgramostin (Schering and Novartis).
Use: Immunomodulator.

l-leucovorin.
Use: Antineoplastic. [Orphan drug]
See: Isovorin (Lederle).

•**leucovorin calcium.** (loo-koe-VORE-in)

U.S.P. 23. (Various Mfr.) **Tab.:** 5 mg. Bot. 30s, 100s, UD 50s.
Use: Antagonist of amithopterin, antianemic (folate-deficiency), antidote to folic acid antagonists, antineoplastic. [Orphan drug]
See: Wellcovorin, Inj., Tab. (GlaxoWellcome).

•**leucovorin calcium.** (loo-koe-VORE-in) U.S.P. 23.
Use: Antianemic (folate-deficiency); antidote to folic acid antagonists.

leucovorin calcium. (Various Mfr.) **Tab.:** 15 mg or 25 mg as calcium. Pkg. 12s, 24s, 25s, UD 50s. **Inj.:** 3 mg/ml as calcium w/ benzyl alcohol 0.9%. Amps 1 ml. **Pow. for Inj.:** 50 mg/vial, 100 mg/vial, 350 mg/vial. *Rx.*
Use: Folic acid antagonist overdosage.

Leukeran. (GlaxoWellcome) Chlorambucil 2 mg/Tab. Bot. 50s. *Rx.*
Use: Antineoplastic.

Leukine. (Immunex) Sargramostin. **Pow. for Inj.:** 250 mcg or 500 mcg. Lyophilized. **Liq.:** 500 mcg/ml Vial. *Rx.*
Use: Bone marrow transplant adjunct.

leukocyte protease inhibitor, recombinant secretory.
Use: Alpha-1 antitrypsin deficiency; cystic fibrosis. [Orphan drug]

leukocyte protease inhibitor, secretory.
Use: Bronchopulmonary dysplasia. [Orphan drug]

•**leukocyte typing serum.** U.S.P. 23.
Use: Diagnositc aid (blood, in vitro).

leupeptin. (Neuromuscular Agents)
Use: Adjunct to nerve repair. [Orphan drug]

•**leuprolide acetate.** (loo-PRO-lide) USAN.
Use: Antineoplastic, LHRH agonist, central precocious puberty [Orphan drug]
See: Lupron, Inj. (TAP Pharm).
Lupron Depot, Microspheres for Inj. (TAP Pharm).
Lupon Depot inj. (TAP Pharm).

leurocristine.
See: Vincristine Sulfate (Eli Lilly).

leurocristine sulfate (1:1) (salt). Vincristine Sulfate, U.S.P. 23.
Use: Antineoplastic.

Leustatin. (Ortho Biotech) Cladribine. Soln. 1 mg/ml. Vial. 20 ml single-use. *Rx.*
Use: Antineoplastic.

leutinizing hormone (recombinant) human.
Use: With recombinant human follicle stimulating hormone for chronic anovulation due to hypogonadotropic hypogonadism. [Orphan drug]

levamfetamine. (LEV-am-FET-ah-meen) F.D.A.
Use: Anorexic.

levamfetamine. (LEV-am-FET-ah-meen)
See: Levamphetamine succinate.

•**levamfetamine succinate.** (LEV-am-FET-ah-meen) USAN.
Use: Anorexic.

•**levamisole hydrochloride.** (lev-AM-ih-sole) U.S.P. 23.
Use: Biological response modifier; antineoplastic.
See: Ergamisol (Janssen).

Levaquin. (Ortho McNeil) Levofloxacin 250 mg and 500 mg/Tab. Bot. 50s, UD 100s. Levofloxacin 500 mg/Inj. Vial. 20 ml. Levofloxacin 250 mg and 500/Inj. (premix). 50 ml flexible containers with 5% Dextrose solution (250 mg). 100 ml flexible containers with 5% Dextrose Solution (500 mg). *Rx.*
Use: Fluoroquinolone.

levarterenol. *Rx.*
Use: Vasoconstrictor.
See: Levophed, Inj. (Sanofi Winthrop).

levarterenol bitartrate.
See: Norepinephrine Bitartate, U.S.P. 23.

Levatol. (Schwarz Pharma) Penbutolol sulfate 20 mg. Tab. Bot. 100s. *Rx.*
Use: Beta-adrenergic blocker.

Levbid. (Schwarz Pharma) Hyoscyamine sulfate 0.375 mg/DR Tab. Bot. 100s. *Rx.*
Use: Anticholinergic.

•**levcromakalim.** (lev-KROE-mah-KAY-lim) USAN.
Use: Antihypertensive; antiasthmatic.

•**levcycloserine.** (LEV-sigh-kloe-SER-een) USAN.
Use: Enzyme inhibitor (Gaucher's disease).

•**levdobutamine lactobionate.** (LEV-dah-BYOOT-ah-meen LACK-toe-BYE-oh-nate) USAN.
Use: Cardiovascular agent.

Leviron. (Health for Life Brands) Desiccated liver 7 gr, iron and ammonium citrate 3 gr, vitamins B_1 1 mg, B_2 0.5 mg, B_6 0.5 mg, calcium pantothenate 0.3 mg, niacinamide 2.5 mg, B_{12} 1 mcg/Cap. Bot. 100s, 1000s. *otc.*
Use: Mineral, vitamin supplement.

Levlen 21 Tablets. (Berlex) Levonorgestrel 0.15 mg, ethinyl estradiol 0.03

mg/Tab. Slidecase 21s, Box 3s. *Rx.*
Use: Contraceptive.

Levlen 28 Tablets. (Berlex) Levonorgestrel 0.15 mg, ethinyl estradiol 0.03 mg/Tab. (21 active, 7 inert). Slidecase 28s, Box 3s. *Rx.*
Use: Contraceptive.

•**levoamphetamine.** (lee-voe-meth-am-FET-uh-meen) U.S.P. 23.
Use: Nasal decongestant.

levo-amphetamine. Alginate (l-isomer) alpha-2-phenylaminopropane succinate.
See: Levamphetamine.

levo-amphetamine succinate.
See: Pedestal, Cap., Tab. (Len-Tag).

•**levobetaxolol hydrochloride.** (LEE-voe-beh-TAX-oh-lahl) USAN.
Use: Antiadrenergic (β-receptor).

levobunolol hydrochloride. (LEE-voe-BYOO-no-lahl) U.S.P. 23.
Use: Antiadrenergic (β-receptor).

levobunolol hydrochloride. (LEE-voe-BYOO-no-lahl) (Various Mfr.) 0.25% or 0.5% Ophth. Soln. Bot. 5 ml, 10 ml, 15 ml. *Rx.*
Use: Beta-adrenergic blocker.
See: AKBeta, Ophth. Soln. (Akorn).
Betagan, Ophth. Soln. (Allergan).

•**levocabastine hydrochloride.** (LEE-voe-cab-ASS-teen) USAN.
Use: Antihistamine.
See: Livostin, Ophth. Susp. (Ciba Vision Ophthalmics).

•**levocarnitine.** (LEE-voe-CAR-nih-teen) U.S.P. 23.
Use: Carnitine replenisher. [Orphan drug]
See: Carnitor, Liq., Tab. (Sigma-Tau Pharmaceuticals).
L-Carnitine, Cap. (R & D Laboratories).
Vitacarn, Liq. (McGaw).

•**levodopa.** (LEE-voe-DOE-puh) U.S.P. 23.
Use: Antiparkinsonian.
See: Bio Dopa, Cap. (Bio-Deriv.).
Dopar, Cap. (Procter & Gamble).
Larodopa, Tab. or Cap. (Roche Laboratories).
Levora, Cap. (Zeneca).
Parda, Cap. (Parke-Davis).

levodopa & carbidopa. (LEE-voe-DOE-puh and CAR-bih-doe-puh)
Use: Antiparkinsonian.
See: Carbidopa and levodopa, Tab. (Lemmon)
Sinemet-10/100, Tab. (DuPont Merck Pharmaceuticals).
Sinemet-25/100, Tab. (DuPont Merck Pharmaceuticals).
Sinemet-25/250, Tab. (DuPont Merck Pharmaceuticals).
Sinemet CR, SR Tab., (DuPont Merck Pharmaceuticals).

Levo-Dromoran. (Roche Laboratories) Levorphanol tartrate. **Amp.:** 2 mg/ml w/methyl and propyl parabens, sodium hydroxide to adjust pH. Amp. 1 ml, Box 10s. **Vial:** 2 mg/ml w/phenol 0.45%, sodium hydroxide to adjust pH. Vial 10 ml. **Tab.:** 2 mg. Bot. 100s. *c-II.*
Use: Analgesic, narcotic.

levo-epinephrine bitartrate.
See: Lyophrin, Soln. (Alcon Laboratories).

•**levofloxacin.** (lee-voe-FLOX-ah-sin) USAN.
Use: Anti-infective.
See: Levaquin, Tab. Inj. (Ortho McNeil).

•**levofuraltadone.** (LEE-voe-fer-AL-tah-dohn) USAN.
Use: Anti-infective, antiprotozoal.

•**levoleucovorin calcium.** (LEE-voe-loo-koe-VORE-in) USAN.
Use: Antidote to folic acid antagonist.
See: Isovorin (Immunex).

•**levomethadyl acetate.** (LEE-voe-METH-uh-dill) USAN.
Use: Analgesic, narcotic.

•**levomethadyl acetate hydrochloride.** (LEE-voe-METH-uh-dill) USAN.
Use: Analgesic, narcotic; treatment of heroin addicts. [Orphan drug]
See: ORLAAM (Biodevelopment Corp.).

•**levonantradol hydrochloride.** (LEE-voe-NAN-trah-DAHL) USAN.
Use: Analgesic.

•**levonordefrin.** U.S.P. 23. (lee-voe-nore-DEFF-rin)
Use: Adrenergic (vasoconstrictor).

•**levonorgestrel.** (LEE-voe-nor-JESS-truhl) U.S.P. 23.
Use: Hormone, progestin.
See: Alesse, Tab. (Wyeth-Ayerst).
Levora, Tab. (SCS).
Norplant (Wyeth Ayerst).

levonorgestrel and ethinyl estradiol tablets.
Use: Contraceptive.
See: Nordette, Tab. (Wyeth Ayerst).

Levophed. (Breon) Norepinephrine bitartrate 1 mg/ml Amp. 4 ml. *Rx.*
Use: Vasoconstrictor.

Levophed Bitartrate. (Sanofi Winthrop) Norepinephrine bitartrate w/sodium Cl, sodium metabisulfite 1 mg or 2 mg/ml. Amp. 4 ml. Box 10s. *Rx.*

Use: Vasoconstrictor.

Levoprome. (ESI Lederle Generics) Methotrimeprazine 20 mg/ml w/benzyl alcohol 0.9%, disodium edetate 0.065%, sodium metabisulfite 0.3%. Vial 10 ml. *Rx.*
Use: Analgesic.

•**levopropoxyphene napsylate.** (lee-voe-pro-POX-ee-feen NAP-sih-late) USAN. U.S.P. XXII.
Use: Antitussive.

•**levopropylcillin potassium.** (lee-voe-pro-pihl-SILL-in) USAN.
Use: Anti-infecive.

Levora. (SCS Pharmaceuticals) Ethinyl estradiol 0.03 mg, levonorgestrel 0.15 mg. Tab. Bot. 21s, 28s. *Rx.*
Use: Contraceptive.

levorenine.
See: Epinephrine, U.S.P. 23. (Various Mfr.).

Levoroxine. (Bariatric) Sodium levothyroxine 0.05 mg, 0.1 mg, 0.2 mg or 0.3 mg/Tab. Bot. 100s, 500s. *Rx.*
Use: Hormone, thyroid.

•**levorphanol tartrate.** (lee-VORE-fah-nole TAR-trate) U.S.P. 23.
Use: Analgesic, narcotic.
See: Levo-Dromoran, Amp., Tab., Vial (Roche Laboratories).

Levo-T. (ESI Lederle Generics) Levothyroxine sodium 0.025, 0.05, 0.075, 0.1, 0.125, 0.15, 0.2 or 0.3 mg. Tab. Bot. 100s (all strengths), 1000s (0.05, 0.1, 0.15 and 0.2 mg only). *Rx.*
Use: Hormone, thyroid.

Levothroid. (Forest Pharmaceutical) Levothyroxine sodium. **Tab.:** 25 mcg, 50 mcg, 75 mcg, 88 mcg, 100 mcg, 112 mcg, 125 mcg, 137 mcg, 150 mcg, 175 mcg, 200 mcg or 300 mcg/Tab. Bot. 100s (all strengths), UD 100s (50 mcg, 100 mcg, 150 mcg, 200 mcg, 300 mcg only). **Inj.:** 200 mcg or 500 mcg. Vial 6 ml. *Rx.*
Use: Hormone, thyroid.

levothyroxine sodium. (lee-voe-thigh-ROX-een) (Various Mfr.) Levothyroxine sodium 200 mcg, 500 mcg/Vial. Pow. for Inj. 6 ml, 10 ml. *Rx.*
Use: Hormone, thyroid.

•**levothyroxine sodium.** (lee-voe-thigh-ROX-een) U.S.P. 23.
Use: Hormone, thyroid.
See: Eltroxin, Tab. (Roberts Pharm).
Levoid, Tab., Vial (Nutrition Control Products).
Levo-T, Tab. (ESI Lederle Generics).
Levothroid, Tab., Inj. (Forest Pharmaceutical).
Levoxine, Inj. (Jones Medical Industries).
Levoxyl, Tab. (Jones Medical Industries).
Synthroid, Tab., Inj. (Boots).
W/Mannitol.
See: Levoxine, Inj. (Jones Medical Industries).
Synthroid, Inj. (Knoll Pharmaceuticals).
W/Sodium liothyronine.
Use: Hormone, thyroid.
See: Thyrolar, Tab. (Rhone-Poulenc Rorer).

levothyroxine sodium. (Various Mfr.) 0.1 mg, 0.15 mg, 0.2 mg, 0.3 mg/Tab. Bot. 100s, 1000s, UD 100s.
Use: Hormone, thyroid.

•**levoxadrol hydrochloride.** (lev-OX-ah-drole) USAN.
Use: Anesthetic, local; muscle relaxant.

Levoxyl. (Jones Medical Industries) Levothyroxine sodium 0.025 mg, 0.05 mg, 0.75 mg, 0.088 mg, 0.1 mg, 0.112 mg, 0.125 mg, 0.137 mg, 0.15 mg, 0.175 mg, 0.2 mg, 0.3 mg/Tab. Bot. 100s, 1000s, UD 100s. *Rx.*
Use: Hormone, thyroid.

Levsin. (Schwarz Pharma) L-hyoscyamine sulfate. **Tab.:** 0.125 mg. Bot. 100s, 500s. **Soln.:** 0.125 mg/ml, alcohol 5%. Bot. 15 ml. **Elix.:** 0.125 mg/5 ml, alcohol 20%. Bot. pt. **Inj.:** 0.5 mg/ml. Vial 1 ml, 10 ml. *Rx.*
Use: Anticholinergic, antispasmodic.

Levsin-PB Drops. (Schwarz Pharma) Hyoscyamine sulfate 0.125 mg, phenobarbital 15 mg/ml, alcohol 5%. Liq. Bot. 15 ml. *Rx.*
Use: Anticholinergic, antispasmodic, hypnotic, sedative.

Levsin/SL. (Schwarz Pharma) Hyoscyamine sulfate 0.125 mg/Tab. Sublingual. Bot. 100s, 500s. *Rx.*
Use: Gastrointestinal anticholinergic.

Levsinex Timecaps. (Schwarz Pharma) L-hyoscyamine sulfate 0.375 mg/TR Cap. Bot. 100s, 500s. *Rx.*
Use: Anticholinergic, antispasmodic.

levulose. Fructose.

levulose-dextrose.
See: Invert Sugar.

•**lexipafant.** (lex-IH-pah-fant) USAN.
Use: Platelet activating factor (PAP) antagonist.

•**lexithromycin.** (lex-ith-row-MY-sin) USAN.
Use: Anti-infective.

Lextron. (Eli Lilly) Liver-stomach concen-

trate 50 mg, iron 30 mg, vitamins B_{12} (activity equivalent) 2 mcg, B_1 1 mg, B_2 0.25 mg w/other factors of vitamin B complex present in the liver-stomach concentrate/Pulv. Bot. 84s. *otc.*
Use: Mineral, vitamin supplement.

Lexxel. (Astra Merck) Enalapril maleate 5 mg, felodipine 5 mg/ER Tab. Bot. 30s, 100s, UD 100s. *Rx.*
Use: Antihypertensive combination.

l-glutathione.
See: Glutathione.

L'Homme. (Armenpharm) Vitamins A 4000 IU, D 400 IU, B_1 1 mg, B_2 1.2 mg, B_{12} 2 mcg, calcium pantothenate 5 mg, B_3 10 mg, C 30 mg, calcium 100 mg, phosphorus 76 mg, iron 10 mg, manganese 1 mg, magnesium 1 mg, zinc 1 mg. Bot. 100s. *otc.*
Use: Mineral, vitamin supplement.

L-5 hydroxytryptophan. (Circa)
Use: Postanoxic intention myoclonus. [Orphan drug]

•**liarozole fumarate.** (lie-AHR-oh-zole) USAN.
Use: Antipsoriatic.

•**liarozole hydrochloride.** (lie-AHR-oh-zole) USAN.
Use: Antineoplastic.

Li Ban Spray. (Pfizer) Synthetic pyrethroid 0.5%, related compounds 0.065%, aromatic petroleum hydrocarbons 0.664%. Bot. 5 oz, Box 6s. *otc.*
Use: Pediculicide, inanimate objects. (Not to be used on humans or animals).

•**libenzapril.** (lie-BENZ-ah-prill) USAN.
Use: ACE inhibitor.

Librax. (Roche Laboratories) Clidinium bromide (Quarzan) 2.5 mg, chlordiazepoxide HCl (Librium) 5 mg, parabens, lactose/Cap. Bot. 100s, 500s, Teledose 100s (10 strips of 10). *Rx.*
Use: Anticholinergic combination.

Libritabs. (Roche Laboratories) Chlordiazepoxide 10 mg or 25 mg/Tab. **10 mg:** Bot. 100s, 500s; **25 mg:** Bot. 100s. *c-IV.*
Use: Anxiolytic.

Librium. (Roche Laboratories) Chlordiazepoxide HCl 5 mg, 10 mg or 25 mg/Cap. Bot. 100s, 500s, Tel-E-Dose (10 strips of 10; 4 cards of 25) in RNP (Reverse Numbered Package). *c-IV.*
Use: Anxiolytic.

Librium Injectable. (Roche Laboratories) Chlordiazepoxide HCl 100 mg/dry filled amp. plus special I.M. diluent, 2 ml for IM administration/compound w/benzyl alcohol 1.5%, polysorbate 80 4%, propylene glycol 20%, w/maleic acid and sodium hydroxide to adjust pH to approx. 3. Amp. 5 ml w/2 ml diluent, Box 10s. *c-IV.*
Use: Anxiolytic.

Lice-Enz. (Copley) Pyrethrins 0.3%, piperonylbutoxide 3%. Shampoo. Bot. 60 g. *otc.*
Use: Pediculicide.

•**licryfilcon a.** (lih-krih-FILL-kahn) USAN.
Use: Contact lens material (hydrophilic).

•**licryfilcon b.** USAN.
Use: Contact lens material (hydrophilic).

Lida-Mantle-HC Creme. (Bayer Corp) Lidocaine 3%, hydrocortisone acetate 0.5% in cream base. Tube oz. *Rx.*
Use: Corticosteroid, anesthetic, local.

•**lidamidine hydrochloride.** (LIE-DAM-ih-deen) USAN.
Use: Antiperistaltic.

Lidex Cream. (Syntex) Fluocinonide 0.05%. Cream. In 15 g, 30 g, 60 g, 120 g. *Rx.*
Use: Corticosteroid, topical.

Lidex-E. (Syntex) Fluocinonide 0.05% in aqueous emollient base. Tube 15 g, 30 g, 60 g, 120 g. *Rx.*
Use: Corticosteroid, topical.

Lidex Gel. (Syntex) Fluocinonide 0.05% in gel base. Tube 15 g, 30 g, 60 g, 120 g. *Rx.*
Use: Corticosteroid, topical.

Lidex Ointment. (Syntex) Fluocinonide 0.05% in ointment base. Tube 15 g, 30 g, 60 g, 120 g. *Rx.*
Use: Corticosteroid, topical.

Lidex Topical Solution. (Syntex) Fluocinonide 0.05%. Soln. Bot. 20 ml, 60 ml. *Rx.*
Use: Corticosteroid, topical.

•**lidocaine.** (LIE-doe-cane) U.S.P. 23.
Use: Anesthetic, local.
See: Dentipatch, Patch (Noven).
Dermaflex, Gel (Schering Plough).
Solarcaine Aloe Extra Burn Relief, Cream, Gel, Spray (Schering Plough).
Xylocaine, Oint. (Astra).
Zilactin-L, Liq. (Zila).

lidocaine and epinephrine injection.
Use: Local anesthetic.
See: L-Caine E, Vial (Century Pharm).
Norocaine 1%, 2% w/Epinephrine. (Vortech).
Xylocaine W/Epinephrine, Soln. (Astra).

•**lidocaine hydrochloride.** (LIE-doe-cane) U.S.P. 23.

Use: Cardiovascular agent; anesthetic, local.
See: Anestacon, Jelly (PolyMedica).
Ardecaine 1%, 2%, Inj. (Burgin-Arden).
Dilocaine, Inj. (Hauck).
Dolicaine, I.M. (Solvay).
Duo-Track Kit, Inj. (Astra).
L-Caine, Inj., Liq. (Century Pharm).
Lidoject-1, Inj. (Merz).
Lidoject-2, Inj. (Merz).
Nervocaine, Inj. (Keene Pharmaceuticals).
Norocaine, Inj. (Vortech).
Octocaine HCl, Inj. (Novocol Chemical).
Xylocaine HCl, Oint., Liq., Soln., Jelly (Astra).
Xylocaine 10% Oral, Spray (Astra).
Xylocaine Viscous, Soln. (Astra).
W/Benzalkonium Cl.
See: Medi-Quik, Aerosol (Reckitt & Colman).
W/Benzalkonium Cl, phenol, menthol, eugenol, thyme oil, eucalyptus oil.
See: Unguentine Spray (Procter & Gamble).
W/Cetyltrimethylammonium bromide, hexachlorophene.
See: Aerosept, Aerosol (Dalin).
W/Hydrocortisone, clioquinol.
See: Bafil, Lot. (Scruggs).
Hil-20 Lot. (Solvay).
W/Dextrose.
W/Methylparaben, sodium Cl.
W/Methyl parasept.
See: L-Caine, Inj. (Century Pharm).
W/Methyl parasept, epinephrine.
See: L-Caine-E, Inj. (Century Pharm).
W/Orthohydroxyphenyl mercuric Cl, menthol, camphor, allantoin.
See: Kip First Aid preps. (Schmid).
W/Parachlorometaxylenol, phenol, zinc oxide.
See: Unguentine Plus, Cream (Procter & Gamble).
W/Polymyxin B sulfate.
See: Lidosporin, Otic soln. (Glaxo-Wellcome).

lidocaine hydrochloride.
(Abbott Laboratories) **0.2%, 0.4%, 0.8%:** w/5% Dextrose. 250 ml single-dose container; **1%, 2%.** Abboject syringe 5 ml; Vial 1 g, 2 g. Premixed: 0.2%, 0.4% in 5% dextrose. Inj. containers (flexible or glass) 500 ml. **1%:** 2 ml, 5 ml single-dose amp. **1.5%:** 20 ml single-dose amp. **2%:** 10 ml/20 ml vial (for dilution to prepare I.V. drip soln.) **5%:** w/ 7.5% Dextrose amp. 2 ml.
(Maurry) 2%. Vial.
Use: Injection for infiltration block anesthesia and I.V. drip for cardiac arrhythmias.

Lidocaine HCl. (Abbott Laboratories) Lidocaine HCl. 1%: 2 ml, 5 ml, 20 ml, 30 ml, 50 ml. 1.5%: 20 ml. w/Epinephrine 1:200,000. 5 ml. 2%: 5 ml, 20 ml, 30 ml, 50 ml. *Rx.*
Use: Anesthetic, local.

lidocaine hydrochloride and dextrose injection.

lidocaine hydrochloride and epinephrine bitartrate injection.

lidocaine hydrochloride and epinephrine injection.

lidocaine patch 5%.
Use: Post-herpetic neuralgia resulting from herpes zoster infection. [Orphan drug]
See: Lidoderm Patch. (Hind Health Care).

Lidocaine 2% Viscous. (Various Mfr.) Lidocaine HCl 2%. Soln. 100 ml, UD 20 ml. *Rx.*
Use: Anesthetic, local.

Lidoderm Patch. (Hind Health Care) Lidocaine 5%.
Use: Post-herpetic neuralgia resulting from herpes zoster infection. [Orphan drug]

•**lidofenin.** (LIE-doe-FEN-in) USAN.
Use: Diagnostic aid (hepatic function determination).

•**lidofilcon a.** (lih-DAH-FILL-kahn A) USAN.
Use: Contact lens material (hydrophilic).

•**lidofilcon b.** (lih-DAH-FILL-kahn B) USAN.
Use: Contact lens material (hydrophilic).

•**lidoflazine.** (LIE-dah-FLAY-zeen) USAN.
Use: Coronary vasodilator.

Lidoject-1. (Merz) Lidocaine HCl 1%. Vial 50 ml. *Rx.*
Use: Anesthetic, local.

Lidoject-2. (Merz) Lidocaine HCl 2%. Vial 50 ml. *Rx.*
Use: Anesthetic, local.

LIdopen Auto-Injector. (Survival Technology) Lidocaine HCl 10%. Auto-injection device. *Rx.*
Use: Antiarrhythmic.

Lidox Caps. (Major) Chlordiazepoxide HCl 10 mg, clidinium bromide 2.5 mg. Cap. Bot. 100s, 500s, 1000s, UD 100s. *Rx.*
Use: Anticholinergic combination.

Lidoxide. (Henry Schein) Chlordiazepoxide HCl 5 mg, clidinium bromide 2.5

mg/Tab. Bot. 100s, 500s. *Rx.*
Use: Anticholinergic combination.

lid scrubs.
Use: Cleanser, ophthalmic.
See: I-Scrub, Soln. (Cooper Pharm).
Lid Wipes-SPF, Soln. (Akorn).
OcuClenz, Soln. (Storz/Lederle).
OCuSOFT, Soln. (Cynacon/OCuSOFT).

Lid Wipes-SPF. (Akorn) PEG-200 glyceryl monotallowate, PEG-80 glyceryl monococoate, laureth-23, cocoamidopropylamine oxide, NaCl, glycerin, sodium phosphate, sodium hydroxide. Soln. Pads UD 30s. *otc.*
Use: Cleanser, ophthalmic.

•**lifarizine.** (lih-FAR-ih-ZEEN) USAN.
Use: Cerebral anti-ischemic; platelet aggregation inhibitor.

Lifer-B. (Burgin-Arden) Cyanocobalamin 30 mcg, liver inj. 0.1 ml, ferrous gluconate 100 mg, riboflavin 1.5 mg, panthenol 2.5 mg, niacinamide 100 mg, citric acid 16.4 mg, sodium citrate 23.6 mg/ml. Vial 30 ml. *Rx.*
Use: Mineral, vitamin supplement.

Life Saver Kit. (Whiteworth Towne) Ipecac syrup two 1 oz bottles, activated charcoal pow. 1 oz, poison treatment instruction booklet. *otc.*
Use: Antidote, poisons.

Life Spanner. (Spanner) Vitamins A 12,500 IU, D 400 IU, E 5 IU, B_1 10 mg, B_2 5 mg, B_6 2 mg, B_{12} 5 mcg, niacinamide 50 mg, calcium pantothenate 10 mg, biotin 10 mcg, C 100 mg, hesperidin complex 10 mg, rutin 20 mg, choline bitartrate 40 mg, inositol 30 mg, betaine anhydrous 15 mg, l-lysine monohydrochloride 25 mg, iron 30 mg, copper 1 mg, manganese 1 mg, potassium 5 mg, calcium 105 mg, phosphorus 82 mg, magnesium 5.56 mg, zinc 1 mg/Cap. Bot. 100s. *otc.*
Use: Mineral, vitamin supplement.

•**lifibrate.** (lih-FIE-brate) USAN.
Use: Antihyperlipoproteinemic.

•**lifibrol.** (lie-FIB-rahl) USAN.
Use: Hypercholesterolemic.

Lifol-B. (Burgin-Arden) Liver inj. 10 mcg, folic acid 1 mg, cyanocobalamin 100 mcg, phenol 0.5%/ml. Inj. Vial 10 ml. *Rx.*
Use: Nutritional supplement.

Lifolex. (Taylor Pharmaceuticals) Liver 10 mcg, cyanocobalamin 100 mcg, folic acid 5 mg/ml. Inj. Vial 10 ml. *Rx.*
Use: Nutritional supplement.

Lilly Bulk Products. (Eli Lilly) The following products are supplied by Eli Lilly under the U.S.P., N.F. or chemical name as a service to the health professions:
Ammoniated Mercury Oint.
Amyl Nitrite.
Analgesic Balm.
Apomorphine HCl.
Aromatic Elix.
Aromatic Ammonia.
Atropine Sulfate.
Bacitracin Oint.
Belladonna Tincture.
Benzoin.
Boric Acid.
Calcium Gluceptate.
Calcium Gluconate.
Calcium Gluconate with Vitamin D.
Calcium Hydroxide.
Calcium Lactate.
Carbarsone.
Cascara, Aromatic, fluidextract.
Cascara Sagrada fluidextract.
Citrated Caffeine.
Cocaine HCl.
Codeine Phosphate.
Codeine Sulfate.
Colchicine.
Compound Benzoin.
Dibasic Calcium Phosphate.
Diethylstilbestrol.
Ephedrine Sulfate.
Ferrous Gluconate.
Ferrous Sulfate.
Folic Acid.
Glucagon for Inj.
Green Soap Tincture.
Heparin Sodium.
Histamine Phosphate.
Ipecac.
Isoniazid.
Isopropyl Alcohol, 91%.
Liver, Vial for Inj.
Magnesium Sulfate.
Mercuric Oxide, Yellow.
Methadone HCl.
Methenamine for Timed Burning.
Methyltestosterone.
Milk of Bismuth.
Morphine Sulfate.
Myrrh.
Neomycin Sulfate.
Niacin.
Niacinamide.
Nitroglycerin.
Opium (Deodorized).
Ox Bile Extract.
Pancreatin.
Papaverine HCl.
Paregoric.
Penicillin G Potassium.
Phenobarbital.

Phenobarbital Sodium.
Potassium Cl.
Potassium Iodide.
Powder Papers (Glassine).
Progesterone.
Propylthiouracil.
Protamine Sulfate.
Pyridoxine HCl.
Quinidine Gluconate.
Quinidine Sulfate.
Quinine Sulfate.
Riboflavin.
Silver Nitrate.
Sodium Bicarbonate.
Sodium Chloride.
Sodium Salicylate.
Streptomycin Sulfate.
Sulfadiazine.
Sulfapyridine.
Sulfur.
Terpin Hydrate.
Terpin Hydrate and Codeine.
Testosterone Propionate.
Thiamine HCl.
Thyroid.
Tubocurarine HCl.
Tylosterone.
Whitfield's Oint.
Wild Cherry Syrup.
Zinc Oxide.
Zinc Oxide Paste.

limarsol.
See: Acetarsone. (City Chemical).

Limbitrol. (Roche Laboratories) Chlordiazepoxide 5 mg, amitriptyline HCl 12.5 mg/Tab. Bot. 100s, 500s, Tel-E-Dose 100s, Prescription pak 50s. *c-IV.*
Use: Psychotherapeutic agent.

Limbitrol DS. (Roche Laboratories) Chlordiazepoxide 10 mg, amitriptyline HCl 25 mg/Tab. Bot. 100s, 500s, Tel-E-Dose 100s, Prescription pak 50s. *c-IV.*
Use: Psychotherapeutic agent.

•**lime.** U.S.P. 23.
Use: Pharmaceutical necessity.

lime solution, sulfurated. U.S.P. XXI.
Use: Scabicide.

lime sulfur solution. Calcium polysulfide, calcium thiosulfate.
Use: Wet dressing.

•**linarotene.** (lin-AHR-oh-teen) USAN.
Use: Antikeratolytic.

Lincocin. (Pharmacia & Upjohn) Lincomycin HCl 500 mg/Cap. Bot. 24s, 100s. **Pediatric:** 250 mg/Cap. Bot. 24s. *Rx.*
Use: Anti-infective.

Lincocin Sterile Solution. (Pharmacia & Upjohn) Lincomycin HCl equivalent to 300 mg or 600 mg lincomycin base, benzyl alcohol 9.45 mg/ml. Vial 2 ml in 5s, 25s, 100s; 10 ml U-Ject. *Rx.*
Use: Anti-infective.

•**lincomycin.** (LIN-koe-MY-sin) USAN. Antibiotic produced by *Streptomyces lincolnensis* variant.
Use: Anti-infecive; infections due to gram-positive organisms.

•**lincomycin hydrochloride.** (LIN-koe-MY-sin) U.S.P. 23.
Use: Anti-infective.
See: Lincocin, Cap., Soln., Syr. (Pharmacia & Upjohn).

•**lindane.** (LIN-dane) U.S.P. 23. Gamma-benzene-hexachloride, hexachlorocyclohexane.
Use: Pediculicide, scabicide.
See: Kwell, Cream, Lot., Shampoo (Schwarz Pharma).

lindane. (Fidelity Lab.) Pow. 50%, Pkg. 1 lb, 5 lb. (Imperial Lab) Pow. 50%, Pkg. 1 lb, 4 lb; 12%, Pkg. 1 lb, 4 lb.
Use: Pediculicide, scabicide.

Lindora. (Westwood Squibb) Sodium laureth sulfate, water, cocamide DEA, sodium Cl, lactic acid, tetra sodium EDTA, benzophenone-4, FD&C Blue No. 1, fragrance. Bot. 8 oz. *otc.*
Use: Dermatologic, cleanser.

•**linezolid.** (lin-EH-zoe-lid) USAN.
Use: Anti-infecive.

Linodil Capsules. (Sanofi Winthrop) Inositol hexanicotinate. *Rx.*
Use: Hyperlipidemic, peripheral vasodilator.

•**linogliride.** (lie-no-GLIE-ride) USAN.
Use: Antidiabetic.

•**linogliride fumarate.** (lih-no-GLIE-ride) USAN.
Use: Antidiabetic.

linolenic acid w/vitamin E.
See: Petropin, Cap. (Lannett).

linomide. (Pharmacia & Upjohn). Roquinimex.
Use: Immunomodulator. [Orphan drug]

•**linopirdine.** (lih-no-PIHR-deen) USAN.
Use: Treatment of Alzheimer's disease (cognition enhancer).

Lioresal. (Novartis Pharmaceuticals) Baclofen 10 mg or 20 mg/Tab. Bot. 100s, UD 100s. *Rx.*
Use: Muscle relaxant.

•**liothyronine I 125.** (lie-oh-THIGH-row-neen) USAN.
Use: Radiopharmaceutical.

•**liothyronine I 131.** (lie-oh-THIGH-row-neen) USAN.
Use: Radiopharmaceutical.

•**liothyronine sodium.** (lie-oh-THIGH-row-neen) U.S.P. 23.
Use: Hormone, thyroid.
See: Cytomel, Tab. (SmithKline Beecham Pharmaceuticals).
Triostat, Inj. (SmithKline Beecham Pharmaceuticals).

liothyronine sodium. (Various Mfr.) 10 mg/ml. Tab. Bot. 100s.
Use: Hormone, thyroid.

liothyronine sodium injection.
Use: Myxedema coma/precoma. [Orphan drug]

•**liotrix tablets.** (LIE-oh-trix) U.S.P. 23.
Use: Hormone, thyroid.
See: Euthroid, Tab. (Parke-Davis).
Thyrolar, Tab. (Rhone-Poulenc Rorer).

lipase.
W/Amylase, Protease.
Use: Digestive enzyme.
W/Amylase, bile salts, wilzyme, pepsin, pancreatin, calcium.
See: Enzyme, Tab. (Barth's).
W/Alpha-amylase W-100, proteinase W-300, cellase W-100, estrone, testosterone, vitamins, minerals.
See: Geramine, Tab. (Zeneca).
W/Alpha-Amylase, proteinase, cellase.
See: Kutrase (Schwarz Pharma).
Ku-Zyme (Schwarz Pharma).
W/Amylolytic, proteolytic, cellulolytic enzymes.
See: Arco-Lase, Tab. (Arco).
W/Amylolytic, proteolytic, cellulolytic enzymes, phenobarbital, hyoscyamine sulfate, atropine sulfate.
See: Arco-Lase Plus, Tab. (Arco).
W/Pancreatin, protease, amylase.
See: Dizymes, Cap. (Recsei).
W/Pepsin, homatropine methylbromide, amylase, protease, bile salts.
See: Digesplen, Tab., Elix., Drops (Med Prod).
Use: Antihyperlipidemic.

lipid/DNA human cystic fibrosis gene. (Genzyme)
Use: Cystic fibrosis. [Orphan drug]

lipids.
Use: Intravenous nutritional therapy.
See: Intralipid 10%, Soln. (Clintec Nutrition).
Intralipid 20%, Soln. (Clintec Nutrition).
Liposyn II 10%, Soln. (Abbott Laboratories).
Liposyn II 20%, Soln. (Abbott Laboratories).
Liposyn III 10%, Soln. (Abbott Laboratories).
Liposyn III 20%, Soln. (Abbott Laboratories).

Lipisorb. (Bristol-Myers) Protein 35 g/L, fat 48 g/L, carbohydrates 115 g/L, Na 733.3 mg/L, K 1250 mg/L, H_2O 320 mOsm/kg. With appropriate vitamins and minerals. 1 calorie/ml. Vanilla flavored. Pow. Can 1 lb. *otc.*
Use: Nutritional supplement.

Lipitor. (Parke-Davis) Atorvastatin calcium 10 mg, 20 mg and 40 mg/Tab. Bot. 90s, 5000s (10 mg only) and UD 100s. *Rx.*
Use: Antihyperlipidemic.

Lipkote by Coppertone. (Schering Plough) Padimate O, oxybenzone. SPF 15. Lip balm 4.2 g. *otc.*
Use: Sunscreen.

Lipkote SPF 15 Ultra Sunscreen Lipbalm. (Schering Plough) Tube 0.15 oz,. *otc.*
Use: Sunscreen.

Lip Medex. (Blistex) Petrolatum, camphor 1%, phenol 0.54%, cocoa butter, lanolin. Oint. 210 g. *otc.*
Use: Fever blisters, lip protectant.

lipocholine. See: Choline dihydrogen citrate. (Various Mfr.).

Lipoflavonoid Caplets. (Numark Laboratories) vitamins C 100 mg, B_1 0.33 mg, B_2 0.33 mg, B_3 3.33 mg, B_6 0.33 mg, B_{12} 1.66 mcg, B_5 1.66 mg, choline 111 mg, bioflavonoids 100 mg, inositol 111 mg. Bot. 100s, 500s. *otc.*
Use: Vitamin supplement.

Lipoflavonoid Capsules. (Numark Laboratories) Choline 111 mg, inositol 111 mg, vitamins B_1 0.3 mg, B_2 0.3 mg, B_3 3.3 mg, B_5 1.7 mg, B_6 0.3 mg, B_{12} 1.7 mcg, C 100 mg, lemon bioflavonoid complex. Cap. Bot. 100s, 500s. *otc.*
Use: Vitamin supplement.

Lipogen Caplets. (Zenith Goldline) Choline 111 mg, inositol 111 mg, vitamins B_1 0.33 mg, B_2 0.33 mg, B_3 3.33 mg, B_5 1.7 mg, B_6 0.33 mg, B_{12} 1.7 mcg, C 20 mg, A 1667 IU, E 10 IU, Zn 30 mg, Cu, Se. Bot. 60s. *otc.*
Use: Mineral, vitamin supplement.

Lipogen Capsules. (Various Mfr.) Choline 111 mg, inositol, vitamins B_1 0.33 mg, B_2 0.33 mg, B_3 3.33 mg, B_5 1.7 mg, B_6 0.33 mg, B_{12} 1.7 mcg, C 100 mg/Cap. Bot. 60s. *otc.*
Use: Vitamin supplement.

lipolytic enzyme.
W/Proteolytic enzyme, amylolytic enzyme, cellulolytic enzyme, methyl polysiloxane, ox bile, betaine HCl.
See: Zymme, Cap. (Scrip).

Lipomul. (Pharmacia & Upjohn) Corn oil

10 g/15 ml w/d-Alpha tocopheryl acetate, butylated hydroxy-anisole, polysorbate 80, glyceride phosphates, sodium saccharin, sodium benzoate 0.05%, benzoic acid 0.05%, sorbic acid 0.07%. Bot. pt. *otc.*
Use: Nutritional supplement.

Lipo-Nicin/300 mg. (Zeneca) Niacin 300 mg, vitamin C 150 mg, B_1 25 mg, B_2 2 mg, B_6 10 mg/TR Cap. 100s. *Rx.*
Use: Vasodilator.

Lipo-Nicin/100 mg. (Zeneca) Nicotinic acid 100 mg, niacinamide 75 mg, vitamins C 150 mg, B_1 25 mg, B_2 2 mg, B_6 10 mg/Tab. Bot. 100s, 500s. *Rx.*
Use: Vasodilator combination.

Liponol Capsules. (Rugby) Choline, inositol 83 mg, methionine 110 mg, vitamins B_1 3 mg, B_2 3 mg, B_3 10 mg, B_5 2 mg, B_6 2 mg, B_{12} 2 mcg, desiccated liver 56 mg, liver concentrate 30 mg, sorbitol, lecithin/Cap. Bot. 60s. *otc.*
Use: Nutritional supplement.

liposomal amphotericin B.
Use: Antiviral. [Orphan drug]
See: AmBisome. (Fujisawa).

liposomal doxorubicin.
See: doxorubicin hydrochloride.

liposomal prostaglandin E-1 injection. (Liposome)
Use: Acute respiratory distress syndrome. [Orphan drug]

liposome encapsulated recombinant interleukin-2. (Biomira)
Use: Antineoplastic. [Orphan drug]

Liposyn. (Abbott Hospital Prods) Intravenous fat emulsion containing safflower oil 10%, egg phosphatides 1.2%, glycerin 2.5% in water for inj. **10%:** Single-dose container 50 ml, 100 ml, 200 ml, 500 ml; Syringe Pump Unit 50 ml single-dose. **20%:** Single-dose container 200 ml, 500 ml Syringe Pump Unit 25 ml or 50 ml single-dose. *Rx.*
Use: Nutritional supplement, parenteral.

Liposyn II. (Abbott Hospital Prods) Intravenous fat emulsion: **10%:** Safflower oil 5%, soybean oil 5%. Bot. 100 ml, 200 ml, 500 ml. **20%:** Safflower oil 10%, soybean oil 10% w/egg phosphatides 1.2%, glycerin 2.5%. 200 ml, 500 ml. Bot. Syringe pump unit 25 ml, 50 ml. *Rx.*
Use: Nutritional supplement, parenteral.

Liposyn III. (Abbott Laboratories) Oil, soybean, egg yolk phospholipids. **10%:** 100, 200, 500 ml. **20%:** 100, 500 ml. *Rx.*
Use: Nutritional supplement, parenteral.

Lipo-Tears. (Spectra) Mineral oil, petrolatum. Preservative free. Drops. Bot. 1 ml (in 30s). *otc.*
Use: Lubricant, ophthalmic.

Lipotriad Caplets. (Numark Laboratories) Zn 30 mg, vitamin A 5000 IU, C 60 mg, E 30 IU, Cu, Se, B_3 20 mg, B_1 1.5 mg, B_2 1.7 mg, B_6 2 mg, B_{12} 6 mcg, B_5 10 mg, choline bitartrate, inositol. Bot. 60s. *otc.*
Use: Mineral, vitamin supplement.

lipotropics with vitamins.
Use: Nutritional supplement.
See: Lipotriad, Liq. (Numark Laboratories).
Lipogen, Cap. (Various Mfr.).
Lipotriad, Cap. (Numark Laboratories).
Lipoflavonoid, Cap. (Numark Laboratories).
Cholinoid, Cap. (Zenith Goldline).
Akoline, C.B., Cap. (Akorn).
Akoline, C.B., Capl. (Akorn).
Liponol, Cap. (Rugby).
Methatropic, Cap. (Zenith Goldline).
Cholidase, Tab. (Freeda Vitamins).

Lipoxide Caps. (Major) Chlordiazepoxide HCl 5 mg, 10 mg or 25 mg/Cap. Bot. 100s, 500s, 1000s. *c-iv.*
Use: Anxiolytic.

Liqua-Gel. (Paddock) Boric acid, glycerine, propylene glycol, methylparaben, propylparaben, Irish moss extract, methylcellulose. Bot. 4 oz, 16 oz. *otc.*

Liquibid. (ION Laboratories) Guaifenesin 600 mg, dye free. SR Tab. Bot. 100s. *Rx.*
Use: Expectorant.

Liquibid-D. (ION) Guaifenesin 600 mg, phenylephrine HCl 40 mg. SR Tab. Bot. 100s. *Rx.*
Use: Expectorant.

Liqui-Char. (Jones Medical Industries) Activated charcoal. **Liq. Bot.:** 12.5 g/60 ml, 15 g/75 ml. **Squeeze container:** 25 g/120 ml, 50 g/240 ml, 30 g/120 ml. *otc.*
Use: Antidote.

Liqui-Doss. (Ferndale Laboratories) Docusate sodium 60 mg, mineral oil. Bot. pt. *otc.*
Use: Laxative.

Liquid Barosperse. (Lafayette Pharm) Barium sulfate 60%. Susp. Bot. 355 ml.
Use: Radiopaque agents.

Liquid Geritonic. (Roberts Pharm) Fe 105 mg, liver fraction 1 375 mg, B_1 3 mg, B_2 3 mg, B_3 30 mg, B_6 0.3 mg, B_{12} 9 mcg, inositol 60 mg, glycine 180 mg,

yeast concentrate 375 mg, Ca, I, K, Mg, Mn, P, alcohol 20%. Liq. Bot. 240 ml, gal. *otc.*
Use: Nutritional supplement.

Liquid Lather. (Ulmer) Gentle wash for hands, body, face, hair. Bot. 8 oz, gal. *otc.*
Use: Cleanser.

liquid petrolatum emulsion.
See: Mineral Oil Emulsion, U.S.P. 23.

Liquid Pred Syrup. (Muro) Prednisone 5 mg/5 ml in syrup base. Alcohol 5%, saccharin, sorbitol. Bot. 120 ml, 240 ml. *Rx.*
Use: Corticosteroid.

Liquifilm Forte. (Allergan) Polyvinyl alcohol 3%, thimerosal 0.002%, EDTA, sodium Cl. Soln. Bot. 15 ml, 30 ml. *otc.*
Use: Artificial tears.

Liquifilm Tears. (Allergan) Polyvinyl alcohol 1.4%, chlorobutanol 0.5%, sodium Cl. Bot. 15 ml, 30 ml. *otc.*
Use: Artificial tears.

Liquifilm Wetting Solution. (Allergan) Polyvinyl alcohol, hydroxypropyl methylcellulose, edetate disodium, sodium Cl, potassium Cl, benzalkonium Cl 0.004%. Bot. 60 ml. *otc.*
Use: Contact lens care.

Liqui-Histine-D Elixir. (Liquipharm) Phenylpropanolamine HCl 12.5 mg, pyrilamine maleate 4 mg, phenyltoloxamine citrate 4 mg, pheniramine maleate 4 mg/5ml. Liq. Bot. 473 ml. *Rx.*
Use: Antihistamine, decongestant.

Liqui-Histine DM. (Liquipharm) Dextromethorphan HBr 10 mg, phenylpropanolamine HCl 12.5 mg, brompheniramine maleate 2 mg/5 ml. Alcohol free. Syr. Bot. 473 ml. *Rx.*
Use: Antihistamine, antitussive, decongestant.

Liquimat. (Galderma) Sulfur 5%, SD alcohol 40 22%, cetyl alcohol in drying makeup base. Plastic Bot. 45 ml. *otc.*
Use: Dermatologic, acne.

Liquipake. (Lafayette Pharm) Barium sulfate suspension 100% w/v for dilution. Bot. 1850 ml, Case 4s.
Use: Radiopaque agent.

Liquiprin. (Menley & James) Acetaminophen 80 mg/1.66 ml, saccharin. Soln. Bot. 35 ml w/dropper. *otc.*
Use: Analgesic.

liquor carbonis detergens.
See: Coal Tar Topical Soln., U.S.P. 23. (Various Mfr.).

•**lisadimate.** (liss-AD-ih-mate) USAN.
Use: Sunscreen.

•**lisinopril.** (lie-SIN-oh-pril) U.S.P. 23.
Use: Antihypertensive.
See: Prinivil, Tab. (Merck).
Zestril, Tab. (Zeneca).
W/Hydrochlorothiazide
See: Prinzide, Tab. (Merck).
Zestorectic, Tab. (Zeneca).

•**lisofylline.** (lie-SO-fih-lin) USAN.
Use: Immunomodulator.

Listerine Antiseptic. (Warner Lambert Consumer Healthcare) Thymol 0.06%, eucalyptol 0.09%, methyl salicylate 0.06%, menthol 0.04%. Alcohol 26.9% (regular flavor), 21.6% (cool mint flavor), sorbitol, saccharin. Bot. 90 ml, 180 ml, 360 ml, 540 ml, 720 ml, 960 ml, 1440 ml. *otc.*
Use: Mouthwash, antiseptic.

Listermint Arctic Mint Mouthwash. (Warner Lambert Consumer Healthcare) Glycerin, poloxamer 335, PEG 600, sodium lauryl sulfate, sodium benzoate, benzoic acid, zinc chloride, saccharin. Liq. 946 ml. *otc.*
Use: Antiseptic, mouthwash.

Lite Pred. (Horizon) Prednisolone sodium phosphate 0.125%. Soln. Bot. 5 ml. *Rx.*
Use: Corticosteroid, ophthalmic.

•**lithium carbonate.** (LITH-ee-uhm CAR-boe-nate) U.S.P. 23.
Use: Antipsychotic, manic depressive state; antimanic; antidepressant.
See: Eskalith, Cap., Tab. (SmithKline Beecham Pharmaceuticals).
Lithobid, Tab. (Novartis Pharmaceuticals).
Lithonate, Cap. (Solvay).
Lithotabs, Tab. (Solvay).

lithium carbonate capsules and tablets. (Roxane) Lithium carbonate. **Tab.:** 300 mg. Bot. 100s, 1000s, UD 100s. **Cap.:** 150 mg, 300 mg or 600 mg. Bot. 100s, 1000s, UD 100s. *Rx.*
Use: Antipsychotic, manic depressive state; antimanic; antidepressant.

•**lithium citrate.** (LITH-ee-uhm) U.S.P. 23.
Use: Antimanic.
See: Cibalith-Si, Liq. (Novartis Pharmaceuticals).
Lithonate-S, Liq. (Solvay).

lithium citrate. (Various Mfr.) Lithium citrate 8 mEq (equivalent to 300 mg lithium carbonate)/5 ml. Syr. Bot. 480 ml, 500 ml, UD 5 ml, 10 ml. *Rx.*
Use: Antipsychotic.

•**lithium hydroxide.** (LITH-ee-uhm high-DROX-ide) U.S.P. 23.
Use: Antipsychotic, manic depressive state; antimanic; antidepressant.

Lithonate. (Solvay) Lithium carbonate 300 mg/Cap. Bot. 100s, 1000s, UD 100s. *Rx.*
Use: Antipsychotic.

Lithostat. (Mission Pharmacal) Acetohydroxamic acid 250 mg/Tab. Bot. 100s. *Rx.*
Use: Anti-infective, urinary.

Lithotabs. (Solvay) Lithium carbonate 300 mg/Tab. Bot. 100s, 1000s, UD 100s. *Rx.*
Use: Antipsychotic.

Livec. (Enzyme Process) Vitamins A 5000 IU, B_1 1.5 mg, B_2 1.7 mg, niacin 20 mg, C 60 mg, B_6 2 mg, pantothenic acid 10 mg, E 30 IU, B_{12} 6 mcg, calcium 250 mg, iron 5 mg, D 400 IU, folacin 0.075 mg/3 Tab. Bot. 100s, 300s. *otc.*
Use: Mineral, vitamin supplement.

Liverbex. (Spanner) Liver 2 mcg, vitamins B_1, B_2, B_6, B_{12}, niacinamide, pantothenate/ml. Vial 30 ml. *otc.*
Use: Nutritional supplement.

Liver Combo No. 5. (Rugby) Liver vitamin B_{12} equivalent 10 mcg, crystalline B_{12} 100 mcg, folic acid 0.4 mg/ml. Inj. Vial 10 ml. *Rx.*
Use: Nutritional supplement, parenteral.

liver derivative complex.
See: Kutapressin, Inj. (Schwarz Pharma).

liver desiccated. Desiccated liver substance.

liver extract. Dry liver extract w/Vitamin B_{12}, folic acid.

liver function agents.
See: Bromsulphalein, Amp. (Becton Dickinson).
Iodophthalein (Various Mfr.).
Sulfobromophthalein Sodium U.S.P. 23 (Gotham).

Livergran. (Rawl) Desiccated whole liver 9 g, vitamins B_1 18 mg, B_2 36 mg, niacinamide 90 mg, choline bitartrate 216 mg, B_6 3.6 mg, calcium pantothenate 3.6 mg, inositol 90 mg, biotin 6 mcg, vitamins B_{12} 5.4 mcg, methionine 198 mg, arginine 242 mg, cystine 72 mg, glutamic acid 675 mg, histidine 99 mg, isoleucine 333 mg, leucine 495 mg, lysine 297 mg, phenylalanine 189 mg, threonine 333 mg, tryptophan 45 mg, tyrosine 180 mg, valine 306 mg/3 Tsp. Bot. 15 oz. *otc.*
Use: Nutritional supplement.

liver injection. (Various Mfr.) Liver extract for parenteral use. *Rx.*
Use: Parenteral liver supplement.

liver injection. (Arcum; Lederle) Vitamin B_{12} 20 mcg/ml. Vial 10 ml. *Rx.*
Use: Nutritional supplement.

Liver Injection, Crude. (Eli Lilly) 2 mcg/ml. Vial 30 ml; (Medwick) 2 mcg/ml. Vial 30 ml. *Rx.*
Use: Liver supplement.

Liver Iron Vitamins Inj. (Arcum) Liver inj. (10 mcg B_{12} activity/ml) 0.1 ml, crude liver inj. (2 mcg B_{12} activity/ml) 0.125 ml, green ferric ammonium citrate 20 mg, niacinamide 50 mg, vitamin B_6 0.3 mg, B_2 0.3 mg, procaine HCl 0.5%, phenol 0.5%/2 ml. Vial 30 ml. *Rx.*
Use: Nutritional supplement.

Liver, Refined. (Medwick) 20 mcg/ml. Vial 10 ml, 30 ml. *Rx.*
Use: Nutritional supplement.

liver vasoconstrictor.
See: Kutapressin, Vial, Amp. (Schwarz Pharma).

Livifol. (Dunhall Pharmaceuticals) Vitamin B_{12} activity from liver inj. equivalent to cyanocobalamin 10 mcg, folic acid 1 mg, cyanocobalamin 100 mcg/ml. Vial 10 ml. *Rx.*
Use: Vitamin supplement.

Livitrinsic-f Capsules. (Zenith Goldline) Iron 110 mg, vitamins B_{12} 15 mcg, C 75 mg, intrinsic factor concentrate 240 mg, folic acid 0.5 mg/Cap. Bot. 100s, 1000s. *Rx.*
Use: Mineral, vitamin supplement.

Livostin. (Ciba Vision Ophthalmics) Levocabastine HCl 0.05%. Susp. Dropper Bot. 2.5 ml, 5 ml, 10 ml. *otc.*
Use: Antiallergic, ophthalmic.

•**lixazinone sulfate.** (lix-AZE-ih-NOHN) USAN.
Use: Cardiotonic (phosphodiesterase inhibitor).

Lixoil. (Lixoil Labs.) Sulfonated fatty oils and one or more esters of higher fatty acids. Bot. 16 oz. *otc.*
Use: Dermatologic.

LKV-Drops. (Freeda Vitamins) Vitamins A 5000 IU, D 400 IU, E 2 mg, B_1 1.5 mg, B_2 1.5 mg, B_3 10 mg, B_5 2 mg, B_6 2 mg, B_{12} 6 mcg, C 50 mg, biotin 50 mcg/0.6 ml. Bot. 60 ml. *otc.*
Use: Vitamin supplement.

LKV Infant Drops. (Freeda Vitamins) Vitamins A 2500 IU, D 400 IU, E 5 IU, B_1 1 mg, B_2 1 mg, B_3 10 mg, B_5 3 mg, B_6 1 mg, B_{12} 4 mcg, C 50 mg, biotin 75 mcg/0.5 ml. Bot. 60 ml. *otc.*
Use: Vitamin supplement.

lld factor.
See: Vitamin B_{12}, Preps. (Various Mfr.).

l-leucovorin.
Use: Antineoplastic.
See: Isovorin.

lm-427. Ribabutin.
Use: CDC anti-infective agent.

LMD. (Abbott Laboratories) Dextran 40 10%. 500 ml. With 0.9% sodium chloride or in 5% dextrose. *Rx.*
Use: Plasma volume expander.

LMWD-Dextran 40. (Pharmachem) Normal saline 0.9%, dextrose 10%. *Rx.*
Use: Plasma volume expander.

Lobac. (Seatrace) Salicylamide 200 mg, phenyltoloxamine 20 mg, acetaminophen 300 mg/Cap. Bot. 100s. *Rx.*
Use: Analgesic, muscle relaxant.

Lobak Tablets. (Sanofi Winthrop) Chlormezanone 250 mg, acetaminophen 300 mg/Tab. In 40s, 100s, 1000s. *Rx.*
Use: Anxiolytic, analgesic.

Lobana Body. (Ulmer) Mineral oil, triethanolamine stearate, stearic acid, lanolin, cetyl alcohol, potassium stearate, propylene glycol parabens. Lot. Bot. 120, 240 ml, gal. *otc.*
Use: Emollient.

Lobana Body Shampoo. (Ulmer) Chloroxylenol. Bot. 240 ml, gal. *otc.*
Use: Dermatologic, hair and skin.

Lobana Conditioning Shampoo. (Ulmer) Bot. 8 oz, gal. *otc.*
Use: Dermatologic, hair and scalp.

Lobana Derm-Ade Cream. (Ulmer) Vitamin A, D, E cream. Jar 2 oz, 8 oz. *otc.*
Use: Dermatologic, counterirritant.

Lobana Liquid Lather. (Ulmer) Sodium laureth sulfate, sodium lauroyl sarcosinate, sodium myristyl sarcosonate, lauramide DEA, linoleamide DEA, octyl hydroxystearate, polyquaternium 7, tetrasodium EDTA, quaternium 15, sodium chloride, citric acid. Liq. Bot. 240 ml, gal. *otc.*
Use: Cleanser.

Lobana Peri-Gard. (Ulmer) Water-resistant ointment containing vitamin A & D. Jar 2 oz, 8 oz. *otc.*
Use: Dermatologic, protectant.

Lobana Perineal Cleanser. (Ulmer) Sprayer 4 oz, 8 oz. Bot. gal. *otc.*
Use: Urine and fecal cleanser.

lobelia fluidextract.
W/Hyoscyamus fluidextract, grindelia fluidextract, potassium iodide.
See: L.S. Mixture, Liq. (Paddock).

lobeline sulfate.
See: Lobidram, Tab. (Dram).
Nikoban, Loz., Gum. (Thompson Medical).

•**lobenzarit sodium.** (low-BENZ-ah-RIT) USAN.
Use: Antirheumatic.

Lobidram. (Dram) Lobeline sulfate 2 mg/Tab. Pkg. 15s, 30s. *otc.*
Use: Smoking cessation aid.

•**lobucavir.** (lah-BYOO-kah-vihr) USAN.
Use: Antiviral.

Locoid. (Ferndale Laboratories) **Cream:** Hydrocortisone butyrate 0.1%. Tube 15 g, 45 g. **Oint.:** Hydrocortisone butyrate 0.1%. Tube 15 g, 45 g. **Soln.:** Hydrocortisone butyrate 0.1%, isopropyl alcohol 50%, glycerin, povidone. Bot. 20 ml, 60 ml. *Rx.*
Use: Corticosteroid, topical.

•**lodelaben.** (low-DELL-ah-ben) USAN.
Formerly Declaben.
Use: Antiarthritic; emphysema therapy adjunct.

Lodine. (Wyeth Ayerst) Etodolac 200, 300 or 400 mg, lactose/Cap. Bot. 100s, UD 100s. *Rx.*
Use: Analgesic, NSAID.

Lodine XL. (Wyeth Ayerst) Etodolac 400 mg and 600 mg, lactose/ER Tab. Bot. 100s and UD 100s. *Rx.*
Use: Analgesic, NSAID.

Lodosyn. (Merck) Carbidopa 25 mg/Tab. Bot. 100s. *Rx.*
Use: Antiparkinsonian.

•**lodoxamide ethyl.** (low-DOX-ah-mide ETH-uhl) USAN.
Use: Antiasthmatic, antiallergic; bronchodilator.

•**lodoxamide tromethamine.** (low-DOX-ah-mide troe-METH-ah-meen) USAN.
Use: Antiasthmatic, antiallergic; bronchodilator; vernal keratoconjunctivitis [Orphan drug]
See: Alomide, Soln. (Alcon Laboratories).

Lodrane LD. (ECR Pharmaceuticals) Brompheniramine maleate 6 mg, pseudoephedrine HCl 60 mg/SR Cap. Bot. 100s. *Rx.*
Use: Antihistamine, decongestant.

Loestrin 21 1/20. (Parke-Davis) Norethindrone acetate 1 mg, ethinyl estradiol 20 mcg Tab. Petipac compact 21 Tab. Ctn. 5 compacts or Ctn. 5 refills. *Rx.*
Use: Contraceptive.

Loestrin 21 1.5/30. (Parke-Davis) Norethindrone acetate 1.5 mg, ethinyl estradiol 30 mcg/Tab. Petipac compact. Ctn. 5 compacts or Ctn. 5 refills. *Rx.*
Use: Contraceptive.

Loestrin Fe 1/20. (Parke-Davis) **White**

Tab.: Norethindrone acetate 1 mg, ethinyl estradiol 20 mcg/Tab.; **Brown Tab.:** Ferrous fumarate 75 mg (7 tabs.) Carton 5 petipac compacts 28 Tab., carton of 5 refills 28 Tab. *Rx.*
Use: Contraceptive.

Loestrin Fe 1.5/30. (Parke-Davis) **Green Tab.:** Norethindrone acetate 1.5 mg, ethinyl estradiol 30 mcg. **Brown Tab.:** Ferrous fumarate 75 mg (7 tabs.). Carton 5 petipac compacts 28 Tab., carton of 5 refills 28 Tab. *Rx.*
Use: Oral contraceptive.

•**lofemizole hydrochloride.** (low-FEM-ih-ZOLE) USAN.
Use: Anti-inflammatory; analgesic; antipyretic.

Lofenalac. (Bristol-Myers) Corn syrup solids 49.2%, casein hydrolysate 18.7% (enzymic digest of casein containing amino acids and small peptides), corn oil 18%, modified tapioca starch 9.57%, protein equivalent 15%, fat 18%, carbohydrate 60%, minerals (ash) 3.6%, phenylalanine 75 mg/100 g pow., Vitamins A 1600 IU, D 400 IU, E 10 IU, C 52 mg, folic acid 100 mcg, B_1 0.5 mg, B_2 0.6 mg, niacin 8 mg, B_6 0.4 mg, B_{12} 2 mcg, biotin 0.05 mg, pantothenic acid 3 mg, Vitamin K-1 100 mcg, choline 85 mg, inositol 30 mg, calcium 600 mg, phosphorus 450 mg, iodine 45 mcg, iron 12 mg, magnesium 70 mg, copper 0.6 mg, zinc 4 mg, manganese 1 mg, chloride 450 mg, potassium 650 mg, sodium 300 mg/qt. at normal dilution of 20 k cal/fl oz, Can 2 1/2 lb. *otc.*
Use: Nutritional supplement.

•**lofentanil oxalate.** (low-FEN-tah-NILL OX-ah-late) USAN.
Use: Analgesic, narcotic.

•**lofepramine hydrochloride.** (low-FEH-prah-MEEN) USAN.
Use: Antidepressant.

•**lofexidine hydrochloride.** (low-FEX-ih-DEEN) USAN.
Use: Antihypertensive.

Logen Liquid. (Zenith Goldline) Diphenoxylate HCl w/atropine sulfate. Bot. 2 oz. *c-v.*
Use: Antidiarrheal.

Logen Tablets. (Zenith Goldline) Diphenoxylate HCl, atropine sulfate. Bot. 100s, 500s, 1000s. *c-v.*
Use: Antidiarrheal.

Lomanate. (Various Mfr.) Diphenoxylate HCl 2.5 mg, atropine sulfate 0.025 mg/5 ml. Bot. 60 ml. *c-v.*
Use: Antidiarrheal.

•**lomefloxacin.** (low-MEH-FLOX-ah-sin) USAN.
Use: Anti-infective.

•**lomefloxacin hydrochloride.** (low-MEH-FLOX-ah-sin) USAN.
Use: Anti-infective.
See: Maxaquin, Tab. (Searle).

•**lomefloxacin mesylate.** (low-MEH-FLOX-ah-sin) USAN.
Use: Anti-infective.

•**lometraline hydrochloride.** (low-MET-rah-LEEN) USAN.
Use: Antipsychotic, antiparkinsonian.

•**lometrexol sodium.** (LOW-meh-TREX-ole) USAN.
Use: Antineoplastic.

•**lomofungin.** (low-moe-FUN-jin) USAN.
Use: Antifungal.

Lomotil. (Searle) Diphenoxylate HCl 2.5 mg, atropine sulfate 0.025 mg/Tab. or 5 ml. **Tab.:** Bot. 100s, 500s, 1000s, 2500s, UD 100s. **Liq.:** Bot. w/dropper 2 oz. *c-v.*
Use: Antidiarrheal.

•**lomustine.** (LOW-muss-teen) USAN.
Use: Antineoplastic.
See: CeeNu, Cap. (Bristol-Myers Squibb).

Lonalac. (Bristol-Myers) Protein as casein 21%, fat as coconut oil 49%, carbohydrate as lactose 30%, vitamins A 1440 IU, B_1 0.6 mg, B_2 2.6 mg, niacin 1.2 mg, calcium 1.69 g, phosphorus 1.5 g, chloride 750 mg, potassium 1.88 g, sodium 38 mg, magnesium 135 mg/qt. Pow. Can 16 oz. *otc.*
Use: Nutritional supplement.

•**lonapalene.** (low-NAP-ah-LEEN) USAN.
Use: Antipsoriatic.

Long Acting Nasal Spray. (Weeks & Leo) Oxymetazoline HCl 0.05%. Soln. Bot. 0.75 oz. *otc.*
Use: Decongestant.

Long Acting Neo-Synephrine II Nose Drops and Nasal Spray. (Sanofi Winthrop) Xylometazoline HCl 0.1% (adult strength) or 0.05% (child strength). Bot. 1 oz, Spray 0.5 oz (adult strength). *otc.*
Use: Decongestant.

Long Acting Neo-Synephrine II Vapor Spray. (Sanofi Winthrop) Xylometazoline HCl 0.1%. Mentholated. Spray Bot. 0.5 fl oz. *otc.*
Use: Decongestant.

Loniten. (Pharmacia & Upjohn) Minoxidil 2.5 mg or 10 mg/Tab. **2.5 mg:** Unit-of-use Bot. 100s. **10 mg:** Bot. 500s, Unit-of-use Bot. 100s. *Rx.*

Use: Antihypertensive.

Lonox. (Geneva Pharm) Diphenoxylate HCl 2.5 mg, atropine sulfate 0.025 mg/Tab. Bot. 100s, 500s, 1000s, UD 100s. *c-v.*
Use: Antidiarrheal.

Lo/Ovral. (Wyeth Ayerst) Norgestrel 0.3 mg, ethinyl estradiol 0.03 mg/Tab. Pilpak dispenser 6s, Tab. 21s. *Rx.*
Use: Contraceptive.

Lo/Ovral-28. (Wyeth Ayerst) Tab. 21s, each containing norgestrel 0.03 mg, ethinyl estradiol 0.03 mg, 7 pink inert. Tab. Pilpak dispenser 6s, Tab 28s. *Rx.*
Use: Contraceptive.

•**loperamide hydrochloride.** (low-PURR-ah-mide) U.S.P. 23.
Use: Antiperistaltic.
See: Imodium, Cap. (Ortho McNeil).
Neo-Diaral, Cap. (Roberts Pharm).

Lopid. (Parke-Davis) Gemfibrozil. 600 mg/Tab. Bot. 60s. *Rx.*
Use: Antihyperlipidemic.

Lopressor. (Novartis Pharmaceuticals) Metoprolol tartrate. **Tab.:** 50 mg or 100 mg. Bot. 100s, 1000s, UD 100s, Gy-Pak 60s, 100s. **Amp.:** 5 mg/5 ml. *Rx.*
Use: Beta-adrenergic blocker.

Lopressor HCT. (Novartis Pharmaceuticals) Metoprolol tartrate, hydrochlorothiazide. **Tab.:** 50/25 mg, 100/25 mg or 100/50 mg. Bot. 100s. *Rx.*
Use: Antihypertensive combination.

Loprox. (Hoechst Marion Roussel) Ciclopirox olamine 1% in cream base. Tube 15 g, 30 g, 90 g. *Rx.*
Use: Antifungal, topical.

Lopurin. (Knoll Pharmaceuticals) Allopurinol 100 mg or 300 mg/Tab. Bot. 100s, 1000s, UD 100s. *Rx.*
Use: Antigout agent.

Lorabid. (Eli Lilly) Loracarbef. **Cap.:** 200 mg, 400 mg. Bot. 30s. **Pow. for Oral Susp.:** 100 mg/5 ml, 200 mg/5 ml, parabens, sucrose. Bot. 50 ml, 75 ml, 100 ml. *Rx.*
Use: Anti-infective, cephalosporin.

•**loracarbef.** (LOW-ra-CAR-beff) U.S.P. 23.
Use: Anti-infective.
See: Lorabid, Cap., Pow. (Eli Lilly).

•**lorajmine hydrochloride.** (lahr-AZH-meen) USAN.
Use: Cardiovascular agent.

•**loratadine.** (lore-AT-uh-DEEN) USAN.
Use: Antihistamine.
See: Claritin, Prods. (Schering Plough).

•**lorazepam.** (lore-AZE-uh-pam) U.S.P. 23.
Use: Anxiolytic.
See: Alzapam, Tab. (Ultra).
Ativan, Tab., Inj. (Wyeth Ayerst).

lorazepam. (lore-AZE-uh-pam) (Purepac) Lorazepam. **0.5 mg:** Tab. Bot. 100s, 500s. **1 mg, 2 mg:** Tab. Bot. 100s, 500s, 1000s. *c-iv.*
Use: Anxiolytic, hypnotic, sedative.

lorazepam. (lore-AZE-uh-pam) (Various Mfr.) Lorazepam, benzyl alcohol 2%. Inj. 2 mg/ml, 4 mg/ml. Vial 1 ml, 10 ml. *c-iv.*
Use: Anxiolytic, hypnotic, sedative.

Lorazepam Intensol. (Roxane) Lorazepam 2 mg/ml. Concentrated oral soln. Alcohol and dye free. Dropper Bot. 30 ml. *c-iv.*
Use: Anxiolytic, hypnotic, sedative.

•**lorbamate.** (lore-BAM-ate) USAN.
Use: Muscle relaxant.

•**lorcainide hydrochloride.** (lahr-CANE-ide) USAN.
Use: Cardiovascular agent; antiarrhythmic.

Lorcet-HD. (Forest Pharmaceutical) Hydrocodone bitartrate 5 mg, acetaminophen 500 mg/Cap. Bot. 500s. *c-iii.*
Use: Analgesic combination, narcotic.

Lorcet Plus. (Forest Pharmaceutical) Hydrocodone bitartrate 7.5 mg, acetaminophen 650 mg/Tab. Bot. 100s., 500s, UD 100s. *c-iii.*
Use: Analgesic combination, narcotic.

Lorcet 10/650. (Forest Pharmaceutical) Hydrocodone bitartrate 10 mg, acetaminophen 650 mg/Tab. Bot. 20s, 100s, UD 100s. *c-iii.*
Use: Analgesic combination, narcotic.

•**lorcinadol.** (LORE-sin-ah-dole) USAN.
Use: Analgesic.

•**loreclezole.** (lahr-EH-kleh-zole) USAN.
Use: Antiepileptic.

Lorelco. (Hoechst Marion Roussel) Probucol 250 mg/Tab. Bot. 120s. *Rx.*
Use: Antihyperlipidemic.

•**lormetazepam.** (LORE-met-AZE-eh-pam) USAN.
Use: Hypnotic, sedative.

•**lornoxicam.** (lore-NOX-ih-kam) USAN.
Use: Anti-inflammatory; analgesic.

Loroxide. (Dermik Laboratories) Benzoyl peroxide 5.5%, cetyl alcohol, parabens, EDTA, 1% silica, 64% calcium phosphate. Lot. Bot. 25 g. *otc.*
Use: Dermatologic, acne.

Lorprn. (UCB Pharmaceuticals) Aspirin 325 mg, caffeine 40 mg, butalbital 50 mg/Cap. Bot. 100s. *c-iii.*
Use: Analgesic combination, narcotic.

Lortab 2.5/500. (UCB Pharmaceuticals) Hydrocodone 2.5 mg, acetaminophen 500 mg/Tab. Bot. 100s, 500s. *c-III.*
Use: Analgesic combination, narcotic.

Lortab 5/500. (UCB Pharmaceuticals) Hydrocodone 5 mg, acetaminophen 500 mg/Tab. Bot. 100s, 500s, UD 100s. *c-III.*
Use: Analgesic combination, narcotic.

Lortab 7/500. (UCB Pharmaceuticals) Hydrocodone 7.5 mg, acetaminophen 500 mg/Tab. Bot. 100s, 500s, UD 100s. *c-III.*
Use: Analgesic combination, narcotic.

Lortab 10/500. (UCB Pharmaceuticals) Hydrocodone bitartrate 10 mg, acetaminophen 500 mg/Tab. Bot. 100s, 500s. *c-III.*
Use: Analgesic combination, narcotic.

Lortab ASA. (UCB Pharmaceuticals) Hydrocodone bitartrate 5 mg, aspirin 500 mg/Tab. Bot. 100s. *c-III.*
Use: Analgesic combination, narcotic.

Lortab Elixir. (UCB Pharmaceuticals) Hydrocodone bitartrate 2.5 mg, acetaminophen 167 mg/5 ml w/alcohol 7%, parabens, saccharin, sorbitol, sucrose. Bot. 473 ml. *c-III.*
Use: Analgesic combination, narcotic.

•**lortalamine.** (lahr-TAHL-ah-MEEN) USAN.
Use: Antidepressant.

•**lorzafone.** (LAHR-zah-FONE) USAN.
Use: Anxiolytic.

•**losartan potassium.** (low-SAHR-tan) USAN.
Use: Antihypertensive; treatment of CHF (angiotensin II receptor blocker).
See: Cozaar, Tab. (Merck).
Hyzaar, Tab. (Merck).

Losec.
See: Prilosec.

Losopan Liquid. (Zenith Goldline) Magaldrate 540 mg/5 ml. Bot. 12 oz. *otc.*
Use: Antacid.

Losopan Plus Liquid. (Zenith Goldline) Magaldrate 540 mg, simethicone 20 mg/5 ml. Bot. 12 oz. *otc.*
Use: Antacid, antiflatulent.

Losotron Plus Liquid. (Various Mfr.) Magaldrate 540 mg, simethicone 20 mg/5 ml. Bot. 360 ml. *otc.*
Use: Antacid, antiflatulent.

•**losoxantrone hydrochloride.** (low-SOX-an-trone) USAN.
Use: Antineoplastic.

•**losulazine hydrochloride.** (low-SULL-ah-zeen) USAN.
Use: Antihypertensive.

Lotawin Capsules. (Sanofi Winthrop) Oxypertine. *Rx.*
Use: Anxiolytic.

Lotemax. (Bausch & Lomb) Loteprednol etabonate 5 mg/ml, EDTA, glycerin, povidone, tyloxapol. Ophth. Susp. Bot. 2.5 ml, 5 ml, 10 ml, 15 ml. *Rx.*
Use: Anti-inflammatory.

Lotensin. (Novartis Pharmaceuticals) Benazepril HCl 5 mg, 10 mg, 20 mg, or 40 mg, lactose/Tab. Bot. 100s, UD 100s. *Rx.*
Use: Antihypertensive.

•**loteprednol etabonate.** (low-TEH-PRED-nole ett-AB-ohn-ate) USAN.
Use: Anti-inflammatory, topical.
Use: Alrex, Ophth. Susp. (Bausch & Lomb).
Lotemax, Ophth. Susp. (Bausch & Lomb).

lotio alba. White lotion. *otc.*
Use: Antiseborrheic; dermatologic, acne.
W/Sulfur, calamine, alcohol.
See: Sulfa-Lo, Lot. (Whorton).

lotio alsulfa. (Doak Dermatologics) Colloidal sulfur 5%. Bot. 4 oz. *otc.*
Use: Antiseborrheic; dermatologic, acne.

Lotion-Jel. (C.S. Dent) Benzocaine in gel base. Tube 0.2 oz. *otc.*
Use: Anesthetic, local.

Lotrel. (Novartis Pharmaceuticals) Amlodipine 2.5 mg or 5 mg, benazepril HCl 10 mg/Cap. or amlodipine 5 mg, benazepril HCl 20 mg/Cap. Bot. 100s. *Rx.*
Use: Antihypertensive combination.

Lotrimin. (Schering Plough) Clotrimazole 1%. **Cream:** Tube 15 g, 30 g, 45 g, 90 g. **Lot.:** Bot. 30 ml. **Soln.:** 1%. Bot. 10 ml, 30 ml. *Rx.*
Use: Antifungal, topical.

Lotrimin AF. (Schering Plough).

Lotrisone. (Schering Plough) Clotrimazole 1%, betamethasone dipropionate 0.05%/g. Tube 15 g, 45 g. *Rx.*
Use: Antifungal, topical.

Lo-Trop. (Vangard) Diphenoxylate HCl 2.5 mg, atropine sulfate 0.025 mg/Tab. Bot. 100s, 1000s. *c-v.*
Use: Antidiarrheal.

•**lovastatin.** (LOW-vuh-STAT-in) U.S.P. 23. *Formerly Mevinolin.*
Use: Antihypercholesteremic; antihyperlipidemic; HMG-CoA reductase inhibitor.
See: Mevacor, Tab. (Merck).

Love Longer. (Schmid) Benzocaine 7.5%

in water-soluble lubricant base. Tube 0.5 oz. *otc.*
Use: Anesthetic, local.

Lovenox. (Rhone-Poulenc Rorer) Enoxaparin sodium. 30 mg/0.3 ml, 40 mg/ 0.4 ml. Inj. Pk. 10 prefilled syringes w/26 guage x ½-inch needle. *Rx.*
Use: Anticoagulant.

•**loviride.** (LOW-vihr-ide) USAN.
Use: Antiviral for chronic oral treatment of HIV-seropositive patients (nonnucleoside reverse transcriptase inhibitor).

Lowila Cake. (Westwood Squibb) Sodium lauryl sulfoacetate, dextrin, boric acid, urea, sorbitol, mineral oil, PEG 14 M, lactic acid, cellulose gum, docusate sodium, water, fragrance. Cake 112.5 g. *otc.*
Use: Dermatologic, cleanser.

Low-Quel. (Halsey) Diphenoxylate HCl 2.5 mg, atropine sulfate 0.025 mg/Tab. Bot. 100s. *c-v.*
Use: Antidiarrheal.

Lowsium. (Rugby) Magaldrate 540 mg/5 ml. Susp. Bot. 360 ml. *otc.*
Use: Antacid.

Lowsium Plus. (Rugby) **Tab.:** Magaldrate 480 mg, simethicone 20 mg. Bot. 60s. **Susp.:** Magaldrate 540 mg, simethicone 40 mg/5 ml. Bot. 360 ml. *otc.*
Use: Antacid, antiflatulent.

•**loxapine.** (LOX-ah-peen) USAN.
Use: Anxiolyitc.

loxapine hydrochloride. *Rx.*
Use: Anxiolytic.
See: Daxolin Concentrate, Liq. (Bayer Corp).
Loxitane-C Oral Concentrate (ESI Lederle Generics).
Loxitane, Inj. (ESI Lederle Generics).

•**loxapine succinate.** (LOX-ah-peen) U.S.P. 23.
Use: Anxiolytic.
See: Loxitane, Preps. (ESI Lederle Generics).

loxapine succinate. (Various Mfr.) 5 mg, 10 mg, 25 mg, 50 mg. Cap. Bot. 30s, 100s, 1000s. *Rx.*
Use: Antipsychotic.

Loxitane C. (ESI Lederle Generics) Loxapine HCl oral concentrate 25 mg/ ml. Bot. 120 ml w/dropper. *Rx.*
Use: Antipsychotic.

Loxitane Capsules. (ESI Lederle Generics) Loxapine succinate. 10 mg, 50 mg/ Cap.: Bot. 100s, 1000s, UD 100s. *Rx.*
Use: Antipsychotic.

Loxitane IM. (ESI Lederle Generics) Loxapine HCl (base equivalent) 50 mg/ ml. Inj. Vial 10 ml. *Rx.*
Use: Antipsychotic.

•**loxoribine.** (LOX-ore-ih-BEAN) USAN.
Use: Immunostimulant; vaccine adjuvant.

L_2-oxothiazolidine$_4$-carboxylic acid.
Use: Treatment of adult respiratory distress syndrome. [Orphan drug]
See: Procysteine (Transcend Therapeutics).

Lozol. (Rhone-Poulenc Rorer) Indapamide 2.5 mg/Tab. Bot. 100s, 1000s, 2500s, Strip dispenser 100s. *Rx.*
Use: Diuretic, antihypertensive.

L-PAM.
See: Alkeran (GlaxoWellcome).

l-sarcolysin.
See: Alkeran, Tab. (GlaxoWellcome).

l-threonine.
Use: Antispasmodic.

l-triiodothyronine sod.
See: Cytomel, Tab. (SmithKline Beecham Pharmaceuticals).
Liothyronine Sod.

Lubafax. (GlaxoWellcome) Surgical lubricant, sterile; water soluble, non-staining. Foil wrapper 2.7 g, 5 g. Box 144s.
Use: Lubricant.

Lubath. (Warner Lambert) Mineral oil, PPG-15, stearyl ether, oleth-2, nonoxynol-5, fragrance, FD&C; Green No. 6. Bot. 4 oz, 8 oz, 16 oz. *otc.*
Use: Emollient.

•**lubeluzole.** (loo-BELL-you-zole) USAN.
Use: Stroke treatment.

Lubinol. (Purepac) Light, heavy and extra heavy mineral oil. Bot. pt, qt, gal. (Extra heavy Bot.) 8 oz, pt, qt, gal. *otc.*
Use: Emollient.

Lubraseptic Jelly. (Guardian Laboratories) Water-soluble amyl phenyl phenol complex 0.12%, phenylmercuric nitrate, 0.007%. Bellows-type tube 10 g, 24s.
Use: Genitourinary aid.

LubraSOL Bath Oil. (Pharmaceutical Specialties) Mineral oil, lanolin oil, PEG-200 dilaurate, oxybenzone. Bot. 240 ml, 480 ml, gal. *otc.*
Use: Emollient.

Lubricating Jelly. (Taro Pharm) Glycerin, propylene glycol. Jelly. 60 g, 125 g. *otc.*
Use: Vaginal agent.

Lubriderm Cream. (Warner Lambert)

Lubriderm Lotion. (Warner Lambert) Water, mineral oil, petrolatum, sorbitol, lanolin, lanolin alcohol, stearic acid, TEA, cetyl alcohol, fragrance (if

scented), butylparaben, methylparaben, propylparaben, sodium Cl. Bot. (scented), 4 oz, 8 oz, 16 oz; (unscented) 8 oz, 16 oz. *otc.*
Use: Emollient.

Lubriderm Lubath Oil. (Warner Lambert) Mineral oil, PPG-15 stearyl ether, oleth-2, nonoxynol-5. Lanolin free. Bot. 240 ml, pt. *otc.*
Use: Emollient.

Lubrin. (Kenwood/Bradley) Glycerin, caprylic/capric triglyceride. Inserts. Pkg. 5s, 12s. *otc.*
Use: Lubricant.

LubriTears. (Bausch & Lomb) White petrolatum, mineral oil, lanolin, chlorobutanol 0.5%. Oint. Tube 3.5 g. *otc.*
Use: Lubricant, ophthalmic.

LubriTears Solution. (Bausch & Lomb) Hydroxypropyl methylcellulose 2906 0.3%, dextran 70 0.1%, EDTA, KCl, NaCl, benzalkonium chloride 0.01%. Bot. 15 ml. *otc.*
Use: Artificial tears.

•**lucanthone hydrochloride.** (LOO-kan-thone) USAN.
Use: Antischistosomal.

Ludens Cough Drops. (Luden's).

Ludiomil. (Novartis Pharmaceuticals) Maprotiline 25 mg, 50 mg or 75 mg/Tab. Bot. 100s, Accu-Pak 100s. *Rx.*
Use: Antidepressant.

•**lufironil.** (loo-FIHR-ah-nill) USAN.
Use: Collagen inhibitor.

Lufyllin. (Wallace Laboratories) Dyphylline. Inj. **Amp.:** (500 mg/2 ml) Box 25s. **Elix.:** 100 mg/15 ml; alcohol 20%. Bot. pt, gal. **Tab.:** 200 mg. Bot. 100s, 1000s, UD 100s. *Rx.*
Use: Bronchodilator.

Lufyllin-400. (Wallace Laboratories) Dyphylline 400 mg/Tab. Bot. 100s, 1000s. *Rx.*
Use: Bronchodilator.

Lufyllin-EPG. (Wallace Laboratories) Ephedrine HCl 16 mg, dyphylline 100 mg, phenobarbital 16 mg, guaifenesin 200 mg/Tab. or 10 ml. Tab. Bot. 100s. *Rx.*
Use: Antiasthmatic combination.

Lufyllin-EPG Elixir. (Wallace Laboratories) Dyphylline 150 mg, ephedrine HCl 24 mg, guaifenesin 300 mg, phenobarbital 24 mg, alcohol 5.5%/15 ml. Elix. Bot. 480 ml. *Rx.*
Use: Antiasthmatic combination.

Lufyllin-GG. (Wallace Laboratories) **Tab.:** Dyphylline 200 mg, guaifenesin 200 mg/Tab. Bot. 100s, 3000s, UD 100s. **Elix.:** Dyphylline 100 mg, guaifenesin 100 mg, alcohol 17%/15 ml. Elix. Bot. pt, gal. *Rx.*
Use: Bronchodilator, expectorant.

Lugol's Solution. Strong iodine soln, U.S.P. 23. (Lyne). Iodine 5 g, potassium iodide 10 g, in purified water to make 100 ml. Bot. 15 ml. (Wisconsin Pharm) Bot. pt. *otc, Rx.*
Use: Antithyroid, antiseptic, topical.

Luminal Injection. (Sanofi Winthrop) Phenobarbital 130 mg/ml. Amp 1 ml. Box 100s.
Use: Hypnotic, sedative.

Lumopaque Capsules. (Sanofi Winthrop) Tyropanoate sodium.
Use: Radiopaque agent.

lung surfactants.
Use: Surfactant replacement therapy in neonatal respiratory distress syndrome.
See: Exosurf (GlaxoWellcome).
Survanta (Ross Laboratories).

Lupron. (TAP Pharm) Leuprolide acetate 5 mg/ml, benzyl alcohol 1.8 mg. Multiple-dose Vial 2.8 ml. *Rx.*
Use: Hormone.

Lupron Depot. (TAP Pharm) Leuprolide acetate 3.75 or 7.5 mg. Lyophilized microspheres for injection. Single-use kit. Preservative free. Microspheres for inj. Kit. Single-dose vials. *Rx.*
Use: Hormone.

Lupron Depot-Ped. (TAP Pharm) Leuprolide acetate 7.5, 11.25 or 15 mg. Preservative free. Microspheres for inj. Kit. *Rx.*
Use: Hormone.

Lupron Depot-3 Month. (TAP Pharm) Leuprolide acetate 11.25 mg/Lyophilized microspheres for injection. Single-use kit. Leuprolide acetate 22.5 mg. Preservative free. Microspheres for inj. *Rx.*
Use: Hormone.

Lupron Depot-4 Month. (TAP Pharm) Leuprolide acetate 30 mg, polylactic acid 264.8 mg, D-mannitol 51.9 mg. Inj. Single-use Kit. *Rx.*
Use: Antineoplastic.

Lupron Injection. (TAP Pharm) Leuprolide acetate 1 mg/0.2 ml. Vial 2.8 ml. *Rx.*
Use: Antineoplastic.

Lupron for Pediatric Use. (TAP Pharm) Leuprolide acetate 5 mg/ml, benzyl alcohol 1.8 mg. Multiple-dose Vial 2.8 ml. *Rx.*
Use: Hormone.

Luramide Tabs. (Major) Furosemide 20 mg, 40 mg or 80 mg/Tab. Bot. 100s, 1000s. *Rx.*
Use: Diuretic.

Luride Drops. (Colgate Oral) Sodium fluoride equivalent to 0.5 mg of fluoride/ Drop. Plastic dropper bot. 50 ml. *Rx.*
Use: Dental caries agent.

Luride Gel. (Colgate) Fluoride (from sodium fluoride and hydrogen fluoride) 1.2%. 7 g. *Rx.*
Use: Dental caries agent.

Luride Lozi-Tabs. (Colgate Oral) Sodium fluoride 0.25 mg/Chew. Tab. Sugar free. Bot. 120s. *Rx.*
Use: Dental caries agent.

Luride-F Lozi Tablets. (Colgate Oral) Sodium fluoride in Lozi base tab. available as fluoride. **0.25 mg:** Bot. 120s; **0.5 mg:** Bot. 120s, 1200s; **1 mg:** Bot. 120s, 1000s, 5000s. *Rx.*
Use: Dental caries agent.

Luride Prophylaxis Paste. (Colgate Oral) Acidulated phosphate sodium fluoride containing 0.4% fluoride ion w/ silicon dioxide abrasive. UD 3 g, Jar 50 g. *otc.*
Use: Dentrifice.

Luride-SF Lozi Tablets. (Colgate Oral) Sodium fluoride 1 mg fluoride/Tab. Bot. 120s. *Rx.*
Use: Dental caries agent.

Luride Topical Gel. (Colgate Oral) Fluoride 1.2%. Tube 7 g. *Rx.*
Use: Dental caries agent.

Luride Topical Solution. (Colgate Oral) Acidulated phosphate sodium fluoride w/pH 3.2. Bot. 250 ml. *otc.*
Use: Dental caries agent.

Lurline PMS. (Fielding) Acetaminophen 500 mg, pamabrom 25 mg, pyridoxine 50 mg/Tab. Bot. 24s, 50s. *otc.*
Use: Analgesic combination.

•**lurosetron mesylate.** (loo-ROW-set-rahn MEH-sih-late) USAN.
Use: Antiemetic.

Lurotin Caps. (BASF Wyandotte) Betacarotene 25 mg/Cap. Bot. 100s. *otc.*
Use: Nutritional supplement.

•**lurtotecan dihyrdochloride.** (lure-toe-TEE-kan die-HIGH-droe-KLOR-ide) USAN.
Use: Antineoplastic (DNA topoisomerase I inhibitor).

luteogan.
See: Progesterone (Various Mfr.).

luteosan.
See: Progesterone (Various Mfr.).

lutocylol. (Novartis Pharmaceuticals) Ethisterone.

Lutolin-F. (Spanner) Progesterone 25 mg or 50 mg/ml. Vial 10 ml.
Use: Hormone, progestin.

Lutolin-S. (Spanner) Progesterone 25 mg/ml. Vial 10 ml. *Rx.*
Use: Hormone, progestin.

•**lutrelin acetate.** (loo-TRELL-in ASS-eh-tate) USAN.
Use: LHRH agonist.

lutren.
See: Progesterone (Various Mfr.).

Lutrepulse. (Ortho McNeil) Gonadorelin acetate 0.8 mg or 3.2 mg/vial. Pow. for reconstitution (lyophilized). Vial 10 ml. *Rx.*
Use: Hormone, gonadotropin-releasing.

lututrin.
See: Lutrexin, Tab. (Becton Dickinson).

Luvox. (Solvay) Fluvoxamine maleate 50 mg or 100 mg/Tab. Bot. 100s, 1000s, UD 100s. *Rx.*
Use: Antidepressant.

•**lyapolate sodium.** (lie-APP-oh-late) USAN.
Use: Anticoagulant.
See: Peson (Hoechst Marion Roussel).

•**lycetamine.** (lie-SEET-ah-meen) USAN.
Use: Antimicrobial, topical.

lycine hydrochloride.
See: Betaine HCl (Various Mfr.).

Lydia E. Pinkham Herbal Compound. (Numark Laboratories) Vitamin C, iron. Bot. 8 fl oz, 16 fl oz.

Lydia E. Pinkham Tablets. (Numark Laboratories) Vitamin C, iron, calcium. 72s, 150s. *otc.*

•**lydimycin.** (lie-dih-MY-sin) USAN.
Use: Antifungal.

Lymphazurin. (Hirsch) Isosulfan blue 10 mg, sodium monohydrogen phosphate 6.6 mg, potassium dihydrogen phosphate 2.7 mg/ml. Vial 5 ml.
Use: Radiopaque agent.

lymphocyte immune globulin.
Use: Management of rejection in renal transplant.
See: Atgam, Inj. (Pharmacia & Upjohn).

LymphoScan. (Immunomedics) Technetium TC-99M murine monoclonal antibody (IgG2a) to B cell.
Use: Diagnostic aid. [Orphan drug]

•**lynestrenol.** (lin-ESS-tree-nahl) USAN.
Use: Hormone, progestin.

lynoestrenol. Lynestrenol.

lyopholized vitamin B complex and vitamin C with B_{12}. (McGuff) B_1 50 mg, B_2 5 mg, B_3 125 mg, B_5 6 mg, B_6 5 mg, B_{12} 1000 mcg, C 50 mg/ml/Inj. Vial 10 ml. *Rx.*

Use: Vitamin supplement, parenteral.

Lyphocin P. (Fujisawa) Vancomycin HCl 500 mg. Vial 10 ml. *Rx.*
Use: Anti-infective.

Lypholyte. (Fujisawa) Multiple electrolye concentrate. Vial 20 ml, 40 ml, Maxivial 100 ml, 200 ml. *Rx.*
Use: Electrolyte supplement.

Lypholyte II. (Fujisawa) Na^+ 35 mEq/L, K^+ 20 mEq/L, Ca^{++} 4.5 mEq/L, Mg^{++} 5 mEq/L, Cl 35 mEq/L, acetate 29.5 mEq/L. Single dose flip-top vial 20 ml, 40 ml; flip-top vial 100 ml, 200 ml. *Rx.*
Use: Nutritional supplement, parenteral.

•**lypressin nasal solution.** (LIE-PRESS-in) U.S.P. 23.
Use: Antidiuretic; vasoconstrictor.
See: Diapid Nasal Spray (Novartis).

lysidin. Methyl glyoxalidin.

•**lysine.** (LIE-SEEN) USAN.
Use: Nutrient, rapid weight gain; amino acid.

l-lysine.
Use: Dietary supplement; amino acid.
See: Enisyl (Person & Covey).
L-Lysine (Various Mfr.).

L-Lysine. (Various Mfr.) 312 mg, 500 mg/Tab. Bot. 100s. 1000 mg/Tab. Bot. 60s. 500 mg/Cap. Bot. 100s and 250s. *otc.*
Use: Dietary supplement; amino acid.

•**lysine acetate.** (LIE-SEEN) U.S.P. 23.
Use: Amino acid.

•**lysine hydrochloride.** (LIE-SEEN) U.S.P. 23.
Use: Amino acid.
See: Enisyl, Tab. (Person & Covey).

lysivane.
See: Parsidol, Tab. (Warner Chilcott).

Lysodase. (Enzon) PEG-glucocerebrosidase.
Use: Gaucher's disease. [Orphan drug]

Lysodren. (Bristol-Myers Oncology/Immunology) Mitotane 500 mg/Tab. Bot. 100s. *Rx.*
Use: Antineoplastic.

•**lysostaphin.** (LIE-so-STAFF-in) USAN. Enzyme produced by *Staphylococcus staphylolyticus.*
Use: Antibiotic; antibacterial enzyme.

Lyteers. (PBH Wesley Jessen).

Lytren. (Bristol-Myers) Water, dextrose, sodium citrate, citric acid, sodium Cl, potassium citrate. Ready-To-Use Bot. 8 fl. oz. *otc.*
Use: Electrolyte, fluid replacement.

M

Maagel. (Health for Life Brands) Aluminum and magnesium hydroxide. Bot. 12 oz, gal. *otc.*
Use: Antacid.

Maalox Antacid. (Rhone-Poulenc Rorer) Calcium carbonate 1000 mg, sodium ≤ 0.4 mEq. Capl. Bot. 50s. *otc.*
Use: Antacid.

Maalox Anti-Diarrheal Caplets. (Rhone-Poulenc Rorer) Loperamide HCl 2 mg/Tab. Pkg. 12s. *otc.*
Use: Antidiarrheal.

Maalox Anti-Gas. (Rhone-Poulenc Rorer) Simethicone 80 mg, sucrose/Chew. Tab. Bot. 12s. *otc.*
Use: Antiflatulent

Maalox Daily Fiber Therapy. (Rhone-Poulenc Rorer) Psyllium hydrophilic mucilloid fiber 3.4 g/dose, sucrose and 35 cal/12 g in regular; aspartame, 21 mg/tsp phenylalanine and 9 cal/5.8 g in sugar free. Pow. Can 283 g (sugar free), 369 g, 3 single-dose (12 g) packets. *otc.*
Use: Laxative.

Maalox Extra Strength Plus Suspension. (Rhone-Poulenc Rorer) Magnesium hydroxide 450 mg, aluminum hydroxide 500 mg, simethicone 40 mg/5 ml. Susp. Bot. 148, 355, 769 ml. *otc.*
Use: Antacid, antiflatulent.

Maalox Extra Strength Plus Tablets. (Rhone-Poulenc Rorer) Magnesium hydroxide 350 mg, aluminum hydroxide 350 mg, simethicone 30 mg. Chew. Tab. Bot. 38s, 75s. *otc.*
Use: Antacid, antiflatulent.

Maalox Extra Strength Suspension. (Rhone-Poulenc Rorer) Aluminum hydroxide 500 mg, magnesium hydroxide 450 mg, simethicone 40 mg, parabens, saccharin, sorbitol/5 ml. Susp. Bot. 148 ml, 355 ml, 769 ml. *otc.*
Use: Antacid, antiflatulent.

Maalox Extra Strength Tablets. (Rhone-Poulenc Rorer) Magnesium hydroxide 350 mg, dried aluminum hydroxide gel 350 mg/Tab. Bot. 38s, 75s. *otc.*
Use: Antacid.

Maalox Heartburn Relief Liquid. (Rhone-Poulenc Rorer) Aluminum hydroxide, magnesium carbonate 140 mg, magnesium carbonate 175 mg, tartrazine, saccharin, magnesium alginate, parabens, sorbitol/5 ml. Bot. 296 ml. *otc.*
Use: Antacid.

Maalox HRF. (Rhone-Poulenc Rorer) Aluminum hydroxide/magnesium carbonate codried gel 280 mg, magnesium carbonate 350 mg/10 ml, saccharin, tartrazine. Liq. Bot. 355 ml. *otc.*
Use: Antacid.

Maalox Plus Tablets. (Rhone-Poulenc Rorer) Magnesium hydroxide 200 mg, dried aluminum hydroxide gel 200 mg, simethicone 25 mg/Tab. Bot. 50s, 100s, 144s. *otc.*
Use: Antacid, antiflatulent.

Maalox Suspension. (Rhone-Poulenc Rorer) Magnesium hydroxide 200 mg, aluminum hydroxide 225 mg/5 ml, Susp. Bot. 148 ml, 355 ml, 769 ml. *otc.*
Use: Antacid.

Maalox Tablets. (Rhone-Poulenc Rorer) Magnesium hydroxide 200 mg, dried aluminum hydroxide gel 200 mg/Tab. Bot. 100s. *otc.*
Use: Antacid.

Maalox Therapeutic Concentrate Suspension. (Rhone-Poulenc Rorer) Magnesium hydroxide 300 mg, aluminum hydroxide 600 mg/5 ml, Susp. Bot. 355 ml. *otc.*
Use: Antacid.

Maalox Therapeutic Concentrate Tablets. (Rhone-Poulenc Rorer) Magnesium hydroxide 300 mg, aluminum hydroxide 600 mg. Tab. Bot. 48s. *otc.*
Use: Antacid.

MacPac. (Procter & Gamble) Nitrofurantoin macrocrystals 50 mg or 100 mg/Cap. UD 28s. *Rx.*
Use: Anti-infective, urinary.

macroaggregated albumin.
See: Albumotope-LS. (Bristol-Myers Squibb).

Macrobid. (Procter & Gamble) Nitrofurantoin 100 mg (as 25 mg nitrofurantoin macrocrystals and 75 mg nitrofurantoin monohydrate). Cap. Bot. 100s. *Rx.*
Use: Anti-infective, urinary.

Macrodantin. (Procter & Gamble) Nitrofurantoin macrocrystals **25 mg/Cap.:** Bot. 100s. **50 mg or 100 mg/Cap.:** Bot. 100s, 500s, 1000s, UD 100s. *Rx.*
Use: Anti-infective, urinary.

Macrodex. (Pharmacia & Upjohn) Dextran 6% w/v in normal saline, 6% w/v in dextrose 5% in water. Bot. 500 ml. *Rx.*
Use: Plasma volume expander.

macrogol stearate 2000. Polyoxyl 40 Stearate.

Macrotec. (Bristol-Myers Squibb) Tech-

netium Tc99m Medronate kit. Vial Kit 10s.
Use: Radiopaque agent.

Macrotin. W/Phenobarbital, hyoscyamus extract, caulophyllin, helonin, pulsatilla extract.

•**maduramicin.** (mad-UHR-ah-MY-sin) USAN.
Use: Anticoccidal.

•**mafenide.** (MAY-feh-NIDE) USAN.
Use: Anti-infective.

•**mafenide acetate.** (MAY-feh-NIDE) U.S.P. 23.
Use: Anti-infective, topical.
See: Sulfamylon Cream (Dow Hickam).

mafenide acetate solution.
Use: Prevent graft loss on burn wounds. [Orphan drug]

•**mafilcon a.** (MAY-fill-kahn A) USAN.
Use: Contact lens material (hydrophilic).

Mafylon Cream. (Sanofi Winthrop) Mafenide acetate. *Rx.*
Use: Burn therapy.

•**magaldrate.** (MAG-al-drate) U.S.P. 23. (Wyeth Ayerst) Monalium Hydrate. Aluminum Magnesium Hydroxide.
Use: Antacid.
See: Iosopan (Zenith Goldline).
Monalium Hydrate.
Riopan, Tab., Susp. (Wyeth-Ayerst).

magaldrate and simethicone.
Use: Antacid, antiflatulant.
See: Lowsium. (Rugby).
Lowsium Plus. (Rugby).
Riopan Plus. (Wyeth-Ayerst).

magaldrate plus suspension. (Various Mfr.) Magaldrate 540 mg, simethicone 40 mg/5 ml. Susp. Bot. 360 ml. *otc.*
Use: Antacid, antiflatulant.

Maalox Plus. (Invamed) Dried aluminum hydroxide 200 mg, magnesium hydroxide 200 mg, simethicone 25 mg, sugar/Chew. Tab. Bot. 100s. *otc.*
Use: Antacid.

Magan. (Pharmacia & Upjohn) Magnesium salicylate (anhydrous) 545 mg/Tab. Bot. 100s, 500s. *Rx.*
Use: Analgesic.

Mag-Cal Tablets. (Fibertone) Calcium 416.7 mg (as carbonate), calcium 166.7 mg (as elemental), vitamin D 66.7 IU, magnesium 83.3 mg, copper 0.167 mg, manganese 0.83 mg, potassium 1.67 mg, zinc 0.167 mg/Tab. Bot. 90s, 180s. *otc.*
Use: Mineral, vitamin supplement.

Mag-Cal Mega. (Freeda Vitamins) Mg 800 mg, Ca 400 mg, kosher, sugar free/Tab. Bot. 100s and 250s. *otc.*
Use: Mineral, vitamin supplement.

Magdrox. (Vita Elixir) Magnesium hydroxide, aluminum hydroxide. *otc.*
Use: Antacid.

Mag-G. (Cypress) Magnesium gluconate dihydrate 500 mg (≈ 27 mg elemental magnesium). Tab. Bot. 100s. *otc.*
Use: Mineral supplement.

Magmalin Lozenge. (Pal-Pak) Magnesium hydroxide 0.2 g, aluminum hydroxide gel, dried 0.2 g/Loz. Bot. 1000s. *otc.*
Use: Antacid.

Magnacal Liquid. (Biosearch Medical Products) Protein-calcium, sodium caseinate, carbohydrate-maltodextrin, sucrose, fat (partially hydrogenated), soy oil, lecithin, mono- and diglycerides. 1.5 Cal/ml, 590 mOsm/kg H_2O. Protein 70 g, CHO 250 g, fat 80 g, sodium 1000 mg, potassium 1250 mg/L. Can 120 ml, 240 ml. *otc.*
Use: Nutritional supplement.

Magnalox Liquid. (Schein Pharmaceutical) Aluminum hydroxide 225 mg, magnesium hydroxide 200 mg/5 ml. Liq. Bot. 360 ml. *otc.*
Use: Antacid.

Magnalum. (Global Source) Magnesium hydroxide 3.75 gr, aluminum hydroxide 2 gr/Tab. Bot. 1000s. *otc.*
Use: Antacid.

Magnaprin Arthritis Strength Tablets. (Rugby) Aspirin 325 mg, dried aluminum hydroxide gel 150 mg, magnesium hydroxide 150 mg/Tab. Bot. 100s, 500s. *otc.*
Use: Analgesic.

Magnaprin Tablets. (Rugby) Aspirin 325 mg, dried aluminum hydroxide gel 75 mg, magnesium hydroxide 75 mg/Tab. Bot. 100s, 500s. *otc.*
Use: Analgesic.

magnesia tablets.
Use: Antacid.

magnesia & alumina oral suspension. (Roxane) Oral Susp. 6 fl oz. 25s.
Use: Antacid.
See: Maalox, Liq. (Rhone-Poulenc Rorer).

magnesia & alumina tablets.
Use: Antacid.
See: Maalox, Tab. (Rhone-Poulenc Rorer).

magnesia magma. Milk of Magnesia, U.S.P. 23.
Use: Antacid, cathartic, laxative.
See: Magnesium Hydroxide, Preps.

magnesium acetylsalicylate. Apyron,

Magnespirin, Magisal, Novacetyl.
Use: Analgesic.

magnesium aluminate hydrated.
Use: Antacid.
See: Riopan, Susp., Tab. (Wyeth Ayerst).

magnesium aluminum hydroxide.
Use: Antacid.
See: Maalox, Susp. (Rhone-Poulenc Rorer).
Malogel, Gel (Quality Formulations).
Medalox, Gel (Med Chem).
W/APC.
See: Buffadyne, Tab. (Teva USA).
W/Calcium carbonate.
See: Camalox, Susp. (Rhone-Poulenc Rorer).
W/Simethicone.
See: Maalox Plus, Susp. (Rhone-Poulenc Rorer).

•**magnesium aluminum silicate.** (mag-NEE-zee-uhm) N.F. 18.
Use: Pharmaceutic aid, suspending agent.

•**magnesium carbonate.** (mag-NEE-zee-uhm) U.S.P. 23.
Use: Antacid.

magnesium carbonate. (Baker, d.T.) Pow. 4 oz, 1 lb, 5 lb.
Use: Antacid.

magnesium carbonate and sodium bicarbonate for oral suspension.
Use: Antacid.

magnesium carbonate w/combinations.
Use: Antacid.
See: Algicon, Tab. (Rhone-Poulenc Rorer).
Alkets, Tab. (Pharmacia & Upjohn).
Antacid No. 2, Tab. (Jones Medical Industries).
Bismatesia, Can (Noyes).
Bufferin, Tab. (Bristol-Myers).
Di-Gel, Tab., Liq. (Schering Plough).
Magnagel, Liq., Tab. (Roberts Pharm).
Marblen, Susp., Tab. (Fleming).

•**magnesium chloride.** U.S.P. 23.
Use: Electrolyte replacement, pharmaceutical necessity for hemodialysis and peritoneal dialysis.
W/Potassium Cl, calcium Cl, red phenol.
See: Electrolytic replenisher, Vial (Invenex).

•**magnesium citrate.** (mag-NEE-zee-uhm) U.S.P. 23.
Use: Cathartic; laxative.

•**magnesium gluconate.** U.S.P. 23.
Use: Vitamin supplement, replacement.
See: Almora, Tab. (Forest Pharmaceutical).
Mag-G, Tab. (Cypress).

magnesium gluconate. (Western Research) Magnesium gluconate 500 mg/Tab. Bot. 1000s. *otc.*
Use: Vitamin supplement.

magnesium glycinate.
W/Gastric mucin, aluminum hydroxide gel.
See: Mucogel, Tab. (Inwood).

•**magnesium hydroxide.** U.S.P. 23.
Use: Antacid, cathartic, laxative.
See: Magnesia Magma (Various Mfr.).
Milk of Magnesia (Various Mfr.).
Phillips' Milk of Magnesia (Bayer Corp).
Phillips' Chewable, Tab. (Bayer Corp).

magnesium hydroxide w/combinations.
See: Aludrox, Susp., Tab., Vial (Wyeth Ayerst).
Ascriptin, Tab. (Rhone-Poulenc Rorer).
Ascriptin A/D, Tab. (Rhone-Poulenc Rorer).
Ascriptin Extra Strength, Tab. (Rhone-Poulenc Rorer).
Ascriptin w/Codeine, Tab. (Rhone-Poulenc Rorer).
Banacid, Tab. (Buffington).
Camalox, Susp., Tab. (Rhone-Poulenc Rorer).
Delcid, Susp. (Hoechst Marion Roussel).
Fermalox, Tab. (Rhone-Poulenc Rorer).
Gas-Ban DS, Liq. (Roberts Pharm).
Kolantyl, Gel, Wafer (Hoechst Marion Roussel).
Laxsil Liquid, Liq. (Schwarz Pharma).
Maalox, Susp., Tab. (Rhone-Poulenc Rorer).
Maalox Plus, Susp., Tab. (Rhone-Poulenc Rorer).
Mylanta, Mylanta II, Liq., Tab. (Zeneca).
Simeco, Liq. (Wyeth Ayerst).
WinGel, Liq., Tab. (Sanofi Winthrop).

•**magnesium oxide.** (mag-NEE-zee-uhm OX-ide) U.S.P. 23.
Use: Pharmaceutic aid (sorbent).

magnesium oxide. (Manne) 420 mg/Tab. Bot. 250s, 1000s. (Stanlabs) 10 gr/Tab. Bot. 100s, 1000s. (Cypress) 400 mg. Tab. 120s. *otc.*
Use: Pharmaceutical aid (sorbant).
See: Mag-Ox, Tab. (Blaine).
Mag-Ox 400, Tab. (Blaine).
Niko-Mag, Cap. (Scruggs).
Par-Mag, Cap. (Parmed).
Uro-Mag, Cap. (Blaine).

W/Calcium, Vitamin D.
See: Elekap, Cap. (Western Research).
W/Glutamic acid magnesium complex, N-acetyl-P-aminophenol, ascorbic acid, dl-methionine, lemon bioflavonoid complex, dl-α-tocopheryl acetate, glycine, soybean flour.
W/Magnesium carbonate, calcium carbonate.
See: Alkets, Tab. (Pharmacia & Upjohn).
W/Ox bile (desiccated), hog bile (desiccated.).
See: Hyper-Cholate, Tab. (Roberts Pharm).
W/Phenobarbital, atropine sulfate.
See: Magnox, Tab. (Jones Medical Industries).

•**magnesium phosphate.** (mag-NEE-zee-uhm FOSS-fate) U.S.P. 23.
Use: Antacid.

•**magnesium salicylate.** U.S.P. 23.
Use: Analgesic, antipyretic, antirheumatic.
See: Analate, Tab. (Winston).
Backache Maximum Strength Relief, Capl. (Bristol-Myers Squibb).
Bayer Select Maximum Strength Backache, Capl. (Sterling Health).
Efficin, Tab. (Pharmacia & Upjohn).
Magan, Tab. (Pharmacia & Upjohn).
Momentum Muscular Backache Formula, Capl. (Whitehall Robins).
Nuprin Backache, Capl. (Bristol-Myers Squibb).
W/Diphenhydramine HCl.
See: Extra Strenght Doan's PM, Capl. (Novartis).
W/Phenyltoloxamine citrate.
See: Mobigesic, Tab. (B.F. Ascher).

•**magnesium silicate.** N.F. 18.
Use: Pharmaceutic aid (tablet excipient).

•**magnesium stearate.** N.F. 18.
Use: Pharmaceutic aid (tablet and capsule lubricant).

•**magnesium sulfate.** (mag-NEE-zee-uhm SULL-fate) U.S.P. 23.
Use: Anticonvulsant, electrolyte replacement, laxative.

magnesium sulfate. (Abbott Laboratories)–50% Amp. 2 ml Box 25s, 100s. Abboject Syringe (20 G X 2.5) 5 ml, 10 ml; 12.5% in Pintop Vial, 8 ml, 20 ml. (Atlas)–10% Amp. 10 ml Box 100s; 1 g/2 ml. Box 100s. (Baxter)–10%. Vial 10 ml, 20 ml. (CMC)–1 g/2 ml, 10% Amp. 10 ml, 20 ml; 25% Amp. 10 ml 50%. Vial 30 ml. (Quality Formulations)–50% Amp. 2 ml, 100s. (Eli Lilly)–10% Amp 20 ml Box 6s, 25s; 50% 1 g Amp. 2 ml, Box 12s, 100s. (Parke-Davis)–50% Amp. 2 ml, 10s. (Trent)–50% Amp. 2 ml, 10 ml. (Various Mfr.) Inj. 12.5% Vial 8 ml; 50% Amps 2 ml, 10 ml; Vial 10 ml, 20 ml, 50 ml; Disp. Syringe 5 ml, 10 ml; 2 ml fill in 5 ml vials.

•**magnesium trisilicate.** U.S.P. 23.
Use: Antacid.

magnesium trisilicate w/combinations.
See: Alsorb Gel C.T., Gel (Standex).
Arcodex Tablets, Tab. (Arcum).
Banacid, Tab. (Buffington).
Gacid, Tab. (Arcum).
Gaviscon, Tab. (Hoechst Marion Roussel).
Maracid 2, Tab. (Marin).

Magnevist. (Berlex) Gadopentetate dimeglumine 469.01 mg, meglumine 0.39 mg, diethylenetriamine pentaacetic acid 0.15 mg. Inj. Vial 20 ml.
Use: Radiopaque agent.

Magonate. (Fleming) Magnesium gluconate 500 mg/Tab. Bot. 100s, 1000s. *otc.*
Use: Vitamin supplement.

Mag-Ox 400. (Blaine) Magnesium oxide 400 mg/Tab. Bot. 100s, 1000s. *otc.*
Use: Antacid, vitamin supplement.

Magsal. (US Pharmaceutical) Magnesium salicylate 600 mg, phenyltoloxamine citrate 25 mg/Tab. Bot. 100s. *Rx.*
Use: Analgesic combination.

Mag-Tab SR. (Niche) Magnesium (as lactate) 84 mg/SR Capl. Bot. 60s, 100s. *otc.*
Use: Vitamin supplement.

Maigret-50. (Ferndale Laboratories) Phenylpropanolamine HCl 50 mg/Tab. Bot. 100s.
Use: Decongestant.

Maintenance Vitamin Formula w/Minerals. (Towne) Vitamins A palmitate 10,000 IU, D 400 IU, B_1 5 mg, B_2 2.5 mg, C 75 mg, niacinamide 40 mg, B_6 1 mg, calcium pantothenate 4 mg, B_{12} 2 mcg, E 2 IU, choline bitartrate 31.4 mg, inositol 15 mg, calcium 75 mg, phosphorus 58 mg, iron 30 mg, magnesium 3 mg, manganese 0.5 mg, potassium 2 mg, zinc 0.5 mg/Cap. Bot. 100s. *otc.*
Use: Mineral, vitamin supplement.

majeptil. Thioproperazine. Psychopharmacologic agent; pending release.

Major-gesic. (Major) Phenyltoloxamine citrate 30 mg, acetaminophen 325 mg/Tab. Bot. 100s. *otc.*
Use: Antihistamine, analgesic.

malagride.
See: Acetarsone.

Malaraquin. (Sanofi Winthrop) Chloroquine phosphate. *Rx.*
Use: Antimalarial.

•**malathion.** (mal-ah-THIGH-ahn) U.S.P. 23.
Use: Pediculicide.

•**malethamer.** (mal-ETH-ah-mer) USAN.
Use: Antidiarrheal, antiperistaltic.

•**malic acid.** (MAL-ik) N.F. 18.
Use: Pharmaceutic aid (acidifying agent).

malic acid with pectin.
See: Mallo-Pectin, Liq. (Roberts Pharm).

Mallamint. (Roberts Pharm) Calcium carbonate 420 mg/Tab. Bot. 100s. *otc.*
Use: Antacid.

Mallazine Drops. (Roberts Pharm) Tetrahydrozoline 0.05%. Soln. 15 ml. *otc.*
Use: Mydriatic, vasoconstrictor.

Mallergan-VC w/Codeine Syrup. (Roberts Pharm) Phenylephrine HCl 5 mg, promethazine HCl 6.25 mg, codeine phosphate 10 mg/5 ml, alcohol 7%. Syr. Bot. 120 ml. *c-v.*
Use: Antihistamine, antitussive, decongestant.

Mallisol. (Roberts Pharm) Povidone-iodine. *otc.*
Use: Antimicrobial, antiseptic.

Malogen Injection Aqueous. (Forest Pharmaceutical) Testosterone. **25 mg/ml:** 10 ml, 30 ml; **50 mg/ml:** 10 ml; **100 mg/ml:** 10 ml. *c-III.*
Use: Androgen.

Malogen 100 L.A. in Oil inj. (Forest Pharmaceutical) Testosterone enanthate 100 mg/ml. 10 ml. *c-III.*
Use: Androgen.

Malogen 200 L.A. in Oil inj. (Forest Pharmaceutical) Testosterone enanthate 200 mg/ml. 10 ml. *c-III.*
Use: Androgen.

Malogen Cyp. (Forest Pharmaceutical) Testosterone cypionate in oil 100 mg or 200 mg/ml. Vial 10 ml. *c-III.*
Use: Androgen.

malonal.
See: Barbital (Various Mfr.).

•**malotilate.** (mal-OH-tih-LATE) USAN.
Use: Liver disorder treatment.

•**maltitol solution.** (MAL-tih-tahl) N.F. 18.
Use: Sweetener.

Malotrone Aqueous Injection. (Bluco) Testosterone, USP 25 mg or 50 mg/ml in aqueous susp. Vial 10 ml. *c-III.*
Use: Androgen.

•**maltodextrin.** N.F. 18.
Use: Pharmaceutic aid (coating agent, tablet binder, tablet and capsule diluent, viscosity-increasing agent).

Maltsupex. (Wallace Laboratories) Laxative derived from natural barley malt extract for relief of constipation in children and adults. **Liq.:** Bot. 8 oz, pt. **Pow.:** Jar 8 oz, lb. **Tab.:** Malt soup extract 750 mg/Tab. Bot. 100s. *otc.*
W/Psyllium seed husks.
Use: Laxative.
See: Syllamalt, Pow. (Wallace Laboratories).

Mammol Ointment. (Abbott Laboratories) Bismuth subnitrate 40%, castor oil 30%, anhydrous lanolin 22%, ceresin wax 7%, balsam Peru 1%. Tube ⅞ oz. Ctn. 12s. *otc.*
Use: Dermatologic-protectant, emollient.

mandameth. (Major) Methenamine mandelate 0.5 g/EC Tab. Bot. 1000s. *Rx.*
Use: Anti-infective, urinary.

mandelic acid.
Use: Anti-infective, urinary.

mandelic acid salts.
See: Calcium mandelate (Various Mfr.).

mandelyltropeine.
See: Homatropine Salts (Various Mfr.).

Mandol. (Eli Lilly) Cefamandole nafate. Vial: **1 g/10 ml:** Traypak 25s; **1 g/100 ml:** Traypak 10s. *Rx.*
Use: Anti-infective, cephalosporin.

Manganese.
Use: Dietary supplement.
See: Chelated manganese (Freeda Vitamins).

•**manganese chloride.** (MANG-ah-neese) U.S.P. 23.
Use: Manganese deficiency treatment, trace mineral supplement.

•**manganese gluconate.** U.S.P. 23.
Use: Manganese deficiency, trace mineral supplement.

manganese glycerophosphate. Glycerol phosphate manganese salt.
Use: Pharmaceutical necessity.

manganese hypophosphite. Manganese (2+) phosphinate.
Use: Pharmaceutical necessity.

•**manganese sulfate.** U.S.P. 23.
Use: Trace mineral supplement.
W/Thyroid, ferrous sulfate, ferrous gluconate, sodium ferric pyrophosphate, extract of nux vomica.
See: Hemocrine, Tab. (Roberts Pharm).

Manga-Pak. (SoloPak) Manganese 0.1 mg/ml. Inj. Vial 10 ml, 30 ml. *Rx.*

Use: Nutritional supplement, parenteral.

mangofodopir trisodium.
Use: Diagnostic aid.
See: Teslascan, Inj. (Nycomed).

Maniron. (Jones Medical Industries) Ferrous fumarate 3 mg/Tab. Bot. 100s, 1000s, 5000s. *otc.*
Use: Mineral supplement.

Mann Astringent Mouth Wash Concentrate. (Manne) Bot. 4 oz, qt, 0.5 gal, gal. Also mint flavored. Bot. 4 oz, qt, 0.5 gal, gal. *otc.*
Use: Mouthwash.

Mann Body Deodorant. (Manne) Bot. 4 oz, 8 oz, pt, qt. *otc.*

Mann Breath Deodorant. (Manne) Bot. 1 oz, 4 oz, 8 oz, pt, qt, 0.5 gal. *otc.*

Mann Emollient. (Manne) Jar. 100 g. *otc.*
Use: Emollient.

Mann Eugenol U.S.P. Extra. (Manne) 0.06 lb, 0.13 lb, 0.25 lb, 0.5 lb, 1 lb. *otc.*
Use: Dermatologic-protectant.

Mann Germicidal Solution. (Manne) **Regular:** Bot. gal, 4 gal. **Conc.:** 12.8%. Bot. pt, qt, 0.5 gal, gal. *otc.*
Use: Antimicrobial.

Mann Hand Lotion. (Manne) Twin pack, gal. *otc.*
Use: Emollient.

Mann Hemostatic. (Manne) Bot. 1 oz, 4 oz, 8 oz, pt, qt. *otc.*
Use: Hemostatic.

Mann Liquid Soap. (Manne) Concentrated cococastile. Bot. qt, 0.5 gal, gal. *otc.*
Use: Emollient.

Mann Lubricant and Cleanser. (Manne) Bot. pt, qt. *otc.*
Use: Emollient.

Mann Superfatted Bar Soap. (Manne) Rich in lanolin. Cake. 12s. *otc.*
Use: Emollient.

Mann Talbot's Iodine. (Manne) Glycerin base. Bot. 1 oz, 4 oz, 8 oz, pt, qt. *otc.*
Use: Antiseptic.

Mann Topical Anesthetic. (Manne) Bot. 1 oz, 4 oz, 8 oz, pt. W/stain to indicate area treated. Bot. 1 oz, 4 oz, 8 oz. *otc.*
Use: Anesthetic, local.

manna sugar.
See: Mannitol (Various Mfr.).

Mannan. (Rugby) Purified glucomannan 500 mg/Cap. Bot. 90s. *otc.*
Use: Nutritional supplement.

Mannest. (Manne) Conjugated estrogens 0.625 mg, 1.25 mg or 2.5 mg/Tab. Bot. 100s, 200s. *Rx.*
Use: Estrogen.

mannite.
See: Mannitol, U.S.P. 23.

•**mannitol.** (MAN-ih-tole) U.S.P. 23.
Use: Diagnostic aid (renal function determination), diuretic.
See: Osmitrol (Baxter).
W/Sorbitol.
See: Cystosol, Liq. (Baxter).
Cytal, Liq. (Bayer Corp).

mannitol injection. (Abbott Laboratories) 15% or 20%. Abbo-Vac Single dose container 500 ml.
Use: Diagnostic aid (renal function determination), diuretic.
See: Mannitol Solution, Amp. (Merck).

mannitol hexanitrate.
Use: Coronary vasodilator.
See: Vascunitol, Tab. (Apco).
W/Reserpine, rutin, ascorbic acid.
See: Ruhexatal W/Reserpine, Tab. (Teva USA).

mannitol hexanitrate & phenobarbital tab. (Jones Medical; Quality Generics) Mannitol hexanitrate 0.5 g, phenobarbital 0.25 g/Tab. Bot. 1000s. *c-IV.*
Use: Vasodilator.

mannitol hexanitrate with phenobarbital combinations.
See: Manotensin,Tab. (Dunhall Pharmaceuticals).
Ruhexatal, Tab. (Teva USA).
Vascused, Tab. (Apco).

mannitol in sodium chloride injection.
Use: Diuretic.

Manotensin. (Dunhall Pharmaceuticals) Mannitol hexanitrate 32 mg, phenobarbital 16 mg/Tab. Bot. 100s, 1000s. *c-IV.*
Use: Vasodilator.

Mantoux Test.
See: Tuberculin, U.S.P. 23. Test.

manvene.
Use: Antineoplastic.

MAOI.
See: Monoamine Oxidase Inhibitors.

Maolate Tablets. (Pharmacia & Upjohn) Chlorphenesin carbamate 400 mg/Tab. Bot. 50s, 500s. *Rx.*
Use: Muscle relaxant, anxiolytic.

Maox 420. (Manne) Magnesium oxide 420 mg/Tab. Bot. 250s, 1000s. *otc.*
Use: Antacid.

Mapap Cold Formula. (Major) Acetaminophen 325 mg, pseudoephedrine HCl 30 mg, dextromethorphan HBr 15 mg, chlorpheniramine maleate 2 mg. Tab. Pkg. 24s. *otc.*
Use: Antitussive combination.

Mapap Extra Strength. (Major) Aceta-

minophen 500 mg/Tab. Bot. 30s, 60s, 100s, 200s, 1000s and UD 100s. *otc.*
Use: Analgesic.

Mapap Infant Drops. (Major) Acetaminophen 100 mg/ml, alcohol free/Drops. Bot. 15 and 30 ml. *otc.*
Use: Analgesic.

Mapap Regular Strength. (Major) Acetaminophen 325 mg/Scored Tab. Bot. 100s, 1000s and UD 100s. *otc.*
Use: Analgesic.

maphenide.
See: Sulfbenzamine HCl.

Maprofix.
See: Gardinol Type Detergents (Various Mfr.).

•**maprotiline.** (map-ROW-tih-leen) USAN.
Use: Antidepressant.
See: Ludiomil, Tab. (Novartis).

•**maprotiline hydrochloride.** (map-ROW-tih-leen) U.S.P. 23.
Use: Antidepressant.

Maracid 2. (Marin) Magnesium trisilicate 150 mg, aluminum hydroxide dried gel 90 mg, aminoacetic acid 75 mg/Tab. Bot. *otc.*
Use: Antacid, adsorbant.

Maranox. (C.S. Dent) Acetaminophen 325 mg/Tab. Bot. 8s. *otc.*
Use: Analgesic.

Marax-DF Syrup. (Roerig) Hydroxyzine HCl 7.5 mg, ephedrine sulfate 18.75 mg, theophylline 97.5 mg/15 ml. Color free, dye free. Bot. pt, gal. *Rx.*
Use: Antiasthmatic combination.

Marax Tab. (Roerig) Hydroxyzine HCl 10 mg, ephedrine sulfate 25 mg, theophylline 130 mg/Tab. Bot. 100s, 500s. *Rx.*
Use: Antiasthmatic combination.

Marbaxin 750. (Vortech) Methocarbamol 750 mg/Tab. Bot. 500s. *Rx.*
Use: Muscle relaxant.

Marblen Liquid. (Fleming) Magnesium carbonate 400 mg, calcium carbonate 520 mg/5 ml. Bot. 473 ml. *otc.*
Use: Antacid.

Marblen Tablets. (Fleming) Calcium carbonate 520 mg, magnesium carbonate 400 mg. Tab. Bot. 100s, 1000s. *otc.*
Use: Antacid.

Marcaine. (Sanofi Winthrop) Bupivacaine in sterile isotonic soln. containing sodium Cl pH adjusted 4.0 to 6.5 w/sodium hydroxide or hydrochloric acid. Multiple-dose vial also contains methylparaben 1 mg/ml as preservative. **0.25%:** Amp. 50 ml. Box 5s. Vial: Single dose 10 ml, 30 ml. Box 10s; multiple dose 50 ml. Box 1s. **0.5%:** Amp. 30 ml. Box 1s. Vial: Single dose 10 ml, 30 ml. Box 10s; multiple dose 50 ml. Box 1s. **0.75%:** Amp. 30 ml. Box 5s. Vial (single dose) 10 ml, 30 ml. Box 10s. *Rx.*
Use: Anesthetic, local.

Marcaine with Epinephrine. (1:200,000). (Sanofi Winthrop) **Bupivacaine 0.25%:** with epinephrine 1:200,000 in sterile isotonic soln. containing sodium Cl. Each 1 ml contains bupivacaine HCl 2.5 mg, epinephrine bitartrate 0.0091 mg, sodium metabisulfite 0.5 mg, monothioglycerol 0.001 ml, ascorbic acid 2 mg and edetate calcium disodium 0.1 mg. In Multiple Dose Vial, each 1 ml also contains methylparaben 1 mg as antiseptic preservative. pH adjusted to between 3.4 and 4.5 with sodium hydroxide or hydrochloric acid. Amp. 50 ml, 5s, Single Dose Vial 10 ml, 30 ml. 10s, Multiple Dose Vial 50 ml 1s. **Bupivacaine 0.5%:** with epinephrine 1:200,000 in sterile isotonic soln. containing sodium Cl. Each 1 ml contains bupivacaine HCl 5 mg and epinephrine bitartrate 0.0091 mg, with sodium metabisulfite 0.5 mg, monothioglycerol 0.001 ml and ascorbic acid 2 mg, edetate calcium disodium 0.1 mg. In Multiple Dose Vial, each 1 ml also contains methylparaben 1 mg antiseptic preservative. pH adjusted to between 3.4 and 4.5 with sodium hydroxide or hydrochloric acid. Amp. 3 ml 10s, 30 ml 5s. Single Dose Vial 10 ml, 30 ml 10s. Multiple Dose Vial 50 ml 1s. **Bupivacaine 0.75%:** with epinephrine 1:200,000 in sterile isotonic soln. containing sodium Cl. Each 1 ml contains bupivacaine HCl 7.5 mg, epinephrine bitartrate 0.0091 mg with sodium metabisulfite 0.5 mg, monothioglycerol 0.001 ml, ascorbic acid 2 mg as antioxidants, edetate calcium disodium 0.1 mg. pH adjusted to between 3.4 and 4.5 with sodium hydroxide or hydrochloric acid. Amp 30 ml in 5s. *Rx.*
Use: Anesthetic, local.

Marcaine Spinal. (Sanofi Winthrop) Bupivacaine HCl 15 mg/2 ml (0.75%) and dextrose 165 mg/2 ml (8.25%). Amp. 2 ml. *Rx.*
Use: Anesthetic, local.

Marcillin. (Marnel) **Cap.:** Ampicillin trihydrate 500 mg. Bot. 100s; **Pow. for Susp.:** Ampicillin trihydrate 250 mg/100 ml. *Rx.*
Use: Anti-infective, penicillin.

Marcof Expectorant. (Marnel) Hydrocodone bitartrate 5 mg, potassium guaiacolsulfonate 300 mg/5 ml. Liq. Bot. 480 ml. *c-III.*
Use: Antitussive; expectorant, narcotic.

Mardon. (Armenpharm) Propoxyphene HCl. **Cap.:** 32 mg Bot. 100s, 1000s. **65 mg:** Bot. 100s, 500s, 1000s. [c-iv] c-iv.
Use: Analgesic, narcotic.

Mardon Compound. (Armenpharm) Propoxyphene compound 65 mg, aspirin 3.5 gr, phenacetin 2.5 gr, caffeine 0.5 gr/Cap. Bot. 100s, 500s, 1000s. *c-IV.*
Use: Analgesic combination, narcotic.

Marezine Tablets. (Himmel) Cyclizine HCl 50 mg/Tab. Bot. 100s. Box 12s. *otc.*
Use: Anticholinergic.
W/Ergotamine tartrate, caffeine.
See: Migral, Tab. (GlaxoWellcome).

marfanil.
See: Sulfbenzamine HCl (Various Mfr.).

Margesic. (Marnel) Butalbital 50 mg, acetaminophen 325 mg, caffeine 40 mg/Cap. Bot. 100s. *Rx.*
Use: Analgesic, hypnotic, sedative.

Margesic H. (Marnel) Hydrocodone bitartrate 5 mg, acetaminophen 500 mg/Cap. Bot. 100s. *c-III.*
Use: Analgesic combination, narcotic.

Margesic No. 3. (Marnel) Codeine phosphate 30 mg, acetaminophen 300 mg/Tab. Bot. 100s. *c-III.*
Use: Analgesic combination, narcotic.

Marhist. (Marlop Pharm) Chlorpheniramine maleate 20 mg, phenylephrine HCl 2.5 mg, methscopolamine nitrate in special base/Cap. Bot. 30s, 100s. Expectorant Bot. 4 oz, pt, gal. *Rx.*
Use: Anticholinergic, antihistamine, decongestant.

•**marimastat.** (mah-RIH-mah-stat) USAN.
Use: Antineoplastic (matrix metalloproteinase inhibitor).

Marine Lipid Concentrate. (Vitaline) Omega-3 1200 mg, EPA 360 mg, DHA 240 mg, E 5 IU/Cap., sodium free. Bot. 90s. *otc.*
Use: Nutritional supplement.

Marinol Capsules. (Roxane) Dronabinol 2.5 mg, 5 mg or 10 mg/Cap. Bot. 25s, 60s, 100s. *c-II.*
Use: Antiemetic.

Marlin Salt System. (Marlin) Sodium Cl 250 mg/Tab. Bot. 200s with bot. 27.7 ml. *otc.*
Use: Contact lens care.

Marlyn Formula 50. (Marlyn) Vitamin B_6 w/18 amino acids/Cap. Bot. 100s, 250s, 1000s. *otc.*
Use: Nutritional supplement.

Marnatal-F. (Marnel) Calcium 250 mg, iron 60 mg, vitamins A 4000 IU, D 400 IU, E 30 mg, B_1 3 mg, B_2 3.4 mg, B_3 20 mg, B_6 5 mg, B_{12} 12 mcg, C 100 mg, folic acid 1 mg, Mg, Zn 25 mg, Cu, I/Tab. Bot. 30s, 100s. *Rx.*
Use: Mineral, vitamin supplement; dental caries agent.

Marthritic. (Marnel) Salsalate 750 mg. Tab. Bot. 100s. *Rx.*
Use: Analgesic.

•**masoprocol.** (mass-OH-prah-KOLE) USAN.
Use: Antineoplastic.
See: Actinex, cream. (Schwarz Pharma).

Masse Breast Cream. (Advanced Care Products) Water, glyceryl monostearate, glycerin, cetyl alcohol, lanolin, peanut oil, Span-60, stearic acid, Tween-60, sodium benzoate, propylparaben, methylparaben, potassium hydroxide. Tube 2 oz. *otc.*
Use: Emollient.

Massengill Baking Soda Freshness. (SmithKline Beecham Pharmaceuticals) Sanitized water, sodium bicarbonate. Soln. Bot. 180 ml. *otc.*
Use: Vaginal agent.

Massengill Disposable Douche. (SmithKline Beecham Pharmaceuticals) Water, S.D. alcohol 40, lactic acid, sodium lactate, octoxymol-9, cetylpyridium Cl, propylene glycol, diazolidinyl urea, EDTA, parabens, fragrance, color. Bot. 180 ml. *otc.*
Use: Vaginal agent.

Massengill Extra Cleansing w/Puraclean. (SmithKline Beecham Pharmaceuticals) Vinegar, water, cetylpyridinium chloride, diazolidinyl urea, EDTA. Soln. Bot. 180 ml. *otc.*
Use: Vaginal agent.

Massengill Feminine Cleansing Wash. (SmithKline Beecham Pharmaceuticals) Sodium laureth sulfate, magnesium oleth sulfate, sodium oleth sulfate, magnesium oleth sulfate, PEG-120 methyl glucose dioleate, parabens. Liq. Bot. 240 ml. *otc.*
Use: Vaginal agent.

Massengill Feminine Deodorant Spray. (SmithKline Beecham Pharmaceuticals) Aerosol Bot. 3 oz. *otc.*
Use: Vaginal agent.

Massengill Liquid. (SmithKline Beecham Pharmaceuticals) Lactic acid,

S.D. alcohol 40, octoxynol-9, water, sodium bicarbonate. Bot. 120 ml. *otc.*
Use: Vaginal agent.

Massengill Medicated. (SmithKline Beecham Pharmaceuticals) Povidone-iodine 0.3% when added to sanitized fluid. Bot. 6 oz. *otc.*
Use: Vaginal agent.

Massengill Medicated Disposable Douche w/Cepticin. (SmithKline Beecham Pharmaceuticals) Povidone-iodine 10%. Liq. Vial 5 ml w/180 ml bot. of sanitized water. *otc.*
Use: Vaginal agent.

Massengill Medicated Douche w/Cepticin. (SmithKline Beecham Pharmaceuticals) Povidone-iodine 12%. Liq. concentrate. Bot. 120 ml, 240 ml. *otc.*
Use: Vaginal agent.

Massengill Powder. (SmithKline Beecham Pharmaceuticals) Ammonium alum, PEG-8, methyl salicylate, eucalyptus oil, menthol, thymol, phenol. Jar 120 g, 240 g, 480 g, 660 g. UD Packette 10s, 12s. *otc.*
Use: Vaginal agent.

Massengill Soft Cloth. (SmithKline Beecham Pharmaceuticals) Hydrocortisone 0.5%, diazolidinyl urea, DMDM hydantoin, isopropyl myristate, methylparaben, polysorbate 60, propylene glycol, propylparaben, sorbitan stearate, steareth-2, steareth-21. Towelettes 10s. *otc.*
Use: Vaginal agent.

Massengill Unscented. (SmithKline Beecham Pharmaceuticals) Water, SD alcohol 40, lactic acid, sodium lactate, octoxynol-9, cetylpyridium chloride, propylene glycol, diazolidinyl urea, parabens, EDTA. Soln. Bot. 180 ml. *otc.*
Use: Vaginal agent.

Massengill Vinegar-Water Disposable Douche. (SmithKline Beecham Pharmaceuticals) Water and vinegar solution. Bot. 180 ml. *otc.*
Use: Vaginal agent.

Massengill Vinegar & Water Extra Cleansing with Puraclean. (SmithKline Beecham Pharmaceuticals) Vinegar, water, cetylpyridinium chloride, diazolidinyl urea, EDTA. Soln. Bot. 180 ml. *otc.*
Use: Vaginal agent.

Massengill Vinegar & Water Extra Mild. (SmithKline Beecham Pharmaceuticals) Vinegar, water, preservative free. Soln. Bot. 180 ml. *otc.*
Use: Vaginal agent.

Master Formula. (Barth's) Vitamins A 10,000 IU, D 400 IU, C 180 mg, B_1 7 mg, B_2 14 mg, niacin 4.6 mg, B_6 292 mcg, pantothenic acid 210 mcg, B_{12} 25 mcg, biotin 2.9 mcg, E 50 IU, calcium 800 mg, phosphorus 387 mg, iron 10 mg, iodine 0.1 mg, choline 7.78 mg, inositol 11.6 mg, aminobenzoic acid 35 mcg, rutin 30 mg, citrus bioflavonoid complex 30 mg/4 Tab. Bot. 120s, 600s, 1200s. *otc.*
Use: Mineral, vitamin supplement.

Mastisol. (Ferndale Laboratories) Nonirritating medical adhesive. Bot. 4 oz.
Use: Adhesive.

matrix metalloproteinase inhibitor.
Use: Corneal ulcers. [Orphan drug]

Matulane. (Roche Laboratories) Procarbazine HCl 50 mg/Cap. Bot. 100s. *Rx.*
Use: Antineoplastic.

Mavik. (Knoll Pharmaceuticals) Trandolapril 1 mg, 2 mg and 4 mg, lactose/Tab. Bot. 100s, UD 100s. *Rx.*
Use: Antihypertensive.

Maxair. (3M) Pirbuterol acetate aerosol 0.2 mg pirbuterol/actuation. Metered dose inhaler 25.6 g (300 inhalations). *Rx.*
Use: Sympathomimetic bronchodilator.

Maxaquin. (Searle) Lomefloxacin HCl 400 mg/Tab. Bot. 20s, UD 100s. *Rx.*
Use: Anti-infective, fluoroquinolone.

Max EPA Capsules. (Various Mfr.) Omega-3 polyunsaturated fatty acids 1000 mg/Cap. containing EPA 180 mg, DHA 60 mg/Cap. Bot. 50s, 60s, 100s. *otc.*
Use: Nutritional supplement.

Maxidex. (Alcon Laboratories) Dexamethasone 0.1%. Soln. Drop-Tainers 5 ml, 15 ml. *Rx.*
Use: Corticosteroid, ophthalmic.

Maxiflor Cream & Ointment. (Allergan) Diflorasone diacetate 0.05%. Tubes 15 g, 30 g, 60 g. *Rx.*
Use: Corticosteroid, topical.

Maxilube. (Mission Pharmacal) Water, silicone oil, glycerin, carbomer 934, triethanolamine, sodium lauryl sulfate, parabens. Jelly 90 g, 150 g. *otc.*
Use: Vaginal agent.

Maximum Bayer Aspirin Tablets and Capsules. (Bayer Corp) Aspirin (Acetylsalicylic Acid; ASA) 500 mg. **Tab.:** 10s, 30s, 60s, 100s. **Capl.:** 60s. *otc.*
Use: Analgesic.

Maximum Blue Label. (Vitaline) Vita-

mins A 2500 IU, D 16.7 IU, E 66.7 mg, B_1 16.7 mg, B_2 8.3 mg, B_3 31.7 mg, B_5 66.7 mg, B_6 16.7 mg, B_{12} 16.7 mcg, C 200 mg, folic acid 0.13 mg, zinc 5 mg, Ca, Cr, Cu, I, K, Mg, Mn, Mo, Se, Si, V, biotin 50 mcg, SOD, l-lysine/Tab. Bot. 180s. *otc.*
Use: Mineral, vitamin supplement.

Maximum Green Label. (Vitaline) Vitamins A 2500 IU, D 16.7 IU, E 66.7 mg, B_1 16.7 mg, B_2 8.3 mg, B_3 31.7 mg, B_5 66.7 mg, B_6 16.7 mg, B_{12} 16.7 mcg, C 200 mg, folic acid 0.13 mg, zinc 5 mg, Ca, Cr, I, K, Mg, Mn, Mo, Se, Si, V, biotin 50 mcg, SOD, l-lysine/Tab. Bot. 180s. *otc.*
Use: Mineral, vitamin supplement.

Maximum Pain Relief Pamprin. (Chattem Consumer Products) Acetaminophen 250 mg, magnesium salicylate 250 mg, pamabrom 25 mg/Capl. Bot. 16s, 32s. *otc.*
Use: Analgesic combination.

Maximum Red Label. (Vitaline) Iron 3.3 mg, vitamins A 2500 IU, D 67 IU, E 66.7 mg, B_1 16.7 mg, B_2 8.3 mg, B_3 31.7 mg, B_5 66.7 mg, B_6 16.7 mg, B_{12} 16.7 mcg, C 200 mg, folic acid 0.13 mg, Zn 5 mg, Ca, Cr, Su, I, K, Mg, Mo, Se, Si, V, biotin 50 mcg, choline, inositol, bioflavonoids, l-lysine, PABA/Tab. Bot. 180s. *otc.*
Use: Mineral, vitamin supplement.

Maximum Strength Allergy Drops. (Bausch & Lomb) Naphazoline HCl 0.03%. Soln. Bot. 15 ml. *otc.*
Use: Mydriatic, vasoconstrictor.

Maximum Strength Anbesol Mouth and Throat. (Whitehall Robins) **Gel:** Benzocaine 20%, alcohol 60%, saccharin. Tube 7.2 g. **Liq.:** Benzocaine 20%, alcohol 60%, saccharin. Bot. 9 ml. *otc.*
Use: Anesthetic, local.

Maximum Strength Aqua-Ban. (Thompson Medical) Pamabrom 50 mg, lactose/Tab. Bot. 30s. *otc.*
Use: Diuretic.

Maximum Strength Arthriten. (Alva/Amco Pharmacal) Acetaminophen 250 mg, magnesium salicylate 250 mg, caffeine anhydrous 32.5 mg, magnesium carbonate, magnesium oxide, calcium carbonate. Sugar free/Tab. Bot. 40s. *otc.*
Use: Analgesic.

Maximum Strength Benadryl. (Parke-Davis) **Cream:** Diphenhydramine HCl 2%, parabens in a greaseless base. Jar 15 g. **Spray, non-aerosol:** Diphenhydramine HCl 2%, alcohol 85%. Bot. 60 ml. *otc.*
Use: Antihistamine, topical.

Maximum Strength Benadryl Itch Relief. (Warner Lambert) Diphenhydramine HCl. **Cream:** 2%, zinc acetate 1%, parabens, aloe vera. 14.2 g. **Stick:** 2%, zinc acetate 1%. Alcohol 73.5%, aloe vera. 14 ml. *otc.*
Use: Antihistamine.

Maximum Strength Clearasil Clearstick.
See: Clearasil.

Maximum Strength Clearasil Clearstick for Sensitive Skin.
See: Clearasil.

Maximum Strength Comtrex.
See: Comtrex.

Maximum Strength Cortaid. (Pharmacia & Upjohn) Hydrocortisone 1% in parabens, mineral oil, white petrolatum. Oint. Tube 15 g, 30 g. *otc.*
Use: Corticosteroid, topical.

Maximum Strength Cortaid Faststick. (Pharmacia & Upjohn) Hydrocortisone 1%, alcohol 55%, methylparaben. Stick, roll-on. 14 g. *otc.*
Use: Corticosteroid, topical.

Maximum Strength Corticaine. (UCB Pharmaceuticals) Hydrocortisone acetate 1%, glycerin, menthol, EDTA, parabens. Cream. Tube 30 g. *otc.*
Use: Corticosteroid, topical.

Maximum Strength Dermarest Dricort Creme. (Del Pharmaceuticals) Hydrocortisone (as acetate) 1%, white petrolatum. Cream. Tube 14 g. *otc.*
Use: Corticosteroid, topical.

Maximum Strength Desenex Antifungal. (Novartis) Miconazole nitrate 2%, EDTA. Cream. Tube 14 g. *otc.*
Use: Antifungal, topical.

Maximum Strength Dexatrim with Vitamin C. (Thompson Medical) Phenylpropanolamine HCl, vitamin C 180 mg/Cap. Bot. 20s. *otc.*
Use: Dietary aid.

Maximum Strength Diet Aid Plus Vitamin C. (Columbia) Phenylpropanolamine HCl 75 mg, vitamin C 180 mg/Cap. Bot. 20s. *otc.*
Use: Dietary aid.

Maximum Strength Dristan. (Whitehall Robins) Pseudoephedrine HCl 30 mg, acetaminophen 500 mg/Cap. Bot. 24s, 48s, 100s. *otc.*
Use: Analgesic, decongestant.

Maximum Strength Dristan Cold. (Whitehall Robins) Pseudoephedrine HCl 30 mg, brompheniramine maleate 2 mg, acetaminophen 500 mg/Capl.

Pkg. 16s, bot. 36s. *otc.*
Use: Analgesic, antihistamine, decongestant.

Maximum Strength Dynafed Plus. (BDI Pharm) Acetaminophen 500 mg, pseudoephedrine 30 mg/Tab. Bot. 30s. *otc.*
Use: Analgesic, decongestant.

Maximum Strength Flexall 454. (Chattem Consumer Products) Menthol 16%, aloe vera gel, eucalyptus oil, methylsalicylate, SD alcohol 38-B, thyme oil. Gel. Tube. 90 g. *otc.*
Use: Liniment.

Maximum Strength Grapefruit Diet Plan w/Diadex. (Columbia) Phenylpropanolamine HCl 37.5 mg, grapefruit extract, sugar/Cap. Bot. 20s. *otc.*
Use: Dietary aid.

Maximum Strength Halls-Plus. (Warner Lambert) Menthol 10 mg, corn syrup, sucrose. Loz. Pkg. 10s, 20s. *otc.*
Use: Anesthetic.

Maximum Strength Kericort-10. (Bristol-Myers Squibb) Hydrocortisone 1%, parabens, cetyl alcohol, stearyl alcohol. Cream. Tube 56.7 g. *otc.*
Use: Corticosteroid, topical.

Maximum Strength Meted. (GenDerm) Sulfur 5%, salicylic acid 3%. Shampoo. Bot. 118 ml. *otc.*
Use: Antiseborrheic combination.

Maximum Strength, Midol Multi-Symptom. (Bayer Corp) Acetaminophen 325 mg, pyrilamine maleate 12.5 mg/Tab. Bot. 30s. *otc.*
Use: Analgesic combination.

Maximum Strength Midol PMS. (Bayer Corp) Acetaminophen 500 mg, pamabrom 25 mg, pyrilamine maleate 15 mg/Capl. Pkg. 8s, 16s. Bot. 32s. Gelcaps. Pkg. 12s, 24s. *otc.*
Use: Analgesic combination.

Maximum Strength Nasal Decongestant. (Taro Pharm) Oxymetazoline HCl 0.05%, 0.002% phenylmercuric acetate, benzalkonium chloride. Spray. Bot. 15 ml, 30 ml. *otc.*
Use: Decongestant.

Maximum Strength Neosporin. (GlaxoWellcome) Polymyxin B sulfate 10,000 units, neomycin 3.5 mg, bacitracin 500 units/g, white petrolatum. Oint. Tube 15 g. *otc.*
Use: Anti-infective, topical.

Maximum Strength No-Aspirin Sinus Medication. (Walgreens) Acetaminophen 500 mg, pseudoephedrine HCl 30 mg/Tab. Bot. 50s. *otc.*
Use: Analgesic, decongestant.

Maximum Strength Nytol. (Block Drug) Diphenhydramine HCl 50 mg/Tab., lactose. Pkg. 8s, 16s. *otc.*
Use: Sleep aid.

Maximum Strength Orajel Gel. (Del Pharmaceuticals) Benzocaine 20%, saccharin. Tube. 9.45 g. *otc.*
Use: Anesthetic, local.

Maximum Strength Orajel Liquid. (Del Pharmaceuticals) Benzocaine 20%, ethyl alcohol 44.2%, phenol, tartrazine, saccharin. Liq. Bot. 13.3 ml. *otc.*
Use: Anesthetic, local.

Maximum Strength Ornex. (Menley & James) Pseudoephedrine HCl 30 mg, acetaminophen 500 mg/Cap. Bot. 24s, 48s. *otc.*
Use: Analgesic, decongestant.

Maximum Strength Sine-Aid. (McNeil Consumer Products) Pseudoephedrine HCl 30 mg, acetaminophen 500 mg/Cap., Tab. or Gelcap. **Cap. & Tab.:** Bot. 50s. **Gelcaps:** Bot. 40s. *otc.*
Use: Analgesic, decongestant.

Maximum Strength Sinutab Nighttime. (Warner Lambert Consumer Healthcare) Pseudo- ephedrine HCl 10 mg, diphenhydramine HCl 8.33 mg, acetaminophen 167 mg/5 ml. Alcohol free. In 120 ml. *otc.*
Use: Analgesic, antihistamine, decongestant.

Maximum Strength Sinutab Without Drowsiness. (Warner Lambert) Pseudoephedrine HCl 30 mg, acetaminophen 500 mg/Tab. or Capl. Bot. 24s, 48s (tab. only). *otc.*
Use: Analgesic, decongestant.

Maximum Strength Sleepinal. (Thompson Medical) **Cap.:** Diphenhydramine HCl 50 mg, lactose. Pkg. 16s. **Soft gel:** diphenhydramine HCl 50 mg, sorbitol. Pkg. 16s. *otc.*
Use: Sleep aid.

Maximum Strength Sudafed Severe Cold Formula. (GlaxoWellcome) Dextromethorphan HBr 15 mg, pseudoephedrine HCl 30 mg, acetaminophen 500 mg/Tab. 10s. *otc.*
Use: Analgesic, antitussive, decongestant.

Maximum Strength Sudafed Sinus. (Warner Lambert) Pseudoephedrine HCl 30 mg, acetaminophen 500 mg/Tab. or Capl. Bot. 24s, 48s. *otc.*
Use: Analgesic, decongestant.

Maximum Strength Thera-Flu Non-Drowsy.

See: Thera-Flu.

Maximum Strength Tylenol Allergy Sinus. (McNeil Consumer Products) Pseudoephedrine HCl 30 mg, chlorpheniramine maleate 2 mg, acetaminophen 500 mg/Tab. Bot. 24s, 60s. *otc.*
Use: Analgesic, antihistamine, decongestant.

Maximum Strength Tylenol Cough Liquid. (McNeil Consumer Products) Dextromethorphan HBr 7.5 mg, acetaminophen 250 mg, alcohol 10%. Bot. 120 ml. *otc.*
Use: Analgesic, antitussive.

Maximum Strength Tylenol Cough w/ Decongestant Liquid. (McNeil Consumer Products) Pseudoephedrine HCl 15 mg, dextromethorphan HBr 7.5 mg, acetaminophen 250 mg, alcohol 10%. Bot. 120 ml. *otc.*
Use: Analgesic, antitussive, decongestant.

Maximum Strength Tylenol Flu Gelcaps. (McNeil Consumer Products) Acetaminophen 500 mg, pseudoephedrine HCl 30 mg, dextromethorphan HBR 15 mg. Tab. Pkg. 10s. *otc.*
Use: Analgesic, antitussive, decongestant.

Maximum Strength Tylenol Flu Night-Time Gelcaps. (McNeil Consumer Products) Pseudoephedrine HCl 30 mg, chlorpheniramine maleate 2 mg, acetaminophen 500 mg/Cap. Pkg. 12s, 20s. *otc.*
Use: Analgesic, antihistamine, decongestant.

Maximum Strength Tylenol Flu Night-Time Powder. (McNeil Consumer Products) Pseudoephedrine HCl 60 mg, diphenhydramine HCl 50 mg, acetaminophen 1000 mg. Powd. Pkt. 6s. *otc.*
Use: Analgesic, antihistamine, decongestant.

Maximum Strength Tylenol Select Allergy Sinus. (McNeil Consumer Products) Pseudoephedrine HCl 30 mg, diphenhydramine HCl 25 mg, acetaminophen 500 mg. Cap. Bot. 24s. *otc.*
Use: Analgesic, antihistamine, decongestant.

Maximum Strength Tylenol Sinus. (McNeil Consumer Products) Pseudoephedrine HCl 30 mg, acetaminophen 500 mg/Tab., Capl. or Gelcap. **Tab. and Capl.:** Bot. 24s, 50s. **Gelcap:** Bot. 24s, 60s. *otc.*
Use: Analgesic, decongestant.

Maximum Strength Unisom SleepGels. (Pfizer) Diphendhydramine HCl 50 mg, sorbitol. Cap. Pkg. 8s. *otc.*
Use: Sleep aid.

Maximum Strength Wart Remover. (Stiefel) Salicylic acid 17%, alcohol 29%, castor oil, flexible collodion. Liq. 13.3 ml. *otc.*
Use: Keratolytic.

Maxipime. (Bristol-Myers Squibb) Cefepime HCl 500 mg/15 ml, 1 g/15 ml or 2 g/20 ml. Pow. for Inj. Vial, piggyback bottle. *Rx.*
Use: Cephalosporin.

maxiton.
See: Amphetamine (Various Mfr.).

Maxitrol Ointment. (Alcon Laboratories) Dexamethasone 0.1%, neomycin 0.35%, polymyxin B sulfate 10,000 units/g. Tube 3.5 g. *Rx.*
Use: Anti-infective, ophthalmic.

Maxitrol Ophthalmic Suspension. (Alcon Laboratories) Dexamethasone 0.1%, neomycin (as sulfate) 0.35%, polymyxin B sulfate 10,000 units/ml. Bot. 5 ml drop-tainer. *Rx.*
Use: Anti-infective, ophthalmic.

Maxivate. (Westwood Squibb) Betamethasone dipropionate 0.05%. Cream, Oint. Tube 15 g, 45 g. *Rx.*
Use: Corticosteroid, topical.

Maxi-Vite. (Zenith Goldline) Vitamins A 10,000 IU, D 400 IU, E 15 mg, B_1 10 mg, B_2 10 mg, B_3 100 mg, B_5 20 mg, B_6 5 mg, B_{12} 5 mcg, C 200 mg, Ca 53.5 mg, iron 1.5 mg, folic acid 0.4 mg, biotin 1 mcg, I, P, Cu, Mg, Mn, Zn 1.5 mg, PABA, rutin, glutamic acid, inositol, choline bitartrate, bioflavonoids, L-lysine, betaine, lecithin/Tab. Bot. 60s. *otc.*
Use: Mineral, vitamin supplement.

Maxolon Tablets. (SmithKline Beecham Pharmaceuticals) Metoclopramide HCl 10 mg/Tab. Bot. 100s. *Rx.*
Use: Antiemetic, gastrointestinal stimulant.

Maxovite. (Tyson and Associates) Vitamins A 2083 IU, D 16.7 IU, E 16.7 mg, B_1 5 mg, B_2 4.2 mg, B_3 4.2 mg, B_5 4.2 mg, B_6 54.2 mg, B_{12} 10.8 mcg, C 250 mg, folic acid 0.33 mg, Zn 5 mg, Ca, Cr, Cu, Fe, I, K, Mg, Mn, Se, biotin 11.7 mcg/Tab. Bot. 120s, 240s. *otc.*
Use: Mineral, vitamin supplement.

Maxzide. (ESI Lederle Generics) Hydrochlorothiazide 50 mg, triamterene 75 mg/Tab. Bot. 100s, 500s, UD 10 × 10s. *Rx.*
Use: Antihypertensive, diuretic.

Maxzide-25MG. (ESI Lederle Generics) Triamterene 37.5 mg, hydrochlorothia-

zide 25 mg/Tab. Bot. 100s, UD 100s. *Rx.*
Use: Diuretic combination.

Mayotic. (Merz) Hydrocortisone 1%, neomycin sulfate 5 mg, polymyxin B sulfate 10,000 units/ml, thimerosal 0.01%. Susp. Bot. 10 ml w/dropper. *Rx.*
Use: Otic.

•**maytansine.** (MAY-tan-SEEN) USAN.
Use: Antineoplastic.

May-Vita Elixir. (Merz) B_3 4.4 mg, B_5 1.1 mg, B_6 0.44 mg, B_{12} 1.33 mcg, FA 0.1 mg, Fe 4 mg, Mn, Zn 1.7 mg, alcohol 13%/Liq. Bot. 473 ml. *Rx.*
Use: Mineral, vitamin supplement.

Mazanor. (Wyeth Ayerst) Mazindol 1 mg/Tab. Bot. 30s. *c-IV.*
Use: Anorexiant.

•**mazapertine succinate.** (mazz-ah-PURR-teen) USAN.
Use: Antipsychotic.

Mazicon. (Roche Laboratories) Flumazenil 0.1 mg/ml. Inj. Vial 5 ml, 10 ml. *Rx.*
Use: Antidote.

•**mazindol.** (MAZE-in-dole) U.S.P. 23.
Use: Anorexic, appetite suppressant, Duchenne muscular dystrophy [Orphan drug]
See: Mazanor, Tab. (Wyeth Ayerst). Sanorex, Tab. (Novartis).

M-Caps. (Mill-Mark) Methionine 200 mg/Cap. Bot. 50s, 1000s. *Rx.*
Use: Diaper rash preparation.

MCT Oil. (Bristol-Myers) Triglycerides of medium chain fatty acids. Lipid fraction of coconut oil; fatty acid shorter than C-8 < 6%, C_8(octanoic) 67%, C_{10}(decanoic) 23%, longer than C_{10} 4%. Bot. qt. *otc.*
Use: Nutritional supplement, enteral.

MD-Gastroview. (Mallinckrodt) Diatrizoate meglumine 66%, diatrizoate sodium 10%. Soln. 120 ml, 240 ml.
Use: Radiopaque agent.

MD-60. (Mallinckrodt) Diatrizoate meglumine 52%, diatrizoate sodium 8% (29.2% iodine). Inj. Vial 30 ml, 50 ml.
Use: Radiopaque agent.

MD-76. (Mallinckrodt) Diatrizoate meglumine 66%, diatrizoate sodium 10% (37% iodine). Inj. Vial 50 ml, 100 ml, 150 ml, 200 ml.
Use: Radiopaque agent.

MDP-Squibb. (Bristol-Myers Squibb) Technetium Tc 99 medronate. Reaction vial pkg. 10s.
Use: Radiopaque agent.

meadinin. Mixture of Amoidin & Amidin alk. of Ammi Majus Linn.

measles prophylactic serum.
See: Immune Globulin (Intramuscular).

measles, mumps and rubella virus vaccine live. (MEE-zuhls, mumps and ru-BELL-uh vaccine)
Use: Immunization.
See: M-M-R II, Inj. (Merck).

measles and rubella virus vaccine live.
See: M-R-Vax II, Inj. (Merck).

•**measles virus vaccine, live.** (MEE-zuhls) U.S.P. 23. Modified live-virus measles vaccine.
Use: Immunization.
See: Attenuvax, Inj. (Merck).
W/Mumps virus vaccine, rubella virus vaccine.
See: M-M-R II (Merck).
W/Rubella virus vaccine.
See: M-R-Vax (Merck).

measles virus vaccine, live attenuated. Moraten line derived from Enders' attenuated Edmonston strain grown in cell cultures of chick embryos.
See: Attenuvax, Inj. (Merck).
W/Mumps virus vaccine, rubella virus vaccine.
See: M-M-R., Vial (Merck).
W/Rubella virus vaccine.
See: M-R-Vax, Inj. (Merck).

Mebaral. (Sanofi Winthrop) Mephobarbital. Tab. **0.5 gr, 0.75 gr or 1.5 gr:** Bot. 250s. *c-IV.*
Use: Anticonvulsant, sedative.

•**mebendazole.** (meh-BEND-uh-zole) U.S.P. 23.
Use: Anthelmintic.
See: Vermox, Tab. (Janssen).

mebendazole. (Copley) 100 mg/Chew. Tab. Pkg. 12s, 36s.
Use: Anthelmintic.

•**mebeverine hydrochloride.** (MEH-BEH-ver-een) USAN.
Use: Spasmolytic agent, muscle relaxant.

•**mebrofenin.** (MEH-broe-FEN-in) U.S.P. 23.
Use: Diagnostic aid (hepatobiliary function determination).

•**mebutamate.** (MEH-byoo-TAM-at) USAN.
Use: Antihypertensive.

•**mecamylamine hydrochloride.** (mek-ah-MILL-ah-meen) U.S.P. 23.
Use: Antihypertensive.

•**mecetronium ethylsulfate.** (MEH-seh-TROE-nee-uhm ETH-ill-SULL-fate) USAN.
Use: Antiseptic.

•**mechlorethamine hydrochloride.** (meh-

klor-ETH-ah-meen) U.S.P. 23.
Use: Antineoplastic.
See: Mustargen, Pow. For Inj. (Merck).

mecholin hydrochloride.
See: Methacholine Cl, U.S.P. 23.

Mecholyl Ointment. (Gordon Laboratories) Methacholine Cl 0.25%, methyl salicylate 10% in ointment base. Jar 4 oz, 1 lb, 5 lb. *otc.*
Use: Analgesic, topical.

Meclan. (Advanced Care Products) Meclocycline sulfosalicylate 1%. Cream Tube 20 g, 45 g. *Rx.*
Use: Dermatologic, acne.

meclastine. Clemastine.

•**meclizine hydrochloride.** (MEK-lih-zeen) U.S.P. 23.
Use: Antinauseant, antiemetic.
See: Antivert, Chew. Tab. (Roerig).
Antrizine (Major).
Bonine, Tab. (Roerig).
Dizmiss (Jones Medical Industries)
Dramamine II, Tab. (Pharmacia & Upjohn).
Meclizine HCl (Various Mfr.).
Meni-D (Seatrace).
Vergon, Cap. (Marnel).

Meclizine HCl. (Various) **Tab.: 12.5 mg:** Bot. 30s, 60s, 100s, 500s, 1000s & UD 100s. **25 mg:** In 12s, 20s, 30s, 60s, 100s, 500s, 1000s & UD 32s & 100s. **50 mg:** 100s. **Chew Tab.: 25 mg:** Bot. 20s, 30s, 60s, 100s, 1000s & UD 100s. *otc, Rx.*
Use: Antinauseant.

•**meclocycline.** (meh-kloe-SIGH-kleen) USAN.
Use: Anti-infective.

•**meclocycline sulfosalicylate.** (meh-kloe-SIGH-kleen SULL-foe-sah-LIH-sih-late) U.S.P. 23.
Use: Anti-infective.
See: Meclan, Cream (Ortho McNeil).

•**meclofenamate sodium.** (mek-loe-FEN-uh-mate) U.S.P. 23.
Use: Anti-inflammatory.

meclofenamate sodium. (Mylan) Meclofenamate sodium 50 mg or 100 mg/Cap. Bot. 100s, 500s.
Use: Anti-inflammatory.

•**meclofenamic acid.** (MEH-kloe-fen-AM-ik Acid) USAN.
Use: Anti-inflammatory.

•**mecloqualone.** (MEH-kloe-KWAH-lone) USAN.
Use: Sedative, hypnotic.

•**meclorisone dibutyrate.** (MEH-KLAHR-ih-sone die-BYOO-tih-rate) USAN.
Use: Anti-inflammatory, topical.

•**mecobalamin.** (MEH-koe-BAHL-ah-min) USAN.
Use: Vitamin (hematopoietic).

mecodrin.
See: Amphetamine (Various Mfr.).

•**mecrylate.** (MEH-krih-late) USAN.
Use: Surgical aid (tissue adhesive).

mecysteine. Methyl Cysteine.

Meda Cap. (Circle) Acetaminophen 500 mg/Cap. Bot. 25s, 60s, 100s. *otc.*
Use: Analgesic.

Medacote. (Dal-Med) Pyrilamine maleate 1%, dimethyl polysiloxane, zinc oxide, menthol, camphor in a greaseless base. Lot. Bot. 120 ml. *otc.*
Use: Antihistamine, topical.

Medadyne. (Dal-Med) **Liq.:** Methylbenzethonium chloride, benzocaine, tannic acid, camphor, chlorothymol, menthol, benzyl alcohol, alcohol 61%. Bot. 15 ml, 30 ml. **Throat Spray:** Lidocaine, cetyl dimethyl ammonium chloride, ethyl alcohol. Bot. 30 ml. *otc.*
Use: Mouth and throat preparation.

Meda-Hist Expectorant. (Medwick) Bot. 4 oz, pt, gal.
Use: Decongestant, antitussive.

Medalox Gel. (Med Chem) Magnesium aluminum hydroxide gel. Bot. 12 oz, pt, gal. *otc.*
Use: Antacid.

Medamint. (Dal-Med) Benzocaine 10 mg/Loz. Pkg. 12s, 24s. *otc.*
Use: Mouth and throat preparation.

Meda Tab. (Circle) Acetaminophen 325 mg/Tab. Bot. 100s. *otc.*
Use: Analgesic.

Medatussin Pediatric. (Dal-Med) Dextromethorphan HBr 5 mg, guaifenesin 50 mg, potassium citrate, citric acid, sorbitol, saccharin. Syr. Bot. 120 ml. *otc.*
Use: Antitussive, expectorant.

Medatussin Plus Cough. (Dal-Med) Phenylpropanolamine HCl 25 mg, chlorpheniramine maleate 2 mg, phenyltoloxamine citrate 25 mg, dextro- methorphan HBr 20 mg, guaifenesin 100 mg. Bot. pt. gal. *otc.*
Use: Antihistamine, antitussive, decongestant, expectorant.

•**medazepam hydrochloride.** (med-AZE-eh-pam) USAN. Under study.
Use: Anxiolytic.

Medent. (Stewart-Jackson) Pseudoephedrine HCl 120 mg, guaifenesin 500 mg/Tab. Bot. 100s.
Use: Decongestant, expectorant.

Medicaine Cream. (Walgreens) Benzocaine 3%, resorcinol 2%. Tube 1.25 oz. *otc.*

Use: Antipruritic.

Medicated Acne Cleanser. (C & M Pharmacal) Sulfur 4%, resorcinol 2%, SD alcohol 40 11.65%, methylparaben. Lot. Bot. 120 ml. *otc.*
Use: Dermatologic, acne.

Medicated Healer. (Walgreens) Strong ammonia soln. 10%, camphor 2.6%. Bot. 6 oz. *otc.*
Use: Emollient.

Medicated Powder. (Johnson & Johnson Consumer Products) Zinc oxide, talc, fragrance, menthol. Plastic container 3 oz, 6 oz, 11 oz. *otc.*
Use: Antipruritic.

Medicone Derma. (Medicone) Benzocaine 2%, zinc oxide 13.73%, 8-hydroxyquinoline sulfate 1.05%, ichthammol 1%, menthol 0.48%, petrolatum-lanolin base 79.87%. Oint. Tube 42.5 g. *otc.*
Use: Anesthetic, local.

Medicone Dressing. (Medicone) Cod liver oil 125 mg, zinc oxide 125 mg, 8-hydroxyquinoline-sulfate 0.5 mg, benzocaine 5 mg, menthol 1.8 mg/g w/ petrolatum, lanolin, talcum, paraffin, perfume. Tube 1 oz, 3 oz, Jar lb. *otc.*
Use: Anesthetic, local.

Medicone Ointment. (EE Dickinson) Benzocaine 20%. Oint. 30 g. *otc.*
Use: Anorectal preparation.

Medicone Rectal. (Medicone) Benzocaine 130 mg, hydroxyquinoline sulfate 16 mg, zinc oxide 195 mg, menthol 9 mg, balsam Peru 65 mg. In a vegetable and petroleum oil base. Supp. 12s, 24s. *otc.*
Use: Anorectal preparation.

Medicone-HC Rectal. (Medicone) Hydrocortisone acetate 10 mg, benzocaine 2 gr, oxyquinoline sulfate 0.25 gr, zinc oxide 3 gr, menthol 1/7 gr, balsam Peru 1 gr, in a cocoa butter base/Supp. Box 12s. *Rx.*
Use: Anorectal preparation.

Medicone Suppositories. (EE Dickinson) Phenylephrine HCl 0.25%, hard fat 88.7%, parabens. Pkg. 12s, 24s. *otc.*
Use: Anorectal preparation.

Medigesic. (US Pharmaceutical) Acetaminophen 325 mg, caffeine 40 mg, butalbital 50 mg/Cap. Bot. 100s. *Rx.*
Use: Analgesic, hypnotic, sedative.

Medihaler-Duo.
See: Duo-Medihaler. (3M).

Medihaler-Iso. (3M) Isoproterenol sulfate 2 mg/ml. Soln. Oral adapter w/ 15 ml. Oral adapter w/22.5 ml vial. Refill vial 15 ml and 22.5 ml. *Rx.*
Use: Antiasthmatic.

Medi-Ject UD Vials. (Century Pharm) Tamper-proof rubber stoppered vial containing 1 ml sterile soln. Single dose use.
See: Ulti-ject disposable syringe prods.
Atropine sulfate 0.4 mg/ml.
Atropine sulfate 1.2 mg/ml.
Scopolamine HBr 400 mcg/ml.

Medilax. (Mission Pharmacal) Phenolphthalein 120 mg, aspartame, phenylalanine 1.5 mg/Chew. Tab. Bot. 24s. *otc.*
Use: Laxative.

Medipak. (Armenpharm) First-aid kit.

Medi-Phite. (Med Chem) Vitamins B_1 and B_{12}. Syr. Bot. 4 oz, pt, gal. *otc.*
Use: Vitamin supplement.

Mediplast. (Beiersdorf) Salicylic acid plaster 40%. Box 25s. *otc.*
Use: Keratolytic.

Mediplex Tabules. (US Pharmaceutical) Vitamins E 60 IU, B_1 25 mg, B_2 10 mg, B_3 100 mg, B_5 25 mg, B_6 10 mg, B_{12} 25 mcg, C 300 mg, Zn 4 mg, Cu, Mg, Mn/Tab. Bot. 100s. *otc.*
Use: Mineral, vitamin supplement.

Mediquell. (Parke-Davis) Dextromethorphan HBr 15 mg/Chewy square. Pkg. 12s, 24s. *otc.*
Use: Antitussive.

Medi-Quik Aerosol. (Mentholatum) Lidocaine 2.5%, benzalkonium Cl 0.1%, ethanol 38%. Aerosol 3 oz. *otc.*
Use: Antiseptic; anesthetic, local.

Medi-Quick Antibiotic Ointment. (Mentholatum) Bacitracin neomycin, polymyxin in ointment base. Tube 0.5 oz. *otc.*
Use: Anti-infective, topical.

Meditussin-X Liquid. (Roberts Pharm) Codeine phosphate 50 mg, ammonium Cl 520 mg, potassium guaiacolsulfonate 520 mg, pyrilamine maleate 50 mg, phenylpropanolamine HCl 50 mg, dl-desoxyephedrine HCl 2 mg, tartar emetic 5 mg, phenyltoloxamine dihydrogen citrate 30 mg/30 ml. Bot. pt, gal. *c-v.*
Use: Antihistamine, antitussive, expectorant.

•**medorinone.** (MEH-doe-RIH-nohn) USAN.
Use: Cardiovascular agent.

Medotar. (Medco Lab) Coal tar 1%, polysorbate 80 0.5%, octoxynol 5, zinc oxide, starch, white petrolatum. Jar lb. *otc.*
Use: Antipsoriatic, antipruritic.

Medotopes. (Bristol-Myers Squibb) Radiopharmaceuticals.
See: A-C-D Solution Modified (Bristol-Myers Squibb).
Acid Citrate Dextrose Anticoagulant Solution Modified (Bristol-Myers Squibb).
Aggregated Albumin (Bristol-Myers Squibb).
Albumotope (Bristol-Myers Squibb).
Angiotensin Immutope Kit (Bristol-Myers Squibb).
Cobalt-Labeled Vitamin B_{12} (Bristol-Myers Squibb).
Cobalt Standards for Vitamin B_{12} (Bristol-Myers Squibb).
Cobatope (Bristol-Myers Squibb).
Digoxin (^{125}I) Immutope Kit (Bristol-Myers Squibb).
Gastrin (^{125}I) Immutope Kit (Bristol-Myers Squibb).
Gold-198 (Bristol-Myers Squibb).
Hipputope (Bristol-Myers Squibb).
Human Serum Albumin (Bristol-Myers Squibb).
Iodine 131: Capsules Diagnostic-Capsules Therapeutic-Solution Therapeutic Oral (Bristol-Myers Squibb).
Iodinated Human Serum Albumin (Bristol-Myers Squibb).
Iodo-hippuric Acid (Bristol-Myers Squibb).
Macroaggregated Albumin (Bristol-Myers Squibb).
Macrotec (Bristol-Myers Squibb).
Minitec (Bristol-Myers Squibb).
Phosphorus-32: Solution Oral, Therapeutic-Sodium Phosphate Solution U.S.P. for oral or IV use therapeutic or diagnostic (Bristol-Myers Squibb).
Red Cell Tagging Solution (Bristol-Myers Squibb).
Renotec (Bristol-Myers Squibb).
Rose Bengal (Bristol-Myers Squibb).
Rubratope-57: Diagnostic Capsules-Diagnostic Kit (Bristol-Myers Squibb).
Rubratope-60: Diagnostic Capsules-Diagnostic Kit (Bristol-Myers Squibb).
Selenomethionine (Bristol-Myers Squibb).
Sethotope (Bristol-Myers Squibb).
Technetium 99m (Bristol-Myers Squibb).
Technetium 99m-Iron-Ascorbate (DTPA) (Bristol-Myers Squibb).
Technetium 99m Sulfur Colloid Kit (Bristol-Myers Squibb).
Tesuloid (Bristol-Myers Squibb).
Thyrostat-FTI (Bristol-Myers Squibb).
Thyrostat-3 (Bristol-Myers Squibb).
Thyrostat-4 FTI (Bristol-Myers Squibb).

Medralone 40. (Keene Pharmaceuticals) Methylprednisolone acetate 40 mg/ml. Vial 5 ml. *Rx.*
Use: Corticosteroid.

Medralone 80. (Keene Pharmaceuticals) Methylprednisolone acetate 80 mg/ml. Vial 5 ml. *Rx.*
Use: Corticosteroid.

•**medrogestone.** (MEH-droe-JEST-ohn) USAN.
Use: Hormone, progestin.
See: Colprone (Wyeth Ayerst).

Medrol. (Pharmacia & Upjohn) Methylprednisolone. **Tab.:** 2 mg. Bot. 100s; 4 mg Bot. 30s, 100s, 500s, UD 100s; 8 mg Bot. 25s; 16 mg Bot. 50s; 24 mg Bot. 25s; 32 mg Bot. 25s. **Dosepak:** 4 mg Pkg. 21s. **Alternate Daypak:** 16 mg Pkg. 14s. *Rx.*
Use: Corticosteroid.

•**medronate disodium.** (MEH-droe-nate die-SO-dee-uhm) USAN. *Formerly Disodium Methylene Diphosphonate; MDP.*
Use: Pharmaceutic aid.

•**medronic acid.** (meh-DRAH-nik acid) USAN.
Use: Pharmaceutic aid.

Medrosphol Hg-197.
See: Merprane.

•**medroxalol.** (meh-DROX-ah-LAHL) USAN.
Use: Antihypertensive.

•**medroxalol hydrochloride.** (meh-DROX-ah-LAHL) USAN.
Use: Antihypertensive.

medroxyprogesterone acetate. (meh-DROX-ee-pro-JESS-tuh-rone) (ESI Lederle Generics) Medroxyprogesterone acetate 10 mg/Tab. Bot. 50s, 250s. *Rx.*
Use: Hormone, progestin.

•**medroxyprogesterone acetate.** (meh-DROX-ee-pro-JESS-tuh-rone) U.S.P. 23.
Use: Hormone, progestin.
See: Amen, Tab. (Carnrick Labs).
Curretab, Tab. (Solvay).
Cycrin, Tab. (ESI Lederle Generics).
depCorlutin (Forest Pharmaceutical).
Depo-Provera, Vial (Pharmacia & Upjohn).
P-Medrate-P.A., Inj. (Solvay).
Provera, Tab. (Pharmacia & Upjohn).

medroxyprogesterone acetate. (meh-

DROX-ee-pro-JESS-tuh-rone) (CMC) 50 mg, 100 mg/ml. Vial 5 ml.
Use: Hormone, progestin.

medroxyprogesterone acetate. (Various Mfr.) Medroxyprogesterone acetate 2.5 mg, 5 mg, 10 mg/Tab. Bot. 30s, 40s (10 mg only), 50s, 90s (2.5 mg only), 100s, 250s, 500s, 1000s (2.5 and 5 mg only). *Rx.*
Use: Hormone, progestin.

MED-Rx. (Iomed Labs) Pseudoephedrine HCl 60 mg, guaifenesin 600 mg/CR Tab. Box 28s. Guaifenesin 600 mg/CR Tab. Box 28s. *Rx.*
Use: Decongestant, expectorant.

MED-Rx DM. (Iomed Labs) Pseudoephedrine 60 mg, guaifenesin 600 mg/CR Tab. Bot. 28s. Dextromethorphan hydrobromide 30 mg, guaifenesin 600 mg/CR Tab. Bot. 28s. *Rx.*
Use: Antitussive, expectorant.

•**medrysone.** (MEH-drih-sone) USAN. U.S.P. XXII.
Use: Corticosteroid, topical.
See: HMS Liquifilm, Ophth. Soln. (Allergan).

•**mefenamic acid.** (MEH-fen-AM-ik) USAN. U.S.P. 23.
Use: Anti-inflammatory, analgesic.
See: Ponstel, Kapseal (Parke-Davis).

•**mefenidil.** (meh-FEN-ih-dill) USAN.
Use: Cerebral vasodilator.

•**mefenidil fumarate.** (meh-FEN-ih-dill) USAN.
Use: Cerebral vasodilator.

•**mefenorex hydrochloride.** (meh-FEN-oh-rex) USAN. Under study.
Use: Anorexic.

•**mefexamide.** (meh-FEX-am-IDE) USAN.
Use: Stimulant (central).

•**mefloquine.** (MEH-flow-kwin) USAN.
Use: Antimalarial.

•**mefloquine hydrochloride.** (MEH-flow-kwin) USAN.
Use: Antimalarial. [Orphan drug]
See: Lariam (Roche Laboratories).

Mefoxin. (Merck) Sterile cefoxitin sodium **Pow. for Inj.:** 1 g, 2 g, 10 g. Vial and Infusion Bot. (1 g, 2 g), Bulk Bot. (10 g). **Inj.:** 1 g, 2 g, dextrose. Premixed, frozen in 50 ml plastic containers. *Rx.*
Use: Anti-infective, cephalosporin.

Mefoxin in 5% Dextrose. (Merck) Cefoxitin sodium 1 g or 2 g in Dextrose in Water 5%. Inj. Containers 50 ml. *Rx.*
Use: Anti-infective, cephalosporin.

•**mefruside.** (MEFF-ruh-side) USAN.
Use: Diuretic.

Mega B. (Arco) Vitamins B_1 100 mg, B_2 100 mg, B_3 100 mg, B_5 100 mg, B_6 100 mg, B_{12} 100 mcg, folic acid 100 mcg, d-biotin 100 mcg, PABA 100 mg/Tab. Bot. 100s. *otc.*
Use: Vitamin supplement.

Megace. (Bristol-Myers) Megestrol acetate 20 mg or 40 mg/Tab. **20 mg/Tab.:** Bot. 100s; **40 mg/Tab.:** Bot. 100s, 250s, 500s. Megestrol acetate 40 mg/ml, alcohol ≤ 0.06%, sucrose. Susp. Bot. 236.6 ml. *Rx.*
Use: Antineoplastic; hormone, progestin.

•**megalomicin potassium phosphate.** (meh-GAL-OH-my-sin) USAN.
Use: Anti-infective.

Megaton. (Hyrex) Vitamins B_3 4.4 mg, B_5 1.1 mg, B_6 0.44 mg, B_{12} 1.33 mcg, FA 0.1 mg, Fe 4 mg, Mn, Zn 1.7 mg, alcohol 13%/Liq. Bot. 473 ml. *Rx.*
Use: Mineral, vitamin supplement.

Mega VM-80. (NBTY) Vitamins A 10,000 IU, D 1000 IU, E 100 mg, B_1 80 mg, B_2 80 mg, B_3 80 mg, B_5 80 mg, B_6 80 mg, B_{12} 80 mcg, C 250 mg, iron 1.2 mg, folic acid 0.4 mg, calcium 4.5 mg, zinc 3.58 mg, choline, inositol, biotin 80 mcg, PABA, bioflavonoids, betaine, hesperidin, Cu, I, K, Mg, Mn. Tab. Bot. 60s, 100s. *otc.*
Use: Mineral, vitamin supplement.

•**megestrol acetate.** (meh-JESS-trole) U.S.P. 23.
Use: Antineoplastic; palliative treatment of advanced carcinoma of the breast or endometrium. AIDS-related weight loss. [Orphan drug]
See: Megace, Susp. (Bristol-Myers).
Pallace, Tab. (Bristol-Myers Squibb).

•**meglumine.** (meh-GLUE-meen) U.S.P. 23.
Use: Diagnostic aid (radiopaque medium).

meglumine, diatrizoate inj.
Use: Diagnostic aid; radiopaque medium.
See: Cardiografin, Vial (Bristol-Myers Squibb).
Cystografin, Vial (Bristol-Myers Squibb).
Gastrografin, Soln. (Bristol-Myers Squibb).
Hypaque-76, Inj. (Sanofi Winthrop).
Hypaque-M 75%, Inj. (Sanofi Winthrop).
Hypaque-M 90%, Inj. (Sanofi Winthrop).
Hypaque Meglumine, Vial (Sanofi Winthrop).

Reno-M-30, -60, Vial (Bristol-Myers Squibb).
Reno-M-Dip, Vial (Bristol-Myers Squibb).
W/Meglumine iodipamide.
See: Sinografin, Soln. (Bristol-Myers Squibb).
W/Sodium diatrizoate.
See: Gastrografin, Soln. (Bristol-Myers Squibb).
Renografin-60, Inj. (Bristol-Myers Squibb).
Renografin-76, Inj. (Bristol-Myers Squibb).
Renovist II, Inj. (Bristol-Myers Squibb).

meglumine, iodipamide inj.
Use: Diagnostic aid; radiopaque medium.
See: Cholografin, Vial (Bristol-Myers Squibb).
W/Meglumine diatrizoate.
See: Sinografin, Soln. (Bristol-Myers Squibb).

meglumine, iothalamate inj. U.S.P. 23.
Use: Diagnostic aid; radiopaque medium.

•**meglutol.** (MEH-glue-tahl) USAN.
Use: Antihyperlipoproteinemic.

mejeptil.

•**melafocon a.** (MEH-lah-FOE-kahn A) USAN.
Use: Contact lens material (hydrophobic).

Melanex. (Neutrogena) Hydroquinone 3% in solution containing alcohol 47.3%. Bot. 1 oz w/Appliderm applicator and pinpoint rod applicator. *Rx.*
Use: Dermatologic.

melanoma vaccine.
Use: Stage III-IV melanoma. [Orphan drug]

melanoma cell vaccine.
Use: Invasive melanoma. [Orphan drug]

melarsoprol. (Mel B)
Use: Anti-infective.
See: Arsobol.

melatonin.
Use: Treatment of circadian rhythm sleep disorders in blind patients. [Orphan drug]

Mel B.
See: Melarsoprol.

•**melengestrol acetate.** (meh-len-JESS-trole ASS-eh-tate) USAN.
Use: Antineoplastic; hormone, progestin.

Melhoral Child Tablet. (Sanofi Winthrop) Acetylsalicylic acid. *otc.*
Use: Analgesic.

melitoxin.
See: Dicumarol (Various Mfr.).

•**melitracen hydrochloride.** (meh-lih-TRAY-sen) USAN.
Use: Antidepressant.

•**melizame.** (MEH-lih-zame) USAN.
Use: Sweetener.

Mellaril Concentrate. (Novartis) Thioridazine HCl 30 mg/ml, alcohol 3%. Soln. Bot. 118 ml. Concentrate 100 mg/ml, alcohol 4.2%. Pk. 4 oz. *Rx.*
Use: Antipsychotic.

Mellaril-S. (Novartis) Thioridazine 25 mg/5 ml or 100 mg/5 ml. Susp. Bot. pt. *Rx.*
Use: Antipsychotic.

Mellaril Tablets. (Novartis) Thioridazine HCl 10 mg, 15 mg, 25 mg, 50 mg, 100 mg, 150 mg or 200 mg/Tab. Bot. 100s, 1000s, UD 100s (except 150 mg). *Rx.*
Use: Antipsychotic.

mellose. Methylcellulose.

Melonex. Metahexamide.
Use: Oral antidiabetic.

Melpaque HP. (Stratus) Hydroquinone 4% in a sunblocking base of talc, EDTA, sodium metabisulfite. Cream. Tinted. Tube 14.2 g, 28.4 g. *Rx.*
Use: Dermatologic.

•**melphalan.** (MELL-fuh-lan) U.S.P. 23.
Use: Antineoplastic. [Orphan drug]
See: Alkeran, Tab. (GlaxoWellcome).
Alkeran, Pow. for Inj. (GlaxoWellcome).

Melquin HP. (Stratus) Hydroquinone 4%, mineral oil, propylparaben, sodium metabisulfite. Vanishing base. Cream. Tube 14.2 g, 28.4 g. *Rx.*
Use: Dermatologic.

•**memotine hydrochloride.** (MEH-moe-teen) USAN.
Use: Antiviral.

•**menabitan hydrochloride.** (meh-NAB-ih-tan) USAN.
Use: Analgesic.

•**menadiol sodium diphosphate.** (men-ah-DIE-ole SO-dee-uhm die-FOSS-fate) U.S.P. 23.
Use: Vitamin (prothrombogenic).

•**menadione.** (men-ah-DIE-ohn) U.S.P. 23.
Use: Oral & IM, Vitamin K therapy, vitamin (prothrombogenic).
W/Ascorbic acid, hesperidin.
See: Hescor-K, Tab. (Madland).
W/Bioflavonoid citrus compound, ascorbic acid.
See: C.V.P. W/Vitamin K, Syr., Tab. (Rhone-Poulenc Rorer).

menadione diphosphate sodium.
See: menadiol sodium diphosphate.

Menadol. (Rugby) Ibuprofen 200 mg/Tab. Bot. 50s, 100s. *otc.*
Use: Analgesic, NSAID.

menaphthene or menaphthone.
See: Menadione (Various Mfr.).

menaquinone.
See: Menadione (Various Mfr.).

Menest. (SmithKline Beecham Pharmaceuticals) Esterified estrogens, conjugated estrogens (equine) **0.3 mg, 0.625 mg or 1.25 mg/Tab.:** Bot. 100s. **2.5 mg/Tab.:** Bot. 50s. *Rx.*
Use: Estrogen combination.

Meni-D. (Seatrace) Meclizine 25 mg/Cap. Bot. 100s. *Rx.*
Use: Antiemetic, antivertigo.

meningococcal polysaccharide vaccine group A, C, Y, W-135. (Pasteur Merieux Connaught) Serogroup A, C, Y and W-135 capsular polysaccharides 50 mcg/0.5 ml. Pow. for Inj.
Use: Immunization.
See: Menomune A/C/Y/W-135 (Pasteur Merieux Connaught).

•**meningococcal polysaccharide vaccine group A.** U.S.P. 23.
Use: Immunization.

•**meningococcal polysaccharide vaccine group C.** U.S.P. 23.
Use: Immunization.

•**menoctone.** (meh-NOCK-tone) USAN. Under study.
Use: Antimalarial.

•**menogaril.** (MEN-oh-gar-ILL) USAN.
Use: Antineoplastic.

Menogen. (Breckenridge) Esterified estrogen 1.25 mg, methyltestosterone 2.5 mg. Tab. Bot. 100s. *Rx.*
Use: Hormone.

Menogen HS. (Breckenridge) Esterified estrogen 0.625 mg, methyltestosterone 1.25 mg. Tab. Bot. 100s. *Rx.*
Use: Hormone.

Menoject L.A. (Merz) Testosterone cypionate, estradiol cypionate. Vial 10 ml. *Rx.*
Use: Androgen, estrogen combination.

Menolyn. (Arcum) Ethinyl estradiol 0.05 mg/Tab. Bot. 100s, 1000s. *Rx.*
Use: Estrogen.

Menomune-A/C/Y/W-135. (Pasteur Merieux Connaught) Serogroup A, C, Y and W-135 capsular polysaccharides 50 mcg/0.5 ml. Pow. for Inj.
Use: Immunization.

Menoplex Tablets. (Fiske) Acetaminophen 325 mg, phenyltoloxamine citrate 30 mg/ Tab. Bot. 20s. *otc.*
Use: Analgesic.

•**menotropins.** (MEN-oh-trope-inz) U.S.P. 23. *Formerly Human Follicle Stimulating Hormone.*
Use: Hormone, gonadotropin; gonad-stimulating principle.
See: Humegon, Inj. (Organon Teknika).
Pergonal, Inj. (Serono Labs).

Mentax. (Schering/Penederm) Butenafine HCl 1%, benzyl and cetyl alcohol/Cream. Tube. 2 g, 15 g, 30 g. *Rx.*
Use: Antifungal.

Mentene. (Hoechst Marion Roussel) Velnacrine.
Use: Cholinesterase inhibitor for Alzheimer's disease.

•**menthol.** (MEN-thole) U.S.P. 23.
Use: Topical antipruritic, local analgesic, nasal decongestant, antitussive.
See: Benzedrex Inhaler (SmithKline Beecham Pharmaceuticals).
Blue Gel Muscular Pain Reliever (Rugby).
Robitussin Liquid Center Cough Drops, Loz. (Robins).
Vicks Cough Silencers, Loz. (Procter & Gamble).
Vicks Formula 44 Cough Control Discs, Loz. (Procter & Gamble).
Vicks Inhaler (Procter & Gamble).
Vicks Blue Mint, Lemon, Regular and Wild Cherry Medicated Cough Drops ().
Vicks Medi-Trating Throat Loz. (Procter & Gamble).
Vicks Oracin Regular and Cherry, Loz. (Procter & Gamble).
Vicks Sinex, Nasal Spray (Procter & Gamble).
Vicks Vaporub, Oint. (Procter & Gamble).
Vicks Vaposteam, Liq. (Procter & Gamble).
Vicks Va-Tro-Nol, Nose Drops (Procter & Gamble).
Victors Regular and Cherry, Loz. (Procter & Gamble).
W/Combinations.
See: Eucalyptamint, Gel (Novartis).
Eucalyptamint Maximum Strength, Oint. (Novartis).
Halls Mentho-Lyptus, Prods. (Warner Lambert).
Listerine Antiseptic, Liq. (Warner Lambert).

Mentholatum. (Mentholatum) Menthol 1.35%, camphor 9%, titanium dioxide and fragrance in ointment base of petrolatum. Tube 0.4 oz, 1 oz. Jar 1 oz, 3 oz. *otc.*

Use: Analgesic, topical.

Mentholatum Deep Heating Lotion. (Mentholatum) Menthol 6%, methyl salicylate 20%, lanolin derivative in lotion base. Bot. 2 oz, 4 oz. *otc.*
Use: Analgesic, topical.

Mentholatum Deep Heating Rub. (Mentholatum) Menthol 5.8%, methyl salicylate 12.7%, eucalyptus oil, turpentine oil, anhydrous lanolin, vehicle and fragrance. Tube 1.25 oz, 3.33 oz, 5 oz. *otc.*
Use: Analgesic, topical.

Mentholin. (Apco) Methyl salicylate 30%, chloroform 20%, hard soap 3%, camphor gum 2.2%, menthol 0.8%, alcohol 35%. Bot. 2 oz. *otc.*
Use: Analgesic, topical.

menthyl valerate. Validol.
Use: Sedative.

•**meobentine sulfate.** (meh-OH-BEN-teen SULL-fate) USAN.
Use: Cardiovascular agent (antiarrhythmic).

mepacrine hydrochloride.
Use: Anthelmintic, antimalarial.
See: Quinacrine HCl, U.S.P. 23.

meparfynol.

•**mepartricin.** (meh-PAR-trih-sin) USAN.
Use: Antifungal, antiprotozoal.

mepavlon.
See: Meprobamate, U.S.P. 23.

mepazine acetate & hydrochloride.

•**mepenzolate bromide.** (meh-PEN-zoe-late BROE-mide) U.S.P. 23.
Use: Anticholinergic.
See: Cantil, Tab., Liq. (Hoechst Marion Roussel).
W/Phenobarbital.
See: Cantil w/phenobarbital (Hoechst Marion Roussel).

mepenzolate methyl bromide. Mepenzolate bromide.
Use: Anticholinergic.

Mepergan. (Wyeth Ayerst) Promethazine HCl 25 mg, meperidine HCl 25 mg/ml. Inj. Vial 10 ml, Tubex 2 ml. Box 10s. *c-II.*
Use: Analgesic combination, narcotic.

Mepergan Fortis. (Wyeth Ayerst) Meperidine HCl 50 mg, promethazine HCl 25 mg/Cap. Bot. 100s. *c-II.*
Use: Analgesic combination, narcotic.

•**meperidine hydrochloride.** (meh-PEHR-ih-deen) U.S.P. 23.
Use: Analgesic, narcotic.

meperidine hydrochloride. (meh-PEHR-ih-deen) (Parke-Davis) 50 mg/ml, 75 mg/ml or 100 mg/ml as 1 ml fill in 2 ml Steri-dose syringe.
Use: Analgesic, narcotic.
See: Demerol HCl, Prods. (Sanofi Winthrop).
W/Acetaminophen.
See: Demerol APAP, Tab. (Sanofi Winthrop).
W/Promethazine HCl.
See: Mepergan, Preps. (Wyeth Ayerst).

meperidine hydrochloride and atropine sulfate.
Use: Anesthetic, general.
See: Atropine and Demerol, Inj. (Sanofi Winthrop).

mephenesin.
Use: Muscle relaxant.
See: Myanesin.
W/Acetaminophen, Vitamin C, butabarbital.
See: T-Caps, Cap. (Burlington).
W/Pentobarbital.
See: Nebralin, Tab. (Novartis).
W/Salicylamide, butabarbital sodium.
See: Metrogesic, Tab. (Lexis).

mephenesin carbamate.
See: Methoxydone.

mephenoxalone.

•**mephentermine sulfate.** (meh-FEN-ter-meen) U.S.P. 23.
Use: Vasoconstrictor; decongestant, nasal. Also IV or IM; adrenergic (vasoconstrictor).
See: Wyamine Sulfate Inj. (Wyeth Ayerst).

•**mephenytoin.** (meh-FEN-ee-TOE-in) U.S.P. 23.
Use: Anticonvulsant.
See: Mesantoin, Tab. (Novartis).

•**mephobarbital.** (meh-foe-BAR-bih-tahl) U.S.P. 23.
Use: Anticonvulsant, hypnotic, sedative.
See: Mebaral, Tab. (Sanofi Winthrop).
W/Acetaminophen.
See: Koly-Tabs (Scrip).
W/Homatropine methylbromide, atropine methylnitrate and hyoscine HBr.

mephone.
See: Mephentermine.

Mephyton. (Merck) Phytonadione (vitamin K_1) 5 mg/Tab. Bot. 100s. *Rx.*
Use: Anticoagulant.

Mepiben. (Schein Pharmaceutical) Methylpiperidyl benzhydryl ether.
Use: Antihistamine.

mepiperphenidol bromide.
Use: Anticholinergic.

•**mepivacaine hydrochloride.** (meh-PIHV-ah-cane) U.S.P. 23.

Use: Anesthetic, local.
See: Carbocaine, Inj. (Sanofi Winthrop).
Carbocaine Dental, Inj. (Cook-Waite).
Carbocaine with Neo-Cobefrin, Inj. (Cook-Waite).
Isocaine HCl, Inj. (Novocol Chemical).
Polocaine, Inj. (Astra).
Polocaine MPF, Inj. (Astra).

mepivacaine hydrochloride. (Zenith Goldline) Mepivacaine HCl 1%, 2%, methylparaben. Inj. Vial 50 ml. *Rx.*
Use: Anesthetic, local.

mepivacaine hydrochloride and levonordefrin inj.
Use: Anesthetic, local.
See: Carbocaine, Cartridge, Vial (Cook-Waite).

•**meprednisone.** (meh-PRED-nih-sone) U.S.P. 23.
Use: Corticosteroid, topical.

•**meprobamate.** (meh-pro-BAM-ate) U.S.P. 23.
Use: Anxiolytic, hypnotic, sedative.
See: Arcoban Tab. (Arcum).
Bamate, Tab. (Century Pharm).
Equanil Tab., Cap., (Wyeth Ayerst).
Meprospan, Cap. (Wallace Laboratories).
Miltown, Tab. (Wallace Laboratories).
Tranmep, Tab. (Solvay).
W/Acetylsalicylic acid.
See: Equagesic, Tab. (Wyeth Ayerst).
W/Benactyzine HCl.
See: Deprol, Tab. (Wallace Laboratories).
W/Estrogens conjugated.
See: Milprem, Tab. (Wallace Laboratories).
W/Pentaerythritol tetranitrate.
See: Miltrate, Tab. (Wallace Laboratories).
W/Premarin.
See: PMB 200, Tab. (Wyeth Ayerst).
W/Tridihexethyl Cl.
See: Milpath, Tab. (Wallace Laboratories).
Pathibamate–200, 400, Tab. (ESI Lederle Generics).

meprobamate/aspirin. (Various Mfr.) Aspirin 325 mg, meprobamate 200 mg/Tab. Bot. 100s, 500s. *Rx.*
Use: Analgesic combination.

meprobamate/benactyzine.
Use: Miscellaneous psychotherapeutic agent.
See: Deprol (Wallace Laboratories).

meprobamate, n-isopropyl.
See: Carisoprodol.

Meprogesic Q. (Various Mfr.) Aspirin 325 mg, meprobamate 200 mg/Tab. Bot. 100s, 500s. *Rx.*
Use: Analgesic combination.

Meprolone Tabs. (Major) Methylprednisolone 4 mg/Tab. Bot. 25s, 100s. *Rx.*
Use: Corticosteroid.

Mepron Suspension. (GlaxoWellcome) Atovaquone 750 mg/5 ml. Bot. 210 ml. *Rx.*
Use: Anti-infective.

meprylcaine hydrochloride. U.S.P. XXII.
Use: Anesthetic, local.

•**meptazinol hydrochloride.** (mep-TAZE-ih-nahl) USAN.
Use: Analgesic.

mepyrapone.
See: Metopirone, Tab., Amp. (Novartis).

•**mequidox.** (MEH-kwih-dox) USAN. Under study.
Use: Anti-infective.

mequinolate. (meh-KWIN-ole-ate) Name used for Proquinolate.

meragidone sodium.

•**meralein sodium.** (MER-ah-leen) USAN.
Use: Anti-infective, topical.
See: Sodium Meralein.

merbaphen.

merbromin. *otc.*
Use: Antiseptic, topical.

•**mercaptopurine.** (mer-cap-toe-PURE-een) U.S.P. 23.
Use: Antineoplastic.
See: Purinethol, Tab. (GlaxoWellcome).

mercarbolid. o-Hydroxy-phenylmercuric Cl.

mercazole.
See: Methimazole, U.S.P. 23.

mercocresols.
See: Mercresin, Tr. (Pharmacia & Upjohn).

•**mercufenol chloride.** (MER-cue-FEEN-ole) USAN.
Use: Anti-infective, topical.

mercupurin.
See: Mercurophylline Inj. (Various Mfr.).

mercuranine.
See: Merbromin.

mercurial, antisyphilitics. Mercuric Oleate Mercuric Salicylate.

mercuric oleate. Oleate of mercury.
Use: Parasitic and fungal skin diseases.

mercuric oxide ophthalmic ointment, yellow.
Use: Local anti-infective, ophthalmic.

mercuric salicylate. Mercury subsalicylate.

Use: Parasitic and fungal skin diseases.

mercuric succinimide. BisSuccinimidato-mercury.

mercuric sulfide, red. W/Colloidal sulfur, urea.
See: Teenac Cream, Oint. (Baxter).

mercurin.

mercurocal.
See: Merbromin Soln. (Premo).

Mercurochrome. (Various Mfr.) Merbromin 2%. Soln. Bot. 15 ml, 30 ml. *otc.*
Use: Antiseptic, topical.

mercurome.
See: Merbromin Soln.

•**mercury, ammoniated.** U.S.P. 23.
Use: Anti-infective, topical.

mercury bichloride.
See: Diamond, Tab. (Eli Lilly).

mercury compounds.
See: Antiseptics, Mercurials.

mercury-197-203.
See: Chlormerodrin (Bristol-Myers Squibb).

mercury oleate. Mercury (2+) oleate. Pharmaceutic aid.

Merdex. (Faraday) Docusate sodium 100 mg/Tab. Vial 60 ml. *otc, Rx.*
Use: Laxative.

Meridia. (Knoll) Sibutramine 5 mg, 10 mg, 15 mg, lactose. Cap. 100s. *c-IV.*
Use: Anorexiant.

•**merisoprol acetate Hg 197.** (mer-EYE-so-prole) USAN.
Use: Radiopharmaceutical.

•**merisoprol acetate Hg 203.** (mer-EYE-so-prole) USAN.
Use: Radiopharmaceutical.

Meritene Powder. (Novartis) Vanilla flavor: Specially processed nonfat dry milk, corn syrup solids, sucrose, fructose, calcium caseinate, sodium Cl, natural and artificial flavors, lecithin, vitamins and minerals. Can 1 lb, 4.5 lb, 25 lb. Packet 1.14 oz. Vanilla, chocolate, eggnog, milk chocolate, plain flavors. *otc.*
Use: Nutritional supplement.

merodicein. Sodium meralein.
W/Saligenin.
See: Thantis, Loz. (Becton Dickinson).

•**meropenem.** (meh-row-PEN-em) USAN.
Use: Anti-infective.
See: Merrem IV. (Zeneca).

meroxapol 105.
Use: Irrigating solution.
See: Saf-Clens, Spray (Calgon Vestal).

merprane. 1-(Hydroxymercuri-197 Hg)-2-propanol.
Use: Diagnostic aid.

Merrem. (Zeneca) Meropenem 500 mg/Pow. for Injection. Vial 20 ml, 100 ml, 15 ml ADD-Vantage. Meropenem 1 g/Pow. for Injection. Vial 30 ml, 100 ml, 15 ml ADD-Vantage. *Rx.*
Use: Anti-infective.

mersol. (Century Pharm) Thimerosal tincture, N.F. 1/1000. 1 oz, 4 oz, pt, gal. *otc.*
Use: Antiseptic.

Merthiolate. (Eli Lilly) Thimerosal.
Soln: 1:1000: 4 fl. oz, 16 fl oz, gal.
Tincture: 1:1000: alcohol 50%, 0.75 oz, 4 fl oz, 16 fl oz, gal. *otc.*
Use: Antiseptic.

Meruvax II. (Merck) Lyophilized, live attenuated rubella virus of the Wistar Institute RA 27/3 strain. Each dose contains approximately 25 mcg of neomycin. Single dose Vial w/diluent. Pkg. 1s, 10s. *Rx.*
Use: Immunization.
W/Attenuvax.
See: M-R-Vax II, Vial (Merck).
W/Attenuvax, Mumpsvax.
See: M-M-R II, Vial (Merck).
W/Mumpsvax.
See: Biavax II, Vial (Merck).

Mervan. (Continental Pharma, Belgium) Alclofenac.
Use: Anti-inflammatory.

•**mesalamine.** (me-SAL-uh-MEEN) USAN.
Use: Anti-inflammatory.
See: Asacol, DR Tab. (Procter & Gamble).
Pentasa, CR Cap. (Hoechst Marion Roussel).
Rowasa, Enema, Supp. (Solvay).

mesantoin. (Novartis) 100 mg/Tab. Bot. 100s. *Rx.*
Use: Anticonvulsant.

Mescolor. (Horizon) Chlorpheniramine maleate 8 mg, pseudoephedrine HCl 120 mg, methscopolamine nitrate 2.5 mg, dye free/Tab. Bot. 100s. *Rx.*
Use: Anticholinergic, antihistamine, decongestant.

mescomine.
See: Methscopolamine bromide (Various Mfr.).

•**meseclazone.** (meh-SAK-lah-zone) USAN.
Use: Anti-inflammatory.

•**mesifilcon a.** (MEH-sih-FILL-kahn A) USAN.
Use: Contact lens material, hydrophilic.

•**mesna.** (MESS-nah) USAN.

Use: Hemorrhagic cystitis prophylactic; detoxifying agent. [Orphan drug]
See: Mesnex, Inj. (Bristol-Myers Oncology/Immunology).

Mesnex. (Bristol-Myers Oncology/Immunology) Mesna 100 mg/ml, 0.25 mg/ml EDTA, benzyl alcohol 10.4 mg (10 ml)/Inj. Vial 2 ml, 10 ml. *Rx.*
Use: Antidote.

•**mesoridazine.** (MESS-oh-RID-ah-zeen) USAN.
Use: Antipsychotic, anxiolytic.

•**mesoridazine besylate.** (MESS-oh-RID-ah-zeen BESS-ih-late) U.S.P. 23.
Use: Antipsychotic.
See: Serentil, Amp., Liq., Tab. (Boehringer Ingelheim).

•**mesterolone.** (MESS-TER-oh-lone) USAN.
Use: Androgen.

mestibol. Monomestrol.

Mestinon. (Zeneca) Pyridostigmine bromide 60 mg/Tab. Bot. 100s, 500s. Timespan 180 mg/Tab. Bot. 100s, 500s. *Rx.*
Use: Muscle stimulant.

Mestinon Injectable. (Zeneca) Pyridostigmine bromide 5 mg/ml, w/methyl and propyl parabens 0.2%, sodium citrate 0.02%, pH adjusted to approximately 5 w/citric acid, sodium hydroxide. Amp. 2 ml. Box 10s. *Rx.*
Use: Muscle stimulant.

Mestinon Syrup. (Zeneca) Pyridostigmine bromide 60 mg/5 ml, alcohol 5%. Bot. pt. *Rx.*
Use: Muscle stimulant.

Mestinon Timespan. (Zeneca) Pyridostigmine bromide 180 mg/Timespan Tab. Bot. 100s. *Rx.*
Use: Muscle stimulant.

•**mestranol.** (MESS-trah-nole) U.S.P. 23.
Use: Contraceptive, estrogen.
W/Ethynodiol Diacetate.
See: Ovulen, Tab. (Searle).
Ovulen-21, Tab. (Searle).
Ovulen-28, Tab. (Searle).
W/Norethindrone.
See: Norinyl, Tab. (Syntex).
Norinyl-1 Fe 28 (Syntex).
Ortho-Novum, Tab. (Ortho McNeil).
W/Norethindrone, ferrous fumarate.
See: Ortho Novum Fe-28, Fe-28, 1 mg Fe-28, Tab. (Ortho McNeil).
W/Norethynodrel.
See: Enovid, Tab. (Searle).
Enovid-E, Tab. (Searle).
Enovid-E 21, Tab. (Searle).

•**mesuprine hydrochloride.** (MEH-suh-PREEN) USAN.
Use: Vasodilator, muscle relaxant.

Metabolin. (Thurston) Vitamins A 833 IU, D 66 IU, B_1 833 mcg, B_2 500 mcg, B_6 0.083 mcg, calcium pantothenate 833 mcg, niacinamide 5 mg, folic acid 0.066 mcg, niacinamide 5 mg, p-aminobenzoic acid 0.416 mcg, inositol 833 mcg, B_{12} 500 mcg, C 5 mg, calcium 33.1 mg, phosphorus 14.6 mg, iron 2.5 mg, iodine 0.15 mg/Tab. Bot. 100s, 500s, 1000s. *otc.*
Use: Mineral, vitamin supplement.

•**metabromsalan.** (MET-ah-BROME-sah-lan) USAN.
Use: Antimicrobial, disinfectant.

metabutethamine hydrochloride.
Use: Anesthetic, local.

metabutoxycaine hydrochloride.
Use: Anesthetic, local.

metacaraphen hydrochloride. Netrin.

metacordralone.
See: Prednisolone. (Various Mfr.).

metacortalone.
See: Meticortelone, Susp. (Schering Plough).

metacortandracin.
See: Prednisone, Tab. (Various Mfr.).

metacortin.
See: Meticorten, Tab. (Schering Plough).

•**metacresol.** (met-ah-KREE-sole) U.S.P. 23.
Use: Antiseptic, topical; antifungal.

meta-delphene. Diethyltoluamide U.S.P. 23.

metaglycodol.
Use: Central nervous system depressant.

Metahydrin. (Hoechst-Marion Roussel) Trichlormethiazide 2 mg or 4 mg/Tab. Bot. 100s. *Rx.*
Use: Diuretic.

•**metalol hydrochloride.** (MEH-ta-lahl) USAN. Under study.
Use: Antiadrenergic β-receptor.

Metalone T.B.A. (Foy) Prednisolone tertiary butylacetate 20 mg, sodium citrate 1 mg, polysorbate 80 1 mg, d-sorbitol 450 mg/ml, benzyl alcohol 0.9%, water for inj. Vial 10 ml. *Rx.*
Use: Corticosteroid.

Metamucil. (Procter & Gamble) Psyllium hydrophilic mucilloid, sodium 1 mg, potassium 31 mg/Dose. **Regular Flavor:** w/ dextrose. Jar 7 oz, 14 oz, 21 oz. Packette 5.4 g. Box 100s. **Orange and Strawberry Flavors:** w/flavoring, sucrose and coloring. Jar 7 oz, 14 oz, 21 oz. *otc.*

Use: Laxative.

Metamucil Instant Mix. (Procter & Gamble) Psyllium hydrophilic mucilloid with citric acid, sucrose, potassium bicarbonate, sodium bicarbonate. Powder when combined with water forms an effervescent, flavored liquid. **Lemon Lime Flavor:** w/calcium carbonate. Cartons of 16, 30 or 100 packets of 3.4 g. **Orange Flavor:** w/flavoring and coloring. Ctn. 16 or 30 packets of 3.4 g. *otc.*
Use: Laxative.

Metamucil, Sugar Free. (Procter & Gamble) Psyllium hydrophilic mucilloid in sugar-free formula. **Regular Flavor:** Jar 3.7 oz, 7.4 oz, 11.1 oz. Packet 3.4 g. Box 100s. **Orange Flavor:** Jar 3.7 oz, 7.4 oz, 11.1 oz. *otc.*
Use: Laxative.

Metandren. (Novartis) Methyltestosterone. **Linguet:** 5 mg or 10 mg Bot. 100s. **Tab.:** 10 mg or 25 mg Bot. 100s. *Rx.*
Use: Androgen.

metaphenylbarbituric acid.
See: Mephobarbital.

metaphyllin.
See: Aminophylline (Various Mfr.).

Metaprel Syrup. (Novartis) Metaproterenol sulfate 10 mg/5 ml. Bot. pt. *Rx.*
Use: Bronchodilator.

•**metaproterenol polistirex.** (MEH-tuh-pro-TEHR-uh-nahl pahl-ee-STIE-rex) USAN.
Use: Bronchodilator.

•**metaproterenol sulfate.** (MEH-tuh-pro-TEHR-uh-nahl) U.S.P. 23.
Use: Bronchodilator.
See: Alupent Inhalation (Novartis).
Metaprel, Tab., Inhalation, Syr. (Novartis).
Prometa, Syr. (Muro).

•**metaraminol bitartrate.** (met-uh-RAM-in-ole by-TAR-trate) U.S.P. 23.
Use: Adrenergic.
See: Aramine, Amp., Vial (Merck).

Metastron. (Medi-Physics/Amersham) Strontium-89 Cl 10.9 to 22.6 mg/ml. Preservative free. Inj. Vial 10 ml.
Use: Radiopharmaceutical.

Metatensin #2 & #4. (Hoechst Marion Roussel) Trichlormethiazide 2 mg or 4 mg, each containing reserpine 0.1 mg/Tab. Bot. 100s. *Rx.*
Use: Antihypertensive.

•**metaxalone.** (mex-TAX-ah-lone) USAN.
Use: Muscle relaxant.
See: Skelaxin (Carnrick Labs).

metcaraphen hydrochloride.

Meted, Maximum Strength. (GenDerm) Sulfur 5%, salicylic acid 3%. Shampoo. Bot. 118 ml. *otc.*
Use: Antiseborrheic combination.

•**meteneprost.** (meh-TEN-eh-PRAHST) USAN.
Use: Oxytocic, prostaglandin.

•**metesind glucuronate.** (MEH-teh-sind glue-CURE-oh-nate) USAN.
Use: Antineoplastic (specific thymidylate synthase inhibitor).

metethoheptazine.
Use: Analgesic.

•**metformin.** (MET-fore-min) USAN.
Use: Oral hypoglycemic; antidiabetic.
See: Glucophage, Tab. (Bristol-Myers Squibb).

•**metformin hydrochloride.** (MET-fore-min) USAN.
Use: Antidiabetic.

methacholine bromide. Mecholin bromide.
Use: Cholinergic.

•**methacholine chloride.** U.S.P. 23.
Use: Cholinergic.
See: Mecholyl Cl, Amp. (Mallinckrodt Baker).
Provocholine, Amp. (Roche Laboratories).

methacholine chloride.
Use: Diagnostic aid.
See: Provocholine, pow. for reconstitution. (Roche Laboratories).

•**methacrylic acid copolymer.** (meth-ah-KRILL-ik ASS-id koe-PAHL-ih-mer) N.F. 18.
Use: Pharmaceutic aid (tablet coating agent).

•**methacycline.** (meth-ah-SIGH-kleen) USAN.
Use: Anti-infective.
See: Rondomycin, Cap., Syr. (Wallace Laboratories).

•**methacycline hydrochloride.** (meth-ah-SIGH-kleen) U.S.P. 23.
Use: Antibacterial.

•**methadone hydrochloride.** (METH-uh-dohn) U.S.P. 23.
Use: Analgesic, narcotic; narcotic abstinence syndrome suppressant.
See: Dolophine HCl, Preps. (Eli Lilly).
Methadose, Tab. (Mallinckrodt).

methadone hydrochloride diskets. (METH-uh-dohn) (Eli Lilly) Methadone HCl 40 mg/Dispersible Tab. Bot. 100s. *c-II.*
Use: Analgesic, narcotic.

methadone hydrochloride intensol.

(METH-uh-dohn) (Eli Lilly) Methadone HCl 10 mg/ml. Oral concentrate. Bot. 30 mg. *c-II.*
Use: Analgesic, narcotic.

Methadose. (Mallinckrodt) Methadone 5 mg, 10 mg. Tab. Bot. 100s. *c-II.*
Use: Analgesic, narcotic.

•**methadyl acetate.** (METH-ah-dill ASS-eh-tate) USAN.
Use: Analgesic, narcotic.

•**methafilcon b.** (METH-ah-FILL-kahn B) USAN.
Use: Contact lens material (hydrophilic).

Methagual. (Gordon Laboratories) Guaiacol 2%, methyl salicylate 8% in petrolatum. Oint. 2 oz, lb. *otc.*
Use: Analgesic, topical.

methalamic acid. Name used for Iothalamic acid, U.S.P. 23.

methalgen. (Alra Laboratories) Camphor, menthol, mustard oil, methyl salicylate in non-greasy cream base. Bot. 2 oz, Jar 4 oz, lb. *otc.*
Use: Analgesic, topical.

methallatal.

•**methalthiazide.** (METH-al-THIGH-ah-zide) USAN.
Use: Antihypertensive, diuretic.

methaminodiazepoxide. Chlordiazepoxide HCl, U.S.P. 23.
See: Librium, Cap., Amp. (Roche Laboratories).

methamoctol.
Use: Adrenergic.

•**methamphetamine hydrochloride.** (meth-am-FET-uh-meen) U.S.P. 23
Use: CNS stimulant.
See: Desoxyn, Gradumets, Tab. (Abbott Laboratories).
Methampex, Tab. (Teva USA).
Methamphetamine HCl, Tab. (Various Mfr.).
W/Pamabrom, pyrilamine maleate, homatropine methylbromide, hyoscyamine sulfate, scopolamine HBr.
See: Aridol, Tab. (MPL).
W/Pentobarbital sodium, vitamins, minerals.
See: Fetamin, Tab. (Mission Pharmacal).

methamphetamine-dl hydrochloride.
See: dl-Methamphetamine HCl.

methampyrone.
See: Dipyrone.

methandriol. Methylandrostenediol. (Various Mfr.)
See: Anabol, Inj. (Keene Pharmaceuticals).

methandriol dipropionate.
See: Andriol Inj. (Solvay).
Arbolic, Inj. (Burgin-Arden).
Crestabolic, Vial (Nutrition).
Probolik (Hickam).

methandrostenolone.
See: Dianabol, Tab. (Novartis).

methantheline bromide. U.S.P. XXII. Sterile, Tab., U.S.P. XXII.
Use: Parasympatholytic, anticholinergic.
See: Banthine, Vial, Tab. (Roberts Pharm).
W/Phenobarbital.
See: Banthine w/Phenobarbital, Tab. (Roberts Pharm).

Methaphor. (Borden) Protein hydrolysate (l-leucine, l-isoleucine, l-methionine, l-phenylalanine, l-tyrosine); methionine, camphor, benzethonium Cl, in Dermabase vehicle/Oint. Tube 1.5 oz. *otc.*
Use: Dermatologic, amino acid supplement.

•**methaqualone.** (METH-ah-kwan-lone) USAN.
Use: Hypnotic, sedative.

Methatropic Capsules. (Zenith Goldline) Choline 115 mg, inositol 83 mg, methionine 110 mg, vitamins B_1 3 mg, B_2 3 mg, B_3 10 mg, B_5 2 mg, B_6 2 mg, B_{12} 2 mcg, desiccated liver 86 mg/Cap. Bot. 100s. *otc.*
Use: Vitamin supplement.

•**methazolamide.** (meth-ah-ZOLE-ah-mide) U.S.P. 23.
Use: Carbonic anhydrase inhibitor.
See: GlaucTabs, Tab. (Akorn).
Neptazane, Tab. (ESI Lederle Generics).

methazolamide. (Various Mfr.) Methazolamide 25 mg or 50 mg/Tab. Bot. 100s. *Rx.*
Use: Carbonic anhydrase inhibitor.

Methblue 65. (Manne) Methylene blue 65 mg/Tab. Bot. 100s, 1000s. *Rx.*
Use: Antidote, cyanide.

Meth-Choline Capsules. (Schein Pharmaceutical) Choline 115 mg, inositol 83 mg, methionine 110 mg, vitamins B_1 3 mg, B_2 3 mg, B_3 10 mg, B_5 2 mg, B_6 2 mg, B_{12} 2 mcg, desiccated liver 56 mg, liver concentrate 30 mg/Cap. Bot. 100s, 250s, 1000s. *otc.*
Use: Vitamin supplement.

Meth-Dia-Mer Sulfa Tablets. Trisulfapyrimidines Tab., U.S.P. 23.
Use: Triple sulfonamide therapy.
See: Chemozine, Tab. (Tennessee Pharmaceutic).
Neotrizine, Tab. (Eli Lilly).

Terfonyl, Susp., (Bristol-Myers Squibb).
Triple Sulfa, Tab. (Various Mfr.).

Meth-Dia-Mer Sulfonamides.
Use: Triple sulfonamide therapy.
W/Sulfacetamide.
See: Sulfa-Plex Vaginal Cream (Solvay).
W/Sulfacetamide, hexestrol.
See: Vagi-Plex, Cream (Solvay).

Meth-Dia-Mer Sulfonamides Suspension. Trisulfapyrimidines Oral Suspension, U.S.P. 23.
Use: Triple sulfonamide therapy.
See: Chemozine, Susp. (Tennessee Pharmaceutic).
Neotrizine, Susp. (Eli Lilly).
Terfonyl, Susp. (Bristol-Myers Squibb).
Triple Sulfa, Susp. (CMC).

•**methdilazine.** U.S.P. 23.
Use: Antipuritic.

•**methenamine.** (meh-THEN-uh-meen) U.S.P. 23. *Formerly Hexamethylenamine.*
Use: Anti-infective, urinary.

methenamine w/combinations. (meh-THEN-uh-meen)
Use: Anti-infective, urinary.
See: Cystamine, Tab. (Tennessee Pharmaceutic).
Cystex, Tab. (Numark Laboratories).
Cystitol, Tab. (Briar).
Cysto, Tab. (Freeport).
Hexalol, Tab. (Schwarz Pharma).
Prosed/DS, Tab. (Star).
Urimar-T, Tab. (Marnel).
Urisan-P, Tab. (Sandia).
Urised, Tab. (PolyMedica).
Urogesic Blue, Tab. (Edwards Pharmaceuticals).
Uro Phosphate, Tab. (ECR Pharmaceuticals).
UTA, Tab. (Bentex).
U-Tract, Tab. (Jones Medical Industries).
U-Tran, Tab. (Scruggs).

methenamine and monobasic sodium phosphate tablets. U.S.P. 23.
Use: Anti-infective, urinary.

methenamine anhydromethylene citrate. Formanol, Uropurgol, Urotropin.

•**methenamine hippurate.** (meth-EE-nah-meen HIP-you-rate) U.S.P. 23.
Use: Anti-infective, urinary.
See: Hiprex, Tab. (Hoechst Marion Roussel).
Urex, Tab. (3M).

•**methenamine mandelate.** (meth-EE-nah-meen MAN-deh-late) U.S.P. 23.
Use: Anti-infective, urinary.
See: Mandelamine, Tab. (Parke-Davis).

methenamine mandelate. (Various Mfr.) **Tab.:** 0.5 g or 1 g/Tab. 100s, 1000s. **Susp.:** 0.5 g/5 ml. Susp. BOt. 480 ml. *Rx.*
Use: Anti-infective, urinary.

methenamine mandelate w/combinations.
Use: Anti-infective, urinary.
See: Mandex, Tab. (Pal-Pak).
Thiacide, Tab. (Beach Pharmaceuticals).
Urisedamine, Tab. (PolyMedica).

•**methenolone acetate.** (meth-EEN-oh-lone) USAN.
Use: Anabolic.

•**methenolone enanthate.** (meth-EEN-oh-lone eh-NAN-thate) USAN.
Use: Anabolic.

Metheponex. (Rawl) Choline 0.54 g, dl-methionine 1.80 g, inositol 0.27 g, whole desiccated liver 8.10 g, vitamins B_1 18 mg, B_2 36 mg, niacinamide 90 mg, B_6 3.6 mg, calcium pantothenate 3.6 mg, biotin 10.8 mcg, B_{12} 5.4 mcg and amino acid/daily therapeutic dose. Cap. Bot. 100s, 500s. *Rx.*
Use: Antidiabetic, nutritional supplement.

metheptazine.
Use: Analgesic.

Methergine. (Novartis) Methylergonovine maleate. **Amp.:** 0.2 mg/ml, tartaric acid 0.25 mg/ml, sodium Cl 3 mg/ml. **Tab.:** 0.2 mg. Bot. 100s, 1000s, Sando-Pak pkgs. 100s. *Rx.*
Use: Oxytocic.

methestrol.
See: Promethestrol (Various Mfr.).

methetharimide bemegride. (METH-eh-toe-in) USAN.
Use: Anticonvulsant.

•**methetoin.** (METH-eh-toe-in) USAN.
Use: Anticonvulsant.

Methibon Capsules. (Barrows) Choline dihydrogen citrate 278 mg, dl-methionine 111 mg, inositol 83.3 mg, vitamin B_{12} 2 mcg, liver concentrate, desiccated liver 86.6 mg/Cap. Bot. 100s. *Rx.*
Use: Antidiabetic, nutritional supplement.

•**methicillin sodium, sterile.** (meth-ih-SILL-in) U.S.P. 23.
Use: Anti-infective.
See: Celbenin, Vial (SmithKline Beecham Pharmaceuticals).

•**methimazole.** (meth-IMM-uh-zole) U.S.P. 23.

Use: Thyroid inhibitor.
See: Tapazole, Tab. (Eli Lilly).

methiodal sodium. U.S.P. XXI. Sodium monoiodomethanesulfonate. Abrodil, Radiographol, Diagnorenol.
Use: Radiopaque medium.

Methiokaps. (Pal-Pak) dl-methionine 200 mg/Cap. Bot. 1000s. *Rx.*
Use: Diaper rash product.

methiomeprazine hydrochloride. (SmithKline Beecham Pharmaceuticals)
Use: Antiemetic.

•**methionine C 11 injection.** (meh-THIGH-oh-NEEN) U.S.P. 23.
Use: Radiopharmaceutical.

•**methionine.** (meh-THIGH-oh-NEEN) U.S.P. 23.
Note: Also see Racemethionine, U.S.P. 23.
Use: Amino acid.

methionyl human stem cell factor (recombinant).
Use: Combination w/filgrastim to decrease the number of phereses required to collect blood progenitor cells following myelosuppressive/myeloblative therapy. [Orphan drug]

methionyl neurotrophic (brain-derived, recombinant) factor.
Use: Amyotrophic lateral sclerosis agent. [Orphan drug]

Methioplex. (Lincoln) Methionine 25 mg, vitamins B_1 50 mg, niacinamide 100 mg, B_2 2 mg, choline 50 mg, B_6 2 mg, panthenol 2 mg, benzyl alcohol 1%, distilled water q.s./ml. Vial 30 ml. *Rx.*
Use: Nutritional supplement.

•**methisazone.** (METH-eye-SAH-zone) USAN.
Use: Antiviral.

methitural sodium.
Use: Hypnotic; sedative.

•**methixene hydrochloride.** (meh-THIX-een) USAN.
Use: Muscle relaxant.

•**methocarbamol.** (meth-oh-CAR-buh-mahl) U.S.P. 23.
Use: Muscle relaxant.
See: Delaxin, Tab. (Ferndale Laboratories).
Robaxin, Prods. (Robins).
W/Aspirin.
See: Robaxisal, Tab. (Robins).

methocarbamol. (Various Mfr.) **Tab.:** 500 mg or 750 mg. Bot. 60s (750 mg only), 100s, 500s, UD 100s. **Inj.:** 100 mg/ml Vial 10 ml.
Use: Muscle relaxant.

Methocarbamol/ASA. (Various Mfr.) Methocarbamol 400 mg, aspirin 325 mg/Tab. Bot. 15s, 30s, 40s, 100s, 500s, 1000. *Rx.*
Use: Muscle relaxant.

methocel. Methylcellulose.

•**methohexital.** (meth-oh-HEX-ih-tahl) U.S.P. 23.
Use: Pharmaceutic necessity for Methohexital Sodium for Injection.

•**methohexital sodium for injection.** U.S.P. 23.
Use: Anesthetic, general; anesthetic (intravenous).
See: Brevital, Amp., Pow. (Eli Lilly).

•**methopholine.** (METH-oh-foe-leen) USAN.
Use: Analgesic.
See: Versidyne.

Methopto 0.25%. (Professional Pharmacal) Methylcellulose pow. 2.5 mg (0.25% soln.), boric acid 12 mg, potassium Cl 7.3 mg, benzalkonium Cl 0.04 mg, glycerin 12 mg/ml w/sodium carbonate to adjust pH and purified water. Bot. 15 ml, 30 ml. *otc.*
Use: Artificial tears.

Methopto Forte 0.5%. (Professional Pharmacal) Methylcellulose pow. 5 mg (0.5% soln.), boric acid 12 mg, potassium Cl 7.3 mg, benzalkonium Cl 0.4 mg, glycerin 12 mg/ml w/sodium carbonate to adjust pH and purified water. Bot. 15 ml. *otc.*
Use: Artificial tears.

Methopto Forte 1%. (Professional Pharmacal) Methylcellulose pow. 10 mg (1% soln.), boric acid 12 mg, potassium Cl 7.3 mg, benzalkonium Cl 0.04 mg, glycerin 12 mg/ml w/sodium carbonate to adjust pH and purified water. Bot. 15 ml. *otc.*
Use: Artificial tears.

methopyraphone.
See: Metopirone, Tab., Amp. (Novartis).

methorate.
See: Dextromethorphan HBr.

Methorbate S.C. (Standex) Methenamine 40.8 mg, atropine sulfate 0.03 mg, hyoscyamine sulfate 0.03 mg, salol 18.1 mg, benzoic acid 4.5 mg, methylene blue 5.4 mg/Tab. Bot. 100s. *Rx.*
Use: Anti-infective, urinary.

d-methorphan hydrobromide.
See: Dextromethorphan HBr (Various Mfr.).

methorphinan. Racemorphan HBr. Dromoran.

•**methotrexate.** (meth-oh-TREK-sate)

U.S.P. 23. *Formerly Amethopterin.*
Use: Leukemia in children, antineoplastic, antipsoriatic, juvenile rheumatoid arthritis [Orphan drug]

methotrexate. (Various Mfr.) Tab. 2.5 mg. Bot. 36s, 100s, UD 20s.
Use: Antineoplastic.

methotrexate. (Immunex) **Inj.:** 25 mg/ml as sodium, benzyl alcohol 0.9%, sodium Cl 0.26% and water for inj. Vials 2 ml or 10 ml. **Pow. for Inj.:** 20 mg or 1 g/vial as sodium. Single-use vials. *Rx.*
Use: Antipsoriatic.

methotrexate sodium for injection. (ESI Lederle Generics) 2.5 mg/ml Vial 2 ml; 25 mg/ml. Vial 2 ml w/preservatives; 20 mg, 50 mg, 100 mg Vial cryodesiccated, preservative free; 50 mg, 100 mg, 200 mg Vial; 25 mg/ml solution preservative free.
Use: Leukemia therapy, psoriasis, osteogenic sarcoma [Orphan drug]
See: Folex, Inj. (Pharmacia & Upjohn)
Folex PFS. Inj. (Pharmacia & Upjohn) Methotrexate, Inj., Pow. (ESI Lederle Generics).
Mexate, Inj. (Bristol-Myers Squibb).

methotrexate USP with laurocapram.
Use: Topical treatment of *Mycosis fungoides.* [Orphan drug]

•**methotrimeprazine.** (METH-oh-trih-MEP-rah-zeen) U.S.P. 23.
Use: Analgesic, anxiolytic.
See: Levoprome, Amp., Vial (Immunex).

methoxamine hydrochloride. U.S.P. XXII.
Use: Vasoconstrictor.
See: Vasoxyl (GlaxoWellcome).

•**methoxsalen.** (meth-OX-ah-len) U.S.P. 23.
Use: Pigmenting agent.
See: Meloxine, (Pharmacia & Upjohn).
Oxsoralen, Cap., Lot. (Baxter).
Oxsoralen-Ultra, Cap. (Baxter).

8-methoxsalen.
Use: Treatment of diffuse systemic sclerosis, rejection of cardiac allografts. [Orphan drug]
See: Uvadex.

methoxsalen topical solution.
Use: Pigmenting agent, topical.

methoxydone.
See: Mephenoxalone (Various Mfr.).

•**methoxyflurane.** (meth-OCK-sih-FLEW-rane) U.S.P. 23.
Use: Anesthetic, general.
See: Penthrane, Liq. (Abbott Laboratories).

methoxyphenamine hydrochloride. U.S.P. XXI.
Use: Adrenergic (bronchodilator).
W/Chlorpheniramine maleate, acetophenetidin, acetylsalicylic acid, caffeine.
See: Pyrroxate, Cap., Tab. (Pharmacia & Upjohn).
W/Dextromethorphan HCl, orthoxine, sodium citrate.
See: Orthoxicol, Syr. (Pharmacia & Upjohn).
W/Dextromethorphan HBr, phenylephrine HCl, chlorpheniramine maleate.
See: Statuss, Syr., Cap. (Baxter).
W/Medrol.
See: Medrol, Tab. (Pharmacia & Upjohn).

methoxypromazine maleate.
Use: CNS depressant.

methoxypsoralen, oral.
Use: Psoralen.
See: Oxsoralen (Baxter).
Oxsoralen-Ultra (Baxter).
8-MOP (Baxter).

methscopolamine bromide. U.S.P. XXII. Tab., U.S.P. XXII.
Use: Anticholinergic.
See: Pamine, Tab., Vial (Pharmacia & Upjohn).
Scoline, Tab. (Westerfield).
W/Amobarbital.
See: Scoline-Amobarbital, Tab. (Westerfield).
W/Butabarbital sodium, dried aluminum hydroxide gel and magnesium trisilicate.
See: Eulcin, Tab. (Leeds Pharmacal).
W/Phenobarbital.
See: Pamine PB, Preps. (Pharmacia & Upjohn).
W/Phenylpropanolamine HCl, chlorpheniramine maleate.
See: Bobid, Cap. (Boyd).
Symptrol, Cap. (Saron).

methscopolamine nitrate. Scopolamine Methyl Nitrate, Preps. (Various Mfr.) Mescomine.
See: Cenahist, Cap. (Century Pharm).
Dallergy, Cap., Tab., Syr. (Laser).
Extendryl, Cap., Tab., Syr. (Fleming).
Histaspan-D, Cap. (Rhone-Poulenc Rorer).
Sanhist T.D. 12, Tab. (Sandia).
Scotnord, Tab. (Scott/Cord).
Sinovan, Timed Cap. (Drug Ind.).

•**methsuximide.** (meth-SUCK-sih-mide) U.S.P. 23.
Use: Anticonvulsant.
See: Celontin Kapseal (Parke-Davis).

Methyclodine. (Rugby) Methyclothiazide

5 mg, deserpidine 0.25 mg/Tab. Bot. 100s. *Rx.*
Use: Antihypertensive, diuretic.

•**methyclothiazide.** (METH-ee-kloe-THIGH-ah-zide) U.S.P. 23.
Use: Antihypertensive, diuretic.
See: Enduron, Tab. (Abbott Laboratories) Methyclodine, Tab. (Rugby).
W/Deserpidine.
See: Enduronyl, Tab. (Abbott Laboratories).
Enduronyl Forte, Tab. (Abbott Laboratories).
W/Pargyline HCl.
See: Eutron, Tab. (Abbott Laboratories).

methylacetylcholine.
See: Methacholine.

•**methyl alcohol.** (METH-ill) N.F. 18.
Use: Pharmaceutic acid (solvent).

methylamphetamine hydrochloride & sulfate.
See: Desoxyephedrine HCl (Various Mfr.).

methylandrostenediol.
See: Hybolin, Vial (Hyrex).
Methandriol.
W/Adrenal cortex extract, Vitamin B_{12}.
See: Geri-Ace, Inj. (Baxter).
W/Carboxymethylcellulose sodium, thimerosal.
See: Cenabolic, Vial (Century Pharm).
W/Pentylenetetrazol, nicotinic acid, l-lysine, dl-methionine, ethinyl estradiol, thiamine, pyridoxine, riboflavin, vitamins B_{12}, A, D, ascorbic acid.
See: Ardiatric, Tab. (Burgin-Arden).

•**methylatropine nitrate.** (METH-ill-AT-row-peen) USAN.
Use: Anticholinergic.

•**methylbenzethonium chloride.** (meth-ill-benz-eth-OH-nee-uhm) U.S.P. 23.
Use: Bactericide, local anti-infective (topical).
See: Ammorid, Oint. (Kinney).
Benephen, Prods. (Halsted).
Cuticura Acne Cream (Purex).
Cuticura Medicated First Aid Cream (Purex).
Diaparene Prods. (Bayer Corp).
Fordustin, Pow. (Sween).
Surgi-Kleen, Liq. (Sween).
W/Cod liver oil.
See: Benephen, Prods. (Halsted).
Sween Cream (Sween).
W/Magnesium stearate.
See: Mennen Baby Pow. (Mennen).
W/Phenol, acetanilid, zinc oxide, calamine and eucalyptol.
See: Taloin, Oint. (Warren-Teed).
W/Phenylmercuric acetate, methylparaben.
See: Lorophyn, Supp. (Eaton Medical).
Norforms, Aerosal, Supp. (Procter & Gamble).
W/Zinc oxide, calamine, eucalyptol.
See: Taloin, Tube (Warren-Teed).

methylbenztropine.
See: Ethybenztropine (Novartis).

methylbromtropin mandelate.
See: Homatropine Methylbromide, U.S.P. 23.

•**methylcellulose.** (METH-ill-SELL-you-lohs) U.S.P. 23.
Use: Pharmaceutic aid (suspending agent).
See: Cellothyl, Tab. (International Drug).
Cologel, Soln. (Eli Lilly)
Isopto-Plain, Liq. (Alcon Laboratories).
Melozets, Wafer (SmithKline Beecham Pharmaceuticals).
W/Boric acid, glycerine, propylene glycol, methylparaben, propylparaben, irish moss extract.
See: Canfield Lubricating Jelly (Paddock).
W/Carboxymethylcellulose.
See: Ex-Caloric, Wafer (Eastern Research).
W/Dicyclomine HCl, magnesium trisilicate, aluminum hydroxide-magnesium carbonate, dried.
See: Triactin Tab. (Procter & Gamble).
W/Dicyclomine HCl, aluminum hydroxide and magnesium hydroxide.
See: Triactin Liq. (Procter & Gamble).
W/Phenylephrine HCl.
W/Phenylephrine HCl, benzalkonium Cl.
See: Efricel % (Professional Pharmacal).
W/Polysorbate 80, boric acid.
See: Lacril Artificial Tears (Allergan).

methyl cysteine hydrochloride. Cysteine methyl ester hydrochloride.
Use: Mucolytic agent.

•**methyldopa.** (meth-ill-DOE-puh) U.S.P. 23. *Formerly Alpha-Methyldopa.*
Use: Antihypertensive.
See: Aldomet, Tab. (Merck).

methyldopa and chlorothiazide tablets.
Use: Antihypertensive.
See: Aldoclor, Tab. (Merck).

methyldopa/hydrochlorothiazide tablets.
Use: Antihypertensive.
See: Aldoril, Tab. (Merck).

methyldopa/hydrochlorothiazide. (Various Mfr.) Methyldopa 250 mg, hydro-

chlorothiazide 15 mg or 25 mg/Tab. Bot. 100s, 500s, 1000s, UD 100s. *Rx.*
Use: Antihypertensive combination.

methyldopa/hydrochlorothiazide. (Various Mfr.) Methyldopa 500 mg, hydrochlorothiazide 30 mg or 50 mg/Tab. Bot. 100s, 250s, 500s. *Rx.*
Use: Antihypertensive combination.

•**methyldopate hydrochloride.** (meth-ill-DOE-pate) U.S.P. 23.
Use: Antihypertensive.
See: Aldomet Ester HCl, Inj. (Merck).

methyldopate hydrochloride. (Fujisawa) Methyldopate HCl 250 mg/5 ml. Inj. Vial. 6 ml. *Rx.*
Use: Antihypertensive.

•**methylene blue.** (METH-ih-leen blue) U.S.P. 23.
Use: Antidote, cyanide.
See: Methblue 65, Tab. (Manne).
Urolene Blue, Tab. (Star).
Wright's Stain, Liq. (Becton Dickinson).

methylene blue. (Various) 10 mg/ml. Inj. Vial 1 ml, 10 ml. *Rx.*
Use: GU antiseptic; antidote, cyanide.

methylene blue w/combinations.
See: Hexalol, Tab. (Schwarz Pharma).
Urised, Tab. (PolyMedica).
U-Tract, Tab. (Jones Medical Industries).

•**methylene chloride.** N.F. 18.
Use: Pharmaceutic aid (solvent).

•**methylergonovine maleate.** (METH-ill-err-go-NO-veen MAL-ee-ate) U.S.P. 23.
Use: Oxytocic.
See: Methergine, Amp., Tab. (Novartis).

methylethylamino-phenylpropanol hydrochloride.
See: Nethamine HCl. (Various Mfr.).

methylglucamine diatrizoate, Inj. A water-soluble radiopaque iodine cpd. N-methylglucamine salt of Diatrizoate.
See: Diatrizoate (Various Mfr.).
Diatrizoate Meglumine Inj., U.S.P. 23.

methulglucamine iodipamide, inj.
See: Meglumine Iodipamide, Inj., U.S.P-. 23. (Various Mfr.).
W/Diatrizoate methylglucamine.
See: Sinografin, Vial (Bristol-Myers Squibb).

methylglyoxal-bis-guanylhydrazone. Methyl GAG.

•**methyl isobutyl ketone.** (METH-ill eye-so-BYOO-till KEE-tone) N.F. 18.
Use: Pharmaceutic aid (alcohol denaturant).

methyliso-octenylamine.
See: Isometheptene HCl (Various Mfr.).

methylmercadone. Name used for Nifuratel.

•**methyl nicotinate.** USAN.
W/Histamine dihydrochloride, oleoresin capsicum, glycomonosalicylate.
See: Akes-N-Pain Rub, Oint. (Moore).
W/methyl salicylate, menthol.
See: Musterole Deep Strength Oint. (Schering Plough).
W/Methyl salicylate, menthol, camphor, dipropylene glycol salicylate, cassia oil, oleoresins capsicum, ginger.
See: Arthaderm, Lot. (Paddock).
Scrip-Gesic, Oint. (Scrip).

Methylone. (Paddock) Methylprednisolone acetate 40 mg/ml. Vial 5 ml. *Rx.*
Use: Corticosteroid.

•**methyl palmoxirate.** (METH-ill pal-MOX-ihr-ate) USAN.
Use: Antidiabetic.

•**methylparaben.** (meth-ill-PAR-ah-ben) N.F. 18.
Use: Pharmaceutic aid (antifungal agent).

•**methylparaben sodium.** (meth-ill-PAR-ah-ben) N.F. 18.
Use: Pharmaceutic aid antimicrobial preservative.

methylparafynol.

methylphenethylamine.
See: Amphetamine HCl (Various Mfr.).

•**methylphenidate hydrochloride.** (meth-ill-FEN-ih-date) U.S.P. 23.
Use: CNS stimulant.
See: Ritalin HCl, Tab., Vial (Novartis).

methylphenidate hydrochloride. (Various Mfr.) **Tab.:** 5 mg, 10 mg or 20 mg. Bot. 100s, 1000s; **SR Tab.:** 20 mg. Bot. 100s.
Use: CNS stimulant.

methylphenidylacetate hydrochloride.
See: Methylphenidate HCl (Various Mfr.).

methylphenobarbital.
See: Mephobarbital.

d-methylphenylamine sulfate.
See: Dextroamphetamine Sulfate, U.S.P. 23. (Various Mfr.).

methyl phenylethylhydantoin.
See: Mesantoin, Tab. (Novartis).

methylphenylsuccinimide.
See: Milontin, Kapseal, Susp. (Parke-Davis).

methylphytyl naphthoquinone.
Use: Vitamin supplement.
See: Phytonadione (Various Mfr.)

methyl polysiloxane.
See: Mylicon, Tab., Drops (Zeneca).
Phasil, Tab. (Schwarz Pharma).
Silain, Tab. (Robins).
Simethicone (Various Mfr.)

methylpred-40. (Seatrace) Methylprednisolone acetate 40 mg/ml. Vial 5 ml, 10 ml. *Rx.*
Use: Corticosteroid.

•**methylprednisolone.** (METH-ill-pred-NIH-suh-lone) U.S.P. 23.
Use: Corticosteroid, topical.
See: A-Methapred, Inj. (Abbott Laboratories).
Dura-Meth, Inj. (Foy).
Medralone 40, Inj. (Keene Pharmaceuticals).
Medralone 80, Inj. (Keene Pharmaceuticals).
Medrol, Tab. (Pharmacia & Upjohn).
W/Neomycin sulfate.
See: Neo-Medrol, Oint. (Pharmacia & Upjohn).
W/Sodium succinate.
See: Solu-Medrol, Vial (Pharmacia & Upjohn).

•**methylprednisolone acetate.** (METH-ill-pred-NIH-suh-lone) U.S.P. 23.
Use: Corticosteroid, topical.
See: Adlone, Inj. (Forest Pharmaceutical).
Depo-Medrol, Inj., Rectal (Pharmacia & Upjohn).
Depo-Pred., Vial (Hyrex).
Mepred-40, Susp. (Savage).
Mepred-80, Susp. (Savage).
Neo-Medrol, Preps. (Pharmacia & Upjohn).
Rep-Pred, Vial (Schwarz Pharma).

•**methylprednisolone hemisuccinate.** (METH-ill-pred-NIH-suh-lone hem-ih-SUCK-sih-nate) U.S.P. 23.
Use: Adrenocortical steroid.

•**methylprednisolone sodium phosphate.** (METH-ill-pred-NIH-suh-lone) USAN.
Use: Corticosteroid, topical.

•**methylprednisolone sodium succinate.** (METH-ill-pred-NIH-suh-lone) U.S.P. 23.
Use: Adrenocorticoid steroid; corticosteroid, topical.
See: Solu-Medrol, Mix-O-Vial (Pharmacia & Upjohn).

•**methylprednisolone suleptanate.** (METH-ill-pred-NIH-suh-lone sull-EPP-tah-NATE) USAN.
Use: Adrenocortical steroid, anti-inflammatory.

methylpromazine.

4-methylpyrazole.
Use: Methanol or ethylene glycol poisoning. [Orphan drug]

methylpyrimal.
See: Sulfamerazine (Various Mfr.).

methylrosaniline chloride.
Use: Anthelmintic, anti-infective.
See: Gentian Violet, U.S.P. 23. (Various Mfr.).

•**methyl salicylate.** (METH-ill sal-ISS-ih-late) N.F. 18.
Use: Pharmaceutic aid (flavor).

methyl salicylate w/combinations.
Use: Rubefacient rub (topical).
See: Analbalm, Liq. (Schwarz Pharma).
Analgesic Balm (Various Mfr.).
Banalg, Liniment (Forest Pharmaceutical).
Chloral-Methylol, Oint. (Ulmer).
Cydonol, Lot. (Gordon Laboratories).
Emul-o-balm, Liq. (Medeva).
Gordobalm, Oint. (Gordon Laboratories).
Listerine Antiseptic, Liq. (Warner Lambert).
Musterole, Oint. (Schering Plough).
Pain Bust-R II, Cream (Continental Consumer Products).
Sloan's Liniment, Liq. (Warner Lambert).
Ziks, Cream (Nnodum).

methyl sulfanil amidoisoxazole. Sulfamethoxazole.
See: Gantanol, Tab., Susp. (Roche Laboratories).

•**methyltestosterone.** (METH-ill-tess-TAHS-ter-ohn) U.S.P. 23.
Use: Androgen.
See: Android-10 or 25, Tab. (Zeneca).
Arcosterone, Tab. (Arcum).
Metandren, Linguet, Tab. (Novartis).
Neo-Hombreol-M, Tab. (Organon Teknika).
Oreton-M, Tab., Buccal Tab. (Schering Plough).
Ostone, Tab. (Solvay).
Testred, Cap. (Zeneca).
Virilon, Cap. (Star).

methyltestosterone. (Various Mfr.) 10 mg, 25 mg/Tab. Bot. 100s, 1000s. 10 mg/Tab., Buccal. Bot. 100s. *c-III.*
Use: Androgen.

methyltestosterone w/combinations.
Use: Androgen.
See: Android-5, 10 or 25, Tab. (Baxter).
Mediatric, Cap., Liq., Tab. (Wyeth Ayerst).
Menogen, Prods. (Breckenridge).

Premarin w/Methyltestosterone, Tab. (Wyeth Ayerst).
Virilon, Cap. (Star).

methylthionine chloride. Name used for Methylene Blue.

methylthionine hydrochloride. Name used for Methylene Blue.

methylthiouracil. U.S.P. XXI.
Use: Antithyroid agent.

methyl violet.
See: Gentian Violet, Crystal Violet, Methylrosaniline Cl.

methyndamine. Name used for Tetrydamine.

•**methynodiol diacetate.** (meh-THIN-oh-die-ole die-ASS-eh-tate) USAN.
Use: Hormone, progestin.

•**methysergide.** (METH-ih-SIR-jide) USAN.
Use: Antimigraine; vasoconstrictor.

•**methysergide maleate.** (METH-ih-SIR-jide) U.S.P. 23.
Use: Antimigraine; vasoconstrictor.
See: Sansert, Tab. (Novartis).

•**metiamide.** (meh-TIE-aim-id) USAN. Histamine H_2 antagonist.
Use: Treatment for peptic ulcer; antiulcerative.

•**metiapine.** (meh-TIE-ah-PEEN) USAN.
Use: Antipsychotic.

meticlopindol. Name used for Clopidol.

Meticorten. (Schering Plough) Prednisone 1 mg/Tab. Bot. 100s. *Rx.*
Use: Corticosteroid.

Metimyd Ophthalmic Oint. Sterile. (Schering Plough) Prednisolone acetate 0.5% (5 mg), sulfacetamide sodium 10%. Tube 3.5 g. *Rx.*
Use: Corticosteroid; sulfonamide, topical.

Metimyd Ophthalmic Susp. Sterile. (Schering Plough) Prednisolone acetate 0.5%, sulfacetamide sodium 10%. Bot. dropper 5 ml. *Rx.*
Use: Corticosteroid; sulfonamide, topical.

•**metioprim.** (meh-TIE-oh-PRIM) USAN.
Use: Anti-infective.

•**metipranolol.** (meh-tih-PRAN-oh-lahl) USAN.
Use: Antihypertensive (β-blocker, ophthalmic).
See: OptiPranolol (Bausch & Lomb).

metipranolol hydrochloride.
Use: Antihypertensive (β-blocker, ophthalmic).

metizoline. (meh-TIH-zoe-leen) F.D.A.
Use: Decongestant.

•**metizoline hydrochloride.** (meh-TIH-zoe-leen) USAN.
Use: Adrenergic vasoconstrictor.

•**metkephamid acetate.** (MET-KEFF-am-id) USAN.
Use: Analgesic.

metoclopramide.

•**metoclopramide hydrochloride.** (MET-oh-kloe-PRA-mide) U.S.P. 23.
Use: Antiemetic, gastrointestinal stimulant.
See: Reclomide, Tab. (Ultra).
Reglan, Amp. (Robins).

metoclopramide intensol. (Roxane) Metoclopramide HCl 10 mg/ml, EDTA, sorbitol/Concentrated Soln. Dropper Bot. 10 ml, 30 ml. *Rx.*
Use: Antiemetic, gastrointestinal stimulant.

•**metocurine iodide.** (MEH-toe-CURE-een) U.S.P. 23. *Formerly Dimethyl Tubocurarine Iodide.*
Use: Neuromuscular blocker.
See: Metubine Iodide, Vial (Eli Lilly).

metofurone. (MET-oh-fyoor-OHN) Name used for Nifurmerone.

•**metogest.** (MET-oh-JEST) USAN.
Use: Hormone.

•**metolazone.** (meh-TOLE-uh-ZONE) U.S.P. 23.
Use: Antihypertensive, diuretic.
See: Mykrox, Tab. (Medeva).
Zaroxolyn, Tab. (Medeva).

•**metopimazine.** (meh-toe-PIH-mazz-EEN) USAN.
Use: Antiemetic.

Metopirone. (Novartis) Metyrapone 250 mg. Softgel Cap. Pkg. 18s. *Rx.*
Use: Diagnostic aid.

•**metoprine.** (MET-oh-preen) USAN.
Use: Antineoplastic.

•**metoprolol.** (meh-TOE-pro-lahl) USAN.
Use: Antiadrenergic β-receptor.

•**metoprolol fumarate.** (meh-TOE-pro-lahl) U.S.P. 23.
Use: Antihypertensive.

•**metoprolol succinate.** (meh-TOE-pro-lahl) USAN.
Use: Antihypertensive; antianginal; treatment of myocardial infarction.
See: Toprol XL, Extended release Tab. (Astra).

•**metoprolol tartrate.** (meh-TOE-pro-lahl TAR-trate) U.S.P. 23.
Use: Antiadrenergic (β-receptor).
See: Lopressor, Tab. (Novartis).

metoprolol tartrate. (Various Mfr.) **Tab.:** 50 mg or 100 mg, lactose. Bot. 100s, 500s, 1000s, UD 100s. **Inj.:** 1 mg/ml. Amp. 5 ml.

Use: Antiadrenergic (β-receptor).

metoprolol tartrate and hydrochlorothiazide.
Use: Antihypertensive combination.
See: Lopressor HCT 100/50, Tab. (Novartis).
Lopressor HCT 100/25, Tab. (Novartis).
Lopressor HCT 50/25, Tab. (Novartis).

metoquine.
Use: Antimalarial.
See: Quinacrine HCl, U.S.P.

•**metoquizine.** (MET-oh-kwih-zeen) USAN.
Use: Anticholinergic, antiulcerative.

Metreton Ophthalmic Solution. (Schering Plough) Prednisolone sodium phosphate 5.5 mg/ml. Bot. 5 ml. *Rx.*
Use: Corticosteroid, ophthalmic.

Metric 21. (Fielding) Metronidazole 250 mg/Tab. Bot. 100s. *Rx.*
Use: Anti-infective.

•**metrizamide.** (meh-TRIH-zam-ide) USAN.
Use: Myelography, diagnostic aid (radiopaque medium).
See: Amipaque, Inj. (Sanofi Winthrop).

•**metrizoate sodium.** (meh-trih-ZOE-ate) USAN.
Use: Diagnostic aid (radiopaque medium).

MetroGel. (Galderma) Metronidazole 0.75%. Gel Tube 28.4 g. *Rx.*
Use: Dermatologic, acne.

MetroGel-Vaginal. (3M Pharm) Metronidazole 0.75%, carbomer 934P, EDTA, parabens and propylene glycol. Gel/Tube (with applicator) 70 g. *Rx.*
Use: Anti-infective, vaginal.

Metrogesic. (Lexis) Salicylamide 325 mg, acetaminophen 162 mg, phenacetin 65 mg/Tab. Bot. 100s.
Use: Analgesic.

metrogestone. (MEH-troe-JEST-ohn)
Use: Hormone, progestin.

Metro I.V. (McGaw) Metronidazole 500 mg/100 ml. Inj. Vial 100 ml. Plastic containers 100 ml. *Rx.*
Use: Anti-infective.

•**metronidazole.** (meh-troe-NID-uh-zole) U.S.P. 23.
Use: Antiprotozoal (trichomonas); antitrichomonal. [Orphan drug]
See: Flagyl, Prods. (Searle).
MetroGel-Vaginal, Gel (3M Pharm)
Metronid, Tab. (B.F. Ascher).
Metryl, Tab., Vial (Teva USA).
Noritate, Cream (Dermik Laboratories).

•**metronidazole hydrochloride.** (meh-troe-NIH-dah-zole) USAN.
Use: Anti-infective.
See: Flagyl I.V. (Searle).

•**metronidazole phosphate.** (meh-troe-NIH-dah-zole FOSS-fate) USAN.
Use: Antibacterial, anti-infective, antiprotozoal.

Metronidazole Redi-Infusion. (ESI Lederle Generics) Metronidazole 500 mg/100 ml Vial. *Rx.*
Use: Amebicide.

Metrozole. (Lexis) Metronidazole 250 mg or 500 mg/Tab. **250 mg:** Bot. 100s, 250s; **500 mg:** Bot. 100s. *Rx.*
Use: Amebicide, anti-infective.

MET-RX. (Met-Rx Substrate Technology) Fat 2 g, sodium 37 mg, potassium 900 mg, carbohydrate 22 g, protein, < 1 g dietary fiber, sugar, vitamins A, D, C, E, B_1, B_5, B_6, B_{12}, biotin, magnesium, zinc, calcium, folate, phosphorus, copper, iron, riboflavin, iodine. Pow. For Drink. 72 g. *otc.*
Use: Nutritional therapy.

MET-RX Food Bar. (Met-Rx Substrate Technology) Fat 4 g, sodium 110 mg, potassium 700 mg, carbohydrate 50 g, protein 27 g, sugar, calcium, vitamins A, D, B_1, B_2, B_3, B_5, B_6, B_{12}, C, E, folate, biotin, phosphorus, magnesium, copper, iron, iodine, zinc. Food Bar. 100 g. *otc.*
Use: Nutritional therapy.

Metryl. (Teva USA) Metronidazole 250 mg/Tab. Bot. 100s, 250s, 500s, UD 100s. *Rx.*
Use: Amebicide, anti-infective.

Metryl 500. (Teva USA) Metronidazole 500 mg/Tab. Bot. 100s, 500s. *Rx.*
Use: Amebicide, anti-infective.

Metubine Iodide. (Eli Lilly) Metocurine iodide 2 mg/ml. Vial 20 ml. *Rx.*
Use: Muscle relaxant.

•**meturedepa.** (meh-TOO-ree-DEH-pah) USAN.
Use: Antineoplastic.

Metussin. (Faraday) Dextromethorphan. Bot. 4 oz. *otc.*
Use: Antitussive.

Metussin Jr. (Faraday) Dextromethorphan. Bot. 4 oz. *otc.*
Use: Antitussive.

•**metyrapone.** (meh-TEER-ah-pone) U.S.P. 23.
Use: Diagnostic aid (pituitary function determination).
Adrenocortical enzyme inhibitor.
See: Metopirone, Cap. (Novartis).

•**metyrapone tartrate.** (meh-TEER-ah-pone) USAN.
Use: Diagnostic aid (pituitary function determination).

metyrapone tartrate injection.
Use: Diagnostic aid.

•**metyrosine.** (meh-TIE-roe-seen) U.S.P. 23.
Use: Antihypertensive.
See: Demser (Merck).

Mevacor. (Merck) Lovastatin Tab. **10 mg:** Bot. 60s; **20 mg:** Bot. 60s, 90s, 100s, 1000s, 10,000s, UD 100s; **40 mg:** Bot. 60s, 90s, 1000s, 10,000s. *Rx.*
Use: Antihyperlipidemic.

mevinolin.
See: Lovastatin.

Mexate-AQ. (Bristol-Myers/Bristol Oncology) Preservative-free liquid. Methotrexate 50 mg, 100 mg or 250 mg/Vial. *Rx.*
Use: Antineoplastic.

•**mexiletine hydrochloride.** (MEX-ih-leh-teen) U.S.P. 23.
Use: Cardiovascular agent (antiarrhythmic).
See: Mexitil, Cap. (Boehringer Ingelheim).

mexiletine hydrochloride. (Various Mfr.) Mexiletine HCl 150 mg, 200 mg or 250 mg/Cap. Bot. 100s, UD 100s (except 250 mg). *Rx.*
Use: Cardiovascular agent (antiarrhythmic).

Mexitil. (Boehringer Ingelheim) Mexiletine HCl 150 mg, 200 mg or 250 mg/ Cap. Bot. 100s, UD 100s. *Rx.*
Use: Antiarrhythmic.

•**mexrenoate potassium.** (mex-REN-oh-ate poe-TASS-ee-uhm) USAN.
Use: Aldosterone antagonist.

Mexsana Medicated Powder. (Schering Plough) Corn starch, kaolin, triclosan, zinc oxide. Can 3 oz, 6.25 oz, 11 oz. *otc.*
Use: Diaper rash preparation.

Meyenberg Goat Milk. (Jackson-Mitchell) Evaporated and powdered cans of goat milk. Foil pack 4 oz. (makes one quart). *otc.*
Use: Cows' milk allergies.

Mezlin. (Bayer Corp) Mezlocillin sodium. Vial 1 g, 2 g, 3 g, 4 g. Infusion Bot. 2 g, 3 g, 4 g. *Rx.*
Use: Anti-infective, penicillin.

•**mezlocillin.** (MEZZ-low-SILL-in) USAN.
Use: Anti-infective.

•**mezlocillin sodium, sterile.** (MEZZ-low-SILL-in) U.S.P. 23.
Use: Anti-infective.
See: Mezlin, Inj. (Bayer Corp).

MG Cold Sore Formula. (Outdoor Recreations) Menthol 1%, lidocaine, propylene glycol in alcohol base. Soln. Bot. 7.5 ml. *otc.*
Use: Cold sores, fever blisters.

MG-Oroate. (Miller) Magnesium (as magnesium orotate) 33 mg/Tab. Bot. 100s. *otc.*
Use: Vitamin supplement.

MG217 Medicated Conditioner. (Triton Consumer Products) Coal tar solution 2%. Bot. 120 ml. *otc.*
Use: Antiseborrheic.

MG217 Medicated Formula. (Triton Consumer Products) Coal tar solution 5%, colloidal sulfur 1.5%, salicylic acid 2% in a special base of cleansers, wetting agents and lanolin. Shampoo 120 ml, 240 ml, 480 ml. *otc.*
Use: Antiseborrheic, antipruritic.

MG400. (Triton Consumer Products) Colloidal sulfur in Guy-Base II 5%, salicylic acid 3%. Shampoo. Bot. 240 ml, pt. *otc.*
Use: Antiseborrheic.

MG-Plus Protein. (Miller) Magnesium-protein complex made w/specially isolated soy protein 133 mg/Tab. Bot. 100s. *otc.*
Use: Vitamin supplement.

Miacalcin. (Novartis) Calcitonin-salmon 200 IU, acetic acid 2.25 mg, phenol 5 mg, sodium acetate trihydrate 2 mg, sodium chloride 7.5 mg/ml. Inj. Vial 2 ml. *Rx.*
Use: Hormone.

Miacalcin Nasal Spray. (Novartis) Calcitonin-salmon/activation (0.9 ml/dose) 200 IU, sodium chloride 8.5 mg/Spray. Bot. 2 ml. *Rx.*
Use: Antihypercalcemic.

Mi-Acid Gelcaps. (Major) Calcium carbonate 311 mg, magnesium carbonate 232 mg, parabens, EDTA. Bot. 50s. *otc.*
Use: Antacid.

Mi-Acid Liquid. (Major) Aluminum hydroxide 200 mg, magnesium hydroxide 200 mg, simethicone 20 mg/5 ml. Bot. 355 ml, 780 ml. *otc.*
Use: Antacid, antiflatulent.

Mi-Acid II Liquid. (Major) Aluminum hydroxide 400 mg, magnesium hydroxide 400 mg, simethicone 40 mg/5 ml. Bot. 355 ml. *otc.*
Use: Antacid, antiflatulent.

miadone.
See: Methadone HCl. (Various Mfr.).

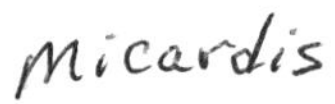

•**mianserin hydrochloride.** (my-AN-ser-in) USAN. Under study.
Use: Serotonin inhibitor, antihistamine.

miaquin.
See: Camoquin, Tab. (Parke-Davis).

•**mibefradil dihydrochloride.** (mih-beh-FRAH-dill-die-HIGH-droe-KLOR-ide) USAN.
Use: Vasodilator.

•**mibolerone.** (my-BOLE-ehr-ohn) USAN.
Use: Anabolic, androgen.

Micanolol. (Bioglan Pharma) Anthralin 1%/Cream. Tube 50 g. *Rx.*
Use: Dermatologic.

micasorb. W/Red Veterinary Petrolatum.
See: RV Plus, Oint. (Baxter).

Micatin. (Advanced Care Products) Miconazole nitrate 2%. **Cream:** Tube 0.5 oz, 1 oz. **Spray powder:** Aerosol 3 oz. **Spray Liquid Aerosol:** Bot. 3.5 oz. *otc.*
Use: Antifungal, topical.

Mi-Cebrin. (Eli Lilly) Vitamins B_1 10 mg, B_2 5 mg, B_6 1.7 mg, pantothenic acid 10 mg, niacinamide 30 mg, B_{12} (activity equiv.) 3 mcg, C 100 mg, E 5.5 IU, A 10,000 IU, D 400 IU, iron 15 mg, copper 1 mg, iodine 0.15 mg, manganese 1 mg, magnesium 5 mg, zinc 1.5 mg/Tab. Pkg. 60s, 100s, 1000s, Blister pkg. 10 × 10s. *otc.*
Use: Mineral, vitamin supplement.

Mi-Cebrin T. (Eli Lilly) Vitamins B_1 15 mg, B_2 10 mg, B_6 2 mg, pantothenic acid 10 mg, niacinamide 100 mg, B_{12} 7.5 mcg, C 150 mg, E 5.5 IU, A 10,000 IU, D 400 IU, iron 15 mg, copper 1 mg, iodine 0.15 mg, manganese 1 mg, magnesium 5 mg, zinc 1.5 mg/Tab. Bot. 30s, 100s, 1000s, Blister pkg. 10 × 10s. *otc.*
Use: Mineral, vitamin supplement.

micofur. Anti 5-Nitro-2-Furaldoxime, Nifuroxime.
Use: Antifungal, anti-infective, topical.
See: Tricofuron, Vaginal Pow., Supp. (Eaton Medical).

Miconal. (Bioglan Pharma) Anthrelin 1% Cream Tube 50 g. *Rx.*
Use: Antipsoriatic.

•**miconazole.** (my-KAHN-uh-zole) U.S.P. 23.
Use: Antifungal.
See: Monistat IV, Inj. (Janssen).

•**miconazole nitrate.** (my-CONE-ah-zole NYE-trate) U.S.P. 23.
Use: Antifungal.
See: Femizol-M, Vag. Cream (Lake Consumer Products).
Fungoid Tincture, Soln. (Pedinol).
Lotrimin AF, Pow., Spray Pow. (Schering Plough).
Maximum Strength Desenex Antifungal, Cream (Novartis).
Monistat, Cream, supp. (Ortho McNeil).
Monistat-3, Vaginal supp. (Ortho McNeil).
Monistat-7, Vaginal cream, supp. (Advanced Care Products).
Monistat-Derm, Prods. (Ortho McNeil).
M-Zole 7 Dual Pack, Supp. Cream (Alpharma).
Nibustat Prods. (Ortho McNeil).
Zeasorb-AF, Pow. (Stiefel).

miconazole nitrate. (Copley) Miconazole nitrate 2%. Cream. Tube 45 g (100 mg/dose for 7 doses). *otc.*
Use: Antifungal, vaginal.

miconazole nitrate. (Taro Pharm) Miconazole nitrate 2%, benzoic acid, mineral oil, apricot kernel oil. Cream. Tube 15 g, 30 g. *otc.*
Use: Antifungal, topical.

micoren. (Novartis) A respiratory stimulant; pending release.

Micrainin. (Wallace Laboratories) Meprobamate 200 mg, aspirin 325 mg/Tab. Bot. 100s, UD 100s. *c-IV.*
Use: Analgesic combination.

MICRhoGAM. (Ortho Diagnostics) Rh_0 (D) immune globulin (Human) micro dose. Single-dose prefilled syringe. *Rx.*
Use: Agent to prevent immunization against Rh antigen.

microbubble contrast agent.
Use: Aid in ID of intracranial tumors. [Orphan drug]

Microcult-GC Test. (Bayer Corp) Miniaturized culture test for the detection of *Neisseria Gonorrhoeae.* Test Kit 25s.
Use: Diagnostic aid.

microfibrillar collagen hemostat.
Use: Hemostatic, topical.
See: Avitene (Alcon Laboratories).
Hemopad (Astra).
Hemotene (Astra).

Micro-Guard. (Sween) Antimicrobial skin cream. Tube 0.5 oz, Jar 2 oz. *otc.*
Use: Antifungal, topical.

Micro-K Extencaps. (Robins) Potassium Cl (8 mEq) 600 mg/Cap. Bot. 100s, 500s, Dis-Co pack 100s. *Rx.*
Use: Electrolyte supplement.

Micro-K 10 Extencaps. (Robins) Potassium Cl 750 mg (10 mEq)/Cap. Bot. 100s, 500s, Dis-co UD 100s. *Rx.*

Use: Electrolyte supplement.

Micro-K LS. (Robins) Potassium Cl 20 mEq (1500 mg). Extended release Susp. Packet 30s, 100s. *Rx.*
Use: Electrolyte supplement.

Microlipid. (Biosearch Medical Products) Fat emulsion 50%, safflower oil, polyglycerol esters of fatty acids, soy lecithin, xanthan gum, ascorbic acid. Cal 4500, fat 500 g/L, 80 mOsm/Kg. H_2O. 120 ml. *Rx.*
Use: Nutritional supplement.

Micronase Tablets. (Pharmacia & Upjohn) Glyburide 1.25, 2.5 or 5 mg/Tab. **1.25 mg:** Bot. 100s. **2.5 mg:** Bot. 30s, 60s, 100s, UD 100s. **5 mg:** Bot. 30s, 60s, 90s, 100s, 500s, 1000s, UD 100s. *Rx.*
Use: Antidiabetic.

microNefrin. (Bird) Racemic methylaminoethanol catechol HCl 2.25 g, sodium Cl, sodium bisulfite, potassium metabisulfite 0.99 g, chlorobutanol 0.5 g, benzoic acid 0.5 g, propylene glycol 8 mg/100 ml. Bot 15 ml, 30 ml. *Rx.*
Use: Antiasthmatic.

Micronized Glyburide. (Copley) 1.5 mg/Tab. Bot. 100s, UD 100s. 3 mg/Tab. Bot. 100s, 500s, 1000s, UD 100s. *Rx.*
Use: Antidiabetic.

Microsol. (Star) Sulfamethizole 0.5 g or 1 g/Tab. Bot. 100s, 1000s. *Rx.*
Use: Anti-infective, urinary.

Microsol-A. (Star) Phenazopyridine 50 mg, sulfamethizole 0.5 g/Tab. Bot. 100s, 1000s. *Rx.*
Use: Anti-infective, urinary.

Microstix Candida. (Bayer Corp) Test for *Candida* species in vaginal specimens. Box 25s.
Use: Diagnostic aid.

Microstix-3 Reagent Strips. (Bayer Corp) For recognition of nitrite in urine and for semi-quantitation of bacterial growth. Bot. 25s w/25 incubation pouches.
Use: Diagnostic aid.

MicroTrak Chlamydia Trachomatis Direct Specimen Test. (Syva) To detect and identify chlamydia trachomatis. Slide test 60s.
Use: Diagnostic aid.

MicroTrak HSV 1/HSV 2 Culture Confirmation/Typing Test. (Syva) For identification and typing of herpes simplex in tissue culture. Test kit 1s.
Use: Diagnostic aid.

MicroTrak Neisseria Gonorrhea Culture Test. (Syva) For endocervical, urethral, rectal and pharyngeal cultures. Test kit 85s.
Use: Diagnostic aid.

Microzide. (Watson) Hydrochlorothiazide 12.5 mg, lactose. Cap. 100s. *Rx.*
Use: Diuretic.

micrurus fulvius antivenin. (Wyeth Ayerst) Inj. Combination package: One vial antivenin, one vial diluent (Bacteriostatic Water for Injection 10 ml.).
Use: Antivenin.

Mictrin Plus. (Johnson & Johnson Consumer Products) Water, S.D. alcohol 38-B, glycerin, poloxamer 407, flavor, sodium saccharin, glutamic acid buffer, cetylpyridinium Cl, FD & C Yellow #5, Blue #1. Bot. 12 oz, 24 oz. *otc.*
Use: Mouth preparation.

•**midaflur.** (MY-dah-flure) USAN.
Use: Hypnotic, sedative.

Midahist Expectorant. (Vangard) Codeine phosphate 10 mg, phenylpropanolamine HCl 18.75 mg, guaifenesin 100 mg/5 ml, alcohol 7.5%. Bot. pt, gal. *c-v.*
Use: Antitussive, decongestant, expectorant.

midamaline hydrochloride.
Use: Anesthetic, local.

Midamor. (Merck) Amiloride 5 mg/Tab. Bot. 100s. *Rx.*
Use: Diuretic, antihypertensive.

Midaneed. (Hanlon) Vitamins A 5000 IU, D 500 IU, B_1 5 mg, B_2 3 mg, B_6 0.5 mcg, B_{12} 5 mcg, C 100 mg, niacinamide 10 mg, calcium pantothenate 5 mg/Cap. Bot. 100s. *otc.*
Use: Mineral, vitamin supplement.

Midatane DC Expectorant. (Vangard) Brompheniramine maleate 2 mg, guaifenesin 100 mg, phenylephrine HCl 5 mg, phenylpropanolamine HCl 5 mg, codeine phosphate 10 mg/5 ml, alcohol 3.5% Bot. pt, gal. *c-v.*
Use: Antihistamine, antitussive, decongestant, expectorant.

Midatapp TR Tablets. (Vangard) Brompheniramine maleate 12 mg, phenylephrine HCl 15 mg, phenylpropanolamine HCl 15 mg/Tab. Bot. 100s, 500s, 1000s. *Rx.*
Use: Antihistamine, decongestant.

•**midazolam hydrochloride.** (meh-DAZE-oh-lam) USAN.
Use: Anesthetic (injectable).
See: Versed, Inj. (Roche Laboratories).

•**midazolam maleate.** (meh-DAZE-oh-lam) USAN.
Use: Anesthetic, intravenous.

Midchlor. (Schein Pharmaceutical) Isometheptene mucate 65 mg, dichloralphenazone 100 mg, acetaminophen 325 mg/Cap. Bot. 100s. *Rx.*
Use: Antimigraine.

•**midodrine hydrochloride.** (MIH-doe-DREEN) USAN.
Use: Antihypotensive, vasoconstrictor.
See: ProAmatine, Tab. (Roberts Pharm).

Midol for Cramps Caplets. (Bayer Corp) Aspirin 500 mg, caffeine 32.4 mg, cinnamedrine HCl 14.9 mg/Tab. In 8s, 16s, 32s. *otc.*
Use: Analgesic combination.

Midol IB. (Bayer Corp) Ibuprofen 200 mg. Tab. Bot. 50s. *otc.*
Use: Analgesic, NSAID.

Midol Maximum Strength. (Bayer Corp) Cinnamedrine HCl 14.9 mg, aspirin 500 mg, caffeine 32.4 mg/Tab. Bot. 12s, 30s, 60s. *otc.*
Use: Analgesic combination.

Midol Multi-Symptom, Maximum Strength. (Bayer Corp) Acetaminophen 500 mg, pyrilamine maleate 15 mg. Capl. Bot. 32s. *otc.*
Use: Analgesic combination.

Midol Multi-Symptom, Regular Strength. (Bayer Corp) Acetaminophen 325 mg, pyrilamine maleate 12.5 mg. Capl. Bot. 32s. *otc.*
Use: Analgesic combination.

Midol Maximum Strength Multi-Symptom Menstrual. (Bayer Corp) Acetaminophen 500 mg, caffeine 60 mg, pyrilamine maleate 15 mg. Capl. Pkg. 8s, 16s, 32s. Gelcaps. Pkg. 12s, 24s. *otc.*
Use: Analgesic combination.

Midol Original Formula. (Bayer Corp) Cinnamedrine HCl 14.9 mg, aspirin 454 mg, caffeine 32.4 mg/Tab. Bot. 30s, 60s. Strip pack 12s. *otc.*
Use: Analgesic combination.

Midol PM. (Bayer Corp) Acetaminophen 500 mg, diphenhydramine 25 mg. Capl. Pkg. 16s. *otc.*
Use: Analgesic combination.

Midol, Teen. (Bayer Corp) Acetaminophen 400 mg, pamabrom 25 mg/Cap. Pkg. 16s, 32s. *otc.*
Use: Analgesic combination.

Midrin. (Carnrick Labs) Isometheptene mucate 65 mg, acetaminophen 325 mg, dichloralphenazone 100 mg/Cap. Bot. 50s, 100s. *Rx.*
Use: Antimigraine.

Midstream Pregnancy Test Kit. (Zenith Goldline) Stick for urine test. Kit 1s. *otc.*
Use: Pregnancy test.

•**mifobate.** (mih-FOE-bate) USAN.
Use: Antiatherosclerotic.

•**miglitol.** (mih-GLIH-tole) USAN.
Use: Antidiabetic.
See: Glyset, Tab. (Bayer Corp).

migraine agents.
See: Sansert, Tab. (Novartis).
Ergostat, Tab. (Parke-Davis).
Medihaler Ergotamine, Aerosol (3M).
D.H.E. 45, Inj. (Novartis).
Imitrex (GlaxoWellcome).

migraine combinations.
See: Isometheptene/Dichloralphenazone/Acetaminophen. (Various Mfr.).
Isocom, Cap. (Nutripharm).
Isopap, Cap. (Geneva Pharm).
Midchlor, Cap. (Schein Pharmaceutical).
Midrin, Cap. (Carnrick Labs).
Migratine, Cap. (Major).

Migranal. (Novartis) Dihydroergotamine mesylate 4 mg/ml, caffeine, dextrose. Nasal spray. Bot. UD 4s. *Rx.*
Use: Antimigraine.

Migratine. (Major) Isometheptene mucate 65 mg, dichloralphenazone 100 mg, acetaminophen 325 mg/Cap. Bot. 100s, 250s. *Rx.*
Use: Antimigraine.

MIH.
Use: Antineoplastic.
See: Matulane (Roche Laboratories).

•**milacemide hydrochloride.** (mill-ASS-eh-mide HIGH-droe-KLOR-ide) USAN.
Use: Anticonvulsant, antidepressant.

•**milameline hydrochloride.** (mill-AM-eh-leen) USAN.
Use: Antidementia (partial muscarinic agonist).

mild silver protein.
See: Silver Protein, Mild.

•**milenperone.** (mih-LEN-per-OHN) USAN.
Use: Antipsychotic.

Miles Nervine. (Bayer Corp) Diphenhydramine HCl 25 mg/Tab. Pkg. 12s, Bot. 30s. *otc.*
Use: Nonprescription sleep aid.

•**milipertine.** (MIH-lih-PURR-teen) USAN.
Use: Antipsychotic.

Milkinol. (Schwarz Pharma) Mineral oil in an emulsifying base. Bot. 240 ml. *otc.*
Use: Laxative.

milk of bismuth. (Various Mfr.) Bismuth hydroxide, bismuth subcarb.
Use: Orally, intestinal disturbances.

•**milk of magnesia.** (milk of mag-NEE-zhuh) U.S.P. 23. *Formerly Magnesia Magma.*
Use: Antacid, laxative.
See: Magnesium hydroxide (Various Mfr.).

milk of magnesia. (Various Mfr.). Magnesia (Magnesium hydroxide) 325 mg, 390 mg. **Tab.:** 250s, 1000s; **Liq.:** 120 ml, 360 ml, 720 ml, pt, qt, gal, UD 10 ml, 15 ml, 20 ml, 30 ml, 100 ml, 180 ml, 400 ml. **Susp.:** Pt, qt, gal, UD 15 and 30 ml.
Use: Antacid, laxative.

Milk of Magnesia-Concentrated. (Roxane) Magnesium hydroxide. Liq. Bot. 100 ml, 180 ml, 400 ml, UD 10 ml, 15 ml, 20 ml, 30 ml.
Use: Antacid.

Millazine. (Major) Thioridazine. **10 mg or 15 mg/Tab.:** Bot. 100s; **25 mg/Tab.:** Bot. 100s, 1000s; **100 mg, 150 mg or 200 mg/Tab.:** Bot. 100s, 500s. *Rx.*
Use: Antipsychotic.

•**milodistim.** (my-low-DIH-stim) USAN.
Use: Immunomodulator (antineutropenic).

Milontin. (Parke-Davis) Phensuximide 0.5 g/Kapseal. Bot. 100s. *Rx.*
Use: Anticonvulsant.

Milpar. (Sanofi Winthrop) Magnesium hydroxide, mineral oil. *otc.*
Use: Antacid, laxative.

•**milrinone.** (MILL-rih-nohn) USAN.
Use: Cardiovascular agent, congestive heart failure.
See: Primacor (Sanofi Winthrop).

Milroy Artificial Tears. (Milton Roy) Bot. 22 ml. *otc.*
Use: Artificial tears.

Miltown. (Wallace Laboratories) Meprobamate. **200 mg/Tab.** Bot. 100s. **400 mg/Tab.** Bot. 100s, 500s, 1000s. **600 mg/Tab.** Bot. 100s. *c-IV.*
Use: Anxiolytic.
See: Meprospan (Wallace Laboratories).

Miltown 600. (Wallace Laboratories) Meprobamate 600 mg/Tab. Bot. 100s. *c-IV.*
Use: Anxiolytic.

•**mimbane hydrochloride.** (MIM-bane) USAN.
Use: Analgesic.

•**minalrestat.** (min-AL-reh-stat) USAN.
Use: Aldose reductase inhibitor.

•**minaprine.** (MIN-ah-preen) USAN.
Use: Psychotherapeutic agent.

•**minaprine hydrochloride.** (MIN-ah-preen) USAN.
Use: Antidepressant.

•**minaxolone.** (min-AX-oh-lone) USAN.
Use: Anesthetic.

mincard.
Use: Diuretic.

Mineral Ice, Therapeutic. (Bristol-Myers Products) Menthol 2%, ammonium hydroxide, carbomer 934, cupric sulfate, isopropyl alcohol, magnesium sulfate, thymol. Gel. Tube 105 g, 240 g, 480 g. *otc.*
Use: Liniment.

mineral-corticoids.
See: Desoxycorticosterone salts (Various Mfr.).

•**mineral oil.** U.S.P. 23.
Use: Laxative, pharmaceutic aid (solvent, oleaginous vehicle).
See: Petrolatum, Liq (Various Mfr.).

mineral oil emulsion.
Use: Cathartic.

mineral oil enema.
Use: Cathartic.

•**mineral oil, light.** N.F. 18.
Use: Pharmaceutic aid (tablet and capsule lubricant, vehicle).

Minibex. (Faraday) Vitamins B_1 6 mg, B_2 3 mg, B_6 0.5 mg, C 50 mg, niacinamide 10 mg, calcium pantothenate 3 mg, B_{12} 2 mcg, folic acid 0.1 mg/Cap. Bot. 100s, 250s, 1000s. *otc.*
Use: Mineral, vitamin supplement.

Minidyne 10%. (Pedinol) Povidone-iodine 10%, citric acid, sodium phosphate dibasic. Soln. Bot. 15 ml. *otc.*
Use: Antimicrobial, antiseptic.

Mini-Gamulin Rh. (Centeon) Rh_o (D) Immune Globulin (Human). Single-dose vial. *Rx.*
Use: Agent to prevent immunization against Rh antigen.

Minipress. (Pfizer) Prazosin HCl 1 mg, 2 mg or 5 mg/Cap. **1 mg, 2 mg:** Bot. 250s, 1000s, UD 100s; **5 mg:** Bot. 250s, 500s, UD 100s. *Rx.*
Use: Antihypertensive.

Minitec. (Bristol-Myers Squibb) Sodium pertechnetate Tc 99 m generator.
Use: Radiopaque agent.

Minitec Generator (Complete with Components). (Bristol-Myers Squibb) Medotopes Kit.
Use: Diagnostic aid.

Mini Thin Asthma Relief. (BDI Pharm) Ephedrine HCl 25 mg, guaifenesin 100 mg or 200 mg/Tab. Bot. 60s (25/100 mg), 100s (25/200 mg). *otc.*
Use: Antiasthmatic.

Mini Thin Pseudo. (BDI Pharm) Pseudoephedrine HCl 60 mg/Tab. Bot. 60s. *otc.*
Use: Decongestant.

Minitran Transdermal Delivery System. (3M Pharm) Nitroglycerin 9 mg, 18 mg, 36 mg or 54 mg. Patch 33s. *Rx.*
Use: Antianginal.

Minit-Rub. (Bristol-Myers) Methyl salicylate 15%, methol 3.5%, camphor 2.3% in anhydrous base. Tube 1.5 oz, 3 oz. *otc.*
Use: Analgesic, topical.

Minizide. (Pfizer) Prazosin HCl and polythiazide. **Minizide 1:** Prazosin 1 mg, polythiazide 0.5 mg/Cap. **Minizide 2:** Prazosin 2 mg, polythiazide 0.5 mg/Cap. **Minizide 5:** Prazosin 5 mg, polythiazide 0.5 mg/Cap. Bot. 100s. *Rx.*
Use: Antihypertensive.

Minocin. (ESI Lederle Generics) Minocycline HCl **Cap., pellet-filled 50 mg:** Bot. 100s, 250s; **100 mg:** Bot. 50s, 250s. **I.V.:** 100 mg/Vial. **Oral Susp.:** 50 mg/5 ml, propylparaben 0.1%, butylparaben 0.06%, alcohol 5% v/v. Bot. 2 oz. *Rx.*
Use: Anti-infective, tetracycline.

•**minocromil.** (MIH-no-KROE-mill) USAN.
Use: Antiallergic (prophylactic).

•**minocycline.** (mihn-oh-SIGH-kleen) USAN.
Use: Anti-infective.
See: Minocyn (ESI Lederle Generics).

•**minocycline hydrochloride.** (mihn-oh-SIGH-kleen) U.S.P. 23.
Use: Anti-infective. [Orphan drug]
See: Dynacin, Cap. (Medicis Dermatologics).
Minocin, Cap., Syr., Vial (ESI Lederle Generics).
Vectrin, Cap. (Warner Chilcott).

minocycline hydrochloride. (Warner Chilcott) Minocycline HCl. Cap. **50 mg:** Bot. 100s; **100 mg:** Bot. 50s.
Use: Anti-infective.

minoxidil. (min-OX-ih-dill) (Schein Pharmaceutical) Minoxidil 2.5 mg/Tab. Bot. 100s, 500s, 1000s. *Rx.*
Use: Antihypertensive.

minoxidil. (min-OX-ih-dill) (Rugby) Minoxidil 10 mg/Tab. Bot. 500s. *Rx.*
Use: Antihypertensive.

•**minoxidil.** (min-OX-ih-dill) U.S.P. 23.
Use: Antihypertensive, vasodilator, hair growth stimulant (topical).
See: Loniten, Tab. (Pharmacia & Upjohn).

Minoxidil for Men. (Lemmon) Minoxidil 2%, alcohol 60%/Soln (topical). Pouches. 60 ml single and twin. *otc.*
Use: Male pattern baldness.

minoxidil, topical.
Use: Antialopecia agent.
See: Rogaine, Soln. (Pharmacia & Upjohn).

Mintezol. (Merck) Thiabendazole. **Susp.:** 500 mg/5 ml. Bot. 120 ml. **Chew. Tab.:** 500 mg. Pkg. 36s. *Rx.*
Use: Anthelmintic.

Minto-Chlor Syrup. (Pal-Pak) Codeine sulfate 10 mg, potassium citrate 219 mg, alcohol 2%. Gal. *c-v.*
Use: Antitussive, expectorant.

Mintox. (Major) Aluminum hydroxide 200 mg, magnesium hydroxide 200 mg. Tab. Bot. 100s. *otc.*
Use: Antacid.

Mintox Plus Extra Strength Liquid. (Major) Aluminum hydroxide 500 mg, magnesium hydroxide 450 mg, simethicone 40 mg/5 ml. Bot. 355 ml. *otc.*
Use: Antacid, antiflatulent.

Mintox Plus Tablets. (Major) Aluminum hydroxide 200 mg, magnesium hydroxide 200 mg, simethicone 25 mg. Chew. Tab. 100s. *otc.*
Use: Antacid, antiflatulent.

Mintox Suspension. (Major) Aluminum hydroxide 225 mg, magnesium hydroxide 200 mg, parabens, saccharin, sorbitol/5 ml. Susp. Bot. 355 ml, 780 ml. *otc.*
Use: Antacid, antiflatulent.

Mint Sensodyne. (Block Drug) Potassium nitrate 5%, saccharin, sorbitol. Toothpaste. Tube 28.3 g. *otc.*
Use: Toothpaste for sensitive teeth.

Minute-Gel. (Oral-B Laboratories) Acidulated phosphate fluoride 1.23% Gel. Bot. 16 oz. *Rx.*
Use: Dental caries agent.

Miochol-E. (Ciba Vision Ophthalmics) Acetylcholine Cl 1:100, mannitol 2.8% when reconstituted. Soln. In 2 ml univials. *Rx.*
Use: Antiglaucoma agent.

•**mioflazine hydrochloride.** (MY-ah-FLAY-zeen) USAN.
Use: Vasodilator (coronary).

Miostat Intraocular Solution. (Alcon Surgical) Carbachol 0.01%. Vial 1.5 ml. Pkg. 12s. *Rx.*
Use: Antiglaucoma agent.

miotics, cholinesterase inhibitors.
Use: Antiglaucoma agents.
See: Humorsol, Soln. (Merck).
Eserine Sulfate, Oint. (Various Mfr.).
Isopto Eserine, Soln. (Alcon Laboratories).

Eserine Salicylate, Soln. (Alcon Laboratories).
Phospholine Iodide, Pow. (Wyeth Ayerst).
Floropryl, Oint. (Merck).

•**mipafilcon a.** (mih-paff-ILL-kahn A) USAN.
Use: Contact lens material (hydrophilic).

Miradon. (Schering Plough) Anisindione 50 mg/Tab. Bot. 100s. *Rx.*
Use: Anticoagulant.

MiraFlow Extra Strength. (Ciba Vision Ophthalmics) Isopropyl alcohol 15.7%, poloxamer 407, amphoteric 10. Thimerosal free. Soln. Bot. 12 ml. *otc.*
Use: Contact lens care.

Miral. (Armenpharm) Dexamethasone 0.75 mg/Tab. Bot. 100s, 1000s. *Rx.*
Use: Corticosteroid.

Mirapex. (Pharmacia & Upjohn) Pramipexole 0.125 mg, 0.25 mg, 1 mg, 1.5 mg. Tab. Bot. 63s (0.125 mg only), 90s. *Rx.*
Use: Antiparkinson agent.

MiraSept. (Alcon Laboratories) **Disinfecting Solution:** Hydrogen peroxide 3%, sodium stannate, sodium nitrate. Bot. 120 ml. **Rinse and neutralizer:** Boric acid, sodium borate, sodium Cl, sodium pyruvate, EDTA. Bot. 120 ml (2s). *otc.*
Use: Contact lens care.

•**mirfentanil hydrochloride.** (MIHR-FEN-tan-ill) USAN.
Use: Analgesic.

•**mirincamycin hydrochloride.** (mihr-IN-kah-MY-sin) USAN.
Use: Anti-infective, antimalarial.

•**mirisetron maleate.** (my-RIH-seh-trahn) USAN.
Use: Antianxiety.

•**mirtazapine.** (mihr-TAZZ-ah-PEEN) USAN.
Use: Antidepressant.
See: Remeron, Tab. (Organon Teknika).

•**misonidazole.** (MY-so-NIH-dah-zole) USAN.
Use: Antiprotozoal (trichomonas).

•**misoprostol.** (MY-so-PRAHST-ole) USAN.
Use: Antiulcerative.
See: Cytotec, Tab. (Searle).

misoprostol and diclofenac sodium.
Use: Arthritis; antiulcerative.
See: Arthrotec, Tab. (Searle).

Mission Prenatal. (Mission Pharmacal) Ferrous gluconate 260 mg (iron 30 mg), vitamins C 100 mg, B_1 5 mg, B_6 3 mg, B_2 2 mg, B_3 10 mg, B_5 1 mg, B_{12} 2 mcg, A 4000 IU, D 400 IU, Ca, zinc 15 mg/Tab. Bot. 100s. *otc.*
Use: Mineral, vitamin supplement.

Mission Prenatal F.A. (Mission Pharmacal) Ferrous gluconate 260 mg (iron 30 mg), vitamins C 100 mg, B_1 5 mg, B_6 10 mg, B_2 2 mg, B_3 10 mg, B_{12} 2 mcg, folic acid 0.8 mg, A acetate 4000 IU, D 400 IU, Ca, B_5 1 mg/Tab. Bot. 100s. *otc.*
Use: Mineral, vitamin supplement.

Mission Prenatal H.P. (Mission Pharmacal) Ferrous gluconate 260 mg (iron 30 mg), vitamins C 100 mg, B_1 5 mg, B_6 25 mg, B_2 2 mg, B_3 10 mg, B_5 1 mg, B_{12} 2 mcg, folic acid 0.8 mg, A 4000 IU, D 400 IU, Ca/Tab. Bot. 100s. *otc.*
Use: Mineral, vitamin supplement.

Mission Prenatal Rx. (Mission Pharmacal) Vitamins A 8000 IU, D 400 IU, C 240 mg, B_1 4 mg, B_2 2 mg, B_3 20 mg, B_5 10 mg, B_6 20 mg, B_{12} 8 mcg, folic acid 1 mg, iron 60 mg, calcium 175 mg, I, zinc 15 mg, Cu/Tab. Bot. 100s. *Rx.*
Use: Mineral, vitamin supplement.

Mission Surgical Supplement. (Mission Pharmacal) Vitamins C 500 mg, B_1 2.5 mg, B_2 2.6 mg, B_3 30 mg, B_5 16.3 mg, B_6 3.6 mg, B_{12} 9 mcg, A 5000 IU, D 400 IU, E 45 IU, iron 27 mg, zinc 22.5 mg/Tab. Bot. 100s. *otc.*
Use: Mineral, vitamin supplement.

Mithracin. (Bayer Corp) Plicamycin 2500 mcg/Vial. Unit vial 10s. *Rx.*
Use: Antineoplastic, antihypercalcemic.

mithramycin. (MITH-rah-MY-sin)
Use: Antineoplastic.
See: Plicamycin.

•**mitindomide.** (my-TIN-doe-MIDE) USAN.
Use: Antineoplastic.

•**mitocarcin.** (MY-toe-CAR-sin) USAN. Antibiotic derived from *Streptomyces* species.
Use: Antineoplastic.

•**mitocromin.** (MY-toe-KROE-min) USAN. Produced by *Streptomyces virdochromogenes.*
Use: Antineoplastic.

•**mitogillin.** (MY-toe-GIH-lin) USAN. An antibiotic obtained from a "unique strain" of *Aspergillus restrictus.*
Use: Antitumorigenic antibiotic; antineoplastic.

mitoguazone. (CTRC Research Foundation)
Use: Treatment of diffuse non-Hodgkin's lymphoma. [Orphan drug]

mitolactol.

Use: Adjuvant therapy in the treatment of primary brain tumors. [Orphan drug]

•**mitomalcin.** (MY-toe-MAL-sin) USAN. Produced by *Streptomyces malayensis*. Under study.
Use: Antineoplastic.

•**mitomycin.** (MY-toe-MY-sin) U.S.P. 23. In literature as Mitomycin C. Antibiotic isolated from *Streptomyces caespitosis*.
Use: Anti-infective; antineoplastic.
See: Mutamycin, Inj. (Bristol-Myers Squibb).

•**mitosper.** (MY-toe-sper) USAN. Substance derived from *Aspergillus* of the glaucus group.
Use: Antineoplastic.

•**mitotane.** (MY-toe-TANE) U.S.P. 23. *Formerly o,p'-DDD.*
Use: Antineoplastic.
See: Lysodren, Tab. (Bristol-Myers Oncology/Immunology).

•**mitoxantrone hydrochloride.** (MY-toe-ZAN-trone) U.S.P. 23.
Use: Antineoplastic. [Orphan drug]
See: Novantrone (ESI Lederle Generics).

Mitran. (Roberts Pharm) Chlordiazepoxide HCl 10 mg/Cap. Bot. 100s. *c-IV.*
Use: Anxiolytic.

Mitrolan. (Robins) Calcium polycarbophil equivalent to polycarbophil 500 mg/ Tab. Blister Pak 36s, 100s. *otc.*
Use: Laxative.

•**mivacurium chloride.** (mih-vah-CURE-ee-uhm) USAN.
Use: Neuromuscular blocker.

•**mivobulin isethionate.** (mih-VOE-byoo-lin eye-seh-THIGH-oh-nate) USAN.
Use: Antineoplastic (microtubule inhibitor).

Mixed Respiratory Vaccine. Each ml contains *Staphylococcus aureus* 1,200 million organisms, *Streptococcus* (both *viridans* and non-hemolytic) 200 million organisms, *Streptococcus (Diplococcus) pneumoniae* 150 million organisms, *Moraxella (Branhamella, Neisseria) catarrhalis* 150 million organisms, *Klebsiella pneumoniae* 150 million organisms, and *Haemophilus influenzae* types a and b 150 million organisms. Vial. 20 ml.
Use: Bacterial vaccine.
See: MRV, Inj. (Bayer Corp).

mixed vespid Hymenoptera venom. *Rx.*
Use: Agent for immunization.
See: Albay (Bayer Corp).
Pharmalgen (ALK Laboratories).
Venomil (Bayer Corp).

•**mixidine.** (MIX-ih-deen) USAN.
Use: Vasodilator (coronary).

mixture 612. Dimethyl Phthalate Solution, Compound.

M-M-R II. (Merck) Lyophilized preparation of live attenuated measles virus vaccine (Attenuvax), live attenuated mumps virus vaccine (Mumpsvax), live attenuated rubella virus vaccine (Meruvax II). See details under Attenuvax, Mumpsvax and Meruvax II. Single dose vial w/diluent. Pkg. 1s, 10s. *Rx.*
Use: Agent for immunization.

Moban. (DuPont Merck Pharmaceuticals) Molindone HCl. **Liq.:** 20 mg/ml concentrate. Bot. 120 ml. **Tab.:** 5 mg, 10 mg, 25 mg, 50 mg or 100 mg, lactose. Tab. Bot. 100s. *Rx.*
Use: Antipsychotic.

mobenol.
See: Tolbutamide, U.S.P. 23.

Mobidin. (B.F. Ascher) Magnesium salicylate, anhydrous 600 mg/Tab. Bot. 100s, 500s. *Rx.*
Use: Antiarthritic.

Mobigesic. (B.F. Ascher) Magnesium salicylate 325 mg, phenyltoloxamine citrate 30 mg/ Tab. Bot. 50s, 100s, Pkg. 18s. *otc.*
Use: Analgesic combination.

Mobisyl Creme. (B.F. Ascher) Trolamine salicylate in vanishing creme base. Tubes 100 g. *otc.*
Use: Analgesic, topical.

moccasin bite.
See: Antivenin (Crotalidae).

•**moclobemide.** (moe-KLOE-beh-mide) USAN.
Use: Antidepressant.

moctanin. (Ethitek Pharmaceuticals) Glyceryl-l-mono-oc- tanoate (80-85%), glyceryl-l-mono-de- canoate (10-15%), glyceryl-l-2-di-oc- tanoate (10-15%), free glyceryl (2.5% maximum). Bot. 120 ml. *Rx.*
Use: Urolithic.

•**modafinil.** (moe-DAFF-ih-nill) USAN.
Use: Analeptic treatment of narcolepsy and hypersomnia. [Orphan drug]

•**modaline sulfate.** (MODE-al-een) USAN
Use: Antidepressant.

Modane. (Pharmacia & Upjohn) Phenolphthalein 130 mg/Tab. Pkg. 10s, 30s. Bot. 100s. *otc.*
Use: Laxative.

Modane Bulk. (Pharmacia & Upjohn) Powdered mixture of equal parts of psyllium and dextrose. Container 14 oz. *otc.*

Use: Laxative.

Modane Mild. (Pharmacia & Upjohn) Phenolphthalein 60 mg/Tab. Bot. 10s, 30s, 100s. *otc.*
Use: Laxative.

Modane Plus. (Pharmacia & Upjohn) Phenolphthalein 60 mg, docusate sodium 100 mg/Tab. Bot. 100s, Box 10s, 30s. *otc.*
Use: Laxative.

Modane Soft. (Pharmacia & Upjohn) Docusate sodium 100 mg/Cap. UD Pkg. 30s. *otc.*
Use: Laxative.

Modane Versabran. (Pharmacia & Upjohn) Psyllium hydrophilic mucilloid in wheat bran base. Dose 3.4 g, Bot. 10 oz. *otc.*
Use: Laxative.

•**modecainide.** (moe-deh-CANE-ide) USAN.
Use: Cardiovascular (antiarrhythmic).

Modicon 21. (Ortho McNeil) Norethindrone 0.5 mg, ethinyl estradiol 35 mcg/Tab. Dialpak 21s. *Rx.*
Use: Contraceptive.

Modicon 28. (Ortho McNeil) Norethindrone 0.5 mg, ethinyl estradiol 35 mcg/Tab., 7 inert Tab. Dialpak 28s. *Rx.*
Use: Contraceptive.

modified burow's solution.
See: Burow's solution.

modinal.
See: Gardinol Type Detergents (Various Mfr.).

Moducal. (Bristol-Myers) Maltodextrin. Pow. Can 13 oz. *otc.*
Use: Nutritional supplement.

Moduretic. (Merck) Hydrochlorothiazide 50 mg, amiloride 5 mg/Tab. Bot. 100s, UD 100s. *Rx.*
Use: Antihypertensive, diuretic.

moenomycin. Phosphorus-containing glycolipide antibiotic. Active against gram-positive organisms. Under study.

•**moexipril hydrochloride.** (moe-EX-ah-prill) USAN.
Use: Antihypertensive, ACE inhibitor.
See: Univasc, Tab. (Schwarz Pharma).

moexipril hydrochloride and hydrochlorothiazide.
Use: Antihypertensive.
See: Uniretic, Tab. (Schwarz Pharma).

•**mofegiline hydrochloride.** (moe-FEH-jih-leen) USAN.
Use: Antiparkinsonian.

Moist Again. (Lake Consumer Products) Aloe vera, EDTA, methylparaben, glycerin. Gel. Tube 70.8 g. *otc.*
Use: Vaginal agent.

Moi-Stir. (Kingswood) Dibasic sodium phosphate, magnesium, calcium, sodium Cl, potassium Cl, sorbitol, sodium carboxymethylcellulose, parabens. Soln. 120 ml with pump spray. *otc.*
Use: Saliva substitute.

Moi-Stir Swabsticks. (Kingswood) Dibasic sodium phosphate, magnesium, calcium, sodium Cl, potassium Cl, sorbitol, sodium carboxymethylcellulose, parabens. Soln. Pkt. 3s. *otc.*
Use: Saliva substitute.

Moisture Drops. (Bausch & Lomb) Hydroxypropyl methylcellulose 0.5%, povidone 0.1%, glycerin 0.2%, benzalkonium Cl 0.01%, EDTA, sodium Cl, boric acid, potassium Cl, sodium borate. Soln. Bot. 0.5 oz, 1 oz. *otc.*
Use: Artificial tears.

molar phosphate.
W/Fluoride ion.
See: Coral Prods. (Young Dental).
Karigel, Gel. (Young Dental).

molecusol-carbamazepine.
See: PR-320.

•**molgramostim.** (mahl-GRAH-moe-STIM) USAN.
Use: Hematopoietic stimulant, antineutropenic.

•**molinazone.** (moe-LEEN-ah-zone) USAN.
Use: Analgesic.

•**molindone hydrochloride.** (moe-LIN-dohn) U.S.P. 23.
Use: Antipsychotic.
See: Lidone, Cap. (Abbott Laboratories).
Lidone Concentrate, Liq. (Abbott Laboratories).
Moban, Tab. (DuPont Merck Pharmaceuticals).

Mollifene Ear Drops. (Pfeiffer) Glycerin, camphor, cajaput oil, eucalyptus oil, thyme oil. Soln. Bot. 24 ml. *otc.*
Use: Otic.

•**molsidomine.** (mole-SIH-doe-meen) USAN.
Use: Antianginal, vasodilator (coronary).

molybdenum solution. (American Quinine) Molybdenum 25 mcg/ml (as 46 mcg/ml ammonium molybdate tetrahydrate). Inj. Vial 10 ml. *Rx.*
Use: Nutritional supplement, parenteral.

Molycu. (Burns) Meprobamate 400 mg, copper 60 mg/ml. *Rx.*
Use: Antidote.

Moly-Pak. (SoloPak) Molybdenum 25

mcg. Inj. Vial 10 ml. *Rx.*
Use: Nutritional supplement, parenteral.

Molypen. (Fujisawa) Ammonium molybdate tetrahydrate 46 mcg/ml. Vial 10 ml. *Rx.*
Use: Nutritional supplement, parenteral.

Momentum. (Whitehall Robins) Aspirin 500 mg, phenyltoloxamine citrate 15 mg/Capl. Bot. 24s, 48s. *otc.*
Use: Analgesic.

Momentum Muscular Backache Formula. (Whitehall Robins) Magnesium salicylate tetrahydrate 580 mg (equivalent to 467 mg magnesium salicylate anhydrous)/Cap. Box. 48s. *otc.*
Use: Analgesic compound.

•**mometasone furoate.** (moe-MET-uh-SONE FYU-roh-ate) U.S.P. 23.
Use: Topical steroid.
See: Elocon Cream, Oint., Lot. (Schering Plough).
Nasonex, Nasal Spray (Schering Plough).

monacetyl pyrogallol. Eugallol. Pyrogallol Monoacetate.
Use: Keratolytic.

Monafed. (Monarch Pharmaceuticals) Guaifenesin 600 mg, lactose/SR Tab. Bot. 100s. *Rx.*
Use: Expectorant.

Monafed DM. (Monarch Pharmaceuticals) Guaifenesin 600 mg, dextromethorphan HBr 30 mg/ER Tab. Bot. 100s. *Rx.*
Use: Antitussive, expectorant.

monalium hydrate. Hydrated magnesium aluminate. Magaldrate.
See: Riopan, Tab., Susp. (Wyeth Ayerst).

•**monatepil maleate.** (moe-NAT-eh-pill) USAN.
Use: Antianginal; antihypertensive.

•**monensin.** (mah-NEN-sin) U.S.P. 23.
Use: Antifungal, anti-infective, antiprotozoal.

•**monensin sodium.** (mah-NEN-sin) U.S.P. 23.
Use: Antifungal, anti-infective, antiprotozoal.

Monistat Dual-Pak. (Ortho McNeil) Miconazole nitrate suppositories and cream. **200 mg/Supp.:** Pkg. 3s w/applicator; **Cream 2%.:** Tube 15 g, 30 g, 90 g. *Rx.*
Use: Antifungal, vaginal.

Monistat 3 Vaginal Suppositories. (Ortho McNeil) Miconazole nitrate 200 mg/Supp. Pkg. 3s w/applicator. *Rx.*
Use: Antifungal, vaginal.

Monistat i.v. (Janssen) Miconazole 10 mg/ml, PEG 40, castor oil, lactate, methylparaben, propylparaben, water. Amp. 20 ml. *Rx.*
Use: Antifungal.

Monistat 7 Vaginal Cream. (Advanced Care Products) Miconazole nitrate 2% in water-miscible cream. Tube 45 g w/dose applicator. *otc.*
Use: Antifungal, vaginal.

Monistat 7 Vaginal Suppositories. (Advanced Care Products) Miconazole nitrate 100 mg/Supp. Pkg. 7s w/applicator. *otc.*
Use: Antifungal, vaginal.

Monistat 7 Combination Pack. (Advanced Care Products) **Vaginal Supp.:** Miconazole nitrate 100 mg. In 7s with applicator; **Topical Cream:** Miconazole nitrate 2%. Tube 9 g. *otc.*
Use: Antifungal, vaginal.

Monistat-Derm Cream. (Ortho McNeil) Miconazole nitrate 2%, pegoxol 7 stearate, peglicol 5 oleate, mineral oil, benzoic acid, butylated hydroxyanisole. Tube 15 g, 30 g, 90 g. *otc.*
Use: Antifungal, topical.

Monistat-Derm Lotion. (Advanced Care Products) Miconazole nitrate 2%, pegoxol 7 stearate, peglicol 5 oleate, mineral oil, benzoic acid, butylated hydroxyanisole. Squeeze bot. 30 ml, 60 ml. *Rx.*
Use: Antifungal, topical.

monoamine oxidase inhibitors.
Use: Antidepressant.
See: Parnate, Tab. (SmithKline Beecham Pharmaceuticals).
Marplan, Tab. (Roche Laboratories).
Nardil, Tab. (Parke-Davis).

•**mono and di-acetylated monoglycerides.** N.F. 18. A mixture of glycerin esterfied mono- and di-esters of edible fatty acids followed by direct acetylation.
Use: Pharmaceutic aid (plasticizer).

•**mono and di-glycerides.** N.F. 18. A mixture of mono- and di-esters of fatty acids from edible oils.
Use: Fatty acids, pharmaceutic aid (emulsifying agent).

•**monobenzone.** (mahn-oh-BEN-zone) U.S.P. 23.
Use: Depigmentor.
See: Benoquin, Oint., Lot. (Zeneca).

monobenzyl ether of hydroquinone.
See: Benoquin, Oint., Lot. (Zeneca).

monobromisovalerylurea.
See: Bromisovalum. (Various Mfr.).

Monocaps Tablets. (Freeda Vitamins) Iron 14 mg, vitamins A 10,000 IU, D 400 IU, E 15 IU, B_1 15 mg, B_2 15 mg, B_3 41 mg, B_5 15 mg, B_6 15 mcg, B_{12} 15 mcg, C 125 mg, folic acid 0.1 mg, biotin 15 mg, PABA, L-lysine, Ca, Cu, I, K, Mg, Mn, Se, Zn 12 mg, lecithin/Tab. Bot. 100s, 250s, 500s. *otc.*
Use: Mineral, vitamin supplement.

Mono-Chlor. (Gordon Laboratories) Monochloroacetic acid 80%. Bot. 15 ml.
Use: Cauterizing agent.

monochloroacetic acid.
Use: Cauterizing agent.
See: Monocete, Soln. (Pedinol).
Mono-Chlor, Soln. (Gordon Laboratories).

monchlorophenol-para.
See: Camphorated para-chlorophenol, Liq. (Novocol Chemical).

Monocid. (SmithKline Beecham Pharmaceuticals) Cefonicid sodium 500 mg, 1 g or 10 g/Vial and piggyback vial. Pharmacy Bulk Vial. *Rx.*
Use: Anti-infective, cephalosporin.

Monoclate. (Centeon) Monoclonal antibody derived stable lyophilized concentrate of Factor VIII: R heat-treated. With albumin (human) 1% to 2%, mannitol 0.8%, histadine 1.2 mM. Inj. Vial 1 ml single dose with diluent. *Rx.*
Use: Antihemophilic.

Monoclate-P. (Centeon). Stable concentrate of Factor VIII: C. ≈ 300 to 450 mmol sodium ions and ≈ 2 to 5 mmol calcium (as chloride) per L. With albumin (human) 1% to 2%, mannitol 0.8%, histadine 1.2 mmol, ≤ 50 ng/100 AHF activity units mouse protein. Pow. for Inj. *Rx.*
Use: Antihemophilic.

monoclonal antibodies (murine) anti-idiotype melanoma associated antigen.
Use: Invasive cutaneous melanoma. [Orphan drug]

monoclonal antibodies (murine or human) B-cell lymphoma. (Idec Pharm)
Use: B-cell lymphoma. [Orphan Drug]

monoclonal antibodies PM-81.
Use: Adjunctive treatment for leukemia. [Orphan drug]

monoclonal antibodies PM-81 and AML-2-23.
Use: Leukemic bone marrow transplantation. [Orphan drug]

monoclonal antibody 17-1A.
Use: Pancreatic cancer. [Orphan drug]

monoclonal antibody to CD4, 5a8. (Biogen)
Use: Post-exposure prophylaxis for HIV. [Orphan drug]

monoclonal antibody (human) against hepatitis B virus.
Use: Prophylaxis in hepatitis B reinfection in liver transplants. [Orphan drug]

monoclonal antibody to lupus nephritis. (Medclone)
Use: Immunization. [Orphan drug]

•**monoctanoin.** (MAHN-ahk-tuh-NO-in) USAN.
Use: Anticholelithic (dissolution of gallstones). [Orphan drug]
See: Moctanin, Inf. (Ethiteck).

monocycline hydrochloride.
See: Minocin I.V., Syr., Cap. (ESI Lederle Generics).

Mono-Diff Test. (Wampole Laboratories).
Use: Diagnostic aid, mononucleosis.

Monodox. (Oclassen) Doxycycline monohydrate equivalent to **50 mg** doxycycline. Cap. Bot. 100s; or **100 mg** doxycycline. Cap. Bot. 50s, 250s. *Rx.*
Use: Anti-infective, tetracycline.

•**monoethanolamine.** (mahn-oh-eth-an-OLE-ah-meen) N.F. 18.
Use: Pharmaceutic aid (surfactant).

Mono-Gesic Tablets. (Schwarz Pharma) Salsalate (salicylsalicylic acid) 750 mg/ Tab. Bot. 100s, 500s. *Rx.*
Use: Analgesic.

monoiodomethanesulfonate sodium.
See: Methiodal Sodium, U.S.P. 23.

Monojel. (Sherwood Medical) Glucose 40% in UD 25 g. *otc.*
Use: Hyperglycemic.

Monoket. (Schwarz Pharma) Isosorbide mononitrate 10 mg or 20 mg. Tab. Bot. 60s, 100s, 180s, UD 100s. *Rx.*
Use: Antianginal.

Mono-Latex. (Wampole Laboratories) Two minute latex agglutination slide test for the qualitative or semiquantitative detection of infectious mononucleosis heterophile antibodies in serum or plasma. Test kit 20s, 50s, 1000s.
Use: Diagnostic aid.

monolaurin.
Use: Treatment of congenital primary ichthyosis. [Orphan drug]
See: Glylorin.

monomercaptoundecahydrocloso-DO decaborate sodium.
Use: Treatment of glioblastoma multiforme. [Orphan drug]

Mononine. (Centeon) Factor IX 100 IU/ ml with nondetectable levels of Factors II, VII and X with histidine ≈ 10 mM, mannitol ≈ 3%, mouse protein ≤ 50

ng/100 IU Factor IX activity units. Pow. for inj. (lyophilized). Single-dose vials with diluent. *Rx.*
Use: Antihemophilic.

mononucleosis tests.
Use: Diagnostic aid.
See: Mono-Diff Test (Wampole Laboratories).
Mono-Latex (Wampole Laboratories).
Mono-Lisa (Orion Diagnostics).
Mono-Plus (Wampole Laboratories).
Monospot (Ortho Diagnostics).
Monosticon (Organon Teknika).
Monosticon Dri-Dot (Organon Teknika).
Mono-Sure Test (Wampole Laboratories).
Mono-Test (Wampole Laboratories).
Mono-Test (FTB) (Wampole Laboratories).

Monopar. Stilbazium Iodide.
Use: Anthelmintic.

monophen.
Use: Orally, cholecystography.

Mono-Plus. (Wampole Laboratories) To diagnose infectious mononucleosis from serum, plasma or fingertip blood. Test kits of 24s.
Use: Diagnostic aid.

Monopril. (Bristol-Myers) Fosinopril sodium. 10 mg, 20 mg, 40 mg, lactose. Tab. In 30s, 90s, 1000s, UD 100s. *Rx.*
Use: Antihypertensive; congestive heart failure.

•**monosodium glutamate.** (mahn-oh-SO-dee-uhm GLUE-tah-mate) N.F. 18.
Use: Pharmaceutic aid (flavor, perfume).

monosodium phosphate.
See: Sodium Biphosphate, U.S.P. 23.

Monospot. (Ortho Diagnostics) Diagnosis of infectious mononucleosis. Test kit 20s.
Use: Diagnostic aid.

monostearin. (Various Mfr.) Glyceryl monostearate.

Monosticon Dri-Dot. (Organon Teknika) Diagnosis of infectious mononucleosis. Test kit 40s, 100s.
Use: Diagnostic aid.

Mono-Sure Test. (Wampole Laboratories) One-minute hemagglutination slide test for the differential qualitative detection and quantitative determination of infectious mononucleosis heterophile antibodies in serum or plasma. Kit 20s.
Use: Diagnostic aid.

Monosyl. (Arcum) Secobarbital sodium 1 gr, butabarbital 0.5 gr/Tab. Bot. 100s, 1000s. *c-II.*
Use: Hypnotic, sedative.

Monotard Human Insulin. (Squibb/Novo) Human insulin zinc 100 units/ml. Susp. Vial 10 ml. *otc.*
Use: Antidiabetic.

•**monothioglycerol.** (mahn-oh-thigh-oh-GLIS-er-ole) N.F. 18.
Use: Pharmaceutic aid (preservative).

Mono-Vacc Test O.T. (Pasteur Merieux Connaught) 5 tuberculin units by the mantoux method. Multiple puncture disposable device. Box 25s (tamper-proof). *Rx.*
Use: Diagnostic aid, tuberculosis.

monoxychlorosene. A stabilized, buffered, organic hypochlorous acid derivative.
See: Oxychlorosene (Guardian Chem.).

Monsel Solution. (Wade) Bot. 2 oz, 4 oz.
Use: Styptic solution.

•**montelukast sodium.** (mahn-teh-LOO-kast) USAN.
Use: Antiasthmatic (leukotriene antagonist).
See: Singulair, Tab., Chew. Tab. (Merck).

Monurol. (Forest Pharmaceutical) Fosfomycin tromethamine 3 g/Granules. Single-dose packet. *Rx.*
Use: Anti-infective, urinary.

•**morantel tartrate.** (moe-RAN-tell) USAN.
Use: Anthelmintic.

moranyl.
See: Suramin Sodium.

Morco. (Archer-Taylor) Cod liver oil ointment, zinc oxide, benzethonium Cl, benzocaine 1%. 1.5 oz, lb. *otc.*
Use: Antiseptic, antipruritic, topical.

More Dophilus. (Freeda Vitamins) Acidophilus-carrot derivative 4 billion units/g Pow. Bot. 120 g. *otc.*
Use: Antidiarrheal, nutritional supplement.

•**moricizine.** (MAHR-IH-sizz-een) USAN.
Use: Cardiovascular agent (antiarrhythmic).
See: Ethmozine (DuPont Merck Pharmaceuticals).

•**morniflumate.** (MAR-nih-FLEW-mate) USAN.
Use: Anti-inflammatory.

Moroline. (Schering Plough) Petrolatum. Jar 1.75 oz, 3.75 oz, 15 oz. *otc.*
Use: Dermatologic, lubricant, protectant.

Morpen Tabs. (Major) Ibuprofen 400 mg or 600 mg/Tab. Bot. 500s. *Rx.*
Use: Analgesic, NSAID.

morphine acetate.
W/Terpin hydrate, ammonium hypophosphite, potassium guaiacol-sulfonate.
See: Broncho-Tussin Soln. (First Texas).

morphine and atropine sulfates tablets.
Use: Analgesic, parasympatholytic.

morphine hydrochloride. (Various Mfr.) Pow. Bot. 1 oz, 5 oz. *c-II.*
Use: Analgesic.

•**morphine sulfate.** (MORE-feen) U.S.P. 23.
Use: Analgesic, narcotic; sedative. [Orphan drug]
See: Infumorph 200 & 500, Inj. (ESI Lederle Generics).
Kadian, SR Cap. (Zeneca).
MS Contin, CR Tab. (Purdue Frederick).
MSIR, Cap. (Purdue Frederick).
MS/S, Supp. (Richwood).
MS/L-Concentrate, Oral Soln. (Richwood).
OMS Concentrate, Soln. (Upsher-Smith Labs).
Oramorph SR Tab. (Roxane).
Roxanol Rescudose, Soln. (Roxane).
W/Tartar emetic, bloodroot, ipecac, squill, wild cherry.
See: Pectoral, Preps. (Noyes).

morphine sulfate. (Various Mfr.) Flake or Pow. Bot. 1/8 oz, 1 oz, 5 oz, H.T. gr, gr, 0.25 gr, 0.5 gr, 1 gr.
Use: Analgesic, narcotic.

morphine sulfate. (IMS) Morphine sulfate **25 mg/ml:** Inj. 4, 10, 20, 40 ml *Select-A-Jet syringe systems.* **50 mg/ml:** Inj. 10, 20, 40 ml *Select-A-Jet syringe systems. c-II.*
Use: Analgesic, narcotic.

•**morrhuate sodium injection.** (MORE-you-ate) U.S.P. 23.
Use: Sclerosing agent.

Morton Salt Substitute. (Morton Grove) Potassium Cl, fumaric acid, tricalcium phosphate, monocalcium phosphate. Sodium: < 0.5 mg/5 g (0.02 mEq/5 g), potassium 2800 mg/5 g (72 mEq/5 g) 88.6 g. *otc.*
Use: Salt substitute.

Morton Seasoned Salt Substitute. (Morton Grove) Potassium chloride, spices, sugar, fumaric acid, triacalcium phosphate, monocalcium phosphate. Sodium < 1 mg/5 g (< 0.04 mEq/5 g), potassium 2165 mg/5 g (56 mEq/5 g). Bot. 85.1 g. *otc.*
Use: Salt substitute.

Mosco. (Medtech) 17.6% Salicylic acid. Jar 10 ml. *otc.*
Use: Keratolytic.

Motilium. (Janssen) Domperidone maleate. *Rx.*
Use: Antiemetic.

Motion Aid Tablets. (Vangard) Dimenhydrinate 50 mg/Tab. Bot. 100s, 1000s, UD 10×10s. *otc, Rx.*
Use: Antiemetic, antivertigo.

Motion Cure. (Wisconsin Pharm) Meclizine 25 mg/Chew. Tab. 12s. *otc, Rx.*
Use: Antiemetic, antivertigo.

motion sickness agents.
See: Antinauseants.
Bucladin, Softab Tab. (Zeneca).
Dramamine, Preps. (Searle).
Emetrol, Liq. (Rhone-Poulenc Rorer).
Marezine, Tab., Amp. (Glaxo-Wellcome).
Scopolamine HBr (Various Mfr.).

Motofen. (Carnrick Labs) Difenoxin HCl 1 mg, atropine sulfate 0.025 mg/Tab. Bot. 100s. *c-IV.*
Use: Antidiarrheal.

•**motretinide.** (MOE-TREH-tih-nide) USAN.
Use: Keratolytic.

Motrin. (Ortho McNeil) Ibuprofen. **Capl.: 100 mg:** Bot. 100s; **Tab: 50 mg or 100 mg:** Bot. 100s; **300 mg:** Bot. 500s, Unit-Of-Use 60s; **400 mg:** Bot. 500s, Unit-of-Use 100s, UD 100s; **600 mg:** Bot. 500s, Unit-of-Use 100s, UD 100s, **800 mg:** Bot. 500s, Unit-of-Use 100s, UD 100s. **Chew. Tab.: 50 mg:** 100s. **100 mg:** 100s. **Susp.:** 100 mg/5 ml, sucrose. 120, 480 ml. *Rx.*
Use: Analgesic, NSAID.

Motrin, Children's. (McNeil Consumer Products) Ibuprofen 100 mg/5 ml, sucrose. Susp. Bot. 120 ml, 480 ml. *otc, Rx.*
Use: Analgesic, NSAID.

Motrin IB. (Pharmacia & Upjohn) Ibuprofen 200 mg. **Tab.** or **Capl.** Bot. 24s, 50s, 100s, 165s. **Gelcaps:** parabens. Bot. 24s, 50s. *otc.*
Use: Analgesic, NSAID.

Motrin IB Sinus. (Pharmacia & Upjohn) Pseudoephedrine HCl 30 mg, ibuprofen 200 mg. Capl. Pkg. 20s, Bot. 40s. *otc.*
Use: Decongestant, NSAID.

Motrin, Junior Strength. (Ortho-McNeil) Ibuprofen 100 mg, aspartame, phenylalanine 5 mg. Chew. Tab. Bot. 24s. *otc.*
Use: Analgesic.

MouthKote. (Unimed) Xylitol, sorbitol, Mucoprotective Factor (MPF), Yerba Santa, saccharin. Alcohol free. Soln. Bot. 60, 240 ml and UD 5 ml. *otc.*
Use: Saliva substitute.

MouthKote O/R Rinse. (Unimed) Benzyl alcohol, menthol, sorbitol. Rinse. Sugar free. Bot. 240 ml. *otc.*
Use: Antiseptic.

MouthKote O/R Solution. (Unimed) Diphenhydramine HCl 1.25%, cetylpyridinium Cl, EDTA, saccharin. Soln. Bot. 40 ml. *otc.*
Use: Antiseptic.

MouthKote P/R. (Parnell) **Oint.:** Diphenhydramine HCl 25%. Tube 15 g. **Soln.:** Diphenhydramine HCl 1.25%, cetylpyridinium Cl, EDTA, saccharin. Bot. 40 ml. *otc.*
Use: Mouth and throat preparation.

•**moxalactam disodium for injection.** (MOX-ah-LACK-tam die-SO-dee-uhm [for injection]) U.S.P. 23.
Use: Anti-infective.
See: Moxam, Inj. (Eli Lilly).

Moxam. (Eli Lilly) Moxalactam disodium. Vial 1 g/10 ml Traypak 10s; Vial 2 g/20 ml Traypak 10s; Vial 10 g/100 ml Traypak 6s. *Rx.*
Use: Anti-infective, cephalosporin.

•**moxazocine.** (MOX-AZE-oh-seen) USAN.
Use: Analgesic, antitussive.

•**moxnidazole.** (MOX-NIH-dazz-ole) USAN.
Use: Antiprotozoal (trichomonas).

Moxy Compound. (Major) Theophylline 130 mg, ephedrine 25 mg, hydroxyzine HCl 10 mg/Tab. Bot. 100s. *Rx.*
Use: Antiasthmatic compound.

Moyco Fluoride Rinse. (Moyco) Fluoride 2%. Flavor. Bot. 128 oz. with pump. *otc, Rx.*
Use: Dental caries agent.

6-MP.
Use: Antimetabolite.
See: Purinethol, Tab. (GlaxoWellcome).

M-Prednisol-40. (Taylor Pharmaceuticals) Methylprednisolone acetate 40 mg/ml. Inj. Susp. Vial 5 ml. *Rx.*
Use: Corticosteroid.

M-Prednisol-80. (Taylor Pharmaceuticals) Methylprednisolone acetate 80 mg/ml. Inj. Susp. Vial 5 ml. *Rx.*
Use: Corticosteroid.

MRV. (Bayer Corp) 2000 million organisms/ml from *Staphylococcus aureus* (1200 million), *Streptococcus*, viradens and non-hemolytic (200 million), *Streptococcus pneumoniae* (150 million), *Branhamella catarrhalis* (150 million), *Klebsiella pneumoniae* (150 million), *Haemophilus influenzae* (150 million). Inj. Vial 20 ml. *Rx.*
Use: Immunization.

M-R-VAX II. (Merck) Live attenuated measles virus vaccine (Attenuvax) and live attenuated rubella virus vaccine (Meruvax II). See details under Attenuvax and Meruvax II. Single dose vial w/diluent. Pkg. 1s, 10s. *Rx.*
Use: Immunization.

MS Contin. (Purdue Frederick) Morphine sulfate. **CR Tab.: 15 mg or 100 mg:** Bot. 100s, 500s, UD 100s. **30 mg:** Bot. 50s, 100s, 250s, Card 25s. **60 mg or 200 mg:** Bot. 100s, UD 25s. *c-II.*
Use: Analgesic, narcotic.

MSIR. (Purdue Frederick) Morphine 15 mg and 30 mg/IR Tab. Bot. 50s. Morphine sulfate 15 mg and 30 mg, lactose, sucrose/Cap. Bot. 50s. *c-II.*
Use: Analgesic, narcotic.

MSL-109. (Novartis) Monoclonal antibody.
Use: Antiviral. [Orphan Drug]

MS/L-Concentrate. (Richwood) Morphine sulfate 100 mg/5 ml. Oral Soln. Bot. 120 ml w/calibrated dropper. *c-II.*
Use: Analgesic, narcotic.

MS/S. (Richwood) Morphine sulfate 5 mg, 10 mg, 20 mg or 30 mg/Supp. 12s. *c-II.*
Use: Analgesic, narcotic.

MSTA. (Pasteur Merieux Connaught) Mumps skin test antigen. Inj. Vial 1 ml. *Rx.*
Use: Diagnostic aid.

MTC. Mitomycin.
Use: Anti-infective.
See: Mutamycin, Pow. (Bristol-Myers Oncology/Immunology).

M.T.E.-4. (Fujisawa) Zinc 1 mg, copper 0.4 mg, chromium 4 mcg, manganese 0.1 mg/ml. Vial 3 ml, 10 ml, MD Vial 30 ml. *Rx.*
Use: Mineral supplement.

M.T.E.-4 Concentrated. (Fujisawa) Zinc 5 mg, copper 1 mg, chromium 10 mcg, manganese 0.5 mg/ml. Vial 1 ml, MD Vial 10 ml. *Rx.*
Use: Mineral supplement.

M.T.E.-5. (Fujisawa) Zinc 1 mg, copper 0.4 mg, chromium 4 mcg, manganese 0.1 mg, selenium 20 mcg/ml. Vial 10 ml. *Rx.*
Use: Mineral supplement.

M.T.E.-5 Concentrated. (Fujisawa) Zinc 5 mg, copper 1 mg, chromium 10 mcg,

manganese 0.5 mg, selenium 60 mcg/ml. Vial 1 ml, MD vial 10 ml. *Rx.*
Use: Mineral supplement.

M.T.E.-6. (Fujisawa) Zinc 1 mg, copper 0.4 mg, chromium 4 mcg, manganese 0.1 mg, selenium 20 mcg, iodide 25 mcg/ml. Vial 10 ml. *Rx.*
Use: Mineral supplement.

M.T.E.-6 Concentrate. (Fujisawa) Zinc 5 mg, copper 1 mg, chromium 10 mcg, manganese 0.5 mg, selenium 60 mcg, iodide 75 mcg/ml. Vial 1 ml. MD vial 10 ml. *Rx.*
Use: Mineral supplement.

M.T.E.-7. (Fujisawa) Zinc 1 mg copper 0.4 mg, manganese 0.1 mg, chromium 4 mcg, selenium 20 mcg, iodide 25 mcg, molybdenum 25 mcg/ml. Vial 10 ml. *Rx.*
Use: Mineral supplement.

MTP-PE. (Novartis) Muramyl-tripeptide.
Use: Immunomodulator.

MTX. *Rx.*
Use: Antineoplastic, antipsoriatic.
See: Methotrexate.

MUC 9 + 4 Pediatric. (Fujisawa) Vitamin A 2300 IU, D 400 IU, E 7 mg, B_1 1.2 mg, B_2 1.4 mg, B_3 17 mg, B_5 5 mg, B_6 1 mg, B_{12} 1 mcg, C 80 mg, biotin 20 mcg, folic acid 0.14 mg, K 200 mcg/5 ml, mannitol 375 mg. Pow. Vial. 10 ml. *Rx.*
Use: Nutritional supplement, parenteral.

mucilloid of psyllium seed.
W/Dextrose.
See: Metamucil, Liq. (Searle).

mucin.
See: Gastric Mucin (Wilson).

mucin, vegetable.
W/Yeast or alkalized.
See: Plantamucin, Granules (Baxter).

Muco-Fen-DM. (Wakefield Pharm) Guaifenesin 600 mg, dextromethorphan HBr 30 mg/TR Tab. Bot. 100s. *Rx.*
Use: Antitussive, expectorant.

Muco-Fen-LA. (Wakefield Pharm) Guaifenesin 600 mg, dye free/TR Tab. Bot. 100s. *Rx.*
Use: Expectorant.

mucolytics.
Use: Respiratory.
See: Mucomyst, Soln. (Bristol-Myers).

Mucomyst. (Bristol-Myers Squibb) A sterile 20% solution of acetylcysteine for nebulization or direct instillation into the lung as a mucolytic agent. Approved as antidote for acetaminophen overdose. Vial. **4 ml:** Ctn. 12s; **10 ml:** Ctn. 3s with dropper; **30 ml:** Ctn. 3s. *Rx.*
Use: Respiratory.

Mucomyst 10. (Bristol-Myers Squibb) A sterile 10% solution of acetylcysteine for nebulization or direct instillation into the lung as a mucolytic agent. Approved as antidote for acetaminophen overdose. Vial. **4 ml:** Ctn. 12s; **10 ml:** Ctn. 3s with dropper; **30 ml:** Ctn. 3s. *Rx.*
Use: Respiratory.

Mucosil-10 & -20 Solution. (Dey Labs) Acetylcysteine sodium salt 10% or 20%. Soln. Vial 4 ml Box 12s. *Rx.*
Use: Respiratory.

Mudd. (Chattem Consumer Products) Natural hydrated magnesium aluminum silicate. Topical preparation. *otc.*
Use: Cleanser.

Mudrane. (ECR Pharmaceuticals) Aminophylline (anhydrous) 130 mg, phenobarbital 8 mg, ephedrine HCl 16 mg, potassium iodide 195 mg/Tab. Bot. 100s. *Rx.*
Use: Antiasthmatic combination.

Mudrane-2. (ECR Pharmaceuticals) Potassium iodide 195 mg, aminophylline (anhydrous) 130 mg/Tab. Bot. 100s. *Rx.*
Use: Antiasthmatic combination.

Mudrane GG. (ECR Pharmaceuticals) Aminophylline (anhydrous) 130 mg, ephedrine HCl 16 mg, guaifenesin 100 mg, phenobarbital 8 mg/Tab. Bot. 100s. *Rx.*
Use: Antiasthmatic combination.

Mudrane GG-2. (ECR Pharmaceuticals) Guaifenesin 100 mg, theophylline 111 mg/Tab. Bot. 100s. *Rx.*
Use: Antiasthmatic combination.

Mudrane GG Elixir. (ECR Pharmaceuticals) Theophylline 20 mg, ephedrine HCl 4 mg, guaifenesin 26 mg, phenobarbital 2.5 mg/5 ml, alcohol 20%. Bot. pt, 0.5 gal. *Rx.*
Use: Antiasthmatic combination.

Multa-Gen 12 + E. (Jones Medical Industries) Vitamin A 5000 IU, D 400 IU, B_1 2 mg, B_2 2 mg, B_6 0.5 mg, B_{12} 3 mcg, C 37.5 mg, E 15 IU, folic acid 0.2 mg, nicotinamide 20 mg/Cap. Bot. 60s, 500s, 1000s. *otc.*
Use: Vitamin supplement.

MulTE-PAK-4. (SoloPak) Zinc 1 mg, copper 0.4 mg, manganese 0.1 mg, chromium 4 mg/ml. Vial 3 ml, 10 ml, 30 ml. *Rx.*
Use: Mineral supplement.

MulTE-PAK -5. (SoloPak) Zinc 1 mg, copper 0.4 mg, manganese 0.1 mg, chromium 4 mg, selenium 20 mcg/ml.

Vial 3 ml, 10 ml. *Rx.*
Use: Mineral supplement.

Multi-B-Plex. (Forest Pharmaceutical) Vitamins B_1 100 mg, B_2 1 mg, nicotinamide 100 mg, pantothenic acid 10 mg, B_6 10 mg/ml. Vial 10 ml, 30 ml. *Rx.*
Use: Mineral, vitamin supplement.

Multi-B-Plex Capsules. (Forest Pharmaceutical) Vitamins B_1 50 mg, B_2 5 mg, niacinamide 50 mg, calcium pantothenate 5.4 mg, B_6 0.2 mg, C 150 mg, B_{12} 1 mcg/Cap. Bot. 100s, 1000s. *otc.*
Use: Mineral, vitamin supplement.

Multi-Day. (NBTY) Vitamins A 5000 IU, D 400 IU, E 30 mg, B_1 1.5 mg, B_2 1.7 mg, B_3 20 mg, B_5 10 mg, B_6 2 mg, B_{12} 6 mcg, C 60 mg, FA 0.4 ml/Tab. Bot. 100s. *otc.*
Use: Vitamin supplement.

Multi-Day Plus Iron. (NBTY) Fe 18 mg, A 5000 IU, D 400 IU, E 15 mg, B_1 1.5 mg, B_2 1.7 mg, B_3 20 mg, B_6 2 mg, B_{12} 6 mcg, C 60 mg, FA 0.4 mg. Tab. Bot. 100s. *otc.*
Use: Vitamin supplement.

Multi-Day Plus Minerals. (NBTY). Fe 18 mg, A 6500 IU, D 400 IU, E 30 mg, B_1 1.5 mg, B_2 1.7 mg, B_3 20 mg, B_5 10 mg, B_6 2 mg, B_{12} 6 mcg, C 60 mg, FA 0.4 mg, Ca, Cl, Cr, Cu, I, K, Mg, Mn, Mo, P, Se, Zn 15 mg, biotin 30 mcg. Tab. Bot. 100s. *otc.*
Use: Vitamin supplement.

Multi-Day with Calcium and Extra Iron Tablets. (NBTY). Fe 27 mg, A 5000 IU, D 400 IU, E 30 mg, B_1 1.5 mg, B_2 1.7 mg, B_3 20 mg, B_5 10 mg, B_6 2 mg, B_{12} 6 mcg, C 60 mg, FA 0.4 mg, Ca, Zn 15 mg, tartrazine/Tab. Bot. 100s. *otc.*
Use: Mineral, vitamin supplement.

Multi-Germ Oil. (Viobin) Corn, sunflower and wheat germ oils. Bot. 4 oz, 8 oz, pt, qt. *otc.*
Use: Nutritional supplement.

Multi-Jets. (Kirkman Sales) Vitamins A 10,000 IU, D_2 400 IU, B_1 20 mg, B_2 8 mg, C 120 mg, niacinamide 10 mg, calcium pantothenate 5 mg, B_6 0.5 mg, E 50 IU, desiccated liver 100 mg, dried debittered yeast 100 mg, choline bitartrate 62 mg, inositol 30 mg, dl-methionine 30 mg, B_{12} 7 mcg, iron 2.6 mg, calcium (dical phosphate) 58 mg, phosphorus (dical phosphate) 45 mg, iodine (potassium iodide) 0.114 mg, magnesium sulfate 1 mg, copper sulfate 1.99 mg, manganese sulfate 1.11 mg, potassium Cl iodide 79 mg/Tab. Bot. 100s. *otc.*
Use: Mineral, vitamin supplement.

Multilex Tablets. (Rugby) Iron 15 mg, vitamins A 10,000 IU, D 400 IU, E 5.5 mg, B_1 10 mg, B_2 5 mg, B_3 30 mg, B_5 10 mg, B_6 1.7 mg, B_{12} 3 mcg, C 100 mg, zinc 1.5 mg, Cu, I, Mg, Mn/Tab. Bot. 100s. *otc.*
Use: Mineral, vitamin supplement.

Multilex T & M Tablets. (Rugby) Iron 15 mg, vitamins A 10,000 IU, D 400 IU, E 5.5 mg, B_1 15 mg, B_2 10 mg, B_3 100 mg, B_5 10 mg, B_6 2 mg, B_{12} 7.5 mcg, C 150 mg, Cu, I, Mg, Mn, Zn 1.5 mg, sugar/Tab. Bot. 100s. *otc.*
Use: Mineral, vitamin supplement.

Multilyte. (Fujisawa) Vitamins A 5000 IU, D 400 IU, E 15 mg, B_1 3 mg, B_2 3.4 mg, B_3 36 mg, B_5 14 mg, B_6 4.4 mg, B_{12} 6 mcg, C 120 mg, FA 0.4 mg, Zn 10.5 mg, biotin 100 mcg, Ca, K, Mg, Mn, phenylalanine. Tab. Pkg. 12s. *otc.*
Use: Mineral, vitamin supplement.

Multilyte-20. (Fujisawa) Sodium 25 mEq/L, potassium 20 mEq/L, calcium 5 mEq/L, magnesium 5 mEq/L, chloride 30 mEq/L, acetate 25 mEq/L, gluconate 5 mEq/L. Vial 25 ml fill in 50 ml. *Rx.*
Use: Electrolyte, fluid replacement.

Multilyte-40. (Fujisawa) Sodium 25 mEq/L, potassium 40.5 mEq/L, calcium 5 mEq/L, magnesium 8 mEq/L, chloride 33.5 mEq/L, acetate 40.6 mEq/L, gluconate 5 mEq/L. Vial 25 ml fill in 50 ml. *Rx.*
Use: Electrolyte, fluid replacement.

Multi-Mineral Tablets. (NBTY) Ca 166.7 mg, P 75.7 mg, I 25 mcg, Fe 3 mg, Mg 66.7 mg, Cu 0.33 mg, Zn 2.5 mg, K 12.5 mg, Mn 8.3 mg/Tab. Bot. 100s. *otc.*
Use: Mineral, vitamin supplement.

Multipals. (Faraday) Vitamins A 5000 IU, D 400 IU, C 50 mg, B_1 3 mg, B_6 0.5 mg, B_2 3 mg, calcium pantothenate 5 mg, niacinamide 20 mg, B_{12} 2 mcg/Tab. Bot. 100s, 250s, 1000s. *otc.*
Use: Mineral, vitamin supplement.

Multipals-M. (Faraday) Vitamins A 6000 IU, D 400 IU, B_1 3 mg, B_2 3 mg, B_6 0.5 mg, B_{12} 5 mcg, C 60 mg, E 2 IU, niacinamide 20 mg, calcium pantothenate 5 mg, iron 10 mg, iodine 0.15 mg, copper 1 mg, magnesium 6 mg, manganese 1 mg, potassium 5 mg/Tab. Bot. 100s, 250s, 1000s. *otc.*
Use: Mineral, vitamin supplement.

Multiple Trace Element. (American Regent) Zinc sulfate 1 mg, copper sulfate 0.4 mg, manganese sulfate 0.1 mg, chromium Cl 4 mg/ml. Inj. Soln. Vial 10 ml. *Rx.*
Use: Mineral supplement.

Multiple Trace Element Concentrated. (American Regent) Zinc sulfate 5 mg, copper sulfate 1 mg, manganese sulfate 0.5 mg, chromium Cl 10 mcg/ml. Inj. Soln. Vial 10 ml. *Rx.*
Use: Mineral supplement.

Multiple Trace Element Neonatal. (American Regent) Zn 1.5 mg, Cu 0.1 mg, Mn 25 mcg, Cr 0.85 mcg/ml. Vial 2 ml single dose. *Rx.*
Use: Mineral supplement.

Multiple Trace Element Pediatric. (American Regent) Zinc sulfate 0.5 mg, copper sulfate 0.1 mg, manganese sulfate 0.03 mg, chromium Cl 1 mcg/ml. Inj. Soln. Vial 10 ml. *Rx.*
Use: Mineral supplement.

Multiple Vitamin Mineral Formula. (Kirkman Sales) Vitamins A 5000 IU, D_2 400 IU, C 50 mg, B_1 2.5 mg, B_2 2.5 mg, B_6 0.5 mg, B_{12} 1 mcg, niacinamide 15 mg, calcium pantothenate 5 mg, E 0.1 IU, calcium 100 mg, iron 7.5 mg, magnesium 2.5 mg, potassium 2.5 mg, zinc 0.15 mg, manganese 0.5 mg, iodine 0.07 mg/Tab. Bot. 100s. *otc.*
Use: Mineral, vitamin supplement.

Multiple Vitamins Chewable. (Kirkman Sales) Vitamins A 5000 IU, D 400 IU, C 50 mg, B_1 3 mg, B_2 2.5 mg, B_6 1 mg, B_{12} 1 mcg, niacinamide 20 mg/Tab. Bot. 100s. *otc.*
Use: Vitamin supplement.

Multiple Vitamins w/Iron. (Kirkman Sales) Vitamins A 5000 IU, D 400 IU, C 50 mg, B_1 3 mg, B_2 2.5 mg, B_6 1 mg, B_{12} 1 mcg, niacinamide 20 mg, iron 10 mg/Tab. Bot. 100s. *otc.*
Use: Mineral, vitamin supplement.

Multi 75. (Fibertone) Vitamins A 25,000 IU, D 500 IU, E 150 IU, B_1 75 mg, B_2 75 mg, B_3 75 mg, B_5 75 mg, B_6 75 mg, B_{12} 75 mcg, C 250 mg, FA 0.4 mg, Ca 50 mg, Fe 10 mg, Biotin, I, Mg, Zn 15 mg, Cu, PABA, K, Mn, Cr, Se, Mo, B, Si, choline bitartrate, inosol, rutin, lemon bioflavonoid complex, hesperidin, betaine, HCl/TR Tab. Bot. 60s, 90s. *otc.*
Use: Mineral, vitamin supplement.

Multistix 2 Reagent Strips. (Bayer Corp) Urinalysis reagent strip test for nitrite and leukocytes. Bot. 100s.
Use: Diagnostic aid.

Multistix 7. (Bayer Corp) Urinalysis reagent strip test for glucose ketone, blood, pH, protein, nitrite and leukocytes. Box 100s.
Use: Diagnostic aid.

Multistix 8. (Bayer Corp) Urinalysis reagent strip test for detecting glucose, ketone, blood, pH, protein, nitrite, bilirubin and leukocytes. Box. 100s.
Use: Diagnostic aid.

Multistix 8 SG Reagent Strips. (Bayer Corp) Urinalysis reagent strip test for glucose, ketone, specific gravity, blood, pH, protein nitrite, leukocytes. Box 100s.
Use: Diagnostic aid.

Multistix 9 Reagent Strips. (Bayer Corp) Urinalysis reagent strip test for glucose, bilirubin, ketone, blood, pH, protein, urobilinogen, nitrite, leukocytes. Box 100s.
Use: Diagnostic aid.

Multistix 9 SG Reagent Strips. (Bayer Corp) Urinalysis reagent strip test for glucose, bilirubin, ketone, specific gravity, blood, pH, protein, nitrite and leukocytes. Box 100s.
Use: Diagnostic aid.

Multistix 10 SG Reagent Strips. (Bayer Corp) Reagent strip test for glucose, bilirubin, ketone, specific gravity, blood, pH, protein, urobilinogen, nitrite and leukocytes in urine. Box 100s.
Use: Diagnostic aid.

Multistix-N. (Bayer Corp) Glucose, protein, pH, blood, ketones, bilirubin, urobilinogen, nitrate, leukocytes. Kit. 100s.
Use: Diagnostic aid.

Multistix-N S.G. Reagent Strips. (Bayer Corp) Urinalysis reagent strip test for pH, protein, glucose, ketones, bilirubin, blood nitrite, urobilinogen and specific gravity. Bot. 100s.
Use: Diagnostic aid.

Multistix Reagent Strips. (Bayer Corp) Urinalysis reagent strip test for pH, protein, glucose, ketone, bilirubin and blood. Box 100s.
Use: Diagnostic aid.

Multistix S. G. Reagent Strips. (Bayer Corp) Urinalysis reagent strip test for pH, glucose, protein, ketones, bilirubin, blood and urobilinogen. Box. 100s.
Use: Diagnostic aid.

Multi-Symptom Tylenol Cold. (McNeil Consumer Products) Pseudoephedrine HCl 30 mg, chlorpheniramine maleate 2 mg, dextromethorphan HBr 15 mg, acetaminophen 325 mg/Capl. or Tab. Bot. 24s, 50s. *otc.*
Use: Analgesic, antihistamine, antitussive, decongestant.

Multi-Symptom Tylenol Cough. (Ortho McNeil) Dextromethorphan HBr 10 mg, acetaminophen 216.7 mg, alcohol 5%/5 ml. Liq. Bot. 120 ml. *otc.*
Use: Analgesic, antititussive.

Multi-Symptom Tylenol Cough with Decongestant. (Ortho McNeil) Dextromethorphan HBr 10 mg, acetaminophen 200 mg, pseudoephedrine HCl 20 mg, alcohol 5%, saccharin, sorbitol/5 ml. Liq. Bot. 120 ml. *otc.*
Use: Analgesic, antititussive, decongestant.

Multitest CMI. (Pasteur Merieux Connaught) One disposable applicator preloaded with seven glycerinated liquid antigens (tetanus toxoid, diphtheria toxoid, *Streptococcus* group C antigen, old tuberculin, *Candida albicans, Trichophyton mentagrophytes, Proteus mirabilis*) and glycerin negative control. 10 units/box.
Use: Diagnostic aid.

Multi-Thera Tablets. (NBTY) Vitamins A 5500 IU, D 400 IU, E 30 mg, B_1 3 mg, B_2 3.4 mg, B_3 30 mg, B_5 10 mg, B_6 3 mg, B_{12} 9 mcg, C 120 mg, folic acid 0.4 mg, biotin 15 mcg/Tab. Bot. 100s. *otc.*
Use: Vitamin supplement.

Multi-Thera-M. (NBTY) Iron 27 mg, vitamins A 5500 IU, D 400 IU, E 30 mg, B_1 3 mg, B_2 3.4 mg, B_3 30 mg, B_5 10 mg, B_6 3 mg, B_{12} 9 mcg, C 120 mg, folic acid 0.4 mg, biotin 15 mcg, zinc 15 mg, Ca, Cl, Cr, Cu, I, K, Mg, Mn, Mo, Se/Tab. Bot. 130s. *otc.*
Use: Mineral, vitamin supplement.

Multitrace-5 Concentrate. (American Regent) Zinc sulfate 5 mg, copper sulfate 1 mg, manganese sulfate 0.5 mg, chromium Cl 10 mcg, selenium 60 mcg, benzyl alcohol 0.9%. Inj. Soln. Vial 1 ml and 10 ml. *Rx.*
Use: Mineral supplement.

Multi-Vit Drops. (Alphalma USPD) Vitamins A 500 IU, D 400 IU, E 5 mg, B_1 0.5 mg, B_2 0.6 mg, B_3 8 mg, B_6 0.4 mg, B_{12} 2 mcg, C 35 mg/ml. Bot. 50 ml. *otc.*
Use: Vitamin supplement.

Multi-Vit Drops w/Iron. (Alphalma USPD) Iron 10 mg, vitamins A 1500 IU, D 400 IU, E 5 IU, B_1 0.5 mg, B_2 0.6 mg, B_3 8 mg, B_6 0.4 mg, C 35 mg/ml. Methylparaben. Bot. 50 ml. *otc.*
Use: Mineral, vitamin supplement.

Multi-Vita. (Rosemont) Vitamins A 1500 IU/ml, D 400 IU, E 5 mg, B_1 0.5 mg, B_2 0.6 mg, B_3 8 mg, B_6 0.4 mg, B_{12} 2 mcg, C 35 mg, alcohol free. Drop. Bot. 50 ml. *otc.*
Use: Vitamin supplement.

Multi-Vita Drops. (Rosemont) Vitamins A 1500 IU, D 400 IU, E 5 mg, B_1 0.5 mg, B_2 0.6 mg, B_3 8 mg, B_6 0.4 mg, B_{12} 2 mcg, C 35 mg/ml. Alcohol free. Bot. 50 ml. *otc.*
Use: Mineral, vitamin supplement.

Multi-Vita Drops w/Fluoride. (Rosemont) Fluoride 0.5 mg, vitamins A 1500 IU, D 400 IU, E 5 mg, B_1 0.5 mg, B_2 0.6 mg, B_3 8 mg, B_6 0.4 mg, B_{12} 2 mcg, C 35 mg/ml. Alcohol free. Bot. 50 ml. *Rx.*
Use: Vitamin supplement; dental caries agent.

Multi-Vita Drops w/Iron. (Rosemont) Iron 10 mg, vitamins A 1500 IU, D 400 IU, E 5 mg, B_1 0.5 mg, B_2 0.6 mg, B_3 8 mg, B_6 0.4 mg, C 35 mg/ml. Alcohol free. Bot. 50 ml. *otc.*
Use: Mineral, vitamin supplement.

Multivitamin with Fluoride Drops. (Major) Fluoride 0.5 mg, vitamins A 1500 IU, D 400 IU, E 5 IU, B_1 0.5 mg, B_2 0.6 mg, B_3 8 mg, B_6 0.4 mg, B_{12} 2 mcg, C 35 mg, F 0.25 mg/Drop. Bot. 50 ml. *Rx.*
Use: Vitamin supplement; dental caries agent.

multi vitamin concentrate injection. (Fujisawa) Vitamins A 10,000 IU, D 1000 IU, E 5 IU, B_1 50 mg, B_2 10 mg, B_3 100 mg, B_5 25 mg, B_6 15 mg, C 500 mg/Inj. Vial 5 ml. *Rx.*
Use: Vitamin supplement.

multivitamin infusion (neonatal formula).
Use: Nutritional supplement for low birth weight infants. [Orphan drug]

Multi-Vitamin Mineral w/Beta Carotene. (Mission Pharmacal) Iron 27 mg, A 5000 IU, D 400 IU, E 30 IU, B_1 2.25 mg, B_2 2.6 mg, B_3 20 mg, B_5 10 mg, B_6 3 mg, B_{12} 9 mcg, C 90 mg, folic acid 0.4 mg, biotin, 0.45 mg, Ca, Cl, Cr, Cu, I, K, Mg, Mn, Mo, P, Se, Zn 15 mg, Vitamin K/Tab. Bot. 130s. *otc.*
Use: Mineral, vitamin supplement.

Multi-Vitamins Capsules. (Forest Pharmaceutical) Vitamins A 5000 IU, D 400 IU, B_1 1.5 mg, B_2 2 mg, B_6 0.1 mg, C 37.5 mg, calcium pantothenate 1 mg, niacinamide 20 mg/Cap. Bot. 100s, 1000s, 5000s. *otc.*
Use: Mineral, vitamin supplement.

Multivitamins Capsules. (Solvay) Vitamins A 5000 IU, D 400 IU, B_1 2.5 mg, B_2 2.5 mg, C 50 mg, B_3 20 mg, B_5 5 mg, B_6 0.5 mg, B_{12} 2 mcg, E 10 IU/Cap. Bot. 100s, UD 100s. *otc.*
Use: Mineral, vitamin supplement.

Multivitamin with Fluoride Drops. (Major) Fluoride 0.5 mg, vitamins A 1500 IU, D 400 IU, E 4.1 IU, B_1 0.5 mg, B_2 0.6

mg, B_3 8 mg, B_6 0.4 mg, B_{12} 2 mg, C 35 mg/Drop. Bot. 50 ml. *Rx.*
Use: Vitamin supplement; dental caries agent.

multizine.
See: Trisulfapyrimidines Tab., U.S.P. 23.

Multorex. (Health for Life Brands) Vitamins A 6000 IU, D 1250 IU, C 50 mg, E 5 IU, B_1 3 mg, B_2 3 mg, B_6 0.5 mg, niacinamide 20 mg, calcium pantothenate 5 mg, B_{12} 5 mcg, calcium 59 mg, phosphorus 45 mg/Cap. Bot. 100s, 250s, 1000s. *otc.*
Use: Mineral, vitamin supplement.

Mulvidren-F Softabs. (Wyeth Ayerst) Fluoride 1 mg, vitamins A 4000 IU, D 400 IU, B_1 1.6 mg, B_2 2 mg, B_3 10 mg, B_5 2.8 mg, B_6 1 mg, B_{12} 3 mcg, C 75 mg, Saccharin/Tab. Bot. 100s. *Rx.*
Use: Mineral, vitamin supplement; dental caries agent.

•**mumps skin test antigen.** U.S.P. 23.
Use: Diagnostic aid (dermal reactivity indicator).
See: MSTA, Inj. (Pasteur Merieux Connaught).

Mumpsvax. (Merck) Live mumps virus vaccine, Jeryl Lynn strain. Single-dose vial w/diluent Pkg. 1s, 10s. *Rx.*
Use: Agent for immunization.
W/Attenuvax, Meruvax II.
See: M-M-R II, Inj. (Merck).
W/Meruvax II.
See: Biavax II (Merck).

•**mumps virus vaccine live.** U.S.P. 23.
Use: Immunization.
See: Mumpsvax, Inj. (Merck).

mumps virus vaccine, live attenuated. Jeryl Lynn (B level) strain.
See: Mumpsvax (Merck).
W/Measles virus vaccine, rubella virus vaccine.
See: M-M-R, Inj. (Merck).

•**mupirocin.** (myoo-PIHR-oh-sin) U.S.P. 23.
Use: Anti-infective (topical and nasal).
See: Bactroban, Oint. (SmithKline Beecham Pharmaceuticals).

•**mupirocin calcium.** (myoo-PIHR-oh-sin KAL-see-uhm) USAN.
Use: Anti-infective, topical.
See: Bactroban, Cream (SmithKline Beecham).

•**muplestim.** (myoo-PLEH-stim) USAN.
Use: Hematopoietic stimulant; antineutropenic.

muriatic acid.
See: Hydrochloric Acid, N.F. 18.

Muri-Lube. (Fujisawa) Mineral Oil "Light." Vial 2 ml, 10 ml. *Rx.*
Use: Lubricant.

Murine Ear Drops. (Ross Laboratories) Carbamide peroxide 6.5% in anhydrous glycerin. Bot. 0.5 oz. *otc.*
Use: Otic.

Murine Ear Wax Removal System. (Ross Laboratories) Carbamide peroxide 6.5% in anhydrous glycerin w/ear washing syringe. Bot. 0.5 oz. and ear washer 1 oz. *otc.*
Use: Otic.

Murine Eye Drops. (Ross Laboratories) Polyvinyl alcohol 0.5%, povidone 0.6%, benzalkonium chloride, dextrose, EDTA, NaCl, sodium bicarbonate, sodium phos- phate. Soln. Bot. 15 ml, 30 ml. *otc.*
Use: Artificial tears.

Murine Plus Eye Drops. (Ross Laboratories) Tetrahydrozoline HCl 0.05%. Drop. Bot. 15 ml, 30 ml. *otc.*
Use: Vasoconstrictor, ophthalmic.

Murine Regular Formula. (Ross Laboratories) Sodium chloride, potassium chloride, sodium phosphate, glycerin, benzalkonium chloride 0.01%, EDTA 0.05%/Drop. Bot. 15, 30 ml. *otc.*
Use: Artificial tears.

Muro 128 Ointment. (Bausch & Lomb) Sodium Cl 5% in sterile ointment base. Tube 3.5 g. *otc.*
Use: Hyperosmolar.

Muro 128 Solution. (Bausch & Lomb) Sodium Cl 2% or 5%. Soln. Bot. 15 ml, 30 ml (5% only). *otc.*
Use: Hyperosmolar.

Murocel Solution. (Bausch & Lomb) Methylcellulose 1%, propylene glycol, sodium Cl, methylparaben 0.046%, propylparaben 0.02%, boric acid, sodium borate. Soln. Bot. 15 ml. *otc.*
Use: Artificial tears.

Murocoll-2. (Bausch & Lomb) Phenylephrine HCl 10%, scopolamine HBR 0.3% Bot. 5 ml. *Rx.*
Use: Cycloplegic, mydriatic.

•**muromonab-CD3.** (MYOO-row-MOE-nab cd3) USAN. *Rx.*
Use: Monoclonal antibody (immunosuppressant).
See: Orthoclone OKT3, Inj. (Ortho McNeil).

Muroptic-5. (Optopics) Sodium Cl, hypertonic 5%. Soln. Bot. 15 ml. *otc.*
Use: Hyperosmolar.

Muro's Opcon A Solution. (Bausch & Lomb) Naphazoline HCl 0.025%, phe-

niramine maleate 0.3%. Bot. 15 ml. *otc.*
Use: Antihistamine (ophthalmic), decongestant.

Muro's Opcon Solution. (Bausch & Lomb) Naphazoline HCl 0.1%. Bot. 15 ml. *otc.*
Use: Decongestant, ophthalmic.

Muro Tears Solution. (Bausch & Lomb) Hydroxypropyl methylcellulose, dextran 40. Soln. Bot. 15 ml. *otc.*
Use: Artificial tears.

muscle adenylic acid. (Various Mfr.) Active form of adenosine 5-monophosphate.
See: Adenosine 5-monophosphate, Preps. (Various Mfr.).

muscle relaxants.
See: Arduan (Organon Teknika).
Curare (Various Mfr.).
Flexeril, Tab. (Merck).
Flaxedil Triethiodide, Vial (Davis & Geck).
Lioresal, Tab. (Novartis).
Mephenesin (Various Mfr.).
Meprobamate (Various Mfr.).
Metubine Iodine, Vial (Eli Lilly).
Neostig, Tab. (Freeport).
Norflex, Tab., Inj. (3M).
Nuromax (GlaxoWellcome).
Parafon Forte, Tab. (Ortho McNeil).
P-A-V, Cap. (T.E. Williams).
Rela, Tab. (Schering Plough).
Robaxin, Tab., Inj. (Robins).
Soma, Tab., Cap. (Wallace Laboratories).
Succinylcholine Cl (Various Mfr.).
d-Tubocurarine Cl (Various Mfr.).

mustaral oil.
See: Allyl Isothiocyanate.

Mustargen. (Merck) Mechlorethamine HCl 10 mg Pow. For Inj. Vial. Treatment set vial 4s. *Rx.*
Use: Antineoplastic.

Musterole. (Schering Plough) **Regular:** Camphor 4%, menthol 2%. Jar 0.9 oz. **Extra Strength:** Camphor 5%, menthol 3%. Jar 0.9 oz., Tube 1 oz, 2.25 oz. *otc.*
Use: Analgesic, topical.

Musterole Deep Strength. (Schering Plough) Methyl salicylate 30%, menthol 3%, methyl nicotinate 0.5%. Jar 1.25 oz, Tube 3 oz. *otc.*
Use: Analgesic, topical.

Musterole Extra Strength. (Schering Plough) Camphor 5%, menthol 3%, methyl salicylate, lanolin, oil of mustard, petrolatum. 27, 30, 67.5 g. *otc.*
Use: Liniment.

mustin.
See: Mechlorethamine HCl, Sterile.

mutalin. (Spanner) Protein and iodine. Vial 30 ml.

Mutamycin. (Bristol-Myers/Bristol Oncology) Mitomycin 5 mg, 20 mg or 40 mg/Vial. *Rx.*
Use: Antineoplastic.

•**muzolimine.** (MYOO-ZOLE-ih-meen) USAN.
Use: Antihypertensive, diuretic.

M.V.I.-12. (Astra) Vitamins A 3300 IU, D 200 IU, E 10 IU, B_1 3 mg, B_2 3.6 mg, B_3 40 mg, B_5 15 mg, B_6 4 mg, B_{12} 5 mcg, C 100 mg, biotin 60 mcg, FA 0.4 mg. Inj. Vials. 5 ml single dose or 50 ml multiple dose; Unit vial: 10 ml two-chambered vials *Rx.*
Use: Nutritional supplement, parenteral.

M.V.I. Pediatric. (Astra) Vitamin A 2300 IU, D 400 IU, E 7 IU, B_1 1.2 mg, B_2 1.4 mg, B_3 17 mg, B_5 5 mg, B_6 1 mg, B_{12} 1 mcg, C 80 mg, biotin 20 mcg, FA 0.14 mg, vitamin K 200 mcg, mannitol 375 mg/Inj. Vial. *Rx.*
Use: Nutritional supplement, parenteral.

M.V.M. (Tyson and Associates) Iron 3.6 mg, vitamins A 400 IU, E 60 IU, B_1 20 mg, B_2 10 mg, B_3 10 mg, B_5 100 mg, B_6 31 mg, B_{12} 160 mcg, C 50 mg, folic acid 0.08 mg, Ca, Cr, Cu, I, K, Mg, Mo, Zn 6 mg, biotin 160 mcg, PABA, Mn, Se, tryptophan/Cap. Bot 150s. *otc.*
Use: Mineral, vitamin supplement.

Myadec. (Parke-Davis) Iron 18 mg, A 5000 IU, D 400 IU, E 30 IU, B_1 1.7 mg, B_2 2 mg, B_3 20 mg, B_5 10 mg, B_6 3 mg, B_{12} 6 mcg, C 60 mg, folic acid 0.4 mg, biotin 30 mcg, vitamin K, Ca, P, I, Mg, Cu, zinc 15 mg, Mn, K, Cl, Cr, Mo, Se, Ni, Si, V, B, Sn/Tab. Bot. 130s. *otc.*
Use: Mineral, vitamin supplement.

myagen. Bolasterone.
Use: Anabolic agent.

Myambutol. (ESI Lederle Generics) Ethambutol HCl. Tab. **100 mg:** Bot. 100s. **400 mg:** Bot. 100s, 1000s, UD 10 × 10s. *Rx.*
Use: Antituberculous.

myanesin.
See: Mephenesin (Various Mfr.).

Myapap Drops. (Rosemont) Acetaminophen 80 mg/0.8 ml. Bot. 15 ml w/dropper. *otc.*
Use: Analgesic.

Myapap Elixir. (Rosemont) Acetaminophen 160 mg/5 ml. Bot. 4 oz, pt, gal. *otc.*
Use: Analgesic.

Myapap with Codeine Elixir. (Rosemont) Acetaminophen 120 mg, codeine phosphate 12 mg/5 ml. Bot. 4 oz, pt, gal. *c-v.*
Use: Analgesic, antitussive.

Mybanil. (Rosemont) Codeine phosphate 10 mg, bromodiphenhydramine HCl 12.5 mg/5 ml, alcohol 5%. Bot. 4 oz, pt, gal. *c-v.*
Use: Antihistamine, antitussive.

Mycadec DM Drops. (Rosemont) Pseudoephedrine 25 mg, carbinoxamine maleate 2 mg, dextromethorphan HBr 4 mg. Bot. 30 ml. *Rx.*
Use: Antihistamine, antitussive, decongestant.

Mycadec DM Syrup. (Rosemont) Carbinoxamine maleate 4 mg, pseudoephedrine HCl 60 mg, dextromethorphan HBr 15 mg/5 ml, alcohol 0.6%. Bot. 4 oz, pt, gal. *Rx.*
Use: Antihistamine, antitussive, decongestant.

Mycadec Drops. (Rosemont) Pseudoephedrine HCl 25 mg, dextromethorphan HBr 4 mg, carbinoxamine maleate 2 mg/ml. Bot. 30 ml. *Rx.*
Use: Antihistamine, antitussive, decongestant.

Mycartal. (Sanofi Winthrop) Pentaerythritol tetranitrate. *Rx.*
Use: Coronary vasodilator.

Mycelex. (Bayer Corp) Clotrimazole. **Topical Cream:** 1%. Tube 15 g, 30 g, 90 g (2 × 45 g). **Topical Soln.:** 1%. Bot. 10 ml, 30 ml. *otc, Rx.*
Use: Antifungal, topical.

Mycelex-7. (Bayer Corp) **Vaginal Tab.:** Clotrimazole 100 mg. Pkg. 7s with applicator; **Vaginal Cream:** Clotrimazole 1%. Tube 45 g (7 day therapy) with applicator. *otc.*
Use: Antifungal, vaginal.

Mycelex-7 Combination Pack. (Bayer Corp) Clotrimazole. **Cream:** 1%. Tube 7 g; **Supp.:** 100 mg. Pkg. 7s w/applicator. *otc.*
Use: Antifungal, vaginal.

Mycelex-G. (Bayer Corp) Clotrimazole. **Vaginal Tab.:** 100 mg. Pkg. 7s w/applicator. **Cream:** 1%. Tube 45 g, 90 g. *Rx.*
Use: Antifungal, vaginal.

Mycelex-G 500. (Bayer Corp) Clotrimazole 500 mg/Vaginal Tab. w/applicator. *Rx.*
Use: Antifungal, vaginal.

Mycelex OTC. (Bayer Corp) Clotrimazole 1%, benzyl alcohol 1%. Cream. Tube 15 g. *otc.*
Use: Anti-infective, topical.

Mycelex Troches. (Bayer Corp) Clotrimazole 10 mg/Troche 70s, 140s. *Rx.*
Use: Antifungal.

Mycelex Twin Pack. (Bayer Corp) Clotrimazole 500 mg/Vaginal Tab. w/applicator. Topical cream 1%. Tube 7 g. *Rx.*
Use: Antifungal, vaginal.

Mychel-S. (Rachelle) Sterile chloramphenicol sodium succinate. Vial 1 g/15 ml. Box 5s. *Rx.*
Use: Anti-infective.

Mycifradin. (Pharmacia & Upjohn) Neomycin sulfate 125 mg/5 ml (equivalent to 87.5 mg neomycin). Oral soln. Bot. pt. *Rx.*
Use: Anti-infective.

Myciguent. (Pharmacia & Upjohn) Neomycin sulfate. **Cream:** 5 mg/g. Tube 0.5 oz. **Oint.:** 5 mg/g. Tube 0.5 oz, 1 oz, 4 oz. *otc.*
Use: Anti-infective, topical.

Mycinette. (Pfeiffer) Benzocaine 15 mg, sorbitol, saccharin, menthol. Loz. 12s. *otc.*
Use: Anesthetic, local; antiseptic, expectorant.

Mycinette Sore Throat. (Pfeiffer) Phenol 1.4%, alum 0.3%, alcohol free, sugar free. Spray 180 ml. *otc.*
Use: Mouth and throat preparation.

Myci-Spray. (Misemer) Phenylephrine HCl 0.25%, pyrilamine maleate 0.15%/ml. Bot. 20 ml. *otc.*
Use: Antihistamine, decongestant.

Mycitracin. (Pharmacia & Upjohn) Bacitracin 500 units, neomycin sulfate 5 mg, polymyxin B sulfate 5000 units/g. Oint.: Tube 0.5 oz. Box 36s; 1 oz; UD 1/32 oz Box 144s. *otc.*
Use: Anti-infective, topical.

Mycitracin Plus. (Pharmacia & Upjohn) Polymyxin B sulfate 5000 units/g, neomycin 3.5 mg/g, bacitracin 500 units/g, lidocaine 40 mg, white petrolatum. Tube Oint. 15 g. *otc.*
Use: Anti-infective, topical.

Mycitracin Triple Antibiotic, Maximum Strength. (Pharmacia & Upjohn) Polymyxin B sulfate 5000 units/g, neomycin 3.5 mg/g, bacitracin 500 units/g, parabens, mineral oil, white petrolatum. Oint. Tube 30 g, UD 0.94 g. *otc.*
Use: Anti-infective, topical.

Mycobutin. (Pharmacia & Upjohn) Rifabutin. 150 mg/Cap. Bot. 100s. *Rx.*
Use: Antituberculous.

Mycocide NS. (Woodward) Benzalkonium Cl, propylene glycol, methyl-

paraben. Soln. Bot. 30 ml. *otc.*
Use: Antimicrobial, antiseptic.

Mycodone Syrup. (Rosemont) Hydrocodone bitartrate 5 mg, homatropine MBr 1.5 mg/5 ml. Bot. 4 oz, pt, gal. *c-III.*
Use: Antitussive.

Mycogen-II Cream. (Zenith Goldline) Nystatin 100,000 units, triamcinolone acetonide 1 mg/g. Cream Tube 15 g, 30 g, 60 g, 120 g, lb. *Rx.*
Use: Antifungal, corticosteroid, topical.

Mycogen-II Ointment. (Zenith Goldline) Nystatin 100,000 units, triamcinolone acetonide 1 mg/g. Oint. Tube 15 g, 30 g, 60 g. *Rx.*
Use: Antifungal, corticosteroid, topical.

Mycolog-II Cream and Ointment. (Bristol-Myers Squibb) Triamcinolone acetonide 1 mg, nystatin 100,000 units/g. Ointment base w/Plastibase (polyethylene, mineral oil). Tube 15 g, 30 g, 60 g, Jar 120 g. *Rx.*
Use: Antifungal, corticosteroid, topical.

Mycomist. (Gordon Laboratories) Chlorophyll, formalin, benzalkonium Cl. Bot. 4 oz, plastic Bot. 1 oz. *otc.*
Use: Antifungal for clothing.

•**mycophenolate mofetil.** (my-koe-FEN-oh-LATE MOE-feh-till) USAN.
Use: Immunomodulator.
See: CellCept, Cap. (Roche Laboratories).

•**mycophenolic acid.** (MY-koe-fen-AHL-ik acid) USAN.
Use: Antineoplastic.

Mycoplasma Pneumonia IFA IgM Test. (Wampole Laboratories) Indirect fluorescent assay for IgM antibodies to *Mycoplasma pneumoniae.* Box test 100s.
Use: Diagnostic aid.

Mycoplasma Pneumonia IFA Test. (Wampole Laboratories) Indirect fluorescent assay for antibodies to *Mycoplasma pneumoniae.* Box test 100s.
Use: Diagnostic aid.

Mycostatin. (Apothecon) Nystatin. **Tab.:** 500,000 units. Bot. 100s. **Cream:** 100,000 units/g in aqueous base. Tube 15 g, 30 g. **Oint.:** 100,000 units/g in Plastibase (polyethylene and mineral oil). Tube 15 g, 30 g. **Susp.:** 100,000 units/ml. In vehicle containing sucrose 50%, saccharin $<$ 1% alcohol. Bot. 60 ml, 473 ml. **Troche:** 200,000 units. 30s. **Vaginal Tab:** 100,000 units, lactose 0.95 g, ethyl cellulose, stearic acid, starch. Pkg. 15s, 30s. **Pow.:** (topical) 100,000 units/g in talc. Shaker bot. 15 g. *Rx.*
Use: Antifungal.

Mycostatin Pastilles. (Bristol-Myers Oncology/Immunology) Nystatin, 200,000 units/Troche. 30s. *Rx.*
Use: Antifungal.

Myco-Triacet. (Various Mfr.) Triamcinolone acetonide 0.1%, neomycin sulfate 0.25%, gramicidin 0.25 mg, nystatin 100,000 units/g. **Cream:** 15 g, 30 g, 60 g, 480 g. **Oint.:** 15 g, 30 g, 60 g. *Rx.*
Use: Antifungal, corticosteroid, topical.

Myco-Triacet II Cream & Ointment. (Teva USA) Nystatin 100,000 units, triamcinolone acetonide 1 mg/g. **Cream:** White petrolatum and mineral oil. Tube 15 g, 30 g, 60 g. **Oint.:** Tube 15 g, 30 g, 60 g. *Rx.*
Use: Antifungal, corticosteroid, topical.

Mycotussin Expectorant. (Rosemont) Pseudoephedrine HCl 60 mg, hydrocodone bitartrate 5 mg, guaifenesin 200 mg/5 ml, alcohol 12.5%. Bot. 4 oz, pt, gal. *c-III.*
Use: Antitussive, decongestant, expectorant.

Mycotussin Liquid. (Rosemont) Pseudoephedrine HCl 60 mg, hydrocodone bitartrate 5 mg/5 ml, alcohol 5%. Bot. 4 oz, pt, gal. *c-III.*
Use: Antitussive, decongestant.

Mydacol. (Rosemont) Vitamins B_1 5 mg, B_2 2.5 mg, niacinamide 50 mg, B_6 1 mg, B_{12} 1 mcg, pantothenic acid 10 mg, iodine 100 mcg, iron 15 mg, magnesium 2 mg, zinc 2 mg, choline 100 mg, manganese 2 mg/30 ml. Bot. pt, gal. *otc.*
Use: Mineral, vitamin supplement.

Mydfrin Ophthalmic 2.5%. (Alcon Laboratories) Phenylephrine HCl 2.5%. Drop-Tainers. 3 ml, 5 ml. *Rx.*
Use: Mydriatic.

Mydriacyl. (Alcon Laboratories) Tropicamide 0.5% or 1%. Soln. 3 ml (1% only), 15 ml Drop-Tainer. *Rx.*
Use: Cycloplegic, mydriatic.

mydriatics.

Parasympatholytic Types

Atropine Salts (Various Mfr.).
Homatropine Hydrobromide (Various Mfr.).
Scopolamine Salts (Various Mfr.).

Sympathomimetic Types

Amphetamine Sulfate 3% (Various Mfr.).
Clopane HCl, Liq. (Eli Lilly).
Ephedrine Sulfate (Various Mfr.).
Epinephrine HCl (Various Mfr.).
Neo-Synephrine HCl, Preps. (Sanofi Winthrop).

Phenylephrine HCl. (Various Mfr.).

myelin.
Use: Multiple sclerosis. [Orphan drug]

Myelo-Kit. (Sanofi Winthrop) Omnipaque 180 or 240 in various sizes and one sterile myelogram tray.
Use: Radiopaque agent.

Myfedrine. (Rosemont) Pseudoephedrine 30 mg/5 ml. Liq. Bot. 473 ml. *otc.*
Use: Decongestant.

Myfedrine Plus Syrup. (Rosemont) Pseudoephedrine HCl 30 mg, chlorpheniramine maleate 2 mg/5 ml. Bot. 4 oz, pt, gal. *otc.*
Use: Antitussive, decongestant.

Myfed Syrup. (Rosemont) Triprolidine HCl 1.25 mg, pseudoephedrine HCl 30 mg/5 ml. Bot. 4 oz, pt, gal. *otc.*
Use: Antihistamine, decongestant.

Mygel Liquid. (Geneva Pharm) Aluminum hydroxide 200 mg, magnesium hydroxide 200 mg, simethicone 20 mg, sodium 1.38 mg/5 ml. Liq. Bot. 360 ml. *otc.*
Use: Antacid, antiflatulent.

Mygel Suspension. (Geneva Pharm) Aluminum hydroxide 200 mg, magnesium hydroxide 200 mg, simethicone 20 mg/5 ml. Bot. 360 ml. *otc.*
Use: Antacid, antiflatulent.

Mygel II Suspension. (Geneva Pharm) Aluminum hydroxide 400 mg, magnesium hydroxide 400 mg, simethicone 40 mg/5 ml. Bot. 360 ml. *otc.*
Use: Antacid, antiflatulent.

Myhistine DH. (Rosemont) Codeine phosphate 10 mg, chlorpheniramine maleate 2 mg, pseudoephedrine HCl 30 mg/5 ml. Liq. Bot. 4 oz, pt, gal. *c-v.*
Use: Antihistamine, antitussive, decongestant.

Myhistine Elixir. (Rosemont) Chlorpheniramine maleate 2 mg, phenylephrine HCl 5 mg/5 ml, alcohol 5%. Liq. Bot. 4 oz, pt, gal. *otc.*
Use: Antihistamine, decongestant.

Myhistine Expectorant. (Rosemont) Codeine phosphate 10 mg, guaifenesin 100 mg, pseudoephedrine HCl 30 mg/5 ml, alcohol 7.5%. Liq. Bot. 4 oz, pt, gal. *c-v.*
Use: Antitussive, decongestant, expectorant.

Myhydromine Pediatric. (Rosemont) Phenylpropanolamine HCl 12.5 mg, hydrocodone bitartrate 2.5 mg/5 ml. Bot. pt, gal. *c-III.*
Use: Antitussive, decongestant.

Myhydromine Syrup. (Rosemont) Phenylpropanolamine HCl 25 mg, hydrocodone bitartrate 5 mg/5 ml. Bot. 4 oz, pt, gal. *c-III.*
Use: Antihistamine, antitussive, decongestive.

Myidone Tabs. (Major) Primidone 250 mg/Tab. Bot. 100s, 1000s. *Rx.*
Use: Anticonvulsant.

Mykacet Cream. (NMC Labs) Nystatin 100,000 units, triamcinolone acetonide 0.1%/g. Tube 15 g, 30 g, 60 g. *Rx.*
Use: Antifungal, corticosteroid, topical.

My-K Elixir. (Rosemont) Potassium 20 mEq/15 ml, alcohol 5%, saccharin. Bot. pt, gal. *Rx.*
Use: Electrolyte supplement.

My-K Formula 77D. (Rosemont) Phenylpropanolamine HCl 12.5 mg, dextromethorphan HBr 10 mg, guaifenesin 100 mg/5 ml, alcohol 10%. Liq. Bot. 180 ml. *otc.*
Use: Antitussive, decongestant, expectorant.

My-K Formula 77 Liquid. (Rosemont) Doxylamine succinate 3.75 mg, dextromethorphan HBr 7.5 mg/5 ml, alcohol 10%. Liq. Bot. 180 ml. *otc.*
Use: Antihistamine, antitussive.

Mykinac Cream. (NMC Labs) Nystatin 100,000 units/g in cream base. Tube 15 g, 30 g. *otc.*
Use: Antifungal, topical.

My-K Nasal Spray. (Rosemont) Oxymetazoline HCl 0.05%. Bot. 0.5 oz. *otc.*
Use: Decongestant.

Mykrox. (Medeva) Metolazone 0.5 mg/Tab. Bot. 100s. *Rx.*
Use: Diuretic.

Mylagen Gelcaps. (Zenith Goldline) Calcium carbonate 311 mg, magnesium carbonate 232 mg. Pkg. 24s. *otc.*
Use: Antacid.

Mylagen Liquid. (Zenith Goldline) Magnesium hydroxide 200 mg, aluminum hydroxide 200 mg, simethicone 20 mg/5 ml. Bot. 355 ml. *otc.*
Use: Antacid, antiflatulent.

Mylagen II Liquid. (Zenith Goldline) Aluminum hydroxide 400 mg, magnesium hydroxide 400 mg, simethicone 40 mg/5 ml. Bot. 355 ml. *otc.*
Use: Antacid, antiflatulent.

Mylanta. (J & J Merck Consumer Pharm) Calcium carbonate 600 mg. Loz. 18s, 50s. *otc.*
Use: Antacid.

Mylanta Double Strength. (J & J Merck Consumer Pharm) **Chew. Tab.:** Magnesium hydroxide 400 mg, aluminum

hydroxide dried gel 400 mg, simethicone 40 mg, Bot. 24s, 60s. **Liq.:** Magnesium hydroxide 400 mg, aluminum hydroxide dried gel 400 mg, simethicone 40 mg, sorbitol/5 ml. Bot. 150 ml, 360 ml. **Susp.:** Magnesium hydroxide 400 mg, aluminum hydroxide dried gel 400 mg, simethicone 40 mg, sodium 0.05 mEq/5 ml. Bot. 150 ml, 360 ml, 720 ml, UD 30, 150 ml. *otc.*
Use: Antacid.

Mylanta Gas. (J & J Merck Consumer Pharm) Simethicone **40 mg:** Chew. Tab. Bot. 100s, UD 100s; **80 mg:** Chew. Tab. Pkg. 12s, Bot. 48s, 100s, UD 100s. *otc.*
Use: Antiflatulent.

Mylanta Gas, Maximum Strength. (J & J Merck Consumer Pharm) Simethicone 125 mg/Chew. Tab. Pkg. 12s, Bot. 60s. *otc.*
Use: Antiflatulent.

Mylanta Gelcaps. (J & J Merck Consumer Pharm) Calcium carbonate 311 mg, magnesium carbonate 232 mg. Bot. 24s, 50s. *otc.*
Use: Antacid.

Mylanta Liquid. (J & J Merck Consumer Pharm) Magnesium hydroxide 200 mg, aluminum hydroxide 200 mg, simethicone 20 mg, sodium 0.68 mg/5 ml. Bot. 150 ml, 360 ml, 720 ml, UD 30 ml. *otc.*
Use: Antacid, antiflatulent.

Mylanta Natural Fiber Supplement. (J & J Merck Consumer Pharm) Psyllium hydrophilic mucilloid fiber 3.4 g/dose, sucrose, orange flavor. Pow. Can 390 g. *otc.*
Use: Laxative.

Mylanta Soothing Antacids. (J & J Merck Consumer Pharm) Calcium carbonate 600 mg, corn syrup, sucrose. Loz. Pkg. 18s. Bot. 50s. *otc.*
Use: Antacid.

Mylanta Tablets. (J & J Merck Consumer Pharm) Magnesium hydroxide 200 mg, aluminum hydroxide 200 mg, simethicone 20 mg, sodium 0.77 mg, sorbitol/ Chew. Tab. Bot. 12s, 40s, 48s, 100s, 180s. *otc.*
Use: Antacid, antiflatulent.

Mylanta-II Liquid. (J & J Merck Consumer Pharm) Magnesium hydroxide 400 mg, aluminum hydroxide 400 mg, simethicone 40 mg, sodium 1.14 mg, sorbitol/5 ml. Bot. 0.5 oz, 12 oz, UD 30 ml, 100s. *otc.*
Use: Antacid, antiflatulent.

Mylanta-II Tablets. (J & J Merck Consumer Pharm) Magnesium hydroxide 400 mg, aluminum hydroxide 400 mg, simethicone 40 mg, sodium 1.3 mg/ Chew. Tab. Box 24s, 60s. *otc.*
Use: Antacid, antiflatulent.

Mylase 100. Alpha-amylase.
See: Diastase.
W/Prolase, cellulase, calcium carbonate, magnesium glycinate.
See: Zylase Tab. (Eon Labs Manufacturing).

Myleran. (GlaxoWellcome) Busulfan 2 mg/Tab. Bot. 25s. *Rx.*
Use: Antineoplastic.

Mylicon. (Zeneca) Simethicone 40 mg. **Chew. Tab.:** Bot. 100s, 500s, UD 100s. **Drops:** 40 mg/0.6 ml. Bot. 30 ml. *otc.*
Use: Antiflatulent.

Mylicon-80. (Zeneca) Simethicone 80 mg/Chew. Tab. Bot. 100s, Box 12s, 48s, UD 100s. *otc.*
Use: Antiflatulent.

Mylicon-125. (Zeneca) Simethicone 125 mg/Chew. Tab. In 12s, 50s. *otc.*
Use: Antiflatulent.

Mylocaine 2% Viscous Solution. (Rosemont) Lidocaine HCl 2%. Bot. 100 ml. *Rx.*
Use: Anesthetic, local.

Mylocaine 4% Solution. (Rosemont) Lidocaine HCl 4%. Bot. 50 ml, 100 ml. *Rx.*
Use: Anesthetic, local.

Mymethasone Elixir. (Rosemont) Dexamethasone 0.5 mg/5 ml, alcohol 5%. Bot. 100 ml, 240 ml. *Rx.*
Use: Corticosteroid.

Myminic Expectorant. (Morton Grove) Phenylpropanolamine HCl 12.5 mg, guaifenesin 100 mg/5 ml, alcohol 5%. Bot. 4 oz, pt, gal. *otc.*
Use: Decongestant, expectorant.

Myminic Pediatric. (Rosemont) Phenylpropanolamine HCl 12.5 mg, guaifenesin 100 mg/5 ml, alcohol 5%. Liq. Bot. 4 oz, pt, gal. *otc.*
Use: Decongestant, expectorant.

Myminic Syrup. (Rosemont) Phenylpropanolamine HCl 12.5 mg, chlorpheniramine maleate 2 mg/5 ml. Alcohol free. Bot. 4 oz, pt, gal. *otc.*
Use: Antihistamine, decongestant.

Myminicol Liquid. (Morton Grove) Phenylpropanolamine HCl 12.5 mg, chlorpheniramine maleate 2 mg, dextromethorphan HBr 10 mg/5 ml. Liq. Bot. 4 oz, pt, gal. *otc.*
Use: Antihistamine, antitussive, decongestant.

Mynatal. (ME Pharm) Ca 300 mg, iron 65 mg, vitamins A 5000 IU, D 400 IU, E 30 mg, B_1 3 mg, B_2 3.4 mg, B_3 20 mg, B_5 10 mg, $B_6$10 mg, B_{12} 12 mcg, C 120 mg, folic acid 1 mg, biotin 30 mcg, Cr, Cu, I, Mg, Mn, Mo, Zn 25 mg/Cap. Bot. 100s, 500s. *Rx.*
Use: Mineral, vitamin supplement.

Mynatal FC. (ME Pharm) Calcium 250 mg, iron 60 mg, vitamin A 5000 IU, D 400 IU, E 30 IU, B_1 3 mg, B_2 3.4 mg, B_3 20 mg, B_5 10 mg, B_6 10 mg, B_{12} 12 mcg, C 100 mg, folic acid 1 mg, biotin 30 mcg, zinc 25 mg, I, Mg, Cr, Cu, Mo, Mn. Capl. Bot. 100s. *Rx.*
Use: Mineral, vitamin supplement.

Mynatal P.N. Captabs. (ME Pharm) Ca 125 mg, iron 60 mg, vitamins A 4000 IU, D 400 IU, B_1 3 mg, B_2 3 mg, B_3 10 mg, B_6 2 mg, B_{12} 3 mcg, C 50 mg, folic acid 1 mg, Zn 18 mg/Tab. Bot. 100s. *Rx.*
Use: Mineral, vitamin supplement.

Mynatal P.N. Forte. (ME Pharm) Iron 60 mg, vitamin A 5000 IU, D 400 IU, E 30 IU, C 80 mg, B_1 3 mg, B_2 3.4 mg, B_3 20 mg, B_6 4 mg, B_{12} 12 mcg, folic acid 1 mg, calcium 250 mg, zinc 25 mg, I, Mg, Cu. Capl. Bot. 100s. *Rx.*
Use: Mineral, vitamin supplement.

Mynatal Rx. (ME Pharm) Calcium 200 mg, iron 60 mg, vitamin A 4000 IU, D 400 IU, E 15 mg, B_1 1.5 mg, B_2 1.6 mg, B_3 17 mg, B_5 7 mg, B_6 4 mg, B_{12} 2.5 mcg, C 80 mg, folic acid 1 mg, biotin 0.03 mg, zinc 25 mg, Mg, Cu. Capl. Bot. 100s. *Rx.*
Use: Mineral, vitamin supplement.

Mynate 90 Plus. (ME Pharm) Calcium 250 mg, iron 90 mg, vitamin A 4000 IU, D 400 IU, E 30 IU, B_1 3 mg, B_2 3.4 mg, B_3 20 mg, B_6 20 mg, B_{12} 12 mcg, C 120 mg, folic acid 1 mg, zinc 25 mg, DSS, I, Cu. Capl. Bot. 100s. *Rx.*
Use: Mineral, vitamin supplement.

Myo-B. (Sigma-Tau Pharmaceuticals) Adenosine-5-monophosphoric acid, vitamin B_{12}. Vial 10 ml. *Rx.*

Myocide NS. (Woodward) Benzalkonium chloride, propylene glycol, methylparaben/Soln. 30 ml. *otc.*
Use: Antiseptic.

myodil.
See: Iophendylate Inj., U.S.P. 23.

Myoflex Creme. (Rhone-Poulenc Rorer) Trolamine salicylate 10% in a vanishing cream base. Tube 2 oz, 4 oz, Jar 8 oz, lb, Pump dispenser 3 oz. *otc.*
Use: Analgesic, topical.

Myolin. (Roberts Pharm) Orphenadrine citrate 30 mg/ml. Inj. Vial 10 ml. *Rx.*
Use: Muscle relaxant.

Myorgal. (Mysuran.) Ambenonium Cl.
Use: Cholinergic.

Myotalis. (Vita Elixir) Digitalis 1.5 gr/EC Tab. *Rx.*
Use: Cardiovascular agent.

Myoscint. (Centocor) Imciromab pentetate 0.5 mg for conjugation with indium-111. Kit. *Rx.*
Use: Radioimmunoscintigraphy agent.

Myotonachol. (Glenwood) Bethanechol Cl 10 mg or 25 mg/Tab. Bot. 100s. *Rx.*
Use: Urinary tract product.

Myotoxin. (Vita Elixir) **#1:** Digitoxin 0.1 mg/Tab. **#2:** Digitoxin 0.2 mg/Tab. *Rx.*
Use: Cardiovascular agent.

Myphentol Elixir. (Rosemont) Phenobarbital 16.2 mg, hyoscyamine SO_4 or HBr 0.1037 mg, atropine sulfate 0.0194 mg, scopolamine HBr 0.0065 mg/5 ml, alcohol 23%. Bot. 4 oz, pt, gal. *Rx.*
Use: Anticholinergic, antispasmodic, hypnotic, sedative.

Myphetane DC Cough Syrup. (Morton Grove) Codeine phosphate 10 mg, brompheniramine maleate 2 mg, phenylpropanolamine HCl 12.5 mg/5 ml, alcohol 1.2%. Bot. 4 oz, gal. *c-v.*
Use: Antihistamine, antitussive, decongestant.

Myphetane DX Cough Syrup. (Various Mfr.) Brompheniramine maleate 2 mg, pseudoephedrine HCl 30 mg, dextromethorphan HBr 10 mg/5 ml, alcohol 0.95%. Bot. 4 oz, pt, gal. *Rx.*
Use: Antihistamine, antitussive, decongestant.

Myphetane Elixir. (Rosemont) Brompheniramine maleate 2 mg/5 ml, alcohol 3%. *otc.*
Use: Antihistamine.

Myphetapp Elixer. (Rosemont) Brompheniramine maleate 2 mg, phenylpropanolamine HCl 12.5 mg/5 ml, alcohol 2.3%. Bot. 4 oz, pt. *otc.*
Use: Antihistamine, decongestant.

Myproic Acid Syrup. (Rosemont) Valproic acid 250 mg (as sodium valproate)/5 ml. Bot. pt. *Rx.*
Use: Anticonvulsant.

Myriatin Drops. (Sanofi Winthrop) Atropine methonitrate BP. *Rx.*
Use: Antispasmodic.

myristica oil.
Use: Flavor.

•**myristyl alcohol.** (mih-RIST-ill) N.F. 18.
Use: Pharmaceutic aid (stiffening agent).

myristyl-picolinium chloride.
See: Wet Tone, Soln. (3M).

Myrj 45. (Zeneca) Mixture of free polyoxyethylene glycol and its mono- and di-stearates. Polyoxyl 8 stearate.
Use: Surface active agent.

Myrj 52 and M2s. (Zeneca) Polyoxyethylene 40 stearate. Mixture of free polyoxyethylene glycol and its mono-and distearates.
Use: Surface active agent.

Myrj 53. (Zeneca) Polyoxyl 50 stearate.
Use: Surface active agent.

Mysoline. (Wyeth Ayerst) Primidone, lactose, saccharin. **Tab.:** 50 mg Bot. 100s, 500s; 250 mg. Bot. 100s, 1000s, UD 100s. **Susp.:** 250 mg/5 ml. Bot. 240 ml. *Rx.*
Use: Anticonvulsant.

Mysuran. Ambenonium Cl.
Use: Muscle stimulant.
See: Mytelase Cl, Cap. (Winthrop-Breon).

Mytelase. (Sanofi Winthrop) Ambenonium Cl 10 mg/Cap. Bot. 100s. *Rx.*
Use: Muscle stimulant.

Myticin G Creme and Ointment.
See: g-myticin creme and ointment.

Mytomycin-C. (IOP)
Use: Antiglaucoma agent. [Orphan drug]

Mytrex. (Savage) Triamcinolone acetonide 0.1%, nystatin 100,000 units/g. Cream, Oint. 15 g, 30 g, 60 g, 120 g. *Rx.*
Use: Antifungal, topical; corticosteroid.

Mytussin AC Cough. (Morton Grove) Guaifenesin 100 mg, codeine phosphate 10 mg/5 ml, alcohol 3.5%. Bot. 4 oz, pt, gal. *c-v.*
Use: Antitussive, expectorant.

Mytussin DM Expectorant. (Morton Grove) Guaifenesin 100 mg, dextromethorphan HBr 10 mg/5 ml, alcohol 1.6%. Bot. 4 oz, pt, gal. *otc.*
Use: Antitussive, expectorant.

Mytussin DAC Syrup. (Rosemont) Guaifenesin 100 mg, pseudoephedrine HCl 30 mg, codeine phosphate 10 mg/5 ml. Bot. 4 oz, pt, gal. *c-v.*
Use: Antitussive, decongestant, expectorant.

Mytussin Syrup. (Rosemont) Guaifenesin 100 mg/5 ml, alcohol 3.5%. Bot. 4 oz, pt, gal. *otc.*
Use: Expectorant.

Myverol. (Eastman Kodak) Glyceryl monostearate.

My-Vitalife. (ME Pharm) Ca 130 mg, iron 27 mg, vitamins A 6500 IU, D 400 IU, E 30 mg, B_1 1.5 mg, B_2 1.7 mg, B_3 20 mg, B_5 10 mg, B_6 2 mg, B_{12} 6 mcg, C 60 mg, folic acid 0.4 mg, Cr, Cu, K, I, Mg, Mn, Mo, P, Se, Zn, 15 mg, vitamin K, biotin 30 mcg/Cap. Bot. 60s. *otc.*
Use: Mineral, vitamin supplement.

My-Zole 7 Dual Pack. (Alpharma) Miconazole nittrate 100 mg. Vag. Supp. Miconazole nitrate 2%. Cream. *otc.*
Use: Vaginal preparation.

N

Na-Ana-Tal. (Churchill) Phenobarbital 0.25 g, phenacetin 2 g, aspirin 3 g, nicotinic acid 50 mg/Tab. Bot. 100s, Liq. Bot. 16 oz. *c-IV.*
Use: Analgesic, hypnotic, sedative.

•**nabazenil.** (nab-AZE-eh-nill) USAN.
Use: Anticonvulsant.

•**nabilone.** (NAB-ih-lone) USAN.
Use: Anxiolytic.

•**nabitan hydrochloride.** (NAB-ih-tan) USAN. *Formerly Nabutan Hydrochloride.*
Use: Analgesic.

•**naboctate hydrochloride.** (NAB-ock-tate) USAN.
Use: Antiglaucoma agent, antinauseant.

•**nabumetone.** (nab-YOU-meh-TONE) USAN.
Use: Anti-inflammatory.
See: Relafen (SmithKline Beecham Pharmaceuticals).

n-acetylcysteine.
See: Acetylcysteine.

n-acetyl-p-aminophenol. Acetaminophen, U.S.P. 23.

n^1-acetylsulfanilamide.
See: Acetylsulfanilamide.

•**nadide.** (NAD-ide) USAN. *Formerly Diphosphopyridine Nucleotide, Nicotinamide Adenine Dinucleotide.*
Use: Antagonist to alcohol and narcotics.

Nadinola (Deluxe) for Oily Skin. (Strickland) Hydroquinone 2%. Bot. 1.25 oz, 2.25 oz. *Rx.*
Use: Dermatologic.

Nadinola for Dry Skin. (Strickland) Hydroquinone 2%. Bot. 1.25 oz, 2.25 oz. *Rx.*
Use: Dermatologic.

Nadinola (Ultra) for Normal Skin. (Strickland) Hydroquinone 2%. Bot. 1.25 oz, 3.75 oz, Tube 1.85 oz. *Rx.*
Use: Dermatologic.

•**nadolol.** (nay-DOE-lahl) U.S.P. 23.
Use: Antihypertensive, antianginal, beta-adrenergic blocker.
See: Corgard, Tab. (Bristol Labs).

nadolol. (nay-DOE-lahl) (Various Mfr.) Tab.: **20 mg:** 100s, UD 100s. **40 mg, 80 mg:** 100s, 1000s, UD 100s. **120 mg:** 100s, 1000s. **160 mg:** 100s. *Rx.*
Use: Beta-adrenergic blocker.

nadolol and bendroflumethiazide.
Use: Antihypertensive, antianginal beta blocker.
See: Corzide (Bristol-Myers).

naepaine hydrochloride.
Use: Anesthetic, local.

•**nafamostat mesylate.** (naff-AM-oh-stat) USAN.
Use: Anticoagulant; antifibrinolytic.

•**nafarelin acetate.** (NAFF-uh-RELL-in) USAN.
Use: LHRH agonist; agonist, hormone [Orphan drug].
See: Synarel (Syntex).

Nafazair. (Bausch & Lomb) Naphazoline HCl 0.1%. Soln. Bot. 15 ml. *Rx.*
Use: Mydriatic, vasoconstrictor.

Nafazair A. (Bausch & Lomb) Naphazoline HCl 0.025%, pheniramine maleate 0.3%, benzalkonium chloride 0.01%, EDTA, boric acid, sodium borate. Bot. 15 ml. *Rx.*
Use: Decongestant combination, ophthalmic.

•**nafcillin, sodium.** (naff-SILL-in) U.S.P. 23.
Use: Anti-infective.
See: Unipen, Vial. (Wyeth Ayerst).

Na-Feen. (Pacemaker) Fluoride 1 mg/ Dose. Tab. Bot. 100s, 500s, 1000s; Liq. 2 oz. *Rx.*
Use: Dental caries agent.

•**nafenopin.** (naff-EN-oh-pin) USAN.
Use: Antihyperlipoproteinemic.

•**nafimidone hydrochloride.** (naff-IH-mih-DOHN) USAN.
Use: Anticonvulsant.

•**naflocort.** (NAFF-lah-cort) USAN.
Use: Adrenocortical steroid (topical).

•**nafomine malate.** (NAFF-oh-meen) USAN.
Use: Muscle relaxant.

•**nafoxidine hydrochloride.** (naff-OX-ih-deen) USAN.
Use: Antiestrogen.

•**nafronyl oxalate.** (NAFF-row-NILL OX-ah-late) USAN.
Use: Vasodilator.

naftalan.
W/Ichthyol, calamine, amber petrolatum.
See: Nagtalan, Oint. (Paddock).

•**naftifine hydrochloride.** (NAFF-tih-FEEN) USAN.
Use: Antifungal.
See: Naftin, Cream (Allergan).

Naftin. (Allergan) Naftifine HCl 1%. Cream. 2 g, 15 g, 30 g. *Rx.*
Use: Antifungal, topical.

naganol.
See: Suramin Sodium. Naphuride Sodium.

Nailicure. (Purepac) Denatonium benzoate in a clear nail polish base. Bot. 0.33 oz. *otc.*
Use: Nail biting deterrent.

Nail Plus. (Faraday) Gelatin Cap. Bot. 100s, 200s.

•**nalbuphine hydrochloride.** (NAL-byoo-FEEN) USAN.
Use: Analgesic, narcotic.
See: Nubain, Vial (DuPont Merck Pharmaceuticals).

Naldecon CX Adult Liquid. (Apothecon) Phenylpropanolamine 12.5 mg, guaifenesin 200 mg, codeine phosphate 10 mg/10 ml. Alcohol free. Bot. 4 oz, pt. *c-v.*
Use: Antitussive, decongestant, expectorant.

Naldecon DX Adult Liquid. (Apothecon) Phenylpropanolamine HCl 12.5 mg, guaifenesin 200 mg, dextromethorphan HBr 10 mg/10 ml, saccharin, sorbitol. Alcohol free. Bot. 4 oz, pt. *otc.*
Use: Antitussive, decongestant, expectorant.

Naldecon DX Children's Syrup. (Apothecon) Phenylpropanolamine HCl 6.25 mg, dextromethorphan HBr 5 mg, guaifenesin 100 mg/5 ml. Bot. 4 oz, 16 oz. *otc.*
Use: Antitussive, decongestant, expectorant.

Naldecon DX Pediatric Drops. (Apothecon) Phenylpropanolamine HCl 6.25 mg, guaifenesin 50 mg, dextromethorphan HBr 5 mg/ml, alcohol free, saccharin, sorbitol. Bot. 30 ml. *otc.*
Use: Antitussive, decongestant, expectorant.

Naldecon EX Children's Syrup. (Apothecon) Phenylpropanolamine HCl 6.25 mg, guaifenesin 100 mg/5 ml, saccharin, sorbitol. Bot. 118 ml, 480 ml. *otc.*
Use: Decongestant, expectorant.

Naldecon EX Pediatric Drops. (Apothecon) Phenylpropanolamine HCl 6.25 mg, guaifenesin 50 mg/ml. Bot. 30 ml. w/dropper. *otc.*
Use: Decongestant, expectorant.

Naldecon Pediatric Drops. (Apothecon) Chlorpheniramine maleate 0.5 mg, phenyltoloxamine citrate 2 mg, phenylpropanolamine HCl 5 mg, phenylephrine HCl 1.25 mg/ml, sorbitol. Bot. 30 ml. *Rx.*
Use: Antihistamine, decongestant.

Naldecon Pediatric Syrup. (Apothecon) Chlorpheniramine maleate 0.5 mg, phenyltoloxamine citrate 2 mg, phenylpropanolamine HCl 5 mg, phenylephrine HCl 1.25 mg/5 ml, sorbitol. Bot. 473 ml. *Rx.*
Use: Antihistamine, decongestant.

Naldecon Senior DX. (Apothecon) Dextromethorphan HBr 10 mg, guaifenesin 200 mg/5 ml, saccharin, sorbitol, alcohol free. Liq. Bot. 118 ml. *otc.*
Use: Antitussive, expectorant.

Naldecon Senior EX. (Apothecon) Guaifenesin 200 mg/5 ml, saccharin, sorbitol. Liq. Bot. 118 ml. *otc.*
Use: Expectorant.

Naldecon Syrup. (Apothecon) Chlorpheniramine maleate 2.5 mg, phenyltoloxamine citrate 7.5 mg, phenylpropanolamine HCl 20 mg, phenylephrine HCl 5 mg/5 ml. Bot. 473 ml. *Rx.*
Use: Antihistamine, decongestant.

Naldecon Tablets. (Apothecon) Phenylephrine HCl 10 mg, phenylpropanolamine HCl 40 mg, phenyltoloxamine citrate 15 mg, chlorpheniramine maleate 5 mg/SR Tab. Bot. 100s, 500s. *Rx.*
Use: Antihistamine, decongestant.

Naldegesic Tablets. (Bristol-Myers Squibb) Pseudoephedrine HCl 15 mg, acetaminophen 325 mg/Tab. Bot. 100s. *otc.*
Use: Analgesic, decongestant.

Naldelate DX Adult Liquid. (Alphalma USPD) Phenylpropanolamine HCl 12.5 mg, dextromethorphan HBr 10 mg, guaifenesin 200 mg. Bot. 120 ml or 480 ml. *otc.*
Use: Antitussive, decongestant, expectorant.

Naldelate Pediatric Syrup. (Various Mfr.) Phenylpropanolamine HCl 5 mg, phenylephrine HCl 1.25 mg, chlorpheniramine maleate 0.5 mg, phenyltoloxamine citrate 2 mg/5 ml. Bot. 120 ml, 473 ml, gal. *Rx.*
Use: Antihistamine, decongestant.

Naldelate Syrup. (Various Mfr.) Phenylpropanolamine HCl 20 mg, phenylephrine HCl 5 mg, chlorpheniramine maleate 2.5 mg, phenyltoloxamine citrate 7.5 mg/5 ml. Syr. Bot. 473 ml, gal. *Rx.*
Use: Antihistamine, decongestant.

Nalfon. (Eli Lilly) Fenoprofen calcium. **Cap.: 200 mg.** Rx Pak 100s. **300 mg.** Rx Pak 100s, Bot. 500s. *Rx.*
Use: Analgesic, NSAID.

Nalgest. (Major) Phenylpropanolamine HCl 40 mg, phenylephrine HCl 10 mg, chlorpheniramine maleate 5 mg, phenyltoloxamine citrate 15 mg/Tab. Bot. 100s, 500s, 1000s. *Rx.*
Use: Antihistamine, decongestant.

Nalgest Pediatric Drops. (Major) Phenylpropanolamine HCl 5 mg, phenylephrine HCl 1.25 mg, chlorpheniramine maleate 0.5 mg, phenyltolox- amine citrate 2 mg, sorbitol/Drop. Bot. 30 ml. *Rx.*
Use: Antihistamine, decongestant.

Nalgest Pediatric Syrup. (Major) Phenylpropanolamine HCl 5 mg, phenylephrine HCl 1.25 mg, chlorpheniramine maleate 0.5 mg, phenyltolox- amine citrate 2 mg/5 ml. Syr. Bot. 473 ml, gal. *Rx.*
Use: Antihistamine, decongestant.

Nalgest Syrup. (Major) Phenylpropanolamine HCl 20 mg, phenylephrine HCl 5 mg, chlorpheniramine maleate 2.5 mg, phenyltoloxamine citrate 7.5 mg/5 ml. Syr. Bot. 473 ml. *Rx.*
Use: Antihistamine, decongestant.

•**nalidixate sodium.** (nal-ih-DIK-sate) USAN. Under study.
Use: Anti-infective.

•**nalidixic acid.** (nal-ih-DIK-sik) U.S.P. 23.
Use: Anti-infective.
See: NegGram, Capl., Susp. (Sanofi Winthrop).

Nallpen. (SmithKline Beecham Pharmaceuticals) Nafcillin sodium monohydrate 500 mg, 1 g or 2 g/Vial. Inj. Piggyback 1 g, 2 g, Bulk 10 g. *Rx.*
Use: Anti-infective, penicillin.

•**nalmefene.** (NAL-meh-FFEN) USAN.
Formerly Naletrene.
Use: Antagonist to narcotics.
See: Revex, Inj. (Ohmeda Pharmaceuticals).

nalmetrene. (NAL-meh-treen)
Use: Antagonist to narcotics.

•**nalmexone hydrochloride.** (NAL-mex-ohn) USAN.
Use: Analgesic, narcotic.

•**nalorphine hydrochloride.** U.S.P. 23.
See: Nalline (Merck).

•**naloxone hydrochloride.** (NAL-ox-ohn) U.S.P. 23.
Use: Narcotic antagonist.
See: Narcan, Amp. (DuPont Merck Pharmaceuticals).

naloxone hydrochloride. (Various Mfr.) **0.02 mg/ml:** Amps 2 ml. **0.4 mg/ml:** Amps 1 ml, syringes 1 ml, vials 1 ml, 2 ml, 10 ml. *Rx.*
Use: Narcotic antagonist.

Nalspan. (Rosemont) Phenylpropanolamine HCl 20 mg, phenylephrine HCl 5 mg, chlorpheniramine maleate 2.5 mg, phenyltoloxamine citrate 7.5 mg/ml, alcohol free. Syr. Bot. pt. *otc.*
Use: Antihistamine, decongestant.

•**naltrexone.** (nal-TREX-ohn) USAN.
Use: Antagonist to narcotics. [Orphan drug]
See: Depade, Tab. (Mallinckrodt).
ReVia, Tab. (DuPont Merck Pharmaceuticals).

namazene. Phenothiazine.

namol xenyrate. (NAY-mahl ZEH-neh-rate)
See: Namoxyrate.

•**namoxyrate.** (nam-OX-ee-rate) USAN.
Use: Analgesic.
See: Namol Xenyrate (Warner Chilcott).

namuron.
See: Cyclobarbital Calcium (Various Mfr.).

•**nandrolone cyclotate.** (NAN-drole-ohn SIH-kloe-tate) USAN.
Use: Anabolic.

•**nandrolone decanoate.** (NAN-drole-ohn deh-KAN-oh-ate) U.S.P. 23.
Use: Androgen.
See: Anabolin LA-100, Vial (Alto Pharmaceuticals).
Androlone-D, Inj. (Keene Pharmaceuticals).
Androlone-D 50, Inj. (Keene Pharmaceuticals).
Deca-Durabolin, Amp., Vial (Organon Teknika).
Hybolin Decanoate, Inj. (Hyrex).

•**nandrolone phenpropionate.** (NAN-droe-lone fen-PRO-pee-oh-nate) U.S.P. 23.
Use: Androgen.
See: Anabolin IM, Vial (Alto Pharmaceuticals).
Androlone, Inj. (Keene Pharmaceuticals).
Androlone 50, Inj. (Keene Pharmaceuticals).
Durabolin Inj. (Organon Teknika).
Hybolin Improved, Vial (Hyrex).
Nandrolin, Inj. (Solvay).

•**nantradol hydrochloride.** (NAN-trah-DAHL) USAN.
Use: Analgesic.

Naotin. (Drug Products) Sodium nicotinate. Amp. (equivalent to 10 mg nicotinic acid/ml) 10 ml, Box 25s, 100s. *Rx.*
Use: Vitamin B_3 supplement.

NAPA. (Medco Research/Parke-Davis) Acecainide hydrochloride.
Use: Cardiovascular agent.

•**napactadine hydrochloride.** (nap-ACK-tah-deen) USAN.
Use: Antidepressant.

•**napamezole hydrochloride.** (nap-am-EH-zole) USAN.
Use: Antidepressant.
Napamide Caps. (Major) Disopyramide phosphate 100 mg or 150 mg/Cap. Bot. 100s, 500s, UD 100s. *Rx.*
Use: Antiarrhythmic.
•**naphazoline hydrochloride.** (naff-AZZ-oh-leen) U.S.P. 23.
Use: Adrenergic (vasoconstrictor).
See: AK-Con, Soln., (Akorn).
Albalon, Soln., (Allergan America).
Allerest Eye Drops, Soln. (Novartis Pharmaceuticals).
Comfort Eye Drops, Soln., (PBH Wesley Jessen).
Clear Eyes, Drops (Abbott Laboratories).
Degest 2, Soln., (PBH Wesley Jessen).
Estivin II, Soln. (Alcon Laboratories).
Maximum Strength Allergy Drops (Bausch & Lomb).
Muro's Opcon, Soln. (Bausch & Lomb).
Nafazair, Soln. (Bausch & Lomb).
Naphcon, Drops (Alcon Laboratories).
Privine HCl, Soln., Spray (Novartis Pharmaceuticals).
VasoClear, Soln., (Ciba Vision Ophthalmics).
Vasocon Regular, Liq. (Ciba Vision Ophthalmics).
W/Antazoline phosphate, boric acid, phenylmercuric acetate, sodium Cl, sodium carbonate anhydrous.
See: Antazoline-V, Soln. (Rugby).
Vasocon-A Ophthalmic, Soln. (Ciba Vision Ophthalmics).
W/Antazoline phosphate, polyvinyl alcohol.
See: Albalon-A Liquifilm, Ophth. (Allergan).
W/Methapyrilene HCl, cetylpyridinum Cl, thimerosal.
See: Vapocyn II Nasal Spray (Solvay).
W/Pheniramine maleate.
See: AK-Con-A, Soln., (Akorn).
Nafazair A, Soln., (Bausch & Lomb).
Naphazole-A, Soln., (Major).
Naphazoline Plus, Soln. (Parmed).
Naphcon A, Liq. (Alcon Laboratories).
Naphoptic-A, Soln. (Optopics).
W/PEG 300, benzalkonium Cl.
See: Allergy Drops (Bausch & Lomb).
W/Phenylephrine HCl, pyrilamine maleate, phenylpropanolamine HCl.
See: 4-Way Nasal Spray (Bristol-Myers).
W/Polyvinyl alcohol.
See: Albalon, Ophth. Soln. (Allergan).
Albalon Liquifilm, Ophth. Soln. (Allergan).
naphazoline hydrochloride. (Various Mfr.) 0.1% Soln. Bot. 15 ml. *Rx.*
Use: Adrenergic (vasoconstrictor).
naphazoline hydrochloride & antazoline phosphate. (Various Mfr.) Naphazoline HCl 0.05%, antazoline phosphate 0.5%. Soln. 5 ml, 15 ml. *otc.*
Use: Antihistamine, decongestant, ophthalmic.
naphazoline hydrochloride & pheniramine maleate. (Various Mfr.) Naphazoline HCl 0.025%, pheniramine maleate 0.3%. soln. bot. 15 ml. *otc.*
Use: Antihistamine, decongestant, ophthalmic.
naphazoline plus. (Parmed) Naphazoline HCl 0.025%, pheniramine maleate 0.3%. Bot. 15 ml. *otc.*
Use: Decongestant combination, ophthalmic.
Naphcon. (Alcon Laboratories) Naphazoline HCl 0.012%, Bot. 15 ml. *otc.*
Use: Mydriatic, vasoconstrictor.
Naphcon-A. (Alcon Laboratories) Naphazoline HCl 0.025%, pheniramine maleate 0.3%. Bot. 15 ml. *otc.*
Use: Decongestant combination, ophthalmic.
Naphcon Forte. (Alcon Laboratories) Naphazoline HCl 0.1%/ml. Drop-Tainer Bot. 15 ml. *Rx.*
Use: Mydriatic, vasoconstrictor.
Napholine. (Horizon) Naphazoline HCl 0.1%. Soln. Bot. 15 ml. *Rx.*
Use: Mydriatic, vasoconstrictor.
Naphoptic-A. (Optopics) Naphazoline HCl 0.025%, pheniramine maleate 0.3%. Bot. 15 ml. *Rx.*
Use: Decongestant combination, ophthalmic.
Naphthyl-B Salicylate. Betol, Naphthosalol, Salinaphthol.
Use: GI & GU, antiseptic.
naphuride sodium. Suramin Sodium.
•**napitane mesylate.** (NAP-ih-tane) USAN.
Use: Antidepressant.
Naprelan. (Wyeth Ayerst) Naproxen 375 or 500 mg/ER Tab. 100s (375 mg), 75s (500 mg). *Rx.*
Use: Analgesic.
•**napitane mesylate.** (NAP-ih-tane) USAN.
Use: Antidepressant.
Naprosyn. (Syntex) Naproxen. **Oral susp.:** 125 mg/5 ml, sorbitol. Bot. 480 ml. **250 mg/Tab.:** Bot. 100s, 500s, UD

100s; **375 mg/Tab.:** Bot. 100s, 500s, UD 100s; **500 mg/Tab.:** Bot. 100s, 500s, UD 100s. *Rx.*
Use: Analgesic, NSAID.

•**naproxen.** (nah-PROX-ehn) U.S.P. 23.
Use: Analgesic, anti-inflammatory, antipyretic.
See: Naprosyn, Susp., Tab. (Syntex).

naproxen. (Various Mfr.) 250, 375, 500 mg/Tab. 100s, 500s, 1000s, UD 100s. *Rx.*
Use: Analgesic, NSAID, antipyretic.

naproxen. (Roxane) 125 mg/5ml, methylparaben, sorbitol, sucrose, pineapple-orange flavor. Oral Susp. 500 ml, UD 15 ml and 20 ml.
Use: Analgesic, NSAID.

•**naproxen sodium.** (nah-PROX-ehn) U.S.P. 23.
Use: Analgesic, anti-inflammatory, antipyretic.
See: Aleve, Tab. (Procter & Gamble).
Anaprox, Tab. (Syntex).
Anaprox DS, Tab. (Syntex).
Naprosyn, Tab., Susp. (Syntex).

naproxen sodium. (Various Mfr.) 200 mg, 250 mg, 500 mg/Tab. 100s, 500s, 1000s, UD 100s. *Rx.*
Use: Analgesic, NSAID.

naproxen sodium. (Zenith Goldline) Naproxen sodium 200 mg (220 mg naproxen sodium). Tab. Bot. 24s. *otc.*
Use: Anti-inflammatory.

•**naproxol.** (nay-PROX-ole) USAN.
Use: Analgesic, anti-inflammatory, antipyretic.

Naqua. (Schering Plough) Trichlormethiazide 2 mg or 4 mg/Tab. Bot. 100s, 1000s. *Rx.*
Use: Diuretic.
W/Reserpine.
See: Naquival, Tab. (Schering Plough).

•**napsagatran.** (nap-sah-GAT-ran) USAN.
Use: Antithrombotic.

•**naranol hydrochloride.** (NARE-ah-nahl) USAN.
Use: Antipsychotic.

•**naratriptan hydrochloride.** (NAHR-ah-trip-tan) USAN.
Use: Antimigraine.
See: Amerge, Tab. (GlaxoWellcome).

Narcan. (DuPont Merck Pharmaceuticals) Naloxone HCl. **0.02 mg/ml:** Amp. 2 ml. **0.4 mg/ml:** Amp. 1 ml, Box 10s. Prefilled syringe 1 ml, Tray 10s; 1 ml, 2 ml, 10 ml multiple dose vials. **1 mg/ml:** Amp. 2 ml, Box 10s; Multiple dose vial 10 ml. *Rx.*
Use: Narcotic antagonist.

Nardil. (Parke-Davis) Phenelzine sulfate 15 mg/Tab. Bot. 100s. *Rx.*
Use: Antidepressant.

Naropin. (Astra USA) Ropivacaine HCL 2, 5, 7.5, and 10 mg/ml concentrations/Inj. Single-dose amps, vials and infusion bottles. *Rx.*
Use: Anesthetic, local.

Nasabid. (Jones Medical) Pseudoephedrine HCl 90 mg, guaifenesin 250 mg, sucrose. Cap., prolonged action. Bot. 100s. *Rx.*
Use: Decongestant, expectorant.

Nasabid SR. (Jones Medical) Pseudoephedrine HCl 90 mg, guaifenesin 500 mg. LA Tab. Bot. 100s. *Rx.*
Use: Decongestant, expectorant.

Nasacort. (Rhone-Poulenc Rorer) Triamcinolone acetonide 55 mcg per actuation. Spray. Cannister 10 mg. *Rx.*
Use: Corticosteroid, nasal.

Nasacort AQ. (Rhone-Poulenc Rorer) Triamcinolone acetonide 55 mcg per actuation, benzalkonium chloride, dextrose, EDTA/Spray. Bot. 16.5 g (120 actuations). *Rx.*
Use: Corticosteroid, nasal.

Nasadent. (Scherer) Sodium metaphosphate, glycerin, distilled water, dicalcium phosphate dihydrate, sodium carboxymethylcellulose, oil of spearmint, sodium benzoate, saccharin. *otc.*
Use: Ingestible dentifrice.

Nasahist Capsules. (Keene Pharmaceuticals) Phenylpropanolamine HCl 40 mg, phenylephrine HCl 10 mg, chlorpheniramine maleate 12 mg/Cap. Bot. 100s. *Rx.*
Use: Antihistamine, decongestant.

NaSal Saline Nasal. (Sanofi Winthrop) Sodium Cl 0.65%. Drops, Spray. Bot. 15 ml. *otc.*
Use: Moisturizer, nasal.

Nasalcrom Nasal Solution. (Ortho McNeil) Cromolyn sodium 40 mg/ml, benzalkonium Cl 0.01%, EDTA 0.01%. Metered dose spray. Delivers 5.2 mg/spray. Complete pkg. 13 ml. Refill 13 ml. *otc.*
Use: Antiallergic, nasal.

Nasalide. (Syntex) Flunisolide 0.025% soln. Pump. Bot. 25 ml. *Rx.*
Use: Corticosteroid, nasal.

Nasal Jelly. (Kondon) Phenol, camphor, menthol, eucalyptus oil, lavender oil. Oint. Tube. 20 g. *otc.*
Use: Decongestant.

Nasal Saline. (Sanofi Winthrop) Nasal spray and drops. Sodium Cl 0.65%

buffered w/phosphates, preservatives. Bot. 15 ml. Spray Bot. 15 ml. *otc.*
Use: Moisturizer, nasal.

Nasarel. (Roche Laboratories) Flunisolide 0.025%/Spray Soln. Bot. 25 ml (200 actuations). *Rx.*
Use: Anti-inflammatory.

Nasatab LA. (ECR Pharmaceuticals) Guaifenesin 500 mg, pseudoephedrine HCl 120 mg/LA Tab. Dye free. Bot. 100s. *Rx.*
Use: Decongestant, expectorant.

Nascobal. (Schwarz Pharma) Cyanocobalamin 500 mcg/0.1 ml, benzal konium chloride. 500 mcg/actuation Intranasal Gel. Bot. 5 ml (≈ 8 doses). *Rx.*
Use: Vitamin supplement.

Nasonex. (Schering Plough) Mometasone furoate monohydrate 50 mcg, glycerin, phenylethyl alcohol. Nasal spray. Bot. 17 g. *Rx.*
Use: Corticosteroid.

Nasophen. (Premo) Phenylephrine HCl 0.25% or 1%. Bot. pt. *otc.*
Use: Decongestant.

Natabec. (Parke-Davis) Vitamins A 4000 IU, D 400 IU, B_1 3 mg, B_2 2 mg, B_6 3 mg, C 50 mg, B_{12} 5 mcg, B_3 10 mg, elemental calcium 240 mg, elemental iron 30 mg/Kapseal. Bot. 100s. *otc.*
Use: Mineral, vitamin supplement.

Natabec-F.A. (Parke-Davis) Vitamins A 4000 IU, D 400 IU, B_1 3 mg, B_2 2 mg, B_6 3 mg, C 50 mg, B_{12} 5 mcg, B_3 10 mg, elemental calcium 240 mg, elemental iron 30 mg, folic acid 0.1 mg/Kapseal, magnesium, bisulfites. Bot. 100s. *otc.*
Use: Mineral, vitamin supplement.

Natabec with Fluoride. (Parke-Davis) Vitamins A 4000 IU, D 400 IU, B_1 3 mg, B_2 2 mg, B_6 3 mg, C 50 mg, B_{12} 5 mcg, B_3 10 mg, elemental calcium 240 mg, elemental iron 30 mg, elemental fluoride 1 mg/Kapseal. Bot. 100s. *Rx.*
Use: Vitamin supplement, dental caries agent.

Natacyn. (Alcon Laboratories) Natamycin 5%. Bot. 15 ml. *Rx.*
Use: Antifungal agent, ophthalmic.

Natalins. (Bristol-Myers Squibb) Ca 200 mg, iron 30 mg, vitamins A 4000 IU, D 400 IU, E 15 IU, B_1 1.5 mg, B_2 1.6 mg, B_3 17 mg, B_6 2.6 mg, B_{12} 2.5 mcg, C 70 mg, folic acid 0.5 mg, Mg, Cu, Zn 15 mg/Tab. Bot. 100s. *otc.*
Use: Mineral, vitamin supplement.

•**natamycin.** (NAT-uh-MY-sin) U.S.P. 23.
Use: Anti-infective, ophthalmic.
See: Natacyn, Susp. (Alcon Laboratories).

Natarex Prenatal. (Major) Ca 200 mg, iron 60 mg, vitamins A 4000 IU, D 400 IU, E 15 mg, B_1 1.5 mg, B_2 1.6 mg, B_3 17 mg, B_5 7 mg, B_6 4 mg, B_{12} 2.5 mcg, C 80 mg, folic acid 1 mg, Cu, Mg, Zn 25 mg, biotin 30 mcg/Tab. Bot 100s. *Rx.*
Use: Mineral, vitamin supplement.

Nata-San. (Sandia) Vitamins A 4000 IU, D 400 IU, B_1 5 mg, B_2 4 mg, B_6 10 mg, nicotinic acid 10 mg, C 100 mg, B_{12} activity 5 mcg, ferrous fumarate 200 mg (elemental iron 65 mg), calcium carbonate 500 mg (calcium 196 mg), copper (sulfate) 0.5 mg, magnesium (sulfate) 0.1 mg, manganese (sulfate) 0.1 mg, potassium (sulfate) 0.1 mg, zinc (sulfate) 0.5 mg/Tab. Bot. 100s, 1000s. *otc.*
Use: Mineral, vitamin supplement.

Nata-San F.A. (Sandia) Vitamins A 4000 IU, D 400 IU, B_1 5 mg, B_2 4 mg, B_6 10 mg, nicotinic acid 10 mg, C 100 mg, B_{12} activity 5 mcg, folic acid 1 mg, iron 65 mg, calcium 200 mg, copper (sulfate) 0.5 mg, magnesium (sulfate) 0.1 mg, manganese (sulfate) 0.1 mg, potassium (sulfate) 0.1 mg, zinc (sulfate) 0.5 mg/Tab. Bot. 100s, 1000s. *Rx.*
Use: Mineral, vitamin supplement.

Natodine. (Faraday) Iodine in organic form as found in kelp 1 mg/Tab. Bot. 100s, 250s. *otc.*

Natrapel. (Tender) Citronella 10% in 15% Aloe Vera base. *otc.*
Use: Insect repellent.

Natrico. (Drug Products) Potassium nitrate 2 g, sodium nitrite 1 g, nitroglycerin 0.25 g, crataegus oxycantha 0.25 gr/Pulvoid. Bot. 100s, 1000s. *Rx.*
Use: Antihypertensive.

Naturacil. (Bristol-Myers) Psyllium seed husks 3.4 g, carbohydrate 9.6 g, sodium 11 mg, 54 cal./2 pieces. Carton 24s, 40s. *otc.*
Use: Laxative.

Natur-Aid. (Scott/Cord) Lactose, pectin and Carob-lemon juice. Pow. 90%. Bot. 8 oz. *otc.*
Use: Increase in normal intestinal flora.

Natural Diuretic Water Tablet. (Amlab) Buchu leaves 1 g, uva ursi 1 g, trilicum 1 g, parsley 1 g, juniper berries 1 g, asparagus 1 g, alfalfa powder 1 gr/ Tab. Bot. 100s. *otc.*
Use: Diuretic.

natural lung surfactant.
See: Survanta (Ross Laboratories).

natural vegetable powder. (Various Mfr.) Psyllium hydrophilic mucilloid 3.4 g,

dextrose, sodium < 10 mg, 14 Cal/ Dose. Pow. 210 g, 420 g, 630 g. *otc.*
Use: Laxative.

natural vitamin a in oil.
See: Oleovitamin A, U.S.P.

Naturalyte. (UBI) Sodium 45 mEq, potassium 20 mEq, chloride 35 mEq, citrate 48 mEq, dextrose 25 g/L. Soln. Bot. 240 ml, 1 L. *otc.*
Use: Electrolyte, mineral supplement.

Nature's Aid Laxative Tabs. (Walgreens) Docusate sodium 100 mg, yellow phenolphthalein 65 mg/Tab. Bot. 60s. *otc.*
Use: Laxative.

Nature's Remedy Tablets. (SmithKline Beecham Pharmaceuticals) Aloe 100 mg, cascara sagrada 150 mg/FC Tab. Foil backed blister pkg. Box 12s, 30s, 60s. *otc.*
Use: Laxative.

Nature's Tears. (Rugby) Hydroxypropyl methylcellulose 2906 0.4%, KCl, NaCl, sodium phosphate, benzalkonium Cl 0.01%, EDTA. Soln. Bot. 15 ml. *otc.*
Use: Artificial tears.

Naturetin. (Bristol-Myers) Bendroflumethiazide. **5 mg/Tab.:** Bot. 100s, 1000s. **10 mg/Tab.:** Bot. 100s. *Rx.*
Use: Diuretic.

Natur-Lax Tablets. (Faraday) Rhubarb root, cape aloes, cascara sagrada extract, mandrake root, parsley, carrot. Protein coated tab. Bot. 100s. *otc.*
Use: Laxative.

Naus-A-Tories. (Table Rock) Pyrilamine maleate 25 mg, secobarbital 30 mg/ Supp. Box 12s. *c-II.*
Use: Antiemetic.

Nausea Relief. (Zenith Goldline) Dextrose 1.87 g, fructose 1.87 g, phosphoric acid 21.5 mg, methylparaben. Soln. Bot. 118 ml. *otc.*
Use: Antiemetic.

Nausetrol. (Qualitest) Fructose, dextrose, orthophosphoric acid with controlled hydrogen ion concentration. Soln. Bot. 118 ml, 473 ml, 3785 ml. *otc.*
Use: Antiemetic, antivertigo.

Navane. (Roerig) Thiothixene. **Cap.:** 1 mg, 2 mg, 5 mg, 10 mg or 20 mg. Bot. 100s, 500s, 1000s, UD 100s. **Liq.:** 5 mg/ml. Bot. 30 ml, 120 ml. *Rx.*
Use: Antipsychotic.

Navelbine. (GlaxoWellcome) Vinorelbine tartrate 10 mg/ml. Inj. Vial 1 ml, 5 ml. *Rx.*
Use: Antineoplastic.

Navidrix. Cyclopenthiazide. 3-Cyclopentylmethyl derivative of hydrochlorothiazide. *Rx.*
Use: Diuretic.

•**naxagolide hydrochloride.** (nax-AH-go-LIDE) USAN.
Use: Antiparkisonian; dopamine agonist.

Nazafair. (Various Mfr.) Naphazoline HCl 0.1%. Soln. Bot. 15 ml. *Rx.*
Use: Mydriatic, vasoconstrictor.

N D Clear. (Seatrace) Chlorpheniramine maleate 8 mg, pseudoephedrine HCl 120 mg/T.D. Cap. Bot. 100s, 1000s. *Rx.*
Use: Antihistamine, decongestant.

n-diethyl meta-toluamide.
W/Red Veterinary Petrolatum.
See: RV Pellent, Oint. (ICN Pharmaceuticals).

n-diethylvanillamide.
See: Ethamivan, Inj. (Various Mfr.).

ND-Gesic. (Hyrex) Acetaminophen 300 mg, pyrilamine maleate 12.5 mg, chlorpheniramine maleate 2 mg, phenylephrine HCl 5 mg/Tab. Bot. 100s, 1000s. *otc.*
Use: Analgesic, antihistamine, decongestant.

NDNA. (Wampole Laboratories) Anti-native DNA test by IFA. Confirmatory test for active SLE. Test 48s.
Use: Diagnostic aid.

•**nebacumab.** (neh-BACK-you-mab) USAN. *Formerly Septomonab.*
Use: Monoclonal antibody (antiendotoxin).

Nebcin. (Eli Lilly) Tobramycin sulfate. **Inj.:** 10 mg/ml (Vial 6 ml, 8 ml), 40 mg/ml (*Hyporets* 1.5 ml, 2 ml). **Pow. for Inj.:** 1.2 g. Vial 1.2 g. **Pediatric Inj.:** 10 mg/ ml Vial 2 ml. *Rx.*
Use: Anti-infective, aminoglycoside.

•**nebivolol.** (neh-BIV-oh-lole) USAN.
Use: Antihypertensive (beta blocker).

•**nebramycin.** (neh-brah-MY-sin) USAN. A complex of antibiotic substances produced by *Streptomyces tenebrarius.*
Use: Anti-infective.

NebuPent. (Fujisawa) Pentamidine isethionate 300 mg. Aerosol single dose vial. *Rx.*
Use: Anti-infective.

Nebu-Prel. (Mahon) Isoproterenol sulfate 0.4%, phenylephrine HCl 2%, propylene glycol 10%. Liq. Vial 10 ml. *Rx.*
Use: Bronchodilator.

Nechlorin. (Henry Schein) Chlorpheniramine 5 mg, phenylpropanolamine 40 mg, phenylephrine 20 mg, phenyltoloxamine 15 mg/Tab. Bot. 100s.

Use: Antihistamine, decongestant.

•**nedocromil.** (NEH-doe-KROE-mill) USAN.
Use: Antiallergic (prophylactic).

•**nedocromil calcium.** (NEH-doe-KROE-mill) USAN.
Use: Antiallergic (prophylactic).
See: Tilade.

•**nedocromil sodium.** (NEH-doe-KROE-mill) USAN.
Use: Antiallergic (prophylactic).
See: Tilade, Aerosol (Fisons).

N.E.E.. (Lexis) Ethinyl estradiol 35 mcg, norethindrone 1 mg/Tab. 6 pcks. 21s, 28s. *Rx.*
Use: Contraceptive.

•**nefazodone hydrochloride.** (neff-AZE-oh-dohn) USAN.
Use: Antidepressant.
See: Serzone, Tab. (Princeton).

•**neflumozide hydrochloride.** (neh-FLEW-moe-ZIDE) USAN.
Use: Antipsychotic.

•**nefocon a.** (NEE-FOE-kahn A) USAN.
Use: Contact lens material (hydrophilic).

•**nefopam hydrochloride.** (NEFF-oh-pam) USAN.
Use: Muscle relaxant; analgesic.

Negacide. (Sanofi Winthrop) Nalidixic acid. *Rx.*
Use: Anti-infective, urinary.

NegGram. (Sanofi Winthrop) Nalidixic acid. **1 g/Capl.:** UD 100s; **250 mg/Capl.:** Bot. 56s. **500 mg/Capl.:** Bot. 56s, 500s. **250 mg/5 ml/Susp:** Bot. 480 ml. *Rx.*
Use: Anti-infective, urinary.

•**nelezaprine maleate.** (neh-LEH-zah-PREEN) USAN.
Use: Muscle relaxant.

•**nelfilcon a.** (nell-FILL-kahn A) USAN.
Use: Contact lens material (hydrophilic).

•**nelfinavir mesylate.** (nell-FIN-ah-veer) USAN.
Use: Antiviral.
See: Viracept, Tab., Pow. (Agouron).

Nelova 0.5/35. (Warner Chilcott) Ethinyl estradiol 35 mcg, norethindrone 0.5 mg/Tab. 6 Pcks. 21 day and 28 day w/ 7 inert tabs. *Rx.*
Use: Contraceptive.

Nelova 1/35E. (Warner Chilcott) Norethindrone 1 mg, ethinyl estradiol 35 mcg/Tab. 21 day and 28 day (with 7 inert tabs.). *Rx.*
Use: Contraceptive.

Nelova 1/50M. (Warner Chilcott) Norethindrone 1 mg, mestranol 50 mcg/Tab. 21 day and 28 day (with 7 inert tabs). *Rx.*
Use: Contraceptive.

Nelova 10/11. (Warner Chilcott) **Phase 1-** Norethindrone 0.5 mg, ethinyl estradiol 35 mcg/Tab., 10 tabs.; **Phase 2-** Norethindrone 1 mg, ethinyl estradiol 35 mcg/Tab., 11 tabs. 21 day and 28 day (with 7 inert tabs). *Rx.*
Use: Contraceptive.

Nelulen. (Watson Laboratories) **1/35 E Tab.:** Ethynodiol diacetate 1 mg, ethinyl estradiol 35 mcg. Pcks 21s, 28s. **1/50 E Tab.:** Ethynodiol diacetate 1 mg, ethinyl estradiol 50 mcg. Pcks. 21s, 28s. *Rx.*
Use: Contraceptive.

nemazine. Under study.
Use: Anti-inflammatory.

•**nemazoline hydrochloride.** (neh-MAZZ-oh-leen) USAN.
Use: Decongestant, nasal.

Nembutal Elixir. (Abbott Laboratories) Pentobarbital 18.2 mg/5 ml, alcohol 18%. Bot. pt, gal. *c-II.*
Use: Hypnotic, sedative.

Nembutal Sodium. (Abbott Laboratories) Pentobarbital sodium. **Inj.:** 50 mg/ml. Amp 2 ml; Vial 20 ml, 50 ml. Box 5s. **Cap.:** 50 mg: Bot. 100s; 100 mg: Bot. 100s, 500s. Display pack 100s. **Supp.:** 30 mg, 60 mg, 120 mg or 200 mg. Box 12s. *c-II.*
Use: Hypnotic, sedative.

neoarsphenamine.

Neo-Benz-All. (Xttrium) Benzalkonium Cl 20.1%. Packet 25 ml 15s. To make gal of 1:750 soln. Also Aqueous Neo-Benz-All 1:750 soln. Packet 20 ml, 50s. *otc.*
Use: Antiseptic, antimicrobial.

Neo Beserol. (Sanofi Winthrop) Aspirin, methocarbamol. *Rx.*
Use: Analgesic, muscle relaxant.

Neocalamine. (Various Mfr.) Red ferric oxide 30 g, yellow ferric oxide 40 g, zinc oxide 930 g. *otc.*
Use: Astringent, antiseptic.

Neo-Calglucon. (Novartis) Glubionate calcium 1.8 g/5 ml. Syr. Bot. pt. *Rx.*
Use: Mineral supplement.

Neocate One +. (SHS) Protein 2.5 g (amino acids 3 g), carbohydrates 14.6 g (maltodextrin, sucrose), fat (fractionated) 3.5 g, coconut, canola, and high oleic sunflower oils, vitamins A, D, E, K, B_1, B_2, B_3, B_5, B_6, B_{12}, folic acid, biotin, C, choline, inositol, Ca, P, Mg, Fe, Zn, Mn, Cu, I, Mo, Cr, Se, Cl, Na 20 mg

(0.9 mEq), K 93 mg (2.4 mEq), 835 mOsm/kg per 100 ml, 100 cal/ml. Liq. Bot. 237 ml. *otc.*
Use: Nutritional supplement, enteral.

Neo-Cholex. (Lafayette Pharm) Fat emulsion containing 40%/w/v pure vegetable oil. Bot. 60 ml.
Use: Cholecystokinetic.

Neocidin. (Major) Polymyxin B sulfate 10,000 units, neomycin sulfate 1.75 mg, gramicidin 0.025 mg/ml. Soln. Bot. 10 ml. *Rx.*
Use: Anti-infective, ophthalmic.

neo-cobefrin.
Use: Vasoconstrictor.

Neo-Cortef Cream. (Pharmacia & Upjohn) Hydrocortisone acetate 10 mg (1%), neomycin sulfate 5 mg (0.5%), methylparaben 1 mg, butylparaben 4 mg, polysorbate 80, propylene glycol, cetyl palmitate, glyceryl monostearate, emulsifier/g. When necessary, pH adjusted with sulfuric acid. Tube 20 g. *Rx.*
Use: Anti-infective, corticosteroid, topical.

Neo-Cortef Ointment. (Pharmacia & Upjohn) **0.5%:** Hydrocortisone acetate 5 mg, neomycin sulfate 5 mg, methylparaben 0.2 mg, butylparaben 1.8 mg in a bland base of white petrolatum, microcrystalline wax, mineral oil, cholesterol/g. Tube 20 g. **1%:** Hydrocortisone acetate 10 mg, neomycin sulfate 5 mg/g. Oint. Tube 5 g, 20 g. *Rx.*
Use: Anti-infective, corticosteroid, topical.

Neo-Cultol. (Fisons) Refined mineral oil jelly. Chocolate flavored. Bot. 6 oz. *otc.*
Use: Laxative.

Neocurb. (Taylor Pharmaceuticals) Phendimetrazine tartrate 35 mg/Tab. Bot. 100s, 1000s. *c-III.*
Use: Anorexient.

Neocylate. (Schwarz Pharma) Potassium salicylate 280 mg, aminobenzoic acid 250 mg/Tab. Bot. 100s, 1000s. *otc.*
Use: Analgesic.

Neocyten. (Schwarz Pharma) Orphenadrine citrate 30 mg/ml. Vial 10 ml. *Rx.*
Use: Muscle relaxant.

NeoDecadron Ophthalmic Solution. (Merck) Dexamethasone sodium phosphate equivalent to 0.1% dexamethasone phosphate, neomycin sulfate equivalent to 0.35% mg neomycin base. Ocumeter ophthalmic dispenser 5 ml. *Rx.*
Use: Anti-infective, corticosteroid, ophthalmic.

Neo-Dexair. (Bausch & Lomb) Dexamethasone sodium phosphate 0.1%, neomycin sulfate 0.35%, polysorbate 80, EDTA, benzalkonium Cl 0.02%, sodium bisulfite 0.1%. Soln. Bot. 5 ml. *Rx.*
Use: Anti-infective, corticosteroid, ophthalmic.

Neo-Dexameth. (Major) Dexamethasone sodium phosphate 0.1%, neomycin sulfate 0.35%. Soln. Bot. 5 ml. *Rx.*
Use: Anti-infective, corticosteroid, ophthalmic.

Neo-Diaral. (Roberts Pharm) Loperamide 2 mg/Cap. Bot. UD 8s, 250s. *otc.*
Use: Antidiarrheal.

neodrenal.
See: Isoproterenol.

Neo-Durabolic. (Roberts Pharm) Nandrolone decanoate injection. **50 mg/ml** or **100 mg/ml:** Vial 2 ml. **200 mg/ml:** Vial 1 ml. *c-III.*
Use: Anabolic steroid.

Neo-fradin. (Pharma-Tek) Neomycin sulfate 125 mg/5 ml. Parabens. Oral Soln. Bot. 480 ml. *Rx.*
Use: Amebicide.

Neogesic Tablets. (Pal-Pak) Aspirin 194.4 mg, acetaminophen 129.6 mg, caffeine 32.4 mg/Tab. Bot. 1000s. *otc.*
Use: Analgesic combination.

Neoloid. (Kenwood Labs) Castor oil 36.4% (emulsified), sodium benzoate 0.1%, potassium sorbate 0.2%. Sugar free. Bot. 118 ml. *otc.*
Use: Laxative.

Neo-Mist Nasal Spray. (A.P.C.) Phenylephrine HCl 0.5%, cetalkonium Cl 0.02%. Spray Bot. 20 ml. *otc.*
Use: Antiseptic, decongestant.

Neo-Mist Pediatric 0.25% Nasal Spray. (A.P.C.) Phenylephrine HCl 0.25%, cetalkonium Cl 0.02%. Squeeze Bot. 20 ml. *otc.*
Use: Antiseptic, decongestant.

Neomixin. (Roberts Pharm) Bacitracin zinc 400 units, neomycin sulfate 3.5 mg, polymyxin B sulfate 5000 units in petrolatum base/g. Tube 15 g. *otc.*
Use: Anti-infective, topical.

neomycin base.
Use: Anti-infective.
W/Combinations.
See: Maxitrol, Oint., Susp. (Alcon Laboratories).
Neo-Cort-Dome, Cream, Lot. (Bayer Corp).
Neotal, Oint. (Roberts Pharm).

•**neomycin palmitate.** (NEE-oh-MY-sin

PAL-mih-tate) USAN.
Use: Anti-infective.
See: Biozyme, Oint. (Centeon).

neomycin and polymyxin B sulfates, bacitracin, and hydrocortisone acetate ointment.
Use: Anti-infective; antifungal; anti-inflammatory, topical.

neomycin and polymyxin B sulfates, bacitracin, and hydrocortisone acetate ophthalmic ointment.
Use: Anti-infective, antifungal, anti-inflammatory, topical.

neomycin and polymyxin B sulfates and bacitracin ointment.
Use: Anti-infective, topical.

neomycin and polymyxin B sulfates and bacitracin ophthalmic ointment.
Use: Anti-infective, topical.

neomycin and polymyxin B sulfates, bacitracin zinc, and hydrocortisone acetate ophthalmic ointment.
Use: Anti-infective, corticosteroid, topical.

neomycin and polymyxin B sulfates, bacitracin zinc, and hydrocortisone ointment.
Use: Anti-infective, corticosteroid, topical.

neomycin and polymyxin B sulfates, bacitracin zinc, and hydrocortisone ophthalmic ointment.
Use: Anti-infective, corticosteroid, topical.

neomycin and polymyxin B sulfates, bacitracin zinc, and lidocaine ointment.
Use: Anti-infective, topical.
See: Lanabiotic, Oint. (Combe).

neomycin and polymyxin B sulfates and bacitracin zinc ointment.
Use: Anti-infective, topical.

neomycin and polymyxin B sulfates and bacitracin zinc ophthalmic ointment.
Use: Anti-infective, ophthalmic.

neomycin and polymyxin B sulfates and bacitracin zinc topical aerosol. U.S.P. XXI.
Use: Anti-infective, topical.

neomycin and polymyxin B sulfates and bacitracin zinc topical powder. U.S.P. XXI.
Use: Anti-infective, topical.

neomycin and polymyxin B sulfates cream.
Use: Anti-infective, topical.

neomycin and polymyxin B sulfates and dexamethasone ophthalmic ointment. (Various Mfr.) Dexamethasone 0.1%, neomycin sulfate 0.35%, polymyxin B sulfate 10,000 units. Tube 3.5 g.
Use: Anti-infective, corticosteroid, ophthalmic.

neomycin and polymyxin B sulfates and dexamethasone ophthalmic suspension. (Various Mfr.) Dexamethasone 0.1%, neomycin sulfate 0.35%, polymyxin B sulfate 10,000 units. Bot. 5 ml, 10 ml.
Use: Anti-infective, corticosteroid, ophthalmic.

neomycin and polymyxin B sulfates and gramicidin cream.
Use: Anti-infective, topical.

neomycin and polymyxin B sulfates, gramicidin, and hydrocortisone acetate cream.
Use: Anti-infective, corticosteroid, topical.

neomycin and polymyxin B sulfates and gramicidin ophthalmic solution.
Use: Anti-infective, ophthalmic.

neomycin and polymyxin B sulfates and hydrocortisone acetate cream.
Use: Anti-infective, corticosteroid, topical.

neomycin and polymyxin B sulfates and hydrocortisone acetate ophthalmic suspension.
Use: Anti-infective, corticosteroid, ophthalmic.

neomycin and polymyxin B sulfates and hydrocortisone ophthalmic suspension. (Various Mfr.) Hydrocortisone 1%, neomycin sulfate 0.35%, polymyxin B sulfate 10,000 units. Bot. 7.5 ml, 10 ml.
Use: Anti-infective, corticosteroid, ophthalmic.

neomycin and polymyxin B sulfates and hydrocortisone otic solution.
Use: Anti-infective, corticosteroid, otic.

neomycin and polymyxin B sulfates and hydrocortisone otic suspension. (Steris) Polymyxin B sulfate equiv. to 10,000 polymyxin B units, neomycin sulfate equiv. to 3.5 mg neomycin base/ml. Hydrocortisone 1%, thimerosal 0.01%, cetyl alcohol, propylene glycol, polysorbate 80. Susp. Bot. 10 ml.
Use: Anti-infective, corticosteroid, otic.

neomycin and polymyxin B sulfates ophthalmic ointment.
Use: Anti-infective, ophthalmic.

neomycin and polymyxin B sulfates and prednisolone acetate ophthal-

mic suspension.
Use: Anti-infective, corticosteroid, ophthalmic.

neomycin and polymyxin B sulfates solution for irrigation.
Use: Irrigant, ophthalmic, anti-infective, topical.
See: Neosporin G.U. Irrigant (GlaxoWellcome).

neomycin and polymyxin B sulfates ophthalmic solution.
Use: Anti-infective, ophthalmic.

•**neomycin sulfate.** (NEE-oh-MY-sin) U.S.P. 23.
Use: Anti-infective.
See: Mycifradin Sulfate, Tab., Soln. (Pharmacia & Upjohn).
Myciguent, Oint., Ophth. Oint., Cream (Pharmacia & Upjohn).
Neo-fradin, Soln. (Pharma-Tek).
Neo-Tabs (Pharma-Tek).
W/Combinations.
See: AK-Spore, Preps. (Akorn).
Bacitracin Neomycin, Oint. (Various Mfr.).
Baximin, Oint. (Quality Formulations).
Biotres HC, Oint. (Schwarz Pharma).
B.N.P., Ophthalmic Oint. (Solvay).
B.P.N., Oint. (Procter & Gamble).
Bro-Parin, Otic Susp. (3M).
Coracin, Oint. (Roberts Pharm).
Cordran-N, Oint., Lot. (Eli Lilly).
Cor-Oticin, Liq. (Maurry).
Cortisporin, Preps. (GlaxoWellcome).
Epimycin A, Oint. (Delta).
Hi-Cort N, Cream (Blaine).
Hysoquen Oint. (Solvay).
Maxitrol, Ophth., Oint., Susp. (Alcon Laboratories).
Mity-Mycin, Oint. (Solvay).
Mycifradin Sulfate Sterile, Vial (Pharmacia & Upjohn).
Mycitracin, Oint., Ophth. Oint. (Pharmacia & Upjohn).
My-Cort, Oint., Cream, Soln. (Scrip).
Neo-Cort Dome, Otic Soln. (Bayer Corp).
Neo-Cortef, Preps. (Pharmacia & Upjohn).
Neo-Decadron, Ophth., Topical (Merck).
Neo-Delta-Cortef, Preps. (Pharmacia & Upjohn).
Neo-Hydeltrasol, Oint., Soln. (Merck).
Neo-Hytone, Cream (Dermick Laboratories).
Neo-Medrol, Preps. (Pharmacia & Upjohn).
Neo-Nysta-Cort, Oint. (Bayer Corp).
Neo-Oxylone, Oint. (Pharmacia & Upjohn).
Neosone, Ophth. Oint. (Pharmacia & Upjohn).
Neosporin, Preps. (GlaxoWellcome).
Neotal, Ophth. Oint. (Roberts Pharm).
Neo-Thrycex, Oint. (Del Pharmaceuticals).
Ocutricin, Preps. (Bausch & Lomb).
Otobione, Soln. (Schering Plough).
Otoreid-HC, Liq. (Solvay).
Spectrocin, Oint. (Squibb Diagnostic).
Statrol Sterile, Ophthalmic Oint. (Alcon Laboratories).
Tigo, Oint. (Burlington).
Tri-Bow, Oint. (Jones Medical Industries).
Tricidin, Oint. (Amlab).
Trimixin, Oint. (Hance).

neomycin sulfate. (Pharmacia & Upjohn) Pow. micronized for compounding. Bot. 100 g.
Use: Anti-infective.

neomycin sulfate and bacitracin ointment.
Use: Anti-infective, topical.

neomycin sulfate and bacitracin zinc ointment.
Use: Anti-infective, topical.

neomycin sulfate and dexamethasone sodium phosphate cream.
Use: Anti-infective, corticosteroid, topical.

neomycin sulfate and dexamethasone sodium phosphate ophthalmic ointment.
Use: Anti-infective, corticosteroid, ophthalmic.

neomycin sulfate and dexamethasone sodium phosphate ophthalmic solution. (Various Mfr.) Dexamethasone sodium phosphate 0.1%, neomycin sulfate 0.35%. Bot. 5 ml.
Use: Anti-infective, corticosteroid, ophthalmic.

neomycin sulfate and fluocinolone acetonide cream.
Use: Anti-infective, corticosteroid, topical.

neomycin sulfate and fluorometholone ointment.
Use: Anti-infective, corticosteroid, topical.

neomycin sulfate and flurandrenolide.
Use: Anti-infective, corticosteroid, topical
See: Cordran Prods. (Eli Lilly).

neomycin sulfate and gramicidin ointment.
Use: Anti-infective, topical.

neomycin sulfate and hydrocortisone.
Use: Anti-infective, corticosteroid, topical.

neomycin sulfate and hydrocortisone acetate.
Use: Anti-infective, corticosteroid.

neomycin sulfate and methylprednisolone acetate cream.
Use: Anti-infective, corticosteroid, topical.

neomycin sulfate, polymyxin B sulfate and gramicidin solution. (Various Mfr.) Polymyxin B sulfate 10,000 units/g, neomycin sulfate 1.75 mg/g, gramicidin 0.025 mg/ml. Bot. 2 ml, 10 ml. *Rx.*
Use: Anti-infective, ophthalmic.

neomycin sulfate, polymyxin B sulfate and lidocaine.
Use: Anti-infective; anesthetic, local.
See: Clomycin, Oint. (Roberts).
Neosporin Plus, Cream, Oint. (GlaxoWellcome).
Tribiotic Plus, Oint. (Thompson).

neomycin sulfate and prednisolone acetate ointment.
Use: Anti-infective, corticosteroid, topical.

neomycin sulfate and prednisolone acetate ophthalmic ointment.
Use: Anti-infective, corticosteroid, topical.

neomycin sulfate and prednisolone acetate ophthalmic suspension.
Use: Anti-infective, corticosteroid, topical.

neomycin sulfate and prednisolone sodium phosphate ophthalmic ointment.
Use: Anti-infective, corticosteroid, topical.

neomycin sulfate, sulfacetamide sodium, and prednisolone acetate ophthalmic ointment.
Use: Anti-infective, corticosteroid, topical.

neomycin sulfate and triamcinolone acetonide cream.
Use: Anti-infective, corticosteroid, topical.

neomycin sulfate and triamcinolone acetonide ophthalmic ointment.
Use: Anti-infective, corticosteroid, ophthalmic.

•**neomycin undecylenate.** (NEE-oh-MY-sin UHN-de-sih-LEN-ate) USAN.
Use: Anti-infective, antifungal.
See: Neodecyllin (Penick).

neomycorsone.
See: Neosone, Oint. (Pharmacia & Upjohn).

Neopap. (PolyMedica) Acetaminophen 125 mg/Supp. In 12s. *otc.*
Use: Analgesic.

Neopham 6.4%. (Pharmacia & Upjohn) Essential and non-essential amino acids 6.4%. Inj. 250 ml, 500 ml. *Rx.*
Use: Nutritional supplement, parenteral.

Neo Picatyl. (Sanofi Winthrop) Glycobiarsoln. *Rx.*
Use: Amebicide.

neoquinophan.
See: Neocinchophen (Various Mfr.).

Neo Quipenyl. (Sanofi Winthrop) Primaquine phosphate. *Rx.*
Use: Antimalarial.

Neoral Capsules. (Novartis) Cyclosporine 25 mg or 100 mg/Soft gelatin Cap. 9.5% dehydrated alcohol. Bot. UD 30s. *Rx.*
Use: Immunosuppressant.

Neoral Oral Solution. (Novartis) Cyclosporine 100 mg/ml. Denatured alcohol 9.5% Bot. 50 ml. *Rx.*
Use: Immunosuppressant.

Neosar. (Pharmacia & Upjohn) Cyclophosphamide. 100 mg, sodium bicarbonate 82 mg. Pow. for Inj. Vial 100 mg, 200 mg, 500 mg, 1 g, 2 g. *Rx.*
Use: Antineoplastic.

neo-skiodan.
Iodopyracet, Diodrast.

Neosporin Cream. (GlaxoWellcome) Polymyxin B sulfate, neomycin sulfate. Tube 0.5 oz, foil packet 1/32 oz. Ctn. 144s. *otc.*
Use: Anti-infective, topical.

Neosporin G.U. Irrigant. (GlaxoWellcome) Neomycin sulfate 40 mg, polymyxin B sulfate 200,000 units/ml. Amp. 1 ml. Box 10s, 50s, Multiple dose vial 20 ml. *Rx.*
Use: Irrigant, genitourinary.

Neosporin Ointment. (GlaxoWellcome) Polymyxin B sulfate 5000 units, bacitracin zinc 400 units, neomycin sulfate 5 mg/g. Tube 0.5 oz, 1 oz. Foil packet 1/32 oz. Box 144s. *otc.*
Use: Anti-infective, topical.

Neosporin Maximum Strength. (GlaxoWellcome) Polymyxin B sulfate 10,000 units, neomycin 3.5 mg, bacitracin 500 units/g, white petrolatum. Oint. Tube 15 g. *otc.*
Use: Anti-infective, topical.

Neosporin Ophthalmic Ointment, Sterile. (GlaxoWellcome) Polymyxin B sulfate 10,000 units, bacitracin zinc 400 units, neomycin sulfate 3.5 mg/g. Tube 3.5 g. *Rx.*

Use: Anti-infective, ophthalmic.

Neosporin Ophthalmic Solution, Sterile. (GlaxoWellcome) Polymyxin B sulfate 10,000 units, neomycin sulfate 1.75 mg, gramicidin 0.025 mg/ml. Bot. 10 ml. Drop-dose. *Rx.*
Use: Anti-infective, ophthalmic.

Neosporin Plus. (GlaxoWellcome) **Cream:** 10,000 polymyxin B sulfate, neomycin 3.5 mg and lidocaine 40 mg/g, methylparaben 0.25%, mineral oil, white petrolatum. Tube 15 g. **Oint.:** Polymyxin B sulfate 10,000 units, bacitracin zinc 500 units, neomycin 3.5 mg and lidocaine 40 mg per g. In a white petrolatum base. Tube 15 g. *otc.*
Use: Anti-infective, topical.

neostibosan. Ethylstibamine.

neostigine and atropine sulfate.
Use: Muscle stimulant.
See: Neostigine Min-I-Mix (IMS).

neostigmine. (nee-oh-STIGG-meen)
Use: Cholinergic.
See: Neostigmine Bromide (Lannett).
Neostigmine Methylsulfate (Various Mfr.).
Prostigmin (Roche Laboratories).

•**neostigmine bromide.** (nee-oh-STIGG-meen BROE-mide) U.S.P. 23.
Use: Cholinergic.
See: Prostigmin Bromide, Tab. (Roche Laboratories).

neostigmine bromide. (Lannett) 15 mg/Tab. 100s and 1000s.
Use: Cholinergic.

•**neostigmine methylsulfate.** (nee-oh-STIGG-meen METH-ill-SULL-fate) U.S.P. 23.
Use: Cholinergic.
See: Prostigmin methylsulfate, Vial (Roche Laboratories).

neostigmine methylsulfate. (Various Mfr.) 1:1000 Inj. In 10 ml vials. 1:2000 Inj. In 1ml amps. and 10 ml vials. 1:4000 Inj. In 1 ml amps.
Use: Cholinergic.

Neostigmine Min-I-Mix. (IMS) Atropine sulfate 1.2 mg, neostigmine methysulfate 2.5 mg. Inj. Vial.
Use: Cholinergic muscle stimulant.
Use: Mydriatic, vasoconstrictor.

Neostrate AHA for Age Spots and Skin Lightening. (NeoStrata) Hydroquinone 2%, glycolic acid, propylene glycol, sodium bisulfite, sodium sulfite, EDTA/Gel. 48 g. *otc.*
Use: Dermatologic.

neo-strepsan.
See: Sulfathiazole (Various Mfr.).

Neo-Synephrine. (Sanofi Winthrop) Phenylephrine HCl 2.5% or 10%. Soln. Bot. 5 ml (10%), 15 ml (2.5%). *Rx.*
Use: Mydriatic, vasoconstrictor.

Neo-Synephrine Hydrochloride. (Sanofi Winthrop) Phenylephrine HCl. **Spray:** 0.25% children and adult, 0.5% adult. **Regular:** Squeeze bot. 0.5 oz. **0.5% mentholated:** Squeeze bot. 0.5 oz. **Drops:** 0.125% infant; 0.25% children and adult; 0.5% adult; 1% adult extra strength. Bot. 1 oz; 0.25% and 1% also bot. 16 oz. **Jelly:** 0.5%. Tube 18.75 g. *otc.*
Use: Decongestant.

Neo-Synephrine Hydrochloride. (Sanofi Winthrop) Phenylephrine HCl. **Amp.:** 1%, Carpuject sterile cartridge-needle unit 10 mg/ml. (1 ml fill in 2 ml cartridge) w/22 gauge, 1.25 inch needle. Dispensing Bin 50s; Vial 1 ml Box 25s. *Rx.*
Use: Vasoconstrictor.

Neo-Synephrine Viscous Ophthalmic. (Sanofi Winthrop) Phenylephrine HCl 10%. Soln. Bot. 5 ml. *Rx.*
Use: Mydriatic, vasoconstrictor.

Neo-Tabs. (Pharma-Tek) Neomycin sulfate 500 mg (equivalent to 350 mg neomycin base)/Tab. Bot. 100s. *Rx.*
Use: Amebicide.

Neotal. (Roberts Pharm) Zinc bacitracin 400 units, polymyxin B sulfate 5000 units, neomycin sulfate 5 mg, petrolatum and mineral oil base/g. Tube 3.5 g. *Rx.*
Use: Anti-infective, ophthalmic.

Neo-Thrycex Oint. (Del Pharmaceuticals) Bacitracin, neomycin sulfate, polymyxin B sulfate. Tube 0.5 oz. *Rx.*
Use: Anti-infective, topical.

Neothylline. (Teva USA) Dyphylline. **200 mg/Tab.:** Bot. 100s, 1000s. **400 mg/Tab.:** Bot. 100s, 500s. *Rx.*
Use: Bronchodilator.

Neothylline-GG. (Teva USA) Dyphylline 200 mg, guaifenesin 200 mg/Tab. Bot. 100s, 1000s. *Rx.*
Use: Bronchodilator, expectorant.

Neotrace-4. (Fujisawa) Zinc 1.5 mg, copper 0.1 mg, chromium 0.85 mcg, manganese 25 mcg/ml. Vial 2 ml. *Rx.*
Use: Mineral supplement.

Neotricin HC. (Bausch & Lomb) Hydrocortisone acetate 1%, neomycin sulfate 0.35%, bacitracin zinc 400 units, polymyxin B sulfate 10,000 units. Oint. Tube 3.5 g. *Rx.*
Use: Anti-infective, corticosteroid, ophthalmic.

Neotricin Ophthalmic Ointment. (Bausch & Lomb) Polymyxin B sulfate 10,000 units, neomycin sulfate 3.5 mg, bacitracin 400 units/g. In 3.5 g. *Rx.*
Use: Anti-infective, ophthalmic.

Neotricin Ophthalmic Solution. (Bausch & Lomb) Polymyxin B sulfate 10,000 units, neomycin sulfate 1.75 mg, gramicidin 0.025 mg/ml. Dropper bot. 10 ml. *Rx.*
Use: Anti-infective, ophthalmic.

Neo-Trobex Injection. (Forest Pharmaceutical) Vitamins B_1 150 mg, B_6 10 mg, riboflavin 5-phosphate sodium 2 mg, niacinamide 150 mg, panthenol 10 mg, choline Cl 20 mg, inositol 20 mg/ml. Vial 30 ml. *Rx.*
Use: Vitamin supplement.

Neotrol. (Horizon) Phenylephrine HCl 0.25%, pyrilamine maleate 0.2%, cetalkonium Cl 0.05%, tyrothricin 0.03%, phenylmercuric acetate 1:50,000. Soln. Squeeze Bot. 20 ml. *otc.*
Use: Antihistamine, decongestant.

Neo-Vadrin Stress Formula Vitamins Plus Zinc. (Scherer) Vitamins E 45 IU, C 600 mg, folic acid 400 mcg, B_1 20 mg, B_2 10 mg, B_{12} 25 mcg, biotin 45 mcg, pantothenic acid 25 mg, copper 3 mg, zinc 23.9 mg/Tab. Bot. 60s. *otc.*
Use: Mineral, vitamin supplement.

Neo-Vadrin Time Release Vit. C. (Scherer) Vitamin C 500 mg/Cap. Bot. 50s, 100s. *otc.*
Use: Vitamin supplement.

Neo-Vadrin Vitamin B_6 TR. (Scherer) Vitamin B_6 100 mg/Cap. Bot. 100s. *otc.*
Use: Vitamin supplement.

Neoval. (Halsey) Vitamins A 10,000 IU, D 400 IU, B_1 10 mg, B_2 5 mg, B_6 2 mg, B_{12} 3 mcg, C 100 mg, E 5 mg, pantothenic acid 10 mg, niacinamide 30 mg, iron 15 mg, copper 1 mg, magnesium 5 mg, manganese 1 mg, zinc 1.5 mg, iodine 0.15 mg/Tab. Bot. 100s. *otc.*
Use: Mineral, vitamin supplement.

Neoval T. (Halsey) Vitamins A 10,000 IU, D 400 IU, B_1 15 mg, B_2 10 mg, B_6 2 mg, C 150 mg, B_{12} 7.5 mcg, E 5 mg, pantothenic acid 10 mg, E 5 mg, niacinamide 100 mg, iron 15 mg, magnesium 5 mg, manganese 1 mg, zinc 1.5 mg, copper 1 mg/Tab. Bot. 1000s. *otc.*
Use: Mineral, vitamin supplement.

Nephplex Rx. (Nephro-Tech) B_1 1.5 mg, B_2 1.7 mg, B_3 20 mg, B_5 10 mg, B_6 10 mg, B_{12} 6 mcg, C 60 mg, folic acid 1 mg, d-biotin 300 mcg/Tab. Bot. 100s. *Rx.*
Use: Mineral, vitamin supplement.

5.4% NephrAmine. (McGaw) Amino acid concentration 5.4%, nitrogen 0.65 g/100 ml. **Essential amino acids:** Isoleucine 560 mg, leucine 880 mg, lysine 640 mg, methionine 880 mg, phenylalanine 880 mg, threonine 400 mg, tryptophan 200 mg, valine 640 mg, histidine 250 mg/100 ml. **Nonessential amino acids:** Cysteine <20 mg/100 ml, sodium 5 mEq, acetate 44 mEq, chloride 3 mEq/L, sodium bisulfite. Inj. 250 ml. *Rx.*
Use: Nutritional supplement, parenteral.

nephridine.
See: Epinephrine (Various Mfr.).

Nephro-Calci. (R & D) Calcium carbonate 1.5 g/Chew. Tab. (600 mg calcium). Bot. 100s, 200s, 500s, 1000s. *otc.*
Use: Mineral supplement.

Nephrocaps Capsules. (Fleming) Vitamins B_1 1.5 mg, B_2 1.7 mg, B_3 20 mg, B_5 5 mg, B_6 10 mg, B_{12} 6 mcg, C 100 mg, folic acid 1 mg, biotin 150 mcg/Cap. Bot. 100s. *Rx.*
Use: Vitamin supplement.

Nephro-Fer. (R & D Laboratories) Ferrous fumarate 350 mg (iron 115 mg)/Tab. Bot. 30s. *otc.*
Use: Mineral supplement.

Nephro-Fer RX. (R & D Labs) Iron 106.9 mg, folic acid 1 mg. Tab. Bot. 120s. *Rx.*
Use: Mineral, vitamin supplement.

Nephron FA. (Nephro-Tech) Fe 200 mg, C 40 mg, B_1 1.5 mg, B_2 1.7 mg, B_3 20 mg, B_5 10 mg, B_6 10 mg, B_{12} 5 mcg, biotin 300 mcg, FA 1 mg, docusate sodium 75 mg/Tab. Bot. 100s. *Rx.*
Use: Mineral, vitamin supplement.

Nephron Inhalant and Vaporizer. (Nephron) Racemic epinephrine HCl 2.25%. Bot. 0.25 oz, 0.5 oz, 1 oz. *otc.*
Use: Bronchodilator.

Nephro-Vite Rx. (R & D Laboratories) Vitamins B_1 1.5 mg, B_2 1.7 mg, B_3 20 mg, B_5 10 mg, B_6 10 mg, B_{12} 6 mcg, C 60 mg, folic acid 1 mg, d-biotin 300 mcg/Tab. Bot. 100s. *Rx.*
Use: Mineral, vitamin supplement.

Nephro-Vite Rx + Fe. (R & D Laboratories) Iron 100 mg, Vitamins B_1 1.5 mg, B_2 1.7 mg, B_3 20 mg, B_5 10 mg, B_6 10 mg, B_{12} 6 mcg, C 60 mg, folic acid 1 mg, d-biotin 300 mcg, lactose/Tab. Bot. 120s. *Rx.*
Use: Mineral, vitamin supplement.

Nephro-Vite Vitamin B Complex & C Supplement. (R & D Laboratories) Vitamins B_1 1.5 mg, B_2 1.7 mg, B_3 20 mg, B_5 10 mg, B_6 10 mg, B_{12} 6 mcg, C

60 mg, folic acid 800 mcg, biotin 300 mcg/Tab. Bot. 100s. *otc.*
Use: Mineral, vitamin supplement.

Nephrox. (Fleming) Aluminum hydroxide 320 mg, mineral oil 10%/5 ml. Bot. pt. *otc.*
Use: Antacid.

Nepro. (Ross Laboratories) Protein 6.6 g (as Ca, Mg and Na caseinates), fat 22.7 g (as 90% high-oleic safflower oil, 10% soy oil), carbohydrate 51.1 g (as sucrose, hydrolyzed corn starch), vitamins A, D, E, K, C, B_1, B_3, B_5, B_6, B_{12}, biotin, FA, Na, K, Cl, Ca, P, Mg, I, Mn, Cu, Zn, Fe 4.5 mg, Se/240 ml. Bot. 59.4 calories. Liq. Can. 240 ml. *otc.*
Use: Nutritional supplement, enteral.

Neptazane. (ESI Lederle Generics) Methazolamide 25 mg or 50 mg/Tab. Bot. 100s. *Rx.*
Use: Carbonic anhydrase inhibitor.

neraval.
Use: Anesthetic, general.

•**nerelimomab.** (neh-reh-LI-moe-mab) USAN.
Use: Monoclonal antibody.

Nervine Nighttime Sleep-Aid. (Bayer Corp) Diphenhydramine HCl 25 mg/Tab. Bot. 12s, 30s, 50s. *otc.*
Use: Sleep aid.

Nervocaine. (Keene Pharmaceuticals) Lidocaine HCl 1%/Inj. Vial 50 ml. *Rx.*
Use: Anesthetic, local.

Nesacaine. (Astra) Chloroprocaine HCl 1% or 2%, methylparaben, EDTA. Inj. Vial 30 ml. *Rx.*
Use: Anesthetic, local.

Nesacaine-CE. (Astra) **Conc. 2%:** Chloroprocaine HCl 20 mg/ml in a sterile soln. containing sodium bisulfite, sodium Cl, HCl. Vial 30 ml. **Conc. 3%:** Chloroprocaine HCl 30 mg/ml in a sterile soln. containing sodium bisulfite, sodium Cl, HCl. Vial 30 ml. *Rx.*
Use: Anesthetic, local.

Nesacaine-MPF. (Astra) Chloroprocaine HCl 2% or 3%. EDTA or preservative-free. Inj. Vial 30 ml. *Rx.*
Use: Anesthetic, local.

Nesa Nine Cap. (Standex) Vitamins A 5000 IU, D 400 IU, C 37.5 mg, B_1 1.5 mg, B_2 2 mg, niacinamide 20 mg, B_6 0.1 mg, calcium pantothenate 1 mg, E 2 IU/Cap. Bot. 100s. *otc.*
Use: Mineral, vitamin supplement.

nesdonal sodium.
See: Thiopental Sodium U.S.P. 23.
Pentothal Sodium, Prods. (Abbott Laboratories).

Nestabs. (Fielding) Vitamins A 5000 IU, D 400 IU, E 30 mg, C 120 mg, B_1 3 mg, B_2 3 mg, B_3 20 mg, B_6 3 mg, B_{12} 8 mcg, calcium 200 mg, iron 36 mg, folic acid 0.8 mg, zinc 15 mg, I/Tab. Bot. 100s. *otc.*
Use: Mineral, vitamin supplement.

Nestabs FA Tablets. (Fielding) Vitamins A 5000 IU, D 400 IU, E 30 mg, C 120 mg, B_1 3 mg, B_2 3 mg, B_3 20 mg, B_6 3 mg, B_{12} 8 mcg, Ca 200 mg, iron 36 mg, folic acid 1 mg, zinc 15 mg, I/Tab. Bot. 100s. *Rx.*
Use: Mineral, vitamin supplement.

Nestrex. (Fielding) Pyridoxine 25 mg/Tab., dextrose. Bot. 100s. *otc.*
Use: Vitamin supplement.

Nethamine.
W/Codeine phosphate, phenylephrine HCl, sodium citrate, doxylamine succinate.
See: Mercodol with Decapryn. Syr. (Hoechst Marion Roussel).

•**netilmicin sulfate.** (neh-TILL-MY-sin SULL-fate) U.S.P. 23.
Use: Anti-infective.
See: Netromycin (Schering Plough).

•**netrafilcon a.** (NET-rah-FILL-kahn A) USAN.
Use: Contact lens material (hydrophilic).

netrin. Under Study.
Use: Anticholinergic.
See: Metcaraphen HCl.

Netromycin. (Schering Plough) Netilmicin 100 mg/ml. Inj. Vial 1.5 ml Box 10s, 25s. Multi-dose vial 15 ml Box 5s. Disposable Syringe 1.5 ml Box 10s. *Rx.*
Use: Anti-infective, aminoglycoside.

neulactil.
See: Pericyazine.

Neumega. (Genetics Institute) Oprelvekin 5 mg. Pow. for Inj. Box. Single-dose Vial with 5 ml diluent. *Rx.*
Use: Antithrombotic.

Neupogen. (Amgen). Filgrastim (G-CSF) 300 mcg/ml. Vial 1 ml, 1.6 ml. *Rx.*
Use: Immunomodulator.

Neurodep-Caps. (Medical Products) Vitamins B_1 125 mg, B_6 125 mg, B_{12} 1000 mcg/Cap. Bot. 50s. *otc.*
Use: Vitamin supplement.

Neurodep Injection. (Medical Products) Vitamins B_1 50 mg, B_2 5 mg, B_3 125 mg, B_5 6 mg, B_6 5 mg, B_{12} 1000 mcg, C 50 mg/ml. Inj. Vial 10 ml. *Rx.*
Use: Vitamin supplement, parenteral.

Neurontin. (Parke-Davis) Gabapentin 100 mg, 300 mg, 400 mg; lactose. Cap.

Bot. 100s, UD 50s. *Rx.*
Use: Anticonvulsant.

neurosin.
See: Calcium glycerophosphate (Various Mfr.).

Neut (sodium bicarbonate 4% additive solution). (Abbott Laboratories) Sodium bicarbonate 4%. Vial (2.4 mEq each of sodium and bicarbonate), disodium edetate anhydrous 0.05% as stabilizer. Pintop Vial 5 ml, 10 ml. Box 25s, 100s. *Rx.*
Use: Nutritional supplement, parenteral.

neutral acriflavin.
See: Acriflavin (Various Mfr.).

Neutralin. (Dover Pharmaceuticals) Calcium carbonate, magnesium oxide/Tab. Sugar, lactose and salt free. UD Box 500s. *otc.*
Use: Antacid.

neutral protamine hagedorn-insulin.
See: Insulin, N.P.H. Iletin (Eli Lilly).

•**neutramycin.** (NEW-trah-MY-sin) USAN. A neutral macrolide antibiotic produced by a variant strain of *Streptomyces rimosus.*
Use: Anti-infective.

Neutrexin. (US Bioscience) Trimetrexate glucuronate 25 mg. Pow. for Inj. (lyophilized). Vial 5 ml w/wo 50 mg leucovorin. *Rx.*
Use: Anti-infective.

neutroflavin.
See: Acriflavine (Various Mfr.).

Neutrogena Acne Mask. (Neutrogena) Benzoyl peroxide 5% in sebum absorbing facial mask vehicle, SD alcohol 40, glycerin, titanium dioxide. Tube 60 g. *otc.*
Use: Dermatologic, acne.

Neutrogena Antiseptic Cleanser for Acne-Prone Skin. (Neutrogena) Benzethonium Cl, butylene glycol, methylparaben, menthol, peppermint oil, eucalyptus oil, cornmint oil, rosemary oil, witch hazel extract, camphor. Liq. Bot. 135 ml. *otc.*
Use: Dermatologic, acne.

Neutrogena Baby Cleansing Formula Soap. (Neutrogena) Triethanolamine, glycerin, stearic acid, tallow, coconut oil, castor oil, sodium hydroxide, oleic acid, laneth-10 acetate, cocamide DEA, nonoxynol 14, PEG-4 octoate. Bar 105 g. *otc.*
Use: Dermatologic, cleanser.

Neutrogena Body Lotion. (Neutrogena) Glyceryl stearate, isopropyl myristate, PEG-100 stearate, butylene glycol, imidazolidinyl urea, carbomer-934, parabens, sodium lauryl sulfate, triethanolamine, cetyl alcohol. Lot. Bot. 240 ml. *otc.*
Use: Emollient.

Neutrogena Body Oil. (Neutrogena) Isopropyl myristate, sesame oil, PEG-40 sorbitan peroleate, parabens. Bot. 240 ml. *otc.*
Use: Emollient.

Neutrogena Chemical-Free Sunblocker. (Neutrogena) Titanium dioxide, parabens, diazolidinyl urea, shea butter. SPF 17. Lot. Bot. 120 ml. *otc.*
Use: Sunscreen.

Neutrogena Cleansing for Acne-Prone Skin. (Neutrogena) TEA-stearate, triethanolamine, glycerin, sodium tallowate, sodium cocoate, TEA-oleate, sodium ricinoleate, acetylated lanolin alcohol, cocamide DEA, TEA lauryl sulfate, tocopherol. Bar 105 g. *otc.*
Use: Dermatologic, cleanser.

Neutrogena Drying. (Neutrogena) Witch hazel, isopropyl alcohol, EDTA, parabens, tartrazine. Gel. Tube 22.5 g. *otc.*
Use: Dermatologic, acne.

Neutrogena Dry Skin Soap. (Neutrogena) Triethanolamine, stearic acid, tallow, glycerin, coconut oil, castor oil, sodium hydroxide, oleic acid, laneth-10 acetate, cocamide DEA, nonoxynol 14, PEG-14 octoate, BHT, O-tolyl biguanide. Bar 105 g, 165 g. Scented or unscented. *otc.*
Use: Dermatologic, cleanser.

Neutrogena Glow Sunless Tanning. (Neutrogena) Octyl methoxycinnamate, cetyl alcohol, diazolidinyl urea, parabens, EDTA. SPF 8. Lot. Bot. 120 ml. *otc.*
Use: Sunscreen.

Neutrogena Intensified Day Moisture. (Neutrogena) Octyl methoxycinnamate, 2-phenylbenzimidazole sulfonic acid, titanium dioxide, cetyl alcohol, diazolidinyl urea, parabens, EDTA. SPF 15. Cream 67.5 g. *otc.*
Use: Dermatologic, moisturizer.

Neutrogena Lip Moisturizer. (Neutrogena) Octyl methoxycinnamate, benzophenone-3, corn oil, castor oil, mineral oil, lanolin oil, petrolatum, lanolin, stearyl alcohol. SPF 15. Lip balm 4.5 g. *otc.*
Use: Lip protectant.

Neutrogena Moisture SPF 5. (Neutrogena) Octyl methoxycinnamate, petrolatum, cetyl alcohol, parabens, diazolidinyl urea, EDTA, cetyl alcohol. Lot.

Bot 60 ml, 120 ml. *otc.*
Use: Dermatologic, moisturizer.

Neutrogena Moisture SPF 15. (Neutrogena) Octyl methoxycinnamate, benzophenone-3, glycerine, PEG 100 stearate, dimethicone, PEG-6000 monostearate, triethanolamine, parabens, imidazolidinyl urea, carbomer 954, PABA free. Lot. Bot. 120 ml. *otc.*
Use: Sunscreen.

Neutrogena Non-Drying Cleansing. (Neutrogena) Glycerin, caprylic/capric triglyceride, PEG-20 almond glycerides, cetyl recinoleate, isohexadecane, TEA-cocoyl glutamate, PEG-20 methyl glucose sesquistearate, stearyl alcohol, cetyl alcohol, EDTA, dipotassium glycyrrhizate, stearyl glycyrrhetinate, bisabolol, parabens, acrylates/C 10-30 alkyl acrylate crosspolymer, triethanolamine, diazolidinyl urea. Lot. Bot. 165 ml. *otc.*
Use: Dermatologic, cleanser.

Neutrogena Norwegian Formula Emulsion. (Neutrogena) Glycerin base 2%. Pump dispenser 5.25 oz. *otc.*
Use: Emollient.

Neutrogena Norwegian Formula Hand Cream. (Neutrogena) Glycerin base 41%. Tube 2 oz. *otc.*
Use: Emollient.

Neutrogena No-Stick Sunscreen. (Neutrogena) SPF 30. Homosalate 15%, octyl methoxycinnamate 7.5%, benzophenone-3 6%, octyl salicylate 5%, EDTA, parabens, diazolidinyl urea/ Cream. Waterproof 118 g. *otc.*
Use: Sunscreen.

Neutrogena Oil-Free Acne Wash. (Neutrogena) Salicylic acid 2%, EDTA, propylene glycol, tartrazine, aloe extract. Liq. Bot. 180 ml. *otc.*
Use: Dermatologic, acne.

Neutrogena Oily Skin Formula Soap. (Neutrogena) Triethanolamine, glycerin, fatty acids. Bar 3.5 oz. *otc.*
Use: Dermatologic, cleanser.

Neutrogena Original Formula Soap. (Neutrogena) Triethanolamine, glycerin, fatty acids. Bar 3.5 oz, 5.5 oz. *otc.*
Use: Dermatologic, cleanser.

Neutrogena Soap. (Neutrogena) TEA-stearate, triethanolamine, glycerin, sodium tallowate, sodium cocoate, sodium ricinoleate, TEA-oleate, cocamide DEA, tocopherol. Bar 105 g, 165 g. *otc.*
Use: Dermatologic, cleanser.

Neutrogena Sunblock. (Neutrogena) **SPF 8:** Octyl methoxycinnamate, menthyl anthranilate, titanium dioxide, mineral oil. Cream 67.5 g. **SPF 15:** Octyl methoxycinnamate, octyl salicylate, menthyl anthranilate, mineral oil, titanium dioxide, propylparaben. Cream 67.5 g. **SPF 25:** Octyl methoxycinnamate, benzophenone-3, octyl salicylate, castor oil, cetearyl alcohol, propylparaben, shea butter. Stick 12.6 g. **SPF30:** Octocrylene, octyl methoxycinnamate, menthyl anthranilate, zinc oxide, mineral oil, vitamin E. Cream 67.5 g. *otc.*
Use: Sunscreen.

Neutrogena Sunscreen. (Neutrogena) Ethylhexyl p-methoxycinnamate 7%, oxybenzone 4%, titanium dioxide 2%. Tube 3 oz. *otc.*
Use: Sunscreen.

Neutrogena T/Gel. (Neutrogena) Coal tar extract 2%. Shampoo. Bot. 132 ml. *otc.*
Use: Antiseborrheic.

Neutrogena T/Sal. (Neutrogena) Salicylic acid 2%, solubilized coal tar extract 2%. Shampoo. Bot. 135 ml. *otc.*
Use: Antiseborrheic.

neutropin-1.
Use: Motor neuron disease/amyothrophic lateral sclerosis. [Orphan drug]

•**nevirapine.** (neh-VIE-rah-peen) USAN.
Use: Antiviral.
See: Viramune, Tab. (Roxane).

New Decongest Pediatric Syrup. (Zenith Goldline) Phenylpropanolamine HCl 5 mg, phenylephrine HCl 1.25 mg, chlorpheniramine maleate 0.5 mg, phenyltoloxamine citrate 2 mg/5 ml. Syr. Bot. pt, gal. *Rx.*
Use: Antihistamine, decongestant.

New Decongestant. (Zenith Goldline) Phenylpropanolamine HCl 40 mg, phenylephrine HCl 10 mg, chlorpheniramine maleate 5 mg/ SR Tab. Bot. 100s, 1000s. *otc, Rx.*
Use: Antihistamine, decongestant.

•**nexeridine hydrochloride.** (NEX-eh-RIH-deen) USAN.
Use: Analgesic.

NG-29.
Use: Diagnostic aid. [Orphan drug]

N.G.T. (Geneva Pharm) Triamcinolone acetonide 0.1%, nystatin 100,000 units/g. Cream. Tube 15 g. *Rx.*
Use: Antifungal, corticosteroid, topical.

Nia-Bid. (Roberts Pharm) Niacin 400 mg/ TR Cap. Bot. 100s. *otc.*
Use: Vitamin supplement.

Niacal. (Jones Medical Industries) Cal-

cium lactate 324 mg, niacin 25 mg/Tab. Peppermint flavor. Bot. 100s, 1000s. *otc.*
Use: Vasodilator, vitamin supplement.

niacamide.
See: Nikethamide (Various Mfr.).

•**niacin.** (NYE-uh-sin) U.S.P. 23.
Use: Antihyperlipidemic; vitamin (enzyme co-factor).
See: Efacin, Tab. (Person & Covey).
Niac, Cap. (Cole).
Niaspan, ER Tab. (KOS).
Nico-400 (Hoechst Marion Roussel).
Ni Cord XL, Cap. (Scott/Cord).
Nicotinex, Elix. (Fleming).
Span Niacin 300, Tab. (Scrip).

niacin w/combinations.
See: Lipo-Nicin, Tab., Cap. (ICN Pharmaceuticals).
Vasostim, Cap. (Dunhall Pharmaceuticals).

•**niacinamide.** (nye-ah-SIN-ah-mide) U.S.P. 23.
Use: Vitamin (enzyme co-factor).
W/Pentylenetetrazol, thiamine HCl, cyanocobalamin, alcohol.
See: Cenalene, Tab., Elix. (Schwarz Pharma).
W/Potassium iodide.
See: Iodo-Niacin, Tab. (Cole).
W/Riboflavin.
See: Riboflavin and Niacinamide, Amp. (Eli Lilly).

Niacor. (Upsher-Smith Labs) Niacin 500 mg/Tab. Bot. 100s. *Rx.*
Use: Vitamin supplement.

Nialexo-C. (Roberts Pharm) Niacin 50 mg, vitamin C 30 mg/Tab. Bot. 100s. *otc.*
Use: Vitamin supplement.

Niarb Super. (Miller) Magnesium 100 mg, vitamin C 200 mg, niacinamide 200 mg (as ascorbate)/Tab. Bot. 100s. *otc.*
Use: Mineral, vitamin supplement.

Niaspan. (KOS) Niacin 375 mg, 500 mg, 750 mg, 1000 mg. ER Tab. Bot. 100s. Starter packs. *Rx.*
Use: Antihyperlipidemic.

Niazide. (Major) Trichlormethiazide 4 mg/Tab. Bot. 100s, 1000s. *Rx.*
Use: Diuretic.

niazo. Neotropin.
Use: Antiseptic, urinary.

•**nibroxane.** (nye-BROX-ane) USAN.
Use: Antimicrobial, topical.

nicamindon.
See: Nicotinamide (Various Mfr.).

•**nicardipine hydrochloride.** (NYE-CAR-dih-peen) USAN.
Use: Vasodilator.
See: Cardene (Syntex).

nicardipine hydrochloride. (Mylan) 20 mg and 30 mg/Cap. 90s and 500s. *Rx.*
Use: Vasodilator.

N'ice. (SmithKline Beecham Pharmaceuticals) Menthol 5 mg/Loz. in sugarless sorbitol base, saccharin. Pkg. 16s. *otc.*
Use: Anesthetic, local.

N'ice 'n Clear. (SmithKline Beecham Pharmaceuticals) Menthol 5 mg, sorbitol. Loz. Pkg. 16s. *otc.*
Use: Anesthetic, local.

N'ice Throat Spray. (SmithKline Beecham Pharmaceuticals) Menthol 0.12%, glycerin 25%, alcohol 23%, glucose, saccharin, sorbitol. Spray. 180 ml. *otc.*
Use: Mouth and throat preparation.

N'ice w/Vitamin C Drops. (SmithKline Beecham Consumer Healthcare) Ascorbic acid 60 mg, menthol, sorbitol, tartrazine/Loz. Pks. 16s. *otc.*
Use: Vitamin supplement, anesthetic, local.

•**nicergoline.** (nice-ERR-go-leen) USAN.
Use: Vasodilator.

Nichols Syphon Powder. (Last) Sodium bicarbonate, sodium Cl, sodium borate. Pouch 12.2 g (add to 32 oz. water to yield isotonic soln.).

•**niclosamide.** (nye-CLOSE-ah-mide) USAN.
Use: Antihelmintic.

Nico-400. (Jones Medical Industries) Niacin 400 mg/Cap. Bot. 100s. *otc.*
Use: Vitamin supplement.

nicobion.
See: Nicotinamide (Various Mfr.).

Nicoderm. (Hoechst Marion Roussel) Total nicotine content 36 mg or 114 mg/patch. 14 systems/box. *Rx.*
Use: Smoking deterrent.

nicoduozide. A mixture of nicothazone and isoniazid.

•**nicorandil.** (NIH-CAR-an-dill) USAN.
Use: Coronary vasodilator.

Ni Cord XL Caps. (Scott/Cord) Nicotinic acid 400 mg/Cap. Bot. 100s, 500s. *otc.*
Use: Vitamin supplement.

Nicorette. (SmithKline Beecham Pharmaceuticals) Nicotine polacrilex 2 mg/Chew. piece. Box 96s. *Rx.*
Use: Smoking deterrent.

nicotamide.
See: Nicotinamide (Various Mfr.).

nicothazone. Nicotinaldehyde thiosemicarbazone.

nicotilamide.
See: Nicotinamide (Various Mfr.).

nicotinamide. Niacinamide, U.S.P. 23. Vitamin B_3, Aminicotin, Dipegyl, Nicamindon, Nicotamide, Nicotilamide, Nicotinic Acid Amide.

nicotinamide adenine dinucleotide. Name used for Nadide.

•**nicotine.** (NIK-oh-TEEN) U.S.P. 23.
Use: Smoking cessation adjunct.
See: Nicotrol NS, Spray (McNeil Consumer Products).

nicotine transdermal systems.
Use: Smoking deterrent.
See: Habitrol (Basel Pharm)
Nicoderm (Hoechst Marion Roussel).
Nicotrol (Parke-Davis).
Prostep (ESI Lederle Generics).

•**nicotine polacrilex.** (NIK-oh-TEEN PAHL-ah-KRILL-ex) U.S.P. 23.
Use: Smoking cessation adjunct.
See: Nicorette (Hoechst Marion Roussel).

nicotine resin complex.
See: nicotine polacrilex.

Nicotinex Elixir. (Fleming) Niacin 50 mg/5 ml, alcohol 14%. Bot. pt, gal.
Use: Vitamin B_3 supplement.

nicotinic acid. Niacin, U.S.P. 23.

nicotinic acid w/combinations.
See: Niacin w/Combinations (Various Mfr.).

nicotinic acid amide. Niacinamide, U.S.P. 23.
See: Niacinamide (Various Mfr.).

•**nicotinyl alcohol.** (NIK-oh-TIN-ill AL-koe-hahl) USAN.
Use: Vasodilator (peripheral).

nicotinyl tartrate. 3-Pyridinemethanol tartrate.
See: Roniacol Timespan, Tab. (Roche Laboratories).

Nicotrol. (McNeil Consumer Products) Total nicotine content 8.3 mg, 16.6 mg or 24.9 mg/patch. 14 systems/box. Nicotine 15 mg/Patch. Kit. 7 patches. *otc.*
Use: Smoking deterrent.

Nicotrol NS. (McNeil Consumer Products) Nicotine 0.5 mg per actuation, methlyparaben, propylparaben, EDTA/Spray, pump. Bot. 10 ml. (200 sprays). *Rx.*
Use: Smoking deterrent.

nidroxyzone.

nieraline.
See: Epinephrine (Various Mfr.).

•**nifedipine.** (nye-FED-ih-peen) U.S.P. 23.
Use: Coronary vasodilator, urinary tract agent. [Orphan drug]
See: Adalat, Cap. (Bayer Corp).
Adalat CC, ER Tab. (Bayer Corp).
Procardia, Cap. (Pfizer).

nifedipine. (Various Mfr.) Nifedipine 10 mg or 20 mg/Tab. In 100s, 300s and UD 100s. *Rx.*
Use: Calcium channel blocker.

Niferex. (Schwarz Pharma) **Elix.:** Iron 100 mg/5 ml polysaccharide-iron complex, alcohol 10%. Sugar and dye free. Bot. 236 ml. **Tab.:** Iron 50 mg. Bot. 100s. *otc.*
Use: Mineral supplement.

Niferex-150. (Schwarz Pharma) Polysaccharide iron complex equivalent to iron 150 mg/Cap. Bot. UD 100s. *otc.*
Use: Mineral supplement.

Niferex-150 Forte Capsules. (Schwarz Pharma) Elemental iron as polysaccharide-iron complex 150 mg, folic acid 1 mg, vitamin B_{12} 25 mcg/Cap. Bot. 100s, 1000s. *Rx.*
Use: Mineral, vitamin supplement.

Niferex-PN. (Schwarz Pharma) Iron 60 mg, folic acid 1 mg, vitamins C 50 mg, B_{12} 3 mcg, A 4000 IU, D 400 IU, B_1 3 mg, B_2 3 mg, B_6 2 mg, B_3 10 mg, Zn 18 mg, Ca, sorbitol/Tab. Bot. 30s, 100s, 1000s. *Rx.*
Use: Mineral, vitamin supplement.

Niferex-PN Forte Tablets. (Schwarz Pharma) Calcium 250 mg, iron 60 mg, vitamins A 5000 IU, D 400 IU, E 30 mg, B_1 3 mg, B_2 3.4 mg, B_3 20 mg, B_6 4 mg, B_{12} 12 mcg, C 80 mg, folic acid 1 mg, Cu, I, Mg, zinc 25 mg/Tab. Bot. 100s. *Rx.*
Use: Mineral, vitamin supplement.

•**nifluridide.** (nye-FLURE-ih-DIDE) USAN.
Use: Ectoparasiticide.

•**nifungin.** (nih-FUN-jin) USAN. Substance derived from *Aspergillus giganteus.*

•**nifuradene.** (NYE-fyoor-ad-EEN) USAN.
Use: Anti-infective.

•**nifuraldezone.** (NYE-fer-AL-dee-zone) USAN. (Eaton Medical).
Use: Anti-infective.

•**nifuratel.** (NYE-fyoor-at-ell) USAN.
Use: Anti-infective, antifungal, antiprotozoal (trichomonas).

•**nifuratrone.** (nye-FYOOR-ah-trone) USAN.
Use: Anti-infective.

•**nifurdazil.** (NYE-fyoor-dazz-ill) USAN.
Use: Anti-infective.

nifurethazone.
Use: Anti-infective.

•**nifurimide.** (nye-FYOOR-ih-MIDE) USAN.

Use: Anti-infective.

•**nifurmerone.** (NYE-fyoor-MER-ohn) USAN.
Use: Antifungal.

nifuroxime.
Use: Antifungal, anti-infective, topical, antiprotozoal.
See: Micofur.
W/Furazolidone.
See: Tricofuron, Pow., Supp. (Eaton Medical).

•**nifurpirinol.** (nye-fer-PIHR-ih-nole) USAN.
Use: Anti-infective.

•**nifurquinazol.** (NYE-fyoor-KWIN-azz-ole) USAN.
Use: Anti-infective.

•**nifurthiazole.** (NYE-fyoor-THIGH-ah-zole) USAN.
Use: Anti-infective.

nifurtimox.
Use: CDC anti-infective agent.
See: Lampit (Bayer Corp 2502).

Night-Time Effervescent Cold Tablets. (Zenith Goldline) Phenylpropanolamine HCl 15 mg, diphenhydramine citrate 38.33 mg, aspirin 325 mg/Tab. Pkg. 20s. *otc.*
Use: Analgesic, antihistamine, decongestant.

Nighttime Pamprin. (Chattem Consumer Products) Diphenhydramine HCl 50 mg, acetaminophen 650 mg. Pow. Pkg. 4s. *otc.*
Use: Sleep aid.

NightTime TheraFlu. (Novartis) Pseudoephedrine HCl 60 mg, chlorpheniramine maleate 4 mg, dextromethorphan HBr 30 mg, acetaminophen 1000 mg. Powd. 6s. *otc.*
Use: Analgesic, antihistamine, antitussive, decongestant.

nigrin. Streptonigrin.
Use: Antineoplastic.

Niko-Mag. (Scruggs) Magnesium oxide 500 mg/Cap. Bot. 100s, 1000s. *otc.*
Use: Antacid.

Nikotime TD Caps. (Major) Niacin 125 mg or 250 mg/TD Cap. Bot. 100s, 1000s. *otc.*
Use: Vitamin supplement.

Nilandron. (Hoechst Marion Roussel) Nilutamide 50 mg/Tab. Bot. 90s. *Rx.*
Use: Antineoplastic.

Nilspasm. (Parmed) Phenobarbital 50 mg, hyoscyamine sulfate 0.31 mg, atropine sulfate 0.06 mg, scopolamine hydrobromide 0.0195 mg/Tab. Bot. 100s, 1000s. *Rx.*
Use: Anticholinergic, antispasmodic, hypnotic, sedative.

Nilstat Ointment & Cream. (ESI Lederle Generics) Nystatin 100,000 units/g. **Cream base** w/Emulsifying wax, isopropyl myristate, glycerin, lactic acid, sodium hydroxide, sorbic acid 0.2%. Tube 15 g, Jar 240 g. **Oint. base:** w/light mineral oil, Plastibase 50 W. Tube 15 g. *Rx.*
Use: Antifungal, topical.

Nilstat Oral. (ESI Lederle Generics) Nystatin 500,000 units/FC Tab. Bot. 100s, UD 10 × 10s. *Rx.*
Use: Antifungal.

Nilstat Oral Suspension. (ESI Lederle Generics) Nystatin 100,000 units/ml, methylparaben 0.12%, propylparaben 0.03%, cherry flavor. Bot. 60 ml w/dropper, 16 fl oz. *Rx.*
Use: Antifungal.

Nilstat Powder. (ESI Lederle Generics) Nystatin pow. 150 million, 1 billion or 2 billion units/Bot. *Rx.*
Use: Antifungal.

Nil Tuss. (Minnesota Pharm) Dextromethorphan HBr 10 mg, chlorpheniramine maleate 1.25 mg, phenylephrine HCl 5 mg, ammonium Cl 83 mg/5 ml. Syr. Bot. pt. *otc.*
Use: Antihistamine, antitussive, decongestant, expectorant.

•**nilutamide.** (nye-LOO-tah-mide) USAN.
Use: Antineoplastic.
See: Nilandron, Tab. (Hoechst Marion Roussel).

Nil Vaginal Cream. (Century Pharm) Sulfanilamide 15%, 9-aminoacridine HCl 0.2%, allantoin 1.5%. Bot. 4 oz. w/applicator. *otc.*
Use: Anti-infective, vaginal.

•**nilvadipine.** (NILL-vah-DIH-peen) USAN.
Use: Antagonist (calcium channel).

•**nimazone.** (nih-mah-ZONE) USAN.
Use: Anti-inflammatory.

Nimbex. (GlaxoWellcome) Cisatracurium besylate 2 mg/ml, Vial 5 ml, 10 ml; 10 mg/ml, Vial 20 ml. Inj. *Rx.*
Use: Nondepolarizing neuromuscular blocker; muscle relaxant.

Nimbus. (Biomerica) Monoclonal antibody-based enzyme immunoassay. Screens for urinary chorionic gonadotropin. Pkg. 10s, 25s, 50s.
Use: Diagnostic aid.

•**nimodipine.** (NYE-MOE-dih-peen) USAN.
Use: Vasodilator.
See: Nimotop, Cap. (Bayer Corp).

Nimotop. (Bayer Corp) Nimodipine 30 mg Liq. Cap. Bot. UD 100s. *Rx.*
Use: Calcium channel blocker.

Nion B Plus C. (Nion) Vitamins B_1 15 mg, B_2 10.2 mg, B_3 50 mg, B_5 10 mg, C 300 mg/Capl. Bot 100s. *otc.*
Use: Vitamin supplement.

Niong. (U.S. Ethicals) Nitroglycerin 2.6 mg or 6.5 mg/CR Tab. Bot. 100s. *Rx.*
Use: Antianginal.

Nipent. (Super Gen) Pentostatin 10 mg/ Pow. Vial. Single dose. *Rx.*
Use: Antineoplastic.

Niratron. (Progress) Chlorpheniramine maleate 4 mg/Tsp. Bot. pt.
Use: Antihistamine.

•**niridazole.** (nye-RIH-dah-ZOLE) USAN.
Use: Antischistosomal.

•**nisbuterol mesylate.** (NISS-BYOO-teh-role) USAN.
Use: Bronchodilator.

•**nisobamate.** (NYE-so-BAM-ate) USAN.
Use: Anxiolytic, hypnotic, sedative.

•**nisoldipine.** (nye-SOLE-idh-peen) USAN.
Use: Vasodilator (coronary).
See: Sular, ER Tab. (Zeneca).

•**nisoxetine.** (NISS-OX-eh-teen) USAN.
Use: Antidepressant.

•**nisterime acetate.** (nye-STEER-eem) USAN.
Use: Androgen.

•**nitarsone.** (NITE-AHR-sone) USAN.
Use: Antiprotozoal (histomonas).

Nite Time Cold Formula. (Alphalma USPD) Pseudoephedrine HCl 10 mg, doxylamine succinate 1.25 mg, dextromethorphan HBr 5 mg, acetaminophen 167 mg, alcohol 25%. Liq. Bot. 180 ml, 300 ml. *otc.*
Use: Analgesic, antihistamine, antitussive, decongestant.

•**nitrafudam hydrochloride.** (NIGH-trah-FEW-dam) USAN.
Use: Antidepressant.

•**nitralamine hydrochloride.** (nye-TRAL-ah-meen) USAN.
Use: Antifungal.

•**nitramisole hydrochloride.** (nye-TRAM-ih-sole) USAN.
Use: Anthelmintic.

•**nitrazepam.** (nye-TRAY-zeh-pam) USAN.
Use: Anticonvulsant, hypnotic, sedative.

Nitrazine Paper. (Bristol-Myers Squibb) Determines pH of a solution, in pH 4.5-7.5 range. 15 ft. roll with dispenser and color chart.
Use: Diagnostic aid.

Nitrek. (Bertek) Nitroglycerin 22.4 mg/8 cm^2 (0.2 mg/hr), 44.8 mg/16cm^2 (0.4 mg/hr), 67.2 mg/24 cm^2 (0.6 mg/hr). Patch. Box 30s. *Rx.*
Use: Antianginal.

•**nitrendipine.** (NIGH-TREN-dih-peen) USAN.
Use: Antihypertensive.

•**nitric acid.** (NYE-trick) N.F. 18.
Use: Pharmaceutic aid (acidifying agent).

nitric acid silver. Silver Nitrate, U.S.P. 23.

nitric oxide. (Ohmeda Pharmaceuticals)
Use: Primary pulmonary hypertension agent. [Orphan drug]

Nitro-Bid IV. (Hoechst Marion Roussel) Nitroglycerin 5 mg/ml. Inj. Vial 1 ml box 10s; 5 ml Box 10s; 10 ml Box 5s. *Rx.*
Use: Antianginal.

Nitro-Bid Ointment. (Hoechst Marion Roussel) Nitroglycerin (glyceryl trinitrate) 2%, in lanolin and petrolatum base. Tube 20 g, 60 g, UD 1 g (100s). *Rx.*
Use: Antianginal.

Nitro-Bid Plateau Caps. (Hoechst Marion Roussel) Nitroglycerin 2.5 mg, 6.5 mg or 9 mg/SR Cap. Bot. 60s, 100s. *Rx.*
Use: Antianginal.

Nitrocap. (Freeport) Nitroglycerin 2.5 mg/ TR Cap. Bot. 100s. *Rx.*
Use: Antianginal.

•**nitrocycline.** (NYE-troe-SIGH-kleen) USAN.
Use: Anti-infective.

•**nitrodan.** (NYE-troe-dan) USAN.
Use: Anthelmintic.

Nitrodisc. (Roberts Pharm) Nitroglycerin. Transcutaneous nitroglycerin discs releasing 16 mg, 24 mg or 32 mg/ Patch. Carton 30s, 100s. *Rx.*
Use: Antianginal.

Nitro-Dur. (Key Pharm) Nitroglycerin. Transdermal system releasing 20 mg, 40 mg, 60 mg, 80 mg, 120 mg or 160 mg/Patch. Carton 30s, 100s, UD 30s, 100s. *Rx.*
Use: Antianginal.

Nitrofan Caps. (Major) Nitrofurantoin 50 mg or 100 mg/Cap. Bot. 100s, 500s. *Rx.*
Use: Anti-infective, urinary.

•**nitrofurantoin.** (nye-troe-FYOOR-an-toyn) U.S.P. 23.
Use: Anti-infective, urinary.
See: Furadantin, Soln. (Procter & Gamble Pharm).

nitrofurantoin macrocrystals. (Various Mfr.) 50 mg or 100 mg/Cap. Bot. 100s, 500s, 1000s. *Rx.*
Use: Anti-infective, urinary.
See: Macrobid, Cap. (Procter & Gamble Pharm)
Macrodantin, Cap. (Procter & Gamble Pharm).

•**nitrofurazone.** U.S.P. 23.
Use: Anti-infective, topical.
See: Furacin, Preps. (Roberts Pharm).
Nitrozone, Oint. (Century Pharm).
W/Allantoin, stearic acid.
See: Eldezol, Oint. (ICN Pharmaceuticals).

nitrofurazone. (Various Mfr.) **Top. Soln:** 0.2%. Bot. Pt., gal. **Oint.:** 0.2%. Tube 480 g.
Use: Anti-infective, topical.

Nitrogard. (Parke-Davis) Transmucosal controlled-released nitroglycerin 1 mg, 2 mg or 3 mg/Tab. Bot. 100s. *Rx.*
Use: Antianginal.

•**nitrogen.** (NYE-troe-jen) N.F. 18.
Use: Pharmaceutic aid (air displacement).

nitrogen monoxide. Laughing Gas, Nitrous Oxide.
Use: Anesthetic, general; analgesic.

nitrogen mustard.
See: Mustargen, Vial (Merck).

nitrogen mustard derivatives.
See: Leukemia Agents.
Leukeran, Tab. (Burroughs-Wellcome).
Mustargen HCl, Vial (Merck).
Triethylene Melamine, Tab. (ESI Lederle Generics).

nitroglycerin. (nye-troe-GLIH-suh-rin) (Various Mfr.) 5 mg/ml. Inj. Vial 5 ml, 10 ml. *Rx.*
Use: Antianginal.

•**nitroglycerin, diluted.** (nye-troe-GLIH-suh-rin) U.S.P. 23. *Formerly Glyceryl Trinitrate.*
Use: Vasodilator (coronary).

nitroglycerin in 5% dextrose. (Various Mfr.) **25 mg, 100 mg:** Inj. Soln. 250 ml. **50 mg:** Inj. Soln. 250, 500 ml. **200 mg:** Inj. Soln. 500 ml. *Rx.*
Use: Antianginal.

nitroglycerin injection. (Abbott Laboratories) 25 mg/ml. Vial 5 ml, 10 ml.
Use: Antianginal, vasodilator.
See: Tridil, Inj. (DuPont Merck Pharmaceuticals).

nitroglycerin, intravenous.
Use: Vasodilator.
See: Nitro-Bid IV (Hoechst Marion Roussel).

nitroglycerin ointment. (Various Mfr.) 2% in lanolin-petrolatum base. Tube 30 g, 60 g. *Rx.*
Use: Vasodilator.

nitroglycerin patch.
Use: Antianginal.
See: Nitrek (Bertek).

nitroglycerin tablets/capsules. (Various Mfr.) Glyceryl Trinitrate, Glonoin, Nitroglycerol, Trinitrin, Trinitroglycerol Tab.
Use: Vasodilator.
See: Niglycon, Tab. (Consoln. Midland).
Niong, Tab. (U.S. Ethicals).
Nitrobid, Cap. (Hoechst Marion Roussel).
Nitrocels, Cap. (Winston).
Nitrodyl, Cap. (Sanofi Winthrop).
Nitrogard (Parke-Davis).
Nitroglyn, Tab. (Key Pharm).
Nitrol Oint. (Kremers Urban).
Nitro-Lyn, Cap. (Lynwood).
Nitrong, Tab. (Wharton).
Nitrospan, Cap. (Rhone-Poulenc Rorer).
Nitro, TD Cap. (Fleming).
Nitro-Time, Cap. (Time-Cap Labs).
Trates, Cap. (Solvay).
Vasoglyn, Unicelles (Solvay).
W/Butabarbital.
See: Nitrodyl-B, Cap. (Sanofi Winthrop).

nitroglycerin transdermal. (Various Mfr.) 16 mg - 62.5 mg, 32 mg - 125 mg or 75 mg - 187.5 mg (some systems have different release rates). Box 30s.
Use: Vasodilator.
See: Deponit 5 and 10 (Wyeth Ayerst).
Nitrodisc (Searle).
NTS (Circa Pharm).
Transderm-Nitro (Novartis Pharmaceuticals).

nitroglycerol.
See: Nitroglycerin (Various Mfr.).

Nitroglyn. (Key Pharm) Nitroglycerin 2.5 mg, 6.5 mg or 9 mg/SR Cap. Bot. 100s. *Rx.*
Use: Antianginal.

Nitrolan. (Elan) Protein 60 g, fat 40 g, carbohydrates 160 g, sodium 690 mg, potassium 1.17 g/L, lactose free. With appropriate vitamins and minerals. Liq. In 237 ml Tetra Pak containers and 1000 ml New Pak closed systems with and without Color Check. *otc.*
Use: Nutritional supplement.

Nitrolin. (Schein Pharmaceutical) Nitroglycerin 2.5 mg or 9 mg/SR Cap. **2.5 mg:** Bot. 100s. **9 mg:** Bot. 60s. *Rx.*
Use: Antianginal.

Nitrolingual Spray. (Rhone-Poulenc Rorer) Nitroglycerin lingual aerosol 0.4

mg/metered dose. Canister 13.8 g containing 200 metered doses. *Rx.*
Use: Antianginal.

Nitrol IV. (Rhone-Poulenc Rorer) Nitroglycerin 0.8 mg/ml. Amp. 1 ml Box 25s; 10 ml Box 10s; 30 ml Box 5s. *Rx.*
Use: Antianginal.

Nitrol IV Concentrate. (Rhone-Poulenc Rorer) Nitroglycerin for infusion 50 mg/10 ml. Amp. Box 10s. *Rx.*
Use: Antianginal.

Nitrol Ointment. (Pharmacia & Upjohn) Nitroglycerin 2% in lanolin and petrolatum base. Tube 30 g, 60 g, Pack 6s. *Rx.*
Use: Antianginal.

Nitrol Ointment. (Savage) Nitroglycerin 2% in a lanolin-petrolatum base. Tube 60 g, UD 3 g (50s). *Rx.*
Use: Antianginal agent.

Nitro-Lyn. (Lynwood) Nitroglycerin 2.5 mg/Cap. Bot. 100s. *Rx.*
Use: Antianginal.

nitromannite.
See: Mannitol Hexanitrate (Various Mfr.).

nitromannitol.
See: Mannitol Hexanitrate (Various Mfr.).

Nitromed. (U.S. Ethicals) Nitroglycerin 2.6 mg or 6.5 mg/CR Tab. Bot. 100s. *Rx.*
Use: Antianginal.

•**nitromersol.** (nye-troe-MER-sole) U.S.P. 23.
Use: Anti-infective, topical.

•**nitromide.** (NYE-troe-mid) USAN.
Use: Anti-infective.

•**nitromifene citrate.** (nye-TROE-mih-feen) USAN.
Use: Antiestrogen.

Nitronet. (U.S. Ethicals) Nitroglycerin 2.6 mg or 6.5 mg/CR Tab. Bot. 100s. *Rx.*
Use: Antianginal.

Nitrong Ointment. (Wharton) Nitroglycerin 2%. Oint. Tube 30 g, 60 g with dose applicator. *Rx.*
Use: Antianginal.

Nitrong Tablets. (Wharton) Nitroglycerin 2.6 mg, 6.5 mg or 9 mg/CR Tab. Bot. 30s, 60s (9 mg), 100s. *Rx.*
Use: Antianginal.

Nitropress. (Abbott Laboratories) Sodium nitroprusside 50 mg/2 ml. Vial. *Rx.*
Use: Antihypertensive.

nitroprusside sodium. (nye-troe-PRUSS-ide SO-dee-uhm)
Use: Antihypertensive.
See: Nitropress, Pow. for Inj. (Abbott Laboratories).
Sodium Nitroprusside, Pow. for Inj. (Various Mfr.).

nitrosoureas.
Use: Alkylating agent (antineoplastic).
See: CeeNu (Bristol Myers Oncology).
BiCNU (Bristol Myers Oncology).
Zanosar (Pharmacia & Upjohn).
Thiotepa (ESI Lederle Generics).

Nitrostat. (Parke-Davis) Nitroglycerin 0.3 mg, 0.4 mg or 0.6 mg/Tab. Bot. 25s, 100s, UD 100s. *Rx.*
Use: Antianginal.

Nitrostat IV. (Parke-Davis) Nitroglycerin for infusion. **0.8 mg/ml:** Amp. 10 ml. **5 mg/ml:** Amp. 10 ml, Vial 10 ml. **10 mg/ml:** Vial 10 ml. *Rx.*
Use: Antianginal.

Nitro-Time. (Time-Cap Labs) Nitroglycerin 2.5 mg, 6.5 mg or 9 mg, lactose, sucrose/ER Cap. Bot. 60s, 90s, 100s. *Rx.*
Use: Antianginal.

nitrous acid, sodium salt. Sodium Nitrite, U.S.P. 23.

•**nitrous oxide.** U.S.P. 23. Laughing Gas. Nitrogen Monoxide.
Use: Anesthesia (inhalation).

•**nivazol.** (NIH-vah-ZOLE) USAN.
Use: Corticosteroid, topical.

Nivea Moisturizing. (Beiersdorf) **Cream:** Mineral oil, petrolatum, lanolin alcohol, glycerin, microcrystalline wax, paraffin, magnesium sulfate, decyloleate, octyl dodecanol, aluminum stearate, citric acid, magnesium stearate. In 120 g, 180 g, 300 g, 480 g. **Lot.:** Mineral oil, lanolin, isopropyl myristate, cetearyl alcohol, glyceryl stearate, acrylamide/sodium acrylate copolymer, simethicone, methychloroisothiazolinone, methylisothiazolinone. In 180 ml, 300 ml, 450 ml. *otc.*
Use: Emollient.

Nivea Moisturizing Creme Soap. (Beiersdorf) Sodium tallowate, sodium cocoate, glycerin, petrolatum, titanium dioxide, NaCl, octyldodecanol, macadamia nut oil, aloe, sodium thiosulfate, lanolin alcohol, pentasodium pentetate, EDTA, BHT, beeswax. Bar 90 g, 150 g. *otc.*
Use: Dermatologic, cleanser.

Nivea Oil. (Beiersdorf) Emulsion of neutral aliphatic hydrocarbons. **Liq.:** Bot. 2 oz, 4 fl oz, pt, qt. **Cream:** Tube 1 oz, 2⅓ oz, Jar 4 oz, 6 oz, 1 lb, 5 lb. tin. **Soap:** Bath or toilet size. *otc.*
Use: Emollient.
See: Basic, soap (Beiersdorf).

Nivea Sun. (Beiersdorf) Octyl methoxycinnamate, octyl salicylate, benzophenone-3, 2-phenylbenzimidazole-5-sulfonic acid. Lot. Bot. 120 ml. *otc.*
Use: Sunscreen.

•**nivimedone sodium.** (nih-VIH-meh-dohn) USAN.
Use: Antiallergic.

Nix Creme Rinse. (GlaxoWellcome) Permethrin 1%. Bot. 2 oz. *otc.*
Use: Pediculicide.

•**nizatidine.** (nye-ZAT-ih-deen) U.S.P. 23.
Use: Antiulcerative.
See: Axid, Prods. (Eli Lilly).

Nizoral Cream. (Janssen) Ketoconazole 2% cream. Tube 15 g, 30 g. *Rx.*
Use: Antifungal, topical.

Nizoral Suspension. (Janssen) Ketoconazole 20 mg/ml. Saccharin. Bot. 4 oz. *Rx.*
Use: Antifungal.

Nizoral Tablets. (Janssen) Ketoconazole 200 mg/Tab. Bot. 100s, UD 100s. *Rx.*
Use: Antifungal.

n-methylhydrazine.
Use: Antineoplastic.
See: Procarbazine.

n-methylisatin beta-thiosemicarbazone. Under study.
Use: Smallpox protection.

N-Multistix. (Bayer Corp) Glucose, protein, pH, blood, ketones, bilirubin, urobilinogen, nitrate, leukocytes. Kit 100s.
Use: Diagnostic aid.

N-Multistix S. G. Reagent Strips. (Bayer Corp) Urinalysis reagent strip test for pH, protein, glucose, ketones, bilirubin, blood, nitrite, urobilinogen and specific gravity. Bot. 100s.
Use: Diagnostic aid.

n, n-diethylvanillamide.
See: Ethamivan, Inj. (Various Mfr.).

No-Aspirin. (Walgreens) Acetaminophen 325 mg/Tab. Bot. 100s. *otc.*
Use: Analgesic.

No-Aspirin Extra Strength. (Walgreens) Acetaminophen 500 mg/Tab. or Cap. **Tab.:** Bot. 60s, 100s. **Cap.:** Bot. 50s, 100s. *otc.*
Use: Analgesic.

•**noberastine.** (no-BER-ast-een) USAN.
Use: Antihistamine.

•**nocodazole.** (no-KOE-DAH-zole) USAN.
Use: Antineoplastic.

NoDoz. (Bristol-Myers) **Tab.:** Caffeine 200 mg, sucrose. Bot. 16s, 36s, 60s. **Chew. Tab.:** Caffeine 100 mg, aspartame, phenylalanine 15 mg, spearmint flavor. Pkg. 12s, 30s. *otc.*
Use: Analeptic.

No Drowsiness Allerest. (Novartis Pharmaceuticals) Pseudoephedrine HCl 30 mg, acetaminophen 500 mg/Tab. Bot. 20s. *otc.*
Use: Analgesic, decongestant.

No Drowsiness Sinarest. (Fisons) Pseudoephedrine HCl 30 mg, acetaminophen 500 mg/Tab. Bot. 24s. *otc.*
Use: Analgesic, decongestant.

nofetumomab merpentan.
See: Verluma (NeoRx, DuPont Merck).

•**nogalamycin.** (no-GAL-ah-MY-sin) USAN.
Use: Antineoplastic.

No-Hist Capsules. (Dunhall Pharmaceuticals) Phenylephrine HCl 5 mg, phenylpropanolamine HCl 40 mg, pseudoephedrine HCl 40 mg/Cap. Bot. 100s. *Rx.*
Use: Decongestant.

No-Hist-S Syrup. (Dunhall Pharmaceuticals) Phenylephrine HCl 5 mg, phenylpropanolamine HCl 40 mg, pseudoephedrine HCl 40 mg/5 ml. Bot. pt. *Rx.*
Use: Decongestant.

Nokane. (Wren) Salicylamide 4 g, N-acetyl-p-aminophenol 4 g, caffeine 0.5 gr/Tab. Bot. 40s. *otc.*
Use: Analgesic combination.

Nolahist. (Carnrick Labs) Phenindamine tartrate 25 mg/Tab. Bot. 100s. *otc.*
Use: Antihistamine.

Nolamine. (Carnrick Labs) Chlorpheniramine maleate 4 mg, phenindamine tartrate 24 mg, phenylpropanolamine HCl 50 mg/Tab. Bot. 100s, 250s. *Rx.*
Use: Antihistamine, decongestant.

Nolex LA. (Carnrick Labs). Phenylpropanolamine 75 mg, guaifenesin 400 mg/ SR Tab. Bot. 100s. *Rx.*
Use: Decongestant, expectorant.

•**nolinium bromide.** (no-LIN-ee-uhm) USAN.
Use: Antisecretory, antiulcerative.

Nolvadex. (Zeneca) Tamoxifen citrate 10 mg: 60s, 250s. 20 mg: 30s. *Rx.*
Use: Antineoplastic.

Nometic. Diphenidol.
Use: Antiemetic.

•**nomifensine maleate.** (NO-mih-FEN-seen) USAN.
Use: Antidepressant.

Nonamin. (Western Research) Calcium 100 mg, chloride 90 mg, magnesium 50 mg, zinc 3.75 mg, iron 4.5 mg, copper 0.5 mg, iodine 37.5 mcg, potassium 49 mg, phosphorus 100 mg/Tab. Bot. 1000s. *otc.*

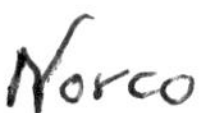

Use: Mineral supplement.

Non-Drowsy Contac Sinus. (SmithKline Beecham Pharmaceuticals) Pseudoephedrine HCl 30 mg, acetaminophen 500 mg. Cap. Bot. 24s. *otc.*
Use: Analgesic, decongestant.

None. (Forest Pharmaceutical) Heparin sodium 1000 units/ml. No preservatives. Amps 5 ml. Box 25s. *Rx.*
Use: Anticoagulant.

nonoxynol. (nahn-OCK-sih-nahl) (Ortho McNeil) *otc.*
Use: Contraceptive, spermicide.
See: Emko, Preps. (Schering Plough).

•**nonoxynol 4.** (NAHN-ox-sih-nahl 4) USAN.
Use: Pharmaceutic aid (surfactant).

•**nonoxynol 9.** (NAHN-ox-sih-nahl 9) U.S.P. 23.
Use: Spermaticide, pharmaceutic aid (wetting and solubilizing agent).
See: Conceptrol, Cream, Gel (Ortho McNeil).
Delfen, Foam (Ortho McNeil).
Encare, Insert (Eaton-Merz).
Gynol II, Jelly (Ortho McNeil).
Ortho-Creme, Cream (Ortho McNeil).
Ortho-Gynol, Jelly (Ortho McNeil).

•**nonoxynol 10.** (nahn-OCK-sih-nahl 10) N.F. 18.
Use: Pharmaceutic aid (surfactant).

•**nonoxynol 15.** (NAHN-ox-sih-nahl 15) USAN.
Use: Pharmaceutic aid (surfactant).

•**nonoxynol 30.** (NAHN-ox-sih-nahl 30) USAN. Under study.
Use: Pharmaceutic aid (surfactant).

nonspecific protein therapy.
See: Protein, Nonspecific Therapy.

nonsteroidal anti-inflammatory agents, ophthalmic.
See: Ocufen (Allergan).
Profenal (Alcon Laboratories).
Voltaren (Ciba Vision Ophthalmics).

nonylphenoxypolyethoxy ethanol. Nonoxynol.
Use: Contraceptive, spermicide.
See: Delfen Vaginal Foam (Ortho McNeil).

No Pain-HP. (Young Again Products) Capsaicin 0.075%. Roll-on. 60 ml. *otc.*
Use: Analgesic, topical.

•**noracymethadol hydrochloride.** (nahr-ASS-ih-METH-ah-dole) USAN.
Use: Analgesic.

•**norbolethone.** (nahr-BOLE-eth-ohn) USAN.
Use: Anabolic.

Norcet Tablets. (Holloway) Hydrocodone bitartrate 5 mg, acetaminophen 500 mg/Tab. Bot. 100s. *c-III.*
Use: Analgesic combination, narcotic.

Norcuron. (Organon Teknika) Vecuronium bromide 10 mg/5 ml. **With diluent:** Vial 5 ml lyophilized powder and 5 ml ampul of sterile water for injection. Box 10s. **Without diluent:** Vial 5 ml lyophilized powder. Box 10s. **Prefilled syringe:** Vial 10 ml lyophilized powder and 10 ml syringe w/bacteriostatic water for injection. Box 10s. *Rx.*
Use: Muscle relaxant.

norcycline.
Use: Anti-infective.

Nordette. (Wyeth Ayerst) Levonorgestrel 0.15 mg, ethinyl estradiol 0.03 mg/Tab. 6 Pilpak dispensers, 21 day and 28 day w/ 7 inert tabs. *Rx.*
Use: Contraceptive.

Norditropin. (Novo Nordisk) Somatropin 4 mg (≈ to 12 IU) or 8 mg (≈ to 24 IU), glycine 8.8 mg, mannitol 44 mg. Pow. for Inj. Benzyl alcohol 1.5%. Vials. *Rx.*
Use: Hormone, growth.

Norel. (US Pharmaceutical) Phenylephrine HCl 5 mg, phenylpropanolamine HCl 45 mg, guaifensin 200 mg. Cap. Bot. 100s. *Rx.*
Use: Decongestant, expectorant.

Norel Plus Capsules. (US Pharmaceutical) Chlorpheniramine maleate 4 mg, phenyltoloxamine dihydrogen citrate 25 mg, phenylpropanolamine HCl 25 mg, acetaminophen 325 mg/Cap. Bot. 100s. *Rx.*
Use: Analgesic, antihistamine, decongestant.

•**norepinephrine bitartrate.** (NOR-eh-pih-NEFF-reen bye-TAR-trate) U.S.P. 23.
Formerly levarterenol bitartrate.
Use: Adrenergic (vasoconstrictor).
See: Levophed Bitartrate, Soln., Amp. (Sanofi Winthrop).

Norethin 1/50M. (Roberts Pharm) Norethindrone 1 mg, mestranol 50 mcg/Tab. 21 day and 28 day (with 7 inert tabs.). *Rx.*
Use: Contraceptive.

Norethin 1/35E. (Roberts Pharm) Norethindrone 1 mg, ethinyl estradiol 35 mg/Tab. 21 day and 28 day (with 7 inert tabs.). *Rx.*
Use: Contraceptive.

•**norethindrone.** (nore-eth-IN-drone) U.S.P. 23.
Use: Progestin.
See: Micronor, Tab. (Ortho McNeil).
Norlutin, Tab. (Parke-Davis).
Nor-QD, Tab. (Syntex).

W/Ethinyl estradiol.
See: Brevicon 21 and 28, Tab. (Syntex).
GenCept, Tab. (Gencon).
Jenest-28, Tab. (Organon Teknika).
Modicon 21 and 28, Tab. (Ortho McNeil).
Ortho-Novum 21 and 28, Prods. (Ortho McNeil).
Ovcon-35, Tab. (Bristol-Myers).
Ovcon-50, Tab. (Bristol-Myers).
W/Mestranol.
See: Norinyl, Prods. (Syntex).
Ortho-Novum, Prods. (Ortho McNeil).
W/Mestranol, ferrous fumarate.
See: Norinyl-l Fe 28, Prods. (Syntex).

•**norethindrone acetate.** U.S.P. 23.
Use: Hormone, progestin.
See: Aygestin, Tab. (Wyeth Ayerst).
Norlutate, Tab. (Parke-Davis).

norethindrone acetate and ethinyl estradiol tablets.
Use: Contraceptive.
See: Brevicon, Tab. (Syntex).
Estrostep, Prods. (Parke-Davis).
Gestest, Tab. (Bristol-Myers Squibb).
Loestrin, Prods. (Parke-Davis).
Norinyl, Prods. (Syntex).
Norlestrin, Prods. (Parke-Davis).

norethindrone and ethinyl estradiol tablets.
Use: Contraceptive.

norethindrone and mestranol tablets.
Use: Contraceptive.

•**norethynodrel.** (nahr-eh-THIGH-no-drell) U.S.P. 23.
Use: Hormone, progestin.
See: Enovid, Prods. (Searle).

Norflex. (3M Pharm) Orphenadrine citrate 100 mg/SR Tab. Bot. 100s, 500s. *Rx.*
Use: Muscle relaxant.

Norflex Injectable. (3M Pharm) Orphenadrine citrate 30 mg, sodium bisulfite 2 mg, sodium Cl 5.8 mg, water for injection qs 2 ml. Amp. 2 ml 6s, 50s. *Rx.*
Use: Muscle relaxant.

•**norfloxacin.** (nor-FLOX-uh-SIN) U.S.P. 23.
Use: Anti-infective.
See: Chibroxin, Ophth. Soln. (Merck).
Noroxin, Tab. (Merck).

•**norflurane.** (nahr-FLEW-rane) USAN. Under study.
Use: Anesthetic, general.

Norgesic Forte Tablets. (3M) Orphenadrine citrate 50 mg, aspirin 770 mg, caffeine 60 mg, lactose/Tab. Bot. 100s, 500s, UD 100s. *Rx.*
Use: Muscle relaxant, analgesic.

Norgesic Tablets. (3M) Orphenadrine citrate 25 mg, aspirin 385 mg, caffeine 30 mg, lactose/Tab. Bot. 100s, 500s, UD 100s. *Rx.*
Use: Muscle relaxant, analgesic.

•**norgestimate.** (nore-JEST-ih-mate) USAN. *Formerly Dexnorgestrel Acetime.*
Use: Hormone, progestin.
W/ Ethinyl estradiol.
See: Ortho-Cyclen, Tab. (Ortho McNeil).
Ortho Tri-Cyclen, Tab. (Ortho McNeil).

•**norgestomet.** (nore-JESS-toe-met) USAN.
Use: Hormone, progestin.

•**norgestrel.** (nahr-JESS-trell) U.S.P. 23.
Use: Contraceptive; hormone, progestin.
See: Ovrette, Tab. (Wyeth Ayerst).

norgestrel and ethinyl estradiol tablets.
Use: Contraceptive.
See: Lo/Ovral, Tab. (Wyeth Ayerst).
Ovral-Prep. (Wyeth Ayerst).

Norinyl 1 + 35. (Syntex) Norethindrone 1 mg, ethinyl estradiol 0.035 mg/Tab. Wallette 21 and 28 day (7 inert tabs). *Rx.*
Use: Contraceptive.

Norinyl 1 + 50. (Syntex) Norethindrone 1 mg, mestranol 0.05 mg/Tab. Wallette 21 and 28 day (7 inert tabs). *Rx.*
Use: Contraceptive.

Norinyl 2 mg. (Syntex) Norethindrone 2 mg, mestranol 0.1 mg/Tab. Memorette Disp. of 20s. Refill folders of 20s. *Rx.*
Use: Contraceptive.

Norisodrine Aerotrol. (Abbott Laboratories) Norisodrine HCl (isoproterenol HCl) 0.25% (2.8 mg/ml) in inert chlorofluorohydrocarbon propellants, alcohol 33%, ascorbic acid 0.1% as preservative. Aerotrol 15 ml. Box 12s. *Rx.*
Use: Bronchodilator.

Norisodrine/Calcium Iodide Syrup. (Abbott Laboratories) Isoproterenol sulfate 3 mg, calcium iodide, anhydrous 150 mg/5 ml, alcohol 6%. Bot. pt. *Rx.*
Use: Bronchodilator.

Noritate. (Dermik Laboratories) Metronidazole 1%. Cream. Tube 30 g. *Rx.*
Use: Dermatologic, acne.

Norlestrin-21 1/50 Tablets. (Parke-Davis) Norethindrone acetate 1 mg, ethinyl estradiol 50 mcg/Tab. (yellow). Compact 21s. Pkg. 5 compacts. Pkg. 5 refills; Ctn. 10×5 refills. *Rx.*

Use: Contraceptive.

Norlestrin-28 1/50 Tablet. (Parke-Davis) Norethindrone acetate 1 mg, ethinyl estradiol 50 mcg/Tab. (yellow). Compact 21 yellow, 7 white (inert) tablets. Pkg. 5 compacts. Pkg. 5 refills; Ctn. 10×5 refills. *Rx.*
Use: Contraceptive.

Norlestrin-21 2.5/50 Tablets. (Parke-Davis) Norethindrone acetate 2.5 mg, ethinyl estradiol 50 mcg/Tab. (pink). Compact 21s. Pkg. 5 compacts. Pkg. 5 refills; Ctn. 10×5 refills. *Rx.*
Use: Contraceptive.

Norlestrin Fe 1/50 Tablets. (Parke-Davis) Norethindrone acetate 1 mg, ethinyl estradiol 50 mcg/Tab. (yellow). Compact 21 yellow tab., 7 brown 75 mg ferrous fumarate tab. Pkg. 5 compacts. Pkg. 5 refills; Ctn. 10×5 refills. *Rx.*
Use: Contraceptive.

Norlestrin Fe 2.5/50 Tablets. (Parke-Davis) Norethindrone acetate 2.5 mg, ethinyl estradiol 50 mcg/Tab. (pink). Compact 21 pink tab., 7 brown 75 mg ferrous fumarate tab. Pkg. 5 compacts. Pkg. 5 refills; Ctn. 10×5 refills. *Rx.*
Use: Contraceptive.

Normaderm Cream & Lotion. (Doak Dermatologics) Buffered lactic acid in vanishing bases. **Cream:** Jar 3¾ oz, 16 oz. **Lot.:** Bot. 4 oz, 16 oz, 128 oz. *otc.*
Use: Dermatologic, emollient.

normal human serum albumin. Albumin Human, U.S.P. 23.

normal human serum albumin. (Immuno-U.S.). 5%/Inj.: 50, 250, 500 ml. 25%/Inj.: 20, 50, 100 ml. *Rx.*
Use: Blood volume supporter.

normal saline.
See: 0.2% Sodium chloride (Solopak).
0.45% sodium chloride (1/2 normal saline) (Various Mfr.).
0.9% Sodium chloride (Normal saline) (Various Mfr.).
3% Sodium chloride (Various Mfr.).
5% Sodium chloride (Various Mfr.).

Normaline Kit. (Apothecary Products) Salt tablets for normal saline 250 mg/Tab. Preservative free. 200s with Bot. 27.7 ml. *otc.*
Use: Ophthalmic.

Normiflo. (Wyeth Ayerst) Ardeparin sodium 5000 anti-Xa U in 0.5 ml, 10,000 anti-Xa U in 0.5 ml/Inj. In 10s w/25 gauge × ⅝ needle. *Rx.*
Use: Prevention of deep vein thrombosis.

Normodyne. (Schering Plough) Labetalol HCl. **Inj.:** 5 mg/ml. Amp. 20 ml. Vial 40 ml, 60 ml. **Tab.:** 100 mg, 200 mg or 300 mg. Bot. 100s, 500s, UD 100s. *Rx.*
Use: Antihypertensive.

Normol. (Alcon Lenscare) Sterile, isotonic solution of thimerosal 0.004%, chlorhexidine gluconate 0.005%, edetate disodium 0.1%. Bot. 8 oz. *otc.*
Use: Contact lens care.

Normosol-M in D5-W. (Abbott Hospital Prods) Dextrose 5 g, sodium Cl 234 mg, potassium acetate 128 mg, magnesium acetate 21 mg, sodium bisulfite 30 mg/100 ml. Bot. 500 ml, 1000 ml in Abbo-Vac (glass) or Life Care (flexible) containers. *Rx.*
Use: Nutritional supplement, parenteral.

Normosol-R; Normosol-R pH 7.4; 500 ml., 1000 ml. Normosol-R D5-W. (Abbott Hospital Prods) Sodium Cl 526 mg, sodium acetate 222 mg, sodium gluconate 502 mg, potassium Cl 37 mg, magnesium Cl 14 mg, pH of Normosol-R and Normosol R in D5-W adjusted with HCl/100 ml. Bot. 1000 ml, 500 ml. in Life Care (flexible) containers. *Rx.*
Use: Nutritional supplement, parenteral.

Normotensin. (Marcen) IM soln. for inj. Mucopolysaccharide 20 mg, sodium nucleate 25 mg, epinephrine-neutralizing factor 25 units, sodium citrate 10 mg, inositol 5 mg, phenol 0.5%/ml. Multi-dose vial 10 ml, 30 ml.
Use: Antihypertensive.

Norolon. (Sanofi Winthrop) Chloroquine phosphate. *Rx.*
Use: Antimalarial.

Noroxin. (Roberts Pharm) Norfloxacin 400 mg/Tab. Bot. 100s, UD 20s, UD 100s. *Rx.*
Use: Urinary anti-infective.

Norpace. (Searle) Disopyramide phosphate 100 mg or 150 mg/Cap. Bot. 100s, 500s, 1000s, UD 100s. *Rx.*
Use: Antiarrhythmic.

Norpace CR. (Searle) Disopyramide phosphate 100 mg or 150 mg/CR Cap. Bot. 100s, 500s, UD 100s. *Rx.*
Use: Antiarrhythmic.

Norphyl. (Vita Elixir) Aminophylline 100 mg/Tab. *Rx.*
Use: Bronchodilator.

Norplant System. (Wyeth Ayerst) Levonorgestrel 36 mg. Implant kit 6s. *Rx.*
Use: Progestin contraceptive system.

Norpramin. (Hoechst Marion Roussel) Desipramine HCl 10 mg, 25 mg, 50 mg, 75 mg, 100 mg or 150 mg/Tab. **10**

mg: Bot. 100s; **25 mg:** Bot. 100s, 1000s, UD 100s; **50 mg:** Bot. 100s, 1000s, UD 100s; **75 mg:** Bot. 100s; **100 mg:** Bot. 100s. **150 mg:** Bot. 50s. *Rx.*
Use: Antidepressant.

nortesterionate.

Nortriptyline. (nor-TRIP-tih-leen) (Schein Pharmaceutical) 10 mg, 25 mg, 50 mg or 75 mg. Cap. Bot. 100s; **25 mg:** Bot. 500s also. *Rx.*
Use: Antidepressant.

nortriptyline. (Various Mfr.) 10, 25, 50 and 75 mg/Cap. 100s, 500s. *Rx.*
Use: Antidepressant.

•**nortriptyline hydrochloride.** (nor-TRIP-tih-leen) U.S.P. 23.
Use: Antidepressant.
See: Aventyl HCl, Liq., Pulvule (Eli Lilly).
Pamelor, Cap., Liq. (Novartis).

Norval. Docusate sodium.
Use: Laxative.

Norvasc. (Pfizer) Amlodipine **2.5 mg:** Bot. 100s; **5 mg:** Bot. 100s, UD 100s; **10 mg:** Bot. 100s, UD 100s. *Rx.*
Use: Calcium channel blocker.

Norvir. (Abbott Laboratories) Ritonavir 100 mg. Soln.: 80 mg/ml ritonavir, saccharin. *Rx.*
Use: Antiviral.

Norwich Extra Strength. (Procter & Gamble) Aspirin 500 mg/Tab. Bot. 150s. *otc.*
Use: Analgesic.

Nosalt. (SmithKline Beecham Pharmaceuticals) Potassium Cl, potassium bitartrate, adipic acid, mineral oil, fumaric acid. Sodium < 10 mg/5 g (0.43 mEq/5 g), potassium 2502 mg/5 g (64 mEq/5 g). Pkg. 330 g. *otc.*
Use: Salt substitute.

Nosalt Seasoned. (SmithKline Beecham Pharmaceuticals) Potassium Cl, dextrose, onion and garlic, spices, lactose, cream of tartar, paprika, silica, disodium inosinate, disodium guanylate, turmeric. Sodium < 5 mg/5 g (0.2 mEq/5 g), potassium 1328 mg/5 g (34 mEq/5 g). Pkg. 240 g. *otc.*
Use: Salt substitute.

•**noscapine.** (NAHS-kah-peen) U.S.P. 23.
Use: Antitussive.

noscapine hydrochloride. l-Narcotine hydrochloride.
Use: Antitussive.
See: Conar Prods. (SmithKline Beecham Pharmaceuticals).
W/Chlorpheniramine maleate, phenylephrine HCl, N-acetyl-p-aminophenol, salicylamide, vitamin C.
See: Noscaps, Cap. (Table Rock).
W/Phenylephrine HCl.
See: Conar Liq. (SmithKline Beecham Pharmaceuticals).
W/Phenylephrine HCl, guaifensin.
See: Conar, Expectorant (SmithKline Beecham Pharmaceuticals).

Noscaps. (Table Rock) Noscapine 7.5 mg, chlorpheniramine maleate 1 mg, phenylephrine HCl 5 mg, N-acetyl-p-aminophenol 150 mg, salicylamide 150 mg, vitamin C 20 mg/Cap. Bot. 100s, 500s. *otc.*
Use: Analgesic, antihistamine, decongestant, vitamin C.

Noskote. (Schering Plough) Oxybenzone 3%, homosalate 8%. SPF 8. Cream 13.2 g, 30 g. *otc.*
Use: Sunscreen.

Noskote Sunblock. (Schering Plough) Padimate O 8%, oxybenzone 3%, benzyl alcohol. SPF 15. Cream. Tube 30 g. *otc.*
Use: Sunscreen.

Nostril. (Boehringer Ingelheim) Phenylephrine HCl 0.25% or 0.5%, benzalkonium Cl 0.004% in buffered aqueous soln. Bot. 15 ml, pump spray. *otc.*
Use: Decongestant.

Novacet. (Genderm) Sodium sulfacetamide 100 mg, sulfur 50 mg, benzyl alcohol, cetyl alcohol, sodium thiosulfate, EDTA. Lot. Bot. 30 ml. *Rx.*
Use: Dermatologic, acne.

Nova-Dec. (Rugby) Iron 18 mg, vitamins A 5000 IU, D 400 IU, E 30 IU, B_1 1.7 mg, B_2 2 mg, B_3 20 mg, B_5 10 mg, B_6 3 mg, B_{12} 6 mcg, C 60 mg, folic acid 0.4 mg, Ca, Cr, Cu, I, Mg, Mo, Mn, P, Se, K, Zn 15 mg, vitamin K, Cl, Ni, Sn, V, B, biotin 30 mcg/Tab. Bot. 130s. *otc.*
Use: Mineral, vitamin supplement.

Novadyne Expectorant. (Various Mfr.) Pseudoephedrine 30 mg, codeine phosphate 10 mg, guaifenesin 100 mg, alcohol 7.5%. Bot. 120 ml, pt, gal. *c-III.*
Use: Antitussive, decongestant, expectorant.

Novagest Expectorant w/Codeine. (Major) Pseudoephedrine HCl 30 mg, codeine phosphate 10 mg, guaifenesin 100 mg/5 ml, alcohol 8.2%. Liq. Bot. 118 ml. *c-v.*
Use: Antitussive, decongestant, expectorant.

Novahistine Elixir. (SmithKline Beecham Pharmaceuticals) Phenylephrine HCl 5 mg, chlorpheniramine maleate 2 mg/5 ml, alcohol 5%, sorbitol. Bot. 118 ml. *otc.*

Use: Decongestant, antihistamine.

novamidon.
See: Aminopyrine (Various Mfr.).

Novamine. (Clintec Nutrition) Amino acid concentration 11.4%, for infusion. Nitrogen 1.8 g/100 ml. Essential amino acids (mg/100 ml): Isoleucine 570, leucine 790, lysine 900, methionine 570, phenylalanine 790, threonine 570, tryptophan 190, valine 730. Nonessential amino acids (mg/100 ml): Alanine 1650, arginine 1120, histidine 680, proline 680, serine 450, tyrosine 30, glycine 790, glutamic acid 570, aspartic acid 330, acetate 114 mEq/L, sodium metabisulfite 30 mg/100 ml. In 250 ml, 500 ml, 1 l. *Rx.*
Use: Parenteral nutritional supplement.

Novamine 15%. (Clintec Nutrition) Amino acids 15%: Lysine 1.18 g, leucine 1.04 g, phenylalanine 1.04 g, valine 960 mg, isoleucine 749 mg, methionine 749 mg, threonine 749 mg, tryptophan 250 mg, alanine 2.17 g, arginine 1.47 g, glycine 1.04 g, histidine 894 mg, proline 894 mg, glutamic acid 749 mg, serine 592 mg, aspartic acid 434 mg, tyrosine 39 mg, nitrogen 2.37 g/100 ml. Inj. 500 ml, 1000 ml. *Rx.*
Use: Nutritional supplement, parenteral.

Novamine Without Electrolytes. (Clintec Nutrition) Amino acid concentration 8.5%, for infusion. Nitrogen 1.35 g/100 ml. Essential amino acids (mg/100 ml): Isoleucine 420, leucine 590, lysine 673, methionine 420, phenylalanine 590, threonine 420, tryptophan 140, valine 550. Nonessential amino acids (mg/100 ml): Alanine 1240, arginine 840, histidine 500, proline 500, serine 340, tyrosine 20, glycine 590, glutamic acid 420, aspartic acid 250, acetate 88 mEq/L, sodium bisulfite 30 mg/100 ml. In 500 ml, 1 L. *Rx.*
Use: Nutritional supplement, parenteral.

Novantrone. (Immunex) Mitoxantrone HCl 2 mg base/ml. Inj. Vial 10 ml, 12.5 ml, 15 ml. *Rx.*
Use: Antineoplastic.

novatophan.
See: Neocinchophen (Various Mfr.).

novatropine.
See: Homatropine Methylbromide (Various Mfr.).

novobiocin calcium. U.S.P. XXII.
Use: Anti-infective.
See: Cathomycin Calcium.

novobiocin monosodium salt.
Use: Anti-infective.
See: Sodium Novobiocin.

•**novobiocin sodium.** U.S.P. 23.
Use: Anti-infective.
See: Albamycin, Cap. (Pharmacia & Upjohn).
Cathomycin Sodium.

Novocain. (Sanofi Winthrop) Procaine HCl. **1%:** 2 ml, 6 ml, 30 ml. **2%:** 30 ml. **10%:** 2 ml/Inj. *Rx.*
Use: Anesthetic, local.

Novocain for Spinal Anesthesia. (Sanofi Winthrop) Procaine HCl 10% soln. Amp. 2 ml. Box 25s. *Rx.*
Use: Anesthetic, spinal.

Novolin 70/30. (Novo Nordisk) Isophane susp. 70% (human), regular insulin 30% (human, semi-synthetic) 100 units/ml. Inj. Vial 10 ml. *otc.*
Use: Antidiabetic.

Novolin 70/30 PenFill. (Novo Nordisk) Isophane insulin suspension and insulin injection 100 U per ml human insulin. Cartridge 1.5 ml. *otc.*
Use: Antidiabetic.

Novolin 70/30 Prefilled. (Novo Nordisk) Isophane Insulin 100 units/ml human insulin (rDNA). Inj. Prefilled syringe 1.5 ml. *otc.*
Use: Antidiabetic.

Novolin L. (Novo Nordisk) Human insulin (semi-synthetic) 100 units/ml. An insulin-zinc suspension (Lente). Inj. Vial 10 ml. *otc.*
Use: Antidiabetic.

Novolin N. (Novo Nordisk) Human insulin NPH (semisynthetic) 100 units/ml. Isophane insulin suspension (insulin w/ protamine and zinc). Inj. Vial 10 ml. *otc.*
Use: Antidiabetic.

Novolin N PenFill. (Novo Nordisk) Isophane insulin suspension (NPH) 100 U per ml human insulin. Cartridge. 1.5 ml. *otc.*
Use: Antidiabetic.

Novolin N Prefilled. (Novo Nordisk) Isophane insulin suspension (NPH) 100 units/ml human insulin (rDNA). Inj. Prefilled syringe 1.5 ml. *otc.*
Use: Antidiabetic.

Novolin R. (Novo Nordisk) Human insulin, regular (semisynthetic) 100 units/ml. Inj. Vial 10 ml. *otc.*
Use: Antidiabetic.

Novolin R PenFill. (Novo Nordisk) Semisynthetic human regular insulin 100 units/ml. Inj. 1.5 ml cartridges. *otc.*
Use: Antidiabetic.

Novolin R Prefilled. (Novo Nordisk) Insulin 100 units/ml human insulin

(rDNA). Inj. Prefilled syringe 1.5 ml. *otc.*
Use: Antidiabetic.

Noxzema Antiseptic Cleanser Sensitive Skin Formula. (Noxell) Benzalkonium Cl 0.13%. Bot. 4 oz, 8 oz. *otc.*
Use: Dermatologic, cleanser.

Noxzema Antiseptic Skin Cleanser. (Noxell) SD-40 alcohol 63%. Bot. 4 oz, 8 oz. *otc.*
Use: Dermatologic, cleanser.

Noxzema Antiseptic Skin Cleanser Extra Strength Formula. (Noxell) SD-40 alcohol 36%, isopropyl alcohol 34%. Bot. 4 oz, 8 oz. *otc.*
Use: Dermatologic, cleanser.

Noxzema Clear Ups. (Noxell) Salicylic acid 0.5% on pads. Jar 50s. *otc.*
Use: Dermatologic, acne.

Noxzema Clear Ups Acne Medicine Maximum Strength Lotion. (Noxell) Benzoyl peroxide 10%. Bot. 1 oz. Vanishing formula. *otc.*
Use: Dermatologic, acne.

Noxzema Clear Ups Maximum Strength. (Noxell) Salicylic acid 2% on pads. Jar 50s. *otc.*
Use: Dermatologic, acne.

Noxzema Medicated Skin Cream. (Noxell) Menthol, camphor, clove oil, eucalyptus oil, phenol. Jar 2.5 oz, 4 oz, 6 oz, 10 oz. Tube 4.5 oz. Bot. 6 oz., 14 oz. Pump Bottle 10.5 oz. *otc.*
Use: Counterirritant.

Noxzema On-The-Spot. (Noxell) Benzoyl peroxide 10% in vanishing and tinted lotion. Bot. 0.25 oz. *otc.*
Use: Dermatologic, acne.

NP-27 Aerosol. (Thompson Medical) Tolnaftate 1%, alcohol 14.9%. Spray Can 100 ml. *otc.*
Use: Antifungal, topical.

NP-27 Cream. (Thompson Medical) Tolnaftate 1% in cream base. Tube 45 g. *otc.*
Use: Antifungal, topical.

NP-27 Liquid. (Thompson Medical) Tolnaftate 1%. Plastic bot. 2 oz. *otc.*
Use: Antifungal, topical.

NPH Iletin I. (Eli Lilly) Insulin from beef and pork. 100 units/ml. Inj. Vial 10 ml. *otc.*
Use: Antidiabetic.

NPH-N. (Novo Nordisk) Purified pork insulin 100 units/ml in isophane insulin suspension (insulin w/protamine and zinc). Inj. Vial 10 ml. *otc.*
Use: Antidiabetic.

NTBC.
Use: Tyrosinemia type 1. [Orphan drug]

N-Trifluoroacetyladriamycin-14-valerate. (Anthra Pharm) *Rx.*
Use: Antineoplastic.

NTS Transdermal System. (Circa Pharm) Nitroglycerin transdermal system 5 mg/24 hours or 15 mg/24 hours. Box 30s. *Rx.*
Use: Antianginal.

NTZ Long-Acting. (Sanofi Winthrop) Oxymetazoline HCl 0.05%, benzalkonium Cl and phenylmercuric acetate 0.002% as preservatives. Drops. Bot. 1 oz. Spray Bot. 1 oz. *otc.*
Use: Decongestant.

Nubain. (DuPont Merck Pharmaceuticals) Nalbuphine HCl, sodium metabisulfite 0.1%. **10 mg/ml:** Amp 1 ml. Vial 10 ml. Box 1s. **20 mg/ml:** Amp 1 ml. Syringe 1 ml calibrated. Vial 10 ml. *Rx.*
Use: Analgesic, narcotic.

Nu-Bolic. (Seatrace) Nandrolone phenpropionate 25 mg/ml. Vial 5 ml. *c-III.*
Use: Anabolic steroid.

nucite.
See: Inositol (Various Mfr.).

Nucofed. (Roberts Pharm) Codeine phosphate 20 mg, pseudoephedrine HCl 60 mg/5 ml or Cap. Syrup is alcohol-free. **Liq.:** Bot. pt. **Cap.:** Bot. 60s. *c-III.*
Use: Antitussive, decongestant.

Nucofed Expectorant. (Roberts Pharm) Codeine phosphate 20 mg, pseudoephedrine HCl 60 mg, guaifenesin 200 mg/5 ml, alcohol 12.5%, saccharin. Bot. 480 ml. *c-III.*
Use: Antitussive, decongestant, expectorant.

Nucofed Pediatric Expectorant. (Roberts Pharm) Codeine phosphate 10 mg, pseudoephedrine HCl 30 mg, guaifenesin 100 mg/5 ml, alcohol 6%. Bot. pt. *c-v.*
Use: Antitussive, decongestant, expectorant.

Nucotuss Expectorant. (Alphalma USPD) Pseudoephedrine HCl 60 mg, codeine phosphate 20 mg, guaifenesin 200 mg/5 ml, alcohol 12.5%, wintergreen flavor. Liq. Bot. 480 ml. *c-III.*
Use: Antitussive, decongestant, expectorant.

Nucotuss Pediatric Expectorant. (Alphalma USPD) Pseudoephedrine HCl 30 mg, codeine phosphate 10 mg, guaifenesin 100 mg/5 ml, strawberry flavor. Liq. Bot. 480 ml. *c-v.*
Use: Antitussive, decongestant, expectorant.

•**nufenoxole.** (NEW-fen-OX-ole) USAN.
Use: Antiperistaltic.

Nu-Iron 150. (Merz) Polysaccharide-iron complex. 150 mg iron. Cap. Bot. 100s, 500s. *otc.*
Use: Mineral supplement.

Nu-Iron 150. (Merz) Polysaccharide-Iron complex 100 mg/5 ml, alcohol 10%. Elix. 237 ml. *otc.*
Use: Mineral supplement.

Nu-Iron Plus Elixir. (Merz) Polysaccharide iron complex 300 mg, folic acid 3 mg, vitamin B_{12} 75 mcg/15 ml. Bot. 237 ml. *Rx.*
Use: Mineral, vitamin supplement.

Nu-Iron-V. (Merz) Polysaccharide iron 60 mg, folic acid 1 mg, vitamins A 4000 IU, C 50 mg, D 400 IU, B_1 3 mg, B_2 3 mg, B_3 10 mg, B_6 2 mg, B_{12} 3 mcg, Ca/Tab. Bot. 100s. *Rx.*
Use: Mineral, vitamin supplement.

Nul-Tach. (Davis & Sly) Potassium 16 mg, magnesium 13 mg, ascorbic acid 250 mg/Tab. Bot. 100s. *Rx.*
Use: Antiarrythmic.

NuLytely. (Braintree Laboratories) PEG 3350 420 g, sodium bicarbonate 5.72 g, sodium chloride 11.2 g, potassium chloride 1.48 g. Pow. Jugs. 4 L. *Rx.*
Use: Laxative.

Numorphan. (DuPont Merck Pharmaceuticals) Oxymorphone HCl. **1 mg/ml.:** Amp. 1 ml. Box 10s. **1.5 mg/ml.:** Amp. 1 ml, Box 10s. Vial 10 ml, Box 1s. **Rectal Supp.:** 5 mg. Box 6s. *c-II.*
Use: Analgesic, narcotic.

Numotizine Cataplasm. (Hobart) Guaiacol 0.26 g, beechwood creosote 1.302 g, methyl salicylate 0.26 g/100 g. Jar 4 oz. *otc.*
Use: Analgesic, topical.

Numotizine Cough Syrup. (Hobart) Guaifenesin 5 g, ammonium Cl 5 g, sodium citrate 20 g, menthol 0.04 g/fl oz. Bot. 3 oz, pt, gal. *otc.*
Use: Expectorant.

Numzident. (Purepac) Benzocaine 10%, PEG-400 NF 47.86%, PEG-3350 NF 10%, saccharin. Gel. 15 g. *otc.*
Use: Anesthetic, local.

Numzit. (Purepac) Benzocaine, menthol, glycerin, methylparaben, alcohol 12%. Liq. Bot. 22.5 ml. *otc.*
Use: Anesthetic, local.

Numzit Gel. (Purepac) Benzocaine, menthol. Tube 10 g. *otc.*
Use: Anesthetic, local.

Numzit Teething Gel. (Goody's) Benzocaine 7.5%, peppermint oil 0.018%, clove leaf oil 0.09%, PEG-400 66.2%, PEG-3350 26.1%, saccharin 0.036%. Tube. 14.1 g. *otc.*
Use: Anesthetic, local.

Numzit Teething Lotion. (Goody's) Benzocaine 0.2%, alcohol 12.1%, saccharin 0.02%, glycerin 2%, kelgin MU 0.5%, methylparaben. Lot. Bot. 15 ml. *otc.*
Use: Anesthetic, local.

nunol.
See: Phenobarbital (Various Mfr.).

Nupercainal. (Novartis Pharmaceuticals) **Oint.:** Dibucaine 1%, acetone, sodium bisulfite, lanolin, mineral oil, white petrolatum. 30 g, 60 g. **Cream:** Dibucaine 0.5%, acetone, sodium bisulfite, glycerin. 42.5 g. **Supp.:** Cocoa butter, zinc oxide, sodium bisulfite. 12s, 24s. *otc.*
Use: Anesthetic, local (Oint., Cream); Anorectal preparation (Supp.).

Nuprin Backache. (Bristol-Myers Squibb) Magnesium salicylate tetrahydrate 580 mg (equivalent to 467 mg anhydrous magnesium salicylate). Capl. Bot. 50s. *otc.*
Use: Anti-inflammatory.

Nuprin Caplets. (Bristol-Myers) Ibuprofen 200 mg/Capl. Bot. 24s, 50s, 100s. *otc.*
Use: Analgesic, NSAID.

Nuprin Tablets. (Bristol-Myers) Ibuprofen 200 mg/Tab. Blister Pak 8s. Bot. 24s, 50s, 100s. *otc.*
Use: Analgesic, NSAID.

Nuquin HP. (Stratus) **Cream:** 4% hydroquinone, 30 mg dioxybenzone, 20 mg oxybenzone per g. Vanishing base. Stearyl alcohol, EDTA, sodium metabisulfite. Tube 14.2 g, 28.4 g, 56.7 g. **Gel:** 4% hydroquinone, 30 mg dioxybenzone per g. Alcohol, sodium metabisulfite, EDTA. Tube 14.2 g, 28.4 g. *Rx.*
Use: Dermatologic.

Nuromax. (GlaxoWellcome) Doxacurium chloride 1 mg/ml. Inj. Vial 5 ml. *Rx.*
Use: Neuromuscular blocker.

Nu-Salt. (Cumberland Pkg) Potassium Cl, potassium bitartrate, calcium silicate, natural flavor derived from yeast. Sodium 0.85 mg/5 g (< 0.04 mEq/5 g), potassium 2640 mg/5 g (68 mEq/5 g). Pkg. 90 g. *otc.*
Use: Salt substitute.

Nu-Tears. (Optopics) Polyvinyl alcohol 1.4%, EDTA, NaCl, benzalkonium chloride, potassium chloride. Soln. Bot. 15 ml. *otc.*
Use: Artificial tears.

Nu-Tears II. (Optopics) Polyvinyl alcohol 1%, PEG-400 1%, EDTA, benzalkonium chloride. Soln. Bot. 15 ml. *otc.*
Use: Artificial tears.

Nu-Thera. (Kirkman Sales) Vitamins A 10,000 IU, D 400 IU, B_1 10 mg, B_2 5 mg, niacinamide 100 mg, B_6 1 mg, B_{12} 5 mcg, C 150 mg, calcium 103 mg, phosphorus 80 mg, iron 10 mg, magnesium 5.5 mg, manganese 1 mg, potassium 5 mg, zinc 1.4 mg/Cap. Bot. 100s. *otc.*
Use: Mineral, vitamin supplement.

nutmeg oil.
Use: Pharmaceutic aid (flavor).

Nutracort. (Galderma) Hydrocortisone 1%. **Cream:** Jar 4 oz. Tube 30 g, 60 g. *Rx.*
Use: Corticosteroid, topical.

Nutraderm. (Galderma) Oil-in-water emulsion. **Lot.:** Plastic bot. 8 oz, 16 oz. **Cream:** Tube 1.5 oz, 3 oz, Jar lb. *otc.*
Use: Emollient.

Nutraderm Bath Oil. (Galderma) Mineral oil, PEG-4 dilaurate, lanolin oil, butylparaben, benzophenone-3, fragrance, D & C Green No. 6. Bot. 8 oz. *otc.*
Use: Emollient.

Nutraloric. (Nutraloric) A chocolate, vanilla or strawberry flavored liquid containing, when mixed with whole milk to make 1 L, 91.7 g protein, 175 g carbohydrates, 125 g fat, 875 mg sodium, 3166.7 mg potassium, 2.2 calories/ml. Pow. Can 480 g. *otc.*
Use: Nutritional supplement.

Nutrament Drink Box. (Drackett) Protein 10 g, fat 7 g, carbohydrate 35 g, vitamins, minerals/240 calories/8 oz. Drink Box. *otc.*
Use: Nutritional supplement.

Nutrament Liquid. (Drackett) Protein 16 g, fat 10 g, carbohydrates 52 g, vitamins, minerals/360 calories/12 oz. Can. *otc.*
Use: Nutritional supplement.

Nutramigen. (Bristol-Myers) Hypoallergenic formula that supplies 640 calories/qt. Protein 18 g, fat 25 g, carbohydrates 86 g, vitamins A 2000 IU, D 400 IU, E 20 IU, C 52 mg, folic acid 100 mcg, B_1 0.5 mg, B_2 0.6 mg, niacin 8 mg, B_6 0.4 mg, B_{12} 2 mcg, biotin 50 mcg, pantothenic acid 3 mg, K-1 100 mcg, choline 85 mg, inositol 30 mg, calcium 600 mg, phosphorus 400 mg, iodine 45 mcg, iron 12 mg, magnesium 70 mg, copper 0.6 mg, zinc 5 mg, manganese 200 mcg, chloride 550 mg, potassium 700 mg, sodium 300 mg/qt of formula (4.9 oz pow.). Can 16 oz, 390 ml concentrate and 1 qt ready-to-use. *otc.*
Use: Nutritional supplement.

Nutramin. (Thurston) Vitamins A 666 IU, D 66 IU, B_1 666 mcg, B_2 333 mcg, niacinamide 2 mg, folic acid 0.0444 mcg, calcium 16.6 mg, phosphorus 8.33 mg, iron 1.33 mg, iodine 0.15 mg/Tab. Bot. 200s, 500s, 1000s. *otc.*
Use: Mineral, vitamin supplement.

Nutramin Granular. (Thurston) Vitamins A 333 IU, D 333 IU, B_1 3.3 mg, B_2 1.6 mg, niacinamide 10 mg, folic acid 0.133 mg, calcium 250 mg, phosphorus 115 mg, iron 6.6 mg, iodine 0.15 mg/5 g. Bot. 10 oz, 32 oz. *otc.*
Use: Mineral, vitamin supplement.

Nutraplus. (Galderma) Urea 10% in emollient cream base or lotion base with preservatives. **Cream:** Tube 3 oz, Jar lb. **Lot.:** Bot. 8 oz, 16 oz. *otc.*
Use: Emollient.

Nutra-Soothe. (Pertussin) Colloidal oatmeal and light mineral oil. Emollient bath preparation. Pow. Pkts. 9s. *otc.*
Use: Dermatologic.

Nutravims. (Health for Life Brands) Vitamins A 6000 IU, D 1250 IU, C 50 mg, E 5 IU, B_{12} 5 mcg, B_1 3 mg, B_2 3 mg, B_6 0.5 mg, niacinamide 20 mg, calcium pantothenate 5 mg, zinc 1.5 mg, manganese 1 mg, iodine 0.15 mg, potassium 5 mg, magnesium 4 mg, iron 15 mg, calcium 59 mg, phosphorus 45 mg/Cap. Bot. 100s, 250s, 1000s. *otc.*
Use: Mineral, vitamin supplement.

Nutren 1.0 Liquid. (Clintec Nutrition) Potassium and sodium caseinate, maltodextrin, sucrose, MCT, corn oil, lecithin, vitamins A, B_1, B_2, B_3, B_5, B_6, B_{12}, C, D, E, K, folic acid, biotin, choline, Ca, Cl, Cu, Fe, I, Mg, Mn, P, Zn. 250 ml. *otc.*
Use: Nutritional supplement.

Nutren 1.5 Liquid. (Clintec Nutrition) Casein, maltodextrin, corn syrup, sucrose, MCT, corn oil, vitamins A, B_1, B_2, B_3, B_5, B_6, B_{12}, C, D, E, K, folic acid, biotin, choline, Ca, Cl, Cu, Fe, I, Mg, Mn, P, Zn. 250 ml. *otc.*
Use: Nutritional supplement.

Nutren 2.0 Liquid. (Clintec Nutrition) Casein, maltodextrin, corn syrup, sucrose, MCT, corn oil, vitamins A, B_1, B_2, B_3, B_5, B_6, B_{12}, C, D, E, K, folic acid, biotin, choline, Ca, Cl, Cu, Fe, I, Mg, Mn, P, Zn. 250 ml. *otc.*
Use: Nutritional supplement.

Nutrex. (Holloway) Calcium 162 mg, iron 27 mg, vitamins A 5000 IU, D 400 IU,

E 30 mg, B_1 2.25 mg, B_2 2.6 mg, B_3 20 mg, B_5 10 mg, B_6 3 mg, B_{12} 9 mcg, C 90 mg, folic acid 0.4 mg, Cu, I, K, Mg, Mn, P, zinc 22.5 mg, biotin 45 mcg/Tab. Bot. 100s. *otc.*
Use: Mineral, vitamin supplement.

Nutricon Tablets. (Taylor Pharmaceuticals) Calcium 200 mg, iron 20 mg, vitamins A 2500 IU, D 200 IU, E 15 mg, B_1 1.5 mg, B_2 1.5 mg, B_3 10 mg, B_5 5 mg, B_6 2 mg, B_{12} 5 mcg, C 50 mg, folic acid 0.4 mg, Cu, I, Mg, zinc 3.75 mg, biotin 150 mcg/Tab. Bot. 120s. *otc.*
Use: Mineral, vitamin supplement.

Nutri-E. (Nutri Lab.) Vitamin E. **Cream:** 200 IU/g. Jar 1 oz, 2 oz. **Oil:** 1 oz. **Oint.:** 200 IU/g. Tube 1 oz, 1.5 oz. **Cap.:** 200 IU. Bot. 80s; 400 IU. Bot. 60s, 100s; 800 IU. Bot. 55s. *otc.*
Use: Vitamin supplement.

Nutrilan. (Elan) A vanilla, chocolate or strawberry flavored liquid containing 38 g protein, 37 g fat, 143 g carbohydrates, 632.5 mg Na, 1.073 g K/L. With appropriate vitamins and minerals. In 237 ml Tetra Pak containers. *otc.*
Use: Nutritional supplement.

Nutrilipid. (McGaw) Soybean oil intravenous fat emulsion. **10%:** Calories 1.1/ml. In 250 ml, 500 ml. **20%:** Calories 2/ml. In 250 ml, 500 ml. *Rx.*
Use: Nutritional supplement, parenteral.

Nutrilyte. (American Regent) Acetate 2.03 mEq, potassium 2.03 mEq, chloride 1.68 mEq, sodium 1.25 mEq, magnesium 0.4 mEq, calcium 0.25 mEq, gluconate 0.25 mEq per ml, ≈ 6212 mOsml/L. Concentrated soln. Bot. 20 ml, 100 ml. *Rx.*
Use: Nutritional supplement, parenteral.

Nutrilyte II. (American Regent) Acetate 1.475 mEq, potassium 1 mEq, chloride 1.75 mEq, sodium 1.75 mEq, magnesium 0.25 mEq, calcium 0.225 mEq per ml, ≈ 6212 mOsml/L. Concentrated soln. Bot. 20 ml, 100 ml. *Rx.*
Use: Nutritional supplement, parenteral.

Nutri-Plex Tablets. (Faraday) Vitamins B_1 5 mg, B_2 5 mg, B_6 5 mg, pantothenic acid 25 mg, B_{12} 12.5 mcg, niacinamide 50 mg, iron gluconate 30 mg, choline bitartrate 50 mg, inositol 50 mg, PABA 15 mg, C 150 mg/2 Tab. Bot. 100s, 250s. *otc.*
Use: Mineral, vitamin supplement.

Nutrisource Modular System. (Novartis) Individual Nutrisource modules available: protein, amino acids, amino acids-high branched chain, carbohydrate, lipid-medium chain triglycerides, lipid-long branched chain triglycerides, vitamins, minerals. Cans of liquid. Packets of powder. *otc.*
Use: Nutritional supplement.

Nutri-Val. (Marcen) Vitamins A 5000 IU, D 500 IU, B_1 10 mg, B_2 5 mg, B_{12} activity 5 mcg, B_6 5 mcg, C 50 mg, hesperidin 5 mg, niacinamide 15 mg, folic acid 0.2 mg, calcium pantothenate 50 mg, choline bitartrate 50 mg, betaine HCl 25 mg, lipo-K 0.4 mg, duodenum substance 50 mg, pancreas substance 50 mg, inositol 25 mg, Cy-yeast hydrolysates 50 mg, rutin 5 mg, 1-lysine HCl 5 mg, E 5 IU, Ossonate (glucuronic complex) 8 mg, glutamic acid 30 mg, lecithin 5 mg, iron 20 mg, iodine 0.15 mg, calcium 50 mg, phosphorus 40 mg, boron 0.1 mg, copper 1 mg, manganese 1 mg, magnesium 1 mg, potassium 5 mg, zinc 0.5 mg, biotin 0.02 mg/Cap. Bot. 100s, 500s, 1000s. *otc.*
Use: Mineral, vitamin supplement.

Nutri-Vite Natural Multiple Vitamin and Minerals. (Faraday) Vitamins A 15,000 IU, D 400 IU, B_1 1.5 mg, B_2 3 mg, B_{12} 15 mcg, niacin 500 mcg, B_6 20 mcg, choline 1.75 mg, folic acid 13 mcg, pantothenic acid 50 mcg, p-aminobenzoic acid 12 mcg, inositol 1.72 mg, C 60 mg, citrus bioflavonoids 15 mg, E 50 IU, iron gluconate 15 mg, calcium 192 mg, phosphorus 85 mg, iodine 0.15 mg, red bone marrow 30 mg/3 Tab. Protein coated Tab. Bot. 100s, 250s. *otc.*
Use: Mineral, vitamin supplement.

Nutrizyme. (Enzyme Process) Vitamins A 5000 IU, D 400 IU, C 60 mg, B_1 1.5 mg, B_2 1.7 mg, niacinamide 20 mg, B_6 2 mg, pantothenate 10 mg, B_{12} 6 mcg, E 30 IU, iron 10 mg, copper 1 mg, zinc 1 mg, Folacin 0.025 mg/Tab. Bot. 90s, 250s. *otc.*
Use: Mineral, vitamin supplement.

Nutropin. (Genentech) Somatropin 5 mg (≈ 13 IU)/vial, 10 mg (≈ 26 IU)/vial. Pow. for inj. (lyophilized). Vials with 10 ml diluent. *Rx.*
Use: Hormone, growth.

Nutropin AQ. (Genentech) Somatropin 10 mg/Inj. (≈ 30 IU) Vial. *Rx.*
Use: Hormone, growth.

Nutrox Capsules. (Tyson and Associates) Vitamins A 10,000 IU, E 150 IU, B_1 25 mg, B_2 25 mg, B_3 50 mg, B_5 22 mg, C 80 mg, L-cysteine, taurine, glutathione, zinc oxide 15 mg, Se/Cap. Bot. 90s. *otc.*
Use: Mineral, vitamin supplement.

Nuzine Ointment. (Hobart) Guaiacol

1.66 g, oxyquinoline sulfate 0.42 g, zinc oxide 2.5 g, glycerine 1.66 g, lanum (anhydrous) 43.76 g, petrolatum 50 g/ 100 g. Tube 1 oz. *otc.*
Use: Anorectal preparation.

Nycoff. (Dover Pharmaceuticals) Dextromethorphan HBr/Tab. UD Box 500s. Sugar, lactose and salt free. *otc.*
Use: Antitussive.

Nyco-White. (Whiteworth Towne) Nystatin, neomycin, gramcidin, triamcinolone. Cream. Tube 15 g, 30 g, 60 g. *Rx.*
Use: Anti-infective, topical.

Nyco-Worth. (Whiteworth Towne) Nystatin. Cream Tube 15 g. *Rx.*
Use: Antifungal, topical.

Nydrazid Injection. (Apothecon) Isoniazid 100 mg/ml, chlorobutanol 0.25%, sodium hydroxide or hydrochloric acid to adjust pH. Vial 10 ml. *Rx.*
Use: Antituberculous.

•**nylestriol.** (NYE-less-TRY-ole) USAN.
Use: Estrogen.

NyQuil Cough/Cold, Children's. (Procter & Gamble) Pseudoephedrine HCl 10 mg, chlorpheniramine maleate 0.67 mg, dextromethorphan HBr 5 mg/5 ml, sucrose, alcohol free, cherry flavor. Liq. 120 ml. *otc.*
Use: Antihistamine, antitussive, decongestant.

NyQuil Hot Therapy. (Procter & Gamble) Pseudoephedrine HCl 60 mg, doxylamine succinate 12.5 mg, dextromethorphan HBr 30 mg, acetaminophen 1000 mg. Powd. 6s. *otc.*
Use: Analgesic, antihistamine, antitussive, decongestant.

NyQuil Liqui-Caps. (Procter & Gamble) Pseudoephedrine HCl 30 mg, diphenhydramine HCl 25 mg, dextromethorphan HBr 15 mg, acetaminophen 250 mg/Cap. Bot. 20s. *otc.*
Use: Analgesic, antihistamine, antitussive, decongestant.

NyQuil Nighttime Cold/Flu Medicine. (Procter & Gamble) Pseudoephedrine HCl 10 mg, doxylamine succinate 2.1 mg, dextromethorphan HBr 5 mg, acetaminophen 167 mg/5 ml, alcohol 10%, sucrose, saccharin (cherry flavor), tartrazine (regular flavor). Liq. Bot. 295 ml. *otc.*
Use: Analgesic, antihistamine, antitussive, decongestant.

NyQuil Nighttime Cold Medicine Liquid. (Procter & Gamble) Dextromethorphan HBr 30 mg, pseudoephedrine HCl 60 mg, doxylamine succinate 7.5 mg, acetaminophen 1000 mg/oz, alcohol 25%. Regular and cherry flavors. Regular flavor contains FDC Yellow #5 tartrazine. Bot. 6 oz, 10 oz, 14 oz. *otc.*
Use: Analgesic, antihistamine, antitussive, decongestant.

NyQuil Nighttime Head Cold Allergy Formula, Children's. (Procter & Gamble) Pseudoephedrine HCl, chlorpheniramine maleate per 5 ml, 0.67 mg, alcohol free, sorbitol, sucrose, grape flavor. Liq. Bot. 120 ml. *otc.*
Use: Antihistamine, decongestant.

Nyral. (Pal-Pak) Cetylpyridinium Cl 0.5 mg, benzocaine 5 mg/Loz. w/parabens. Pkg. 100s, 1000s. *otc.*
Use: Antiseptic.

•**nystatin.** (nye-STAT-in) U.S.P. 23.
Use: Antifungal.
See: Mycostatin Preps. (Apothecon).
Nilstat, Tab., Cream, Oint., Pow. (ESI Lederle Generics).
Nilstat, Oral Drops (ESI Lederle Generics).
Nilstat, Vaginal Tab. (ESI Lederle Generics).
Nystatin, Bulk Pow. (Paddock).
Nystex, Cream, Oint., Susp. (Savage).
O-V Statin, Tab. (Squibb Diagnostic).
Pedi-Dri, Pow. (Pedinol).
W/Clioquinol.
See: Nystaform, Oint. (Bayer Corp).
W/Demethylchlortetracycline.
See: Declostatin, Tab., Cap. (ESI Lederle Generics).
W/Gramicidin, neomycin, triamcinolone.
See: Mycolog, Cream, Oint. (Bristol-Myers Squibb).
W/Tetracycline phosphate buffered.
See: Achrostatin-V, Cap. (ESI Lederle Generics).
W/Tetracycline phosphate complex.
See: Tetrex-F, Cap. (Bristol-Myers Squibb).

nystatin. (Various Mfr.) 100,000 units/ml.
Oral Susp. Bot. 5 ml, 60 ml, 480 ml.
Vaginal Tab. Pkg. 15s or 30s.
Use: Antifungal.

nystatin and triamcinolone acetonide cream.
Use: Antifungal, corticosteroid, topical.

nystatin and triamcinolone acetonide ointment.
Use: Antifungal, corticosteroid, topical.

nystatin, neomycin sulfate, gramicidin and triamcinolone acetonide.
Use: Antifungal, anti-infective, corticosteroid, topical.
See: Mycolog, Prods. (Bristol-Myers Squibb).

Nystex Cream & Ointment. (Savage) Nystatin 100,000 units/g. Tube 15 g, 30 g. *Rx.*
Use: Antifungal, topical.

Nystex Oral Suspension. (Savage) Nystatin 100,000 units/ml in suspension. Bot. 60 ml. *Rx.*
Use: Antifungal, topical.

Nytcold Medicine. (Rugby) Pseudoephedrine HCl 10 mg, doxylamine succinate 1.25 mg, dextromethorphan HBr 5 mg, acetaminophen 167 mg, alcohol 25%, glucose, saccharin, sucrose, cherry flavor. Liq. Bot. 177 ml. *otc.*
Use: Analgesic, antihistamine, antitussive, decongestant.

Nytime Cold Medicine. (Rugby) Acetaminophen 1000 mg, doxylamine succinate 7.5 mg, pseudoephedrine HCl 60 mg, dextromethorphan HBr 30 mg/30 ml, alcohol 25%. Bot. 6 oz, 10 oz. *otc.*
Use: Analgesic, antihistamine, antitussive, decongestant.

Nytol. (Block Drug) Diphenhydramine HCl 25 mg/Tab. Bot. 16s, 32s, 72s. *otc.*
Use: Sleep aid.

Nytol, Maximum Strength. (Block Drug) Diphenhydramine HCl 50 mg, lactose. Tab. Bot. 8s. *otc.*
Use: Sleep aid.

O

O.A.D. (Sween) Ostomy. Bot. 1.25 oz, 4 oz, 8 oz. *otc.*
Use: Deodorant-ostomy.

Oasis. (Zitar) Artificial saliva. Bot. 6 oz. *otc.*
Use: Antixerostomia agent.

•**oatmeal, colloidal.** U.S.P. 23.
Use: Antipruritic, topical.

oatmeal, gum fraction.
See: Aveeno, Preps. (Rydelle).

Obe-Nix 30. (Holloway) Phentermine HCl 30 mg/Cap. (equivalent to 24 mg base) Bot. 100s. *c-IV.*
Use: Anorexiant.

Obepar. (Tyler) Vitamins A 3000 IU, D 300 IU, B_1 3 mg, B_2 2 mg, nicotinamide 10 mg, B_6 3 mg, calcium pantothenate 2 mg, B_{12} 3 mcg, C 37.5 mg, calcium 150 mg, iron 5 mg, magnesium 1 mg, manganese 0.1 mg, potassium 1 mg, zinc 0.15 mg/Cap. Bot. 100s. *otc.*
Use: Mineral, vitamin supplement.

Obe-Tite. (Scott/Cord) Phendimetrazine tartrate 35 mg/Tab. Bot. 100s, 500s. *c-III.*
Use: Anorexiant.

Obezine. (Western Research) Phendimetrazine tartrate 35 mg/Tab. Handicount 28 (36 bags of 28s). *c-III.*
Use: Anorexiant.

•**obidoxime chloride.** (OH-bih-DOX-eem) USAN.
Use: Cholinesterase reactivator.

Obrical. (Canright) Calcium lactate 500 mg, vitamins D 400 IU, ferrous sulfate exsiccated 35 mg, B_1 1 mg, B_2 1 mg, C 10 mg/Tab. Bot. 100s, 1000s. *otc.*
Use: Mineral, vitamin supplement.

Obrical-F. (Canright) Ferrous sulfate 50 mg, calcium lactate 500 mg, vitamins D 400 IU, B_1 1 mg, B_2 1 mg, C 10 mg, folic acid 0.67 mg/Tab. Bot. 100s, 1000s. *otc.*
Use: Mineral, vitamin supplement.

Obrite. (Milton Roy) Contact lens and eye glass cleaner. Plastic spray Bot. 30 ml, 55 ml. *otc.*
Use: Contact lens and eye glass care.

OB-Tinic. (Roberts Pharm) Iron 65 mg, vitamins A 6000 IU, D 400 IU, E 30 IU, B_1 1.1 mg, B_2 1.8 mg, B_3 15 mg, B_6 2.5 mg, B_{12} 5 mcg, C 60 mg, folic acid 1 mg, Ca/Tab. Bot. 100s. *Rx.*
Use: Mineral, vitamin supplement.

O-Cal f.a. (Pharmics) **Tab.:** Ca 200 mg, iron 66 mg, vitamins A 5000 IU, D 400 IU, E 30 mg, B_1 3 mg, B_2 3 mg, B_3 20 mg, B_6 4 mg, B_{12} 12 mcg, C 90 mg, folic acid 1 mg, fluoride 1.1 mg, Mg, I, Cu, Zn 15 mg. Bot. 100s. *Rx.*
Use: Mineral, vitamin supplement.

•**ocaperidone.** (oke-ah-PURR-ih-dohn) USAN.
Use: Antipsychotic.

Occlusal HP. (Genderm) Salicylic acid 17%. Bot. 10 ml. *otc.*
Use: Keratolytic.

Occucoat. (Storz Ophthalmics) Hydroxypropyl methylcellulose 2%. Soln. Syringe 1 ml with cannula. *Rx.*
Use: Ophthalmic.

Ocean. (Fleming) Sodium Cl 0.65%, benzyl alcohol. Bot. 45 ml, pt. *otc.*
Use: Moisturizer, nasal.

Ocean Plus. (Fleming) Caffeine 2.5%, benzyl alcohol. Bot. 15 ml. *otc.*

•**ocfentanil hydrochloride.** (ock-FEN-tah-NILL) USAN.
Use: Analgesic, narcotic.

•**ocinaplon.** (oh-SIN-ah-plahn) USAN.
Use: Anxiolytic.

OCL Solution. (Abbott Hospital Prods) Oral colonic lavage soln. Sodium Cl 146 mg, sodium bicarbonate 168 mg, sodium sulfate decahydrate 1.29 g, potassium Cl 75 mg, PEG-3350 6 g, polysorbate-80 30 ml/100 ml. 1.35 L 3-pack units. *Rx.*
Use: Laxative.

•**ocrylate.** (AH-krih-late) USAN.
Use: Surgical aid (tissue adhesive).

•**octabenzone.** (OCK-tah-BEN-zone) USAN.
Use: Ultraviolet screen.

octadecanoic acid.
See: Stearic Acid, N.F. 18.

octadecanoic acid, sodium salt.
See: Sodium Stearate, N.F. 18.

octadecanoic acid, zinc salt.
See: Zinc Stearate, N.F. 18.

octadecanol-l.
See: Stearyl Alcohol, N.F. 18.

Octamide. (Pharmacia & Upjohn) Metoclopramide 10 mg/Tab. Bot. 100s, 500s. *Rx.*
Use: Gastrointestinal stimulant, antiemetic.

Octamide PFS. (Pharmacia & Upjohn) Metoclopramide HCl 5 mg/ml, preservative free. Vial. Single dose; 2, 10, 30 ml. *Rx.*
Use: Antiemetic, gastrointestinal stimulant.

•**octanoic acid.** (OCK-tah-NO-ik) USAN.
Use: Antifungal.

octapeptide sequence.
Use: Antiviral.
See: Flumadine (Roche Laboratories).

Octarex. (Health for Life Brands) Vitamins A 5000 IU, D 1000 IU, B_1 1.5 mg, B_2 2 mg, B_6 0.1 mg, calcium pantothenate 1 mg, niacinamide 20 mg, C 37.5 mg, E 1 IU, B_{12} 1 mcg/Cap. Bot. 100s, 1000s. *otc.*
Use: Mineral, vitamin supplement.

Octavims. (Health for Life Brands) Vitamins A 6000 IU, D 1250 IU, C 50 mg, E 5 IU, B_1 3 mg, B_2 3 mg, B_6 0.5 mg, niacinamide 20 mg, calcium pantothenate 5 mg, B_{12} 5 mcg, calcium 59 mg, phosphorus 45 mg/Cap. Bot. 100s, 250s, 1000s. *otc.*
Use: Mineral, vitamin supplement.

•**octazamide.** (OCK-TAY-zah-mide) USAN.
Use: Analgesic.

•**octenidine hydrochloride.** (OCK-TEN-ih-deen) USAN.
Use: Anti-infective, topical.

•**octenidine saccharin.** (OCK-TEN-ih-deen SACK-ah-rin) USAN.
Use: Dental plaque inhibitor.

•**octicizer.** (OCK-tih-SIGH-zer) USAN. Santicizer 141
Use: Pharmaceutic aid (plasticizer).

Octocaine HCl. (Novocol Chemical) Lidocaine HCl 2%, epinephrine 1:50,000 or 1:100,000. Inj. Dent. Cartridge 1.8 ml. *Rx.*
Use: Anesthetic, local.

•**octocrylene.** (OCK-toe-KRIH-leen) USAN.
Use: Ultraviolet screen.

•**octodrine.** (OCK-toe-DREEN) USAN. Under study.
Use: Adrenergic (vasoconstrictor); anesthetic, local.

octofollin.
See: Benzestrol, U.S.P. 23.

•**octoxynol 9.** (ock-TOXE-ih-nahl 9) N.F. 18.
Use: Pharmaceutic aid (surfactant).

OctreoScan. (Mallinckrodt Chemical) Oxidronate sodium 2 mg, stannous chloride (anhydrous) 0.16 mg, gentisic acid 0.56 mg, sodium chloride 30 mg/vial. Powd. lyophilized. In kits containing 5 ml or 30 ml vials and additive-free sodium pertechnate Tc-99m (for reconstitution). *Rx.*
Use: Diagnostic aid, radiopaque agent.

•**octreotide.** (ock-TREE-oh-tide) USAN.
Use: Antisecretory (gastric).

•**octreotide acetate.** (ock-TREE-oh-tide) USAN.
Use: Antidiarrheal, gastrointestinal tumor; antihypotensive, carcinoid crisis; growth hormone suppressant, acromegaly, antisecretory (gastric).

•**octreotide pamoate.** (ock-TREE-oh-tide PAM-oh-ate) USAN.
Use: Antineoplastic.

•**octriptyline phosphate.** (ock-TRIP-tih-leen FOSS-fate) USAN.
Use: Antidepressant.

•**octrizole.** (OCK-TRY-zole) USAN.
Use: Ultraviolet screen.

n-octyl bicyalohephene dicarbosimide.
See: Bansum, Bot. (Summers).

•**octyldodecanol.** N.F. 18.
Use: Pharmaceutic aid (oleaginous vehicle).

octylphenoxy polyethoxyethanol. A mono-ether of a polyethylene glycol. Igepal CA 630 (Antara).
W/Phenylmercuric acetate, methylparaben, sodium borate.
See: Lorophyn jelly, Supp. (Eaton Medical).
W/Lactic acid, sodium lactate.
See: Jeneen premeasured liquid douche (Procter & Gamble).

OcuClear. (Schering Plough) Oxymetazoline HCl 0.025%. Bot. 30 ml. *otc.*
Use: Mydriatic, vasoconstrictor.

OcuCoat. (Storz Ophthalmics) Hydroxypropyl methylcellulose 2%. Soln. Syringe 1 ml. *Rx.*
Use: Lubricant, ophthalmic.

OcuCoat PF. (Storz Ophthalmics) Dextran 70 0.1%, hydroxypropyl methylcellulose, NaCl, KCl, dextrose, sodium phosphate. Preservative free. Drops. In 0.5 ml single-dose containers. *otc.*
Use: Lubricant, ophthalmic.

Ocufen. (Allergan) Flurbiprofen sodium 0.03%. Bot. 2.5 ml, 5 ml, 10 ml w/dropper. *Rx.*
Use: NSAID, ophthalmic.

•**ocufilcon A.** (OCK-you-FILL-kahn A) USAN.
Use: Contact lens material (hydrophilic).

•**ocufilcon B.** (OCK-you-FILL-kahn B) USAN.
Use: Contact lens material (hydrophilic).

•**ocufilcon C.** (OCK-you-FILL-kahn C) USAN.
Use: Contact lens material (hydrophilic).

•**ocufilcon D.** (OCK-you-FILL-kahn D) USAN.
Use: Contact lens material (hydrophilic).

•**ocufilcon E.** (OCK-you-FILL-kahn E) USAN.
Use: Contact lens material (hydrophilic).

Ocuflox. (Allergan) Ofloxacin 3 mg/ml. Soln. Bot. 1 ml, 5 ml. *Rx.*
Use: Anti-infective, ophthalmic.

ocular lubricants.
Use: Ophthalmic.
See: Akwa Tears (Akorn).
Artificial Tears (Rugby).
Dey-Lube (Dey Labs).
Dry Eyes (Bausch & Lomb).
Duolube (Bausch & Lomb).
Duratears Naturale (Alcon Laboratories).
Hypotears (Novartis Vision).
Lacri-Lube NP (Allergan).
Lacri-Lube S.O.P. (Allergan).
Lipo-Tears (Spectra).
LubriTears (Bausch & Lomb).
OcuCoat PF (Storz Ophthalmics).
Puralube (E. Fougera).
Refresh PM (Allergan).
Tears Renewed (Akorn).
Vit-A-Drops (Vision Pharm).

Ocu-Lube. (Bausch & Lomb) Petrolatum sterile, preservative and lanolin free. Tube 3.5 g. *otc.*
Use: Lubricant, ophthalmic.

Ocumeter.
See: Decadron Phosphate, Preps. (Merck).
Humorsol, Ophth. Soln. (Merck).
Neo-Decadron, Preps. (Merck).

Ocupress. (Otsuka America) Carteolol HCl 1%. Soln. Bot. 5 ml, 10 ml. *Rx.*
Use: Beta-adrenergic blocker, antiglaucoma agent.

Ocusert. (Alza) Pilocarpine ocular therapeutic system. *Rx.*
Pilo-20: Releases 20 mcg pilocarpine/hour for one week. Pkg. 8s.
Pilo-40: Releases 40 mcg pilocarpine/hour for one week. Pkg. 8s.
Use: Antiglaucoma agent.

OCuSOFT. (OCuSOFT) PEG-80 sorbitan laurate, sodium trideceth sulfate, PEG-150 distearate, cocoamido propyl hydroxysultaine, lauroamphocarboxyglycinate, sodium laureth-13 carboxylate, PEG-15 tallow polyamine, quaternium-15. Soln. Pads UD 30s, Bot. 30 ml, 120 ml, 240 ml, Compliance kit (120 ml and 100 pads). *otc.*
Use: Cleanser, ophthalmic.

OCuSOFT VMS. tab.: Vitamins A 5000 IU, E 30 IU, C 60 mg, Cu, Se, Zn 40 mg. Bot. 60s. *otc.*
Use: Mineral, vitamin supplement.

Ocusulf-10. (Optopics) Sodium sulfacetamide 10%. Soln. Bot. 2 ml, 5 ml, 15 ml. *Rx.*
Use: Anti-infective, ophthalmic.

Ocutricin. (Bausch & Lomb) **Oint.:** Polymyxin B sulfate 10,000 units, bacitracin zinc 400 units, neomycin sulfate 3.5 mg. Tube 3.5 g. *Rx.*
Use: Antibiotic-ophthalmic.

Ocuvite. (Bausch & Lomb) Formerly distributed by Storz. Vitamins A 5000 IU, E 30 IU, C 60 mg, Zn 40 mg, Cu, Se 40 mcg, lactose/Tab. Bot. 60s. *otc.*
Use: Mineral, vitamin supplement.

Ocuvite Extra. (Bausch & Lomb) Vitamin A 6000 IU, C 200 mg, E 50 IU, Zn 40 mg, B_3 40 mg, B_2 3 mg, Cu, Se, Mn, l-glutathione. 50s. Tab. Bot. *otc.*
Use: Vitamin supplement.

Odara. (Lorvic) Alcohol 48%, carbolic acid less than 2%, zinc Cl, potassium iodide, glycerin, methyl salicylate, oil eucalyptus, tincture myrrh. Concentrated Liq. Bot. 8 oz. *otc.*
Use: Mouthwash.

oestergon.
See: Estradiol (Various Mfr.).

Oesto-Mins. (Tyson and Associates) Ascorbic acid 500 mg, Ca 250 mg, Mg 250 mg, K 45 mg, vitamin D 100 IU/ 4.5 g. Powd. 200 g. *otc.*
Use: Vitamin Supplement.

oestradiol.
See: Estradiol (Various Mfr.).

oestrasid.
See: Dienestrol (Various Mfr.).

oestrin.
See: Estrone (Various Mfr.).

oestroform.
See: Estrone (Various Mfr.).

oestromenin.
See: Diethylstilbestrol (Various Mfr.).

oestromon.
See: Diethylstilbestrol (Various Mfr.).

OFF-Ezy Corn & Callous Remover. (Del Pharmaceuticals) Salicylic acid 17% in a collodion-like vehicle of 65% ether and 21% alcohol. Kit. 13.5 ml with callous smoother and 3 corn cushions. *otc.*
Use: Keratolytic.

OFF-Ezy Corn Remover. (Del Pharmaceuticals) Salicylic acid 13.57% in flexible collodion base, ether 65%, alcohol 21%. Bot. 0.45 oz. *otc.*
Use: Keratolytic.

OFF-Ezy Wart Remover. (Del Pharmaceuticals) Salicylic acid 17% in flexible collodion base, ether 65%, alcohol 21%. Bot. 13.5 ml. *otc.*
Use: Keratolytic.

•**ofloxacin.** (oh-FLOX-uh-SIN) U.S.P. 23.
Use: Anti-infective. [Orphan drug]

See: Floxin (Daiichi).
Ocuflox, Ophth. Soln. (Allergan).

•**ofornine.** (ah-FAR-neen) USAN.
Use: Antihypertensive.

Ogen. (Abbott Laboratories) Estropipate. **Tab. 0.625:** Estropipate 0.75 mg/Tab. Bot. 100s. **Tab. 1.25:** Estropipate 1.5 mg/Tab. Bot. 100s. **Tab. 2.5:** Estropipate 3 mg/Tab. Bot. 100s. *Rx.*
Use: Estrogen.

Ogen Vaginal Cream. (Pharmacia & Upjohn) Estropipate 1.5 mg/g. Cream. Tube 42.5 g w/applicator. *Rx.*
Use: Estrogen.

Oilatum Soap. (Stiefel) Polyunsaturated vegetable oil 7.5%. Bar 120 g, 240 g. *otc.*
Use: Dermatologic, cleanser.

oil of camphor w/combinations.
See: Sloan's Liniment, Liq. (Warner Lambert).

oil of cloves w/alcohol.
See: Buckley "Z.O.", Liq. (Crosby).

Oil of Olay Daily UV Protectant. (Procter & Gamble) SPF 15. **Cream:**Titanium dioxide, ethylhexyl p-methoxycinnamate, 2-phenylbenzimidazole- 5-sulfonic acid, glycerin, triethanolamine, imidazolidinyl urea, parabens, carbomer, PEG-10, EDTA, castor oil, tartrazine. Scented and unscented. 51 g. **Lot.:** Ethylhexyl p-methoxycinnamate, 2-phenylbenzimidazole-5sulfonic acid, titanium dioxide, cetyl alcohol, imidazolidinyl urea, parabens, EDTA, castor oil, tartrazine. Bot. 105 g, 157.7 g. *otc.*
Use: Sunscreen.

Oil of Olay Foaming Face Wash. (Procter & Gamble) Potassium cocoyl hydrolyzed collagen, glycerin, EDTA. Liq. Bot. 90 ml, 210 ml. *otc.*
Use: Dermatologic, acne.

oil of pine w/combinations.
See: Sloan's Liniment, Liq. (Warner Lambert).

ointment base, washable.
See: Absorbent Base (Upsher-Smith Labs).
Cetaphil, Cream, Lot. (Galderma).
Velvachol, Cream (Galderma).

•**ointment, bland lubricating ophthalmic.** U.S.P 23.
Use: Lubricant, ophthalmic.

•**ointment, hydrophilic.** U.S.P. 23.
Use: Pharmaceutic aid (oil-in-water emulsion ointment base).

•**ointment, rose water.** U.S.P 23.
Use: Pharmaceutic aid (emollient, ointment base).

•**ointment, white.** U.S.P. 23.
Use: Pharmaceutical aid (oleaginous ointment base).

•**ointment, yellow.** U.S.P. 23.
Use: Pharmaceutic aid (ointment base).

•**olaflur.** (OH-lah-flure) USAN.
Use: Dental caries agent.

olamine.
See: Ethanolamine.

•**olanzapine.** (oh-LAN-zah-PEEN) USAN.
Use: Antipsychotic.
See: Zyprexa, Tab. (Eli Lilly).

old tuberculin.
See: Mono-Vacc Test (OT), Box (Connaught).
Tuberculin, Old, Tine Test, Jar (Wyeth Ayerst).

oleandomycin phosphate. Phosphate of an antibacterial substance produced by *Streptomyces antibioticus.*
Use: Anti-infective.

oleandomycin salt of penicillin.
See: Pen-M (Pfizer) Under study.

oleandomycin, triacetyl. Troleandomycin, U.S.P. XX.

•**oleic acid.** (oh-LAY-ik) N.F. 18.
Use: Pharmaceutic aid (emulsion adjunct).

•**oleic acid I 125.** USAN.
Use: Radiopharmaceutical.

•**oleic acid I 131.** USAN.
Use: Radiopharmaceutical.

oleovitamin A. Vitamin A, U.S.P. 23.

•**oleovitamin A & D.** U.S.P. 23.
Use: Vitamin supplement.
See: Super-D, Perles, Liq. (Pharmacia & Upjohn).

oleovitamin D, synthetic.
Use: Vitamin supplement.
See: Viosterol in Oil.

•**oleyl alcohol.** (oh-LAY-il) N.F. 18.
Use: Pharmaceutic aid (emulsifying agent, emollient).
See: Patanol, Soln. (Alcon Laboratories).

•**olive oil.** N.F. 18.
Use: Emollient, pharmaceutic aid (setting retardant for dental cements).

•**olopatadine hydrochloride.** (oh-low-pat-AD-een) USAN.
Use: Antiallergic (allergic rhinitis, urticria, allergic conjunctivitis, asthma).
See: Patanol, Soln. (Alcon Laboratories).

•**olsalazine sodium.** (OLE-SAL-uh-zeen) *Formerly Sodium azodisalicylate, azodisal sodium.* USAN.
Use: Maintenance of remission of ulcertiave colitis in patients intolerant of

sulfasalazine; anti-inflammatory (gastrointestinal).
See: Dipentum (Pharmacia & Upjohn).

•**olvanil.** (OLE-van-ill) USAN.
Use: Analgesic.

OM 401.
Use: Sickle cell disease. [Orphan drug]

omega-3 (n-3) polyunsaturated fatty acids. From cold water fish oils.
Use: Dietary supplement to reduce risk of coronary artery disease.
See: Cardi-Omega 3, Cap. (Thompson Medical).
Marine 500, 1000, Cap. (Murdock).
Max EPA, Cap. (Various Mfr.).
Promega, Cap. (Parke-Davis).
Proto-Chol, Cap. (Bristol-Myers Squibb).
Sea-Omega 50, Cap. (Rugby).

Omega Oil. (Block Drug) Methyl nicotinate, methyl salicylate, capsicum oleoresin, histamine dihydrochloride, isopropyl alcohol 44%. Bot. 2.5 oz, 4.85 oz. *otc.*
Use: Analgesic, topical.

•**omeprazole.** (oh-MEH-pray-ZAHL) U.S.P. 23. (Astra Merck)
Use: Depressant (gastric acid secretory).
Agent for gastroesophageal reflux disease.
See: Prilosec, Cap. (Merck).

•**omeprazole sodium.** (oh-MEH-pray-ZOLE) USAN.
Use: Antisecretory (gastric).

OmniCef. (Parke-Davis) **Cap.:** Cefdinir 300 mg. Bot. 60s. **Oral Susp.:** 125 mg/5 ml, sucrose. Bot. 60 ml, 100 ml. *Rx.*
Use: Anti-infective, cephalosporin.

Omnicol. (Delta) Dextromethorphan HBr 15 mg, chlorpheniramine maleate 4 mg, phenylephrine HCl 5 mg, phenindamine tartrate 4 mg, salicylamide 227 mg, acetaminophen 100 mg, caffeine alkaloid 10 mg, ascorbic acid 25 mg/Tab. Bot. 100s. Bot. pt. *otc.*
Use: Antitussive, antihistamine, decongestant, analgesic.

Omnihemin. (Delta) Iron 110 mg, vitamins C 150 mg, B_{12} 7.5 mcg, folic acid 1 mg, zinc 1 mg, copper 1 mg, manganese 1 mg, magnesium 1 mg/Tab. or 5 ml. **Cap.:** Bot. 100s; **Soln.:** Bot. pt. *Rx.*
Use: Mineral, vitamin supplement.

OmniHIB. (SmithKline Beecham Pharmaceuticals) Purified *Haemophilus influenza* type b capsular polysaccharide 10 mcg, tetanus toxoid 24 mcg/0.5 ml, sucrose 8.5%. Pow. for Inj. (lyophilized). Vial w/0.6 ml syringe of diluent. *Rx.*
Use: Immunization.

OMNIhist L.A. (WE Pharm) Phenylephrine 20 mg, chlorpheniramine maleate 8 mg, methscopolamine nitrate 2.5 mg/Tab. Bot. 100s. *Rx.*
Use: Anticholinergic, antihistamine, decongestant.

Omninatal. (Delta) Iron 60 mg, copper 2 mg, zinc 15 mg, vitamins A 8000 IU, D 400 IU, C 90 mg, calcium 200 mg, folic acid 1.5 mg, B_1 2.5 mg, B_2 3 mg, niacinamide 20 mg, pyridoxine HCl 10 mg, pantothenic acid 15 mg, B_{12} 8 mcg/Tab. Bot. 100s. *Rx.*
Use: Mineral, vitamin supplement.

Omnipaque. (Sanofi Winthrop) Iohexol (46.4% iodine). Nonionic contrast medium. **180 mg/ml:** Vial 10 ml, 20 ml. **240 mg/ml:** Vial 10 ml, 100 ml. Bot. 200 ml. **300 mg/ml:** Vial 10 ml, 30 ml, 50 ml, 100 ml. **350 mg/ml:** Vial 50 ml, 100 ml. Bot. 200 ml.
Use: Radiopaque agent.

Omnipen. (Wyeth Ayerst) Ampicillin, anhydrous 250 mg or 500 mg/Cap. Bot. 100s, 500s. *Rx.*
Use: Anti-infective, penicillin.

Omnipen. (Wyeth Ayerst) Ampicillin trihydrate 125 mg or 250 mg/5 ml when reconstituted. Pow. for oral susp. **125 mg/5 ml:** Bot. 100 ml, 150 ml, 200 ml. **250 mg/5 ml:** Bot. 100 ml, 150 ml, 200 ml, UD 5 ml × 20. *Rx.*
Use: Anti-infective, penicillin.

Omnipen-N. (Wyeth Ayerst) Ampicillin sodium pow. for inj. 125 mg, 250 mg, 500 mg, 1 g or 2 g/Vial. Pkg. 10s. Piggyback units 500 mg, 1 g, 2 g, Bulk 10 g/Vial. Pkg. 1s. *Rx.*
Use: Anti-infective, penicillin.

Omniscan. (Sanofi Winthrop) Gadodiamide 287 mg, caldiamide sodium 12 mg/ml. Inj. Vial 10 ml, 20 ml, 15 ml fill in 20 ml vials. *Rx.*
Use: Radiopaque agent.

Omnitabs. (Halsey) Vitamins A 5000 IU, D 400 IU, C 50 mg, B_1 3 mg, B_2 2.5 mg, niacin 20 mg, B_6 1 mg, B_{12} 1 mcg, pantothenic acid 0.9 mg/Tab. Bot. 100s. *otc.*
Use: Vitamin supplement.

Omnitabs with Iron. (Halsey) Vitamins A 5000 IU, D 400 IU, B_1 3 mg, B_2 2.5 mg, B_6 1 mg, B_{12} 1 mcg, C 50 mg, niacinamide 20 mg, calcium pantothenate 1 mg, iron 15 mg/Tab. Bot. 100s. *otc.*
Use: Mineral, vitamin supplement.

•**omoconazole nitrate.** (oh-moe-KAHN-ah-zole) USAN.
Use: Antifungal.

OMS Concentrate. (Upsher-Smith Labs) Morphine sulfate 20 mg/ml. Soln. Bot. 30 ml, 120 ml. *c-II.*
Use: Analgesic, narcotic.

Oncaspar. (Enzon) Pegaspargase 750 IU/ml in a phosphate buffered saline solution. Inj. In single-use vials. *Rx.*
Use: Antineoplastic agent.

Oncet. (Wakefield Pharm) Hydrocodone bitartrate 5 mg, acetaminophen 500 mg/Cap. Bot. 100s. *c-III.*
Use: Analgesic, antitussive.

oncorad ov103.
Use: Antineoplastic. [Orphan drug]

OncoScint CR/OV. (Cytogen) Satumomab pendetide labeled with indium-111, obtained separately. Kit with 1 mg/2 ml satumomab vial, vial of sodium acetate buffer, and filter.

Oncovin Solution. (Eli Lilly) Vincristine sulfate for inj. 1 mg/ml, 2 mg/2 ml or 5 mg/5 ml. Ctn. 10s. Hyporets 1 mg/Pkg 3s; 2 mg/Pkg 3s. *Rx.*
Use: Antineoplastic.

Oncovite. (Mission) Vitamin A 10,000 IU, C 500 mg, D_3 400 IU, E 200 IU, B_1 0.37 mg, B_2 0.5 mg, B_6 25 mg, B_{12} 1.5 mg, folate 0.4 mg, Zn 7.5 mg, sugar. Tab. Bot. 120s. *otc.*
Use: Vitamin supplement.

•**ondansetron hydrochloride.** (ahn-DAN-SEH-trahn) USAN.
Use: Anxiolytic, antiemetic, antischizophrenic.
See: Zofran, Preps. (GlaxoWellcome).

Ondrox. (Unimed) **Tab.:** Ca 25 mg, iron 3 mg, vitamins A 2000 IU, D 100 IU, E 17 mg, B_1 0.25 mg, B_2 0.28 mg, B_3 3.33 mg, B_5 1.67 mg, B_6 0.33 mg, B_{12} 1 mcg, C 41.7 mg, folic acid 0.67, biotin 0.5 mcg, I, Mg, Cu, P, vitamin K, Cr, Mn, Mo, Se, V, B, Si, Zn 2.5 mg, inositol, bioflavonoids, N-acetylcysteine, L-glutathione, L-methionine, L-glutamine, taurine. Bot. 60s, 180s. *otc.*
Use: Mineral, vitamins supplements.

One-A-Day Essential. (Bayer Corp) Vitamins A 5000 IU, E 30 IU, C 60 mg, folic acid 0.4 mg, B_1 1.5 mg, B_2 1.7 mg, B_3 20 mg, B_6 2 mg, B_{12} 6 mcg, B_5 10 mg, D 400 IU/Tab. Sodium free. Bot. 75s, 130s. *otc.*
Use: Vitamin supplement.

One-A-Day Extras Antioxidant. (Bayer Corp) Vitamin E 200 IU, C 250 mg, A 5000 IU, Zn 7.5 mg, Cu, Se, Mn, tartrazine/Softgel cap. Bot. 50s. *otc.*
Use: Vitamin Supplement.

One-A-Day Extras Vitamin C. (Bayer Corp) Vitamin C 500 mg/Tab. Bot. 100s. *otc.*
Use: Vitamin supplement.

One-A-Day Extras Vitamin E. (Bayer Corp) Vitamin E 400 IU/Softgel Cap. Bot. 60s. *otc.*
Use: Vitamin supplement.

One-A-Day Maximum Formula. (Bayer Corp) Iron 18 mg, vitamins A 5000 IU, D 400 IU, E 30 IU, B_1 1.5 mg, B_2 1.7 mg, B_3 20 mg, B_5 10 mg, B_6 2 mg, B_{12} 6 mcg, C 60 mg, folic acid 0.4 mg, Ca, Cl, Cr, Cu, I, K, Mg, Mn, Mo, P, Se, Zn 15 mg, biotin 30 mcg/Tab. Bot. 60s, 100s. *otc.*
Use: Mineral, vitamin supplement.

One-A-Day Men's Vitamins. (Bayer Corp) Vitamin A 5000 IU, C 200 mg, B_1 2.25 mg, B_2 2.55 mg, B_3 20 mg, D 400 IU, E 45 IU, B_6 3 mg, folic acid 0.4 mg, B_{12} 9 mcg, B_5 10 mg/Tab. Bot. 60s, 100s. *otc.*
Use: Mineral, vitamin supplement.

One-A-Day 55 Plus. (Bayer Corp) Vitamin A 6000 IU, C 120 mg, B_1 4.5 mg, B_2 3.4 mg, B_3 20 mg, D 400 IU, E 60 IU, B_6 6 mg, folic acid 0.4 mg, biotin 30 mcg, B_5 20 mg, K 25 mcg, Ca 220 mg, I, Mg, Cu, Zn 15 mg, Cr, Se, Mo, Mn, K, Cl/Tab. Bot. 50s, 80s. *otc.*
Use: Mineral, vitamin supplement.

One-A-Day Women's Formula. (Bayer Corp) **Tab.:** Ca 450 mg, iron 27 mg, vitamins A 5000 IU, D 400 IU, E 30 mg, B_1 1.5 mg, B_2 1.7 mg, B_3 20 mg, B_5 10 mg, B_6 2 mg, B_{12} 6 mcg, C 60 mg, folic acid 0.4 mg, Zn 15 mg, tartrazine. Bot. 60s, 100s. *Rx.*
Use: Mineral, vitamin supplement.

One-Tablet-Daily. (Various Mfr.) Vitamins A 5000 IU, D 400 IU, E 30 mg, B_1 1.5 mg, B_2 1.7 mg, B_3 20 mg, B_5 10 mg, B_6 2 mg, B_{12} 6 mcg, C 60 mg, folic acid 0.4 mg. Tab. Bot. 30s, 100s, 250s, 365s, 1000s. *otc.*
Use: Vitamin supplement.

One-Tablet-Daily. (Various Mfr.) Vitamins A 5000 IU, D 400 IU, E 30 mg, B_1 1.5 mg, B_2 1.7 mg, B_3 20 mg, B_5 10 mg, B_6 2 mg, B_{12} 6 mcg, C 60 mg, folic acid 0.4 mg/Tab. Bot. 365s, 1000s. *otc.*
Use: Vitamin supplement.

One-Tablet-Daily Plus Iron. (Various Mfr.) Iron 18 mg, vitamins A 5000 IU, D 400 IU, E 15 mg, B_1 1.5 mg, B_2 1.7 mg, B_3 20 mg, B_6 2 mg, B_{12} 6 mcg, C

60 mg, folic acid 0.4 mg/Tab. Bot. 100s, 250s, 365s. *otc.*
Use: Mineral, vitamin supplement.

One-Tablet-Daily with Iron. (Zenith Goldline) Iron 18 mg, A 5000 IU, D 400 IU, E 30 mg, B_1 1.5 mg, B_2 1.7 mg, B_3 20 mg, B_5 10 mg, B_6 2 mg, B_{12} 6 mcg, C 60 mg, folic acid 0.4 mg. Bot. 100s. *otc.*
Use: Mineral, viatmin supplement.

One-Tablet-Daily with Minerals. (Zenith Goldline) Iron 18 mg, vitamins A 5000 IU, D 400 IU, E 30 IU, B_1 1.5 mg, B_2 1.7 mg, B_3 20 mg, B_5 10 mg, B_6 2 mg, B_{12} 6 mcg, C 60 mg, folic acid 0.4 mg, Ca, Cl, Cr, Cu, I, K, Mg, Mn, Mo, P, Se, Zn 15 mg, biotin 30 mcg/Tab. Bot. 100s, 1000s. *otc.*
Use: Mineral, vitamin supplement.

1000-BC, IM or IV. (Solvay) Vitamins B_1 25 mg, B_2 2.5 mg, B_6 5 mg, panthenol 5 mg, B_{12} 500 mcg, niacinamide 75 mg, C 100 mg/ml. Vial 10 ml. *Rx.*
Use: Vitamin supplement.

1+1-F Creme. (Dunhall Pharmaceuticals) Hydrocortisone 1%, pramoxine HCl 1%, iodochlorhydroxyquin 3%. Tube 30 g. *Rx.*
Use: Corticosteroid; anesthetic, local; antifungal, topical.

1-2-3 Ointment No. 20. (Durel) Burow's solution, lanolin, zinc oxide (Lassar's paste). Jar oz, 1 lb, 6 lb. *otc.*
Use: Anti-inflammatory, topical.

1-2-3 Ointment No. 21. (Durel) Burow's solution 1 part, lanolin 2, zinc oxide (Lassar's paste) 1.5, cold cream 1.5. Jar oz, 1 lb, 6 lb. *otc.*
Use: Anti-inflammatory agent, topical.

Onoton Tablets. (Sanofi Winthrop) Pancreatin, hemicellulose, ox bile extracts. *otc.*
Use: Digestive aid.

•**ontazolast.** (ahn-TAH-zoe-last) USAN.
Use: Antiasthmatic (leukotriene antagonist).

ontosein.
See: Orgotein (Diagnostic Data).

Ony-Clear. (Pedinol) Benzalkonium chloride. Soln. Bot. 1 oz w/applicator. *otc.*
Use: Antiseptic.

Opcon. (Bausch & Lomb) Naphazoline HCl 0.1%. Bot. 15 ml. *otc.*
Use: Mydriatic, vasoconstrictor.

Opcon-A. (Bausch & Lomb)**Soln.:** 0.027% nephazoline HCl, 0.315% pheniramine maleate, 0.5% hydroxypropyl methylcellulose, 0.01% benzalkonium chloride, 0.1% EDTA, NaCl, boric acid, sodium buffers. 15 ml. *otc.*
Use: Mydriatic, vasoconstrictor, antihistamine.

o,p'-DDD.
Use: Miscellaneous antineoplastic.
See: Lysodren (Bristol-Myers Oncology/Immunology).

Operand. (Aplicare) **Aerosal:** Iodine 0.5%. 90 ml. **Skin cleanser:** Iodine 1%. 90 ml. **Oint.:** Iodine 1%. 30 g, lb, packette 1.2 g and 2.7 g. **Perineal wash conc.:** Iodine 1%. 240 ml. **Prep soln.:** Iodine 1%. 60 ml, 120 ml, 240 ml, pt, qt. **Soln:** Prep pad 100s, swab stick 25s. **Surgical scrub:** Povidone-iodine 7.5%. 60 ml, 120 ml, 240 ml, pt, qt, gal, packette 22.5 ml. **Whirlpool conc.:** Iodine 1%. gal. *otc.*
Use: Antiseptic, antimicrobial.

Operand Douche. (Aplicare) Povidone-iodine. Soln. 60 ml, 240 ml, UD 15 ml. *otc.*
Use: Vaginal agent.

o-phenylphenol. W/Amyl complex, phenylmercuric nitrate.
See: Lubraseptic Jelly (Gordon Laboratories).

Ophthacet. (Vortech) Sodium sulfacetamide 10%. Soln. 15 ml. *Rx.*
Use: Anti-infective, ophthalmic.

Ophthaine Hydrochloride. (Apothecon) Proparacaine HCl 0.5%. Soln. Bot. w/dropper 15 ml. *Rx.*
Use: Anesthetic, ophthalmic.

Ophthalgan. (Wyeth Ayerst) Glycerin ophthalmic soln. w/chlorobutanol 0.55% as preservative. Bot. 7.5 ml. *Rx.*
Use: Hyperosmolar.

Ophtha P/S. (Misemer) Prednisolone acetate 0.5%, sodium sulfacetamide 10%, hydroxyethylcellulose, EDTA, polysorbate 80, sodium thiosulfate, benzalkonium chloride 0.025%. Susp. Bot. 5 ml. *Rx.*
Use: Corticosteroid; anti-infective, ophthalmic.

Ophtha P/S Ophthalmic Suspension. (Misemer) Sodium sulfacetamide 10%, prednisolone acetate 0.5%. Bot. 5 ml w/dropper. *Rx.*
Use: Corticosteroid; anti-infective, ophthalmic.

Ophthetic. (Allergan) Proparacaine HCl 0.5%. Bot. 15 ml. *Rx.*
Use: Anesthetic, ophthalmic.

•**opipramol hydrochloride.** (oh-PIH-prahmole) USAN.
Use: Antipsychotic, antidepressant, tranquilizer.

•**opium.** (OH-pee-uhm) U.S.P. 23.
Use: Pharmaceutic necessity for powdered opium.

opium alkaloids, total, as the hydrochloride salt.
See: Pantopon, Amp. (Roche Laboratories).

opium and belladonna. (Wyeth Ayerst) Powdered opium 60 mg, extract of belladonna 15 mg/Supp. Box 20s. *c-II.*
Use: Analgesic, narcotic; anticholinergic; antispasmodic.

•**opium powdered.** U.S.P. 23.
Use: Pharmaceutical necessity for Paregoric.
W/Albumin tannate, colloidal kaolin, pectin.
See: Ekrised, Tab. (Roberts Pharm).
W/Atropine sulfate, alcohol.
W/Belladonna extract.
See: B & O, Supp. (PolyMedica).
W/Bismuth subgallate, kaolin, pectin, zinc phenolsulfonate.
See: Diastay, Tab. (ICN Pharmaceuticals).
W/Kaolin, pectin, bismuth subcarbonate.
See: KBP/O, Cap. (Cole).
W/Kaolin, pectin, hyoscyamine sulfate, atropine sulfate, hyoscine HBr.
See: Donnagel-PG, Susp. (Robins).

opium tincture.
W/Homatropine MBr, Pectin.
See: Dia-Quel, Liq. (I.P.C.).
W/Pectin.
See: Opecto, Elix. (Jones Medical Industries).
Parelixir, Liq. (Purdue Frederick).

opium tincture, camphorated.
Use: Antidiarrheal.
See: Paregoric, U.S.P. 23.
W/Glycyrrhiza fluid extract, tartar emetic, glycerin.
See: Brown Mixture.

•**oprelvekin.** (oh-PRELL-veh-kin) USAN.
Use: Hematopoietic stimulant.
See: Neumega, Pow. For Inj. (Genetics Institute).

Opti-Bon Eye Drops. (Barrows) Phenylephrine HCl, berberine sulfate, boric acid, sodium Cl, sodium bisulfite, glycerine, camphor water, peppermint water, thimerosal 0.004%. Bot. 1 oz. *otc.*
Use: Ophthalmic.

Opticaps. (Health for Life Brands) Vitamins A 32,500 IU, D 3250 IU, B_1 15 mg, B_2 5 mg, B_6 0.5 mg, C 150 mg, E 5 IU, calcium pantothenate 3 mg, niacinamide 150 mg, B_{12} 20 mcg, iron 11.26 mg, choline bitartrate 30 mg, inositol 30 mg, pepsin 32.5 mg, diastase 32.5 mg, calcium 30 mg, phosphorus 25 mg, magnesium 0.7 mg, Fr. dicalcium phosphate 110 mg, manganese 1.3 mg, potassium 0.68 mg, zinc 0.45 mg, hesperidin compound 25 mg, biotin 20 mcg, Brewer's yeast 50 mg, wheat germ oil 20 mg, hydrolized yeast 81.25 mg, protein digest. 47.04 mg, amino acids 34.21 mg/Cap. Bot. 30s, 60s, 90s, 1000s. *otc.*
Use: Mineral, vitamin supplement.

Opticare PMS. (Standard Drug) Iron 2.5 mg, vitamins 2083 IU, D 17 IU, E 14 IU, B_1 4.2 mg, B_2 4.2 mg, B_3 4.2 mg, B_5 4.2 mg, B_6 50 mg, B_{12} 10.4 mcg, C 250 mg, folic acid 0.03 mg, Cr, Cu, I, K, Mg, Mn, Se, Zn 4.2 mg, biotin 10.4 mcg, choline bitartrate, bioflavonoids, inositol, PABA, rutin, Ca, amylase activity, protease activity, lipase activity, betaine, tartrazine. Bot. 150s. *otc.*
Use: Mineral, vitamin supplement.

Opti-Clean. (Alcon Laboratories) Tween 21, polymeric cleaners, hydroxyethylcellulose, thimerosal 0.004%, EDTA 0.1%. Bot 12 ml, 20 ml. *otc.*
Use: Contact lens care.

Opti-Clean II. (Alcon Laboratories) Polymeric cleaning agent, Tween 21, EDTA 0.1%, polyquaternium-1 0.001%. Thimerosal free. Bot. 12 ml, 20 ml. *otc.*
Use: Contact lens care.

Opti-Clean II Especially For Sensitive Eyes. (Alcon Laboratories) EDTA 0.1%, polyquaternium-1 0.001%, polymeric cleaners, Tween 21. Thimerosal free. Bot. 12 ml, 20 ml. *otc.*
Use: Contact lens care.

Opticyl. (Optopics) Tropicamide 0.5%, 1%. Soln. Bot. 2 ml, 15 ml. *Rx.*
Use: Cycloplegic, mydriatic.

Opti-Free Enzymatic Cleaner. (Alcon Laboratories) Highly purified pork pancrentin. Tab. Pkg. 6s, 12s, 18s. *otc.*
Use: Contact lens care.

Opti-Free Non-Hydrogen Peroxide-Containing System. (Alcon Laboratories) Citrate buffer, NaCl, EDTA 0.05%, polyquaternium-1 0.001%. Soln. 118 ml, 237 ml, 355 ml. *otc.*
Use: Ophthalmic.

Opti-Free Rewetting Solution. (Alcon Laboratories) Citrate buffer, sodium Cl, EDTA 0.05%, polyquaternium-1 0.001%. Soln. Bot. 10 ml, 20 ml. *otc.*
Use: Contact lens care.

Opti-Free Surfactant Cleaning Solution. (Alcon Laboratories) EDTA 0.01%, polyquaternium-1 0.001%, microclens polymeric cleaners, Tween 21.

Thimerosal free. Soln. Bot. 12 ml, 20 ml. *otc.*
Use: Contact lens care.

Optigene. (Pfeiffer) Sodium Cl, sodium phosphate mono- and dibasic, benzalkonium Cl, EDTA. Soln. Bot. 118 ml. *otc.*
Use: Irrigant, ophthalmic.

Optigene 3. (Pfeiffer) Tetrahydrozoline HCl 0.05%. Soln. Bot. 15 ml. *otc.*
Use: Mydriatic, vasoconstrictor.

Optilets-500. (Abbott Laboratories) Vitamins B_1 15 mg, B_2 10 mg, B_3 100 mg, B_5 20 mg, B_6 5 mg, C 500 mg, A 10,000 IU, D 400 IU, E 30 IU, B_{12} 12 mcg/Filmtab. Bot. 120s. *otc.*
Use: Mineral, vitamin supplement.

Optilets-M-500. (Abbott Laboratories) Vitamins C 500 mg, B_3 100 mg, B_5 20 mg, B_1 15 mg, A 5000 IU, B_2 10 mg, B_6 5 mg, D 400 IU, B_{12} 12 mcg, E 30 IU, iron 20 mg, Mg, zinc 1.5 mg, Cu, Mn, I/Filmtab. Bot. 120s. *otc.*
Use: Mineral, vitamin supplement.

Optimine. (Schering Plough) Azatadine maleate 1 mg/Tab. Bot. 100s. *Rx.*
Use: Antihistamine.

Optimoist. (Colgate Oral) Xylitol, calcium phosphate monobasic, citric acid, sodium hydroxide, sodium benzoate, acesulfame potassium, hydroxyethyl cellulose, sodium monofluoro phosphate, 2 ppm fluoride. Soln. Bot. 60 ml and 330 ml. Spray. *otc.*
Use: Saliva substitute.

Optimox Prenatal. (Optimox) **Tab.:** Ca 100 mg, iron 5 mg, vitamins A 833 IU, D 67 IU, E 2 mg, B_1 0.5 mg, B_2 0.6 mg, B_3 6.7 mg, B_5 3.3 mg, B_6 0.73 mg, B_{12} 0.87 mcg, C 30 mg, folic acid 0.13 mg, Cr, Cu, I, K, Mg, Mn, Se, Zn 3.17 mg. Bot. 360s. *otc.*
Use: Mineral, vitamin supplement.

Optimyd. (Schering Plough) Prednisolone phosphate 0.5%, sodium sulfacetamide 10%, sodium thiosulfate. Soln-Sterile. Drop bot. 5 ml. *Rx.*
Use: Anti-infective, corticosteroid, ophthalmic.

Opti-One. (Alcon Laboratories) EDTA 0.05%, polyquaternium-1 0.001%, sodium chloride, sodium citrate. Buffered, isotonic. Soln. 120 ml. *otc.*
Use: Contact lens care.

Opti-One Multi-Purpose. (Alcon Laboratories) **Soln.:** 0.05% EDTA, 0.001% polyquaternium-1, NaCl. Buffered, isotonic. 118, 237, 355, 473 ml. *otc.*
Use: Contact lens care.

Opti-One Rewetting. (Alcon Laboratories) EDTA 0.05%, polyquaternium-1 0.001%, sodium chloride, citrate buffer, isotonic. Drops. Bot. 10 ml. *otc.*
Use: Contact lens care.

OptiPranolol. (Bausch & Lomb) Metipranolol HCl 0.3%. Bot. 5 ml, 10 ml. *Rx.*
Use: Antiglaucoma agent.

Optiray. (Mallinckrodt Chemical) Ioversol.
Use: Radiopaque agent.

Optiray 350. (Mallinckrodt Medical) Ioversol 74%, iodine 35%, tromethamine 3.6 mg, EDTA 0.2 mg/ml. Inj. 30 and 50 ml glass vials, 75 ml fill in 150 ml glass bottles, 100 ml fill in 150 ml glass bottles, 150 ml glass bottles, 200 ml fill in 250 ml glass bottles, 30 and 50 ml handheld plastic syringes, 50 ml fill in 125 ml power injector plastic syringes, 100 ml fill in 125 ml power injector plastic syringes and 125 ml power injector plastic syringes.
Use: Radiopaque agent.

Opti-Soft. (Alcon Laboratories) Isotonic soln of sodium Cl, borate buffer, EDTA 0.1%, polyquaternium-1 0.001%. Thimerosal free. Soln. Bot. 237 ml, 355 ml. *otc.*
Use: Contact lens care.

Opti-Soft Especially for Sensitive Eyes. (Alcon Laboratories) Buffered, isotonic. EDTA 0.1%, polyquaternium-1 0.001%, NaCl, borate buffer. For lenses w/ $\leq$ 45% water content. Soln. Bot. 118 ml, 237 ml, 355 ml. *otc.*
Use: Contact lens care.

Opti-Tears. (Alcon Laboratories) Isotonic solution with dextran, sodium Cl, potassium Cl, hydroxypropyl methylcellulose, EDTA 0.1%, polyquaternium-1 0.001%. Thimerosal and sorbic acid free. Soln. Bot. 15 ml. *otc.*
Use: Contact lens care.

Optivite for Women. (Optimox) Vitamins A 2083 IU, D 16.7 IU, E 14 mg, B_1 4.2 mg, B_2 4.2 mg, B_3 4.2 mg, B_5 4.2 mg, B_6 50 mg, B_{12} 10.4 mcg, C 250 mg, iron 2.5 mg, folic acid 0.03 mg, zinc 4.2 mg, choline 52 mg, inositol 10 mg, Cr, Cu, I, K, Mg, Mn, Se, citrus bioflavonoids, PABA, rutin, pancreatin, biotin/Tab. Bot. 180s. *otc.*
Use: Mineral, vitamin supplement.

Optivite P.M.T. (Optimox) Vitamins A 2083 IU, D, E 16.7 mg, B_1 4.2 mg, B_2 4.2 mg, B_3 4.2 mg, B_5 4.2 mg, B_6 50 mg, B_{12} 10.4 mcg, C 250 mg, iron 2.5 mg, FA 0.03 mg, Zn 4.2 mg, choline, Ca, Cr, Cu, I, K, Mg, Mn, Se, bioflavonoids, betaine, PABA, rutin, pancreatin,

biotin, inositol/Tab. Bot. 180s. *otc.*
Use: Mineral, vitamin supplement.

Opti-Zyme Enzymatic Cleaner Especially For Sensitive Eyes. (Alcon Laboratories) Pork pancreatin tablets. Pak 8s, 24s, 36s, 56s. *otc.*
Use: Contact lens care.

ORA5. (McHenry) Copper sulfate, iodine, potassium iodide, alcohol 1.5%. Liq. Bot. 3.75 ml, 30 ml. *otc.*
Use: Mouth preparation.

Orabase. (Colgate Oral) Gelatin, pectin, sodium carboxymethylcellulose in hydrocarbon gel w/polyethylene and mineral oil. 0.75 g Packet Box 100s. Tube 5 g, 15 g. *otc.*
Use: Mouth preparation.

Orabase-B. (Colgate Oral) Benzocaine 20%, mineral oil. Paste. 5 g, 15 g. *otc.*
Use: Mouth and throat preparation.

Orabase Baby. (Colgate Oral) Benzocaine 7.5%, alcohol free, fruit flavor. Gel. 7.2 g. *otc.*
Use: Anesthetic, local.

Orabase Gel. (Colgate-Palmolive) Benzocaine 15%, ethyl alcohol, tannic acid, salicylic acid, saccharin. Gel. 7 g. *otc.*
Use: Anesthetic, local.

Orabase HCA. (Colgate Oral) Hydrocortisone acetate 0.5%, polyethylene 5%, mineral oil. Tube 5 g. *Rx.*
Use: Corticosteroid, dental.

Orabase Lip. (Colgate Oral) Benzocaine 5%, allantoin 1.5%, menthol 0.5%, petrolatum, lanolin, parabens, camphor, phenol. Cream. 10 g. *otc.*
Use: Anesthetic, local.

Orabase Plain. (Colgate Oral) Gelatin, pectin & sodium carboxymethyl cellulose in polyethylene and mineral gel. Paste. 5, 15 g. *otc.*
Use: Mouth and throat preparation.

Orabase with Benzocaine. (Colgate Oral) Benzocaine 20% in gel base. Packet 0.75 g, Box 100s. Tube 5 g, 15 g. *otc.*
Use: Anesthetic, local.

Oracap Capsules. (Vangard) Phenylpropanolamine HCl 75 mg, chlorpheniramine maleate 12 mg/Cap. Bot. 100s, 1000s. *Rx.*
Use: Antihistamine, decongestant.

Oracit. (Carolina Medical Products) Sodium citrate 490 mg, citric acid 640 mg/5 ml, (sodium 1 mEq/ml equivalent to 1 mEq bicarbonate), alcohol 0.25%. Soln. Bot. pt, UD 15, 30 ml. *Rx.*
Use: Alkalinizer, systemic.

Oraderm Lip Balm. (Schattner) Sodium phenolate, sodium tetraborate, phenol, base containing an anionic emulsifier. ⅛ oz. *otc.*
Use: Anesthetic; antiseptic, local.

Orafix Medicated. (SmithKline Beecham Pharmaceuticals) Allantoin 0.2%, benzocaine 2%. Tube 0.75 oz. *otc.*
Use: Anesthetic, local; denture adhesive.

Orafix Original. (SmithKline Beecham Pharmaceuticals) Tube 1.5 oz, 2.5 oz, 4 oz. *otc.*
Use: Denture adhesive.

Orafix Special. (SmithKline Beecham Pharmaceuticals) Tube 1.4 oz, 2.4 oz. *otc.*
Use: Denture adhesive.

Oragrafin Calcium Granules. (Bristol-Myers Squibb) Ipodate calcium (61.7% iodine) 3 g/8 g Pkg. 25 × 1 dose pkg.
Use: Radiopaque agent.

Oragrafin Sodium Capsules. (Bristol-Myers Squibb) Ipodate sodium (61.4% iodine) 0.5 g/Cap. Bot. 100s, 144s. Unimatic pkg. 100s. Card 6s. Box 25s.
Use: Radiopaque agent.

Orahesive Powder. (Colgate Oral) Gelatin, pectin, sodium carboxymethylcellulose. Bot. 25 g. *otc.*
Use: Denture adhesive.

Orajel. (Del Pharmaceuticals) Benzocaine 10% in a special base. Tube 0.2 oz, 0.5 oz. *otc.*
Use: Anesthetic, local.

Orajel D. (Del Pharmaceuticals) Benzocaine 10%, saccharin. Tube 9.45 g. *otc.*
Use: Anesthetic, local.

Orajel Mouth-Aid. (Del Pharmaceuticals) Benzocaine 20%.
Liq.: Cetylpyridinium 0.1%, ethyl alcohol 70%, tartrazine, saccharin, 13.5 ml.
Gel: Benzalkonium Cl 0.02%, zinc Cl 0.1%, EDTA, saccharin. 5.6 g, 10 g. *otc.*
Use: Anesthetic, local.

Orajel Perioseptic. (Del Pharmaceuticals) Carbamide peroxide 15% in anhydrous glycerin, saccharin, methylparaben, EDTA. Liq. Bot. 13.3 ml. *otc.*
Use: Mouth preparation.

Oral-B Muppets Fluoride Toothpaste. (Oral-B Laboratories) Fluoride 0.22%. Pump 4.3 oz. *otc.*
Use: Dental caries agent.

oralcid.
See: Acetarsone.

oral contraceptives.
See: Demulen, Tab. (Searle).
Desogen, Tab. (Organon Teknika).
Enovid-E, Tab. (Searle).
GenCept, Tab. (Gencon).
Jenest-28, Tab. (Organon Teknika).
Loestrin, Prods. (Parke-Davis).
Lo/Ovral, Prods. (Wyeth Ayerst).
Micronor, Tab. (Ortho McNeil).
Modicon, Prods. (Ortho McNeil).
Nelulen, Tab. (Watson Laboratories).
Norethin 1/35 E Tab. (Roberts Pharm).
Norethin 1/50 M Tab. (Roberts Pharm).
Nordette, Tab. (Wyeth Ayerst).
Norinyl, Prods. (Syntex).
Norlestrin, Prods. (Parke-Davis).
Norquen, Tab. (Syntex).
Ortho Cept, Tab. (Ortho McNeil).
Ortho-Cyclen, Tab. (Ortho McNeil).
Ortho Tri-Cyclen, Tab. (Ortho McNeil).
Ortho-Novum, Prods. (Ortho McNeil).
Ovcon-35, Tab. (Bristol-Myers).
Ovcon-50, Tab. (Bristol-Myers).
Ovral, Tab. (Wyeth Ayerst).
Ovrette, Tab. (Wyeth Ayerst).
Ovulen, Tab. (Searle).
Triphasil, Tab. (Wyeth Ayerst).

Oral Drops/Canker Sore Relief. (Weeks & Leo) Carbamide peroxide 10% in anhydrous glycerin base. Bot. 30 ml. *otc.*
Use: Mouth preparation.

Oralone Dental. (Thames) Triamcinolone acetonide 0.1%. Paste 5 g. *Rx.*
Use: Corticosteroid, dental.

oral rehydration salts.
Use: Electrolyte combination.

Oramide. (Major) Tolbutamide 0.5 g/Tab. Bot. 100s, 1000s. *Rx.*
Use: Antidiabetic.

Oraminic II. (Vortech) Brompheniramine maleate 10 mg per ml/Inj. Vial. 10 ml multidose. *Rx.*
Use: Antihistamine.

Oramorph SR. (Roxane) Morphine sulfate 30 mg, 60 mg, 100 mg, lactose. SR Tab. Bot. 50s (30 mg only), 100s, 250s (30 mg only), UD 25s (60 mg & 100 mg only), 100s (30 mg only). *c-II.*
Use: Analgesic, narcotic.

orange flower oil. N.F. XVII.
Use: Flavor, perfume, vehicle.

orange flower water. N.F. XVI.
Use: Flavor, perfume.

orange oil. N.F. XVI.
Use: Flavor.

orange peel tincture, sweet. N.F. XVI.
Use: Flavor.

orange spirit, compound. N.F. XVI.
Use: Flavor.

orange syrup. N.F. XVI.
Use: Flavored vehicle.

Orap. (Ortho McNeil) Pimozide 2 mg/Tab. Bot. 100s. *Rx.*
Use: Antipsychotic.

Oraphen-PD. (Great Southern) Acetaminophen 120 mg per 5 ml, alcohol 5%, cherry flavor. Elix. 120 ml. *otc.*
Use: Analgesic.

orarsan.
See: Acetarsone.

Orasept. (Pharmakon Labs) Tannic acid 12.16%, methylbenzethonium HCl 1.53%, ethyl alcohol 53.31%, camphor, menthol, benzyl alcohol, spearmint oil, cassia oil. Liq. Bot. 15 ml. *otc.*
Use: Mouth and throat preparation.

Orasept, Throat. (Pharmakon Labs) Benzocaine 0.996%, methylbenzethonium Cl 1.037%, sorbitol 70%, menthol, peppermint, saccharin. Throat spray. 45 ml. *otc.*
Use: Mouth and throat preparation.

Orasol. (Zenith Goldline) Benzocaine 6.3%, phenol 0.5%, alcohol 70%, povidone-iodine. Liq. Bot. 14.79 ml. *otc.*
Use: Anesthetic, local.

Orasone. (Solvay) Prednisone **1 mg, 5 mg, 10 mg or 20 mg/Tab.:** Bot. 100s, 1000s, UD 100s. **50 mg/Tab.:** Bot. 100s, UD 100s. *Rx.*
Use: Corticosteroid.

OraSure HIV-1. (Epitope) Collection kit: Cotton fiber on a stick with collection vial. Device for oral specimen collection. For professional use only.
Use: Diagnostic aid.

Oratuss TR. (Vangard) Caramiphen edisylate 20 mg, chlorpheniramine maleate 8 mg, phenylpropanolamine HCl 50 mg, isopropamide iodide 2.5 mg/TR Cap. Bot. 100s, 500s. *Rx.*
Use: Anticholinergic, antihistamine, antispasmodic, antitussive, decongestant.

Orazinc. (Mericon) Zinc sulfate 220 mg/Cap. Bot. 100s, 1000s. *otc.*
Use: Mineral supplement.

orbenin. Sodium cloxacillin.
Use: Anti-infective.
See: Cloxapen (SmithKline Beecham Pharmaceuticals).

Orbiferrous. (Orbit) Ferrous fumarate 300 mg, vitamins B_{12} 12 mcg, C 50 mg, B_1 3 mg, defatted desiccated liver 50 mg/Tab. Bot. 60s, 500s. *otc.*
Use: Mineral, vitamin supplement.

Orbit. (Spanner) Vitamins A 6250 IU, D 400 IU, B_1 3 mg, B_2 3 mg, B_6 2 mg, B_{12} 5 mcg, C 75 mg, niacinamide 20 mg, calcium pantothenate 10 mg, E 15 IU, biotin 15 mcg, iron 20 mg/Tab. Bot. 100s. *otc.*
Use: Mineral, vitamin supplement.

•**orbofiban acetate.** (ore-boe-FIE-ban) USAN.
Use: Fibrinogen receptor antagonist; platelet aggregation inhibitor, antithrombotic.

•**orconazole nitrate.** (ahr-KOE-nah-zole NYE-trate) USAN.
Use: Antifungal.

Ordrine. (Eon Labs Manufacturing) Chlorpheniramine maleate 12 mg, phenylpropanolamine HCl 75 mg/SR Cap. Bot. 100s, 1000s. *Rx.*
Use: Antihistamine, decongestant.

Ordrine AT Extended Release. (Eon Labs Manufacturing) Phenylpropanolamine HCl 75 mg, caramiphen edisylate 40 mg/Cap. Bot. 50s, 100s, 500s. *Rx.*
Use: Cough preparation.

Oretic. (Abbott Laboratories) Hydrochlorothiazide 25 mg or 50 mg/Tab. Bot. 100s, 1000s, UD 100s. *Rx.*
Use: Diuretic.

Oreton Methyl. (Schering Plough) Methyltestosterone. **Buccal Tab.:** 10 mg, Bot. 100s. **Tab.:** 10 mg or 25 mg. Bot. 100s. *c-III.*
Use: Androgen.

Orexin. (Roberts Pharm) Vitamins B_1 8.1 mg, B_6 4.1 mg, B_{12} 25 mcg/Chew-Tab. Bot. 100s. *otc.*
Use: Vitamin supplement.

Organidin. (Wallace Laboratories) **Tab.:** 30 mg. Rose, scored. In 100s. **Elix.:** 60 mg/5 ml. 21.75% alcohol, glucose, saccharin. In pt and gal. **Sol.:** 50 mg/ml. In 30 ml w/dropper.
Use: Expectorant.

Organidin NR. (Wallace Laboratories) **Tab:** guaifenesin 200 mg/Tab. Bot. 100s. **Liq:** guaifenesin 100 mg/5 ml. Liq. Bot. pt, gal. *Rx.*
Use: Expectorant.

Orgaran. (Organon Teknika) Danaparoid sodium 750 anti-Xa units/0.6 ml, sodium sulfite/Inj. Box. Single-dose ampules and pre-filled syringes. 10s. *Rx.*
Use: Anticoagulant.

Orglagen Tablets. (Zenith Goldline) Orphenadrine citrate 100 mg/Tab. Bot. 100s, 1000s. *Rx.*
Use: Muscle relaxant.

•**orgotein.** (ORE-go-teen) USAN. A group of soluble metalloproteins isolated from liver, red blood cells, and other mammalian tissues.
Use: Anti-inflammatory, antirheumatic.

orgotein. (Diagnostic Data) Pure water soluble protein with a compact conformation maintained by 4 g atoms of chelated divalent metals, produced from bovine liver as a Cu-Zn mixed chelate having superoxide dismutase activity. Ontosein, Palosein.

orgotein for injection.
Use: Familial amyotrophic lateral sclerosis. [Orphan drug]

Original Alka-Seltzer Effervescent. (Bayer Corp) **Tab.:** 1700 mg sodium bicarbonate, 325 mg aspirin, 1000 mg citric acid, 9 mg phenylalanine, 506 mg sodium, aspartame. 24s. *otc.*
Use: Antacid.

Original Eclipse Sunscreen. (Tri Tec Laboratories) Padimate O, glyceryl PABA, SPF 10. Lot. Bot. 120 ml. *otc.*
Use: Sunscreen.

Original Sensodyne. (Block Drug) Strontium chloride hexahydrate 10%, saccharin, sorbitol. Toothpaste. Tube 59.5 g. *otc.*
Use: Mouth and throat preparation.

Orimune. (Wyeth Ayerst) Poliovirus vaccine. Live, Oral, Trivalent. Sabin strains Types 1, 2, and 3. Dose of 0.5 ml Dispette disposable pipette 1 dose. 10s and 50s. *Rx.*
Use: Immunization.

Orinase. (Pharmacia & Upjohn) Tolbutamide 500 mg/Tab. Bot. 200s, 500s, 1000s, unit-of-use 100s. *Rx.*
Use: Antidiabetic.

Orinase Diagnostic. (Pharmacia & Upjohn) Tolbutamide sodium 1 g/Vial. Pow. for inj. Vial with 20 ml amp diluent.
Use: Diagnostic aid.

Orisul. (Novartis Pharmaceuticals) Sulfaphenazole. A sulfonamide under study.

ORLAAM. (Biodevelopment) Levomethadyl acetate HCl 10 mg, methylparaben 1.8 mg and propylparaben 0.2 mg/ml. Soln. Bot. 474 ml. *c-II.*
Use: Analgesic, narcotic.

•**orlistat.** (ORE-lih-stat) USAN.
Use: Inhibitor (pancreatic lipase).

•**ormaplatin.** (ORE-mah-PLAT-in) USAN.
Use: Antineoplastic.

•**ormetoprim.** (ore-MEH-toe-PRIM) USAN.
Use: Anti-infective.

Ornade. (SmithKline Beecham Pharma-

ceuticals) Phenylpropanolamine HCl 75 mg, chlorpheniramine maleate 12 mg/ Spansule. Bot. 50s, 500s. *Rx.*
Use: Antihistamine, decongestant.

Ornex. (Menley & James) Acetaminophen 325 mg, phenylpropanolamine HCl 12.5 mg/Capl. Blister Pak 24s, 48s. Bot. 100s. Dispensary pak 792s. *otc.*
Use: Analgesic, decongestant.

Ornex Maximum Strength. (Menley & James) Pseudoephedrine HCl, acetaminophen 500 mg. Cap. Bot. 24s, 30s, 48s. *otc.*
Use: Analgesic, decongestant.

Ornex No Drowsiness. (Menley & James) Pseudoephedrine HCl 30 mg, acetaminophen 325 mg. Tab. Cap. Bot. 24s, 48s. *otc.*
Use: Analgesic, decongestant.

•**ornidazole.** (ahr-NIH-DAH-zole) USAN.
Use: Anti-infective.

Ornidyl. (Hoechst Marion Roussel) Eflornithine HCl 200 mg/ml. Inj. Vial. 100 ml. *Rx.*
Use: Antiprotozoal.

•**orpanoxin.** (AHR-pan-OX-in) USAN.
Use: Anti-inflammatory.

Orpeneed VK. (Hanlon) Penicillin, buffered 400,000 units/Tab. Bot. 100s. *Rx.*
Use: Anti-infective, penicillin.

•**orphenadrine citrate.** (ore-FEN-uh-dreen) U.S.P. 23.
Use: Antihistamine, muscle relaxant.
See: Banflex (Forest Pharmaceutical).
Flexoject (Merz).
Flexon, Inj. (Keene Pharmaceuticals).
Myolin (Roberts Pharm).
Norflex, Tab., Amp. (3M Pharm).
Orphanate, Inj. (Hyrex).
W/Aspirin, phenacetin, caffeine.
See: Norgesic, Tab. (3M).
Norgesic Forte, Tab. (3M).

orphenadrine citrate. (Various Mfr.) **Inj.:** 30 mg/ml. Amps 2 ml, vial 10 ml. **Tab.:** 100 mg. Bot. 30s, 100s, 500s, 1000s.
Use: Antihistamine, muscle relaxant.

orphenadrine hydrochloride.
See: Disipal, Tab. (3M).
W/Comb.
See: Estomul, Liq., Tab. (3M).

Orphengesic. (Various Mfr.) Orphenadrine citrate 25 mg, aspirin 385 mg, caffeine 30 mg/Tab. Bot. 100s, 500s, UD 100s. *Rx.*
Use: Analgesic, muscle relaxant.

Orphengesic Forte. (Various Mfr.) Orphenadrine citrate 50 mg, aspirin 770 mg, caffeine 60 mg/Tab. Bot. 100s, 500s. *Rx.*
Use: Analgesic, muscle relaxant.

Ortac-DM Liquid. (ION Laboratories) Dextromethorphan 10 mg, phenylephrine HCl 5 mg, guaifenesin 100 mg/ 5 ml. Bot. 4 oz. *otc.*
Use: Antitussive, decongestant, expectorant.

ortal sodium. Sodium 5-ethyl-5-hexylbarbiturate. Hexethal sodium.

ortedrine.
See: Amphetamine (Various Mfr.).

orthesin.
See: Benzocaine.

Ortho All-Flex Diaphragm. (Ortho McNeil) Diaphragm kit (all flex arcing spring) in plastic compact, sizes 55, 60, 65, 70, 75, 80, 85, 90, 95 mm. *Rx.*
Use: Contraceptive.

orthocaine.
See: Orthoform.

Ortho-Cept. (Ortho McNeil) Desogestrel 0.15 mg, ethinyl estradiol 0.03 mg. Tab. Pkg. 28s w/ 7 inert tab. and 21s. *Rx.*
Use: Contraceptive.

Orthoclone OKT3. (Ortho McNeil) Muromonab-CD3 5 mg per 5 ml. Inj. 5 ml amps. *Rx.*
Use: Immunosuppressant.

Ortho-Cyclen. (Ortho McNeil) Norgestimate 250 mcg, ethinyl estradiol 35 mcg. Tab. Pkg. 21s, 28s. *Rx.*
Use: Contraceptive.

Ortho Diaphragm. (Ortho McNeil) Diaphragm kit, coil spring sizes 50, 55, 60, 65, 70, 75, 80, 85, 90, 95, 100, 105 mm. *Rx.*
Use: Contraceptive.

Ortho Diaphragm-White. (Ortho McNeil) Diaphragm kit, flat spring sizes 55, 60, 65, 70, 75, 80, 85, 90, 95 mm. *Rx.*
Use: Contraceptive.

Ortho Dienestrol Vaginal Cream. (Ortho McNeil) Dienestrol 0.01%. Tube 78 g with or without applicator. *Rx.*
Use: Estrogen.

Ortho-Est. (Ortho McNeil) **Tab.:** 0.625 or 1.25 mg estropipate, lactose. 100s. *Rx.*
Use: Estrogen.

Orthoflavin. (Enzyme Process) Vitamins C 150 mg, E 25 mg/Tab. Bot. 100s, 250s. *otc.*
Use: Vitamin supplement.

Orthoform. Menthyl 3-amino-4-hydroxybenzoate.
Use: Anesthetic, local.
W/Tyrothricin. (Columbus) Tyrothricin 0.5 mg, tetracaine HCl 0.5%, epinephrine 1/ 1000 Soln. 2%/g. Oint., Tube oz.

Use: Anti-infective, ophthalmic.

Ortho-Gynol Contraceptive. (Advanced Care Products) Oxtoxynol 9. Gel. Tube. 75 g w/applicator and 75 g, 114 g refills. *otc.*
Use: Contraceptive.

ortho-hydroxybenzoic acid. Salicylic Acid, U.S.P. 23.

orthohydroxyphenylmercuric chloride.
Use: Antiseptic.
W/Benzocaine, ephedrine HCl.
See: Myrimgacaine, Liq. (Pharmacia & Upjohn).
W/Benzocaine, parachlorometaxylenol, benzalkonium Cl, phenol.
See: Unguentine Aerosol (Procter & Gamble).
W/Benzoic acid, salicylic acid.
See: NP-27 Liq. (Procter & Gamble).
W/Benzoic acid, salicylic acid, sec.-amyltricresols
W/Zinc acetate, salicylic acid, phenol.
See: Zemacol, Medicated Skin Lotion (Procter & Gamble).

Ortho-Novum 1/35-21. (Ortho McNeil) Norethindrone 1 mg, ethinyl estradiol 0.035 mg/Tab. Dialpak 21s. *Rx.*
Use: Contraceptive.

Ortho-Novum 1/35-28. (Ortho McNeil) Norethindrone 1 mg, ethinyl estradiol 0.035 mg/Tab. w/ 7 inert Tab. Dialpak 28s. *Rx.*
Use: Contraceptive.

Ortho-Novum 1/50-21. (Ortho McNeil) Norethindrone 1 mg, mestranol 50 mcg/Tab. Dialpak 21s. *Rx.*
Use: Contraceptive.

Ortho-Novum 1/50-28. (Ortho McNeil) Norethindrone 1 mg, mestranol 50 mcg/Tab. w/ 7 inert Tab. Dialpak 28s. *Rx.*
Use: Contraceptive.

Ortho-Novum 7/7/7-21 Tablets. (Ortho McNeil) Norethindrone 0.5 mg, ethinyl estradiol 0.035 mg/Tab.; norethindrone 0.75 mg, ethinyl estradiol 0.035 mg/Tab.; norethindrone 1 mg, ethinyl estradiol 0.035 mg/Tab. Dialpak 21s. *Rx.*
Use: Contraceptive.

Ortho-Novum 7/7/7-28 Tablets. (Ortho McNeil) Same as Ortho-Novum 7/7/7/-21 w/ 7 inert tab. Dialpak 28s. *Rx.*
Use: Contraceptive.

Ortho-Novum 10/11-21 Tablets. (Ortho McNeil) Norethindrone 0.5 mg, ethinyl estradiol 0.035 mg/Tab; norethindrone 1 mg, ethinyl estradiol 0.035 mg/Tab. Dialpak 21s. *Rx.*
Use: Contraceptive.

Ortho-Novum 10/11-28 Tablets. (Ortho McNeil) Norethindrone 0.5 mg, ethinyl estradiol 0.035 mg/Tab; norethindrone 1 mg, ethinyl estradiol 0.035 mg/Tab; w/ inert tab. Dialpak 28s. *Rx.*
Use: Contraceptive.

Ortho Personal Lubricant. (Advanced Care Products) Greaseless, water soluble and non-staining aqueous hydrocolloid gel. Acid buffered to vaginal pH. Tube 2 oz, 4 oz. *otc.*
Use: Lubricant.

Ortho Tri-Cyclen. (Ortho McNeil) 7 white tablets containing norgestimate 0.18 mg, ethinyl estradiol 35 mcg; 7 light blue tablets containing norgestimate 0.215 mg, ethinyl estradiol 35 mcg; 7 blue tablets containing norgestimate 0.25 mg, ethinyl estradiol 35 mcg. Tab. Pkg. 21s, 28s. *Rx.*
Use: Contraceptive.

Orthoxicol Cough Syrup. (Roberts Pharm) Phenylpropanolamine HCl 8.3 mg, chlorpheniramine maleate 1.3 mg, dextromethorphan HBr 6.7 mg, alcohol 8%, sorbitol, parabens. Bot. 60 ml, 120 ml, 480 ml. *otc.*
Use: Antihistamine, antitussive, decongestant.

orthoxine. Methoxyphenamine.

orticalm.
Use: Hypotensive, tranquilizer.
See: Serpasil, Prod. (Bristol-Myers Squibb).

Orudis. (Wyeth Ayerst) Ketoprofen 25 mg, 50 mg or 75 mg/Cap. Bot. **25 mg or 50 mg:** 100s; **75 mg:** 100s, 500s, UD 100s. *Rx.*
Use: Analgesic, NSAID.

Orudis KT. (Whitehall Robins) **Tab.:** 12.5 mg ketoprofen, tartrazine, sugar. In 50s. *otc.*
Use: Analgesic, NSAID.

Oruvail. (Wyeth Ayerst) **SR Tab.:** Ketoprofen 100 mg, 150 mg or 200 mg/SR Tab. Bot. 100s, Redipak 100s. **SR Cap.:** 100 mg, 150 mg. 100s, Redipak 100s. *Rx.*
Use: Analgesic, NSAID.

orvus.
See: Gardinol Type Detergents (Various Mfr.).

osarsal.
See: Acetarsone.

Os-Cal 250. (Hoechst Marion Roussel) Oyster shell powder as calcium 250 mg, vitamin D 125 IU and trace minerals (Cu, Fe, Mg, Mn, Zn, silica)/Tab. Bot. 100s, 240s, 500s, 1000s. *otc.*

Use: Mineral, vitamin supplement.

Os-Cal 500. (SmithKline Beecham Pharmaceuticals) Calcium 500 mg/Tab. Bot. 60s, 120s. *otc.*
Use: Mineral supplement.

Os-Cal 250 + D. (SmithKline Beecham Pharmaceuticals) Calcium carbonate 625 mg, vitamin D 125 units/Tab. Bot. 100s. *otc.*
Use: Mineral, vitamin supplement.

Os-Cal 500 + D. (SmithKline Beecham Pharmaceuticals) Calcium carbonate 1250 mg, vitamin D 125 units/Tab. Bot. 60s. *otc.*
Use: Mineral, vitamin supplement.

Os-Cal 500 Chewable Tablets. (SmithKline Beecham Pharmaceuticals) Calcium 500 mg/Tab. Bot. 60s. *otc.*
Use: Mineral supplement.

Os-Cal Fortified. (SmithKline Beecham Pharmaceuticals) Calcium 250 mg, iron 5 mg, Mg, Mn, zinc 0.5 mg, vitamin A 1668 IU, D 125 IU, B_1 1.7 mg, B_2 1.7 mg, B_3 15 mg, B_6 2 mg, C 50 mg, E 0.8 IU, parabens/Tab. Bot. 100s. *otc.*
Use: Mineral, vitamin supplement.

Os-Cal Fortified Multivitamin & Minerals. (SmithKline Beecham Pharmaceuticals) **Tab.:** 1668 IU vitamin A, 125 IU D, 0.8 IU E, 1.7 mg B_1, 1.7 mg B_2, 15 mg B_3, 2 mg B_6, 50 mg C, 5 mg Fe, 250 mg Ca, 0.5 mg Zn, Mn, Mg, EDTA, parabens. In 100s. *otc.*
Use: Mineral, vitamin supplement.

Os-Cal Plus. (SmithKline Beecham Pharmaceuticals) Calcium 250 mg, vitamins D 125 IU, A 1666 IU, C 33 mg, B_2 0.66 mg, B_1 0.5 mg, B_6 0.5 mg, niacinamide 3.33 mg, zinc 0.75 mg, manganese 0.75 mg, iron 16.6 mg/Tab. Bot. 100s. *otc.*
Use: Mineral, vitamin supplement.

Osmitrol. (Baxter) Mannitol in water. **5%:** 1000 ml; **10%:** 500 ml, 1000 ml; **15%:** 150 ml, 500 ml; **20%:** 250 ml, 500 ml. Mannitol in 0.3% sodium **5%:** 1000 ml. Mannitol in 0.45% sodium **20%:** 500 ml. *Rx.*
Use: Diuretic.
See: Mannitol.

Osmoglyn. (Alcon Surgical) Glycerin 50% in flavored aqueous vehicle. Plastic bot. 6 oz. *Rx.*
Use: Diuretic.

Osmolite. (Ross Laboratories) Isotonic liquid food containing 1.06 calories/ml. Two quarts (2000 calories) provides 100% US RDA vitamins and minerals for adults and children. Osmolality: 300 mOsm/kg water. Ready-to-Use: Bot. Can 8 fl oz, 32 fl oz. *otc.*
Use: Nutritional supplement.

Osmolite HN. (Ross Laboratories) High nitrogen isotonic liquid food containing 1.06 calories/ml; 1400 calories provides 100% US RDA vitamins and minerals for adults and children. Osmolality: 300 mOsm/kg water. Ready-to-Use: Bot. 8 fl oz. Can 8 fl oz, 32 fl oz. *otc.*
Use: Nutritional supplement.

Osmotic Diuretics.
See: Mannitol (Various Mfr.).
Osmitrol (Baxter).
Ureaphil (Abbott Laboratories).
Glyrol (Ciba Vision Ophthalmics).
Osmoglyn (Alcon Laboratories).
Ismotic (Alcon Laboratories).

ospolot.
Use: Anticonvulsant drug; pending release.

Ossonate Capsule. (Marcen) Cartilage mucopolysaccharide extract, chondroitin sulfate 50 mg/Cap. Bot. 100s, 500s, 1000s.

Ossonate-Plus, Caps. (Marcen) Ossonate-mucopolysaccharide extract 50 mg, acetaminophen 300 mg, salicylamide 200 mg/Cap. Bot. 100s, 500s, 1000s. *otc.*
Use: Antiarthritic.

Ossonate-Plus, Inj. (Marcen) Ossonate cartilage mucopolysaccharide extract 12.5 mg, casein hydrolysates 80 mg, sulfur 20 mg, sodium citrate 5 mg, benzyl alcohol 0.5%, phenol 0.5%/ml. Multidose 10 ml vial. *Rx.*
Use: Muscle relaxant, pain reliever.

Ossonate-75. (Marcen) Chondroitin sulfate 37.5 mg, benzyl alcohol 0.5%, phenol 0.5%, sodium citrate 5 mg/ml. Vial 10 ml. *Rx.*
Use: Infantile and atopic eczemas, drug allergies, dermatoses associated with intestinal toxemias.

Osteocalcin. (Arcola Laboratories) Calcitonin-salmon 200 IU, phenol 5 mg/ml. Inj. Vial 2 ml. *Rx.*
Use: Hormone.

Osteo-D. (Teva USA)
See: Secalciferol.

Osteolate Injection. (Fellows) Sodium thiosalicylate 50 mg, benzyl alcohol 2%/ml. Vial 30 ml. *Rx.*
Use: Analgesic.

Osteo-Mins. (Tyson and Associates) **Powd.:** 500 mg vitamin C, 250 mg Ca, 250 mg Mg, 45 mg K, 100 IU D/4.5 g. Sugar free. 200 g. *otc.*
Use: Vitamin supplement.

Osteon/D. (Taylor Pharmaceuticals) Calcium 600 mg, phosphorus 400 mg, magnesium 240 mg, vitamin D 400 IU/ 6 Tab. Bot. 180s. *Rx.*
Use: Mineral, vitamin supplement.

Osti-Derm Lotion. (Pedinol) Aluminum sulfate, zinc oxide. Lot. Bot. 42.5 g. *otc.*
Use: Antipruritic; astringent, topical.

Ostiderm Roll-On. (Pedinol) Aluminum chlorohydrate, camphor, alcohol, EDTA, diazolidinyl urea. Bot. 88.7 ml. *otc.*
Use: Antipruritic; astringent, topical.

Osto-K. (Parthenon) Potassium 1 mEq (39 mg from gluconate, Cl and citrate), vitamin C 25 mg, sodium 0.52 mg/Tab. Bot. 60s. *otc.*
Use: Mineral, vitamin supplement.

osvarsan.
See: Acetarsone.

Otic-Care. (Parmed) Hydrocortisone 1%, neomycin sulfate 5 mg, polymyxin B sulfate 10,000 units/ml, glycerin, hydrochloric acid, propylene glycol, potassium metabisulfite. Soln. *Rx.*
Use: Otic.

Otic Domeboro. (Bayer Corp) Acetic acid 2%, aluminum acetate solution. Plastic dropper bot 2 oz. *Rx.*
Use: Otic.

Otic-HC. (Roberts Pharm) Chloroxylenol 1 mg, pramoxine HCl 10 mg, hydrocortisone alcohol 10 mg, benzalkonium Cl 0.2 mg/ml. Bot. 12 ml. *Rx.*
Use: Otic.

Otic-Neo-Cort Dome.
See: Neo-Cort Dome Otic Soln. (Bayer Corp).

Otic-Plain. (Roberts Pharm) Chloroxylenol 1 mg, pramoxine HCl 10 mg, benzalkonium Cl 0.2 mg/ml. Bot. 12 ml. *Rx.*
Use: Otic.

Otic Solution No. 1. (Foy) Hydrocortisone alcohol 10 mg, pramoxine HCl 10 mg, benzalkonium Cl 0.2 mg, acetic acid glacial 20 mg/ml w/propylene glycol q.s. *Rx.*
Use: Otic.

Oti-Med. (Hyrex) Chloroxylenol 1 mg, pramoxine HCl 10 mg, hydrocortisone 10 mg/ml, propylene glycol, benzalkonium chloride. Drops. Vial 10 ml. *Rx.*
Use: Otic.

Otobiotic Otic Solution. (Schering Plough) Polymyxin B, hydrocortisone in propylene glycol and glycerin vehicle w/edetate disodium, sodium bisulfite, anhydrous sodium sulfite, purified water. Bot. w/dropper 15 ml. *Rx.*
Use: Otic.

Otocain. (Holloway) Benzocaine 20%, benzethonium Cl 0.1%, glycerin 1%, polyethylene glycol. Soln. Bot. 15 ml. *Rx.*
Use: Otic.

Otocalm-H Ear Drops. (Parmed) Pramoxine HCl 10 mg, hydrocortisone alcohol 10%, p-Chloro-m-Xylenol 1 mg, benzalkonium Cl 0.2 mg, acetic acid glacial 20 mg, propylene glycol/ml. Bot. 10 ml. *Rx.*
Use: Otic.

Otocort Sterile Solution. (Teva USA) Neomycin sulfate equivalent to 3.5 mg neomycin base, polymyxin B sulfate 10,000 units, hydrocortisone 10 mg/ml, propylene glycol, glycerin, potassium metabisulfite, HCl, purified water. Bot. 10 ml. *Rx.*
Use: Otic.

Otocort Sterile Suspension. (Teva USA) Neomycin sulfate equivalent to 3.5 mg neomycin base, polymyxin B sulfate 10,000 units, hydrocortisone 10 mg/ml, cetyl alcohol, propylene glycol, polysorbate 80, thimerosal, water for injection. Bot. 10 ml. *Rx.*
Use: Otic.

Otogesic HC Solution. (Lexis) Polymyxin B sulfate 10,000 IU, neomycin sulfate 3.5 mg, hydrocortisone 10 mg/ ml, potassium metabisulfite 0.1%. Bot. 10 ml. *Rx.*
Use: Otic.

Otogesic HC Suspension. (Lexis) Polymyxin B sulfate 10,000 units, neomycin sulfate 3.5 mg, hydrocortisone 10 mg/ ml, benzalkonium Cl 0.01%. Bot. 10 ml. *Rx.*
Use: Otic.

Otomar-HC. (Marnel) Chloroxylenol 1 mg, hydrocortisone 10 mg, pramoxine HCl/ml. Otic Soln. Plastic dropper vials. *Rx.*
Use: Otic preparation.

Otomycin-HPN. (Misemer) Polymyxin B sulfate 10,000 units, neomycin sulfate 3.5 mg, hydrocortisone 10 mg/ml. Bot. w/dropper 10 ml. *Rx.*
Use: Otic.

Otrivin. (Novartis Pharmaceuticals) Xylometazoline HCl. **Nasal Drops:** 0.1% w/ sodium Cl, phenylmercuric acetate 1:50,000. Dropper bot. 20 ml. **Nasal Spray:** 0.1% w/potassium phosphate monobasic, potassium Cl, sodium phosphate dibasic, sodium Cl, benzalkonium Cl 1:5000. Plastic squeeze

spray 15 ml. **Ped. Nasal Soln. Drops:** 0.05%. Bot. 20 ml. *otc.*
Use: Decongestant.

ouabain octahydrate. Ouabain, U.S.P. 23.

ovarian extract. Aqueous extract of whole ovaries of cattle.
Use: Estrogen.

ovarian substance. (Various Mfr.) Whole ovarian substance from cattle, sheep or swine. *Rx.*
Use: Estrogen.

Ovastat. (Medac)
See: Treosulfan.

Ovcon-35. (Bristol-Myers) Norethindrone 0.4 mg, ethinyl estradiol 0.035 mg/Tab. Ctn. 6×21s. *Rx.*
Use: Contraceptive.

Ovcon-35, 28 Day. (Bristol-Myers) Norethindrone 0.4 mg, ethinyl estradiol 0.035 mg, w/7 inert tab/Carton 6×28s. *Rx.*
Use: Contraceptive.

Ovcon-50. (Bristol-Myers) Norethindrone 1 mg, ethinyl estradiol 0.05 mg/Tab. Ctn. 6×21s. *Rx.*
Use: Contraceptive.

Ovcon-50, 28 Day. (Bristol-Myers) Norethindrone 1 mg, ethinyl estradiol 0.05 mg, w/7 inert tab/Carton. 6×28s. *Rx.*
Use: Contraceptive.

Ovide. (Medicis Dermatologics, Inc.) Malathion 0.5%. Lot. Bot. 59 ml. *Rx.*
Use: Pediculicide, scabicide.

ovifollin.
See: Estrone (Various Mfr.).

Ovlin. (Sigma-Tau Pharmaceuticals) **Tab.:** Ethinyl estradiol 0.02 mg, conjugated estrogens 0.2 mg/Tab. Bot. 100s, 1000s. **Inj.:** Estrone 2 mg, estradiol 0.05 mg, vitamin B_{12} 1000 mcg/ml. Vial 30 ml. *Rx.*
Use: Estrogen.

Ovocylin Dipropionate. (Novartis Pharmaceuticals) Estradiol dipropionate. *Rx.*
Use: Estrogen.

Ovral. (Wyeth Ayerst) Norgestrel 0.5 mg, ethinyl estradiol 0.05 mg/Tab. 6 Pilpak dispensers, 21 Tab. Tripak 63s. *Rx.*
Use: Contraceptive.

Ovral-28. (Wyeth Ayerst) Norgestrel 0.5 mg, ethinyl estradiol 0.05 mg/Tab. w/7 inert Tab. Pilpak dispenser 6s containing 21 Tab, 7 inert Tab. *Rx.*
Use: Contraceptive.

Ovrette. (Wyeth Ayerst) Norgestrel 0.075 mg/Tab. 6 Pilpak dispenser, Tab. 28s. *Rx.*
Use: Contraceptive.

OvuGen. (BioGenex) In vitro diagnostic test for measurement of LH urine to determine ovulation. Kits. 6s, 10s.
Use: Diagnostic aid, ovulation.

OvuKIT Self-Test. (Monoclonal Antibodies) Monoclonal antibody-based enzyme immunoassay test for hLH in urine. Kit 6, 9 day.
Use: Diagnostic aid, ovulation.

ovulation stimulants.
See: Clomid (Merrell Dow).
Serophene (Serono Labs).
Metrodin (Serono Labs).

ovulation tests.
See: Answer Ovulation (Carter Products).
Clearplan Easy (Whitehall Robins).
OvuQUICK Self-Test (Monoclonal Antibodies).
Color Ovulation Test (Biomerica).
Conceive Ovulation Predictor (Quidel).
First Response Ovulation Predictor Test Kit (Carter Products).
Fortel Home Ovulation Test (Biomerica).
OvuGen (BioGenex).
OvuKIT Self-Test (Monoclonal Antibodies).

Ovulen-21. (Searle) Ethynodiol diacetate 1 mg, mestranol 0.1 mg/Tab. Compack Disp. 21s, 6×21, 24 ×21. Refill 21s, 12×21. *Rx.*
Use: Contraceptive.

Ovulen-28. (Searle) Ethynodiol diacetate 1 mg, mestranol 0.1 mg/Tab. w/7 inert Tab. Compack 28s: 21 active tab., 7 placebo tab. Compack dispenser 28s. Box 6×28. Refill 28s, Box 12×28. *Rx.*
Use: Contraceptive.

Ovustick Self-Test. (Monoclonal Antibodies) Home test for ovulation. Test kit 10s.
Use: Diagnostic aid.

Oxabid. (Jamieson-McKames) Magnesium oxide 140 mg or magnesium oxide heavy 400 mg/Cap. Bot. 100s. *otc.*
Use: Antacid.

•**oxacillin sodium.** (ox-uh-SILL-in) U.S.P. 23.
Use: Anti-infective.
See: Bactocill, Vial (SmithKline Beecham Pharmaceuticals).
Prostaphlin, Preps. (Bristol-Myers Squibb).
Sodium oxacillin.

oxadimedine hydrochloride.
Use: Antiarrhythmic.

oxafuradene. Name used for Nifuradene. (OX-ah-FYOOR-ah-deen)
Use: Platelet aggregation agent.

•**oxagrelate.** (OX-ah-greh-LATE) USAN.
Use: Platelet aggregation inhibitor.

oxaliplatin. (Axion)
Use: Antineoplastic. [Orphan drug]

•**oxamarin hydrochloride.** (OX-ah-mah-rin) USAN.
Use: Hemostatic.

•**oxamisole hydrochloride.** (ox-AM-ih-sole) USAN.
Use: Immunoregulator.

•**oxamniquine.** (ox-AM-nih-kwin) U.S.P. 23.
Use: Antischistosomal, treatment of schistosomiasis.
See: Vansil, Cap. (Pfizer).

oxanamide.
Use: Anxiolytic.

Oxandrin. (Bio-Technology General) **Tab.:** 2.5 mg oxandrolone, lactose. In 100s. *c-III.*
Use: Anabolic steroid.

•**oxandrolone.** (ox-AN-droe-lone) U.S.P. 23.
Use: Androgen, anabolic. [Orphan drug]
See: Anavar, Tab. (Searle).

•**oxantel pamoate.** (OX-an-tell PAM-oh-ate) USAN.
Use: Anthelmintic.

•**oxaprotiline hydrochloride.** (OX-ah-PRO-tih-leen) USAN.
Use: Antidepressant.

•**oxaprozin.** (OX-ah-pro-zin) USAN.
Use: Anti-inflammatory.
See: Daypro, Capl. (Searle).

•**oxarbazole.** (ox-AHR-bah-zole) USAN.
Use: Antiasthmatic.

•**oxatomide.** (ox-AT-ah-mid) USAN.
Use: Antiallergic, antiasthmatic.

•**oxazepam.** (ox-AZE-uh-pam) U.S.P. 23.
Use: Anxiolytic, sedative.
See: Serax, Cap., Tab. (Wyeth Ayerst).

oxazolindinediones.
See: Paradione (Abbott Laboratories).
Tridione (Abbott Laboratories).

ox bile extract. Purified oxgall.
See: Bile Extract, Ox.

•**oxendolone.** (OX-en-doe-LONE) USAN.
Use: Antiandrogen (benign prostatic hypertrophy).

•**oxethazaine.** (OX-ETH-ah-zane) USAN.
Use: Anesthetic, local.

•**oxetorone fumarate.** (ox-EH-toe-rone) USAN.
Use: Antimigraine.

•**oxfendazole.** (ox-FEN-DAH-zole) USAN.
Use: Anthelmintic.
See: Synanthic (Syntex).

•**oxfenicine.** (OX-FEN-ih-seen) USAN.
Use: Vasodilator.

ox gall.
See: Bile Extract, Ox.

•**oxibendazole.** (ox-ee-BEND-ah-zole) USAN.
Use: Anthelmintic.

•**oxiconazole nitrate.** (ox-ee-KAHN-ah-zole) USAN.
Use: Antifungal.
See: Oxistat Cream, Lot. (Glaxo-Wellcome).

oxidized bile acids.
See: Bile Acids, Oxidized.

oxidized cellulose. Absorbable cellulose. Cellulosic acid.
Use: Hemostatic.
See: Oxycel, **Pad, Pledg., Strip.** (Becton Dickinson).
Surgicel, **Stip, Nu-knid.** (Johnson & Johnson Consumer Products).

•**oxidopamine.** (OX-ih-DOE-pah-meen) USAN.
Use: Adrenergic (ophthalmic).

•**oxidronic acid.** (OX-ih-DRAHN-ik) USAN.
Use: Regulator (calcium).

Oxi-Freeda. (Freeda Vitamins) Vitamin A 5000 IU, E 150 mg, B_3 40 mg, C 100 mg, B_1 20 mg, B_2 20 mg, B_5 20 mg, B_6 20 mg, B_{12} 10 mcg, Zn 15 mg, Se, glutathione, L-cysteine. Tab. Bot. 100s, 250s. *otc.*
Use: Mineral, vitamin supplement.

•**oxifungin hydrochloride.** (OX-ih-FUN-jin) USAN.
Use: Antifungal.

•**oxilorphan.** (ox-ih-LORE-fan) USAN.
Use: Narcotic antagonist.

•**oximonam.** (OX-ih-MOE-nam) USAN.
Use: Anti-infective.

•**oximonam sodium.** (OX-ih-MOE-nam) USAN.
Use: Anti-infective.

oxine.
See: Oxyquinoline sulfate (Various Mfr.).

•**oxiperomide.** (ox-ih-PURR-oh-mide) USAN.
Use: Antipsychotic.

Oxipor VHC Psoriasis Lotion. (Whitehall Robins) **Lot.:** Coal tar soln: 25%, alcohol 79%. 56 ml. *otc.*
Use: Antipsoriatic.

•**oxiramide.** (ox-EER-am-ide) USAN.
Use: Cardiovascular agent.

Oxistat. (GlaxoWellcome) Oxiconazole nitrate 1%. **Cream:** Tube 15 g, 30 g, 60 g; **Lotion:** Bot. 30 ml. *Rx.*
Use: Antifungal, topical.

•**oxisuran.** (OX-ih-SUH-ran) USAN.
Use: Antineoplastic.

•**oxmetidine hydrochloride.** (ox-MEH-tih-DEEN) USAN.
Use: Antiulcerative.

•**oxmetidine mesylate.** (ox-MEH-tih-DEEN) USAN.
Use: Antiulcerative.

•**oxogestone phenpropionate.** (ox-oh-JESS-tone fen-PRO-pih-oh-nate) USAN.
Use: Hormone, progestin.

Oxolamine. (Arcum) Crystalline hydroxycobalamin 1000 mcg/ml. Vial 10 ml. *Rx.*
Use: Vitamin supplement.

•**oxolinic acid.** (ox-oh-LIH-nik acid) USAN.
Use: Anti-infective.

oxophenarsine hydrochloride.

l-2-oxothiazolidine$_4$-carboxylic acid.
Use: Treatment of adult respiratory distress syndrome. [Orphan drug]
See: Procysteine.

Oxothiazolidine Carboxylate. (Clintec Nutritional/Ben Venise Labs) Phase I restoration of glutathione depletion in HIV, ARC, AIDS; prevention of inflammation-induced HIV replication. *Rx.*
Use: Immunomodulator.

oxpheneridine. 1-(β-phenyl-βhydroxyethyl)-4-carbethoxy-4- phenylpiperidine.

•**oxprenolol hydrochloride.** (ox-PREH-no-lole) U.S.P. 23. Under study.
Use: Beta-adrenergic receptor blocker, vasodilator (coronary).

Oxsoralen Lotion. (ICN Pharmaceuticals) Methoxsalen 1% in an inert lotion vehicle of alcohol 71%, propylene glycol, acetone, water. Bot. oz. *Rx.*
Use: Dermatologic.

Oxsoralen Ultra. (ICN Pharmaceuticals) **Soft Cap.:** 10 mg methoxsalen. 50s, 100s. *Rx.*
Use: Dermatologic.

•**oxtriphylline.** (ox-TRY-fih-lin) U.S.P. 23.
Use: Bronchodilator.
See: Choledyl, Tab., Elix. (Parke-Davis).
W/Guaifenesin.
See: Brondecon, Tab., Elix. (Parke-Davis).

oxtriphylline and guaifenesin elixir. (Alphalma USPD) Oxtriphylline 300 mg, guaifenesin 150 mg, alcohol 20%/15 ml. Elix. Bot. pt, gal. *Rx.*
Use: Bronchodilator, expectorant.

Oxy-5 Acne-Pimple Medication. (SmithKline Beecham Pharmaceuticals) Benzoyl peroxide 5% in lotion base. Bot. fl oz. *otc.*
Use: Dermatologic, acne.

Oxy 5 Tinted. (SmithKline Beecham Pharmaceuticals) Benzoyl peroxide 5%, titanium dioxide, sodium PCA, cetyl alcohol, silica, iron oxides, propylene glycol, citric acid, sodium laurel sulfate, stearyl alcohol, parabens. Lot. Bot. 30 ml. *otc.*
Use: Dermatologic, acne.

Oxy 10 Maximum Strength Advanced Formula. (SmithKline Beecham Pharmaceuticals) Benzoyl peroxide 10%, EDTA. Gel. 30 g. *otc.*
Use: Dermatologic, acne.

•**oxybenzone.** (ox-ee-BEN-zone) U.S.P. 23. Cyasorb UV 9 (ESI Lederle Generics).
Use: Ultraviolet screen.
W/Dioxybenzone, benzophenone.
See: Solbar, Lot. (Person & Covey).

oxybenzone with combinations.
See: Coppertone, Prods. (Schering Plough).
Noskote, Cream (Schering Plough).
Shade, Prods. (Schering Plough).
Sunger, Prods. (Schering Plough).
Super Shade, Lot. (Schering Plough).

•**oxybutynin chloride.** (OX-ee-BYOO-tih-nin) U.S.P. 23.
Use: Anticholinergic.
See: Ditropan Syr., Tab. (Hoechst Marion Roussel).

oxybutynin chloride. (Various Mfr.) **Tab.:** 5 mg. Bot. 100s, 500s, 1000s, UD 100s. **Syr.:** 5 mg/5 ml, sorbitol, sucrose, methylparaben. Bot. 473 ml. *Rx.*
Use: Antispasmodic.

Oxycel. (Becton Dickinson) Cellulosic acid in absorbable hemostatic agent prepared from cellulose. Resembles ordinary surgical gauze or cotton. Pledget 2 × 1 × 1 in. 10s. Pad 3 × 3 in. 8 ply. 10s. Strip 5 × 0.5 in. 4 ply. 18 × 2 in. 4 ply. 10s. 36 × 0.5 in. 4 ply. *Rx.*
Use: Hemostatic, topical.

Oxycet. (Halsey) Oxycodone HCl 5 mg, acetaminophen 325 mg/Tab. Bot. 100s, 500s, Hospital pack 250s. *c-II.*
Use: Narcotic analgesic combination.

Oxy-Chinol. (Ferndale Laboratories) Potassium oxyquinoline sulfate 1 gr/Tab. Bot. 100s, 1000s. *otc.*
Use: Antimicrobial, deodorant.

•**oxychlorosene.** (OCK-sih-KLOR-ah-seen) USAN. Monoxychlorosene. Hydrocarbon derivative containing four-

teen carbons and hypochlorous acid. The hydrocarbon chain also has a phenyl substituent which in turn holds a sulfonic acid group.
Use: Anti-infective, topical.
See: Clorpactin, Prod. (Scrip).

•**oxychlorosene sodium.** (OCK-sih-KLOR-ah-seen) USAN. Sodium salt of the complex derived from hypochlorous acid and tetradecylbenzene sulfonic acid. Action of active chlorine.
Use: Anti-infective, topical.

Oxy Clean Lathering Facial. (SmithKline Beecham Pharmaceuticals) Sodium tetraborate decahydrate dissolving particles in a base of surfactant cleaning agents. Soap free. Scrub 79.5 g. *otc.*
Use: Dermatologic, acne.

Oxy Clean Medicated Cleanser and Pads. (SmithKline Beecham Pharmaceuticals) **Cleanser and reg. strength pads:** Salicylic acid 0.5%, SD alcohol 40 B 40%, citric acid, menthol, sodium lauryl sulfate. **Max. strength pads:** Salicylic acid 2%, SD alcohol 40 B 50%, citric acid, menthol, sodium lauryl sulfate. Cleanser 120 ml Pad. 50s. *otc.*
Use: Dermatologic, acne.

Oxy Clean Medicated Pads for Sensitive Skin. (SmithKline Beecham Pharmaceuticals) Salicylic acid 0.5%, SD alcohol 40B 16%. Jar 50s. *otc.*
Use: Dermatologic, acne.

Oxy Clean Scrub. (SmithKline Beecham Pharmaceuticals) Sodium tetraborate decahydrate dissolving particles in a base of surfactant cleaning agents, soap free. Lot. Bot. 79.5 g. *otc.*
Use: Dermatologic, acne.

Oxy Clean Soap. (SmithKline Beecham Pharmaceuticals) Salicylic acid 3.5%, sodium borate. Bar 97.5 g. *otc.*
Use: Dermatologic, acne.

•**oxycodone.** (OX-ee-KOE-dohn) USAN.
Use: Analgesic, narcotic.

oxycodone and aspirin. (Various Mfr.) Oxycodone HCl 4.5 mg, oxycodone terephthalate 0.38 mg, aspirin 325 mg/Tab. Bot. 100s, 500s, 1000s, UD 25s. *c-II.*
Use: Analgesic combination, narcotic.

oxycodone and acetaminophen capsules. (OX-ee-KOE-dohn and ass-cet-ah-MEE-noe-fen) (Various Mfr.) Oxycodone HCl 5 mg, acetaminophen 500 mg/Cap. Bot. 100s, 500s, 1000s, UD 25s. *c-II.*
Use: Analgesic combination, narcotic.

oxycodone and acetaminophen tablets. (OX-ee-KOE-dohn and ass-cet-ah-MEE-noe-fen) (Various Mfr.) Oxycodone HCl 5 mg, acetaminophen 325 mg/Tab. Bot. 100s, 500s, 1000s, UD 25s. *c-II.*
Use: Analgesic combination, narcotic.

•**oxycodone hydrochloride.** (OX-ee-KOE-dohn) U.S.P. 23.
Use: Analgesic, narcotic.
See: Dihydrohydroxycodeinone HCl.
OxyContin, CR Tab. (Purdue Frederick).
OxyIR, IR Cap. (Purdue Frederick).
W/Acetaminophen, oxycodone terephthalate.
See: Percocet-5, Tab. (DuPont Merck Pharmaceuticals).
Tylox, Cap. (Ortho McNeil).

•**oxycodone terephthalate.** (OX-ee-KOE-dohn teh-REFF-thah-late) U.S.P. 23.
Use: Analgesic, narcotic.

OxyContin. (Purdue Frederick) Oxycodone HCl 10 mg, 20 mg, 40 mg, 80 mg, lactose. CR Tab. Bot. 100s, UD 25s (80 mg only). *c-II.*
Use: Analgesic, narcotic.

Oxy Cover. (SmithKline Beecham Pharmaceuticals) Benzoyl peroxide 10%. Cream. 30 g. *otc.*
Use: Dermatologic, acne.

oxyethylated tertiary octylphenol-formaldehyde polymer.
See: Triton WR-1339 (Rohm and Haas).

oxyethylene oxypropylene polymer.
See: Poloxalkol.
W/Danthron, B_1, carboxymethyl cellulose.
See: Evactol, Cap. (Delta).

•**oxyfilcon A.** (OX-ee-FILL-kahn A) USAN.
Use: Contact lens material (hydrophilic).

•**oxygen.** U.S.P. 23.
Use: Gas, medicinal.

•**oxygen 93 percent.** U.S.P. 23.
Use: Gas, medicinal.

OxyIR. (Purdue Frederick) Oxycodone HCl 5 mg/IR Cap. Bot. 100s. *c-II.*
Use: Analgesic, narcotic.

Oxy Medicated Cleanser and Regular Strength Pads. (SmithKline Beecham Pharmaceuticals) Salicylic acid 0.5%, SD alcohol 28%, citric acid, menthol, propylene glycol. Cleanser. Bot. 120 ml. Pads 50s, 90s. *otc.*
Use: Dermatologic, acne.

Oxy Medicated Cleanser and Maximum Strength Pads. (SmithKline Beecham Pharmaceuticals) Salicylic acid 2%, SD alcohol 44%, citric acid,

menthol, propylene glycol. Cleanser. Bot. 120 ml. Pads 50s, 90s. *otc.*
Use: Dermatologic, acne.

Oxy Medicated Cleanser and Sensitive Skin Pads. (SmithKline Beecham Pharmaceuticals) Salicylic acid 0.5%, alcohol 22%, disodium lauryl sulfosuccinate, menthol, trisodium EDTA. Cleanser. Bot. 120 ml. Pads 50s, 90s. *otc.*
Use: Dermatologic, acne.

Oxy Medicated Soap. (SmithKline Beecham Pharmaceuticals) Triclosan 1%, bentonite, cocoamphodipropionate, iron oxides, glycerin, magnesium silicate, sodium borohydride, sodium cocoate, sodium tallowate, talc, EDTA, titanium dioxide. Bar. 97.5 g. *otc.*
Use: Dermatologic, acne.

oxymetazoline hydrochloride.
Use: Mydriatic, vasoconstrictor.
See: Ocuclear (Schering Plough).
Visine (Pfizer).

•**oxymetazoline hydrochloride.** (OX-ee-MET-azz-oh-leen) U.S.P. 23.
Use: Decongestant, adrenergic (vasoconstrictor).
See: Afrin, Nasal Spray, Soln. (Schering Plough).
Cheracol Nasal, Spray (Roberts Pharm).
Dristan 12-Hr Nasal, Spray (Whitehall Robins).
Duration Nasal Spray (Schering Plough).
Duration Nose Drops (Schering Plough).
Duration Nose Drops for Children (Schering Plough).
St. Joseph Nasal Spray for Children (Schering Plough).
St. Joseph Nose Drops for Children (Schering Plough).

•**oxymetholone.** (OCK-sih-METH-oh-lone) U.S.P. 23.
Use: Androgen.
See: Anadrol, Tab. (Syntex).

•**oxymorphone hydrochloride.** (ox-ee-MORE-fone) U.S.P. 23.
Use: Analgesic, narcotic. [Orphan drug]
See: Numorphan Amp., Vial, Supp. (DuPont Merck Pharmaceuticals).

Oxy Night Watch. (SmithKline Beecham Pharmaceuticals) Salicylic acid 1%, cetyl alcohol, silica, propylene glycol, stearyl alcohol, sodium laureth sulfate, parabens, EDTA. Lot. Bot. 60 ml. *otc.*
Use: Dermatologic, acne.

Oxy Night Watch Maximum Strength. (SmithKline Beecham Pharmaceuticals) Salicylic acid 2%, cetyl alcohol, EDTA, parabens, stearyl alcohol. Lot. Bot. 60 ml. *otc.*
Use: Dermatologic, acne.

Oxy Night Watch Sensitive Skin. (SmithKline Beecham Pharmaceuticals) Salicylic acid 1%, cetyl alcohol, EDTA, stearyl alcohol, parabens. Lot. Bot. 60 ml. *otc.*
Use: Dermatologic, acne.

•**oxypertine.** (OX-ee-PURR-teen) USAN. Integrin hydrochloride.
Use: Psychotherapeutic agent, antidepressant.

•**oxyphenbutazone.** (ox-ee-fen-BYOO-tah-zone) U.S.P. 23.
Use: Analgesic, antiarthritic, anti-inflammatory, antipyretic, antirheumatic.
See: Oxalid, Tab. (Rhone-Poulenc Rorer).

oxyphenisatin acetate. (OX-ee-fen-EYE-sah-tin) USAN.
Use: Laxative.
See: Endophenolphthalein (Roche Laboratories).
Isacen (No Mfr. currently lists).
Prulet, Tab. (Mission Pharmacal).
Prulet Liquitab. (Mission Pharmacal).

•**oxyphenudrine.**

•**oxypurinol.** (OX-ee-PYOO-ree-nahl) USAN.
Use: Xanthine oxidase inhibitor.

•**oxyquinoline.** (OX-ih-KWIN-oh-lin) USAN.
Use: Disinfectant.

oxyquinoline benzoate. (Merck) Pkg. lb. 8-Hydroxyquinoline benzoate.
W/Alkyl aryl sulfonate, disodium edetate, aminacrine HCl, copper sulfate, sodium sulfate.
See: Triva, Vaginal Jelly, Pow. (Boyle).
W/Benzoic acid, salicylic acid, sodium tetradecyl sulfate.
See: NP-27 Cream (Procter & Gamble).

•**oxyquinoline sulfate.** (OX-ih-KWIN-oh-lin) N.F. 18.
Use: Disinfectant, pharmaceutic aid (complexing agent).
See: Chinosol, Tab., Pow., Vial (Vernon).

oxyquinoline sulfate w/combinations.
See: Oxyzal Wet Dressing, Soln. (Gordon Laboratories).
Rectal Medicone, Oint. (Medicone).
Rectal Medicone-HC, Oint. (Medicone).
Rectal Medicone Unguent, Oint. (Medicone).
Triticoll, Tab. (Western Research).
Triva, Douche Pow. (Boyle).

Oxy Residon't Medicated Face Wash. (SmithKline Beecham Pharmaceuticals) Cocamidopropyl betaine, sodium laureth sulfate, sodium cocoyl isethionate, triclosan, diazolidinyl urea. Liq. Bot. 240 ml. *otc.*
Use: Dermatologic, acne.

Oxy-Scrub. (SmithKline Beecham Pharmaceuticals) Abradant cleanser containing dissolving abradant particles of sodium tetraborate decahydrate. Tube 2.65 oz. *otc.*
Use: Dermatologic, acne.

Oxysept. (Allergan) **Disinfecting Soln.:** Hydrogen peroxide 3%, sodium stannate, sodium nitrate, phosphate buffer. Bot. 240 ml or 360 ml. **Neutralizer Tab.:** Catalase, buffering agents. In 12s (w/Oxy-Tab cup) or 36s. *otc.*
Use: Contact lens care.

Oxysept 1. (Allergan) Microfiltered hydrogen peroxide 3% w/sodium stannate and sodium nitrate, preservative free, buffered. Soln. Bot. 355 ml. *otc.*
Use: Contact lens care.

Oxysept 2. (Allergan) Catalytic neutralizing agent, EDTA, sodium Cl, mono- and dibasic sodium phosphates. Buffered, preservative free. Soln. In 15 ml single-use containers (25s). *otc.*
Use: Contact lens care.

•**oxytetracycline.** (ox-ee-teh-trah-SIGH-kleen) U.S.P. 23.
Use: Anti-infective.
See: Terramycin, Prods. (Pfizer).

oxytetracycline and hydrocortisone acetate ophthalmic suspension.
Use: Anti-infective, anti-inflammatory.

oxytetracycline and nystatin capsules.
Use: Anti-infective, antifungal.

oxytetracycline and nystatin for oral suspension.
Use: Anti-infective, antifungal.

oxytetracycline and phenazopyridine hydrochlorides and sulfamethizole capsules.
Use: Analgesic; anti-infective; antispasmodic, urinary.

•**oxytetracycline calcium.** U.S.P. 23.
Use: Anti-infective.

•**oxytetracycline hydrochloride.** U.S.P. 23. An antibiotic from *Streptomyces rimosus.*
Use: Anti-infective, antirickettsial.
See: Dalimycin, Cap. (Dalin).
Oxlopar, Cap. (Parke-Davis).
Oxy-Kesso-Tetra, Cap. (McKesson).
Terramycin HCl, Preps. (Pfizer Laboratories, Pfipharmecs).
Uri-tet, Cap. (American Urologicals).
Urobiotic (Roerig).

oxytetracycline hydrochloride and hydrocortisone ointment.
Use: Anti-infective, anti-inflammatory.

oxytetracycline hydrochloride and polymyxin B sulfate.
Use: Anti-infective.

oxytetracycline hydrochloride and polymyxin B sulfate ophthalmic ointment.
Use: Anti-infective.

oxytetracycline hydrochloride and polymyxin B sulfate topical powder.
Use: Anti-infective.

oxytetracycline hydrochloride and polymyxin B sulfate vaginal tablets.
Use: Anti-infective.

oxytetracycline-polymyxin B. Mix of oxytetracycline HCl and polymyxin B sulfate.
Use: Anti-infective.
See: Terramycin HCl w/Polymyxin B. Sulfate, Tab. (Pfizer Laboratories, Pfipharmecs).

oxytocics.
See: Ergotrate Maleate, **Inj.** (Bedford Labs).
Methergine, **Inj.** (Novartis).

•**oxytocin.** (ox-ih-TOE-sin) U.S.P. 23.
Use: Oxytocic.
See: Pitocin, Amp. (Parke-Davis).

oxytocin nasal solution. (ox-ih-TOE-sin)
Use: Oxytocic.

oxytocin, synthetic. (ox-ih-TOE-sin)
See: Pitocin, Amp. (Parke-Davis).
Syntocinon, Amp. (Novartis).

Oxy Wash. (SmithKline Beecham Pharmaceuticals) Benzoyl peroxide 10%. Liq. Bot. 120 ml. *otc.*
Use: Dermatologic, acne.

Oxyzal Wet Dressing. (Gordon Laboratories) Benzalkonium Cl 1:2000, oxyquinoline sulfate, distilled water. Dropper bot. 1 oz, 4 oz. *otc.*
Use: Dermatologic, counterirritant.

Oysco. (Rugby) Elemental calcium 500 mg/Tab. Bot. 60s. *otc.*
Use: Mineral supplement.

Oysco D. (Rugby) Ca 250 mg, D 125 IU. Tab. Bot. 100s, 250s, 1000s. *otc.*
Use: Mineral, vitamin supplement.

Oyst-Cal 500. (Zenith Goldline) Calcium carbonate 1.25 g (calcium 500 mg)/Tab. Bot. 60s, 120s. *otc.*
Use: Mineral supplement.

Oyst-Cal-D. (Zenith Goldline) Calcium 250 mg, vitamin D 125 IU/Tab. Bot. 100s, 1000s. *otc.*

Use: Mineral, vitamin supplement.

Oyster Calcium. (NBTY) Ca 275 mg, D 200 IU, A 800 IU. Tab. Bot. 100s. *otc.*
Use: Mineral, vitamin supplement.

Oyster Shell Calcium-500. (Vangard) Calcium carbonate 1.25 g, (calcium 500 mg). Tab. Bot. 100s, UD 100s, 640s. *otc.*
Use: Mineral supplement.

oyster shells.
See: Os-Cal, Tab. (Hoechst Marion Roussel).
W/Vitamin D-2.
See: Ostrakal, Tab. (ICN Pharmaceuticals).

Oystercal 500. (NBTY) Calcium carbonate 1.25 g (calcium 500 mg)/Tab. Bot. 100s. *otc.*
Use: Mineral supplement.

Oystercal-D. (NBTY) Calcium 250 mg, vitamin D 125 IU/Tab. Bot. 100s, 250s. *otc.*
Use: Mineral, vitamin supplement.

•**ozolinone.** (oh-ZOE-lih-NOHN) USAN.
Use: Diuretic.

P

P_1E_1; P_2E_1; P_3E_1; P_4E_1; P_6E_1. (Alcon Laboratories) Pilocarpine HCl 1%, 2%, 3%, 4% or 6% respectively, with epinephrine bitartrate 1%. Plastic dropper vial 15 ml. *Rx.*
Use: Antigout agent.

P and S Liquid. (Baker/Cummins) Bot. 4 oz, 8 oz. *otc.*
Use: Antiseborrheic.

P and S Shampoo. (Baker/Cummins) Salicylic acid 2%, lactic acid 0.5% Bot. 4 oz. *otc.*
Use: Antiseborrheic.

Pabalate. (Robins) Sodium salicylate 300 mg, sodium aminobenzoate 300 mg/ EC Tab. Bot. 100s, 500s. *otc.*
Use: Antirheumatic.

Pabalate-SF. (Robins) Potassium salicylate 300 mg, potassium aminobenzoate 300 mg/Tab. Bot. 100s, 500s. *otc.*
Use: Antirheumatic.

PABA-Salicylate. (Various Mfr.) Sodium salicylate, p-aminobenzoate, vitamin C/ Tab. Bot. 100s, 500s. *otc.*
Use: Analgesic, vitamin combination.

PABA sodium. (Various Mfr.). Sodium p-aminobenzoate. *otc.*
Use: Vitamin supplement.

Pabasone. (Pinex) Sodium salicylate 5 gr, para-aminobenzoic acid 5 gr, ascorbic acid 20 mg/Tab. Bot. 100s. *otc.*
Use: Analgesic, vitamin supplement.

P-A-C. Preparations of phenacetin, aspirin, caffeine.
See: A.P.C. Preparations, Empirin Preparations.

p-acetylaminobenzaldehyde thiosemicarbazone. (Amithiozone, Antib, Berculon A, Benzothiozon, Conteben, Myuizone, Neustab, Tebethion, Thiomicid, Thioparamizone, Thiacetazone)
Use: Antituberculous.

P-A-C Revised Formula Analgesic. (Pharmacia & Upjohn) Aspirin 400 mg, caffeine 32 mg/Tab. Bot. 100s, 1000s. *otc.*
Use: Analgesic.

Pacemaker Prophylaxis Pastes with Fluoride. (Pacemaker) Silicone dioxide and diatomaceous earth, sodium fluoride 4.4%. Light abrasive, cinnamon/cherry. Medium abrasive, orange. Heavy abrasive, mint. Paste Bot. 8 oz.
Use: Dental caries agent.

Packer's Pine Tar Liquid Shampoo. (Rydelle) Pine tar. Bot. 6 fl oz. *otc.*
Use: Antiseborrheic.

Packer's Pine Tar Soap. (Rydelle) Bar 3.3 oz. *otc.*
Use: Dermatologic.

Paclin VK. (Armenpharm) Penicillin phenoxymethyl 125 mg or 250 mg/Tab. Bot. 100s, 1000s. *Rx.*
Use: Anti-infective, penicillin.

•**paclitaxel.** (pak-lih-TAX-uhl) USAN.
Use: Antineoplastic.
See: Taxol, Inj. (Bristol-Myers Squibb).

•**padimate a.** (PAD-ih-mate A) USAN.
Use: Ultraviolet screen.

•**padimate O.** (PAD-ih-mate O) U.S.P. 23.
Use: Ultraviolet screen.
See: Coppertone Prods. (Schering Plough).
Eclipse Prods. (Novartis).
Escalol 506 (Van Dyk).
Noskote Prods. (Schering Plough).
Pabafilm (Galderma).
Shade Prods. (Schering Plough).
Sunger Prods. (Schering Plough).
Super Shade, Prods. (Schering Plough).
Tropical Blend Sunscreen Lot. (Schering Plough).

•**pagoclone.** (PAG-oh-klone) USAN.
Use: Anxiolytic.

PAH.
See: Sodium Aminohippurate Inj. (Various Mfr.).

Pain-a-Lay. (Glessner) Antiseptic, anesthetic soln. Bot. 4 oz w/sprayer, Bot. 4 oz, 8 oz, 1 pt.
Use: Mouth and throat preparation.

Pain and Fever Capsules. (ESI Lederle Generics) Acetaminophen 500 mg/Cap. Bot. 50s, 100s. *otc.*
Use: Analgesic.

Pain and Fever Liquid. (ESI Lederle Generics) Acetaminophen 160 mg/5 ml (children's strength). Unit-of-use 4 oz, Bot. 16 oz. *otc.*
Use: Analgesic.

Pain and Fever Tablets. (ESI Lederle Generics) Acetaminophen 325 mg or 500 mg/Tab. **325 mg:** Bot. 100s, 1000s; **500 mg:** Bot. 50s, 100s. *otc.*
Use: Analgesic.

Pain Bust-R II. (Continental Consumer Products) Methyl salicylate 17%, menthol 12%. Cream. Jar 90 g. *otc.*
Use: Liniment.

Pain Doctor. (E. Fougera) Capsaicin 0.025%, methyl salicylate 25%, menthol 10%, parabens, propylene glycol. Cream. Tube. 60g. *otc.*
Use: Anesthetic, local.

Pain Gel Plus. (Mentholatum) Menthol

4%, aloe, vitamin E. Gel. Tube 57 g. *otc.*
Use: Liniment.

Pain Relief, Aspirin Free. (Hudson) Acetaminophen 325 mg/Tab. Bot. 100s, 200s. *otc.*
Use: Analgesic, local.

Pain Relief Ointment. (Walgreens) Methyl salicylate 15%, menthol 10%. Tube 1.5 oz, 3 oz. *otc.*
Use: Analgesic, topical.

Pain Reliever. (Rugby) Acetaminophen 250 mg, aspirin 250 mg, caffeine 65 mg/Tab. Bot. 100s, 1000s. *otc.*
Use: Analgesic combination.

Pain Relievers-Tension Headache Relievers. (Weeks & Leo) Acetaminophen 325 mg, phenyltoloxamine citrate 30 mg/Tab. Bot. 40s, 100s. *otc.*
Use: Analgesic combination.

Pain-X. (BF Ascher) Capsaicin 0.05%, menthol 5%, camphor 4%, alcohols, parabens. Gel. Tube. 42.5 g. *otc.*
Use: Topical pain reliever.

Palbar No. 2. (Roberts Pharm) Atropine sulfate 0.012 mg, scopolamine HBr 0.005 mg, hyoscyamine HBr 0.018 mg, phenobarbital 32.4 mg/Tab. Bot. 100s. *Rx.*
Use: Anticholinergic, antispasmodic, sedative, hypnotic.

•**paldimycin.** (pal-dih-MY-sin) USAN.
Use: Anti-infective.

palestrol.
See: Diethylstilbestrol (Various Mfr.).

•**palinavir.** (pal-LIH-nah-veer) USAN.
Use: Antiviral.

palinum.
Use: Hypnotic, sedative.
See: Cyclobarbital Calcium (Various Mfr.).

palmidrol. N-(2-Hydroxyethyl) palmitamide.

Palmitate-A 5000. Vitamin A 5000 IU. Tab. Bot. 100s. *otc.*
Use: Vitamin supplement.

•**palmoxirate sodium.** (pal-MOX-ihr-ate) USAN.
Use: Antidiabetic.

•**palonosetron hydrochloride.** (pal-oh-NO-seh-trahn) USAN.
Use: Antiemetic, antinauseant.

PALS. (Palisades Pharm) Chlorophyllin copper complex 100 mg. Tab. Bot. 30s, 100s, 1000s, UD 30s. *otc.*
Use: Deodorant, systemic.

PAM.
See: Melphalan.

•**pamabrom.** USAN.
See: Maximum Strength Aqua-Ban, Tab. (Thompson).
W/Acetaminophen.
See: Pamprin, Tab. (Chattem Labs.).
W/Acetaminophen, pyrilamine maleate.
See: Cardui, Tab. (Chattem Labs.).
Fem-1, Tab. (BDI).
Sunril, Cap. (Schering Plough).
W/Pyrilamine maleate, homatropine methylbromide, hyoscyamine sulfate, scopolamine HBr, methamphetamine HCl.
See: Aridol, Tabs. (MPL).

•**pamaqueside.** (pam-ah-KWEH-side) USAN.
Use: Antiatherosclerotic, hypocholesterolemic.

•**pamatolol sulfate.** (PAM-ah-TOE-lole) USAN.
Use: Anti-adrenergic (β-receptor).

Pamelor. (Novartis) Nortriptyline HCl. Cap or Liq. **Cap.:** 10 mg, 25 mg, 50 mg or 75 mg base. **10 mg:** Bot. 100s, SandoPak 100s; **25 mg:** Bot. 100s, 500s, SandoPak 100s; **50 mg:** Bot. 100s, SandoPak 100s. **75 mg:** Bot. 100s. **Liq.:** Nortriptyline HCl equivalent to 10 mg base/5 ml. Bot. pt. *Rx.*
Use: Antidepressant.

•**pamidronate disodium.** (pam-IH-DROE-nate) USAN.
Use: Bone resorption inhibitor.
See: Aredia, Inj. (Novartis).

Pamine. (Kenwood/Bradley) Methscopolamine bromide 2.5 mg/Tab. Bot. 100s, 500s. *Rx.*
Use: Anticholinergic, antispasmodic.

p-aminobenzene-sulfonylacetylimide.
See: Sulfacetamide.

p-aminobenzoic acid, salts.
See: p-Aminobenzoate potassium and p-Aminobenzoate sodium.

p-aminosalicylic acid salts.
See: Aminosalicylic Acid Salts.

Pamprin. (Chattem Consumer Products) Acetaminophen 400 mg, pamabrom 25 mg, pyrilamine maleate 15 mg/Tab. Bot. 24s, 48s. *otc.*
Use: Analgesic combination.

Pamprin Extra Strength Multi-Symptom Relief Formula Tablets. (Chattem Consumer Products) Acetaminophen 400 mg, pamabrom 25 mg, pyrilamine maleate 15 mg/Tab. Bot. 12s, 24s, 48s. *otc.*
Use: Analgesic combination.

Pamprin Maximum Cramp Relief Formula Caplets. (Chattem Consumer

Products) Acetaminophen 500 mg, pamabrom 25 mg, pyrilamine maleate 15 mg/Tab. Bot. 8s, 16s, 32s. *otc.*
Use: Analgesic combination.

Pamprin Multi-Symptom Caplets and Tablets. (Chattem Consumer Products) Acetaminophen 500 mg, pamabrom 25 mg, pyrilamine maleate 15 mg. Capl. Bot. 24s, 48s, Tab. Bot. 12s, 24s, 48s. *otc.*
Use: Analgesic combination.

Panacet 5/500. (ECR Pharmaceuticals) Hydrocodone bitartrate 5 mg, acetaminophen 500 mg. Tab. Bot. 100s. *c-III.*
Use: Analgesic combination, narcotic.

•**panadiplon.** (pan-ad-IH-pione) USAN.
Use: Anxiolytic.

Panadol. (Bayer Corp) Acetaminophen 500 mg/Tab. or Cap. **Tab:** Bot. 2s, 30s, 60s, 100s; **Cap:** Bot. 10s, 24s, 48s. *otc.*
Use: Analgesic.

Panadol, Children's. (Bayer Corp) Acetaminophen. **Tab.:** 80 mg. Bot. 30s. **Liq.:** 80 mg/0.8 ml. Bot. 2 oz, 4 oz. **Drops:** 80 mg/0.5 oz. Bot. 0.5 oz. *otc.*
Use: Analgesic.

Panadol, Infants' Drops. (Bayer Corp) Acetaminophen 100 mg/ml. Bot. 15 ml with 0.8 ml dropper. *otc.*
Use: Analgesic.

Panadol , Jr. (Bayer Corp) Acetaminophen 160 mg/Caplet. Box. 30s. *otc.*
Use: Analgesic.

Panadyl. (Misemer) Pyrilamine maleate 25 mg, phenylpropanolamine HCl 50 mg, pheniramine maleate 25 mg/Tab. Bot. 100s, 1000s. *Rx.*
Use: Antihistamine, decongestant.

Panadyl Forte. (Misemer) Phenylpropanolamine HCl 50 mg, phenylephrine HCl 25 mg, chlorpheniramine maleate 8 mg/Tab. Bot. 100s. *Rx.*
Use: Antihistamine, decongestant.

Panafil. (Rystan) Papain pow. 10%, urea 10%, chlorophyllin copper complex 0.5%, hydrophilic base. Oint. Tube oz, Jar lb. *Rx.*
Use: Enzyme, topical.

Panafil White Ointment. (Rystan) Papain 10,000 units enzyme activity, hydrophilic base/g, urea 10%. Tube oz. *Rx.*
Use: Enzyme, topical.

Panalgesic Cream. (ECR Pharmaceuticals) Methyl salicylate 35%, menthol 4%. Jar 4 oz. *otc.*
Use: Analgesic, topical.

Panalgesic Liquid. (ECR Pharmaceuticals) Methyl salicylate 55.01%, menthol 1.25%, camphor 3.1%, in alcohol 22%, emollients, color. Bot. 4 oz, pt, 0.5 gal. *otc.*
Use: Analgesic, topical.

Panasal 5/500. (E.C. Robins) Hydrocodone bitartrate 5 mg, aspirin 500 mg. Tab. Bot. 100s. *c-III.*
Use: Analgesic combination, narcotic.

Panasol. (Seatrace) Prednisone 5 mg/ Tab. Bot. 100s. *Rx.*
Use: Corticosteroid.

Panasol-S. (Seatrace) Prednisone 1 mg/ Tab. Bot. 100s, 1000s. *Rx.*
Use: Corticosteroid.

Pan C-500. (Freeda Vitamins) Hesperidin 100 mg, citrus bioflavonoids 100 mg, rutin 50 mg, vitamin C 500 mg/Tab. Bot. 100s, 250s, 500s. *otc.*
Use: Vitamin supplement.

Pancof-HC. (Pan Am Labs) Hydrocodone bitartrate 2.5 mg, chlorpheniramine 2 mg, pseudoephedrine 15 mg/5 ml, dye and alcohol free. Liq. Bot. 25 ml, pt. *c-III.*
Use: Antihistamine, antitussive, decongestant.

•**pancopride.** (PAN-koe-pride) USAN.
Use: Antiemetic, anxiolytic, peristaltic stimulant.

Pancrease. (Ortho McNeil) Enteric coated pancrelipase capsules. **Regular:** Lipase 4500 units, amylase 20,000 units, protease 25,000 units/Cap. Sugar. Dye free. Bot. 100s, 250s; **MT4:** Lipase 4500 units, amylase 12,000 units, protease 12,000 units/Cap. Bot. 100s; **MT10:** Lipase 10,000 units, amylase 30,000 units, protease 30,000 units/Cap. Bot. 100s; **MT16:** Lipase 16,000 units, amylase 48,000 units, protease 48,000 units/Cap. Bot. 100s; **MT20:** Lipase 20,000 units, amylase 56,000 units, protease 44,000 units/ Cap. Bot. 100s. **MT 25:** Lipase 25,000 units, amylase 70,000 units, protease 55,000 units. Cap. Bot. 100s; **MT 32:** Lipase 32,000 units, amylase 90,000 units, protease 70,000 units. Cap. Bot. 100s. *Rx.*
Use: Digestive enzyme.

pancreatic enzyme.
W/Pepsin, ox bile.
See: Nu' Leven, Nu' Leven Plus, Tab. (Teva USA).

pancreatic substance. Substance from fresh pancreas of hog or ox, containing the enzymes amylopsin, trypsin, steapsin.
W/Bile extract, dl-methionine, choline bitartrate.

See: Licoplex, Tab. (Mills).
W/Bile salts, lipase.
See: Cotazym-B, Tab. (Organon Teknika).
W/Bile, whole (desiccated), oxidized bile acids, homatropine methylbromide.
See: Pancobile, Tab. (Solvay).
W/Lipase.
See: Cotazym, Cap., Packet (Organon Teknika).

•**pancreatin.** (PAN-kree-ah-tin) U.S.P. 23. Pancreatic enzymes obtained from hog or cattle pancreatic tissue.
Use: Enzyme (digestant adjunct).
See: Depancol, Tab. (Warner Chilcott).
Elzyme, Tab. (ICN Pharmaceuticals).
Panteric, Tab. (Parke-Davis).

pancreatin w/combinations.
See: Entozyme, Tab. (Robins).
Nu'Leven, Tab. (Teva USA).
Ro-Bile, Tab. (Solvay).
Sto-Zyme, Tab. (Jalco).
Zypan, Tab. (Standard Process).

•**pancrelipase.** (pan-KREE-lih-pace) U.S.P. 23. Preparation of hog pancreas with high content of steapsin and adequate amounts of pancreatic enzymes.
Use: Enzyme (digestant adjunct).
See: Accelerase, Cap. (Organon Teknika).
Cotazym, Cap., Packet (Organon Teknika).
Viokase, Pow., Tab. (Robins).
W/Mixed conjugated bile salts, cellulase.
See: Accelerase, Cap. (Organon Teknika).
Cotazym-B, Tab. (Organon Teknika).

Pancretide. (Baxter) Pancreatic polypeptide in normal saline.
Use: Fibrinolytic conditions.

pancuronium. (PAN-cue-ROW-nee-uhm)
See: Pancuronium Bromide (Organon Teknika).

•**pancuronium bromide.** (PAN-cue-ROW-nee-uhm) USAN.
Use: Neuromuscular blocker.
See: Pavulon, Inj. (Organon Teknika).

pancuronium bromide. (Various Mfr.) **1 mg/ml:** Vials 10 ml; **2 mg/ml:** Vials, amps, syringes 2 ml or 5 ml.
Use: Neuromuscular blocker.

Pandel. (Savage) Hydrocortisone buteprate 0.1%. Cream. Tube 15 g, 45 g. *Rx.*
Use: Corticosteroid, topical.

Panex. (Roberts Pharm) Acetaminophen 325 mg/Tab. Bot. 1000s. *otc.*
Use: Analgesic.

Panex 500. (Roberts Pharm) Acetaminophen 500 mg/Tab. Bot. 1000s. *otc.*
Use: Analgesic.

Panhematin. (Abbott Laboratories) Hemin 301 mg/2 ml when reconstituted, 300 mg sorbitol. Inj. Vial 2 ml. *Rx.*
Use: Hematinic.

Panitol. (Wesley Pharmacal) Allylisobutyl barbituric acid 15 mg, acetaminophen 300 mg/Tab. Bot. 100s, 1000s. *Rx.*
Use: Analgesic, hypnotic, sedative.

Panmist JR. (Pan Am Labs) Pseudoephedrine 45 mg, guaifenesin 600 mg, dye free. LA Tab. Bot. 100s. *Rx.*
Use: Decongestant, expectorant.

Panmycin. (Pharmacia & Upjohn) Tetracycline HCl 250 mg/Cap. Bot. 100s, 1000s. *Rx.*
Use: Anti-infective, tetracycline.
See: Panmycin, Cap. (Pharmacia & Upjohn).

Pannaz. (Pan Am Labs) Phenylpropanolamine 75 mg, chlorpheniramine 6 mg, methscopolamine 2.5 mg. Tab. 100s. *Rx.*
Use: Anticholinergic, antihistamine, decongestant.

PanOxyl 5, 10 Acne Gel. (Stiefel) Benzoyl peroxide 5% or 10%, alcohol 20% in a hydroalcoholic gel base. Tube 56.7 g, 113.4 g. *Rx.*
Use: Dermatologic, acne.

PanOxyl AQ 2.5, 5, 10 Acne Gel. (Stiefel) Benzoyl peroxide 2.5%, 5% or 10%, methylparaben, EDTA in an aqueous gel base. Tube 56.7 g, 113.4 g. *Rx.*
Use: Dermatologic, acne.

PanOxyl Bar. (Stiefel) Benzoyl peroxide 5% cetostearyl alcohol, EDTA, glycerin, castor oil, mineral oil in a rich-lathering, mild surfactant cleansing base. Bar 113 g. *otc.*
Use: Dermatologic, acne.

PanOxyl-10 Bar. (Stiefel) Benzoyl peroxide 10% cetostearyl alcohol, castor oil, mineral oil, soap free in rich-lathering, mild surfactant cleansing base. Bar 113 g. *otc.*
Use: Dermatologic, acne.

panparnit hydrochloride. Caramiphen HCl.
Use: Antiparkinsonian.

Panscol. (Baker/Cummins) Salicylic acid 3%, lactic acid 2%, phenol (less than 1%). **Oint.:** Jar 3 oz. **Lot.:** Bot. 4 oz. *otc.*
Use: Emollient.

•**panthenol.** (PAN-theh-nahl) U.S.P. 23.

Alcohol corresponding to pantothenic acid. Pantothenol. Pantothenylol.
Use: Treatment of paralytic ileus and postoperative distention; vitamin.
See: Ilopan, Amp., Vial (Warren-Teed).
Panadon, Cream (Gordon Labs.).
Panthoderm Cream (Rhone-Poulenc Rorer).

panthenol w/combinations.
See: Lifer-B, Liq. (Burgin-Arden).
Nutricol, Cap., Inj. (Nutrition Control).

Panthoderm Cream. (Rhone-Poulenc Rorer) Dexpanthenol 2% in water-miscible cream. Tube 1 oz, Jar 2 oz, lb. *otc.*
Use: Emollient.

pantocaine.
See: Tetracaine HCl. (Various Mfr.).

Pantocrin-F. (Spanner) Plurigland, ovarian, anterior and posterior pituitary, adrenal, thyroid extracts. Vial 30 ml. *Rx.*
Use: Hormone.

Pantopaque. (Alcon Surgical) Iophendylate, ethyl iodophenylundecanoate. Amp. 3 ml 3s; 6 ml 6s; 1 ml 2s.
Use: Radiopaque agent.

•**pantoprazole.** (pahn-TOE-prazz-ole) USAN.
Use: Antiulcerative.

pantothenic acid. As calcium or sodium salt.
Use: Vitamin B_5 supplement.
See: Vitamin preparations.

pantothenic acid salts.
See: Calcium Pantothenate.
Sodium Pantothenate.

pantothenol.
See: Panthenol, Preps. (Various Mfr.).

pantothenyl alcohol.
See: Panthenol, Preps. (Various Mfr.).

pantothenylol.
See: Panthenol, Preps. (Various Mfr.).

Panvitex Geriatric Capsules. (Forest Pharmaceutical) Safflower oil 340 mg, vitamins A 10,000 IU, D 400 IU, B_1 5 mg, B_6 1 mg, B_2 2.5 mg, B_{12} activity 2 mcg, C 75 mg, niacinamide 40 mg, calcium pantothenate 4 mg, E 2 IU, inositol 15 mg, choline bitartrate 31.4 mg, calcium 75 mg, phosphorus 58 mg, iron 30 mg, manganese 0.5 mg, potassium 2 mg, zinc 0.5 mg, magnesium 3 mg/Cap. Bot. 100s, 1000s. *otc.*
Use: Mineral, vitamin supplement.

Panvitex Plus Minerals Capsules. (Forest Pharmaceutical) Vitamins A 5000 IU, D 400 IU, B_1 3 mg, B_2 2.5 mg, niacinamide 20 mg, B_6 1.5 mg, calcium pantothenate 5 mg, B_{12} 2.5 mcg, C 50 mg, E 3 IU, calcium 215 mg, phosphorus 166 mg, iron 13.4 mg, magnesium 7.5 mg, manganese 1.5 mg, potassium 5 mg, zinc 1.4 mg/Cap. Bot. 100s, 1000s. *otc.*
Use: Mineral, vitamin supplement.

Panvitex Prenatal Capsules. (Forest Pharmaceutical) Ferrous fumarate 150 mg, cobalamin concentration 2 mcg, vitamins A 6000 IU, D 400 IU, B_1 1.5 mg, B_2 2.5 mg, niacinamide 15 mg, B_6 3 mg, C 100 mg, calcium 250 mg, calcium pantothenate 5 mg, folic acid 0.2 mg/Cap. Bot. 100s, 1000s. *otc.*
Use: Mineral, vitamin supplement.

Panvitex T-M. (Forest Pharmaceutical) Vitamins A 10,000 IU, D 400 IU, B_1 10 mg, B_6 1 mg, B_2 5 mg, B_{12} 5 mcg, C 150 mg, niacinamide 100 mg, calcium 103 mg, phosphorus 80 mg, iron 10 mg, manganese 1 mg, potassium 5 mg, zinc 1.4 mg, magnesium 5.56 mg/Cap. Bot. 100s, 1000s. *otc.*
Use: Mineral, vitamin supplement.

PAP. (Abbott Diagnostics) Enzyme immunoassay for measurement of prostatic acid phosphatase. Test kit 100s.
Use: Diagnostic aid.

Papadeine #3. (Vangard) Codeine phosphate 30 mg, acetaminophen 300 mg/Tab. Bot. 100s, 1000s. *c-III.*
Use: Analgesic combination, narcotic.

•**papain.** (pap-ANE) U.S.P. 23. A proteolytic substance derived from *Carlica papaya.*
Use: Proteolytic enzyme.
See: Papase, Tab. (Parke-Davis).

papain w/combinations.
See: Bilate, Tab. (Schwarz Pharma).
Cerophen, Tab. (Wendt-Bristol).
Digenzyme, Tab. (Burgin-Arden).
Panafil, Oint. (Rystan).

Pap-a-Lix. (Freeport) n-Acetyl-aminophenol 120 mg, alcohol 10%/5 ml. Bot. 4 oz, gal. *otc.*
Use: Analgesic.

•**papaverine hydrochloride.** (pap-PAV-uhr-een) U.S.P. 23.
Use: Muscle relaxant.
See: BP-Papaverine, Cap. (Burlington).
Cerespan, Cap. (Rhone-Poulenc Rorer).
Cirbed, Cap. (Boyd).
Delapav, Time Cap. (Dunhall Pharmaceuticals).
Myobid, Cap. (Laser).
P-200, Cap. (Knoll Pharmaceuticals).
Pavabid, Cap. (Hoechst Marion Roussel).
Pavacap, Unicells (Solvay).

Pavacaps, Cap. (Freeport).
Pavacen Cenules, Cap. (Schwarz Pharma).
Pavaclor, Cap. (Taylor Pharmaceuticals).
Pavadel, Cap. (Canright).
Pavadyl, Cap. (Sanofi Winthrop).
Pavakey 300, Cap. (Key Pharm).
Pavakey S.A., Cap. (Key Pharm).
Pava-lyn, Cap. (Lynwood).
Pava Par, Cap. (Parmed).
Pavasule, Cap. (Jalco).
Pavatest T.D., Cap. (Fellows-Testagar).
Pavatym, Cap. (Everett Laboratories).
Pavatran T.D. Cap. (Merz).
Vasocap, Cap. (Keene Pharmaceuticals).
Vazosan, Tab. (Sandia).

W/Codeine sulfate.
See: Copavin, Pulvule, Tab. (Eli Lilly).

W/Codeine sulfate, aloin, sodium salicylate.
See: Copavin Compound, Elix. (Eli Lilly).

W/Codeine sulfate, emetine HCl, ephedrine HCl.
See: Golacol, Syr. (Arcum).

W/Phenobarbital.
See: Pavadel-PB, Cap. (Canright).

Paplex Ultra. (Medicis Dermatologics) Salicylic acid 26% in flexible collodion. Bot. 15 ml. *otc.*
Use: Keratolytic.

para-aminobenzoic acid. (Various Mfr.). **Tab.:** 100 mg or 500 mg. Bot. 100s, 250s (100 mg only); **Pow.:** 120 g. *otc.*
Use: Sunscreen, agent for scleroderma.
See: Potaba, Tab., Cap., Powd., envules. (Glenwood).

para-aminosalicylic acid. Aminosalicylic Acid, U.S.P. 23. *Rx.*
Use: Antituberculosis.

Parabaxin. (Parmed) Methocarbamol 500 mg or 750 mg/Tab. Bot. 100s. *Rx.*
Use: Muscle relaxant.

parabrom.
See: Pyrabrom.

parabromidylamine.
See: Brompheniramine, Dimetane, Preps. (Robins).

paracain.
See: Procaine Hydrochloride (Various Mfr.).

paracarbinoxamine maleate. Carbinoxamine.

Paracet Forte Tabs. (Major) Chlorzoxazone, acetaminophen. Bot. 100s, 1000s. *Rx.*
Use: Muscle relaxant.

paracetaldehyde.
See: Paraldehyde, U.S.P. 23.

parachloramine hydrochloride. Meclizine HCl, U.S.P. 23.
See: Bonine, Tab. (Pfizer).

parachlorometaxylenol.
Use: Phenolic antiseptic.
See: D-Seb, Liq. (Rydelle).
Nu-Flow, Liq. (Rydelle).

W/9-aminoacridine HCl, methyl-dodecylbenzyl-trimethyl ammonium Cl, pramoxine HCl, hydrocortisone, acetic acid.
See: Drotic No. 2, Drops (B.F. Ascher).

W/Benzocaine.
See: TPO 20 (DePree).

W/Coconut oil, pine oil, castor oil, lanolin, cholesterols, lecithin.
See: Sebacide, Liq. (Paddock).

W/Hydrocortisone, pramoxine HCl, benzalkonium Cl, acetic acid.
See: Oto Drops (Solvay).

W/Lidocaine, phenol, zinc oxide.
See: Unguentine Plus, Cream (Procter & Gamble Pharm).

W/Pramoxine HCl, hydrocortisone, benzalkonium Cl, acetic acid.
See: My Cort Otic #2, Drops (Scrip).
Steramine Otic, Drops (Merz).

W/Resorcinol, sulfur.
See: Rezamid, Lot. (Dermik Laboratories).

•**parachlorophenol.** (par-ah-KLOR-oh-feh-nole) U.S.P. 23.
Use: Anti-infective, topical.

•**parachlorophenol, camphorated.** U.S.P. 23.
Use: Anti-infective, topical.

paracodin.
See: Dihydrocodeine.

Paraeusal Liquid. (Paraeusal) Liq. Bot. 2 oz, 6 oz, 12 oz.
Use: Minor skin irritations.

Paraeusal Solid. (Paraeusal) Oint. Jar 1 oz, 2 oz, 16 oz.
Use: Dermatologic, counterirritant.

•**paraffin.** (PAR-ah-fin) N.F. 18.
Use: Pharmaceutic aid (stiffening agent).

•**paraffin, synthetic.** N.F. 18.
Use: Pharmaceutic aid (stiffening agent).

Paraflex. (Ortho McNeil) Chlorzoxazone 250 mg/Tab. Bot. 100s. *Rx.*
Use: Muscle relaxant.

Parafon Forte DSC. (Ortho McNeil) Chlorzoxazone 500 mg/Capl. Bot. 100s, 500s, UD 100s. *Rx.*
Use: Muscle relaxant.

paraform. Paraformaldehyde. (No Mfr. listed).

paraformaldehyde.
Use: Essentially the same as formaldehyde.
See: Formaldehyde (Various Mfr.).
Trioxymethylene (an incorrect term for paraformaldehyde).

paraglycylarsanilic acid. N-Carbamylmethyl-p-aminobenzenearsonic acid, the free acid of tryparsamide.

Parahist HD Liquid. (Pharmics) Phenylephrine HCl 5 mg, chlorpheniramine maleate 2 mg, hydrocodone bitartrate 1.67 mg, alcohol free. Bot. 473 ml. *c-III.*
Use: Antihistamine, antitussive, decongestant.

Para-Jel. (Health for Life Brands) Benzocaine 5%, cetyl dimethyl benzyl ammonium Cl. Tube 0.25 oz. *otc.*
Use: Anesthetic, local.

•**paraldehyde.** (par-AL-deh-hide) U.S.P. 23.
Use: Hypnotic, sedative.
See: Paral, Cap., Liq., Amp. (Forest Pharmaceutical).

Paral Oral. (Forest Pharmaceutical) Paraldehyde 30 ml. Bot. 12s, 25s. *c-IV.*
Use: Hypnotic, sedative.

paramephrin.
See: Epinephrine (Various Mfr.).

•**paramethasone acetate.** (PAR-ah-meth-ah-zone) U.S.P. 23.
Use: Corticosteriod, topical.
See: Haldrone, Tab. (Eli Lilly).

para-monochlorophenol.
See: Camphorated para-chlorophenol, Liq. (Novocol Chemical).

•**paranyline hydrochloride.** (PAR-ah-NYE-leen) USAN.
Use: Anti-inflammatory.

•**parapenzolate bromide.** (pa-rah-PEN-zoe-late BROE-mide) USAN.
Use: Anticholinergic.

Paraplatin. (Bristol-Myers Oncology) Carboplatin 50 mg, 150 mg or 450 mg. Inj. Vial. *Rx.*
Use: Antineoplastic.

pararosaniline embonate. Pararosaniline pamoate.

•**pararosaniline pamoate.** (par-ah-row-ZAN-ih-lin PAM-oh-ate) USAN.
Use: Antischistosomal.

parasympatholytic agents. Cholinergic blocking agents.
See: Anticholinergic Agents.
Antispasmodics.
Mydriatics.
Parkinsonism.

parasympathomimetic agents.
See: Cholinergic Agents.

Paratrol Liquid. (Walgreens) Pyrethrins 0.2%, piperonyl butoxide technical 2%, deodorized kerosene 0.8%. Bot. 2 oz. *otc.*
Use: Pediculicide.

Parazone. (Henry Schein) Chlorzoxazone 250 mg, acetaminophen 300 mg/Tab. Bot. 100s, 1000s. *Rx.*
Use: Muscle relaxant, analgesic.

•**parbendazole.** (par-BEN-dah-ZOLE) USAN. Under study.
Use: Anthelmintic.

parbutoxate.

Parcillin. (Parmed) Crystalline potassium penicillin G 240 mg, 400,000 units/Tab. Bot. 100s, 1000s. Pow. for syr. 400,000 units/Tsp. 80 ml. *Rx.*
Use: Anti-infective, penicillin.

•**parconazole hydrochloride.** (par-KOE-nah-zole) USAN.
Use: Antifungal.

Par Decon. (Par Pharm) Phenylpropanolamine HCl 40 mg, phenylephrine HCl 10 mg, chlorpheniramine maleate 5 mg, phenyltoloxamine citrate 15 mg/Tab. Bot. 100s, 500s, 1000s. *Rx.*
Use: Antihistamine, decongestant.

Paredrine. (Pharmics) Hydroxyamphetamine HBr 1%. Bot. 15 ml. *Rx.*
Use: Mydriatic.

•**paregoric.** (par-eh-GORE-ik) U.S.P. 23.
Use: Antiperistaltic.

paregoric. (Various Mfr.) Morphine equivalent 2 mg/5 ml, 45% alcohol. Liq. Bot. 60 ml, pt, gal, UD 5 ml (40s, 50s, 100s). *c-III.*
Use: Antiperistaltic.

Paremyd. (Allergan) Hydroxyamphetamine HBr 1%, tropicamide 0.25%. Soln. Bot. 5 ml, 15 ml. *Rx.*
Use: Cycloplegic, mydriatic.

parenabol. Boldenone undecylenate.

•**pareptide sulfate.** (PAR-epp-tide) USAN.
Use: Antiparkinsonian.

Par Estro. (Parmed) Conjugated estrogens 1.25 mg/Tab. Bot. 100s. *Rx.*
Use: Estrogen.

parethoxycaine hydrochloride.
W/Zirconium oxide, calamine.
See: Zotox, Spray, Cream (Del Pharmaceuticals).

Par-F. (Pharmics) Iron 60 mg, calcium 250 mg, vitamins C 120 mg, A 5000 IU, D 400 IU, B_1 3 mg, B_2 3.4 mg, B_{12} 12 mcg, B_6 12 mg, B_3 20 mg, Cu, I, Mg, Zn 15 mg, E 30 IU, folic acid 1 mg/Tab. Bot. 100s. *Rx.*
Use: Mineral, vitamin supplement.

Par Glycerol. (Par Pharm) Iodinated glycerol 60 mg/5 ml. Alcohol 21.75%, peppermint oil, corn syrup, saccharin. Caramel-mint flavor. Elixir. Bot. Pt. *Rx.*
Use: Expectorant.

•**pargyline hydrochloride.** (PAR-jih-leen) USAN. U.S.P. XXII
Use: Antihypertensive.

Parhist SR. (Parmed) Phenylpropanolamine HCl 75 mg, chlorpheniramine maleate 12 mg/Cap. Bot. 100s, 1000s. *Rx.*
Use: Antihistamine, decongestant.

paricalcitol.
Use: Vitamin supplement.
See: Zemplar, Inj. (Abbott).

Parkelp. (Phillip R. Park) Pacific sea kelp. **Tab.:** Bot. 100s, 200s, 500s, 800s. **Gran.:** Bot. 2 oz, 7 oz, 1 lb, 3 lb. *otc.*
Use: Nutritional supplement.

parkinsonism, agents for. Parasympatholytic agents.
See: Akineton, Tab., Inj. (Knoll Pharmaceuticals).
Artane, Elix., Tab., Sequels (ESI Lederle Generics).
Benztropine Mesylate, Tab. (Various Mfr.).
Caramiphen HCl.
Cogentin, Tab., Amp. (Merck).
Dopar, Cap. (Procter & Gamble Pharm).
Eldepryl, Tab. (Somerset).
Kemadrin, Tab. (GlaxoWellcome).
Larodopa, Tab. (Roche Laboratories).
Lodosyn, Tab. (Merck).
Parlodel, Tab., Cap. (Novartis).
Permax, Tab. (Eli Lilly).
Sinemet, Tab. (DuPont Pharma).
Symmetrel, Cap., Syr. (DuPont Merck Pharmaceuticals).
Trihexyphenidyl HCl (Various Mfr.).
Trihexy-2 (Geneva Pharm).

Parlodel. (Novartis) Bromocriptine mesylate. Lactose. **Tab.:** 2.5 mg. Bot. 30s, 100s. **Cap.:** 5 mg. Bot. 30s, 100s. *Rx.*
Use: Antiparkinsonian.

Parmeth. (Parmed) Promethazine HCl 50 mg/Cap. Bot. 100s, 1000s. *Rx.*
Use: Antiemetic, antihistamine, antivertigo.

parminyl. W/Salicylamide, phenacetin, caffeine, acetaminophen.
See: Dolopar, Tab. (O'Neal).

Par-Natal-FA. (Parmed) Vitamins A 4000 IU, D 400 IU, thiamine HCl 2 mg, riboflavin 2 mg, pyridoxine HCl 0.8 mg, ascorbic acid 50 mg, niacinamide 10 mg, iodine 0.15 mg, folic acid 0.1 mg, cobalamin concentrate 2 mcg, iron 50 mg, calcium 240 mg/Cap. Bot. 100s, 1000s. *otc.*
Use: Mineral, vitamin supplement.

Par-Natal Plus 1 Improved. (Parmed) Elemental calcium 200 mg, elemental iron 65 mg, vitamins A 4000 IU, D 400 IU, E 11 mg, B_1 1.5 mg, B_2 3 mg, B_3 20 mg, B_6 10 mg, B_{12} 12 mcg, C 120 mg, folic acid 1 mg, zinc 25 mg, Cu/Tab. Bot. 500s. *Rx.*
Use: Mineral, vitamin supplement.

Parnate. (SmithKline Beecham Pharmaceuticals) Tranylcypromine sulfate 10 mg/Tab. Bot. 100s. *Rx.*
Use: Antidepressant.

parodyne.
See: Antipyrine (Various Mfr.).

paroleine.
See: Petrolatum Liquid (Various Mfr.).

•**paromomycin sulfate.** (par-oh-moe-MY-sin) U.S.P. 23. An antibiotic substance obtained from cultures of certain *Streptomyces* species, one of which is *Streptomyces rimosus.*
Use: Antiamebic.

parothyl. (Henry Schein) Meprobamate 400 mg, tridihexethyl Cl 25 mg/Tab. Bot. 100s. *c-IV.*
Use: Anticholinergic, anxiolytic, antispasmodic.

•**paroxetine.** (puh-ROX-eh-teen) USAN.
Use: Antidepressant.

paroxetine hydrochloride.
Use: Antidepressant.
See: Paxil, Tab. (SmithKline Beecham Pharmaceuticals).

paroxyl.
See: Acetarsone (Various Mfr.).

parpanit.
See: Caramiphen HCl (Various Mfr).

parsley concentrate. *Rx.*
W/Garlic concentrate.
See: Allimin, Tab. (Mosso).

Par-Supp. (Parmed) Estrone 0.2 mg, lactose 50 mg/Vaginal Supp. Pkg. 12s.
Use: Estrogen.

Partapp TD. (Parmed) Phenylpropanolamine HCl 15 mg, phenylephrine HCl 15 mg, brompheniramine maleate 12 mg/TD Tab. Bot. 1000s.

Parten. (Parmed) Acetaminophen 10 gr/Tab. Bot. 100s, 1000s. *otc.*
Use: Analgesic.

•**partricin.** (PAR-trih-sin) USAN. Antibiotic produced by *Streptomyces aureofaciens.*
Use: Antifungal, antiprotozoal.

Partuss. (Parmed) Dextromethorphan hydrobromide 60 mg, potassium

guaiacolsulfonate 8 gr, chlorpheniramine maleate 6 mg, ammonium Cl 8 gr, tartar emetic 1/12 gr, chloroform 2 min/30 ml. Bot. 4 oz, pt, gal. *Rx.*
Use: Antihistamine, antitussive, expectorant.

Partuss A.C. (Parmed) Guaifenesin 100 mg, pheniramine maleate 7.5 mg, codeine phosphate 10 mg, alcohol 3.5%/5 ml. Bot 4 oz. *c-v.*
Use: Antihistamine, antitussive, expectorant.

Partuss LA. (Parmed) Phenylpropanolamine HCl 75 mg, guaifenesin 400 mg/LA Tab. Bot. 100s, 500s. *Rx.*
Use: Decongestant, expectorant.

Parvlex. (Freeda Vitamins) Iron 100 mg, vitamins B_1 20 mg, B_2 20 mg, B_3 20 mg, B_5 1 mg, B_6 10 mg, B_{12} 50 mcg, C 50 mg, folic acid 0.1 mg, Cu, Mn/Tab. Bot. 100s, 250s. *otc.*
Use: Mineral, vitamin supplement.

Pas-C. (Hellwig) Pascorbic. p-aminosalicylic acid 0.5 g with vitamin C/Tab. Bot. 1000s. *Rx.*
Use: Antituberculous.

Paser. (Jacobus) Aminosalicylic acid 4 g/packet. Gran. Pkt. 30s. *Rx.*
Use: Adjunctive tuberculosis agent.

passiflora. Dried flowering and fruiting tops of Passiflora incarnata.
W/Phenobarbital, valerian, hyoscyamus.
See: Aluro, Tab. (Foy).

Patanol. (Alcon Laboratories) Olopatadine HCl 0.1%/Soln. Drop-Tainer. 5 ml. *Rx.*
Use: Antihistamine, ophthalmic.

Path. (Parker) Buffered neutral formalin soln. 10%. Bot. 1 gal, 5 gal. Jar 4 oz.
Use: Tissue specimen fixative.

Pathilon. (ESI Lederle Generics) Tridihexethyl chloride 25 mg/Tab. Bot. 100s. *Rx.*
Use: Anticholinergic, antispasmodic.

Pathocil. (Wyeth Ayerst) Sodium dicloxacillin monohydrate. **250 mg/Cap.:** Bot. 100s. **500 mg/Cap.:** Bot. 50s. **Pow. for oral susp.:** 62.5 mg/5 ml. Bot. to make 100 ml. *Rx.*
Use: Anti-infective, penicillin.

•**paulomycin.** (PAW-low-MY-sin) USAN.
Use: Anti-infective.

Pavabid Plateau. (Hoechst Marion Roussel) Papaverine HCl 150 mg/TR Cap. Bot. 100s, 250s, 1000s, UD 100s. *Rx.*
Use: Vasodilator.

Pavacaps. (Freeport) Papaverine HCl 150 mg/TR Cap. Bot. 1000s. *Rx.*
Use: Vasodilator.

Pavacen Cenules. (Schwarz Pharma) Papaverine HCl 150 mg/TR Cap. Bot. 100s. *Rx.*
Use: Vasodilator.

Pavadel. (Canright) Papaverine HCl 150 mg/Cap. Bot. 100s, 1000s. *Rx.*
Use: Vasodilator.

Pavadel PB. (Canright) Papaverine HCl 150 mg, phenobarbital 45 mg/Cap. Bot. 100s. *Rx.*
Use: Vasodilator.

Pavadyl Capsules. (Sanofi Winthrop) Papaverine HCl 150 mg/Cap. Bot. 100s. *Rx.*
Use: Vasodilator.

Pavagen. (Rugby) Papaverine 150 mg/TR Cap. Bot. 500s, 1000s, UD 100s. *Rx.*
Use: Vasodilator.

Pava-Lyn. (Lynwood) Papaverine HCl 150 mg/Cap. Bot. 100s. *Rx.*
Use: Vasodilator.

Pavatine Tabs. (Major) Papaverine 300 mg/Tab. Bot. 100s. *Rx.*
Use: Vasodilator.

Pavatine T.D. Caps. (Major) Papaverine 150 mg/TD Cap. Bot. 100s, 1000s. *Rx.*
Use: Vasodilator.

Pavulon. (Organon Teknika) Pancuronium bromide. **1 mg/ml:** Vial 10 ml, Box 25s. **2 mg/ml:** Amp. 2 ml, 5 ml, Box 25s. *Rx.*
Use: Muscle relaxant, adjunct to anesthesia.

Paxarel. (Circle) Acetylcarbromal 250 mg/Tab. Bot. 100s. *Rx.*
Use: Hypnotic, sedative.

Paxil. (SmithKline Beecham Pharmaceuticals) Paroxetine 20 mg or 30 mg. Tab. **20 mg:** Bot. 30s, 100s, UD 100s; **30 mg:** Bot. 30s. *Rx.*
Use: Antidepressant.

•**pazinaclone.** (pah-ZIN-ah-klone) USAN.
Use: Anxiolytic.

Pazo Hemorrhoid Ointment. (Bristol-Myers) Zinc oxide 5%, ephedrine sulfate 0.2%, camphor 2% in lanolin-petrolatum base. Tube 28 g. *otc.*
Use: Anorectal preparation.

•**pazoxide.** (pay-ZOX-ide) USAN.
Use: Antihypertensive.

PB 100. (Schlicksup) Phenobarbital 1.5 gr/Tab. Bot. 1000s. *c-IV.*
Use: Hypnotic, sedative.

PBZ. (Novartis) Tripelennamine HCl 25 mg, 50 mg Tab. Bot. 100s. *Rx.*
Use: Antihistamine.

PBZ-SR. (Novartis) Tripelennamine HCl 100 mg/SR Tab. Bot. 100s. *Rx.*

Use: Antihistamine.

PCE Dispertab Tablets. (Abbott Laboratories) Erythromycin particles 333 mg/Tab. Bot. 60s, 500s. *Rx.*
Use: Anti-infective, erythromycin.

p-chlorometaxylenol.
W/Benzocaine, benzyl alcohol, propylene glycol.
See: 20-Caine Burn Relief (Alto Pharmaceuticals).
W/Hydrocortisone, pramoxine HCl.
See: Orlex HC, Otic (Baylor).

p-chlorophenol.
See: Parachlorophenol.

PCMX.
See: Parachlorometaxylenol.

PDP Liquid Protein. (Wesley Pharmacal) Protein 15 g (from protein hydrolysates), cal 60/30 ml. Bot. pt, qt, gal. *otc.*
Use: Protein supplement.

Peacock's Bromides. (Natcon) **Liq.:** Potassium bromide 6 gr, sodium bromide 6 gr, ammonium bromide 3 gr/5 ml. Bot. 8 oz. **Tab.:** Potassium bromide 3 gr, sodium bromide 3 gr, ammonium bromide 1.5 gr. Bot. 100s. *Rx.*
Use: Hypnotic, sedative.

•**peanut oil.** N.F. 18.
Use: Pharmaceutic aid (solvent).

Pectamol. (British Drug House) Diethylaminoethoxyethyl-a,a-diethylphenylacetate citrate. Bot. 4 fl oz, 16 fl oz, 80 fl oz, 160 fl oz.
Use: Antitussive.

•**pectin.** (PECK-tin) U.S.P. 23.
Use: Protectant, pharmaceutic aid (suspending agent).

pectin w/combinations.
See: Donnagel Susp. (Robins).
Donnagel-PG, Susp. (Robins).
Furoxone, Liq., Tab. (Eaton Medical).
Infantol Pink, Liq. (Scherer).
Kaopectate, Liq. (Pharmacia & Upjohn).
Kapigam, Liq. (Solvay).
KBP/O, Cap. (Cole).
Parepectolin, Susp. (Rhone-Poulenc Rorer).
Pectokay, Liq. (Jones Medical Industries).

Pedameth. (Forest Pharmaceutical) Racemethionine. **Cap.:** 200 mg. Bot. 50s, 500s. **Liq.:** 75 mg/5 ml. Bot. pt. *Rx.*
Use: Diaper rash preparation.

Pedenex. (Health for Life Brands) Caprylic acid, zinc undecylenate, sodium propionate. Tube 1.5 oz. Foot pow. spray 5 oz. *otc.*
Use: Antifungal, topical.

Pedia Care Allergy Formula. (McNeil Consumer Products) Chlorpheniramine maleate 1 mg/5 ml, sorbitol, sucrose. Alcohol free. Grape flavor. Syr. Bot. 120 ml. *otc.*
Use: Antihistamine.

Pedia Care Cold Allergy Chewable Tablets. (McNeil Consumer Products) Pseudoephedrine HCl 15 mg, chlorpheniramine maleate 1 mg, aspartame, phenylalanine 8 mg/Tab. Pkg. 18s. *otc.*
Use: Antihistamine, decongestant.

Pedia Care Cough-Cold. (McNeil Consumer Products) **Chew. Tab.:** Pseudoephedrine HCl 15 mg, chlorpheniramine maleate 1 mg, dextromethorphan HBr 5 mg, aspartame (phenylalanine 6 mg), dextrose, sucrose. Fruit flavor. Pkg. 16s. **Liq.:** Pseudoephedrine HCl 15 mg, chlorpheniramine maleate 1 mg, dextromethorphan HBr 5 mg/5 ml, sorbitol, sucrose. Alcohol free. Cherry flavor. Syr. Bot. 120 ml. *otc.*
Use: Antihistamine, antitussive, decongestant.

Pedia Care Infants' Decongestant. (McNeil Consumer Products) Pseudoephedrine HCl 7.5 mg/0.8 ml. Cherry flavor. Syr. Bot. 15 ml. *otc.*
Use: Decongestant.

Pedia Care NightRest Liquid. (McNeil Consumer Products) Pseudoephedrine HCl 15 mg, chlorpheniramine maleate 1 mg, dextromethorphan HBr 7.5 mg/5 ml, sorbitol, sucrose. Alcohol free. Cherry flavor. Syr. Bot. 120 ml. *otc.*
Use: Antihistamine, antitussive, decongestant.

Pediacof Syrup. (Sanofi Winthrop) Codeine phosphate 5 mg, phenylephrine HCl 2.5 mg, chlorpheniramine maleate 0.75 mg, potassium iodide 75 mg/5 ml, sodium benzoate 0.2%, alcohol 5%. Syr. Bot. 16 fl oz. *c-v.*
Use: Antihistamine, antitussive, decongestant, expectorant.

Pediacon DX Children's. (Zenith Goldline) Phenylpropanolamine HCl 6.25 mg, guaifenesin 100 mg, dextromethorphan HBr 5 mg, alcohol 5%/5 ml. Syrup. Bot. 118 ml. *otc.*
Use: Antitussive, decongestant, expectorant.

Pediacon DX Pediatric. (Zenith Goldline) Phenylpropanolamine HCl 6.25 mg, guaifenesin 50 mg, dextromethorphan HBr 5 mg/ml. 5% alcohol. Sugar free. Drops. Bot. 30 ml. *otc.*
Use: Antitussive, decongestant, expectorant.

Pediacon EX. (Zenith Goldline) Phenylpropanolamine 6.25 mg, guiafenesin 50 mg/ml. Sugar free. Drops. Bot. 30 ml. *otc.*
Use: Decongestant, expectorant.

Pediaflor Fluoride Drops. (Ross Laboratories) Fluoride 0.5 mg/ml as sodium fluoride 1.1 mg/ml. Bot. 50 ml. *Rx.*
Use: Dental caries agent.

Pedialyte. (Ross Laboratories) Sodium 45 mEq, potassium 20 mEq, chloride 35 mEq, citrate 30 mEq, dextrose 25 g/L. 100 calories/L. **Plastic Bot.:** 8 fl oz. (unflavored), 32 fl oz. (unflavored, fruit). **Nursing Bot.:** Hospital use. Bot. 8 fl oz. *otc.*
Use: Electrolytes, mineral supplement.

Pedialyte Freezer Pops. (Ross Laboratories) Na 45 mEq/L, K 20 mEq/L, Cl 35 mEq/L, citrate 30 mEq/L, dextrose 25 g/L, phenylalanine, aspartame/Liq. 2.1 fl oz. Box. 16s. *otc.*
Use: Electrolytes, mineral supplement.

Pediamycin Drops. (Ross Laboratories) Erythromycin ethylsuccinate for oral suspension 100 mg/2.5 ml. Bot. 50 ml (Dropper enclosed). *Rx.*
Use: Anti-infective, erythromycin.

Pediapred Oral Liquid. (Medeva) Prednisolone sodium phosphate 6.7 mg/5 ml. Bot. 4 oz. *Rx.*
Use: Corticosteroid.

PediaSure. (Ross Laboratories) Protein 30 g (Na caseinate, whey protein concentrate), carbohydrate 109.8 g (hydrolyzed cornstarch, sucrose), fat 49.8 g (hi-oleic safflower oil, soy oil, MCT [fractionated coconut oil], mono- and diglycerides, soy lecithin), sodium 380 mg, potassium 1308 mg/L, vitamins A, B_1, B_2, B_3, B_5, B_6, B_{12}, C, D, E, K, inositol, Cl, Ca, P, Mg, I, Mn, Cu, Zn, Fe, biotin, choline, folic acid. < 310 mosm/kg H_2O, 1 cal/ml. Gluten free. Vanilla flavor. Ready-to-use can 240 ml. *otc.*
Use: Nutritional supplement.

Pediatric Advil Drops. (Whitehall-Robins) Ibuprofen 100 mg/2.5 ml, EDTA, glycerin, sorbitol, sucrose. Oral Susp. Bot. 15 ml. *otc.*
Use: Anti-inflammatory.

Pediatric Cough Syrup. (Weeks & Leo) Ammonium Cl 300 mg, sodium citrate 600 mg/oz. Bot. 4 oz. *otc.*
Use: Expectorant.

Pediatric Electrolyte. (Zenith Goldline) Dextrose 25 g, K 20 mEq, Cl 35 mEq, Na 45 mEq, citrate 48 mEq, calories 100/L. Soln. Bot. 1 L. *otc.*
Use: Nutritional supplement, enteral.

Pediatric Maintenance Solution. (Abbott Laboratories) I.V. solution w/dose calculated according to age, weight, clinical condition. Bot. 250 ml. *Rx.*
Use: Fluid, electrolyte, nutrient replacement.

Pediatric Multiple Trace Element. (American Regent) Zinc (as sulfate) 0.5 mg, copper (as sulfate) 0.1 mg, manganese (as sulfate) 0.03 mg, chromium (as chloride) 1 mcg/ml. Soln. Vial 10 ml. *Rx.*
Use: Nutritional supplement, parenteral.

Pediatric Triban. (Great Southern) Trimethobenzamide HCl 100 mg, benzocaine 2%/Supp. Pkg. 10s. *Rx.*
Use: Antiemetic, antivertigo.

Pediatric Vicks 44d Dry Hacking Cough and Head Congestion. (Procter & Gamble) Dextromethorphan HBr 15 mg/15 ml (1 mg/ml), sorbitol, sucrose, cherry flavor, alcohol free. Syr. Bot. 120 ml. *otc.*
Use: Antitussive.

Pediazole Suspension. (Ross Laboratories) Erythromycin ethylsuccinate 200 mg, sulfisoxazole acetyl 600 mg/5 ml. Bot. Granules reconstituted to 100 ml, 150 ml, 200 ml. *Rx.*
Use: Anti-infective, erythromycin.

Pedi-Boot Mist Kit. (Pedinol) Cetyl pyridinium Cl, triacetin, chloroxylenol. Bot. 2 oz. *otc.*
Use: Antifungal, antiseptic, deodorant.

Pedi-Boro Soak Paks. (Pedinol) Astringent wet dressing w/aluminum sulfate, calcium acetate, coloring agent. Box 12s, 100s. *otc.*
Use: Dermatologic, counterirritant.

Pedi-Cort V Creme. (Pedinol) Clioquinol 3%, hydrocortisone 1%. Tube 20 g. *Rx.*
Use: Antifungal, corticosteroid, topical.

Pedicran with Iron. (Scherer) Vitamin B_{12} (crystallized) 25 mcg, ferric pyrophosphate, soluble (elemental iron 30 mg) 250 mg, thiamine mononitrate 10 mg, nicotinamide 10 mg, alcohol 1%/5 ml. Bot. 4 oz, pt. *otc.*
Use: Mineral, vitamin supplement.

pediculicides/scabicides.
See: A-200, Shampoo (SmithKline Beecham Pharmaceuticals).
A-200 Pyrinate, Gel (SmithKline Beecham Pharmaceuticals).
Barc, Liq. (Del Pharmaceuticals).
Blue, Gel (Various Mfr.).
Elimite, Cream (Allergan).
Eurax, Preps. (Westwood Squibb).
G-well, Preps. (Zenith Goldline).

Kwell, Preps. (Schwarz Pharma).
Licetrol 400, Liq. (Republic).
Lindane, Preps. (Various Mfr.).
Nix, Liq. (GlaxoWellcome).
Ovide, Lot. (GenDerm).
Pronto Concentrate, Shampoo (Del Pharmaceuticals).
Pyrinyl, Liq. (Various Mfr.).
R & C, Shampoo (Schwarz Pharma).
RID, Liq. (Pfizer).
Scabene, preps. (Stiefel).
Step 2, Liq. (GenDerm).
Tisit, Preps. (Pfeiffer).
Tisit Blue, Gel (Pfeiffer).
Triple X Kit, Liq. (Carter Products).

Pedi-Dri. (Pedinol) Nystatin 100,000 u/g, corn starch, aluminum chlorhydroxide, menthol. Bot. 56.7 g. *Rx.*
Use: Antifungal, antiperspirant, deodorant, foot powder.

Pediotic. (GlaxoWellcome) Hydrocortisone 1%, neomycin 3.5 mg (as sulfate), polymyxin B sulfate 10,000 units/ml. Susp. Bot 7.5 ml with dropper. *Rx.*
Use: Otic.

Pedi-Pro Foot Powder. (Pedinol) Aluminum chlorhydroxide, menthol, zinc undecylenate, chloroxylenol. Bot. 2 oz. *otc.*
Use: Antifungal, antiperspirant, deodorant.

Pedituss Cough. (Major) Phenylephrine HCl 2.5 mg, chlorpheniramine maleate 0.75 mg, codeine phosphate 5 mg, potassium iodide 75 mg/5 ml, alcohol 5%, saccharin, sorbitol, sucrose. Syr. Bot. pt., gal. *c-v.*
Use: Antihistamine, antitussive, decongestant, expectorant.

Pedolatum. (King Pharm) Salicylic acid, sodium salicylate. Oint. Pkg. 0.5 oz. *otc.*
Use: Analgesic, topical.

Pedric Senior. (Pal-Pak) Acetaminophen 320 mg. *otc.*
Use: Analgesic.

PedTE-PAK-4. (SoloPak) Zinc 1 mg, copper 0.1 mg, manganese 0.025 mg, chromium 1 mcg. Vial 3 ml. *Rx.*
Use: Nutritional supplement, parenteral.

Pedtrace-4. (Fujisawa) Zinc 0.5 mg, copper 0.1 mg, chromium 0.85 mcg, manganese 0.25 mg/ml. Vial 3 ml, 10 ml. *Rx.*
Use: Nutritional supplement, parenteral.

PedvaxHIB. (Merck) Purified capsular polysaccharide of *Haemophilus influenzae* type b, *Neisseria meningitidis* OMPC 250 mcg/dose when reconstituted, sodium chloride 0.9%, lactose 2 mg, thimerosal 1:20,000. Pow. for Inj. or Soln. Single-dose vial with vial of aluminum hydroxide diluent or single-dose vial. *Rx.*
Use: Immunization.

•**pefloxacin.** (PEH-FLOX-ah-sin) USAN.
Use: Anti-infective.

•**pefloxacin mesylate.** (PEH-FLOX-ah-sin) USAN.
Use: Anti-infective.

•**pegademase bovine.** (peg-AD-ah-MASE BOE-vine) USAN.
Use: Replacement therapy (adenosine deaminase deficiency); modified enzyme for use in ADA deficiency. [Orphan drug]
See: Adagen (Enzon).

Peganone. (Abbott Laboratories) Ethotoin 250 mg/Tab. or 500 mg/Cap. Bot. 100s. *Rx.*
Use: Anticonvulsant.

•**pegaspargase.** (peh-ASS-par-jase) USAN.
Use: Antineoplastic. [Orphan drug]
See: Oncaspar, Inj. (Enzon).

•**peglicol 5 oleate.** (PEG-lih-kahl 5 OH-lee-ate) USAN.
Use: Pharmaceutic aid (emulsifying agent).

PEG-glucocerebrosidase. (Enzon)
Use: Treatment of Gaucher's disease. [Orphan drug]

PEG-interleukin-2. (Cetus)
Use: Immunomodulator. [Orphan drug]

PEG-L-asparaginase. (Enzon) *Rx.*
Use: Antineoplastic.

PEG Ointment. (Medco Lab) Polyethylene glycol. Jar 16 oz. *otc.*
Use: Pharmaceutical aid, ointment base.

•**pegorgotein.** (peg-AHR-gah-teen) USAN.
Use: Free oxygen radical scavenger.

•**pegoterate.** (PEG-oh-TEER-ate) USAN.
Use: Pharmaceutic aid (suspending agent).

•**pegoxol 7 stearate.** (peg-OX-ole 7 STEE-ah-rate) USAN.
Use: Pharmaceutic aid (emulsifying agent).

•**pelanserin hydrochloride.** (peh-LAN-ser-in) USAN.
Use: Antihypertensive; vasodilator (serotonin S_2 and α_1 adrenergic receptor blocker).

•**peldesine.** (PELL-deh-seen) USAN.
Use: Antineoplastic, antipsoratic.

pelentan. Ethyl Biscoumacetate. (No Mfr. currently lists).

•**peliomycin.** (PEE-lee-oh-MY-sin) USAN. An antibiotic derived from *Streptomycin luteogriseus.*
Use: Antineoplastic.

•**pelretin.** (PELL-REH-tin) USAN.
Use: Antikeratinizer.

•**pelrinone hydrochloride.** (PELL-rih-nohn) USAN.
Use: Cardiovascular agent.

•**pemedolac.** (peh-MEH-doe-LACK) USAN.
Use: Analgesic.

•**pemerid nitrate.** (PEM-eh-rid) USAN.
Use: Antitussive.

•**pemirolast potassium.** (peh-mihr-OH-last) USAN.
Use: Antiallergic; inhibitor (mediator release).

•**pemoline.** (PEM-oh-leen) USAN.
Use: Stimulant (central); childhood attention-deficit syndrome (hyperkinetic syndrome).
See: Cylert Prods. (Abbott Laboratories).

Penagen-VK. (Grafton) Penicillin V. **Tab.:** 250 mg. Bot. 100s. **Pow.:** 250 mg/100 ml. *Rx.*
Use: Anti-infective, penicillin.

•**penamecillin.** (PEN-ah-meh-SILL-in) USAN.
Use: Anti-infective.

•**penbutolol sulfate.** (pen-BYOO-toe-lole) U.S.P. 23.
Use: Beta-adrenergic blocking agent.
See: Levatol (Schwarz Pharma).

•**penciclovir.** (pen-SIGH-kloe-VEER) USAN.
Use: Antiviral.
See: Denavir, Cream. (SmithKline Beecham Pharmaceuticals).

Penecare. (Schwarz Pharma) **Cream:** Isostearic acid, lactic acid, stearic acid, PPG-12/SMDI copolymer, steareth-21, steareth-2, mineral oil, magnesium aluminum silicate, imidurea. Tube. 120 g. **Lot.:** Isostearic acid, lactic acid, stearic acid, steareth-21, PPG-12/SMDI copolymer, steareth-2, magnesium aluminum silicate, imidurea. Bot. 240 ml. *otc.*
Use: Emollient.

Penecort Cream. (Allergan) Hydrocortisone 1% or 2.5%, benzyl alcohol, petrolatum, stearyl alcohol, propylene glycol, isopropyl myristate, polyoxyl 40 stearate, carbomer 934, sodium lauryl sulfate, edetate disodium w/sodium hydroxide to adjust pH, purified water. **1%:** Tube 30 g, 60 g. **2.5%:** Tube 30 g. *Rx.*
Use: Corticosteroid, topical.

Penetrex. (Rhone-Poulenc Rorer) Enoxacin 200 mg or 400 mg/Tab. Bot. 50s. *Rx.*
Use: Anti-infective, fluoroquinolone.

•**penfluridol.** (pen-FLEW-rih-dahl) USAN.
Use: Antipsychotic.

penfonylin.
See: Pentid, Prods. (Bristol-Myers Squibb).

•**penicillamine.** (PEN-ih-SILL-ah-meen) U.S.P. 23.
Use: Chelating agent; metal complexing agent, cystinuria, rheumatoid arthritis.
See: Cuprimine, Cap. (Merck).
Depen, Tab. (Wallace Laboratories).

penicillin. (pen-ih-SILL-in) Unless clarified, it means an antibiotic substance or substances produced by growth of the molds *Penicillium notatum* or *P. chrysogenum. Rx.*
Use: Anti-infective.

penicillin aluminum. *Rx.*
Use: Anti-infective, penicillin.

penicillin calcium. U.S.P. XIII. *Rx.*
Use: Anti-infective, penicillin.

penicillin, dimethoxy-phenyl. Methicillin Sodium.
Use: Anti-infective, penicillin.
See: Staphcillin, Vial (Bristol-Myers).

•**penicillin g benzathine.** (pen-ih-SILL-in G BENZ-ah-theen) U.S.P. 23.
Use: Anti-infective.
See: Bicillin, Tab. (Wyeth Ayerst).
Bicillin Long-Acting (Wyeth Ayerst).
Permapen, Aqueous Susp. (Pfizer).

penicillin G benzathine & procaine combined. (pen-ih-SILL-in G BENZ-ah-theen and PRO-cane)
Use: Anti-infective, penicillin.
See: Bicillin C-R, Inj. (Wyeth Ayerst).
Bicillin C-R 900/300, Inj. (Wyeth Ayerst).

•**penicillin G potassium.** (pen-ih-SILL-in G peo-TASS-ee-uhm) U.S.P. 23.
Use: Anti-infective.
See: Pfizerpen, Syr. (Pfizer).

penicillin G potassium w/combinations.
See: Pentid, Prods. (Bristol-Myers Squibb).

•**penicillin G procaine.** (pen-ih-SILL-in G PRO-cane) U.S.P. 23.
Use: Anti-infective.

penicillin G procaine combinations.
See: Bicillin C-R, Tubex (Wyeth Ayerst).
Bicillin C-R 900/300 Inj. (Wyeth Ayerst).

Duracillin F.A., Amp. (Eli Lilly).
Duracillin Fortified, Vial (Eli Lilly).

penicillin G procaine and dihydrostreptomycin sulfate intramammary infusion.
Use: Anti-infective.

penicillin G procaine, dihydrostreptomycin sulfate, chlorpheniramine maleate and dexamethasone suspension, sterile. (pen-ih-SILL-in G PRO-cane, die-HIGH-droe-STREP-toe-MY-sin klor-fen-EAR-ah-meen MAL-ee-ate and DEX-ah-METH-ah-sone)
Use: Anti-infective, antihistamine, anti-inflammatory.

penicillin G procaine, dihydrostreptomycin sulfate, and prednisolone suspension, sterile.
Use: Anti-infective, anti-inflammatory.

penicillin G procaine and dihydrostreptomycin sulfate suspension, sterile.
Use: Anti-infective.

penicillin G procaine, neomycin and polymyxin B sulfates, and hydrocortisone acetate topical suspension.
Use: Anti-infective, anti-inflammatory.

penicillin G procaine and novobiocin sodium intramammary infusion.
Use: Anti-infective.

penicillin G procaine w/aluminum stearate suspension, sterile.
Use: Anti-infective.

penicillin G, procaine, sterile. Sterile Susp., Intramammary infusion, U.S.P. 23. Procaine Penicillin.
Use: Anti-infective.
W/Parenteral, aqueous susp., (Procaine Penicillin, for Aqueous Inj.,) Procaine Penicillin and buffered Penicillin for aqueous, Inj.
See: Crysticillin A.S., Vial (Bristol-Myers Squibb).
Diurnal-Penicillin (Pharmacia & Upjohn).
Duracillin A.S., Preps. (Eli Lilly).
Pfizerpen-A.S. (Roerig).
Tu-Cillin, Inj. (Solvay).
Wycillin, Susp. (Wyeth Ayerst).
W/Parenteral, in oil w/aluminum monostearate. Penicillin Procaine in Oil Inj.

•**penicillin G sodium for injection.** (pen-ih-SILL-in G so-dee-uhm) U.S.P. 23.
Use: Anti-infective.

penicillin hydrabamine phenoxymethyl.
Use: Anti-infective.

penicillin O chloroprocaine.
Use: Anti-infective, penicillin.

penicillin O, sodium. Allylmercaptomethyl penicillin.
Use: Anti-infective.

penicillin, phenoxyethyl.
Use: Anti-infective, penicillin.
See: Phenethicillin, Penicillin potassium 152.

penicillin phenoxymethyl benzathine.
Use: Anti-infective, penicillin.
See: Penicillin V Benzathine.

penicillin phenoxymethyl hydrabamine.
Use: Anti-infective, penicillin.
See: Penicillin V Hydrabamine.

penicillin S benzathine and penicillin G procaine suspension, sterile.
Use: Anti-infective.

•**penicillin V.** (pen-ih-SILL-in V) U.S.P. 23. *Formerly Penicillin Phenoxymethyl.* A biosynthetic penicillin formed by fermentation, with suitable precursors of *Penicillin notatum.*
Use: Anti-infective.
See: Biotic Pow. (Scrip).
Compocillin-V, Water, Susp. (Ross Laboratories).
Penagen-VK, Tab., Pow. (Gafton).
Robicillin-VK (Robins).
Uticillin VK (Pharmacia & Upjohn).
V-Cillin, Preps. (Eli Lilly).
V-Pen, Tab. (Century Pharm).

•**penicillin V benzathine.** (pen-ih-SILL-in V BEN-zah-theen) U.S.P. 23. *Formerly Penicillin Benzathine Phenoxymethyl.*
Use: Anti-infective.
See: Pen-Vee, Prods. (Wyeth Ayerst).

•**penicillin V hydrabamine.** (pen-ih-SILL-in V HIGH-drah-BAM-een) USAN. U.S.P. XX. *Formerly Penicillin Hydrabamine Phenoxymethyl.*
Use: Anti-infective.
See: Compocillin-V Hydrabamine, Oral Susp. (Ross Laboratories).

•**penicillin V potassium.** (pen-ih-SILL-in V poe-TASS-ee-uhm) U.S.P. 23. *Formerly Penicillin Potassium Phenoxymethyl.*
Use: Anti-infective.
See: Beepen VK, Tab., Syr. (SmithKline Beecham Pharmaceuticals).
Betapen VK., Soln., Tab. (Bristol-Myers).
Biotic-V-Powder (Scrip).
Bopen, V-K, Tab. (Boyd).
Dowpen VK, Tab. (Hoechst Marion Roussel).
Ledercillin VK, Oral Soln., Tab. (ESI Lederle Generics).
LV, Tab (ICN Pharmaceuticals).

Pen-Vee-K, Soln., Tab. (Wyeth Ayerst).
Pfizerpen VK, Pow., Tab. (Pfizer).
Phenethicillin Potassium.
Repen-VK, Tab., Oral Susp. (Solvay).
Ro-Cillin VK, Soln., Tab. (Solvay).
SK-Penicillin VK, Soln., Tab. (SmithKline Beecham Pharmaceuticals).
Suspen, Liq. (Circle).
Uticillin VK, Tab., Soln. (Pharmacia & Upjohn).
V-Cillin K, Tab., Oral Soln. (Eli Lilly).
Veetids, Soln., Tab. (Squibb Diagnostic).

penidural.
Use: Anti-infective.

Pen-Kera Creme with Keratin Binding Factor. (B.F. Ascher) Bot. 8 oz. *otc.*
Use: Emollient.

Penntuss. (Medeva) Codeine (as polistirex) 10 mg, chlorpheniramine maleate 4 mg/5 ml. Bot. pt. *c-v.*
Use: Antitussive, antihistamine.

•**pentabamate.** (PEN-tah-BAM-ate) USAN.
Use: Anxiolytic.

Pentacarinat. (Centeon) Pentamidine isethionate 300 mg. Inj. Single-dose vial. *Rx.*
Use: Anti-infective.

pentacosactride.
Use: Corticotrophic peptide.
See: Norleusactide (I.N.N.).

•**pentaerythritol tetranitrate diluted.** (pen-tuh-eh-Rith-rih-tole teh-truh-NYE-trate) U.S.P. 23.
Use: Vasodilator.
See: Arcotrate Nos. 1 and 2, Tab. (Arcum).
Dilac-80, Cap. (B.F. Ascher).
Duotrate-45, Cap. (Hoechst Marion Roussel).
Kortrate, Cap. (Amide Pharmaceuticals).
Maso-Trol, Tab. (Mason).
Metranil, Cap. (Meyer).
Nitrin, Tab. (Pal-Pak).
Penta-E, Tab. (Recsei).
Pentafin, Granucap, Tab. (Solvay).
Pentetra, Tab. (Paddock).
Peritrate, Tab. (Parke-Davis).
Petro-20 mg, Tab. (Foy).
Tetracap-30, Cap. (Freeport).
Tetracap-80, Cap. (Freeport).
Tetratab, Tab. (Freeport).
Tetratab No. 1, Tab. (Freeport).
Vasolate, Cap. (Parmed).
Vasolate-80, Cap. (Parmed).

pentaerythritol tetranitrate, diluted. U.S.P. 23.
Use: Vasodilator.

pentaerythritol tetranitrate w/combinations.
See: Arcotrate No. 3, Tab. (Arcum).
Bitrate, Tab. (Arco).
Dimycor, Tab. (Standard Drug).
Pentetra w/Phenobarbital, Tab. (Paddock).
Peritrate w/Nitroglycerin, Tab. (Parke-Davis).

•**pentafilcon a.** (PEN-tah-FILL-kahn A) USAN.
Use: Contact lens material (hydrophilic).

•**pentagastrin.** (PEN-tah-ASS-trin) USAN.
Use: Diagnostic aid (gastric secretion indicator).
See: Peptavlon, Amp. (Wyeth Ayerst).

•**pentalyte.** (PEN-tah-lite) USAN.
Use: Electrolyte combination.

Pentam 300. (Fujisawa) Pentamidine isethionate 300 mg/Vial. *Rx.*
Use: Anti-infective.

pentamethylenetetrazol.
See: Pentylenetetrazol, U.S.P.

pentamidine isethionate. (pen-TAM-ih-deen ice-uh-THIGH-uh-nate) (Abbott Laboratories) 300 mg. Inj., lyophilized. Single-dose fliptop vials. *Rx.*
Use: Anti-infective. [Orphan drug]
See: Pentam 300, Inj. (Fujisawa).
Pentacarinat, Inj. (Armour).

pentamidine isethionate (inhalation).
Use: Anti-infective. [Orphan drug]

•**pentamorphone.** (PEN-tah-MORE-fone) USAN.
Use: Analgesic (narcotic).

pentamoxane hydrochloride.
Use: Anxiolytic.

•**pentamustine.** (PEN-tah-MUSS-teen) USAN.
Use: Antineoplastic.

pentaphonate. Dodecyltriphenylphosphonium pentachlorophenolate.
Use: Anti-infective.

•**pentapiperium methylsulfate.** (PEN-tah-PIP-ehr-ee-uhm METH-ill-SULL-fate) USAN.
Use: Anticholinergic.

pentapyrrolidinium bitartrate.
See: Pentolinium Tartrate.

pentaquine phosphate.

Pentasa. (Hoechst Marion Roussel) Mesalamine 250 mg. CR Cap. Bot. 240s, UD 80s. *Rx.*
Use: Anti-inflammatory.

pentasodium colistinmethanesulfonate. Sterile Colistimethate Sodium, U.S.P. 23.

•**pentastarch.** (PEN-tah-starch) USAN.
Use: Leukopheresis adjunct (red cell sedimenting agent). [Orphan drug]

Penta-Stress. (Penta) Vitamins A 10,000 IU, D 500 IU, B_1 10 mg, B_2 10 mg, B_6 1 mg, calcium pantothenate 5 mg, niacinamide 50 mg, C 100 mg, E 2 IU, B_{12} 3.3 mcg/Cap. Bot. 90s, 1000s, Jar 250s. *otc.*
Use: Mineral, vitamin supplement.

Penta-Viron. (Penta) Calcium carbonate 500 mg, ferrous fumarate 100 mg, vitamins C 50 mg, D 167 IU, A 3.333 IU, B_1 3.3 mg, B_2 3.3 mg, B_6 2 mg, calcium pantothenate 1.6 mg, niacinamide 16.7 mg, E 2 IU/Cap. Bot. 100s, 1000s, Jar 250s. *otc.*
Use: Mineral, vitamin supplement.

Pentazine Inj. (Century Pharm) Promethazine 50 mg/ml. Inj. Vial 10 ml. *Rx.*
Use: Antihistamine.

Pentazine w/Codeine. (Century Pharm) Promethazine expectorant. Bot. 4 oz, 16 oz, gal.
Use: Antihistamine.

Pentazine VC w/Codeine Liquid. (Century Pharm) Promethazine HCl 6.25 mg, codeine phosphate 10 mg. Liq. Bot. 118 ml, pt, gal. *c-v.*
Use: Antihistamine, antitussive.

•**pentazocine.** (pen-TAZ-oh-seen) U.S.P. 23.
Use: Analgesic.

•**pentazocine hydrochloride.** (pen-TAZ-oh-seen) U.S.P. 23.
Use: Analgesic.
W/ Acetaminophen.
See: Talacen, Cap. (Sanofi Winthrop).

pentazocine hydrochloride and aspirin tablets.
Use: Analgesic.
See: Talwin Compound, Tab. (Sanofi Winthrop).

•**pentazocine lactate injection.** (pen-TAZ-oh-seen LACK-tate) U.S.P. 23.
Use: Analgesic.
See: Talwin Injection, Inj. (Sanofi Winthrop).

pentazocine and naloxone hydrochloride tablets. (Royce) Pentazocine 50 mg, naloxone HCl 0.5 mg/Tab. Box. 100s, 500s, 1000s. *Rx.*
Use: Analgesic.
See: Talwin NX, Tab. (Sanofi Winthrop).

•**pentetate calcium trisodium.** (PEN-teh-tate KAL-see-uhm try-SO-dee-uhm) USAN.
Use: Chelating agent (plutonium).

•**pentetate calcium trisodium Yb 169.** (PEN-teh-tate KAL-see-uhm TRY-SO-dee-uhm Yb 169) USAN.
Use: Radiopharmaceutical.

•**pentetate indium disodium In 111.** (PEN-teh-tate IN-dee-uhm) USAN.
Use: Diagnostic aid, radiopharmaceutical.

•**pentetic acid.** (PEN-teh-tick) U.S.P. 23.
Use: Diagnostic aid.

Pentetra-Paracote. (Paddock) Pentaerythritol tetranitrate 30 mg or 80 mg/Cap. Bot. 100s, 500s, 1000s. *Rx.*
Use: Antianginal.

penthienate bromide.

Penthrane. (Abbott Hospital Prods) Methoxyflurane. Bot. 15 ml, 125 ml. *Rx.*
Use: Anesthetic, general.

•**pentiapine maleate.** (pen-TIE-ah-PEEN) USAN.
Use: Antipsychotic.

•**pentigetide.** (pent-EYE-jeh-TIDE) USAN.
Use: Antiallergic.

Pentina. (Freeport) Rauwolfia serpentina, 100 mg/Tab. Bot. 1000s. *Rx.*
Use: Antihypertensive.

•**pentisomicin.** (pent-IH-so-MY-sin) USAN.
Use: Anti-infective.

•**pentizidone sodium.** (pen-TIH-ZIH-dohn) USAN.
Use: Anti-infective.

•**pentobarbital.** (pen-toe-BAR-bih-tahl) U.S.P. 23.
Use: Hypnotic, sedative.
See: Nembutal, Elix., Gradumets (Abbott Laboratories) Penta, Tab. (Dunhall Pharmaceuticals).

pentobarbital combinations.
Use: Sedative/hypnotic.
See: Cafergot-PB, Supp., Tab. (Novartis).
Nembutal, Preps. (Abbott Laboratories).

•**pentobarbital, sodium.** (pen-toe-BAR-bih-tahl) U.S.P. 23.
Use: Hypnotic, sedative.
See: Maso-Pent, Tab. (Mason).
Nembutal Sodium, Preps. (Abbott Laboratories).
Night-Caps, Cap. (Jones Medical Industries).
W/Adiphenine HCl, phamasorb, aluminum hydroxide.
See: Spasmasorb, Tab. (Roberts Pharm).
W/Atropine sulfate, hyoscine HBr, hyoscyamine sulfate.
See: Eldonal, Elix., Tab., Cap. (Canright).

W/Ephedrine.
See: Ephedrine and Nembutal-25, Cap. (Abbott Laboratories).
W/Ergotamine tartrate, caffeine alkaloid, bellafoline.
See: Cafergot-P.B., Tab. (Novartis).
W/Homatropine methylbromide, dehydrocholic acid, ox bile extract.
See: Homachol, Tab. (Teva USA).
W/Pyrilamine maleate.
See: A-N-R, Rectorette (Roberts Pharm).
W/Seco-, buta-, phenobarbital.
W/Vitamin compounds, d-methamphetamine HCl.
See: Fetamin, Tab. (Mission Pharmacal).

pentobarbital sodium. (Various Mfr.) 100 mg/Cap. Bot. 100s.
Use: Hypnotic, sedative.

pentobarbital sodium. (Wyeth Ayerst) 50mg/ml. Inj. Tubex 2 ml. *c-II.*
Use: Hypnotic, sedative.

pentobarbital, soluble.
See: Pentobarbital Sodium, U.S.P.

Pentol Tabs. (Major) Pentaerythritol tetranitrate. **10 mg/Tab.:** Bot. 1000s; **20 mg/Tab.:** Bot. 100s, 1000s; **80 mg/SA Tab.:** Bot. 250s, 1000s. *Rx.*
Use: Antianginal.

Pentolair. (Bausch & Lomb) Cyclopentolate HCl 1%. Soln. Squeeze Bot. 2 ml, 15 ml. *Rx.*
Use: Cycloplegic mydriatic.

pentolinium tartrate. Pentamethylene-1:5-bis (1'-methylpyrrolidinium bitartrate).
Use: Antihypertensive.

•**pentomone.** (PEN-toe-MONE) USAN.
Use: Prostate growth inhibitor.

•**pentopril.** (PEN-toe-prill) USAN.
Use: Enzyme inhibitor (angiotensin-converting).

•**pentosan polysulfate sodium.** (PEN-toe-san PAHL-in-SULL-fate SO-dee-uhm) USAN.
Use: Anti-inflammatory (interstitial cystitis).

pentosan sodium polysulfate.
Use: Treatment of interstitial cystitis. [Orphan drug]
See: Elmiron, Cap. (Ivax).

•**pentostatin.** (PEN-toe-STAT-in) USAN.
Use: Potentiator; leukemia. [Orphan drug]

Pentothal. (Abbott Laboratories) **Pow. for Inj.:** Thiopental sodium 20 mg/ml. In 1, 2.5, 5 g kits, 400 mg syringes; 25 mg/ml. In 1, 2.5, 5 g, 500 mg kits, 250, 400, 500 mg syringes. **Rectal Susp.:** Thiopental sodium 400 mg/g. In 2 g syringe. *Rx.*
Use: Anesthetic.

•**pentoxifylline.** (pen-TOX-IH-fill-in) USAN.
Use: Hemorrheologic, vasodilator.
See: Trental (Hoechst Marion Roussel).

pentoxifylline. (Copley) Pentoxifylline 400 mg. Tab. Bot. 100s, 500s, 5000s. *Rx.*
Use: Hemorrheologic, vasodilator.

pentoxifyline extended release. (Purepac) Pentoxifylline 400 mg. Tab. Bot. 100s, 500s, 1000s. *Rx.*
Use: Hemorrheologic, vasodilator.

Pentrax Gold. (GenDerm) Solubilized coal tar extract 4%. Shampoo. Bot. 168 ml. *otc.*
Use: Antiseborrheic.

Pentrax Shampoo. (Rydelle) Tar extract 8.75%, detergents, conditioning agents. Bot. 4 oz, 8 oz. *otc.*
Use: Antiseborrheic.

•**pentrinitrol.** (pen-TRY-nye-TROLE) USAN.
Use: Vasodilator (coronary).

Pent-T-80. (Mericon) Pentaerythritol tetranitrate 80 mg/T.D. Cap. Bot. 100s, 1000s. *Rx.*
Use: Antianginal.

Pen-V. (Zenith Forest Pharmaceutical) Penicillin 250 mg or 500 mg/Tab. Bot. 100s, 1000s. *Rx.*
Use: Anti-infective, penicillin.

Pen-Vee K. (Wyeth Ayerst) Potassium phenoxymethyl penicillin. 250 mg Tab. Bot. 100s, 500s, Redipak 100s. *Rx.*
Use: Anti-infective, penicillin.

Pen-Vee K for Oral Solution. (Wyeth Ayerst) Penicillin V potassium. **125 mg/5 ml:** Bot. 100 ml, 200 ml. **250 mg/5 ml:** Bot. 100 ml, 150 ml, 200 ml. *Rx.*
Use: Anti-infective, penicillin.

Pepcid. (Merck) Famotidine. **Tab.:** 20 mg or 40 mg. Bot. 30s, 90s, 100s, UD 100s. **Oral Susp.:** 40 mg/5 ml. Bot. 400 mg. **I.V. Inj. Premixed:** 20 mg/50 ml in 0.9% NaCl. 50 ml *Galaxy* container. *Rx.*
Use: Antiulcerative.

Pepcid AC Acid Controller. (J & J Merck Consumer Pharm) Famotidine 10 mg/Tab. Pkg. 12s. *otc.*
Use: Antiulcerative.

Pepcid RPD. (Merck) Famotidine 20 mg, 40 mg, aspartame, mint flavor, gelatin, mannitol. Orally disintegrating Tab. UD 30s, 100s. *Rx.*

Use: Histamine H_2 agonist.

•**peplomycin sulfate.** (PEP-low-MY-sin) USAN.
Use: Antineoplastic.

•**peppermint.** N.F. 18.
Use: Pharmaceutic aid (flavor, perfume), antitussive, expectorant, nasal decongestant.
See: Vicks Prods. (Procter & Gamble).

•**peppermint oil.** N.F. 18.
Use: Pharmaceutic aid (flavor).

•**peppermint spirit.** U.S.P. 23.
Use: Pharmaceutic aid (flavor, perfume).

•**peppermint water.** N.F. 18.
Use: Pharmaceutic aid (vehicle, flavored).

Pepsamar Comp. Tablets. (Sanofi Winthrop) Aluminum hydroxide, magnesium hydroxide. *otc.*
Use: Antacid.

Pepsamar Esp Liquid. (Sanofi Winthrop) Aluminum hydroxide, glycerin. *otc.*
Use: Antacid.

Pepsamar Esp Tablets. (Sanofi Winthrop) Aluminum hydroxide, magnesium hydroxide, mannitol powder. *otc.*
Use: Antacid.

Pepsamar HM Tablets. (Sanofi Winthrop) Aluminum hydroxide, starch. *otc.*
Use: Antacid.

Pepsamar Liquid. (Sanofi Winthrop) Aluminum hydroxide. *otc.*
Use: Antacid.

Pepsamar Suspension. (Sanofi Winthrop) Aluminum hydroxide, magnesium hydroxide, sorbitol. *otc.*
Use: Antacid.

Pepsamar Tablets. (Sanofi Winthrop) Aluminum hydroxide. *otc.*
Use: Antacid.

Pepsicone Gel. (Sanofi Winthrop) Aluminum hydroxide, magnesium hydroxide, simethicone. *otc.*
Use: Antacid, antiflatulent.

Pepsicone Tablet. (Sanofi Winthrop) Aluminum hydroxide, magnesium hydroxide, simethicone. *otc.*
Use: Antacid, antiflatulent.

pepsin.
Use: Digestive aid.

pepsin w/combinations.
See: Biloric, Cap. (Arcum).
Digipepsin, Tab. (Kenwood/Bradley).
Donnazyme, Tab. (Robins).
Entozyme, Tab. (Robins).
Enzobile, Tab. (Roberts Pharm).
Gourmase-PB, Cap. (Solvay).
Kanulase, Tab. (Novartis).
Leber Taurine, Liq. (Paddock).
Nu'Leven, Tab. (Teva USA).
Ro-Bile, Tab. (Solvay).
Zypan, Tab. (Standard Process).

pepsin lactated, elixir.
See: Peptalac, Liq. (Jones Medical Industries).

•**pepstatin.** (pep-STAT-in) USAN.
Use: Enzyme inhibitor (pepsin).

Peptamen Liquid. (Clintec Nutrition) Enzymatically hydrolyzed whey proteins, maltodextrin, starch, MCT, sunflower oil, lecithin, vitamins A, B_1, B_2, B_3, B_5, B_6, B_{12}, C, D, E, K, folic acid, biotin, choline, Ca, Cl, Cu, Fe, I, Mg, Mn, P, Zn. Can 500 ml. *otc.*
Use: Nutritional supplement.

Peptavlon. (Wyeth Ayerst) Pentagastrin 0.25 mg, sodium Cl/ml. For evaluation of gastric acid secretion. Amp. 2 ml, Ctn. 10s.
Use: Diagnostic aid.

Peptenzyme. (Schwarz Pharma) Alcohol 16%. Pleasantly aromatic. Bot. pt.
Use: Pharmaceutic aid.

Pepto-Bismol Caplets. (Procter & Gamble Company) Bismuth subsalicylate 262 mg, < 2 mg sodium/Capl. Sugar free. Bot. 24s, 40s. *otc.*
Use: Antidiarrheal.

Pepto-Bismol Liquid. (Procter & Gamble Company) Bismuth subsalicylate 262 mg/15 ml. Bot. 4 oz, 8 oz, 12 oz, 16 oz. *otc.*
Use: Antidiarrheal.

Pepto-Bismol Maximum Strength Liquid. (Procter & Gamble Company) 524 mg/15 ml. Bot. 120 ml, 240 ml, 360 ml. *otc.*
Use: Antidiarrheal.

Pepto-Bismol Tablets. (Procter & Gamble Company) Bismuth subsalicylate 262.5 mg/Chew. Tab. Pkg. 24s, 42s. *otc.*
Use: Antidiarrheal.

Perandren Phenylacetate. (Novartis) Testosterone phenylacetate. *c-III.*
Use: Androgen.

percaine.
Use: Local anesthetic.
See: Dibucaine HCl, U.S.P.

Perchloracap. (Mallinckrodt) Potassium perchlorate 200 mg/Cap. Bot. 100s.
Use: Radiographic adjunct.

perchlorethylene.
See: Tetrachlorethylene, U.S.P. 23.

perchlorperazine.
See: Compazine, Preps. (SmithKline Beecham Pharmaceuticals).

Percocet. (DuPont) Oxycodone HCl 5 mg, acetaminophen 325 mg/Tab. Bot. 100s, 500s, UD 100s. *c-II.*
Use: Analgesic combination, narcotic.

Percodan. (DuPont) Oxycodone HCl 4.5 mg, oxycodone terephthalate 0.38 mg, aspirin 325 mg/Tab. Bot. 100s, 500s, 1000s, UD 250s. *c-II.*
Use: Analgesic combination, narcotic.
W/Hexobarbital.
See: Percobarb, Cap. (DuPont).

Percodan-Demi. (DuPont) Oxycodone HCl 2.25 mg, oxycodone terephthalate 0.19 mg, aspirin 325 mg/Tab. Bot. 100s. *c-II.*
Use: Analgesic combination, narcotic.

Percogesic. (Procter & Gamble) Acetaminophen 325 mg, phenyltoloxamine citrate 30 mg/Tab. Bot. 24s, 50s, 90s. *otc.*
Use: Analgesic, antihistamine.

Percomorph Liver Oil. (May be blended with 50% other fish liver oils; each g contains vitamins A 60,000 IU & D 8500 IU).
See: Oleum Percomorphum.

Percy Medicine. (Merrick Medicine) Bismuth subnitrate 959 mg, calcium hydroxide 21.9 mg/10 ml, alcohol 5%. *otc.*
Use: Antidiarrheal.

Perdiem. (Rhone-Poulenc Rorer) Blend of psyllium 82%, senna 18% as active ingredients in granular form. Sodium content (0.08 mEq) 1.8 mg/rounded tsp. (6 g). Canister 100 g, 250 g, UD 6 g. *otc.*
Use: Laxative.

Perdiem Fiber. (Rhone-Poulenc Rorer) Psyllium 100% as active ingredient in granular form. Sodium content (0.08 mEq) 1.8 mg/rounded tsp. (6 g). Canister 100 g, 250 g, UD 6 g. *otc.*
Use: Laxative.

Pere-Diosate. (Towne) Docusate sodium 100 mg, casanthranol 30 mg/Cap. Bot. 100s. *otc.*
Use: Laxative.

Perestan. (Henry Schein) Docusate sodium 100 mg, casanthranol 30 mg/Cap. Bot. 100s, 1000s. *otc.*
Use: Laxative.

•**perfilcon a.** (per-FILL-kahn A) USAN.
Use: Contact lens material (hydrophilic).
See: Permalens (Ciba Vision Ophthalmics).

•**perflenapent.** (per-FLEN-ah-pent) USAN.
Use: Diagnostic aid (ultrasound contrast agent).

•**perflisopent.** USAN.
Use: Diagnostic aid (ultrasound contrast agent).

•**perflubron.** (per-FLEW-brahn) U.S.P. 23.
Use: Contrast agent; blood substitute.

•**perfosfamide.** (per-FOSS-fam-ide) USAN.
Use: Antineoplastic. [Orphan drug]

pergalen.
See: Sodium Apolate.

•**pergolide mesylate.** (PURR-go-lide) USAN.
Use: Dopamine agonist.
See: Permax, Tab. (Athena Neurosciences).

Pergonal (menotropins). (Serono Labs) Follicle stimulating hormone (FSH) and luteinizing hormone (LH) 75 IU or 150 IU. Inj. Amp 2 ml. *Rx.*
Use: Hormone, gonadotropin.

Pergrava. (Arcum) Vitamins A 2000 IU, D 300 IU, B_1 2 mg, B_2 2 mg, nicotinamide 10 mg, B_6 2 mg, B_{12} 5 mcg, C 60 mg, calcium 40 mg/Cap. Bot. 100s, 1000s. *otc.*
Use: Mineral, vitamin supplement.

Pergrava No. 2. (Arcum) Vitamins A 2000 IU, D 300 IU, B_1 2 mg, B_2 2 mg, nicotinamide 10 mg, B_6 2 mg, C 60 mg, calcium lactate monohydrate 200 mg, ferrous gluconate 31 mg, folic acid 0.1 mg/Cap. Bot. 100s, 1000s. *otc.*
Use: Mineral, vitamin supplement.

perhexiline. (per-HEX-ih-leen)
Use: Antianginal.

•**perhexiline maleate.** (per-HEX-ih-leen) USAN.
Use: Vasodilator (coronary).

perhydrol.
See: Hydrogen Peroxide 30% (Various Mfr.).

Peri Sofcap. (Alton) Docusate sodium with peristim. Bot. 100s, 1000s. *otc.*
Use: Laxative.

Periactin. (Merck) Cyproheptadine HCl 4 mg/Tab. Bot. 100s. *Rx.*
Use: Antihistamine.

Periactin Syrup. (Merck) Cyproheptadine HCl 2 mg/5 ml, alcohol 5%, sucrose, saccharin. Bot. 473 ml. *Rx.*
Use: Antihistamine.

Peri-Care. (Sween) Vitamins A and D in petroleum ointment base. Tube 0.5 oz, 1.75 oz. Jar 2 oz, 5 oz, 8 oz. *otc.*
Use: Emollient.

Peri-Colace. (Bristol-Myers) **Cap.:** Docusate sodium 100 mg, casanthranol 30 mg/Cap. Bot. 30s, 60s, 250s, 1000s, UD 100s. **Syr.:** Docusate sodium 60

mg, casanthranol 30 mg/15 ml, ethyl alcohol 10%. Bot. 8 oz, pt. *otc.*
Use: Laxative.

Peridex. (Procter & Gamble Pharm) Chlorhexidine gluconate 0.12%, alcohol 11.6%, glycerin, PEG-40 sorbitan diisostearate, flavor, sodium saccharin, FD&C blue No. 1, water. Bot. 480 ml. *Rx.*
Use: Mouth preparation.

Peridin-C. (Beutlich) Hesperidin methyl chalcone 50 mg, hesperidin complex 150 mg, ascorbic acid 200 mg/Tab. Bot. 100s, 500s. *otc.*
Use: Vitamin supplement.

Peri-Dos. (Zenith Forest Pharmaceutical) Docusate sodium 100 mg, casanthranol 30 mg/Cap. Bot. 30s, 60s, 100s, 1000s. *otc.*
Use: Laxative.

Peries. (Xttrium) Medicated pads w/witch hazel, glycerin. Jar pad 40s. *otc.*
Use: Hygienic wipe and local compress.

•**perindopril.** (per-IN-doe-prill) USAN.
Use: ACE inhibitor.

•**perindopril erbumine.** (per-IN-doe-prill ehr-BYOO-meen) USAN.
Use: Antihypertensive.
See: Aceon, Tab. (Ortho McNeil).

Perio-Eze-20. (Moyco) Oral paste.
Use: Analgesic, topical.

PerioGard. (Colgate Oral) Chlorhexidine gluconate 0.12%, alcohol 11.6%, glycerin, PEG-40, sorbitol diisostearnate, saccharin. Rinse. 473 ml w/ 15 ml dose cup. *Rx.*
Use: Anesthetic.

peristomal covering.

Peritinic. (ESI Lederle Generics) Elemental iron 100 mg, docusate sodium 100 mg, vitamins B_1 7.5 mg, B_2 7.5 mg, B_6 7.5 mg, B_{12} 50 mcg, C 200 mg, niacinamide 30 mg, folic acid 0.05 mg, pantothenic acid 15 mg/Tab. Bot. 60s. *otc.*
Use: Mineral, vitamin supplement; laxative.

Peritrate. (Parke-Davis) Pentaerythritol tetranitrate. **10 mg/Tab.:** Bot. 100s, 1000s. **20 mg/Tab.:** Bot. 100s, 1000s, UD 100s. **40 mg/Tab.:** Bot. 100s. *Rx.*
Use: Antianginal.

Peritrate S.A. (Parke-Davis) Pentaerythritol tetranitrate 80 mg (20 mg in immediate release layer, 60 mg in sustained release base)/Tab. Bot. 100s, 1000s, UD 100s. *Rx.*
Use: Antianginal.

Peri-Wash. (Sween) Bot. 4 oz, 8 oz, 1 gal, 5 gal, 30 gal, 55 gal.
Use: Anorectal preparation.

Peri-Wash II. (Sween) Bot. 4 oz, 8 oz, 1 gal, 5 gal, 30 gal, 55 gal.
Use: Anorectal preparation.

•**perlapine.** (PURR-lah-peen) USAN.
Use: Hypnotic, sedative.

perlatan.
See: Estrone (Various Mfr.).

permanganic acid, potassium salt. Potassium permanganate, U.S.P. 23.

Permapen. (Roerig) Benzathine penicillin G 1,200,000 units/ml. Disp. syringe 2 ml. *Rx.*
Use: Anti-infective, penicillin.

Permax. (Athena Neurosciences) Pergolide mesylate. 0.05 mg, 0.25 mg, 1 mg. Tab. Bot. 30s (0.05 mg only), 100s. *Rx.*
Use: Antiparkinsonian.

•**permethrin.** (per-METH-rin) USAN. Synthetic pyrethrin.
Use: Pediculicide for treatment of head lice, ectoparasiticide.
See: Acticin, Cream (Alpharma USPD). Nix, Cream (GlaxoWellcome).

Permitil. (Schering Plough) Fluphenazine HCl. **2.5 mg or 5 mg/Tab:** Bot. 100s. **10 mg/Tab.:** Bot. 1000s. *Rx.*
Use: Antipsychotic.

Permitil Oral Concentrate. (Schering Plough) Fluphenazine HCl 5 mg/ml, alcohol 1%, parabens. Dropper Bot. 118 ml. *Rx.*
Use: Antipsychotic.

Pernox Lathering Abradant Scrub. (Westwood Squibb) Sulfur, salicylic acid. Lot. Bot. 141 g. *otc.*
Use: Dermatologic, acne.

Pernox Lotion. (Westwood Squibb) Microfine granules of polyethylene 20%, sulfur 2%, salicylic acid 2% in a combination of soapless cleansers and wetting agents. Bot. 6 oz. *otc.*
Use: Dermatologic, acne.

Pernox Medicated Lathering Scrub Cleanser. (Westwood Squibb) Polyethylene granules 26%, sulfur 2%, salicylic acid 1.5% w/soapless surface-active cleansers and wetting agents. Regular or lemon. Tube 2 oz, 4 oz. *otc.*
Use: Dermatologic, acne.

Pernox Scrub for Oily Skin. (Westwood Squibb) Sulfur, salicylic acid, EDTA. Cleanser. 56 g, 113 g. *otc.*
Use: Dermatologic, acne.

Pernox Shampoo. (Westwood Squibb) Sodium laureth sulfate, water, lauramide DEA, quaternium 22, PEG-75

lanolin/hydrolyzed animal protein, fragrance, sodium Cl, lactic acid, sorbic acid, disodium EDTA, FD&C yellow No. 6 and blue No. 1. Bot. 8 oz. *otc.*
Use: Cleanser, conditioner.

peroxidase. W/Glucose oxidase, potassium, iodide.
See: Diastix Reagent Strips (Bayer Corp).

peroxide, dibenzoyl. Benzoyl Peroxide, Hydrous.

peroxides.
See: Hydrogen Peroxide (Various Mfr.).
Urea Peroxide.
Zinc Peroxide.

Peroxin A5. (Dermol Pharmaceuticals) Benzoyl peroxide 5%. Gel. Tube 45 g. *Rx.*
Use: Dermatologic, acne.

Peroxin A10. (Dermol Pharmaceuticals) Benzoyl peroxide 10%. Gel. Tube 45 g. *Rx.*
Use: Dermatologic, acne.

Peroxyl Dental Rinse. (Colgate Oral) Hydrogen peroxide 1.5% in mint flavored base, alcohol 6%. Bot. 240 ml, pint. *otc.*
Use: Mouth preparation.

Peroxyl Gel. (Colgate Oral) Hydrogen peroxide 1.5% in a mint flavored base. Tube. 15 g. *otc.*
Use: Mouth preparation.

•**perphenazine.** (per-FEN-uh-ZEEN) U.S.P. 23.
Use: Antiemetic, antipsychotic, anxiolytic.
See: Trilafon, Prods. (Schering Plough).

perphenazine. (Various Mfr.) Perphenazine 2 mg, 4 mg, 8 mg, 16 mg. Tab. Bot. 100s, 250s (8 mg only), 500s. *Rx.*
Use: Antipsychotic.

perphenazine/amitriptyline tablets. (per-FEN-uh-zeen am-ee-TRIP-tih-leen) (Various, eg, Bolar, Geneva, Forest Pharmaceutical, Lemmon, Par, Rugby, Schein Pharmaceutical, Zenith). Perphenazine (mg): 2, 2; Amitriptyline (mg): 10, 25. Bot. 21s, 100s, 500s, 1000s; Bot. 100s, 500s, 1000s.
Use: Miscellaneous psychotherapeutic.
See: Etrafon, Prods. (Schering Plough).

Persa-Gel. (Advanced Care Products) Benzoyl peroxide 5% or 10%, acetone base. Tube 45 g, 90 g. *Rx.*
Use: Dermatologic, acne.

Persa-Gel W 5%, 10%. (Advanced Care Products) Benzoyl peroxide 5% or 10% in water base. Tube 45 g, 90 g. *Rx.*
Use: Dermatologic, acne.

Persangue. (Arcum) Ferrous gluconate 192 mg, vitamins C 150 mg, B_1 3 mg, B_2 3 mg, B_{12} 50 mcg/Cap. Bot. 100s, 500s. *otc.*
Use: Mineral, vitamin supplement.

Persantine. (Boehringer Ingelheim) Dipyridamole 25 mg, 50 mg or 75 mg/Tab. **25 mg or 50 mg:** Bot. 100s, 1000s, UD 100s. **75 mg:** Bot. 100s, 500s, UD 100s. *Rx.*
Use: Antiplatelet.

Persantine IV. (DuPont Merck Pharmaceuticals) Dipyridamole. Inj. For evaluation of coronary artery disease.
Use: Diagnostic aid.

persic oil. N.F. XVII.
Use: Vehicle.

pertechnetic acid, sodium salt. Sodium Pertechnetate Tc 99 m Solution.

Pertscan-99m. (Abbott Diagnostics) Radiodiagnostic. Inj. Tc-99m.
Use: Diagnostic aid.

Pertussin All-Night PM. (Pertussin Labs) Acetaminophen 167 mg, doxylamine succinate 1.25 mg, pseudoephedrine HCl 10 mg, dextromethorphan HBr 5 mg/5 ml, alcohol 25%. Liq. Bot. 240 ml. *otc.*
Use: Analgesic, antihistamine, antitussive, decongestant.

Pertussin CS. (Pertussin) Dextromethorphan HBr 3.5 mg, guaifenesin 25 mg/5 ml, 8.5% alcohol. Bot. 90 ml. *otc.*
Use: Antitussive, expectorant.

Pertussin ES. (Pertussin) Dextromethorphan HBr 15 mg/5 ml, alcohol 9.5%, sugar, sorbitol. Liq. Bot. 120 ml. *otc.*
Use: Antitussive.

Pertussin Syrup. (Pertussin) Dextromethorphan HBr 15 mg/5 ml, alcohol 9.5%. Bot. 3 oz, 6 oz. *otc.*
Use: Antitussive.

•**pertussis immune globulin.** (per-TUSS-iss) U.S.P. 23. *Formerly Pertussis Immune Human Globulin.*
Use: Immunization.

•**pertussis vaccine.** U.S.P. 23.
Use: Immunization.
W/diphtheria and tetanus toxoids.
See: Acel-Imune, Vial (Wyeth Ayerst).
Infanrix (SKB).
Tri-Immunol, Vial (Wyeth Ayerst).
Tripedia, Vial (Pasteur Merieux Connaught).

pertussis vaccine. (Michigan Department of public Health). Vial 5 mL.
Use: Immunization.

•**pertussis vaccine adsorbed.** U.S.P. 23.

Use: Immunization.

pertussis vaccine and diphtheria and tetanus toxoids, combined.
Use: Immunization.
See: Acel-Imune, Vial (Wyeth Ayerst).
Infanrix (SKB).
Tri-Immunol, Vial (Wyeth Ayerst).
Tripedia, Vial (Pasteur Merieux Connaught).

peruvian balsam.
Use: Local protectant, rubefacient.
W/Benzocaine, zinc oxide, bismuth subgallate, boric acid.
See: Anocaine, Supp. (Roberts Pharm).
W/Benzocaine, zinc oxide, 8-hydroxyquinoline benzoate, menthol. Unit-of-Use 90s. **50 mg:** Bot. 100s, 1000s, UD 100s. **75 mg:** Bot. 100s.
See: Hemorrhoidal Oint. (Towne).
W/Ephedrine sulfate, belladonna extract, zinc oxide, boric acid, bismuth oxyiodide, subcarbonate.
See: Wyanoids, Preps. (Wyeth Ayerst).
W/Lidocaine, bismuth subgallate, zinc oxide, aluminum subacetate.
See: Xylocaine, Supp. (Astra).
W/Oxyquinoline sulfate, pramoxine HCl, zinc oxide.

peson. Sodium Lyapolate. Polyethylene sulfonate sodium.
Use: Anticoagulant.

Peterson's Ointment. (Peterson) Carbolic acid, camphor, tannic acid, zinc oxide. Tube w/pipe 1 oz. Jar 16 oz. Can 1.4 oz, 3 oz. *otc.*
Use: Anorectal preparation.

Pethadol Tablets. (Halsey) Meperidine HCl 50 mg or 100 mg/Tab. Bot. 100s, 1000s. *c-II.*
Use: Analgesic, narcotic.

pethidine hydrochloride.
See: Meperidine HCl, U.S.P. 23.

PETN.
See: Pentaerythritol tetranitrate.

petrichloral. Pentaerythritol chloral.
Use: Sedative.

Petro-20. (Foy) Pentaerythritol tetranitrate 20 mg/Tab. Bot. 100s, 1000s. *Rx.*
Use: Antianginal.

•**petrolatum.** (pen-troe-LAY-tum) U.S.P. 23.
Use: Pharmaceutic aid (ointment base).
See: Lipkote, Stick (Schering Plough).

petrolatum gauze.
Use: Surgical aid.

•**petrolatum, hydrophilic.** U.S.P. 23.
Use: Pharmaceutic aid (absorbent, oihtment base) topical protectant.
See: Lipkote (Schering Plough).

petrolatum, liquid. Mineral Oil, U.S.P. 23. Light Mineral Oil, U.S.P. 23. Adepsine Oil, Glymol, Liquid Paraffin, Parolein, White Mineral Oil, Heavy Liquid Petrolatum.
Use: Laxative.
See: Clyserol Oil Retention Enema (Fuller Labs).
Fleet Mineral Oil Enema (C.B. Fleet).
Mineral Oil (Various Mfr.).
Nujol, Liq. (Schering Plough).
Saxol (Various Mfr.).

petrolatum, liquid, emulsion.
Use: Lubricant, laxative.
See: Milkinol, Liq. (Kremers Urban).
W/Agar-Gel.
See: Agoral Plain, Liq. (Parke-Davis).
Petrogalar, Preps. (Wyeth Ayerst).
W/Cascara.
See: Petrogalar w/Cascara, Emulsion (Wyeth Ayerst).
W/Docusate sodium.
See: Milkinol, Liq. (Kremers Urban).
W/Irish moss, casanthranol.
See: Neo-Kondremul (Medeva).
W/Milk of magnesia.
See: Haley's M. O., Liq. (Sanofi Winthrop).
W/Phenolphthalein.
See: Agoral, Emulsion (Parke-Davis).
Petrogalar w/Phenolphthalein, Emulsion (Wyeth Ayerst).
Phenolphthalein in liquid Petrolatum Emulsion.

petrolatum, red veterinarian. (Zeneca) Also known as RVP.
W/Micasorb.
See: RV Plus, Oint. (ICN Pharmaceuticals).
W/N-diethyl metatoluamide.
See: RV Pellent, Oint. (Zeneca).
W/Zinc oxide, 2-ethoxyethyl p-methoxycinnamate.
See: RV Paque, Oint. (ICN Pharmaceuticals).

•**petrolatum, white.** U.S.P. 23.
Use: Pharmaceutic aid (oleaginous ointment base) topical protectant.
See: Moroline, Oint. (Schering Plough).

Petro-Phylic Soap. (Doak Dermatologics) Hydrophilic Petrolatum. Cake 4 oz.
Use: Emollient, anti-infective, topical.

PF4RIA. (Abbott Diagnostics) Platelet factor 4 radioimmunoassay for the quantitative measurement of total PF4 levels in plasma.
Use: Diagnostic aid.

Pfeiffer's Cold Sore. (Pfeiffer) Gum benzoin 7%, camphor, menthol, thymol, eucalyptol, alcohol 85%. Lot. Bot. 15 ml. *otc.*

Use: Cold sores, fever blisters, moisturizer.

Pfizerpen VK Tablets. (Pfizer) Penicillin V potassium 250 mg or 500 mg/Tab. **250 mg:** Bot. 1000s. **500 mg:** Bot. 100s. *Rx.*
Use: Anti-infective, penicillin.

PGA.
See: Folic Acid, U.S.P. 23.

PGE.
Use: Prostaglandin.
See: Alprostadil.

pHacid. (Baker/Cummins) Bot. 8 oz.
Use: Dermatologic.

Phadiatop RIA Test. (Pharmacia & Upjohn) Determination of IgE antibodies specific to inhalant allergens in human serum. Kit 60s.
Use: Diagnostic aid.

Phanacol Cough. (Pharmakon Labs) Phenylpropanolamine HCl 25 mg, dextromethorphan HBr 10 mg, guaifenesin 100 mg, acetaminophen 325 mg/5 ml. Syrup. Bot. 118 ml, 236 ml. *otc.*
Use: Antitussive, decongestant, expectorant.

Phanadex Cough Syrup. (Pharmakon Labs) Phenylpropanolamine HCl 25 mg, pyrilamine maleate 40 mg, dextromethorphan HBr 15 mg, guaifenesin 100 mg/5 ml, sugar, potassium citrate, citric acid. Syr. Bot. 118 ml, 236 ml. *otc.*
Use: Antihistamine, antitussive, decongestant, expectorant.

Phanatuss Cough Syrup. (Pharmakon Labs) Dextromethorphan HBr 10 mg, guaifenesin 85 mg, potassium citrate 75 mg, citric acid 35 mg/5 ml, sorbitol, menthol. Syr. Bot. 118 ml. *otc.*
Use: Antitussive, expectorant.

pH Antiseptic Skin Cleanser. (Walgreens) Alcohol 63%. Bot. 16 oz. *otc.*
Use: Astringent, cleanser.

Pharazine. (Halsey) Bot. 4 oz, 16 oz, gal.
Use: A series of cough and cold products.

Pharmadine. (Sherwood Medical) Povidone-iodine. **Oint.:** Pkt. 1 g, 1.5 g, 2 g, 30 g, 1 lb. **Perineal wash:** 240 ml. **Skin cleanser:** 240 ml. **Soln.:** 15 ml, 120 ml, 240 ml, pt, qt. **Soln., swabs:** 100s. **Soln., swabsticks:** 1 or 3/packet in 250s. **Spray:** 120 g. **Surgical scrub:** 30 ml, pt, qt, gal, foil-pack 15 ml. **Surgical scrub sponge/brush:** 25s. **Swabsticks, lemon glycerin:** 100s. **Whirlpool soln.:** gal. *otc.*
Use: Antiseptic.

Pharmaflur. (Pharmics) Sodium fluoride 2.21 mg. Tab. Bot. 1000s. *Rx.*
Use: Dental caries agent.

Pharmalgen Hymenoptera Venoms. (ALK Laboratories) Freeze-dried venom or venom protein. Vials of 120 mcg or 1100 mcg for each of honey bee, white-faced hornet, yellow hornet, yellow jacket, or wasp. Vials of 360 mcg or 3300 mcg for mixed vespids (white-faced hornet, yellow hornet, yellow jacket). Diagnostic kit: 5 × 1 ml vial. Treatment kit: 6 × 1 ml vial or 1 × 1.1 mg multiple dose vial. Starter Kit: 6 × 1 ml, pre-diluted 0.01 mcg to 100 mcg/ml.
Use: Antivenim.

Pharmalgen Standardized Allergenic Extracts. (ALK Laboratories) 100,000 allergenic units/Vial. Box 5 x 1 ml.
Use: Diagnostic aid.

Phazyme. (Schwarz Pharma) Simethicone 60 mg/Tab. Bot. 50s, 100s, 1000s. *otc.*
Use: Antiflatulent.

Phazyme 95. (Schwarz Pharma) Simethicone 95 mg/Tab. Bot. 100s. *otc.*
Use: Antiflatulent.

Phazyme 125. (Schwarz Pharma) Simethicone 125 ml. Cap. Bot. 50s. *otc.*
Use: Antiflatulent.

Phazyme Drops. (Schwarz Pharma) Simethicone 40 mg/0.6 ml, saccharin. Bot. 30 ml w/dropper. *otc.*
Use: Antiflatulent.

•**phemfilcon a.** (FEM-fill-kahn A) USAN.
Use: Contact lens material (hydrophilic).

phenacaine hydrochloride. U.S.P. XXI.
Use: Anesthetic, local.
W/Cod liver oil.
See: Morusan Oint. (SmithKline Beecham Pharmaceuticals).
W/Ephedrine. (Pharmacia & Upjohn) Phenacaine HCl 1%, epinephrine 1:25,000. Ophth. oint. Tube 1 dr.
W/Mercarbolide. (Pharmacia & Upjohn) Holocaine HCl 2%, mercarbolide 1:3000. Ophth. oint., Tube w/applicator tip, 1 dr.

Phenacal. (NeuroGenesis/Matrix) D,L-phenylalanine 500 mg, L-glutamine 15 mg, L-tyrosine 25 mg, L-carnitine 10 mg, L-arginine pyroglutamate 10 mg, L-ornithine/L-aspartate 10 mg, chromium 0.033 mg, selenium 0.012 mg, vitamin B_1 0.33 mg, B_2 5 mg, B_3 3.3 mg, B_5 0.33 mg, B_6 0.33 mg, B_{12} 1 mcg, E 5 IU, biotin 0.05 mg, folic acid 0.066 mg, iron 1 mg, zinc 2.5 mg, calcium 35 mg, io-

dine 0.25 mg, copper 0.33 mg, magnesium 25 mg/Cap. Bot. 42s, 180s. *otc.*
Use: Nutritional supplement.

phenacetin. Acetophenetidin. Ethoxyacetanilide.
Use: Antipyretic, analgesic.
Note: This drug has been withdrawn from the market due to liver and kidney toxicity. This drug is no longer official in the U.S.P.

phenacetylcarbamide.
See: Phenurone, Tab. (Abbott Laboratories).

phenacetylurea.
See: Phenurone, Tab. (Abbott Laboratories).

phenacridane. (9(p-Hexloxphenyl)-10-methyl-acridinium Cl).
See: Micridium (Johnson & Johnson Consumer Products).

Phenadex Senior. (Barre-National) Dextromethorphan HBr 10 mg, guaifenesin 200 mg/5 ml. Liq. Bot. 118 ml. *otc.*
Use: Antitussive, expectorant.

Phenahist Injectable. (T.E. Williams) Atropine sulfate 0.2 mg, phenylpropanolamine HCl 12.5 mg, chlorpheniramine maleate 5 mg/ml. Vial 10 ml. *Rx.*
Use: Anticholinergic, antihistamine, antispasmodic, decongestant.

Phenahist-TR Tablets. (T.E. Williams) Phenylephrine HCl 25 mg, phenylpropanolamine HCl 50 mg, chlorpheniramine maleate 8 mg, hyoscyamine sulfate 0.19 mg, atropine 0.04 mg, scopolamine HBr 0.01 mg. Tab. Bot. 100s. *Rx.*
Use: Anticholinergic, antihistamine, antispasmodic, decongestant.

phenamazoline hydrochloride. 2-(Anilinomethyl)-2-imidazoline HCl.
Use: Vasoconstrictor.

Phenameth DM. (Major) Promethazine HCl 6.25 mg, dextromethorphan HBr 15 mg/5 ml, alcohol. Syr. Bot. 120 ml. *Rx.*
Use: Antihistamine, antitussive.

Phenameth Tablets. (Major) Promethazine 25 mg. Tab. Bot. 1000s. *Rx.*
Use: Antiemetic, antihistamine.

Phenameth VC w/Codeine. (Major) Phenylephrine HCl 5 mg, promethazine HCl 6.25 mg, codeine phosphate 10 mg/5 ml, alcohol 7%. Syr. Bot. pt, gal. *c-v.*
Use: Antihistamine, antitussive, decongestant.

Phenameth w/Codeine. (Major) Promethazine HCl 6.25 mg, codeine phosphate 10 mg/5 ml, alcohol 7%. Syr. Bot. 4 oz, pt, gal. *c-v.*
Use: Antihistamine, antitussive.

phenantoin. Mephenytoin. N-Methyl-5,5-phenylethylhydantoin.
See: Mesantoin, Tab. (Novartis).

Phenapap Sinus Headache & Congestion. (Rugby) Pseudoephedrine HCl 30 mg, chlorpheniramine 2 mg, acetaminophen 325 mg. Tab. Bot. 30s, 100s, 1000s. *otc.*
Use: Analgesic, antihistamine, decongestant.

Phenaphen w/Codeine No. 3. (Robins) Codeine phosphate 30 mg, acetaminophen 325 mg/Tab. *c-III.*
Use: Analgesic combination, narcotic.

phenaphthazine. Sodium dinitro phenylazonaphthol disulfonate.
See: Nitrazine Paper, Roll (Bristol-Myers Squibb).

phenarsone sulfoxylate. (5-Arsono-2-hydroxyanilino)methanesulfinic acid disodium salt.
Use: Antiamebic.

Phenaspirin Compound. (Davis & Sly) Phenobarbital 0.25 gr, aspirin 3.5 gr. Cap. Bot. 1000s. *Rx.*
Use: Analgesic, hypnotic, sedative.

Phenate. (Roberts Pharm) Phenylpropanolamine HCl 40 mg, chlorpheniramine maleate 4 mg, acetaminophen 325 mg. CR Tab. Bot. 100s, 1000s. *Rx.*
Use: Analgesic, antihistamine, decongestant.

phenazocine hydrobromide.
Use: Analgesic.

phenazone.
See: Antipyrine (Various Mfr.).

•**phenazopyridine hydrochloride.** (fen-AZZ-oh-PIH-rih-deen) U.S.P. 23.
Use: Analgesic, urinary.
See: Azogesic, Tab. (Century Pharm).
Azo-Pyridon, Tab. (Solvay).
Azo-Standard, Tab. (PolyMedica).
Azo-Sulfizin (Solvay).
Phen-Azo, Tab. (Vangard).
Pyridium, Tab. (Warner Chilcott).
Uri-Pak (Westerfield).

phenazopyridine hydrochloride w/ combinations.
See: Azo Gantanol, Tab. (Roche Laboratories).
Azo Gantrisin, Tab. (Roche Laboratories).
Azosulfisoxazole (Various Mfr.).
Thiosulfil-A, Tab. (Wyeth Ayerst).
Thiosulfil-A Forte, Tab. (Wyeth Ayerst).

Triurisul, Tab. (Sheryl).
Uridium, Tab. (Ferndale; Pharmex).
Urisan-P, Tab. (Sandia).
Uritral, Cap. (Schwarz Pharma).
Urobiotic, Cap. (Pfizer).
Urogesic, Tab. (Edwards Pharmaceuticals).
Urotrol, Tab. (Mills).

•**phenbutazone sodium glycerate.** (fen-BYOO-tah-zone so-dee-uhm GLIH-seh-rate) USAN.
Use: Anti-inflammatory.

•**phencarbamide.** (FEN-car-BAM-id) USAN.
Use: Anticholinergic, spasmolytic.
See: Escorpal (Farben-Fabriken).

Phenchlor-Eight. (Freeport) Chlorpheniramine maleate 8 mg. TR Cap. Bot. 1000s. *Rx.*
Use: Antihistamine.

Phenchlor S.H.A. (Rugby) Phenylpropanolamine HCl 50 mg, phenylephrine HCl 25 mg, chlorpheniramine maleate 8 mg, hyoscyamine sulfate 0.19 mg, atropine sulfate 0.04 mg, scopolamine HBr 0.01mg/SR. Tab. Bot. 100s, 500s. *Rx.*
Use: Anticholinergic, antihistamine, decongestant.

Phenchlor-Twelve. (Freeport) Chlorpheniramine maleate 12 mg. TR Cap. Bot. 1000s. *Rx.*
Use: Antihistamine.

•**phencyclidine hydrochloride.** (fen-SIGH-klih-deen) USAN.
Use: Anesthetic.

•**phendimetrazine tartrate.** (fen-die-MEH-trah-zeen TAR-trate) U.S.P. 23.
Use: Appetite suppressant (systemic).
See: Adipost, Cap. (B.F. Ascher).
Adphen, Tab. (Ferndale Laboratories).
Anorex, Cap., Tab. (Dunhall Pharmaceuticals).
Bacarate, Tab. (Solvay).
Bontril PDM, Tab. (Carnrick Labs).
Bontril Slow Release, Cap. (Carnrick Labs).
Delcozine, Tab. (Delco).
Di-Ap-Trol, Tab. (Foy).
Elphemet, Tab. (Canright).
Limit, Tab. (Sanofi Winthrop).
Melfiat, Tab. (Solvay).
Obepar, Tab. (Parmed).
Obe-Tite, Tab. (Scott/Cord).
Phen-70, Tab. (Parmed).
Phenzine, Tab. (Roberts Pharm).
Prelu-2, Cap. (Boehringer Ingelheim).
Reducto, Tab. (Arcum).
Rexigen Forte, SR Cap. (ION Laboratories).
Slim-Tabs, Tab. (Wesley Pharmacal).
Statobex, Prods. (Teva USA).

Phendry. (LuChem) Diphenhydramine HCl 12.5 mg/5 ml, alcohol 14%. Elix. Bot. pt, gal. *otc.*
Use: Antihistamine.

Phendry Children's Allergy Medicine. (LuChem) Diphenhydramine HCl 12.5 mg/5 ml, alcohol 14%. Elix. Bot. 120 ml. *otc.*
Use: Antihistamine.

phenelzine dihydrogen sulfate.
See: Nardil, Tab. (Parke-Davis).

•**phenelzine sulfate.** (FEN-uhl-zeen) U.S.P. 23.
Use: Antidepressant.
See: Nardil, Tab. (Parke-Davis).

Phenerbel-S. (Rugby) Phenobarbital 40 mg, ergotamine tartrate 0.6 mg, l-alkaloids of belladonna 0.2 mg. Tab. Bot. 100s. *Rx.*
Use: Anticholinergic, hypnotic, sedative.

Phenergan-D. (Wyeth Ayerst) Promethazine HCl 6.25 mg, pseudoephedrine HCl 60 mg. Tab. Bot. 100s. *Rx.*
Use: Antihistamine, decongestant.

Phenergan Fortis. (Wyeth Ayerst) Promethazine HCl 25 mg/5 ml, alcohol 1.5%, saccharin. Bot. 473 ml. *Rx.*
Use: Antihistamine.

Phenergan Injection. (Wyeth Ayerst) Promethazine HCl 25 mg or 50 mg/ml, EDTA, phenol Inj. Amp. 1 mg. *Rx.*
Use: Antihistamine.

Phenergan Plain. (Wyeth Ayerst) Promethazine HCl 6.25 mg/5 ml, alcohol 7%, saccharin. Syr. Bot. 118 ml, 473 ml. *Rx.*
Use: Antihistamine.

Phenergan Suppositories. (Wyeth Ayerst) Promethazine HCl 12.5 mg, 25 mg or 50 mg. Supp. Box. 12s. *Rx.*
Use: Antihistamine.

Phenergan Syrup Plain. (Wyeth Ayerst) Promethazine HCl 6.25 mg/5 ml. Bot. 4 oz, 6 oz, 8 oz, pt, gal. *Rx.*
Use: Antihistamine.

Phenergan Tablets. (Wyeth Ayerst) Promethazine HCl 12.5 mg, 25 mg or 50 mg. Tab. Bot. 100s. Redipak 100s. *Rx.*
Use: Antihistamine.

Phenergan VC. (Wyeth Ayerst) Promethazine HCl 6.25 mg, phenylephrine HCl 5 mg/5 ml. Syr. Bot. 118 ml, 473 ml. *Rx.*
Use: Antihistamine, decongestant.

Phenergan VC with Codeine. (Wyeth Ayerst) Promethazine HCl 6.25 mg,

codeine phosphate 10 mg, phenylephrine HCl 5 mg/5 ml, alcohol 7%. Bot. 4 oz, 6 oz, 8 oz, pt, gal. *c-v.*
Use: Antihistamine, antitussive, decongestant.

Phenergan with Codeine. (Wyeth Ayerst) Promethazine HCl 6.25 mg, codeine phosphate 10 mg/5 ml. Bot. 4 oz, 6 oz, 8 oz, pt, gal. *c-v.*
Use: Antihistamine, antitussive.

Phenergan with Dextromethorphan. (Wyeth Ayerst) Promethazine HCl 6.25 mg, dextromethorphan HBr 15 mg/5 ml, alcohol 7%. Bot. 4 oz, 6 oz, pt, gal. *Rx.*
Use: Antihistamine, antitussive.

pheneridine.
Use: Analgesic.

i-phenethylbiguanide monohydrochloride. Phenformin HCl.

Phenex-1. (Ross Laboratories) Protein 15 g, fat 23.9 g, carbohydrates 46.3 g, linoleic acid 1800 mg, Fe 9 mg, Na 190 mg, K 675 mg, Cal 480/100 g. With appropriate vitamins and minerals. Phenylalanine free. Pow. Can 350 g. *otc.*
Use: Nutritional supplement.

Phenex-2. (Ross Laboratories) Protein 30 g, fat 15.5 g, carbohydrates 30 g, Na 880 mg, K 1370 mg, Cal 410/ml. With appropriate vitamins and minerals. Phenylalanine free. Pow. Can 325 g. *otc.*
Use: Nutritional supplement.

phenformin hydrochloride. *Rx.*
Use: Hypoglycemic.
Note: Withdrawn from market in 1978. Available under IND exemption.

Phenhist DH w/Codeine. (Rugby) Pseudoephedrine HCl 30 mg, chlorpheniramine maleate 2 mg, codeine phosphate 10 mg/5 ml, alcohol 5%. Liq. Bot. 120 ml, 480 ml. *c-v.*
Use: Antihistamine, antitussive, decongestant.

Phenhist Expectorant. (Rugby) Pseudoephedrine HCl 30 mg, codeine phosphate 10 mg, guaifenesin 100 mg/5 ml, alcohol 7.5%. Liq. Bot. 118 ml, pt, gal. *c-v.*
Use: Antihistamine, antitussive, decongestant.

pheniform.
See: Phenformin HCl.

•**phenindamine tartrate.** USAN.
Use: Antihistamine.
See: Nolahist, Tab. (Carnrick Labs).
W/Chlorpheniramine maleate, phenylpropanolamine HCl.
See: Nolamine, Tab. (Carnrick Labs).
W/Phenylephrine HCl, aspirin, caffeine, aluminum hydroxide, magnesium carbonate.
See: Dristan, Tab. (Whitehall Robins).
W/Phenylephrine HCl, caramiphen ethanedisulfonate.
See: Dondril, Tab. (Whitehall Robins).
W/Phenylephrine HCl, chlorpheniramine maleate, drytane.
See: Comhist, Tab., Elix. (Baylor).
W/Phenylephrine HCl, chlorpheniramine maleate, belladonna alkaloids.
See: Comhist L.A., Cap. (Baylor Labs).
W/Phenylephrine HCl, pyrilamine maleate, chlorpheniramine maleate, dextromethorphan HBr.
See: Histalet, Histalet-DM, Histalet-Forte, Syr. (Solvay).

pheniodol.
See: Iodoalphionic Acid (Various Mfr.).

pheniprazine hydrochloride. (α-Methylphenethyl)-hydrazine monohydrochloride.
Use: Antihypertensive.

•**pheniramine maleate.** USAN.
Use: Antihistamine.
See: Inhiston, Tab. (Schering Plough).
W/Combinations.
Allerstat, Cap. (Teva USA).
Chexit, Tab. (Novartis).
Citra Forte, Cap., Syr. (Boyle).
Partuss AC (Parmed).
Poly-Histine Cap., Elix., Lipospan (Sanofi Winthrop).
T.A.C., Cap. (Towne).
Thor, Cap. (Towne).
Tritussin, Syr. (Towne).
Vetuss HC, Syr. (Cypress).

•**phenmetrazine hydrochloride.** (fen-MEH-trah-zeen) U.S.P. 23.
Use: Anorexic.

•**phenobarbital.** (fee-no-BAR-bih-tahl) U.S.P. 23.
Use: Anticonvulsant, hypnotic, sedative.
See: Henomint, Elix. (Jones Medical Industries).
Hypnette, Supp., Tab. (Fleming).
Orprine, Liq. (Medeva).
Pheno-Square, Tab. (Roberts Pharm).
Solfoton, Tab., Cap. (ECR Pharmaceuticals).

phenobarbital. (Various Mfr.) **Tab.: 15 mg, 30 mg:** Bot. 100s, 1000s, 5000s, UD 100s; **60 mg:** Bot. 100s, 1000s, UD 100s; **100 mg:** 100s, 1000s. **Elixir:** 20 mg/5 ml. Bot. Pt, gal, UD 5 ml, UD 7.5 ml.
Use: Anticonvulsant, hypnotic, sedative.

phenobarbital. (Pharmaceutical Associates) 15 mg/5 ml. Elixir. Bot. Pt, UD 5 ml, 10 ml, 20 ml. *c-iv.*
Use: Anticonvulsant, hypnotic, sedative.

phenobarbital w/aminophylline.
See: Aminophylline (Various Mfr.).

phenobarbital w/atropine sulfate.
See: Atropine Sulfate (Various Mfr.).
P.A., Tab. (Scrip).

phenobarbital w/belladonna.
See: Belladonna Products and Phenobarbital Combinations.

phenobarbital with central nervous system stimulants.
See: Arcotrate No. 3, Tab. (Arcum).
Bronkolixir, Elix. (Sanofi Winthrop).
Bronkotab, Tab. (Sanofi Winthrop).
Quadrinal, Susp., Tab. (Knoll Pharmaceuticals).
Sedamine, Tab. (Dunhall Pharmaceuticals).
Spabelin, Elix., Tab. (Arcum).

phenobarbital combinations.
See: Aminophylline w/Phenobarbital, Combinations.
Aspirin-Barbiturate, Combinations.
Atropine-Hyoscine-Hyoscyamine Combinations.
Atropine Sulfate w/Phenobarbital.
Belladonna Extract Combinations.
Belladonna Products and Phenobarbital Combinations.
Bellatal, Tab. (Richwood).
Folergot-DF, Tab. (Marnel).
Homatropine Methylbromide and Phenobarbital Combinations.
Hyoscyamus Products and Phenobarbital Combinations.
Mannitol Hexanitrate w/Phenobarbital Combinations.
Mephenesin and Barbiturates Combinations.
Phenobarbital w/Central Nervous System Stimulants.
Secobarbital Combinations.
Sodium Nitrite Combinations.
Theobromine w/Phenobarbital Combinations.
Theophylline w/Phenobarbital Combinations.
Veratrum Viride w/Phenobarbital Combinations.

phenobarbital w/homatropine methylbromide.
See: Homatropine Methylbromide and Phenobarbital Combinations.

phenobarbital w/hyoscyamus.
See: Hyoscyamus Products and Phenobarbital Combinations.

phenobarbital w/mannitol hexanitrate.
Use: Anticonvulsant, sedative, hypnotic.
See: Mannitol Hexanitrate w/Phenobarbital Combinations.

•**phenobarbital sodium.** U.S.P. 23.
Use: Anticonvulsant, hypnotic, sedative.
See: Luminal Sodium, Inj. (Sanofi Winthrop).

phenobarbital sodium. (Wyeth Ayerst) Inj. **30 mg/ml, 60 mg/ml:** Tubex 1 ml; **65 mg/ml:** Vial 1 ml; **130 mg/ml:** Tubex 1 ml, vial 1 ml. *c-iv.*
Use: Anticonvulsant, hypnotic, sedative.

phenobarbital sodium in propylene glycol. Vitarine. Amp. 0.13 g: 1 ml, Box 25s, 100s. *c-iv.*
Use: Anticonvulsant, hypnotic, sedative.

phenobarbital and theobromine combinations.
See: Theobromine w/Phenobarbital Combinations.

phenobarbital w/theophylline.
See: Theophylline w/Phenobarbital Combinations.

phenobarbital w/veratrum viride.
See: Veratrum Viride w/Phenobarbital Combinations.

Pheno-Bella. (Ferndale Laboratories) Belladonna extract 10.8 mg, phenobarbital 16.2 mg/Tab. Bot. 100s, 1000s. *Rx.*
Use: Anticholinergic, antispasmodic, hypnotic, sedative.

•**phenol.** (FEE-nole) U.S.P. 23.
Use: Pharmaceutic aid (preservative), topical antipruritic.
W/Aluminum hydroxide, zinc oxide, camphor, eucalyptol, ichthammol, thyme oil.
See: Almophen, Oint. (Jones Medical Industries).
W/Benzocaine, triclosan.
See: Solarcaine Pump Spray (Schering Plough).
W/Dextromethorphan.
See: Chloraseptic DM Lozenges (Eaton Medical).
W/Resorcinol.
See: Black & White Ointment (Schering Plough).
W/Resorcinol, boric acid, basic fuchsin, acetone.
See: Castellani's Paint, Liq. (Various Mfr.).

•**phenol, liquefied.** U.S.P. 23.
Use: Topical antipruritic.

•**phenolate sodium.** (FEEN-oh-late) USAN.
Use: Disinfectant.

Phenolax. (Pharmacia & Upjohn) Phenolphthalein 64.8 mg/Wafer. Bot. 100s. *otc.*
Use: Laxative.

•**phenolphthalein.** (fee-nahl-THAY-leen) U.S.P. 23.
Use: Laxative.
See: Espotabs, Tab. (Combe).
Evac-U-Lax, Wafer (Roberts Pharm).
Evasof, Tab. (Teva USA).
Ex-Lax, Prods. (Novartis).
Feen-A-Mint, Tab., Gum (Schering Plough).
Phenolax, Wafer (Pharmacia & Upjohn).
Veracolate, Tab. (Numark Laboratories).

phenolphthalein. (Various Mfr.) Pkg. 1 oz, 0.25 lb, 1 lb.
Use: Laxative.

phenolphthalein w/combinations.
See: Correctol, Tab. (Schering Plough).
Dialose Plus, Cap. Tab. (Merck).
Evac-Q-Kit, Tab., Supp. (Warren-Teed).
Dual Formula Feen-A-Mint Pills (Schering Plough).
Feen-A-Mint, Gum, Mint, Pill (Schering Plough).
4-Way Cold Tab. (Bristol-Myers).
Phillips' Laxative Gel-Caps (Sterling Health).
Veracolate, Tab. (Numark).

phenolphthalein in liquid petrolatum emulsion. (Various Mfr.).
See: Petrolatum, Liq.

phenolphthalein. (Various Mfr.). Pkg. 1 oz, 0.25 lb., 1 lb.
Use: Laxative.

•**phenolphthalein yellow.** (fee-nahl-THAY-leen) U.S.P. 23.
Use: Laxative.

phenolsulfonates.
See: Sulfocarbolates.

phenolsulfonic acid. Sulfocarbolic acid.
Note: Used in Sulphodine, Tab. (Strasenburgh).

phenoltetrabromophthalein. Disulfonate Disodium.
See: Sulfobromophthalein Sodium, U.S.P. 23.

phenolzine sulfate.

Pheno Nux Tablets. (Pal-Pak) Phenobarbital 16.2 mg, nux vomica extract 8.1 mg, calcium carbonate 194.4 mg/Tab. Bot. 1000s. *c-IV.*
Use: Sedative, hypnotic, antacid.

Phenoptic. (Optopics) Phenylephrine HCl 2.5%. Soln. Bot. 2 ml, 5 ml, 15 ml. *Rx.*
Use: Mydriatic, vasoconstrictor.

phenothiazine. Thiodiphenylamine.

Phenoturic. (Truett) Phenobarbital 40 mg/5 ml. Elix. Bot. pt, gal. *c-IV.*
Use: Hypnotic, sedative.

•**phenoxybenzamine hydrochloride.** (fen-ox-ee-BEN-zuh-meen) U.S.P. 23.
Use: Antihypertensive.
See: Dibenzyline, Cap. (SmithKline Beecham Pharmaceuticals).

phenoxymethyl penicillin.
See: Penicillin V.

phenoxymethyl penicillin potassium.
See: Penicillin V Potassium.

phenoxynate. Mixture of phenylphenols 17-18%, octyl and related alkylphenols 2-3%.

•**phenprocoumon.** (fen-PRO-koo-mahn) USAN.
Use: Anticoagulant.
See: Liquamar, Tab. (Organon Teknika).

Phen-70. (Parmed) Phendimetrazine tartrate 70 mg/Tab. Bot. 100s, 1000s. *c-III.*
Use: Anorexiant.

•**phensuximide.** (fen-SUCK-sih-mide) U.S.P. 23.
Use: Anticonvulsant.
See: Milontin, Preps. (Parke-Davis).

Phental. (Armenpharm) Belladonna alkaloids, phenobarbital 0.25 gr/Tab. Bot. 1000s. *c-IV.*
Use: Anticholinergic, antispasmodic, hypnotic, sedative.

Phentamine. (Major) Phentermine HCl 30 mg/Cap. (equivalent to 24 mg base). Bot. 100s. *c-IV.*
Use: Anorexiant.

•**phentermine.** (FEN-ter-meen) USAN.
Use: Anorexic.
See: Adipex, Tab. (Teva USA).
Adipex-8 C.T., Cap. (Teva USA).
Adipex-P, Cap. (Teva USA).
Fastin, Cap. (SmithKline Beecham Pharmaceuticals).
Parmine, Cap. (Parmed).
Tora, Tab. (Solvay).
Wilpowr, Cap. (Foy).

phentermine as resin complex.
See: Ionamin, Cap. (Medeva).

•**phentermine hydrochloride.** (Fen-ter-meen) U.S.P. 23. Benzeneethanamine, α,α-dimethyl-, HCl.
Use: Appetite suppressant (systemic).
See: Zantryl, Cap. (ION Laboratories).

phentetiothalein sodium. Iso-Iodeikon.
Use: Radiopaque agent.

phentolamine hydrochloride. (fen-TOLE-uh-meen)
Use: Antihypertensive.
See: Regitine HCl, Tab. (Novartis).

•**phentolamine mesylate.** (fen-TOLE-uh-meen) U.S.P. 23. *Formerly Phentolamine Methanesulfonate.*
Use: Antiadrenergic.
See: Regitine Inj. (Novartis).

phentolamine methanesulfonate. Phentolamine mesylate, U.S.P. 23.

Phentolox w/APAP. (Global Source) Phenyltoloxamine citrate 30 mg, acetaminophen 325 mg/Tab. Bot. 1000s. *Rx.*
Use: Antihistamine, analgesic.

Phentox Compound. (Rosemont) Phenylpropanolamine HCl 20 mg, phenylephrine HCl 5 mg, chlorpheniramine maleate 2.5 mg, phenyltoloxamine citrate 7.5 mg/5 ml. Bot. pt, gal. *Rx.*
Use: Decongestant, antihistamine.

phentydrone.
Use: Systemic fungicide.

n-phenylacetamide.
See: Acetanilid (Various Mfr.).

phenylacetylurea.
See: Phenurone, Tab. (Abbott Laboratories).

phenylalanine ammonia-lyase.
Use: Hyperphenylalaninemia. [Orphan drug]

•**phenyl aminosalicylate.** (FEN-ill ah-MEE-no-sah-LIH-sih-late) USAN.
Use: Anti-infective.

•**phenylalanine.** (fen-ill-AL-ah-NEEN) U.S.P. 23.
Use: Amino acid.
See: Phenylketonuria therapy.

phenylalanine mustard.
See: Melphalan, U.S.P. 23. analgesic.

phenylazo-diamino-pyridine.
See: Phenazopyridine (Various Mfr.).

phenylazo-diamino-pyridine hcl or hbr.
See: Phenazopyridine HCl or HBr (Various Mfr.).

phenylazo-diaminopyridine hydrochloride.

phenylazo sulfisoxazole. (A.P.C.) Sulfisoxazole 0.5 g, phenylazopyridine 50 mg/Tab. Bot. 1000s. *Rx.*
Use: Anti-infective, sulfonamide.

phenylazo tablets. (A.P.C.) Phenylazodiamino-pyridine HCl 1.5 gr/Tab. Bot. 1000s. *Rx.*
Use: Analgesic, urinary.

•**phenylbutazone.** (fen-ill-BYOO-tah-zone) U.S.P. 23.
Use: Antirheumatic.

phenylbutyrate sodium.
Use: Treatment of blood disorders. [Orphan drug]

phenylcarbinol.
See: Benzyl Alcohol, N.F. 18.

phenylcinchoninic acid. Name used for cinchophen.

•**phenylephrine hydrochloride.** (fen-ill-EFF-rin) U.S.P. 23.
Use: Adrenergic, mydriatic, sympathomimetic, vasoconstrictor.
See: AH-Chew D, Chew. Tab. (WE Pharm).
AK-Dilate (Akorn).
AK-Nefrin (Akorn).
Alcon-Efrin, Soln. (PolyMedica).
Allerest Nasal Spray (Novartis).
Coricidin Decongestant Nasal Mist (Schering Plough).
Ephrine, Spray (Walgreens).
Isopto Frin (Alcon Laboratories).
Mydfrin 2.5% (Alcon Laboratories).
Neo-Synephrine HCl, Preps. (Sanofi Winthrop).
Phenoptic (Optopics).
Prefrin Liquifilm Ophth. Soln. (Allergan).
Pyracort-D, Spray (Teva USA).
Relief (Allergan).
Sinarest, Nasal Spray (Novartis).
Super-Anahist Nasal Spray (Warner Lambert).

W/Combinations.
See: Acotus, Liq. (Whorton).
Anodynos Forte, Tab. (Buffington).
Atuss DM, Syr. (Atley).
Atuss G, Syr. (Atley).
Atuss HD, Liq. (Atley).
Bur-Tuss Expectorant (Burlington).
Cenahist, Cap. (Century Pharm).
Cenaid, Tab. (Century Pharm).
Chlor-Trimeton Expectorant (Schering Plough).
Chlor-Trimeton Expectorant w/Codeine (Schering Plough).
Coldloc, Elix. (Flemming).
Conar, Susp., Expectorant (SmithKline Beecham Pharmaceuticals).
Conar-A, Tab., Susp. (SmithKline Beecham Pharmaceuticals).
Congespirin, Tab. (Bristol-Myers).
Coricidin Demilets (Schering Plough).
Dallergy, Syr., Cap., Tab., Inj. (Laser).
Demazin, Syr. (Schering Plough).
Diabetic Tussin, Liq. (Roberts Pharm).
Dimetane Decongestant, Tab., Elix. (Robins).

Dimetane Expectorant, Liq. (Robins).
Dimetane Expectorant-DC, Liq. (Robins).
Dimetapp, Elix., Extentabs (Robins).
Doktors, Drops, Spray (Scherer).
Eldatapp, Tab., Liq. (ICN Pharmaceuticals).
Entex, Prods. (Procter & Gamble Pharm).
Ex-Histine, Syr. (WE Pharma).
Eye-Gene, Soln. (Pearson).
4 Way Tab., Spray (Bristol-Myers).
Furacin Nasal Soln. (Eaton Medical).
Guaifenex, Liq. (Ethex).
Guiatex, Preps. (Rugby).
Histabid, Cap. (Meyer).
Histapp Prods. (Upsher-Smith Labs).
Histaspan-D, Cap. (Rhone-Poulenc Rorer).
Histaspan-Plus, Cap. (Rhone-Poulenc Rorer).
Histinex HC, Syr. (Ethex).
Hydrocodone CP, Liq. (Morton Grove).
Hydrocodone HD, Liq. (Morton Grove).
Iodal HD, Liq. (Iomed).
Iotussin HC, Syr. (Iomed).
Liquibid-D, SR Tab. (ION).
Mydfrin Ophthalmic, Liq. (Alcon Laboratories).
Nasahist, Cap. (Keene Pharmaceuticals).
Norel, Cap. (US Pharmaceutical).
Pediacof, Syr. (Sanofi Winthrop).
Phenoptic, Soln. (Muro).
Phenylzin Drops, Ophth. Soln. (Ciba Vision Ophthalmics).
Prefrin-A Ophth. Soln. (Allergan).
Prefrin-Z Ophth. Soln. (Allergan).
Pyristan, Cap., Elix. (Arcum).
Rhinall, Liq. (Scherer).
Rhinex DM, Tab. (Teva USA).
Rymed, Prods. (Edwards Pharmaceuticals).
Sil-Tex, Liq. (Silarx).
Sinex, Nasal Spray (Procter & Gamble).
Singlet, Tab. (Hoechst Marion Roussel).
Spec-T Sore Throat-Decongestant Loz. (Bristol-Myers Squibb).
Sucrets Cold Decongestant Loz. (SmithKline Beecham Pharmaceuticals).
Trind, Liq. (Bristol-Myers).
Trind-DM, Liq. (Bristol-Myers).
Tri-Ophtho, Soln. (Maurry).
Turbilixir, Liq. (Burlington).
Turbispan Leisurecaps, Cap. (Burlington).
Tussar-DM, Liq. (Rhone-Poulenc Rorer).
Tympagesic, Liq. (Pharmacia & Upjohn).
Unituss HC, Syr. (URL).
Vasocidin, Ophth. Soln. (Ciba Vision Ophthalmics).
Vasosulf, Ophth. Soln. (Novartis).
Vetuss HC, Syr. (Cypress).

phenylephrine hydrochloride. (Various Mfr.) **Ophth. Soln. 2.5%:** Bot. 15 ml; **10%:** Bot. 2 ml, 5 ml. **Inj. 1%:** Vial 5 ml. *Rx.*
Use: Adrenergic, mydriatic, sympathomimetic, vasoconstrictor.

Phenylephrine tannate, chlorpheniramine tannate and pyrilamine tartrate. (Zenith Forest Pharmaceutical) Phenylephrine tannate 25 mg, chlorpheniramine tannate 8 mg, pyrilamine tannate 25 mg/Tab. Bot. 100s, 500s. *Rx.*
Use: Antihistamine, decongestant.

•**phenylethyl alcohol.** (fen-ill-ETH-ill) U.S.P. 23.
Use: Pharmaceutic aid (antimicrobial).

phenyl-ethyl-hydrazine, beta. Phenelzine dihydrogen sulfate.
See: Nardil, Tab. (Parke-Davis).

phenylethylmalonylurea.
See: Phenobarbital (Various Mfr.).

Phenylfenesin L.A. (Zenith Forest Pharmaceutical) Phenylpropanolamine HCl 75 mg, guaifenesin 400 mg/ER Tab. Bot. 100s, 500s. *Rx.*
Use: Decongestant, expectorant.

Phenylgesic Tabs. (Zenith Forest Pharmaceutical) Phenyltoloxamine citrate 30 mg, acetaminophen 325 mg/ Bot. 100s, 1000s. *otc.*
Use: Analgesic, antihistamine.

phenylic acid.
See: Phenol, U.S.P. 23.

•**phenylmercuric acetate.** (fen-ill-mer-CURE-ik ASS-eh-tate) N.F. 18.
Use: Pharmaceutic aid (antimicrobial), preservative (bacteriostatic).

W/9-Aminoacridine HCl, tyrothricin, urea, lactose.
See: Trinalis, Vaginal Supp. (Poly-Medica).

W/Benzocaine, chlorothymol, resorcin.
See: Lanacane Creme (Combe).

W/Boric acid, polyoxyethylenenonylphenol or oxyquinoline benzoate.
See: Koromex, Preps. (Holland-Rantos).

W/Methylbenzethonium Cl.
See: Norforms, Aerosol, Supp. (Procter & Gamble Pharm).

phenylmercuric acetate. (Various Mfr.) Bot. 1 lb, 5 lb, 10 lb.
Use: Pharmaceutic aid (antimicrobial), preservative (Bacteriostatic).

phenylmercuric borate. (F. W. Berk) Pkg. Custom packed.
W/Benzyl alcohol, benzocaine, butyl p-aminobenzoate.
See: Dermathyn, Oint. (Davis & Sly).

phenylmercuric chloride. Chlorophenylmercury.

•**phenylmercuric nitrate.** N.F. 18.
Use: Pharmaceutic aid (antimicrobial); preservative (bacteriostatic).
See: Preparation H, Oint., Supp. (Whitehall Robins).
W/Amyl, phenylphenol complex.
See: Lubraseptic Jelly (Guardian Laboratories).
W/Undecylenic acid.
See: Bridex, Oint. (Briar).

phenylmercuric nitrate. (A.P.L.) **Oint. 1:1500**, 1 oz, 4 oz, lb. (Chicago Pharm) Loz. w/benzocaine. Bot. 100s, 1000s. **Ophth. Oint., 1:3000**, Tube ⅛ oz. **Soln. 1:20,000**, Bot. pt, gal. **Vaginal supp., 1:5000**, Box 12s.
Use: Pharmaceutic aid (antimicrobial), preservative (bacteriostatic).

phenylmercuric picrate.
Use: Antimicrobial.

phenylphenol-o.
W/Amyl complex, phenylmercuric nitrate.
See: Lubraseptic Jelly. (Guardian Laboratories).

•**phenylpropanolamine bitartrate.** (fen-ill-pro-pan-OLE-uh-meen bye-TAR-trate) U.S.P. 23.

•**phenylpropanolamine hydrochloride.** (fen-ill-pro-pan-OLE-uh-meen) U.S.P. 23.
Use: Adrenergic (vasoconstrictor).
See: Maximum Strength Dexatrim, ER Tab. (Thompson Medical).
Obestat, Cap. (Teva USA).
Obestat 150, Cap. (Teva USA).
Propadrine HCl, Preps. (Merck).
Propagest, Tab. (Carnrick Labs).
Spray-U-Thin (Caprice Greystoke).

phenylpropanolamine hydrochloride w/combinations.
See: Allerest, Prods. (Novartis).
Allerstat, Cap. (Teva USA).
Alka-Seltzer Plus Sinus, Tab. (Bayer).
Antihist-D, Tab. (Zenith-Goldline).
A.R.M., Tab. (SmithKline Beecham Pharmaceuticals).
Bayer, Prods. (Bayer Corp).
BQ Cold, Tab. (Bristol-Myers).
Breacol Cough Medication, Liq. (Bayer Corp).
Bur-Tuss Expectorant (Burlington).
Chexit, Tab. (Novartis).
Coldloc, Elix. (Flemming).
Coldloc-LA, SR Capl. (Flemming).
Comtrex, Cap., Liq., Tab. (Bristol-Myers).
Congespirin, Liq., Tab. (Bristol-Myers).
Contac, Prods. (SmithKline Beecham Pharmaceuticals).
Cophene No. 2, Cap. (Dunhall Pharmaceuticals).
Coricidin Cough Formula (Schering Plough).
Coricidin "D" Decongestant, Tab. (Schering Plough).
Coricidin Sinus Headache, Tab. (Schering Plough).
Coryban-D, Cap. (Pfizer).
Dex-A-Diet, Prods. (Columbia).
Detatrim Plus Viatmins, TR Capl. (Thompson).
Dezest, Cap. (Geneva Pharm).
Dimetane Expectorant, Liq. (Robins).
Dimetapp, Elix., Extentabs (Robins).
Dynafed Asthma Relief, Tab. (BDI).
Entex, Cap., Liq. (Procter & Gamble Pharm).
Entex LA, Tab. (Procter & Gamble Pharm).
Guaifenex, Liq. (Ethex).
Guaifenex PPA 75, ER Tab. (Ethex).
Guiatex, Prods. (Rugby).
Halls Mentho-Lyptus Cough Formula, Liq. (Warner Lambert).
Histabid, Cap. (GlaxoWellcome).
Histalet Forte T. D., Tab. (Solvay).
Hista-Vadrin, Syr., Tab., Cap. (Scherer).
Hydrocodone PA Pediatric, Syr. (Morton Grove).
Iohist DM, Syr. (Iomed).
Kleer Compound, Tab. (Scrip).
Liquibid-D, SR Tab. (ION).
Liqui-Histine DM, Syr. (Liquipharm).
Meditussin-X, Liq. (Roberts Pharm).
Naldecon, Drop, Syr., Tab. (Bristol-Myers).
Nasahist, Cap., Inj. (Keene Pharmaceuticals).
Nolamine, Tab. (Carnrick Labs).
Norel, Cap. (US Pharmaceutical).
Ornade, Cap. (SmithKline Beecham Pharmaceuticals).
Ornex, Cap. (SmithKline Beecham Pharmaceuticals).
Panadyl, Tab., Cap. (Misemer).
Pannaz, Tab. (Pan Am Labs).
Partuss-A, Tab. (Parmed).

Partuss T.D., Tab. (Parmed).
Pediacon DX Children's, Syr. (Zenith Goldline).
Pediacon DX Pediatric, Drops (Zenith Goldline).
Pediacon EX, Drops (Zenith Goldline).
Phenadex Children's Cough/Cold, Syr. (Barre-National).
Phenadex Pediatric Cough/Cold, Drops (Barre-National).
Phenylfenesin LA, EA Tab. (Zenith Goldline).
Profen LA, TR Tab. (Wakefield).
Profen II DM, TR Tab. (Wakefield).
Pyristan, Cap., Elix. (Arcum).
Rhinex DM, Liq. (Teva USA).
Rymed, Prods. (Edwards Pharmaceuticals).
Sanhist TD, Tab., Vial (Sandia).
Santussin, Cap., Susp. (Sandia).
Silaminic Expectorant, Liq. (Silarx).
Sildicon-E, Ped. Drops (Silarx).
Siltapp with Dextromethoprphan HBr Cold & Cough, Elix. (Silarx).
Sil-Tex, Liq. (Silarx).
Siltussin-CF, Liq. (Silarx).
Sinarest, Tab. (Pharmcraft).
Sine-Off, Tab. (SmithKline Beecham Pharmaceuticals).
Sinulin, Tab. (Carnrick Labs).
Spec-T Sore Throat-Decongestant, Loz. (Bristol-Myers Squibb).
St. Joseph Cold Tablets for Children (Schering Plough).
Sto-Caps, Cap. (Jalco).
Sucrets Cold Decongestant Loz. (SmithKline Beecham Pharmaceuticals).
Triaminic, Preps. (Novartis).
Triaminicin, Chew. Tab. (Novartis).
Triaminicol, Syr. (Novartis).
Turbilixir, Liq. (Burlington).
Turbispan Leisurecaps, Cap. (Burlington).
Tusquelin, Syr. (Circle).
Tussagesic, Susp., Tab. (Novartis).
U.R.I., Cap., Liq. (ICN Pharmaceuticals).
Vanex Forte-R, ER Cap. (Schwarz Pharma).

phenylpropanolamine hydrochloride & chlorpheniramine maleate capsules. (Various Mfr.) Chlorpheniramine maleate 12 mg, pseudoephedrine HCl 75 mg/Cap. Bot. 50s, 100s, 1000s. *otc, Rx.*
Use: Antihistamine, decongestant.

phenylpropanolamine hydrochloride & guaifenesin tablets. (fen-ill-pro-pan-OLE-uh-meen HIGH-droe-KLOR-ide & GWH-fen-ah-sin) (Various Mfr.) Phenylpropanolamine HCl 75 mg, guaifenesin 400 mg. Tab. Bot. 100s, 500s. *c-III.*
Use: Decongestant, expectorant.

phenylpropanolamine hydrochloride & hydrocodone syrup. (Rosemont) Phenylpropanolamine HCl 25 mg, hydrocodone bitartrate 5 mg. Bot. 480 ml.
Use: Antitussive, decongestant.

•**phenylpropanolamine polistirex.** (fen-ill-pro-pan-OLE-ah-meen pahl-ee-STIE-rex) USAN.
Use: Adrenergic (vasoconstrictor).

phenylpropylmethylamine hydrochloride. Vonedrine HCl.

phenyl salicylate. Salol.
W/Atropine sulfate, hyoscyamine, methenamine, methylene blue, gelsemium, benzoic acid.
See: U-Tract, Tab. (Jones Medical Industries).
W/Euphorbia extract and various oils.
See: Rayderm Oint. (Velvet Pharmacal).
W/Methenamine, methylene blue, benzoic acid, hyoscyamine alkaloid, atropine sulfate.
See: Urised, Tab. (PolyMedica).
UTA, Tab. (ICN Pharmaceuticals).
W/Methenamine, sodium biphosphate, methylene blue, hyoscyamine, alkaloid.
See: Urostat Forte, Tab. (ICN Pharmaceuticals).

phenyl-tert-butylamine.
See: Phentermine.

phenylthilone.
Use: Anticonvulsant.

phenyltoloxamine citrate.
Use: Antihistamine.

phenyltoloxamine citrate w/combinations.
See: Dengesic, Tab. (Scott-Alison).
Dilone, Tab. (Procter & Gamble).
Meditussin-X, Liq. (Roberts Pharm).
Myocalm, Tab. (Parmed).
Naldecon, Preps. (Bristol-Myers).
Poly-histine Prods. (Sanofi Winthrop).
S.A.C. Sinus, Tab. (Towne).
Scotgesic, Elix., Cap. (Scott/Cord).

phenyltoloxamine resin w/combinations.
See: Tussionex, Cap., Liq., Tab. (Medeva).

Phenylzin. (Ciba Vision Ophthalmics) Zinc sulfate 0.25%, phenylephrine HCl 0.12%. Bot. 15 ml. *Rx.*
Use: Decongestant, ophthalmic.

•**phenyramidol hydrochloride.** (FEN-ih-

RAM-ih-dole) USAN.
Use: Analgesic; muscle relaxant.

phenythilone.

•**phenytoin.** (FEN-ih-toe-in) U.S.P. 23. *Formerly Diphenylhydantoin.*
Use: Anticonvulsant.
See: Dilantin Prods. (Parke-Davis).
Di-phenyl, TR Cap. (Drug. Ind.).
Ekko, Cap. (Fleming).

phenytoin. (Alpharma) Phenytoin 125 mg/5 ml. Oral Susp. Bot. 240 ml. *Rx.*
Use: Anticonvulsant.

•**phenytoin sodium.** (FEN-in-toe-in) U.S.P. 23. *Formerly Diphenylhydantoin Sodium.*
Use: Anticonvulsant, cardiac depressant (antiarrhythmic).
See: Dilantin Sodium, Preps. (Parke-Davis).
Ekko Jr. and Sr., Cap. (Fleming).

phenytoin sodium with phenobarbital.
Use: Anticonvulsant.
See: Dilantin with Phenobarbital Kapseals, Cap. (Parke-Davis).

pheochromocytoma, agents for.
See: Demser, Cap. (Merck).
Dibenzyline, Cap. (SmithKline Beecham Pharmaceuticals).
Regitine, Inj. (Novartis) Pharm).

Pherazine DM. (Halsey) Promethazine 6.25 mg, dextromethorphan HBr 15 mg, alcohol 7%/5 ml. Bot. 4 oz, 6 oz, pt, gal. *Rx.*
Use: Antihistamine, antitussive.

Pherazine VC with Codeine Syrup. (Halsey) Phenylephrine HCl 5 mg, promethazine HCl 6.25 mg, codeine phosphate 10 mg, alcohol 7%/5 ml. Bot. pt, gal. *c-v.*
Use: Antihistamine, antitussive, decongestant.

Pherazine VC Syrup. (Halsey) Phenylephrine HCl 5 mg, promethazine HCl 6.25 mg, alcohol 7%/5 ml. Bot. pt, gal. *Rx.*
Use: Antihistamine, decongestant.

Pherazine w/Codeine. (Halsey) Promethazine HCl 6.25 mg, codeine phosphate 10 mg/5 ml, alcohol 7%, sorbitol, sucrose. Syr. Bot. 120 ml, pt, gal. *c-v.*
Use: Antihistamine, antitussive.

phetharbital.

phethenylate. Also sodium salt.

Phicon. (T.E. Williams) Pramoxine HCl 0.5%, vitamin A 7500 IU, E 2000 IU/30 g. Cream. Tube 60 g. *otc.*
Use: Anesthetic, local.

Phicon F. (T.E. Williams) Undecylenic acid 8%, pramoxine HCl 0.05%. Cream. 60 g. *otc.*
Use: Anesthetic, local; antifungal,.

Phillips' Chewable. (Bayer Corp) Magnesium hydroxide 311 mg. Tab. 100s, 200s.
Use: Laxative, antacid.

Phillips' Laxcaps. (Bayer Corp) Docusate sodium 83 mg, phenolphthalein 90 mg/Cap. Bot. 8s, 24s, 48s. *otc.*
Use: Laxative.

Phillips' Milk of Magnesia. (Bayer Corp) Magnesium hydroxide. Reg. and Mint. Bot. 4 oz, 12 oz, 26 oz; Tab. Bot. 30s, 100s, 200s. *otc.*
Use: Laxative, antacid.

Phillips' Milk of Magnesia Concentrated. (Bayer Corp) Magnesium hydroxide 800 mg/5 ml, sorbitol, sugar. Liq. Bot. 240 ml. *otc.*
Use: Antacid.

Phish Omega. (Pharmics) Natural salmon oil concentrate containing EPA 120 mg, DHA 100 mg/Cap. Bot. 60s. *otc.*
Use: Vitamin Supplement.

Phish Omega Plus. (Pharmics) Natural fish oil concentrate containing EPA 300 mg, DHA 200 mg/Cap. Bot. 60s. *otc.*
Use: Vitamin supplement.

pHisoDerm. (Chattem Consumer Products) Sodium octoxynol-2 ethane sulfonate, white petrolatum, water, mineral oil (with lanolin alcohol and oleyl alcohol), sodium benzoate, octoxynol-3, tetrasodium EDTA, methylcellulose, cocamide MEA, imidazolidinyl urea.
Regular: 150 ml, 270 ml, 480 ml, gal.
Oily skin: 150 ml, 480. *otc.*
Use: Dermatologic, cleanser.

pHisoDerm for Baby. (Chattem Consumer Products) Sodium octoxynol-2 ethane sulfonate, petrolatum, octoxynol-3, mineral oil (with lanolin alcohol and oleyl alcohol), cocamide MEA, imidazolidinyl urea, sodium benzoate, tetrasodium EDTA, methylcellulose, hydrochloric acid. Liq. Bot. 150 ml, 270 ml. *otc.*
Use: Dermatologic, cleanser.

pHisoDerm Gentle Cleansing Bar. (Chattem Consumer Products) Sodium tallowate, sodium cocoate, petrolatum, glycerin, lanolin, sodium Cl, BHT, trisodium EDTA, titanium dioxide. Bar 99 g. *otc.*
Use: Dermatologic, cleanser.

pHisoHex. (Sanofi Winthrop) Entsufon sodium, hexachlorophene 3%, petrolatum, lanolin cholesterols, methylcellu-

lose, polyethylene glycol, polyethylene glycol monostearate, lauryl myristyl diethanolamide, sodium benzoate, water, pH adjusted with hydrochloric acid. Emulsion, Bot. 5 oz, pt, gal. Wall dispensers pt. Unit packets 0.25 oz. Box 50s, Pedal operated dispenser 30 oz. *otc.*
Use: Antimicrobial, antiseptic.

pHisoMed. (Sanofi Winthrop) Hexachlorophene. *otc.*
Use: Antimicrobial, antiseptic.

pHisoPuff. (Sanofi Winthrop) Nonmedicated cleansing sponge. Box sponge 1s. *otc.*
Use: Dermatologic, cleanser.

PhosChol. (American Lecithin) Phosphatidycholine (highly purified lecithin). **Softgel:** 565 mg or 900 mg. Bot. 100s, 300s. **Liq. Conc.:** 3000 mg/5 ml. Bot. 240 ml, 480 ml. *otc.*
Use: Nutritional supplement.

phoscolic acid.
Use: Adjuvant.

Phos-Flur Oral Rinse Supplement. (Colgate Oral) Acidulated phosphate sodium fluoride 0.05%, fluoride 1 ml/5 ml. Bot. 250 ml, 500 ml, gal. *Rx.*
Use: Dental caries preventative.

PhosLo. (Braintree Laboratories) Calcium acetate 667 mg (calcium 169 mg)/Tab. Bot. 200s. *Rx.*
Use: Electrolytes, mineral supplement.

phosphate.
See: Potassium Phosphate, Inj. (Abbott Laboratories).
Sodium Phosphate, Inj. (Abbott Laboratories).

phosphentaside. Adenosine-5-monophosphate. Adenylic acid.
W/Vitamin B_{12}, niacin.
See: Denylex Gel, Vial (Westerfield).
W/Vitamin B_{12}, niacin, B_1.
See: Adenolin, Vial (Lincoln).

phosphocol P32. (Mallinckrodt) Chromic phosphate P32: 15 mCi with a concentration of up to 5 mCi/ml and specific activity of up to 5 mCi/mg at time of standardization. Susp. Vial 10 ml.
Use: Radiopharmaceutical.

phosphocysteamine.
Use: Cystinosis. [Orphan drug]

Phospholine Iodide. (Wyeth Ayerst) Echothiophate Iodide for Ophthalmic Solution. 0.03%, 0.06%, 0.125% and 0.25% potencies/5 ml of sterile eye drops. Package: 1.5 mg for 0.03%; 3 mg for 0.06%; 6.25 mg for 0.125%; 12.5 mg for 0.25% w/5 ml diluent. *Rx.*
Use: Antiglaucoma.

phospholipids, soy.
See: Granulestin Concentrate, Gran. (Associated Concentrates).

phosphonoformic acid.
See: Foscarnet sodium.

phosphorated carbohydrate solution.
See: Emetrol, Liq. (Sanofi Winthrop).
Naus-A-Way, Soln. (Roberts Pharm).
Nausea Relief, Soln. (Zenith Goldline).
Nausetrol, Soln. (Various Mfr.).

•**phosphoric acid.** (foo-FORE-ik) N.F. 18.
Use: Pharmaceutic aid (solvent).

phosphoric acid, diluted.
Use: Pharmaceutic aid (solvent).

phosphorus.
Use: Phosphorus replacement.
See: Uro-KP-Neutral, Tab. (Star).
K-Phos Neutral, Tab. (Beach Pharmaceuticals).
Neutra-Phos, Cap., Pow. (Baker Norton).
Neutra-Phos-K, Cap., Pow. (Baker Norton).

Phospho-Soda. (C.B. Fleet) Sodium biphosphate 48 g, sodium phosphate 18 g/100 ml. Bot. 1.5 oz, 3 oz, 8 oz. Flavored, unflavored. *otc.*
Use: Laxative.

Phosphotec. (Bristol-Myers Squibb) Technetium Tc 99m pyrophosphate kit. 10 vials/kit.
Use: Radiodiagnostic.

Photofrin. (QLT Photo) Porfimer sodium 75 mg. Freeze-dried cake or powder. *Rx.*
Use: Antineoplastic.

Photoplex Sunscreen. (Allergan) Butyl methoxydibenzoylmethane 3%, padimate O 7%. Lot. 120 ml. *otc.*
Use: Sunscreen.

Phrenilin Forte Capsules. (Schwarz Pharma) Acetaminophen 650 mg, butalbital 50 mg/Cap. Bot. 100s, 500s. *Rx.*
Use: Analgesic, hypnotic, sedative.

Phrenilin Tablets. (Schwarz Pharma) Butalbital 50 mg, acetaminophen 325 mg/Tab. Bot. 100s. *Rx.*
Use: Analgesic, hypnotic, sedative.

Phrenilin with Codeine #3. (Schwarz Pharma) Acetaminophen 325 mg, butalbital 50 mg, codeine phosphate 30 mg/Cap. Bot. 100s. *c-III.*
Use: Analgesic combination, hypnotic, sedative.

Phresh 3.5 Finnish Cleansing Liquid. (3M Products) Water, cocamidopropyl betaine, lactic acid, polyoxyethylene

distearate, polyoxyethylene monostearate, hydroxyethyl cellulose, sodium phosphate, methylparaben. Bot. 6 oz. *otc.*
Use: Soapless cleansing agent.

pH-Stabil Cream. (Hermal) Skin protection cream. Bot. 8 oz. Tube 2 oz. *otc.*
Use: Dermatologic.

Phthalamaquin. (Penick) Quinetolate.
Use: Antiasthmatic.

phthalazine, i-hydrazino-, monohydrochloride. Hydralazine Hydrochloride, U.S.P. 23.

phylcardin.
See: Aminophylline (Various Mfr.).

phyllindon.
See: Aminophylline (Various Mfr.).

Phyllocontin. (Purdue Frederick) Aminophylline 225 mg/CR Tab. Bot. 100s. *Rx.*
Use: Bronchodilator.

phylloquinone. 2-Methyl-3-phytyl-1,4-naphthoquinine, vitamin K.
See: Phytonadione, U.S.P., Inj., Tab. (Various Mfr.).
Vitamin K-1 (Various Mfr.).

Phylorinol Liquid. (Schaffer) Phenol 0.6%, boric acid, strong iodine solution, sorbitol 70% solution, sodium copper chlorophyll. 240 ml. *otc.*
Use: Mouth and throat preparation.

Phylorinol Mouthwash. (Schaffer) Phenol 0.6%, methyl salicylate, sorbitol. Mouthwash. 240 ml. *otc.*
Use: Mouth and throat preparation.

physiological irrigating solution.
See: TIS-U-SOL, Soln. (Baxter).
Physiosol, Soln. (Abbott Laboratories).
Physiolyte, Soln. (American McGaw).

Physiolyte. (American McGaw) Sodium Cl 530 mg, sodium acetate 370 mg, sodium gluconate 500 mg, potassium Cl 37 mg, magnesium Cl 30 mg/100 ml. Soln. Bot. 500 ml, 2 L, 4 L. *Rx.*
Use: Irrigant, ophthalmic.

PhysioSol Irrigation. (Abbott Hospital Prods) Bot. 250 ml, 500 ml, 1000 ml glass or Aqualite (semi-rigid) containers. *Rx.*
Use: Irrigant, ophthalmic.

•**physostigmine.** (fie-zoe-STIG-meen) U.S.P. 23. An alkaloid.
Use: Cholinergic (ophthalmic).

•**physostigmine salicylate.** U.S.P. 23.
Use: Cholinergic (ophthalmic); parasympathomimetic agent, Friedreich's and other inherited ataxias [Orphan drug]
See: Antilirium, Amp. (Forest Pharmaceutical).
Isopto-Eserine, Ophthalmic, Soln. (Alcon Laboratories).
W/l-Hyoscyamine HBr.
See: Phyatromine-H, Amp., Vial (Kremers Urban).
W/Pilocarpine, methylcellulose.
See: Isopto P-ES, Soln. (Alcon Laboratories).

physostigmine salicylate. (Forest Pharmaceutical) Pow., Tube 1 gr, 5 gr, 15 gr.
Use: Cholinergic (ophthalmic).

•**physostigmine sulfate.** U.S.P. 23.
Use: Cholinergic (ophthalmic).

•**phytate persodium.** (FIE-tate per-SO-dee-uhm) USAN.
Use: Pharmaceutic aid.

•**phytate sodium.** (FIE-tate) USAN. Sodium salt of inositol hexaphosphoric acid.
Use: Chelating agent (calcium).

phytic acid. Inositol hexophosphoric acid.

phytonadiol sodium diphosphate.

•**phytonadione.** (fye-toe-nuh-DIE-ohn) U.S.P. 23.
Use: Vitamin (prothrombogenic).
See: Aquamephyton, Inj. (Merck).
Konakion, Amp. (Roche Laboratories).
Mephyton, Tab. (Merck).

phytonadione. (IMS, Ltd.) 2 mg/ml (Vitamin K_1). Inj. 0.5 ml, Min-I-ject prefilled syringes. *Rx.*
Use: Vitamin (prothrombogenic).

•**picenadol hydrochloride.** (pih-SEN-AID-ole) USAN.
Use: Analgesic.

•**piclamilast.** (pih-KLAM-ill-ast) USAN.
Use: Antiasthmatic (type IV phosphodiesterase inhibitor).

•**picotrin diolamine.** (PIH-koe-trin die-OH-lah-meen) USAN.
Use: Keratolytic.

picric acid, trinitrophenol.
See: Butesyn Picrate, Oint. (Abbott Laboratories).
Silver Salts (Various Prods.).

picrotoxin. Cocculin.
Use: Respiratory.

•**picumeterol fumarate.** (PIKE-you-MEH-teh-role) USAN.
Use: Bronchodilator.

P.I.D.
See: Phenindione (Various Mfr.).

•**pifarnine.** (pih-FAR-neen) USAN.
Use: Antiulcerative (gastric).

Pilagan. (Allergan) Pilocarpine nitrate 1%, 2% or 4%. Soln. Bot. 15 ml. *Rx.*
Use: Antiglaucoma.

Pilocar. (Ciba Vision Ophthalmics) Pilocarpine HCl 0.5%, 1%, 2%, 3%, 4% or 6%. Bot. 15 ml; Twinpack 2 × 15 ml 0.5%, 1%, 2%, 3%, 4% or 6%; 1 ml Dropperettes 1%, 2% or 4%. *Rx.*
Use: Antiglaucoma.

•**pilocarpine.** (pie-low-CAR-peen) U.S.P. 23.
Use: Antiglaucoma, ophthalmic cholinergic, miotic.
See: Ocusert Pilo-20 and Pilo-40 (Novartis).

•**pilocarpine hydrochloride.** (pie-low-CAR-peen) U.S.P. 23.
Use: Cholinergic (ophthalmic), topically as a miotic, xerostomia and keratoconjunctivitis sicca [Orphan drug]
See: Almocarpine (Wyeth Ayerst).
Mi-Pilo, Soln. (PBH Wesley Jessen).
Pilocar, Soln. (Ciba Vision Ophthalmics).
Pilomiotin, Soln. (Ciba Vision Ophthalmics).
Piloptic, Soln. (Muro).
Salagen, Tab. (MGI Pharma).
W/Epinephrine HCl.
See: E-Carpine, Inj. (Alcon Laboratories).
Epicar, Ophthalmic Soln. (PBH Wesley Jessen).
W/Epinephrine bitartrate, mannitol, benzalkonium Cl.
See: E-Pilo, Soln. (Ciba Vision Ophthalmics).
W/Physostigmine salicylate, methylcellulose.
See: Isopto P-ES, Soln. (Alcon Laboratories).

pilocarpine hydrochloride. (Various Mfr.) Pilocarpine HCl. **0.5%:** 15 ml, 30 ml; **1%:** 2 ml, 15 ml, 30 ml, UD 1 ml; **2% and 4%:** 2 ml, 15 ml, 30 ml; **6%:** 15 ml; **8%:** 2 ml.
Use: Cholinergic (ophthalmic), topically as a miotic, xerostomia and keratoconjunctivitis sicca [Orphan drug]

•**pilocarpine nitrate.** (pie-low-CAR-peen) U.S.P. 23.
Use: Cholinergic (ophthalmic).
See: P.V. Carpine (Allergan).
W/Phenylephrine HCl.
Use: Parasympathomimetic agent.
See: Pilofrin Liquifilm, Ophthalmic (Allergan).

Pilopine. (International Pharm) Pilocarpine HCl 1%, 2% or 4%. Soln. Bot. 15 ml. *Rx.*
Use: Antiglaucoma.

Pilopine HS Gel. (Alcon Laboratories) Pilocarpine HCl 4%. Tube 3.5 g. *Rx.*
Use: Antiglaucoma.

Piloptic. (Optopics) Pilocarpine HCl 0.5%, 1%, 2%, 3%, 4% or 6%. Soln. Bot. 15 ml. *Rx.*
Use: Antiglaucoma.

Pilostat. (Bausch & Lomb) Pilocarpine HCl 0.5%, 1%, 2%, 3%, 4% or 6%. Soln. Bot. 15 ml, twin pack 2 x 15 ml. *Rx.*
Use: Antiglaucoma.

Pima Syrup. (Fleming) Potassium iodide 5 gr/5 ml. Bot. pt, gal. *Rx.*
Use: Expectorant.

•**pimagedine hydrochloride.** (pih-MAH-jeh-deen) USAN.
Use: Inhibitor (advanced glycosylation end-product formation inhibitors).

•**pimetine hydrochloride.** (PIM-eh-teen) USAN.
Use: Antihyperlipoproteinemic.

piminodine esylate.
Use: Analgesic.

piminodine ethanesulfonate.
Use: Analgesic, narcotic.

•**pimobendan.** (pie-MOE-ben-dan) USAN.
Use: Cardiovascular agent.

•**pimozide.** (pih-moe-ZIDE) U.S.P. 23.
Use: Antipsychotic.
See: Orap, Tab. (Ortho McNeil).

•**pinacidil.** (pie-NASS-ih-DILL) USAN.
Use: Antihypertensive.

•**pinadoline.** (pih-nah-DOE-leen) USAN.
Use: Analgesic.

•**pindolol.** (PIN-doe-lahl) U.S.P. 23.
Use: Beta-adrenergic blocking agent, vasodilator.
See: Visken (Novartis).

pine needle oil. N.F. XVI.
Use: Perfume; flavor.

pine tar. U.S.P. XXI.
Use: Local antieczematic; rubefacient.

Pinex Concentrate Cough Syrup. (Last) Dextromethorphan HBr 7.5 mg/5 ml (after diluting 3 oz. concentrate to make 16 oz. solution). Bot. 3 oz. *otc.*
Use: Antitussive.

Pinex Cough Syrup. (Last) Dextromethorphan HBr 7.5 mg/5 ml. Bot. 3 oz, 6 oz. *otc.*
Use: Antitussive.

Pinex Regular. (Pinex) Potassium guaiacolsulfonate, oil of pine and eucalyptus, extract of grindelia, alcohol 3%/30 ml. Syr. Bot. 3 oz, 8 oz. Also cherry flavored 3 oz. Super and concentrated 3 oz. *otc.*
Use: Expectorant.

Pink Bismuth. (Zenith Forest Pharmaceutical) 130 mg/15 ml. Liq. Bot. 240 ml. *otc.*

Use: Antidiarrheal.

•**pinoxepin hydrochloride.** (pih-NOX-eh-PIN) USAN.
Use: Antipsychotic.

Pin-Rid. (Apothecary Products) **Soft gelcap:** Pyrantel pamoate 180 mg (equivalent to 62.5 mg pyrantel base). Pkg. 24s; **Liq.:** Pyrantel pamoate 144 mg/ml (equivalent to 50 mg/ml pyrantel base), saccharin, sucrose. Bot. 30 ml. *otc.*
Use: Anthelmintic.

Pin-X. (Effcon) Pyrantel base (as pamoate) 50 mg/ml, sorbitol. Liq. Bot. 30 ml. *otc.*
Use: Anthelmintic.

•**pioglitazone hydrochloride.** (PIE-oh-GLIH-tah-zone) USAN.
Use: Antidiabetic.

•**pipamperone.** (pih-PAM-peer-OHN) USAN. *Formerly Floropipamide.*
Use: Antipsychotic.

•**pipazethate.** (pip-AZZ-eh-thate) USAN.
Use: Cough suppressant; antitussive.

pipazethate hydrochloride.
Use: Antitussive.

•**pipecuronium bromide.** (pih-peh-cure-OH-nee-uhm) USAN.
Use: Neuromuscular blocker.

•**piperacetazine.** (pih-PURR-ah-SET-ah-zeen) USAN.
Use: Antipsychotic.

•**piperacillin.** (PIH-per-uh-SILL-in) U.S.P. 23.
Use: Anti-infective.

•**piperacillin sodium.** (PIH-per-uh-SILL-in) U.S.P. 23.
Use: Anti-infective.
W/ Tazobactam
See: Zosyn, Inj. (ESI Lederle Generics).

•**piperamide maleate.** (PIH-per-ah-mid) USAN.
Use: Anthelmintic.

•**piperazine.** (pie-PEAR-ah-zeen) U.S.P. 23.
Use: Anthelmintic.

•**piperazine citrate.** (pie-PEAR-ah-zeen) U.S.P. 23. Piperazine Citrate Telra Hydrous Tripiperazine Dicitrate.
Use: Anthelmintic.
See: Bryrel, Syr. (Sanofi Winthrop).
Ta-Verm, Syr., Tab. (Table Rock).

•**piperazine edetate calcium.** (pie-PEAR-ah-zeen EH-deh-tate) USAN.
Use: Anthelmintic.

piperazine estrone sulfate. (pie-PEAR-ah-zeen)
See: Estropipate.

piperazine hexahydrate. Tivazine.

piperazine phosphate.
Use: Anthelmintic.

piperazine tartrate.

piperidine phosphate.
Use: Psychiatric drug.

piperidinoethyl benzilate hydrochloride. No products listed.

piperidolate hydrochloride.
Use: Anticholinergic.

piperoxan hydrochloride. Fourneau 933. Benzodioxane. Diagnosis of hypertension.
Use: Diagnostic aid.

piperphenidol hydrochloride.

pipethanate hydrochloride.
Use: Anxiolytic.

•**piposulfan.** (PIP-oh-SULL-fan) USAN.
Use: Antineoplastic.

•**pipotiazine palmitate.** (PIP-oh-TIE-ah-zeen PAL-mih-tate) USAN.
Use: Antipsychotic.
See: Piportil (Ives).

•**pipoxolan hydrochloride.** (pih-POX-oh-lan) USAN.
Use: Muscle relaxant.

Pipracil. (ESI Lederle Generics) Piperacillin sodium 2 g, 3 g, 4 g or 40 g/Vial; 2 g, 3 g or 4 g/Infusion Bottle. Sterile. *Rx.*
Use: Anti-infective, penicillin.

•**piprozolin.** (PIP-row-ZOE-lin) USAN.
Use: Choleretic.

•**piquindone hydrochloride.** (PIH-kwin-dohn) USAN.
Use: Antipsychotic.

•**piquizil hydrochloride.** (PIH-kwih-zill) USAN.
Use: Bronchodilator.

•**piracetam.** (PIHR-ASS-eh-tam) USAN.
Use: Cognition adjuvant, cerebral stimulant, myoclonus [Orphan drug]

•**pirandamine hydrochloride.** (pih-RAN-dah-meen) USAN.
Use: Antidepressant.

•**pirazmonam sodium.** (pihr-AZZ-moe-nam SO-dee-uhm) USAN.
Use: Antimicrobial.

•**pirazolac.** (PIHR-AZE-oh-lack) USAN.
Use: Antirheumatic.

•**pirbenicillin sodium.** (pihr-ben-IH-SILL-in) USAN.
Use: Anti-infective.

•**pirbuterol acetate.** (pihr-BYOO-tuh-role) USAN.
Use: Bronchodilator.
See: Maxair, Aerosol (3M Pharm).

•**pirbuterol hydrochloride.** USAN.

Use: Bronchodilator.

•**pirenperone.** (PIHR-en-PURR-ohn) USAN.
Use: Anxiolytic.

•**pirenzepine hydrochloride.** (PIHR-en-zeh-PEEN) USAN.
Use: Antiulcerative.

•**piretanide.** (pihr-ETT-ah-nide) USAN.
Use: Diuretic.
See: Arlix, Prods. (Hoechst Marion Roussel).

•**pirfenidone.** (PEER-FEN-ih-dohn) USAN.
Use: Analgesic, anti-inflammatory, anti-pyretic.

piridazol.
See: Sulfapyridine, Tab. (Various Mfr.).

•**piridicillin sodium.** (pihr-RIH-dih-SILL-in) USAN.
Use: Anti-infective.

piridocaine hydrochloride.

•**piridronate sodium.** (pihr-IH-DROE-nate) USAN.
Use: Regulator (calcium).

•**piriprost.** (PIHR-ih-prahst) USAN.
Use: Antiasthmatic.

•**piriprost potassium.** (PIHR-ih-prahst) USAN.
Use: Antiasthmatic.

piriton.
See: Chlorpheniramine (Various Mfr.).

•**piritrexim isethionate.** (pih-rih-TREX-im eye-seh-THIGH-oh-nate) USAN.
Use: Antiproliferative. [Orphan drug]

•**pirlimycin hydrochloride.** (PIHR-lih-MY-sin) USAN.
Use: Anti-infective.

•**pirmagrel.** (PIHR-mah-GRELL) USAN.
Use: Inhibitor (thromboxane synthetase).

•**pirmenol hydrochloride.** (PIHR-MEH-nahl) USAN.
Use: Cardiovascular agent, antiarrhythmic.

•**pirnabine.** (PIHR-NAH-bean) USAN.
Use: Antiglaucoma agent.

•**piroctone.** (pihr-OCK-TONE) USAN.
Use: Antiseborrheic.

•**piroctone olamine.** (pihr-OCK-TONE OH-lah-meen) USAN.
Use: Antiseborrheic.

•**pirodavir.** (pih-ROW-dav-ihr) USAN.
Use: Antiviral.

•**pirogliride tartrate.** (PIHR-oh-GLIE-ride) USAN.
Use: Antidiabetic.

•**pirolate.** (PIHR-oh-late) USAN.
Use: Antiasthmatic.

•**pirolazamide.** (PIHR-ole-aze-ah-mide) USAN.
Use: Cardiovascular agent, antiarrhythmic.

•**piroxantrone hydrochloride.** (PIH-row-ZAN-trone) USAN.
Use: Antineoplastic.

•**piroxicam.** (pihr-OX-ih-kam) U.S.P. 23.
Use: Anti-inflammatory.
See: Feldene, Cap. (Pfizer).

piroxicam. (Various Mfr.) 10 mg, 20 mg. Cap. Bot. 100s, 500s, 1000s.
Use: Anti-inflammatory.

•**piroxicam betadex.** (pihr-OX-ih-kam BAY-tah-dex) USAN.
Use: Analgesic, anti-inflammatory, anti-rheumatic.

•**piroxicam cinnamate.** (pihr-OX-ih-kam SIN-ah-mate) USAN.
Use: Anti-inflammatory.

•**piroxicam olamine.** (pihr-OX-ih-kam OH-lah-meen) USAN.
Use: Anti-inflammatory, analgesic.

•**piroximone.** (PIHR-ox-ih-MONE) USAN.
Use: Cardiovascular agent.

•**pirprofen.** (pihr-PRO-fen) USAN.
Use: Anti-inflammatory.

•**pirquinozol.** (PIHR-KWIN-oh-zole) USAN.
Use: Antiallergic.

•**pirsidomine.** (pihr-SIH-doe-meen) USAN.
Use: Vasodilator.

Piso's. (Pinex) Ipecac, ammonium Cl, menthol in syrup base. Bot. 3 oz, 5 oz. *otc.*
Use: Expectorant.

pitayine.
See: Quinidine, Preps. (Various Mfr.).

Pitocin. (Monarch) Oxytocin w/chlorobutanol 0.5%, acetic acid to adjust pH. Amp. 5 units/0.5 ml; 10 units/1 ml. Box 10s, Steri-dose syringe; 10 units/1 ml 10s. *Rx.*
Use: Oxytocic.

Pitressin Synthetic. (Parke-Davis) Vasopressin w/chlorobutanol 0.5%, pH adjusted with acetic acid. Amp. 0.5 ml, 1 ml (20 pressor units). Box 10s. *Rx.*
Use: Hormone.

Pitts Carminative. (Del Pharmaceuticals) Bot. 2 oz.
Use: Antiflatulent.

pituitary, anterior. The anterior lobe of the pituitary gland supplies protein hormones classified under following headings.
See: Corticotropin, Preps. (Various Mfr.).

Gonadotropin, Preps. (Various Mfr.).
Growth Hormone.
Thyrotropic Principle.

Pituitary Function Test.
See: Metopirone, Tab. (Novartis).

pituitary, posterior, hormones.
(a) Vasopressin. Pressor principle, β-hypophamine, postlobin-V.
See: Pitressin, Amp. (Parke-Davis).
(b) Oxytocin. Oxytocic principle. α-hypophamine, postiobin-O.
See: Oxytocin, Inj. (Various Mfr.).
Pitocin, Amp. (Parke-Davis).
Syntocinon, Amp. (Novartis).

•**pituitary, posterior, injection.** U.S.P. 23.
Use: Hormone (antidiuretic).
See: Pituitrin, Obstetrical, Amp. (Parke-Davis).
Pituitrin, Surgical, Amp. (Parke-Davis).

•**pivampicillin hydrochloride.** (pihv-AM-pih-SILL-in) USAN.
Use: Anti-infective.

•**pivampicillin pamoate.** (pihv-AM-pih SILL-in PAM-oh-ate) USAN.
Use: Anti-infective.

•**pivampicillin probenate.** (pihv-AM-pih-SILL-in PRO-ben-ate) USAN.
Use: Anti-infective.

•**pivopril.** (PIH-voe-PRILL) USAN.
Use: Antihypertensive.

pix carbonis.
See: Coal Tar, Preps. (Various Mfr.).

pix juniperi.
Use: Sunscreen, moisturizer.
See: Juniper Tar, Comp. (Various Mfr.).

•**pizotyline.** (pih-ZOE-tih-leen) USAN.
Use: Anabolic, antidepressant, serotonin inhibitor (migraine).

placebo capsules. (Cowley) No. 3 orange red; No. 4 yellow. Bot. 1000s.
Use: Placebo.

placebo tablets. (Cowley) 1 gr white; 2 gr white; 3 gr white, red or yellow, pink, orange; 4 gr white; 5 gr white. Bot. 1000s.
Use: Placebo.

Placidyl. (Abbott Laboratories) Ethchlorvynol. **200 mg/Cap.:** Bot. 100s. **500 mg/Cap.:** Bot. 100s, 500s, UD 100s. **750 mg/Cap.:** Bot. 100s. *c-iv.*
Use: Hypnotic, sedative.

•**plague vaccine.** U.S.P. 23.
Use: Immunization.

plague vaccine. (Greer Laboratories) 2000 million killed *Pasteurella pestis*/ml. Vial 20 ml.
Use: Immunization.

planocaine.
See: Procaine HCl, Preps. (Various Mfr.).

planochrome.
See: Merbromin, Soln. (Various Mfr.).

plantago, ovata coating.
See: Effersyllium, Prods. (Zeneca).
Konsyl, Pow. (Burton, Parsons).
L.A. Formula, Pow. (Burton, Parsons).
Metamucil, Pow. (Searle).
W/Psyllium seed, gum karaya, Brewer's yeast.
See: Plantamucin, Gran. (ICN Pharmaceuticals).
W/Vitamin B_1.
See: Siblin, Gran. (Parke-Davis).

•**plantago seed.** (PLAN-tah-go seed) U.S.P. 23.
Use: Laxative.

plant protease concentrate.
See: Ananase, Tab. (Rhone-Poulenc Rorer).

Plaquenil Sulfate. (Sanofi Winthrop) Hydroxychloroquine sulfate 200 mg/Tab. (equivalent to base 155 mg). Bot. 100s. *Rx.*
Use: Antimalarial, antirheumatic.

Plaquenil Tablet. (Sanofi Winthrop) Hydroxychloroquine sulfate. *Rx.*
Use: Antimalarial, antirheumatic.

Plasbumin-5. (Bayer Corp) Normal serum albumin (Human) 5% U.S.P. fractionated from normal serum plasma, heat treated against hepatitis virus. Albumin 12.5 g/250 ml. Vial 50 ml. Bot. with IV set 250 ml, 500 ml. *Rx.*
Use: Plasma protein fraction.

Plasbumin-25. (Bayer Corp) Normal serum albumin (Human) 25% U.S.P. fractionated from normal serum plasma, heat treated against hepatitis virus. Albumin 12.5 g/50 ml. Vial 20 ml. Bot. with IV set 50 ml, 100 ml. *Rx.*
Use: Plasma protein fraction.

plasma.
See: Normal Human Plasma (Various Mfr.).

plasma expanders or substitutes.
See: Dextran 6% and LMD 10% (Abbott Laboratories).
Macrodex, Soln. (Pharmacia & Upjohn).

Plasma-Lyte A Injection. (Baxter) Sodium 140 mEq, potassium 5 mEq, magnesium 3 mEq, chloride 98 mEq, acetate 27 mEq, gluconate 23 mEq/L w/ pH adjusted to 7.4. Plastic bot. 500 ml, 1000 ml. *Rx.*
Use: Nutritional supplement, parenteral.

Plasma-Lyte 148 Injection. (Baxter) Sodium 140 mEq, potassium 5 mEq, magnesium 3 mEq, chloride 98 mEq, acetate 27 mEq, gluconate 23 mEq/L. Plastic bot. 500 ml, 1000 ml. *Rx.*
Use: Nutritional supplement, parenteral.

Plasma-Lyte M and 5% Dextrose Injection. (Baxter) Sodium 40 mEq, potassium 16 mEq, calcium 5 mEq, magnesium 3 mEq, chloride 40 mEq, acetate 12 mEq, lactate 12 mEq/L. Plastic bot. 500 ml, 1000 ml. *Rx.*
Use: Nutritional supplement, parenteral.

Plasma-Lyte R and 5% Dextrose Injection. (Baxter) Sodium 140 mEq, potassium 10 mEq, calcium 5 mEq, magnesium 3 mEq, chloride 103 mEq, acetate 47 mEq, lactate 8 mEq/L. Bot. 500 ml, 1000 ml. *Rx.*
Use: Nutritional supplement, parenteral.

Plasma-Lyte 56 and 5% Dextrose. (Baxter) Sodium 40 mEq, potassium 13 mEq, magnesium 3 mEq, chloride 40 mEq, acetate 16 mEq/L. Plastic bot. 500 ml, 1000 ml. *Rx.*
Use: Nutritional supplement, parenteral.

Plasma-Lyte 148 and 5% Dextrose. (Baxter) Dextrose 50 g, calories 190, sodium 140 mEq, potassium 5 mEq, magnesium 3 mEq, chloride 98 mEq, acetate 27 mEq, 547 mOsm, gluconate 23 mEq/L. Soln. Bot. 500 ml, 1000 ml. *Rx.*
Use: Nutritional supplement, parenteral.

Plasma-Lyte 56 in Water. (Baxter) Sodium 40 mEq, potassium 13 mEq, magnesium 3 mEq, chloride 40 mEq, acetate 16 mEq/L. Plastic bot. 500 ml, 1000 ml. *Rx.*
Use: Nutritional supplement, parenteral.

Plasma-Lyte R Injection. (Baxter) Sodium 140 mEq, potassium 10 mEq, calcium 5 mEq, magnesium 3 mEq, chloride 103 mEq, acetate 47 mEq, lactate 8 mEq/L. Bot. 1000 ml. *Rx.*
Use: Nutritional supplement, parenteral.

Plasmanate. (Bayer Corp) Plasma protein fraction (Human) 5%. U.S.P. Vial 50 ml. Bot. 250 ml, 500 ml with set. *Rx.*
Use: Plasma protein fraction.

Plasma-Plex. (Centeon) Plasma protein fraction 5%. Inj. Vial 250 ml, 500 ml. *Rx.*
Use: Plasma protein fraction.

•**plasma protein fraction.** U.S.P. 23. *Formerly Plasma Protein Fraction, Human.*
Use: Blood-volume supporter.
See: Plasmanate, Soln. (Bayer Corp).
Plasma-Plex, Soln. (Centeon).
Plasmatein, Soln. (Abbott Laboratories).
Protenate, Soln. (Baxter).

plasma protein fraction. (Baxter) For the plasma protein preparation obtained from human plasma using the Cohn fractionation technique Bot. 250 ml.
Use: Blood volume supporter.

Plasmatein. (Alpha Therapeutics) Plasma protein fraction 5%. Inj. Vial w/ injection set 250 ml, 500 ml. *Rx.*
Use: Plasma protein fraction.

plasmochin naphthoate. Pamaquine naphthoate.
Use: Antimalarial.

•**platelet concentrate.** U.S.P. 23.
Use: Platelet replenisher.

Platelet Factor 4. (Abbott Diagnostics) Radioimmunoassay for quantitative measurement of total PF4 levels in plasma. Test kit 100s.
Use: Diagnostic aid.

Platinol-AQ. (Bristol-Myers Oncology) Cisplatin (CDDP) 1 mg/ml. Inj. Vial. 50 ml, 100 ml. *Rx.*
Use: Antineoplastic.

Plavix. (Sanofi Winthrop) Clopidogrel 75 mg (as bisulfate), lactose. Tab. Bot. 100s, 500s, UD 100s. *Rx.*
Use: Antiplatelet.

Plegisol. (Abbott Hospital Prods) Calcium Cl dihydrate 17.6 mg, magnesium Cl hexahydrate 325.3 mg, potassium Cl 119.3 mg, sodium Cl 643 mg/ 100 ml. Approximately 260 mOsm/L. Single Dose Container 1000 ml without sodium bicarbonate. *Rx.*
Use: Cardiovascular agent.

Plendil. (Astra Merck) Felodipine 2.5 mg, 5 mg or 10 mg/ER Tab. Bot. 30s, 100s, UD 100s. *Rx.*
Use: Calcium channel blocker.

Plewin Tablets. (Sanofi Winthrop) Glycobiarsol, chloroquine phosphate. *Rx.*
Use: Amebicide.

Plexolan Cream. (Last) Zinc oxide, lanolin. Tube 1.25 oz, 3 oz. Jar 16 oz. *otc.*
Use: Dermatologic.

Plexon. (Sigma-Tau Pharmaceuticals) Testosterone 10 mg, estrone 1 mg, liver 2 mcg, pyridoxine HCl 10 mg, panthenol 10 mg, inositol 20 mg, choline Cl 20 mg, vitamin B_2 2 mg, B_{12} 100 mcg, procaine HCl 1%, niacinamide 100 mg/ml. Vial 10 ml.
Use: Hormone, mineral, vitamin supplement.

Pliagel. (Alcon Laboratories) Sodium Cl, potassium Cl, poloxamer 407, sorbic acid 0.25%, EDTA 0.5%. Soln. Bot. 25 ml. *otc.*

Use: Contact lens care.

•**plicamycin.** (PLY-kae-MY-sin) U.S.P. 23. Antibiotic derived from *Streptomyces agrillaceus* & *S. tanashiensis. Formerly Mithramycin.*
Use: Antineoplastic.
See: Mithracin, Pow. (Bayer Corp).

•**plomestane.** (PLOE-mess-TANE) USAN.
Use: Antineoplastic (aromatase inhibitor).

Plova. (Washington Ethical) Psyllium mucilloid. Pow. (flavored) 12 oz., (plain) 10 0.5 oz. *otc.*
Use: Laxative.

Pluravit Drops. (Sanofi Winthrop) Multivitamin.
Use: Vitamin supplement.

PMB 200. (Wyeth Ayerst) Conjugated estrogens 0.45 mg, meprobamate 200 mg, lactose, sucrose/Tab. Bot. 60s. *Rx.*
Use: Anxiolytic, estrogen.

PMB 400. (Wyeth Ayerst) Conjugated estrogens 0.45 mg, meprobamate 400 mg, lactose, sucrose/Tab. Bot. 100s. *Rx.*
Use: Anxiolytic, estrogen.

P.M.P. Compound. (Mericon) Chlorpheniramine maleate 4 mg, phenylephrine HCl 15 mg, salicylamide 300 mg, scopolamine methylnitrate 0.8 mg/ Tab. Bot. 100s, 1000s. *Rx.*
Use: Analgesic, antihistamine, decongestant.

PMP Expectorant. (Mericon) Codeine phosphate 10 mg, phenylephrine HCl 10 mg, guaifenesin 40 mg, chlorpheniramine maleate 2 mg/5 ml. Bot. gal. *c-v.*
Use: Antihistamine, antitussive, decongestant, expectorant.

pneumococcal vaccine, polyvalent. (new-moe-KAH-kuhl) Purified capsular polysaccharides from 23 pneumococcal types. 25 mcg each of 23 polysaccharides per 0.5 ml.
Use: Immunization.

Pneumomist. (ECR Pharmaceuticals) Guaifenesin 600 mg. SR Tab. Bot. 100s. *Rx.*
Use: Expectorant.

Pneumotussin HC. (ECR Pharmaceuticals) Hydrocodone bitartrate 5 mg, guaifenesin 100 mg/5 ml Syrup. Bot. 120 ml, 480 ml. *c-III.*
Use: Antitussive, expectorant.

PNS Unna Boot. (Pedinol) Non-sterile gauze bandage 10 yds × 3″. Box 12s.
Use: Ambulatory procedure in treatment of leg ulcers and varicosities.

Pnu-Imune 23. (Wyeth Ayerst) Pneumococcal vaccine 0.5 ml dose. 5-dose vials. Lederject disposable syringe 5 × 1 dose. *Rx.*
Use: Immunization.

•**pobilukast edamine.** (poe-BIH-loo-kast EH-dah-meen) USAN.
Use: Antiasthmatic (leukotriene antagonist).

pochlorin. Prophyrinic and chlorophyllic compound.
Use: Antihypercholesteremic agent.

Pod-Ben-25. (C & M Pharmacal) Podophyllin 25% in benzoin tincture. Bot. 1 oz. *Rx.*
Use: Keratolytic.

Podoben. (American) Podophyllum resin extract 25%. Bot. 5 ml. *Rx.*
Use: Keratolytic.

Podocon-25. (Paddock) Podophyllum resin 25% in benzoin tincture. Soln. 15 ml. *Rx.*
Use: Keratolytic.

•**podofilox.** (pah-dah-FILL-ox) USAN.
Use: Antimitotic.
See: Condylox (Oclassen).

podophyllin.
See: Podophyllum resin.

•**podophyllum.** (poe-doe-FILL-uhm) U.S.P. 23.
Use: Pharmaceutic necessity.
W/Oxgall, cascara sagrada, dandelion root, tincture nux vomica.
See: Oxachol, Liq. (Roxane).

•**podophyllum resin.** U.S.P. 23.
Use: Caustic.
See: Podoben, Liq. (Maurry).
W/Salicylic acid.
See: Ver-Var, Soln. (Galderma).

podophyllum resin. (Various Mfr.) Podophyllin. Pkg. 1 oz, 0.25 lb, 1 lb.
Use: Caustic

Point-Two Mouthrinse. (Colgate Oral) Sodium fluoride 0.2% in a flavored neutral liquid. Bot. 120 ml. *Rx.*
Use: Dental caries agent.

Poison Antidote Kit. (Jones Medical Industries) Charcoal suspension. Bot. 60 ml, 4s. Ipecac syrup, Bot. 30 ml, 1/ Kit. *otc.*
Use: Antidote.

•**poison ivy extract, alum precipitated.** (poly-zuhn EYE-vee EX-tract, AL-uhm pree-SIP-ih-lay-tehd) USAN.
Use: Ivy poisoning counteractant.

Poison Oak-N-Ivy Armor. (Tec Labs) Trioctyl citrate, mineral oil, monostearyl citrate, beeswax, 4-chloro-3,5-xylenol. Lot. Bot. 59.1 ml. *otc.*

Use: Dermatologic, poison ivy.

•**polacrilin.** (pahl-ah-KRILL-in) USAN. Methacrylic acid with divinylbenzene. A synthetic ion-exchange resin, supplied in the hydrogen or free acid form. Amberlite IRP-64.
Use: Pharmaceutic aid.

•**polacrilin potassium.** N.F. 18. A synthetic ion-exchange resin, prepared through the polymerization of methacrylic acid and divinylbenzene, further neutralized with potassium hydroxide to form the potassium salt of methacrylic acid and divinylbenzene. Supplied as a pharmaceutical-grade ion-exchange resin in a particle size of 100- to 500-mesh.
Use: Pharmaceutic aid (tablet disintegrant).
See: Amberlite IRP-88 (Rohm and Haas).

Poladex Tabs. (Major) Dexchlorpheniramine maleate. **4 mg/Tab.:** Bot. 100s, 250s, 1000s; **6 mg/Tab.:** Bot. 100s, 1000s. *Rx.*
Use: Antihistamine.

polamethene resin caprylate. The physiochemical complex of the acid-binding ion exchange resin, polyamine-methylene resin and caprylic acid.

Polaramine. (Schering Plough) Dexchlorpheniramine maleate **Tab.:** 2 mg, Bot. 100s. **Repetab:** 4 mg, 6 mg/Tab. Bot. 100s. **Syr.:** 2 mg/5 ml alcohol 6%. Bot. 473 ml. *Rx.*
Use: Antihistamine.

Polaramine Expectorant. (Schering Plough) Dexchlorpheniramine maleate 2 mg, pseudoephedrine sulfate 20 mg, guaifenesin 100 mg/5 ml, alcohol 7.2%. Bot. 16 oz. *Rx.*
Use: Antihistamine, decongestant, expectorant.

Poldeman AD Suspension. (Sanofi Winthrop) Kaolin. *otc.*
Use: Antidiarrheal.

Poldeman Suspension. (Sanofi Winthrop) Kaolin. *otc.*
Use: Antidiarrheal.

Poldemicina Suspension. (Sanofi Winthrop) Kaolin. *otc.*
Use: Antidiarrheal.

•**poldine methylsulfate.** (POLE-deen METH-ill-SULL-fate) USAN. U.S.P. XX.
Use: Anticholinergic.

•**policapram.** (PAH-lee-CAP-ram) USAN.
Use: Pharmaceutic aid (tablet binder).

Polident Dentu-Grip. (Block Drug) Carboxymethylcellulose gum, ethylene oxide polymer. Pkg. 0.675 oz, 1.75 oz, 3.55 oz. *otc.*
Use: Denture adhesive.

•**polifeprosan 20.** (pahl-ee-FEH-pro-SAHN 20) USAN.
Use: Pharmaceutic aid (biodegradable polymer for controlled drug delivery).

•**poligeenan.** (PAHL-ih-JEE-nan) USAN. Polysaccharide produced by extensive hydrolysis of carragheen from red algae.
Use: Pharmaceutic aid (dispersing agent).

•**poliglecaprone 25.** (poe-lih-GLEH-kah-prone 25) USAN.
Use: Surgical aid (surgical suture material, absorbable).

•**poliglecaprone 90.** (poe-lih-GLEH-kah-prone 90) USAN.
Use: Surgical aid (surgical suture coating, absorbable).

•**poliglusam.** (pahl-ee-GLUE-sam) USAN.
Use: Antihemorrhagic, hemostatic, dermatologic, wound therapy.

•**polignate sodium.** (poe-LIG-nate) USAN.
Use: Enzyme inhibitor (pepsin).

Poli-Grip. (Block Drug) Karaya gum, magnesium oxide in petrolatum mineral oil base, peppermint and spearmint flavor. Tube 0.75 oz, 1.5 oz, 2.5 oz. *otc.*
Use: Denture adhesive.

poliomyelitis vaccine, inactivated. (Pasteur Merieux Connaught) (Purified, Salk Type IPV) Amp. 5 x 1 ml. Vial 10 dose. *Rx.*
Use: Immunization.
See: IPOL.
Poliovirus vaccine, inactivated.

poliomyelitis vaccine inactivated.
See: Immunization.

•**poliovirus vaccine, inactivated.** (POE-lee-oh-VYE-russ) U.S.P. 23. *Formerly Poliomyelitis Vaccine. Rx.*
Use: Immunization.
See: IPOL.

poliovirus vaccine, inactivated. (Pasteur Merieux Connaught) Amp. 1 ml. Box 5s. Vial 10 dose. Subcutaneous administration.
Use: Agent for immunization (active).

•**poliovirus vaccine live oral.** (POE-lee-oh-VYE-russ) U.S.P. 23. Poliovirus vaccine, live, oral, type I, II or III. Poliovirus vaccine, live, oral, trivalent.
Use: Immunization.
See: Orimune Trivalent I, II & III, Vial (Wyeth Ayerst).

poliovirus vaccine, live, oral, trivalent.

Immunization against polio strains 1, 2 & 3. *Rx.*
Use: Immunization.
See: Orimune (Wyeth Ayerst).

•**polipropene 25.** (pahl-ee-PRO-peen 25) USAN.
Use: Pharmaceutic aid (tablet excipient).

•**polixetonium chloride.** (pahl-ix-eh-TOE-nee-uhm) USAN.
Use: Pharmaceutic aid (preservative).

Polocaine. (Astra) Mepivacaine. **1%, 2%:** Inj. Vial 50 ml. **3%:** Inj. Dental cartridge 1.8 ml. **2% w/levonordefrin 1:20,000:** Sodium bisulfite. Inj. Dental cartridge 1.8 ml.*Rx.*
Use: Anesthetic, local.

Polocaine MPF. (Astra) Mepivacaine HCl. **1%, 1.5%:** Inj. Vial 30 ml. **2%:** Inj. Vial 20 ml. *Rx.*
Use: Anesthetic. local.

Poloris Poultices. (Block Drug) Benzocaine 7.5 mg, capsicum 4.6 mg in poultice base. Pkg. 5 unit, 12 unit. *Rx.*
Use: Anesthetic, local.

•**poloxalene.** (PAHL-OX-ah-leen) USAN. Liquid nonionic surfactant polymer of polyoxypropylene polyoxyethylene type.
Use: Pharmaceutic aid (surfactant).

poloxalkol. Polyoxyethylene polyoxypropylene polymer.
See: Magcyl, Cap. (ICN Pharmaceuticals).
W/Casanthrol.
See: Casakol, Cap. (Pharmacia & Upjohn).
W/Phenylephrine HCl, dextrose soln.
See: Isohalent, Soln. (ICN Pharmaceuticals).

•**poloxamer.** (pahl-OX-ah-mer) N.F. 18.
Use: Pharmaceutic aid (ointment and suppository base, surfactant, tablet binder and coating agent, emulsifying agent).

poloxamer 182 d. (pahl-OX-ah-mer 182D)
Use: Pharmaceutic aid (surfactant).

poloxamer 182 lf. (pahl-OX-ah-mer 182LF)
Use: Food additive; pharmaceutic aid.

poloxamer 188. (pahl-OX-ah-mer 188)
Use: Cathartic; sickle cell crisis, severe burns [Orphan drug]

poloxamer 188 lf. (pahl-OX-ah-mer 188LF)
Use: Pharmaceutic aid (surfactant).

poloxamer 331. (pahl-OX-ah-mer 331)
Use: Food additive (surfactant); AIDS-related toxoplasmosis [Orphan drug]

poloxamer-iodine.
See: Prepodyne, Soln. (West).

polyamine-methylene resin.
See: Exorbin (Various Mfr.).

polyamine resin.
See: Polyamine-Methylene Resin (Various Mfr.).

polyanethol sulfonate, sodium.
See: Grobax, Vial (Roche Laboratories).

polyanhydroglucose. Polyanhydroglucuronic acid.
See: Dextran, Inj., Soln. (Various Mfr.).

Polybase. (Paddock) Preblended polyethylene glycol suppository base for incorporation of medications where a water soluble base is indicated. Jar 1 lb, 5 lb.
Use: Pharmaceutical aid, suppository base.

polybenzarsol. Benzocal.

Poly-Bon Drops. (Barrows) Vitamins A 3000 IU, D 400 IU, C 60 mg, B_1 1 mg, B_2 1.2 mg, niacinamide 8 mg/0.6 ml. Bot. 50 ml. *otc.*
Use: Vitamin supplement.

•**polybutester.** (PAHL-ee-byoot-ESS-ter) USAN.
Use: Surgical aid (surgical suture material).

•**polybutilate.** (PAHL-ee-BYOO-tih-late) USAN.
Use: Surgical aid (surgical suture coating).

•**polycarbophil.** U.S.P. 23. A synthetic, loosely crosslinked, hydrophilic resin of the polycarboxylic type. Sorboquel.
Use: Laxative.

Polycillin. (Bristol-Myers) Ampicillin trihydrate. **250 mg/Cap.:** Bot. 100s, 500s, 1000s, UD 100s. **500 mg/Cap.:** Bot. 100s, 500s, UD 100s. **Pediatric Drops:** 100 mg/ml. Dropper bot. 20 ml. *Rx.*
Use: Anti-infective, penicillin.

Polycillin Oral Suspension. (Bristol-Myers) Ampicillin trihydrate. **125 mg/5 ml:** Bot. 80 ml, 100 ml, 150 ml, 200 ml, UD 5 ml. **250 mg/5 ml:** Bot. 80 ml, 100 ml, 150 ml, 200 ml, UD 5 ml. **500 mg/5 ml:** Bot. 100 ml, UD 5 ml. *Rx.*
Use: Anti-infective, penicillin.

Polycitra K. (Baker Norton) Potassium citrate monohydrate 1100 mg, citric acid monohydrate 334 mg, potassium ion 10 mEq/5 ml. Bot. 4 oz, pt. *Rx.*
Use: Alkalinizer, systemic.

Polycitra K Crystals. (Baker Norton) Potassium citrate monohydrate 3300 mg,

citric acid 1002 mg, potassium ion 30 mEq, equivalent to 30 mEq bicarbonate/ UD pkg. Sugar free. Box 100s. *Rx.*
Use: Alkalinizer, systemic.

Polycitra LC. (Baker Norton) Potassium citrate monohydrate 550 mg, sodium citrate dihydrate 500 mg, citric acid monohydrate 334 mg, potassium ion 5 mEq, sodium ion 5 mEq/5 ml. Bot. 4 oz, pt. *Rx.*
Use: Alkalinizer, systemic.

Polycitra Syrup. (Baker Norton) Potassium citrate monohydrate 550 mg, sodium citrate dihydrate 500 mg, citric acid monohydrate 334 mg, potassium ion 5 mEq, sodium ion 5 mEq/5 ml. Bot. 4 oz, pt. *Rx.*
Use: Alkalinizer, systemic.

Polycose. (Ross Laboratories) **Pow.:** Glucose polymers derived from controlled hydrolysis of corn starch. Calories 380, carbohydrate 94 g, water 6 g, sodium 110 mg, potassium 10 mg, chloride 223 mg, calcium 30 mg, phosphorus 5 mg/100 g. Can 12.3 oz. Case 6s. **Liq.:** Calories 200, carbohydrate 50 g, water 70 g, sodium 70 mg, potassium 6 mg, chloride 140 mg, calcium 20 mg, phosphorus 3 mg/100 ml. Bot. 4 oz. Case 48s. *otc.*
Use: Nutritional supplement.

polycycline intravenous.
See: Bristacycline, Cap., Vial (Bristol-Myers).

•**polydextrose.** (PAH-lee-DEX-trose) USAN.
Use: Food additive.

polydimethylsiloxane (silicone oil).
Use: Ophthalmic.
See: AdatoSil 5000, Inj. (Escalon Ophthalmics).

Polydine Ointment. (Century Pharm) Povidone-iodine in ointment base. Jar 1 oz, 4 oz, lb. *otc.*
Use: Anti-infective, topical.

Polydine Scrub. (Century Pharm) Povidone-iodine in scrub solution. Bot. 1 oz, 4 oz, 8 oz, pt, gal. *otc.*
Use: Antiseptic.

Polydine Solution. (Century Pharm) Povidone-iodine solution. Bot. 1 oz, 4 oz, 8 oz, pt, gal. *otc.*
Use: Antiseptic.

•**polydioxanone.** (PAHL-ee-die-OX-ah-nohn) USAN.
Use: Surgical aid (surgical suture material, absorbable).

Poly ENA Test System for RNP and SM. (Wampole Laboratories) Qualitative identification of auto antibodies to extractable nuclear antigens in human serum by gel precipitation technique. Aid in the diagnosis of SLE, MCTD, PSS, SS. Box test 48s.
Use: Diagnostic aid.

Poly ENA Test System for RNP, SM, SSA and SSB. (Wampole Laboratories) Qualitative identification of auto antibodies to extractable nuclear antigens in human serum by gel precipitation techniques. Aid in the diagnosis of SLE, MCTD, PSS, SS. Box test 96s.
Use: Diagnostic aid.

Poly ENA Test System for SSA and SSB. (Wampole Laboratories) Qualitative identification of auto antibodies to extractable nuclear antigens in human serum by gel precipitation techniques. Aid in the diagnosis of SLE, MCTD, PSS, SS. Box test 48s.
Use: Diagnostic aid.

polyestradiol phosphate.
See: Estradurin, Amp. (Wyeth Ayerst).

•**polyethadene.** (PAHL-ee-ETH-ah-DEEN) USAN.
Use: Antacid.

polyethylene excipient. N.F. XVII.
Use: Pharmaceutic aid (stiffening agent).

•**polyethylene glycol.** (poli-eth-uh-leen gli-cawl) N.F. 18.
Use: Pharmaceutic aid (ointment and suppository base, tablet excipient, solvent, tablet and capsule lubricant).
See: P.E.G., Oint. (Medco).

polyethylene glycol 3350 and electrolytes for oral solution. (poli-eth-uh-leen gli-cawl)
Use: Rehydration.

•**polyethylene glycol monomethyl ether.** (PAHL-ee-ETH-ah-LEEN EETH-ehr) N.F. 18.
Use: Pharmaceutic aid (excipient).

•**polyethylene oxide.** (PAHL-ee-ETH-ah-LEEN) N.F. 18.
Use: Pharmaceutic aid (suspending and viscosity agent, tablet binder).

•**polyferose.** (PAHL-ee-feh-rohs) USAN. An iron carbohydrate chelate containing approximately 45% of iron in which the metallic (Fe) ion is sequestered within a polymerized carbohydrate derived from sucrose.
Use: Hematinic.

Poly-F Fluoride Drops. (Major) Fluoride 0.5 mg, vitamins A 1500 IU, D 400 IU, E 5 mg, B_1 0.5 mg, B_2 0.6 mg, B_3 8 mg, B_6 0.4 mg, B_{12} 2 mcg, C 35 mg/

ml. Drops. Bot. 50 ml. *Rx.*
Use: Mineral, vitamin supplement.

Polygam S/D. (American Red Cross) Protein 50 mg (90% gamma globulin). Inj. Single-use vials 2.5 g, 5 g, 10 g. *Rx.*
Use: Immunization.

•**polyglactin 370.** (PAHL-ee-GLAHK-tin 370) USAN. Lactic acid polyester with glycolic acid.
Use: Surgical aid (surgical suture coating, absorbable).

•**polyglactin 910.** (PAHL-ee-GLAHK-tin 910). USAN.
Use: Surgical aid (surgical suture coating, absorbable).

•**polyglycolic acid.** (PAHL-ee-glie-KAHL-ik) USAN.
Use: Surgical aid (surgical suture material).
See: Dexone Sterile Suture (David & Geck).

•**polyglyconate.** (PAHL-ee-GLIE-koe-nate) USAN.
Use: Surgical aid (surgical suture material, absorbable).

Poly-Histine. (Bock) Pheniramine maleate 4 mg, pyrilamine maleate 4 mg, phenyltoloxamine citrate 4 mg, alcohol 4%/5 ml. Elix. Bot. 473 ml. *Rx.*
Use: Antihistamine.

Poly-Histine CS. (Sanofi Winthrop) Brompheniramine maleate 2 mg, phenylpropanolamine HCl 12.5 mg, codeine phosphate 10 mg/5 ml, alcohol 0.95%. Bot. pt. *c-v.*
Use: Antihistamine, antitussive, decongestant.

Poly-Histine-D Capsules. (Sanofi Winthrop) Phenylpropanolamine HCl 50 mg, phenyltoloxamine citrate 16 mg, pyrilamine maleate 16 mg, pheniramine maleate 16 mg/Cap. Bot. 100s. *Rx.*
Use: Antihistamine, decongestant.

Poly-Histine-D Elixir. (Sanofi Winthrop) Phenylpropanolamine HCl 12.5 mg, phenyltoloxamine citrate 4 mg, pyrilamine maleate 4 mg, pheniramine 4 mg/5 ml. Bot. 473 ml. *Rx.*
Use: Antihistamine, decongestant.

Poly-Histine DM. (Sanofi Winthrop) Dextromethorphan HBr 10 mg, phenylpropanolamine HCl 12.5 mg, brompheniramine maleate 2 mg/5 ml. Bot. pt. *Rx.*
Use: Antihistamine, antitussive, decongestant.

Poly-Histine-D Ped Caps. (Sanofi Winthrop) Phenylpropanolamine HCl 25 mg, phenyltoloxamine citrate 8 mg, pheniramine maleate 8 mg, pyrilamine maleate 8 mg/Cap. Bot. 100s. *Rx.*
Use: Antihistamine, decongestant.

Poly-Histine Elixir. (Sanofi Winthrop) Phenyltoloxamine citrate 4 mg, pyrilamine maleate 4 mg, pheniramine maleate 4 mg/5 ml, alcohol 4%. Elix. Bot. pt. *Rx.*
Use: Antihistamine.

poly I; poly C12U.
Use: AIDS, antineoplastic. [Orphan drug]

•**polymacon.** (PAHL-ee-MAY-kahn) USAN.
Use: Contact lens material (hydrophilic).

polymeric oxygen.
Use: Sickle cell disease. [Orphan drug]

•**polymetaphosphate P 32.** (pahl-ee-met-ah-FOSS-fate) USAN.
Use: Radiopharmaceutical.

polymethine blue dye.

polymonine.

Polymox. (Bristol-Myers) Amoxicillin trihydrate. **Cap.:** 250 mg. Bot. 100s, 500s, UD 100s; 500 mg. Bot. 50s, 100s, 500s, UD 100s. **Oral Susp.:** 125 mg or 250 mg/5 ml. Bot. 80 ml, 100 ml, 150 ml. **Ped. Drops:** 50 mg/ml. Bot. 15 ml. *Rx.*
Use: Anti-infective, penicillin.

polymyxin B. (Various Mfr.) (No pharmaceutical form available) Antimicrobial substances produced by *Bacillus polymyxa.*
W/Bacitracin zinc, neomycin sulfate, benzalkonium Cl.
See: Biotres, Oint. (Schwarz Pharma).

•**polymyxin B sulfate.** (pahl-ee-mix-in) U.S.P. 23.
Use: Anti-infective.
See: Aerosporin, Pow., Soln. (Glaxo-Wellcome).

polymyxin B sulfate and bacitracin zinc topical aerosol.
Use: Anti-infective, topical.

polymyxin B sulfate and bacitracin zinc topical powder.
Use: Anti-infective, topical.

polymyxin B sulfate and hydrocortisone otic solution.
Use: Anti-infective, anti-inflammatory, otic.

polymyxin B sulfate sterile. (Roerig) Polymyxin B sulfate 500,000 units Ophth Soln. Vial 20 ml for reconstitution. *Rx.*
Use: Anti-infective.

polymyxin B sulfate w/combinations.
See: AK-Poly-Bac Oint. (Akorn).

AK-Spore, Preps. (Akorn).
Aquaphor, Oint. (Beiersdorf).
Cortisporin, Preps. (GlaxoWellcome).
Epimycin A, Oint. (Delta).
Maxitrol, Oint., Ophthalmic Oint. (Pharmacia & Upjohn).
Mycitracin, Oint., Ophthalmic Oint. (Pharmacia & Upjohn).
Neomixin, Oint. (Roberts Pharm).
Neosporin, Preps. (GlaxoWellcome).
Neosporin G.U. Irrigant, Amp. (GlaxoWellcome).
Neotal, Oint. (Roberts Pharm).
Neo-Thrycex, Oint. (Del Pharmaceuticals).
Ocutricin, Preps. (Bausch & Lomb).
Otobiotic, Soln. (Schering Plough).
Otoreid-HC, Liq. (Solvay).
Polysporin, Oint., Ophthalmic Oint. (GlaxoWellcome).
Polytrim Ophth. Soln. (Allergan).
Pyocidin-Otic, Soln. (Berlex).
Statrol, Liq. (Alcon Laboratories).
Statrol Sterile Ophthalmic Oint. (Alcon Laboratories).
Terramycin, Preps. w/Oxytetracycline (Pfizer).
Tigo, Oint. (Burlington).
Tribiotic Plus, Oint. (Thompson Medical).
Trimixin, Oint. (Hance).

polymyxin-neomycin-bacitracin ointment. (Various Mfr.). *otc.*
Use: Anti-infective, topical.

polynoxylin. Poly[methylenedi(hydroxymethyl)urea]. Anaflex.

polyoxyethylene 8 stearate. Myrj 45. (Zeneca), Polyoxyl 8 Stearate.

polyoxyethylene (20) sorbitan monoleate.
See: Polysorbate 80, U.S.P. 23. (Various Mfr.).

polyoxyethylene 20 sorbitan trioleate. Tween 85. (Zeneca), Polysorbate 85.

polyoxyethylene 20 sorbitan tristearate. Tween 65. (Zeneca), Polysorbate 65.

polyoxyethylene 40 monostearate. Polyoxyl 40 Stearate.
See: Myrj 52 & Myrj 52S (Zeneca).

polyoxyethylene 50 stearate.
See: Polyoxyl 50 stearate.

polyoxyethyleneonylphenol.
W/Alkylbenzyldimethylammonium Cl, methylrosaniline Cl, polyethylene glycol tert-dodecylthioether.
See: Hyva, Vaginal Tab. (Holland-Rantos).

polyoxyethylene lauryl ether.
W/Benzoyl peroxide, ethyl alcohol.
See: Benzagel, Gel (Dermik Laboratories).
Desquam-X, Preps. (Westwood Squibb).
W/Hydrocortisone, sulfur.
See: Fostril HC, Lot. (Westwood Squibb).
W/Sulfur.
See: Fostril, Lot. (Westwood Squibb).
Proseca, Oint. (Westwood Squibb).

polyoxyethylene nonyl phenol.
W/Sodium edetate, docusate sodium, 9-aminoacridine HCl.
See: Vagisec Plus, Supp. (Schmid).

polyoxyethylene sorbitan monolaurate. Polysorbate 20, N.F. 18.
W/Ferrous gluconate.
See: Simron, Cap. (Hoechst Marion Roussel).
W/Ferrous gluconate, vitamins.
See: Simron Plus, Cap. (Hoechst Marion Roussel).

•**polyoxyl 8 stearate.** (PAHL-ee-OX-ill 8 STEE-ah-rate) USAN.
Use: Pharmaceutic aid (surfactant).
See: Myrj 45 (Atlas).

•**polyoxyl 10 oleyl ether.** (PAHL-ee-OX-ill 10 EETH-ehr) N.F. 18.
Use: Pharmaceutic aid (surfactant).

•**polyoxyl 20 cetostearyl ether.** (PAHL-ee-OX-ill 20 SEE-toe-STEE-rill EETH-ehr) N.F. 18.
Use: Pharmaceutic aid (surfactant).

•**polyoxyl 35 castor oil.** (PAHL-ee-OX-ill) N.F. 18.
Use: Pharmaceutic aid (surfactant, emulsifying agent).

•**polyoxyl 40 hydrogenated castor oil.** (PAHL-ee-OX-ill 40 high-DRAH-jen-ATE-ehd) N.F. 18.
Use: Pharmaceutic aid (surfactant, emulsifying agent).

•**polyoxyl 40 stearate.** (PAHL-ee-OX-ill 40 STEE-ah-rate) N.F. 18. Macrogic Stearate 2,000 (I.N.N.) Polyoxyethylene 40 monostearate.
Use: Pharmaceutic aid (surfactant).
Use: Hydrophilic oint., surfactant; surface-active agent.
See: Myrj 52 (Atlas).
Myrj 52S (Atlas).
W/Polyethylene glycol, chlorobutanol.
See: Blink-N-Clean (Allergan).

•**polyoxyl 50 stearate.** (PAHL-ee-OX-ill 50 STEE-ah-rate) N.F. 18. *Formerly Polyxyethylene 50 stearate.*
Use: Pharmaceutic aid (surfactant, emulsifying agent).

•**polyoxypropylene 15 stearyl ether.** USAN. *Formerly PPG-15 Stearyl Ether.*

Use: Pharmaceutic aid (solvent).

Poly-Pred Suspension. (Allergan) Prednisolone acetate 0.5%, neomycin sulfate equivalent to 0.35% neomycin base, polymyxin B sulfate 10,000 units/ml. Dropper bot. 5 ml, 10 ml. *Rx.*
Use: Anti-infective; corticosteroid, ophthalmic.

polypropylene glycol. An addition polymer of propylene oxide and water.
Use: Pharmaceutic aid (suspending agent).

polysaccharide iron complex. (Various Mfr.) Iron 50 mg/Cap. Bot. 100s. *otc.*
Use: Mineral supplement.
See: Hytinic, Preps. (Hyrex).
Niferex, Prods. (Schwarz Pharma).
Nu-Iron, Prods. (Merz).

polysonic lotion. (Parker) Multi-purpose ultrasound lotion with high coupling efficiency. Bot. 8.5 oz, gal.
Use: Diagnostic aid, therapeutic aid.

•**polysorbate 20.** (PAHL-ee-SORE-bate 20) N.F. 18.
Use: Pharmaceutic aid (surfactant).

•**polysorbate 40.** (PAHL-ee-SORE-bate 40) N.F. 18.
Use: Pharmaceutic aid (surfactant).

•**polysorbate 60.** (PAHL-ee-SORE-bate 60) N.F. 18.
Use: Pharmaceutic aid (surfactant).

•**polysorbate 65.** (PAHL-ee-SORE-bate 65) USAN.
Use: Pharmaceutic aid (surfactant).

•**polysorbate 80.** (PAHL-ee-SORE-bate 80) N.F. 18.
Use: Pharmaceutic aid (surfactant).

•**polysorbate 85.** (PAHL-ee-SORE-bate 85) USAN.
Use: Pharmaceutic aid (surfactant).

Polysorb Hydrate. (E. Fougera) Sorbitan sesquinoleate in a wax and petrolatum base. Cream. Tube 56.7 g, lb. *otc.*
Use: Emollients.

Polysporin Ointment. (GlaxoWellcome) Polymyxin B sulfate 10,000 units, bacitracin zinc 500 units/g in special white petrolatum base. Tube 3.75 g. *otc.*
Use: Anti-infective, topical.

Polysporin Ophthalmic Ointment. (GlaxoWellcome) Polymyxin B sulfate, 10,000 units, bacitracin zinc 500 units. Tube 3.5 g. *Rx.*
Use: Antibiotic, ophthalmic.

Polysporin Powder. (GlaxoWellcome) Polymyxin B 10,000 units, zinc bacitracin 500 units, lactose base/g. Shaker vial 10 g. *Rx.*
Use: Anti-infective, topical.

polysulfides. Polythionate.

Polytabs-F Chewable Vitamin. (Major) Fluoride 1 mg, vitamins A 2500 IU, D 400 IU, E 15 mg, B_1 1.05 mg, B_2 1.2 mg, B_3 13.5 mg, B_6 1.05 mg, B_{12} 4.5 mcg, C 60 mg, folic acid 0.3 mg/Tab. Bot. 100s, 1000s. *Rx.*
Use: Mineral, vitamin supplement.

Polytar Shampoo. (Stiefel) A neutral soap containing 1% Polytar in a surfactant shampoo. Buffered. Plastic Bot. 6 fl oz, 12 fl oz, gal. *otc.*
Use: Antiseborrheic.

Polytar Soap. (Stiefel) A neutral soap containing 1% Polytar. Cake 4 oz. *otc.*
Use: Dermatologic.

•**polytef.** (PAHL-ee-teff) USAN.
Use: Prosthetic aid.

•**polythiazide.** (PAHL-ee-THIGH-azz-ide) U.S.P. 23.
Use: Antihypertensive, diuretic.
See: Renese Tab. (Pfizer).
W/Prazosin.
See: Minizide, Cap. (Pfizer).
W/Reserpine.
See: Renese-R, Tab. (Pfizer).

Polytinic. (Pharmics) Elemental iron 100 mg, vitamin C 300 mg, folic acid 1 mg/tab. Bot. 100s. *Rx.*
Use: Mineral, vitamin supplement.

Polytrim. (Allergan) Polymyxin B sulfate 10,000 units/g or ml, trimethoprim 1 mg/ml. Drop. Bot. 10 ml. *Rx.*
Use: Anti-infective, ophthalmic.

Polytuss-DM. (Rhode) Dextromethorphan HBr 15 mg, chlorpheniramine maleate 1 mg, guaifenesin 25 mg/5 ml. Bot. 4 oz, 8 oz. *otc.*
Use: Antihistamine, antitussive, expectorant.

•**polyurethane foam.** (PAHL-ih-you-ree-thane foam) USAN.
Use: Prosthetic aid (internal bone splint).

polyvidone.
See: Polyvinylpyrrolidone.

Poly-Vi-Flor 0.25 mg. (Bristol-Myers Squibb) **Drops:** Vitamins A 1500 IU, D 400 IU, E 5 IU, C 35 mg, B_1 0.5 mg, B_2 0.6 mg, B_6 0.4 mg, B_3 8 mg, B_{12} 2 mcg, fluoride 0.25 mg/ml. Dropper bot. 50 ml. **Tab.:** Vitamins A 2500 IU, D 400 IU, E 15 IU, B_1 1.05 mg, B_2 1.2 mg, B_3 13.5 mg, B_6 1.05 mg, B_{12} 4.5 mcg, C 60 mg, folic acid, 0.3 mg, fluoride 0.25 mg, lactose, sucrose. Chewable. Bot. 100s. *Rx.*
Use: Mineral, vitamin supplement; dental caries agent.

Poly-Vi-Flor 0.5 mg Chewable Tabs. (Bristol-Myers Squibb) Vitamins A 2500 IU, D 400 IU, E 15 IU, C 60 mg, B_1 1.05 mg, B_2 1.2 mg, B_3 13.5 mg, B_6 1.05 mg, B_{12} 4.5 mcg, fluoride 0.5 mg, folic acid 0.3 mg/Chew. tab. Bot. 100s. **With Iron:** Above formula plus iron 12 mg, copper, zinc 10 mg/Tab. Bot. 100s. *Rx.*
Use: Mineral, vitamin supplement; dental caries agent.

Poly-Vi-Flor 1 mg Chewable Tablets. (Bristol-Myers Squibb) Vitamins A 2500 IU, D 400 IU, E 15 IU, C 60 mg, B_1 1.05 mg, B_2 1.2 mg, B_3 13.5 mg, B_6 1.05 mg, B_{12} 4.5 mcg, fluoride 1 mg, folic acid 0.3 mg, sucrose/Chew. tab. Bot. 100s, 1000s. **With Iron:** Above formula plus iron 12 mg, copper 1 mg, zinc 10 mg/Tab. *Rx.*
Use: Mineral, vitamin supplement; dental caries agent.

Poly-Vi-Flor 0.5 mg Drops. (Bristol-Myers Squibb) Vitamins A 1500 IU, D 400 IU, E 5 IU, C 35 mg, B_1 0.5 mg, B_2 0.6 mg, B_6 0.4 mg, niacin 8 mg, B_{12} 2 mcg, fluoride 0.5 mg/ml. Dropper bot. 30 ml, 50 ml. *Rx.*
Use: Mineral, vitamin supplement; dental caries agent.

Poly-Vi-Flor 0.25 mg w/Iron. (Bristol-Myers Squibb) **Drops:** Vitamins A 1500 IU, D 400 IU, E 5 IU, C 35 mg, B_1 0.5 mg, B_2 0.6 mg, B_6 0.4 mg, niacin 8 mg, fluoride 0.25 mg, iron 10 mg/ml. Bot. 50 ml. **Tab.:** Vitamins A 2500 IU, D 400 IU, E 15 IU, B_1 1.05 IU, B_2 1.2 mg, B_3 13.5 mg, B_6 1.05 mg, B_{12} 4.5 mcg, C 60 mg, folic acid 0.3 mg, fluoride 0.25 mg, Cu, iron 12 mg, zinc 10 mg, lactose, sucrose. Chewable. Bot. 100s. *Rx.*
Use: Mineral, vitamin supplement; dental caries agent.

Poly-Vi-Flor 0.5 mg w/Iron. (Bristol-Myers) **Drops:** Vitamins A 1500 IU, D 400 IU, E 5 IU, C 35 mg, B_1 0.5 mg, B_2 0.6 mg, B_3 8 mg, B_6 0.4 mg, fluoride 0.5 mg, iron 10 mg/ml. Dropper bot. 50 ml. **Tab.:** Vitamins A 2500 IU, D 400 IU, E 15 IU, B_1 1.05 mg, B_2 1.2 mg, B_3 13.5 mg, B_6 1.05 mg, B_{12} 4.5 mcg, C 60 mg, folic acid 0.3 mg, fluoride 0.5 mg, iron 12 mg, Cu, zinc 10 mg, lactose, sucrose. Chewable. Bot. 100s. *Rx.*
Use: Mineral, vitamin supplement; dental caries agent.

Poly-Vi-Flor 0.5 Tabs. (Bristol-Myers Squibb) Fluoride 0.5 mg, vitamins A 2500 IU, D 400 IU, E 15 mg, B_1 1.05 mg, B_2 1.2 mg, B_3 13.5 mg, B_6 1.05 mg, B_{12} 4.5 mcg, C 60 mg, folic acid 0.3 mg, Cu, iron 12 mg, zinc 10 mg, sucrose. Tab. Bot. 100s. *Rx.*
Use: Mineral, vitamin supplement; dental caries agent.

•**polyvinyl acetate phthalate.** (pahl-ee-VYE-nil) N.F. 18.
Use: Pharmaceutic aid (coating agent).

•**polyvinyl alcohol.** U.S.P. 23. Ethanol, homopolymer.
Use: Pharmaceutic aid (viscosity-increasing agent).
See: Liquifilm Forte (Allergan).
Liquifilm Tears (Allergan).
Puralube Tears, Drops (Fougera).
W/Hydroxypropyl methylcellulose.
See: Liquifilm Wetting Soln. (Allergan).

polyvinylpyrrolidone, polyvidone, povidone.
W/Acetrizoate Sodium
See: Salpix, Vial (Ortho McNeil).

polyvinylpyrrolidone vinylacetate copolymers.
See: Ivy-Rid, Spray (Roberts Pharm).
W/Benzalkonium.
See: Ivy-Chex, Aerosol (Jones Medical Industries).

Poly-Vi-Sol Drops. (Bristol-Myers Squibb) Vitamins A 1500 IU, D 400 IU, C 35 mg, B_1 0.5 mg, B_2 0.6 mg, E 5 IU, B_6 0.4 mg, B_3 8 mg, B_{12} 2 mcg/ml. Bot. 50 ml. *otc.*
Use: Vitamin supplement.

Poly-Vi-Sol Tablets. (Bristol-Myers Squibb) Vitamins A 2500 IU, E 15 IU, D 400 IU, C 60 mg, B_1 1.05 mg, B_2 1.2 mg, B_3 13.5 mg, B_6 1.05 mg, B_{12} 4.5 mcg, folic acid 0.3 mg/Chew. Tab. Bot. 100s. **With Iron:** Above formula plus iron 12 mg, zinc 8 mg/Tab. Bot. 100s. Circus shape Tab. Bot. 100s. *otc.*
Use: Mineral, vitamin supplement.

Poly-Vi-Sol w/Iron Drops. (Bristol-Myers Squibb) Vitamins A 1500 IU, D 400 IU, E 5 IU, C 35 mg, B_1 0.5 mg, B_2 0.6 mg, B_3 8 mg, B_6 0.4 mg, iron 10 mg/ml. Bot. 50 ml. *otc.*
Use: Mineral, vitamin supplement.

Poly-Vi-Sol w/Iron Tablets, Chewable. (Bristol-Myers Squibb) Iron 12 mg, vitamins A 2500 IU, D 400 IU, E 15 mg, B_1 1.05 mg, B_2 1.2 mg, B_3 13.5 mg, B_6 1.05 mg, B_{12} 4.5 mcg, C 60 mg, folic acid 0.3 mg, Cu, zinc 8 mg, sugar/Tab. Bot. 100s. *otc.*
Use: Mineral, vitamin supplement.

Poly-Vi-Sol w/Minerals. (Bristol-Myers) Iron 12 mg, vitamins A 2500 IU, D 400 IU, E 15 mg, B_1 1.05 mg, B_2 1.2 mg, B_3 13.5 mg, B_6 1.06 mg, B_{12} 4.5 mcg, C

60 mg, folic acid 0.3 mg, Cu, zinc 8 mg/ Chew. tab. Bot. 60s, 100s. *otc.*
Use: Mineral, vitamin supplement.

poly-vitamin drops. (Schein Pharmaceutical) Vitamins A 1500 IU, D 400 IU, E 5 IU, B_1 0.5 mg, B_2 0.6 mg, B_3 8 mg, B_6 0.4 mg, B_{12} 1.5 mcg, C 35 mg/ml. Drop. Bot. 50 ml. *otc.*
Use: Vitamin supplement.

Polyvitamin Drops with Iron. (Various Mfr.) Iron 10 mg, vitamins A 1500 IU, D 400 IU, E 5 mg, B_1 0.5 mg, B_2 0.6 mg, B_3 8 mg, B_6 0.4 mg, C 35 mg/ml. Bot. 50 ml. *otc.*
Use: Mineral, vitamin supplement.

polyvitamin drops w/iron and fluoride. (Various Mfr.) Fluoride 0.25 mg, vitamins A 1500 IU, D 400 IU, E 5 IU, B_1 0.5 mg, B_2 0.6 mg, B_3 8 mg, B_6 0.4 mg, C 35 mg, iron 10 mg. Bot. 50 ml. *Rx.*
Use: Mineral, vitamin supplement; dental caries agent.

polyvitamin fluoride. (Various Mfr.) Fluoride 0.25 mg, Vitamins A 1500 IU, D 400 IU, E 5 IU, B_1 0.5 mg, B_2 0.6 mg, B_3 8 mg, B_6 0.4 mg, B_{12} 2 mcg, C 35 mg/ml. Drop. Bot. 50 ml. *Rx.*
Use: Mineral, vitamin supplement; dental caries agent.

poly-vitamins w/fluoride 0.5 mg. (Various Mfr.) **Drops:** Fluoride 0.5 mg, vitamins A 1500 IU, D 400 IU, E 5 IU, B_1 0.5 mg, B_2 0.6 mg, B_3 8 mg, B_6 0.4 mg, B_{12} 2 mcg, C 35 mg/ml. Bot. 50 ml. **Tab.:** Fluoride 0.5 mg, vitamins A 2500 IU, D 400 IU, E 15 mg, B_1 1 mg, B_2 1.2 mg, B_3 13.5 mg, B_6 1 mg, B_{12} 4.5 mcg, C 60 mg, folic acid 0.3 mg/Tab. Bot. 100s, 1000s. *Rx.*
Use: Mineral, vitamin supplement; dental caries agent.

poly-vitamins w/fluoride tablets chewable. (Various Mfr.) Fluoride 1 mg, vitamins A 2500 IU, D 400 IU, E 15 mg, B_1 1.05 mg, B_2 1.2 mg, B_3 13.5 mg, B_6 1.05 mg, B_{12} 4.5 mcg, C 60 mg, folic acid 0.3 mg. Bot. 100s, 1000s. *Rx.*
Use: Mineral, vitamin supplement; dental caries agent.

Polyvitamin Fluoride w/Iron. (Various Mfr.) Fluoride 1 mg, vitamins A 2500 IU, D 400 IU, E 15 mg, B_1 1.05 mg, B_2 1.2 mg, B_3 13.5 mg, B_6 1.05 mg, B_{12} 4.5 mcg, C 60 mg, folic acid 0.3 mg, iron 12 mg, Cu, zinc 10 mg/Tab. Bot. 100s, 1000s. *Rx.*
Use: Mineral, vitamin supplement; dental caries agent.

Polyvitamin w/Fluoride. (Rugby) Fluoride 0.5 mg, vitamins A 1500 IU, D 400 IU, E 5 mg, B_1 0.5 mg, B_2 0.6 mg, B_3 8 mg, B_6 0.4 mg, B_{12} 2 mcg, C 35 mg/ml. Dropper bot. 50 ml. *Rx.*
Use: Mineral, vitamin supplement; dental caries agent.

polyvitamins w/fluoride 0.5 mg and iron. (Rugby) Fluoride 0.5 mg, vitamins A 2500 IU, D 400 IU, E 15 IU, B_1 1.05 mg, B_2 1.2 mg, B_3 13.5 mg, B_6 1.05 mg, B_{12} 4.5 mcg, C 60 mg, folic acid 0.3 mg, Cu, iron 12 mg, zinc 10 mg, sucrose/Tab. Bot. 100s. *Rx.*
Use: Mineral, vitamin supplement; dental caries agent.

Polyvite with Fluoride. (Geneva Pharm) Fluoride 0.25 mg, vitamins A 1500 IU, D 400 IU, E 5 mg, B_1 0.5 mg, B_2 0.6 mg, B_3 8 mg, B_6 0.4 mg, B_{12} 2 mcg, C 35 mg/ml. Dropper bot. 50 ml. *Rx.*
Use: Mineral, vitamin supplement; dental caries agent.

•**ponalrestat.** (poe-NAHL-ress-TAT) USAN.
Use: Antidiabetic.

Ponaris. (Jamol) Nasal emollient of mucosal lubricating and moisturizing botanical oils. Cajeput, eucalyptus, peppermint in iodized cottonseed oil. Bot. 1 oz w/dropper. *otc.*
Use: Moisturizer, nasal.

Ponstel Kapseals. (Parke-Davis) Mefenamic acid 250 mg/Cap. Bot. 100s. *Rx.*
Use: Analgesic, NSAID.

Pontocaine. (Sanofi Winthrop) **Cream:** Tetracaine HCl 1%, glycerin, light mineral oil, methylparaben, sodium metabisulfite. Tube 28.35 g. **Oint.:** Tetracaine 0.5%, menthol, white petrolatum. Tube 28.35 g. *otc.*
Use: Anesthetic, topical.

Pontocaine Hydrochloride. (Sanofi Winthrop) Tetracaine HCl. **Inj. 0.2%:** Dextrose 6%. Amp 2 ml. **0.3%:** Dextrose 6%. Amp 5 ml. **1%:** Acetone sodium bisulfite. Amp 2 ml. **Powd. for reconstitution:** Niphanoid (instantly soluble) amps 20 mg. *Rx.*
Use: Anesthetic, topical.

Pontocaine Hydrochloride 0.5% Solution for Ophthalmology. (Sanofi Winthrop) Tetracaine HCl 0.5%. Bot. 15 ml, 59 ml. *Rx.*
Use: Anesthetic, local.

Pontocaine Hydrochloride in Dextrose (Hyperbaric). (Sanofi Winthrop) **0.2%:** Tetracaine HCl 2 mg/ml in a sterile solution containing dextrose 6%. Amp. 2 ml, 10s. **0.3%:** Tetracaine HCl 3 mg/ml in a sterile solution containing dextrose 6%. Amp. 5 ml, 10s. *Rx.*

Use: Anesthetic, local.

Pontocaine Ointment. (Sanofi Winthrop) Tetracaine 0.5% and menthol in an ointment consisting of white petrolatum and white wax. Tube 1 oz. *Rx.*
Use: Anesthetic, local.

Pontocaine 2% Aqueous Solution. (Sanofi Winthrop) Tetracaine HCl 20 mg, chlorobutanol 4 mg/ml of 2% soln. Bot. 30 ml, Box 12s. Bot. 118 ml, Box 6s. *Rx.*
Use: Anesthetic, local.

Po-Pon-S. (Shionogi) Vitamins A 2000 IU, D 100 IU, E 5 mg, B_1 5 mg, B_2 3 mg, B_3 35 mg, B_5 15 mg, B_6 4 mg, B_{12} 6 mcg, C 100 mg, Ca, P/Tab. Bot. 60s, 240s. *otc.*
Use: Vitamin/mineral supplement.

poppy-seed oil. The ethyl ester of the fatty acids of the poppy w/iodine.
See: Lipiodol, Ascendant & Lafay, Amps., Vial (Savage).

Porcelana Skin Bleaching Agent. (DEP) **Regular:** Hydroquinone 2%. Jar 2 oz, 4 oz. **Sunscreen:** Hydroquinone 2%, octyl dimethyl PABA 2.5%. Jar 4 oz. *Rx.*
Use: Dermatologic.

porcine islet preparation, encapsulated.
Use: For Type I diabetic patients already on immunosuppression. [Orphan drug]

•**porfimer sodium.** (PORE-fih-muhr) USAN.
Use: Antineoplastic. [Orphan drug]
See: Photofrin, Inj. (QLT Photo).

•**porfiromycin.** (par-FIH-row-MY-sin) USAN.
Use: Anti-infective, antineoplastic.

Pork NPH Iletin II. (Eli Lilly) Purified pork insulin 100 units/ml in isophane insulin suspension (insulin w/ protamine and zinc). Inj. Bot. 10 ml.
Use: Antidiabetic.

Pork Regular Iletin II. (Eli Lilly) Insulin 100 units/ml. Purified pork. Inj. Vial 10 ml.
Use: Antidiabetic.

pork thyroid, defatted.

•**porofocon a.** (PAR-oh-FOE-kahn A) USAN.
Use: Contact lens material (hydrophobic).

•**porofocon b.** (PAR-oh-FOE-kahn B) USAN.
Use: Contact lens material (hydrophobic).

Portabiday. (Washington Ethical) Concentrated soln. of alkylamine lauryl sulfate, a mild detergent with pH approx. 6 for use with Portabiday Vaginal Cleansing Kit. Bot. 3 oz. *otc.*
Use: Vaginal agent.

Portagen. (Bristol-Myers) A nutritionally complete dietary powder containing as a % of the calories protein 14% as caseinate, fat 41% (medium chain triglycerides 86%, corn oil 14%), carbohydrate 45% as corn syrup solids and sucrose, vitamins A 5000 IU, D 500 IU, E 20 IU, C 52 mg, B_1 1 mg, B_2 1.2 mg, B_6 1.4 mg, B_{12} 4 mcg, niacin 13 mg, folic acid 0.1 mg, choline 83 mg, biotin 0.05 mg, calcium 600 mg, phosphorus 450 mg, magnesium 133 mg, iron 12 mg, iodine 47 mcg, copper 1 mg, zinc 6 mg, manganese 0.8 mg, chloride 550 mg, sodium 300 mg, potassium 800 mg, pantothenic acid 6.7 mg, K-1 0.1 mg/Qt. 20 Kcal/fl oz. Can 1 lb. *otc.*
Use: Nutritional supplement, enteral.

porton asparaginase.
See: Erwinia asparaginase.

Posicor. (Roche) Mibefradil dihydrochloride 50 mg, 100 mg, lactose. Tab. Bot. 100s, 300s, Tel-E-Dose 100s. *Rx.*
Use: Antihypertensive.

positive and negative hcg urine controls. (Wampole Laboratories) Positive and negative human urine controls for Wampole urine pregnancy tests. 1 set, 1 vial each.
Use: Diagnostic aid.

Poslam Psoriasis Ointment. (Last) Sulfur 5%, salicylic acid 2%. Jar 1 oz.
Use: Antipsoriatic.

postafene.
See: Bonamine, Tab. (Pfizer).

posterior pituitary hormones.
See: Pituitrin (S) (Parke-Davis).
Pitressin Synthetic (Parke-Davis).
Pitressin Tannate in Oil (Parke-Davis).
Diapid (Novartis).
Concentraid (Ferring Pharmaceuticals).
DDAVP (Rhone-Poulenc Rorer).

posterior pituitary injection.
Use: Hormone (antidiuretic).

postlobin-o.
See: Pituitary, Posterior, Hormone (b).

postlobin-v.
See: Pituitary, Posterior, Hormone (a).

Posture. (Wyeth Ayerst) Calcium phosphate 300 mg or 600 mg/Tab. Bot. 60s. *otc.*
Use: Mineral supplement.

Posture D 600. (Wyeth Ayerst) Calcium phosphate 600 mg, vitamin D 125 IU/Tab. Bot. 60s. *otc.*

Use: Mineral supplement.

Potaba. (Glenwood) Potassium p-aminobenzoate. **Cap.:** 0.5 g. Bot. 250s, 1000s. **Pow.:** 100 g. 1 lb. **Tab.:** 0.5 g. Bot. 100s, 1000s. **Envule:** 2 g. Box 50s. *Rx.*
Use: Nutritional supplement.

Potable Aqua Kit. (Wisconsin Pharm) Tetraglycine hydroperiodide 16.7% (6.68% titrable iodine). Tab. Bot. 50s with collapsible gallon container. *otc.*
Use: Water purifier.

Potachlor 10%. (Rosemont) Potassium and chloride 20 mEq/15 ml. With alcohol 5%. Bot. pt, gal. With alcohol 3.8%. Bot. pt, gal, UD 15 ml and 30 ml. *Rx.*
Use: Electrolyte supplement.

Potachlor 20%. (Rosemont) Potassium and chloride 40 mEq/15 ml, alcohol free. Liq. Bot. pt, gal. *Rx.*
Use: Electrolyte supplement.

•**potash, sulfurated.** U.S.P. 23.
Use: Source of sulfide.

potassic saline lactated injection.
Use: Fluid, electrolyte replacement.

•**potassium acetate.** (poe-TASS-ee-uhm ASS-eh-tate) U.S.P. 23. Acetic acid, potassium salt.
Use: Electrolyte replacement; to avoid Cl when high concentration of potassium is needed.

potassium acetate. (Various Mfr.) **Inj.:**40 mEq, 20 ml in 50 ml Vial.
Use: Electrolyte replacement; to avoid Cl when high concentration of potassium is needed.

potassium acid phosphate.
See: K-Phos, Tab. (Beach Pharmaceuticals).
Uro-K, Tab. (Star).

potassium acid phosphate/sodium acid phosphate.
Use: Genitourinary.
See: K-Phos M.F. (Beach Pharmaceuticals).
K-Phos No. 2 (Beach.

•**potassium aspartate and magnesium aspartate.** (poe-TASS-ee-uhm ass-PAR-tates and mag-NEE-zee-uhm ass-PAR-tate) USAN.
Use: Nutrient.

•**potassium benzoate.** (poe-TASS-ee-uhn) N.F. 18.
Use: Pharmaceutic aid (preservative).

•**potassium bicarbonate.** (poe-TASS-ee-uhm) U.S.P. 23.
Use: Pharmaceutic necessity; electrolyte replacement.

potassium bicarbonate effervescent tablets for oral solution.
Use: Electrolyte supplement.

potassium bicarbonate and potassium chloride for effervescent oral solution.
Use: Electrolyte supplement.

potassium bicarbonate and potassium chloride effervescent tablets for oral solution.
Use: Electrolyte supplement.

potassium bicarbonate and sodium bicarbonate and citric acid effervescent tablets for oral solution.
Use: Electrolyte supplement.

•**potassium bitartrate.** (poe-TASS-ee-uhm bye-TAR-trate) U.S.P. 23.
Use: Cathartic.

•**potassium carbonate.** U.S.P. 23.
Use: Potassium therapy; pharmaceutic aid (alkalizing agent).

•**potassium chloride.** (poe-TASS-ee-uhm KLOR-ide) U.S.P. 23.
Use: Electrolyte replacement, potassium deficiency, hypopotassemia.

potassium chloride. (Abbott Laboratories) **Ampules:** 20 mEq, 10 ml; 40 mEq, 20 ml. **Pintop Vials:** 10 mEq, 5 ml in 10 ml; 20 mEq, 10 ml in 20 ml; 30 mEq, 12.5 ml in 30 ml; 40 mEq, 12.5 ml in 30 ml. **Fliptop Vials:** 20 mEq, 10 ml in 20 ml; 40 mEq, 20 ml in 50 ml. **Univ. Add. Syr.:** 5 mEq/5 ml, 20 mEq/10 ml, 30 mEq/20 ml, 40 mEq/20 ml (Eli Lilly) Amp. (40 mEq) 20 ml, 6s, 25s.
Capsules:
See: K-Norm, Cap. (Medeva). Micro-K Extencaps, Cap. (Robins). **Liquid:**
See: Cena-K, Liq. (Century Pharm).
Choice 10 and 20, Soln. (Whiteworth Towne).
Kaochlor, Preps. (Pharmacia & Upjohn).
Kaon-C1 20%, Liq. (Pharmacia & Upjohn).
Kay Ciel, Elix. (Berlex).
Klor-Con, Liq. (Upsher-Smith Labs).
Klotrix, Tab. (Bristol-Myers).
Klowess (Novartis).
K-Lyte/C1, Tab. (Bristol-Myers).
Pan-Kloride, Liq. (U.S. Products).
Potassine, Liq. (Recsei).
Powder:
See: Kaochlor-Eff, Gran. (Pharmacia & Upjohn).
Kato, Pow. (Ingram).
Kay Ciel, Pow. (Berlex).
K-Lor, Pow. (Abbott Laboratories).
K-Lyte/Cl, Pow. (Bristol-Myers).
Potage, Pow. (Teva USA).
Tablets:

See: K+8, ER Tab. (Alra Laboratories).
Kaon, Tab. (Pharmacia & Upjohn).
Kaon Controlled Release Tab. (Pharmacia & Upjohn).
Klorvess Effervescent Tab. (Novartis).
K-Lyte/Cl 50, Tab. (Bristol-Myers).
K-Tab, Tab. (Abbott Laboratories).
Micro-K Extencap (Robins).
Slow-K, Tab. (Novartis).
Ten-K, Cap. (Novartis).

potassium chloride. (Roxane) **Oral soln.:** Potassium Cl, sugar free. 40 mEq/30 ml. Bot. 6 oz, 500 ml, 1 L, 5 L 20%. 80 mEq/30 ml. Bot. 500 ml, 1 L, 5 L. **Pow.:** 20 mEq/4 g. Pkt. 30s, 100s. *Rx.*
Use: Electrolyte supplement.

potassium chloride in dextrose and sodium chloride injection.
Use: Electrolyte supplement.

potassium chloride in lactated ringer's and dextrose injection.
Use: Electrolyte supplement.

potassium chloride in sodium chloride injection.
Use: Electrolyte supplement.

•**potassium chloride K 42.** (poe-TASS-ee-uhm KLOR-ide K 42) USAN.
Use: Radiopharmaceutical.

potassium chloride with potassium gluconate.
See: Kolyum, Prods. (Medeva).

potassium chloride, potassium bicarbonate, and potassium citrate effervescent tablets for oral solution.

potassium chloride solution. (ESI Lederle Generics) Potassium Cl 10% or 20%. Sugar free. Bot. 16 oz, gal. *Rx.*
Use: Electrolyte supplement.

•**potassium citrate.** (poe-TASS-ee-uhm SIH-trate) U.S.P. 23. Tripotassium Citrate.
Use: Alkalizer. [Orphan drug]
See: Urocit-K, Tab. (Mission Pharmacal).
W/Sodium citrate.
See: Bicitra, Liq. (Baker Norton).
W/Sodium citrate, citric acid.
See: Cytra, Prods. (Cypress).
Polycitra-K, Crystals, Liq. (Baker Norton).
Polycitra-LC, Liq. (Baker Norton).

potassium citrate and citric acid oral solution.
Use: Alkalizer, systemic.

potassium clavulanate/amoxicillin.
Use: Anti-infective, penicillin.
See: Amoxicillin and Potassium Clavulanate.

potassium clavulanate/ticarcillin.
Use: Anti-infective, penicillin.
See: Ticarcillin and Clavulanate Potassium.

potassium estrone sulfate.
W/Micro crystalline estrone.
See: Estrones Duo-Action, Vial (Med Chem).

•**potassium glucaldrate.** (poe-TASS-ee-uhm glue-KAL-drate) USAN.
Use: Antacid.

•**potassium gluconate.** U.S.P. 23.
Use: Electrolyte replacement.
See: Kalinate, Elix. (Sanofi Winthrop).
Kaon, Elixir, Tab. (Warren-Teed).

potassium gluconate and potassium chloride oral solution.
Use: Replacement therapy.

potassium gluconate and potassium chloride for oral solution.
Use: Replacement therapy.

potassium gluconate elixir. (Various Mfr.) Potassium 40 mEq provided by potassium gluconate 9.36 g/30 ml, alcohol 5%. Bot. pt, Patient-Cup 15 ml. *Rx.*
Use: Electrolyte supplement.

potassium gluconate, potassium citrate, and ammonium chloride oral solution.
Use: Electrolyte supplement.

potassium gluconate and potassium citrate oral solution.
Use: Electrolyte supplement.

potassium glutamate. The monopotassium salt of l-glutamic acid.

potassium G penicillin.
See: Penicillin G Potassium, U.S.P. 23.

•**potassium guaiacolsulfonate.** (poe-TASS-ee-uhm gwie-ah-kole-SULL-foe-nate) U.S.P. 23. Sulfoguaiacol. Potassium Hydroxymethoxybenzenesulfonate. Used in many cough preps.
Use: Expectorant.
See: Conex, Liq. (Westerfield).
Pinex Regular, Syr. (Pinex).

potassium guaiacolsulfonate w/combinations.
See: Cherralex, Syr. (Alphalma USPD).
Guahist, Vial (Hickam).
Partuss, Liq. (Parmed).
Protuss, Liq. (Horizon).
Protuss-D, Liq. (Horizon).
Tusquelin, Syr. (Circle).

potassium hetacillin.
See: Versapen K, Inj., Cap. (Bristol-Myers).

•**potassium hydroxide.** N.F. 18.
Use: Pharmaceutic aid (alkalinizing agent).

potassium in sodium chloride. (Various Mfr.) Potassium Cl 0.15%, 0.22% or 0.3% in sodium Cl 0.9%. Soln. for Inj. 1000 ml. *Rx.*
Use: Intravenous replenishment solution, nutritional supplement.

•**potassium iodide.** (poe-TASS-ee-uhm EYE-oh-dide) U.S.P. 23.
Use: Expectorant, antifungal, supplement (iodine).
See: Pima, Syr., Expectorant (Fleming).
SSKI, Liq. (Upsher-Smith Labs).

potassium iodide w/combinations.
See: Diastix, Reagent Strips (Bayer Corp).
Elixophyllin-KI, Elix. (Berlex).
Iodo-Niacin, Tab. (Cole).
KIE, Syr., Tab. (Laser).
Mudrane, Tab. (ECR Pharmaceuticals).
Mudrane-2, Tab. (ECR Pharmaceuticals).
Quadrinal, Tab., Susp. (Knoll Pharmaceuticals).

potassium iodide and niacinamide.
See: Iodo-Niacin, Tab. (Cole).

•**potassium metabisulfite.** N.F. 18.
Use: Pharmaceutic aid (antioxidant).

•**potassium metaphosphate.** N.F. 18.
Use: Pharmaceutic aid (buffering agent).

•**potassium nitrate.** (poe-TASS-ee-uhm NYE-trate) U.S.P. 23.

potassium p-aminobenzoate.
See: Potaba, Preps. (Glenwood).
W/Potassium salicylate.
See: Pabalate-SF, Tab. (Robins).
W/Pyridoxine.
See: Potaba Plus 6, Cap., Tab. (Glenwood).

potassium p-aminosalicylate.
See: Paskalium, Preps. (Glenwood).

potassium penicillin G.
Use: Anti-infective, penicillin.
See: Penicillin G, Potassium U.S.P. 23.

potassium penicillin V.
Use: Anti-infective, pencillin.
See: Phenoxymethyl Penicillin Potassium, U.S.P. 23.

potassium perchlorate.
Use: Radiopaque agent.
See: Perchloracap (Mallinckrodt).

•**potassium permanganate.** (poe-TASS-ee-uhm per-MANG-gah-nate) U.S.P. 23. Permanganic acid, potassium salt.
Use: Anti-infective, topical.

potassium phenethicillin. Phenethicillin Potassium, U.S.P. 23.
Use: Anti-infective.

potassium phenoxymethyl penicillin.
Use: Anti-infective.
See: Penicillin V Potassium, U.S.P. 23.

•**potassium phosphate, dibasic.** (poe-TASS-ee-uhm FOSS-fate) U.S.P. 23.
Use: Calcium regulator.

•**potassium phosphate, monobasic.** (poe-TASS-ee-uhm Foss-fate) N.F. 18. Dipotassium hydrogen phosphate.
Use: Pharmaceutic aid (buffering agent), source of potassium.

potassium phosphate, monobasic. (Abbott Laboratories) 15 mM, 5 ml in 10 ml Vial; 45 mM, 15 ml in 20 ml/Inj. Vial.
Use: Pharmaceutic aid (buffering agent), source of potassium.

potassium reagent strips. (Bayer Corp) Quantitative dry reagent strip test for potassium in serum or plasma. Bot. 50s.
Use: Diagnostic aid.

potassium-removing resins.
See: Sodium Polystyrene Sulfonate (Various Mfr.).
SPS (Carolina Medical Products Co.).
Kayexalate (Sanofi Winthrop)

potassium rhodanate.
See: Potassium Thiocyanate.

potassium salicylate.
See: Neocylate, Tab. (Schwarz Pharma).
W/Mephenesin, colchicine alkaloid.
W/Potassium bromide, methapyrilene HCl, vitamins.
See: Alva-Tranquil, Cap., Tab., T.D. Tab. (Alva/Amco).
W/Potassium p-aminobenzoate.
See: Pabalate-SF, Tab. (Robins).

potassium salt.
See: Potassium Sorbate, N.F. 18.

•**potassium sodium tartrate.** (poe-TASS-ee-uhm so-dee-uhm TAR-trate) U.S.P. 23.
Use: Laxative.

•**potassium sorbate.** N.F. 18.
Use: Pharmaceutic aid (antimicrobial).

potassium sulfocyanate. Potassium Rhodanate.
See: Potassium Thiocyanate (Various Mfr.).

potassium thiocyanate. Potassium sulfocyanate, Potassium Rhodanate.

potassium thiphencillin. (poe-TASS-ee-uhm thigh-FEN-sill-in)
Use: Anti-infective.

potassium troclosene. (poe-TASS-ee-uhm TROE-kloe-seen) (Monsanto) Potassium dichloroisocyanurate.
Use: Anti-infective.

•**povidone.** (POE-vih-dohn) U.S.P. 23. *Formerly Polyvidone, Polyvinylpyrrolidone.*
Use: Pharmaceutic aid (dispersing and suspending agent).

•**povidone I 125.** (POE-vih-dohn) USAN.
Use: Radiopharmaceutical.

•**povidone I 131.** (POE-vih-dohn) USAN.
Use: Radiopharmaceutical.

•**povidone-iodine.** (POE-vih-dohn-EYE-uh-dine) U.S.P. 23.
Use: Anti-infective, topical.
See: Betadine, Preps. (Purdue-Fredrick).
Efo-Dine (E. Fougera).
Isodine, Preps. (Blair Laboratories).
Massengill Medicated, Liq. (SmithKline Beecham Pharmaceuticals).

povidone-iodine complex.
See: Betadine, Preps. (Purdue Frederick).
Isodine, Preps. (Blair Laboratories).

PowerMate. (Green Turtle Bay) Vitamins A 5000 IU, E 100 IU, B_3 12.5 mg, C 250 mg, zinc 2.5 mg, Se, n-acetyl-L-cysteine/Tab. Bot. 50s. *otc.*
Use: Mineral, vitamin supplement.

PowerVites. (Green Turtle Bay) Vitamin A 2500 IU, D 150 IU, E 12.5 IU, C 125 mg, B_1 6.3 mg, B_2 6.3 mg, B_3 25 mg, B_5 25 mg, B_6 12.5 mg, B_{12} 6.3 mcg, biotin, folic acid 0.15 mg, B, Ca, Mg, Cu, Zn 2.5 mg, Cr, Mn, K, Se, betaine, hesperidin/Tab. Bot. 40s, 100s, 200s. *otc.*
Use: Mineral, vitamin supplement.

Poyaliver Stronger. (Forest Pharmaceutical) Liver inj. (equivalent to 10 mcg B_{12}), vitamin B_{12} 100 mcg, folic acid 10 mcg, niacinamide 1%/ml. Vial 10 ml. *Rx.*
Use: Nutritional supplement, parenteral.

Poyamin Jel Injection. (Forest Pharmaceutical) Cyanocobalamin 1000 mcg/ml. Vial 10 ml.
Use: Nutritional supplement, parenteral.

Poyaplex. (Forest Pharmaceutical) Vitamins B_1 100 mg, niacinamide 100 mg, B_6 10 mg, B_2 1 mg, panthenol 10 mg, B_{12} 5 mcg/ml. Vial 10 ml, 30 ml. *Rx.*
Use: Nutritional supplement, parenteral.

P.P.D. tuberculin.
See: Tuberculin, Purified Protein Derivative, U.S.P. (Various Mfr.).

P.P. factor (pellagra preventive factor).
See: Nicotinic Acid, Preps. (Various Mfr.)

ppg-15 stearyl ether. (PPG-15 STEE-rill EE-ther)
Use: Pharmaceutic aid (surfactant).

PPI-002.
Use: Malignant mesothelioma. [Orphan drug]

PR-122 (redox-phenytoin). (Pharmos)
Use: Anticonvulsant. [Orphan drug]

PR-225 (redox-acyclovir). (Pharmos)
Use: Treatment of Herpes simplex encephalitis in AIDS. [Orphan drug]

PR-239 (redox-penicillin g). (Pharmos)
Use: Treatment of AIDS-associated neurosyphilis. [Orphan drug]

PR-320 (molecusol-carbamazepine). (Pharmos)
Use: Anticonvulsant. [Orphan drug]

•**practolol.** (PRAK-toe-lole) USAN.
Use: Antiadrenergic (β-receptor).

•**pralidoxime chloride.** (pra-lih-DOCK-seem) U.S.P. 23.
Use: Cholinesterase reactivator.
See: Protopam Chloride, Tab., Inj. (Wyeth Ayerst).

pralidoxime chloride. (Survival Technology) 600 mg. Benzyl alcohol, aminocaproic acid. Inj. Vial 2 ml. *Rx.*
Use: Antidote.

•**pralidoxime iodide.** (pral-ih-DOX-eem EYE-oh-dide) USAN.
Use: Cholinesterase reactivator.
See: Protopam Iodide (Wyeth Ayerst).

•**pralidoxime mesylate.** (pral-ih-DOX-eem) USAN.
Use: Cholinesterase reactivator.

pralidoxime methiodide.
See: Pralidoxime Iodide (Various Mfr.).

pralmorelin dihydrochloride. (pral-more-ELL-in die-HIGH-droe-KLOR-ide) USAN.
Use: Growth hormone releasing factor.

PrameGel. (GenDerm) Pramoxine HCl 1%, menthol 0.5% in base w/benzyl alcohol. Gel. Bot. 118 g. *otc.*
Use: Anesthetic, local.

Pramilet FA. (Ross Laboratories) Vitamins A 4000 IU, B_1 3 mg, B_2 2 mg, B_6 3 mg, B_{12} 3 mcg, C 60 mg, D 400 IU, B_5 1 mg, B_3 10 mg, calcium 250 mg, Cu, I, iron 40 mg, Mg, zinc, folic acid 1 mg/Filmtab. Bot. 100s. *Rx.*
Use: Mineral, vitamin supplement.

•**pramipexole.** (pram-ih-PEX-ole) USAN. (Pharmacia & Upjohn).
Use: Antidepressant (dopamine agonist), antiparkinsonian, antischizophrenic.
See: Mirapex, Tab. (Pharmacia & Upjohn).

•**pramiracetam hydrochloride.** (PRAM-ih-RASS-eh-tam) USAN. *Formerly Amacetam Hydrochloride.*

Use: Cognition adjuvant.

•**pramiracetam sulfate.** (PRAM-ih-RASS-eh-tam) USAN. *Formerly Amacetam Sulfate.*
Use: Cognition adjuvant.

•**pramlintide.** (PRAM-lin-tide) USAN.
Use: Antidiabetic.

Pramosone Cream 0.5%. (Ferndale Laboratories) Hydrocortisone acetate 0.5%, pramoxine HCl 1% in cream base. Tube 1 oz, 4 oz. Jar 4 oz, lb.
Use: Corticosteroid; anesthetic, local.

Pramosone Cream 1%. (Ferndale Laboratories) Hydrocortisone acetate 1%, pramoxine HCl 1% in cream base. Tube 1 oz, 4 oz. Jar 4 oz, lb. *Rx.*
Use: Corticosteroid; anesthetic, local.

Pramosone Cream 2.5%. (Ferndale Laboratories) Hydrocortisone acetate 2.5%, pramoxine HCl 1% in cream base. Tube 1 oz, 4 oz. Jar lb. *Rx.*
Use: Corticosteroid; anesthetic, local.

Pramosone Lotion 0.5%. (Ferndale Laboratories) Hydrocortisone acetate 0.5%, pramoxine HCl 1% in lotion base. Bot. 1 oz, 4 oz, 8 oz. *Rx.*
Use: Corticosteroid; anesthetic, local.

Pramosone Lotion 1%. (Ferndale Laboratories) Hydrocortisone acetate 1%, pramoxine HCl 1% in lotion base. Bot. 2 oz, 4 oz, 8 oz. *Rx.*
Use: Corticosteroid; anesthetic, local.

Pramosone Lotion 2.5%. (Ferndale Laboratories) Hydrocortisone acetate 2.5%, pramoxine HCl 1% in lotion base. Bot 2 oz, gal. *Rx.*
Use: Corticosteroid; anesthetic, local.

Pramosone Ointment 1%. (Ferndale Laboratories) Hydrocortisone acetate 1%, pramoxine HCl 1% in ointment base. Tube 1 oz, 4 oz. Jar 4 oz, lb. *Rx.*
Use: Corticosteroid; anesthetic, local.

Pramoxine HC. (Rugby) Pramoxine HCl 1%, hydrocortisone acetate 1%. Aerosol foam. 10 g w/applicator. *Rx.*
Use: Anorectal preparation.

•**pramoxine hydrochloride.** (pram-OX-een) U.S.P. 23.
Use: Anesthetic, topical.
See: Itch-X, Gel, Spray (B. F. Ascher & Co.).
Prax, Cream, Lot. (Ferndale Laboratories).
Proctofoam, Aerosol (Schwarz Pharma).
Tronothane HCl, Cream, Jel (Abbott Laboratories).

pramoxine hydrochloride w/combinations.
See: Anti-Itch, Lot. (Towne).
Caladryl, Prods. (Parke-Davis).
Dermarex, Cream (Hyrex).
Gentz, Jelly, Wipes (Roxane).
1 + 1 Creme (Dunhall Pharmaceuticals).
1 + 1-F Creme (Dunhall Pharmaceuticals).
Oti-Med, Drops (Hyrex Pharmaceuticals).
Otocalm-H Ear Drops (Parmed).
Perifoam, Aerosol (Rowell Labs.).
Proctofoam-HC, Aerosol (Reed-Carnrick).
Sherform-HC, Oint. (Sheryl).
Steramine Otic, Drops (Merz).
Tri-Otic, Drops (Pharmics).
Zoto-HC, Drops (Horizon).

Prandin. (Novo Nordisk) Repaglinide 0.5 mg, 1 mg, 2 mg. Tab. Bot. 100s, 500s, 1000s. *Rx.*
Use: Antidiabetic.

•**pranolium chloride.** (pray-NO-lee-uhm) USAN.
Use: Cardiovascular agent, antiarrhythmic.

Pravachol. (Bristol-Myers Squibb) Pravastatin sodium 10 mg, 20 mg, 40 mg. Tab. Bot. 90s, 1000s (20 mg only), UD 100s. *Rx.*
Use: Antihyperlipidemic.

•**pravadoline maleate.** (pray-AH-doe-leen) USAN.
Use: Analgesic.

•**pravastatin sodium.** (PRUH-vuh-stuh-tin) USAN.
Use: Antihyperlipidemic.
See: Pravachol, Tab. (Bristol-Myers Squibb).

Prax. (Ferndale Laboratories) Pramoxine HCl 1%. **Cream:** Glycerin, cetyl alcohol, white petrolatum. Jar 13.4 g. **Lot.:** Potassium sorbate, sorbic acid, mineral oil, cetyl alcohol, glycerin, lanolin. Bot. 15 ml, 120 ml, 240 ml. *otc.*
Use: Anesthetic, local.

prazepam. (Various Mfr.) Prazepam. **Tab.:** 5 mg, 10 mg. Bot. 100s, 500s. **Cap.:** 5 mg, 10 mg. Bot. 100s, 500s. *c-iv.*
Use: Anxiolytic.

•**prazosin hydrochloride.** (PRAY-zoe-sin) U.S.P. 23.
Use: Antihypertensive.
See: Minipress, Cap. (Pfizer).

prazosin hydrochloride. (Various Mfr.) 1 mg, 2 mg, 5 mg. Cap. Bot. 30s, 60s, 90s, 100s, 120s, 250s, 500s, 1000s, UD 100s.
Use: Antihypertensive.

Pre-Attain Liquid. (Sherwood Medical) Sodium caseinate, maltodextrin, corn oil, soy lecithin, vitamins A, B_1, B_2, B_3, B_5, B_6, B_{12}, C, D, E, K, folic acid, Ca, Cl, Cu, Fe, I, Mg, Mn, P, Zn. Can 250 ml, closed system 1000 ml. *otc.*
Use: Nutritional supplement.

Precef for Injection. (Bristol-Myers) Ceforanide 500 mg or 1 g/Vial or piggyback. *Rx.*
Use: Anti-infective, cephalosporin.

Precision High Nitrogen Diet. (Novartis) Vanilla flavor: Maltodextrin, pasteurized egg white solids, sucrose, natural and artificial flavors, medium chain triglycerides, partially hydrogenated soybean oil, polysorbate 80, mono and diglycerides, vitamins, minerals. Pow. Packet 2.93 oz. *otc.*
Use: Nutritional supplement.

Precision LR Diet. (Novartis) Orange flavor: Maltodextrin, pasteurized egg white solids, sucrose, medium chain triglycerides, partially hydrogenated soybean oil with BHA, citric acid, natural and artificial flavors, mono- and diglycerides, polysorbate 80, FD & C Yellow No. 5 and No. 6, vitamins, minerals. Pow. Packet 3 oz. *otc.*
Use: Nutritional supplement.

Precose. (Bayer Corp) Acarbose 50 mg or 100 mg/Tab. Bot. 100s, UD 100s. *Rx.*
Use: Antidiabetic.

Predalone 50. (Forest Pharmaceutical) Prednisolone acetate 50 mg/ml. Vial 10 ml. *Rx.*
Use: Corticosteroid.

Predamide Ophthalmic. (Maurry) Sodium sulfacetamide 10%, prednisolone acetate 0.5%, hydroxyethyl cellulose, polysorbate 80, sodium thiosulfate, benzalkonium Cl 0.025%. Bot. 5 ml, 15 ml. *Rx.*
Use: Anti-infective, corticosteroid, ophthalmic.

Predcor-50 Injection. (Roberts Pharm) Prednisolone acetate 50 mg/ml. Vial 10 ml. *Rx.*
Use: Corticosteroid.

Pred Forte. (Allergan) Prednisolone acetate 1%. Susp. Bot. 1 ml, 5 ml, 10 ml, 15 ml. *Rx.*
Use: Corticosteroid, ophthalmic.

Pred-G. (Allergan) Prednisolone acetate 1%, gentamicin sulfate 0.3%. Bot. 2 ml, 5 ml, 10 ml. *Rx.*
Use: Corticosteroid, anti-infective, ophthalmic.

Pred-G S.O.P. (Allergan) Prednisolone acetate 0.6%, gentamicin sulfate 0.3%, chlorobutanol 0.5%. Oint. Tube 3.5 g. *Rx.*
Use: Anti-infective, corticosteroid, ophthalmic.

Predicort-AP. (Dunhall Pharmaceuticals) Prednisolone sodium phosphate 20 mg, prednisolone acetate 80 mg/ml. Vial 10 ml. *Rx.*
Use: Corticosteroid.

Predicort-RP. (Dunhall Pharmaceuticals) Prednisolone sodium phosphate equivalent to prednisolone phosphate 20 mg, niacinamide 25 mg/ml. Vial 10 ml. *Rx.*
Use: Corticosteroid.

Pred Mild. (Allergan) Prednisolone acetate 0.12%. Susp. Bot. 5 ml, 10 ml. *Rx.*
Use: Corticosteroid, ophthalmic.

•**prednazate.** (PRED-nah-zate) USAN.
Use: Anti-inflammatory.

•**prednicarbate.** (PRED-nih-CAR-bate) USAN.
Use: Corticosteroid, topical.
See: Dermatop, Cream (Hoechst Marion Roussel).

Prednicen-M. (Schwarz Pharma) Prednisone 5 mg/Tab. Bot. 100s, 1000s. *Rx.*
Use: Corticosteroid.

•**prednimustine.** (PRED-nih-MUSS-teen) USAN.
Use: Antineoplastic. [Orphan drug]

•**prednisolone.** (pred-NISS-oh-lone) U.S.P. 23. Metacortandralone.
Use: Corticosteroid, topical.
See: Cordrol, Tab. (Vita Elixir).
Delta-Cortef, Tab. (Pharmacia & Upjohn).
Fernisolone, Tab., Inj. (Ferndale Laboratories).
Orasone, Tab. (Solvay).
Orasone 50, Tab. (Solvay).
Prednis, Tab. (Rhone-Poulenc Rorer).
W/Aluminum hydroxide gel, dried.
See: Predoxide, Tab. (Roberts Pharm).
W/Chloramphenicol.
See: Chloroptic-P, Ophthalmic Oint. (Allergan).
W/Neomycin sulfate.
Neo-Deltef, Drops (Pharmacia & Upjohn).
W/Sulfacetamide sodium, methylcellulose.
See: Isopto Cetapred, Susp. (Alcon Laboratories).
W/Sulfacetamide sodium.
See: Cetapred Ophthalmic Oint. (Alcon Laboratories).

•**prednisolone acetate.** (pred-NISS-oh-lone ASS-eh-tate) U.S.P. 23.
Use: Corticosteroid, topical.
See: Econopred, Susp. (Alcon Laboratories).
Key-Pred, Inj. (Hyrex).
Nisolone, Vial (B.F. Ascher).
Predicort, Amp. (Dunhall Pharmaceuticals).
Pred, Preps. (Allergan).
Pred-Forte, Ophthalmic Susp. (Allergan).
Savacort-50, 100, Vial (Savage).
Sigpred, Inj. (Sigma-Tau Pharmaceuticals).
Steraject, Vial (Merz).
Sterane, Inj. (Pfizer).

prednisolone acetate. (Various Mfr.) 1% Susp. Bot. 5 ml, 10 ml.
Use: Corticosteroid, topical.

prednisolone acetate w/combinations.
See: Blephamide Liquifilm, Soln. (Allergan).
Blephamide S.O.P., Ophthalmic, Oint. (Allergan).
Cetapred Opthalmic Oint. (Alcon Laboratories).
Dua-Pred, Inj. (Solvay).
Isopto Cetapred Susp. (Alcon Laboratories).
Metimyd, Ophthalmic Susp., Oint. (Schering Plough).
Neo-Delta-Cortef, Preps. (Pharmacia & Upjohn).
Panacort R-P, Vial (Ferndale Laboratories).
Prednefrin, Mild, Susp. (Allergan).
Sulphrin Ophth. Oint. (Bausch & Lomb).
Tri-Ophtho, Ophthalmic (Maurry).
Vasocidin, Preps. (Novartis).

prednisolone acetate and prednisolone sodium phosphate. (Various Mfr.) Prednisolone acetate 80 mg, prednisolone sodium phosphate 20 mg/ml. Inj. Susp. Vial 10 ml. *Rx.*
Use: Corticosteroid.

prednisolone acetate ophthalmic suspension. (Falcon Ophthalmics) Prednisolone 1%, benzalkonium Cl 0.01%, EDTA. Susp. Bot. 5 ml, 10 ml. *Rx.*
Use: Corticosteroid.

prednisolone butylacetate. 1,4-Pregnadiene-3,20-dione-11β,17α,21-triol-tert-butyl-acetate.
Use: Corticosteroid.
See: Hydeltra-T.B.A., Vial (Merck).

prednisolone cyclopentylpropionate.
Use: Corticosteroid.

•**prednisolone hemisuccinate.** U.S.P. 23.
Use: Corticosteroid, topical.

•**prednisolone sodium phosphate.** (pred-NISS-oh-lone So-dee-uhm FOSS-fate) U.S.P. 23.
Use: Corticosteroid, topical.
See: AK-Pred, Soln. (Akorn).
Alto-Pred Soluble, Vial (Alto Pharmaceuticals).
Hydeltrasol, Inj. (Merck).
Inflamase Forte, Ophthalmic Soln. (Novartis).
Inflamase, Ophthalmic Soln. (Novartis).
Key-Pred SP, Inj. (Hyrex).
Liquid Pred, Inj. (Muro).
Metreton, Ophthalmic Soln. Sterile (Schering Plough).
Pediapred, Liq. (Medeva).
P.S.P. IV (Four), Inj. (Solvay).
Savacort-S, Inj. (Savage).
W/Neomycin sulfate.
See: Neo-Hydeltrasol, Ophthalmic Soln., Ophthalmic Oint. (Merck).
W/Niacinamide, disodium edetate, sodium bisulfite, phenol.
See: P.S.P. IV, Inj. (Solvay).
W/Prednisolone acetate.
See: Panacort R-P, Vial (Ferndale Laboratories).
W/Sodium Sulfacetamide.
See: Optimyd, Soln. (Schering Plough).
Vasocidin, Liq. (Novartis).

prednisolone sodium phosphate. (Various Mfr.) 0.125%, 1% Soln. Bot. 5 ml, 10 ml, 15 ml.
Use: Corticosteroid, topical.

•**prednisolone sodium succinate for injection.** (pred-NISS-oh-lone So-dee-uhm SUCK-sih-nate) U.S.P. 23.
Use: Corticosteroid, topical.

prednisolone tertiary-butylacetate.
See: Prednisolone Tebutate, U.S.P. 23.

Prednisol TBA. (Taylor Pharmaceuticals) Prednisolone tebutate 20 mg/ml. Vial 10 ml. *Rx.*
Use: Corticosteroid.

•**prednisolone tebutate.** U.S.P. 23.
Use: Corticosteroid, topical.
See: Hydeltra-T.B.A., Vial (Merck).
Metalone, Vial (Foy).

•**prednisone.** (PRED-nih-sone) U.S.P. 23.
Use: Corticosteroid, topical.
See: Delta-Dome, Tab. (Bayer Corp).
Deltasone, Tab. (Pharmacia & Upjohn).
Keysone, Tab. (Hyrex).
Meticorten, Tab. (Schering Plough).
Maso-Pred, Tab. (Mason).
Orasone, Tab. (Solvay).
Sterapred, Tab. (Merz).

W/Chlorpheniramine maleate.
See: Histone, Tab. (Blaine).
W/Phenylephrine HCl.
See: Prednefrin-S, Soln. (Allergan).

prednisone. (Various Mfr.) 1 mg, 5 mg, 20 mg/Tab. Bot. 100s, 1000s, UD 100s. *Rx.*
Use: Corticosteroid, topical

Prednisone Intensol Oral Solution. (Roxane) Prednisone concentrated oral solution 5 mg/ml. Bot. 30 ml w/calibrated dropper. *Rx.*
Use: Corticosteroid.

•**prednival.** (PRED-nih-val) USAN.
Use: Corticosteroid.

Predsulfair. (Bausch & Lomb) **Drops:** Prednisolone acetate 0.5%, sodium sulfacetamide 10%, hydroxypropyl methylcellulose, polysorbate 80 0.5%, sodium thiosulfate, benzalkonium Cl 0.01%. Bot. 5 ml, 15 ml. **Oint.:** Prednisolone acetate 0.5%, sodium sulfacetamide 10%, mineral oil, white petrolatum, lanolin, parabens. In 3.5 g. *Rx.*
Use: Anti-infective; corticosteroid, ophthalmic.

Preflex Daily Cleaning Especially for Sensitive Eyes. (Alcon Laboratories) Isotonic, aqueous solution of sorbic acid, sodium phosphates, sodium Cl, tyloxapol, hydroxyethyl cellulose, polyvinyl alcohol, EDTA. Bot. 30 ml. *otc.*
Use: Contact lens care.

Prefrin Liquifilm. (Allergan) Phenylephrine HCl 0.12%. Bot. 20 ml. *otc.*
Use: Mydriatic, vasoconstrictor.

Pregestimil. (Bristol-Myers) Protein hydrolysate formula supplies 640 calories/qt. protein 18 g, fat 26 g, carbohydrate 86 g, vitamins A 2000 IU, D 400 IU, E 15 IU, C 52 mg, folic acid 100 mcg, thiamine 0.5 mg, riboflavin 0.6 mg, niacin 8 mg, B_6 0.4 mg, B_{12} 2 mcg, biotin 0.05 mg, pantothenic acid 3 mg, K-1 100 mcg, choline 85 mg, inositol 30 mg, calcium 600 mg, phosphorus 400 mg, iodine 45 mcg, iron 12 mg, magnesium 70 mg, copper 0.6 mg, zinc 4 mg, manganese 0.2 mg, chloride 550 mg, potassium 700 mg, sodium 300 mg/Qt. (20 Kcal/fl oz.). Pow. Can lb. *otc.*
Use: Nutritional supplement, enteral.

Pregnaslide Latex hCG Test with Fast Trak Slides. (Wampole Laboratories) Latex agglutination slide test for the qualitative detection of human chorionic gonadotropin in urine. Test 24s. Test kit 96s.
Use: Diagnostic aid.

pregneninolone.
See: Ethisterone.

•**pregnenolone.** (preg-NEN-oh-lone) F.D.A.
Use: Treatment of rheumatoid arthritis.

•**pregnenolone succinate.** (PREG-neh-no-lone SUCK-sih-nate) USAN.
Use: Non-hormonal sterol derivative.

Pregnosis Slide Test. (Roche Laboratories) Latex agglutination inhibition slide test. 50s, 200s.
Use: Diagnostic aid.

Pregnyl. (Organon Teknika) Human chorionic gonadotropin 10,000 IU/Vial w/diluent 10 ml, mannitol, benzyl alcohol. Vial 10 ml. *Rx.*
Use: Hormone, chorionic gonadotropin.

Pre-Hist-D. (Marnel) Phenylephrine HCl 20 mg, chlorpheniramine maleate 8 mg, methscopolamine nitrate 2.5 mg/S.R. Tab. or Capl. Bot. 100s. *Rx.*
Use: Anticholinergic, antihistamine, decongestant.

Preject Preinjection Topical Anesthetic. (Colgate Oral) Benzocaine 20% in polyethylene glycol base. Jar 2 oz. *otc.*
Use: Anesthetic, local.

Prelestrin. (Taylor Pharmaceuticals) Conjugated estrogens 0.625 mg or 1.25 mg/Tab. Bot. 100s, 1000s. *Rx.*
Use: Estrogen.

Prelone Syrup. (Muro) Prednisolone 15 mg/5 ml, alcohol 5%, saccharin. Cherry flavor. 240 ml. *Rx.*
Use: Corticosteroid.

Prelu-2. (Boehringer Ingelheim) Phendimetrazine tartrate 105 mg/Cap. Bot. 100s. *c-III.*
Use: Anorexiant.

Premarin. (Wyeth Ayerst) Conjugated estrogens tablets. Water-soluble conjugated estrogens derived from natural sources. Sucrose. 0.3 mg, 0.625 mg, 0.9 mg, 1.25 mg or 2.5 mg/Tab.: Bot. 100s, 1000s. 0.625 mg or 1.25 mg: 5000s, UD 100s. Cycle packs 25s. *Rx.*
Use: Estrogen.

Premarin Intravenous. (Wyeth Ayerst) Conjugated Estrogens U.S.P., for Injection. Vial 25 mg/5 ml w/diluent. (Vial also contains lactose 200 mg, sodium citrate 12.5 mg, simethicone 0.2 mg). Diluent contains benzyl alcohol 2%, Water for Injection, U.S.P. *Rx.*
Use: Estrogen.

Premarin Vaginal Cream. (Wyeth Ayerst) Conjugated Estrogens, U.S.P. 0.625 mg/1 g w/cetyl esters wax, cetyl

alcohol, white wax, glyceryl monostearate, propylene glycol monostearate, methyl stearate, phenylethyl alcohol, sodium lauryl sulfate, glycerin, mineral oil. Tube w/applicator 1.5 oz. (42.5 g). Tube refill. *Rx.*
Use: Estrogen.

Premarin w/Meprobamate.
See: PMB 200 and 400, Tab. (Wyeth Ayerst).

Premarin w/Methyltestosterone. (Wyeth Ayerst) Premarin (Conjugated Estrogens, U.S.P.) 1.25 mg, methyltestosterone 10 mg/Yellow Tab. Premarin 0.625 mg, methyltestosterone 5 mg/ Red Tab. Bot. 100s. *Rx.*
Use. Androgen, estrogen combination.

W/Methyltestosterone, methamphetamine HCl, vitamins.
See: Mediatric, Cap., Liq., Tab. (Wyeth Ayerst).

Premate-200. (Major) Meprobamate 200 mg, tridihexethyl Cl 25 mg/Tab. Bot. 100s. *Rx.*
Use: Anticholinergic, anxiolytic.

Premate-400. (Major) Meprobamate 400 mg, tridihexethyl Cl 25 mg/Tab. Bot. 100s. *Rx.*
Use: Anticholinergic, anxiolytic.

Premphase. (Wyeth Ayerst) Conjugated estrogens 0.625 mg/Tab. Medroxyprogesterone acetate 5 mg, conjugated estrogens 0.625 mg/Tab. Blister-card 28s (14 of each). *Rx.*
Use: Estrogen, progestin combination.

Prempro. (Wyeth Ayerst) Conjugated estrogen 0.625 mg, medroxyprogesterone acetate 2.5 mg, lactose, sucrose/Tab. Blister-card 14s (2s). *Rx.*
Use: Estrogen, progestin combination.

Premsyn PMS Caplets. (Chattem Consumer Products) Acetaminophen 500 mg, pamabrom 25 mg, pyrilamine maleate 15 mg/Capl. Bot. 20s, 40s. *otc.*
Use: Analgesic, antihistamine, diuretic.

•**prenalterol hydrochloride.** (PREE-NAL-teh-role) USAN.
Use: Adrenergic.

Prenatal Folic Acid + Iron. (Everett Laboratories) Vitamins, minerals, folic acid 1 mg/Tab. Bot. 100s. *Rx.*
Use: Mineral, vitamin supplement.

Prenatal MR 90. (Ethex) Calcium 250 mg, iron 90 mg, vitamin A 4000 IU, D 400 IU, E 30 mg, B_1 3 mg, B_2 3.4 mg, B_3 20 mg, B_6 20 mg, B_{12} 12 mcg, C 120 mg, folic acid 1 mg, Zn 25 mg, I, Cu, DSS. Tab. Bot. 100s. *Rx.*
Use: Mineral, vitamin supplement.

Prenatal-S. (Zenith Forest Pharmaceutical) Calcium 200 mg, iron 60 mg, vitamins A 4000 IU, D 400 IU, E 11 mg, B_1 1.5 mg, B_2 1.7 mg, B_3 18 mg, B_6 2.6 mg, B_{12} 4 mcg, C 100 mg, folic acid 0.8 mg, zinc 25 mg/Tab. Bot. UD 100s. *otc.*
Use: Mineral, vitamin supplement.

Prenatal with Folic Acid. (Geneva Pharm) Calcium 200 mg, iron 60 mg, vitamins A 4000 IU, D 400 IU, E 11 mg, B_1 1.5 mg, B_2 1.7 mg, B_3 18 mg, B_6 2.6 mg, B_{12} 4 mcg, C 100 mg, folic acid 0.8 mg, Zn 25 mg/Tab. Bot. 100s. *otc.*
Use: Mineral, vitamin supplement.

Prenatal with Folic Acid. (Eon Labs Manufacturing) Vitamins A 6000 IU, D 400 IU, E 30 IU, folic acid 1 mg, C 60 mg, B_1 1.1 mg, B_2 1.8 mg, B_6 2.5 mg, B_{12} 5 mcg, niacin 15 mg, calcium 125 mg, iron 65 mg/Tab. Bot. 100s, 1000s. *Rx.*
Use: Mineral, vitamin supplement.

Prenatal H.P. (Mission) Vitamin A 4000 IU, C 100 mg, D_3 400 IU, B_1 4 mg, B_2 2 mg, B_3 10 mg, B_5 1 mg, B_6 20 mg, B_{12} 2 mcg, folate 0.8 mg, Ca 50 mg, Fe 30 mg, sugar. Tab. Bot. 100s. *otc.*
Use: Mineral, vitamin supplement.

Prenatal Maternal. (Ethex) Ca 250 mg, iron 4 mg, $B_2$60 mg, vitamins A 5000 IU, D 400 IU, E 30 mg, B_1 2.9 mg, B_2 3.4 mg, B_3 20 mg, B_5 10 mg, B_6 12.2 mg, B_{12} 12 mcg, C 100 mg, folic acid 1 mg, Cr, Cu, I, Mg, Mn, Mo, zinc 25 mg, biotin 30 mcg/Tab. Bot. 100s. *Rx.*
Use: Mineral, vitamin supplement.

Prenatal-1 + Iron. (Various Mfr.) Ca 200 mg, iron 65 mg, vitamins A 4000 IU, D 400 IU, E 11 mg, B_1 1.5 mg, B_2 3 mg, B_3 20 mg, B_6 10 mg, B_{12} 12 mcg, C 120 mg, folic acid 1 mg, Cu, zinc 25 mg/ Tab. Bot. 100s, 500s. *Rx.*
Use: Mineral, vitamin supplement.

Prenatal Plus. (Zenith Forest Pharmaceutical) Vitamin A (as acetate and carotene) 4000 IU, D IU 400, E 22 mg, C 120 mg, folic acid 1 mg, B_1 1.84 mg, B_2 3 mg, B_3 20 mg, B_6 10 mg, B_{12} 12 mcg, calcium 200 mg, Fe 65 mg, Cu 2 mg, Zn 25 mg/Tab. Bot. 100s. *Rx.*
Use: Mineral, vitamin supplement.

Prenatal Plus with Beta Carotene. (Rugby) Ca 200 mg, iron 65 mg, vitamins A 4000 IU, D 400 IU, E 11 mg, B_1 1.84 mg, B_2 3 mg, B_3 20 mg, B_6 10 mg, B_{12} 12 mcg, C 120 mg, folic acid 1 mg, Cu, zinc 25 mg/Tab. Bot. 100s, 500s. *Rx.*
Use: Mineral, vitamin supplement.

Prenatal Plus-Improved. (Rugby) Ca 200 mg, iron 65 mg, vitamins A 4000 IU, D 400 IU, E 11 mg, B_1 1.5 mg, B_2 3 mg, B_3 20 mg, B_6 10 mg, B_{12} 12 mcg, C 120 mg, folic acid 1 mg, Cu, zinc 25 mg/Tab. Bot. 100s. *Rx.*
Use: Mineral, vitamin supplement.

Prenatal Rx. (Mission) Vitamin A 3000 IU (as acetate), D_3 400 IU, C 240 mg (as ascorbic and calcium ascorbate), B_1 4 mg, B_2 2 mg, B_3 20 mg, B_5 10 mg, B_6 20 mg, B_{12} 8 mcg, folic acid 1 mg, Fe 29.5 mg (as ferrous fumarate), Ca 175 mg (as carbonate and ascorbate), I 0.3 mg (as potassium iodide), Zn 15 mg (as dried zinc sulfate), Cu 2 mg (as cupric oxide). Tab. Bot. 100s. *Rx.*
Use: Mineral, vitamin supplement.

Prenatal Rx with Beta Carotene. (Various Mfr.) Ca 200 mg, iron 60 mg, vitamins A 4000 IU, D 400 IU, E 15 mg, B_1 1.5 mg, B_2 1.6 mg, B_3 17 mg, B_5 7 mg, B_6 4 mg, B_{12} 2.5 mcg, C 80 mg, folic acid 1 mg, biotin 30 mcg, Cu, Mg, zinc 25 mg/Tab. Bot. 100s, 500s. *Rx.*
Use: Mineral, vitamin supplement.

Prenatal Z. (Ethex) Ca 300 mg, iron 65 mg, vitamins A 5000 IU, D 400 IU, E 30 mg, B_1 3 mg, B_2 3 mg, B_3 20 mg, B_6 12.2 mg, B_{12} 12 mcg, C 80 mg, folic acid 1 mg, zinc 20 mg, I, Mg/Tab. Bot. 100s. *Rx.*
Use: Mineral, vitamin supplement.

Prenatal Z Advanced Formula. (Ethex) Vitamin A 3000 IU, ascorbic acid 70 mg, calcium carbonate 200 mg, ferrous fumarate 65 mg, cholecalciferol 400 IU, dl-alpha tocopheryl acetate 10 IU, B_1 1.5 mg, B_2 1.6 mg, B_3 17 mg, B_6 2.2 mg, folic acid 1 mg, B_{12} 2.2 mcg, potassium iodide 175 mcg, magnesium oxide 100 mg, zinc oxide 15 mg. Tab. Bot. 100s. *Rx.*
Use: Mineral, vitamin supplement.

Prenate 90 Tablets. (Sanofi Winthrop) Vitamins A 4000 IU, D 400 IU, E 30 mg, C 120 mg, folic acid 1 mg, B_1 3 mg, B_2 3.4 mg, B_6 20 mg, B_{12} 12 mcg, B_3 20 mg, DSS, calcium 250 mg, iodine, iron 90 mg, Cu, zinc 20 mg/FC Tab. Bot. 100s, 1000s. *Rx.*
Use: Mineral, vitamin supplement.

Prenavite. (Rugby) Ca 200 mg, iron 60 mg, vitamins A 4000 IU, D 400 IU, E 11 mg, B_1 1.5 mg, B_2 1.7 mg, B_3 18 mg, B_6 2.6 mg, B_{12} 4 mcg, C 100 mg, folic acid 0.8 mg, zinc 25 mg/Tab. Bot. 100s, 500s. *otc.*
Use: Mineral, vitamin supplement.

•**prenylamine.** (PREH-nill-ah-meen) USAN. Segontin; Synadrin lactate.
Use: Coronary vasodilator.

Preparation H. (Whitehall Robins) Shark liver oil 3%, cocoa butter 79%, corn oil, EDTA, parabens, tocopherol. Supp. 12s, 24s, 36s, 48s. *otc.*
Use: Anorectal preparation.

Preparation H Cream. (Whitehall Robins) Petrolatum 78%, glycerin 12%, shark liver oil 3%, phenylephrine HCl 0.25%, cetyl and stearyl alcohol, EDTA, parabens, lanolin, tocopherol. Tube 27 g, 54 g. *otc.*
Use: Anorectal preparation.

Preparation H Ointment. (Whitehall Robins) Petrolatum 71.9%, mineral oil 14%, shark liver oil 3%, phenylephrine HCl 0.25%, corn oil, glycerin, lanolin, lanolin alcohol, parabens, tocopherol. Oint. 30 g, 60 g. *otc.*
Use: Anorectal preparation.

Prepcat. (Lafayette Pharm) Barium sulfate 1.2% w/w suspension. Bot. 480 ml, Case Bot. 24s.
Use: Radiopaque agent.

Prepcat 2000. (Lafayette Pharm) Barium sulfate 1.2% w/w suspension. Bot. 2000 ml, Case Bot. 4s.
Use: Radiopaque agent.

Prepcort Cream. (Whitehall Robins) Hydrocortisone 0.5%. Tube 0.5 oz, 1 oz.
Use: Corticosteroid.

Pre-Pen. (Kremers Urban) Benzylpenicilloyl-polylysine 0.25 ml/Amp. *Rx.*
Use: Diagnostic aid.

Pre-Pen/MDM. (Kremers Urban)
See: Benzylpenicillin, Benzylpenicilloic, Benzylpenilloic Acid.

Prepidil. (Pharmacia & Upjohn) Dinoprostone 0.5 mg/Gel. Syringes (with 2 shielded catheters 10 and 20 mm tip) 3 g. *Rx.*
Use: Cervical ripening.

Prepodyne. (West) Titratable iodine. **Soln.:** 1%. Bot. pt, gal. **Scrub:** 0.75%. Bot. 6 oz, gal. **Swabs:** Saturated with soln. Pkt. 1s, Box 100s. **Swabsticks:** Saturated with soln. Pkt. 1s, Box 50s. Pkt. 3s, Box 75s.
Use: Antiseptic, topical.

Presalin. (Roberts Pharm) Aspirin 260 mg, salicylamide 120 mg, acetaminophen 120 mg, aluminum hydroxide 100 mg/Tab. Bot. 50s. *otc.*
Use: Analgesic combination, antacid.

Prescription Strength Desenex. (Novartis) **Spray Liquid:** Miconazole nitrate 2%. 105 ml. **Spray Powder:** Miconazole nitrate 2%. 90 ml. **Cream:** Clo-

trimazole 1%. Tube 15 g. *otc.*
Use: Antifungal, topical.

pressor agents.
See: Sympathomimetic agents.

Pressorol. (Baxter) Metaraminol bitartrate. Vial 10 ml (10 mg/ml). *Rx.*
Use: Vasoconstrictor.

PreSun 4 Creamy. (Bristol-Myers Squibb) Padimate O 1.4%, alcohol, titanium dioxide. Waterproof lotion. Bot. 4 oz. *otc.*
Use: Sunscreen.

PreSun 8 Creamy. (Bristol-Myers Squibb) Padimate O 5%, oxybenzone 2%. Waterproof. Bot. 4 oz. *otc.*
Use: Sunscreen.

PreSun 8 Lotion. (Bristol Myers Squibb) Padimate O 7.3%, oxybenzone 2.3%, SD alcohol 40 60%. Bot. 4 oz. *otc.*
Use: Sunscreen.

PreSun 15 Creamy. (Bristol-Myers Squibb) Padimate O 8%, oxybenzone 3%, benzyl alcohol. Waterproof. Bot. 4 oz. *otc.*
Use: Sunscreen.

PreSun 15 Facial Sunscreen. (Bristol-Myers Squibb) Padimate O (Octyl dimethyl PABA) 8%, oxybenzone 3%. Bot. 2 oz. *otc.*
Use: Sunscreen.

PreSun 15 Facial Sunscreen Stick. (Bristol-Myers Squibb) Octyl dimethyl PABA 8%, oxybenzone 3%. Stick 0.42 oz. *otc.*
Use: Sunscreen.

PreSun 15 Lip Protector. (Bristol-Myers Squibb) Padimate O 8%, oxybenzone 3%. Stick 4.5 g. *otc.*
Use: Sunscreen.

PreSun 15 Lotion. (Bristol-Myers Squibb) Padimate O 5%, PABA 5%, oxybenzone 3%, SD alcohol 40 58%. Bot. 4 oz. *otc.*
Use: Sunscreen.

PreSun 15 Sensitive Skin Sunscreen. (Bristol-Myers Squibb) Octyl methoxycinnamate, oxybenzone, octyl salicylate, cetyl alcohol, PABA free, waterproof, SPF 15. Cream. Bot. 120 ml. *otc.*
Use: Sunscreen.

PreSun 23. (Bristol-Myers Squibb) Padimate O, octyl methoxycinnamate, oxybenzone, octyl salicylate, SD alcohol 40 19%, waterproof. Spray mist. Bot. 105 ml. *otc.*
Use: Sunscreen.

PreSun 29 Sensitive Skin Sunscreen. (Bristol-Myers Squibb) Octyl methoxycinnamate, oxybenzone, octyl salicylate. SPF 29. Waterproof. Bot. 4 oz. *otc.*
Use: Sunscreen.

PreSun 39 Creamy Sunscreen. (Bristol-Myers Squibb) Padimate O, oxybenzone, cetyl alcohol, waterproof. Cream. Bot. 120 ml. *otc.*
Use: Sunscreen.

PreSun Active. (Bristol-Myers Squibb) Octyl methoxycinnamate, oxybenzone, octyl salicylate, 69% SD alcohol 40. PABA free. Waterproof. SPF 15, 30. Gel. 120 g. *otc.*
Use: Sunscreen.

PreSun for Kids Cream. (Bristol-Myers Squibb) Octyl methoxycinnamate, oxybenzone, octyl salicylate, cetyl alcohol, PABA free, waterproof SPF 29. Cream. Bot. 120 ml. *otc.*
Use: Sunscreen.

PreSun for Kids Spray. (Bristol-Myers Squibb) Padimate O, octyl methoxycinnamate, oxybenzone, octyl salicylate, SD alcohol 40 19%, waterproof, SPF 23. Spray Bot. 105 ml. *otc.*
Use: Sunscreen.

PreSun Moisturizing. (Bristol-Myers Squibb) Octyl dimethyl PABA, oxybenzone, cetyl alcohol, diazolidinyl urea. SPF 46. Lot. Bot. 120 ml. *otc.*
Use: Sunscreen.

PreSun Moisturizing Sunscreen with Keri, SPF 15. (Bristol-Myers Squibb) Octyl dimethyl PABA, oxybenzone, cetyl alcohol, diazolidinyl urea. Waterproof. Lot. 120 ml. *otc.*
Use: Sunscreen.

PreSun Moisturizing Sunscreen with Keri, SPF 25. (Bristol-Myers Squibb) Octyl methoxycinnamate, oxybenzone, octyl salicylate, petrolatum, cetyl alcohol, diazolidinyl urea. Waterproof. Lot. 120 ml. *otc.*
Use: Sunscreen.

PreSun Spray Mist. (Bristol-Myers Squibb) Octyl dimethyl PABA, octyl methoxycinnamate, oxybenzone, octyl salicylate, 19% SD alcohol 40, C12-15 alcohols benzoate. Waterproof. SPF 23. 120 ml. *otc.*
Use: Sunscreen.

PreSun Ultra. (Bristol-Myers Squibb) Avobenzone 3%, octyl methoxycinnamate 7.5%, octyl salicylate 5%, oxybenzone 3%. Lotion, Clear Gel. SPF 30. 4 oz. *otc.*
Use: Sunscreen.

Pretend-U-Ate. (Vitalax) Enriched candy-appetite pacifier. Pkg. 20s. *otc.*
Use: Dietary aid.

prethcamide. Mixture of crotethamide and cropropamide.
See: Micoren (Novartis).

Pretts Diet Aid. (Milance Lab) Alginic acid 200 mg, sodium carboxymethylcellulose 100 mg, sodium bicarbonate 70 mg/Chew. Tab. Bot. 60s. *otc.*
Use: Dietary aid.

Pretty Feet & Hands. (B.F. Archer) Paraffin, triethanolamine, parabens. Cream 90 g. *otc.*
Use: Emollient.

PretzPak. (Parnell) Benzyl alcohol 3.5%, polyethylene glycols, carboxymethylcellulose, urea, poloxamer, *Mucoprotective Factor* yerba santa, allantoin, aluminum chlorhydroxy allantoin. Oint. Tube 15 g. *otc.*
Use: Operative and postoperative care in intranasal and endoscopic surgery; local anesthetic.

Prevacid. (TAP Pharm) Lansoprazole 15 mg or 30 mg/SR Cap. Bot. 100s, 1000s, unit-of-use 30s, UD 100s. *Rx.*
Use: Proton pump inhibitor.

Prevalite. (Upsher-Smith Labs) Cholestyramine 4 g, phenylalanine 14.1 mg/dose/Pow. Box. 5.5 g single dose packets. 60s. *Rx.*
Use: Antihyperlipidemic agent.

Prevident Disclosing Drops. (Colgate Oral) Erythrosine sodium 1%. Bot. 1 oz.
Use: Diagnostic aid, dental plaque.

Prevident Disclosing Tablet. (Colgate Oral) Erythrosine sodium 1%/Tab. UD strip 1000s.
Use: Diagnostic aid, dental plaque.

Prevident Prophylaxis Paste. (Colgate Oral) Sodium fluoride containing 1.2% fluoride ion w/pumice and alumina abrasives. Cup 2 g, Box 200s. Jar 9 oz. *Rx.*
Use: Dental caries agent.

Prevident Rinse. (Colgate Oral) Neutral sodium fluoride 0.2%, alcohol 6%. Sol. Bot. 250 ml, gal (w/pump dispenser). *Rx.*
Use: Dental caries agent.

Preview. (Lafayette Pharm) Barium sulfate 60% w/v suspension. Bot. 355 ml, Case 24 bot.
Use: Radiopaque agent.

Preview 2000. Barium sulfate 60% w/v suspension. Bot. 2000 ml, Case 4 Bot.
Use: Radiopaque agent.

Prevision. Mestranol, U.S.P. 23.

Prexonate Tablets. (Tennessee Pharmaceutic) Vitamins A acetate 5000 IU, D 500 IU, B_6 2 mg, B_1 5 mg, B_2 2 mg, C 100 mg, B_{12} 2.5 mcg, calcium pantothenate 1 mg, niacinamide 15 mg, folic acid 1 mg, iron 45 mg, calcium 500 mg, intrinsic factor 3 mg/Tab. Bot. 100s, 1000s. *Rx.*
Use: Mineral, vitamin supplement.

•**prezatide copper acetate.** (PREH-zat-IDE KAH-per) USAN.
Use: Immunomodulator.

Prid Salve. (Walker Pharmacal) Ichthammol, Phenol, Lead Oleate, Rosin, Beeswax, Lard. Tin 20 g. *otc.*
Use: Drawing salve.

•**pridefine hydrochloride.** (PRIH-deh-FEEN) USAN.
Use: Antidepressant.

•**prifelone.** (PRIH-feh-LONE) USAN.
Use: Anti-inflammatory (dermatologic).

•**priliximab.** (prih-LICK-sih-mab) USAN.
Use: Monoclonal antibody (autoimmune lymphoproliferative diseases, organ transplantation).

prilocaine. (PRILL-oh-cane) USAN,
Use: Anesthetic, local.

prilocaine and epinephrine injection.
Use: Anesthetic, local.

•**prilocaine hydrochloride.** (PRILL-oh-cane) U.S.P. 23.
Use: Anesthetic, local.
See: Citanest Hydrochloride, Vial, Amp. (Astra).

Prilosec. (Astra Merck) Omeprazole 10 mg or 20 mg, lactose/DR Cap. 100s, 1000s, unit-of-use 30s, UD 100s. *Rx.*
Use: Antiulcerative.

primacaine.
Use: Anesthetic, local.

Primacor. (Sanofi Winthrop) Milrinone lactate. **Inj.:** 1 mg/ml. Single-dose vial 10 ml, 20 ml; Carpuject units 5 ml. **Inj., Premixed:** 200 mcg/ml in dextrose 5%. Vial 100 ml. *Rx.*
Use: Cardiovascular agent.
See: Milrinone.

•**primaquine phosphate.** (PRIM-uh-kween) U.S.P. 23.
Use: Antimalarial.

primaquine phosphate. (PRIM-uh-kween) (Sanofi Winthrop). 26.3 mg/Tab. Bot. 100s.
Use: Antimalarial.

primaquine phosphate. (PRIM-uh-kween) (Sterling Winthrop)
Use: Treatment of PCP associated with AIDS. [Orphan drug]

Primatene. (Whitehall Robins) Theophylline 130 mg, ephedrine HCl 24 mg, phenobarbital 7.5 mg/Tab. Bot. 24s. *otc.*

Use: Antiasthmatic combination.

Primatene Dual Action. (Whitehall Robins) Theophylline 60 mg, ephedrine HCl 12.5 mg, guaifenesin 100 mg/Tab. Bot. 24s. *otc.*
Use: Antiasthmatic combination.

Primatene Mist Solution. (Whitehall Robins) Epinephrine 0.2 mg, alcohol 34%. Bot. 0.5 oz. Spray. *otc.*
Use: Bronchodilator.

Primatene Mist Suspension. (Whitehall Robins) Epinephrine bitartrate 0.3 mg. Bot. 10 ml w/mouthpiece. Spray. *otc.*
Use: Bronchodilator.

Primatene M. Tablets. (Whitehall Robins) Theophylline 118 mg, ephedrine HCl 24 mg, pyrilamine maleate 16.6 mg/Tab. Bot. 24s, 60s. *otc.*
Use: Antihistamine, bronchodilator.

Primatene P Tablets. (Whitehall Robins) Theophylline 118 mg, ephedrine HCl 24 mg, phenobarbital 8 mg/Tab. Bot. 24s, 60s. *otc.*
Use: Bronchodilator, hypnotic, sedative.

Primatuss Cough Mixture 4 Liquid. (Rugby) Doxylamine succinate 3.75 mg, dextromethorphan HBr 7.5 mg/5 ml, alcohol 10% Liq. Bot. 180 ml. *otc.*
Use: Antihistamine, antitussive.

Primatuss Cough Mixture 4D Liquid. (Rugby) Pseudoephedrine HCl 20 mg, dextromethorphan HBr 10 mg, guaifenesin 67 mg/5 ml, alcohol 10%. Liq. Bot. 120 ml. *otc.*
Use: Antitussive, decongestant, expectorant.

Primaxin. (Merck) Imipenem (anhydrous equivalent), cilastatin w/sodium bicarbonate buffer. **250-250:** ADD-Vantage Vial, Tray 10s, 25s. Tray 10 infusion bottles. **500-500:** ADD-Vantage Vial, Tray 10s, 25s. Tray 10 infusion bottles. *Rx.*
Use: Anti-infective.

Primaxin I.M. (Merck) Imipenem (anhydrous equivalent), cilastatin w/ sodium bicarbonate buffer. Pow. for Inj. Vials 500 mg/500 mg, 750 mg/750 mg. *Rx.*
Use: Anti-infective.

Primaxin I.V. (Merck) Imipenem (anhydrous equivalent), cilastatin w/ sodium bicarbonate buffer. Pow. for Inj. Vials, infusion bot., ADD-Vantage vials 250 mg/250 mg, 500 mg/500 mg. *Rx.*
Use: Anti-infective.

•**primidolol.** (prih-MID-oh-lahl) USAN.
Use: Antianginal; antihypertensive; cardiovascular agent, antiarrhythmic.

•**primidone.** (PRIM-ih-dohn) U.S.P. 23.
Use: Anticonvulsant.

primidone. (Various Mfr.) 250 mg. Tab. Bot. 100s, 500s, 1000s, UD 100s.
Use: Anticonvulsant.

primostrum. A prep. of primiparous colostrum.

Principen "125" for Oral Suspension. (Bristol-Myers Squibb) Ampicillin trihydrate 125 mg/5 ml, saccharin. Reconstitution to 80 ml, 100 ml, 150 ml, 200 ml, UD 5 ml 100s. *Rx.*
Use: Anti-infective, penicillin.

Principen "250" Capsules. (Bristol-Myers Squibb) Ampicillin 250 mg/Cap. Bot. 100s, 500s, UD 100s. *Rx.*
Use: Anti-infective, penicillin.

Principen "250" for Oral Suspension. (Bristol-Myers Squibb) Ampicillin trihydrate 250 mg/5 ml, saccharin. Reconstitution to 80 ml, 100 ml, 150 ml, 200 ml, UD 5 ml 100s. *Rx.*
Use: Anti-infective, penicillin.

Principen "500" Capsules. (Bristol-Myers Squibb) Ampicillin trihydrate 500 mg/Cap. 100s, 500s, UD 100s. *Rx.*
Use: Anti-infective, penicillin.

Principen with Probenecid. (Bristol-Myers Squibb) Ampicillin (as trihydrate) 3.5 g, probenecid 1 g/regimen. Single dose bot., 9s. *Rx.*
Use: Anti-infective, penicillin.

Prinivil. (Merck) Lisinopril **2.5 mg/Tab.:** Bot. 30s, 100s, UD 100s. **5 mg/Tab.:** Bot. 1000s, Unit-of-Use 90s, 100s, UD 100s. **10 mg or 20 mg/Tab.:** Bot. 1000s, Unit-of-Use 30s, 90s, 100s, UD 100s. **40 mg/Tab.:** Bot. 100s. *Rx.*
Use: Antihypertensive.

•**prinomide tromethamine.** (PRIH-no-MIDE troe-METH-ah-meen) USAN.
Use: Antirheumatic.

•**prinoxodan.** (prin-OX-oh-dan) USAN.
Use: Cardiovascular agent.

Prinzide. (Merck) Lisinopril 10 or 20 mg, hydrochlorothiazide 12.5 mg/Tab or lisinopril 20 mg, hydrochlorothiazide 25 mg/Tab. Bot. 30s, 100s. *Rx.*
Use: Antihypertensive.

Priscoline. (Novartis) Tolazoline HCl 25 mg/ml, tartaric acid 0.65%, hydrous sodium citrate 0.65%. Vial 4 ml. *Rx.*
Use: Antihypertensive.

prisilidene hydrochloride.
See: Alphaprodine HCl (Various Mfr.).

privadorn.
See: Bromisovalum (Various Mfr.).

Privine. (Novartis) Naphazoline HCl. **Nasal Soln.:** 0.05%. Bot. 20 ml w/drop-

per. **Nasal Spray:** 0.05%. Bot. 15 ml. *otc.*
Use: Decongestant.

•**prizidilol hydrochloride.** (PRIH-zie-DILL-ole) USAN.
Use: Antihypertensive.

Pro-Acet Douche Concentrate. (Pro-Acet) Lactic, citric, and acetic acids, sodium lauryl sulfate, lactose, dextrose and sodium acetate. Pkg. polyethylene envelope 10 ml. Contents of 1 envelope to be diluted with 2 quarts of water. Douche 6 oz, 12 oz. Travel Packet 10 ml. *otc.*
Use: Vaginal agent.

•**proadifen hydrochloride.** (pro-AD-ih-fen) USAN.
Use: Synergist (non-specific).

ProAmatine. (Roberts Pharm) Midodrine HCl 2.5 mg and 5 mg/Tab. Bot. 100s. *Rx.*
Use: Orthostatic hypotension.

Pro-Banthine. (Schiapparelli Searle) Propantheline bromide **7.5 mg/Tab.:** Bot. 100s. **15 mg/Tab.:** Bot. 100s, 500s, UD 100s.
Use: Anticholinergic, antispasmodic.

Probarbital Sodium. 5-Ethyl-5-isopropylbarbiturate sodium.

Probax. (Fischer) Propolis 2%, petrolatum, mineral oil, lanolin. Gel. Tube 3.5 g. *otc.*
Use: Mouth and throat preparation.

Probec-T. (Roberts Pharm) Vitamins B_1 12.2 mg, B_2 10 mg, B_3 100 mg, B_5 18.4, B_6 4.1 mg, B_{12} 5 mcg, C 600 mg/Tab. Bot. 60s. *otc.*
Use: Mineral, vitamin supplement.

Proben-C. (Rugby) Probenecid 500 mg, colchicine 0.5 mg/Tab. Bot. 100s, 1000s. *Rx.*
Use: Anitgout agent.

•**probenecid.** (pro-BEN-uh-sid) U.S.P. 23.
Use: Uricosuric.
See: Benemid, Tab. (Merck).
W/Ampicillin.
See: Amcill-GC, Oral Susp. (Parke-Davis).
Polycillin-PRB, Liq. (Bristol-Myers).
Principen w/Probenecid, Cap. (Bristol-Myers Squibb).
W/Ampicillin trihydrate.
See: Probampacin (Biocraft).

probenecid and colchicine. (Various Mfr.) Probenecid 500 mg, colchicine 0.5 mg/Tab. Bot. 100s, 1000s. *Rx.*
Use: Uricosuric combination for chronic gouty arthritis.
See: Colbenemid, Tab. (Merck).
Col-Probenecid, Tab. (Various Mfr.).

probenzamide. 0-Propoxybenzamide. (Warner Lambert).

•**probicromil calcium.** (pro-BYE-KROE-mill) USAN.
Use: Antiallergic (prophylactic).

Pro-Bionate. (Natren) *Lactobacillus acidophilus* strain NAS 2 billion units/g. **Pow.** 52.5 g, 90 g. **Cap.** Bot. 30s, 60s. *otc.*
Use: Antidiarrheal, nutritional supplement.

•**probucol.** (PRO-byoo-kahl) U.S.P. 23.
Use: Antihyperlipidemic.
See: Lorelco, Tab. (Hoechst Marion Roussel).

•**procainamide hydrochloride.** (pro-CANE-uh-mide) U.S.P. 23.
Use: Cardiovascular agent, antiarrhythmic.
See: Procamide SR, Tab. (Solvay).
Procanbid, SR Tab. (Parke-Davis).
Pronestyl, Cap., Vial (Bristol-Myers).

procaine base.
W/Benzyl alcohol, propyl-p-aminobenzoate.
Use: Anesthetic, local.
See: Rectocaine, Vial (Moore-Kirk).
W/Butyl-p-aminobenzoate, benzyl alcohol, in sweet almond oil.
See: Anucaine, Amp. (Calvin).

procaine butyrate. p-Aminobenzoyl-diethylaminoethanol butyrate.

•**procaine hydrochloride.** (pro-CANE) U.S.P. 23. Bernocaine, Chlorocaine, Ethocaine, Irocaine, Kerocaine, Syncaine.
Use: Anesthetic, local.
See: Novocain, Inj. (Sanofi Winthrop).

procaine hydrochloride. (Abbott Laboratories) 1% or 2% solution. Multiple-dose Vial 30 ml.
Use: Anesthetic, local.

procaine hydrochloride and epinephrine injection.
Use: Anesthetic, local.

procaine hydrochloride and levonordefrin injection.
Use: Anesthetic, local.

procaine penicillin g suspension, sterile.
Use: Anti-infective, penicillin.
See: Crysticillin, Vial (Bristol-Myers Squibb).
Penicillin G, Procaine (Various Mfr.).
Pfizerpen For Injection (Pfipharmecs).

procaine, penicillin g w/aluminum stearate suspension, sterile.
Use: Anti-infective, penicillin.

See: Penicillin G Procaine with Aluminum Stearate, Sterile, U.S.P. 23.

procaine and phenylephrine hydrochlorides injection.
Use: Anesthetic, local.

procaine and tetracaine hydrochlorides and levonordefrin injection.
Use: Anesthetic, local.

procaine, tetracaine and nordefrin hydrochlorides injection.
Use: Anesthetic, local.

procaine, tetracaine and phenylephrine hydrochlorides injection.
Use: Anesthetic.

ProcalAmine Injection. (McGaw) Injection of amino acid 3%, glycerin 3%, electrolytes. Bot. 1000 ml. *Rx.*
Use: Nutritional supplement, parenteral.

Pro-Cal-Sof. (Vangard) Docusate calcium 240 mg/Cap. Bot. 100s, 1000s, UD 100s. *otc.*
Use: Laxative.

Procanbid. (Parke-Davis) Procainamide 500 mg or 1000 mg/ER Tab. Bot. 60s, UD 100s. *Rx.*
Use: Antiarrhythmic.

•**procarbazine hydrochloride.** (pro-CAR-buh-ZEEN) U.S.P. 23. (Roche Laboratories) Natulan.
Use: Cytostatic, antineoplastic.
See: Matulane, Cap. (Roche Laboratories).

Procardia. (Pfizer) Nifedipine 10 mg or 20 mg/Cap. Bot. 100s, 300s, UD 100s. *Rx.*
Use: Calcium channel blocker.

Procardia XL. (Pfizer) Nifedipine 30 mg, 60 mg or 90 mg/SR Tab. **30 mg or 60 mg:** Bot. 100s, 300s, 5000s, UD 100s. **90 mg:** Bot 100s. *Rx.*
Use: Calcium channel blocker.

•**procaterol hydrochloride.** (PRO-CAT-ehr-ole) USAN.
Use: Bronchodilator.

Proception Sperm Nutrient Douche. (Milex) Ringer type glucose douche. Bot. ample for 10 douches. *otc.*
Use: Vaginal agent.

•**prochlorperazine.** (pro-klor-PURR-uh-zeen) U.S.P. 23.
Use: Antiemetic.
See: Compazine, Preps. (SmithKline Beecham Pharmaceuticals).
W/Isopropamide.
See: Iso-Perazine, Cap. (Teva USA).

prochlorperazine maleate. (Various Mfr.) Prochlorperazine maleate 5 mg, 10 mg, 25 mg. Tab. Bot. 30s (except 25 mg), 100s, 1000s, UD 100s. *Rx.*
Use: Antipsychotic.

prochlorperazine edisylate. (Various Mfr.) Prochlorperazine edisylate 5 mg/ml. Inj. Amp. 2 ml. Vial 10 ml. Tubex 1 ml, 2 ml. *Rx.*
Use: Antipsychotic.

prochlorperazine. (G & W Labs) Prochlorperazine 25 mg, coconut oil, palm kernel oil. Supp. 12s. *Rx.*
Use: Antiemetic.

•**prochlorperazine edisylate.** (pro-klor-PURR-uh-zeen) U.S.P. 23.
Use: Antipsychotic, antiemetic.
See: Compazine, Preps. (SmithKline Beecham Pharmaceuticals).

prochlorperazine ethanedisulfonate. Prochlorperazine Edisylate, U.S.P. 23.
Use: Anxiolytic.

prochlorperazine/isopropamide. (Various Mfr.) Isopropamide iodide 5 mg, prochlorperazine maleate 10 mg/Cap. Bot. 100s, 500s, 1000s, UD 100s. *Rx.*
Use: Anticholinergic, antispasmodic, antiemetic, antivertigo.

•**prochlorperazine maleate.** (pro-klor-PURR-uh-zeen) U.S.P. 23.
Use: Antiemetic, antipsychotic.
See: Compazine, Preps. (SmithKline Beecham Pharmaceuticals).

•**procinonide.** (pro-SIN-oh-nide) USAN.
Use: Adrenocortical steroid.

•**proclonol.** (PRO-klah-nole) USAN. Under study.
Use: Anthelmintic, antifungal.

Pro Comfort Athlete's Foot Spray. (Scholl) Tolnaftate 1%. Aerosol Can 4 oz. *otc.*
Use: Antifungal, topical.

Pro Comfort Jock Itch Spray Powder. (Scholl) Tolnaftate 1%. Aerosol can 3.5 oz. *otc.*
Use: Antifungal, topical.

Procort. (Roberts Pharm) Hydrocortisone 1%. **Cream:** Tube. 30 g. **Spray:** Can. 45 ml. *otc.*
Use: Corticosteroid, topical.

Procrit. (Ortho Biotech) Epoetin alfa 2000, 3000, 4000 or 10,000 units. Inj. Vial. 1 ml. *Rx.*
Use: Hematopoietic.

Proctocort. (Monarch Pharmaceuticals) Hydrocortisone Cream 30 g w/rectal applicator. Hydrocortisone acetate 30 mg. Supp. Box. 12s. *Rx.*
Use: Corticosteroid.

ProctoCream-HC. (Schwarz Pharma) Hydrocortisone acetate 1% or 2.5%, pramoxine HCl 1%. Cream 30 g. *Rx.*
Use: Corticosteroid; anesthetic, local.

Proctofoam. (Schwarz Pharma) Pramoxine HCl 1% in an anesthetic mucoadhesive foam base. Foam. Can. 15 g. *otc.*
Use: Anorectal preparation.

ProctoFoam-HC. (Schwarz Pharma) Hydrocortisone acetate 1%, pramoxine HCl 1% in hydrophilic foam base. Bot. aerosol container, Aerosol foam 10 g w/ applicator. *Rx.*
Use: Corticosteroid, anesthetic, local.

Proctofoam NS. (Schwarz Pharma) Pramoxine HCl 1%. Aerosol Bot. 15 g w/applicator. *otc.*
Use: Anesthetic, local.

Pro-Cute Cream. (Ferndale Laboratories) Silicone, hexachlorophene, lanolin. 2 oz, lb. *otc.*
Use: Emollient.

ProCycle Gold. (Cyclin Pharm) Vitamins A 833.3 IU, D 66.7 IU, E 66.7 IU, C 30 mg, B_1 1.7 mg, B_2 1.7 mg, B_3 3.3 mg, B_5 1.7 mg, B_6 3.3 mg, B_{12} 21 mcg, folic acid 66.7 mg, Ca 166.7 mg, iron 3 mg, zinc 2.5 mg, B, Cu, Cr, I, Mg, Mn, Se, PABA, inositol, rutin, biotin, hesperidin, pancreatin, betaine/Tab. Sugar free. Bot. 100s. *otc.*
Use: Mineral, vitamin supplement.

•**procyclidine hydrochloride.** (pro-SI-klih-deen) Sigma-Tau Pharmaceuticals U.S.P. 23.
Use: Muscle relaxant; antiparkinsonian.
See: Kemadrin, Tab. (Glaxo-Wellcome).

Procysteine. (Free Radical Sciences)
See: L_2-Oxothiazolidine$_4$-carboxylic acid.

Proderm Topical Dressing. (Hickam) Castor oil 650 mg, peruvian balsam 72.5 mg/0.82 cc. Aerosol 4 oz. *otc.*
Use: Dermatologic, wound therapy.

•**prodilidine hydrochloride.** (pro-DIH-lih-deen) USAN.
Use: Analgesic.

Prodium. (Breckenridge Pharmaceuticals) Phenazopyramide HCl 90 mg/ Tab. Pkg. 12s, Bot. 30s. *otc.*
Use: Analgesic.

•**prodolic acid.** (PRO-dole-ik acid) USAN.
Use: Anti-inflammatory.

Pro-Est. (Burgin-Arden) Progesterone 25 mg, estrogenic substance 25,000 IU, sodium carboxymethylcellulose 1 mg, sodium Cl 0.9%, benzalkonium Cl 1:10,000, sodium phosphate dibasic 0.1% in water. *Rx.*
Use: Estrogen, progestin combination.

•**profadol hydrochloride.** (PRO-fah-dahl) USAN.
Use: Analgesic.

profamina.
See: Amphetamine (Various Mfr.).

Profasi. (Serono Labs) Chorionic gonadotropin 5000 units or 10,000 units/Vial. Vial 10 ml. *Rx.*
Use: Chorionic gonadotropin.

Profenal. (Alcon Laboratories) Suprofen 1% soln. Drop-Tainer 2.5 ml. *Rx.*
Use: NSAID, ophthalmic.

Profen LA. (Wakefield Pharm) Phenylpropanolamine HCl 75 mg, guaifenesin 600 mg/TR Tab. Dye free. Bot. 100s. *Rx.*
Use: Decongestant, expectorant.

Profen II. (Wakefield Pharm) Phenylpropanolamine HCl 37.5 mg, guaifenesin 600 mg/TR Tab. Dye free. Bot. 100s. *Rx.*
Use: Decongestant, expectorant.

Profen II DM. (Wakefield) Phenylpropanolamine HCl 37.5 mg, guaifenesin 600 mg, dextromethorphan HBr 30 mg. TR Tab. Bot. 100s. *Rx.*
Use: Antihistamine, decongestant, expectorant.

Professional Care Lotion, Extra Strength. (Walgreens) Zinc oxide 0.25% in a lotion base. Bot. 16 oz. *otc.*
Use: Astringent, antiseptic, dermatologic.

Profiber Liquid. (Sherwood Medical) Sodium caseinate, dietary fiber from soy, calcium caseinate, hydrolyzed cornstarch, corn oil, soy lecithin, vitamins A, B_1, B_2, B_3, B_5, B_6, B_{12}, C, D, E, K, folic acid, biotin, choline, Ca, Cl, Cr, Cu, Fe, I, Mg, Mn, Mo, P, Se, Zn. Can 250 ml, closed system 1000 ml. *otc.*
Use: Nutritional supplement.

Profilnine Heat-Treated. (Alpha Therapeutics) Dried plasma fraction of coagulation factors II, VII, IX and X. Heparin free. Vial, single dose with diluent. *Rx.*
Use: Antihemophilic.

Profilnine SD. (Alpha Therapeutics) Dried plasma fraction of coagulation factors II, VII, IX and X. Heparin free. Solvent detergent treated. Inj. Single dose vials with diluent. *Rx.*
Use: Antihemophilic.

proflavine.
Use: Antiseptic, topical.

proflavine dihydrochloride. 3,6-Diaminoacridine dihydrochloride.

proflavine sulfate. 3,6-Diaminoacridine sulfate.

ProFree/GP Weekly Enzymatic

Cleaner. (Allergan) Papain, sodium Cl, sodium borate, sodium carbonate, edetate disodium. Kit 16s or 24s with vials. *otc.*
Use: Contact lens care.

•**progabide.** (pro-GAB-ide) USAN.
Use: Anticonvulsant, muscle relaxant.

Progens Tabs. (Major) Conjugated estrogens. **0.625 mg/Tab.:** Bot. 100s, 1000s; **1.25 mg/Tab.:** Bot. 1000s; **2.5 mg/Tab.:** Bot. 100s, 1000s. *Rx.*
Use: Estrogen.

Pro-Gesic. (Nastech) Trolamine salicylate 10%, propylene glycol, methylparahydroxybenzoic acid, propyl parahydroxybenzoic acid, EDTA. Liq. Bot. 75 ml. *otc.*
Use: Liniment.

Progestasert. (Alza) T-shaped intrauterine device (IUD) unit containing a reservoir of progesterone 38 mg with barium sulfate dispersed in medical grade silicone fluid. In 6s w/inserter. *Rx.*
Use: Contraceptive.

•**progesterone.** (pro-JESS-ter-ohn) U.S.P. 23. Flavolutan, Luteogan, Luteosan, Lutren.
Use: Hormone, progestin. [Orphan drug]
W/Aqueous. Susp.
See: Prorone, Inj. (Sigma-Tau Pharmaceuticals).
W/In Oil
See: Crinone 8%, Gel (Wyeth Labs).
Femotrone, Inj. (Bluco).
Lipo-Lutin, Amp. (Parke-Davis).
Progestin, Vial (Various Mfr.).
Prorone, Inj. (Sigma-Tau Pharmaceuticals).
W/Estradiol, testosterone, procaine HCl, procaine base.
See: Hormo-Triad, Vial (Bell).
W/Estrogenic substance.
See: Profoygen Aqueous (Foy).
Progex, Inj. (Taylor Pharmaceuticals).

progesterone. (Various Mfr.) Pow. 1 g, 10 g, 25 g, 100 g, 1000g.
Use: Hormone, progestin.

progesterone in oil. (Various Mfr.) 50 mg/ml. In sesame or peanut oil with benzyl alcohol. Inj. Vial 10 ml. *Rx.*
Use: Hormone, progestin.

progesterone intrauterine contraceptive system.
Use: Contraceptive.

progestin. Progesterone (Various Mfr.).
See: Hydroxyprogesterone.
Medroxyprogesterone.
Megestrol.
Norethindrone.

•**proglumide.** (pro-GLUE-mid) USAN. (Wallace Laboratories).
Use: Anticholinergic.

Proglycem. (Baker Norton) **Cap.:** Diazoxide 50 mg/Cap. Bot. 100s. **Oral Susp.:** Diazoxide 50 mg/ml. Bot. 30 ml w/calibrated dropper. *Rx.*
Use: Hyperglycemic.

Prograf. (Fujisawa) **Cap.:** Tacrolimus 1 mg or 5 mg. Bot. 100s; **Inj.:** Tacrolimus 5 mg/ml. In 1 ml amps (10s). *Rx.*
Use: Immunosuppressant.

proguanil hydrochloride.
See: Chloroguanide Hydrochloride.
Paludrine, Tab. (Wyeth Ayerst).

ProHance. (Bracco Diagnostics) Gadoteridol 279.3 mg, calteridol calcium 0.23 mg, tromethamine 1.21 mg/ml. Inj Vials. 15 ml, 30 ml. *Rx.*
Use: Radiopaque agent.

ProHIBIT. (Pasteur Merieux Connaught) Purified capsular polysaccharide of *Haemophilus influenzae* type b 25 mcg, conjugated diphtheria toxoid protein 18 mcg/0.5 ml dose. Also called PRP-D. Inj. Vial 0.5 ml, 2.5 ml, 5 ml. Syr. 0.5 ml. *Rx.*
Use: Immunization.

•**proinsulin human.** (PRO-in-suh-LIN HYOO-muhn) USAN.
Use: Antidiabetic.

Prolactin RIA. (Abbott Diagnostics) Quantitative measurement of total circulating human prolactin. Test unit 50s, 100s.
Use: Diagnostic aid.

Prolactin RIAbead. (Abbott Diagnostics) Radioimmunoassay for the quantitative measurement of prolactin in human serum and plasma.
Use: Diagnostic aid.

proladyl. Pyrrobutamine. 1-Pyrrolidyl-3-phenyl-4-(p-chlorophenyl)-2-butene phosphate.
Use: Antihistamine.

prolase. Proteolytic enzyme from *Carica papaya.*
See: Papain.

Prolastin. (Bayer Corp) Alpha$_1$-proteinase inhibitor $\geq$ 20 mg alpha$_1$-PI/ml when reconstituted. W/polyethylene glycol, sucrose and small amounts of other plasma proteins. Inj. Vial, single dose. *Rx.*
Use: Alpha$_1$-proteinase inhibitor.

Proleukin. (Chiron Therapeutics) Aldesleukin, interleukin-2. Pow. for Inj. 22 million IU/Vial (1.1 mg when reconstituted). Single-use Vial. *Rx.*

Use: Antineoplastic.

•**proline.** (PRO-leen) U.S.P. 23.
Use: Amino acid.

•**prolintane hydrochloride.** (pro-LIN-tane) USAN.
Use: Antidepressant.

Prolixin. (Bristol-Myers Squibb) Fluphenazine HCl. **Tab.:** 1 mg, 2.5 mg, 5 mg, 10 mg. Bot. 50s, 100s, 500s, 1000s, UD 100s. **Elixir:** 2.5 mg/5 ml, alcohol 14%. Dropper Bot. 60 ml. Bot. 473 ml. **Conc.:** 5 mg/ml, alcohol 14%, Dropper Bot. 120 ml. **Inj.:** 2.5 mg/ml. Vial 10 ml w/methyl and propyl parabens. *Rx.*
Use: Antipsychotic.

Prolixin Decanoate. (Bristol-Myers Squibb) Fluphenazine decanoate 25 mg/ml (in sesame oil with benzyl alcohol). Unimatic syringe 1 ml. Vial 5 ml. *Rx.*
Use: Antipsychotic.

Prolixin Enanthate. (Bristol-Myers Squibb) Fluphenazine enanthate 25 mg/ml (in sesame oil with benzyl alcohol). Vial 5 ml. *Rx.*
Use: Antipsychotic.

Proloprim. (GlaxoWellcome) Trimethoprim 100 mg/Tab. Bot. 100s, UD 100s (in sesame oil with benzyl alcohol). *Rx.*
Use: Anti-infective, urinary.

Promachlor. (Geneva Pharm) Chlorpromazine HCl 10 mg, 25 mg, 50 mg, 100 mg or 200 mg/Tab. Bot. 100s, 1000s. *Rx.*
Use: Antiemetic, antivertigo, antipsychotic.

•**promazine hydrochloride.** (PRO-mah-zeen) U.S.P. 23.
Use: Antipsychotic, anticholinergic, ataraxic.
See: Sparine, Tab. (Wyeth Ayerst).

promazine hydrochloride. (Various Mfr.) Promazine HCl 25 mg/ml, 50 mg/ml. Inj. Vial 10 ml. *Rx.*
Use: Antipsychotic.

Promega. (Parke-Davis) Omega-3 (N-3) polyunsaturated fatty acids 1000 mg, containing EPA 350 mg, DHA 150 mg, vitamins E (3% RDA), A, B_1, B_2, B_3, Ca, Fe (< 2% RDA)/Cap., cholesterol and sodium free. Bot. 30s. *otc.*
Use: Mineral, vitamin supplement.

Promega Pearls. (Parke-Davis) EPA 168 mg, DHA 72 mg, < cholesterol 2 mg, E 1 IU, < 2% RDA of A, B_1, B_2, B_3, Fe, Ca. Cap. Bot. 60s, 90s. *otc.*
Use: Vitamin supplement.

Prometa. (Muro) Metaproterenol sulfate 10 mg/5 ml, with saccharin and sorbitol, strawberry flavor. Syr. Bot. 480 ml. *Rx.*
Use: Bronchodilator.

Promethazine DM. (Various Mfr.) Promethazine HCl 6.25 mg, dextromethorphan HBr 15 mg/5 ml, alcohol. Syr. Bot. 120 ml, pt, gal. *Rx.*
Use: Antihistamine, antitussive.

Prometh VC Plain Liquid. (Various Mfr.) Phenylephrine HCl 5 mg, promethazine HCl 6.25 mgm/5 ml. Liq. Bot. 120 ml, 473 ml, gal. *Rx.*
Use: Antihistamine, decongestant.

promethazine. (pro-METH-uh-zeen) **Tab.:** 25 mg, 50 mg. Bot. 100s, 1000s. **Syr.:** 6.25 mg/ 5 ml, alcohol. Bot. 118 ml, pt. **Supp.:** 50 mg, cocoa butter. Pkg. 12s. **Inj.:** 25 mg/ml, 50 mg/ml. Amp. 1 ml, Multi-dose Vial 10 ml. *Rx.*
Use: Antiemetic, antihistamine, sedative.

•**promethazine hydrochloride.** (pro-METH-uh-zeen) U.S.P. 23.
Use: Antiemetic, antihistamine.
See: Pentazine, Expectorant, Vial (Century Pharm).
Phenergan, Prods. (Wyeth Ayerst).
Phenerject, Vial (Merz).
Prorex, Vial, Amp. (Hyrex).
Provigan, Inj. (Solvay).
Remsed, Tab. (DuPont).
Sigazine, Inj. (Sigma-Tau Pharmaceuticals).

promethazine hydrochloride with codeine. (pro-METH-uh-zeen) (Various Mfr.) Promethazine HCl 6.25 mg, codeine phosphate 10 mg/5 ml, alcohol 7%. Syr. Bot. 120 ml, pt, gal. *c-v.*
Use: Antihistamine, antitussive.

promethazine hydrochloride w/combinations. (pro-METH-uh-zeen)
Use: Antiemetic, antihistamine, antivertigo.
See: Mepergan, Vial, Cap. (Wyeth Ayerst).
Phenergan-D, Tab. (Wyeth Ayerst).
Phenergan VC Expectorant (Wyeth Ayerst).

Promethazine VC. (Various Mfr.) Promethazine HCl 6.25 mg, phenylephrine HCl 5 mg/5 ml. 120 ml, 240 ml, 473 ml, gal. *Rx.*
Use: Antihistamine, decongestant.

Promethazine VC with Codeine. (Various Mfr.) Promethazine HCl 6.25 mg, phenylephrine HCl 5 mg, codeine 10 mg/5 ml, alcohol 7%. Bot. 4 oz, pt, gal. *c-v.*
Use: Antihistamine, antitussive, decongestant.

Promethazine VC Plain. (Various Mfr.) Phenylephrine HCl 5 mg, promethazine HCl 6.25 mg/5 ml. Syr. Bot. 473 ml. *Rx.*
Use: Antihistamine, decongestant.

promethestrol dipropionate.
Use: Estrogen.
See: Meprane Dipropionate, Tab. (Schwarz Pharma).
W/Phenobarbital.
See: Meprane-Phenobarbital, Tab. (Schwarz Pharma).

Prometol. (Viobin) Concentrated wheat germ oil. **3 min/Cap.:** Bot. 100s, 250s. **10 min/Cap.:** Bot. 100s. *otc.*
Use: Supplement.

prominal.
See: Mephobarbital.

Prominol. (MCR American Pharm) Butalbital 50 mg, acetaminophen 650 mg/Tab. Bot. 100s. *Rx.*
Use: Analgesic.

Promine. (Major) Procainamide 250 mg, 375 mg or 500 mg/Cap. Bot. 100s, 250s, 1000s, UD 100s (375 mg/Cap. w/500s instead of 250s). *Rx.*
Use: Antiarrhythmic.

Promine S.R. (Major) Procainamide. **SR Tab.:** 250 mg. Bot. 100s, 250s; 500 mg. Bot. 100s, 250s, 1000s; 750 mg. Bot. 100s, 250s. **SR Cap.:** 250 mg, 375 mg or 500 mg. *Rx.*
Use: Antiarrhythmic.

Promist HD. (UCB Pharmaceuticals) Hydrocodone bitartrate 2.5 mg, pseudoephedrine HCl 30 mg, chlorpheniramine maleate 2 mg/5 ml, alcohol 5%, menthol, saccharin, sorbitol. Bot. pt. *c-III.*
Use: Antihistamine, antitussive, decongestant.

Promist LA. (UCB Pharmaceuticals) Pseudoephedrine HCl 120 mg, guaifenesin 500 mg/Tab. Bot. 100s. *Rx.*
Use: Decongestant, expectorant.

Promit. (Pharmacia & Upjohn) Dextran 1 150 mg/ml Inj. Vial 20 ml. *Rx.*
Use: Antiallergic.

Pro-Mix R.D.P. (Navaco) Protein 15 g (from whey protein), fat 0.8 g, carbohydrate 1 g, sodium 46 mg, potassium 165 mg, chloride 46 mg, calcium 73.6 mg, phosphorus 64.4 mg, iron 0.3 mg, Cr, Cu, Mg, Mn, Mo, Se, Zn, 72 Cal./5 Tbsp. (20 g). Pow. Packet 20 g, can 300 g. *otc.*
Use: Nutritional supplement.

ProMod. (Ross Laboratories) Protein supplement. Nine scoops provides protein 45 g, 100% U.S. RDA. Pow. Can 9.7 oz. *otc.*
Use: Nutritional supplement.

Promylin Enteric Coated Microzymes. (Shear/Kershman) Enteric coated pancrelipase. Lipase 4000 units, amylase 20,000 units, protease 25,000 units. *Rx.*
Use: Digestive enzymes.

Pro-Nasyl. (Progonasyl) o-Iodobenzoic acid 0.5%, triethanolamine 5.5% in a special neutral hydrophilic base compounded from oleic acid, mineral oil, vegetable oil. Bot. 15 ml, 60 ml.
Use: Treatment of sinusitis.

Pronemia Hematinic. (ESI Lederle Generics) Iron 115 mg, B_{12} 15 mcg, IFC 75 mg, C 150 mg, folic acid 1 mcg. Cap. Bot. 30s. *Rx.*
Use: Iron w/B_{12} and intrinsic factor.

Pronestyl. (Bristol-Myers) Procainamide. **Cap.:** 250 mg. Bot. 100s, 1000s; 375 mg. Bot. 100s; 500 mg. Bot. 100s, 1000s. **Inj.:** 100 mg/ml w/benzyl alcohol 0.9%, sodium bisulfite 0.09%. Vial 10 ml; 500 mg/ml w/methylparaben 0.1%, sodium bisulfite 0.2%. Vial 2 ml. **Tab.:** 250 mg. Bot. 100s, 1000s, Unimatic 100s; 375 mg. Bot. 100s; 500 mg. Bot. 100s, 1000s, Unimatic 100s. *Rx.*
Use: Antiarrhythmic.

Pronestyl-SR. (Bristol-Myers) Procainamide 500 mg/Tab. Bot. UD 100s. *Rx.*
Use: Antiarrhythmic.

pronethelol. (Zeneca) Adrenergic beta-receptor antagonist; pending release.

Pronto Concentrate Lice Killing Shampoo Kit. (Del Pharmaceuticals) Pyrethrins 0.33%, piperonyl butoxide technical 4%. Bot. 2 oz, 4 oz. *otc.*
Use: Pediculicide.

Pronto Lice Killing Spray. (Del Pharmaceuticals) Spray cans 5 oz. *otc.*
Use: Pediculicide for inanimate objects.

Propac. (Biosearch Medical Products) Protein 3 g (from whey protein), carbohydrate 0.2 g, fat 0.3 g, chloride 3 mg, potassium 20 mg, sodium 9 mg, calcium 24 mg, phosphorus 12 mg, 16 Cal./Tbsp. (4 g). Pow. Packet 19.5 g, Can 350 g. *otc.*
Use: Nutritional supplement.

Propacet 100. (Teva USA) Propoxyphene napsylate 100 mg, acetaminophen 650 mg/Tab. Bot. 100s, 500s. *c-IV.*
Use: Analgesic combination, narcotic.

propaesin. Propyl p-Aminobenzoate. (Various Mfr.).

•**propafenone hydrochloride.** (pro-pah-FEN-ohn) U.S.P. 23.

Use: Cardiovascular agent, antiarrhythmic.
See: Rythmol, Tab. (Knoll Pharmaceuticals).

Propagest Tablets. (Schwarz Pharma) Phenylpropanolamine HCl 25 mg/Tab. Bot. 100s. *otc.*
Use: Decongestant.

Propagon-S. (Spanner) Estrone 2 mg or 5 mg/ml. Vial 10 ml. *Rx.*
Use: Estrogen.

Propain HC. (Springbok) Acetaminophen 500 mg, hydrocodone bitartrate 5 mg/Cap. Bot. 100s, 500s. *c-III.*
Use: Analgesic combination, narcotic.

propamidine isethionate 0.1% ophthalmic soln.
Use: Acanthamoeba keratitis. [Orphan drug]

•**propane.** N.F. 18.
Use: Aerosol propellant.

propanediol diacetate, 1,2.
See: VoSoL, Liq. (Wampole Laboratories).

1,2,3-propanetriol, trinitrate. Nitroglycerin Tab., U.S.P. 23.

•**propanidid.** (pro-PAN-ih-did) USAN.
Use: Anesthetic (intravenous).

propanolol. Propranolol.

•**propantheline bromide.** (pro-PAN-thuh-leen) U.S.P. 23.
Use: Anticholinergic.
See: Pro-Banthine, Preps. (Searle).
W/Phenobarbital.
See: Probital, Tab. (Searle).
W/Thiopropazate dihydrochloride.
See: Pro-Banthine W/Dartal, Tab. (Searle).

PROPApH Cleansing Lotion for Normal/Combination Skin. (Del Pharmaceuticals) Salicylic acid 0.5%, SD alcohol 40, EDTA. Lot. Bot. 180 ml. Pads. 45s. *otc.*
Use: Antiacne.

PROPApH Cleansing for Oily Skin. (Del Pharmaceuticals) Salicylic acid 0.6%, SD alcohol 40, EDTA, menthol. Lot. Bot. 180 ml. *otc.*
Use: Dermatologic, acne.

PROPApH Cleansing for Sensitive Skin. (Del Pharmaceuticals) Salicylic acid 0.5%, SD alcohol 40, aloe vera gel, EDTA, menthol. Pads. In 45s. *otc.*
Use: Dermatologic, acne.

PROPApH Cleansing Maximum Strength. (Del Pharmaceuticals) Salicylic acid 2%, SD alcohol 40, aloe vera gel, EDTA, propylene glycol, menthol. Pads. In 45s. *otc.*
Use: Dermatologic, acne.

PROPApH Cleansing Pads. (Del Pharmaceuticals) Salicylic acid 0.5%, SD alcohol 40, EDTA, menthol. Pads. 45s. *otc.*
Use: Dermatologic, ance.

PROPApH Foaming Face Wash. (Del Pharmaceuticals) Salicylic acid 2%, aloe vera gel, EDTA, menthol. Alcohol, oil and soap free. Liq. Bot. 180 ml. *otc.*
Use: Dermatologic, acne.

PROPApH Maximum Strength Acne Cream. (Del Pharmaceuticals) Salicylic acid 2%, acetylated lanolin alcohol, cetearyl alcohol, stearyl alcohol, EDTA, menthol. Cream. Tube 19.5 g. *otc.*
Use: Dermatologic, acne.

PROPApH Medicated Acne Cream with Aloe. (Del Pharmaceuticals) Salicylic acid 2%. Tube 1 oz. *otc.*
Use: Dermatologic, acne.

PROPApH Medicated Acne Stick with Aloe. (Del Pharmaceuticals) Salicylic acid 2%. Stick 0.05 oz. *otc.*
Use: Dermatologic, acne.

PROPApH Medicated Cleansing Pads with Aloe. (Del Pharmaceuticals) Salicylic acid 0.5%, SD alcohol 40 25%, aloe. Jar containing 45 pads. *otc.*
Use: Dermatologic, acne.

PROPApH Peel-Off Acne Mask. (Del Pharmaceuticals) Salicylic acid 2%, tartrazine, parabens, polyvinyl alcohol, vitamin E acetate, SD alcohol 40. In 60 ml. *otc.*
Use: Dermatologic, acne.

PROPApH Skin Cleanser with Aloe. (Del Pharmaceuticals) Salicylic acid USP 0.5%, SD alcohol 40 25%. Bot. 6 oz, 10 oz. *otc.*
Use: Dermatologic, acne.

•**proparacaine hydrochloride.** (pro-PAR-ah-cane) U.S.P. 23.
Use: Anesthetic local, ophthalmic.
See: Alcaine Ophthalmic Soln. (Alcon Laboratories).
AK-Taine, Soln. (Akorn).
Fluoracaine, Soln. (Akorn).
Ophthaine HCl, Soln. (Squibb Diagnostic).
Ophthetic, Ophthalmic Soln. (Allergan).

proparacaine hydrochloride. (Various Mfr.) 0.5% Soln. Bot. 2 ml, 15 ml, UD 1 ml.
Use: Anesthetic local, ophthalmic.

proparacaine hydrochloride & fluorescein sodium. (Taylor Pharmaceuticals) Proparacaine HCl 0.5%, fluore-

scein sodium 0.25%, thimerosal 0.01%, EDTA. Soln. Bot. 5 ml. *Rx.*
Use: Anesthetic local, ophthalmic.

proparacaine hydrochloride/procaine hydrochloride.
Use: Anesthetic.
See: Ravocaine and novocain w/Levophed (Cook-Waite).
Ravocaine and novocain w/neocobefrin (Cook-Waite).

•**propatyl nitrate.** (PRO-pah-till) USAN. Investigational drug in U.S. but available in England.
Use: Coronary vasodilator.

Propecia . (Merck) Finasteride 1 mg, lactose. Tab. Unit-of-use 30s, UD 30s. *Rx.*
Use: Androgen hormone inhibitor, hair growth.

•**propenzolate hydrochloride.** (pro-PEN-zoe-late) USAN.
Use: Anticholinergic.

propesin. Name used for Risocaine.

Prophene 65. (Halsey) Propoxyphene HCl 65 mg/Cap. Bot. 100s, 500s, 1000s. *c-IV.*
Use: Analgesic, narcotic.

prophenpyridamine.
See: Pheniramine (Various Mfr.).

prophenpyridamine maleate.
See: Pheniramine Maleate.

prophenpyridamine maleate w/combinations.
See: Panadyl, Tab., Cap. (Misemer).
Polyectin, Liq. (Amide Pharmaceuticals).
Trimahist Elix., Liq. (Tennessee Pharmaceutic).
Vasotus, Liq. (Sheryl).

Pro-Phree. (Ross Laboratories) Fat 31 g, carbohydrate 60 g, linoleic acid 2250 mg, Fe 11.9 mg, Na 250 mg, K 875 mg, with appropriate vitamins and minerals, 520 Cal/100 g. Protein free. Pow. Can 350 g. *otc.*
Use: Nutritional supplement.

Prophyllin. (Rystan) Sodium propionate 5%, chlorophyll derivatives 0.0125%. Tube 1 oz. *Rx.*
Use: Anti-infective, topical.

•**propikacin.** (PRO-pih-KAY-sin) USAN.
Use: Anti-infective.

Propimex-1. (Ross Laboratories) Protein 15 g, fat 23.9 g, carbohydrate 46.3 g, linoleic acid 1800 mg, Fe 9 mg, Na 190 mg, K 675 mg, with appropriate vitamins and minerals, 480 Cal/100 g. Methionine and valine free. Pow. Can 350 g. *otc.*
Use: Nutritional supplement.

Propimex-2. (Ross Laboratories) Protein 30 g, fat 15.5 g, carbohydrate 30 g, Na 880 mg, K 1370 mg, with appropriate vitamins and minerals, 410 Cal/ml. Methionine and valine free. Pow. Can 325 g. *otc.*
Use: Nutritional supplement for propionic or methylmalonic acidemia.

Propine Sterile Ophthalmic Solution. (Allergan) Dipivefrin HCl 0.1%. Soln. Bot. 5 ml, 10 ml, 15 ml. *Rx.*
Use: Antiglaucoma.

propiodal.
See: Entodon.

•**propiolactone.** (PRO-pee-oh-LACK-tone) USAN.
Use: Disinfectant, sterilizing agent of vaccines and tissue grafts.

•**propiomazine.** (PRO-pee-oh-MAY-zeen) USAN.
Dorevane; Indorm.
Use: Sedative (pre-anesthetic).
See: Largon, Amp. (Wyeth Ayerst).

propiomazine. (PRO-pee-oh-MAY-zeen)
Use: Sedative.
See: Largon, Inj. (Wyeth Ayerst).

propiomazine hydrochloride. (PRO-pee-oh-MAY-zeen)
Use: Sedative.
See: Largon, Inj. (Wyeth Ayerst). Propion Gel (Wyeth Ayerst).

•**propionic acid.** (pro-pee-AHN-ik) N.F. 18.
Use: Antimicrobial; pharmaceutic aid (acidifying agent).
W/Sodium propionate, docusate sodium, salicylic acid.
See: Prosal, Liq. (Gordon Laboratories).
Propionate-Caprylate Mixtures.

propionyl erythromycin lauryl sulfate.
See: Erythromycin Propionate Lauryl Sulfate.

•**propiram fumarate.** (PRO-pih-ram) USAN.
Use: Analgesic.

propisamine.
See: Amphetamine (Various Mfr.).

propitocaine. Prilocaine.
See: Citanest, Soln., Vial, Amp. (Astra).

Proplex. (Baxter) Factor IX Complex (Human), clotting Factor II (prothrombin), VII (proconvertin), IX (PTC, antihemophilic factor B) and X (Stuart-Prower factor) all dried and concentrated. Vial 30 ml w/Diluent. *Rx.*
Use: Antihemophilic.

Proplex T. (Baxter) Factor IX complex,

heat treated. W/Factors II, VII, IX and X. W/heparin. Dried concentrate. Vial w/ diluent. *Rx.*
Use: Antihemophilic.

•**propofol.** (PRO-puh-FOLE) USAN.
Use: Anesthetic (intravenous).
See: Diprivan, Inj. (Zeneca).

Proponade Capsules. (Halsey) Chlorpheniramine maleate 8 mg, phenylpropanolamine HCl 50 mg, isopropamide 2.5 mg/Cap. Bot. 100s. *Rx.*
Use: Antihistamine, decongestant.

Propoquin. Amopyroquin HCl.
Use: Antimalarial.

propoxamide.

•**propoxycaine hydrochloride.** (pro-POX-ih-cane) U.S.P. 23.
Use: Anesthetic, local.

propoxycaine and procaine hydrochlorides and levonordefrin injection.
Use: Anesthetic, local.

propoxycaine and procaine hydrochlorides and norepinephrine bitartrate injection.
Use: Anesthetic, local.
See: Ravocaine and Novocain w/levophed, Inj. (Cook-Waite).

propoxychlorinol. Toloxychlorinol.

•**propoxyphene hydrochloride.** (pro-POX-ih-feen) U.S.P. 23.
Use: Analgesic.
See: Darvon, Pulvules (Eli Lilly).
Dolene, Cap. (ESI Lederle Generics).
Progesic, Cap. (Ulmer).
SK-65, Cap. (SmithKline Beecham Pharmaceuticals).

propoxyphene hydrochloride w/combinations.
Use: Analgesic.
See: Darvon Compound, Pulvule (Eli Lilly).
Darvon Compound-65, Cap. (Eli Lilly).
Darvon With A.S.A., Cap. (Eli Lilly).
Dolene, AP-65, Tab. (ESI Lederle Generics).
Dolene Compound-65, Cap. (ESI Lederle Generics).
Wygesic, Tab. (Wyeth Ayerst).

propoxyphene hydrochloride and acetaminophen tablets. (pro-POX-ee-feen HIGH-droe-KLOR-ide & ass-cet-ah-MEE-noe-fen tablets)
Use: Analgesic.

propoxyphene hydrochloride and acetaminophen tablets. (Various Mfr.) Propoxyphene HCl 65 mg, acetaminophen 650 mg/Tab. Bot. 500s. *c-IV.*
Use: Analgesic.

propoxyphene hydrochloride and APC capsules.
Use: Analgesic.

propoxyphene hydrochloride, aspirin and caffeine capsules.
Use: Analgesic.

propoxyphene hydrochloride compound capsules. (Various Mfr.) Propoxyphene HCl 65 mg, aspirin 389 mg, caffeine 32.4/Cap. Bot. 100s, 500s. *c-IV.*
Use: Analgesic.

•**propoxyphene napsylate.** (pro-POX-ih-feen NAP-sill-ate) U.S.P. 23.
Use: Analgesic.
See: Darvocet-N (Eli Lilly).
Darvon-N, Tab. (Eli Lilly).
W/Acetaminophen.
See: Darvocet-N, Tab. (Eli Lilly).

propoxyphene napsylate and acetaminophen tablets. (Various Mfr.) Propoxyphene napsylate 50 mg, acetaminophen 325 mg/Tab. Bot. 100s, 500s, 550s, 1000s, UD 100s. Propoxyphene napsylate 100 mg, acetaminophen 650 mg/Tab. Bot. 30s, 50s, 100s, 500s, 1000s, UD 100s. *c-IV.*
Use: Analgesic.

propoxyphene napsylate and aspirin tablets.
Use: Analgesic.

•**propranolol hydrochloride.** (pro-PRAN-oh-lahl) U.S.P. 23.
Use: Cardiovascular agent (antiarrhythmic), antiadrenergic (beta-receptor).
See: Betachron E-R, Cap. (Inwood).
Inderal, Tab., Inj. (Wyeth Ayerst).

proprandol hydrochloride SR capsules. (Various Mfr.) Propranolol HCl 60 mg, 80 mg, 120 mg, 160 mg. Bot. 100s, 250s, 500s, 1000s. *Rx.*
Use: Cardiovascular agent (antiarrhythmic), antiadrenergic (beta-receptor).

propanol hydrochloride tablets. (Various Mfr.) Propranolol HCl 10 mg, 20 mg, 40 mg, 60 mg, 80 mg, 90 mg. Bot. 100s, 500s, 1000s, UD 100s. *Rx.*
Use: Cardiovascular agent (antiarrhythmic), antiadrenergic (beta-receptor).

propranolol hydrochlorlde solution. (Roxane) **Oral Soln.**: 20 mg or 40 mg/ 5 ml. Patient cups UD 5 ml (10s). **Concentrated Oral Soln.**: 80 mg/ml. Bot. 30 ml w/calibrated dropper.
Use: Cardiovascular agent (antiarrhythmic), antiadrenergic (β-receptor).

propranolol hydrochloride and hydrochlorothiazide tablets. (Various Mfr.) Propanolol HCl 40 mg or 80 mg, hydrochlorothiazide 25 mg/Tab. Bot. 100s, 1000s. *Rx.*

Use: Antihypertensive.
See: Inderide, Tab. (Wyeth Ayerst).

Propranolol Hydrochloride Intensol. (Roxane) Propranolol HCl 80 mg/ml concentrated oral soln. Bot. 30 ml with dropper. *Rx.*
Use: Beta-adrenergic blocker.

Propulsid. (Janssen) Cisapride. **Tab.:** 10 mg or 20 mg, lactose. Bot. 100s, 500s (10 mg only). **Susp.:** 1 mg/ml, parabens, sorbitol. Bot. 450 ml. *Rx.*
Use: Gastrointestinal.

•**propyl gallate.** (PRO-pill GAL-ate) N. F. 18.
Use: Pharmaceutic aid (antioxidant).

propyl p-aminobenzoate. (Various Mfr.) Propaesin.
Use: Anesthetic, local.
W/Procaine base, benzyl alcohol, phenol.
See: Rectocaine, Vial (Moore-Kirk).

•**propylene carbonate.** (PRO-pih-leen CAR-boe-nate) N.F. 18.
Use: Pharmaceutic aid (gelling agent).

•**propylene glycol.** U.S.P. 23.
Use: Pharmaceutic aid (humectant, solvent, suspending agent).

•**propylene glycol alginate.** N.F. 18.
Use: Pharmaceutic aid (suspending, viscosity-increasing agent).

•**propylene glycol diacetate.** N.F. 18.
Use: Pharmaceutic aid (solvent).

•**propylene glycol monostearate.** N.F. 18.
Use: Pharmaceutic aid (emulsifying agent).

•**propylhexedrine.** (pro-pill-HEX-ih-dreen) U.S.P. 23.
Use: Adrenergic (vasoconstrictor), appetite suppressant, antihistamine.
See: Benzedrex, Inhalant (SmithKline Beecham Pharmaceuticals).

•**propyliodone.** (pro-pill-EYE-oh-dohn) U.S.P. 23.
Use: Diagnostic aid (radiopaque medium).
See: Dionosil Oily (GlaxoWellcome).

propylnoradrenaline-iso.
See: Isoproterenol.

•**propylparaben.** (pro-pill-PAR-ah-ben) N.F. 18. Propyl Chemosept (Chemo Puro).
Use: Pharmaceutic aid (antifungal agent).

•**propylparaben sodium.** (pro-pill-PAR-ah-ben) N.F. 18.
Use: Pharmaceutic aid (antimicrobial preservative).

•**propylthiouracil.** (pro-puhl-thigh-oh-YOU-rah-sill) U.S.P. 23.
Use: Antithyroid agent.

propylthiouracil. (Abbott Laboratories) 50 mg/Tab. Bot. 100s, 1000s. (Eli Lilly) 50 mg/Tab. Bot. 100s, 1000s. (ESI Lederle Generics) 50 mg/Tab. Bot. 100s, 1000s. 50 mg/Tab. Bot. 100s, 1000s, UD 100s.
Use: Antithyroid agent.

•**proquazone.** (PRO-kwah-zone) USAN.
Use: Anti-inflammatory.

•**prorenoate potassium.** (pro-REN-oh-ate) USAN.
Use: Aldosterone antagonist.

Prorone. (Sigma-Tau Pharmaceuticals) Progesterone 25 mg/ml. Aqueous or oil susp Vial 10 ml. *Rx.*
Use: Hormone, progestin.

•**proroxan hydrochloride.** (pro-ROCK-san) USAN. *Formerly Pyrroxane, Pirrousan.*
Use: Anti-adrenergic (α-receptor).

Proscar. (Merck) Finasteride 5 mg/Tab. Unit-of-use 30s, 100s, UD 100s. *Rx.*
Use: Androgen inhibitor.

•**proscillaridin.** (pro-sih-LARE-ih-din) USAN. Talusin, Tradenal.
Use: Cardiovascular agent.

Prosed/DS. (Star) Methenamine 81.6 mg, phenyl salicylate 36.2 mg, methylene blue 10.8 mg, benzoic acid 9 mg, atropine sulfate 0.06 mg, hyoscyamine sulfate 0.06 mg. Tab. Bot. 100s, 1000s. *Rx.*
Use: Anti-infective, urinary.

Pro Skin. (Marlyn) Vitamins A 6250 IU, E 100 IU, C 100 mg, B_5 10 mg, zinc 10 mg, Se/Cap. Bot, 60s. *otc.*
Use: Mineral, vitamin supplement.

ProSobee. (Bristol-Myers) Milk free formula supplies 640 cal./qt, protein 19.2 g, fat 34 g, carbohydrate 64 g, vitamins A 2000 IU, D 400 IU, E 20 IU, C 52 mg, folic acid 100 mcg, B_1 0.5 mg, B_2 0.6 mg, niacin 8 mg, B_6 0.4 mg, B_{12} 2 mcg, biotin 50 mg, pantothenic acid 3 mg, K-1 100 mcg, choline 50 mg, inositol 30 mg, calcium 600 mg, phosphorus 475 mg, iodine 65 mcg, iron 12 mg, magnesium 70 mg, copper 0.6 mg, zinc 5 mg, manganese 1.6 mg, chloride 530 mg, potassium 780 mg, sodium 230 mg/Qt. (20 Kcal/fl oz). Concentrated liq. can 13 fl oz; Ready-to-use liq. can 8 fl oz, 32 fl oz. Pow., can 14 oz. *otc.*
Use: Nutritional supplement.

ProSobee Concentrate. (Bristol-Myers) P-soy protein isolate, l-methionine.

CHO. corn syrup solids, soy and coconut oil, lecithin, mono- and diglycerides. Protein 20.3 g, CHO 65.4 g, fat 33.6 g, iron 12 mg, 640 cal./serving. Concentrate 390 ml. *otc.*
Use: Nutritional supplement.

Pro-Sof Plus. (Vangard) Docusate sodium 100 mg, casanthranol 30 mg/ Cap. Bot. 100s, 1000s, UD 32s, 100s. *otc.*
Use: Laxative.

Pro-Sof w/Casanthranol SG. (Vangard) Casanthranol 30 mg, docusate sodium 100 mg/Cap. Bot. 100s, 1000s.
Use: Laxative.

ProSom. (Abbott Laboratories) Estazolam 1 mg or 2 mg/Tab. Bot. 100s, UD 100s. *c-IV.*
Use: Hypnotic, sedative.

prostaglandins.
Use: Abortifacient, agent for impotence, agent for cervical ripening, patent ductus arteriosus.
See: Caverject, Inj. (Pharmacia & Upjohn).
Cervidil, Inj. (Forest Pharmaceutical).
Hemabate, Inj. (Pharmacia & Upjohn).
Prepidil , Gel. (Pharmacia & Upjohn).
Prostin E2, Supp. (Pharmacia & Upjohn).
Prostin VR Pediatric, Inj. (Pharmacia & Upjohn).

prostaglandin E_1.
See: Alprostadil.

prostaglandin E_2.
See: Dinoprostone.

•**prostalene.** (PRAHST-ah-leen) USAN.
Use: Prostaglandin.

ProstaScint. (Cytogen) Pendetide 0.5 mg for conjugation w/indium-111. Kit. *Rx.*
Use: Radioimmunoscintigraphy agent.

ProStep. (ESI Lederle Generics) Transdermal nicotine 11 or 22 mg/day. Patch 7s. *Rx.*
Use: Smoking deterrent.

Prostigmin. (Zeneca) Injectable neostigmine methylsulfate. **1:1000:** 1 mg/ml w/ phenol 0.45%. Vial 10 ml. Box 10s. **1:2000:** 0.5 mg/ml. Amp. 1 ml w/methyl and propylparabens 0.2%. Box 10s. Vial 10 ml w/phenol 0.45%. Box 10s. **1:4000:** 0.25 mg/ml Amp. 1 ml w/methyl and propylparabens 0.2%. Box 10s. *Rx.*
Use: Muscle stimulant.

Prostigmin Bromide Tablets. (Zeneca) Neostigmine bromide 15 mg/Tab. Bot. 100s, 1000s. *Rx.*
Use: Muscle stimulant.

Prostin E2. (Pharmacia & Upjohn) Dinoprost 20 mg. Supp. Containers of 1 each. *Rx.*
Use: Abortifacient.

Prostin VR Pediatric. (Pharmacia & Upjohn) Alprostadil 500 mcg/ml. Amp. 1 ml. *Rx.*
Use: Arterial patency agent.

Prostonic. (Seatrace) Thiamine HCl 10 mg, alanine 130 mg, glutamic acid 130 mg, amino-acetic acid 130 mg/Cap. Bot. 100s. *Rx.*
Use: Palliative relief of benign prostatic hypertrophy

Protabolin. (Taylor Pharmaceuticals) Methandriol dipropionate 50 mg/ml. Vial 10 ml. *Rx.*
Use: Hormone.

•**protamine sulfate.** (PRO-tuh-meen) U.S.P. 23.
Use: Antidote, heparin.

protamine sulfate. (Eli Lilly) Amp. 1%, 5 ml; 1s, 25s; 25 ml 6s.
Use: Antidote, heparin.

protargin mild.
See: Silver Protein, Mild (Various Mfr.).

Protargol. (Sterwin) Strong silver protein. Pow. Bot. 25 g. *Rx.*
Use: Antiseptic.

protease.
W/Pancreatin, amylase.
See: Dizymes, Cap. (Recsei).
W/Vitamins B_1, B_{12}.
See: Arcoret, Tab. (Arco).
W/Vitamins B_1, B_{12}, iron.
See: Arcoret W/Iron, Tab. (Arco).

Protectol Medicated Powder. (Jones Medical Industries) Calcium undecylenate 15%. Bot. 2 oz. *otc.*
Use: Diaper rash preparation.

Protegra Softgels. (ESI Lederle Generics) Vitamins E 200 IU, C 250 mg, beta carotene 3 mg, zinc 7.5 mg, copper, selenium, manganese. Cap. Bot. 50s. *otc.*
Use: Vitamin supplement.

proteinase inhibitor, alpha 1.
See: Prolastin (Bayer Corp).

protein c concentrate.
Use: Protein C deficiency. [Orphan drug]

•**protein hydrolysate injection.** U.S.P. 23.
Use: Fluid, nutrient replacement.
See: Amigen, Inj. (Baxter Lab.).
Aminogen, Amp., Vial (Christina).
Lacotein, Vial (Christina).

protein hydrolysates oral.

Use: Enteral nutritional supplement.
See: Lofenalac, Pow. (Bristol-Myers).
Nutramigen, Pow. (Bristol-Myers).
Pregestimil, Pow. (Bristol-Myers).
Stuart Amino Acids, Pow. (Zeneca).
W/Vitamin B_{12}.
See: Stuart Amino Acids and B_{12}, Tab. (Zeneca).

Protenate. (Baxter) Plasma protein fraction (Human) 5%. Inj. Vial 250 ml, 500 ml w/administration set. *Rx.*
Use: Plasma protein fraction.

proteolytic enzymes.
See: Papase, Tab. (Parke-Davis).
W/Amylolytic enzyme, cellulolytic enzyme, lipolytic enzyme.
See: Arco-Lase, Tab. (Arco).
Kutrase, Cap. (Kremers Urban).
Kuzyme, Cap. (Kremers Urban).
Zymme, Cap. (Scrip). W/Amylolytic enzyme, lipolytic enzyme, cellulolytic enzyme, belladonna extract.
See: Mallenzyme, Tab. (Roberts Pharm).
W/Amylolytic, cellulolytic enzymes, lipase, phenobarbital, hyoscyamine sulfate, atropine sulfate.
See: Arco-Lipase Plus, Tab. (Arco).
W/Amylolytic enzyme, homatropine methylbromide, d-sorbitol. (Papain).
See: Converzyme, Liq. (B.F. Ascher).
W/Calcium carbonate, glycine, amylolytic and cellulolytic enzymes.
See: Co-Gel, Tab. (Arco).
W/Neomycin palmitrate, hydrocortisone acetate, water-miscible base.
See: Biozyme, Oint. (Centeon).

Prothers. (ICN Pharmaceuticals) Soap Free. White petrolatum, disodium cocamido MIPA-sulfosuccinate, pentane, ammonium laureth sulfate, PEG-150 distearate, hydroxypropyl methylcellulose, imidazolidinyl urea, parabens, propylene glycol stearate, hydrogenated soy glyceride, sodium stearyl lactylate. Liq. Bot. 180 ml. *otc.*
Use: Dermatologic, cleanser.

prothipendyl hydrochloride.
Use: Sedative.

Proticuleen. (Spanner) Vitamin B_{12} activity 10 mcg, folic acid 10 mg, B_{12} crystalline 50 mcg, niacinamide 75 mg/ml. Multiple dose vial 10 ml. I.M. inj. *Rx.*
Use: Nutritional supplement, parenteral.

•**protirelin.** (PRO-tie-reh-lin) USAN. *Formerly Lopremone.*
Use: Prothyrotropin.
See: Thypinone, Inj. (Abbott Laboratories).

protirelin. (UCB Pharmaceuticals)
Use: Diagnostic aid, thyroid. [Orphan drug]

Protopam Chloride. (Wyeth Ayerst) **Hospital package:** Six 20 ml vials of 1 g each of sterile Protopam Cl powder, without diluent or syringe. *Rx.*
Use: Antidote.

Protosan. (Recsei) Protein 87.5%, lactose 0.5%, fat 1.3%, ash 3.5%, sodium 0.02%. Jar 1 lb, 5 lb. *otc.*
Use: Nutritional supplement.

Prot-O-Sea. (Barth's) Protein 90%, containing amino acids and minerals. Bot. 100s, 500s. *otc.*
Use: Nutritional supplement.

Protostat. (Ortho McNeil) Metronidazole 250 mg or 500 mg/Tab. **250 mg:** Bot. 100s. **500 mg:** Bot. 50s. *Rx.*
Use: Anti-infective.

protoveratrine A.
See: Pro-Amid, Tab. (Amide Pharmaceuticals).

protoveratrines a & b maleate.

Protran Plus. (Vangard) Meprobamate 150 mg, ethoheptazine citrate 75 mg, aspirin 250 mg/ Tab. Bot. 100s. 500s. *Rx.*
Use: Analgesic, anxiolytic combination.

•**protriptyline hydrochloride.** (pro-TRIP-tih-leen) U.S.P. 23.
Use: Antidepressant.
See: Vivactil, Tab. (Merck).

Protropin. (Genentech) Somatrem. Vial 5 mg (13 IU), 10 mg (26 IU). Contains 2 vials somatrem and 2 10 ml vials diluent. *Rx.*
Use: Hormone, growth.

Protuss. (Horizon) Hydrocodone bitartrate 5 mg, potassium guaiacolsulfonate 300 mg/5 ml, saccharin, sorbitol. Alcohol free. Liq. Bot. 20 ml, 120 ml, 480 ml. *c-III.*
Use: Antitussive, expectorant.

Protuss-D. (Horizon) Hydrocodone bitartrate 5 mg, pseudoephedrine HCl 30 mg, potassium guaiacolsulfonate 300 mg/5 ml. Alcohol free, dye free. Liq. Bot. 120 ml, 480 ml. *c-III.*
Use: Antitussive, decongestant, expectorant.

Protuss DM. (Horizon) Guaifenesin 600 mg, pseudoephedrine HCl 60 mg, dextromethorphan HBr 30 mg. Tab. Bot. 14s, 100s. *Rx.*
Use: Antitussive, decongestant, expectorant.

Proval #3. (Horizon) Guafenesin 600 mg, pseudoephedrine HCl 60 mg, dextromethorphan HBr 30 mg. Tab. Bot. 14s, 100s. *Rx.*

Use: Antitussive, decongestant, expectorant. (Solvay) Acetaminophen 325 mg, codeine phosphate 30 mg/Tab. Bot. 100s, 500s. *c-III.*
Use: Analgesic combination, narcotic.

Proventil. (Schering Plough) Albuterol sulfate 2 mg or 4 mg/Tab. Bot. 100s, 500s. *Rx.*
Use: Bronchodilator.

Proventil HFA. (Key Pharm) Albuterol 90 mcg per actuation/Aerosol. Can. 6.7 g/200 inhalations). *Rx.*
Use: Bronchodilator.

Proventil Inhaler. (Schering Plough) Metered dose aerosol unit containing albuterol in propellants. Each actuation delivers 90 mcg of albuterol. Canister 17 g with oral adapter. Box 1s. *Rx.*
Use: Bronchodilator.

Proventil Repetabs. (Schering Plough) Albuterol 4 mg, lactose/Tab. Bot. 100s, 500s. *Rx.*
Use: Bronchodilator.

Proventil Solution. (Schering Plough) Albuterol sulfate solution. **0.5%:** Albuterol sulfate 6 mg/ml. Bot. 20 ml. Box 1s. **0.083%:** Albuterol sulfate 0.83 mg/ml. Bot. 3 ml. Box 100s. *Rx.*
Use: Bronchodilator.

Proventil Syrup. (Schering Plough) Albuterol sulfate 2 mg/5 ml. Bot. 16 oz. *Rx.*
Use: Bronchodilator.

Provera. (Pharmacia & Upjohn) Medroxyprogesterone acetate 2.5 mg, 5 mg or 10 mg/Tab. Bot. 30s, 100s; 500s, UD 10s (10 mg only). *Rx.*
Use: Hormone, progestin.

Provocholine. (Roche Laboratories) Methacholine Cl for inhalation 100 mg/5 ml for reconstitution. Vial 5 ml. *Rx.*
Use: Diagnostic aid.

Prox/APAP. (Forest Pharmaceutical) Propoxyphene HCl 65 mg, acetaminophen 650 mg/Tab. Bot. 100s, 500s. *c-IV.*
Use: Analgesic combination, narcotic.

•**proxazole.** (PROX-ah-zole) USAN.
Use: Analgesic, anti-inflammatory, muscle relaxant.

•**proxazole citrate.** (PROX-ah-zole) USAN.
Use: Relaxant (smooth muscle), analgesic, anti-inflammatory.

•**proxicromil.** (prox-ih-KROE-mill) USAN.
Use: Antiallergic.

Proxigel. (Schwarz Pharma) Carbamide peroxide 10% in a water free gel base. Tube 34 g w/applicator. *otc.*
Use: Antiseptic, cleanser.

•**proxorphan tartrate.** (PROX-ahr-fan TAR-trate) USAN.
Use: Analgesic; antitussive.

Proxy 65. (Parmed) Propoxyphene HCl 65 mg, acetaminophen 650 mg/Tab. Bot. 100s, 500s. *c-IV.*
Use: Narcotic analgesic combination.

Prozac. (Eli Lilly) Fluoxetine HCl **Pulvules:** 10 mg or 20 mg Bot. 100s. **Liq.:** 20 mg/5 ml Bot. 120 ml. *Rx.*
Use: Antidepressant.

Prudents. (Bariatric) Acetylphenylisatin 5 mg/Tab. Bot. 30s, 100s. Chewable protein and amino acid. *otc.*
Use: Laxative.

Prulet. (Mission Pharmacal) White phenolphthalein 60 mg/Tab. Strips 12s, 40s. *otc.*
Use: Laxative.

prune concentrate. W/cascarin.

prune powder concentrated dehydrated.
See: Diacetyldihydroxyphenylisatin.
W/Cascara fluidextract aromatic and psyllium husk powder.
See: Casyllium, Pow. (Pharmacia & Upjohn).

Prurilo. (Whorton) Menthol 0.25%, phenol 0.25%, calamine lotion in special lubricating base. Bot. 4 oz, 8 oz. *otc.*
Use: Dermatologic, counter irritant.

Pseudo-Car DM. (Geneva Pharm) Pseudoephedrine HCl 60 mg, carbinoxamine maleate 4 mg, dextromethorphan HBr 15 mg/5 ml, alcohol < 0.6%. Bot. pt, gal. *Rx.*
Use: Antihistamine, antitussive, decongestant.

Pseudo-Chlor. (Various Mfr.) Pseudoephedrine HCl 120 mg, chlorpheniramine maleate 8 mg/Cap. Bot. 100s, 250s. *Rx.*
Use: Antihistamine, decongestant.

•**pseudoephedrine hydrochloride.** (SUE-doe-eh-FED-rin) U.S.P. 23.
Use: Adrenergic (vasoconstrictor).
See: Allerest No Drowsiness, Tab. (Novartis).
Anatuss DM, Syr. (Mayrand).
Aspirin-Free Cayer Select Head & Chest Cold, Capl. (Bayer).
Benylin Multi-Symptom, Liq. (Glaxo-Wellcome).
Bromfenax, ER Cap. (Ethex).
Cenafed, Tab., Syr. (Century Pharm).
Children's Silfedrine, Liq. (Silarx).
Claritin, Prods. (Schering Plough).
Coldrine, Tab. (Roberts).
Cycofed Pediatric, Syr. (Cypress).
D-Feda, Cap., Syr. (Dooner).
Dynafed Pseudo, Tab. (Novartis).
Efidac 124, Tab. (Novartis).

Iofed, ER Cap. (Iomed).
Mini-Thin Pseudo, Tab. (BDI).
Pseudo, Tab. (Novartis).
Novafed, Cap., Liq. (Hoechst Marion Roussel).
Ornex No Drowsiness, Tab. (Menley & James).
Sinufed, Cap. (Roberts Pharm).
Sinus-Relief, Tab. (Major).
Sudafed, Tab., Syr. (GlaxoWellcome).
Sudafed S.A., Cap. (Glaxo-Wellcome).
Sudal, Prods. (Alley Pharm).
Triaminic AM Decongestant Formula, Syr. (Novartis).
Ursinus, Inlay Tab. (Novartis).

pseudoephedrine hydrochloride w/ combinations.

See: Actifed, Tab., Syr. (Glaxo-Wellcome).
Actifed Allergy, Cap. (Glaxo-Wellcome).
Ambenyl-D, Liq. (Hoechst Marion Roussel).
Anatuss DM, Syr., Tab. (Merz).
Aspirin-Free Bayer Select Head & Chest Cold, Capl. (Bayer).
Atridine, Tab. (Henry Schein).
Banophen, Cap. (Major).
Benylin Multi-Symptom, Liq. (Glaxo-Wellcome).
Brexin, Cap., Liq. (Savage).
Bromadine-DM, Syr. (Cypress).
Bromfenex PD, ER Cap. (Ethex).
Carbinoxamine, Prods. (Morton Grove).
Congestac, Tab. (SmithKline Beecham Pharmaceuticals).
CoTylenol, Tab. (Ortho McNeil).
CoTylenol Liquid Cold Formula (Ortho McNeil).
Cycofed Pediatric, Syr. (Cypress).
Deconamine, Cap., Tab., Elix., Syr. (Berlex).
Deconsal Pediatric, Syr. (Adams).
Defen-LA, SR Tab. (Horizon).
Dimacol, Cap., Liq. (Robins).
Dorcol, Prods. (Novartis).
Drixomed, SR Tab. (Iomed).
Fedahist Expectorant (Schwarz Pharma).
Fedrazil, Tab. (GlaxoWellcome).
Guaifenesin DAC, Liq. (Cypress).
Guaifenex PSE 60, ER Tab (Ethex).
Guaifenex PSE 120, ER Tab. (Ethex).
Guaifenex Rx DM, Tab. (Ethex).
Guiatex PSE, Tab. (Rugby).
Guaivent, Cap. (Ethex).
Guaivent PD, Cap. (Ethex).
Guai-Vent/PSE, SR Tab. (Dura).
Histinex PV, Syr. (Ethex).
Histussin D, Liq. (Bock).
H-Tuss-D, Liq. (Cypress).
Iosal II, ER Tab. (Iomed).
Isoclor, Preps. (DuPont Merck Pharmaceuticals).
Kronofed-A, Cap. (Ferndale Laboratories).
Mapap Cold Formula, Tab. (Major).
Maximum Strength Tylenol Flu, Tab. (McNeil Consumer Products).
MED-Rx, CR. Tab. (Iomed).
Multi-Symptom Tylenol Cough with Decongestant, Liq. (Ortho McNeil).
Nasabid, PA Cap. (Jones Medical).
Nasabid SR, LA Tab. (Jones Medical).
Nasatab LA, LA Tab. (ECR Pharmaceuticals).
Novafed A, Liq., Cap. (Hoechst Marion Roussel).
Novahistine Sinus, Tab. (Hoechst Marion Roussel).
Pancof-HC, Liq. (Pan-Am Labs).
Panmist JR, LA Tab. (Pan Am Labs).
Phenergan-D, Tab. (Wyeth Ayerst).
Protuss-D, Liq. (Horizon). Protuss DM, Tab. (Horizon).
Respa-1st, SR Tab. (Respa).
Robitussin Cold & Cough, Cap. (Robins).
Robitussin-DAC, Liq. (Robins).
Robitussin-PE, Liq. (Robins).
Robitussin Severe Congestion, Cap. (Robins).
Rondec D, Drops; C, Tab.; S, Syr.; T, Filmtab (Ross Laboratories).
Rondec DM, Drops, Syr. (Ross Laboratories).
Sine-Aid IB, Cap. (McNeil Consumer Products).
Sine-Off, Prods. (SmithKline Beecham Pharmaceuticals).
Sinutab Non-Drying, Cap., Liq. (GlaxoWellcome).
Sudafed Plus, Tab., Syr. (Glaxo-Wellcome).
Sudal, Prods. (Atley Pharm).
Syn-Rx, CR Tab. (Adams).
Touro LA, LA Capl. (Dartmouth).
Triaminic AM Cough & Decongestant Formula, Liq. (Novartis).
Triphed, Tab. (Teva USA).
Tussafed Expectorant Liq. (Cavital).
Tussend, Syr. (Monarch).
Tylenol Cold Night Time, Liq. (McNeil Consumer Products).
Tyrodone, Liq. (Major).
Vicks 44D Cough & Head Congestion, Liq. (Procter & Gamble).
Vicks NyQuil Multi-Symptom Cold Flu Relief, Liq. (Procter & Gamble).

pseudoephedrine hydrochloride and triprolidine hydrochloride. (Various Mfr.) Pseudoephedrine HCl 60 mg, triprolidine HCl 2.5 mg/Tab. Bot. 100s, 1000s, UD 100s. *Rx.*
Use: Antihistamine, decongestant.

•**pseudoephedrine polistirex.** (sue-doe-ee-FED-rin pahl-ee-STIE-rex) USAN.
Use: Decongestant, nasal.

•**pseudoephedrine sulfate.** (sue-do-eh-FED-rin) U.S.P. 23.
Use: Bronchodilator.
See: Afrinol Repetabs (Schering Plough).
W/Chlorpheniramine maleate.
See: Chlor-trimeton Decongestant, Tab. (Schering Plough).
W/Dexbrompheniramine.
See: Disophrol Chronotabs, Tab. (Schering Plough).
Drixoral S.A., Tab. (Schering Plough).
W/Dexchlorpheniramine.
See: Polaramine Expectorant (Schering Plough).

Pseudo-Gest. (Major) Pseudoephedrine HCl 30 mg or 60 mg/Tab. Bot. 24s, 100s. *otc.*
Use: Decongestant.

Pseudo-Gest Plus. (Major) Pseudoephedrine HCl 60 mg, chlorpheniramine maleate 4 mg/Tab. In 24s, 100s, 200s. *otc. [use]Use:, Antihistamine, decongestant.*

Pseudo-Hist. (Holloway) Pseudoephedrine HCl 30 mg, chlorpheniramine maleate 10 mg/Cap. Bot. 100s. *otc.*
Use: Antihistamine, decongestant.

Pseudo-Hist Expectorant. (Holloway) Pseudoephedrine 15 mg, hydrocodone bitartrate 2.5 mg, guaifenesin 100 mg, alcohol 5%. Bot. 480 ml. *c-III.*
Use: Antitussive, decongestant, expectorant.

pseudomonas hyperimmune globulin (mucoid exopolysaccharide).
Use: Pulmonary infection in cystic fibrosis. [Orphan drug]

pseudomonas test.
Use: Urine test.
See: Isocult for *Pseudomonas aeruginosa* (SmithKline Diagnostics).

pseudomonic acid A.
Use: Anti-infective, topical.
See: Bactroban (SmithKline Beecham Pharmaceuticals).

Pseudo-Phedrine. (Whiteworth Towne) Pseudoephedrine HCl 30 mg/Tab. Bot. 100s, 1000s. *otc.*
Use: Decongestant.

Pseudo Plus. (Weeks & Leo) Pseudoephedrine HCl 60 mg, chlorpheniramine maleate 4 mg/Tab. Bot. 40s. *otc.*
Use: Antihistamine, decongestant.

Pseudo Syrup. (Major) Pseudoephedrine 30 mg/5 ml. Liq. Bot. 120 ml, pt, gal. *otc.*
Use: Decongestant.

psoralens.
See: Methoxsalen.
Trioxsalen.

Psor-a-set. (Hogil Pharm) Salicylic acid 2%. Soap. Bar 97.5 g. *otc.*
Use: Keratolytic.

Psorcon. (Dermik Laboratories) Diflorasone diacetate (0.05%) 0.5 mg/g. **Oint.:** Tube 15 g, 30 g, 60 g. **Cream:** Tube 15 g, 30 g, 60 g. *Rx.*
Use: Corticosteroid, topical.

PsoriGel. (Galderma) Coal tar soln. 7.5%, alcohol 33% in hydroalcoholic gel vehicle. Tube 4 oz. *otc.*
Use: Dermatologic.

Psorinail. (Summers) Coal tar solution w/ isopropyl alcohol 2.5%, 3-butylene glycol I, acetyl mandelic acid. Liq. Bot. 30 ml. *otc.*
Use: Antipsoriatic, topical.

Psorion Cream. (ICN Pharmaceuticals) Betamethasone dipropionate 0.05%, mineral oil, white petrolatum, propylene glycol. Cream. Tube 15 g, 45 g. *Rx.*
Use: Corticosteroid, topical.

psychotherapeutic agents.
See: Ataraxic Agents.
Tranquilizers.

psyllium granules.
Use: Laxative.
See: Perdiem Fiber, Gran. (Rhone-Poulenc Rorer).
W/Dextrose.
See: Muci-lax, Granules (Shionogi).
W/Senna.
See: Perdiem, Granules (Rhone-Poulenc Rorer).

•**psyllium husk.** (SILL-ee-uhm husk) U.S.P. 23.
Use: Laxative.
W/Cascara fluidextract aromatic, prune powder.
Use: Cathartic.
See: Casyllium, Pow. (Pharmacia & Upjohn).

psyllium hydrocolloid.
Use: Laxative.
See: Effersyllium, Pow. (Zeneca).

psyllium hydrophilic mucilloid for oral suspension.
Use: Laxative.

See: Konsyl, Pow. (Lafayette Pharm).
Modane Versabran, Pow. (Pharmacia & Upjohn).
Mucillium, Pow. (Whiteworth Towne).
Mylanta Natural Fiber Supplement, Pow. (J & J Merck Consumer Pharm).
Restore (Inagra).
W/Dextrose.
See: Hydrocil Plain (Solvay).
Konsyl-D Pow. (Lafayette Pharm).
V-lax, Pow. (Century Pharm).
W/Dextrose, casanthranol.
See: Hydrocil Fortified (Solvay).
W/Oxyphenisatin acetate.
See: Plova, Pow. (WEL).
W/Standardized senna concentrate.
See: Senokot w/Psyllium, Pow. (Purdue Frederick).

psyllium seed gel.
Use: Laxative.
W/Planta Ovata, gum Karaya, Brewer's yeast.
See: Plantamucin, Granules (ICN Pharmaceuticals).

PTE-4. (Fujisawa) Zinc 1 mg, copper 0.1 mg, chromium 1 mcg, manganese 25 mcg/ml. Vial 3 ml. *Rx.*
Use: Mineral supplement.

PTE-5. (Fujisawa) Zinc 1 mg, copper 0.1 mg, chromium 1 mcg, manganese 25 mcg, selenium 15 mcg/ml. Vial 3 ml, 10 ml. *Rx.*
Use: Mineral supplement.

pteroic acid. The compound formed by the linkage of carbon 6 of 2-amine-4-hydroxypteridine by means of a methylene group with the nitrogen of p-aminobenzoic acid.

pteroylglutamic acid.
See: Folic Acid, Preps. (Various Mfr.).

pteroylmonoglutamic acid. Pteroylglutamic acid.
See: Folic Acid, Preps. (Various Mfr.).

PTFE. (Ethicon) Polytef.

PTU.
See: Propylthiouracil.

Pulmicort Turbuhaler. (Astra) Budesonide ≈ 160 mg per metered dose. Dry Pow. for Inh. 200 doses per device. *Rx.*
Use: Respiratory inhalant.

Pulmocare. (Ross Laboratories) High-fat, low-carbohydrate liquid diet for pulmonary patients containing 1500 calories/Liter; 1420 calories provides 100% U.S. RDA vitamins and minerals. Calorie:Nitrogen ratio is 150:1. Osmolarity: 490 mosm/Kg water. Can 8 fl oz. *otc.*
Use: Nutritional supplement.

pulmonary surfactant replacement. (Scios Nova)
Use: Diagnostic aid, thyroid. [Orphan drug]

pulmonary surfactant replacement, porcine.
Use: Diagnostic aid, thyroid. [Orphan drug]
See: Curosurf.

Pulmosin. (Spanner) Guaiacol 0.1 g, eucalyptol 0.08 g, camphor 0.05 g, iodoform 0.02 g/2 ml. Multiple dose vial 30 ml. Inj. I.M. *Rx.*

Pulmozyme. (Genentech) Dornase alfa 1 mg, calcium chloride dihydrate 0.15 mg, NaCl 8.77 mg/ml. Soln. for inhalation. Amps. Single-use 2.5 ml. *Rx.*
Use: Anti-infective.

•**pumice.** (PUM-iss) U.S.P. 23.
Use: Abrasive (dental).

punctum plug. (Eagle Vision) Silicone plug. 0.5 mm, 0.6 mm, 0.7 mm or 0.8 mm. Pkg. 2 plugs, one inserter tool. *Rx.*
Use: Punctal plug.

Pura. (D'Franssia) High potency vitamin E cream.
Use: Emollient.

Puralube. (E. Fougera) White petrolatum, light mineral oil. Oint. Tube 3.5 g. *otc.*
Use: Lubricant, ophthalmic.

Puralube Tears. (E. Fougera) Polyvinyl alcohol 1%, polyethylene glycol 400 1%, EDTA, benzalkonium Cl. Drops. Bot. 15 ml. *otc.*
Use: Lubricant, ophthalmic.

Purebrom Compound Elixir. (Purepac) Brompheniramine maleate 4 mg/5 ml, phenylephrine HCl, phenylpropanolamine HCl, alcohol. Bot. pt, gal. *Rx.*
Use: Antihistamine, decongestant.

Puresept Murine Saline. (Ross Laboratories) **Disinfecting soln.:** Sterile hydrogen peroxide solution 3%, sodium stannate, sodium nitrate, phosphate buffers, thimerosal free. 237 ml. **Murine Saline Soln.:** Buffered isotonic solution w/borate buffers, NaCl, sorbic acid 0.1%, EDTA 0.1%. 60, 237, 355 ml. Includes cups and lens holder. *otc.*
Use: Contact lens care.

Purge Evacuant. (Fleming) Castor oil 95%. Bot. 1 oz, 2 oz. *otc.*
Use: Laxative.

Puri-Clens. (Sween) UD 2 oz. Bot. 8 oz.
Use: Dermatologic, wound therapy.

purified oxgall.
See: Bile Extract, Ox (Various Mfr.).

purified protein derivative of tuber-

culin.
Use: Mantoux TB test.
See: Aplisol, Vial (Parke-Davis).
Aplitest, Jar (Parke-Davis).
Tubersol, Vial (Pasteur Merieux Connaught).

purified type II collagen.
Use: Juvenile rheumatoid arthritis. [Orphan drug]

Purinethol. (GlaxoWellcome) Mercaptopurine 50 mg/Tab. Bot. 25s, 250s. *Rx.*
Use: Antineoplastic.

•**puromycin.** (PURE-oh-MY-sin) USAN.
Use: Antineoplastic; antiprotozoal (trypanosoma).

•**puromycin hydrochloride.** (PURE-oh-MY-sin) USAN.
Use: Antineoplastic; antiprotozoal (trypanosoma).

purple foxglove.
See: Digitalis, Preps. (Various Mfr.).

Purpose Shampoo. (Advanced Care Products) Water, amphoteric-19, PEG-44 sorbitan laurate, PEG-150 distearate, sorbitan laurate, boric acid, fragrance, benzyl alcohol. Bot. 8 oz. *otc.*
Use: Dermatologic.

Purpose Soap. (Johnson & Johnson Consumer Products) Sodium tallowate, sodium cocoate, glycerin, NaCl, BHT, EDTA. Bar 108 g, 180 g. *otc.*
Use: Dermatologic, cleanser.

Pursettes Premenstrual Tablets. (DEP) Acetaminophen 500 mg, pamabrom 25 mg, pyrilamine maleate 15 mg/Tab. Bot. 24s. *otc.*
Use: Analgesic, antihistamine, diuretic.

P.V. Carpine Liquifilm. (Allergan) Pilocarpine nitrate 1%, 2% or 4%, polyvinyl alcohol 1.4%, sodium acetate, sodium Cl, citric acid, menthol, camphor, phenol, eucalyptol, chlorobutanol 0.5%, purified water. Dropper bot. 15 ml. *Rx.*
Use: Antiglaucoma agent.

PVP-I Ointment. (Day-Baldwin) Povidone-iodine. Tube 1 oz, Jar lb, Foilpac 1.5 g. *otc.*
Use: Antiseborrheic, antiseptic.

P-V-Tussin. (Solvay) Hydrocodone bitartrate 2.5 mg, pseudoephedrine HCl 30 mg, chlorpheniramine maleate 2 mg, alcohol 5%. Syrup. Bot. pt, gal. *c-III.*
Use: Antihistamine, antitussive, decongestant.

P-V-Tussin Tablets. (Solvay) Hydrocodone bitartrate 5 mg, phenindamine tartrate 25 mg, guaifenesin 200 mg/Tab. Bot. 100s. *c-III.*
Use: Antihistamine, antitussive, expectorant.

Py-Co-Pay Tooth Powder. (Block Drug) Sodium Cl, sodium bicarbonate, calcium carbonate, magnesium carbonate, tricalcium phosphate, eugenol, methyl salicylate. Can 7 oz. *otc.*
Use: Dentifrice.

9-[3-pydidylmethyl]-9-deazaguanine. (Briocryst Pharm)
Use: Antineoplastic. [Orphan drug]

Pyma. (Forest Pharmaceutical) **TR Cap.:** Pyrilamine maleate 50 mg, chlorpheniramine maleate 6 mg, pheniramine maleate 20 mg, phenylephrine HCl 15 mg. Bot. 30s, 100s, 1000s. **Inj.:** Chlorpheniramine maleate 5 mg, phenylpropanolamine HCl 12.5 mg, atropine sulfate 0.2 mg/ml. Vial 10 ml. *Rx.*
Use: Anticholinergic, antihistamine, antispasmodic, decongestant.

Pyocidin-Otic Solution. (Forest Pharmaceutical) Hydrocortisone 5 mg, polymyxin B sulfate 10,000 USP units/ml in a vehicle containing water and propylene glycol. Bot. 10 ml w/sterile dropper. *Rx.*
Use: Anti-infective, corticosteroid, otic.

•**pyrabrom.** (PEER-ah-brahm) USAN.
Use: Antihistamine.

Pyracol. (Davis & Sly) Pyrathyn HCl 0.08 g, ammonium Cl 0.778 g, citric acid 0.52 g, menthol 0.006 g/fl oz. Bot. pt.

pyradone.
See: Aminopyrine (Various Mfr.).

pyraminyl.
See: Pyrilamine Maleate (Various Mfr.).

pyranilamine maleate.
See: Pyrilamine Maleate, Preps. (Various Mfr.).

pyranisamine bromotheophyllinate.
See: Pyrabrom (Various Mfr.).

pyranisamine maleate.
See: Pyrilamine Maleate, Preps. (Various Mfr.).

•**pyrantel pamoate.** (pie-RAN-tell PAM-oh-ate) U.S.P. 23.
Use: Anthelmintic.
See: Antiminth, Oral Susp. (Pfizer).
Pin Rid, Cap., Liq. (Apothecary Products).
Pin-X, Liq. (Effcon).

•**pyrantel tartrate.** (pie-RAN-tell) USAN.
Use: Anthelmintic.

pyrathiazine hydrochloride.

•**pyrazinamide.** (peer-uh-ZIN-uh-mide) U.S.P. 23. Aldinamide, Zinamide.
Use: Anti-infective, tuberculostatic.

pyrazinamide. (ESI Lederle Generics) 500 mg/Tab. Bot. 500s.
Use: Anti-infective, tuberculostatic.

pyrazinecarboxamide. Pyrazinamide, U.S.P. 23.

•**pyrazofurin.** (pihr-AZZ-oh-FYOO-rin) USAN.
Use: Antineoplastic.

pyrazoline.
See: Antipyrine (Various Mfr.).

pyrbenzindole.
See: Benzindopyrine Hydrochloride (Various Mfr.).

•**pyrethrum extract.** U.S.P. 23.
Use: Pediculicide.

pyribenzamine.
See: PBZ, Prods. (Novartis).

pyricardyl.
See: Nikethamide, Inj. (Various Mfr.).

Pyridamole Tabs. (Major) Dipyridamole 25 mg, 50 mg or 75 mg/Tab. **25 mg:** Bot. 1000s, 2500s; **50 mg or 75 mg:** 100s, 1000s. *Rx.*
Use: Antianginal, antiplatelet.

Pyridate Tabs. (Major) Phenazopyridine 100 mg or 200 mg/Tab. Bot. 1000s. *Rx.*
Use: Analgesic, anti-infective, urinary.

Pyridene. (Health for Life Brands) Phenylazo Diamino Pyridine HCl 100 mg/Tab. Bot. 24s, 100s, 1000s. *Rx.*
Use: Analgesic, urinary.

pyridine-beta-carboxylic acid diethyl amide.
See: Nikethamide, Inj. (Various Mfr.).

Pyridium. (Warner Chilcott) Phenazopyridine HCl 100 mg or 200 mg/Tab. Bot. 100s, 1000s, UD 100s. *Rx.*
Use: Analgesic, anti-infective, urinary.
W/Hyoscyamine HBr, butabarbital.
See: Pyridium Plus, Tab. (Parke-Davis).

•**pyridostigmine bromide.** (pihr-id-oh-STIG-meen BROE-mide) U.S.P. 23.
Use: Cholinergic.
See: Mestinon, Tab., Syr., Amp. (Roche Laboratories).
Regonol (Organon Teknika).

Pyridox. (Oxford) **No. 1:** Pyridoxine HCl 100 mg/Tab. *otc.* **No. 2:** Pyridoxine HCl 200 mg/Tab. Bot. 100s. *otc.*
Use: Vitamin supplement.

pyridoxal. Vitamin B_6. *otc.*
Use: Vitamin supplement.

pyridoxamine. Vitamin B_6. *otc.*
Use: Vitamin supplement.
See: Pyridoxine.

•**pyridoxine hydrochloride.** (peer-ih-DOX-een) U.S.P. 23.
Use: Enzyme co-factor vitamin.
See: Hexa Betalin, Amp., Tab., Vial (Eli Lilly).
Hexavibex, Vial (Parke-Davis).
Pan B_6, Tab. (Panray).

pyridoxol.
See: Pyridoxine, Vitamin B_6.

pyrilamine bromotheophyllinate.
See: Pyrabrom.
W/2-amino-2-methyl-1-propanol.
See: Bromaleate.

•**pyrimethamine.** (pihr-ih-METH-ah-meen) U.S.P. 23.
Use: Antimalarial.
See: Daraprim, Tab. (GlaxoWellcome).
W/Sulfadoxine.
See: Fansidar, Tab. (Roche Laboratories).

Pyrinex Pediculicide. (Ambix Laboratories) Pyrethrins 0.2%, piperonyl butoxide technical 2%, deodorized kerosene 0.8%. Shampoo. Bot. 118 ml. *otc.*
Use: Pediculicide.

•**pyrinoline.** (PIHR-ih-NO-leen) USAN.
Use: Cardiovascular agent, antiarrhythmic.

pyrinyl. (Various Mfr.) Pyrethrins 0.2%, piperonyl butoxide technical 2%, deodorized kerosene 0.8%. Liq. Bot. 60, 120 ml. *otc.*
Use: Pediculicide.

Pyristan. (Arcum) Phenylephrine HCl 8 mg, phenylpropanolamine HCl 15 mg, chlorpheniramine maleate 3 mg, pyrilamine maleate 10 mg/Cap. Bot. 50s, 500s. Elix. Bot. 4 oz, pt, gal. *otc.*
Use: Antihistamine, decongestant.

pyrithen.
See: Chlorothen Citrate (Various Mfr.).

•**pyrithione sodium.** (PEER-ih-THIGH-ohn) USAN.
Use: Antimicrobial, topical.

•**pyrithione zinc.** (PEER-ih-THIGH-ohn zingk) USAN. Zinc Omadine.
Use: Antifungal, anti-infective, antiseborrheic.
See: Zincon Shampoo (ESI Lederle Generics).

Pyrogallic Acid Ointment. (Gordon Laboratories) Pyrogallic acid 25%, chlorobutanol. Jar 1 oz, 1 lb.
Use: Dermatologic, wart therapy.

pyrogallol. Pyrogallic acid.

Pyrohep Tabs. (Major) Cyproheptadine HCl 4 mg/Tab. Bot. 250s, 500s. *Rx.*
Use: Antihistamine.

pyrophenindane. (Bristol-Myers).

•**pyrovalerone hydrochloride.** (PIE-row-val-EH-rone) USAN.
Use: Central stimulant.

•**pyroxamine maleate.** (pihr-OX-ah-meen) USAN.
Use: Antihistamine.

•**pyroxylin.** (pihr-OX-ih-lin) U.S.P. 23. Soluble guncotton. Cellulose nitrate.
Use: Pharmaceutic necessity for Collodion.

pyrrobutamine phosphate. U.S.P. XXI.
Use: Antihistamine.
W/Clopane HCl, Histadyl.
See: Co-Pyronil, Preps. (Eli Lilly).

•**pyrrocaine.** (PIHR-oh-cane) USAN.
Use: Anesthetic, local.

pyrrocaine hydrochloride.
Use: Anesthetic, local.

pyrrocaine hydrochloride and epinephrine inj.
Use: Anesthetic, local.

•**pyrroliphene hydrochloride.** (pihr-OLE-ih-feen) USAN.
Use: Analgesic.

•**pyrrolnitrin.** (pihr-OLE-nye-trin) USAN. Under study.
Use: Antifungal.

Pyrroxate. (Roberts Pharm) Chlorpheniramine maleate 4 mg, phenylpropanolamine HCl 25 mg, acetaminophen 650 mg/Cap. Blister pkg. 24s. Bot. 500s. *otc.*
Use: Analgesic, antihistamine, decongestant.

•**pyrvinium pamoate.** (pihr-VIN-ee-uhm PAM-oh-ate) U.S.P. 23.
Use: Anthelmintic.

PYtest. (TRi-Med) 1mCi^{14}C-urea. Cap. UD 1s, 10s, 100s. *Rx.*
Use: Diagnostic aid.

PYtest Kit. (Tri-Med) Breath test for detecting *H. pylori.* Kit. 1 PYtest Cap. and breath collection equipment. *Rx.*
Use: Diagnostic aid.

Q

QB Liquid. (Major) Theophylline 150 mg, guaifenesin 90 mg. Bot. pt, gal. *Rx.*
Use: Bronchodilator, expectorant.

Q.T. Quick Tanning Suntan by Coppertone. (Schering Plough) Ethylhexyl p-methoxycinnamate, dihydroxyacetone. SPF 2. Lot. Bot. 120 ml. *otc.*
Use: Sunscreen, tanning.

Qua-Bid. (Quaker City Pharmacal) Papaverine HCl 150 mg. TR Cap. Bot. 100s, 1000s. *otc.*
Use: Vasodilator.

•**quadazocine mesylate.** (kwad-AZE-oh-SEEN) USAN.
Use: Opioid antagonist.

Quadramet. (DuPont Pharma) Samarium SM 153 lexidronam 1850 MBq/ml (50 mCi/ml) at calibration. Inj. Frozen, single-dose 10 ml vials. In 2 ml fill (3700 MBq) and 3 ml fill (5550 MBq). *Rx.*
Use: Treatment for bone lesions.

quadrodide.
See: Quadrinal, Susp., Tab. (Knoll Pharmaceuticals).

quadruple sulfonamides.
See: Sulfonamide.

Quarzan. (Roche Laboratories) Clidinium bromide 2.5 mg or 5 mg. Cap. Bot. 100s. *Rx.*
Use: Anticholinergic, antispasmodic.

•**quazepam.** (KWAY-zuh-pam) USAN.
Use: Hypnotic, sedative.
See: Doral (Baker Norton).

•**quazinone.** (KWAY-zih-NOHN) USAN.
Use: Cardiovascular agent.

•**quazodine.** (KWAY-zoe-deen) USAN.
Use: Cardiovascular agent.

•**quazolast.** (KWAY-ZOLE-ast) USAN.
Use: Antiasthmatic mediator release inhibitor.

Quelicin. (Abbott Hospital Prods) Succinylcholine Cl. **20 mg/ml:** Fliptop vial 10 ml, Abboject Syringe 5 ml; **50 mg/ml:** Amp. 10 ml; **100 mg/ml:** Amp. 10 ml; **Quelicin-500:** 5 ml in Pintop vial 10 ml; **Quelicin-1000:** 10 ml in Pintop vial 20 ml. *Rx.*
Use: Muscle relaxant.

Quelidrine Cough Syrup. (Abbott Laboratories) Dextromethorphan HBr 10 mg, chlorpheniramine maleate 2 mg, ephedrine HCl 5 mg, phenylephrine HCl 5 mg, ammonium Cl 40 mg, ipecac fluidextract 0.005 ml, ethyl alcohol 2%/5 ml. Bot. 4 oz. *Rx.*
Use: Antihistamine, antitussive, bronchodilator, decongestant, expectorant.

Quercetin. Active constituent of rutin. Quertine.

Quertine.
Use: Bioflavonoid supplement.

Questran. (Bristol-Myers Squibb) Cholestyramine resin 4 g active ingredient/9 g Powder Packet. Box packet 60s. Can 378 g (42 dose). *Rx.*
Use: Antihyperlipidemic, antipruritic.

Questran Light. (Bristol-Myers Squibb) Anhydrous cholestyramine 4 g/Packet or scoopful. Pow. for Oral Susp. Can 210 g (42 doses), carton packet 5 g (60s). *Rx.*
Use: Antihyperlipidemic.

•**quetiapine fumarate.** (cue-TIE-ah-peen) USAN.
Use: Antipsychotic.
See: Seroquel, Tab. (Zeneca).

Quiagel. (Rugby) Kaolin 6 g, pectin 142.8 mg, hyoscyamine sulfate 0.1037 mg, atropine sulfate 0.0194 mg, scopolamine HBr 0.0065 mg/30 ml. Susp. Bot. pt, gal. *Rx.*
Use: Antidiarrheal.

quetiapine hydrochloride. (cue-TIE-ah-peen)
Use: Antipsychotic.

Quibron. (Roberts Pharm) Theophylline (anhydrous) 150 mg, guaifenesin 90 mg. Cap. Bot. 100s, 1000s, UD 100s. *Rx.*
Use: Bronchodilator, expectorant.

Quibron-300. (Roberts Pharm) Theophylline (anhydrous) 300 mg, guaifenesin 180 mg. Cap. Bot. 100s. *Rx.*
Use: Bronchodilator, expectorant.

Quibron Plus. (Bristol-Myers Squibb) Ephedrine HCl 25 mg, theophylline (anhydrous) 150 mg, butabarbital 20 mg, guaifenesin 100 mg. Bot. 100s. *Rx.*
Use: Antiasthmatic combination.

Quibron Plus Elixir. (Bristol-Myers Squibb) Theophylline 150 mg, ephedrine HCl 25 mg, guaifenesin 100 mg, butabarbital 20 mg, alcohol 15%. Elix. Bot. Pt. *Rx.*
Use: Antiasthmatic combination.

Quibron-T Dividose Tablets. (Roberts Pharm) Theophylline anhydrous 300 mg. Tab. Dividose design breakable into 100, 150 or 200 mg portions. Immediate release. Bot. 100s. *Rx.*
Use: Bronchodilator.

Quibron-T/SR Dividose Tablets. (Roberts Pharm) Theophylline anhydrous 300 mg. Tab. Dividose design breakable into 100 mg, 150 mg or 200 mg portions. Sustained release. Bot. 100s. *Rx.*

Use: Bronchodilator.

Quick CARE. (Novartis Pharmaceuticals) **Disinfecting solution:** Isopropanol, sodium Cl, polyoxypropylene-polyoxyethylene block copolymer, disodium lauroamphodiacetate. Bot. 15 ml. **Rinse and neutralizer:** Sodium borate, boric acid, sodium perborate (generating up to 0.006% hydrogen peroxide), phophoric acid. Bot. 360 ml. *otc.*
Use: Contact lens care.

Quick-K. (Western Research) Potassium bicarbonate 650 mg (6.5 mEq) potassium. Tab. Bot. 30s, 100s. *Rx.*
Use: Electrolyte supplement.

Quick Pep. (Thompson Medical) Caffeine 150 mg, dextrose, sucrose 300 mg. Tab. Bot. 32s. *otc.*
Use: CNS stimulant.

Quiebar. (Nevin) Butabarbital sodium. **Spantab:** 1.5 gr. TR Spantab. Bot. 50s, 500s. **Elix.:** 30 mg/5 ml. Bot. pt, gal. **Tab.:** 15 mg. Bot. 100s, 1000s; 30 mg. Bot. 1000s. **A.C. Cap.:** Bot. 100s, 500s. *c-III.*
Use: Hypnotic, sedative.

Quiebel. (Nevin) Butabarbital sodium 15 mg, belladonna extract 15 mg. Cap. Bot. 100s, 1000s. Elix. pt, gal. *c-III.*
Use: Anticholinergic, antispasmodic, hypnotic, sedative.

Quiecof. (Nevin) Dextromethorphan HBr 7.5 mg, chlorpheniramine maleate 0.75 mg, guaiacol glyceryl ether 25 mg. Bot. 4 oz, pt, gal. *otc.*
Use: Antitussive, antihistamine, expectorant.

Quiet Night. (Rosemont) Pseudoephedrine HCl 10 mg, doxylamine succinate 1.25 mg, dextromethorphan HBr 5 mg, acetaminophen 167 mg/5 ml. Liq. Bot. 180 ml, 300 ml. *otc.*
Use: Analgesic, antihistamine, antitussive, decongestant.

Quiet Time. (Whiteworth Towne) Acetaminophen 600 mg, ephedrine sulfate 8 mg, dextromethorphan HBr 15 mg, doxylamine succinate 7.5 mg, alcohol 25 mg/30 ml. Bot. 180 ml. *otc.*
Use: Analgesic, antihistamine, antitussive, decongestant.

Quiet World. (Whitehall Robins) Acetaminophen 2.5 gr, aspirin 3.5 gr, pyrilamine maleate 25 mg. Tab. Bot. 12s, 30s. *otc.*
Use: Analgesic combination, antihistamine.

•**quiflapon sodium.** (KWIH-flap-ahn) USAN.
Use: Antiasthmatic, inflammatory bowel disease suppressant.

Quik-Cept. (Laboratory Diagnostics) Slide test for pregnancy, rapid latex inhibition test. Kit 25s, 50s, 100s.
Use: Diagnostic aid.

Quik-Cult. (Laboratory Diagnostics) Slide test for fecal occult blood. Kit 150s, 200s, 300s and tape test.
Use: Diagnostic aid.

•**quilostigmine.** (Kwill-oh-STIG-meen) USAN.
Use: Cholinergic (cholinesterase inhibitor); treatment of Alzheimer's disease.

Quinaglute Dura-Tabs. (Berlex) Quinidine gluconate 324 mg. Tab. Bot. 100s, 250s, 500s, UD 100s. Unit-of-use 90s, 120s. *Rx.*
Use: Antiarrhythmic.

•**quinaldine blue.** (kwin-AL-deen) USAN.
Use: Diagnostic agent (obstetrics).

•**quinapril hydrochloride.** (KWIN-uh-PRILL) USAN.
Use: Antihypertensive, enzyme inhibitor (angiotensin-converting)
See: Accupril, Tab. (Parke-Davis).

•**quinaprilat.** (KWIN-ah-PRILL-at) USAN.
Use: Antihypertensive, enzyme inhibitor (angiotensin-converting).

•**quinazosin hydrochloride.** (kwin-AZZ-oh-sin) USAN.
Use: Antihypertensive.

•**quinbolone.** (KWIN-bole-ohn) USAN.
Use: Anabolic.

•**quindecamine acetate.** (kwin-DECK-ah-meen) USAN.
Use: Anti-infective.

•**quindonium bromide.** (kwin-DOE-nee-uhn) USAN.
Use: Cardiovascular agent. (antiarrhythmic).

•**quinelorane hydrochloride.** (kwih-NELL-oh-RANE) USAN.
Use: Antihypertensive, antiparkinsonian.

quinethazone, U.S.P. XXII.
Use: Diuretic.
See: Hydromox, Tab. (ESI Lederle Generics).

W/Reserpine.
See: Hydromox R, Tab. (ESI Lederle Generics).

•**quinetolate.** (Kwin-EH-toe-late) USAN.
Use: Muscle relaxant.

•**quinfamide.** (KWIN-fah-mide) USAN.
Use: Antiamebic.

•**quingestanol acetate.** (kwin-JESS-tan-ahl) USAN.
Use: Hormone, progestin.

•**quingestrone.** (kwin-JESS-trone) USAN.
Use: Hormone, progestin.

Quinidex Extentabs. (Robins) Quinidine sulfate 300 mg. Tab. Bot. 100s, 250s. Dis-co pack 100s. *Rx.*
Use: Antiarrhythmic.

Quinidex L-A.
See: Quinidex Extentabs (Robins).

•**quinidine gluconate,** (KWIN-ih-deen) U.S.P. 23.
Use: Cardiovascular agent (antiarrhythmic).
See: Duraquin, Tab. (Parke-Davis). Quinaglute, Dura-Tab. (Berlex).

quinidine polygalacturonate.
See: Cardioquin Tab. (Purdue Frederick).

•**quinidine sulfate,** (KWIN-ih-deen) U.S.P. 23.
Use: Cardiovascular agent (antiarrhythmic).
See: Quinidex Extentabs (Robins). Quinora, Tab. (Key Pharm).

quinidine sulfate. (Various, eg, Copley) 300 mg. Tab., SR Tab. Bot. 100s, 250s, 1000s *Rx.*
Use: Cardiovascular agent.

•**quinine ascorbate.** (KWIE-nine ass-CORE-bate) USAN. *Formerly quinine biascorbate.*
Use: Smoking deterrent.

quinine bisulfate. (KWIE-nine)
Use: Analgesic, antimalarial, antipyretic.

quinine dihydrochloride. (KWIE-nine)
Use: Antimalarial.

quinine ethylcarbonate.
See: Euquinine (Various Mfr.).

quinine glycerophosphate. Quinine compound with glycerol phosphate.

•**quinine sulfate,** (KWIE-nine) U.S.P. 23.
Use: Antimalarial.
See: Quinamm, Tab. (Hoechst Marion Roussel).
W/Aminophylline.
See: Strema, Cap. (Foy).
W/Atropine sulfate, emetine HCl, aconitine, camphor monobromate.
See: Coryza, Tab. (Jones Medical Industries).
W/Niacin, vitamin E.
See: Myodyne, Tab. (Paddock).

quinine and urea hydrochloride.
Use: Sclerosing agent.

quinisocaine.
See: Dimethisoquin HCl, USAN.

quinophan.
See: Cinchophen (Various Mfr.).

Quinora. (Key Pharm) Quinidine sulfate 300 mg. Tab. Bot. 100s, 1000s, UD 100s. *Rx.*
Use: Antiarrhythmic.

quinoxyl.
See: Chiniofon

•**quinpirole hydrochloride.** (KWIN-pihr-ole) USAN.
Use: Antihypertensive.

quinprenaline. Quinterenol Sulfate.

Quin-Release. (Major) Quinidine gluconate 324 mg. SR Tab. Bot. 100s, 250s, 500s, UD 100s. *Rx.*
Use: Antiarrhythmic.

Quinsana Plus. (Stephan) Tolnafate 1%, cornstarch, talc. Pow. In 90 g. *otc.*
Use: Antifungal, topical.

Quintabs. (Freeda Vitamins) Vitamins A 10,000 IU, D 400 IU, E 29 mg, B_1 25 mg, B_2 25 mg, B_3 100 mg, B_5 25 mg, B_6 25 mg, B_{12} 25 mcg, C 300 mg, folic acid 0.1 mg, inositol, PABA/Tab. Bot. 100s, 250s. *otc.*
Use: Vitamin supplement.

Quintabs-M. (Freeda Vitamins) Iron 15 mg, Vitamins A 10,000 IU, D 400 IU, E 50 mg, B_1 30 mg, B_2 30 mg, B_3 150 mg, B_5 30 mg, B_6 30 mg, B_{12} 30 mcg, C 300 mg, folic acid 0.4 mg, Ca, Cu, K, Mg, Mn, Se, Zn 30 mg., PABA./Tab. Bot. 100s, 250s, 500s. *otc.*
Use: Mineral, vitamin supplement.

•**quinterenol sulfate.** (kwin-TER-en-ahl) USAN.
Use: Bronchodilator.

•**quinuclium bromide.** (kwih-NEW-klee-uhm) USAN.
Use: Antihypertensive.

•**quinupristin.** (kwih-NEW-priss-tin) USAN.
Use: Anti-infective.

•**quipazine maleate.** (KWIP-ah-zeen) USAN.
Use: Antidepressant, oxytocic.

quipenyl naphthoate.
See: Pamaquine naphthoate. Plasmochin naphthoate.

R

R-3 Screen Test. (Wampole Laboratories) A three-minute latex-eosin slide test for the qualitative detection of rheumatoid factor activity in serum. Kit 100s.
Use: Diagnostic aid.

RabAvert. (Chiron) Rabies antigen 2.5 IU, < 1 mcg neomycin, < 20 ng chlortetracycline, < 2 ng amphotericin B, < 3 ng ovalbumin. Inj. *Rx.*
Use: Immunization.

•**rabeprazole sodium.** (rab-EH-pray-zahl) USAN.
Use: Antiulcerative, gastric acid pump inhibitor.

rabies antigen.
Use: Immunization.

•**rabies immune globulin.** (RAY-beez-ih-MYOON GLAB-byoo-lin) U.S.P. 23.
Use: Immunization.
See: Bayrab (Bayer Corp).
Imogam Rabies (Pasteur Merieux Connaught).

rabies immune globulin (RIG), human.
See: rabies immune globulin.

•**rabies vaccine.** (RAY-beez vaccine) U.S.P. 23.
Use: Immunization.
See: Imovax Rabies, Syr. (Connaught).
RabAvert (Chiron).
rabies vaccine adsorbed, vial (Michigan Department of Public Health).

rabies vaccine (adsorbed). (Michigan Department of Public Health) Challenge virus standard (CVS) Kissling/MDPH Strain. Inj. Vial 1 ml. *Rx.*
Use: Immunization.

•**racemethionine.** (RAY-see-meh-THIGH-oh-neen) USAN. U.S.P. XXI *Formerly Methionine.*
Use: Acidifier, urinary.
See: Amurex, Cap. (Solvay).
Pedameth. Cap., Liq. (Forest Pharmaceutical).

racemethionine w/combinations.
See: Aminomin, Vial (Pharmex).
Aminovit, Vial (Hickam).
Ardiatric, Tab. (Burgin-Arden).
Limvic, Tab. (Briar).
Lipo-K, Cap. (Marcen).
Lychol-B, Inj. (Burgin-Arden).
Minoplex, Vial (Savage).
Vio-Geric, Tab. (Solvay).
Vio-Geric-H, Tab. (Solvay).

racemic amphetamine sulfate.
See: Amphetamine sulfate.

racemic calcium pantothenate.
See: Calcium Pantothenate, Racemic.

racemic desoxy-nor-ephedrine.
See: Amphetamine (Various Mfr.).

racemic ephedrine hydrochloride. Racephedrine HCl.

racemic pantothenic acid.
See: Vitamin, Preps.

•**racephedrine hydrochloride.** USAN.
Use: Vasoconstrictor; decongestant, nasal.
See: Ephedrine Combinations
W/Aminophylline, phenobarbital.
See: Amodrine, Tab. (Searle).
W/Theophylline sodium glycinate, phenobarbital.
See: Synophedal, Tab. (Schwarz Pharma).

racephedrine hydrochloride. (Pharmacia & Upjohn) **Cap.:** 3/8 gr. Bot. 40s, 250s, 1000s. **Soln.:** 1%. Bot. 1 fl oz, pt, gal.
Use: Vasoconstrictor; decongestant, nasal.

•**racephenicol.** (ray-see-FEN-ih-KAHL) USAN.
Use: Anti-infective.

•**racepinephrine hydrochloride,** (race-epp-ih-NEFF-rin) U.S.P. 23
Use: Bronchodilator.

•**raclopride C11,** (RACK-low-pride) U.S.P. 23.
Use: Radiopharmaceutical.

radioactive isotopes.
See: Aggregated Radioiodinated Albumin, Human I-131.
Chlormerodrin Hg-197, Inj.
Chlormerodrin Hg-203, Inj.
Cyanocobalamin Co-57, Cap.
Cyanocobalamin Co-60, Cap.
Gold Au-198, Inj.
Medotope, Prods. (Bristol-Myers Squibb).
Radio-Gold, Soln.
Radio-Iodinated Serum Albumin (Human).
Sodium Radio-Chromate, Inj.
Sodium Radio-Iodide, Soln.
Sodium Radio Phosphate, Soln.
Radiodinated Serum Albumin, Human I-125.
Radiodinated Serum Albuminia, Human I-131.
Selenomethionine Se-75, Inj.
Sodium Chromate Cr-51, Inj.
Sodium Iodide I-125, Soln., Cap.
Sodium Iodide I-131, Soln., Cap.
Sodium Phosphate P-32, Cap., Inj.
Sodium Rose Bengal I-131, Inj.
Strontium Nitrate Sr-85, Inj.
Technetium Tc-99m, Kit, Inj.

Triolein I-131, Cap., Soln.
Xenon Xe-133, Inj.

radiogold (^{198}Au), solution. Gold Au-198 Injection, U.S.P. 23.
Use: Irradiation therapy.
See: Auretope, Vial (Bristol-Myers Squibb).

radio-iodide (^{131}I), sodium.
Use: Radiopharmaceutical.
See: Iodotope (Bristol-Myers Squibb).

radio-iodinated (^{131}I) serum albumin. (Human), Iodinated I-131 Albumin Injection, U.S.P. 23.

radio-iodinated serum albumin (human), (^{125}I).
See: Albumotope (^{125}I) (Bristol-Myers Squibb).

radiopaque polyvinyl chloride.
Use: Radiopaque agent, gastrointestinal.
See: Sitzmarks (Lafayette Pharm).

radio-phosphate (^{32}P), sodium.
Use: Radiopharmaceutical.

radioselenomethionine 75 Se. Selenomethionine Se 75.

radiotolpovidone I-131. Tolpovidone I-131.
See: Raovin (Abbott Laboratories).

•**rafoxanide.** (ray-FOX-ah-nide) USAN.
Use: Anthelmintic.

Ragus. (Miller) Magnesium 27 mg, vitamins C 100 mg, calcium 580 mg, phosphorus 450 mg, l-lysine 25 mg, dl-methionine 50 mg, A 5000 IU, D 400 IU, E 10 mg, B_1 20 mg, B_2 3 mg, B_6 5 mg, B_{12} 9 mcg, niacinamide 80 mg, pantothenic acid 5 mg, iron 20 mg, copper 1 mg, manganese 2 mg, potassium 10 mg, zinc 2 mg, iodine 0.1 mg/3 Tab. Bot. 100s. *otc.*
Use: Mineral, vitamin supplement.

•**ralitoline.** (rah-LIT-oh-leen) USAN.
Use: Anticonvulsant.

R A Lotion. (Medco Lab) Resorcinol 3%, alcohol 43%. Plastic Bot. 120 ml, 240 ml, 480 ml. *otc.*
Use: Dermatologic, acne.

•**raloxifene hydrochloride.** (ral-OX-ih-FEEN) USAN. Formerly Keoxifene hydrochloride.
Use: Antiestrogen.
See: Evista, Tab. (Eli Lilly).

•**raltitrexed.** USAN. (ral-tih-TREX-ehd)
Use: Advanced colorectal cancer treatment (thymidylate synthase inhibitor), antineoplastic.

•**raluridine.** (ral-YOUR-ih-deen) USAN.
Use: Antiviral.

•**ramipril.** (ruh-MIH-prill) USAN.
Use: Antihypertensive, enzyme inhibitor (angiotensin-converting), congestive heart failure.
See: Altace, Cap. (Hoechst Marion Roussel, Pharmacia & Upjohn).

•**ramoplanin.** (ram-oh-PLAN-in) USAN.
Use: Anti-infective.

Ramses. (Schmid) Nonoxynol 9 5%. Vaginal jelly. 150 g. *otc.*
Use: Contraceptive, spermicide.

Ramses Bendex. (Schmid) Flexible cushioned diaphragm; arcing spring. 65-90 mm. Pkg. w/Ramses Vaginal Jelly Tube 1 oz, 3 oz. *Rx.*
Use: Contraceptive.

Ramses Diaphragm. (Schmid) Flexible cushioned diaphragm 50-95 mm. Pkg. diaphragm, tube of Ramses Vaginal Jelly. Pkg. diaphragm alone. *Rx.*
Use: Contraceptive.

Ramses Extra. (Schmid) Condom with nonoxynol 9 15%. In 3s, 12s, 24s, 36s. *otc.*
Use: Contraceptive.

Ramses Jelly. (Schmid) Nonoxynol 9 5%. Tube w/applicator 150 g. *otc.*
Use: Contraceptive.

Randolectil. (Farbenfabriken Bayer Corp) Butaperazine. *Rx.*
Use: Psychotherapeutic agent.

ranestol. Triclofenol piperazine.
Use: Anthelmintic.

•**ranimycin.** (ran-ih-MY-sin) USAN.
Use: Anti-infective.

•**ranitidine.** (ran-EYE-tih-DEEN) USAN.
Use: Antiulcerative.
See: Zantac, Tab., Inj., Syr. (Glaxo and Roche).

ranitidine. (Zenith Goldline) Ranitidine 150 mg, 300 mg. Tab. Bot. 30s (300 mg only), 60s (150 mg only), 100s, 250s (300 mg only), 500s (150 mg only). *Rx.*
Use: Antiulcerative.

•**ranitidine bismuth citrate.** (ran-EYE-tih-DEEN BIZZ-muth SIH-trate) USAN.
Use: Antiulcerative.
See: Tritec, Tab. (GlaxoWellcome).

•**ranitidine hydrochloride,** (ran-EYE-tih-DEEN) U.S.P. 23.
Use: Antiulcerative.
See: Zantac, Inj., Tab., Syr. (GlaxoWellcome).

ranitidine hydrochloride. (UDL) 15 mg/ml. Syr. Bot. UD 10 ml.
Use: Antiulcerative.

ranitidine hydrochloride in sodium chloride injection.

Use: Antiulcerative.
See: Zantac Inj. Premixed (Glaxo-Wellcome).

•**ranolazine hydrochloride.** (RAY-no-lah-ZEEN) USAN.
Use: Antianginal.

Rapid Test Strep. (SmithKline Diagnostics) Latex slide agglutination test for identification of group A Streptococci. In 25s, 100s.
Use: Diagnostic aid.

•**rasagiline mesylate.** (rass-AH-jih-leen MEH-sih-late) USAN.
Use: Antiparkinsonian.

rastinon. Tolbutamide, U.S.P. 23.
Use: Antidiabetic.

rattlesnake bite therapy.
See: Antivenin, (crotalidae) (Wyeth Ayerst).

Rauneed. (Hanlon) Rauwolfia 50 mg or 100 mg/Tab. Bot. 100s. *Rx.*
Use: Antihypertensive.

Raunescine. (Penick) An alkaloid of Rauwolfia serpentina. Under study.
Use: Antihypertensive.

Raunormine. (Penick) 11-Desmethoxy reserpine. *Rx.*

Raurine. (Westerfield) Reserpine. **Tab.:** 0.1 mg. Bot. 100s. **Delayed Action Cap.:** 0.5 mg. Bot. 100s. *Rx.*
Use: Antihypertensive.

Rauserfia. (New Eng. Phr. Co.) Rauwolfia serpentina 50 mg or 100 mg/Tab. Bot. 100s. *Rx.*
Use: Antihypertensive.

Rautina. (Fellows) Rauwolfia serpentina whole root 50 mg or 100 mg/Tab. Bot. 1000s. *Rx.*
Use: Antihypertensive.

Rauval. (Pal-Pak) Rauwolfia whole root 50 mg or 100 mg/Tab. Bot. 100s, 500s, 1000s. *Rx.*
Use: Antihypertensive.

rauwolfia/bendroflumethiazide. (Various Mfr.) Bendroflumethiazide 4 mg, powdered rauwolfia serpentina 50 mg/Tab. Bot. 100s. *Rx.*
Use: Antihypertensive.
See: Rauzide, Tab. (Bristol-Myers Squibb).

rauwolfia canescens alkaloid.
See: Harmonyl, Tab. (Abbott Laboratories).

rauwolfia serpentina active principles (alkaloids). Deserpidine, Rescinnamine.
See: Reserpine, Inj. (Various Mfr.).

rauwolfia serpentina alkaloidal extract.
See: Alseroxylon (Various Mfr.).

•**rauwolfia serpentina.** (rah-WOOL-fee-ah ser-pen-TEE-nah) U.S.P. 23.
Use: Antihypertensive.
See: Raudixin, Tab. (Bristol-Myers).
Rauneed, Tab. (Hanlon).
Rauval, Tab. (Pal-Pak).
Rawfola, Tab. (Foy).
T-Rau, Tab. (Tennessee Pharmaceutic).
Wolfina, Tab. (Westerfield).
W/Bendroflumethiazide.
See: Rautrax-N, Tab. (Bristol-Myers).
Rauzide, Tab. (Bristol-Myers).
W/Bendroflumethiazide, potassium Cl (400).
See: Rautrax, Tab. (Bristol-Myers).
W/Mannitol hexanitrate, rutin.
See: Maxitate W/Rauwolfia, Tab. (Fisons).

rauwolscine. An alkaloid of *Rauwolfia canescens*. Under study.
Use: Antihypertensive.

Rauzide. (Bristol-Myers Squibb) Rauwolfia serpentina pow. 50 mg, bendroflumethiazide 4 mg, tartrazine/Tab. Bot. 100s. *Rx.*
Use: Antihypertensive.

Ravocaine. (Cook-Waite) Propoxycaine HCl 4 mg, procaine 20 mg, norepinephrine bitartrate equivalent to 0.033 mg levophed base, sodium Cl 3 mg, acetone sodium bisulfite not more than 2 mg. Cartridge 1.8 ml. *Rx.*
Use: Anesthetic, local.

Ravocaine and Novocain with Levophed. (Cook-Waite) Propoxycaine HCl 7.2 mg, procaine 36 mg, norepinephrine 0.12 mg, acetone sodium bisulfite 1.8 ml. Inj. Dental Cartridge. *Rx.*
Use: Anesthetic, local.

Rawfola. (Foy) Rauwolfia serpentina 50 mg/Tab. Bot. 1000s. *Rx.*
Use: Antihypertensive.

Rawl Vite. (Rawl) Vitamins A 10,000 IU, D 500 IU, B_1 10 mg, B_2 5 mg, B_6 1 mg, calcium pantothenate 5 mg, nicotinamide 50 mg, C 125 mg, E 2.5 IU/Tab. Bot. 100s. *otc.*
Use: Mineral, vitamin supplement.

Rawl Whole Liver Vitamin B Complex. (Rawl) Whole liver 500 mg, amino acids found in the whole liver, vitamins B_1 1 mg, B_2 2 mg, niacinamide 5 mg, choline Cl 12 mg, B_6 0.2 mg, calcium pantothenate 0.2 mg, inositol 5 mg, biotin 0.6 mcg, B_{12} 0.3 mcg/Cap. Bot. 100s, 500s.
Use: Mineral, vitamin supplement.

Raxar. (GlaxoWellcome) Levofloxacin HCl 200 mg. Tab. Bot. 60s, UD 60s. *Rx.*

Use: Anti-infective.

Ray Block. (Del-Ray) Octyl dimethyl PABA 5%, benzophenone-3 3%, SD alcohol. Lot. Bot. 118.3 ml. *otc.*
Use: Sunscreen.

Ray-D. (Nion) Vitamin D 400 IU, thiamine mononitrate 1 mg, riboflavin 2 mg, niacin 10 mg, iodine 0.1 mg, calcium 375 mg, phosphorus 300 mg/6 Tab. In base of brewer's yeast. Bot. 100s, 500s. *otc.*
Use: Mineral, vitamin supplement.

Rayderm Ointment. (Velvet Pharmacal) Euphorbia extract, phenyl salicylate, neatsfoot oil, olive oil, lanolin in emulsion base preserved with methyl and propylparabens. Tube 1.5 oz, Jar lb. *otc.*
Use: Burn therapy.

•**rayon, purified,** (RAY-ahn) U.S.P. 23.
Use: Surgical aid.

raythesin. (Raymer).
See: Propyl p-Aminobenzoate.

Razepam. (Major) Temazepam 15 mg or 30 mg/Cap. Bot. 100s. *c-iv.*
Use: Hypnotic, sedative.

RCF. (Ross Laboratories) Carbohydrate free low iron soy protein formula base. Carbohydrate and water must be added. For infants unable to tolerate the amount or type of carbohydrate in conventional formulas. Can 14 fl oz. (Concentrated liq.). *otc.*
Use: Nutritional supplement.

R & C Shampoo. (Schwarz Pharma) Pyrethrin shampoo. Bot. 2 oz, 4 oz. *otc.*
Use: Pediculicide.

R & C Spray III. (Schwarz Pharma) Spray containing pyrethroid (sumethrin) 0.382%, other isomers 0.018%, petroleum distillate 4.255%. Aerosol Container 5 oz. *otc.*
Use: Pediculicide.

Reabilan. (Elan) Protein 31.5 g, fat 39 g, carbohydrates 131.5 g, Na 702 mg, K 1.252 g/L, lactose free. With appropriate vitamins and minerals. Liq. Bot. 375 ml. *otc.*
Use: Nutritional supplement.

Reabilan HN. (Elan) Protein 58.2 g, fat 52 g, carbohydrates 158 g, Na 1000 mg, K 1661 mg/L, lactose free. With appropriate vitamins and minerals. Liq. Bot. 375 ml. *otc.*
Use: Nutritional supplement.

Rea-Lo. (Whorton) Urea in water soluble moisturizing oil base. **Lot.:** 15%. Bot. 4 oz, pt. **Cream:** 30%. Jar 2 oz, 16 oz. *otc.*
Use: Emollient.

•**recainam hydrochloride.** (reh-CANE-am) USAN.
Use: Cardiovascular agent (antiarrhythmic).

•**recainam tosylate.** (reh-CANE-am TAH-sill-ate) USAN.
Use: Cardiovascular agent (antiarrhythmic).

•**reclazepam.** (reh-CLAY-zeh-pam) USAN.
Use: Hypnotic, sedative.

Reclomide. (Major) Metoclopramide HCl 10 mg/Tab. Bot. 100s, 500s, 1000s, UD 100s. *Rx.*
Use: Antiemetic, gastrointestinal stimulant.

recombinant human insulin-like growth factor I.
Use: Antibody-mediated growth hormone resistance. [Orphan drug]

recombinant tissue plasminogen activator. *Rx.*
See: Activase (Genentech).

recombinant vaccinia (human papillomavirus).
Use: Cervical cancer. [Orphan drug]

Recombinate. (Hyland) Concentrated recombinant antihemophilic factor, contains albumin (human) 12.5 mg/ml, polyethylene glycol 1.5 mg, sodium 180 mEq/L, histidine 55 mm, polysorbate-80 1.5 mcg/AHF IU, calcium 0.2 mg/ml. Pow. for inj. Single dose bot. 250 IU, 500 IU, 1000 IU. *Rx.*
Use: Antihemophilic.

Recombivax HB. (Merck) Hepatitis B vaccine recombinant. **Pediatric:** 2.5 mcg/0.5 ml. Single-dose vials 0.5 ml and 3 ml, prefilled, single-dose syringes 0.5 ml. **Adolescent/High Risk Infant:** 5 mcg/0.5 ml. single-dose vials 0.5 ml. **Adult:** 10 mcg/ml. Vials 1 ml, 3 ml, prefilled, single-dose syringes 1 ml. **Dialysis:** 40 mcg/ml. Vial 1 ml. *Rx.*
Use: Immunization.

Recortex 10X in Oil. (Forest Pharmaceutical) 1000 mcg/ml. Vial 10 ml. *Rx.*

Recover. (Dermik Laboratories) Bot. 2.25 oz. *otc.*
Use: Dermatologic.

Rectagene. (Pfeiffer) Live yeast cell derivative supplying 2000 units Skin Respiratory Factor/oz, shark liver oil in a cocoa butter base. Supp. 12s. *otc.*
Use: Anorectal preparation.

Rectagene Medicated Rectal Balm. (Pfeiffer) Live yeast cell derivative that supplies 2000 units Skin Respiratory Factor/30 g, refined shark liver oil 3%, white petrolatum, lanolin, thyme oil, 1:10,000 phenyl mercuric nitrate. Oint. 56.7 g. *otc.*

Use: Anorectal preparation.

Rectal Medicone. (Medicone) Benzocaine 2 gr, balsam peru 1 gr, hydroxyquinoline sulfate 0.25 gr, menthol 1/7 gr, zinc oxide 3 gr/Supp. Box 12s, 24s. *otc.*
Use: Anesthetic; antiseptic, topical.

Rectal Medicone Unguent. (Medicone) Benzocaine 20 mg, oxyquinoline sulfate 5 mg, menthol 4 mg, zinc oxide 100 mg, balsam peru 12.5 mg, petrolatum 625 mg, lanolin 210 mg/g. Tube 1.5 oz. *otc.*
Use: Anorectal preparation.

Rectules. (Forest Pharmaceutical) Chloral hydrate 10 or 20 gr in water-soluble base. Supp. Pkg. 12s.
Use: Hypnotic, sedative.

red blood cells. Human red blood cells given by IV infusion.
Use: Blood replenisher.

red cell tagging solution.
See: A-C-D Solution (Bristol-Myers Squibb).

Red Cross Toothache Kit. (Mentholatum) Eugenol 85%, sesame oil. Drops. Bot. 3.7 ml w/cotton pellets and tweezers. *otc.*
Use: Anesthetic, local.

red ferric oxide.
Use: Pharmaceutic aid (color).

red mercuric iodide.
See: Auralcaine, Liq. (Truett).

Reditemp-C. (Wyeth Ayerst) Ammonium nitrate, water and special additives. Pkg. large and small sizes. 4 × 10s.
Use: Cold compress.

Reducto, Improved. (Arcum) Phendimetrazine bitartrate 35 mg/Tab. Bot. 100s, 1000s. *c-III.*
Use: Anorexiant.

Redutemp. (Inter. Ethical Labs) Acetaminophen 500 mg/Tab. Bot. 60s. *otc.*
Use: Analgesic.

Reese's Pinworm. (Reese Pharmaceutical) Pyrantel pamoate 144 mg. Liq. 30 ml. *otc.*
Use: Anthelmintic.

Refludan. (Hoechst Marion Roussel) Lepirudin (rDNA) 50 mg, sodium hydroxide, mannitol. Pow. for Inj. Vial 50 mg. Box 10s. *Rx.*
Use: Anticoagulant.

Refresh. (Allergan) Polyvinyl alcohol 1.4%, povidone 0.6%, sodium Cl. UD 30s or 50s (0.3 ml single dose container). *otc.*
Use: Artificial tears.

Refresh Plus. (Allergan) Carboxymethylcellulose sodium 0.5%, KCl, NaCl. Preservative free. Soln. 0.3 ml/single use container. 30s, 50s. *otc.*
Use: Artificial tears.

Refresh PM. (Allergan) White petrolatum 56.8%, mineral oil 41.5%, lanolin alcohol, sodium Cl. Tube 3.5 g. *otc.*
Use: Lubricant, opthalmic.

Regain. (NCI) Protein 15 g, carbohydrates 52 g, fat 7 g, sodium 45 mg, K 75 mg, Ca 200 mg, P 100 mg, Ca, Fe, vitamin B_{12}, Mg, folic acid, fructose. With dietary fiber. 300 calories. Lactose free. Vanilla, strawberry and malt flavors. Bar 85 g. *otc.*
Use: Nutritional supplement.

Regitine. (Novartis) Phentolamine mesylate 5 mg/Vial (w/mannitol 25 mg in lyophilized form). Pkg. 2s, 6s.
Use: Diagnostic aid.

Reglan. (Robins) Metoclopramide HCl. **Inj.: 10 mg/2 ml:** Amp. 2 ml, 10 ml; **5 mg/ml:** Vial 2 ml, 10 ml, 30 ml. **Syr.:** 5 mg (as monohydrochloride monohydrate)/5 ml. Bot. pt, Dis-Co Pack 10×10s. **Tab.: 5 mg:** Bot. 100s. **10 mg:** Bot. 100s, 500s, Dis-co Pak 100s. *Rx.*
Use: Antiemetic, gastrointestinal stimulant.

Regonol. (Organon Teknika) Pyridostigmine bromide 5 mg/ml. Amp 2 ml, Vial 5 ml. *Rx.*
Use: Muscle stimulant.

•**regramostim.** (reh-GRAH-moe-STIM) USAN.
Use: Biological response modifier; antineoplastic adjunct; antineutropenic; hematopoietic stimulant.

Regranex. (Ortho-McNeil) Becaplermin 100 mcg, parabens. Gel. Tube 2 g, 7.5 g, 15 g. *Rx.*
Use: Diabetic neuropathic ulcers.

Regroton. (Rhone-Poulenc Rorer) Chlorthalidone 50 mg, reserpine 0.25 mg/Tab. Bot. 100s. *Rx.*
Use: Antihypertensive.

Regroton Demi. (Rhone-Poulenc Rorer) Chlorthalidone 25 mg, reserpine 0.125 mg/Tab. Bot. 100s, 1000s. *Rx.*
Use: Antihypertensive.

Regular Iletin I. (Eli Lilly) Insulin 100 units/ml. Beef and pork. Inj. Bot. 10 ml. *otc.*
Use: Antidiabetic agent.

regular purified pork insulin. (Novo Nordisk) Insulin 100 units/ml. Purified pork. Inj. Vial. 10 ml. *otc.*
Use: Antidiabetic.

Regular Strength Bayer Enteric Coated

Caplets. (Bayer Corp) Aspirin 325 mg. Bot. 50s, 100s. *otc.*
Use: Analgesic.

Regular Strength Midol Multisymptom. (Bayer Corp) Acetaminophen 325 mg, pyrilamine maleate 12.5 mg. Tab. Bot. 30s. *otc.*
Use: Analgesic combination.

Reguloid, Orange. (Rugby) Psyllium mucilloid 3.4 g, sucrose 70%/rounded tsp. Pow. 420 g, 630 g. *otc.*
Use: Laxative.

Reguloid Sugar Free. (Rugby) Psyllium hydrophilic mucilloid 3.4 g, sodium ≤ 0.01 g, aspartame, phenylalanine 6 mg. Pow. 222, 333 g. *otc.*
Use: Laxative.

Rehydralyte. (Ross Laboratories) Sodium 75 mEq, potassium 20 mEq, chloride 65 mEq, citrate 30 mEq, dextrose 25 g/L, 100 calories/L. Ready-to-use Bot. 8 oz. *Rx.*
Use: Fluid, electrolyte replacement.

Relafen. (SmithKline Beecham Pharmaceuticals) Nabumetone 500 mg/Tab. Bot. 100s, 500s, UD 100s. Nabumetone 750 mg/Tab. Bot. 100s, 500s, UD 100s. *Rx.*
Use: Analgesic, NSAID.

relaxin. A purified ovarian hormone of pregnancy (obtained from sows) responsible for pubic relaxation or separation of the symphysis pubis in mammals.
See: Lutrexin, Tab. (Becton Dickinson).

Relief Eye Drops. (Allergan) Phenylephrine HCl 0.12%, antipyrine 0.1%, polyvinyl alcohol 1.4%, edetate disodium. Bot. UD 0.3 ml. *otc.*
Use: Decongestant, ophthalmic.

relief solution. (Allergan) Phenylephrine HCl 0.12%, antipyrine 0.1%. soln. Bot. 20 ml. *otc.*
Use: Decongestant combination, ophthalmic.

•**relomycin.** (REE-low-MY-sin) USAN. A macrolide antibiotic produced by a variant strain of *Streptomyces hygroscopicus.*
Use: Anti-infective.

•**remacemide hydrochloride.** (rem-ASS-eh-MIDE) USAN.
Use: Anticonvulsant (neuroprotective).

Rem Cough Medicine. (Last) Dextromethorphan HBr 5 mg/5 ml. Bot. 3 oz, 6 oz. *otc.*
Use: Antitussive.

Remegel Soft Chewable Antacid Tablets. (Warner Lambert) Aluminum hydroxide-magnesium carbonate 476.4 mg/Chew. Tab. Pkg. 8s, 24s. *otc.*
Use: Antacid.

Remeron. (Organon Teknika) Mirtazapine 15 mg, 30 mg, lactose/Tab. Bot. 30s, 100s. *Rx.*
Use: Antidepressant.

•**remifentanil hydrochloride.** (reh-mih-FEN-tah-nill) USAN.
Use: Analgesic.
See: Ultiva, Pow. for inj. (Glaxo-Wellcome).

•**remiprostol.** (reh-mih-PROSTE-ole) USAN.
Use: Antiulcerative.

Remivox. (Janssen) Lorcainide HCl. *Rx.*
Use: Antiarrhythmic.

•**remoxipride.** (reh-MOX-ih-PRIDE) USAN.
Use: Antipsychotic.

•**remoxipride hydrochloride.** (reh-MOX-ih-PRIDE) USAN.
Use: Antipsychotic.

Remular-S. (Inter. Ethical Labs) Chlorzoxazone 250 mg/Tab. Bot. 100s. *Rx.*
Use: Muscle relaxant.

Renacidin. (Guardian Laboratories) The composition of this powder, as manufactured, is in terms of 156 to 171 g citric acid (anhydrous) and 21 to 30 g d-gluconic acid (as the lactone) w/purified magnesium hydroxycarbonate 75 to 87 g, magnesium acid citrate 9 to 15 g, calcium (as carbonate) 2 to 6 g, water 17 to 21 g per 300 g. Bot. 25 g 6s; 150 g, 300 g. *Rx.*
Use: Irrigant, genitourinary.

Renaltabs-S.C. (Forest Pharmaceutical) Methenamine 40.8 mg, benzoic acid 4.5 mg, phenyl salicylate 18.1 mg, hyoscyamine sulfate 1/2000 gr, atropine sulfate 0.03 mg, methylene blue 5.4 mg, gelsemium 6.1 mg/Tab. Bot. 1000s. *Rx.*
Use: Anti-infective, urinary.

RenAmin. (Clintec Nutrition) Sterile hypertonic soln. of essential and nonessential amino acids. Bot. 250 ml, 500 ml. *Rx.*
Use: Nutritional supplement, parenteral.

renanolone. *Rx.*
Use: Steroid anesthetic.

Renbu. (Wren) Butabarbital sodium 32.4 mg/Tab. Bot. 100s, 1000s. *c-III.*
Use: Hypnotic, sedative.

Renese. (Pfizer) Polythiazide 1 mg, 2 mg or 4 mg/Tab. Bot. 100s, 1000s. *Rx.*
Use: Antihypertensive, duretic.

Renese-R Tablets. (Pfizer) Polythiazide 2 mg, reserpine 0.25 mg/Tab. Bot. 100s, 1000s. *Rx.*

Use: Antihypertensive.

Rengasil. (Novartis) Pirprofen. Investigational drug.
Use: Anti-inflammatory.

renoform.
See: Epinephrine, Preps. (Various Mfr.).

Renografin-60, -76. (Bracco Diagnostics) **-60:** Diatrizoate meglumine 52%, sodium diatrizoate 8%, iodine 29.2%. Vial 10 ml, 100 ml, 10s; 30 ml, 50 ml, 25s. **-76:** Diatrizoate meglumine 66%, sodium diatrizoate 10%, iodine 37%. Vial 20 ml, 50 ml, 25s; 100 ml, 200 ml, 10s.
Use: Radiopaque agent.

Reno-M-Dip. (Bracco Diagnostics) Diatrizoate meglumine, iodine 14.1%. 30% for drip infusion pyelography. Inj. Bot. 300 ml. Also w/soln. admin. sets. (Formerly Renografin-Dip).
Use: Radiopaque agent.

Reno-M-30. (Bracco Diagnostics) Diatrizoate meglumine 30%, iodine 14.1%. Vial 50 ml, 100 ml, Box 25s.
Use: Radiopaque agent.

Reno-M-60. (Bracco Diagnostics) Diatrizoate meglumine 60%, iodine 28%. Vial 10 ml, 30 ml, 50 ml, 100 ml.
Use: Radiopaque agent.

Renormax. (Novartis) Spirapril 3 mg, 6 mg, 12 mg or 24 mg/Tab. *Rx.*
Use: ACE inhibitor.

Reno-Sed. (Vita Elixir) Methenamine 2 gr, salol 0.5 gr, methylene blue 1/10 gr, benzoic acid 1/8 gr, atropine sulfate 1/1000 gr, hyoscyamine sulfate 1/2000 gr/Tab. *Rx.*
Use: Anti-infective, urinary.

Renova. (Ortho McNeil) Tretinoin 0.05%, water in oil emulsion. Cream 40 g, 60 g. *Rx.*
Use: Dermatologic.

Renovist Inj. (Bracco Diagnostics) Diatrizoate methylglucamine 34.3%, diatrizoate sodium 35%, iodine 37%. Vial 50 ml, Box 25s.
Use: Radiopaque agent.

Renovist II. (Bracco Diagnostics) Diatrizoate sodium 29.1%, meglumine diatrizoate 28.5%, iodine 31%. Inj. Vial 30 ml, 60 ml, Box 25s.
Use: Radiopaque agent.

Renovue-65. (Bracco Diagnostics) Iodamide meglumide 65%, organically bound iodine 30%, edetate disodium. Vial 50 ml.
Use: Radiopaque agent.

Renovue-Dip. (Bracco Diagnostics) Iodamide meglumide 24%, iodine 11.1%. Infusion Bot. 300 ml.
Use: Radiopaque agent.

Renpap. (Wren) Acetaminophen 4 gr, salicylamide 3 gr, caffeine 2/3 gr, allylisobutylbarbituric acid gr/Tab. Bot. 100s, 1000s. *otc.*
Use: Analgesic.

Rentamine Pediatric. (Major) Phenylephrine tannate 5 mg, chlorpheniramine tannate 4 mg, carbetapentane tannate, saccharin, sucrose. Pt.
Use: Antihistamine, antitussive, decongestant.

ReNu Effervescent Enzymatic Cleaner. (Bausch & Lomb) Subtilisin, polyethylene glycol, sodium carbonate, sodium Cl, tartaric acid. Tab. In 10s, 20s, 30s. *otc.*
Use: Contact lens care.

ReNu Liquid. (Biosearch Medical Products) P-Ca and Na caseinates, CHO-maltodextrin sucrose, F-partially hydrogenated soy oil, mono and diglycerides, soy lecithin, protein 35 g, CHO 125 g, fat 40 g, sodium 500 mg, potassium 1250 mg/L, 1 Cal/ml, 300 mOsm/kg, H_2O. In 250 ml ready to use. *otc.*
Use: Nutritional supplement.

ReNu Multi-Purpose. (Bausch & Lomb) Isotonic soln. w/sodium Cl, sodium borate, boric acid, poloxamine, polyaminopropyl biguanide 0.00005%, EDTA. Soln. Bot. 118 ml, 237 ml, 355 ml. *otc.*
Use: Contact lens care.

ReNu Saline. (Bausch & Lomb) Isotonic buffered soln. of sodium Cl, boric acid, polyaminopropyl biguanide 0.00003%, EDTA. Soln. Bot. 355 ml. *otc.*
Use: Contact lens care.

ReNu Thermal Enzymatic Cleaner. (Bausch & Lomb) Subtilisin, sodium carbonate, sodium Cl, boric acid. Tab. 16s. *otc.*
Use: Contact lens care.

ReoPro. (Eli Lilly) Abciximab 2 mg/ml. Inj. Vial 5 ml. *Rx.*
Use: Antiplatelet, monoclonal antibody (antithrombotic).

repaglinide.
Use: Antidiabetic.
See: Prandin, Tab. (Novo Nordisk).

Repan. (Everett Laboratories) Butalbital 50 mg, caffeine 40 mg, acetaminophen 325 mg/Tab. Bot. 100s. *Rx.*
Use: Analgesic, hypnotic, sedative.

Repan CF. (Everett Laboratories) Acetaminophen 650 mg, butalbital 50 mg/Tab. Bot. 100s. *Rx.*
Use: Analgesic combination.

•**repirinast.** (reh-PIRE-ih-nast) USAN.
Use: Antiallergic; antiasthmatic.

Replens. (Warner Lambert) Purified water, glycerin, mineral oil, methylparaben. Gel. Appl. 3, 8 pre-filled. *otc.*
Use: Vaginal agent.

Replete Liquid. (Clintec Nutrition) K caseinate, Ca caseinate, maltodextrin, sucrose, corn oil, lecithin, vitamins A, B_1, B_2, B_3, B_5, B_6, B_{12}, C, D, E, K, folic acid, biotin, choline, Ca, Cl, Cu, Fe, I, Mg, Mn, P, Zn. In 250 ml. *otc.*
Use: Nutritional supplement.

Reposans-10. (Wesley Pharmacal) Chlordiazepoxide HCl 10 mg/Cap. Bot. 1000s. *c-IV.*
Use: Anxiolytic.

Reprieve. (Mayer) Caffeine 32 mg, salicylamide 225 mg, vitamin B_1 50 mg, homatropine methylbromide 0.5 mg/ Tab. Bot. 8s, 16s. *Rx.*
Use: Analgesic combination.

•**repromicin.** (rep-ROW-MY-sin) USAN.
Use: Anti-infective.

Repronex. (Ferring) FSH activity 75 IU or 150 IU, luteinizing hormone (LH) activity 75 IU or 150 IU, lactose. Inj. Box 1 or 5 Vials. *Rx.*
Use: Ovulation inducer.

•**reproterol hydrochloride.** (rep-ROW-TEE-role) USAN.
Use: Bronchodilator.

Reptilase-R. (Abbott Diagnostics) Diagnostic for the investigation of fibrin formation and disturbances in fibrin formation due to causes other than thrombin inhibition.
Use: Diagnostic aid.

Requa's Charcoal Tablets. (Requa) Wood charcoal 10 gr/Tab. Pkg. 50s. Can 125s. *otc.*
Use: Antiflatulent.

Requip. (SmithKline Beecham) Ropinirole HCl 0.25 mg, 0.5 mg, 1 mg, 2 mg, 5 mg, lactose. Tab. Bot. 30s, 100s. *Rx.*
Use: Antiparkinson agent.

Resa. (Vita Elixir) Reserpine 0.25 mg/ Tab. *Rx.*
Use: Antihypertensive.

Resaid. (Geneva Pharm) Phenylpropanolamine HCl 75 mg, chlorpheniramine maleate 12 mg/Cap. Bot. 100s, 1000s. *Rx.*
Use: Antihistamine, decongestant.

Resaid S.R. (Geneva Pharm) Phenylpropanolamine HCl 75 mg, chlorpheniramine maleate 12 mg/SR Cap. Bot. 100s, 1000s. *Rx.*
Use: Antihistamine, decongestant.

Rescaps-D S.R. (Geneva Pharm) Phenylpropanolamine HCl 75 mg, caramiphen edisylate 40 mg/Cap. Bot. 100s. *Rx.*
Use: Antitussive, decongestant.

Rescon Capsules. (ION Laboratories) Pseudoephedrine 120 mg, chlorpheniramine maleate 12 mg/TR Cap. Bot. 100s. *Rx.*
Use: Antihistamine, decongestant.

Rescon-DM. (ION Laboratories) Dextromethorphan HBr 10 mg, pseudoephedrine HCl 30 mg, chlorpheniramine maleate 2 mg, sugar free. Liq. Bot. 120 ml. *otc.*
Use: Antihistamine, antitussive, decongestant.

Rescon-ED. (ION Laboratories) Chlorpheniramine maleate 8 mg, pseudoephedrine HCl 120 mg/Cap. Bot. 100s. *Rx.*
Use: Antihistamine, decongestant.

Rescon-GG Capsules. (ION Laboratories) Pseudoephedrine HCl 120 mg, chlorpheniramine maleate 8 mg/Cap. Bot. 100s. *otc.*
Use: Antihistamine, decongestant.

Rescon-GG Liquid. (ION Laboratories) Phenylephrine HCl 5 mg, guaifenesin 100 mg/5 ml Bot. 4 oz. *otc.*
Use: Decongestant, expectorant.

Rescon JR. (ION Laboratories) Pseudoephedrine HCl 60 mg, chlorpheniramine maleate 4 mg/SR Cap. Bot. 100s. *Rx.*
Use: Antihistamine, decongestant.

Rescon Liquid. (ION Laboratories) Phenylpropanolamine HCl 12.5 mg, chlorpheniramine maleate 2 mg/5 ml. Bot. 120 ml, 473 ml. *otc.*
Use: Antihistamine, decongestant.

Rescriptor. (Pharmacia & Upjohn) Delavirdine mesylate 100 mg, lactose. Tab. Bot. 360s. *Rx.*
Use: Antiviral.

Resectisol. (McGaw) Mannitol soln. 5 g/ 1000 ml in distilled water (275 mOsm/ L.). In 2000 ml. *Rx.*
Use: Irrigant, genitourinary.

Reserpaneed. (Hanlon) Reserpine 0.25 mg/Tab. Bot. 100s, 1000s. *Rx.*
Use: Antihypertensive.

•**reserpine,** (reh-SER-peen) U.S.P. 23.
Use: Antihypertensive.
See: Arcum R-S, Tab. (Arcum).
Broserpine, Tab. (Brothers).
De Serpa, Tab. (De Leon).
Elserpine, Tab. (Canright).
Maso-Serpine, Tab. (Mason).

Raurine, Tab. (Westerfield).
Reserpaneed, Tab. (Hanlon).
Serpasil Preps. (Novartis).
Sertabs, Tab. (Table Rock).
T-Serp, Tab. (Tennessee Pharmaceutic).
Vio-Serpine, Tab. (Solvay).
Zepine, Tab. (Foy).

reserpine w/combinations.
See: Demi-Regroton, Tab. (Rhone-Poulenc Rorer).
Diupres, Tab. (Merck).
Harbolin, Tab. (Arcum).
Hydromox R, Tab. (ESI Lederle Generics).
Hydropres-25 or -50, Tab. (Merck).
Hydroserp, Tab. (Zenith Goldline).
Hydroserpine, Tab. (Geneva Pharm).
Hydrotensin-50, Tab. (Merz).
Mallopress, Tab. (Roberts Pharm).
Metatensin, Tab. (Hoechst Marion Roussel).
Naquival, Tab. (Schering Plough).
Regroton, Tab. (Rhone-Poulenc Rorer).
Renese-R, Tab. (Pfizer).
Salutensin, Tab. (Bristol-Myers).
Ser-Ap-Es, Tab. (Novartis).
Serpasil-Apresoline, Tab. (Novartis).
Serpasil-Esidrix, Tab. (Novartis).
Unipres, Tab. (Solvay).

reserpine and chlorothiazide tablets.
Use: Antihypertensive.

reserpine and hydrochlorothiazide tablets. (Various Mfr.) Hydrochlorothiazide 25 mg or 50 mg, reserpine 0.125 mg/Tab. Bot. 100s, 1000s. *Rx.*
Use: Antihypertensive.

reserpine, hydralazine hydrochloride and hydrochlorothiazide.
Use: Antihypertensive.

Resinol Medicinal Ointment. (Mentholatum) Zinc oxide 12%, calamine 6%, resorcinol 2% in a lanolin and petrolatum base. Jar 3.5 oz, 1.25 oz. *otc.*
Use: Dermatologic, protectant.

resin uptake kit with liothyronine i-125 buffer solution.
See: Thyrostat-3 (Bristol-Myers Squibb).

resins, antacid.
See: Polyamine methylene Resins. .

•**resocortol butyrate.** (reh-so-CORE-tole BYOO-tih-rate) USAN.
Use: Corticosteroid; anti-inflammatory, topical.

Resol. (Wyeth Ayerst) Sodium 50 mEq, potassium 20 mEq, Cl 50 mEq, citrate 34 mEq, calcium 4 mEq, magnesium 4 mEq, phosphate 5 mEq, glucose 20 g/L. Contains 80 calories/L. Ctn. 32 fl oz. *Rx.*
Use: Fluid, electrolyte replacement.

Resolve/GP Daily Cleaner. (Allergan) Buffered solution with cocoamphocarboxyglycinate, sodium lauryl sulfate, hexylene glycol, alkyl ether sulfate, fatty acid amide surfactant cleaning agents, preservative free. Soln. Bot. 30 ml. *otc.*
Use: Contact lens care.

Resonium-A. (Sanofi Winthrop) Sodium polystyrene sulfonate. *Rx.*
Use: Potassium removing resin.

resorcin.
See: Resorcinol (Various Mfr.).

•**resorcinol.** (reh-SORE-sih-nole) U.S.P. 23.
Use: Keratolytic.

resorcinol and sulfur lotion.
Use: Antifungal, parasiticide, scabicide.

resorcinol w/combinations.
See: Acnomel, Cake, Cream. (SmithKline Beecham Pharmaceuticals).
Bicozene, Cream (Ex-Lax).
Black and White Ointment (Schering Plough).
Clearasil, Stick (Procter & Gamble Company).
Lanacane Creme (Combe).
Mazon, Oint. (SmithKline Beecham Pharmaceuticals).
RA Lot. (Medco).
Rezamid Lot. (Del Pharmaceuticals).

•**resorcinol monoacetate.** U.S.P. 23.
Use: Antiseborrheic, keratolytic.
See: Euresol, Liq. (Knoll Pharmaceuticals).
W/Salicylic acid, ethyl alcohol, castor oil.
W/Salicylic acid, LCD, betanaphthol, castor oil, isopropyl alcohol.
See: Neomark, Liq. (C & M Pharmacal).

resorcinolphthalein sodium.
See: Fluorescein Sodium, U.S.P. 23. (Various Mfr.).
W/Oil. Resorcinol monoacetate 1.5%, salicylic acid 1.5%, castor oil 1.5%, ethyl alcohol 81%. Bot. 8 fl oz.
Use: Antiseborrheic, topical.

Resource. (Novartis) Ca and Na caseinates, soy protein isolate 37 g, sugar, hydrolyzed cornstarch 140 g, corn oil, soy lecithin 37 g, Na 890 mg, K 1600 mg, A, B_1, B_2, B_3, B_5, B_6, B_{12}, C, D, E, K, Ca, P, I, Fe, Mg, Cu, Zn, Mn, Cl, gluten free, vanilla, chocolate, strawberry flavor. Liq. Bot. 237 ml. *otc.*
Use: Nutritional supplement.

Resource Instant Crystals. (Novartis) Vanilla flavor: maltodextrin, sucrose,

hydrogenated soy oil, sodium caseinate, calcium caseinate, soy protein isolate, potassium citrate, polyglycerol esters of fatty acids, artificial flavors, vitamins and minerals. Instant Crystals 1.5 oz. or 2 oz. packets. *otc.*
Use: Nutritional supplement.

Resource Plus. (Novartis) Ca and Na caseinates, soy protein isolate 54.9 g, maltodextrin, sucrose 200 g, corn oil, lecithin 53.3 g, Na 899 mg, K 1740 mg, A, B_1, B_2, B_3, B_5, B_6, B_{12}, C, D, E, K, biotin, choline, Ca, P, I, Fe, Mg, Cu, Zn, Cl, Mn, gluten free, vanilla, chocolate, strawberry flavor. Liq. Bot. 8 oz. *otc.*
Use: Nutritional supplement.

Respa-1st. (Respa) Pseudoephedrine HCl 60 mg, guaifenesin 600 mg. SR Tab. Bot. 100s. *Rx.*
Use: Decongestant, expectorant.

Respa-DM. (Respa) Dextromethorphan HBr 30 mg, guaifenesin 600 mg. SR Tab. Bot. 100s. *Rx.*
Use: Antitussive, expectorant.

Respa-GF. (Respa) Guaifenesin 600 mg, lactose. SR Tab. Bot. 100s. *Rx.*
Use: Expectorant.

Respahist. (Respa). Pseudoephedrine HCl 60 mg, brompheniramine maleate 6 mg/SR Cap. Bot 100s. *Rx.*
Use: Antihistamine, decongenstant.

Respaire-60 SR. (Laser) Pseudoephedrine HCl 60 mg, guaifenesin 200 mg/ S.R. Cap. Bot. 100s, 1000s. *Rx.*
Use: Decongestant, expectorant.

Respaire-120 SR. (Laser) Pseudoephedrine HCl 120 mg, guaifenesin 250 mg/ SR Cap. Bot. 100s, 1000s. *Rx.*
Use: Decongestant, expectorant.

Respalor. (Bristol-Myers) Protein 75 g, carbohyrate 146 g, fat 70 g, Na 1248 mg, K 1456 mg, Fe 12.5 mg, cal/L 1498. Lactose free. Vanilla flavor. With appropriate vitamins and minerals. Liq. Bot. 237 ml. *otc.*
Use: Nutritional supplement.

Respbid. (Boehringer Ingelheim) Theophylline 250 mg or 500 mg/Tab. Bot. 100s. *Rx.*
Use: Bronchodilator.

RespiGam. (MedImmune) RSV immunoglobulin (human) 2500 mg, sucrose 5%, albumin (human) 1% w/sodium 1 to 1.5 mEq/50 ml. Preservative free. I.V. Vial 2500 mg/50 ml. *Rx.*
Use: Immunization.

Respihaler Decadron Phosphate. (Merck).
See: Decadron phosphate, respihaler (Merck).

Respiracult. (Orion Diagnostica) Culture test for group A beta-hemolytic streptococci. In 10s.
Use: Diagnostic aid.

Respiralex. (Orion Diagnostica) Latex agglutination test to detect group A streptococci in throat and nasopharynx. Kit 1s.
Use: Diagnostic aid.

respiratory syncytial virus immune globulin (human) (RSV-IG).
Use: Prophylaxis against respiratory tract infection. [Orphan drug]
See: RespiGam, Inj. (MedImmune).

respiratory syncytial virus immune globulin intravenous (human) (RSV-IVIG).
Use: Respiratory syncytial virus immune serum.
See: RespiGam (MedImmune).

Rest Easy. (Walgreens) Acetaminophen 1000 mg, pseudoephedrine HCl 60 mg, dextromethorphan HBr 30 mg, doxylamine succinate 7.5 mg/30 ml. Bot. 6 oz, 16 oz. *otc.*
Use: Analgesic, antihistamine, antitussive, decongestant.

Restore. (Inagra) Psyllium hydrophilic mucilloid fiber 3.4 g/12 g dose, orange flavor, saccharin, sucrose. Pow. 390 g, 538 g. Also available sugar free with aspartame, phenylalanine 30 mg/tsp, saccharin. Pow. 300 g, 425 g. *otc.*
Use: Laxative.

Restoril. (Novartis) Temazepam 7.5 mg, lactose. Cap. Bot. 100s. ControlPak 25s, UD 100s. *c-iv.*
Use: Hypnotic, sedative.

Retavase. (Boehringer Mannheim) Reteplase 10.8 IU (18.8 mg)/Pow. for inj. Kit. *Rx.*
Use: Management of acute myocardial infarction.

•**reteplase.** USAN.
Use: Management of acute myocardial infarction, plasminogen activator.
See: Retavase, Pow. for inj. (Boehringer Mannheim).

Retin-A Cream. (Ortho McNeil) Tretinoin 0.1%, 0.05% or 0.025%. Tube 20 g, 45 g. *Rx.*
Use: Dermatologic, acne.

Retin-A Gel. (Ortho McNeil) Tretinoin 0.01% or 0.025%, alcohol 90%. Tube 15 g, 45 g. *Rx.*
Use: Dermatologic, acne.

Retin-A Liquid. (Ortho McNeil) Tretinoin (retinoic acid, Vitamin A acid) 0.05%, polyethylene glycol 400, butylated hy-

droxytoluene and alcohol 55%. Bot. 28 ml. *Rx.*
Use: Dermatologic, acne.

Retin-A Micro. (Ortho McNeil) Tretinoin 0.1%, glycerin, propylene glycol, benzyl alcohol, EDTA. Gel. Tube 20 g, 45 g. *Rx.*
Use: Dermatologic, acne.

retinoic acid. Tretinoin, U.S.P. 23.
Use: Keratolytic.
See: Retin A Prods. (Ortho McNeil).

retinoic acid, 9-cis.
Use: Acute promyelocytic leukemia. [Orphan drug]

retinoin.
Use: Squamous metaplasia of the ocular surface epithelia with mucus deficiency and keratinization. [Orphan drug]

Retinol. (NBTY) Vitamin A 100,000 IU, glycol stearate, mineral oil, propylene glycol, lanolin oil, propylene glycol stearate SE, lanolin alcohol, retinol, parabens, EDTA. Cream. Tube 60 g. *otc.*
Use: Emollient.

Retinol-A. (Young Again Products) Vitamin A palmitate 300,000 IU/30 g. Cream. 60 g. *otc.*
Use: Emollient.

Retrovir. (GlaxoWellcome) Zidovudine **Tab.:** 300 mg. Bot. 60s. **Cap:** 100 mg/Cap. Bot. 100s. **Syrup:** 50 mg/5 ml. Bot. 240 ml. **Inj:** 10 mg/ml. Vial 20 ml. *Rx.*
Use: Antiviral.

Reversol. (Organon Teknika) Edrophonium chloride 10 mg/ml. Inj. Vial. 10 ml. *Rx.*
Use: Muscle stimulant.

Revex. (Ohmeda Pharmaceuticals) Nalmefene 100 mcg/ml or 1 mg/ml. Inj. **100 mcg/ml:** Amp 1 ml; **1 mg/ml:** Amp 2 ml. *Rx.*
Use: Narcotic antagonist, antidote.

Rēv-Eyes. (Storz/Lederle) Dapiprazole HCl 25 mg. Pow. Vial. 5 ml. *Rx.*
Use: Alpha-adrenergic blocker, ophthalmic.

ReVia. (DuPont Merck Pharmaceuticals) Naltrexone HCl 50 mg/Tab. Bot. 50s. *Rx.*
Use: Antagonist, narcotic.

Revs Caffeine T.D. Capsules. (Eon Labs Manufacturing) Caffeine 250 mg/Cap. Bot. 100s, 1000s. *otc.*
Use: CNS stimulant.

Rexahistine. (Econo Med Pharmaceuticals) Phenylephrine HCl 5 mg, chlorpheniramine maleate 1 mg, menthol 1 mg, sodium bisulfite 0.1%, alcohol 5%/5 ml. Bot. Gal. *otc.*
Use: Antihistamine, decongestant.

Rexahistine DH. (Econo-Rx) Codeine phosphate 10 mg, phenylephrine HCl 10 mg, chlorpheniramine maleate 2 mg, menthol 1 mg, alcohol 5%/5 ml. Bot. gal. *c-v.*
Use: Antihistamine, antitussive, decongestant.

Rexahistine Expectorant. (Econo-Rx) Codeine phosphate 10 mg, phenylephrine HCl 10 mg, chlorpheniramine maleate 2 mg, guaifenesin 100 mg, menthol 1 mg, alcohol 5%/5 ml. Bot. Gal. *c-v.*
Use: Antihistamine, antitussive, decongestant, expectorant.

Rexigen. (ION Laboratories) Phendimetrazine tartrate 35 mg/Tab. Bot. 100s. *c-III.*
Use: Anorexiant.

Rexigen Forte Capsules. (ION Laboratories) Phendimetrazine tartrate 105 mg/SR Cap. Bot. 100s. *c-III.*
Use: Anorexiant.

Rezamid Lotion. (Summers) Sulfur 5%, resorcinol 2%, SD-40 alcohol 28%. Lot. 56.7 ml. *otc.*
Use: Dermatologic, acne.

Rezulin. (Parke-Davis) Troglitazone 200 mg, 300 mg, 400 mg/Tab. Bot. 30s, 90s, UD 100s (200 mg, 400 mg), 60s, 120s (300 mg). *Rx.*
Use: Antidiabetic.

Rezine. (Marnel) Hydroxyzine HCl 10 mg or 25 mg. Tab. Bot. 100s. *Rx.*
Use: Anxiolytic.

RF Latex Test. (Laboratory Diagnostics) Rapid latex agglutination test for the qualitative screening and semi-quantitative determination of rheumatoid factor. Kit 100s.
Use: Diagnostic aid.

R-Frone. (Serono Labs)
See: Interferon Beta (Recombinant).

R-Gel. (Healthline Labs) Capsaicin 0.025%, EDTA. Gel. Tube 15 g, 30 g. *otc.*
Use: Analgesic, topical.

R-Gen. (Galderma) Purified water, amphoteric 2, hydrolyzed animal protein, lauramine oxide, methylparaben, benzalkonium Cl, tetrasodium, EDTA, propylparaben, fragrance. Bot. 8 oz. *otc.*
Use: Dermatologic, hair.

R-Gen. (Zenith Goldline) Iodinated glycerol 60 mg/5 ml, alcohol 21.75%. Elixir. Bot. pt.

Use: Expectorant.

R-Gene 10. (Pharmacia & Upjohn) Arginine HCl 10% (950 mOsm/L) with Cl ion 47.5 mEq/100 ml. Inj. 300 ml. *Rx.*
Use: Diagnostic aid, pituitary (growth hormone) function test.

R-HCTZ-H. (ESI Lederle Generics) Reserpine 0.1 mg, hydrochlorothiazide 15 mg, hydralazine HCl 25 mg/Tab. Bot. 100s, 500s. *Rx.*
Use: Antihypertensive.

Rheaban Maximum Strength. (Pfizer) Activated attapulgite 750 mg. Capl. Pkg. 12s. *otc.*
Use: Antidiarrheal.

Rheomacrodex. (Medisan) Dextran 40 10% in sodium Cl 0.9% or in dextrose 5%. Soln. Bot. 500 ml. *Rx.*
Use: Plasma expander.

Rheumatex. (Wampole Laboratories) Latex agglutination test for the qualitative detection and quantitative determination of rheumatoid factor in serum. Kit 100s.
Use: Diagnostic aid.

rheumatoid factor tests.
See: Rheumanosticon Dri-Dot (Organon Teknika).

Rheumaton. (Wampole Laboratories) Two-minute hemagglutination slide test for the qualitative and quantitative determination of rheumatoid factor in serum or synovial fluid. Test kit 20s, 50s, 150s.
Use: Diagnostic aid.

Rheumatrex Dose Pack. (ESI Lederle Generics) Methotrexate 2.5 mg. Tab. Pkg. 5, 7.5, 10, 12.5, 15 mg/week dose packs. *Rx.*
Use: Antipsoriatic.

Rhinall Drops. (Scherer) Phenylephrine HCl 0.25%, sodium bisulfite. Bot. oz. *otc.*
Use: Decongestant.

Rhinall Spray. (Scherer) Phenylephrine HCl 0.25%. Bot. oz. *otc.*
Use: Decongestant.

Rhinall 10. (Scherer) Phenylephrine HCl 0.2%. Drop. Bot. oz. *otc.*
Use: Decongestant.

Rhinatate. (Major) Phenylephrine tannate 25 mg, chlorpheniramine tannate 8 mg, pyrilamine tannate 25 mg/Tab. Bot. 100s, 250s. *Rx.*
Use: Antihistamine, decongestant.

Rhinocort. (Astra) Budesonide 32 mcg/actuation (200 sprays). Can 7 g. *Rx.*
Use: Corticosteroid, nasal.

Rhinolar-EX. (McGregor) Phenylpropanolamine HCl 75 mg, chlorpheniramine maleate 8 mg/SR Cap. Dye free. Bot. 60s. *Rx.*
Use: Antihistamine, decongestant.

Rhinolar-EX 12. (McGregor) Phenylpropanolamine HCl 75 mg, chlorpheniramine maleate 12 mg/SR Cap. Dye free. Bot. 60s. *Rx.*
Use: Antihistamine, decongestant.

Rhinosyn. (Great Southern) Pseudoephedrine HCl 60 mg, chlorpheniramine maleate 4 mg, alcohol 0.45%, sucrose. Liq. Bot. 120 ml, 473 ml. *otc.*
Use: Antihistamine, cecongestant.

Rhinosyn-DM Liquid. (Great Southern) Pseudoephedrine HCl 30 mg, chlorpheniramine maleate 2 mg, dextromethorphan HBr 15 mg, alcohol 1.4%, sucrose. Bot. 120 ml. *otc.*
Use: Antihistamine, antitussive, decongestant.

Rhinosyn-DMX Syrup. (Great Southern) Dextromethorphan HBr 15 mg, guaifenesin 100 mg, alcohol 1.4%. Bot. 120 ml. *otc.*
Use: Antitussive, expectorant.

Rhinosyn-PD Liquid. (Great Southern) Pseudoephedrine HCl 30 mg, chlorpheniramine maleate 2 mg. Liq. Bot. 120 ml. *otc.*
Use: Antihistamine, decongestant.

Rhinosyn-X Liquid. (Great Southern) Pseudoephedrine HCl 30 mg, dextromethorphan HBr 10 mg, guaifenesin 100 mg, alcohol 7.5%. Bot. 120 ml. *otc.*
Use: Antitussive, decongestant, expectorant.

rhodanate.
See: Potassium Thiocyanate.

rhodanide. More commonly Rhodanate, same as thiocyanate.
See: Potassium thiocyanate.

•**rh_o (d) immune globulin.** (RH_0D ih-MYOON GLAB-byoo-lin) U.S.P. 23. *Formerly Rh_o (D) Immune Globulin.*
Use: Immunizination.
See: Gamulin Rh, Vial (Centeon).
Mini-Gamulin Rh (Centeon).
$MICRh_0GAM$ (Ortho McNeil).
$BayRh_0D$ (Bayer Corp).
RhoGAM (Ortho McNeil).
WinRho SD (Univax Biologics).

rh_o(d) immune globulin. (RH_0D ih-MYOON GLAB-byoo-lin) *Formerly RH_o Immune Human Globulin.*
Use: Immune thrombocytopenic purpura, immunizing agent (passive). [Orphan drug]
See: WinRho SD (Univax Biologics).

RhoGAM. (Ortho Diagnostics) Rh_o (D) immune globulin (human). Single-dose vial Pkg. 5s; Prefilled syringe Pkg. 5s, 25s. *Rx.*
Use: Immunization.

Rhuli Gel. (Rydelle) Phenylcarbinol 2%, menthol 0.3%, camphor 0.3%, SD alcohol 23A 31%. Gel 60 g. *otc.*
Use: Dermatologic, poison ivy.

Rhuli Spray. (Rydelle) Phenylcarbinol 0.67%, calamine 4.7%, menthol 0.025%, camphor 0.25%, benzocaine 1.15%, alcohol 28.8%. Aerosol 120 g. *otc.*
Use: Dermatologic, poison ivy.

Rhythmin. (Sidmak) Procainamide 250 mg or 500 mg/SR Tab. Bot. 100s, 500s, 1000s. *Rx.*
Use: Antiarrhythmic.

•**ribaminol.** (rye-BAM-ih-nahl) USAN.
Use: Memory adjuvant.

•**ribavirin,** (rye-buh-VIE-rin) U.S.P. 23.
Use: Antiviral. [Orphan drug]
See: Virazole, Inj. (ICN Pharmaceuticals).

•**riboflavin,** (RYE-boh-FLAY-vin) U.S.P. 23.
Use: Vitamin (enzyme co-factor).
W/Nicotinamide. (Eli Lilly) Riboflavin 5 mg, nicotinamide 200 mg/ml Amp. 1 ml, Box 100s.
Use: IM, IV; Vitamin B therapy.
W/Vitamins.
See: Vitamin Preparations.

•**riboflavin 5'-phosphate sodium,** (RYE-boh-FLAY-vin 5'-FOSS-fate so-dee-oum) U.S.P. 23.
Use: Vitamin.

•**riboprine.** (RYE-boe-PREEN) USAN.
Use: Antineoplastic.

Ribozyme Injection. (Fellows) Riboflavin-5-Phosphate Sodium 50 mg/ml Vial 10 ml. *Rx.*

ricin (blocked) conjugated murine mca. (Immunogen)
Use: Antineoplastic. [Orphan drug]

ricin (blocked) conjugated murine moab.
Use: Antineoplastic. [Orphan drug]

ricinoleate sodium.
See: Preceptin, Gel (Ortho McNeil).

Ricolon Solution. (Sanofi Winthrop) Ricolon concentrate. *Rx.*
Use: Leucocytotic preparation.

RID. (Pfizer) Piperonyl butoxide 3%, pyrethrins 0.3%, petroleum distillate 1.2%, benzyl alcohol 2.4%. Bot. 2 oz, 4 oz. *otc.*
Use: Pediculicide.

Ridaura. (SmithKline Beecham Pharmaceuticals) Auranofin 3 mg/Cap. Bot. 60s. *Rx.*
Use: Antirheumatic.

Ridenol. (R.I.D.) Acetaminophen 80 mg/5 ml. Syr. Bot. 120 ml. *otc.*
Use: Analgesic.

Rid Lice Control Spray. (Pfizer) Synthetic pyrethroids 0.5%, related compounds 0.065%, aromatic petroleum hydrocarbons 0.664%. Can 5 oz. *otc.*
Use: Pediculicide.

Rid Lice Elimination System. (Pfizer) Rid lice killing shampoo, nit removal comb, Rid lice control spray and instruction booklet/unit. *otc.*
Use: Pediculicide.

Rid Lice Shampoo-Kit. (Pfizer) Pyrethrins 0.3%, piperonyl butoxide 3%. Bot. 2 oz, 4 oz. *otc.*
Use: Pediculicide.

Ridaura Capsules. (SmithKline Beecham Pharmaceuticals) Auranofin 3 mg/Cap. Bot. 60s. *Rx.*
Use: Antirheumatic.

•**ridogrel.** (RYE-doe-grell) USAN.
Use: Thromboxane synthetase inhibitor.

•**rifabutin.** (RIFF-uh-BYOO-tin) U.S.P. 23.
Use: Anti-infective (antimycobacterial), MAC disease [Orphan drug]
See: Mycobutin.

Rifadin. (Hoechst Marion Roussel) Rifampin. **150 mg/Cap.:** Bot. 30s. **300 mg/Cap.:** Bot. 30s, 60s, 100s. **600 mg/Inj.:** Vials. *Rx.*
Use: Antituberculous.

Rifamate. (Hoechst Marion Roussel) Rifampin 300 mg, isoniazid 150 mg/Cap. Bot. 60s. *Rx.*
Use: Antituberculous.

•**rifametane.** (RIFF-ah-met-ane) USAN.
Use: Anti-infective.

•**rifamexil.** (riff-ah-MEX-ill) USAN.
Use: Anti-infective.

•**rifamide.** (RIFF-am-ide) USAN.
Use: Anti-infective.

•**rifampin.** (RIFF-am-pin) U.S.P. 23.
Use: Anti-infective.
See: Rifadin, Cap, Inj. (Hoechst Marion Roussel).
Rifater, Tab. (Hoechst Marion Roussel).
Rimactane, Cap. (Novartis).

rifampin and isoniazid capsules.
Use: Anti-infective (tuberculostatic).

rifampin, isoniazid, pyrazinamide.
Use: Anti-infective (tuberculostatic). [Orphan drug]

Rifapentine.
Use: Pulmonary tuberculosis; mycobacterium avium complex in AIDS patients. [Orphan drug]

•**rifapentine.** (RIFF-ah-pen-teen) USAN.
Use: Anti-infective.

Rifater. (Hoechst Marion Roussel) Rifampin 120 mg, isoniazid 50 mg, pyrazinamide 300 mg. Tab. 60s, UD 100s. *Rx.*
Use: Antituberculous.

•**rifaximin.** (riff-AX-ih-min) USAN.
Use: Anti-infective.

r-IFN-beta. (Biogen)
See: Interferon Beta (Recombinant).

RIG.
Use: Immunization, rabies.
See: Bayrab (Bayer).
Imogam (Merieux).

Rilutek. (Rhone-Poulenc Rorer) Riluzole 50 mg/Tab. *Rx.*
Use: Amyotrophic lateral sclerosis agent.

•**riluzole.** (RILL-you-zole) USAN.
Use: Amyotrophic lateral sclerosis agent. [Orphan drug]
See: Rilutek, Tab. (Rhone-Poulenc Rorer).

Rimactane. (Novartis) Rifampin 300 mg/Cap. Bot. 30s, 60s, 100s. *Rx.*
Use: Antituberculous.

Rimadyl. (Roche Laboratories) *Rx.*
Use: Analgesic, NSAID.
See: Carprofen.

•**rimantadine hydrochloride.** (rih-MAN-tuh-deen) USAN.
Use: Antiviral.
See: Flumadine, Tab., Syr. (Forest Pharmaceutical).

•**rimcazole hydrochloride.** (RIM-kazz-OLE) USAN.
Use: Antipsychotic.

•**rimexolone.** (rih-MEX-oh-lone) USAN.
Use: Anti-inflammatory.
See: Vexol, Susp. (Alcon Laboratories).

•**rimiterol hydrobromide.** (RIH-mih-TER-ole) USAN.
Use: Bronchodilator.

Rimso-50. (Research Industries) Dimethyl sulfoxide in a 50% aqueous soln. Bot. 50 ml. *Rx.*
Use: Urinary tract agent.

Rinade. (Econo Med Pharmaceuticals) Chlorpheniramine maleate 8 mg, phenylephrine HCl 20 mg, methscopolamine nitrate 2.5 mg/Cap. Bot. 120s. *Rx.*
Use: Anticholinergic, antihistamine, decongestant.

Rinade-B.I.D. (Econo Med Pharmaceuticals) Chlorpheniramine maleate 8 mg, pseudoephedrine HCl 120 mg/SR Cap. Bot. 100s. *Rx.*
Use: Antihistamine, decongestant.

ringer's-dextrose injection. (Various Mfr.) Dextrose 50 g/l, Na 147, K 4, C 4.5, Cl 156. 500, 1000 ml. *Rx.*
Use: Nutritional supplement, parenteral.

•**ringer's injection.** U.S.P. 23.
Use: Fluid, electrolyte replacement; irrigant, ophthalmic.
W/Dextrose. (Bayer Corp) 5% soln. Bot. 1000 ml.

ringer's injection. (Abbott Laboratories) 250 ml, 500 ml, 1000 ml; (Invenex) 250 ml, 500 ml, 1000 ml; Abbo-Vac glass or flexible containers, Vial 50 ml Pkg. 25s. (Eli Lilly) Amp. 20 ml, Pkg. 6s. (Bayer Corp) Bot. 500 ml, 1000 ml.
Use: Fluid, electrolyte replacement; irrigant.

ringer's injection, lactated.
Use: Fluid, electrolyte replacement.

ringer's irrigation. (Various Mfr.) Sodium chloride 0.86 g, potassium chloride 0.03 g, calcium chloride 0.033 g/100 ml. Bot. 1 L. *Rx.*
Use: Irrigant, ophthalmic.

Riopan. (Whitehall Robins) Magaldrate 540 mg, sodium 0.1 mg/5 ml. Bot. 6 oz, 12 oz. Individual Cup 30 ml each. *otc.*
Use: Antacid.

Riopan Plus Double Strength Suspension. (Whitehall Robins) Magaldrate 1080 mg, simethicone 40 mg/5 ml. Bot. 360 ml. *otc.*
Use: Antacid, antiflatulent.

Riopan Plus Double Strength Tablets. (Whitehall Robins) Magaldrate 1080 mg, simethicone 20 mg. Chew. Tab. Bot. 60s. *otc.*
Use: Antacid, antiflatulent.

Riopan Plus Tablets. (Whitehall Robins) Magaldrate 480 mg, simethicone 20 mg. Chew. Tab. Bot. 50s, 100s. *otc.*
Use: Antacid, antiflatulent.

•**rioprostil.** (RYE-oh-PRAHS-till) USAN.
Use: Gastric antisecretory.

•**ripazepam.** (rip-AZE-eh-pam) USAN.
Use: Anxiolytic.

•**risedronate sodium.** (riss-ED-row-nate) USAN.
Use: Regulator (calcium).

•**rismorelin porcine.** (riss-more-ELL-in PORE-sine) USAN.
Use: Hormone, growth hormone-releasing.

•**risocaine.** (RIZZ-oh-cane) USAN.
Use: Anesthetic, local.

•**risotilide hydrochloride.** (rih-SO-tih-LIDE) USAN.
Use: Cardiovascular agent (antiarrhythmic).

Risperdal. (Janssen) Risperidone 1 mg, 2 mg, 3 mg, 4 mg. Tab. Bot. 60s, 500s, blister pack 100s. Risperidone 1 mg/ml/Oral Soln. Bot. 100 ml w/calibrated pipette. *Rx.*
Use: Antipsychotic.

•**risperidone.** (RISS-PURR-ih-dohn) USAN.
Use: Antipsychotic, neuroleptic.
See: Risperdal, Oral Soln. (Janssen).

•**ristianol phosphate.** (riss-TIE-ah-NOLE) USAN.
Use: Immunoregulator.

Ritalin Hydrochloride. (Novartis) Methylphenidate HCl. 5 mg, 10 mg, 20 mg. Tab. Bot. 100s. *c-II.*
Use: CNS stimulant.

Ritalin-SR. (Novartis) Methylphenidate HCl 20 mg/SR Tab. Bot. 100s. *c-II.*
Use: CNS stimulant.

•**ritanserin.** (rih-TAN-ser-in) USAN.
Use: Serotonin antagonist.

•**ritodrine.** (RIH-toe-DREEN) USAN.
Use: Muscle relaxant.
See: Yutopar, Inj. (Astra).

•**ritodrine hydrochloride,** (RIH-toe-dreen) U.S.P. 23.
Use: Muscle relaxant.

ritodrine hydrochloride. (Abbott Laboratories) Ritodrine HCl 10 mg/ml, 15 mg/ml or 0.3 mg/ml. **10 mg/ml:** Amp. 5 ml. **15 mg/ml:** Vial 10 ml. **0.3 mg/ml:** In 15% dextrose. LifeCare flexible container 500 ml. *Rx.*
Use: Uterine relaxant.

•**ritolukast.** (rih-tah-LOO-kast) USAN.
Use: Antiasthmatic (leukotriene antagonist).

•**ritonavir.** (rih-TON-a-veer) USAN.
Use: Antiviral.
See: Norvir, Cap., Susp. (Abbott Laboratories).

Rituxan. (IDEC Pharmaceuticals) Rituximab 10 mg/ml. Inj. Single-unit Vial 10 ml, 50 ml. *Rx.*
Use: Antineoplastic.

•**rituximab.** (rih-TUCK-sih-mab) USAN.
Use: Antineoplastic (microtubule inhibitor), monoclonal antibody.
See: Rituxan, Inj. (IDEC Pharmaceuticals).

•**rizatriptan benzoate.** (rye-zah-TRIP-tan BENZ-oh-ate) USAN.
Use: Antimigraine.

•**rizatriptan sulfate.** (rye-zah-TRIP-tan) USAN.
Use: Antimigraine.

RMS Suppositories. (Upsher-Smith Labs) Morphine sulfate 5 mg, 10 mg, 20 mg or 30 mg/Supp. Box 12s. *c-II.*
Use: Analgesic, narcotic.

Robafen. (Major) Guaifenesin 100 mg/5 ml, alcohol 3.5%. Syr. Bot. 118 ml, 240 ml, pt, gal. *otc.*
Use: Expectorant.

Robafen AC Cough. (Major) Guaifenesin 100 mg, codeine phosphate 10 mg/5 ml, alcohol 3.5%, parabens. Syrup. Bot. 473 ml. *c-v.*
Use: Antitussive; expectorant, narcotic.

Robafen CF. (Major) Phenylpropanolamine HCl 12.5 mg, dextromethorphan HBr 10 mg, guaifenesin 100 mg, alcohol 4.75%. Bot. 118 ml. *otc.*
Use: Antitussive, decongestant, expectorant.

Robafen DAC. (Major) Pseudoephedrine 30 mg, codeine phosphate 10 mg, guaifenesin 100 mg, alcohol 1.4%. Bot. Pt. *c-v.*
Use: Antitussive, decongestant, expectorant.

Robafen DM. (Major) Dextromethorphan HBr 10 mg, guaifenesin 100 mg/5 ml, alcohol 1.4%. Syrup. Bot. 473 ml. *otc.*
Use: Antitussive, expectorant.

robanul.
See: Robinul, Preps. (Robins).

RoBathol Bath Oil. (Pharmaceutical Specialties) Cottonseed oil, alkyl aryl polyether alcohol. Lanolin free. Bot. 240 ml, 480 ml, gal. *otc.*
Use: Dermatologic.

Robaxin. (Robins) Methocarbamol. **Tab.:** 500 mg, Bot. 100s, 500s, UD 100s. **Inj.:** 100 mg/ml of a 50% aqueous soln. of polyethylene glycol 300. Vial 10 ml. *Rx.*
Use: Muscle relaxant.

Robaxin-750. (Robins) Methocarbamol 750 mg/Tab. Bot. 100s, 500s, Dis-Co Pak 100s. *Rx.*
Use: Muscle relaxant.

Robaxisal. (Robins) Methocarbamol (Robaxin) 400 mg, aspirin 325 mg/Tab. Bot. 100s, 500s, Dis-Co pack 100s. *Rx.*
Use: Muscle relaxant, analgesic.

Robimycin. (Robins) Erythromycin 250 mg/Tab. Bot. 100s, 500s. *Rx.*
Use: Anti-infective, erythromycin.

Robinul. (Robins) Glycopyrrolate 1 mg/Tab. Bot. 100s, 500s. *Rx.*
Use: Anticholinergic.

Robinul Forte Tablets. (Robins) Glycopyrrolate 2 mg/Tab. Bot. 100s. *Rx.*
Use: Anticholinergic.

Robinul Injectable. (Robins) Glycopyrrolate 0.2 mg/ml, benzyl alcohol 0.9%. Vial 1 ml, 2 ml, 5 ml, 20 ml. *Rx.*
Use: Anticholinergic.

Robitussin. (Robins) Guaifenesin 100 mg/5 ml, alcohol 3.5%. Bot 1 oz, 4 oz, 8 oz, 1 pt, gal. UD 5 ml, 10 ml, 15 ml. *otc.*
Use: Expectorant.

Robitussin A-C. (Robins) Guaifenesin 100 mg, codeine phosphate 10 mg/5 ml, alcohol 3.5%, saccharin, sorbitol. Bot. 2 oz, 4 oz, pt, gal. *c-v.*
Use: Antitussive, expectorant.

Robitussin-CF. (Robins) Guaifenesin 100 mg, phenylpropanolamine HCl 12.5 mg, dextromethorphan HBr 10 mg/10 ml, alcohol 4.75%, saccharin, sorbitol. Syr. Bot. 4 oz, 8 oz, 12 oz, pt. *otc.*
Use: Antitussive, decongestant ,expectorant.

Robitussin Cold & Cough Liqui-Gels. (Robins) Guaifenesin 200 mg, pseudoephedrine HCl 30 mg, dextromethorphan HBr 10 mg, sorbitol. Cap. Bot. 20s. *otc.*
Use: Antitussive, expectorant, decongestant.

Robitussin Cough Calmers. (Robins) Dextromethorphan HBr 5 mg, corn syrup, sucrose, cherry flavor. Loz. Pkg. 16s. *otc.*
Use: Antitussive.

Robitussin Cough Drops. (Robins) Menthol 7.4 mg and 10 mg, eucalyptus oil, sucrose, corn syrup. Loz. Pkg. 9s, 25s, menthol 10 mg, eucalyptus oil, sucrose, corn syrup, honey-lemon flavor. Loz. Pkg. 9s, 25s. *otc.*
Use: Antitussive.

Robitussin-DAC. (Robins) Guaifenesin 100 mg, pseudoephedrine HCl 30 mg, codeine phosphate 10 mg/5 ml, alcohol 1.9%, saccharin, sorbitol. Syr. Bot. 4 oz, pt. *c-v.*
Use: Antitussive, expectorant, decongestant.

Robitussin Dis-Co. (Robins) Guaifenesin 100 mg, alcohol 3.5%/5 ml. Syr. UD pack 5 ml, 10 ml, 15 ml; (10 × 10s). *otc.*
Use: Expectorant.

Robitussin-DM. (Robins) Guaifenesin 100 mg, dextromethorphan HBr 10 mg/5 ml. Syr. Bot. 4 oz, 8 oz, pt, gal, UD 5 ml, 10 ml (100s). *otc.*
Use: Antitussive, expectorant.

Robitussin Liquid Center Cough Drops. (Robins) Menthol 10 mg, eucalyptus oil, corn syrup, honey, lemon oil, high fructose, parabens, sorbitol, sucrose. Loz. Pkg. 20s. *otc.*
Use: Mouth and throat preparation.

Robitussin Maximum Strength Cough & Cold Formula. (Robins) Dextromethorphan HBr 15 mg, pseudoephedrine HCl 30 mg, alcohol 1.4%, glucose. Liq. Bot. 240 ml. *otc.*
Use: Antitussive, decongestant.

Robitussin Night Relief. (Robins) Acetaminophen 108.3 mg, pseudoephedrine HCl 10 mg, pyrilamine maleate 8.3 mg, dextromethorphan HBr 5 mg, alcohol-free, saccharin, sorbitol. Bot. 300 ml. *otc.*
Use: Analgesic, antihistamine, antitussive, decongestant.

Robitussin-PE. (Robins) Guaifenesin 100 mg, pseudoephedrine HCl 30 mg/5 ml, alcohol 1.4%, saccharin. Syr. Bot. 4 oz, 8 oz, pt. *otc.*
Use: Decongestant, expectorant.

Robitussin Pediatric. (Robins) Dextromethorphan HBr 7.5 mg/5 ml, alcohol free, saccharin, sorbitol, cherry flavor. Liq. Bot. 120, 240 ml. *otc.*
Use: Antitussive.

Robitussin Pediatric Cough & Cold Formula. (Robins) Dextromethorphan HBr 7.5 mg, pseudoephedrine HCl 15 mg/5 ml. Liq. Bot. 120 ml. *otc.*
Use: Antitussive, decongestant.

Robitussin Severe Congestion Liqui-Gels. (Robins) Guaifenesin 200 mg, pseudoephedrine HCl 30 mg, sorbitol. Cap. Pkg. 24s. *otc.*
Use: Decongestant, expectorant.

Robomol/ASA Tabs. (Major) Methocarbamol w/ASA. Bot. 100s, 500s. *Rx.*
Use: Muscle relaxant, analgesic.

Rocaltrol. (Roche Laboratories) Calcitriol 0.25 mcg or 0.5 mcg/Cap. **0.25 mcg:** Bot. 30s, 100s. **0.5 mcg:** Bot. 100s. *Rx.*
Use: Antihypocalcemic.

•**rocastine hydrochloride.** (row-KASS-teen) USAN.
Use: Antihistamine.

Rocephin. (Roche Laboratories) Ceftriaxone sodium **Pow. for Inj.:** 250 mg, 500 mg, 1 g, 2 g, or 10 g Vial. **250 mg, 500 mg:** Vial. **1 g, 2 g:** Vial, piggyback vial, ADD-Vantage vial. **10 g:** Bulk Containers. **Inj.: 1 g, 2 g, Frozen Premixed:** 50 ml plastic containers. *Rx.*
Use: Anti-infective, cephalosporin.

•**rocuronium bromide.** (row-kuhr-OH-nee-uhm) USAN.
Use: Neuromuscular blocker.
See: Zemuron, Inj. (Organon Teknika).

•**rodocaine.** (ROW-doe-cane) USAN.
Use: Anesthetic, local.

roentgenography.
See: Iodine Products, Diagnostic.

Roferon-A. (Roche Laboratories) Interferon alfa-2a, recombinant as 3 million, 6 million, 9 million, or 36 million IU/Vial in injectable soln. Available as Sterile Pow. yielding 18 million IU/3 ml when reconstituted. Subcutaneous or intramuscular Inj. 3 million IU/ml. 6 million IU/ml. 9 million IU/0.9 ml. 18 million IU/3 ml. 36 million IU/1 ml. Single-dose vial (3, 6 million IU/ml); multidose vial (9, 18, 36 million IU). *Rx.*
Use: Antineoplastic agent.

•**roflurane.** (row-FLEW-rane) USAN.
Use: Anesthetic, general.

Rogaine. (Pharmacia & Upjohn) Minoxidil 2% Topical Soln. Bot. 60 ml w/applicator. *otc.*
Use: Antialopecia agent.

•**rogletimide.** (row-GLETT-ih-MIDE) USAN.
Use: Antineoplastic (aromatase inhibitor).

Rolaids Calcium Rich. (Warner Lambert) Calcium carbonate 412 mg, magnesium hydroxide 80 mg. Chew. Tab. 12s, 36s, 75s, 150s. *otc.*
Use: Antacid.

Rolatuss Expectorant Liquid. (Huckaby Pharmacal) Phenylephrine HCl 5 mg, chlorpheniramine maleate 2 mg, codeine phosphate 9.85 mg, ammonium Cl 33.3 mg, alcohol 5%. Bot. 480 ml. *c-v.*
Use: Antihistamine, antitussive, decongestant, expectorant.

Rolatuss w/Hydrocodone. (Major) Phenylpropanolamine HCl 3.3 mg, phenylephrine HCl 5 mg, pyrilamine maleate 3.3 mg, pheniramine maleate 3.3 mg, hydrocodone bitartrate 1.67 mg. Liq. Bot. 480 ml. *c-III.*
Use: Antihistamine, antitussive, decongestant.

Rolatuss Plain Liquid. (Major) Phenylephrine HCl 5 mg, chlorpheniramine maleate 2 mg/5 ml. Liq. Bot. 473 ml. *otc.*
Use: Antihistamine, decongestant.

•**roletamide.** (row-LET-am-ide) USAN.
Use: Hypnotic, sedative.

•**rolgamidine.** (role-GAM-ih-deen) USAN.
Use: Antidiarrheal.

Rolicap. (Arcum) Vitamins A acetate 5000 IU, D_2 400 IU, B_1 3 mg, B_2 2.5 mg, B_6 10 mg, C 50 mg, niacinamide 20 mg, B_{12} 1 mcg/Chew. Tab. Bot. 100s, 1000s. *otc.*
Use: Vitamin supplement.

•**rolicyprine.** (ROW-lih-SIGH-preen) USAN.
Use: Antidepressant.

•**rolipram.** (ROLE-ih-pram) USAN.
Use: Anxiolytic.

•**rolitetracycline.** (ROW-lee-tet-rah-SIGH-kleen) USAN.
Use: Anti-infective.

•**rolitetracycline nitrate.** (ROW-lee-tet-rah-SIGH-kleen) USAN. Tetrim.
Use: Anti-infective.

•**rolodine.** (ROW-low-deen) USAN.
Use: Muscle relaxant.

Romach Antacid Tablets. (Last) Magnesium carbonate 400 mg, sodium bicarbonate 250 mg/Tab. Strip pack 60s, 500s. *otc.*
Use: Antacid.

•**romazarit.** (row-MAZZ-ah-rit) USAN.
Use: Anti-inflammatory, antirheumatic.

Romazicon. (Roche Laboratories) Flumazenil 0.1 mg/ml, parabens, EDTA. Inj. vials 5 and 10 ml. *Rx.*
Use: Antidotes.

Romex Cough & Cold Capsules. (APC) Guaifenesin 65 mg, dextromethorphan HBr 10 mg, chlorpheniramine maleate 1.5 mg, pyrilamine maleate 12.5 mg, phenylephrine HCl 5 mg, acetaminophen 160 mg/Cap. Bot. 21s. *otc.*
Use: Antihistamine, antitussive, decongestant, expectorant.

Romex Cough & Cold Tablets. (APC) Dextromethorphan HBr 7.5 mg, phenylephrine HCl 2.5 mg, ascorbic acid 30 mg. Box 15s. *otc.*
Use: Antitussive, decongestant.

Romex Troches & Liquid. (APC) **Troche:** Polymyxin B sulfate 1000 units, benzocaine 5 mg, cetalkonium Cl 2.5 mg, gramicidin 100 mcg, chlorpheniramine maleate 0.5 mg, tyrothricin 2 mg. Pkg. 10s. **Liq.:** Guaifenesin 200 mg, dextromethorphan HBr 60 mg, chlorpheniramine maleate 12 mg, phenylephrine HCl 30 mg/fl oz. Bot. 4 oz. *Rx.*
Use: Antihistamine, anti-infective, antitussive, decongestant, expectorant.

Rondamine-DM. (Major) Pseudoephedrine 25 mg/ml, carbinoxamine maleate 2 mg/ml, dextromethorphan HBr 4 mg/ml. Drop. 30 ml. *Rx.*
Use: Antihistamine, antitussive, decongestant.

Rondec Chewable Tablets. (Dura Pharm) Brompheniramine maleate 4 mg, pseudoephedrine HCl 60 mg, aspartame, phenylalanine 30.9 mg. Chew. Tab. Bot. 100s. *Rx.*
Use: Antihistamine, decongestant.

Rondec-DM Oral Drops. (Dura Pharm) Carbinoxamine maleate 2 mg, pseudoephedrine HCl 25 mg, dextromethorphan HBr 4 mg/ml, alcohol 6%. Bot. 30 ml w/dropper. *Rx.*
Use: Antihistamine, antitussive, decongestant.

Rondec-DM Syrup. (Dura Pharm) Carbinoxamine maleate 4 mg, pseudoephedrine HCl 60 mg, dextromethorphan HBr 15 mg/5 ml, alcohol 6%. Bot. 4 oz, pt. *Rx.*
Use: Antihistamine, antitussive, decongestant.

Rondec Oral Drops. (Dura Pharm) Carbinoxamine maleate 2 mg, pseudoephedrine HCl 25 mg/ml. Bot. 30 ml. *Rx.*
Use: Antihistamine, decongestant.

Rondec Syrup. (Dura Pharm) Carbinoxamine maleate 4 mg, pseudoephedrine HCl 60 mg/5 ml. Syr. Bot. 120 ml, 473 ml. *Rx.*
Use: Antihistamine, decongestant.

Rondec Tablets. (Dura Pharm) Pseudoephedrine HCl 60 mg, carbinoxamine maleate 4 mg, lactose/Tab. Bot. 100s, 500s. *Rx.*
Use: Antihistamine, decongestant.

Rondec-TR. (Dura Pharm) Carbinoxamine 8 mg, pseudoephedrine HCl 120 mg/SR Tab. Bot. 100s. *Rx.*
Use: Antihistamine, decongestant.

•**ronidazole.** (row-NYE-dazz-OLE) USAN.
Use: Antiprotozoal.

•**ronnel.** (RAHN-ell) USAN. Fenchlorphos.
Use: Insecticide (systemic).
See: Korlan (Dow).

Ronvet. (Armenpharm) Erythromycin stearate 250 mg/Tab. Bot. 100s. *Rx.*
Use: Anti-infective, erythromycin.

•**ropinirole hydrochloride.** (row-PIN-ih-role) USAN.
Use: Antiparkinsonian (D_2 receptor agonist).
See: Requip, Tab. (SmithKline Beecham).

•**ropitoin hydrochloride.** (ROW-pih-toe-in) USAN.
Use: Cardiovascular agent (antiarrhythmic).

ropivacaine HCl.
Use: Anesthetic.
See: Naropin, Inj. (Astra USA).

•**ropizine.** (row-PIH-zeen) USAN.
Use: Anticonvulsant.

•**roquinimex.** (row-KWIH-nih-mex) USAN.
Use: Biological response modifier; immunomodulator; antineoplastic. [Orphan drug]
See: Linomide.

rosa gallical.
See: Estivin, Soln. (Alcon Laboratories).

rosaniline dyes.
See: Fuchsin, Basic (Various Mfr.).
Methylrosaniline Cl, Soln., Inj. (Various Mfr.).

•**rosaramicin.** (row-ZAR-ah-MY-sin) USAN. *Formerly Rosamicin.*
Use: Anti-infective.

•**rosaramicin butyrate.** (row-ZAR-ah-MY-sin BYOO-tih-rate) USAN. *Formerly Rosamicin Butyrate.*
Use: Anti-infective.

•**rosaramicin propionate.** (row-ZAR-ah-MY-sin PRO-pee-oh-nate) USAN. *Formerly Rosamicin Propionate.*
Use: Anti-infective.

•**rosaramicin sodium phosphate.** (row-ZAR-ah-MY-sin) USAN. *Formerly Rosamicin Sodium Phosphate.*
Use: Anti-infective.

•**rosaramicin stearate.** (row-ZAR-ah-MY-sin STEE-ah-rate) USAN. *Formerly Rosamicin Stearate.*
Use: Anti-infective.

rose bengal. (Akorn) Rose bengal 1%. Bot. 5 ml.
Use: Diagnostic, tissue staining.

•**rose bengal sodium I 125.** (rose BEN-gal) USAN.
Use: Radiopharmaceutical.

•**rose bengal sodium I 131 injection.** U.S.P. 23.
Use: Diagnostic aid (hepatic function), radiopharmaceutical.

rose bengal strips. (PBH Wesley Jessen) Rose bengal 1.3 mg. Strip box 100s. *otc.*
Use: Diagnostic aid.

Rose-C Liquid. (Barth's) Vitamin C 300 mg, rose hip extract/Tsp. Dropper Bot. 2 oz, 8 oz. *otc.*
Use: Vitamin supplement.

rose hips. (Burgin-Arden) Vitamin C 300 mg, in base of sorbitol. Bot. 4 oz, 8 oz. *otc.*
Use: Vitamin supplement.

rose hips vitamin C. (Kirkman Sales) Vitamin C. **100 mg/Tab:** Bot. 100s, 250s. **250 mg or 500 mg/Tab:** Bot. 100s, 250s, 500s. *otc.*

Use: Vitamin supplement.

•**rose oil,** N.F. 18.
Use: Pharmaceutic aid (perfume).

Rosets. (Akorn) Rose bengal 1.3 mg/strip. Pkg. 100s. *Rx.*
Use: Diagnostic agent, ophthalmic.

•**rose water, stronger,** N.F. 18.
Use: Pharmaceutic aid (perfume).

rose water ointment.
Use: Emollient, ointment base.

rosin, U.S.P. XXI.
Use: Stiffening agent, pharmaceutical necessity.

•**rosoxacin.** (row-SOX-ah-sin) USAN.
Use: Anti-infective.
See: Rosoxacin, Pow. (Sanofi Winthrop).

Ross SLD. (Ross Laboratories) Low-residue nutritional supplement for patients restricted to a clear liquid feeding or with fat malabsorption disorders. Packet 1.35 oz. Ctn. 6s. Case 4 ctn. Can 13.5 oz. Case 6s. *otc.*
Use: Nutritional supplement.

Rotalex Test. (Orion Diagnostica) Latex slide agglutination test for detection of rotavirus in feces. Kit 1s.
Use: Diagnostic aid.

Rotazyme II. (Abbott Diagnostics) Enzyme immunoassay for detection of rotavirus antigen in feces. Test kit 50s.
Use: Diagnostic aid.

•**rotoxamine.** (row-TOX-ah-meen) USAN.
Use: Antihistamine.

Rowasa. (Solvay) **Rectal Susp.:** Mesalamine 4 g/60 ml. In units of 7 disposable bot. **Supp.:** Mesalamine 500 mg. Box 12s, 24s. *Rx.*
Use: Anti-inflammatory.

•**roxadimate.** (rox-AD-ih-mate) USAN.
Use: Sunscreen.

Roxanol Oral Solution. (Roxane) Morphine sulfate concentrated oral soln, sugar-free and alcohol free. **20 mg/ml:** Bot. 30 ml or 120 ml w/calibrated dropper. **100 mg/5 ml:** Bot. 240 ml w/calibrated spoon. *c-II.*
Use: Analgesic, narcotic.

Roxanol Rectal. (Roxane) Morphine sulfate 5, 10, 20, 30 mg. Supp. 12s. *c-II.*
Use: Analgesic, narcotic.

Roxanol 100. (Roxane) Morphine sulfate 100 mg/5 ml. Soln. Bot. 240 ml. *c-II.*
Use: Analgesic, narcotic.

Roxanol Rescudose. (Roxane) Morphine sulfate 10 mg/2.5 ml. Oral Soln. UD 2.5 ml. *c-II.*
Use: Analgesic, narcotic.

Roxanol SR Tablets. (Roxane) Morphine sulfate 30 mg/SR Tab. Bot. 50s, 250s, UD 100s. *c-II.*
Use: Analgesic, narcotic.

Roxandol UD. (Roxane) Morphine sulfate 20 mg/5 ml. Soln. Bot. 100, 500 ml. *c-II.*
Use: Analgesic, narcotic.

•**roxarsone.** (ROX-AHR-sone) USAN.
Use: Anti-infective.

•**roxatidine acetate hydrochloride.** (ROX-ah-tih-DEEN) USAN.
Use: Antiulcer.

Roxicet Oral Solution. (Roxane) Oxycodone HCl 5 mg, acetaminophen 325 mg/5 ml. Bot. UD 5 ml, 500 ml. *c-II.*
Use: Analgesic combination, narcotic.

Roxicet 5/500. (Roxane) Oxycodone HCl 5 mg, acetaminophen 500 mg/Cap. Bot. 100s, UD 100s. *c-II.*
Use: Analgesic combination, narcotic.

Roxicet Tablets. (Roxane) Oxycodone HCl 5 mg, acetaminophen 325 mg, 0.4% alcohol/Tab. Bot. 100s, 500s, UD 100s. *c-II.*
Use: Analgesic combination, narcotic.

Roxicodone. (Roxane) **Liq.:** Oxycodone HCl 5 mg/5 ml. Bot. 500 ml. **Tab.:** Oxycodone HCl 5 mg. Bot. 100s, UD 4 × 25s. *c-II.*
Use: Analgesic, narcotic.

•**roxifiban acetate.** (rox-ih-FIE-ban) USAN.
Use: Antithrombotic, fibrinogen receptor antagonist.

Roxilox. (Roxane) Oxycodone HCl 5 mg, acetaminophen 500 mg/Cap. Bot. 100s. *c-II.*
Use: Narcotic analgesic combination.

Roxiprin Tablets. (Roxane) Oxycodone HCl 4.5 mg, oxycodone terephthalate 0.38 mg, aspirin 325 mg/Tab. Bot. 100s, 1000s, UD 100s. *c-II.*
Use: Analgesic combination, narcotic.

•**roxithromycin.** (ROX-ith-row-MY-sin) USAN.
Use: Anti-infective.

R/S Lotion. (Summers) Sulfur 5%, resorcinol 2%, alcohol 28%. Lot. Bot. 56.7 ml. *otc.*
Use: Dermatologic, acne.

R-S Lotion. (Hill) No. 2: Sulfur 8%, resorcinol monoacetate 4%. Bot. 2 oz. *otc.*
Use: Drying medication, topical.

R-Tannamine. (Qualitest) Phenylephrine tannate 25 mg, chlorpheniramine tannate 8 mg, pyrilamine tannate 25 mg/Tab. Bot. 100s. *Rx.*
Use: Anithistamine, decongestant.

R-Tannamine Pediatric. (Qualitest) Phenylephrine tannate 5 mg, chlorpheniramine tannate 2 mg, pyrilamine tannate 12.5 mg, 120 ml, 473 ml. *Rx.*
Use: Antihistamine, decongestant.

R-Tannate Tablets. (Various Mfr.) Phenylephrine tannate 25 mg, chlorpheniramine tannate 8 mg, pyrilamine tannate 25 mg. In 100s. *Rx.*
Use: Antihistamine, decongestant.

R-Tannate Pediatric Suspension. (Various Mfr.) Phenylephrine tannate 5 mg, chlorpheniramine tannate 2 mg, pyrilamine tannate 12.5 mg, saccharin. In 473 ml. *Rx.*
Use: Antihistamine, decongestant.

RII Retinamide.
Use: Myelodysplastic syndromes. [Orphan drug]

rt-PA.
Use: Tissue plasminogen.
See: Activase (Genentech).

RU 486.
Use: Antiprogesterone.
See: Mifepristone.

Rubacell. (Abbott Diagnostics) Passive hemagglutination (PHA) test for the detection of antibody to rubella virus in serum or recalcified plasma.
Use: Diagnostic aid.

Rubacell II. (Abbott Laboratories) Passive hemagglutination (PHA) test to detect antibody to rubella in serum or recalcified plasma. In 100s, 1000s.
Use: Diagnostic aid.

Rubaquick Diagnostic Kit. (Abbott Diagnostics) Rapid passive hemagglutination (PHA) for the detection of antibodies to rubella virus in serum specimens.
Use: Diagnostic aid.

Ruba-Tect. (Abbott Diagnostics) Hemagglutination inhibition test for the detection and quantitation of rubella antibody in serum. In 100s.
Use: Diagnostic aid.

Rubazyme. (Abbott Diagnostics) Enzyme immunoassay for 1 gG antibody to rubella virus. Test kit 100s, 1000s.
Use: Diagnostic aid.

Rubazyme-M. (Abbott Diagnostics) Enzyme immunoassay for IgM antibody to rubella virus in serum. Test kit 50s.
Use: Diagnostic aid.

rubella & measles vaccine. (Merck) M-R-VAX II. Inj. Vial. *Rx.*
Use: Immunization.

rubella & mumps virus vaccine, live.
Use: Immunization.
See: Biavax II, Inj. (Merck).

•**rubella virus vaccine, live.** (roo-BELL-ah) U.S.P. 23.
Use: Immunization.
See: Meruvax II, Inj. (Merck).
W/Measles vaccine.
See: M-R-Vax II, Inj. (Merck).
W/Measles vaccine, mumps vaccine.
See: M-M-R Vax II, Inj. (Merck).

Rubex. (Bristol-Myers Oncology/Immunology) Doxorubicin HCl 10 mg, 50 mg or 100 mg. **10 mg:** w/lactose 50 mg. **50 mg:** w/lactose 250 mg. **100 mg:** w/ lactose 500 mg. Pow. for Inj. Vial. *Rx.*
Use: Antineoplastic.

•**rubidium chloride Rb 82 injection,** (roo-BIH-dee-uhm) U.S.P. 23.
Use: Diagnostic aid (radioactive, cardiac disease), radiopharmaceutical.

•**rubidium chloride Rb 86.** (roo-BIH-dee-uhm) USAN.
Use: Radiopharmaceutical.

Rubratope-57. (Bristol-Myers Squibb) Cyanocobalamin Co 57 Capsules; Soln U.S.P. *otc.*
Use: Vitamin supplement.

Ru-lets M 500. (Rugby) Vitamin C 500 mg, B_3 100 mg, B_5 20 mg, B_1 15 mg, B_2 10 mg, B_6 5 mg, A 10,000 IU, B_{12} 12 mcg, D 400 IU, E 30 mg, magnesium, iron 20 mg, copper, zinc 1.5 mg, manganese, iodine/Tab. Bot. 100s. *otc.*
Use: Mineral, vitamin supplement.

Rulox. (Rugby) **#1 Tab.:** Aluminum hydroxide 200 mg, magnesium hydroxide 200 mg. **#2 Tab.:** Aluminum hydroxide 400 mg, magnesium hydroxide 400 mg. Bot. 100s, 1000s. *otc.*
Use: Antacid.

RuLox Plus Suspension. (Rugby) Aluminum hydroxide 500 mg, magnesium hydroxide 450 mg, simethicone 40 mg/ 5 ml. Bot. 355 ml. *otc.*
Use: Antacid, antiflatulent.

RuLox Plus Tablets. (Rugby) Aluminum hydroxide 200 mg, magnesium hydroxide 200 mg, simethicone 25 mg. Chew. Tab. Bot. 50s. *otc.*
Use: Antacid, antiflatulent.

RuLox Suspension. (Rugby) Aluminum hydroxide 225 mg, magnesium hydroxide 200 mg/5 ml. Susp. Bot. 360 ml, 769 ml, gal. *otc.*
Use: Antacid.

Rum-K. (Fleming) Potassium Cl 10 mEq/ 5 ml in butter/rum flavored base. Bot. pt, gal. *Rx.*
Use: Electrolyte supplement.

rust inhibitor.
See: Anti-Rust, Tab. (Sanofi Winthrop).

Sodium Nitrite, Tab. (Various Mfr.).

•**rutamycin.** (ROO-tah-MY-sin) USAN. From strain of *Streptomyces rutgersensis*. Under study.
Use: Antifungal.

rutgers 612.
See: Ethohexadiol. (Various Mfr.).

rutin. (Various Mfr.) 3-Rhamnoglucoside of 5,7,3',4-tetrahydroxyflavonol. Eldrin, globulariacitrin, myrticalorin, oxyritin, phytomelin, rutoside, sophorin. Tab. 20 mg, 50 mg, 60 mg, 100 mg. *Rx.*
Use: Vascular disorders.

rutin combinations.
See: Hexarutan, Tab. (Westerfield).
Vio-Geric-H, Tab. (Solvay).

rutoside.
See: Rutin, Tab. (Various Mfr.).

Ru-Tuss DE. (Knoll Pharmaceuticals) Pseudoephedrine HCl 120 mg, guaifenesin 600 mg/Tab. Bot. 100s. *Rx.*
Use: Decongestant, expectorant.

Ru-Tuss II. (Knoll Pharmaceuticals) Phenylpropanolamine HCl 75 mg, chlorpheniramine maleate 12 mg/Cap. Bot. 100s. *Rx.*
Use: Antihistamine, decongestant.

Ru-Tuss Expectorant. (Knoll Pharmaceuticals) Pseudoephedrine HCl 30 mg, dextromethorphan HBr 10 mg, guaifenesin 100 mg/5 ml, alcohol 10%. Bot. pt. *otc.*
Use: Antitussive, decongestant, expectorant.

Ru-Tuss Liquid. (Knoll Pharmaceuticals) Phenylephrine HCl 5 mg, chlorpheniramine maleate 2 mg/5 ml, alcohol 5%. Bot. 473 ml. *otc.*
Use: Antihistamine, decongestant.

Ru-Tuss w/Hydrocodone. (Knoll Pharmaceuticals) Hydrocodone bitartrate 1.67 mg, phenylephrine HCl 5 mg, phenylpropanolamine HCl 3.3 mg, pheniramine maleate 3.3 mg, pyrilamine maleate 3.3 mg/5 ml, alcohol 5%. Bot. 473 ml. *c-III.*
Use: Antihistamine, antitussive, decongestant.

RVPaque. (ICN Pharmaceuticals) Red petrolatum, zinc oxide, cinoxate, in water-resistant base. Tube 15 g, 37.5 g. *otc.*
Use: Sunscreen.

Rymed. (Edwards Pharmaceuticals) Pseudoephedrine HCl 30 mg, guaifenesin 250 mg/Cap. Bot. 100s. *otc.*
Use: Decongestant, expectorant.

Rymed Liquid. (Edwards Pharmaceuticals) Pseudoephedrine HC1 30 mg, guaifenesin 100 mg/5 ml, alcohol 1.4%. Bot. pt. *otc.*
Use: Decongestant, expectorant.

Rymed-TR. (Edwards Pharmaceuticals) Phenylpropanolamine HCl 75 mg, guaifenesin 400 mg/Tab. Bot. 100s. *otc.*
Use: Decongestant, expectorant.

Ryna. (Wallace Laboratories) Chlorpheniramine 2 mg, pseudoephedrine HCl 30 mg/5 ml. Bot. 118 ml, 473 ml. *otc.*
Use: Antihistamine, decongestant.

Ryna-C. (Wallace Laboratories) Codeine phosphate 10 mg, pseudoephedrine HCl 30 mg, chlorpheniramine maleate 2 mg, saccharin, sorbitol/5 ml. Bot. 4 oz, pt. *c-v.*
Use: Antihistamine, antitussive, decongestant.

Ryna-CX. (Wallace Laboratories) Guaifenesin 100 mg, pseudoephedrine HCl 30 mg, codeine phosphate 10 mg, alcohol 7.5%, saccharin, sorbitol/5 ml. Bot. 4 oz, pt. *c-v.*
Use: Antitussive, decongestant, expectorant.

Rynatan. (Wallace Laboratories) **Tab.:** Phenylephrine tannate 25 mg, chlorpheniramine tannate 8 mg, pyrilamine tannate 25 mg. Bot. 100s, 500s, 2000s. **Pediatric Susp.:** Phenylephrine tannate 5 mg, chlorpheniramine tannate 2 mg, pyrilamine tannate 12.5 mg/5 ml. Bot. 473 ml. *Rx.*
Use: Antihistamine, decongestant.

Rynatan-S Pediatric Suspension. (Wallace Laboratories) Phenylephrine tannate 5 mg, chlorpheniramine tannate 2 mg, pyrilamine tannate 12.5 mg/5 ml. Susp. Bot. 120 ml w/syringe. *Rx.*
Use: Antihistamine, decongestant.

Rynatuss. (Wallace Laboratories) Carbetapentane tannate 60 mg, chlorpheniramine tannate 5 mg, ephedrine tannate 10 mg, phenylephrine tannate 10 mg/Tab. Bot. 100s. *Rx.*
Use: Antihistamine, antitussive, decongestant.

Rynatuss Pediatric Suspension. (Wallace Laboratories) Carbetapentane tannate 30 mg, chlorpheniramine tannate 4 mg, ephedrine tannate 5 mg, phenylephrine tannate 5 mg, saccharin, tartrazine/5 ml. Susp. Bot. 8 oz, pt. *Rx.*
Use: Antihistamine, antitussive, decongestant.

Rythmol. (Knoll Pharmaceuticals) Propafenone HCl 150 mg, 225 mg or 300 mg. Tab. **50 mg or 300 mg:** Bot. 100s, 500s. **225 mg:** Bot. 100s, UD 100s. *Rx.*
Use: Antiarrhythmic.

S

S-2 Inhalant & Nebulizers. (Nephron) Racemic epinephrine HCl 1.25%. Bot. 0.25 oz, 0.5 oz, 1 oz. *Rx.*
Use: Bronchodilator.

Saave+. (NeuroGenesis/Matrix) Vitamin D 40 mg, L-phenylalanine, L-glutamine 25 mg, vitamins A 333.3 IU, B_1 2.417 mg, B_2 0.85 mg, B_3 33 mg, B_5 15 mg, B_6 3 mg, B_{12} 5 mcg, folic acid 0.067 mg, C 100 mg, E 5 IU, biotin 0.05 mg, calcium 25 mg, chromium 0.01 mg, iron 1.5 mg, magnesium 25 mg, zinc 2.5 mg/Cap. Yeast and preservative free. Bot. 42s, 180s. *otc.*
Use: Mineral, vitamin supplement.

•**sabeluzole.** (sah-BELL-you-zole) USAN.
Use: Anticonvulsant; antihypoxic.

Sabin vaccine.
Use: Immunization.
See: Orimune (ESI Lederle Generics).

Sac-500. (Western Research) Vitamin C 500 mg/Timed Release Cap. Bot. 1000s. *otc.*
Use: Vitamin supplement.

•**saccharin.** (SACK-ah-rin) N.F. 18.
Use: Pharmaceutic aid (flavor).
See: Necta Sweet, Tab. (Procter & Gamble).

saccharin. (Merck) Pkg. 1 oz, 0.25 lb, 1 lb. (Bristol-Myers Squibb) Tabs. 0.25, 0.5 gr. Bot. 500s, 1000s; 1 gr. Bot. 1000s.
Use: Pharmaceutic aid (flavor).

•**saccharin calcium.** U.S.P. 23.
Use: Non-nutritive sweetener.

•**saccharin sodium.** U.S.P. 23.
Use: Sweetener (non-nutritive).
See: Crystallose, Crystals, Liq. (Jamieson).
Ril Sweet, Liq. (Schering Plough).
Sweeta (Squibb Diagnostic).

saccharin sodium. (Various Mfr.) Pow., Bot. 1 oz, 0.25 lb, 1 lb. Tab.
Use: Sweetener (non-nutritive).

saccharin soluble.
See: Saccharin Sodium, Tab., Pow. (Various Mfr.).

sacrosidase.
Use: Nutritional therapy.
See: Sucraid, Soln. [Orphan drug]

Saf-Clens. (Calgon Vestal) Meroxapol 105, NaCl, potassium sorbate NF, DMDM hydantoin/Spray. Bot. 177 ml. *otc.*
Use: Dermatologic, wound therapy.

Safeskin. (C & M Pharmacal) A dermatologically acceptable detergent for patients who are sensitive to ordinary detergents. No whiteners, brighteners or other irritants. Bot. qt.
Use: Laundry detergent for sensitive skin.

Safe Suds. (Ar-Ex) Hypoallergenic, all-purpose detergent for patients whose hands or respiratory membranes are irritated by soaps or detergents. pH 6.8. No enzymes, phosphates, lanolin, fillers, bleaches. Bot. 22 oz.
Use: Detergent.

Safe Tussin 30. (Kramer) Guaifenesin 100 mg, dextromethorphan HBr 15 mg/5 ml. Liq. Bot. 120 ml. *otc.*
Use: Antitussive, expectorant.

Safety-Coated Arthritis Pain Formula. (Whitehall Robins) Enteric coated aspirin 500 mg/Tab. Bot. 24s, 60s. *otc.*
Use: Analgesic.

safflower oil.
Use: Nutritional supplement.
See: Microlipid (Sherwood Medical).

•**safflower oil.** U.S.P. 23.
Use: Pharmaceutic aid (vehicle, oleaginous).
See: Safflower Oil Caps. (Various Mfr.).
W/Choline bitartrate, soybean lecithin, inositol, natural tocopherols, B_6, B_{12}, and panthenol.
See: Nutricol, Cap., Vial (Nutrition).

•**safingol.** (saff-IN-gole) USAN.
Use: Antineoplastic (adjunct); antipsoriatic.

•**safingol hydrochloride.** (saff-IN-gole) USAN.
Use: Antineoplastic (adjunct); antipsoriatic.

safrole.

Saizeno. (Serono) Somatropin 5 mg, sucrose. Pow. For Inj., lyophilized. Vial ≈ 15 IU. *Rx.*
Use: Hormone, growth.

SalAc Cleanser. (GenDerm) Salicylic acid 2%, benzyl alcohol, glyceryl cocoate. Liq. Bot. 177 ml. *otc.*
Use: Dermatologic, acne.

salacetin.
See: Acetylsalicylic Acid (Various Mfr.).

Sal-Acid. (Pedinol) Salicylic acid 40% in collodion-like vehicle. Plaster. Pkg. 14s. *otc.*
Use: Keratolytic.

Salacid 25%. (Gordon Laboratories) Salicylic acid 25% in ointment base. Jar 2 oz, lb. *otc.*
Use: Keratolytic.

Salacid 60%. (Gordon Laboratories) Salicylic acid 60% in ointment base. Jar 2 oz. *otc.*

Use: Keratolytic.

Salactic Film. (Pedinol) Salicylic acid 16.7% in flexible collodion w/color. Applicator bot. 0.5 oz. *otc.*
Use: Keratolytic.

Salagen. (SAL-an-tell) (MGI Pharma) Pilocarpine HCl 5 mg. Tab. Bot. 100s. *Rx.*
Use: Mouth and throat preparation.

Salazide-Demi Tablets. (Major) Hydroflumethiazide 25 mg, reserpine 0.125 mg/Tab. Bot. 100s. *Rx.*
Use: Antihypertensive combination.

Salazide Tabs. (Major) Hydroflumethiazide 50 mg, reserpine 0.125 mg/Tab. Bot. 100s, 500s, 1000s. *Rx.*
Use: Antihypertensive combination.

salbutamol.
See: albuterol.

Salcegel. (Apco) Sodium salicylate 5 gr, calcium ascorbate 25 mg, calcium carbonate 1 gr, dried aluminum hydroxide gel 2 gr/Tab. Bot. 100s. *otc.*
Use: Analgesic.

Sal-Clens Acne Cleanser Gel. (C & M Pharmacal) Salicylic acid 2%. Gel. Tube 240 g. *otc.*
Use: Dermatologic, acne.

•**salcolex.** (SAL-koe-lex) USAN.
Use: Analgesic, anti-inflammatory, antipyretic.

•**salethamide maleate.** (sal-ETH-ah-MIDE) USAN. Under study.
Use: Analgesic.

saletin.
See: Acetylsalicylic Acid (Various Mfr.).

Saleto. (Roberts Pharm) Aspirin 210 mg, acetaminophen 115 mg, salicylamide 65 mg, caffeine anhydrous 16 mg/Tab. Bot. 50s, 100s, 1000s, Sani-Pak 1000s. *otc.*
Use: Analgesic.

Saleto-200. (Roberts Pharm) Ibuprofen 200 mg/Tab. Bot. 1000s, UD 50s. *otc.*
Use: Analgesic, NSAID.

Saleto-400. (Roberts Pharm) Ibuprofen 400 mg/Tab. Bot. 100s, 500s. *Rx.*
Use: Analgesic, NSAID.

Saleto-600. (Roberts Pharm) Ibuprofen 600 mg/Tab. Bot. 100s, 500s. *Rx.*
Use: Analgesic, NSAID.

Saleto-800. (Roberts Pharm) Ibuprofen 800 mg/Tab. Bot. 100s, 500s. *Rx.*
Use: Analgesic, NSAID.

Saleto CF. (Roberts Pharm) Phenylpropanolamine 12.5 mg, dextromethorphan HBr 10 mg, acetaminophen 325 mg/Tab. Bot. UD 8s, 1000s. *otc.*
Use: Analgesic, antitussive, decongestant.

Saleto-D. (Roberts Pharm) Acetaminophen 240 mg, salicylamide 120 mg, caffeine 16 mg, phenylpropanolamine HCl 18 mg/Cap. Bot. 50s, 1000s, Sani-Pak 500s. *otc.*
Use: Analgesic, decongestant.

Salflex. (Carnrick Labs) Salsalate 500 mg or 750 mg/Tab. Bot. 100s. *Rx.*
Use: Analgesic.

•**salicyl alcohol.** (SAL-ih-sill AL-koe-hahl) USAN. *Formerly Saligenin, Saligenol, Salicain.*
Use: Anesthetic-local.

•**salicylamide.** U.S.P. 23.
Use: Analgesic.

salicylamide w/combinations.
See: Anodynos, Tab. (Buffington).
Anodynos Forte, Tab. (Buffington).
Arthol, Tab. (Towne).
Cenaid, Tab. (Century Pharm).
Centuss, MLT Tab. (Century Pharm).
Dapco, Tab. (Mericon).
Decohist, Cap. (Towne).
Dengesic, Tab. (Scott-Alison).
Duoprin, Tab. (Dunhall Pharmaceuticals).
Emersal, Liq. (Medco Research).
F.C.A.H., Cap. (Scherer).
Lobac, Cap. (Seatrace).
Myocalm, Tab. (Parmed).
Nokane, Tab. (Wren).
Partuss-A, Tab. (Parmed).
Partuss T.D., Tab. (Parmed).
P.M.P. Compound, Tab. (Mericon).
Presalin, Tab. (Roberts Pharm).
Renpap, Tab. (Wren).
Rhinex, Tab. (Teva USA).
S.A.C., Preps. (Towne).
Saleto, Preps. (Roberts Pharm).
Salipap, Tab. (Freeport).
Salocol, Tab. (Roberts Pharm).
Salphenyl, Liq., Cap. (Roberts Pharm).
Scotgesic, Cap., Elix. (Scott/Cord).
Sinulin, Tab. (Schwarz Pharma).
Sleep, Tab. (Towne).
Triaprin-DC, Cap. (Dunhall Pharmaceuticals).

salicylanilide.
Use: Antifungal.

•**salicylate meglumine.** (suh-LIH-sih-late) USAN.
Use: Antirheumatic, analgesic.

salicylated bile extract. Chologestin.

salicylazosulfapyridine.
See: Sulfasalazine, U.S.P. 23.

•**salicylic acid.** (sal-ih-SILL-ik) U.S.P. 23.
Use: Keratolytic.
See: Calicylic, Creme (Gordon Laboratories).

Listrex Scrub, Liq. (Warner Lambert).
Maximum Strength Wart Remover, Liq. (Stiefel).
OFF-Ezy Corn & Callous Remover, Kit (Del Pharmaceuticals).
Sal-Acid, Plaster (Pedinol).
Salactic Film, Liq. (Pedinol).
Salicylic Acid Acne Treatment, Bar (Stiefel)
Sal-Plant, Gel (Pedinol).
Sebulex, Cream (Westwood Squibb).
Trans-Plantar, Transdermal patch (Tsumura Medical).
Wart-Off, Liq. (Pfizer).

Salicylic Acid Cleansing Bar. (Stiefel) Salicylic acid 2%, EDTA. Cake 113 g. *otc.*
Use: Antiseborrheic, keratolytic.

salicylic acid combinations.
See: Acnaveen, Bar (Rydelle).
Acno (Baker Norton).
Akne Drying Lotion, Liq. (Alto Pharmaceuticals).
Clearasil, Preps (Procter & Gamble).
Cuticura (Purex).
Duofilm, Liq. (Stiefel).
Duo-WR, Soln. (Whorton).
Fostex, Cream, Liq. (Westwood Squibb).
Ionax, Liq. (Galderma).
Ionil, Liq. (Galderma).
Ionil T, Liq. (Galderma).
Keralyt, Gel (Westwood Squibb).
Komed, Lot. (PBH Wesley Jessen).
Neutrogena T/Sal, Shampoo (Neutrogena).
Occlusal HP, Liq. (GenDerm).
Oxy Clean Medicated Pads for Sensitive Skin (SmithKline Beecham Pharmaceuticals).
Oxy Night Watch, Lot. (SmithKline Beecham Pharmaceuticals).
Pernox, Lot. (Westwood Squibb).
Pragmatar, Oint. (Menley & James).
Propa pH, Preps (Del Pharmaceuticals).
Sal-Dex, Liq. (Scrip).
Salicylic Acid Soap (Stiefel).
Salsprin, Tab. (Seatrace).
Sebaveen, Shampoo (Rydelle).
Sebucare, Liq. (Westwood Squibb).
Sebulex Shampoo, Liq. (Westwood Squibb).
Therac, Lot. (C & M Pharm).
Tinver, Lot. (PBH Wesley Jessen).
Vanseb, Dandruff Shampoo (Allergan).
Vanseb-T Tar Shampoo (Allergan).
Ver-Var, Soln. (Galderma).
Zemacol, Lot. (Procter & Gamble).

Salicylic Acid & Sulfur Soap. (Stiefel) Salicylic acid 3%, sulfur 10%, EDTA. Cake 116 g. *otc.*
Use: Antiseborrheic, keratolytic.

salicylic acid topical foam.
Use: Keratolytic.

salicylsalicylic acid. Salsalate. USAN.
Use: Analgesic.
See: Arcylate, Tab. (Roberts Pharm)
Disalcid, Tab. (3M).
W/Aspirin.
See: Duragesic, Tab. (Meyer).
Persistin, Tab. (Medeva).

salicylsulphonic acid. Sulfosalicylic acid.
See: Dextrotest (Bayer Corp).

Saligenin. (City Chemical) Salicyl alcohol. Bot. 25 g, 100 g.
W/Merodicein.
See: Thantis, Loz. (Becton Dickinson).

Saline. (Bausch & Lomb) Buffered isotonic. Thimerosal 0.001%, boric acid, NaCl, EDTA. Soln. Bot. 355 ml. *otc.*
Use: Contact lens care.

Saline Solution. (Americal) Saline solution, isotonic, preserved. Bot. 12 oz. *otc.*
Use: Contact lens care, soaking.

Saline Spray. (Americal) Isotonic nonpreserved saline aerosol soln. Bot. 2 oz, 8 oz, 12 oz. *otc.*
Use: Contact lens care.

Salinex Nasal Drops. (Muro) Buffered nasal isotonic saline drops. Bot. 15 ml w/dropper. *otc.*
Use: Moisturizer, nasal.

Salinex Nasal Mist. (Muro) Sodium Cl 0.4%. Drops 15 ml, spray 50 ml. *otc.*
Use: Moisturizer, nasal.

Salipap. (Freeport) Salicylamide 5 gr, acetaminophen 5 gr/Tab. Bot. 1000s. *otc.*
Use: Analgesic.

Salithol Liquid. (Madland) Balm of methyl salicylate, menthol, camphor. Bot. pt, gal. Oint. Jar 1 lb, 5 lb. *otc.*
Use: Analgesic, topical.

Salivart. (Gebauer) Sodium carboxymethylcellulose 1%, sorbitol 3%, sodium Cl 0.084%, potassium Cl 0.12%, calcium Cl 0.015%, magnesium Cl 0.005%, dibasic potassium phosphate 0.034% and nitrogen (as propellant). Soln. Spray can 25 ml, 75 ml. *otc.*
Use: Mouth preparation.

Saliva Substitute. (Roxane) Sorbitol, sodium carboxymethylcellulose. Soln. 5 ml and 120 ml vials. *otc.*
Use: Mouth preparation.

Salix. (Scandinavian Natural Health and Beauty) Sorbitol, dicalcium phosphate, hydroxypropyl methylcellulose, carboxy methylcellulose, malic acid, hydrogenated cottonseed oil, sodium citrate, citric acid, silicon dioxide. Loz. 100s. *otc.*
Use: Saliva substitute.

Salk vaccine.
See: IPOL (Pasteur Merieux Connaught).
Poliovirus vaccine, inactivated.

•**salmeterol.** (sal-MEH-teh-role) USAN.
Use: Bronchodilator.

•**salmeterol xinafoate.** (sal-MEH-teh-role zin-AF-oh-ate) USAN.
Use: Bronchodilator.

•**salnacedin.** (sal-NAH-seh-din) USAN.
Use: Anti-inflammatory, topical.

Salocol. (Roberts Pharm) Acetaminophen 115 mg, aspirin 210 mg, salicylamide 65 mg, caffeine 16 mg/Tab. Bot. 1000s. *Rx.*
Use: Analgesic combination.

Salpaba w/Colchicine. (Madland) Sodium salicylate 0.25 g, para-aminobenzoic acid 0.25 g, vitamin C 20 mg, colchicine 0.25 mg/Tab. Bot. 100s, 1000s. *Rx.*
Use: Antigout.

Sal-Plant. (Pedinol) Salicylic acid 17% in flexible collodion vehicle. Gel. Tube 14 g. *otc.*
Use: Keratolytic.

•**salsalate.** (SAL-sah-late) U.S.P. 23.
Use: Analgesic; anti-inflammatory.
See: Marthritic, Tab. (Marnel).

Salsitab. (Upsher-Smith Labs) Salsalate 500 mg or 750 mg/Tab. Bot. 100s, 500s, UD 100s. *Rx.*
Use: Analgesic.

Salten. (Wren) Salicylamide 10 gr/Tab. Bot. 100s, 1000s. *otc.*
Use: Analgesic.

Sal-Tropine. (Hope Pharmaceuticals) Atropine sulfate 0.4 mg. Tab. Bot. 100s. *Rx.*
Use: Anticholinergic.

salt replacement products.
See: Slo-Salt (Mission Pharmacal).
Slo-Salt-K (Mission Pharmacal).
Sodium Chloride (Various Mfr.).

•**salts, rehydration, oral.** U.S.P. 23.
Use: Electrolyte combination.

salt substitutes.
Use: Sodium-free seasoning agent.
See: Adolph's Salt Substitute (Adolph's).
Adolph's Seasoned Salt Substitute (Adolph's).
Morton Salt Substitute (Morton Grove).
Morton Seasoned Salt Substitute (Morton Grove).
NoSalt (SmithKline Beecham Pharmaceuticals).
Nu-Salt (Cumberland Pkg).

salt tablets. (Cross) Sodium Cl 650 mg/Tab. Dispenser 500s. *otc.*
Use: Salt replenisher.

Saluron. (Bristol-Myers) Hydroflumethiazide 50 mg/Tab. Bot. 100s. *Rx.*
Use: Diuretic.

Salutensin. (Roberts Pharm) Hydroflumethiazide 50 mg, reserpine 0.125 mg/Tab. Bot. 100s, 1000s. *Rx.*
Use: Antihypertensive combination.

Salutensin-Demi. (Roberts Pharm) Hydroflumethiazide 25 mg, reserpine 0.125 mg/Tab. Bot. 100s, 1000s. *Rx.*
Use: Antihypertensive combination.

Salvarsan.
Use: Antisyphilitic.

Salvite-B. (Faraday) Sodium chloride 7 gr, dextrose 3 gr, vitamin B_1 1 mg/Tab. Bot. 100s, 1000s. *otc.*

•**samarium Sm 153 lexidronam pentasodium.** (sah-MARE-ee-uhm Sm 153 lex-IH-drah-nam pen-tah-SO-dee-uhm) USAN.
Use: Antineoplastic, radiopharmaceutical.
See: Quadramet, Inj. (DuPont).

Sancura. (Thompson Medical) Benzocaine, chlorobutanol, chlorothymol, benzoic acid, salicylic acid, benzyl alcohol, cod liver oil, lanolin in a washable petrolatum base. Oint. 30 g, 90 g.
Use: Anesthetic, local.

•**sancycline.** (SAN-SIGH-kleen) USAN.
Use: Anti-infective.

Sandimmune. (Novartis) Cyclosporine. **Oral soln.:** 100 mg/ml. Bot. 50 ml with syringe. **IV Soln.:** 50 mg/ml Amp. 5 ml. **Cap.:** 25 mg, 50 mg, 100 mg/Cap. Bot. Sorbitol. UD 30s. *Rx.*
Use: Immunosuppressant.

Sandoglobulin. (Novartis) Reconstitution fluid 1 g, 3 g, 6 g, 12g NaCl 0.9%/lyophilized pow. for inj. Vials or kits. Also available as bulk packs without diluent. *Rx.*
Use: Immunization.

sandoptal. Isobutyl allylbarbituric acid.
See: Butalbital.
W/Caffeine, aspirin, phenacetin.
See: Fiorinal, Tab., Cap. (Novartis).
W/Caffeine, aspirin, phenacetin, codeine phosphate.

See: Fiorinal w/codeine, Cap. (Novartis).

sandoptal sodium.
W/Sodium diethylbarbiturate, sodium phenylethylbarbiturate, scopolamine HBr, dihydroergotamine methanesulfonate.
See: Plexonal (Novartis).

Sandostatin. (Novartis) Octreotide acetate. **0.05 mg, 0.1 mg, 0.5 mg/ml:** Inj. Amp 1 ml. **0.2 mg, 1 mg/ml:** 5 ml multidose vials. *Rx.*
Use: Antineoplastic, adjunctive.

Sanestro. (Sandia) Estrone 0.7 mg, estradiol 0.35 mg, estriol 0.14 mg/Tab. Bot. 100s, 1000s. *Rx.*
Use: Estrogen.

•**sanfetrinem cilexitil.** (san-FEH-trih-nem sigh-LEX-eh-till) USAN.
Use: Anti-infective.

•**sanfetrinem sodium.** (san-FEH-trih-nem) USAN.
Use: Anti-infective.

•**sanguinarium chloride.** (san-gwih-NARE-ee-uhm) USAN. *Formerly Sanguinarine Chloride.*
Use: Antimicrobial, anti-inflammatory, antifungal.

Sanguis. (Sigma-Tau Pharmaceuticals) Liver 10 mcg, vitamin B_{12} 100 mcg, folic acid 1 mcg/ml. Vial 10 ml. *Rx.*
Use: Nutritional supplement.

Sanhist T.D. 5. (Sandia) Phenylpropanolamine HCl 50 mg, chlorpheniramine maleate 5 mg, ascorbic acid 100 mg/Tab. Bot. 100s, 1000s. *Rx.*
Use: Decongestant, antihistamine.

Sanhist T.D. 12. (Sandia) Phenylpropanolamine HCl 50 mg, chlorpheniramine maleate 12 mg, ascorbic acid 100 mg, methscopolamine nitrate 4 mg/Tab. Bot. 100s, 1000s. *Rx.*
Use: Decongestant, antihistamine combination.

Sani-Supp. (G & W Laboratories) Glycerin, sodium stearate. Supp. 10s, 12s, 24s, 25s, 48s, 50s, 100s, 1000s. *otc.*
Use: Laxative.

sanluol.
See: Arsphenamine (Various Mfr.).

Sanorex. (Novartis) Mazindol 1 mg or 2 mg/Tab. Bot. 100s. *c-IV.*
Use: Anorexiant.

Sansert. (Novartis) Methysergide maleate 2 mg/Tab. Bot. 100s. *Rx.*
Use: Antimigraine.

Sanstress. (Sandia) Vitamins A 25,000 IU, D 400 IU, B_1 10 mg, B_2 5 mg, niacinamide 100 mg, B_6 1 mg, B_{12} 5 mcg, C 150 mg, calcium 103 mg, phosphorus 80 mg, iron 10 mg, copper 1 mg, iodine 0.1 mg, magnesium 5.5 mg, manganese 1 mg, potassium 5 mg, zinc 1.4 mg/Cap. Bot. 100s, 1000s. *otc.*
Use: Mineral, vitamin supplement.

Santiseptic Lotion. (Santiseptic) Menthol, phenol, benzocaine, zinc oxide, calamine. Bot. 4 oz. *otc.*
Use: Dermatologic, counterirritant.

Santyl. (Knoll Pharmaceuticals) Proteolytic enzyme derived from *Clostridium histolyticum.* 250 units/g Oint. Tube 15 g, 30 g. *Rx.*
Use: Enzyme, topical.

•**saperconazole.** (SAP-ehr-KOE-nah-zole) USAN.
Use: Antifungal.

saponated cresol solution.
See: Cresol (Various Mfr.).

saponins, water soluble.

•**saprisartan potassium.** (sap-rih-SAHR-tan) USAN.
Use: Antihypertensive.

•**saquinavir mesylate.** (sack-KWIN-uh-vihr) USAN.
Use: Antiviral.
See: Invirase, Cap. (Roche Laboratories).

•**sarafloxacin hydrochloride.** (sa-rah-FLOX-ah-SIN) USAN.
Use: Anti-infective (DNA gyrase inhibitor).

•**saralasin acetate.** (sare-AL-ah-sin) USAN.
Use: Antihypertensive.

Saratoga. (Blair Laboratories) Boric acid, zinc oxide, eucalyptol, white petrolatum. Oint. Tube 1 oz, 2 oz. *otc.*
Use: Dermatologic, counterirritant.

Sardo Bath Oil Concentrate. (Schering Plough) Mineral oil, isopropyl palmitate. Bot. 3.75 oz, 7.75 oz. *otc.*
Use: Emollient.

Sardo Bath & Shower. (Schering Plough) Mineral oil, tocopherol. Oil. Bot. 112.5 ml. *otc.*
Use: Emollient.

Sardoettes. (Schering Plough) Mineral oil, tocopherol, beta carotene. Towelettes. Box 25s. *otc.*
Use: Emollient.

Sardoettes Moisturizing Towelettes. (Schering Plough) Mineral oil, isopropyl palmitate, impregnated towelling material. Individual packets. Box 25s. *otc.*
Use: Emollient.

•**sargramostim.** (sar-GRUH-moe-STIM) USAN.

Use: Antineutropenic, hematopoietic stimulant, leukopoietic (granulocyte macrophage colony-stimulating factor). [Orphan drug]
See: Leukine, Preps. (Immunex).

Sarisol No. 2. (Halsey) Butabarbital sodium 30 mg/Tab. Bot. 100s, 1000s. *c-III.*
Use: Hypnotic, sedative.

•**sarmoxicillin.** (sar-MOX-ih-SILL-in) USAN.
Use: Anti-infective.

Sarna. (Stiefel) Camphor 0.5%, menthol 0.5%, phenol 0.5% in a soothing emollient base. Bot. 7.4 oz. *otc.*
Use: Emollient.

Sarna Anti-Itch. (Stiefel) Camphor 5%, menthol 5%, carbomer 940, cetyl alcohol, DM DM hydantoin. Foam. Bot. 105 ml. *otc.*
Use: Emollient.

•**sarpicillin.** (sahr-PIH-SILL-in) USAN.
Use: Anti-infective.

SAStid soap. (Stiefel) Precipitated sulfur 10%. Bar 116 g. *otc.*
Use: Dermatologic, acne.

satumomab pendetide.
Use: Detection of ovarian cancer. [Orphan drug]
See: Oncoscint CR/OV.

saxol.
See: Petrolatum Liquid (Various Mfr.).

scabicides.
See: Benzyl Benzoate (Various Mfr.).
Cuprex, Liq. (SmithKline Beecham Pharmaceuticals).
Eurax, Cream, Lot. (Novartis Pharmaceuticals).
Kwell, Lot., Cream, Shampoo (Schwarz Pharma).

Scalpicin. (Combe) Hydrocortisone 1%, menthol, SD alcohol 40. Liq. Bot. 45 ml, 75 ml, 120 ml. *otc.*
Use: Corticosteroid, topical.

Scan. (Parker) Water soluble gel. Bot. 8 oz, gal.
Use: Ultrasound aid.

Scarlet Red Ointment Dressings. (Sherwood Medical) 5% scarlet red, lanolin, olive oil, petrolatum. Gauze. 5"×9" strips. *Rx.*
Use: Dermatologic, wound therapy.

Schamberg's. (C & M Pharmacal) Menthol 0.15%, phenol 1%, zinc oxide, peanut oil, lime water. Bot. pt, gal. *otc.*
Use: Antipruritic, counterirritant.

•**schick test control.** U.S.P. 23. *Formerly Diphtheria Toxin, Inactivated Diagnostic.*
Use: Diagnostic aid (dermal reactivity indicator).

Schirmer Tear Test. (Various Mfr.) Sterile tear test strips. 250s. *otc.*
Use: Diagnostic aid, ophthalmic.

Schlesinger's Solution.
See: Morphine HCl (Various Mfr.).

Sclerex. (Miller) Inositol 2 g, magnesium complex 34 mg, vitamins C 100 mg, calcium succinate 25 mg, A 2500 IU, D 200 IU, E 100 IU, B_1 5 mg, B_2 5 mg, B_6 5 mg, B_{12} 5 mcg, niacin 10 mg, niacinamide 30 mg, pantothenic acid 7.5 mg, folic acid 0.1 mg, iron 10 mg, copper 1 mg, manganese 2 mg, zinc 9 mg, iodine 0.10 mg/3 Tab. Bot. 60s. *otc.*
Use: Mineral, vitamin supplement.

Scleromate. (Palisades Pharm) Morrhuate sodium 50 mg/ml. Inj. Vial 30 ml. *Rx.*
Use: Sclerosing agent.

sclerosing agents.
See: Morrhuate Sodium (Taylor Pharmaceuticals).
Scleromate (Palisades Pharm).
Sotradecol (ESI Lederle Generics).

Scopace. (Hope Pharm) Scopolamine hydrobromide. 0.4 mg. Tab. Bot. 100s. *Rx.*
Use: Antiparkinson.

•**scopafungin.** (SKOE-pah-FUN-jin) USAN.
Use: Antifungal, anti-infective.

Scope. (Procter & Gamble) Cetylpyridinium Cl, tartrazine, saccharin, SD alcohol 38F 67.9%. Liq. Bot. 90 ml, 180 ml, 360 ml, 720 ml, 1080 ml, 1440 ml. *otc.*
Use: Mouthwash.

scopolamine. (skoe-PAHL-uh-meen) Hyoscine, l-Scopolamine, Epoxytropine tropate.
See: Hyoscine, Preps. (Various Mfr.).

scopolamine aminoxide hydrobromide.
W/Acetylcarbromal and bromisovalum.

•**scopolamine hydrobromide.** (skoe-PAHL-uh-meen) U.S.P. 23. *Formerly Hyoscine Hydrobromide.*
Use: Anticholinergic (ophthalmic), cycloplegic, hypnotic, mydriatic, sedative.
See: Scopace, Tab. (Hope Pharm).
W/Atropine and hyoscyamine.
See: Atropine sulfate tab.
Belladonna alkaloids.
W/Butabarbital, chlorpheniramine maleate.
See: Pedo-Sol, Elix., Tab. (Warren).

W/Hydroxypropyl methylcellulose.
See: Isopto HBr, Soln. (Alcon Laboratories).
W/Hyoscyamine sulfate, atropine sulfate, phenobarbital.
See: Hyonal C.T., Tab. (Paddock).
Hytrona, Tab. (PolyMedica).
Nilspasm, Tab. (Parmed).
Sedamine, Tab. (Dunhall Pharmaceuticals).
Sedapar, Tab. (Parmed).
Spasaid, Cap. (Century Pharm).
W/Pamabrom, pyrilamine maleate, homatropine methylbromide, hyoscyamine sulfate, methamphetamine HCl.
See: Aridol, Tab. (MPL).

scopolamine hydrobromide. (Invenex) Scopolamine HBr 0.3 mg/ml. Inj. Vial 1 ml. *Rx.*
Use: Amnestic, anxiolytic, sedative.

scopolamine hydrobromide. (Glaxo-Wellcome) Scopolamine HBr 0.86 mg/ml. Inj. amp. 0.5 ml. *Rx.*
Use: Amnestic, anxiolytic, sedative.

scopolamine hydrobromide. (Various Mfr.) Scopolamine HBr 0.4 mg and 1 mg/ml. Inj. Amp., Vial 1 ml. *Rx.*
Use: Amnestic, anxiolytic, sedative.

scopolamine hydrobromide combinations.
See: Belladonna Products.
Hyoscine HBr. (Various Mfr.).

scopolamine methobromide.
See: Methscopolamine Bromide, Preps. (Various Mfr.).

scopolamine methyl nitrate.
See: Methscopolamine Nitrate, Prep. (Various Mfr.).

scopolamine salts.
See: Belladonna Products.
Hyoscine salts.

Scorbex/12. (Taylor Pharmaceuticals) Vitamins B_1 20 mg, B_2 3 mg, B_3 75 mg, B_5 5 mg, B_6 5 mg, B_{12} 1000 mcg, C 100 mg/ml. Vial dual compartment 10 ml. *Rx.*
Use: Vitamin supplement.

Scotavite. (Scott/Cord) Vitamins A 25,000 IU, D 400 IU, B_1 10 mg, B_2 10 mg, B_6 5 mg, B_{12} 5 mcg, niacinamide 100 mg, calcium pantothenate 20 mg, C 200 mg, d-alpha tocopheryl 15 IU, acid succinate iodine 0.15 mg/Tab. Bot. 100s, 500s. *otc.*
Use: Mineral, vitamin supplement.

Scotcil. (Scott/Cord) **Tab.:** Potassium penicillin 400,000 units w/calcium carbonate/Tab. Bot. 100s, 500s. **Pow.:** 80 ml, 150 ml. *Rx.*
Use: Anti-infective; penicillin.

Scotcof. (Scott/Cord) Dextromethorphan HBr 6.85 mg, chlorpheniramine maleate 1.8 mg, phenylephrine HCl 4.4 mg, guaifenesin 66 mg, ammonium Cl 30 mg, chloroform 0.125 mg, alcohol 4.1%/5 ml. Bot. 4 oz, pt, gal. *otc.*
Use: Antihistamine, antitussive, decongestant, expectorant.

Scotnord. (Scott/Cord) Chlorpheniramine maleate 8 mg, phenylephrine HCl 20 mg, methscopolamine nitrate 2.5 mg/Cap. Bot. 100s, 500s. *Rx.*
Use: Anticholinergic, antihistamine, decongestant.

Scotonic. (Scott/Cord) Vitamins B_1 10 mg, B_2 5 mg, B_6 1 mg, niacinamide 50 mg, choline Cl 100 mg, inositol 100 mg, B_{12} 25 mcg, calcium 19 mg, iron 50 mg, folic acid 0.15 mg, alcohol 15%, sodium benzoate 0.1%/45 ml. Bot. pt, gal. *otc.*
Use: Mineral/vitamin supplement.

Scotrex. (Scott/Cord) Tetracycline 250 mg/Cap. or 5 ml. Cap. Bot. 16s, 100s, 500s. Syr. 2 oz, pt. *Rx.*
Use: Anti-infective, tetracycline.

Scott's Emulsion. (SmithKline Beecham Pharmaceuticals) Vitamins A 1250 IU, D 1400 IU/4 tsp. Bot. 6.25 oz, 12.5 oz. *otc.*
Use: Vitamin supplement.

Scot-Tussin Allergy DM. (Scot-Tussin Pharmacal) Diphenhydramine HCl 12.5 mg/5 ml, parabens, menthol. Liq. Bot. 118.3 ml. *otc.*
Use: Antihistamine.

Scot-Tussin Pharmacal Allergy. (Scot-Tussin Pharmacal) Diphenhydramine HCl 12.5 mg/5 ml, parabens, menthol. Liq. Dye free, sugar free. Bot. 120 ml. *otc.*
Use: Antihistamine.

Scot-Tussin Pharmacal DM Cough Chasers. (Scot-Tussin Pharmacal) Dextromethorphan HBr 2.5 mg, dye free, sorbitol. Loz. Pkg. 20s. *otc.*
Use: Antitussive.

Scot-Tussin Pharmacal DM Liquid. (Scot-Tussin Pharmacal) Dextromethorphan HBr 15 mg, chlorpheniramine maleate 2 mg/5 ml, alcohol 10%. Bot. 4 oz, 8 oz. Sugar free. *otc.*
Use: Antihistamine.

Scot-Tussin Pharmacal DM2 Syrup. (Scot-Tussin Pharmacal) Dextromethorphan HBr 15 mg, guaifenesin 100 mg, alcohol 1.4%/5 ml. Bot. 120 ml, 240 ml. *otc.*
Use: Antitussive, expectorant.

Scot-Tussin Pharmacal Expectorant. (Scot-Tussin Pharmacal) Guaifenesin 100 mg/5 ml, alcohol 3.5%, saccharin, menthol, sorbitol, dye free. Syr. Bot. pt, gal, 120 ml. *otc.*
Use: Expectorant.

Scot-Tussin Pharmacal Original 5-Action. (Scot-Tussin Pharmacal) Phenylephrine HCl 4.2 mg, pheniramine maleate 13.33 mg, sodium citrate 83.33 mg, sodium salicylate 83.33 mg, caffeine citrate 25 mg/5 ml, non-alcoholic. Bot. 118 ml, 473 ml, gal. *otc.*
Use: Analgesic combination, antihistamine, decongestant.

Scot-Tussin Pharmacal Original 5-Action Cold Formula. (Scot-Tussin Pharmacal) Phenylephrine HCl 4.2 mg, pheniramine maleate 13.3 mg, sodium citrate 83.3 mg, sodium salicylate 83.3 mg, caffeine citrate 25 mg/5 ml, sugar. Alcohol free. Grape flavor. Syr. Bot. 118 ml, 473 ml, gal. *otc.*
Use: Analgesic, antihistamine, decongestant.

Scot-Tussin Pharmacal Senior Clear. (Scot-Tussin Pharmacal) Guaifenesin 200 mg, dextromethorphan HBr 15 mg per 5 ml, parabens, phenylalanine, menthol, aspartame/Liq. Alcohol and sugar free. Bot 118.3 ml. *otc.*
Use: Antitussive, expectorant.

Scot-Tussin Pharmacal Sugar-Free. (Scot-Tussin Pharmacal) Dextromethorphan HBr 15 mg, chlorpheniramine maleate 2 mg/5 ml. Bot. 4 oz, 8 oz, 16 oz, gal. *otc.*
Use: Antitussive, antihistamine.

Scot-Tussin Pharmacal Sugar Free Expectorant. (Scot-Tussin Pharmacal) Guaifenesin 100 mg/5 ml w/alcohol 3.5%. Dye free, sodium free, sugar free. *otc.*
Use: Expectorant.

Scot-Tussin Pharmacal with Sugar. (Scot-Tussin Pharmacal) Phenylephrine HCl 4.17 mg, pheniramine maleate 13.3 mg, sodium citrate 83.33 mg, sodium salicylate 83.33 mg, caffeine citrate 25 mg/5 ml. Bot. 4 oz, 8 oz, 16 oz, gal. *otc.*
Use: Analgesic combination, antihistamine, decongestant.

Scot-Tussin Senior Clear. (Scot-Tussin Pharmacal) Guaifenesin 200 mg, dextromethorphan HBr 15 mg/5 ml, parabens, phenylalanine, aspartame, menthol, alcohol free. Liq. Bot. 118.3 ml. *otc.*

scurenaline.
See: Epinephrine, Prep. (Various Mfr.).

scuroforme.
See: Butyl Aminobenzoate (Various Mfr.).

S.D.M. #5. (Zeneca) Mannitol hexanitrate 7% in lactose. *Rx.*
Use: Vasodilator.

S.D.M. #17. (Zeneca) Nitroglycerin 10% in lactose. *Rx.*
Use: Vasodilator.

S.D.M. #23. (Zeneca) Pentaerythritol tetranitrate 20% in lactose. *Rx.*
Use: Vasodilator.

S.D.M. #27. (Zeneca) Nitroglycerin 10% in propylene glycol. *Rx.*
Use: Vasodilator.

S.D.M. #35. (Zeneca) Pentaerythritol tetranitrate 35% in mannitol. *Rx.*
Use: Vasodilator.

S.D.M. #37. (Zeneca) Nitroglycerin 10% in ethanol. *Rx.*
Use: Vasodilator.

S.D.M. #40. (Zeneca) Isosorbide dinitrate 25% in lactose. *Rx.*
Use: Vasodilator.

S.D.M. #50. (Zeneca) Isosorbide dinitrate 50% in lactose. *Rx.*
Use: Vasodilator.

SDZ MSL-109. (Novartis)
Use: Antiparkinson. [Orphan drug]

Sea Greens. (Modern) Iodine 0.25 mg/Tab. Bot. 220s, 460s. *otc.*

Sea Master. (Barth's) Vitamins A 10,000 units, D 400 units/Cap. Bot. 100s, 500s. *otc.*
Use: Vitamin supplement.

Sea-Omega 30. (Rugby) N-3 fat content (mg) EPA 180, DHA 140. 100s. *otc.*
Use: Nutritional supplement.

Sea-Omega 50. (Rugby) Omega-3 polyunsaturated fatty acid 1000 mg/Cap. containing EPA 300 mg, DHA 200 mg, vitamin E 1 IU Bot. 30s, 50s. *otc.*
Use: Nutritional supplement.

Sea & Ski Baby Lotion Formula. (Carter Products) Octyl-dimethyl PABA. SPF 2. Lot. Bot. 120 ml. *otc.*
Use: Sunscreen.

Sea & Ski Golden Tan. (Carter Products) Padimate O. SPF 4. Lot. Bot. 120 ml. *otc.*
Use: Sunscreen.

Seba-Lo. (Whorton) Acetone-alcohol cleanser. Bot. 4 oz. *otc.*
Use: Skin cleanser.

Sebana Shampoo. (Myers) Salicylic acid 2%. Bot. 4 oz, 8 oz, pt, qt, 0.5 gal. *otc.*
Use: Antiseborrheic.

Sebanatar Shampoo. (Myers) Salicylic acid 2%, liquor carbonis detergens 3%. Bot. 4 oz, 8 oz, pt, qt, 0.5 gal, gal. *otc.*
Use: Antiseborrheic.

Seba-Nil Cleansing Mask. (Galderma) Astringent face mask containing SD alcohol-40, sulfated castor oil, methylparaben. Tube 105 g. *otc.*
Use: Dermatologic, acne.

Seba-Nil Liquid. (Galderma) Alcohol 49.7%, acetone, polysorbate 20. Liq. Bot. 240 ml, pt. *otc.*
Use: Dermatologic, acne.

Seba-Nil Oily Skin Cleanser. (Galderma) SD alcohol, acetone. Liq. Bot. 240 ml, 473 ml. *otc.*
Use: Dermatologic, acne.

Sebasorb Lotion. (Summers) Activated attapulgite 10%, salicylic acid 2%. Bot. 45 ml. *otc.*
Use: Dermatologic, acne.

Sebizon Lotion. (Schering Plough) Sulfacetamide sodium 100 mg, methylparaben 1 mg w/trisodium edetate, sodium thiosulfate, propylene glycol, isopropyl myristate, propylene glycol monostearate, polyethylene glycol 400 monostearate, water. Tube 3 oz. *otc.*
Use: Antiseborrheic.

Sebucare Scalp Lotion. (Westwood Squibb) Laureth-4, salicylic acid 1.5%, alcohol 61%, water, PPG 40 butyl ether, dihydroabietyl alcohol, fragrance. Bot. 4 oz. *otc.*
Use: Antiseborrheic.

Sebulex with Conditioners. (Westwood Squibb) Sulfur 2%, salicylic acid 2%. Bot. 4 oz, 8 oz. *otc.*
Use: Antiseborrheic.

•**secalciferol.** (seh-kal-SIFF-eh-ROLE) USAN.
Use: Regulator (calcium); treatment of familial hypophosphatemic rickets. [Orphan drug]
See: Osteo-D (Tera, Israel).

•**seclazone.** (SEK-lah-zone) USAN.
Use: Anti-inflammatory; uricosuric.

•**secobarbital.** (see-koe-BAR-bih-tahl) U.S.P. 23.
Use: Hypnotic, sedative.

secobarbital combinations.
See: Efed, Syr., Tab. (Alto Pharmaceuticals).
Monosyl, Tab. (Arcum).

secobarbital elixir.
See: Seconal Elix. (Eli Lilly).

•**secobarbital sodium.** (see-koe-BAR-bih-tahl) U.S.P. 23.
Use: Hypnotic, sedative.
See: Seconal Sodium, Prep. (Eli Lilly).

secobarbital sodium. (Wyeth Ayerst) 50 mg/ml. Inj. Tubex 2 ml. *c-II.*
Use: Hypnotic, sedative.

secobarbital sodium and amobarbital sodium capsules.
Use: Hypnotic, sedative.
See: Tuinal, Cap. (Eli Lilly).

Seconal Sodium Pulvules. (Eli Lilly) Secobarbital sodium 100 mg. Cap. Bot. 100s, UD 100s. *c-II.*
Use: Hypnotic, sedative.

Secran Liquid. (Scherer) Vitamins B_1 10 mg, B_3 10 mg, B_{12} 25 mcg, alcohol 17%. Bot. 480 ml. *otc.*
Use: Vitamin supplement.

Secretin Ferring Powder. (Ferring Pharmaceuticals) Secretin 75 cu/10 ml Vial. 10 cu/ml when reconstituted with 7.5 ml.
Use: Diagnostic aid.

Sectral. (Wyeth Ayerst) Acebutolol HCl 200 or 400 mg/ Cap. Bot. 100s, UD 100s. *Rx.*
Use: Antihypertensive.

sedaform.
See: Chlorobutanol (Various Mfr.).

Sedamine. (Health for Life Brands) Phosphorated carbohydrate soln. Bot. 4 oz. *otc.*
Use: Antinauseant.

Sedamine. (Dunhall Pharmaceuticals) Hyoscyamine sulfate 0.1037 mg, atropine sulfate 0.0194 mg, hyoscine HBr 0.0065 mg, phenobarbital 16.2 mg/Tab. Bot. 100s, 1000s. *Rx.*
Use: Antispasmodic, sedative.

Sedapap. (Merz) Acetaminophen 650 mg, butalbital 50 mg. Tab. 100s. *Rx.*
Use: Analgesic.

Sedapap #3 Capsules. (Merz) Acetaminophen 500 mg, butalbital 50 mg, codeine phosphate 30 mg/Cap. Bot. 100s. *c-III.*
Use: Analgesic combination, narcotic.

Sedapap-10 Tablets. (Merz) Acetaminophen 10 gr, butabarbital 50 mg/Tab. Bot. 100s. *Rx.*
Use: Analgesic, sedative.

Sedapar. (Parmed) Atropine sulfate 0.0195 mg, hyoscine HBr 0.0065 mg, hyoscyamine sulfate 0.1040 mg, phenobarbital 0.25 gr/Tab. Bot. 1000s. *Rx.*
Use: Antispasmodic, sedative.

sedative/hypnotic agents.
See: Bromides (Various Mfr.).
Barbiturates (Various Mfr.).
Butisol Sodium (Ortho McNeil).
Carbamide (Urea) Compounds (Various Mfr.).

Chloral Hydrate, Preps. (Various Mfr.).
Chlorobutanol (Various Mfr.).
Dalmane, Cap. (Roche Laboratories).
Intasedol, Elix. (Zeneca).
Largon, Inj. (Wyeth Ayerst).
Lotusate, Cap. (Sanofi Winthrop).
Noludar, Tab., Cap. (Roche Laboratories).
Paraldehyde, Preps. (Various Mfr.).
Phenergan HCl, Preps. (Wyeth Ayerst).
Placidyl, Cap. (Abbott Laboratories).
Plexonal, Tab. (Novartis).
Restoril, Cap. (Novartis).
Triazolam, Tab. (Various Mfr.).
Valmid, Tab. (Eli Lilly).

sedeval.
See: Barbital (Various Mfr.).

•**sedoxantrone trihydrochloride.** (sed-OX-an-trone try-HIGH-droe-KLOR-ide) USAN.
Use: Antineoplastic (DNA topoisomerase II inhibitor).

Sedral. (Vita Elixir) Phenobarbital ⅛ gr, theophylline 2 gr, ephedrine gr/Tab. *Rx.*
Use: Bronchodilator, sedative.

•**seglitide acetate.** (SEH-glih-TIDE) USAN.
Use: Antidiabetic.

selegiline hydrochloride.
Use: Antiparkinson agent.
See: Carbex, Tab. (DuPont Pharma).
Eldepryl, Cap. (Somerset).

selegiline hydrochloride. (Apothecon) Selegiline HCl 5 mg, lactose. Tab. Bot. 60s, 500s. *Rx.*
Use: Antiparkinson agent.

Selenicel. (Taylor Pharmaceuticals) Selenium yeast complex 200 mcg, vitamins C 100 mg, E 100 mg/Cap. Bot. 90s. *otc.*
Use: Vitamin supplement.

•**selenious acid.** (seh-LEE-nee-us) U.S.P. 23.
Use: Supplement (trace mineral).

selenium. (Nion) Selenium 50 mcg/Tab. Bot. 100s. *Rx.*
Use: Nutritional supplement, parenteral.

selenium disulfide.
See: Selenium Sulfide, Deterg., Susp. (Various Mfr.).

•**selenium sulfide.** (seh-LEE-nee-uhm SULL-fide) U.S.P. 23.
Use: Antidandruff; antifungal, antiseborrheic.
See: Iosel 250, Liq. (Galderma).
Selsun, Susp. (Abbott Laboratories).

•**selenomethionine Se 75.** (seh-LEE-no-meh-THIGH-oh-neen Se 75) USAN. U.S.P. XXII.
Use: Diagnostic aid (pancreas function determination), radiopharmaceutical.
See: Sethotope, Inj. (Bristol-Myers Squibb).

Sele-Pak. (SoloPak) Selenium 40 mcg/ml. Inj. Vial 10 ml, 30 ml. *Rx.*
Use: Nutritional supplement, parenteral.

Selepen. (Fujisawa) Selenium 40 mcg/ml. Vial 3 ml, 10 ml. *Rx.*
Use: Nutritional supplement, parenteral.

•**selfotel.** (SELL-fah-tell) USAN.
Use: NMDA antagonist.

Selora Powder. (Sanofi Winthrop) Potassium Cl. *otc.*
Use: Salt substitute.

Selsun Blue. (Ross Laboratories) Selenium sulfide 1% in lotion base. Bot. 4 oz, 7 oz, 11 oz. Dry, oily, normal extra conditioning, and extra medicated (contains 0.5% menthol) formulas. *otc.*
Use: Antiseborrheic.

Selsun Suspension. (Abbott Laboratories) Selenium sulfide 2.5%. Bot. 4 fl oz. *Rx.*
Use: Antiseborrheic.

•**sematilide hydrochloride.** (SEH-may-tih-LIDE) USAN.
Use: Cardiovascular agent (antiarrhythmic).

•**semduramicin.** (sem-DER-ah-MY-sin) USAN.
Use: Coccidiostat.

•**semduramicin sodium.** (sem-DER-ah-MY-sin) USAN.
Use: Coccidiostat.

Semicid. (Whitehall Robins) Nonoxynol-9 100 mg/Vag. Supp. Box 9s, 18s. *otc.*
Use: Contraceptive.

Semprex-D. (GlaxoWellcome) Acrivastine 8 mg, pseudoephedrine HCl 60 mg. Cap. Bot. 100s. *Rx.*
Use: Decongestant.

•**semustine.** (SEH-muss-teen) USAN.
Use: Antineoplastic.

Senexon. (Rugby) Senna concentrate 5.6 mg/Tab. Sugar. Bot. 100s, 1000s. *otc.*
Use: Laxative.

Senilavite. (Defco) Vitamins A 5000 IU, C 100 mg, B_1 2.5 mg, B_2 2 mg, nicotinamide 10 mg, B_6 1 mg, calcium pantothenate 5 mg, B_{12} w/intrinsic factor concentrate 0.133 IU, ferrous fumarate 150 mg, glutamic acid HCl 150 mg, docusate sodium 50 mg/Cap. Bot. 100s. *otc.*
Use: Nutritional supplement.

Senilezol. (Edwards Pharmaceuticals) Vitamins B_1 0.42 mg, B_2 0.42 mg, B_3

1.67 mg, B_5 0.83 mg, B_6 0.17 mg, B_{12} 0.83 mcg, ferric pyrophosphate 3.3 mg, alcohol 15%. Bot. 473 ml. *otc.*
Use: Mineral, vitamin supplement.

•**senna.** (SEN-ah) U.S.P. 23.
Use: Laxative.
See: Senokot (Purdue Frederick).

senna conc., standardized.
Use: Cathartic.
See: Senokot, Gran., Tab., Supp. (Purdue Frederick).
X-Prep. Pow. (Gray).
W/Docusate sodium.
See: Gentlax S. Tab. (Blair Laboratories).
Senokap-DSS, Cap. (Purdue Frederick).
Senokot S., Tab. (Purdue Frederick).
W/Guar gum.
See: Gentlax B Tab., Gran. (Blair Laboratories).
W/Psyllium.
See: Perdiem, Gran. (Rhone-Poulenc Rorer).
Senokot W/Psyllium Pow. (Purdue Frederick).

senna fruit extract, standarized.
Use: Cathartic.
See: Senokot, Syr. (Purdue Frederick).
X-Prep, Liq. (Gray).

Senna-Gen. (Zenith Goldline) Sennosides 8.6 mg, lactose. Tab. Bot. 1000s. *otc.*
Use: Laxative.

•**sennosides.** (SEN-oh-sides) U.S.P. 23.
Use: Laxative.
See: Gentle Nature (Novartis).
Senna-Gen, Tab. (Zenith Goldline).

sennosides a & b.
Use: Laxative.
See: Ex-Lax Gentle Nature (Novartis).

Senokot Tablets and Granules. (Purdue Frederick) **Gran.:** Standardized senna concentrate. Canister 2 oz, 6 oz, 12 oz. **Tab.:** Bot. 50s, 100s, 1000s, Unit strip pack 100s, Box 20s. *otc.*
Use: Laxative.

Senokot-S Tablets. (Purdue Frederick) Standardized senna concentrate w/ docusate sodium. Tab. Bot. 30s, 60s, 1000s. *otc.*
Use: Laxative.

Senokot Suppositories. (Purdue Frederick) Standardized senna concentrate. Pkg. 6s. *otc.*
Use: Laxative.

Senokot Syrup. (Purdue Frederick) Standardized extract senna fruit. Bot. 2 oz, 8 oz. *otc.*
Use: Laxative.

Senokotxtra. (Purdue Frederick) Senna concentrate 374 mg/Tab. Bot. 12s. *otc.*
Use: Laxative.

Sensitive Eyes. (Bausch & Lomb) Sorbic acid 0.1%, EDTA 0.025%, sodium Cl, boric acid, sodium borate. Soln. Bot. 118 ml, 237 ml, 355 ml. *otc.*
Use: Contact lens care.

Sensitive Eyes Daily Cleaner. (Bausch & Lomb) Sorbic acid 0.25%, EDTA 0.5%, sodium Cl, hydroxypropyl methylcellulose, poloxamine, sodium borate. Soln. Bot. 20 ml. *otc.*
Use: Contact lens care.

Sensitive Eyes Drops. (Bausch & Lomb) Isotonic solution, sorbic acid 0.1%, EDTA 0.025%, sodium Cl, boric acid, sodium borate. Soln. Bot. 30 ml. *otc.*
Use: Contact lens care.

Sensitive Eyes Plus. (Bausch & Lomb) Boric acid, sodium borate, potassium chloride, sodium chloride, polyaminopropyl biguanide 0.00003%, EDTA 0.025%. Soln. Bot. 118 ml, 355 ml. *otc.*
Use: Contact lens care.

Sensitive Eyes Saline. (Bausch & Lomb) Sodium Cl, borate buffer, sorbic acid 0.1%, EDTA. Soln. Bot. 118 ml, 237 ml, 355 ml. *otc.*
Use: Contact lens care.

Sensitive Eyes Saline/Cleaning Solution. (Bausch & Lomb) Isotonic solution w/borate buffer, NaCl, poloxamine, sorbic acid 0.15%, sodium borate, boric acid, EDTA 0.1%. Soln. Bot. 237 ml. *otc.*
Use: Contact lens care.

Sensodyne Fresh Mint Toothpaste. (Block Drug) Potassium nitrate 5%, sodium monofluorophosphate 0.76%, saccharin, sorbitol, mint flavor. Tube 2.4 oz, 4.6 oz. *otc.*
Use: Dentrifice.

Sensodyne-SC Toothpaste. (Block Drug) Glycerin, sorbitol, sodium methyl cocoyltaurate, PEG-40 stearate, strontium Cl hexahydrate 10%, methyl and propylparabens, tint. Tube 2.1 oz, 4.0 oz. *otc.*
Use: Dentrifice.

SensoGARD. (Block Drug) Benzocaine 20%. Gel. Parabens. Tube 0.5 g. *otc.*
Use: Anesthetic, local.

Sensorcaine. (Astra) Bupivacaine HCl 0.25%: w/methylparaben. 50 ml. w/epinephrine 1:200,000 methylparaben. 50 ml. 0.5%: w/methylparaben. 50 ml. w/ epinephrine 1:200,000, methylparaben. 50 ml. 0.75%: 30 ml. Inj. *Rx.*
Use: Anesthetic, local.

Sensorcaine MPF. (Astra) Bupivacaine HCl. 0.25%: 10 or 30 ml. w/epinephrine 1:200,000, sodium metabisulfite. 10 ml, 30 ml. 0.5%: 10 or 30 ml. w/epinephrine 1:200,000, sodium metabisulfite. 5, 10 or 30 ml. 0.75%: 10 or 30 ml. w/epinephrine 1:200,000, sodium metabisulfite. 10 or 30 ml. Inj. *Rx.*
Use: Anesthetic, local.

Sensorcaine MPF Spinal. (Astra) Bupivacaine HCl 0.75%, dextrose 8.25%. Inj. 2 ml. *Rx.*
Use: Anesthetic, local.

Sensorcaine MPF Spinal. (Astra) Bupivacaine HCl 0.75%, dextrose 8.25%/ Inj. Bot. 2ml. *Rx.*
Use: Anesthetic, local.

•**sepazonium chloride.** (SEP-ah-ZOE-nee-uhm) USAN.
Use: Anti-infective, topical.

•**seperidol hydrochloride.** (seh-PURR-ih-dahl) USAN.
Use: Neuroleptic, antipsychotic.

•**seprilose.** (SEH-prih-LOHS) USAN.
Use: Antirheumatic.

•**seproxetine hydrochloride.** (sep-ROX-eh-teen) USAN.
Use: Antidepressant.

Septa. (Circle) Bacitracin 400 units, neomycin sulfate 5 mg, polymyxin B sulfate 5000 units/g in ointment base. Tube oz. *otc.*
Use: Anti-infective, topical.

Septi-Chek. (Roche Laboratories) Blood culture and simultaneous sub-culture system with three media to support clinically significant pathogens. Quick and easy assembly forms a closed system to protect sub-cultures from contamination.
Use: Diagnostic aid.

Septiphene. (SEP-tih-feen) (Monsanto)
Use: Disinfectant.

Septi-Soft. (SmithKline Beecham Pharmaceuticals) Hexachlorophene 0.25%. Liq. Bot. 240 ml, pt, gal. *otc.*
Use: Antimicrobial, antiseptic.

Septisol. (SmithKline Beecham Pharmaceuticals) **Soln.:** Hexachlorophene 0.25%. Bot. 240 ml, qt, gal. **Foam:** Hexachlorophene 0.23%, alcohol 46%. In 180 ml, 600 ml. *otc.*
Use: Antimicrobial, antiseptic.

Septo. (Vita Elixir) Methylbenzethonium Cl, ethanol 2%, menthol. *otc.*
Use: Antimicrobial, antiseptic.

Septra. (GlaxoWellcome) Sulfamethoxazole 400 mg, trimethoprim 80 mg/Tab. Bot. 100s. *Rx.*
Use: Anti-infective.

Septra DS. (GlaxoWellcome) Trimethoprim 160 mg, sulfamethoxazole 800 mg/Tab. Bot. 100s, 250s, UD 100s. *Rx.*
Use: Anti-infective.

Septra Grape Suspension. (GlaxoWellcome) Trimethoprim 40 mg, sulfamethoxazole 200 mg/5 ml. Bot. 473 ml. *Rx.*
Use: Anti-infective.

Septra I.V. (GlaxoWellcome) **80/400:** Trimethoprim 80 mg, sulfamethoxazole 400 mg/5 ml. Amp. 5 ml, Vial 10 ml, 20 ml, multidose vials 20 ml. *Rx.*
Use: Anti-infective.

Septra Suspension. (GlaxoWellcome) Trimethoprim 40 mg, sulfamethoxazole 200 mg/5 ml. Bot. 20 ml, 100 ml, 150 ml, 200 ml, 473 ml. *Rx.*
Use: Anti-infective.

•**seractide acetate.** (seer-ACK-tide) USAN.
Use: Corticotrophic peptide, hormone (adrenocorticotropic).

Ser-A-Gen. (Zenith Goldline) Hydrochlorothiazide 15 mg, reserpine 0.1 mg, hydralazine HCl 25 mg/Tab. Bot. 100s, 1000s. *Rx.*
Use: Antihypertensive combination.

Seralyzer. (Bayer Corp) A system for the measurement of enzymes, potassium levels, blood chemistries and therapeutic drug assays consisting of a reflectance photometer and a series of solid-phase reagent strips.
Use: Diagnostic aid.

Ser-Ap-Es. (Novartis Pharmaceuticals) Reserpine 0.1 mg, hydralazine HCl 25 mg, hydrochlorothiazide 15 mg/Tab. Bot. 100s, 1000s. *Rx.*
Use: Antihypertensive combination.

•**seratrodast.** (seh-RAH-troe-dast) USAN.
Use: Anti-inflammatory (non-antihistaminic), antiasthmatic (thromboxane receptor antagonist).

Serax. (Wyeth Ayerst) Oxazepam. **Cap.:** 10 mg, 15 mg, 30 mg. Bot. 100s, 500s, Redipak 25s, 100s. **Tab.:** 15 mg. Bot. 100s. *c-IV.*
Use: Anxiolytic.

•**serazapine hydrochloride.** (ser-AZE-ah-PEEN) USAN.
Use: Anxiolytic.

Sereen. (Foy) Chlordiazepoxide HCl 10 mg/Cap. Bot. 500s, 1000s. *c-IV.*
Use: Anxiolytic.

Sereine Cleaning Solution. (Optikem) Cocoamphodiacetate and glycols, EDTA 0.1%, benzalkonium Cl 0.01%.

Soln. Bot. 60 ml. *otc.*
Use: Contact lens care.

Sereine Wetting Solution. (Optikem) EDTA 0.1%, benzalkonium chloride 0.01%. Soln. Bot. 60 ml, 120 ml. *otc.*
Use: Contact lens care.

Sereine Wetting/Soaking Solution. (Optikem) EDTA 0.1%, benzalkonium Cl 0.01%. Soln. Bot. 120 ml. *otc.*
Use: Contact lens care, soaking, wetting.

Serene. (Health for Life Brands) Salicylamide 2 gr, scopolamine aminoxide HBr 0.2 mg/Cap. Bot. 24s, 60s. *Rx.*
Use: Analgesic, sedative.

Serentil. (Boehringer Ingelheim) Mesoridazine besylate. **Inj.:** 25 mg/ml Amp. 1 ml **Tab.:** 10 mg, 25 mg, 50 mg, 100 mg. Bot. 100s. **Oral Conc.:** 25 mg/ml dropper. *Rx.*
Use: Antipsychotic.

Serevent. (GlaxoWellcome) Salmeterol xinafoate 25 mcg from actuator/actuation. Aerosol. Canister 60 actuations, refills 120 actuations. *Rx.*
Use: Bronchodilator.

•**sergolexole maleate.** (SER-go-LEX-ole) USAN.
Use: Antimigraine.

sericinase. A proteolytic enzyme.

•**serine.** (SER-een) U.S.P. 23.
Use: Amino acid.

•**sermetacin.** (ser-MET-ah-sin) USAN.
Use: Anti-inflammatory.

•**sermorelin acetate.** (SER-moe-REH-lin) USAN.
Use: Growth hormone-releasing factor, diagnostic aid. [Orphan drug]

Seromycin. (Dura Pharm) Cycloserine 250 mg/Pulv. Bot. 40s. *Rx.*
Use: Antituberculous.

Serophene. (Serono Labs) Clomiphene citrate 50 mg/Tab. Bot. 10s, 30s. *Rx.*
Use: Ovulation inducer.

Seroquel. (Zeneca) Quetiapine fumarate 25 mg, 100 mg, 200 mg. Tab. 100s, UD 100s. *Rx.*
Use: Antipsychotic.

Serostim. (Serono) Somatropin 5 mg (≈ 15 IU/Vial), 6 mg (≈ 18 IU/ml). Sucrose. Pow. for Injection, lyophilized. Vial. IV. *Rx.*
Use: Hormone, growth.

serotonin reuptake inhibitors, selective.
Use: Antidepressant.
See: Paxil, Tab. (SmithKline Beecham Pharmaceuticals).
Prozac, Liq., Pulv. (Eli Lilly).
Zoloft, Tab. (Roerig).

Serpasil-Apresoline. (Novartis Pharmaceuticals) **#1:** Reserpine 0.1 mg, hydralazine HCl 25 mg/Tab. Bot. 100s. **#2:** Reserpine 0.2 mg, hydralazine HCl 50 mg/Tab. Bot. 100s. *Rx.*
Use: Antihypertensive combination.

Serpasil-Esidrix. (Novartis Pharmaceuticals) **#1:** Reserpine 0.1 mg, hydrochlorothiazide 25 mg/Tab. **#2:** Reserpine 0.1 mg, hydrochlorothiazide 50 mg/Tab. Bot. 100s, 1000s. *Rx.*
Use: Antihypertensive combination.

Serpazide Tablets. (Major) Reserpine 0.1 mg, hydralazine HCl 25 mg, hydrochlorothiazide 15 mg. Bot. 100s, 1000s. *Rx.*
Use: Antihypertensive combination.

serratia marcescens extract (polyribosomes).
Use: Primary brain malignancies. [Orphan drug]

Sertabs. (Table Rock) Reserpine 0.25 mg or 0.5 mg/Tab. Bot. 100s, 500s. *Rx.*
Use: Antihypertensive.

Sertina. (Fellows) Reserpine 0.25 mg/Tab. Bot. 1000s, 5000s. *Rx.*
Use: Antihypertensive.

•**sertindole.** (ser-TIN-dole) USAN.
Use: Antipsychotic; neuroleptic.

•**sertraline hydrochloride.** (SIR-truh-leen) USAN.
Use: Antidepressant.
See: Zoloft, Tab. (Roerig)

serum, albumin, normal human.
See: Albumin Human, U.S.P. 23. (Various Mfr.).

serum, albumin, human, radioiodinated.
See: Iodinated. I-125
Albumin Injection, U.S.P. 23

serum, globulin (human), immune.
Use: Immunization.

Serutan. (SmithKline Beecham Pharmaceuticals) Psyllium. **Gran.:** Pkg. 6 oz, 18 oz. **Pow.:** 7 oz, 14 oz, 21 oz. Fruit flavored: 6 oz, 12 oz, 18 oz. *otc.*
Use: Laxative.

Serzone. (Bristol-Myers Squibb) Nefazodone 50 mg,100 mg, 150 mg, 200 mg or 250 mg/Tab. Bot. 60s, 100s (except 250 mg). *Rx.*
Use: Antidepressant.

•**sesame oil.** N.F. 18.
Use: Pharmaceutic aid (solvent; vehicle, oleaginous).

Sesame Street Complete. (McNeil Consumer Products) Ca 80 mg, iron 10 mg,

vitamins A 2750 IU, D 200 IU, E 10 mg, B_1 0.75 mg, B_2 0.85 mg, B_3 10 mg, B_5 5 mg, B_6 0.7 mg, B_{12} 3 mcg, C 40 mg, folic acid 0.2 mg, biotin 15 mg, Cu, I, Mg, Zn 8 mg, lactose/Tab. Bot. 50s. *otc.*
Use: Mineral,vitamin supplement.

Sesame Street Plus Extra C. (McNeil Consumer Products) Vitamins A 2750 IU, D 200 IU, E 10 IU, B_1 0.75 mg, B_2 0.85 mg, B_3 10 mg, B_5 5 mg, B_6 0.7 mg, B_{12} 3 mcg, C 80 mg, folic acid 0.2 mg/Tab. Bot. 50s. *otc.*
Use: Vitamin supplement.

Sesame Street Plus Iron. (McNeil Consumer Products) Iron 10 mg, vitamins A 2750 IU, D 200 IU, E 10 IU, B_1 0.75 mg, B_2 0.85 mg, B_3 10 mg, B_5 5 mg, B_6 0.7 mg, B_{12} 3 mcg, C 40 mg, folic acid 0.2 mg/Chew. Tab. Bot. 50s *otc.*
Use: Mineral,vitamin supplement.

Sesame Street Vitamins. (McNeil Consumer Products) **For ages 4 and older:** Vitamins A 5000 IU, B_1 1.5 mg, B_{12} 6 mcg, C 60 mg, D 400 IU, E 30 IU, folic acid 400 mcg, biotin 300 mcg/Chew Tab. Bot. 60s. **For ages 2-3:** Vitamins A 2500 IU, B_1 0.7 mg, B_2 0.8 mg, B_3 9 mg, B_5 5 mg, B_6 0.7 mg, B_{12} 3 mcg, C 40 mg, D 400 IU, E 10 IU, folic acid 200 mcg, biotin 150 mcg/Chew Tab. Bot. 60s. *otc.*
Use: Vitamin supplement.

Sesame Street Vitamins and Minerals. (McNeil Consumer Products) **For ages 4 and older:** Vitamins A 5000 IU, B_1 1.5 mg, B_2 1.7 mg, B_3 20 mg, B_5 10 mg, B_6 2 mg, B_{12} 6 mcg, C 60 mg, D 400 IU, E 30 IU, folic acid 400 mcg, biotin 300 mcg, calcium 100 mg, iron 18 mg, iodine 150 mcg, zinc 15 mg, copper 2 mg/Chew Tab. Bot. 60s. **For ages 2-3:** Vitamins A 2500 IU, B_1 0.7 mg, B_{12} 3 mcg, C 40 mg, D 400 IU, E 10 IU, folic acid 200 mcg, biotin 150 mcg, calcium 80 mg, iron 10 mg, iodine 70 mcg, zinc 8 mg, copper 1 mg/Chew Tab. Bot. 60s. *otc.*
Use: Mineral,vitamin supplement.

sestron. (Smith & Nephew United, Miller & Patch).

Sethotope. (Bristol-Myers Squibb) Selenomethionine selenium 75; available as 0.25, 1 mCi.

•**setoperone.** (SEE-toe-per-OHN) USAN.
Use: Antipsychotic.

•**sevelamer hydrochloride.** (seh-VELL-ah-mer) USAN.
Use: Antihyperphosphatemic, control of hyperphosphatemia in end-stage renal disease (phophate binder).

•**sevirumab.** (seh-VIE-roo-mab) USAN.
Use: Monoclonal antibody (antiviral).

•**sevoflurane.** (SEE-voe-FLEW-rane) USAN.
Use: Anesthetic, general.
See: Ultane, Soln. for Inh. (Abbott Laboratories).

•**sezolamide hydrochloride.** (seh-ZOLE-ah-MIDE) USAN.
Use: Carbonic anhydrase inhibitor.

SFC Lotion. (Stiefel) Soap free. Stearyl alcohol, PEG-75, sodium cocoyl isethionate, parabens. Bot. 237 ml, 480 ml. *otc.*
Use: Dermatologic, cleanser.

Shade. (Schering Plough) SPF 15. Contains one or more of the following ingredients: Padimate O, oxybenzone, ethylhexyl-p-methoxycinnamate. Bot. 118 ml, 120 ml, 240 ml. *otc.*
Use: Sunscreen.

Shade Cream. (O'Leary) Jar 0.25 oz. *otc.*
Use: Contouring cream.

Shade Sunblock Gel, 15 SPF. (Schering Plough) Ethylhexyl p-methoxycinnamate, octyl salicylate, oxybenzone, SD alcohol 40. PABA free. SPF 15. Waterproof. Gel. Bot. 120 g. *otc.*
Use: Sunscreen.

Shade Sunblock Gel, 25 SPF. (Schering Plough) Ethylhexyl p-methoxycinnamate, octyl salicylate, homosalate, oxybenzone, SD alcohol 40. PABA free. Gel. Bot. 120 g. *otc.*
Use: Sunscreen.

Shade Sunblock Gel, 30 SPF. (Schering Plough) Ethylhexyl p-methoxycinnamate, homosalate, oxybenzone, 73% SD alcohol 40. Bot. 120 g. *otc.*
Use: Sunscreen.

Shade Sunblock Lotion, 15 SPF. (Schering Plough) Ethylhexyl p-methoxycinnamate, oxybenzone, benzyl alcohol, phenethyl alcohol. PABA free. Waterproof. Lot. Bot. 120 ml. *otc.*
Use: Sunscreen.

Shade Sunblock Lotion, 30 SPF. (Schering Plough) Ethylhexyl p-methoxycinnamate, 2-ethylhexyl salicylate, homosalate, oxybenzone, benzyl alcohol, phenethyl alcohol. PABA free. Waterproof. Lot. Bot. 120 ml. *otc.*
Use: Sunscreen.

Shade Sunblock Lotion, 45 SPF. (Schering Plough) Ethylhexyl p-methoxycinnamate, oxybenzone, 2-ethylhexyl salicylate, benzyl alcohol, phenethyl alcohol. PABA free. Waterproof. Lot. Bot. 120 ml. *otc.*

Use: Sunscreen.

Shade Sunblock Stick, 30 SPF. (Schering Plough) Ethylhexyl p-methoxycinnamate, oxybenzone, 2-ethylhexyl salicylate, homosalate. PABA free. Waterproof. Stick. 18 g. *otc.*
Use: Sunscreen.

Shade UvaGuard. (Schering Plough) Octyl methoxycinnamate 7.5%, avobenzone 3%, oxybenzone 3%. Waterproof. SPF 15. Lot. 120 ml. *otc.*
Use: Sunscreen.

Sheik Elite. (Schmid) Condom with nonoxynol 9 15%. In 3s, 12s, 24s, 36s. *otc.*
Use: Contraceptive.

•**shellac.** N.F. 18.
Use: Pharmaceutic aid (tablet coating agent).

Shepard's Cream Lotion. (Dermik Laboratories) Creamy lotion with no lanolin or mineral oil, for entire body. Scented or unscented. Bot. 8 oz, 16 oz. *otc.*
Use: Emollient.

Sherform-HC Creme. (Sheryl) Hydrocortisone 1%, pramoxine HCl 0.5%, clioquinol 3%. Oint. Tube 0.5 oz. *Rx.*
Use: Corticosteroid, anesthetic, local, antifungal, topical.

Sherhist. (Sheryl) Phenylephrine HCl, pyrilamine maleate/Tab. 100s. Liq. pt.
Use: Decongestant, antihistamine.

Shernatal Tablets. (Sheryl) Phosphorus free calcium, non-irritating iron, trace minerals and essential vitamins. Tab. 100s.
Use: Mineral, vitamin supplement.

Shertus Liquid. (Sheryl) Dextromethorphan HBr, chlorpheniramine maleate, phenylephrine HCl, ammonium Cl. Liq. pt.
Use: Antihistamine, antitussive, decongestant, expectorant.

Shohl's Solution. Sodium Citrate and Citric Acid Oral Soln, U.S.P. 23.
Use: Alkalizer, systemic.

short chain fatty acid solution.
Use: Ulcerative colitis. [Orphan drug]

Shur-Clens. (SmithKline Beecham Pharmaceuticals) Poloxamer 188 20%. Soln. Bot. UD 100, 200 ml. *otc.*
Use: Dermatologic.

Shur Seal Gel. (Milex) Nonoxynol-9 2%. In 24 UD gel paks. *otc.*
Use: Contraceptive, spermicide.

Sibelium. (Janssen) Flunarizine HCl. *Rx.*
Use: Vasodilator.

•**sibopirdine.** (sih-BOE-pihr-deen) USAN.
Use: Nootropic; cognition enhancer (Alzheimer's disease).

•**sibrafran.** (sib-rah-FIE-ban) USAN.
Use: Antithrombotic, fibrinogen receptor antagonist, platelet aggregation inhibitor.

•**sibutramine hydrochloride.** (sih-BYOO-trah-meen) USAN.
Use: Antidepressant, anorexic.
See: Meridia, Cap. (Knoll).

sickle cell test.
Use: Diagnostic aid.
See: Sickledex Test (Ortho Diagnostics).

Sickledex. (Ortho Diagnostics) Test kit 12s, 100s.
Use: Diagnostic aid.

Sigamine. (Sigma-Tau Pharmaceuticals) Cyanocobalamin injection 1000 mcg/ml. Vial 10 ml, 30 ml. Also Sigamine L.A. Vial 10 ml. *Rx.*
Use: Vitamin supplement.

Sigazine. (Sigma-Tau Pharmaceuticals) Promethazine HCl 50 mg/ml. Vial 10 ml. *Rx.*
Use: Antihistamine.

Signa Creme. (Parker) Conductive cosmetic quality electrolyte cream. Bot. 5 oz, 2 L, 4 L.
Use: Diagnostic aid.

Signa Gel. (Parker) Conductive saline electrode gel. Tube 250 g.
Use: Diagnostic aid-gel.

Signa Pad. (Parker) Pre-moistened electrode pads.
Use: Diagnostic aid, pad.

Signatal C. (Sigma-Tau Pharmaceuticals) Calcium 230 mg, iron 49.3 mg, vitamins A 4000 IU, D 400 IU, B_1 2 mg, B_2 2 mg, B_6 1 mg, B_{12} 2 mcg, folic acid 0.1 mg, niacinamide 10 mg, C 50 mg, iodine 0.15 mg/S.C. Tab. Bot. 100s, 1000s. *otc.*
Use: Mineral, vitamin supplement.

Signate. (Sigma-Tau Pharmaceuticals) Dimenhydrinate 50 mg, propylene glycol 50%, benzyl alcohol 5%/ml. Vial 10 ml. *Rx.*
Use: Antiemetic, antivertigo.

Signef "Supps". (Fellows) Hydrocortisone 15 mg/Supp. 12s. w or w/out appl. *Rx.*
Use: Corticosteroid, vaginal.

Sigpred. (Sigma-Tau Pharmaceuticals) Prednisolone acetate. Vial 10 ml. *Rx.*
Use: Corticosteroid.

Sigtab. (Roberts Pharm) Vitamins A 5000 IU, D 400 IU, B_1 10.3 mg, B_2 10 mg, C 333 mg, B_3 100 mg, B_6 6 mg, B_5 20 mg, folic acid 0.4 mg, B_{12} 18 mcg, E 15 mg/Tab. Bot. 90s, 500s. *otc.*

Use: Vitamin supplement.

Sigtab-M. (Roberts Pharm) Vitamins A 6000 IU, D_3 400 IU, E 45 mg, C 100 mg, B_3 25 mg, B_1 5 mg, B_2 5 mg, B_6 3 mg, folic acid 400 mcg, B_5 0.015 mg, biotin 45 mcg, Ca 200 mg, P, iron 18 mg, Mg, Cu, zinc 15 mg, Mn, K, Cl, Mo, Se, Cr, Ni, Sn, V, Si, B, vitamin K, I/ Tab. Bot.100s. *otc.*
Use: Mineral, vitamin supplement.

Silace. (Silarx) Docusate sodium 20 mg/ 5 ml. ≤ 1% alcohol. Syrup. Bot. 473 ml. *otc.*
Use: Laxative.

Silace-C. (Silarx) Docusate sodium 60 mg, casanthranol 30 mg/15 ml. 10% alcohol. Syrup. Bot. 473 ml. *otc.*
Use: Laxative combination.

Siladryl. (Silarx) Diphenhydramine HCl 12.5 mg/5 ml, alcohol 5.6%. Elixir. Bot. 118 ml. *otc.*
Use: Antihistamine.

Silafed. (Silarx) Pseudoephedrine HCl 30 mg, triprolidine HCl 1.25 mg/5 ml. Syrup. Bot. 120 ml, 240 ml, 473 ml, gal. *otc.*
Use: Antihistamine, decongestant.

•**silafilcon a.** (SIH-lah-FILL-kahn A) USAN.
Use: Contact lens material (hydrophilic).

•**silafocon a.** (SIH-lah-FOH-kahn A) USAN.
Use: Contact lens material (hydrophobic).

Silaminic Cold. (Silarx) Phenylpropanolamine HCl 12.5 mg, chlorpheniramine maleate 2 mg/5 ml. 5% alcohol. Bot. 118 ml. *otc.*
Use: Antihistamine, decongestant.

Silaminic Expectorant. (Silarx) Phenylpropanolamine HCl 12.5 mg, guaifenesin 100 mg/5 ml, alcohol 5%. Liq. Bot. 118 ml. *otc.*
Use: Decongestant, expectorant.

•**silandrone.** (sil-AN-drone) USAN.
Use: Androgen.

Sildec-DM. (Silarx) **Drops, Pediatric:** Carbinoxamine maleate 2 mg, pseudoephedrine HCl 25 mg, dextromethorphan HBr 4 mg/ml. Alcohol and sugar free. Bot. 30 ml. **Syrup:** Carbinoxamine maleate 4 mg, pseudoephedrine HCl 60 mg, dextromethorphan HBr 15 mg/5 ml. Bot. 473 ml. *Rx.*
Use: Antihistamine, antitussive, decongestant.

•**sildenafil citrate.** (sill-DEN-ah-fil SIH-trate) USAN.
Use: Anti-impotence agent.
See: Viagra, Tab. (Pfizer).

Sildicon-E. (Silarx) Phenylpropanolamine HCl 6.25 mg, guaifenesin 30 mg. Pediatric drops. 0.6% alcohol. Bot. 30 ml. *otc.*
Use: Decongestant, expectorant.

•**silica, dental-type.** (SILL-ih-kah) N.F. 18.
Use: Pharmaceutic aid.

•**siliceous earth, purified.** (sih-LIH-shus) N.F. 18.
Use: Pharmaceutic aid (filtering medium).

•**silicon dioxide.** (SILL-ih-kahn die-OX-ide) N.F. 18. *Formerly Silica Gel.*
Use: Pharmaceutic aid (dispersing and suspending agent).

•**silicon dioxide, colloidal.** N.F. 18.
Use: Pharmaceutic aid (tablet/capsule diluent, suspending and thickening agent).

Silicone. (Dow Chemicals) Dimethicone. Liq., Bot. oz. Bulk Pkg. Oint.
See also:
W/Nitro-Cellulose, castor oil.
See: Covicone, Cream (Abbott Laboratories).
W/Triethylene glycol, mineral oil.
See: Allergex, Liq., Spray (Bayer Corp).

silicone oil.
See: polydimethylsiloxane (silicone oil).

silicone ointment. Dimethicone Dimethyl polysiloxane.
See: Covicone Cream (Abbott Laboratories).

Silicone Ointment No. 2. (C & M Pharmacal) High viscosity silicone 10% in a blend of petrolatum and hydrophobic starch. Jar 2 oz, lb. *otc.*
Use: Protective agent.

Silicone Powder. (Gordon Laboratories) Talc with silicone. Pkg. 4 oz, 1 lb, 5 lb. *otc.*
Use: Dusting powder.

•**silodrate.** (SILL-oh-drate) USAN.
Use: Antacid.

Silphen Cough. (Silarx) Diphenhydramine HCl 12.5 mg/5 ml, alcohol 5%, menthol, sucrose. Syrup. Bot. 118 ml. *otc.*
Use: Antihistamine.

Silphen DM. (Silarx) Dextromethorphan HBr 10 mg/5 ml. Syrup. 5% alcohol. Bot. 118 ml. *otc.*
Use: Antitussive.

Siltapp with Dextromethorphan HBr Cold & Cough. (Silarx) Brompheniramine maleate 2 mg, phenylpropanolamine HCl 12.5 mg, dextromethorphan HBr 10 mg/5 ml. Elix. 2.3% alcohol,

sorbitol, saccharin. Bot. 118 ml. *otc.*
Use: Antihistamine, antitussive, decongestant.

Sil-Tex. (Silarx) Phenylephrine HCl 5 mg, phenylpropanolamine HCl 20 mg, guaifenesin 100 mg/5 ml. Liq. 5% alcohol, saccharin, sorbitol, sucrose. In 473 ml. *Rx.*
Use: Expectorant.

Siltussin. (Silarx) Guaifenesin 100 mg/5 ml, alcohol 3.5%. Syrup. Bot. 473 ml. *otc.*
Use: Expectorant.

Siltussin-CF. (Silarx) Phenylpropanolamine HCl 12.5 mg, dextromethorphan HBr 10 mg, guaifenesin 100 mg/5 ml. Liq. 4.75% alcohol. Bot. 118 ml. *otc.*
Use: Antitussive, decongestant, expectorant.

Siltussin DM. (Silarx) Dextromethorphan HBr 10 mg, guaifenesin 100 mg/5 ml. Syrup. Alcohol free. Saccharin, sucrose. Bot. 118 ml. *otc.*
Use: Antitussive, expectorant.

Silvadene. (Hoechst Marion Roussel) Silver sulfadiazine (10 mg/Gm) 1%, base w/white petrolatum, stearyl alcohol, isopropyl myristate, sorbitan monooleate, polyoxyl 40 stearate, propylene glycol, water, methylparaben. Cream Jar 50 g, 85 g, 400 g, 1000 g. Tube 20 g. *Rx.*
Use: Antimicrobial, topical.

silver compounds.
See: Silver Iodide, Colloidal.
Silver Nitrate, Preps. (Various Mfr.).
Silver Protein, Mild (Various Mfr.).
Silver Protein, Strong (Various Mfr.).

•**silver nitrate.** (SILL-ver NYE-trate) U.S.P. 23.
Use: Anti-infective (topical).

silver nitrate ointment. (Gordon Laboratories) Silver nitrate 1% in ointment base. Jar oz. *Rx.*
Use: Astringent, epithelial stimulant.

silver nitrate ophthalmic solution. *Rx.*
Use: Astringent, anti-infective.
Generic Products:
(Gordon Laboratories)–Soln. 10%, 25%, 50%. Bot. oz.
(Eli Lilly)–Amp. 1%, 100s.
(Parke-Davis)–Cap. 1%, 100s.

silver nitrate topical sticks. (Graham Field) Silver nitrate, potassium nitrate 25%. Appl. 100s. *Rx.*
Use: Cauterizing agent.

•**silver nitrate, toughened.** (SILL-ver NYE-trate) U.S.P. 23.
Use: Caustic.

silver protein, mild. Argentum Vitellinum, Cargentos, Mucleinate Mild, Protargin Mild.
See: Argyrol Prods. (Ciba Vision Ophthalmics).

silver protein, strong.
See: Protargol, Pow. (Sterling Health).

silver sulfadiazine. (SILL-ver SULL-fah-DIE-ah-zeen)
Use: Anti-infective, topical.
See: Silvadene, Cream (Hoechst Marion Roussel).
SSD Cream (Knoll Pharmaceuticals).
SSD AF Cream (Knoll Pharmaceuticals).
Thermazene, Cream (Sherwood Medical).

Simaal Gel. (Schein Pharmaceutical) Aluminum hydroxide 200 mg, magnesium hydroxide 200 mg, simethicone 20 mg/5 ml. Liq. Bot. 360 ml. *otc.*
Use: Antacid, antiflatulant.

Simaal Gel 2. (Schein Pharmaceutical) Aluminum hydroxide 500 mg, magnesium hydroxide 400 mg, simethicone 40 mg/5 ml. Liq. Bot. 360 ml. *otc.*
Use: Antacid, antiflatulant.

•**simethicone.** (sih-METH-ih-cone) U.S.P. 23. Mixture of liquid dimethyl polysiloxanes with silica aerogel.
Use: Antiflatulent.
See: Degas, Chew. Tab. (Invamed).
Gas-X Extra Strength, Softgel Cap. (Novartis).
Maalox Anti-Gas, Chew. Tab. (Rhone-Poulenc Rorer).
Mylicon, Tab., Liq. (J & J Merck Consumer Pharm).
Mylicon-80, Tab. (J & J Merck Consumer Pharm).
Silain, Tab. (Robins).
Ingredients of:
Mylanta, Tab., Liq. (J & J Merck Consumer Pharm).
Phazyme, Tab. (Reed & Carnick).
W/Aluminum hydroxide, magnesium hydroxide.
See: Di-Gel, Liq., Tab. (Schering Plough).
Mylanta, Mylanta II, Tab., Liq. (J & J Merck Consumer Pharm).
Silain-Gel, Liq. (Robins).
Simeco, Liq. (Wyeth Ayerst).
W/Enzymes.
See: Phazyme, Tab. (Schwarz Pharma).
W/Hyoscyamine sulfate, atropine sulfate, hyoscine HBr, butabarbital sodium.
See: Sidonna, Tab. (Schwarz Pharma).
W/Hyoscyamine sulfate, atropine sulfate, scopolamine HBr, phenobarbital.

See: Kinesed, Chew. Tab. (J & J Merck Consumer Pharm).
W/Magnesium aluminum hydroxide.
See: Maalox Plus, Susp. (Rhone-Poulenc Rorer).
W/Magnesium carbonate.
See: Di-Gel, Tab., Liq. (Schering Plough).
W/Magnesium hydroxide.
See: Laxsil, Liq. (Schwarz Pharma).
W/Magnesium hydroxide, dried aluminum hydroxide gel.
See: Maalox Plus, Tab. (Rhone-Poulenc Rorer).
W/Pancreatin.
See: Phazyme, Tab. (Schwarz Pharma). Phazyme-95, Tab. (Reed & Carnrick).
W/Pancreatin, phenobarbital.
See: Phazyme-PB, Tab. (Schwarz Pharma).

Similac 13/Similac 13 with Iron. (Ross Laboratories) Milk-based infant formula ready-to-feed containing 13 calories/ fl oz, 1.8 mg iron/100 calories. Bot. 4 fl. oz. *otc.*
Use: Nutritional supplement.

Similac 20/Similac with Iron 20. (Ross Laboratories) Milk-based infant formula. Standard dilution (20 cal/fl oz). Similac with iron: iron 1.8 mg/100 cal. **Pow.:** Can lb. **Concentrated Liq.:** Can 13 fl oz. **Ready-to-feed:** Can 8 fl oz, 32 fl oz. Bot. 4 fl oz, 8 fl oz. *otc.*
Use: Nutritional supplement.

Similac 24 LBW. (Ross Laboratories) Low-iron infant formula, ready-to-feed, 24 calories/fl oz. Bot. 4 fl oz. *otc.*
Use: Nutritional supplement.

Similac 24/Similac 24 with Iron. (Ross Laboratories) Milk-based infant formula ready-to-feed (24 cal/fl oz), iron 1.8 mg/100 calories. Bot. 4 fl oz. *otc.*
Use: Nutritional supplement.

Similac 27. (Ross Laboratories) Milk-based ready-to-feed infant formula (27 cal/fl oz). Bot. 4 fl oz. *otc.*
Use: Nutritional supplement.

Similac Low-Iron Liquid & Powder. (Ross Laboratories) Protein 14.3 g, carbohydrates 72 g, fat 36 g, iron 1.5 mg, with appropriate vitamins and minerals. **Liq.:** 390 ml concentrate, 240 ml and 1 qt. ready-to-use, 120 ml and 240 ml nursettes. **Pow.:** 1 lb. *otc.*
Use: Nutritional supplement.

Similac Natural Care Human Milk Fortifier. (Ross Laboratories) Liquid fortifier designed to be mixed with human milk or fed alternately with human milk to low-birth-weight infants. Supplied as 24 cal/fl oz. Bot. 4 fl oz. *otc.*
Use: Nutritional supplement.

Similac PM 60/40. (Ross Laboratories) Milk-based formula ready-to-feed or powder with 60:40 whey to casein ratio (20 cal/fl oz). **Bot.:** Hospital use 4 fl oz. ready-to-feed. **Pow.:** Can lb. *otc.*
Use: Nutritional supplement.

Similac Special Care 20. (Ross Laboratories) Infant formula ready-to-feed (20 cal/fl oz). Bot. 4 fl oz. *otc.*
Use: Nutritional supplement.

Similac Special Care 24. (Ross Laboratories) Infant formula ready-to-feed (24 Cal/fl oz). Bot. 4 fl oz. *otc.*
Use: Nutritional supplement.

Simplet. (Major) Pseudoephedrine HCl 60 mg, chlorpheniramine maleate 4 mg, acetaminophen 650 mg/Tab. Bot. 100s. *otc.*
Use: Analgesic, antihistamine, decongestant.

Simron Plus. (SmithKline Beecham Pharmaceuticals) Iron 10 mg, vitamins B_{12} 3.33 mcg, C 50 mg, B_6 1 mg, folic acid 0.1 mg/Cap. Parabens. Bot. 100s. *otc.*
Use: Mineral supplement.

•**simtrazene.** (SIM-trah-seen) USAN.
Use: Antineoplastic.

•**simvastatin.** (SIM-vuh-STAT-in) U.S.P. 23. *Formerly Synvinolin.*
Use: Antihyperlipidemic.
See: Zocor, Tab. (Merck).

Sinapils. (Pfeiffer) Phenylpropanolamine HCl 12.5 mg, chlorpheniramine maleate 2 mg, acetaminophen 325 mg, caffeine 32.5 mg/Tab. Bot. 36s. *otc.*
Use: Analgesic, antihistamine, decongestant.

Sinarest 12 Hour. (Novartis Consumer Health) Oxymetazoline HCl 0.05%. Spray Bot. 15 ml. *otc.*
Use: Decongestant.

Sinarest Decongestant Nasal Spray. (Novartis Consumer Health) Oxymetazoline HCl 0.05%. Bot. 0.5 oz. *otc.*
Use: Decongestant.

Sinarest Extra-Strength. (Novartis Consumer Health) Acetaminophen 500 mg, chlorpheniramine maleate 2 mg, pseudoephedrine HCl 30 mg/Tab. 24s. *otc.*
Use: Analgesic, antihistamine, decongestant.

Sinarest No Drowsiness. (Novartis Consumer Health) Pseudoephedrine HCl 30 mg, acetaminophen 500 mg/Tab. Pkg. 20s. *otc.*

Use: Analgesic, decongestant.

Sinarest Sinus. (Novartis Consumer Health) Acetaminophen 325 mg, chlorpheniramine maleate 2 mg, pseudoephedrine HCl 30 mg/Tab. Pkg. 20s, 40s, 80s. *otc.*
Use: Analgesic, antihistamine, decongestant.

•**sincalide.** (SIN-kah-lide) USAN.
Use: Choleretic.

Sine-Aid IB. (McNeil Consumer Products) Pseudoephedrine 30 mg, ibuprofen 200 mg. Capl. Pkg. 20s. *otc.*
Use: Analgesic, decongestant.

Sine-Aid Maximum Strength. (McNeil Consumer Products) Pseudoephedrine HCl 30 mg, acetaminophen 500 mg/Tab.or Cap. **Tab.:** Bot. 24s, 100s. **Cap.:** Bot. 24s, 50s. *otc.*
Use: Analgesic, decongestant.

Sine-Aid Sinus Headache Caplets, Extra Strength. (McNeil Consumer Products) Acetaminophen 500 mg, pseudoephedrine HCl 30 mg/Capl. Bot. 24s, 50s. *otc.*
Use: Analgesic, decongestant.

Sine-Aid Sinus Headache Tablets. (McNeil Consumer Products) Acetaminophen 325 mg, pseudoephedrine HCl 30 mg/Tab. Bot. 24s, 50s, 100s. *otc.*
Use: Analgesic, decongestant.

•**sinefungin.** (sih-neh-FUN-jin) USAN.
Use: Antifungal.

Sinemet CR. (DuPont Pharma) Carbidopa 25 or 50 mg, levodopa 100 or 200 mg/SR Tab. Bot. 100s, UD 100s. *Rx.*
Use: Antiparkinsonian.

Sinemet 10/100. (DuPont Merck Pharmaceuticals) Carbidopa 10 mg, levodopa 100 mg/Tab. Bot. 100s, UD 100s. *Rx.*
Use: Antiparkinsonian.

Sinemet 25/100. (DuPont Merck Pharmaceuticals) Carbidopa 25 mg, levodopa 100 mg/Tab. Bot. 100s, UD 100s. *Rx.*
Use: Antiparkinsonian.

Sinemet 25/250. (DuPont Merck Pharmaceuticals) Carbidopa 25 mg, levodopa 250 mg/Tab. Bot. 100s, UD 100s. *Rx.*
Use: Antiparkinsonian.

Sine-Off Maximum Strength No Drowsiness Formula Caplets. (SmithKline Beecham Pharmaceuticals) Pseudoephedrine HCl 30 mg, acetaminophen 500 mg/Cap. Pkg. 24s. *otc.*
Use: Decongestant, analgesic.

Sine-Off Sinus Medicine. (SmithKline Beecham Pharmaceuticals) Chlorpheniramine maleate 2 mg, pseudoephedrine HCl 30 mg, acetaminophen 500 mg/Cap. Pkg. 24s. *otc.*
Use: Analgesic, antihistamine, decongestant.

Sine-Off Tablets. (SmithKline Beecham Pharmaceuticals) Chlorpheniramine maleate 2 mg, phenylpropanolamine HCl 12.5 mg, aspirin 325 mg. Tab. Pkg. 24s, 48s, 100s. *otc.*
Use: Analgesic, antihistamine, decongestant.

Sinequan. (Roerig) Doxepin HCl. **Cap.:** 10 mg, 25 mg, 50 mg, 75 mg, 100 mg, 150 mg. Bot. 50s (150 mg only), 100s; 500s (150 mg only), 1000s, 5000s. **Oral Concentrate:** 10 mg/ml. Bot. 120 ml. *Rx.*
Use: Antidepressant.

Sinex. (Procter & Gamble) Phenylephrine HCl 0.5%, cetylpyridinium Cl 0.04% w/ thimerosal 0.001% preservative. Nasal spray. Bot. 0.5 oz, 1 oz. *otc.*
Use: Decongestant.

Singlet for Adults. (SmithKline Beecham Pharmaceuticals) Pseudoephedrine HCl 60 mg, chlorpheniramine maleate 4 mg, acetaminophen 650 mg/Tab. Bot. 100s. *otc.*
Use: Analgesic, antihistamine, decongestant.

Singulair. (Merck) Montelukast sodium 10 mg, lactose. Tab. 5 mg, aspartame. Chew. Tab. Unit-of-use 30s, 90s, UD 100s. *Rx.*
Use: Antiasthmastic.

Sinocon TR. (Vangard) Phenylpropanolamine HCl 20 mg, phenylephrine HCl 5 mg, phenyltoloxamine citrate 7.5 mg, chlorpheniramine maleate 2.5 mg/Tab. Bot. 100s, 1000s. *Rx.*
Use: Antihistamine, decongestant.

Sino-Eze MLT. (Global Source) Salicylamide 3.5 gr, acetaminophen 100 mg, phenylephrine HCl 5 mg, chlorpheniramine maleate 2 mg/Tab. Bot. 1000s. *Rx.*
Use: Analgesic, antihistamine, decongestant.

Sinografin. (Bristol-Myers Squibb) Meglumine diatrizoate 52.7%, meglumine iodipamide 26.8%. Vial 10 ml.
Use: Diagnostic aid.

Sinucol. (Tennessee Pharmaceutic) Chlorpheniramine maleate 8 mg, phenylephrine HCl 20 mg, methscopolamine nitrate 2.5 mg/Cap. Bot. 100s, 500s. Inj. Vial 10 ml. *Rx.*
Use: Antihistamine, decongestant combination.

Sinufed Timecelle. (Roberts Pharm) Pseudoephedrine HCl 60 mg, guaifenesin 300 mg/Cap. Bot. 100s. *Rx.*
Use: Decongestant, expectorant.

Sinulin Tablets. (Carnrick Labs) Phenylpropanolamine HCl 25 mg, chlorpheniramine maleate 4 mg, acetaminophen 650 mg/Tab. Bot. 20s, 100s. *otc.*
Use: Analgesic, antihistamine, decongestant.

Sinumist-SR. (Roberts Pharm) Guaifenesin 600 mg/Tab. Bot. 100s. *Rx.*
Use: Expectorant.

Sinupan. (ION Laboratories) Phenylephrine HCl 40 mg, guaifenesin 200 mg/SR Cap. Bot. 100s. *Rx.*
Use: Decongestant, expectorant.

Sinuseze. (Amlab) Acetaminophen 325 mg, phenylpropanolamine HCl 25 mg, phenyltoloxamine citrate 22 mg/Tab. Bot. 36s. *otc.*
Use: Analgesic, antihistamine, decongestant.

Sinus Excedrin Extra Strength. (Bristol-Myers Squibb) Pseudoephedrine HCl 30 mg, acetaminophen 500 mg/Tab or Cap. Bot. 50s. *otc.*
Use: Decongestant, analgesic.

Sinus Headache & Congestion Tablets. (Rugby) Pseudoephedrine HCl 30 mg, chlorpheniramine maleate 2 mg, acetaminophen 500 mg/Tab. Bot. 100s, 1000s. *otc.*
Use: Decongestant, antihistamine, analgesic.

Sinus Pain Formula Allerest. (Medeva) Pseudoephedrine HCl 30 mg, chlorpheniramine maleate 2 mg, acetaminophen 500 mg. **Cap.:** Bot. 24s, 50s. **Gelcap:** Bot. 20s, 40s. *otc.*
Use: Analgesic, antihistamine, decongestant.

Sinus Relief. (Major) Pseudoephedrine HCl 30 mg, acetaminophen 325 mg/Tab. Bot. 24s, 100s, 1000s. *otc.*
Use: Decongestant, analgesic.

Sinus Tablets. (Walgreens) Acetaminophen 325 mg, chlorpheniramine maleate 2 mg, pseudoephedrine HCl mg/Tab. Bot. 30s. *otc.*
Use: Analgesic, antihistamine, decongestant.

Sinutab Maximum Strength Sinus Allergy. (Warner Lambert) Acetaminophen 500 mg, pseudoephedrine HCl 30 mg, chlorpheniramine maleate 2 mg/Tab., Capl. Blister pack 24s. *otc.*
Use: Analgesic, antihistamine, decongestant.

Sinutab Non-Drying. (Warner Lambert) Pseudoephedrine HCl 30 mg, guiafenesin 200 mg/Cap.(Liq.) Pkg. 24s. *otc.*
Use: Decongestant, expectorant.

Sinutab Sinus Maximum Strength Without Drowsiness Formula. (Warner Lambert) Acetaminophen 500 mg, pseudoephedrine HCl 30 mg/Tab or Cap. Pack 24s. *otc.*
Use: Analgesic, decongestant.

Sinutab Sinus Regular Strength Without Drowsiness. (Warner Lambert) Pseudoephedrine HCl 30 mg, acetaminophen 325 mg/Tab. Bot. 24s. *otc.*
Use: Analgesic, decongestant.

Sinutrol. (Weeks & Leo) Phenylpropanolamine HCl 25 mg, phenyltoloxamine citrate 22 mg, acetaminophen 325 mg/Tab. Bot. 40s, 90s. *otc.*
Use: Analgesic, antihistamine, decongestant.

SINUvent. (WE Pharm) Phenylpropanolamine 75 mg, guaifenesin 600 mg. LA Tab. Bot. 100s. *Rx.*
Use: Decongestant, expectorant.

Siroil. (Siroil) Mercuric oleate, cresol, vegetable and mineral oil. Emulsion, Bot. 8 oz. *otc.*
Use: Antiseptic.

sir-o-lene. (Siroil) Tube 4 oz.
Use: Emollient.

•**sirolimus.** (SER-oh-lih-muss) USAN. *Formerly Rapamycin.*
Use: Immunosuppressant.

•**sisomicin.** (SIS-oh-MY-sin) USAN.
Use: Anti-infective.

•**sisomicin sulfate.** (SIS-oh-MY-sin) U.S.P. 23.
Use: Anti-infective.

Sitabs. (Canright) Lobeline sulfate 1.5 mg, benzocaine 2 mg, aluminum hydroxide–magnesium carbonate co-dried gel 150 mg/Loz. Bot. 100s. *otc.*
Use: Smoking deterrent.

•**sitogluside.** (SIGH-toe-GLUE-side) USAN.
Use: Antiprostatic hypertrophy.

Sitzmarks. (Konsyl Pharm) Radiopaque rings 20/Cap. Bot. 10s.
Use: Radiopaque agent, gastrointestinal.

Sixameen. (Spanner) Vitamins B_1 100 mg, B_6 100 mg/ml. Vial 10 ml. *otc.*
Use: Vitamin supplement.

Skeeter Stik. (Outdoor Recreation) Lidocaine 4%, phenol 2%, isopropyl alcohol 45.5% in a propylene glycol base. Stick 1s. *otc.*
Use: Anesthetic, local.

Skelaxin. (Carnrick Labs) Metaxalone 400 mg/Tab. Bot. 100s, 500s. *Rx.*
Use: Muscle relaxant.

skeletal muscle relaxants.
See: Anectine, Soln., Pow. (GlaxoWellcome).
Flexeril, Tab. (Merck).
Mephenesin (Various Mfr.).
Metubine Iodide, Vial (Eli Lilly).
Neostig, Tab. (Freeport).
Paraflex, Tab. (Ortho McNeil).
Parafon Forte, Tab. (Ortho McNeil).
Quelicin, Fliptop & Pintop Vials, Syringe w/lancet, Amp. (Abbott Laboratories).
Rela, Tab. (Schering Plough).
Robaxin, Tab., Inj. (Robins).
Skelaxin, Tab. (Carnrick Labs).
Soma, Preps. (Wallace Laboratories).
Sucostrin, Vial, Amp. (Bristol-Myers Squibb).
Syncurine, Vial (GlaxoWellcome).
Trancopal, Cap. (Sanofi Winthrop).
d-Tubocurarine Chloride (Various Mfr.).

Skelid. (Sanofi Winthrop) Tiludronate sodium 240 mg/lactose/Tab. Foil Strips 5s. *Rx.*
Use: Treatment of Paget's disease.

SK&F 110679. (SmithKline Beecham Pharmaceuticals)
Use: Hormone, growth. [Orphan drug]

Skin Degreaser. (Health & Medical Techniques) Freon 100%. Bot. 2 oz, 4 oz. *otc.*
Use: Dermatologic, degreaser.

Skin Shield. (Del Pharmaceuticals) Dyclonine HCl 0.75%, benzethonium Cl 0.2%, acetone, castor oil, SD alcohol 40 10%. Waterproof. Liq. 13.3 ml. *otc.*
Use: Dermatologic, protectant.

skin test antigen, multiple.
See: Multitest CMI (Pasteur Merieux Connaught).

Sleep II. (Walgreens) Diphenhydramine HCl 25 mg/Tab. Bot. 16s, 32s, 72s. *otc.*
Use: Sleep aid.

Sleep Cap. (Weeks & Leo) Diphenhydramine HCl 50 mg/Cap. Bot. 25s, 50s. *otc.*
Use: Sleep aid.

Sleep-Eze Tablets. (Whitehall Robins) Diphenhydramine HCl 25 mg/Tab. Pkg. 12s, 26s, 52s. *otc.*
Use: Sleep aid.

Sleep-Eze 3. (Whitehall Robins) Diphenhydramine HCl 25 mg/Tab. Pkg. 12s, 24s. *otc.*
Use: Sleep aid.

Sleep Tabs. (Towne) Scopolamine aminoxide HBr 0.2 mg, salicylamide 250 mg/Tab. Bot. 36s, 90s. *Rx.*
Use: Sleep aid.

Sleepwell 2-Nite. (Rugby) Diphenhydramine HCl 25 mg. Tab. Bot. 72s. *otc.*
Use: Sleep aid.

Slender. (Carnation) Skim milk, vegetable oils, caseinates, vitamins, minerals. **Liq.:** 220 cal/ 10 oz. Can. **Pow.:** 173 or 200 cal mixed w/6 oz skim or low fat milk. Pkg oz. *otc.*
Use: Dietary aid.

Slender-X. (Progressive Drugs) Phenylpropanolamine, methylcellulose, caffeine, vitamins/Tab. Pkg. 21s, 42s, 84s. Gum 20s, 60s. *otc.*
Use: Dietary aid.

Slimettes. (Halsey) Phenylpropanolamine HCl 35 mg, caffeine 140 mg/Cap. Box 20s. *otc.*
Use: Dietary aid.

Slim-Fast. (Thompson Medical) Meal replacement powder mixed with milk to replace 1, 2 or 3 meals a day. *otc.*
Use: Dietary aid.

Slim-Line. (Thompson Medical) Benzocaine, dextrose/Chewing gum. Box 24s. *otc.*
Use: Dietary aid.

Slim Plan Plus Without Caffeine. (Whiteworth Towne) Phenylpropanolamine HCl 75 mg/Tab. Box 40s. *otc.*
Use: Dietary aid.

Slim-Tabs. (Wesley Pharmacal) Phendimetrazine tartrate 35 mg/Tab. Bot. 1000s. *c-III.*
Use: Anorexiant.

Sloan's Liniment. (Warner Lambert) Capsicum oleoresin 0.62%, methyl salicylate 2.66%, oil of camphor 3.35%, turpentine oil 46.76%, oil of pine 6.74%. Bot. 2 oz, 7 oz. *otc.*
Use: Analgesic, topical.

Slo-Niacin. (Upsher-Smith Labs) Niacin **250 mg/Tab.** Bot. 100s, 1000s. **500 mg/Tab.** Bot. 100s, UD 100s. **750 mg/Tab.** Bot. 100s. *otc.*
Use: Vitamin supplement.

Slo-Phyllin 80 Syrup. (Rhone-Poulenc Rorer) Theophylline anhydrous 80 mg/15 ml. Nonalcoholic. Bot. 4 oz, pt, gal, UD 15 ml. *Rx.*
Use: Bronchodilator.

Slo-Phyllin GG. (Rhone-Poulenc Rorer) Theophylline anhydrous 150 mg, guaifenesin 90 mg/Cap. or 15 ml syr. **Cap.:** Bot. 100s. **Syr.:** Bot. 480 ml. *Rx.*
Use: Bronchodilator, expectorant.

Slo-Phyllin Gyrocaps. (Rhone-Poulenc Rorer) Theophylline anhydrous 60 mg, 125 mg, 250 mg/TR Cap. Bot. 100s, 1000s, UD 100s. *Rx.*
Use: Bronchodilator.

Slo-Phyllin Tablets. (Rhone-Poulenc Rorer) Theophylline anhydrous 100 mg, 200 mg/Tab. Bot. 100s, 1000s, UD 100s. *Rx.*
Use: Bronchodilator.

Slo-Salt-K. (Mission Pharmacal) Potassium Cl 150 mg, sodium Cl 410 mg/Tab. Bot. 1000s. Strip 100s. *otc.*
Use: Salt substitute.

Slow Fe. (Novartis Pharmaceuticals) Dried ferrous sulfate 160 mg/Tab. Bot. 30s, 100s. *otc.*
Use: Mineral supplement.

Slow Fe Slow Release Iron With Folic Acid. (Novartis Pharmaceuticals) Iron 50 mg, folic acid 0.4 mg/SR Tab. Bot. 20s. *otc.*
Use: Mineral, vitamin supplement.

Slow-K. (Novartis Pharmaceuticals) Potassium Cl. Bot. 100s, 1000s, Accu-Pak units 100s. Consumer Pack 100s. *Rx.*
Use: Electrolyte supplement.

Slow-Mag. (Searle) Magnesium 64 mg/DR Tab. Bot. 60s. *otc.*
Use: Vitamin supplement.

SLT. (Western Research) Sodium levothyroxine 0.1 mg, 0.2 mg or 0.3 mg/Tab. Bot. 1000s.
Use: Hormone, thyroid.

SLT Lotion. (C & M Pharmacal) Salicylic acid 3%, lactic acid 5%, coal tar soln. 2%. Bot. 4.3 oz. *otc.*
Use: Antiseborrheic.

Small Fry Chewable Tabs. (Health for Life Brands) Vitamins A 5000 IU, D 1000 IU, B_{12} 5 mcg, B_1 3 mg, B_2 2.5 mg, B_6 1 mg, C 50 mg, niacinamide 20 mg, calcium pantothenate 1 mg, E 1 IU, l-lysine 15 mg, biotin 10 mg/Tab. Bot. 100s, 250s, 365s. *otc.*
Use: Mineral, vitamin supplement.

•**smallpox vaccine.** U.S.P. 23.
Use: Immunization.

smallpox vaccine. (ESI Lederle Generics) Tube 100 vaccinations.
Use: Immunization.

SN-13, 272.
See: Primaquine Phosphate, U.S.P. 23. (Various Mfr.).

snakebite antivenins.
See: Antivenin (Crotalidae) (Wyeth Ayerst).
Antivenin (Micurus fulvius) (Wyeth Ayerst).

snake venom.
Use: SC, IM, orally; trypanosomiasis.

Snaplets-D. (Baker Norton) Pseudoephedrine HCl 6.25 mg, chlorpheniramine maleate 1 mg, taste free. Granules 30s. *otc.*
Use: Antihistamine, decongestant.

Snaplets-DM. (Baker Norton) Phenylpropanolamine HCl 6.25 mg, dextromethorphan HBr 5 mg, taste free. Granules. 30s. *otc.*
Use: Antitussive, decongestant.

Snaplets-EX. (Baker Norton) Phenylpropanolamine HCl 6.25 mg, guaifenesin 50 mg, taste free. Granules 30s. *otc.*
Use: Expectorant, decongestant.

Snaplets-FR. (Baker Norton) Acetaminophen 80 mg. Granules Pks. 32 premeasured. *otc.*
Use: Analgesic.

Snaplets-Multi. (Baker Norton) Phenylpropanolamine HCl 6.25 mg, chlorpheniramine maleate 1 mg, dextromethorphan HBr 5 mg, taste free. Granules 30s. *otc.*
Use: Antitussive, decongestant.

Snootie by Sea & Ski. (Carter Products) Padimate O. SPF 10. Lot. Bot. 30 ml. *otc.*
Use: Sunscreen.

Snooze Fast. (BDI) Diphenhydramine HCl 50 mg. Tab. Bot. 36s. *otc.*
Use: Sleep aid.

Sno-Strips. (Akorn) Sterile tear flow test strips, 100s. *otc.*
Use: Diagnostic aid, ophthalmic. *otc.*

Soac-Lens. (Alcon Laboratories) Thimerosal 0.004%, EDTA 0.1%, wetting agents. Soln. Bot. 118 ml. *otc.*
Use: Contact lens care.

Soakare. (Allergan) Benzalkonium Cl 0.01%, edetate disodium, NaOH to adjust pH, purified water. Bot. 4 fl oz. *otc.*
Use: Contact lens care.

•**soap, green.** U.S.P. 23.
Use: Detergent.

soaps, germicidal.
See: Dial, Preps. (Centeon).
Fostex, Cake, Cream, Liq. (Westwood Squibb).
pHisoHex, Liq. (Sanofi Winthrop).
Thylox, Shampoo, Soap (Dent).

soap substitutes.
See: Acne-Dome, Cleanser (Bayer Corp).
Domerine, Shampoo (Bayer Corp).
Lowila, Cleanser (Westwood Squibb).
pHisoDerm, Preps. (Sanofi Winthrop).

•**soda lime.** N.F. 18.
Use: Carbon dioxide absorbant.

Soda Mint. (Jones Medical Industries) Sodium bicarbonate 5 gr, peppermint oil q.s./Tab. Bot. 100s, 1000s. *otc.*
Use: Antacid.

Soda Mint. (Eli Lilly) Sodium bicarbonate 5 gr, peppermint oil q.s./Tab. Bot. 100s. *otc.*
Use: Antacid.

Sodasone. (Fellows) Prednisolone sodium phosphate 20 mg, niacinamide 25 mg/ml. Vial 10 ml. *Rx.*
Use: Corticosteroid.

•**sodium acetate.** (SO-dee-uhm ASS-eh-tate) U.S.P. 23.
Use: Pharmaceutic aid (in dialysis solutions).

sodium acetate & theophylline.

•**sodium acetate c 11 injection.**] (SO-dee-uhm ASS-eh-tate) U.S.P. 23.
Use: Radiopharmaceutical.

sodium acetosulfone. (SO-dee-uhm ah-SEE-toe-sull-FONE)
Use: Leprostatic agent.
See: Promacetin, Tab. (Parke-Davis).

sodium acid phosphate.
See: Sodium Biphosphate (Various Mfr.).

sodium actinoquinol. (SO-dee-uhm ack-TIH-no-kwin-OLE)
Use: Treatment of flash burns (ophthalmic).
See: Uviban.

•**sodium alginate.** (SO-dee-uhm AL-jih-nate) N.F. 18.
Use: Pharmaceutic aid (suspending agent).

sodium aminobenzoate.
Use: Dermatomyositis and scleroderma.

sodium aminopterin. Aminopterin sodium.

sodium aminosalicylate.
See: Aminosalicylate Sodium, U.S.P. 23.

sodium amobarbital. Amobarbital Sodium, U.S.P. 23.

•**sodium amylosulfate.** (SO-dee-uhm AM-ill-oh-sull-fate) USAN.
Use: Enzyme inhibitor.

sodium anazolene. (SO-dee-uhm an-AZE-oh-leen)
Use: Diagnostic aid.

sodium antimony gluconate. (Pentostam)
Use: Anti-infective.

•**sodium arsenate As 74.** (SO-dee-uhm AHR-seh-nate) USAN.
Use: Radiopharmaceutical.

•**sodium ascorbate.** (SO-dee-uhm ass-CORE-bate) U.S.P. 23.
Use: Vitamin (antiscorbutic).
See: Cenolate, Inj. (Abbott Laboratories).
Vitac Injection, Vial (Hickman).

sodium aurothiomalate.
See: Gold Sodium Thiosulfate, U.S.P. 23.

•**sodium benzoate.** (SO-dee-uhm BEN-zoe-ate) N.F. 18.
Use: Pharmaceutic aid (antifungal, preservative); antihyperammonemic.

sodium benzoate and sodium phenylacetate.
Use: Antihyperammonemic. [Orphan drug]
See: Ucephan Soln. (Ucyclyd Pharma)

sodium benzylpenicillin. Penicillin G Sodium, U.S.P. 23. Sodium Penicillin G. *Rx.*
Use: Anti-infective, penicillin.

•**sodium bicarbonate.** (SO-dee-uhm by-CAR-boe-nate) U.S.P. 23.
Use: Alkalizer-systemic, antacid, electrolyte replacement.
W/Bismuth subcarbonate and Magnesia.
W/Sodium Bitartrate.
See: Ceo-Two, Supp. (Beutlich).
W/Sodium carboxymethylcellulose, alginic acid.
See: Pretts, Tab. (Hoechst Marion Roussel).

sodium bicarbonate. (Abbott Laboratories) Inj. **4.2%:** (5 mEq) Infant 10 ml Syringe (21 G × 1.5 in. needle). **7.5%:** (44.6 mEq) 50 ml Syringe (18 G × 1.5 in. needle) or 50 ml Amp. **8.4%:** (10 mEq) Pediatric 10 ml Syringe (21 G × 1.5 in. needle) or (50 mEq) 50 ml Syringe (18 G × 1.5 in. needle) or 50 ml Vial.
Use: Alkalizer-systemic, antacid, electrolyte replacement.

sodium biphosphate.
Use: Cathartic.
See: Sodium Phosphate Monobasic, U.S.P. 23.

sodium biphosphate/ammonium phophate sodium acid.
See: Ammonium biphosphate, sodium biphosphate and sodium acid pyrophosphate.

sodium bismuth tartrate.
See: Bismuth Sodium Tartrate, Preps.

sodium bisulfite. Sulfurous acid, monosodium salt. Monosodium sulfite.
Use: Antioxidant.

•**sodium borate.** N.F. 18.
Use: Pharmaceutic aid (alkalizing agent).

sodium butabarbital.
See: Butabarbital Sodium, U.S.P. 23.

sodium calcium edetate.
See: Calcium Disodium Versenate, Amp., Tab. (3M).

•**sodium carbonate.** N.F. 18.
Use: Pharmaceutic aid (alkalizing agent).

sodium carboxymethylcellulose. Carboxymethylcellulose Sodium, U.S.P. 23. CMC. Cellulose Gum.

sodium cellulose glycolate.
See: Carboxymethylcellulose, sodium (Various Mfr.).

sodium cephalothin. (SO-dee-uhm SEFF-ah-low-thin) Cephalothin Sodium, U.S.P. 23.
Use: Anti-infective.

•**sodium chloride.** (SO-dee-uhm KLOR-ide) U.S.P. 23.
Use: Pharmaceutic aid (tonicity agent).

sodium chloride and dextrose tablets.
Use: Electrolyte, nutrient replacement.

sodium chloride injection. U.S.P. 23. (Abbott Laboratories) Normal saline 0.9% in 150 ml, 250 ml, 500 ml, 1,000 ml cont.; **Partial-fill:** 50 ml in 200 ml, 50 ml in 300 ml, 100 ml in 300 ml; **Flip-top vial:** 10 ml, 20 ml, 50 ml, 100 ml; **Bacteriostatic vial:** 10 ml, 20 ml, 30 ml; 50 mEq, 20 ml in 50 ml fliptop or pintop vial; 100 mEq, 40 ml in 50 ml fliptop vial; 50 mEq, 20 ml univ. add. syr.; sodium Cl 0.45%, 500 ml, 1,000 ml; sodium Cl 5%, 500 ml; sodium Cl irrigating solution, 250 ml, 500 ml, 1,000 ml, 3,000 ml; (Pharmacia & Upjohn) sodium Cl 9 mg/ml w/benzyl alcohol 9.45 mg. Vial 20 ml (Sanofi Winthrop) **Carpuject:** 2 ml fill cartridge, 22 gauge 1 1/4 inch needle or 25 gauge 5/8 inch needle.
Use: Fluid and irrigation, electrolyte replacement, isotonic vehicle.

•**sodium chloride Na 22.** (So-dee-uhm KLOR-ide) USAN.
Use: Radioactive agent.

sodium chloride substitutes.
See: Salt substitute.

sodium chloride tablets. (Parke-Davis) Sodium Cl 15 1/2 gr/Tab. Bot. 1000s.
Use: Normal saline.

sodium chloride therapy.

sodium chlorothiazide for injection. (SO-dee-uhm KLOR-oh-thigh-AZZ-ide) Chlorothiazide Sodium For Injection, U.S.P. 23.
Use: Diuretic.

•**sodium chromate Cr 51 injection.** (So-dee-uhm KROE-mate) U.S.P. 23.
Use: Diagnostic aid (blood volume determination); radiopharmaceutical.
See: Radio Chromate Cr 51 Sodium.

•**sodium citrate.** (SO-dee-uhm SIH-trate) U.S.P. 23.
Use: Alkalizer-systemic.
See: Anticoagulant Citrate Dextrose Solution, U.S.P. 23.
Anticoagulant Citrate Phosphate Dextrose Solution, U.S.P. 23.

sodium citrate and citric acid oral solution. Shohl's Solution.
Use: Alkalinizer-systemic.

sodium cloxacillin. (SO-dee-uhm CLOX-ah-SILL-in)
See: Cloxacillin Sodium, U.S.P. 23.

sodium colistimethate. Colistimethane Sodium, Sterile, U.S.P. 23. Antibiotic produced by *Aerobacillus colistinus.*

sodium colistin methanesulfonate. Colistimethane Sodium, U.S.P. 23. The sodium methanesulfonate salt of an antibiotic substance elaborated by *Aerobacillus colistinus.*
Use: Anti-infective.

•**sodium dehydroacetate.** (SO-dee-uhm) N.F. 18.
Use: Pharmaceutic aid (antimicrobial preservative).

sodium dextrothyroxine. (SO-dee-uhm DEX-troe-thigh-ROCK-seen) Sodium D-3,3',5,5-tetraiodothyronine. Sodium D-3-(4-(4-Hydroxy-3,5-diiodophenoxy)-3,5-diiodophenyl)-alanine.
Use: Anticholesteremic.

sodium diatrizoate. Diatrizoate Sodium, U.S.P. 23.
Use: Radiopaque medium.

sodium dichloroacetate.
Use: Treatment of lactic acidosis and familial hypercholesterolemia. [Orphan drug]

sodium dicloxacillin. (SO-dee-uhm die-KLOX-ass-IH-lin) Dicloxacillin Sodium, U.S.P. 23.
Use: Anti-infective.

sodium dicloxacillin monohydrate.
Use: Anti-infective.
See: Pathocil, Prep. (Wyeth Ayerst).

sodium dihydrogen phosphate. Sodium Biphosphate, U.S.P. 23.

sodium dimethoxyphenyl penicillin.
See: Methicillin Sodium (Various Mfr.).

sodium dioctyl sulfosuccinate.
See: Docusate Sodium, U.S.P. 23.

sodium diphenylhydantoin. Phenytoin Sodium, U.S.P. 23. Diphenylhydantoin Sodium.
Use: Anticonvulsant.

sodium edetate. (SO-dee-uhm eh-deh-TATE) Edetate Disodium, U.S.P. 23. Tetrasodium ethylenediaminetetraacetate.
Use: Chelating agent.
See: Vagisec products (Julius Schmid).

sodium ethacrynate. (SO-dee-uhm ETH-ah-krih-nate) Ethacrynate Sodium for Injection, U.S.P. 23.
Use: Diuretic.

•**sodium ethasulfate.** (SO-dee-uhm ETH-ah-SULL-fate) USAN.
Use: Detergent.

sodium ethyl-mercuri-thio-salicylate.
See: Thimerosal (Various Mfr.).
Merthiolate, Preps. (Eli Lilly).

sodium fluorescein. Fluorescein Sodium U.S.P. 23. Resorcinolphthalein sodium.
Use: Diagnostic aid (corneal trauma indicator).

•**sodium fluoride.** (SO-dee-uhm) U.S.P. 23.
Use: Dental caries agent.
See: Fluoride, Tab. (Kirkman Sales).
Fluoride Loz. (Kirkman Sales).
Flura Drops, Drops (Kirkman Sales).
Flura-Loz, Loz. (Kirkman Sales).
Karidium, Liq., Tab. (Young Dental).
Kari-Rinse, Liq. (Young Dental).
Luride, Tab. (Colgate Oral).
Mouthkote F/R, Rinse (Parnell).
NaFeen, Tab., Liq. (Pacemaker).
Pediaflor, Drops (Ross Laboratories).
T-Fluoride, Tab. (Tennessee Pharmaceutic).
W/Vitamins.
See: Fluorac, Tab. (Rhone-Poulenc Rorer).
Mulvidren-F, Tab. (Zeneca).
So-Flo, Tab., Drops (Professional Pharm).
W/Vitamins A, D, C.
See: Tri-Vi-Flor, Drops, Tab. (Bristol-Myers).

sodium fluoride and phosphoric acid gel.
Use: Dental caries agent.

sodium fluoride and phosphoric acid topical solution.
Use: Dental caries agent.

•**sodium fluoride F 18.** (SO-dee-uhm) Injection., U.S.P. 23.
Use: Radiopharmaceutical.

sodium folate. Monosodium folate.
Use: Water-soluble, hematopoietic vitamin.

•**sodium formaldehyde sulfoxylate.** (SO-dee-uhm) N.F. 18.
Use: Pharmaceutic aid (preservative).

sodium-free salt.
See: Co-Salt, Bot. (Rhone-Poulenc Rorer).
Diasal, Prep. (Savage).

sodium gamma-hydroxybutyric acid. Under study.
Use: Anesthetic adjuvant, sleep disorders. [Orphan drug]

sodium gentisate.
See: Gentisate Sodium.

•**sodium gluconate.** (SO-dee-uhm) U.S.P. 23.
Use: Electrolyte, replacement.

sodium glucosulfone inj.
Use: Leprostatic.

sodium glutamate.
See: Glutamate.

sodium glycerophosphate. Glycerol phosphate sodium salt.
Use: Pharmaceutic necessity.

sodium glycocholate, a bile salt.
See: Bile Salts.
W/Phenolphthalein, cascara sagrada extract, sodium taurocholate, aloin.
See: Oxiphen, Tab. (PolyMedica).
W/Sodium nitrite, blue flag.
See: So-Nitri-Nacea, Cap. (Scrip).
W/Sodium taurocholate, sodium salicylate, phenolphthalein, bile extract, cascara sagrada extract.
See: Glycols, Tab. (Jones Medical Industries).

sodium heparin. Heparin Sodium, U.S.P. 23.
Use: Anticoagulant.

sodium hexacyclonate.

sodium hexobarbital.
Use: Intravenous general anesthetic.

sodium hyaluronate.
Use: Ophthalmic.
See: Amo Vitrax (Allergan).
Amvisc (Chiron Therapeutics).
Amvisc Plus (Chiron Therapeutics).
Healon (Pharmacia & Upjohn).
W/Chondroitin sulfate.
See: Viscoat, Soln. (Alcon Laboratories).

sodium hyaluronate and fluorescein sodium.
Use: Surgical aid, ophthalmic.
See: Healon Yellow (Pharmacia & Upjohn).

sodium hydrogen citrate. (Various Mfr.).

•**sodium hydroxide.** (SO-dee-uhm) N.F. 18.
Use: Pharmaceutic aid (alkalizing agent).

sodium hydroxydione succinate. Sodium 21-hydroxypregnane-3,20-dione succinate.

•**sodium hypochlorite solution.** (SO-dee-uhm high-poe-KLOR-ite) U.S.P. 23.
Use: Anti-infective, local, disinfectant.
See: Antiformin.
Dakin's Soln.
Hyclorite.

sodium hypophosphite. Sodium phosphinate.
Use: Pharmaceutic necessity.

sodium hyposulfite.
See: Sodium Thiosulfate (Various Mfr.).
W/Potassium guaiacolsufonate.
See: Guaiadol Aqueous, Vial (Medical Chem.).
W/Potassium guaiacolsulfonate, chlorpheniramine maleate, sodium bisulfite.
See: Gomahist, Inj. (Burgin-Arden).
W/Sulfur, sodium citrate, phenol, benzyl alcohol.
See: Sulfo-Iodide, Inj. (Marcen).

•**sodium iodide.** (SO-dee-uhm) U.S.P. 23.
Use: Nutritional supplement.

•**sodium iodide I 123 capsules.** U.S.P. 23.
Use: Diagnostic aid (thyroid function determination), radiopharmaceutical.

•**sodium iodide I 125.** USAN.
Use: Diagnostic aid (thyroid function determination), radiopharmaceutical.

•**sodium iodide I 131 capsules.** U.S.P. 23.
Use: Antineoplastic, diagnostic aid (thyroid function determination), radiopharmaceutical.
See: Iodotope, Cap., Soln. (Bristol-Myers Squibb).

Sodium iodide I 131. (Mallinckrodt Chemical) 0.75 to 100 mCi/Cap. 3.5 to 150 mCi/Vial. *Rx.*
Use: Antithyroid agent.

sodium iodipamide. Disodium 3,3'- (Adipoyl-diimino) bis-[2,4,6- tri-iodobenzoate].
Use: Radiopaque medium.

sodium iodomethamate.

sodium iodomethane sulfonate. Methiodal Sodium, U.S.P. 23.

sodium iothalamate. Iothalmate Sodium Inj., U.S.P. 23.
Use: Radiopaque medium.

sodium iothiouracil.

sodium ipodate. (SO-dee-uhm EYE-poe-date) Ipodate Sodium, U.S.P. 23.
Use: Radiopaque.
See: Biloptin.
Oragrafin Sodium, Cap. (Bristol-Myers Squibb).

sodium isoamylethylbarbiturate.
See: Amytal Sodium, Prep. (Eli Lilly).

•**sodium lactate injection.** (SO-dee-uhm LACK-tate) U.S.P. 23.
Use: Fluid and electrolyte replacement.

sodium lactate injection. (Abbott Laboratories) 1/6 Molar, 250 ml, 500 ml, 1,000 ml; 50 mEq, 10 ml in 20 ml flip-top vial.
Use: Electrolyte replacement.

sodium lactate solution.
Use: Electrolyte.

•**sodium lauryl sulfate.** (SO-dee-uhm LAH-rill SULL-fate) N.F. 18. Sulfuric acid monododecyl ester sodium salt. Sodium monododecyl sulfate.
Use: Pharmaceutic aid (surfactant).
See: Duponol.
W/Hydrocortisone.
See: Nutracort, Cream, Lot. (Galderma).

sodium levothyroxine. Levothyroxine Sodium, U.S.P. 23.

sodium liothyronine. Liothyronine Sodium, U.S.P. 23.
Use: Hormone, thryoid.

sodium lyapolate. (LIE-app-OLE-ate) Polyethylene sulfonate sodium. Peson (Hoechst Marion Roussel).
Use: Anticoagulant.

sodium malonylurea.
See: Barbital Sodium (Various Mfr.).

sodium mercaptomerin. Mercaptomerin Sodium, U.S.P. 23.
Use: Diuretic.

•**sodium metabisulfite.** (SO-dee-uhm) N.F. 18.
Use: Pharmaceutic aid (antioxidant).

sodium methiodal. Methiodal Sodium, U.S.P. 23. Sodium monoiodomethanesulfonate. Sodium Iodomethanesulfonate, Inj.
Use: Radiopaque medium.

sodium methohexital for injection. Methohexital Sodium for Injection, U.S.P. 23.
Use: Anesthetic, general.
See: Brevital Sod., Pow. (Eli Lilly).

sodium methoxycellulose. Mixture of methylcellulose and sodium.

•**sodium monofluorophosphate.** (SO-dee-uhm mahn-oh-flure-oh-FOSS-fate) U.S.P. 23.
Use: Dental caries agent.

sodium morrhuate, inj. Morrhuate Sodium Inj., U.S.P. 23.
Use: Sclerosing agent.

sodium nafcillin. (SO-dee-uhm naff-SILL-in) Nafcillin Sodium, U.S.P. 23.

Use: Anti-infective.

sodium nicotinate. (Various Mfr.).

W/Adenosine 5 monophosphoric acid.
Use: IV nicotinic acid therapy.

sodium nitrate combinations.

•**sodium nitrite.** (SO-dee-uhm NYE-trite) U.S.P. 23.
Use: Antidote to cyanide poisoning, antioxidant.

W/Sodium thiosulfate, amyl nitrite.
Use: Vasodilator and antidote-cyanide.
See: Cyanide Antidote Pkg. (Eli Lilly).

sodium nitrite. (Various Mfr.) Gran., Bot. 0.25 lb, 1 lb.
Use: Antidote-cyanide.

•**sodium nitroprusside.** (SO-dee-uhm NYE-troe-PRUSS-ide) U.S.P. 23.
Use: Antihypertensive.
See: Keto-Diastix (Bayer Corp).
Nipride, Vial (Roche Laboratories).
Nitropress, Vial (Abbott Laboratories).

sodium nitroprusside. (ESI Lederle Generics) 50 mg/Pow. for Inj. 5 ml. *Rx.*
Use: Antihypertensive.

sodium novobiocin. Sodium salt of antibacterial substance produced by *Streptomyces niveus*. Novobiocin monosodium salt.
Use: Anti-infective.
See: Albamycin, Cap., Syr., Vial (Pharmacia & Upjohn).

sodium ortho-iodohippurate. Iodohippurate Sodium, I-131 Injection, U.S.P. 23.
See: Hipputope (Bristol-Myers Squibb).

•**sodium oxybate.** (SO-dee-uhm OX-ee-bate) USAN.
Use: Adjunct to anesthesia.

sodium pantothenate.
Use: Orally, dietary supplement.

sodium para-aminobenzoate.
See: p-Aminobenzoate, Sodium (Various Mfr.).

sodium para-aminohippurate injection.
Use: IV, to determine kidney tubular excretion function.

sodium para-aminosalicylate.
See: p-Aminosalicylate, Sodium (Various Mfr.).

sodium penicillin G. Penicillin G Sodium, Sterile, U.S.P. 23. Sodium benzylpenicillin.

sodium penicillin O.

sodium pentobarbital. Pentobarbital Sodium, U.S.P. 23.
Use: Hypnotic.

•**sodium perborate monohydrate.** (SO-dee-uhm) USAN.

sodium peroxyborate.
See: Sodium Perborate. (Various Mfr.).

sodium peroxyhydrate.
See: Sodium Perborate. (Various Mfr.).

•**sodium pertechnetate Tc 99m injection.** (SO-dee-uhm per-TEK-neh-tate) U.S.P. 23. Pertechnetic acid, sodium salt.
Use: Radiopharmaceutical.
See: Minitec (Bristol-Myers Squibb).

sodium phenobarbital. Phenobarbital Sodium, U.S.P. 23.
Use: Anticonvulsant, hypnotic.

•**sodium phenylacetate.** (SO-dee-uhm FEN-ill-ASS-eh-tate) USAN.
Use: Antihyperammonemic.

•**sodium phenylbutyrate.** (SO-dee-uhm fen-ill-BYOOT-ih-rate) USAN.
Use: Antihyperammonemic.
See: Buphenyl (Ucyclyd Pharma).

sodium phenylethylbarbiturate. Phenobarbital Sodium, U.S.P. 23.

sodium phosphate. Disodium hydrogen phosphate. (Abbott Laboratories) 3 mM P and 4 mEq sodium. 15 ml in 30 ml fliptop vial.
Use: Cathartic, buffering agent, source of phosphate.

W/Gentamicin sulfate, monosodium phosphate, sodium Cl, benzalkonium Cl.
See: Garamycin Ophthalmic, Soln. (Schering Plough).

W/Sodium biphosphate.
See: Enemeez, Enema (Centeon).
Fleet Enema (C.B. Fleet).
Phospho-Soda, Liq. (C.B. Fleet).
Saf-tip, Enemas (Fuller).

sodium phosphate, dibasic. (SO-dee-uhm FOSS-fate) U.S.P. 23.
Use: Laxative.

•**sodium phosphate, dried.** U.S.P. 23.
Use: Cathartic.

•**sodium phosphate, monobasic.** (SO-dee-uhm FOSS-fate) U.S.P. 23.
Use: Cathartic.

W/Gentamicin sulfate, disodium phosphate, sodium Cl, benzalkonium Cl.
See: Garamycin Ophthalmic Soln. (Schering Plough).

W/Methenamine.
See: Uro-Phosphate, Tab. (ECR Pharmaceuticals).

W/Methenamine mandelate, levo-hyoscyamine sulfate.
See: Levo-Uroquid, Tab. (Beach Pharmaceuticals).

W/Methenamine, phenyl salicylate, methylene blue, hyoscyamine, alkaloid.
See: Urostat Forte, Tab. (Zeneca).

W/Sodium acid pyrophos, sodium bicarbonate.
W/Sodium phosphate.
See: Enemeez Enema (Centeon).
Fleet Enema (C.B. Fleet).
Phospho-Soda, Liq. (C.B. Fleet).
Saf-tip Enemas (Fuller).

sodium phosphates enema.
Use: Cathartic.

sodium phosphates oral solution.
Use: Cathartic.

sodium phosphate P32. (Mallinckrodt Chemical) 0.67 mCi/ml. Vial. 5 mCi Inj. *Rx.*
Use: Antineoplastic.

•**sodium phosphate P32 solution.** (SO-dee-uhm FOSS-fate) U.S.P. 23.
Use: Antineoplastic; antipolycythemic; diagnostic aid (neoplasm); radiopharmaceutical.

sodium phytate. (FYE-tate) Nonasodium phytate: Sodium cyclohexanehexyl (hexaphosphate).
Use: Chelating agent.

•**sodium polyphosphate.** (SO-dee-uhm pahl-ee-FOSS-fate) USAN.
Use: Pharmaceutic aid.

•**sodium polystyrene sulfonate.** (SO-dee-uhm pah-lee-STYE-reen SULL-fuhnate) U.S.P. 23.
Use: Ion exchange resin (potassium).
See: Kayexalate, Pow. (Sanofi Winthrop).

sodium polystyrene sulfonate. (Roxane) 15 g, sorbitol 14.1 g, alcohol 0.1%/60 ml. Susp. Bot. 60 ml, 120 ml, 200 ml, 500 ml. *Rx.*
Use: Ion exchange resin (potassium).

sodium polystyrene sulfonate. (Crookes-Barnes) 5% Soln. Eye-drops. Lacrivial 15 ml.
Use: Ion exchange resin (potassium).

•**sodium propionate.** (SO-dee-uhm PRO-pee-oh-nate) N.F. 18.
Use: Pharmaceutic aid (preservative).
W/Chlorophyll "a"
See: Prophyllin, Pow., Oint. (Rystan).
W/Neomycin sulfate.
See: Otobiotic, Ear Drops (Schering Plough).
W/Propionic acid, docusate sodium, salicylic acid.
See: Prosal, Liq. (Gordon Laboratories).

sodium psylliate.
Use: Sclerosing agent.

•**sodium pyrophosphate.** (SO-dee-uhm pie-row-FOSS-fate) USAN.
Use: Pharmaceutic aid.

sodium radio chromate inj. Sodium Chromate Cr 51 Inj., U.S.P. 23.

sodium radio iodide solution. Sodium Iodide I-131 Solution, U.S.P. 23.
Use: Thyroid tumors, hyperthyroidism, cardiac dysfunction.

sodium radio-phosphate, P-32. Soln. Radio-Phosphate P32 Solution. Sodium phosphate P-32 Solution, U.S.P. 23.

sodium removing resins.
See: Resins.

sodium rhodanate.
See: Sodium Thiocyanate.

sodium rhodanide.
See: Sodium Thiocyanate.

sodium saccharin. Saccharin Sodium, U.S.P. 23.
Use: Noncaloric sweetener.

•**sodium salicylate.** (SO-dee-uhm) U.S.P-. 23.
Use: Analgesic.
W/Iodide (Various Mfr.).
Use: Intravenous injection.
W/Iodide and colchicine. (Various Mfr.).
Use: I.V., gout.

sodium salicylate, natural.
Use: Analgesic.
See: Alysine, Elix. (Hoechst Marion Roussel).

sodium salicylate combinations.
See: Apcogesic, Tab. (Apco).
Bisalate, Tab. (Allison).
Bufosal, Gran. (Table Rock).
Corilin, Liq. (Schering Plough).
Nucorsal, Tab. (Westerfield).
Pabalate, Tab. (Robins).
pHisoDan, Liq. (Sanofi Winthrop).

sodium secobarbital. Secobarbital Sodium, U.S.P. 23.
Use: Hypnotic.

sodium secobarbital and sodium amobarbital capsules.
Use: Sedative.
See: Tuinal, Cap. (Eli Lilly).

•**sodium starch glycolate.** (SO-dee-uhm) N.F. 18.
Use: Pharmaceutic aid (tablet excipient).

•**sodium stearate.** (SO-dee-uhm) N.F. 18.
Use: Pharmaceutic aid (emulsifying and stiffening agent).

•**sodium stearyl fumarate.** N.F. 18.
Use: Pharmaceutic aid (tablet/capsule lubricant).

sodium stibogluconate.
Use: CDC anti-infective agent.

sodium succinate.
Use: Alkalinize urine & awaken patients

following barbiturate anesthesia.

Sodium Sulamyd Ophthalmic Oint. 10% Sterile. (Schering Plough) Sulfacetamide sodium 10%. Tube 3.5 g. *Rx.*
Use: Anti-infective, ophthalmic.

Sodium Sulamyd Ophthalmic Soln. 10% Sterile. (Schering Plough) Sulfacetamide sodium 10%. Bot. 5 ml, 15 ml. *Rx.*
Use: Anti-infective, ophthalmic.

Sodium Sulamyd Ophthalmic Soln. 30% Sterile. (Schering Plough) Sulfacetamide sodium 30%. Bot. 15 ml. Box 1s. *Rx.*
Use: Anti-infective, ophthalmic.

sodium sulfabromomethazine.
Use: Anti-infective.

sodium sulfacetamide.
See: Sulfacetamide Sodium Preps. (Various Mfr.).

sodium sulfadiazine.
See: Sulfadiazine Sodium Preps. (Various Mfr.).

sodium sulfamerazine.
See: Sulfamerazine Sodium Preps. (Various Mfr.).

sodium sulfapyridine.
See: Sulfapyridine Sodium Pow. (Pfaltz & Bauer).

•**sodium sulfate.** (SO-dee-uhm SULL-fate) U.S.P. 23.
Use: Regulator (calcium).

•**sodium sulfate S 35.** (SO-dee-uhm SULL-fate) USAN.
Use: Radiopharmaceutical.

sodium sulfathiazole.
Use: Anti-infective.
See: Sulfathiazole Sodium, Inj. (Various Mfr.).

sodium sulfoacetate. W/Sodium alkyl aryl polyether sulfonate, docusate sodium, kerohydric, sulfur, salicylic acid, hexachlorophene.
See: Sebulex, Liq., Cream (Westwood Squibb).

sodium sulfobromophthalein. Sulfobromophthalein Sodium, U.S.P. XXII.
Use: Diagnostic aid (hepatic function determination).

sodium sulfocyanate.
See: Sodium Thiocyanate. (Various Mfr.).

sodium sulfoxone. Sulfoxone Sodium, U.S.P. 23. Disodium sulfonyl-bis(p-phenyleneimino)dimethanesulfonate.
See: Diasone Sodium, Tab. (Abbott Laboratories).

sodium suramin.
See: Suramin Sodium.

sodium taurocholate, a bile salt.
See: Bile Salts.
W/Phenolphthalein, cascara sagrada extract, sodium glycocholate, aloin.
See: Oxiphen, Tab. (PolyMedica).

sodium tetradecyl sulfate.
Use: Bleeding esophageal varices. [Orphan drug]
See: Sotradecol, Inj. (ESI Lederle Generics).

sodium tetraiodophenolphthalein.
See: Iodophthalein Sodium (Various Mfr.).

sodium thiacetphenarsamide. (Abbott Laboratories).

sodium thiamylal for injection. Thiamylal Sodium For Injection, U.S.P. 23.
Use: Anesthetic-general.
See: Surital, Inj. (Parke-Davis).

sodium thiocyanate. Sodium Sulfocyanate. Sodium Rhodanide.

sodium thiopental.
See: Thiopental Sodium, U.S.P. 23.

sodium thiosalicylate.
See: Rexolate, Vial (Hyrex).
Th-Sal, Vial (Foy).

•**sodium thiosulfate.** (SO-dee-uhm thigh-oh-SULL-fate) U.S.P. 23.
Use: For argyria, cyanide and iodine poisoning, arsphenamine reactions; prevention of spread of ringworm of feet; antidote to cyanide poisoning.
W/Salicylic acid, hydrocortisone acetate, alcohol.
See: Komed HC, Lot. (PBH Wesley Jessen).
W/Salicylic acid, isopropyl alcohol.
See: Tinver, Lot. (PBH Wesley Jessen).
Versiclear, Lot. (Hope Pharmaceuticals).
W/Salicylic acid, resorcinol, alcohol.
See: Mild Komed, Lot. (PBH Wesley Jessen).
Komed, Lot. (PBH Wesley Jessen).
W/Sodium nitrite, amyl nitrite.
See: Cyanide Antidote Pkg. (Eli Lilly).

sodium thiosulfate. (Various Mfr.) 250 mg/ml. KCl 4.4 mg, boric acid 2.8 mg/ Inj. 50 ml. *Rx.*
Use: Antidote.

sodium l-thyroxine.
See: Letter, Tab. (Centeon).
Levoid, Inj., Tab. (Nutrition Control).
Synthroid, Tab., Inj. (Knoll Pharmaceuticals).

sodium tolbutamide. Tolbutamide Sodium, U.S.P. 23.
Use: Diagnostic aid (diabetes).

sodium triclofos. (SO-dee-uhm TRY-kloe-foss) Sodium trichloroethylphosphate.
Use: Sedative, hypnotic.

•**sodium trimetaphosphate.** (SO-dee-uhm try-met-AH-FOSS-fate) USAN.
Use: Pharmaceutic aid.

sodium valproate.
See: Valproate sodium.

sodium vinbarbital injection.
Use: Sedative.

sodium warfarin. Warfarin Sodium, U.S.P. 23.
Use: Anticoagulant.

Sod-Late 10. (Schlicksup) Sodium salicylate 10 gr/Tab. Bot. 1000s. *otc.*
Use: Analgesic.

Sodol Compound. (Major) Carisoprodol 200 mg, aspirin 325 mg/Tab. Bot. 100s, 500s. *Rx.*
Use: Muscle relaxant.

Sofcaps. (Alton) Docusate sodium 100 mg or 250 mg/Cap. Bot. 100s, 1000s. *otc.*
Use: Laxative.

Sofenol 5. (C & M Pharmacal) Moisturizing lotion formulation. Bot. 8 oz. *otc.*
Use: Emollient.

Soflens Enzymatic Contact Lens Cleaner. (Allergan) Papain, sodium Cl, sodium carbonate, sodium borate, edetate disodium/Tab. Vial 12s, 24s, 48s, Refill 24s, 36s. *otc.*
Use: Contact lens care.

Sof/Pro Clean SA. (Sherman) Hypertonic solution: salt buffers, copolymers of ethylene and propylene oxide, octylphenoxypolyethoxyethanol, lauryl sulfate salt of imidazoline, sodium bisulfite 0.1%, sorbic acid 0.1%, trisodium EDTA 0.25%, thimerosal free. Bot. 30 ml. *otc.*
Use: Contact lens care.

Sof/Pro-Clean. (Sherman) Buffered, hypertonic solution with thimerosal 0.004%, EDTA 0.1%, ethylene and propylene oxide, octylphenoxypolyethoxyethanol, lauryl sulfate salt of imidazoline. Bot. 30 ml. *otc.*
Use: Contact lens care.

Soft Mate Comfort Drops for Sensitive Eyes. (PBH Wesley Jessen) Borate buffered, potassium sorbate 0.13%, EDTA 0.1%, sodium Cl, hydroxyethylcellulose, octylphenoxyethanol. Drop. Bot. 15 ml. *otc.*
Use: Contact lens care.

Soft Mate Consept 1. (PBH Wesley Jessen) Hydrogen peroxide 3% w/polyoxyl 40 stearate, sodium stannate, sodium nitrate, phosphate buffer. 240 ml. *otc.*
Use: Contact lens care.

Soft Mate Consept 2. (PBH Wesley Jessen) **Soln:** Isotonic solution of sodium thiosulfate 0.5%, borate buffers, chlorhexidine gluconate 0.001%. Bot. 360 ml. **Spray:** Isotonic sodium thiosulfate 0.5%, borate buffers. Aerosol 360 ml. *otc.*
Use: Contact lens care.

Soft Mate Daily Cleaning for Sensitive Eyes. (PBH Wesley Jessen) Isotonic solution w/NaCl, octylphenoxy (oxyethylene) ethanol hydroxyethylcellulose w/potassium sorbate 0.13%, EDTA 0.2%. Soln. Bot. 1 or 30 ml. *otc.*
Use: Contact lens care.

Soft Mate Daily Cleaning Solution. (PBH Wesley Jessen) Sterile aqueous isotonic solution w/sodium Cl, octylphenoxy (oxyethylene) ethanol, hydroxyethylcellulose, thimerosal 0.004%, edetate disodium 0.2%. Bot. 30 ml. *otc.*
Use: Contact lens care.

Soft Mate Disinfecting Solution For Sensitive Eyes. (PBH Wesley Jessen) Sterile, aqueous, isotonic solution w/ sodium Cl, povidone, octylphenoxy (oxyethylene) ethanol, chlorhexidine gluconate 0.005%, borate buffer, edetate disodium 0.1%. Thimerosal free. Bot. 240 ml. *otc.*
Use: Contact lens care.

Soft Mate Disinfection and Storage Solution. (PBH Wesley Jessen) Sterile aqueous isotonic solution w/sodium Cl, povidone, octylphenoxl (oxyethylene) ethanol with a borate buffer, thimerosal 0.001%, edetate disodium 0.1%, chlorhexidine gluconate 0.005%. Bot. 8 oz. *otc.*
Use: Contact lens care.

Soft Mate Enzyme Plus Cleaner. (PBH Wesley Jessen) Subtilisin, poloxamer 338, povidone, citric acid, potassium bicarbonate, sodium carbonate, sodium benzoate. Tab. Pkg. 8s. *otc.*
Use: Contact lens care.

Soft Mate Lens Drops. (PBH Wesley Jessen) Sterile aqueous isotonic solution w/sodium Cl, potassium sorbate 0.13%, edetate disodium 0.025%. Thimerosal free. Bot. 2 oz. *otc.*
Use: Contact lens care.

Soft Mate Preservative-Free Saline Solution. (PBH Wesley Jessen) Sterile aqueous isotonic solution w/sodium Cl, borate buffer. Contains no preserva-

tives. Bot. 0.5 oz, 30 single use. *otc.*
Use: Contact lens care.

Soft Mate PS Comfort Drops. (PBH Wesley Jessen) Sterile aqueous isotonic solution w/potassium sorbate 0.13%, edetate disodium 0.1%. Bot. 15 ml. *otc.*
Use: Contact lens care.

Soft Mate PS Daily Cleaning Solution. (PBH Wesley Jessen) Sterile aqueous isotonic solution w/sodium Cl, octylphenoxy (oxyethylene) ethanol, hydroxyethyl cellulose, potassium sorbate 0.13%, edetate disodium 0.2%. Bot. 30 ml. *otc.*
Use: Contact lens care.

Soft Mate PS Saline Solution. (PBH Wesley Jessen) Sterile aqueous isotonic solution w/sodium Cl, potassium sorbate 0.13%, edetate disodium 0.025%. Bot. 8 oz, 12 oz. *otc.*
Use: Contact lens care.

Soft Mate Rinsing Solution. (PBH Wesley Jessen) Sterile aqueous isotonic solution w/sodium Cl, thimerosal 0.001%, edetate disodium 0.1%, chlorhexidine gluconate 0.005%. Bot. 8 oz. *otc.*
Use: Contact lens care.

Soft Mate Saline for Sensitive Eyes. (PBH Wesley Jessen) Isotonic, sorbic acid 0.1%, EDTA 0.1%, NaCl, borate buffer. Bot. 360 (2s) or 480 ml. *otc.*
Use: Contact lens care.

Soft Mate Saline Preservative-Free. (PBH Wesley Jessen) Sodium Cl w/borate buffer. Soln. Bot. 15 ml. *otc.*
Use: Contact lens care.

Soft Mate Saline Solution. (PBH Wesley Jessen) Sterile aqueous isotonic solution of sodium Cl. Preservative free. Bot. 8 oz, 12 oz. *otc.*
Use: Contact lens care.

Soft Mate Soft Lens Cleaners. (PBH Wesley Jessen) Kit containing: Soft Mate daily cleaning solution II (4 oz.); soft mate weekly cleaning solution (1.2 oz.); Hydra-Mat II cleaning and storage unit. *otc.*
Use: Contact lens care.

Soft'n Soothe. (B.F. Ascher) Benzocaine, menthol, moisturizers. Tube 50 g. *otc.*
Use: Anesthetic, local.

Soft Sense. (Bausch & Lomb) Lot.: Petrolatum, vitamin E, aloe, parabens. Non-greasy. 444 ml. Body Lot.: Petrolatum, vitamin E, parabens. Non-greasy. 444 ml. *otc.*
Use: Emollient.

SoftWear. (Ciba Vision Ophthalmics) Isotonic, sodium Cl, boric acid, sodium borate, sodium perborate (generating up to 0.006% hydrogen peroxide stabilized with phosphoric acid). Soln. Bot. 120 ml, 240 ml, 360 ml. *otc.*
Use: Contact lens care.

Solaneed. (Hanlon) Vitamin A 25,000 units/Cap. Bot. 100s. *Rx.*
Use: Vitamin supplement.

Solaquin. (Zeneca) Hydroquinone 2%, ethyl dihydroxypropyl PABA 5%, dioxybenzone 3%, oxybenzone 2%. Tube oz. *otc.*
Use: Dermatologic.

Solaquin Forte Cream. (Zeneca) Hydroquinone 4%, ethyl dihydroxypropyl PABA 5%, dioxybenzone 3%, oxybenzone 2% in a vanishing cream base. Tube 0.5 oz, 1 oz. *otc.*
Use: Dermatologic.

Solaquin Forte Gel. (Zeneca) Hydroquinone 4%, ethyl dihydroxypropyl PABA 5%, dioxybenzone 3%, oxybenzone 2%. Tube 0.5 oz, 1 oz. *Rx.*
Use: Dermatologic.

Solarcaine. (Schering Plough). **Lot.:** Benzocaine, triclosan, mineral oil, alcohol, aloe extract, tocoheryl acetate, menthol, camphor, parabens, EDTA. 120 ml. **Spray (aerosol):** Benzocaine 20%, triclosan 0.13%, SD alcohol 40 35%, tocopheryl acetate. 90 or 120 ml. *otc.*
Use: Anesthetic, local.

Solarcaine Aloe Extra Burn Relief. (Schering Plough) Cream: Lidocaine 0.5%, aloe, EDTA, lanolin oil, lanolin, camphor, propylparaben, eucalyptus oil, menthol, tartrazine. 120 g. Gel: Lidocaine 0.5%, aloe vera gel, glycerin, EDTA, isopropyl alcohol, menthol, diazolidinyl urea, tartrazine. 120 or 240 g. Spray: Lidocaine 0.5%, aloe vera gel, glycerin, EDTA, diazolidinyl urea, vitamin E, parabens. 135 ml. *otc.*
Use: Anesthetic, local.

Solar Cream. (Doak Dermatologics) PABA, titanium dioxide, magnesium stearate in a flesh-colored, water-repellent base. Tube oz. *otc.*
Use: Sunscreen.

solargentum.
See: Mild silver protein (Various Mfr.).

Solar Shield 15 SPF. (Akorn) Ethylhexyl-p-methoxy-cinnamate 7.5%, oxybenzone in a moisturizing base 5%, PABA free, waterproof. Lot. Bot. 120 ml. *otc.*
Use: Sunscreen.

Solar Shield 30 SPF. (Akorn) Ethylhexyl-p-methoxycinnamate 7.5%, oxyben-

zone 6%, 2-ethylhexyl salicylate 5%, 3-diphenylacrylate 7.5%, 2-ethylhexyl-2-cyano-3 in a moisturizing base, PABA free, waterproof. Lot. Bot. 120 ml. *otc.*
Use: Sunscreen.

SolBar PF Cream 50 SPF. (Person & Covey) Oxybenzone, octyl methoxycinnamate, octocrylene, PABA free, waterproof. Cream. 120 g. *otc.*
Use: Sunscreen.

SolBar PF Liquid. (Person & Covey) Octyl methoxycinnamate 7.5%, oxybenzone 6%, SD alcohol 40 76%, PABA free. SPF 30. Liq. 120 ml. *otc.*
Use: Sunscreen.

SolBar PF 15 Cream. (Person & Covey) Octyl methoxycinnamate 7.5%, oxybenzone 5%. Bot. 1 oz, 4 oz. *otc.*
Use: Sunscreen.

SolBar PF 50. (Person & Covey) Oxybenzone, octyl methoxycinnamate, octocrylene, PABA free. Waterproof. Cream 120 ml. *otc.*
Use: Sunscreen.

SolBar PF Paba Free 15. (Person & Covey) Oxybenzone 5%, octyl methoxycinnamate 7.5%. Sunscreen SPF 15. Tube 2.5 oz. *otc.*
Use: Sunscreen.

SolBar Plus 15. (Person & Covey) Padimate 6%, oxybenzone 4%, dioxybenzone 2%. Tube 1 oz, 4 oz. *otc.*
Use: Sunscreen.

Solex A15 Clear Lotion Sunscreen. (Dermol Pharmaceuticals) SPF 15. Octyl dimethyl PABA 5%, benzophenone 33%, SD alcohol. Lot. Bot. 120 ml. *otc.*
Use: Sunscreen.

Solfoton. (ECR Pharmaceuticals) Phenobarbital 16 mg/Tab. or Cap. Bot. 100s, 500s. *c-IV.*
Use: Hypnotic, sedative.

Solfoton S/C Tabs. (ECR Pharmaceuticals) Phenobarbital 16 mg/SC Tab. Bot. 100s. *c-IV.*
Use: Hypnotic, sedative.

Solganal. (Schering Plough) Aurothioglucose 50 mg/ml. Vial 10 ml. *Rx.*
Use: IM, gold therapy, antiarthritic.

Soliwax. Docusate Sodium, U.S.P. 23. Docusate Sodium, Solasulfone (I.N.N.).

Soltice Quick-Rub. (Chattem Consumer Products) Methyl salicylate, camphor, menthol, eucalyptol. Cream. Bot. 1.33 oz, 3.75 oz. *otc.*
Use: Analgesic, topical.

Solu-Barb 0.25 Tablets. (Forest Pharmaceutical) Phenobarbital 0.25 gr/Tab. Bot. 24s. *c-IV.*
Use: Hypnotic, sedative.

soluble complement receptor (recombinant human) type 1.
Use: Prevention or reduction of adult respiratory distress syndrome. [Orphan drug]

Solu-Cortef. (Pharmacia & Upjohn) **100 mg:** Hydrocortisone sodium succinate, w/benzyl alcohol. Plain vial, 5s, 25s. 100 mg/2 ml Mix-O-Vial. **250 mg:** Hydrocortisone sodium succinate, benzyl alcohol. Mix-O-Vial 2 ml, 5s, 25s. 25-Pack, 25s, 50s, etc. **500 mg:** Hydrocortisone sodium succinate, benzyl alcohol. Mix-O-Vial, 5s, 25s. **1000 mg:** Hydrocortisone sodium succinate, benzyl alcohol. Mix-O-Vial, 5s, 25s. *Rx.*
Use: Corticosteroid.

Solu-Eze. (Forest Pharmaceutical) Hydroxyquinoline 0.12%, carbitol acetate 12.10%. Bot. 3 oz. *Rx.*
Use: Dermatologic.

Solu-Medrol. (Pharmacia & Upjohn) **40 mg:** Methylprednisolone sodium succinate, benzyl alcohol. Univial 1 ml. **125 mg:** Methylprednisolone sodium succinate, benzyl alcohol. Act-O-Vial 2 ml, 5s, 25s. 25-Pack, 25s, 50s etc. **500 mg:** Methylprednisolone sodium succinate, benzyl alcohol. Vial 8 ml, vials w/diluent 8 ml. **1000 mg:** Methylprednisolone sodium succinate, benzyl alcohol. Vial 16 ml, vial w/diluent 16 ml. **2000 mg:** Methylprednisolone sodium succinate powder for injection, benzyl alcohol. Vial 30.6 ml, vial w/diluent 30.6 ml. *Rx.*
Use: Corticosteroid.

Solumol. (C & M Pharmacal) Petrolatum, mineral oil, cetyl-stearyl alcohol, sodium lauryl sulfate, glycerin, propylene glycol, sorbic acid, purified water. Jar lb. *otc.*
Use: Pharmaceutical aid, ointment base.

Solurex. (Hyrex) Dexamethasone sodium phosphate 4 mg/ml.
W/methyl and propyl parabens, sodium bisulfite. Vial 5 ml, 10 ml, 30 ml. *Rx.*
Use: Corticosteroid.

Solurex LA. (Hyrex) Dexamethasone acetate 8 mg/ml w/polysorbate 80, carboxymethylcellulose, sodium bisulfite, EDTA, benzyl alcohol. Susp. Vial 5 ml. *Rx.*
Use: Corticosteroid.

Soluvite C.T. (Pharmics) Vitamins A 2500 IU, D 400 IU, B_1 1.05 mg, B_2 1.2 mg, B_6 1.05 mg, B_{12} 4.5 mcg, C 60 mg, B_3 13.5 mg, E 15 IU, fluoride 1 mg, folic acid 0.3 mg/Tab. Bot. 100s, 1000s. *Rx.*

Use: Mineral, vitamin supplement.

Soluvite-f Drops. (Pharmics) Vitamins A 1500 IU, D 400 IU, C 35 mg, fluoride 0.25 mg/0.6 ml. Bot. 57 ml. *Rx.*
Use: Mineral, vitamin supplement.

Solvisyn-A. (Towne) Water soluble vitamin A 10,000 units, 25,000 units or 50,000 units/Cap. Bot. 100s, 1000s. *otc, Rx.*
Use: Vitamin supplement.

•**solypertine tartrate.** (SAHL-ee-PURR-teen) USAN.
Use: Antiadrenergic.

Soma. (Wallace Laboratories) Carisoprodol 350 mg/Tab. Bot. 100s, 500s, UD 500s. *Rx.*
Use: Muscle relaxant.

Soma Compound Tabs. (Wallace Laboratories) Carisoprodol 200 mg, aspirin 325 mg/Tab. Bot. 100s, 500s, UD 500s. *Rx.*
Use: Muscle relaxant.

Soma Compound w/Codeine. (Wallace Laboratories) Carisoprodol 200 mg, aspirin 325 mg, codeine phosphate 16 mg/Tab. Sodium metabisulfite. Bot. 100s. *c-III.*
Use: Muscle relaxant.

Somagard. (Roberts Pharm)
See: Deslorelin.

•**somantadine hydrochoride.** (sah-MAN-tah-deen) USAN.
Use: Antiviral.

somatostatin.
Use: Digestive aid. [Orphan drug]
See: Zecnil.

•**somatrem.** (so-muh-TREM) USAN.
Use: Hormone, growth.
See: Protropin, Inj. (Genentech).

•**somatropin.** (SO-muh-TROE-pin) USAN. Growth hormone derived from the anterior pituitary gland.
Use: Hormone, growth. [Orphan drug]
See: Humatrope, Inj. (Eli Lilly).
Norditropin, Pow. for Inj. (Novo Nordisk).
Nutropin, Inj. (Genentech).
Saizen, Inj. (Serono).
Serostim, Inj. (Serono).

Sominex. (SmithKline Beecham Pharmaceuticals) Diphenhydramine HCl 25 mg/Tab. Blister pack 16s, 32s, 72s. *otc.*
Use: Sleep aid.

Sominex Caplets. (SmithKline Beecham Pharmaceuticals) Diphenhydramine HCl 50 mg. Tab. Blister pack 8s, 16s, 32s. *otc.*
Use: Sleep aid.

Sominex Pain Relief Formula. (SmithKline Beecham Pharmaceuticals) Diphenhydramine HCl 25 mg, acetaminophen 500 mg/Tab. Blister pack 16s. Bot. 32s. *otc.*
Use: Sleep aid, analgesic.

Sonacide. (Wyeth Ayerst) Potentiated acid glutaraldehyde. Bot. 1 gal, 5 gal. *otc.*
Use: Disinfectant, sterilizing agent.

Sonekap. (Eastwood) Cap. Bot. 100s.

soneryl.
See: Butethal (Various Mfr.).

Soothaderm. (Pharmakon Labs) Pyrilamine maleate 2.07 mg, benzocaine 2.08 mg, zinc oxide 41.35 mg/ml, camphor, menthol. Lot. Bot. 118 ml. *otc.*
Use: Antihistamine, anesthetic, local.

Soothe. (Alcon Laboratories) Tetrahydrozoline 0.05%, benzalkonium Cl 0.004%, adsorbobase. Bot. 15 ml. *otc.*
Use: Decongestant, ophthalmic.

Soothe. (Walgreens) Bismuth subsalicylate 100 mg/Tsp. Bot. 9 oz. *otc.*
Use: Antidiarrheal.

Soquette. (PBH Wesley Jessen) Polyvinyl alcohol w/benzalkonium Cl 0.01%, EDTA 0.2%. Bot. 4 fl oz. *otc.*
Use: Contact lens care.

Sorbase Cough Syrup. (Fort David) Dextromethorphan HBr 10 mg, guaifenesin 100 mg/5 ml in sorbitol base. Bot. 4 oz, pt, gal. *otc.*
Use: Antitussive, expectorant.

•**sorbic acid.** (SORE-bik) N.F. 18.
Use: Pharmaceutic aid (antimicrobial).

Sorbide T.D. (Merz) Isosorbide dinitrate 40 mg/TR Cap. Bot. 100s. *Rx.*
Use: Antianginal.

Sorbidon Hydrate. (Gordon Laboratories) Water-in-oil ointment. Jar 2 oz, 0.5 oz, 1 lb, 5 lb. *otc.*
Use: Emollient.

sorbimacrogol oleate 300.
See: Polysorbate 80.

•**sorbinil.** (SORE-bih-nill) USAN.
Use: Enzyme inhibitor (aldose reductase).

•**sorbitan monolaurate.** (SORE-bih-tan MAHN-oh-LORE-ate) N.F. 18.
Use: Pharmaceutic aid (surfactant).
See: Span 20 (Zeneca).

•**sorbitan monooleate.** (SORE-bih-tan MAHN-oh-OH-lee-ate) N.F. 18.
Use: Pharmaceutic aid (surfactant).
See: Span 80 (Zeneca).

sorbitan monooleate polyoxyethylene derivatives.
See: Polysorbate 80, N.F. 18.

•**sorbitan monopalmitate.** (SORE-bih-tan MAHN-oh-PAL-mih-tate) N.F. 18.
Use: Pharmaceutic aid (surfactant).
See: Span 40 (Zeneca).

•**sorbitan monostearate.** (SORE-bih-tan MAHN-oh-STEE-ah-rate) N.F. 18.
Use: Pharmaceutic aid (surfactant).
See: Span 60 (Zeneca).

•**sorbitan sesquioleate.** (SORE-bih-tan SESS-kwih-OH-lee-ate) N.F. 18.
Use: Pharmaceutic aid (surfactant).
See: Arlacel C (Zeneca).

•**sorbitan trioleate.** (SORE-bih-tan TRY-OH-lee-ate) N.F. 18.
Use: Pharmaceutic aid (surfactant).
See: Span 85 (Zeneca).

•**sorbitan tristearate.** (SORE-bih-tan TRY-STEE-ah-rate) USAN.
See: Span 65 (Zeneca).
Use: Pharmaceutic aid (surfactant).

sorbitans.
See: Polysorbate 80, U.S.P.

•**sorbitol.** N.F. 18.
Use: Diuretic, dehydrating agent, humectant, pharmaceutic aid (sweetening agent, tablet excipient, flavor).
See: Sorbo (Zeneca).
W/Homatropine methylbromide.
See: Probilagol Liq. (Purdue Frederick).
W/Mannitol.
See: Sorbitol-mannitol Irrigation (Abbott Laboratories).

•**sorbitol solution.** U.S.P. 23.
Use: Pharmaceutic aid (flavor, tablet excipient).

Sorbitol-Mannitol. (Abbott Laboratories) Mannitol 0.54 g, sorbitol/100 ml 2.7 g. 1500 ml, 3000 ml. *Rx.*
Use: Irrigant, genitourinary.

Sorbitrate. (Zeneca) Isosorbide dinitrate. **Tab.:** 5 mg Bot. 100s, 500s, UD 100s; 10 mg Bot. 100s, 500s, UD 100s; 20 mg, 30 mg Bot. 100s, UD 100s. **SA Tab.:** 40 mg Bot. 100s, UD 100s; **Sublingual Tab.:** 2.5 mg, 5 mg, 10 mg Bot. 100s. **Chew. Tab.:** 5 mg Bot. 100s, 500s; 10 mg Bot. 100s. *Rx.*
Use: Antianginal.

Sorbitrate SA. (Zeneca) Isosorbide dinitrite, oral 40 mg/SR Tab. Bot. 100s, UD 100s. *Rx.*
Use: Antianginal.

Sorbo. (Zeneca) Sorbitol Solution, U.S.P. 23.

Sorbsan. (Dow Hickam) Calcium alginate fiber 2"×2", 3"×3", 4"×4", 4"×8". 1s. Wound packing fibers-calcium alginate fiber ¼" × 12". 1s. *Rx.*
Use: Dermatologic, wound therapy.

sorethytan (20) mono-oleate.
See: Polysorbate 80 (Various Mfr.).

Soriatane. (Roche) Acitretin 10 mg, 25 mg. Cap. Bot. 30s. *Rx.*
Use: Antipsoriatic.

Sosegon Solution. (Sanofi Winthrop) Pentazocine. *c-IV.*
Use: Analgesic.

Sosegon Suspension. (Sanofi Winthrop) Pentazocine. *c-IV.*
Use: Analgesic.

Sosegon Tablets. (Sanofi Winthrop) Pentazocine. *c-IV.*
Use: Analgesic.

Soss-10. (Roberts Pharm) Sodium sulfacetamide 10%. Soln. Bot. 15 ml. *Rx.*
Use: Anti-infective, ophthalmic.

•**sotalol hydrochloride.** (SOTT-uh-lahl) USAN.
Use: Beta-adrenergic blocker.
See: Betapace, Tab. (Berlex).

•**soterenol hydrochloride.** (so-TER-en-ole) USAN.
Use: Bronchodilator.

Sotradecol. (ESI Lederle Generics) Sodium tetradecyl sulfate 1% or 3%. Inj. Dosette amp. 2 ml. *Rx.*
Use: Sclerosing agent.

Soxa-Forte. (Vita Elixir) Sulfisoxazole 0.5 g, phenazopyridine 50 mg/Tab. *Rx.*
Use: Anti-infective.

Soxa Tablets. (Vita Elixir) Sulfisoxazole 0.5 g/Tab. Bot. 100s, 1000s. *Rx.*
Use: Anti-infective.

Soyalac. (Mt. Vernon Foods) Infant formula based on an extract from whole soybeans containing all essential nutrients. **Ready to Serve Liq.:** Can 32 fl oz. **Double Strength Conc.:** Can 13 fl oz. **Pow.:** Can 14 oz. *otc.*
Use: Nutritional supplement.

Soyalac-I. (Mt. Vernon Foods) Soy protein isolate infant formula containing no corn derivatives and a negligible amount of soy carbohydrates. Contains all essential nutrients in various forms. **Ready to Serve Liq.:** Can 32 fl oz. **Double Strength Conc.:** Can 13 fl oz. *otc.*
Use: Nutritional supplement.

soya lecithin. Soybean extract. 100s.
Use: Phosphorus therapy.
See: Neo-Vadrin (Scherer).

soybean lecithin.
W/Safflower oil, choline bitartrate, whole liver, inositol, methionine, natural tocopherols, vitamins B_6, B_{12}, panthenol.
See: Nutricol, Cap., Vial (Nutrition Control).

•**soybean oil.** U.S.P. 23.
Use: Pharmaceutic necessity.

Spabelin No. 1. (Arcum) Phenobarbital 15 mg, belladonna powdered extract 1/8 gr/Tab. Bot. 100s, 1000s. *Rx.*
Use: Hypnotic, sedative.

Spabelin No. 2. (Arcum) Phenobarbital 30 mg, belladonna powdered extract 1/8 gr/Tab. Bot. 100s, 1000s. *Rx.*
Use: Hypnotic, sedative.

Spabelin Elixir. (Arcum) Hyoscyamine sulfate 81 mcg, atropine sulfate 15 mcg, scopolamine HBr 5 mcg, phenobarbital 16.2 mg/5 ml. Bot. 16 oz, gal. *Rx.*
Use: Anticholinergic, antispasmodic, hypnotic, sedative.

Span 20. (Zeneca) Sorbitan Monolaurate, N.F. 18.

Span 40. (Zeneca) Sorbitan Monopalmitate, N.F. 18.

Span 60. (Zeneca) Sorbitan Monostearate, N.F. 18.

Span 65. (Zeneca) Sorbitan tristearate. Mixture of stearate esters of sorbitol and its anhydrides.
Use: Surface active agent.

Span 80. (Zeneca) Sorbitan mono-oleate, N.F. 18.

Span 85. (Zeneca) Sorbitan trioleate. Mixture of oleate esters of sorbitol and its anhydrides.
Use: Surface-active agent.

Span C. (Freeda Vitamins) Citrus bioflavonoids 300 mg, rutin 50 mg, vitamin C 200 mg/Tab. Bot. 100s, 250s, 500s. *otc.*
Use: Vitamin supplement.

Span PD. (Lexis) Phentermine HCl 37.5 mg/Cap. Bot. 100s. *c-iv.*
Use: Anorexiant.

Span-RD. (Lexis) d-Methamphetamine HCl 12 mg, dl-methamphetamine HCl 6 mg, butabarbital 30 mg/Tab. Bot. 100s, 1000s. *c-iii.*
Use: Amphetamine, hypnotic, sedative.

•**sparfloxacin.** (spar-FLOX-ah-sin) USAN.
Use: Anti-infective.
See: Zagam, Tab. (Rhone-Poulenc Rorer)

•**sparfosate sodium.** (spar-FOSS-ate) USAN.
Use: Antineoplastic.

Sparkles Effervescent Granules. (Lafayette Pharm) Sodium bicarbonate 2000 mg, citric acid 1500 mg, simethicone. Bot. UD 50s. *otc.*
Use: Antacid.

Sparkles Granules. (Lafayette Pharm) Effervescent granules 4 g/Packet or 6 g/Packet. Each 6 g produces 500 ml of carbon dioxide gas. Ctn. 25 packets. Pkg. 2 Ctn.
Use: Diagnostic aid.

Sparkles Tablets. (Lafayette Pharm) Effervescent tablets. Each 4.3 g of tablets produces 250 ml of carbon dioxide gas. Tab. Bot. 43 g (10 doses).
[use]Use Diagnostic aid.

•**sparsomycin.** (SPAR-so-MY-sin) USAN.
Use: Antineoplastic.

•**sparteine sulfate.** (SPAR-teh-een SULL-fate) USAN.
Use: Oxytocic.
W/Sodium Cl.
See: Tocosamine sulfate, Amp. (Trent).

Spasmatol. (Pharmed) Homatropine MBr 3 mg, pentobarbital 12 mg, mephobarbital 8 mg/Tab. Bot. 100s, 1000s. *Rx.*
Use: Anticholinergic, antispasmodic, hypnotic, sedative.

Spasmolin. (Global Source) Phenobarbital 16.2 mg, hyoscyamine sulfate 0.1037 mg, atropine sulfate 0.0194 mg, hyoscine HBr 0.0065 mg/Tab. Bot. 1000s. *Rx.*
Use: Anticholinergic, antispasmodic, hypnotic, sedative.

spasmolytic agents.
See: Antispasmodics.

Spasno-Lix. (Freeport) Phenobarbital 16.2 mg, hyoscyamine sulfate 0.1037 mg, atropine sulfate 0.0194 mg, hyoscine HBr 0.0065 mg, alcohol 21%-23%/5 ml. Bot. 4 oz. *Rx.*
Use: Anticholinergic, antispasmodic, hypnotic, sedative.

S.P.B. Tablet. (Sheryl) Therapeutic B complex formula with ascorbic acid 300 mg/Tab. Bot. 100s. *otc.*
Use: Vitamin supplement.

SPD. (A.P.C.) Methyl salicylate, methyl nicotinate, dipropylene glycol salicylate, oleoresin capsicum, camphor, menthol. Cream Bot. 4 oz, Tube 1.5 oz. *otc.*
Use: Analgesic, topical.

spearmint. N.F. XVI.
Use: Flavor.

spearmint oil. N.F. XVI.
Use: Flavor.

Special Shampoo. (Del-Ray) Non medicated shampoo. *otc.*
Use: Cleanser.

Spectazole. (Ortho McNeil) Econazole nitrate 1% in a water miscible base. Tube 15 g, 30 g, 85 g. *Rx.*

Use: Antifungal, topical.

spectinomycin. (speck-TIN-oh-MY-sin) Formerly Actinospectocin. An antibiotic isolated from broth cultures of *Streptomyces spectabilis. Rx.*
Use: Anti-infective.
See: Trobicin, Vial, Amp. (Pharmacia & Upjohn).

•**spectinomycin hydrochloride, sterile.** (speck-TIN-oh-MY-sin) U.S.P. 23.
Use: Anti-infective.

Spectra 360. (Parker) Salt-free electrode gel. Tube 8 oz.
Use: T.E.N.S. application, ECG pediatric, and long-term procedures.

Spectrobid Tablets. (Roerig) Bacampicillin HCl 400 mg/Tab. Bot. 100s. *Rx.*
Use: Anti-infective, penicillin.

Spectro-Biotic. (A.P.C.) Bacitracin 400 units, neomycin sulfate 5 mg, polymyxin B sulfate 5000 units/g Oint. 0.5 oz, 1 oz. *otc.*
Use: Anti-infective, topical.

Spectrocin Plus. (Numark Laboratories) Polymyxin B sulfate 5000 units/g or ml, neomycin 3.5 mg/g or ml, bacitracin 400 units/g or ml, lidocaine 5 mg, mineral oil, white petrolatum. Oint. Tube 15 g, 30 g. *otc.*
Use: Anti-infective, topical.

Spectro-Jel. (Recsei) Soap free. Iodomethylcellulose, carboxypolymethylene, cetyl alcohol, sorbitan mono-oleate, fumed silica, triethanolamine stearate, glycol polysiloxane, propylene glycol, glycerin, isopropyl alcohol 5%. Bot. 127.5 ml, pts, gal. *otc.*
Use: Dermatologic, cleanser.

Spec-T Sore Throat Anesthetic Lozenges. (Apothecon) Benzocaine 10 mg/Loz. Box 10s. *otc.*
Use: Anesthetic, local.

Spec-T Sore Throat/Cough Suppressant Lozenges. (Apothecon) Benzocaine 10 mg, dextromethorphan HBr 10 mg w/tartrazine. *otc.*
Use: Anesthetic, local; antitussive.

Spec-T Sore Throat/Decongestant Lozenges. (Apothecon) Benzocaine 10 mg, phenylephrine HCl 5 mg, phenylpropanolamine HCl 10.5 mg w/tartrazine. Loz. Pkg. 10s. *otc.*
Use: Anesthetic, local; decongestant.

spermaceti.
Use: Stiffening agent; pharmaceutic necessity for cold cream.

spermine. Diaminopropyltetramethylene.

Sperti Ointment. (Whitehall Robins) Live yeast cell derivative supplying 2000 units skin respiratory factor/g w/shark liver oil 3%, phenylmercuric nitrate 1:10,000. Tube oz. *otc.*
Use: Dermatologic, wound therapy.

Spherulin. (ALK Laboratories) Coccidioidin: 1:100 equivalent, vial 1 ml, 1:10 equivalent, Vial 0.5 ml. *Rx.*
Use: Diagnostic aid, skin test.

spider-bite antivenin.
See: Antivenin, Latrodectus Mactans (Merck).

Spider-Man Children's Chewable Vitamin. (NBTY) Vitamins A 2500 IU, D 400 IU, E 15 mg, B_1 1.05 mg, B_2 1.2 mg, B_3 13.5 mg, B_6 1.05 mg, B_{12} 4.5 mcg, C 60 mg, folic acid 0.3 mg/Tab., xylitol, sorbitol. Bot. 75s, 130s. *otc.*
Use: Vitamin supplement.

•**spiperone.** (spih-per-OHN) USAN.
Use: Antipsychotic.

•**spiradoline mesylate.** (spy-RAH-doe-leen) USAN.
Use: Analgesic.

•**spiramycin.** (SPIH-rah-MY-sin) USAN. Antibiotic substance from cultures of *Streptomyces ambofaciens.*
Use: Anti-infective.

•**spirapril hydrochloride.** (SPY-rah-prill) USAN.
Use: ACE inhibitor.
See: Renormax, Tab. (Novartis).

•**spiraprilat.** (SPY-rah-PRILL-at) USAN.
Use: ACE inhibitor.

spirobarbital sodium.

•**spirogermanium hydrochloride.** (SPY-row-JER-MAY-nee-uhm) USAN.
Use: Antineoplastic.

•**spiromustine.** (SPY-row-MUSS-teen) USAN. *Formerly spirohydantoin mustard.*
Use: Antineoplastic.

spironazide. (Schein Pharmaceutical) Spironolactone 25 mg, hydrochlorothiazide 25 mg/Tab. Bot. 100s, 1000s, UD 100s. *Rx.*
Use: Diuretic combination.

•**spironolactone.** (SPEER-oh-no-LAK-tone) U.S.P. 23.
Use: Diuretic, aldosterone antagonist.
See: Aldactone, Tab. (Searle).
W/Hydrochlorothiazide.
See: Aldactazide, Tab. (Searle).

spironolactone w/hydrochlorothiazide. (Various Mfr.) Spironolactone 25 mg, hydrochlorothiazide 25 mg. Tab. Bot. 30s, 60s, 100s, 250s, 500s, 1000s, UD 32s, 100s. *Rx.*
Use: Diuretic combination.

spiropitan. (SPY-row-PLAT-in) (Jans-

sen) Spiperone. *Rx.*
Use: Antipsychotic.

•**spiroplatin.** (SPY-row-PLAT-in) USAN.
Use: Antineoplastic.

spirotriazine hydrochloride.
Use: Anthelmintic.

•**spiroxasone.** (spy-ROX-ah-sone) USAN.
Use: Diuretic.

Spirozide. (Rugby) Spironolactone 25 mg, hydrochlorothiazide 25 mg/Tab. Bot. 100s, 500s, 1000s. *Rx.*
Use: Diuretic combination.

SPL-Serologic Types I and III. (Delmont Labs) Staphylococcus aureus 120 to 180 million units, staphylococcus bacteriophage plaque forming units 100 to 1000 million/ml. Inj. Amp. 1 ml, Vial 10 ml. *Rx.*
Use: Anti-infective.

Sporanox. (Janssen) Itraconazole 100 mg, sucrose. Cap. Sugar. Bot. 30s, UD 30s. *Rx.*
Use: Antifungal.

Sportscreme. (Thompson Medical) Triethanolamine salicylate 10% in a nongreasy base. Cream. 37.5 g, 90 g. *otc.*
Use: Analgesic, topical.

Sports Spray Extra Strength. (Mentholatum) Methyl salicylate 35%, menthol 10%, camphor 5%, alcohol 58%, isobutane. Spray. 90 ml. *otc.*
Use: Analgesic, topical.

Spray Skin Protectant. (Morton International) Isopropyl alcohol, polyvinylpyrolidone, vinyl alcohol, plasticizer & propellant. Aerosol can 6 oz. *otc.*
Use: Dermatologic, protectant.

Spray-U-Thin. (Caprice Greystoke) Phenylpropanolamine HCl 6.58 mg, sorbitol, saccharin. Spray. Bot. 44 ml. *otc.*
Use: Dietary aid.

spreading factor.
See: Hyaluronidase (Various Mfr.).

•**sprodiamide.** (sprah-DIE-ah-mide) USAN.
Use: Diagnostic aid (paramagnetic).

SPRX-105. (Reid-Provident) Phendimetrazine tartrate 105 mg/Cap. S.R. Bot. 28s, 500s. *c-III.*
Use: Anorexiant.

SPS. (Carolina Medical Products) Sodium polystyrene sulfonate 15 g, sorbitol solution 21.5 ml, alcohol 0.3%/60 ml. Susp. Bot. 120 ml, 480 ml, UD 60 ml. *Rx.*
Use: Potassium-removing resin.

S-P-T. (Fleming) Pork thyroid, desiccated 1 gr, 2 gr, 3 gr, 5 gr/Cap. Bot. 100s, 1000s. *Rx.*
Use: Hypothyroidism.

•**squalane.** (SKWAH-lane) N.F. 18.
Use: Pharmaceutic aid (vehicle, oleaginous).

SRC Expectorant. (Edwards Pharmaceuticals) Hydrocodone bitartrate 5 mg, pseudoephedrine HCl 60 mg, guaifenesin 200 mg w/alcohol 12.5%. Bot. pt. *c-III.*
Use: Antitussive, decongestant, expectorant.

SSD AF. (Knoll Pharmaceuticals) Silver sulfadiazine 1% in a cream base containing white petrolatum, stearyl alcohol, isopropyl myristate, sorbitan mono-oleate, polyoxyl 40 stearate, sodium hydroxide, propylene glycol, methylparaben 3%. Cream. 50 g, 400 g, 1000 g. *Rx.*
Use: Burn therapy.

SSD Cream. (Knoll Pharmaceuticals) Silver sulfadiazine cream 1%. Jar 50 g, 85 g, 400 g, 1000 g. Tube 25 g. *Rx.*
Use: Burn therapy.

SSKI. (Upsher-Smith Labs) Potassium iodide 300 mg/0.3 ml. Soln. Dropper Bot. 1 oz, 8 oz.
Use: Expectorant.

S-Spas. (Southern States) Pentobarbital 16.2 mg, atropine sulfate 0.0194 mg, hyoscyamine sulfate 0.1037 mg, hyoscine HBr 0.0065 mg/Tab. or 5 ml **Liq.:** Bot. pt. **Tab.:** Bot. 100s, 1000s. *Rx.*
Use: Anticholinergic, antispasmodic, hypnotic, sedative.

Stadol. (Bristol-Myers Squibb) Butorphanol tartrate 1 mg/ml; Vial 1 ml. 2 mg/ml; Vial 1 ml, 2 ml, 10 ml. *c-IV.*
Use: Analgesic.

Staftabs. (Modern) Fine bone flour containing calcium, phosphorus, iron, iodine, vitamin D, magnesium/Tab. Bot. 85s, 160s. *otc.*
Use: Mineral, vitamin supplement.

Stagesic. (Huckaby Pharmacal) Hydrocodone bitartrate 5 mg, acetaminophen 500 mg/Cap. Bot. 100s. *c-III.*
Use: Analgesic combination, narcotic.

Stahist. (Huckaby Pharmacal) Phenylpropanolamine HCl 50 mg, phenylephrine HCl 25 mg, chlorpheniramine maleate 8 mg, hyoscyamine sulfate 0.19 mg, atropine sulfate 0.04 mg, scopolamine HBr 0.01 mg/SR Tab. Bot. 100s *Rx.*
Use: Antihistamine, anticholinergic, decongestant.

stainless iodized ointment. (Day-Baldwin) Jar lb.

stainless iodized ointment with methyl salicylate 5%. (Day-Baldwin) Jar lb.

•**stallimycin hydrochloride.** (stal-IH-MY-sin) USAN.
Use: Anti-infective.

Stamoist E. (Huckaby Pharmacal) Pseudoephedrine HCl 120 mg, guaifenesin 500 mg. SR Tab. Bot. 100s. *Rx.*
Use: Decongestant, expectorant.

Stamoist LA. (Huckaby Pharmacal) Phenylpropanolamine HCl 75 mg, guaifenesin 400 mg. SR Tab. Bot. 100s. *Rx.*
Use: Decongestant, expectorant.

Stamyl Tablets. (Sanofi Winthrop) Pancreatin.
Use: Digestive aid.

•**stannous chloride.** (STAN-uhs KLOR-ide) USAN.
Use: Pharmaceutic aid.

•**stannous fluoride.** (STAN-uhs FLOR-ide) U.S.P. 23.
Use: Dental caries agent.

•**stannous pyrophosphate.** (STAN-uhs PIE-row-FOSS-fate) USAN.
Use: Diagnostic aid (skeletal imaging).

•**stannous sulfur colloid.** (STAN-uhs SULL-fer KAHL-oyd) USAN.
Use: Diagnostic aid (bone, liver, and spleen imaging).

•**stanozolol.** (STAN-oh-zole-ahl) U.S.P. 23. *Formerly Androstanazole.*
Use: Androgen.
See: Stromba.
Winstrol Tab. (Sanofi Winthrop).

staphage lysate (SPL). (Delmont Labs) Phage-lysed staphylococci 120-180 million/ml Amp. 1 ml, package 10s for Inj.; multidose Vial 10 ml for other methods of administration. *Rx.*
Use: Anti-infective.

staphylococcus bacteriophage lysate.
See: Staphage Lysate (Delmont Labs).

staphylococcus test.
See: Isocult for Staphylococcus Aureus (SmithKline Diagnostics).

•**starch.** N.F. 18.
Use: Dusting powder, pharmaceutic aid.

starch glycerite.
Use: Emollient.

•**starch, pregelatinized.** N.F. 18.
Use: Pharmaceutic aid (tablet excipient).

•**starch, topical.** U.S.P. 23.
Use: Dusting powder.

Star-Otic. (Star) Burrows soln. 10%, acetic acid 1%, boric acid 1%. Drop bot. 15 ml. *otc.*
Use: Otic.

Staticin. (Westwood Squibb) Erythromycin 1.5%, alcohol 55%. Soln. Bot. 60 ml. *Rx.*
Use: Dermatologic, acne.

•**statolon.** (STAY-toe-lone) USAN. Antiviral agent derived from *Penicillium stoloniferum.*
Use: Antiviral.

Statomin Maleate II. (Jones Medical Industries) Chlorpheniramine maleate 2 mg, acetaminophen 324 mg, caffeine 32 mg/Tab. Bot. 1000s. *Rx.*
Use: Antihistamine, analgesic.

Statuss Expectorant. (Huckaby Pharmacal) Phenylpropanolamine HCl 12.5 mg, codeine phosphate 10 mg, guaifenesin 100 mg, alcohol 5%, menthol, saccharin, sorbitol/5 ml. Dye free. Liq. Bot. 473 ml. *c-v.*
Use: Antitussive, decongestant, expectorant.

Statuss Green. (Huckaby Pharmacal) Phenylpropanolamine HCl 3.3 mg, phenylephrine HCl 5 mg, pheniramine maleate 3.3 mg, pyrilamine maleate 3.3 mg, hydrocodone bitartrate 1.67 mg/5 ml, alcohol 5%, saccharin, parabens, sorbitol, glucose. Liq. Bot. 480 ml. *c-III.*
Use: Antihistamine, antitussive, decongestant,.

•**stavudine.** (STAHV-you-deen) USAN.
Use: Antiviral.
See: Zerit, Preps. (Bristol-Myers Squibb).

Sta-Wake Dextabs. (Health for Life Brands) Caffeine 1.5 gr, dextrose 3 gr/Tab. Bot. 36s, 1000s. *otc.*
Use: CNS stimulant.

Stay Awake Capsules. (Whiteworth Towne) Caffeine 250 mg/Cap. Bot. 30s. *otc.*
Use: CNS Stimulant.

Stay-Brite. (Sherman) EDTA 0.25%, benzalkonium Cl 0.01%. Spray 30 ml. *otc.*
Use: Contact lens care.

Stay Moist Lip Conditioner. Padimate O, oxybenzone, aloe vera, vitamin E, tropical fruit flavor. SPF 15. Lip Balm: 48 g. *otc.*
Use: Emollient.

Stay Trim. (Schering Plough) Phenylpropanolamine. **Gum:** 8.33 mg. Pkg. 20s. **Mints:** 12.5 mg. Pkg. 36s. *otc.*
Use: Dietary aid.

Stay-Wet. (Sherman) Polyvinyl alcohol, hydroxyethylcellulose, povidone, sodium Cl, potassium Cl, sodium carbonate, benzalkonium Cl 0.01%, EDTA

0.025%. Soln. Bot. 30 ml. *otc.*
Use: Contact lens care.

Stay-Wet 3. (Sherman) Sodium and potassium Cl salts containing polyvinyl pyrrolidone, polyvinyl alcohol, hydroxyethylcellulose, sodium bisulfite 0.02%, benzyl alcohol 0.1%, sorbic acid 0.05%, EDTA 0.1%. Soln. 30 ml. *otc.*
Use: Lubricant, ophthalmic.

Stay Wet 4. (Sherman) Benzyl alcohol 0.15%, EDTA 0.1%, NaCl, KCl, polyvinyl alcohol, hydroxyethyl cellulose. Thimerosol free. Soln. 30 ml. *otc.*
Use: Contact lens care (RGP lenses).

Stay-Wet Rewetting. (Sherman) Polyvinyl alcohol, hydroxyethycellulose, povidone, NaCl, KCL, sodium carbonate, benzalkonium Cl 0.01%, EDTA 0.025%. *otc.*
Use: Lubricant-ophthalmic.

Stay-Wet 3 Wetting. (Sherman) Polyvinyl alcohol, hydroxyethycellulose, povidone, sodium Cl, potassium Cl, sodium carbonate, benzalkonium Cl 0.01%, EDTA 0.025%. Soln. 30 ml. *otc.*
Use: Lubricant, ophthalmic.

Staze. (Del Pharmaceuticals) Karaya gum. Tube 1.75 oz, 3.5 oz. *otc.*
Use: Denture adhesive.

S-T Cort Cream. (Scot-Tussin Pharmacal) Hydrocortisone 0.5%, water-washable base, parabens. 120 g. *Rx.*
Use: Corticosteroid, topical.

S-T Cort Lotion. (Scot-Tussin Pharmacal) Hydrocortisone 0.5%, water-washable, lanolin alcohol, mineral oil base. 60 ml, 120 ml. *Rx.*
Use: Corticosteroid, topical.

•**stearic acid.** (STEER-ik) N.F. 18. Octadecanoic acid.
Use: Pharmaceutic aid (emulsion adjunct, tablet/capsule lubricant).

•**stearyl alcohol.** (STEE-rill AL-koe-hahl) N.F. 18.
Use: Pharmaceutic aid (emulsion adjunct).

•**steffimycin.** (steh-fih-MY-sin) USAN.
Use: Anti-infective, antiviral.

Stelazine. (SmithKline Beecham Pharmaceuticals) Trifluoperazine HCl. **Tab.:** 1 mg, 2 mg, 5 mg, 10 mg. Bot. 100s, 500s, 100s, UD 100s. **Inj.:** 2 mg/ml. Vial 10 ml. Box 1s, 20s. **Oral Conc.:** 10 mg/ml. Bot. 60 ml. *Rx.*
Use: Antipsychotic.

•**stenbolone acetate.** (STEEN-bow-lone) USAN.
Use: Anabolic.

Step 2. (GenDerm) Benzyl alcohol, cetyl alcohol, formic acid 8%, glyceryl stearate, PEG-100 stearate, polyquaterium-10. Creme rinse. 60 ml. *otc.*
Use: Pediculicide, nit removal.

Steraject. (Merz) Prednisolone acetate 25 mg or 50 mg/ml. Vial 10 ml. *Rx.*
Use: Corticosteroid.

Sterapred DS. (Merz) Prednisone 10 mg/Tab. Uni-pak 21s. *Rx.*
Use: Corticosteroid.

Sterapred-Unipak. (Merz) Prednisone 5 mg/Tab. Dosepak 21 tab. *Rx.*
Use: Corticosteroid.

Sterculia Gum.
See: Karaya Gum (Various Mfr.).
W/Vitamin B_1.
See: Imbicoll W/Vitamin B_1 (Pharmacia & Upjohn).

Stericol. (Alton) Isopropyl alcohol 91%. Bot. 16 oz, 32 oz, gal. *otc.*
Use: Anti-infective, topical.

sterile aurothioglucose suspension. Aurothioglucose Injection. Gold thioglucose.
Use: Antirheumatic.
See: Solganal, Vial (Schering Plough).

sterile erythromycin gluceptate. Erythromycin monoglucoheptonate (salt). Erythromycin glucoheptonate (1:1) (salt).
Use: Anti-infective.

Sterile Lens Lubricant. (Blairex Labs) Isotonic w/borate buffer system, sodium Cl, hydroxypropyl methylcellulose, glycerin, sorbic acid 0.25%, EDTA 0.1%, thimerosol free. Soln. 15 ml. *otc.*
Use: Lubricant, ophthalmic.

Sterile Saline. (Bausch & Lomb) Sodium Cl, borate buffer, EDTA, thimerosal free. Soln. 60 ml. *otc.*
Use: Lubricant, ophthalmic

sterile thiopental sodium. Thiopental sodium, U.S.P. 23.
See: Pentothal Sodium, Amp. (Abbott Laboratories).

sterile water for irrigation. (Various Mfr.) 0.45% or 0.9%. Soln. Bot. 150 ml, 250 ml, 500 ml, 1000 ml, 1500 ml, 2000 ml, 4000 ml. *Rx.*
Use: Irrigant, genitourinary.

Steri-Unna Boot. (Pedinol) Glycerin, gum acacia, zinc oxide, white petrolatum, amylum in an oil base. 10 yds. × 3.5 in. sterilized bandage.
Use: Treatment of leg ulcers, varicosities, sprains, strains & to reduce swelling after surgery.

S-T Forte 2 Liquid. (Scot-Tussin Pharmacal) Chlorpheniramine maleate 2

mg, hydrocodone bitartrate 2.5 mg, 99.7% glycerin, menthol, parabens. Alcohol and dye free. Bot. Pt. or gal. *c-III.*
Use: Antihistamine, antitussive.

S-T Forte Sugar Free Liquid. (Scot-Tussin Pharmacal) Hydrocodone bitartrate 2.5 mg, phenylephrine HCl 5 mg, phenylpropanolamine HCl 5 mg, pheniramine maleate 13.33 mg, guaifenesin 80 mg/5 ml w/alcohol 5%. Bot. 4 oz, 8 oz, pt, gal. *c-III.*
Use: Antitussive, antihistamine, decongestant, expectorant.

S-T Forte Syrup. (Scot-Tussin Pharmacal) Hydrocodone bitartrate 2.5 mg, phenylephrine HCl 5 mg, phenylpropanolamine HCl 5 mg, pheniramine maleate 13.33 mg, guaifenesin 80 mg/5 ml, w/alcohol 5%. Bot. 4 oz, 8 oz, pt. gal. *c-III.*
Use: Antitussive, antihistamine, decongestant, expectorant.

stilbamidine isethionate. 2-Hydroxyethane-sulfonic acid compound with 4, 4'-stilbenedicarboxamidine.
Use: Antiprotozoal.

•**stilbazium iodide.** (still-BAY-zee-uhm EYE-oh-dide) USAN.
Use: Anthelmintic.

stilbestrol.
See: Diethylstilbestrol, U.S.P. 23. (Various Mfr.).

stilbestronate.
See: Diethylstilbestrol Dipropionate (Various Mfr.).

stilboestrol.
See: Diethylstilbestrol (Various Mfr.).

Stilboestrol DP.
See: Diethylstilbestrol Dipropionate (Various Mfr.).

Stillman's. (Stillman) Cream Jar. ⅞ oz, oz, Cream Bella Aurora oz.

•**stilonium iodide.** (STILL-oh-nee-uhm EYE-oh-dide) USAN.
Use: Antispasmodic.

Stilphostrol. (Bayer Corp) Diethylstilbestrol diphosphate. Amp. (250 mg/5 ml as sodium salt) 5 ml. Box 20s. Tab. 50 mg, Bot. 50s. *Rx.*
Use: Antineoplastic.

Stilronate.
See: Diethylstilbestrol Dipropionate (Various Mfr.).

Stimate. (centeon) Desmopressin acetate 1.5 mg, chlorobutanol 5 mg, sodium Cl 9 mg/ml. Nasal spray. Vial 2.5 ml. *Rx.*
Use: Hormone.

Sting-Eze. (Wisconsin Pharm) Diphenhydramine HCl, camphor, phenol, benzocaine, eucalyptol. Bot. 15 ml. *otc.*
Use: Antihistamine, topical.

Sting-Kill. (Milance Lab) Benzocaine 18.9%, menthol 0.9%. Swab 14 ml, 0.5 ml (5s). *otc.*
Use: Anesthetic, local.

•**stiripentol.** (STY-rih-PEN-tole) USAN.
Use: Anticonvulsant.

St. Joseph Adult Chewable Aspirin. (Schering Plough) Aspirin 81 mg, saccharin. Chew. Tab. Bot. 36s. *otc.*
Use: Analgesic.

St. Joseph Aspirin for Adults. (Schering Plough) Aspirin 5 gr/Tab. Bot. 36s, 100s, 200s. *otc.*
Use: Analgesic.

St. Joseph Aspirin-Free Cold for Children. (Schering Plough) Phenylpropanolamine HCl 3.125 mg, acetaminophen 80 mg, fruit flavor. Chew. Tab. Bot. 30s. *otc.*
Use: Decongestant combination.

St. Joseph Aspirin-Free Elixir for Children. (Schering Plough) Acetaminophen 160 mg/5 ml. Alcohol Free. Bot. 2 oz, 4 oz. *otc.*
Use: Analgesic.

St. Joseph Aspirin-Free for Children Chewable. (Schering Plough) Acetaminophen 80 mg, fruit flavor. Tab. Bot. 30s. *otc.*
Use: Analgesic.

St. Joseph Aspirin-Free Infant Drops. (Schering Plough) Acetaminophen 100 mg/ml/0.8 ml dropper. Aspirin and sugar free. Bot. 0.5 oz. *otc.*
Use: Analgesic.

St. Joseph Aspirin-Free Tablets for Children. (Schering Plough) Acetaminophen 80 mg/Tab. Bot. 30s. *otc.*
Use: Analgesic.

St. Joseph Cold Tablets for Children. (Schering Plough) Aspirin 80 mg, phenylpropanolamine HCl 3.125 mg/Tab. Bot. 30s. *otc.*
Use: Analgesic, decongestant.

St. Joseph Cough Suppressant. (Schering Plough) Dextromethorphan HBr 7.5 mg/5 ml, alcohol free, sucrose, cherry flavor. Liq. Bot. 60 ml, 120 ml. *otc.*
Use: Antitussive.

St. Joseph Cough Syrup for Children. (Schering Plough) Dextromethorphan HBr 7.5 mg/5 ml. Bot. 2 oz, 4 oz. *otc.*
Use: Antitussive.

Stomal. (Foy) Phenobarbital 16.2 mg,

hyoscyamine sulfate 0.1037 mg, atropine sulfate 0.0194 mg, scopolamine HBr 0.0065 mg/Tab. Bot. 1000s. *Rx.*
Use: Anticholinergic, antispasmodic, hypnotic, sedative.

ST1-RTA immunotoxin (SR44163).
Use: Leukemia, graft-v-host disease in bone marrow transplants. [Orphan drug]

Stool Softener. (Amlab) Docusate sodium 100 mg, 250 mg/Cap. Bot. 100s. *otc.*
Use: Laxative.

Stool Softener. (Weeks & Leo) Docusate sodium 100 mg, 250 mg/Cap. Bot. 30s, 100s. Calcium docusate 240 mg/ Cap. Bot. 100s. *otc.*
Use: Laxative.

Stop. (Oral-B Laboratories) Stannous fluoride 0.4%. Tube 2 oz. *Rx.*
Use: Dental caries agent.

Stopayne Capsules. (Springbok) Codeine phosphate 30 mg, acetaminophen 357 mg/Cap. Bot. 100s, 500s, UD 100s. *c-III.*
Use: Analgesic, antitussive.

Stopayne Syrup. (Springbok) Acetaminophen 120 mg, codeine phosphate 12 mg/5 ml. Bot. 4 oz, 16 oz. *c-v.*
Use: Analgesic, antitussive.

Stop-Zit. (Purepac) Denatonium benzoate in a clear nail polish base. Bot. 0.75 oz. *otc.*
Use: Nail biting deterrent.

•**storax.** (STORE-ax) U.S.P. 23.
Use: Pharmaceutic necessity for Benzoin Tincture compound.

Stovarsol.
Use: Trichomonas vaginalis vaginitis, amebiasis, Vincent's angina.
See: Acetarsone, Tab.

Strema. (Foy) Quinine sulfate 260 mg/ Cap. Bot. 100s, 500s, 1000s.
Use: Antimalarial.

Stren-Tab. (Barth's) Vitamins C 300 mg, B_1 10 mg, B_2 10 mg, niacin 33 mg, B_6 2 mg, pantothenic acid 20 mg, B_{12} 4 mcg/Tab. Bot. 100s, 300s, 500s. *otc.*
Use: Vitamin supplement.

Streptase. (Astra) Streptokinase IV infusion. Ctn. Vial 10s. 250,000 IU/Vial 6.5 ml; 750,000 IU/Vial 6.5 ml. *Rx.*
Use: Thrombolytic.

streptococcus immune globulin group B.
Use: Immunization. [Orphan drug]

streptokinase.
Use: Thrombolytic.
See: Kabikinase (SKF).
Streptase (Hoechst-Roussell).

Streptolysin O Test. (Laboratory Diagnostics) Reagent 6 × 10 ml, buffer 6 × 40 ml, Control Serum, 6 × 10 ml or Kit.
Use: Diagnosis of "Group A" Streptococcal infections.

streptomycin calcium chloride. Streptomycin Calcium Chloride Complex.

streptomycin isoniazid.
See: Streptohydrazid.

streptomycylidene isonicotinyl hydrazine sulfate.
See: Streptohydrazid.

Streptonase B. (Wampole Laboratories) Tube test for determination of streptococcal infection by serum DNase-B antibodies. Kit 1.
Use: Diagnostic aid.

•**streptonicozid.** (STREP-toe-nih-KOE-zid) USAN.
Use: Anti-infective.
See: Streptohydrazid.

•**streptonigrin.** (strep-toe-NYE-grin) USAN. Antibiotic isolated from both filtrates of *Streptomyces flocculus.*
Use: Antineoplastic.
See: Nigrin (Pfizer).

streptovaricin. An antibiotic composed of several related components derived from cultures of *Streptomyces variabilis.* Dalacin (Pharmacia & Upjohn).

•**streptozocin.** (STREP-toe-ZOE-sin) USAN.
Use: Antineoplastic.
See: Zanosar, Powder (Pharmacia & Upjohn).

Streptozyme. (Wampole Laboratories) Rapid hemagglutination slide test for the qualitative detection and quantitative determination of streptococcal extracellular antigens in serum, plasma and peripheral blood. Kit 15s, 50s, 150s.
Use: Diagnostic aid, streptococcus.

Stress "1000". (NBTY) Vitamins E 22 mg, B_1 15 mg, B_2 15 mg, B_3 100 mg, B_5 20 mg, B_6 5 mg, B_{12} 12 mcg, C 1000 mg/Tab. Bot. 60s. *otc.*
Use: Vitamin supplement.

Stress B-Complex. (Moore) Vitamins E 30 IU, B_1 15 mg, B_2 15 mg, B_3 100 mg, B_5 20 mg, B_6 20 mg, B_{12} 12 mcg, C 500 mg, folic acid 0.4 mg, Zn 23.9 mg, Cu, biotin 45 mcg/Tab. Bot. 60s. *otc.*
Use: Mineral, vitamin supplement.

Stress B Complex with Vitamin C. (Mission Pharmacal) Vitamins B_1 13.8 mg, B_2 10 mg, B_3 50 mg, B_6 4.1 mg, C

300 mg, Zn 15 mg/Tab. Bot. 60s. *otc.*
Use: Mineral, vitamin supplement.

Stress-Bee Capsules. (Rugby) Vitamins B_1 10 mg, B_2 10 mg, B_3 100 mg, B_5 20 mg, B_6 2 mg, B_{12} 6 mcg, C 300 mg/Cap. Bot. 100s. *otc.*
Use: Vitamin supplement.

Stressform "605" With Iron. (NBTY) Iron 27 mg, vitamins E 30 mg, B_1 15 mg, B_2 15 mg, B_3 100 mg, B_5 20 mg, B_6 5 mg, B_{12} 12 mcg, C 605 mg, folic acid 0.4 mg, biotin 45 mg/Tab. Bot. 60s. *otc.*
Use: Vitamin supplement.

Stress Formula. (Various Mfr.) Vitamins E 30 mg, B_1 15 mg, B_2 15 mg, B_3 100 mg, B_5 20 mg, B_6 5 mg, B_{12} 12 mcg, C 600 mg, folic acid 0.4 mg, biotin 45 mcg/Cap., Tab. **Cap.:** Bot. 60s, 100s, 1000s. **Tab.:** Bot. 30s, 60s, 100s, 250s, 300s, 400s, 1000s, UD 100s. *otc.*
Use: Vitamin supplement.

Stress Formula 600. (Vangard). Vitamins E 30 IU, B_1 15 mg, B_2 10 mg, B_3 100 mg, B_5 20 mg, B_6 5 mg, B_{12} 12 mcg, C 500 mg, folic acid 0.4 mg, biotin 45 mcg/Tab. Bot. UD 100s. *otc.*
Use: Vitamin supplement.

Stress Formula 600 w/Iron. (Halsey).
Use: Vitamin supplement.

Stress Formula 600 Plus Iron. (Schein Pharmaceutical) Iron 27 mg, vitamins E 30 IU, B_1 15 mg, B_2 15 mg, B_3 100 mg, B_5 20 mg, B_6 5 mg, B_{12} 12 mcg, C 600 mg, folic acid 0.4 mg, biotin 45 mcg/Tab. Bot. 60s, 250s. *otc.*
Use: Mineral, vitamin supplement.

Stress Formula 600 Plus Zinc. (Schein Pharmaceutical) Vitamins E 30 mg, B_1 20 mg, B_2 10 mg, B_3 100 mg, B_5 25 mg, B_6 5 mg, B_{12} 12 mcg, C 600 mg, folic acid 0.4 mg, zinc 23.9 mg, Cu, Mg, biotin 45 mcg/Tab. Bot. 60s, 250s. *otc.*
Use: Mineral, vitamin supplement.

Stress Formula 600 w/Zinc. (Halsey).
Use: Dietary supplement.

Stress Formula "605". (NBTY) Vitamins E 30 mg, B_1 15 mg, B_2 15 mg, B_3 100 mg, B_5 20 mg, B_6 5 mg, B_{12} 12 mcg, C 605 mg, folic acid 0.4 mg, biotin 45 mg/Tab. Bot. 60s. *otc.*
Use: Vitamin supplement.

Stress Formula "605" with Zinc. (NBTY) Vitamins E 30 mg, B_1 20 mg, B_2 10 mg, B_3 100 mg, B_5 25 mg, B_6 5 mg, B_{12} 12 mcg, C 605 mg, folic acid 0.4 mg, zinc 23.9 mg, copper, biotin 45 mcg/Tab. Bot. 60s. *otc.*
Use: Mineral, vitamin supplement.

Stress Formula Vitamins. (Various Mfr.) Vitamins E 30 mg, B_1 10 mg, B_2 10 mg, B_3 100 mg, B_5 20 mg, B_6 5 mg, B_{12} 12 mcg, C 500 mg, folic acid 0.4 mg, biotin 45 mcg. Cap. Bot. 100s/Tab. Bot. 60s. *otc.*
Use: Vitamin supplement.

Stress Formula with Iron. (NBTY) Vitamins C 500 mg, B_1 10 mg, B_2 10 mg, B_3 100 mg, B_5 20 mg, B_6 5 mg, B_{12} 12 mcg, E 30 IU, iron 27 mg, folic acid 0.4 mg, biotin 45 mcg. Tab. Bot. 60s. *otc.*
Use: Mineral, vitamin supplement.

Stress Formula w/Zinc. (Various Mfr.) Vitamins E 30 IU, B_1 10 mg, B_2 10 mg, B_3 100 mg, B_5 20 mg, B_6 5 mg, B_{12} 12 mcg, C 500 mg, folic acid 0.4 mg, biotin 45 mcg, zinc 23.9 mg, Cu/Tab. Bot. 60s. *otc.*
Use: Mineral, vitamin supplement.

Stress Formula with Zinc. (Towne) Vitamins E 45 IU, C 600 mg, folic acid 400 mcg, B_1 20 mg, B_2 10 mg, niacinamide 100 mg, B_6 10 mg, B_{12} 25 mcg, biotin 40 mcg, pantothenic acid 25 mg, copper 3 mg, zinc 23.9 mg/Tab. Bot. 60s. *otc.*
Use: Mineral, vitamin supplement.

Stress 600 w/Zinc. (Nion) Vitamins E 45 IU, B_1 20 mg, B_2 10 mg, B_3 100 mg, B_5 25 mg, B_6 10 mg, B_{12} 25 mcg, C 600 mg, folic acid 0.4 mg, Zn 5.5 mg, Cu, biotin 45 mcg/Tab. Bot. 60s. *otc.*
Use: Mineral, vitamin supplement.

Stresstabs. (ESI Lederle Generics) Vitamins E 30 mg, B_1 10 mg, B_2 10 mg, B_3 100 mg, B_5 20 mg, B_6 5 mg, B_{12} 12 mcg, C 500 mg, folic acid 0.4 mg, biotin 45 mcg/Tab. Bot. 60s. *otc.*
Use: Vitamin supplement.

Stresstabs + Iron. (ESI Lederle Generics) Iron 18 mg, E 30 IU, B_1 10 mg, B_2 10 mg, B_3 100 mg, B_5 20 mg, B_6 5 mg, B_{12} 12 mcg, C 500 mg, folic acid 0.4 mg, biotin 45 mcg/Tab. Bot. 60s. *otc.*
Use: Mineral, vitamin supplement.

Stresstabs + Zinc. (ESI Lederle Generics) Vitamins E 30 mg, B_1 10 mg, B_2 10 mg, B_3 100 mg, B_5 20 mg, B_6 5 mg, B_{12} 12 mcg, C 500 mg, folic acid 0.4 mg, zinc 23.9 mg, copper, biotin 45 mcg/Tab. Bot. 60s. *otc.*
Use: Mineral, vitamin supplement.

Stresstabs 600. (ESI Lederle Generics) Vitamins B_1 15 mg, B_2 10 mg, B_6 5 mg, B_{12} 12 mcg, C 600 mg, niacinamide 100 mg, vitamin E 30 IU, biotin 45 mcg, folic acid 400 mcg, calcium pantothenate 20 mg/Tab. Bot. 30s, 60s. UD 10 × 10s. *otc.*

Use: Vitamin supplement.

Stresstabs 600 with Iron Tablets. (ESI Lederle Generics) Ferrous fumerate 27 mg, vitamins E 30 IU, B_1 15 mg, B_2 15 mg, B_3 100 mg, B_5 20 mg, B_6 5 mg, B_{12} 12 mcg, C 600 mg, folic acid 0.4 mg, biotin 45 mcg/Tab. Bot. 30s, 60s. *otc.*
Use: Mineral, vitamin supplement.

Stresstabs 600 with Zinc. (ESI Lederle Generics) Vitamins B_1 15 mg, B_2 10 mg, B_3 100 mg, B_5 20 mg, B_6 5 mg, B_{12} 12 mcg, C 600 mg, E 30 IU, folic acid 0.4 mg, biotin 45 mcg, Cu, zinc 23.9 mg/Tab. Bot. 30s, 60s. *otc.*
Use: Mineral, vitamin supplement.

Stresstein. (Novartis) Maltodextrin, medium chain triglycerides, l-leucine, soybean oil, l-isoleucine, l-valine, l-glutamic acid, l-arginine, l-lysine acetate, l-alanine, l-threonine, l-phenylalanine, l-aspartic acid, l-histidine, l-methionine, glycine, polyglycerol esters of fatty acids, l-serine, l-proline, sodium Cl, l-tryptophan, l-cysteine, sodium citrate, vitamins and minerals. Powder 3.4 oz. packets. *otc.*
Use: High-protein, branched chain enriched tube feeding.

Stri-dex Antibacterial Cleansing. (Bayer Corp) Triclosan 1%, acetylated lanolin alcohol, EDTA. Bar. 105 g. *otc.*
Use: Dermatologic, acne.

Stri-dex B.P. (Bayer Corp) Benzoyl peroxide 10%. in greaseless, vanishing cream base. *otc.*
Use: Dermatologic, acne.

Stri-dex Clear. (Bayer Corp) Salicylic acid 2%, SD alcohol 9.3%, EDTA. Gel: 30 g. *otc.*
Use: Dermatologic, acne.

Stridex Face Wash. (Bayer Corp) Triclosan 1%, glycerin, EDTA, alcohol free. Soln.: 237 ml. *otc.*
Use: Dermatologic, acne.

Stri-dex Lotion. (Bayer Corp) Salicylic acid 0.5%, alcohol 28%, sulfonated alkyl benzenes, citric acid, sodium carbonate, simethicone, water. Bot. 4 oz. *otc.*
Use: Dermatologic, acne.

Stri-dex Maximum Strength Pads. (Bayer Corp) Salicylic acid 2%, SD alcohol 44%, citric acid, menthol. In pads 55s, 90s, dual-textured 32s. *otc.*
Use: Anti-acne.

Stri-dex Oil Fighting Formula Pads. (Bayer Corp) Salicylic acid 2%, citric acid, menthol, SD alcohol 54%. Super Scrub Pads 55s. *otc.*
Use: Dermatologic, acne.

Stri-dex Regular Strength Pads. (Bayer Corp) Salicylic acid 0.5%, SD alcohol 28%, citric acid, menthol. In 55s. *otc.*
Use: Dermatologic, acne.

Stri-dex Sensitive Skin Pads. (Bayer Corp) Salicylic acid 0.5%, citric acid, aloe vera gel, menthol, SD alcohol 28%. In 50s, 90s. *otc.*
Use: Dermatologic, acne.

Stromba Ampules. (Sanofi Winthrop) Stanozolol. *c-III.*
Use: Anabolic steroid.

strong iodine tincture. (Various Mfr.) Iodine 7%, potassium iodide 5%, alcohol 83%. Soln. Bot. 500 ml, 4000 ml. *otc.*
Use: Antimicrobial, antiseptic.

strontium bromide. Cryst. or Granule, Bot. 0.25 lb, 1 lb. Amp. 1 g/10 ml. *Rx.*
Use: Antiepileptic, sedative.

•**strontium chloride Sr 85.** (STRAHN-shee-uhm) USAN.
Use: Radiopharmaceutical.

•**strontium chloride Sr 89 injection.** (STRAHN-shee-uhm) U.S.P. 23.
Use: Antineoplastic; radiopharmaceutical.
See: Metastron, Inj. (Amersham).

strontium lactate trihydrate.

•**strontium nitrate Sr 85.** (STRAHN-shee-uhm) USAN.
Use: Radiopharmaceutical.

strontium Sr 85 injection.
Use: Diagnostic aid (bone scanning).

strophanthin. K-strophanthin.

Strovite Plus. (Everett Laboratories) Vitamins A 5000 IU, E 30 mg, B_1 20 mg, B_2 20 mg, B_3 100 mg, B_5 25 mg, B_6 25 mg, B_{12} 50 mcg, C 500 mg, iron 9 mg, folic acid 0.8 mg, zinc 22.5 mg, biotin 150 mcg, Cr, Cu, Mg, Mn. Bot. 100s. *otc.*
Use: Mineral, vitamin supplement.

Strovite Tablets. (Everett Laboratories) Vitamins B_1 15 mg, B_2 15 mg, B_3 100 mg, B_5 18 mg, B_6 4 mg, B_{12} 5 mcg, C 500 mg, folic acid 0.5 mg. Bot. 100s. *otc.*
Use: Mineral, vitamin supplement.

S.T. 37. (SmithKline Beecham Pharmaceuticals) Hexylresorcinol 0.1% in glycerin aqueous soln. Bot. 5.5 oz, 12 oz. *otc.*
Use: Antiseptic, topical.

Stuart Formula. (J & J Merck Consumer Pharm) Vitamins A 5000 IU, B_1 1.5 mg, B_2 1.7 mg, B_3 20 mg, B_6 1 mg, B_{12} 3 mcg, C 50 mg, D 400 IU, E 10 IU, iron 5 mg, Cu, folic acid 0.4 mg, Ca, I, P/Tab. Bot. 100s. *otc.*

Use: Mineral, vitamin supplement.

Stuartnatal Plus. (Wyeth Ayerst) Vitamins A 4000 IU, D 400 IU, E 22 mg, C 120 mg, B_1 1.84 mg, B_2 3 mg, B_3 20 mg, B_6 10 mg, B_{12} 12 mcg, calcium 200 mg, folic acid 1 mg, iron 65 mg, zinc 25 mg, Cu 2 mg. Tab. Bot. 100s. *Rx.*
Use: Mineral, vitamin supplement.

Stuart Prenatal. (Wyeth Ayerst) Vitamins A 4000 IU, B_1 1.8 mg, B_2 1.7 mg, B_6 2.6 mg, B_{12} 4 mcg, C 100 mg, D 400 IU, E 11 mg, B_3 18 mg, iron 60 mg, calcium 200 mg, copper 2 mg, zinc 25 mg, folic acid 0.8 mg/Tab. Bot. 100s. *otc.*
Use: Mineral, vitamin supplement.

Stulex. (Jones Medical Industries) Docusate sodium 250 mg/Tab. Bot. 100s, 1000s. *otc.*
Use: Fecal softener.

Stye. (Del Pharmaceuticals) White petrolatum 55%, mineral oil 32%, boric acid, wheat germ oil, stearic acid. Oint. Bot. 3.5 g. *otc.*
Use: Lubricant, ophthalmic.

Stypt-Aid. (Pharmakon Labs) Benzocaine 28.71 mg, methylbenzethonium HCl 9.95 mg, aluminum Cl hexahydrate 55.43 mg, ethyl alcohol 70.97%/ml in a glycerine, menthol base. Spray. In 60 ml. *otc.*
Use: Anesthetic, local.

styptirenal.
See: Epinephrine (Various Mfr.).

Stypto-Caine Solution. (Pedinol) Hydroxyquinoline sulfate, tetracaine HCl, aluminum Cl, aqueous glycol base. Bot. 2 oz. *Rx.*
Use: Hemostatic solution.

styrene polymer, sulfonated, sodium salt. Sodium Polystyrene Sulfonate, U.S.P. 23.

styronate resins. Ammonium and potassium salts of sulfonated styrene polymers.
Use: Conditions requiring sodium restriction.

Sublimaze. (Janssen) Fentanyl 0.05 mg as citrate/ml. Amp. 2 ml, 5 ml, 10 ml, 20 ml. *c-II.*
Use: Analgesic, narcotic.

Sublingual B Total Liquid. (Pharmaceutical Labs) Vitamins B_2 1.7 mg, B_3 20 mg, B_5 30 mg, B_6 2 mg, B_{12} 1000 mcg, C 60 mg. Liq. Bot. 30 ml. *otc.*
Use: Vitamin supplement.

Suby's Solution G. (Various Mfr.) Citric acid 3.24 g, sodium carbonate 0.43 g, magnesium oxide 0.38 g/100 ml. Soln. Bot. 1000 ml. *Rx.*
Use: Irrigant, genitourinary.

•**succimer.** (SUX-ih-mer) USAN.
Use: Diagnostic aid; cystine kidney stones, mercury and lead poisoning [Orphan drug]
See: Chemet (McNeil Consumer Products).

succinchlorimide. N-Chlorosuccinimide.

•**succinylcholine chloride.** (suck-sin-ill-KOE-leen KLOR-ide) U.S.P. 23.
Use: Neuromuscular blocker.
See: Anectine Cl, Amp. (Glaxo-Wellcome).
Quelicin, Amp., Additive Syringes, Fliptop & Pintop Vials (Abbott Laboratories).
Sucostrin, Amp., Vial (Squibb Marsam).

succinylsulfathiazole.
Use: Anti-infective, intestinal.

Succus Cineraria Maritima. (Walker Corp) Aqueous and glycerin solution of senecio compositae, hamamelis water and boric acid. Soln. Bot. 7 ml. *Rx.*
Use: Ophthalmic.

Sucostrin. (Apothecon) Succinylcholine Cl 20 mg/ml Inj. Vial 10 ml. *Rx.*
Use: Neuromuscular blocker.

Sucostrin Chloride. (Marsam Pharmaceuticals) Succinylcholine Cl 20 mg/ml w/methylparaben 0.1%, propylparaben 0.01%. Vial 10 ml; High potency 100 mg/ml. Vial 10 ml. *Rx.*
Use: Muscle relaxant.

Sucraid. (Orphan Medical) Sacrosidase 8500 IU/ml. Soln. Bot. 118 ml. *Rx.*
Use: Nutritional therapy.

•**sucralfate.** (sue-KRAL-fate) U.S.P. 23.
Use: Antiulcerative, oral complications of chemotherapy [Orphan drug]
See: Carafate, Tab., Susp. (Hoechst Marion Roussel).

sucralfate. (Biocraft) Sucralfate 1 g/Tab. Bot. 30s, 100s and 500s. *Rx.*
Use: Antiulcerative.

Sucrets Children's Sore Throat Lozenges. (SmithKline Beecham) Dyclonine HCl 1.2 mg/lozenge. Corn syrup, sucrose, cherry flavor. Tin 24s. *otc.*
Use: Sore throat treatment for children 3 years and over.

Sucrets Cold Decongestant Lozenge. (SmithKline Beecham) Phenylpropanolamine HCl 25 mg/lozenge. Box 24s. *otc.*
Use: Decongestant.

Sucrets Cough Control Lozenge. (SmithKline Beecham) Dextromethorphan HBr 5 mg/lozenge. Tin 24s. *otc.*

Use: Antitussive.

Sucrets 4-Hour Cough. (SmithKline Beecham) Dextromethorphan 15 mg/lozenge. Menthol, sucrose, corn syrup. Pkg. 20s. *otc.*
Use: Antitussive.

Sucrets Maximum Strength. (SmithKline Beecham) Dyclonine HCl 3 mg/lozenge. Corn syrup, menthol, sucrose. Tin 24s, 48s, 55s. *otc.*
Use: Mouth and throat preparation.

Sucrets Sore Throat Lozenge. (SmithKline Beecham) Hexylresorcinol 2.4 mg/loz. Tin 24s. *otc.*
Use: Mouth and throat preparation.

Sucrets Sore Throat Spray. (SmithKline Beecham) Dyclonine HCl 0.1%, alcohol 10%, sorbitol spray. Bot. 90 ml, 120 ml. *otc.*
Use: Mouth and throat preparation.

Sucrets Wintergreen. (SmithKline Beecham) Dyclonine HCl 0.1%, alcohol 10%, sorbitol. Spray bot. 90 ml. *otc.*
Use: Mouth and throat preparation.

•**sucrose.** (SUE-krose) N.F. 18.
Use: IV; diuretic & dehydrating agent; pharmaceutic aid (flavor, tablet excipient).

•**sucrose octaacetate.** N.F. 18.
Use: Pharmaceutic aid (alcohol denaturant).

•**sucrosofate potassium.** (sue-KROE-so-FATE) USAN.
Use: Antiulcerative.

Sudafed 12 Hour Capsules. (Warner Lambert) Pseudoephedrine HCl 120 mg/Sustained Action Cap. Box 10s, 20s, 40s. *otc.*
Use: Decongestant.

Sudafed Cold & Cough Liquid Caps. (Warner Lambert) Dextromethorphan HBr 10 mg, pseudoephedrine HCl 30 mg, acetaminophen 250 mg, guaifenesin 100 mg. Pkg. 10s, 20s. *otc.*
Use: Analgesic, antitussive, decongestant, expectorant.

Sudafed Plus. (Warner Lambert) **Tab.:** Pseudoephedrine HCl 60 mg, chlorpheniramine maleate 4 mg/Tab. Box 24s, 48s. *otc.*
Use: Antihistamine, decongestant.

Sudafed, Severe Cold. (Warner Lambert) Pseudoephedrine HCl 30 mg, dextromethorphan HBr 15 mg, acetaminophen 500 mg/Tab. Pkg. 10s, 20s. *otc.*
Use: Analgesic, antitussive, decongestant.

Sudafed Sinus Maximum Strength. (Warner Lambert) Pseudoephedrine HCl 30 mg, acetaminophen 500 mg. Caplets: In 24s. *otc.*
Use: Analgesic, decongestant.

Sudafed Tablets. (Warner Lambert) Pseudoephedrine HCL 30 mg or 60 mg/Tab. **30 mg:** Box 24s, 48s. Bot. 100s, 1000s. **60 mg:** Bot. 100s, 1000s. *otc.*
Use: Decongestant.

Sudal 60/500. (Atley Pharm) Pseudoephedrine HCl 60 mg, guaifenesin 500 mg. TR Tab. Bot. 100s. *Rx.*
Use: Decongestant, expectorant.

Sudal 120/600. (Atley Pharm) Pseudoephedrine HCl 120 mg, guaifenesin 600 mg. SR Tab. Bot. 100s. *Rx.*
Use: Decongestant, expectorant.

Sudanyl. (Dover Pharmaceuticals) Pseudoephedrine HCl/Tab. Sugar, lactose and salt free. UD Box 500s.
Use: Decongestant.

Sudden Tan Lotion. (Schering Plough) Padimate O, dihydroxyacetone, Bot. 4 oz. *otc.*
Use: Artificial tanning, moisturizer, sunscreen.

•**sudoxicam.** (sue-DOX-ih-kam) USAN.
Use: Anti-inflammatory.

Sudrin. (Jones Medical Industries) Pseudoephedrine HCl 30 mg/Tab. Bot. 100s, 1000s. *otc.*
Use: Decongestant.

Sufenta. (Janssen) Sufentanil citrate 50 mcg/ml. Amps. 1 ml, 2 ml, 5 ml. *c-II.*
Use: Analgesic-narcotic.

•**sufentanil.** (sue-FEN-tuh-nill) USAN.
Use: Analgesic.

•**sufentanil citrate.** (sue-FEN-tuh-nill SIH-trate) U.S.P. 23.
Use: Analgesic, narcotic.
See: Sufenta (Janssen).

sufentanil citrate. (ESI Lederle Generics) 50 mcg/ml. Inj. Amp. 1, 2, 5 ml. *c-II.*
Use: Analgesic, narcotic.

•**sufotidine.** (sue-FOE-tih-DEEN) USAN.
Use: Antiulcerative.

Sufrex. (Janssen) Ketanserin tartrate. *Rx.*
Use: Serotonin antagonist.

•**sugar, compressible.** N.F. 18.
Use: Pharmaceutic aid (flavor; tablet excipient).

•**sugar, confectioner's.** N.F. 18.
Use: Pharmaceutic aid (flavor; tablet excipient).

•**sugar, invert, injection.** U.S.P. 23.
Use: Replenisher (fluid and nutrient).

•**sugar spheres.** N.F. 18.
Use: Pharmaceutic aid (vehicle, solid carrier).

Sulamyd Sodium.
Use: Sulfonamide, ophthalmic.
See: Sodium Sulamyd, Ophth. Soln. (Schering Plough).

Sular. (Zeneca) 10, 20, 30, 40 mg nisoldipine, lactose/E.R. Tab. 100s, UD 100s. *Rx.*
Use: Calcium channel blocker.

•**sulazepam.** (sull-AZE-eh-pam) USAN.
Use: Anxiolytic.

Sulazo. (Freeport) Sulfisoxazole 500 mg, phenylazodiaminopyridine HCl 50 mg/Tab. Bot. 1000s. *Rx.*
Use: Analgesic, anti-infective.

•**sulbactam benzathine.** (sull-BACK-tam BENZ-ah-theen) USAN.
Use: Synergistic (penicillin/cephalosporin), inhibitor (β-lactamase).

•**sulbactam pivoxil.** (sull-BACK-tam pihv-OX-ill) USAN.
Use: Inhibitor (β-lactamase), synergist (penicillin/cephalosporin).

•**sulbactam sodium sterile.** (sull-BACK-tam) U.S.P. 23.
Use: Inhibitor (β-lactamase), synergist (penicillin/cephalosporin).

sulbactam sodium/ampicillin sodium.
Use: Anti-infective, penicillin.
See: Unasyn (Roerig).

•**sulconazole nitrate.** (SULL-CONE-ah-zole) U.S.P. 23.
Use: Antifungal.
See: Exelderm (Syntex).

•**sulesomab.** (sue-LEH-so-mab) USAN.
Use: Monoclonal antibody (diagnostic aid for detection of infectious lesions).

Sulf-10. (Ciba Vision Ophthalmics) Sodium sulfacetamide 10%. Bot. 15 ml; Dropperette 1 ml. *Rx.*
Use: Anti-infective, ophthalmic.

Sulf-15. (Ciba Vision Ophthalmics) Sodium sulfacetamide 15%. Soln. Bot. 5 ml, 15 ml. *Rx.*
Use: Anti-infective, ophthalmic.

Sulfa-10 Ophthalmic. (Maurry) Sodium sulfacetamide 10%, hydroxyethylcellulose, sodium borate, boric acid, disodium edetate, sodium metabisulfite, sodium thiosulfate 0.2%, chlorobutanol 0.2%, methyl paraben 0.015%. Bot. 15 ml. *Rx.*
Use: Anti-infective, ophthalmic.

•**sulfabenz.** (SULL-fah-benz) USAN.
Use: Anti-infective.

•**sulfabenzamide.** (SULL-fah-BENZ-ah-mid) U.S.P. 23.
Use: Anti-infective.
See: Sultrin, Vag. Tab., Cream (Ortho McNeil).

sulfabromethazine sodium.
Use: Anti-infective.

Sulfacet. (Dermik Laboratories).
See: Sulfacetamide.

Sulfacet-R. (Dermik Laboratories) Sulfur 5%, sulfacetamide sodium 10%, parabens. Lot. Bot. 25 ml. *Rx.*
Use: Dermatologic, acne.

•**sulfacetamide.** (sull-fah-SEE-tah-mide) U.S.P. 23.
Use: Anti-infective.

sulfacetamide w/combinations.
See: Acet-Dia-Mer Sulfonamides.
Cetapred, Oint. (Alcon Laboratories).
Chero-Trisulfa (V), Susp. (Vita Elixir).
Sulf-10, Ophth. Soln. (Ciba Vision Ophthalmics).
Sulster, Soln. (Akorn).
Sultrin, Tab., Cream (Ortho McNeil).
Triurisul, Tab. (Sheryl).

•**sulfacetamide sodium.** U.S.P. 23.
Use: Anti-infective.
See: AK-Sulf, Preps. (Akorn).
Bleph 10, Liquifilm (Allergan).
Cetamide, Ophth. Oint. (Alcon Laboratories).
Isopto Cetamide, Ophth. Soln. (Alcon Laboratories).
Ocusulf-10, Ophth. Soln. (Optopics).
Sebizon Lotion (Schering Plough).
Sodium Sulamyd Ophthalmic Ointment 30% (Schering Plough).
Sulf-10, Drops (Maurry).
Sulf-10, Soln., Drops (Ciba Vision Ophthalmics).
Sulf-15, Ophth. Soln. (Ciba Vision Ophthalmics).

W/Fluorometholone.
See: FML-S Susp. (Allergan).

W/Methylcellulose.
See: Sodium Sulamyd Ophth. Soln. 10% (Schering Plough).

W/Phenylephrine HCl, methylparaben, propylparaben.
See: Vasosulf, Liq. (Ciba Vision Ophthalmics).

W/Prednisolone.
See: Cetapred Ophthalmic Ointment (Alcon Laboratories).
Vasocidin, Soln. (Ciba Vision Ophthalmics).

W/Prednisolone acetate.
See: Blephamide S.O.P., Ophth. Oint. and Susp. (Allergan).
Metimyd, Ophth. Oint. and Susp. (Schering Plough).

W/Prednisolone, methylcellulose.

See: Isopto Cetapred, Susp. (Alcon Laboratories).
W/Prednisolone acetate, phenylephrine.
See: Blephamide Liquifilm, Ophth. Susp. (Allergan).
Tri-Ophtho, Ophth. Drops (Maurry).
W/Prednisolone phosphate.
See: Optimyd Soln., Sterile (Schering Plough).
W/Prednisolone sodium phosphate, phenylephrine, sulfacetamide sodium.
Vasocidin, Ophth. Soln. (Ciba Vision Ophthalmics).
W/Sulfur.
See: Novacet, Lot. (Genderm).
Sulfacet-R, Lot. (Dermik Laboratories).

sulfacetamide sodium. (Various Mfr.) **Soln.: 10% or 30%:** Bot. 15 ml; **Oint.:** 10% Tube 3.5 g.
Use: Anti-infective.

sulfacetamide sodium and prednisolone acetate ophthalmic ointment.
Use: Anti-infective, anti-inflammatory.
See: AK-Cide (Akorn).
Blephamide S.O.P. (Allergan).
Cetapred (Alcon Laboratories).
Metimyd (Schering Plough).
Predsulfair (Bausch & Lomb).
Sulphrin (Bausch & Lomb).
Vasocidin (Ciba Vision Ophthalmics).

sulfacetamide sodium and prednisolone sodium phosphate. (Schein Pharmaceutical) Sulfacetamide sodium 10%, prednisolone sodium phosphate 0.25%. Soln. 5 ml, 10 ml. *Rx.*
Use: Anti-infective, ophthalmic.

Sulfacetamide Sodium 10% and Sulfur 5%. (Glades) Sulfur 5%, sodium sulfacetamide 10%, cetyl alcohol, benzyl alcohol, EDTA. Bot. 25 ml. Tube 30 ml. *Rx.*
Use: Dermatologic, acne.

sulfacetamide, sulfadiazine, & sulfamerazine oral suspension.
See: Acet-Dia-Mer-Sulfonamides.

Sulfacet-R Lotion. (Dermik Laboratories) Sodium sulfacetamide 10%, sulfur 5%, in flesh-tinted base. Bot. 25 g. *Rx.*
Use: Dermatologic, acne; seborrhea.

•**sulfacytine.** (SULL-fah-SIGH-teen) USAN.
Use: Anti-infective.

sulfadiasulfone sodium. Acetosulfone sodium.

•**sulfadiazine.** (SULL-fah-DIE-ah-zeen) U.S.P. 23.
Use: Anti-infective. [Orphan drug]

sulfadiazine. (Various Mfr.) Sulfadiazine 500 mg. Tab. Bot. 100s, 1000s, UD 100s. *Rx.*
Use: Anti-infective.

sulfadiazine combinations. (SULL-fah-DIE-ah-zeen)
See: Acet-Dia-Mer-Sulfonamides. (Various Mfr.).
Chemozine, Tab., Susp. (Tennessee Pharmaceutic).
Chero-Trisulfa, Susp. (Vita Elixir).
Dia-Mer-Sulfonamides (Various Mfr.).
Dia-Mer-Thia-Sulfonamide (Various Mfr.).
Meth-Dia-Mer-Sulfonamides (Various Mfr.).
Silvadene (Hoechst Marion Roussel).
Terfonyl, Liq., Tab. (Bristol-Myers Squibb).
Triple Sulfa, Tab. (Various Mfr.).

sulfadiazine and sulfamerazine. Citrasulfas.
See: Dia-Mer-Sulfonamides.

•**sulfadiazine, silver.** (sull-fah-DIE-ah-zeen) U.S.P. 23.
Use: Anti-infective, topical.

•**sulfadiazine sodium.** (SULL-fah-DIE-ah-zeen) U.S.P. 23.
Use: Anti-infective.
W/Sod. bicarbonate.
(Pitman-Moore)–Tab. 5 gr, Bot. 1000s; 2.5 gr, Bot. 100s, 500s, 1000s.

sulfadiazine, sulfamerazine & sulfacetamide suspension.
See: Acet-Dia-Mer-Sulfonamides.
Coco Diazine (Eli Lilly).

sulfadimetine. (Novartis Pharmaceuticals).

sulfadimidine.
See: Sulfamethazine.

sulfadine.
See: Sulfadimidine.
Sulfamethazine.
Sulfapyridine, Tab. (Various Mfr.).

•**sulfadoxine.** (SULL-fah-DOX-een) U.S.P. 23.
Use: Anti-infective.
W/Pyrimethamine.
See: Fansidar, Tab. (Roche Laboratories).

sulfadoxine and pyrimethamine tablets.
Use: Anti-infective, antimalarial.

sulfaethylthiadiazole.

sulfaguanidine.
Use: GI tract infections.
W/Sulfamethazine, sulfamerazine & sulfadiazine.
See: Quadetts, Tab. (Zeneca).

Quad-Ramoid, Susp. (Zeneca).
Sulfair 15. (Bausch & Lomb) Sodium sulfacetamide 15%. Soln. Bot. 15 ml. *Rx.*
Use: Anti-infective, ophthalmic.
Sulfalax Calcium. (Major) Docusate calcium 240 mg/Cap. Bot. 500s. *otc.*
Use: Laxative.
•**sulfalene.** (SULL-fah-leen) USAN.
Use: Anti-infective.
•**sulfamerazine.** (sull-fah-MER-ah-zeen) U.S.P. 23.
Use: Anti-infective.
sulfamerazine combinations.
Use: Anti-infective.
See: Chemozine Tab., Susp. (Tennessee Pharmaceutic).
Chero-Trisulfa-V, Susp. (Vita Elixir).
Terfonyl, Liq., Tab. (Bristol-Myers Squibb).
Triple Sulfa, Tab. (Various Mfr.).
sulfamerazine sodium.
Use: Anti-infective.
sulfamerazine & sulfadiazine.
See: Dia-Mer-Sulfonamides.
sulfamerazine, sulfadiazine & sulfamethazine.
Use: Anti-infective.
See: Meth-Dia-Mer-Sulfonamides.
sulfamerazine, sulfadiazine & sulfathiazole.
Use: Anti-infective.
See: Dia-Mer-Thia-Sulfonamides.
•**sulfameter.** (SULL-fam-EE-ter) USAN.
Use: Anti-infective.
•**sulfamethazine.** (sull fa-METH-ah zeen) U.S.P. 23.
Use: Anti-infective.
See: Neotrizine, Susp., Tab. (Eli Lilly).
W/Sulfacetamide, sulfadiazine, sulfamerazine.
See: Sulfa-Plex, Vaginal Cream (Solvay).
W/Sulfadiazine, sulfamerazine.
See: Sulfaloid, Susp. (Westerfield).
Terfonyl, Liq., Tab. (Bristol-Myers Squibb).
Triple Sulfa, Tab. (Various Mfr.).
•**sulfamethizole.** (sull-fah-METH-ih-zole) U.S.P. 23.
Use: Anti-infective.
See: Bursul, Tab. (Burlington).
Microsul, Tab. (Star).
Proklar-M, Liq., Tab. (Westerfield).
Sulfurine, Tab. (Table Rock).
Thiosulfil, Forte, Tab. (Wyeth Ayerst).
Urifon, Tab. (T.E. Williams).
sulfamethizole w/combinations.
Use: Anti-infective.
See: Microsul-A, Tab. (Star).
Thiosulfil-A, Tab. (Wyeth Ayerst).
Thiosulfil-A Forte, Tab. (Wyeth Ayerst).
Triurisul, Tab. (Sheryl).
Urobiotic, Cap. (Pfizer).
Urotrol, Tab. (Mills).
sulfamethoprim. (Par Pharm) Sulfamethoxazole 400 mg, trimethoprim 80 mg/Tab. Bot. 100s, 500s. *Rx.*
Use: Anti-infective.
•**sulfamethoxazole.** (sull-fah-meth-OX-ah-zole) U.S.P. 23.
Use: Anti-infective.
See: Gantanol, Prep. (Roche Laboratories).
W/Trimethoprim.
See: Bactrim, Prods. (Roche Laboratories).
Septra, Tab. (GlaxoWellcome).
Septra DS, Tab. (GlaxoWellcome).
sulfamethoxazole and phenazopyridine hydrochloride.
Use: Anti-infective, urinary.
See: Azo-Gantanol, Tab. (Roche Laboratories).
sulfamethoxazole and trimethoprim for injection concentrate. (SULL-fah-meth-OX-ah-zole and try-METH-oh-prim)
Use: Anti-infective, urinary.
sulfamethoxazole and trimethoprim oral suspension. (Various Mfr.) Trimethoprim 40 mg, sulfamethoxazole 200 mg/5 ml. Bot. 150 ml, 200 ml, 480 ml. *Rx.*
Use: Anti-infective, urinary.
sulfamethoxazole and trimethoprim tablets. (Various Mfr.) Trimethoprim 80 mg, sulfamethoxazole 400 mg/Tab. Bot. 100s, 500s. *Rx.*
Use: Anti-infective, urinary.
sulfamethoxazole/trimethoprim DS. (Various Mfr.) Trimethoprim 160 mg, sulfamethoxazole 800 mg. Tab, double strength. Bot. 100s, 500s. *Rx.*
Use: Anti-infective.
sulfamethoxydiazine. Sulfameter.
Use: Anti-infective.
sulfamethoxypyridazine acetyl.
Use: Anti-infective.
sulfamethylthiadiazole.
Use: Anti-infective.
See: Sulfamethizole Preps.
sulfametin. N^1-(5-Methoxy-2-pyrimidinyl) sulfanilamide. (Formerly sulfamethoxydiazine).
Use: Anti-infective.
sulfamezanthene.
Use: Anti-infective.

See: Sulfamethazine.

Sulfamide Suspension. (Rugby) Prednisolone acetate 0.5%, sodium sulfacetamide, hydroxypropyl methylcellulose, polysorbate 80, sodium thiosulfate, benzalkonium Cl 0.01%. Susp. Bot. 5 and 15 ml. *Rx.*
Use: Anti-infective, ophthalmic.

•**sulfamonomethoxine.** (SULL-fah-mahn-oh-meh-THOCK-seen) USAN.
Use: Anti-infective.

•**sulfamoxole.** (sull-fah-MOX-ole) USAN.
Use: Anti-infective.

p-sulfamoylbenzylamine hydrochloride. Sulfbenzamide.

Sulfamylon Cream. (Dow Hickam) Mafenide acetate equivalent to 85 mg of base/g. w/cetyl alcohol, stearyl alcohol, cetyl esters wax, polyoxyl 40 stearate, polyoxyl 8 stearate, glycerin, water w/methylparaben and propylparaben, sodium metabisulfite, edetate disodium. Tube 2 oz, 4 oz. Can 14.5 oz. *Rx.*
Use: Burn therapy adjunct.

sulfanilamide. p-Aminobenzene sulfonamide.
Use: Anti-infective.

sulfanilamide. (Various Mfr.) Sulfanilamide 15%. Vaginal Cream. Tube 120 g with applicator. *Rx.*
Use: Anti-infective, vaginal.

sulfanilamide combinations.
Use: Anti-infective.
See: AVC/Dienestrol Cream, Supp. (Hoechst Marion Roussel).
AVC, Cream, Supp. (Hoechst Marion Roussel).
Par Cream (Parmed).
Vagisan Creme (Sandia).
Vagisul, Creme (Sheryl).
Vagitrol, Cream, Supp. (Teva USA).

2-sulfanilamidopyridine. Sulfadiazine, U.S.P. 23.
Use: Anti-infective.

•**sulfanilate zinc.** (sull-FAN-ih-late) USAN.
Use: Anti-infective.

n-sulfanilylacetamide.
Use: Anti-infective.
See: Sulfacetamide, Tab. (Various Mfr.).

sulfanilylbenzamide.
Use: Anti-infective.
See: Sulfabenzamide.

•**sulfanitran.** (SULL-fah-NYE-tran) USAN.
Use: Anti-infective.

•**sulfapyridine.** (sull-fah-PEER-ih-deen) U.S.P. 23.
Use: Dermatitic herpetiformis suppressant. [Orphan drug]

sulfarsphenamine.

•**sulfasalazine.** (SULL-fuh-SAL-uh-zeen) U.S.P. 23. *Formerly Salicylazosulfapyridine.*
Use: Anti-infective.
See: Azulfidine, Preps. (Pharmacia & Upjohn).
Salazopyrin.
Salicylazosulfapyridine.
Salazopyrin.
S.A.S.-50, Tab. (Solvay).
S.A.S.P., Tab. (Zenith Goldline).
Sulfapyridine (I.N.N.).

sulfasalazine. (Various Mfr.) Sulfasalazine 500 mg. Tab. Bot. 50s, 100s, 500s, 1000s. *Rx.*
Use: Anti-infective.

•**sulfasomizole.** (SULL-fah-SAHM-ih-zole) USAN.
Use: Antibacterial, anti-infective, sulfonamide.
See: Bidizole.

sulfasymasine.
Use: Anti-infective sulfonamide.

Sulfa-Ter-Tablets. (A.P.C.) Trisulfapyrimidines, U.S.P. Bot. 1000s.

•**sulfathiazole.** (sull-fah-THIGH-ah-zole) U.S.P. 23.
Use: Anti-infective.
W/Chlorophyllin.

sulfathiazole combinations.
See: Sultrin, Tab. & Cream (Ortho McNeil).

sulfathiazole carbamide.
See: Otosmosan, Liq. (Wyeth Ayerst).

sulfathiazole, sulfacetamide, and sulfabenzamide vaginal cream.
See: Dayto Sulf (Dayton).
Triple Sulfa Vaginal Cream.

sulfathiazole, sulfacetamide, and sulfabenzamide vaginal tablets.
See: Triple Sulfa Vaginal Tablets.

Sulfatrim. (Various Mfr.) Trimethoprim 40 mg, sulfamethoxazole 200 mg/5 ml Susp. Bot. 473 ml. *Rx.*
Use: Anti-infective.

Sulfatrim DS Tabs. (Zenith Goldline) Trimethoprim 800 mg, sulfamethoxazole 160 mg/Tab. Bot. 100s, 500s. *Rx.*
Use: Anti-infective.

Sulfatrim SS Tabs. (Zenith Goldline) Trimethoprim 400 mg, sulfamethoxazole 80 mg/Tab. Bot. 100s. *Rx.*
Use: Anti-infective.

Sulfa-Trip. (Major) Sulfathiazole 3.42%, sulfacetamide 2.86%, sulfabenzamide 3.7%, urea 0.64%. Cream. In 82.5 g. *Rx.*
Use: Anti-infective, vaginal.

Sulfa Triple No. 2. (Global Source) Sulfadiazine 162 mg, sulfamerizine 162 mg, sulfamethazine 162 mg/Tab. Bot. 1000s. *Rx.*
Use: Anti-infective.

•**sulfazamet.** (sull-FAZE-ah-MET) USAN.
Use: Anti-infective.

sulfhydryl ion.
See: Hydrosulphosol (Lientz).

•**sulfinalol hydrochloride.** (SULL-FIN-ah-lahl) USAN.
Use: Antihypertensive.

•**sulfinpyrazone.** (sull-fin-PEER-uh-zone) U.S.P. 23.
Use: Uricosuric.
See: Anturane, Tab., Cap. (Novartis Pharmaceuticals).

•**sulfisoxazole.** (sull-fih-SOX-uh-zole) U.S.P. 23.
Use: Anti-infective.
See: Gantrisin Preps. (Roche Laboratories).
Soxa, Tab. (Vita Elixir).
Sulfisoxazole, Tab. (Purepac).
Sulfizin, Tab. (Solvay).
W/Aminoacridine HCl, allantoin.
See: Vagilia, Cream (Teva USA).
W/Phenazopyridine.
See: Azo-Gantrisin, Tab. (Roche Laboratories).
Azo-Soxazole, Tab. (Quality Formulations).
Azo-Sulfisoxazole, Tab. (Global Pharms; Century).
W/Phenylazo Diamino Pyridine HCl.
See: Azo-Sulfizin (Solvay).

sulfisoxazole. (Various Mfr.) Sulfisoxazole 500 mg. Tab. Bot. 100s, 1000s. *Rx.*
Use: Anti-infective.

•**sulfisoxazole, acetyl.** (sull-fih-SOX-uh-zole, ASS-eh-till) U.S.P. 23.
Use: Anti-infective.
W/Erythromycin Ethylsuccinate.
See: Pediazol, Susp. (Ross Laboratories).

sulfisoxazole diethanolamine. Sulfisoxazole Diolamine.

•**sulfisoxazole diolamine.** (sull-fin-SOX-azz-ole die-OLE-ah-meen) U.S.P. 23.
Use: Anti-infective.
See: Gantrisin, Ophth. Soln. & Oint. (Roche Laboratories).

Sulfoam Medicated Antidandruff Shampoo. (Kenwood/Bradley) Sulfur 2% with cleansers & conditioners. Bot. 4 oz, 8 oz, 15.5 oz. *otc.*
Use: Control dandruff.

sulfobromophthalein sodium. U.S.P. XXII.
Use: Liver function test.

sulfocarbolates. Salts of Phenolsulfonic Acid, Usually Ca, Na, K, Cu, Zn.

sulfocyanate.
See: Potassium Thiocyanate.

Sulfo-Ganic. (Marcen) Thioglycerol 20 mg, sodium citrate 5 mg, phenol 0.5%, benzyl alcohol 0.5%/ml. Vial 10 ml, 30 ml.
Use: Antiarthritic.

sulfoguaiacol.
See: Pot. Guaiacolsulfonate.

Sulfoil. (C & M Pharmacal) Sulfonated castor oil, water. Bot. pt, Gal. *otc.*
Use: Dermatologic-hair and skin.

Sulfolax Calcium. (Major) Docusate calcium 240 mg/Cap. Bot. 100s. *otc.*
Use: Laxative.

Sulfo-Lo. (Whorton) Sublimed sulfur, freshly precipitated polysulfides of zinc, potassium, sulfate, and calamine in aqueous-alcoholic suspension. **Lotion:** Bot. 4 oz, 8 oz, **Soap:** 3 oz. *otc.*
Use: Dermatologic, acne.

•**sulfomyxin.** (SULL-foe-MIX-in) USAN.
Use: Anti-infective.

sulfonamide, doubles.
See: Dia-Mer-Sulfonamides.

sulfonamide preps.
See: Acet-Dia-Mer (Various Mfr.).
Dayto Sulf, Vag. cream (Dayton).
Dia-Mer Sulfonamides (Various Mfr.).
Dia-Mer-Thia (Various Mfr.).
Gyne-Sulf, Vag. cream (G & W Laboratories).
Meth-Dia-Mer, Preps. (Various Mfr.).
Sultrin Triple Sulfa, Vag. cream, Tab. (Ortho McNeil).
Triple Sulfa, Vag. cream (Various Mfr.).
Trysul, Vag. cream (Savage).
V.V.S., Vag. cream (Econo Med Pharmaceuticals).

sulfonamides, quadruple.
See: Quadetts, Tab. (Zeneca).
Quad-Ramoid, Susp. (Zeneca).

sulfonamides, triple.
See: Acet-Dia-Mer Sulfonamides.
Dia-Mer-Thia Sulfonamides.
Meth-Dia-Mer Sulfonamides.

sulfones.
See: Avlosulfon, Tab. (Wyeth Ayerst).
Dapsone.
Diasone, Enterabs (Abbott Laboratories).
Glucosulfone Sodium.
Promacetin, Tab. (Parke-Davis).

sulfonethylmethane. 2,2-Bis-(ethylsulfonyl)butane.

sulfonithocholylglycine.
See: S.L.C.G., Kit (Abbott Laboratories).

sulfonmethane.

sulfonphthal.
See: Phenolsulfonphthalein, Prep. (Various Mfr.).

•**sulfonterol hydrochloride.** (sull-FAHN-teer-ole) USAN.
Use: Bronchodilator.

sulfonylureas.
See: DiaBeta (Hoechst Marion Roussel).
Diabinese, Tab. (Pfizer).
Dymelor, Tab. (Eli Lilly).
Glucotrol (Roerig).
Glynase PresTab (Pharmacia & Upjohn).
Micronase (Pharmacia & Upjohn).
Orinase, Tab., Vial (Pharmacia & Upjohn).
Tolinase, Tab. (Pharmacia & Upjohn).

Sulforcin Lotion. (Galderma) Sulfur 5%, resorcinol 2%, SD alcohol 40 11.65%, methylparaben. Bot. 120 ml. *otc.*
Use: Dermatologic.

sulformethoxine. Name used for Sulfadoxine.

sulforthomidine. Name used for Sulfadoxine.

sulfosalicylate w/methenamine.
See: Hexalen, Tab. (PolyMedica).

sulfosalicylic acid. Salicylsulphonic acid.

sulfoxone sodium. U.S.P. XXII.

sulfoxyl regular. (Stiefel) Benzoyl peroxide 5%, sulfur 2% Bot. 60 ml. *Rx.*
Use: Dermatologic, acne.

sulfoxyl strong. (Stiefel) Benzoyl peroxide 10%, sulfur 5% Bot. 60 ml. *Rx.*
Use: Dermatologic, acne.

Sulfur-8 Hair & Scalp Conditioner. (Schering Plough) Sulfur 2%, menthol 1%, triclosan 0.1%. Jar 2 oz, 4 oz, 8 oz. *otc.*
Use: Antiseborrheic.

Sulfur-8 Light Formula Hair & Scalp Conditioner. (Schering Plough) Sulfur, triclosan, menthol. Jar 2 oz, 4 oz. *otc.*
Use: Antiseborrheic.

Sulfur-8 Shampoo. (Schering Plough) Triclosan 0.2%. Bot. 6.85 oz, 10.85 oz. *otc.*
Use: Antiseborrheic.

sulfur, antiarthritic.
See: Thiocyl, Amp. (Torigian).

sulfurated lime topical solution. Vleminckx Lotion.
Use: Scabicide, parasiticide.

sulfur combinations.
See: Acnaveen, Bar (Rydelle).
Acne-Aid, Cream, Lot. (Stiefel).
Akne Oral Kapsulets, Cap. (Alto Pharmaceuticals).
Acnomel, Cake, Cream (SmithKline Beecham Pharmaceuticals).
Acno, Soln., Lot. (Baker Norton).
Acnotex, Liq. (C & M Pharmacal).
Akne, Drying Lot. (Alto Pharmaceuticals).
Antrocol, Tab., Cap. (ECR Pharmaceuticals).
Aracain Rectal Oint. (Del Pharmaceuticals).
Bensulfoid, Cream (ECR Pharmaceuticals).
Clearasil, Stick (Procter & Gamble).
Epi-clear, Lotion (Bristol-Myers Squibb).
Exzit, Preps. (Bayer Corp).
Fomac, Cream (Dermik Laboratories).
Fostex, Liq. Cream, Bar (Westwood Squibb).
Fostex, Cream, Liq. (Westwood Squibb).
Fostex CM, Cream (Westwood Squibb).
Fostril, Cream (Westwood Squibb).
Hydro Surco, Lot. (Almo).
Klaron, Lot. (Dermik Laboratories).
Liquimat, Liq. (Galderma).
Lotio-P (Alto Pharmaceuticals).
Neutrogena Disposables (Neutrogena).
Pernox, Lot. (Westwood Squibb).
pHisoDan, Liq. (Sanofi Winthrop).
Postacne, Lot. (Dermik Laboratories).
Pragmatar, Oint. (Menley & James).
Proseca, Liq. (Westwood Squibb).
Rezamid, Lot. (Summers).
SAStid Soap (Stiefel).
Sebaveen, Shampoo (Rydelle).
Sebulex Shampoo, Liq. (Westwood Squibb).
Sulfacet-R, Lot. (Dermik Laboratories).
Sulfo-lo, Lot. (Wharton).
Sulforcin, Pow., Lot. (Galderma).
Sulfur-8, Prods. (Schering Plough).
Sulpho-Lac, Cream (Kenwood/Bradley).
Teenac, Cream (Zeneca).
Vanseb, Cream (Allergan).
Vanseb-T Tar Shampoo (Allergan).
Xerac, Oint. (Person & Covey).

•**sulfur dioxide.** (SULL-fer die-OX-ide) N.F. 18.
Use: Pharmaceutic aid (antioxidant).

sulfur ointment.
Use: Scabicide, parasiticide.

•**sulfur, precipitated.** U.S.P. 23.
Use: Scabicide; parasiticide.
See: Bensulfoid, Pow., Lot. (ECR Pharmaceuticals).
Epi-Clear, Lot. (Bristol-Myers Squibb).
Ramsdell's Sulfur Cream (E. Fougera).
SAStid Soap, Bar (Stiefel).
Sulfur Soap (Steifel Labs).

sulfur, salicyl diasporal. (Doak Dermatologics).
See: Diasporal, Cream (Doak Dermatologics).

sulfur soap. (Stiefel) Precipitated sulfur 10%, EDTA. Cake 116 g. *otc.*
Use: Dermatologic, acne.

•**sulfur, sublimed.** U.S.P. 23. Flowers of Sulfur.
Use: Parasiticide, scabicide.

sulfur, topical.
See: Thylox, Liq., Soap (Dent).

•**sulfuric acid.** N.F. 18.
Use: Pharmaceutic aid (acidifying agent).

Sulfurine. (Table Rock) Sulfamethizole 0.5 g/Tab. Bot. 100s & 500s. *Rx.*
Use: Anti-infective, urinary.

•**sulindac.** (sull-IN-dak) U.S.P. 23.
Use: Anti-inflammatory.
See: Clinoril Tab. (Merck).

•**sulisobenzone.** (sul-EYE-so-BEN-zone) USAN.
Use: Ultraviolet screen.
See: Uval Lotion (Novartis).
Uvinul MS-40 (General Aniline & Film).

•**sulmarin.** (SULL-mah-rin) USAN.
Use: Hemostatic.

Sulmasque. (C & M) Sulfur 6.4%, isopropyl alcohol 15%, methylparaben. Mask 150 g. *otc.*
Use: Dermatologic, acne.

Sulnac. (NMC Labs) Sulfathiazole 3.42%, sulfacetamide 2.86%, sulfabenzamide 3.7%, urea 0.64% in cream base. Tube 2.75 oz. *Rx.*
Use: Anti-infective.

•**sulnidazole.** (sull-NIH-dah-zole) USAN.
Use: Antiprotozoal (trichomonas).

sulocarbilate. 2-Hydroxyethyl-p-sulfamylcarbanilate.

•**suloctidil.** (sull-OCK-tih-dill) USAN.
Use: Vasodilator (peripheral).

•**sulofenur.** (SUE-low-FEN-ehr) USAN.
Use: Antineoplastic.

•**sulopenem.** (sue-LOW-PEN-em) USAN.
Use: Anti-infective.

•**sulotroban.** (suh-LOW-troe-ban) USAN.
Use: Treatment of glomerulonephritis.

•**suloxifen oxalate.** (sull-OX-ih-fen OX-ah-late) USAN.
Use: Bronchodilator.

suloxybenzone. (ESI Lederle Generics).

sulphabenzide.
See: Sulfabenzamide.

Sulpho-Lac Acne Medication. (Doak Dermatologics) Sulfur 5%, zinc sulfate 27%, Vleminckx's Soln. 53%. Cream. Tube 28.35 g, 50 g. *otc.*
Use: Dermatologic, acne.

Sulpho-Lac Soap. (Doak Dermatologics) Sulfur 5%, a coconut and tallow oil soap base. Bar 85 g. *otc.*
Use: Dermatologic, acne.

sulphomyxin. Penta-(N-sulphomethyl) polymyxin B.

•**sulpiride.** (SULL-pih-ride) USAN.
Use: Antidepressant.

•**sulprostone.** (sull-PRAHST-ohn) USAN.
Use: Prostaglandin.

Sul-Ray Acne Cream. (Last) Sulfur 2% in cream base. Jars 1.75 oz, 6.75 oz, 20 oz. *otc.*
Use: Dermatologic, acne.

Sul-Ray Aloe Vera Analgesic Rub. (Last) Camphor 3.1%, menthol 1.25%. Bot. 4 oz, 8 oz. *otc.*
Use: Analgesic-topical.

Sul-Ray Aloe Vera Skin Protectant Cream. (Last) Zinc oxide 1%, allantoin 0.5%. Jar 1 oz. *otc.*
Use: Dermatologic, protectant.

Sul-Ray Shampoo. (Last) Sulfur shampoo 2%. Bot. 8 oz. *otc.*
Use: Antidandruff.

Sul-Ray Soap. (Last) Sulfur soap. Bar 3 oz. *otc.*
Use: Dermatologic, acne.

Sulster. (Akorn) Sulfacetamide sodium 1%, prednisolone sodium phosphate. 0.25% Soln. Bot. 5 ml, 10 ml. *Rx.*
Use: Ophthalmic preparation.

•**sultamicillin.** (SULL-TAM-ih-sill-in) USAN.
Use: Anti-infective.

•**sulthiame.** (sull-THIGH-aim) USAN.
Use: Anticonvulsant.

Sultrin Triple Sulfa Vaginal Tablets. (Ortho McNeil) Sulfathiazole 172.5 mg, sulfacetamide 143.75 mg, sulfabenzamide 184 mg/Vag. Tab. Pkg. 20s w/appl. *Rx.*
Use: Treatment of *H. vaginalis* (Gardnerella) vaginitis.

Sultrin Triple Sulfa Cream. (Ortho McNeil) Sulfathiazole 3.42%, sulf-

acetamide 2.86%, sulfabenzamide 3.7%, urea 0.64%. Tube 78 g. with measured dose applicator. *Rx.*
Use: Treatment of *H. vaginalis* (Gardnerella) vaginitis.

•**sulukast.** (suh-LOO-kast) USAN.
Use: Antiasthmatic (leukotriene antagonist).

Sumacal Powder. (Biosearch Medical Products) CHO 95 g, 380 Cal., Na 100 mg, Chloride 210 mg, K < 39 mg, Ca 20 mg/100 g. Pwd. In 400 g. *otc.*
Use: Glucose polymer.

•**sumarotene.** (sue-MAHR-oh-teen) USAN.
Use: Keratolytic.

•**sumatriptan succinate.** (SUE muh-TRIP-tan SOOS-in-ate) USAN.
Use: Antimigraine, treatment of cluster headaches.
See: Imitrex, Preps. (GlaxoWellcome).

Summer's Eve Disposable Douche. (C.B. Fleet) **Soln.:** Vinegar. 135 ml (1s, 2s). **Soln. Reg.:** Citric acid, sodium benzoate. **Soln. Scented:** Citric acid, sodium benzoate, octoxynol 9, EDTA. 135 ml (1s, 2s, 4s). *otc.*
Use: Douche.

Summer's Eve Disposable Douche Extra Cleansing. (C.B. Fleet) Vinegar, sodium Cl, benzoic acid. Soln. 135 ml (1s, 2s, 4s). *otc.*
Use: Douche.

Summer's Eve Feminine Bath. (Fleet) Ammonium laureth sulfate, EDTA. Liq. Bot. 45 ml, 345 ml. *otc.*
Use: Vaginal preparation.

Summer's Eve Feminine Powder. (Fleet) Cornstarch, octoxynol-9, benzethonium chloride. Pow. Bot. 30 g, 210 g. *otc.*
Use: Vaginal preparation.

Summer's Eve Feminine Wash. (Fleet) **Wipes:** Octoxynol-9, EDTA. Box 16s. **Liq.:** ammonium laureth sulfate, PEG-75, lanolin, EDTA. Bot. 60 ml, 240 ml, 450 ml. *Rx.*
Use: Vaginal preparation.

Summer's Eve Medicated Disposable Douche. (C.B. Fleet) Contains povidone-iodide 0.3%. Single or twin 135 ml disposable units. *otc.*
Use: Temporary relief of minor vaginal irritation and itching.

Summer's Eve Post Menstrual Disposable Douche. (C.B. Fleet) Sodium lauryl sulfate, parabens, monosodium and disodium phosphates, EDTA. Soln. 135 ml (2s). *otc.*
Use: Douche.

Sumycin. (Apothecon) Tetracycline HCl. **Cap.** 250 mg/Cap. Bot. 100s, 1000s, Unimatic 100s; 500 mg/Cap. Bot. 100s, 500s, Unimatic 100s. **Tab.** 250 mg/Tab. Bot. 100s, 1000s; 500 mg/Tab. Bot. 100s, 500s. *Rx.*
Use: Anti-infective, tetracycline.

•**suncillin sodium.** (SUN-SILL-in SO-dee-uhm) USAN.
Use: Anti-infective.

Sundown. (Johnson & Johnson Consumer Products) A series of products marketed under the Sundown name including: **Moderate** (SPF 4) Padimate O, oxybenzone. **Extra** (SPF 6) Oxybenzone, Padimate O. **Maximal** (SPF 8) Oxybenzone, Padimate O. **Ultra** (SPF 15, 30) oxybenzone, Padimate O, Octyl Methoxycinnamate. *otc.*
Use: Sunscreen.

Sundown Sport Sunblock. (Johnson & Johnson) Titanium dioxide, zinc oxide. Waterproof. PABA free. SPF 15. Lot. 90 ml. *otc.*
Use: Sunscreen.

Sundown Sunblock Cream Ultra SPF 24. (Johnson & Johnson Consumer Products) Padimate O, oxybenzone. *otc.*
Use: Sunscreen.

Sundown Sunblock Stick SPF 15. (Johnson & Johnson) Octyl dimethyl PABA, oxybenzone. Stick 0.35 oz. *otc.*
Use: Sunscreen.

Sundown Sunblock Stick SPF 20. (Johnson & Johnson Consumer Products) Octyl dimethyl PABA, octyl methoxycinnamate, oxybenzone and titanium dioxide. *otc.*
Use: Sunscreen.

Sundown Sunblock Ultra Lotion 30 SPF. (Johnson & Johnson Consumer Products) Octyl methoxycinnamate, octyl salicylate, oxybenzone, titanium dioxide, cetyl alcohol, PABA free, waterproof. Lot. Bot. 120 ml. *otc.*
Use: Sunscreen.

Sundown Sunblock Ultra SPF 20. (Johnson & Johnson Consumer Products) Octyl dimethyl PABA, octyl methoxycinnamate, oxybenzone, titanium dioxide. *otc.*
Use: Sunscreen.

Sundown Sunscreen Stick SPF 8. (Johnson & Johnson Consumer Products) Octyl Dimethyl PABA, oxybenzone. Stick 0.35 oz. *otc.*
Use: Sunscreen.

Sundown Sunscreen Ultra. (Johnson & Johnson Consumer Products) Octyl methoxycinnamate, octyl salicylate, oxybenzone, titanium dioxide, stearyl alcohol, cetyl alcohol, PABA free, waterproof. SPF 15. Cream. Tube 60 g. *otc.*
Use: Sunscreen.

Sunice. (Citroleum) Allantoin 0.25%, menthol 0.25%, methyl salicylate 10%/ Cream. 3 oz. *otc.*
Use: Burn therapy.

Sunkist Multivitamins Complete, Children's. (Novartis Pharmaceuticals) Iron 18 mg, vitamin A 5000 IU, D_3 400 IU, E 30 IU, B_1 1.5 mg, B_2 1.7 mg, B_3 20 mg, B_5 10 mg, B_6 2 mg, B_{12} 6 mcg, C 60 mg, folic acid 400 mcg, Ca 100 mg, Cu, I, K, Mg, Mn, P, zinc 10 mg, biotin 40 mcg, K_1 10 mcg, sorbitol, aspartame, phenylalanine, tartrazine. Chew. Tab. Bot. 60s. *otc.*
Use: Mineral, vitamin supplement.

Sunkist Multivitamins + Extra C, Children's. (Novartis Pharmaceuticals) Vitamin A 2500 IU, E 15 IU, D_3 400 IU, B_1 1.05 mg, B_2 1.2 mg, B_3 13.5 mg, B_6 1.05 mg, B_{12} 4.5 mcg, C 250 mg, folic acid 0.3 mg, vitamin K 5 mcg, sorbitol, aspartame, phenylalanine/Chew. Tab. Bot. 60s. *otc.*
Use: Vitamin supplement.

Sunkist Multivitamins + Iron, Children's. (Novartis Pharmaceuticals) Iron 15 mg, vitamin A 2500 IU, E 15 IU, D_3 400 IU, E 30 IU, B_1 1.05 mg, B_2 1.2 mg, B_3 13.5 mg, B_6 1.05 mg, B_{12} 4.5 mcg, C 60 mg, folic acid 0.3 mg, K_1 5 mcg, sorbitol, aspartame, phenylalanine, tartrazine. Chew. Tab. Bot. 60s. *otc.*
Use: Vitamin/mineral supplement.

Sunkist Vitamin C. (Novartis Pharmaceuticals) Vitamin C (as ascorbic acid) 500 mg. Capl. Bot. 60s. *otc.*
Use: Vitamin supplement.

Sunkist Vitamin C. (Novartis Pharmaceuticals) Vitamin C (as ascorbic acid) 60 mg, sorbitol, sucrose, lactose. Chew. Tab. Pkg. 11s. *otc.*
Use: Vitamin supplement.

Sunkist Vitamin C. (Novartis Pharmaceuticals) Vitamin C (as sodium ascorbate and ascorbic acid) 250 mg or 500 mg, fructose, sorbitol, sucrose, lactose. Chew. Tab. Bot. 60s. *otc.*
Use: Vitamin supplement.

SUNPRuF 15. (C & M) SPF 15. Octyl methoxycinnamate 7.5%, benzopherone-3 5%. PABA free. Waterproof. Lot. Bot. 240 ml. *otc.*
Use: Sunscreen.

SUNPRuF 17. (C & M Pharmacal) SPF 17. Octyl methoxycinnamate 7.8%, octyl salicylate 5.2%, oil-free, water-resistant. Lot. Bot. 120 g. *otc.*
Use: Sunscreen.

Sunshine Chewable Tablets. (Fibertone) Iron 5 mg, vitamins A 5000 IU, D 400 IU, E 67 mg, B_1 15 mg, B_2 15 mg, B_3 25 mg, B_5 20 mg, B_6 15 mg, B_{12} 15 mcg, C 150 mg, folic acid 0.1 mg, Ca, Cu, Mn, Zn, K, iodide, biotin, betaine, PABA, choline bitartrate, inositol, lecithin, hesperidin, rutin, bioflavonoids, sorbitol, aspartame, citrus flavor/Tab. Bot. 60s. *otc.*
Use: Mineral, vitamin supplement.

Sunstick. (Rydelle) Lip and face protectant containing digalloyl trioleate 2.5% in emollient base. Plas. swivel container 0.14 oz. *otc.*
Use: Lip protectant.

SU-101.
Use: Malignant glioma. [Orphan drug]

Supac. (Mission Pharmacal) Acetaminophen 160 mg, aspirin 230 mg, caffeine 33 mg, calcium gluconate 60 mg/Tab. Bot. 100s. *otc.*
Use: Analgesic.

Super Aytinal Tablets. (Walgreens) Vitamins A 7000 IU, B_1 5 mg, B_2 5 mg, B_5 10 mg, B_6 3 mg, B_{12} 9 mcg, C 90 mg, pantothenic acid 10 mg, D 400 IU, E 30 IU, niacin 30 mg, biotin 55 mcg, folic acid 0.4 mg, iron 30 mg, calcium 162 mg, P 125 mg, iodine 150 mcg, copper 3 mg, manganese 7.5 mg, magnesium 100 mg, potassium 7.7 mg, zinc 24 mg, Cl 7 mg, chromium 15 mcg, selenium 15 mcg, choline bitartrate 1000 mcg, inositol 1000 mcg, PABA 1000 mcg, rutin 1000 mcg, yeast 12 mg. Bot. 50s, 100s, 365s. *otc.*
Use: Mineral, vitamin supplement.

Super-B. (Towne) Vitamins B_1 50 mg, B_2 20 mg, B_6 5 mg, B_{12} 15 mcg, C 300 mg, liver dessic. 100 mg, dried yeast 100 mg, niacinamide 25 mg, Ca pantothenate 5 mg, iron 10 mg/Captab. Bot. 50s, 100s, 150s, 250s. *otc.*
Use: Mineral, vitamin supplement.

Super Calicaps M-Z. (Nion) Calcium 1200 mg, magnesium 400 mg, zinc 15 mg, Vitamins A 5000 IU, Vitamins D 400 IU, selenium 15 mcg/3 Tabs. Bot. 90s. *otc.*
Use: Mineral, vitamin supplement.

Super Calcium 1200. (Schiff) Calcium carbonate 1512 mg (600 mg calcium)/ Cap. Bot. 60s, 120s. *otc.*

Use: Mineral supplement.

Super Citro Cee. (Marlyn) Lemon bioflavonoids 500 mg, rutin 50 mg, ascorbic acid 500 mg, rosehips powder. 500 mg. Tab. Bot. 50s, 100s, 200s. *otc.*
Use: Vitamin supplement.

Super Complex C-500. (Health for Life Brands) Citrus hesperidin complex 25 mg, citrus bioflavonoid complex 100 mg, rutin 50 mg, ascorbic acid 500 mg, rose hips 100 mg, acerola, green pepper & black currant concentrate, sodium free. Tab. Bot. 100s. *otc.*
Use: Vitamin supplement.

Super D. (Pharmacia & Upjohn) Vitamins A 10,000 IU, D 400 IU/Perle. Bot. 100s. *otc.*
Use: Vitamin supplement.

Superdophilus. (Natren) *Lactobacillus acidophilus* strain DDS-1.2 billion/g Pow. 37.5 g, 75 g, 135 g. *otc.*
Use: Antidiarrheal, nutritional supplement.

Super D Perles. (Pharmacia & Upjohn) Vitamins A 10,000 IU, D 400 IU/Cap. Bot. 100s. *otc.*
Use: Vitamins A and D.

SuperEPA. (Advanced Nutritional Technology) Omega-3 polyunsaturated fatty acids 1200 mg/Cap. containing EPA 360 mg, DHA 240 mg. Bot. 60s, 90s. *otc.*
Use: Nutritional supplement.

Superepa 2000. (Advanced Nutritional Technology) EPA 563 mg, DHA 312 mg, vitamin E 20 IU. Cap. Bot. 30s, 60s, 90s. *otc.*
Use: Nutritional supplement.

Supere-Pect. (Barth's) Alpha tocopherol 400 IU, apple pectin 100 mg/Cap. Bot. 50s, 100s, 250s. *otc.*
Use: Nutritional supplement.

Super Hi Potency. (Nion) Vitamins A 10,000 IU, D 400 IU, E 150 IU, B_1 75 mg, B_2 75 mg, B_3 75 mg, B_5 75 mg, B_6 75 mg, B_{12} 75 mcg, C 250 mg, folic acid 0.4 mg, Zn 15 mg, betaine, biotin 75 mcg, Ca, Fe, hesperidin, I, K, Mg, Mn, Se/Tab. Bot. 100s. *otc.*
Use: Mineral, vitamin supplement.

Super Hydramin Protein Powder. (Nion) Protein 41%, carbohydrate 21.8%, fat 1% in powder form. Cans 1 lb. *otc.*
Use: Nutritional supplement.

superinone. Tyloxapol.
See: Triton Consumer Products WR-1339 (Rohm and Haas).

Super Nutri-Vites. (Faraday) Vitamins A 36,000 IU, D 400 IU, B_1 25 mg, B_2 25 mg, B_6 50 mg, B_{12} 50 mcg, niacinamide 50 mg, Ca pantothenate 12.5 mg, choline bitartrate 150 mg, inositol 150 mg, betaine HCl 25 mg, PABA 15 mg, glutamic acid 25 mg, dessic. liver 50 mg, C 150 mg, E 12.5 IU, Mn gluconate 6.15 mg, bone meal 162 mg, Fe gluconate 50 mg, Cu gluconate 0.25 mg, Zn gluconate 2.2 mg, K iodide 0.1 mg, Ca 53.3 mg, P 24.3 mg, Mg gluconate 7.2 mg/Protein Coated Tab. Bot. 60s, 100s. *otc.*
Use: Mineral, vitamin supplement.

superoxide dismutase (human, recombinant human).
Use: Protection of donor organ tissue. [Orphan drug]

Super Plenamins Multiple Vitamins and Minerals. (Rexall) Vitamins A 8000 IU, D_2 400 IU, Vitamins B_1 2.5 mg, B_2 2.5 mg, C 75 mg, niacinamide 20 mg, B_6 1 mg, B_{12} 3 mcg, biotin 20 mcg, E 10 IU, pantothenic acid 3 mg, liver conc. 100 mg, iron 30 mg, calcium 75 mg, phosphorus 58 mg, iodine 0.15 mg, copper 0.75 mg, manganese 1.25 mg, magnesium 10 mg, zinc 1 mg/Tab. Bot. 36s, 72s, 144s, 288s, 365s. *otc.*
Use: Mineral, vitamin supplement.

Superplex T. (Major) Vitamins B_1 15 mg, B_2 10 mg, B_3 100 mg, B_5 20 mg, B_6 5 mg, B_{12} 10 mcg, C 500 mg/Tab. Bot. 100s. *otc.*
Use: Vitamin supplement.

Super Poli-Grip/Wernet's Cream. (Block Drug) Carboxymethylcellulose gum, ethylene oxide polymer, petrolatum-mineral oil base. Tube 0.7, 1.4, 2.4 oz. *otc.*
Use: Denture adhesive.

Super Quints-50. (Freeda Vitamins) Vitamins B_1 50 mg, B_2 50 mg, B_3 50 mg, B_5 50 mg, B_6 50 mg, B_{12} 50 mcg, folic acid 0.4 mg, PABA 30 mg, d-biotin 50 mcg, inositol 50 mg. Tab. Bot. 100s, 250s, 500s. *otc.*
Use: Vitamin supplement.

Super Shade SPF-25. (Schering Plough) Ethylhexyl p-methoxycinnamate, padimate O oxybenzone, SPF-25. Bot. 4 fl. oz. *otc.*
Use: Sunscreen.

Super Shade Sunblock Stick SPF-25. (Schering Plough) Ethylhexyl p-methoxycinnamate, oxybenzone, padimate O in stick, SPF-25. Tube 0.43 oz. *otc.*
Use: Sunscreen.

Super Stress. (Towne) Vitamins C 600 mg, E 30 IU B_1 15 mg, B_2 15 mg, niacin 100 mg, B_6 5 mg, B_{12} 12 mcg,

pantothenic acid 20 mg/Tab. Bot. 60s. *otc.*
Use: Vitamin supplement.

Super Thera 46. (Faraday) Vitamin A 36,000 IU, essential vitamins, minerals, amino acids w/nutrient factors, digestive enzymes, B_{12} 25 mcg/Tab. Bot. 100s.

Super Troche. (Weeks & Leo) Benzocaine 5 mg, cetalkonium Cl 1 mg/lozenge. Bot. 15s, 30s. *otc.*
Use: Mouth and throat preparation.

Super Troche Plus. (Weeks & Leo) Benzocaine 10 mg, cetalkonium Cl. 2 mg/loz. Bot. 12s. *otc.*
Use: Mouth and throat preparation.

Super-T with Zinc. (Towne) Vitamins A 10,000 IU, D 400 IU, E 15 IU, C 200 mg, B_1 10 mg, B_2 10 mg, B_6 5 mg, B_{12} 6 mcg, niacinamide 50 mg, iron 18 mg, iodine 0.1 mg, copper 2 mg, manganese 1 mg, zinc 15 mg/Cap. Bot. 130s. *otc.*
Use: Mineral, vitamin supplement.

Supervim Tablets. (U.S. Ethicals) Vitamins and minerals. Bot. 100s.
Use: Mineral, vitamin supplement.

Super Wernet's Powder. (Block Drug) Carboxymethylcellulose gum, ethylene oxide polymer. Bot. 0.63, 1.75, 3.55 oz. *otc.*
Use: Denture adhesive.

Suplena. (Ross Laboratories) A vanilla flavored liquid containing 29.6 g protein, 252.5 g carbohydrates, 95 g fat per liter. With appropriate vitamins and minerals. Cans 240 ml. *otc.*
Use: Nutritional supplement.

Suplical. (Parke-Davis) Calcium 600 mg/Square. Bot. 30s, 60s. *otc.*
Use: Mineral supplement.

Suppap-120. (Raway) Acetaminophen 120 mg/Supp. 12s, 50s, 100s, 500s, 1000s. *otc.*
Use: Analgesic.

Suppap-650. (Raway) Acetaminophen 650 mg/Supp. 50s, 100s, 500s, 1000s. *otc.*
Use: Analgesic.

Supprelin. (Roberts Pharm) Histrelin acetate 200 mcg, 300 mcg or 600 mcg/ml. Vials 0.6 ml. *Rx.*
Use: Hormone.

Suppress. (Ferndale Laboratories) Dextromethorphan HBr 7.5 mg/loz. 1000s. *otc.*
Use: Antitussive.

Supra Min. (Towne) Vitamins A 10,000 IU, D 400 IU, E 30 IU, C 250 mg, folic acid 0.4 mg, B_1 10 mg, B_2 10 mg, niacin 100 mg, B_6 5 mg, B_{12} 6 mcg, pantothenic acid 20 mg, iodine 150 mcg, iron 100 mg, magnesium 2 mg, copper 20 mg, manganese 1.25 mg/Tab. Bot. 130s. *otc.*
Use: Mineral, vitamin supplement.

Suprane. (Ohmeda Pharmaceuticals) Desflurane. 240 ml. Bot. *Rx.*
Use: Anesthetic, general.

Suprarenal. Dried, partially defatted and powdered adrenal gland of cattle, sheep or swine.

Suprax. (ESI Lederle Generics) Cefixime **Tab.:** 200 mg, Bot. 100s or 400 mg, 50s, 100s UD 10s, unit-of-use 10s. **Pow. for Oral Susp.:** (strawberry flavor) 100 mg/5 ml. Bot. 50 ml, 75 ml, 100 ml. *Rx.*
Use: Anti-infective, cephalosporin.

Suprazine Tabs. (Major) Trifluoperazine 1 mg/Tab. Bot. 100s, 250s, 1000s; 2 mg/Tab. Bot. 100s, 250s, 1000s, UD 100s; 5 mg/Tab. Bot. 100s, 250s, 1000s; 10 mg/Tab. Bot. 100s, 250s, 1000s. *Rx.*
Use: Anxiolytic.

Suprins. (Towne) Vitamins A palmitate 10,000 IU, D 400 IU, B_1 10 mg, B_2 10 mg, B_6 5 mg, B_{12} 6 mcg, C 250 mg, calcium pantothenate 20 mg, niacinamide 100 mg, biotin 25 mcg, vitamins E 15 IU, calcium 103 mg, phosphorus 80 mg, iron 10 mg, iodine 0.1 mg, copper 1.0 mg, zinc 20 mg, manganese 1.25 mg/Captab. Bot. 100s. *otc.*
Use: Mineral, vitamin supplement.

•**suproclone.** (SUH-pro-klone) USAN.
Use: Sedative, hypnotic.

•**suprofen.** (sue-PRO-fen) U.S.P. 23.
Use: Anti-inflammatory.
See: Profenal (Alcon Laboratories).

•**suramin hexasodium.** (SOOR-ah-min hex-ah-SO-dee-uhm) USAN. U.S.P. XVII.
Use: Antineoplastic.

Suramin Sodium.

Surbex Filmtab. (Abbott Laboratories) B_1 6 mg, B_2 6 mg, B_3 30 mg, B_6 2.5 mg, B_5 10 mg, B_{12} 5 mcg/Filmtab. Bot. 100s. *otc.*
Use: Mineral, vitamin supplement.

W/Vitamins C. (Abbott Laboratories) Same as Surbex Filmtab, except vitamins C 250 mg/Filmtab. Bot. 100s, 500s.

Surbex-T Filmtab. (Abbott Laboratories) Vitamins B_1 15 mg, B_2 10 mg, B_3 100 mg, B_6 5 mg, B_{12} 10 mcg, B_5 20 mg, C

500 mg/Filmtab. Bot. 100s. *otc.*
Use: Mineral, vitamin supplement.

Surbex with C Filmtabs. (Abbott Laboratories) Vitamins B_1 6 mg, B_2 6 mg, B_3 30 mg, B_5 10 mg, B_6 2.5 mg, B_{12} 5 mg, C 500 mg/Film coated. Tab. Bot. 100s. *otc.*
Use: Vitamin supplement.

Surbex 750 with Iron. (Abbott Laboratories) Vitamins B_1 15 mg, B_2 15 mg, B_6 25 mg, B_{12} 12 mcg, C 750 mg, B_5 20 mg, E 30 IU, B_3 100 mg, iron 27 mg, folic acid 0.4 mg/Tab. Bot. 50s. *otc.*
Use: Mineral, vitamin supplement.

Surbex 750 with Zinc. (Abbott Laboratories) B_1 15 mg, B_2 15 mg, B_6 20 mg, B_{12} 12 mcg, C 750 mg, E 30 IU, B_5 20 mg, niacin 100 mg, folic acid 0.4 mg, zinc 22.5 mg/Tab. Bot. 50s. *otc.*
Use: Mineral, vitamin supplement.

Surbu-Gen-T. (Zenith Goldline) Vitamins B_1 15 mg, B_2 10 mg, B_3 100 mg, B_5 20 mg, B_6 5 mg, B_{12} 10 mcg, C 500 mg/ Tab. Bot. 100s. *otc.*
Use: Vitamin supplement.

SureCell HCG-Urine Test. (Kodak) Polyclonal/monoclonal antibody sandwich-based ELISA to detect human chorionic gonadotropin in urine. Kit 10s, 25s, 100s.
Use: Diagnostic aid.

SureCell Herpes (HSV) Test. (Kodak) Monoclonal antibody-based ELISA to detect HSV 1 & 2 antigens from lesions. Kit 10s, 25s.
Use: Diagnostic aid.

SureCell Strep A Test. (Kodak) ELISA to detect Group A streptococci. Kit 10s, 25s, 100s.
Use: Diagnostic aid.

SureLac. (Caraco) 3000 FCC lactase units, sorbitol or mannitol. Chew. Tab. Bot. 60s. *otc.*
Use: Nutritional supplement.

surface active extract of saline lavage of bovine lungs.
Use: Respiratory failure in preterm infants. [Orphan drug]

surfactant, natural lung.
Use: Surfactant replacement therapy in neonatal respiratory distress syndrome.
See: Survanta (Ross Laboratories).

surfactant, synthetic lung.
Use: Surfactant replacement therapy in neonatal respiratory distress syndrome.
See: Exosurf Neonatal (Glaxo-Wellcome).

Surfak. (Pharmacia & Upjohn) Docusate calcium. 50 mg: 30s, 100s. 240 mg: 30s, 100s, 500s, UD 100s. Cap. *otc.*
Use: Laxative.

•**surfilcon a.** (SER-FILL-kahn A) USAN.
Use: Hydrophilic contact lens material.

Surfol Post-Immersion Bath Oil. (Stiefel) Mineral oil, isopropyl myristate, isostearic acid, PEG-40, sorbitan peroleate. Bot. 8 oz. *otc.*
Use: Dermatologic.

•**surfomer.** (SER-foe-mer) USAN.
Use: Hypolipidemic.

Surgasoap. (Wade) Castile vegetable oils. Bot. qt., gal. *otc.*
Use: Dermatologic, cleanser.

Surgel. (Ulmer) Propylene glycol, glycerin. Gel. 120 ml, 240 ml, gal. *otc.*
Use: Lubricant.

Surgel Liquid. (Ulmer) Patient lubricant fluid. Bot. 4 oz, 8 oz, gal.
Use: Lubricant.

•**surgibone.** (SER-jih-bone) USAN. Bone and cartilage obtained from bovine embryos and young calves.
Use: Prosthetic aid (internal bone splint).
See: Unilab Surgibone (Unilab).

Surgical Simplex P. (Howmedica) Methyl methacrylate 20 ml poly 6.7 g, methyl methacrylate-styrene copolymer 33.3 g. **Pow.** 40 g. **Liq.** 20 ml.
Use: Bone cement.

Surgical Simplex P Radiopaque. (Howmedica) Methyl methacrylate 20 ml, poly 6 g, methyl methacrylate-styrene copolymer 30 g. **Pow.** 40 g. **Liq.** 20 ml.
Use: Bone cement.

Surgicel. (Johnson & Johnson Consumer Products) Sterile absorbable knitted fabric prepared by controlled oxidation of regenerated cellulose. Sterile strips 2"×14", 4"×8", 2"×3", 0.5"×2". Surgical Nu-knit: 1"×1", 3"×4", 6"×9". 1s.
Use: Hemostatic.

Surgidine. (Continental Consumer Products) Iodine 0.8% in iodine complex. Germicide. Bot. 8 oz, gal. Foot operated dispenser 8 oz, gal. *otc.*
Use: Antiseptic.

Surgi-Kleen. (Sween) Bot. 2 oz, 8 oz, 16 oz, 21 oz, gal., 5 gal., 30 gal., 55 gal.
Use: Dermatologic, cleanser.

Surgilube. (Day-Baldwin) Sterile-bacteriostatic. Foilpac: 3 g, 5 g, Tube: 5 g, 2 oz, 4.5 oz.
Use: Lubricant.

Surgilube. (E. Fougera) Sterile surgical lubricant. Foilpac: 3 g, 5 g; Tube 5 g, 2 oz, 4.25 oz.
Use: Lubricant.

•**suricainide maleate.** (ser-ih-CANE-ide) USAN.
Use: Cardiovascular agent (antiarrhythmic).

•**suritozole.** (suh-RIH-tah-ZOLE) USAN.
Use: Antidepressant.

Surmontil. (Wyeth Ayerst) Trimipramine maleate 25 mg, 50 mg or 100 mg/Cap. Bot. 100s. Redipaks. *Rx.*
Use: Antidepressant.

surofene. Hexachlorophene.

•**suronacrine maleate.** (SUE-row-NAH-kreen) USAN.
Use: Cholinergic, cholinesterase inhibitor.

Survanta. (Ross Laboratories) Beractant 25 mg/ml. Inj. Vial 8 ml. *Rx.*
Use: Lung surfactant.

Susano Elixir. (Halsey) Phenobarbital 0.25 gr, hyoscyamine sulfate 0.1037 mg, atropine sulfate 0.0194 mg, scopolamine HBr 0.0065 mg/5 ml. 23% alcohol, tartrazine. Bot. 16 oz, gal. *Rx.*
Use: Antispasmodic, sedative.

Suspen. (Circle) Penicillin V potassium 250 mg/5 ml. Bot. 100 ml. *Rx.*
Use: Anti-infective, penicillin.

Sus-Phrine Injection. (Forest Pharmaceutical) Epinephrine 1:200 Amp. 0.3 ml, 12s, 25s. Multiple Dose Vial 5 ml, 1s. *Rx.*
Use: Bronchial asthma.

sus scrofa linne var domesticus. W/Proteolytic enzyme, autolyzed.

Sustacal Basic. (Bristol-Myers) A vanilla, strawberry or chocolate flavored liquid containing 36.6 g protein, 34.6 g fat, 145.8 g carbohydrate, 833 mg Na, 1583 mg K/L. 1.04 Cal/ml, with appropriate vitamin and mineral levels to meet 100% of the US RDAs. Liq. Can 240 ml. *otc.*
Use: Nutritional supplement.

Sustacal HC. (Bristol-Myers) High calorie nutritionally complete food. Protein 16%, fat 34%, carbohydrate 50%. Cans 8 oz. Vanilla, chocolate or eggnog. *otc.*
Use: Nutritional supplement.

Sustacal Plus. (Bristol-Myers) A vanilla, eggnog or chocolate flavored liquid containing 61 g protein, 58 g fat, 190 g carbohydrate, 15.2 mg Fe, 850 mg Na, 1480 mg K, 1520 cal/L, with appropriate vitamin and mineral levels to meet 100% of the US RDAs. Liq. Bot. 237 ml, 960 ml. *otc.*
Use: Nutritional supplement.

Sustacal Powder. (Bristol-Myers) Caloric distribution and nutritional value when added to milk are similar to that of Sustacal liquid except lactose. Contains vanilla: Pow. 1.9 oz. packets 4's, 1 lb. can; Chocolate 1.9 oz. packets 4s. *otc.*
Use: Nutritional supplement.

Sustacal Pudding. (Bristol-Myers) Ready-to-eat fortified pudding containing at least 15% of the US RDAs for protein, vitamins and minerals, in a 240 calorie serving. As a % of the calories, protein 11%, fat 36%, carbohydrate 53%. Flavors: chocolate, vanilla, and butterscotch. Tins, 5 oz, 110 oz. *otc.*
Use: Nutritional supplement.

Sustagen. (Bristol-Myers) High-calorie, high-protein supplement containing as a % of the calories, 24% protein, 8% fat, 68% carbohydrate. Contains all known essential vitamins and minerals. Prepared from nonfat milk, corn syrup solids, powdered whole milk, calcium caseinate, and dextrose. Vanilla: Can 1 lb, 5 lb. Chocolate: Can 1 lb. *otc.*
Use: Nutritional supplement.

Sustaire. (Pfizer) Theophylline 100 mg, 300 mg/Sust. Released Tab. Bot. 100s. *Rx.*
Use: Bronchospasm therapy.

•**suture, absorbable surgical.** U.S.P. 23.
Use: Surgical aid.

•**suture, nonabsorbable surgical.** U.S.P. 23.
Use: Surgical aid.

Suvaplex Tablet. (Tennessee Pharmaceutic) Vitamins A 5000 IU, D 500 IU, B_1 2.5 mg, B_2 2.5 mg, B_6 0.5 mg, B_{12} 1 mcg, C 37.5 mg, Ca pantothenate 5 mg, niacinamide 20 mg, folic acid 0.1 mg/Tab. Bot. 100s. *otc.*
Use: Mineral, vitamin supplement.

•**suxemerid sulfate.** (sux-EM-er-rid) USAN.
Use: Antitussive.

swamp root. Compound of various organic roots in an alcohol base.
Use: Diuretic to the kidney.

Sween-A-Peel. (Sween) Wafer 4×4. Box 5s, 20s; Sheets 1212. Box 2s, 12s.
Use: Dermatologic, protectant.

Sween Cream. (Sween) Vitamin A and D cream. Tube 0.5 oz, 2 oz, 5 oz. Jar 2 oz, 9 oz. *otc.*
Use: Dermatologic.

Sween Kind Lotion. (Sween) Bot. 21 oz, gal.

Use: Dermatologic, cleanser.

Sween Prep. (Sween) Box wipes 54s. Dab-o-matic 2 oz. Spray top 4 oz.
Use: Dermatologic, protectant, medicated.

Sween Soft Touch. (Sween) Bot. 2 oz, 16 oz, 21 oz, 32 oz, 1 gal., 5 gal.
Use: Dermatologic-protectant, medicated.

Sweeta. (Squibb Diagnostic) Saccharin sodium and sorbitol. Bot. 24 ml, 2 oz, 4 oz. *otc.*
Use: Sweetening Agent.

Sweetaste. (Purepac) Saccharin 0.25 g, 0.5 g, 1 g/Tab. w/Sodium bicarbonate. Bot. 1000s. *otc.*
Use: Sugar substitute.

sweetening agents.
See: Ril-Sweet (Schering Plough).
Saccharin, Preps. (Various Mfr.).
Sucaryl, Preps. (Abbott Laboratories).
Sweetaste, Tab. (Purepac).

Sweet'n Fresh Clotrimazole-7. (Nutra-Max Products) **Cream:** Clotrimazole 1%, benzyl and cetostearyl alcohol. 45 g. **Vaginal inserts:** Clotrimazole 100 mg. 7s. *otc.*
Use: Antifungal-vaginal.

Swim-Ear. (E. Fougera) 2.75% boric acid in isopropyl alcohol. Bot. 1 oz. *otc.*
Use: Otic.

Swiss Kriss. (Modern) Senna leaves, herbs. Coarse cut mixture. Can 1.5 oz, 3.25 oz, Tab. 24s, 120s, 250s. *otc.*
Use: Laxative.

Syllact. (Wallace Laboratories) Psyllium seed husks 3.3 g/tsp., saccharin. Pow. Bot. 11 oz. *otc.*
Use: Laxative.

Syllamalt. (Wallace Laboratories) Malt soup extract 4 g, psyllium seed husks 3 g, calories/rounded tsp 13. Pow. 300 g. *otc.*
Use: Laxative.

•**symclosene.** (SIM-kloe-seen) USAN.
Use: Anti-infective, topical.

•**symetine hydrochloride.** (SIM-eh-teen) USAN.
Use: Antiamebic.

Symmetrel. (DuPont Merck Pharmaceuticals) Amantadine HCl. 50 mg/5 ml. Syr. Bot. pt. *Rx.*
Use: Antiviral, antiparkinsonian, treatment of drug-induced extrapyramidal symptoms.

sympatholytic agents.
See: Adrenergic-Blocking Agents.
D.H.E. 45, Amp. (Novartis).
Dibenzyline, Cap. (SmithKline Beecham Pharmaceuticals).
Dihydroergotamine.
Ergotamine Tartrate.
Gynergen, Amp., Tab. (Novartis).

sympathomimetic agents.
See: Adrenalin (Parke-Davis).
Adrenergic agents.
Aerolate Sr. & Jr., Cap. (Fleming).
Aerolone Cpd. (Eli Lilly).
Afrin, Preps. (Schering Plough).
Miles Diagnostic, Enseal, Pulvule (Eli Lilly).
Aramine, Amp., Vial (Merck).
Arlidin HCl, Tab. (Rhone-Poulenc Rorer).
Brethine, Amp., Tab (Novartis Pharmaceuticals).
Bronkephrine, Amp., (Sanofi Winthrop).
Bronkometer (Sanofi Winthrop).
Bronkosol Soln. (Sanofi Winthrop).
Delcobese, Tab. (Delco).
Demazin, Tab., Syr. (Schering Plough).
Desoxyn, Gradumet, Tab. (Abbott Laboratories).
Dexamyl Tab. (SmithKline Beecham Pharmaceuticals).
Dexedrine, Elix., Spansule, Tab. (SmithKline Beecham Pharmaceuticals).
D-Feda, Cap., Liq. (Dooner).
Didrex, Liq., Tab. (Pharmacia & Upjohn).
Dipivefrin HCl, Soln. (Schein Pharmaceutical).
Duovent, Tab. (3M).
Ectasule Minus Sr. & Jr., Cap. (Fleming).
Ectasule III, Cap. (Fleming).
Ephedrine preps.
Epinephrine salts.
Extendryl, Cap., Syr., Tab. (Fleming).
Fedrazil, Tab. (GlaxoWellcome).
Fiogesic, Tab. (Novartis).
Histabid, Cap. (GlaxoWellcome).
Isoephedrine HCl.
Isuprel HCl, Preps. (Sanofi Winthrop).
Levophed Bitartrate, Amp. (Sanofi Winthrop).
Metaproterenol Sulfate (Various Mfr.).
Napril, Cap. (Hoechst Marion Roussel).
Neo-Synephrine HCl, Preps. (Sanofi Winthrop).
Nolamine, Tab. (Carnrick Labs).
Norisodrine Sulfate, Soln. (Abbott Laboratories).
Obedrin-LA, Tab. (SmithKline Beecham Pharmaceuticals).
Obetrol, Tab. (Obetrol).

Orthoxine, Orthoxine & Aminophylline (Pharmacia & Upjohn).
Orthoxine HCl, Tab., Syr. (Pharmacia & Upjohn).
Otrivin, Soln., Spray (Novartis Pharmaceuticals).
Phenylephrine HCl, Preps.
Phenylpropanolamine HCl.
Pseudoephedrine HCl, Syr., Tab.
Rondec DSC & T (Ross Laboratories).
Slo-Fedrin & Slo-Fedrin A (Dooner).
Sudafed, Tab., Syr. (GlaxoWellcome).
Triaminic, Prep. (Novartis).
Triaminicol, Syr. (Novartis).
Tussagesic, Susp., Tab. (Novartis).
Tussaminic, Tab. (Novartis).
Ursinus, Tab. (Novartis).
Vasoxyl HCl, Amp., Vial (Glaxo-Wellcome).
Wyamine Sulfate, Amp., Vial (Wyeth Ayerst).

Syna-Clear. (Pruvo) Decongestant plus Vitamins C. 25 mg/Tab. Bot. 12s, 30s.
Use: Decongestant.

Synacol CF. (Roberts Pharm) Dextromethorphan HBr 15 mg, guiafenesin 200 mg/Tab. Bot. UD 8s, 500s. *otc.*
Use: Antitussive, expectorant.

Synacort. (Syntex) Hydrocortisone cream. **1%:** Tube 15 g, 30 g, 60 g. **2.5%:** Tube 30 g. *Rx.*
Use: Corticosteroid, topical.

Synalar. (Syntex) Fluocinolone acetonide. **Cream: 0.01%** Tube 15 g, 30 g, 45 g, 60 g, 120 g. Jar 425 g. **0.025%** Tube 15 g, 30 g, 60 g, 120 g. Jar 425 g. **Oint.: 0.025%:** Tube 15 g, 30 g, 60 g, 120 g. Jar 425 g. **Soln. 0.01%:** Bot. 20 ml, 60 ml. *Rx.*
Use: Corticosteroid, topical.

Synalar-HP Cream. (Syntex) Fluocinolone acetonide 0.2% in water-washable aqueous base. Tube 12 g. *Rx.*
Use: Corticosteroid, topical.

Synalgos-DC Capsules. (Wyeth Ayerst) Dihydrocodeine bitartrate 16 mg, aspirin 356.4 mg, caffeine 30 mg/Cap. Bot. 100s, 500s. *c-III.*
Use: Analgesic combination, narcotic.

Synapp-R. (Halsey) Acetaminophen 325 mg, phenylpropanolamine HCl 25 mg, phenyltoloxamine citrate 22 mg/Tab. Bot. 40s. *otc.*
Use: Analgesic, decongestant.

Synarel. (Syntex) Nafarelin acetate 2 mg/ml (as nafarelin base). Nasal solution. Bottle 10 ml with metered pump spray. *Rx.*
Use: Endometriosis.

Synatuss-One. (Freeport) Guaifenesin 100 mg, dextromethorphan HBr. 15 mg, alcohol 1.4%/5 ml. Bot. 4 oz. *otc.*
Use: Antitussive.

Syncaine.
See: Procaine Hydrochloride, Inj., Tab. (Various Mfr.).

Syncort.
See: Desoxycorticosterone Acetate, Inj., Pellets (Various Mfr.).

Syncortyl.
See: Desoxycorticosterone Acetate, Inj., Pellets (Various Mfr.).

Syndolor Capsules. (Knight) Bot. 100s, 1000s.
Use: Analgesic.

Synemol. (Syntex) Fluocinolone acetonide 0.025% in water-washable aqueous emollient base. Tube 15 g, 30 g, 60 g, 120 g. *Rx.*
Use: Corticosteroid-topical.

synkonin.
See: Hydrocodone (Various Mfr.).

Synophylate. (Schwarz Pharma) Theophylline sodium glycinate. **Elix.:** Theophylline 165 mg/15 ml w/alcohol 20%. Bot. pt, gal. **Tab.:** Theophylline 165 mg/Tab. Bot. 100s, 1000s. *Rx.*
Use: Bronchodilator.

Synophylate-GG. (Schwarz Pharma) Theophylline sodium glycinate 300 mg, guaifenesin 100 mg. **Syr.** 10% alcohol, pt, gal. *Rx.*
Use: Bronchodilator.

Syn-Rx. (Adams Labs) **AM:** Pseudoephedrine HCl 60 mg, guiafenesin 600 mg/CR Tab. Bot. 28s. **PM:** Guaifenesin 600 mg/CR Tab. Bot. 28s. In 14-day treatment regimen of 56 tablets. *Rx.*
Use: Decongestant, expectorant.

Synsorb Pk.
Use: Verocytotoxogenic *E. coli* infections. [Orphan drug]

Synthaloids. (Buffington) Benzocaine, calcium-iodine complex/lozenge. Salt free. Bot. 100s, 1000s. Unit boxes 8s, 16s. Box 24s. Dispens-A-Kit 500s. Aidpaks 100s. Medipaks 200s. *otc.*
Use: Sore throat relief.

synthetic lung surfactant.
See: Exosurf Neonatal (Glaxo-Wellcome).

synthoestrin.
See: Diethylstilbestrol, Preps. (Various Mfr.).

Synthroid. (Knoll Pharmaceuticals) Sodium levothyroxine 25 mcg, 50 mcg, 75 mcg, 88 mcg, 100 mcg, 112 mcg, 125 mcg, 137 mcg, 150 mcg, 200 mcg,

300 mcg/Tab. Bot. 100s (all), 1000s (except 88 mcg, 200 mcg), UD 100s (except 25 mcg, 88 mcg, 200 mcg). *Rx.*
Use: Hormone, thyroid.

Synthroid Injection. (Knoll Pharmaceuticals) Lyophilized sodium levothyroxine 200 mcg or 500 mcg/vial. (100 mcg/ml when reconstituted.) Vial 10 ml. *Rx.*
Use: Hormone, thyroid.

Synvisc. (Wyeth-Ayerst) Sodium hyaluronate/hylan G-F 20 16 mg/2 ml. Glass syringe 2.25 ml. *Rx.*
Use: Antiarthritic.

Syphilis (FTA-ABS) Fluoro Kit. (Clinical Sciences).
Use: Test for syphilis.

Syprinc. (Merck) Trientine HCl 250 mg/Cap. Bot. 100s. *Rx.*
Use: Chelating agent.

Syracol. (Roberts Pharm) Phenylpropanolamine HCl 12.5 mg, dextromethorphan 7.5 mg Liq. 60 and 120 ml. *otc.*
Use: Antitussive, decongestant.

Syracol CF. (Roberts Pharm) Dextromethorphan HBr 15 mg, guaifenesin 200 mg/Tab. Bot. 500s. *otc.*
Use: Antitussive, expectorant.

Syroxine Tabs. (Major) Sodium levothyroxine 0.1 mg, 0.2 mg, or 0.3 mg/Tab. Bot. 100s, 250s, 1000s, UD 100s. (3 mg 1000s.). *Rx.*
Use: Hormone, thyroid.

Syrpalta. (Emerson) Syr. containing comb. of fruit flavors. Bot. 1 pt, 1 gal.
Use: Pharmaceutical aid.

•**syrup.** N.F. 18.
Use: Pharmaceutic aid (flavor).

Syrvite. (Various Mfr.) Vitamins A 2500 IU, D 400 IU, E 15 mg, B_1 1.05 mg, B_2 1.2 mg, B_3 13.5 mg, B_6 1.05 mg, B_{12} 4.5 mcg, C 60 mg/5 ml Liq. Bot. 480 ml. *otc.*
Use: Vitamin supplement.

T

T-3 RIAbead. (Abbott Diagnostics) Test kit 50s, 100s.
Use: Diagnostic aid, thyroid.

T4.
See: levothyroxine sodium.

T4 endonuclease v, liposome encapsulated.
Use: Xeroderma pigmentosum. [Orphan drug]

T-4 RIA (PEG). (Abbott Diagnostics) Diagnostic kit 50s, 100s, 500s.
Use: For quantitative measurement of total circulating serum thyroxine.

T4, soluble, human recombinant. (Biogen) Phase I/II HIV.
Use: Antiviral.

TA. (Wampole Laboratories) Antithyroid antibodies by IFA. Test 48s.
Use: Diagnostic aid, thyroid.

Tabasyn. (Freeport) Chlorpheniramine maleate 2 mg, phenylephrine HCl 10 mg, acetaminophen 5 gr, salicylamide 5 gr/Tab. Bot. 1000s. *Rx.*
Use: Analgesic, antihistamine, decongestant.

Tab-A-Vite. (Major) Vitamins A 5000 IU, D 400 IU, E 30 IU, B_1 1.5 mg, B_2 1.7 mg, B_3 20 mg, B_5 10 mg, B_6 2 mg, B_{12} 6 mcg, C 60 mg, FA 0.4 mg/Tab. Bot. 30s, 100s, 250s, 1000s, UD 100s. *otc.*
Use: Mineral, vitamin supplement.

Tab-A-Vite + Iron. (Major) Iron 18 mg, vitamins A 5000 IU, D 400 IU, E 30 IU, B_1 1.5 mg, B_2 1.7 mg, B_3 20 mg, B_5 10 mg, B_6 2 mg, B_{12} 6 mcg, C 60 mg, FA 0.4 mg, tartrazine/Tab. Bot. 100s. *otc.*
Use: Mineral, vitamin supplement.

Tac-3. (Allergan). Triamcinolone acetonide 3 mg/ml. Susp. Vial 5 ml. *Rx.*
Use: Corticosteroid.

Tac-40. (Parnell) Triamcinolone acetonide 40 mg/ml. Inj. Susp. Vial 5 ml. *Rx.*
Use: Corticosteroid.

Tacaryl Chewable Tab. (Westwood Squibb) Methdilazine 3.6 mg/Tab. Bot. 100s. *Rx.*
Use: Antipruritic.

tachysterol.
See: Dihydrotachysterol, Tab. (Roxane).

Tacitin. (Novartis) Under study. Benzoctamine, B.A.N.

•**taclamine hydrochloride.** (TACK-lah-meen) USAN.
Use: Anxiolytic.

TA Cream. (C & M Pharmacal) Triamcinolone acetonide 0.025% or 0.05%. Jar 2 oz., 8 oz., 1 lb. *Rx.*
Use: Corticosteroid, topical.

•**tacrine hydrochloride.** (TACK-reen) USAN.
Use: Cognition adjuvant.
See: Cognex, Cap. (Parke-Davis).

•**tacrolimus.** (tack-CROW-lih-muss) USAN.
Use: Immunosuppressant.
See: Prograf (Fujisawa).

Tagamet. (SmithKline Beecham Pharmaceuticals) Cimetidine **FC Tab.: 200 mg** Bot. 100s. **300 mg** Bot. 100s, UD 100s. **400 mg** Bot. 60s, UD 100s. **800 mg** Bot. 30s, UD 100s. **Liq.:** 300 mg (as HCl)/5 ml 2.8% alcohol. Bot. 240 ml, UD 5 ml (10s). **Inj.: 300 mg** (as HCl)/ 2 ml with phenol in an aqueous solution. Single-dose vials, disp. syringes, ADD-Vantage vials and 8 ml vials. **300 mg** (as HCl) in 50 ml 0.9% sodium chloride. Single-dose container. *Rx.*
Use: Antiulcerative.

Tagamet HB. (SmithKline Beecham Pharmaceuticals) Cimetidine 100 mg/ Tab. Bot. 16s, 32s, 64s. *otc.*
Use: Antiulcerative.

Talacen. (Sanofi) Pentazocine HCl 25 mg, acetaminophen 650 mg/Caplet. Bot. 100s. UD 250s. (10 × 25s). *c-IV.*
Use: Analgesic combination, narcotic.

•**talampicillin hydrochloride.** (TAL-AM-pih-sill-in) USAN.
Use: Anti-infective.

•**talc.** U.S.P. 23. A native hydrous magnesium silicate.
Use: Dusting powder, pharmaceutic aid (tablet/capsule lubricant).

•**taleranol.** (TAL-ehr-ah-nole) USAN.
Use: Enzyme inhibitor (gonadotropin).

•**talisomycin.** (tal-EYE-so-MY-sin) USAN.
Formerly Tallysomycin A.
Use: Antineoplastic.

•**talmetacin.** (TAL-MET-ah-sin) USAN.
Use: Analgesic, antipyretic, anti-inflammatory.

•**talniflumate.** (tal-NYE-FLEW-mate) USAN.
Use: Anti-inflammatory, analgesic.

Taloin. (Pharmacia & Upjohn) Methylbenzethonium chloride, zinc oxide, calamine, eucalyptol in a water-repellent base. Oint.: Tube 2 oz.
Use: Skin protectant & antiseptic.

•**talopram hydrochloride.** (TAY-low-pram) USAN.
Use: Potentiator (catecholamine).

•**talosalate.** (TAL-oh-SAL-ate) USAN.
Use: Analgesic, anti-inflammatory.

•**talsaclidine fumarate.** (tale-SACK-lih-deen) USAN.

Use: Alzheimer's disease treatment (muscarinic M_1-agonist).

Talwin Compound. (Sanofi) Pentazocine HCl 12.5 mg, aspirin 325 mg/Tab. Bot. 100s. *c-IV.*
Use: Analgesic, narcotic.

Talwin Injection. (Sanofi) Pentazocine lactate injection. 30 mg/ml. **Vials:** 10 ml. **Uni-Amps:** 1, 1.5, 2 ml. **Uni-Nest amps:** 1 ml, 2 ml. **Carpujects:** 1, 1.5, 2 ml. *c-IV.*
Use: Analgesic, narcotic.

Talwin NX. (Sanofi) Pentazocine HCl 50 mg, naloxone 0.5 mg/Tab. Bot. 100s. UD 250s. *c-IV.*
Use: Analgesic, narcotic.

Tambocor. (3M) Flecainide acetate 50 mg, 100 mg or 150 mg/Tab. Bot. 100s, UD 100s. *Rx.*
Use: Antiarrhythmic.

•**tametraline hydrochloride.** (tah-MET-rah-leen) USAN.
Use: Antidepressant.

Tamine S.R. (Geneva Pharm) Phenylpropanolamine HCl 15 mg, phenylephrine HCl 15 mg, brompheniramine maleate 12 mg. Sugar coated. Tab. Bot. 100s, 1000s. *Rx.*
Use: Antihistamine, decongestant.

tamoxifen. (Barr Laboratories) Tamoxifen citrate 10 mg. Tab. Bot. 60s, 250s. *Rx.*
Use: Antineoplastic, antiestrogen.

•**tamoxifen citrate.** (ta-MOX-ih-fen) U.S.P. 23.
Use: Treatment of mammary carcinoma, antiestrogen.
See: Nolvadex, Tab. (Zeneca).
Tamoxifen, Tab. (Barr Laboratories).

•**tampramine fumarate.** (TAM-prah-MEEN) USAN.
Use: Antidepressant.

Tamp-R-Tel. (Wyeth Ayerst) A tamper-resistant package for narcotic drugs which includes the following:
Codeine phosphate 30 mg, 60 mg/1 ml.
Hydromorphone HCl 1 mg, 2 mg, 3 mg, 4 mg/Tubex.
Meperidine HCl 25 mg/ml and **Promethazine HCl** 25 mg/ml 2 ml.
Meperidine HCl 25 mg/1 ml, 50 mg/1 ml, 75 mg/1 ml, 100 mg/1 ml.
Morphine Sulfate 2 mg, 4 mg, 8 mg, 10 mg, 15 mg/1 ml.
Pentobarbital, Sodium 100 mg/2 ml.
Phenobarbital, Sodium 30 mg, 60 mg, 130 mg/1 ml.
Secobarbital, Sodium 100 mg/2 ml.

•**tamsulosin hydrochloride.** USAN.
Use: Benign prostatic hyperplasia therapy.
See: Flomax, Cap. (Boehringer Ingelheim).

Tanac Gel. (Del Pharmaceuticals) Dyclonine HCl 1%, allantoin 0.5%, petrolatum, lanolin. Tube. 9.45 g. *otc.*
Use: Cold sores, fever blisters, moisturizer.

Tanac Liquid. (Del Pharmaceuticals) Benzalkonium Cl 0.12%, benzocaine 10%, tannic acid 6%. Saccharin. Bot. 13 ml. *otc.*
Use: Mouth and throat preparation.

Tanac Stick. (Del Pharmaceuticals) Benzocaine 7.5%, tannic acid 6%, octyl dimethyl PABA 0.75%, allantoin 0.2%, benzalkonium Cl. 7.5%. Saccharin. Stick 0.1 oz. *otc.*
Use: Cold sores, fever blisters, moisturizer.

Tanadex. (Del Pharmaceuticals) Tannic acid 2.86%, phenol 1.05%, benzocaine 0.47%. Bot. 3 oz. *otc.*
Use: Throat preparation.

Tan-a-Dyne. (Archer-Taylor) Tannic acid compound w/iodine. Bot. 4 oz., pt., gal. *otc.*
Use: Gargle.

Tanafed. (Horizon) Chlorpheniramine tannate 4.5 mg, pseudoephedrine tannate 75 mg/5 ml. Susp. Bot. 20 ml, 118 ml, 473 ml. *Rx.*
Use: Antihistamine, decongestant.

tanbismuth.
See: Bismuth Tannate.

•**tandamine hydrochloride.** (TAN-dah-meen) USAN.
Use: Antidepressant.

•**tandospirone citrate.** (tan-DOE-spy-rone) USAN.
Use: Anxiolytic.

•**tannic acid.** U.S.P. 23. Gallotannic acid. Glycerite. Tannin.
Use: Astringent.
See: Amertan, Oint. (Eli Lilly).
Zilactin Medicated, Gel (Zila Pharm).

W/Benzocaine, phenol, thymol iodide, ephedrine HCl, zinc oxide, peru balsam.
See: Hemocaine, Oint. (Roberts Pharm).

W/Bisacodyl.
See: Clysodrast, Packet (PBH Wesley Jessen).

W/Boric acid, salicylic acid, isopropyl alcohol.
See: Sal Dex Boro, Liq. (Scrip).

W/Cyanocobalamin, zinc acetate, glutathione, phenol.

See: Depinar, Amp. (Centeon).
W/Merthiolate.
See: Amertan, Oint. (Eli Lilly).
W/Salicylic acid, boric acid.
See: Tan-Bor-Sal, Liq. (Gordon Laboratories).

Tannic Spray. (Gebauer) Tannic acid 4.5%, chlorobutanol 1.3%, menthol < 1%, benzocaine < 1%, propylene glycol 33%, ethanol 60%. Bot. 2 oz. & 4 oz. *otc.*
Use: Relief of sunburn and other minor burns.

Tanoral. (Pharmed) Phenylephrine tannate 25 mg, chlorpheniramine tannate 8 mg, pyrilamine tannate 25 mg/Tab. Bot. 100s. *Rx.*
Use: Antihistamine, decongestant.

tanphetamin.
See: Dextroamphetamine tannate.

Tao. (Roerig) Troleandomycin equivalent to 250 mg oleandomycin/Cap. Bot. 100s. *Rx.*
Use: Anti-infective.

Tapar Tablets. (Warner Chilcott) Acetaminophen 325 mg/Tab. Bot. 100s. *otc.*
Use: Analgesic.

Tapazole. (Eli Lilly) Methimazole. 1-methyl-2-mercaptoimidazole. 5 mg or 10 mg/Tab. Bot. 100s. *Rx.*
Use: Hyperthyroidism.

•**tape, adhesive.** U.S.P. 23.
Use: Surgical aid.

Ta-Poff. (Ulmer) Adhesive tape remover. Bot. 1 pt. Aerosol. Can 6 oz.

Tapuline. (Wesley Pharmacal) Activated attapulgite 600 mg, pectin 60 mg, homatropine methylbromide 0.5 mg/Chew. Tab. Bot. 100s, 1000s. *otc.*
Use: Antidiarrheal.

tar.
See: Coal Tar, Preps.

Tar Distillate. (Doak Dermatologics) Decolorized fractional distillate of crude coal tar. Each ml equiv. to 1 g whole crude coal tar. Bot. 2 oz., 16 oz.
Use: Dermatologic.

Tarka. (Knoll Pharmaceuticals) Trandolapril maleate 2 mg, verapamil HCl 180 mg or trandolapril 1 mg, verapamil HCl 240 or trandolapril 2 mg, verapamil 240 mg or trandolapril 4 mg, verapamil 240 mg/Tab. Bot. 100s. *Rx.*
Use: Antihypertensive.

Tarnphilic. (Medco Lab) Coal tar 1%, polysorbate 0.5% in aquaphilic base. Jar 16 oz. *otc.*
Use: Dermatologic.

Tarpaste. (Doak Dermatologics) Coal tar distilled 5% in zinc paste. Tube 1 oz, Jar 4 oz, w/Hydrocortisone 0.5%. Tube 1 oz. *otc.*
Use: Dermatitis.

Tarsum Shampoo/Gel. (Summers) Coal tar 10%, salicylic acid 5% in shampoo base. Bot. 4 oz. *otc.*
Use: Antiseborrheic, dermatologic, hair and scalp.

tartar emetic.
See: Antimony Potassium Tartrate, U.S.P.

•**tartaric acid.** N.F. 18.
Use: Pharmaceutic aid (buffering agent).

Tashan. Skin Cream. (Block Drug) Vitamin A palmitate, D_2, D-panthenol, Vit. E. Tube 1 oz. *otc.*
Use: Emollient.

Tasmar. (Roche) Tolcapone 100 mg, 200 mg, lactose. Tab. Bot. 90s. *Rx.*
Use: Antiparkinson.

•**tasosartan.** (tass-OH-sahr-tan) USAN.
Use: Antihypertensive.

Taste Function Test, Accusens T. (Westport Pharmaceuticals) Tastant 60 ml. Kit. 15 Bot.
Use: Diagnostic aid.

taurocholic acid.
W/Pancreatin, pepsin.
See: Enzymet, Tabs. (Westerfield).

Ta-Verm. (Table Rock) Piperazine citrate 100 mg/ml Syr. Bot. 1 pt., 1 gal. Tabs. 500 mg Bot. 100s, 500s. *Rx.*
Use: Anthelmintic.

Tavilen Plus. (Table Rock) Liver solution 1 g, ferric pyrophosphate soluble 500 mg, vitamins B_1 6 mg, B_2 7.2 mg, B_6 3 mg, B_{12} 24 mcg, panthenol 3 mg, niacinamide 60 mg, l-lysine HCl 300 mg, 5% alcohol/ml. Bot. 16 oz., 1 gal. *otc.*
Use: Hematinic.

Tavist. (Novartis) Clemastine fumarate 2.68 mg/Tab. Bot. 100s. *Rx.*
Use: Antihistamine.

Tavist Syrup. (Novartis) Clemastine fumarate 0.67 mg/5 ml. Bot. 118 ml. *Rx.*
Use: Antihistamine.

Tavist-D. (Novartis) Clemastine fumarate 1.34 mg, phenylpropanolamine HCl 75 mg/SR Tab. Pkg. 8s, 16s. *otc.*
Use: Antihistamine, decongestant.

Taxol. (Bristol-Myers Squibb) Paclitaxel. 30 mg/5 ml. Inj. Vial 5 ml, 16.7 ml. *Rx.*
Use: Antineoplastic.

Taxotere. (Rhone-Poulenc Rorer) 20 mg/0.5 ml single-dose vial. 80 mg/2 ml single-dose vial. Inj. with diluent.
Use: Antineoplastic (breast cancer).

•**tazadolene succinate.** (TAZZ-ah-DOE-leen) USAN.
Use: Analgesic.

•**tazarotene.** (tazz-AHR-oh-teen) USAN.
Use: Keratolytic.
See: Tazorac, Gel (Allergan).

Tazicef Injection. (Abbott Laboratories) Ceftazidime. Vial: 1 g/20 ml, 2 g/60 ml or 6 g/100 ml. Piggyback: 1 g/100 ml or 2 g/100 ml. IM or IV Pharmacy Bulk: 6 g/100 ml. *Rx.*
Use: Anti-infective, cephalosporin.

Tazidime. (Eli Lilly) Ceftazidime dry powder. 1 g/20 ml Traypak 10s; 1 g/100 ml; 2 g/50 ml Traypack 10s; 2 g/100 ml Traypack 10s; 6 g/100 ml Traypak 6s. ADD-Vantage Vials 1 g or 2 g Traypak 10s. *Rx.*
Use: Anti-infective, cephalosporin.

•**tazifylline hydrochloride.** (TAY-zih-FIH-lin) USAN.
Use: Antihistamine.

•**tazobactam.** (TAZZ-oh-BACK-tam) USAN.
Use: Inhibitor (beta-lactamase).

•**tazobactam sodium.** (TAZZ-oh-BACK-tam) USAN.
Use: Inhibitor (beta-lactamase).

tazobactam sodium/piperacillin sodium.
See: piperacillin sodium, sterile w/tazobactam.

•**tazofelone.** (TAY-zah-feh-lone) USAN.
Use: Suppressant (inflammatory bowel disease).

•**tazolol hydrochloride.** (TAY-zoe-lole) USAN.
Use: Cardiotonic.

•**tazomeline citrate.** (tazz-OH-meh-leen SIH-trate) USAN.
Use: Alzheimer's disease treatment (cholinergic agonist).

Tazorac. (Allergan) Tazarotene 0.05%, 0.1%. Gel Tube 30 g, 100 g. *Rx.*
Use: Antiacne, antipsoriatic.

TBA-Pred. (Keene Pharmaceuticals) Prednisolone tebutate 10 mg/ml Susp. Vial 10 ml. *Rx.*
Use: Corticosteroid.

TC Suspension. (Rhone-Poulenc Rorer) Aluminum hydroxide 600 mg, magnesium hydroxide 300 mg/5 ml, sorbitol, sodium 0.8 mg Liq. In UD 15 ml, 30 ml (100s). *otc.*
Use: Antacid.

T/Derm Tar Emollient. (Neutrogena) Neutar solubilized coal tar extract 5% in oil base. Bot. 4 oz. *otc.*
Use: Antipsoriatic; antipruritic.

T-Dry. (Jones Medical Industries) Pseudoephedrine HCl 120 mg, chlorpheniramine maleate 12 mg/Cap. S.R. Bot. 100s. *Rx.*
Use: Antihistamine, decongestant.

T-Dry Jr. (Jones Medical Industries) Pseudoephedrine HCl 60 mg, chlorpheniramine maleate 4 mg/Cap. S.R. Bot. 100s. *otc.*
Use: Antihistamine, decongestant.

TDX Cortisol. (Abbott Diagnostics) Fluorescence polarization immunoassay for the quantitative determination of cortisol in serum, plasma or urine.
Use: Diagnostic aid.

TDX Thyroxine. (Abbott Diagnostics) Automated assay for quantitation of unsaturated thyroxine binding sites in serum or plasma.
Use: Diagnostic aid.

TDX Total Estriol. (Abbott Diagnostics) Fluorescence polarization immunoassay for the quantitative determination of total estriol in serum, plasma or urine.
Use: Diagnostic aid.

TDX Total T3. (Abbott Diagnostics) Automated assay for quantitation of total circulating triiodothyronine (T3) in serum or plasma.
Use: Diagnostic aid.

TDX T-Uptake. (Abbott Diagnostics) Automated assay for the determination of thyroxine binding capacity in serum or plasma.
Use: Diagnostic aid.

Te Anatoxal Berna. (Berna Products) Tetanus toxoid adsorbed, 10 Lf units/0.5 ml. Vial 5 ml, Syr. 0.5 ml. *Rx.*
Use: Immunization.

Tear Drop. (Parmed) Benzalkonium Cl 0.01%, polyvinyl alcohol, NaCl, EDTA. Soln. Drop. bot. 15 ml. *otc.*
Use: Artificial tears.

TearGard. (KM Lee) Hydroxyethylcellulose, sorbic acid 0.25%, EDTA 0.1%. Soln. Bot. 15 ml. *otc.*
Use: Lubricant, ophthalmic.

Teargen. (Zenith Goldline) Benzalkonium Cl 0.01%, EDTA, NaCl, polyvinyl alcohol. Soln. Bot. 15 ml. *otc.*
Use: Artificial tears.

Teargen II. (Zenith Goldline) Hydroxypropyl methylcellulose 0.3%, dextran 70 0.1%, benzalkonium Cl 0.01%, EDTA 0.05%. Bot. 15 ml. *otc.*
Use: Artificial tears.

Tearisol. (Ciba Vision Ophthalmics) Hydroxypropyl methylcellulose 0.5%, edetate disodium, benzalkonium chlor-

ide 0.01%, boric acid, potassium chloride. Bot. 15 ml. *otc.*
Use: Artificial tears.

Tears Naturale. (Alcon Laboratories) Dextran 70 0.1%, benzalkonium Cl 0.01%, hydroxypropyl methylcellulose 0.3%, sodium Cl, EDTA, hydrochloric acid, sodium HCl, potassium Cl. Bot. 15 ml, 30 ml. *otc.*
Use: Artificial tears.

Tears Naturale II. (Alcon Laboratories) Dextran 70 0.1%, hydroxypropyl methylcellulose 2910 0.3%, polyquaternium-1 0.001%, sodium Cl, potassium Cl, sodium borate. Droptainer 15 ml, 30 ml. *otc.*
Use: Artificial tears.

Tears Naturale Free. (Alcon Laboratories) Hydroxypropyl methylcellulose 2910 0.3%, dextran 70 0.1%, NaCl, KCl, sodium borate. Soln. Single-use containers 0.6 ml. *otc.*
Use: Artificial tears.

Tears Plus. (Allergan) Polyvinyl alcohol 1.4%, NaCl, povidone 0.6%, chlorobutanol 0.5%. *otc.*
Use: Artificial tears.

Tears Renewed Ointment. (Akorn) White petrolatum, light mineral oil. Ophth. Tube 3.5 g. *otc.*
Use: Lubricant, ophthalmic.

Tears Renewed Solution. (Akorn) Dextran 70 0.1%, sodium chloride, hydroxypropyl methylcellulose 2906, benzalkonium chloride 0.01%, EDTA. Soln. Bot. 2 ml, 15 ml, 30 ml. *otc.*
Use: Artificial tears.

tea tree oil. (Metabolic Prod.) Australian oil of Melaleuca alternifolia 100% pure. Bot. 1 oz, 4 oz, 8 oz, 16 oz. **Cream** Bot. 8 oz. **Oint.** Tube 1 oz, 3 oz. *otc.*
Use: Antiseptic, antifungal, topical.

Tebamide. (G & W Laboratories) Trimethobenzamide HCl 100 mg/Supp. In 10s. *Rx.*
Use: Antiemetic, antivertigo.

•**tebufelone.** (teh-BYOO-feh-LONE) USAN.
Use: Analgesic, anti-inflammatory.

•**tebuquine.** (TEH-buh-KWIN) USAN.
Use: Antimalarial.

T.E.C. (Invenex) Zinc 1 mg, copper 0.4 mg, chromium 4 mcg, manganese 0.1 mg. Vial 10 ml. *Rx.*
Use: Trace element supplement.

•**teceleukin.** (teh-see-LOO-kin) USAN.
Use: Immunostimulant.

Technescan MAA. (Mallinckrodt Medical). Aggregated albumin (human).
Use: Preparation of Tc 99m Aggregated Albumin (Human).

Techneplex. (Bristol-Myers Squibb) Technetium Tc 99m penetate kit. 10 vials/kit.
Use: Radiopaque agent.

•**technetium Tc 99m albumin aggregated injection.** (tek-NEE-shee-uhm Tc 99m al-BYOO-min AGG-reh-GAY-tuhd) U.S.P. 23.
Use: Diagnostic aid (lung imaging), radioactive agent.

•**technetium Tc 99m albumin colloid injection.** (tek-NEE-shee-uhm TC99m al-BYOO-min) U.S.P. 23.
Use: Radiopharmaceutical.

•**technetium Tc 99m albumin injection.** (tek-NEE-shee-uhm Tc 99m al-BYOO-min) U.S.P. 23.
Use: Radiopharmaceutical.

•**technetium Tc 99m albumin microaggregated.** (tek-NEE-shee-uhm TC 99m al-BYOO-min) USAN.
Use: Radiopharmaceutical.

technetium Tc 99m antimelanoma murine monoclonal antibody. (tek-NEE-shee-uhm)
Use: Diagnostic aid. [Orphan drug]

•**technetium Tc 99m antimony trisulfide colloid.** (tek-NEE-shee-uhm) USAN.
Use: Radiopharmaceutical.

•**technetium Tc 99m bicisate.** (tek-NEE-shee-uhm Tc 99m bye-SIS-ate) USAN.
Use: Diagnostic aid (brain imaging), radiopharmaceutical.

•**technetium Tc 99m disofenin injection.** (tek-NEE-shee-uhm) U.S.P. 23.
Use: Radiopharmaceutical; diagnostic aid (hepatobiliary function determination).

•**technetium Tc 99m etidronate injection.** (tek-NEE-shee-uhm) U.S.P. 23.
Use: Radiopharmaceutical.

•**technetium Tc 99m exametazime injection.** (tek-NEE-shee-uhm Tc 99m ex-ah-MET-ah-zeem) U.S.P. 23.
Use: Radiopharmaceutical.

technetium Tc 99m ferpentetate injection. (tek-NEE-shee-uhm) U.S.P. XXII.
Use: Radiopharmaceutical.

•**technetium Tc 99m furifosmin.** (tek-NEE-shee-uhm Tc 99m fyoor-ih-FOSS-min) USAN.
Use: Diagnostic aid (radioactive, cardiac disease), radiopharmaceutical.

technetium Tc 99m generator solution. (tek-NEE-shee-uhm) (New England Nuclear) Pertechnetate sodium Tc 99 m.

Use: Radiopharmaceutical, radiopaque agent.

•**technetium Tc 99m glucepate injection.** (tek-NEE-shee-uhm) U.S.P. 23.
Formerly Technetium Tc 99m Sodium Gluceptate.
Use: Radiopharmaceutical.

•**technetium Tc 99m lidofenin injection.** (tek-NEE-shee-uhm) U.S.P. 23.
Use: Radiopharamceutical.

•**technetium Tc 99m mebrofenin injection.** (tek-NEE-shee-uhm) U.S.P. 23.
Use: Radiopharmaceutical.

•**technetium Tc 99m medronate injection.** (tek-NEE-shee-uhm) U.S.P. 23.
Use: Diagnostic aid (skeletal imaging), radiopharmaceutical.
See: Macrotec, Inj. (Bristol-Myers Squibb).

•**technetium Tc 99m medronate disodium.** (tek-NEE-shee-uhm) USAN.
Use: Radiopharmaceutical.

•**technetium Tc 99m mertiatide injection.** (tek-NEE-shee-uhm Tc 99m MEER-TIE-ah-tide) U.S.P. 23.
Use: Diagnostic aid (renal function); radiopharmaceutical.

technetium Tc 99m murine monoclonal antibody to hCG. (tek-NEE-shee-uhm)
Use: Diagnostic aid. [Orphan drug]

technetium Tc 99m murine monoclonal antibody to human afp. (tek-NEE-shee-uhm)
Use: Diagnostic aid. [Orphan drug]

technetium Tc 99m murine monoclonal antibody (IgG2a) to BCE.
Use: Diagnostic aid. [Orphan drug]

•**technetium Tc 99m oxidronate injection.** (tek-NEE-shee-uhm) U.S.P. 23.
Use: Diagnostic aid (skeletal imaging), radiopharmaceutical.

•**technetium Tc 99m pentetate injection.** (tek-NEE-shee-uhm) U.S.P. 23.
Formerly Technetium Tc 99m Pentetate Sodium.
Use: Radiopharmaceutical.

•**technetium Tc 99m pentetate calcium trisodium.** (tek-NEE-shee-uhm KAL-see-uhm try-so-dee-uhm) USAN.
Use: Radiopharmaceutical.

•**technetium Tc 99m pyrophosphate injection.** (tek-NEE-shee-uhm) U.S.P. 23.
Use: Radiopharmaceutical.

•**technetium Tc 99m (pyro- and trimetra-) phosphates injection.** (tek-NEE-shee-uhm) U.S.P. 23.
Use: Radiopharmaceutical.

•**technetium Tc 99m red blood cells injection.** (tek-NEE-shee-uhm) U.S.P. 23.
Use: Radiopharmaceutical.

•**technetium Tc 99m sestamibi.** (tek-NEE-shee-uhm Tc 99 m SESS-tah-MIH-bih) U.S.P. 23.
Use: Diagnostic aid (radiopaque medium, cardiac perfusion); radiopharmaceutical.

•**technetium Tc 99m siboroxime.** (tek-NEE-shee-uhm Tc 99m sih-boe-ROX-eem) USAN.
Use: Diagnostic aid (brain imaging), radiopharmaceutical.

•**technetium Tc 99m succimer injection.** (tek-NEE-shee-uhm) U.S.P. 23.
Use: Radiopharmaceutical, diagnostic aid (renal function determination).

technetium Tc 99m sulfur colloid kit. (tek-NEE-shee-uhm)
Use: Radiopharmaceutical.
See: Tesuloid (Bristol-Myers Squibb).

•**technetium Tc 99m sulfur colloid injection.** (tek-NEE-shee-uhm) U.S.P. 23.
Use: Radiopharmaceutical.

•**technetium Tc 99m teboroxime.** (tek-NEE-shee-uhm Tc 99m teh-boe-ROX-eem) USAN.
Use: Diagnostic aid (radiopaque medium, cardiac perfusion), radiopharmaceutical.

teclosine. Under study.
Use: Amebicide.

•**teclozan.** (TEH-kloe-zan) USAN.
Use: Antiamebic.
See: Falmonox (Sanofi).

Tecnu Poison Oak-N-Ivy. (Tec Labs) Deodorized mineral spirits, propylene glycol, polyethylene glycol, octylphenoxypolyethoxyethanol, mixed fatty acid soap. Liq. Bot. 118.3 ml. *otc.*
Use: Dermatologic, poison ivy.

•**tecogalan sodium.** (TEE-koe-gay-lan) USAN.
Use: Antineoplastic adjunct.

Teczem. (Hoechst Marion Roussel) Enalapril maleate 5 mg, diltiazem maleate 180 mg, sucrose/ER Tab. Bot. Unit-of-use 100s. *Rx.*
Use: Antihypertensive.

Tedral. (Parke-Davis) **Tab.:** Theophylline 118 mg, ephedrine HCl 24 mg, phenobarbital 8 mg/Tab. Bot. 24s, 100s, 1000s. UD 100s. **Susp. (Pediatric Pharmaceuticals):** Theophylline 65 mg, ephedrine HCl 12 mg, phenobarbital 4 mg/5 ml. Bot. 8 oz. *Rx.*
Use: Antiasthmatic.

Tedral Elixir. (Parke-Davis) Theophylline 32.5 mg, ephedrine HCl 6 mg, pheno-

barbital 2 mg/5 ml. Alcohol 15%. Pediatric. Bot. pt. *Rx.*
Use: Antiasthmatic.

Tedral-SA. (Parke-Davis) Theophylline 180 mg, ephedrine HCl 48 mg, phenobarbital 25 mg/S.A. Tab. Bot. 100s, 1000s. *Rx.*
Use: Antiasthmatic.

Tedrigen. (Zenith Goldline) Theophylline 120 mg, ephedrine HCl 22.5 mg, phenobarbital 7.5 mg/Tab. Bot. 100s, 1000s. *otc.*
Use: Antiasthmatic.

Teebacin. (CMC) Sod. p-aminosalicylate **Tab.** 0.5 g Bot. 1000s. **Pow.** Bot. lb. *Rx.*
Use: Antituberculosis.

Teebaconin. (CMC) Isoniazid 50, 100, 300 mg/Tab. Bot. 100s, 1000s. *Rx.*
Use: Antituberculosis.

Teebaconin w/Vitamin B_6. (CMC) Isoniazid 100 mg, 10 mg pyridoxine HCl/ Tab. Bot. 100s, 500s, 1000s. Isoniazid 300 mg, 30 mg pyridoxine HCl/Tab. Bot. 100s and 1000s. *Rx.*
Use: Antituberculosis.

Teen Midol. (Bayer Corp) Acetaminophen 400 mg, pamabrom 25 mg. Cap. Bot. 16s. *otc.*
Use: Analgesic combination.

Teev. (Keene Pharmaceuticals) Estradiol valerate 4 mg, testosterone enanthate 90 mg/ml Inj. Vial 10 ml. *Rx.*
Use: Androgen, estrogen combination.

•**teflurane.** (TEH-flew-rane) USAN.
Use: Anesthetic, general.

tegacid.
See: Glyceryl monostearate.

•**tegafur.** (TEH-gah-fer) USAN.
Use: Antineoplastic.

Tegamide. (G & W) Trimethobenzamide HCl 100 mg, or 200 mg/ Supp. Boxes 10s, 50s.
Use: Antiemetic.

Tegretol. (Novartis) Carbamazepine **Tab.:** 200 mg. Bot. 100s, 1000s. UD 100s. **Chew. Tab.:** 100 mg/Tab. Bot. 100s. UD 100s; **Susp.:** 100 mg/5 ml, sorbitol. Sucrose. Bot. 450 ml. *Rx.*
Use: Anticonvulsant.

Tegretol-XR. (Novartis) Carbamazepine 100 mg, 200 mg and 400 mg, mannitol/ Tabs, extended release. Bot. 100s, UD 100s. *Rx.*
Use: Anticonvulsant.

Tegrin Cream. (Block Drug) Allantoin 2%, coal tar ext. 5% in cream base. Tube 2 oz., 4.4 oz. *otc.*
Use: Antipsoriatic.

Tegrin Medicated. (Block Drug) **Shampoo:** Crude coal tar 7%, sodium lauryl sulfate, ammonium lauryl sulfate, alcohol 6.4%. Cream 110 ml. *otc.*
Use: Antiseborrheic.

Tegrin Medicated Extra Conditioning. (Block Drug) Coal tar solution 7%, alcohol 6.4%. Shampoo. Bot. 110 ml, 198 ml. *otc.*
Use: Antiseborrheic.

T.E.H. Compound. (Various Mfr.) Theophylline 130 mg, ephedrine sulfate 25 mg, hydroxyzine HCl 10 mg/Tab. Bot. 100s, 500s. *Rx.*
Use: Antiasthmatic.

•**teicoplanin.** (teh-kah-PLAN-in) USAN.
Use: Anti-infective.

Telachlor TD Caps. (Major) Chlorpheniramine maleate 8 mg or 12 mg/T.D. Tab. Bot. 1000s. *Rx.*
Use: Antihistamine.

Teldrin Maximum Strength Capsules. (SmithKline Beecham Pharmaceuticals) Chlorpheniramine maleate 12 mg/ Spansule. Pkg. 12s, 24s, 48s. *otc.*
Use: Antihistamine.

Teldrin Tablets. (SmithKline Beecham Pharmaceuticals) Chlorpheniramine maleate 4 mg/Tab. *otc.*
Use: Antihistamine.

Teldrin 12-Hour Allergy Relief. (SmithKline Beecham Pharmaceuticals) Chlorpheniramine maleate 8 mg, pseudoephedrine HCl 75 mg/Cap. Pkg. 12s, 24s. Bot. 48s. *otc.*
Use: Antihistamine, decongestant.

Telepaque. (Sanofi) Iopanoic acid. 0.5 g/ Tab. Bot. 30s and 150s.
Use: Radiopaque agent.

•**telinavir.** (teh-LIN-ah-veer) USAN.
Use: Antiviral.

•**telmisartan.** (tell-mih-SAHR-tan) USAN,
Use: Angiotensin II receptor antagonist; antihypertensice.

Telodron. (Norden) Chlorpheniramine maleate.
Use: Antihistamine.

•**teloxantrone hydrochloride.** (teh-LOX-an-trone) USAN.
Use: Antineoplastic.

•**teludipine hydrochloride.** (teh-LOO-dih-peen) USAN.
Use: Antihypertensive; calcium channel antagonist.

•**temafloxcin hydrochloride.** (teh-mah-FLOX-ah-SIN) USAN.
Use: Anti-infective (microbial DNA topoisomerase inhibitor).

•**tematropium methylsulfate.** (teh-mah-TROE-pee-UHM METH-ill-SULL-fate) USAN.

Use: Anticholinergic.

•**temazepam.** (tem-AZE-uh-pam) U.S.P. 23.
Use: Anxiolytic.
See: Restoril, Cap. (Novartis).

temazepam. (Various Mfr.) 7.5 mg/Cap. 100s, UD 100s. *c-iv.*
Use: Hypnotic, sedative.

•**temelastine.** (teh-mell-ASS-teen) USAN.
Use: Antihistamine.

Temetan. (Nevin) Acetaminophen 324 mg/Tab. Bot. 100s, 500s. Elixir (324 mg/5 ml) Bot. pt. *otc.*
Use: Analgesic.

•**temocapril hydrochloride.** (teh-MOE-cap-RILL) USAN.
Use: Antihypertensive.

•**temocillin.** (TEE-moe-SIH-lin) USAN.
Use: Anti-infective.

•**temoporfin.** (teh-moe-PORE-fin) USAN.
Use: Antineoplastic.

Temovate Cream. (GlaxoWellcome) Clobetasol propionate 0.05%. Tube 15 g, 30 g, 45 g. *Rx.*
Use: Corticosteroid, topical.

Temovate Emollient. (GlaxoWellcome) Clobetasol propionate 0.05%. Cream. 15 g, 30 g, 60 g. *Rx.*
Use: Corticosteroid, topical.

Temovate Gel. (GlaxoWellcome) Clobetasol propionate 0.05%/Gel. 15, 30, 60 g. *Rx.*
Use: Corticosteroid, topical.

Temovate Ointment. (GlaxoWellcome) Clobetasol propionate 0.05%. Tube 15 g, 30 g; 45 g. *Rx.*
Use: Corticosteroid, topical.

Temovate Scalp. (GlaxoWellcome) **Oint.:** Clobetasol propionate 0.05%, white petro base. 15 g, 30 g, 45 g. **Cream:** Clobetasol propionate 0.03%, 15 g, 30 g, 45 g. **Scalp application:** Clobetasol propionate 0.05%, carbomer 934 P. 25 ml, 50 ml. *Rx.*
Use: Corticosteroid, topical.

Tempo. (Thompson Medical) Calcium carbonate 414 mg, aluminum hydroxide 133 mg, magnesium hydroxide 81 mg, simethicone 20 mg. Chew. Tab. Bot. 10s, 30s, 60s. *otc.*
Use: Antacid, antiflatulent.

Temporary Punctal/Canalicular Collagen Implant. (Eagle Vision) In 0.2 mm, 0.3 mm, 0.4 mm, 0.5 mm, 0.6 mm. Box 72s. *Rx.*
Use: Collagen implant, ophthalmic.

Tempra. (Bristol-Myers) Acetaminophen. **Drops:** Grape flavor. 80 mg/0.8 ml. Bot. w/dropper 15 ml. **Red syrup:** Cherry flavor. 160 mg/5 ml. Bot. 4 oz. **Tab.:** 80 mg/Chewable Grape flavor Tab. Bot 30s. 160 mg/Chewable Grape flavor Tab. Bot. 30s. *otc.*
Use: Analgesic.

•**temurtide.** (teh-MER-TIDE) USAN.
Use: Vaccine adjuvant.

Tencet Capsules. (Hauck) Acetaminophen 500 mg, butalbital 50 mg, caffeine 40 mg. Cap. Bot. 100s, UD 1000s. *Rx.*
Use: Analgesic, hypnotic, sedative.

Tencon. (Inter. Ethical Labs) Acetaminophen 650 mg, butalbital 50 mg. Cap. Bot. 100s. *Rx.*
Use: Analgesic, hypnotic, sedative.

Tenex. (Robins) Guanfacine HCl 1 mg, 2 mg/Tab. Bot. 100s, 500s (1 mg only), UD 100s (1 mg only). *Rx.*
Use: Antihypertensive.

•**tenidap.** (TEH-nih-DAP) USAN.
Use: Anti-inflammatory (osteoarthritis and rheumatoid arthritis).

•**tenidap sodium.** (TEH-nig-DAP) USAN.
Use: Anti-inflammatory (osteoarthritis and rheumatoid arthritis).

•**teniposide.** (TEN-ih-POE-side) USAN.
Use: Antineoplastic. [Orphan drug]
See: Vumon (Bristol-Myers Oncology/Immunology)

Ten-K. (Novartis) Potassium Cl 750 mg (10 mEq)/Controlled Release Cap. Bot. 100s, 500s. UD, blister pak 100s. *Rx.*
Use: Electrolyte supplement.

Tenol. (Vortech) Acetaminophen 325 mg/Tab. Bot. 1000s. *otc.*
Use: Analgesic.

Tenol Liquid. (Vortech) Acetaminophen 120 mg, NAPA alcohol 7%/5 ml. Bot. 3 oz., 4 oz., Gal. *otc.*
Use: Analgesic.

Tenol-Plus. (Vortech) Acetaminophen 250 mg, aspirin 250 mg, caffeine 65 mg/Tab. Bot. 1000s. *otc.*
Use: Analgesic.

Tenoretic Tablets. (Zeneca) **50 mg:** Atenolol 50 mg, Chlorthalidone 25 mg/Tab. Bot. 100s. **100 mg:** Atenolol 100 mg, Chlorthalidone 25 mg/Tab Bot. 100s. *Rx.*
Use: Antihypertensive, diuretic.

Tenormin. (Zeneca) **Oral:** Atenolol 50 mg or 100 mg/Tab. Bot. 100s. UD 100s. **Parenteral:** 5 mg/10 ml. Amp. 10 ml. *Rx.*
Use: Antihypertensive.

•**tenoxicam.** (ten-OX-ih-kam) USAN.
Use: Anti-inflammatory.

Tensilon. (Zeneca) Edrophonium chlor-

ide. **Vial:** 10 mg/ml, w/phenol 0.45%, sodium sulfite 0.2% 10 ml. **Amp.** 10 mg/ml, w/sodium sulfite 0.2%. 1 ml.
Use: Diagnostic aid, myasthenia gravis.

Tensive Conductive Adhesive Gel. (Parker) Non-flammable conductive adhesive electrode gel, eliminates tape and tape irritation. Tube 60 g.
Use: Therapeutic aid.

Tensocaine Tablets. (Sanofi) Acetaminophen. *otc.*
Use: Analgesic.

Tensolate. (Apco) Phenobarbital 0.25 gr, hyoscyamine sulfate 0.1037 mg, atropine sulfate 0.0194 mg, hyoscine HBr 0.0065 mg/Tab. Bot. 100s. *Rx.*
Use: Antispasmodic.

Tensolax Tablets. (Sanofi) Chlormezanone. *Rx.*
Use: Muscle relaxant.

Tensopin. (Apco) Phenobarbital 0.25 gr, homatropine methylbromide 2.5 mg/Tab. Bot. 100s. *Rx.*
Use: Antispasmodic.

Tenuate. (Hoechst Marion Roussel) Diethylpropion HCl 25 mg/Tab. Bot. 100s. *c-IV.*
Use: Anorexiant.

Tenuate Dospan. (Hoechst Marion Roussel) Diethylpropion HCl 75 mg/SR Tab. Bot. UD 100s, 250s. *c-v.*
Use: Anorexiant.

T.E.P. (Geneva Pharm) Phenobarbital 8 mg, theophylline 130 mg, ephedrine HCl 24 mg/Tab. Bot. 100s. *Rx.*
Use: Antiasthmatic combination.

Tepanil. (3M) Diethylpropion HCl. Tab. 25 mg Bot. 100s. *c-IV.*
Use: Anorexiant.

Tepanil Ten-Tab. (3M) Diethylpropion 75 mg/Tab. Bot. 30s, 100s, 250s. *c-IV.*
Use: Anorexiant.

•**tepoxalin.** (teh-POX-ah-lin) USAN.
Use: Antipsoriatic.

•**teprotide.** (TEH-pro-tide) USAN.
Use: Angiotensin converting-enzyme inhibitor.

tequinol sodium. Name used for Actinoquinol Sodium.

Terak Ointment. (Akorn) Polymyxin B sulfate 10,000 units/g or ml, oxytetracycline HCl 5 mg/g. Tube 3.5 g. *Rx.*
Use: Anti-infective, ophthalmic.

teralase. W/Pancreatin, polysorbate-80.
See: Digolase, Cap. (Boyle).

Terazol 3. (Ortho McNeil) **Cream, Vaginal:** Terconazole 0.8%. Tube 20 g with applicator. **Vaginal Supp.:** Terconazole 80 mg. Pks. 3s with applicator. *Rx.*
Use: Antifungal, vaginal.

Terazol 7. (Ortho McNeil) Terconazole 0.4% Cream. In 45 g. *Rx.*
Use: Antifungal, vaginal.

•**terazosin hydrochloride.** (ter-AZE-oh-sin) USAN.
Use: Antihypertensive.
See: Hytrin, Cap. (Abbott).

•**terbinafine.** (TER-bin-ah-feen) USAN.
Use: Antifungal.
See: Lamisil (Novartis).

•**terbutaline sulfate.** (ter-BYOO-tuh-leen) U.S.P. 23.
Use: Bronchodilator.
See: Brethine, Amp., Tab. (Novartis).

Tercodryl. (Health for Life Brands) Codeine phos. 3/4 gr, pyrilamine maleate 25 mg/fl. oz. Bot. 4 oz. *c-v.*
Use: Antihistamine, antitussive.

•**terconazole.** (ter-CONE-uh-zole) USAN.
Formerly Triaconazole.
Use: Antifungal.
See: Terazol 3, Vag. Cream, Supp. (Ortho McNeil).
Terazol 7, Vag. Cream. (Ortho McNeil).

Terg-a-Zyme. (Alconox) Alconox with enzyme action. Box 4 lb. Ctn. 9×4 lb., 25 lb., 50 lb., 100 lb., 300 lb. *otc.*
Use: Biodegradable detergent and wetting agent.

Teridol Jr. (Health for Life Brands) Terpin hydrate, cocillana, potassium guaiacolsulfonate, ammonium chloride. Bot. 3 oz. *otc.*
Use: Expectorant.

•**teriparatide.** (TER-pin HIGH-drate) USAN.
Use: Bone resorption inhibitor, osteoporosis therapy adjunct, diagnostic aid, thyroid function. [Orphan drug]
See: Parathar.

•**teriparatide acetate.** (TEH-rih-PAR-ah-TIDE) USAN.
Use: Diagnostic aid (hypocalcemia).

•**terlakiren.** (ter-lah-KIE-ren) USAN.
Use: Antihypertensive.

terlipressin.
Use: Treatment of bleeding esophageal varices. [Orphan drug]
See: Glypressin.

•**terodiline hydrochloride.** (TEH-row-DIE-leen) USAN.
Use: Vasodilator (coronary).

•**teroxalene hydrochloride.** (ter-OX-ah-leen) USAN.
Use: Antischistosomal.

•**teroxirone.** (TER-OX-ih-rone) USAN.
Use: Antineoplastic.

Terpex Jr. (Health for Life Brands) d-Methorphan 25 mg, terpin hydrate, pot. guaiacolsulfonate, cocillana, ammonium chloride. Bot. 4 oz. *otc.*
Use: Expectorant.

Terphan Elixir. (Pal-Pak) Terpin hydrate 85 mg, dextromethorphan hydrobromide 10 mg/5 ml w/alcohol 40% Bot. Gal. *otc.*
Use: Antitussive, expectorant.

•**terpin hydrate.** (TER-pin HIGH-drate) U.S.P. 23.
Use: Expectorant for chronic cough.
See: Terp, Liq. (Scrip).

terpin hydrate w/combinations.
See: Histogesic, Tab. (Century Pharm).
Prunicodeine, Liq. (Eli Lilly).
W/Dextromethorphan, phenylpropanolamine HCl, pheniramine maleate, pyrilamine maleate.
See: Tussaminic, Tab. (Novartis).
W/Dextromethorphan, phenylpropanolamine HCl, pheniramine maleate, pyrilamine maleate, acetaminophen.
See: Chexit, Tab. (Novartis).
Tussagesic, Tab., Liq. (Novartis).

terpin hydrate and dextromethorphan hydrobromide elixir.
Use: Antitussive, expectorant.

Terra-Cortril. (Roerig) Hydrocortisone 1.5%, oxytetracycline HCl 0.5%. Ophth. Susp. Bot. 5 ml. *Rx.*
Use: Anti-infective, corticosteroid, ophthalmic.

Terramycin. (Pfizer) Oxytetracycline. **Cap.:** HCl salt 250 mg. Bot. 100s, 500s. **Oint., Ophth.:** Ocytetracycline HCl 5 mg, polymyxin B sulfate 1 mg/g. Tube 3.75 g. **Oint., Topical:** Oxytetracycline HCl 100 mg, polymyxin B sulfate 10,000 units/g. Tube 0.5 oz., 1 oz. **Tab., Oral:** Oxytetracycline HCl 250 mg/Tab. Bot. 100s. **Tab., Vaginal:** Oxytetracycline HCl 100 mg, polymyxin B sulfate 100,000 units/Tab. Box 10s. *Rx.*
Use: Anti-infective.

Terramycin Capsules. (Pfizer) Oxytetracycline HCl 250 mg/Cap. Bot. 100s, 500s. *Rx.*
Use: Anti-infective.

Terramycin w/Polymyxin B Ointment. (Roerig) Polymyxin B sulfate 10,000 units/g or ml, oxytetracycline HCl 5 mg/g. Oint. Tube 3.5 g. *Rx.*
Use: Anti-infective.

Tersaseptic. (Doak Dermatologics) DEA-lauryl sulfate, lauramide DEA, propylene glycol, ethoxydiglycol, PEG-12 distearate, EDTA, triclosan, citric acid/Shampoo/cleanser. Soapless. 473 ml. *otc.*
Use: Dermatologic, acne.

tersavid.
Use: Monoamine oxidase inhibitor.

tertiary amyl alcohol.
See: Amylene Hydrate. (Various Mfr.).

Tesamone. (Dunhall Pharmaceuticals) Testosterone aqueous suspension. 25 mg/ml, 50 mg/ml or 100 mg/ml. Amp. 10 ml. *c-III.*
Use: Androgen.

•**tesicam.** (TESS-ih-kam) USAN.
Use: Anti-inflammatory.

•**tesimide.** (TESS-ih-mide) USAN.
Use: Anti-inflammatory.

Teslac. (Squibb Diagnostic) Testolactone 50 mg, lactose/Tab. Bot. 100s. *c-III.*
Use: Antineoplastic, androgen.

Teslascan. (Nycomed) Mangofodipir trisodium 37.9 mg/ml. Inj. Vial 10 ml. *Rx.*
Use: Diagnostic aid.

Tesogen. (Sigma-Tau Pharmaceuticals) Testosterone 25 mg, estrone 2mg/ml. Vial 10 ml. *c-III.*
Use: Androgen.

Tesogen L.A. (Sigma-Tau Pharmaceuticals) Testosterone enanthate 180 mg, 90 mg, 50 mg, estradiol valerate 8 mg, 4 mg and 2 mg respectively/ml. Vial 10 ml. *Rx.*
Use: Androgen, estrogen combination.

Tesone. (Sigma-Tau Pharmaceuticals) Testosterone 25 mg, 50 mg, 100 mg/ml. Vial 10 ml. *c-III.*
Use: Androgen.

Tesone L.A. (Sigma-Tau Pharmaceuticals) Testosterone enanthate 200 mg/ml. Vial 10 ml. *c-III.*
Use: Androgen.

tespa.
Use: Antineoplastic.
See: Thiotepa (ESI Lederle Generics).

Tessalon Perles. (Forest Pharmaceutical) Benzonatate 100 mg/Cap. Bot. 100s. *Rx.*
Use: Antitussive.

Testamone. (Dunhall Pharmaceuticals) Testosterone 100 mg/ml. Inj. Vial 10 ml. *c-III.*
Use: Androgen.

Test-Estro Cypionates. (Rugby) Estradiol cypionate 2 mg, testosterone cypionate 50 mg/ml. Inj. Vial 10 ml. *Rx.*
Use: Androgen, estrogen combination.

Testex. (Taylor Pharmaceuticals) Testosterone propionate in sesame oil 50 mg, 100 mg/ml. Vial 10 ml. *c-III.*
Use: Androgen.

Testoderm. (Alza) Testosterone 10 mg or 15 mg per 40 or 60 cm^2, respec-

tively. Transdermal system. Box 30s. *c-III.*
Use: Hormone, androgen.

Testoject. (Merz) Testosterone cypionate 100 mg/ml. Vial 10 ml. *c-III.*
Use: Androgen.

Testoject-50. (Merz) Testosterone 50 mg/ml. Vial 10 ml. *c-III.*
Use: Androgen.

Testoject-LA. (Merz) Testosterone cypionate 200 mg/ml in oil. Vial 10 ml. *c-III.*
Use: Androgen.

•**testolactone.** (TESS-toe-LAK-tone) U.S.P. 23.
Use: Antineoplastic.
See: Teslac, Vial, Tab. (Squibb Diagnostic).

Testolin. (Taylor Pharmaceuticals) Testosterone suspension 25 mg, 50 mg, 100 mg/ml. Vial 10 ml 25 mg/ml. Vial 30 ml. *c-III.*
Use: Androgen.

Testopel. (Bartor Pharmacal) Testosterone 75 mg, stearic acid 0.2 mg, polyvinylpyrrolidone 2 mg/pellet. 1 Pellet/Vial. *c-III.*
Use: Androgen.

•**testosterone.** (tess-TAHS-ter-ohn) U.S.P. 23.
Use: Androgen.
See: Androderm, Transderm. Patch (SmithKline Beecham Pharmaceuticals).
Android-T, Vial (Zeneca).
Andronaq, Aq. Susp., Vial (Schwarz Pharma).
Depotest, Vial (Hyrex).
Homogene-S, Inj., Vial (Spanner).
Malotrone Aqueous Injection (Bluco).
Neo-Hombreol-F, Aq. Susp., Vial (Organon Teknika).
Tesone, Inj. (Sigma-Tau Pharmaceuticals).
Testoderm, Transdermal patch (Alza).
Testolin, Vial (Taylor Pharmaceuticals).
Testopel, Pellet (Bartor Pharmacal).

testosterone aqueous. (Various Mfr.) Testosterone (in aqueous suspension) 25 mg, 50 mg or 100 per ml/Inj. Vial 10 ml, 30 ml.
Use: Androgen, parenteral.
See: Histerone 100, Inj. (Roberts Pharm).
Tesamone, Inj. (Dunhall Pharmaceuticals).

testosterone w/combinations.
See: Andesterone, Vial (Lincoln).
Angen, Vial (Davis & Sly).
Depo-Testadiol, Vial (Pharmacia & Upjohn).
Glutest, Vial (Zeneca).
Tesogen, Inj. (Sigma-Tau Pharmaceuticals).

testosterone cyclopentane propionate. Testosterone Cypionate, U.S.P. 23.

•**testosterone cypionate.** (tess-TAHS-ter-ohn) U.S.P. 23.
Use: Androgen.
See: Andro-Cyp 100, Inj. (Keene Pharmaceuticals).
Andro-Cyp 200, Inj. (Keene Pharmaceuticals).
depAndro, Inj. (Forest Pharmaceutical).
Depo-Testosterone, Inj. (Pharmacia & Upjohn).
Dep-Test, Inj. (Sigma-Tau Pharmaceuticals).
Depotest, Vial (Hyrex).
D-Test 100, 200, Inj. (Burgin-Arden).
Durandro, Inj. (B.F. Ascher).
Duratest, Inj. (Roberts Pharm).
Testoject, Vial (Merz).
W/Combinations.
See: D-Diol, Inj. (Burgin-Arden).
Depotestogen, Vial (Hyrex).
Depo-Testadiol, Soln. (Pharmacia & Upjohn).
Duo-Cyp (Keene Pharmaceuticals).
Duracrine, Inj. (B.F. Ascher).
Menoject-L.A. Vial (Kay).
T.E. Ionate P.A., Inj. (Solvay).

testosterone cypionate. (Various Mfr.) 100 mg/ml or 200 mg/ml. Inj. Vial 10 ml.
Use: Androgen.

testosterone cypionate/estradiol cypionate.
See: Estradiol cypionate w/testosterone cypionate.

testosterone cypionate and estradiol cypionate. (Schein Pharmaceutical) Testosterone cypionate 50 mg, estradiol cypionate 2 mg/ml. Vials 10 ml. *Rx.*
Use: Androgen, estrogen combination.

•**testosterone enanthate.** (tess-TAHS-ter-ohn) U.S.P. 23.
Use: Androgen.
See: Andryl, Inj. (Keene Pharmaceuticals).
Andropository-200, Inj. (Rugby).
Arderone 100, 200, Inj. (Burgin-Arden).
Delatest, Inj. (Dunhall Pharmaceuticals).
Delatestryl, Inj., Vial (Bristol-Myers Squibb).
Everone 200 mg, Vial (Hyrex).
Tesone L. A., Inj. (Sigma-Tau Pharmaceuticals).

Testate, Inj. (Savage).
Testrin-P.A., Inj. (Taylor Pharmaceuticals).
W/Chlorobutanol.
See: Anthatest, Vial (Kay).
Andro L.A. 200, Inj. (Forest Pharmaceutical).
Delatestryl, Inj. (Gynex).
Durathate-200, Inj. (Roberts Pharm).
Everone 200, Inj. (Hyrex).
W/Estradiol valerate.
See: Valertest No. 1, Amp., Vial (Hyrex).

testosterone enanthate. (Various Mfr.) 100 mg/ml or 200 mg/ml. Inj. Vial 10 ml.
Use: Androgen.

testosterone heptanoate.
Use: Androgen.
See: Testosterone enanthate.

•**testosterone ketolaurate.** (tess-TAHS-ter-ohn KEY-toe-LORE-ate) USAN. Testosterone 3-oxododecanoate.
Use: Androgen.

testosterone ointment 2%.
Use: Vulvar dystrophies. [Orphan drug]

•**testosterone phenylacetate.** (tess-TAHS-ter-ohn fen-ill-ASS-ah-tate) USAN. Perandren phenylacetate.
Use: Androgen.

•**testosterone propionate.** (tess-TAHS-ter-ohn) U.S.P. 23.
Use: Androgen.

testosterone propionate. (Various Mfr.) Testosterone propionate (in oil) 100 mg per ml. Inj. Vial 10 ml.
Use: Androgen.

testosterone sublingual.
Use: Delay of growth and puberty in boys. [Orphan drug]

Testred. (ICN Pharmaceuticals) Methyltestosterone 10 mg/Cap. Bot. 100s. *c-III.*
Use: Androgen.

Testred Cypionate.
Use: Androgen inhibitor.
See: Proscar (Merck).

Testred Cypionate 200. (Zeneca) Testosterone cypionate 200 mg/ml. Vial 10 ml. *c-III.*
Use: Androgen.

Testrin-P.A. (Taylor Pharmaceuticals) Testosterone enanthate 200 mg, in sesame oil with chlorobutanol/ml. Vial 10 ml. *c-III.*
Use: Androgen.

Testuria. (Wyeth Ayerst) Combination kit containing 5 × 20 sterile dip strips and 5 × 20 culture trays of trypticase soy agar.
Use: Diagnostic aid.

Tesuloid. (Bristol-Myers Squibb) Technetium Tc 99m sulfur colloid. 5 vials/kit.
Use: Radiopaque agent.

tetanus and diphtheria toxoids adsorbed for adult use. (TET-ah-nus and diff-THEER-ee-uh TOX-oyds) U.S.P. 23.
Use: Immunization.
Generic Products:
(Pasteur Merieux Connaught) Vial 5 ml for IM use.
(Wyeth Ayerst) Vial 5 ml.

•**tetanus antitoxin.** (TET-n-us) U.S.P. 23.
Use: Immunization.

tetanus, diphtheria toxoids, and aluminum phosphate adsorbed. (Wyeth Ayerst) Vial 5 ml, Tubex 0.5 ml. *Rx.*
Use: Immunization.

tetanus, diphtheria & pertussis vaccine.
Use: Immunization.
See: Acel-Immune, Vial (Wyeth Ayerst)
Diphtheria and Tetanus Toxoids and Whole Cell Pertussis Vaccine, Vial (Pasteur Merieux Connaught).
Infanrix (SKB).
Tri-Immunol, Vial (Wyeth Ayerst).
Tripedia, Vial (Pasteur Merieux Connaught).

tetanus and diphtheria toxoids adsorbed purogenated. (Wyeth Ayerst) Adult Lederject disposable syringe 10 × 0.5 ml. Vial 5 ml New package. *Rx.*
Use: Immunization.

•**tetanus immune globulin.** (TET-ah-nus ih-MYOON GLAH-byoo-lin) U.S.P. 23. *Formerly Tetanus Immune Human Globulin.* Gamma globulin fraction of the plasma of persons who have been hyperimmunized with tetanus toxoid, 16.5%. Vial 250 units.
Use: Prophylaxis of injured, against tetanus (passive immunizing agent).
See: Baytet Injection Vial, 250 u. (Bayer Corp).

tetanus immune globulin, human. 250 units/Tubex, 1 ml Dissolved in glycine 0.3 M; contains thimerosal 0.01%. *Rx.*
Use: Immunization.
See: Baytet (Bayer).

•**tetanus toxoid.** (TET-n-us TOX-oyd) U.S.P. 23.
Use: Immunization.

•**tetanus toxoid, adsorbed.** (TET-n-us TOX-oyd) U.S.P. 23.
Use: Immunization.
See: Te Anatoxal Berna, Vial, Syr. (Berna Products).

tetanus toxoid, adsorbed. 20 Lf purified tetanus toxoid, 0.01% thimerosal as preservative/ml. Box 2 ampuls of 0.5 ml. Vial 5 ml, 7.5 ml, 0.5 ml. Amp. for booster injection. (Pasteur Merieux Connaught)
See: Te Anatoxal (Berna). Vial 5 ml for IM use. (Wyeth Ayerst) Vial 5 ml, disp. syringes 0.5 ml. *Rx.*
Use: Immunization.

tetanus toxoid adsorbed purogenated. (Wyeth Ayerst) Vial 5 ml. Lederject disposable syringe 0.5 ml. Box 10s, 100s. *Rx.*
Use: Immunization.

tetanus toxoid, aluminum phosphate adsorbed. *Rx.*
Use: Immunization.
See: (Wyeth Ayerst) Vial 5 ml 10s. Lederject Disp. Syr. 10 0.5 ml.

tetanus toxoid, fluid. (Pasteur Merieux Connaught) Vial 7.5 ml for IM or SC use. (Wyeth Ayerst) Vial 7.5 ml, Tubex 0.5 ml. *Rx.*
Use: Immunization.

tetanus toxoid, fluid purogenated. (Wyeth Ayerst) Vial 7.5 ml Lederject disposable syringe. 0.5 ml. Box 10s, 100s. *Rx.*
Use: Immunization.

tetanus toxoid purified, fluid. (Wyeth Ayerst) Vial 7.5 ml, Tubex 0.5 ml. *Rx.*
Use: Immunization.

tetiothalein sodium.
See: Iodophthalein Sodium. (Var. Mfr.).

Tetrabead. (Abbott Diagnostics) Solid phase radioimmunoassay for the quantitative measurement of total circulating serum thyroxine.

Tetrabead-125. (Abbott Diagnostics) T-3 uptake radioassay for the measurement of thyroid function by indirectly determining the degree of saturation of serum thyroxine binding globulin (TBG).

•**tetracaine.** (TEH-trah-cane) U.S.P. 23.
Use: Anesthetic (topical).
See: Pontocaine, Oint., Cream (Sanofi).
Viractin, Preps. (J. B. Williams).

tetracaine and menthol ointment.
Use: Anesthetic, local.

•**tetracaine hydrochloride.** U.S.P. 23.
Use: Spinal anesthetic, local.
See: Bristacycline, Cap. (Bristol-Myers).
Pontocaine Hydrochloride Inj., Pow. (Sanofi).
W/Benzocaine, butyl aminobenzoate.
See: Cetacaine, Liq., Oint., Spray (Cetylite Industries).
W/Hexachlorophene, dimethyl polysiloxane, methyl salicylate, pyrilamine maleate, zinc oxide.
W/Isocaine, benzalkonium Cl.
See: Isotraine Oint. (Roxane).

tetracaine hydrochloride 0.5%. (Alcon Laboratories) 0.5%/1 ml Drop-Tainer, Ophth. 15 ml Steri-Unit, 2 ml (Ciba Vision Ophthalmics) Dropperettes 1 ml in 10s. *Rx.*
Use: Anesthetic, ophthalmic.

Tetracap. (Circle) Tetracycline HCl 250 mg/Cap. Bot. 100s. *Rx.*
Use: Anti-infective, tetracycline.

tetrachlorethylene. U.S.P. XXI. Perchlorethylene, tetrachlorethylene.
Use: Anthelmintic (hookworms and some trematodes).

Tetracon. (Professional Pharmacal) Tetrahydrozoline HCl 0.5 mg, disodium edetate 1 mg, boric acid 12 mg, benzalkonium Cl 0.1 mg, sodium Cl 2.2 mg, sodium borate 0.5 mg/ml w/water. Liq. Bot. 15 ml. *otc.*
Use: Anti-irritant, ophthalmic.

•**tetracycline.** (teh-truh-SIGH-kleen) U.S.P. 23.
Use: Antiamebic, anti-infective, antirickettsial.
See: Sumycin, Syrup (Bristol-Myers Squibb).
W/N-acetyl-para-amino-phenol, phenyltoloxamine citrate.
Use: Anti-infective, tetracycline.
See: Paltet, Cap. (Roberts Pharm).
Tetrex, Bid Cap., Cap., Vial (Bristol-Myers).

tetracycline and amphotericin B. U.S.P. XXI.

•**tetracycline hydrochloride.** (teh-trah-SIGH-kleen) U.S.P. 23.
Use: Anti-infective, antiamebic, antirickettsial.
See: Achromycin, Preps. (Storz/Lederle).
Bicycline, Caps. (Knight).
Centet 250, Tab. (Schwarz Pharma).
Cyclopar, Cap. (Parke-Davis).
G-Mycin, Cap. & Syr. (Coast).
Maso-Cycline, Cap. (Mason).
Panmycin, Cap. (Pharmacia & Upjohn).
Scotrex, Caps. (Scott/Cord).
Sumycin, Cap., Tab., Syr. (Squibb Diagnostic).
Tetracap 250, Cap. (Circle).
Tetracyn, Cap. (Pfizer).
Tetram, Cap., Syr. (Dunhall Pharmaceuticals).
Topicycline, Liq. (Procter & Gamble).

W/Citric Acid.
See: Achromycin V, Cap., Drop, Susp., Syr. (ESI Lederle Generics).
W/Nystatin.
See: Comycin, Cap. (Pharmacia & Upjohn).

tetracycline hydrochloride fiber.
Use: Anti-infective, tetracycline.
See: Actisite (Alza).

tetracycline hydrochloride and nystatin capsules.
Use: Anti-infective, tetracycline.
See: Comycin, Cap. (Pharmacia & Upjohn)

tetracycline oral suspension.
Use: Anti-infective, tetracycline.
See: Brand names under Tetracycline.

•**tetracycline phosphate complex.** (teh-truh-SIGH-kleen FOSS-fate) U.S.P. 23.
Use: Anti-infective.

Tetracyn. (Pfizer) Tetracycline HCl. 250 mg or 500 mg/Cap. **250 mg:** Cap. Bot. 1000s. **500 mg:** Bot. 100s. *Rx.*
Use: Anti-infective, tetracycline.

tetradecyl sulfate, sodium.
Use: Sclerosing agent.
See: Sotradecol (ESI Lederle Generics).

tetraethylammonium bromide (teab).
Use: Diagnostic & therapeutic agent in peripheral vascular disorders. Diagnostic in hypertension.

tetraethylammonium chloride.
Use: Ganglionic blocking.

tetraethylthiuram disulfide.
See: Disulfiram.

•**tetrafilcon a.** (teh-trah-FILL-kahn) USAN.
Use: Contact lens material (hydrophilic).

tetrahydroaminoacridine.
Use: A cholinergic agent for Alzheimer's disease.
See: Cognex (Warner Lambert).

tetrahydrophenobarbital calcium.
See: Cyclobarbital Calcium, Prep.

tetrahydroxyquinone. Name used for Tetroquinone.

•**tetrahydrozoline hydrochloride.** (teh-trah-high-DRAHZ-ah-leen) U.S.P. 23.
Use: Adrenergic (vasoconstrictor).
See: Collyrium Fresh Eye Drops (Wyeth Ayerst).
Eyesine, Soln., (Akorn).
Geneye Extra, Drops (Zenith Goldline).
Mallazine Eye Drops (Roberts Pharm).
Murine Plus (Abbott Laboratories).
Optigene 3, Soln. (Pfeiffer).
Soothe, Soln., (Alcon Laboratories).
Tetrasine, Soln., (Optopics).
Tyzine, Soln. (Key Pharm).
Visine, Soln. (Pfizer).

tetraiodophenolphthalein sodium.
See: Iodophthalein Sodium.

tetraiodophthalein sodium.
See: Iodophthalein Sodium.

tetramethylene dimethanesulfonate.
See: Busulfan, U.S.P. 23.

tetramethylthiuram disulfide. Thiram.
Use: Anti-infective, antifungal.

•**tetramisole hydrochloride.** (teh-TRAM-ih-sole) USAN.
Use: Anthelmintic.

Tetramune. (Wyeth Ayerst) 12.5 Lf units of tetanus toxoid, 5 Lf units of diphtheria toxoid, 4 units of pertussis vaccine and 10 mcg *Haemophilus influenzae* type b oligosaccharide, each per 0.5 ml. Vial, 5 ml. *Rx.*
Use: Immunization.

Tetraneed. (Hanlon) Pentaerythritol tetranitrate 80 mg/Time Cap. Bot. 100s. *Rx.*
Use: Antianginal.

tetrantoin.
Use: Anticonvulsant.

Tetrasine. (Optopics) Tetrahydrozoline HCl 0.05%. Bot. 15 ml, 22.5 ml. *otc.*
Use: Ophthalmic vasoconstrictor/mydriatic.

Tetrasine Extra. (Optopics) Polyethylene glycol 400 1%, tetrahydrozoline HCl 0.05%. Bot. 15 ml. *otc.*
Use: Mydriatic, vasoconstrictor.

Tetratab. (Freeport) Pentaerythritol tetranitrate 10 mg/Tab. Bot. 1000s. *Rx.*
Use: Antianginal.

Tetratab No. 1. (Freeport) Pentaerythritol tetranitrate 20 mg/Tab. Bot. 1000s. *Rx.*
Use: Antianginal.

•**tetrazolast meglumine.** (teh-TRAZZ-oh-last meh-GLUE-meen) USAN.
Use: Antiallergic; antiasthmatic.

Tetrazyme. (Abbott Diagnostics) Test kit 100s, 500s.
Use: Enzyme immunoassay for quantitative measurement of total circulating serum thyroxine (free and protein bound).

•**tetrofosmin.** (teh-troe-FOSS-min) USAN.
Use: Diagnostic aid.

•**tetroquinone.** (TEH-troe-kwih-NOHN) USAN.
Use: Treat keloids, keratolytic (systemic).
See: Kelox (Zeneca).

•**tetroxoprim.** (tet-ROX-oh-prim) USAN.
Use: Anti-infective.

•**tetrydamine.** (teh-TRID-ah-meen) USAN.
Use: Analgesic, anti-inflammatory.

Tetterine. (Shuptrine) **Oint.:** Antifungal agents in green petrolatum base. Tin oz.; Antifungal agents in white petroleum base. Tube oz. **Powder:** Fungicide, germicide formula powder for heat and diaper rash. Can 2.25 oz. **Soap:** Bar 3.25 oz.
Use: Dermatologic, counterirritant.

Texacort Scalp Lotion. (GenDerm) Hydrocortisone 1%, alcohol 33%. Lipid free. Dropper Bot. 1 fl. oz. *Rx.*
Use: Corticosteroid.

T-Fluoride. (Tennessee Pharmaceutic) Sodium fluoride 2.21 mg/Tab. Bot. 100s, 1000s. *Rx.*
Use: Dental caries preventative.

TG.
Use: Antineoplastic.
See: Thioguanine (GlaxoWellcome).

T/Gel Scalp Solution. (Neutrogena) Neutar coal tar extract 2%, salicyclic acid 2%. Bot. 2 oz. *otc.*
Use: Antipsoriatic, antiseborrheic.

T/Gel Therapeutic Conditioner. (Neutrogena) Neutar coal tar extract 1.5% in oil free conditioner base. Bot. 1.4 oz. *otc.*
Use: Antipsoriatic, antiseborrheic.

T/Gel Therapeutic Shampoo. (Neutrogena) Neutar coal tar extract 2% in mild shampoo base. Bot. 4.4 oz., 8.5 oz. *otc.*
Use: Antipsoriatic, antiseborrheic.

T-Gen Suppositories. (Zenith Goldline) Trimethobenzamide HCl 100 mg/Pediatric Supp. or 200 mg/Adult Supp. Box 10s, 50s. *Rx.*
Use: Antiemetic.

T-Gesic Capsule. (T.E. Williams) Hydrocodone bitartrate 5 mg, acetaminophen 500 mg/Cap. Bot. 100s. *c-III.*
Use: Analgesic combination, narcotic, hypnotic, sedative.

•**thalidomide.** (the-LID-oh-mide) USAN.
Use: Anti-infective, hypnotic, sedative. [Orphan drug]

Thalitone. (Horus Therapeutics) Chlorthalidone 15 or 25 mg, lactose/Tab. Bot. 100s. *Rx.*
Use: Diuretic.

•**thallous chloride Tl 201 injection.** (THAL-uhs) U.S.P. 23.
Use: Diagnostic aid (radiopaque medium), radioactive agent.

Tham-E. (Abbott Laboratories) Tromethamine 36 g, sodium Cl. 30 mEq/L, potassium Cl. 5 mEq/L, chloride 35 mEq/L. Total osmolarity 367 mOsm/L. Single dose container 150 ml. *Rx.*
Use: Nutritional supplement.

Tham Solution. (Abbott Laboratories) Tromethamine 18 g, acetic acid 2.5 g single-dose container. *Rx.*
Use: Nutritional supplement.

THC.
Use: Antiemetic, antivertigo.
See: Marinol (Roxane).

theamin. Monoethanolamine salt of theophylline.
See: Monotheamin, Supp. (Eli Lilly).
W/Amobarbital.
See: Monotheamin and Amytal, Pulvule (Eli Lilly).

thenalidine tartrate.
Use: Antihistamine; antipruritic.

thenyldiamine hydrochloride.
Use: Antihistamine.

thenylpyramine.
See: Methapyrilene Hydrochloride, Preps.

Theo-24. (UCB Pharmaceuticals) Theophylline anhydrous 100 mg, 200 mg, or 300 mg/Controlled Release Cap. 100 mg Bot. 100s. UD 100s; 200 mg Bot. 100s, 500s. UD 100s; 300 mg Bot. 100s, 500s. UD 100s. *Rx.*
Use: Antiasthmatic, bronchodilator.

Theobid Duracap. (Ross Laboratories) Theophylline anhydrous 260 mg/TR Cap. Bot. 60s, 500s. *Rx.*
Use: Antiasthmatic, bronchodilator.

theobroma oil. Cocoa Butter, N.F. 18.
Use: Pharmaceutical aid, suppository base.

theobromine with phenobarbital combinations.
See: Harbolin, Tab. (Arcum).
T.P. KI, Tab. (Wendt-Bristol).

theobromine calcium gluconate. (Bates) Tab., Bot. 100s, 1000s. Also available w/phenobarbital. (Grant) Tab., Bot. 100s, 500s, 1000s.

theobromine sodium acetate. Theobromine calcium salt mixture with calcium salicylate.
Use: Diuretic; muscle relaxant.

theobromine sodium salicylate.
See: Doan's Pills (Purex).
W/Cal. lactate, Phenobarbital.
See: Theolaphen, Tab. (Zeneca).

Theochron. (Various Mfr.) Theophylline anhydrous 100 mg, 200 mg, 300 mg. ER Tab. 100s, 500s, 1000s. *Rx.*
Use: Bronchodilator.

Theochron. (Forest Pharmaceutical)

Theophylline 200 mg/Tab. T.R. Bot. 100s, 500s, 1000s. 300 mg/Tab. T.R. Bot. 100s, 500s. *Rx.*
Use: Bronchodilator.

Theoclear 80 Syrup. (Schwarz Pharma) Theophylline 80 mg/15 ml. Bot. Pt., Gal. *Rx.*
Use: Bronchodilator.

Theoclear L.A.-130. (Schwarz Pharma) Theophylline 130 mg/Cenule. Bot. 100s. *Rx.*
Use: Bronchodilator.

Theoclear L.A.-260. (Schwarz Pharma) Theophylline 260 mg/Cenule Bot. 100s, 1000s. *Rx.*
Use: Bronchodilator.

Theocolate. (Rosemont) Theophylline 150 mg, guaifenesin 90 mg/15 ml Liq. Bot. pt., gal. *Rx.*
Use: Antiasthmatic.

Theodrine. (Rugby) Theophylline 120 mg, ephedrine HCl 22.5 mg/Tab. Bot. 1000s. *otc.*
Use: Antiasthmatic.

Theo-Dur. (Schering Plough) Theophylline 450 mg/Tab. S.R. Bot. 100s, UD 100s. *Rx.*
Use: Bronchodilator.

Theo-Dur Tablets. (Key Pharm) Theophylline 100 mg, 200 mg or 300 mg/SA Tab. Bot. 100s, 500s, 1000s, 5000s. UD 100s. *Rx.*
Use: Bronchodilator.

•**theofibrate.** (THEE-oh-FIH-brate) USAN.
Use: Antihyperlipoproteinemic.

Theogen. (Sigma-Tau Pharmaceuticals) Conjugated estrogens 2 mg/ml. Vial 10 ml, 30 ml. *Rx.*
Use: Estrogen.

Theogen I.P. (Sigma-Tau Pharmaceuticals) Estrone 2 mg, potassium estrone sulfate 1 mg/ml. Vial 10 ml. *Rx.*
Use: Estrogen.

Theolair. (3M) Theophylline 125, 250 mg/Tab. Box 100s, 250s as foil strip 10s. Bot. 100s. *Rx.*
Use: Bronchodilator.

Theolair Liquid. (3M) Theophylline 80 mg/15 ml. Bot. pt. *Rx.*
Use: Bronchodilator.

Theolair-SR 200. (3M) Theophylline 200 mg/Tab. (slow release). Bot. 100s. Box 100s as foil strip 10s. *Rx.*
Use: Bronchodilator.

Theolair-SR 250. (3M) Theophylline 250 mg/Tab. (slow release). Bot. 100s, 250s. *Rx.*
Use: Bronchodilator.

Theolair-SR 300. (3M) Theophylline 300 mg/Tab. (slow release). Bot. 100s. Box 100s as foil strip 10s. *Rx.*
Use: Bronchodilator.

Theolair-SR 500. (3M) Theophylline 500 mg/Tab. (slow release). Bot. 100s, 250s. *Rx.*
Use: Bronchodilator.

Theolate Liquid. (Various Mfr.) Theophylline 150 mg, guaifenesin 90 mg/15 ml. Liq. Bot. 118 ml, pt, gal. *Rx.*
Use: Antiasthmatic.

Theomax DF Syrup. (Various Mfr.) Theophylline 97.5 mg, ephedrine sulfate 18.75 mg, alcohol 5%, hydroxyzine HCl 7.5 mg/15 ml. Bot. pt. gal. *Rx.*
Use: Antiasthmatic.

Theo-Organidin. (Wallace Laboratories) Theophylline anhydrous 120 mg, iodinated glycerol 30 mg/15 ml w/alcohol 15%, saccharin. Bot. pt., gal. *Rx.*
Use: Antiasthmatic.

Theophenyllin. (H.L. Moore) Theophylline 130 mg, ephedrine HCl 24 mg, phenobarbital 8 mg/Tab. Bot. 1000s. *Rx.*
Use: Antiasthmatic.

Theophyl-SR. (Ortho McNeil) Theophylline 125 mg. Bot. 100s. *Rx.*
Use: Bronchodilator.

•**theophylline.** (thee-AHF-ih-lin) U.S.P. 23.
Use: Bronchodilator; coronary vasodilator, diuretic; pharmaceutic necessity for Aminophylline Injection.
See: Accurbron, Liq. (Hoechst Marion Roussel).
Aerolate, Cap., Elix. (Fleming).
Aquaphyllin, Syr. (Ferndale Laboratories).
Bronkodyl, Cap. (Sanofi).
Duraphyl, Tab. (Ortho McNeil).
Elixicon, Susp. (Berlex).
Elixophyllin, Elix., Cap. (Berlex).
Elixophyllin SR, Cap. (Berlex).
Lodrane, Cap. (ECR Pharmaceuticals).
Optiphyllin, Elix. (E. Fougera).
Oralphyllin, Liq. (Consol. Midland).
Quibron-T Dividose, Tab. (Roberts).
Quibron-T/SR Dividose, Tab. (Roberts).
Slo-bid, Caps. (Rhone-Poulenc Rorer).
Slo-Phyllin, Cap., Syr., Tab. (Dooner).
Somophyllin, Cap. (Medeva).
Sustaire, Tab. (Pfizer)
Theo-II, Elix. (Fleming).
Theobid, Cap. (Ross Laboratories).
Theobid Jr, Cap. (Ross Laboratories).
Theochron, ER Tab. (Various Mfr.)
Theoclear 80, Liq. (Schwarz Pharma).

Theoclear L.A., Cenule (Schwarz Pharma).
Theo-Dur, Tab. (Key Pharm).
Theolair, Tab., Liq. (3M).
Theolair SR, Tab. (3M).
Theospan, Cap. (Laser).
Theostat, Prods. (Laser).
Theovent Long-Acting, Cap. (Schering Plough).
Theo-X, CR Tab. (Schwarz Pharma).
Uni-Dur, ER. Tab. (Key).
Uniphyl, TR Tab. (Purdue Frederick).

theophylline. (Various Mfr.) 100 mg, 125 mg, 200 mg, 300 mg/ER Cap. Bot. 100s. *Rx.*
Use: Bronchodilator.

theophylline, 8-chloro, diphenhydramine. Dimenhydrinate, U.S.P. 23.
See: Dramamine, Prep. (Searle).

theophylline aminoisobutanol. Theophylline w/2-amino-2-methyl-1-propanol.
See: Butaphyllamine (Var. Mfr.).

theophylline-calcium salicylate.
W/Ephedrine HCl, phenobarbital, pot. iodide.
See: Quadrinal, Tab., Susp. (Knoll Pharmaceuticals).
W/Phenobarbital, ephedrine HCl, guaifenesin.
See: Verequad, Tab., Susp. (Knoll Pharmaceuticals).
W/Potassium iodide.

theophylline choline salt.
See: Choledyl, Tab., Elix. (Parke-Davis).

Theophylline and 5% Dextrose. (Abbott and Baxter) Inj. 200 mg/Cont.: 50 ml and 100 ml. 400 mg/Cont.: 100 ml, 250 ml, 500 ml and 1000 ml. 800 mg/ Cont.: 250 ml, 500 ml and 1000 ml.
Use: Bronchodilator.

theophylline, ephedrine hydrochloride, and phenobarbital tablets.
Use: Bronchodilator, sedative.

theophylline ethylenediamine.
See: Aminophylline, Prep., (Var. Mfr.).

theophylline extended release. (Dey) Theophylline 100 mg, 200 mg, 300 mg. ER Tab. Bot. 100s, 500s, 1000s. *Rx.*
Use: Bronchodilator.

theophylline extended-release. (Sidmak) Theophylline anhydrous 450 mg, lactose (SL 518). ER Tab. Bot. 100s, 250s, 500s. *Rx.*
Use: Bronchodilator.

theophylline extended-release capsules.
Use: Bronchodilator.

theophylline w/combinations.
See: Asma-lief, Tab., Susp. (Quality Formulations).
B.A. Prods. (Federal).
Bronkaid, Tab. (Brew).
Co-Xan, Liq. (Schwarz Pharma).
Elixophyllin-KI, Elix. (Berlex).
Liquophylline, Liq. (Paddock).
Marax DF, Syr. (Roerig).
Quibron, Cap., Liq. (Bristol-Myers).
Quibron-300, Cap. (Bristol-Myers).
Quibron Plus, Cap. (Bristol-Myers).
Slo-Phyllin Gg, Cap., Syr. (Dooner).
Synophylate, Liq. (Schwarz Pharma).
Tedral SA, Tab. (Parke-Davis).
Theofenal, Tab. (Cumberland).
Theolair Plus, Tab., Liq. (3M).
Theo-Organidin, Elix. (Wampole Laboratories).

theophylline and guaifenesin capsules.
Use: Bronchodilator, expectorant.

theophylline and guaifenesin oral solution.
Use: Bronchodilator, expectorant.

theophylline KI. (Various Mfr.) Theophylline 80 mg, potassium iodide 130 mg/ 15 ml. Elix. 480 ml, gal. *Rx.*
Use: Antiasthmatic combination.

theophylline olamine. Theophylline compound with 2-amino-ethanol (1:1).
Use: Bronchodilator.

theophylline with phenobarbital combinations.
See: Asma-Lief, Tab., Susp. (Quality Formulations).
Bronkolixir, Elix. (Sanofi).
Bronkotab, Tab. (Sanofi).
Ceepa, Tab. (Geneva Pharm).

theophylline reagent strips. (Bayer Corp) Seralyzer reagent strip. Bot. 25s.
Use: Diagnostic aid, theophylline.

•**theophylline sodium glycinate.** (thee-AHF-ih-lin so-dee-uhm) U.S.P. 23.
Use: Bronchodilator.
See: Synophylate, Elix., Tab. (Schwarz Pharma).
W/Guaifenesin.
See: Asbron G, Tab., Elix. (Novartis).
Synophylate-GG, Tab., Syr. (Schwarz Pharma).
W/Phenobarbital.
See: Synophylate w/Phenobarbital, Tab. (Schwarz Pharma).
W/Potassium iodide.
See: TSG-KI, Elix. (Zeneca).
W/Potassium iodide, ephedrine HCl, codeine phosphate.
See: TSG Croup Liquid. (Zeneca).
W/Racephedrine & phenobarbital.
See: Synophedal, Tab. (Schwarz Pharma).

Theo-Sav. (Savage) Theophylline 100 mg/Tab. Bot. 100s. 200 mg or 300 mg/Tab. Bot. 100s, 500s, 1000s. *Rx.*
Use: Bronchodilator.

Theospan-SR 130. (Laser) Theophylline anhydrous 130 mg/Cap. Bot. 100s, 1000s. *Rx.*
Use: Bronchodilator.

Theospan-SR 260. (Laser) Theophylline anhydrous 260 mg/Cap. Bot. 100s, 1000s. *Rx.*
Use: Bronchodilator.

Theostat 80 Syrup. (Laser) Theophylline anhydrous 80 mg/15 ml. Bot. Pt., Gal. *Rx.*
Use: Bronchodilator.

Theotal. (Major) Theophylline 125 mg, ephedrine HCl 25 mg, phenobarbital 8 mg, lactose. Tab. Bot. 1000s. *Rx.*
Use: Antiasthmatic combination.

Theo-Time. (Major) Theophylline 100 mg, 200 mg and 300 mg/Tab. T.R. Bot. 100s, 500s. *Rx.*
Use: Bronchodilator.

Theo-Time SR Tabs. (Major) Theophylline 100 mg, 200 mg, or 300 mg/S.R. Tab. Bot. 100s, 500s.
Use: Bronchodilator.

Theovent Long-Acting. (Schering Plough) Theophylline anhydrous 125 mg or 250 mg/Cap. Bot. 100s. *Rx.*
Use: Bronchodilator.

Theo-X. (Schwarz Pharma) Theophylline anhydrous 100 mg, 200 mg or 300 mg/Tab. Dye free, lactose. CR Tab. Bot. 100s, 500s, 1000s. *Rx.*
Use: Bronchodilator.

Thera Bath. (Walgreens) Mineral oil 90%. Bot. 16 oz. *otc.*
Use: Emollient.

Thera Bath with Vitamin E. (Walgreens) Mineral oil 91%, Vit E 2000 IU/16 oz. *otc.*
Use: Emollient.

Therabid. (Mission Pharmacal) Vitamins C 500 mg, B_1 15 mg, B_2 10 mg, B_3 100 mg, B_5 20 mg, B_6 10 mg, B_{12} 5 mcg, A 5000 IU, D 200 IU, E 30 mg/Tab. Bot. 60s. *otc.*
Use: Mineral, vitamin supplement.

Therabloat. (Norden) Poloxalene.

Therabrand. (Health for Life Brands) Vitamins A 25,000 IU, D 1000 IU, B_1 10 mg, B_2 10 mg, niacinamide 100 mg, C 200 mg, B_6 5 mg, calcium pantothenate 20 mg, B_{12} 5 mcg/Cap. Bot. 100s, 1000s. *otc.*
Use: Mineral, vitamin supplement.

Therabrand-M. (Health for Life Brands) Vitamins A 25,000 IU, D 1000 IU, C 200 mg, B_1 10 mg, B_2 10 mg, B_6 5 mg, niacinamide 100 mg, calcium pantothenate 20 mg, E 5 IU, B_{12} 5 mcg, iodine 0.15 mg, iron 15 mg, copper 1 mg, calcium 125 mg, manganese 1 mg, magnesium 6 mg, zinc 1.5 mg/Cap. Bot. 100s, 1000s. *otc.*
Use: Mineral, vitamin supplement.

Therac. (C & M Pharmacal) Colloidal sulfur 4% in lotion base. Bot. 60 ml. *otc.*
Use: Antiacne.

Theracap. (Arcum) Vitamins A 10,000 IU, D 400 IU, B_1 10 mg, B_2 5 mg, niacinamide 150 mg, C 150 mg/Cap. Bot. 100s, 1000s. *otc.*
Use: Vitamin supplement.

Thera-Combex H-P. (Parke-Davis) Vitamins C 500 mg, B_1 25 mg, B_2 15 mg, B_{12} 5 mcg, niacinamide 100 mg, panthenol 20 mg/Cap. Bot. 100s. *otc.*
Use: Vitamin supplement.

TheraCys. (Pasteur Merieux Connaught) 81 mg dry weight per vial, 1.7 to 19.2 $\times 10^8$ CFU per vial. Vial with 3 ml vial of diluent; 50 ml vials of phosphate-buffered sodium chloride are available for use as final diluent. *Rx.*
Use: Antineoplastic.

TheraFlu, Flu and Cold Medicine. (Novartis) Pseudoephedrine HCl 60 mg, chlorpheniramine maleate 4 mg, acetaminophen 650 mg, sucrose, lemon flavor. Pow. Pks. 6, 12. *otc.*
Use: Analgesic, antihistamine, decongestant.

TheraFlu, Flu Cold & Cough Medicine. (Novartis) Pseudoephedrine HCl 60 mg, chlorpheniramine maleate 4 mg, dextromethorphan HBr 20 mg, acetaminophen 650 mg. Pow. Pks. 6s. *otc.*
Use: Analgesic, antihistamine, antitussive, decongestant.

Thera-Flu Non-Drowsy Flu, Cold & Cough Maximum Strength. (Novartis) Pseudoephedrine HCl 60 mg, dextromethorphan HBr 30 mg, acetaminophen 1000 mg. Pow. 6s, 12s. *otc.*
Use: Analgesic, antitussive, decongestant.

Thera-Flu Non-Drowsy Formula, Maximum Strength. (Novartis) Pseudoephedrine HCl 30 mg, dextromethorphan HBr 15 mg, acetaminophen 500 mg. Capl. Pkg. 24s. *otc.*
Use: Antitussive, decongestant.

Thera-Flur. (Colgate Oral) Fluoride 0.5% (from sod. fluoride 1.1%). pH 4.5. Gel-Drops. Bot. 24 and 60 ml. *Rx.*
Use: Dental caries agent.

Thera-Flur-N. (Colgate Oral) Neutral sodium fluoride 1.1% Bot. 24 ml, 60 ml. *Rx.*
Use: Dental caries agent.

Therafortis. (General Vitamin) Vitamins A 12,500 IU, D 1000 IU, B_1 5 mg, B_2 5 mg, B_6 1 mg, B_{12} 3 mcg, niacinamide 50 mg, pantothenic acid salt 10 mg, C 150 mg, folic acid 0.5 mg/Cap. Bot. 100s, 1000s. *otc.*
Use: Vitamin supplement.

Theragenerix. (Zenith Goldline) Vitamins A 5500 IU, D 400 IU, E 30 mg, B_1 3 mg, B_2 3.4 mg, B_3 30 mg, B_5 10 mg, B_6 3 mg, B_{12} 9 mcg, C 120 mg, folic acid 0.4 mg, biotin 15 mcg, betacarotene 2500 IU. Tab. Bot. 130s, 1000s. *otc.*
Use: Vitamin supplement.

Theragenerix-H. (Zenith Goldline) Iron 66.7 mg, vitamins A 8333 IU, D 133 IU, E 5 IU, B_1 3.3 mg, B_2 3.3 mg, B_3 33.3 mg, B_5 11.7 mg, B_6 3.3 mg, B_{12} 50 mcg, C 100 mg, folic acid 0.33 mg, Cu, Mg/Tab. Bot. 100s, 1000s. *otc.*
Use: Mineral, vitamin supplement.

Theragenerix-M. (Zenith Goldline) Iron 27 mg, vitamins A 5000 IU, D 400 IU, E 30 mg, B_1 3 mg, B_2 3.4 mg, B_3 30 mg, B_5 10 mg, B_6 3 mg, B_{12} 9 mcg, C 120 mg, folic acid 0.4 mg, Ca, Cl, Cr, Cu, I, K, biotin 15 mcg, Mg, Mn, Mo, P, Se, zinc 15 mg, beta carotene 2500 IU. Tab. Bot. 130s, 1000s. *otc.*
Use: Mineral, vitamin supplement.

Thera-Gesic. (Mission Pharmacal) Methylsalicylate, menthol. Balm. In 90 g, 150 g. *otc.*
Use: Analgesic, topical.

Theragran. (Bristol-Myers Squibb) Vitamins A 5000 IU, D 400 IU, E 30 IU, B_1 3 mg, B_2 3.4 mg, B_3 20 mg, B_5 10 mg, B_6 3 mg, B_{12} 9 mcg, C 90 mg, folic acid 0.4 mg, biotin 30 mcg/Capl. Bot. 100s. *otc.*
Use: Vitamin supplement.

Theragran AntiOxidant. (Bristol-Myers Squibb) Vitamins A 5000 IU, C 250 mg, E 200 IU, Mn, Cu, Zn, Se/Softgel Cap. Bot. 50s. *otc.*
Use: Mineral, vitamin supplement.

Theragran Jr. with Iron. (Bristol-Myers Squibb) Iron 18 mg, vitamins A 5000 IU, D 400 IU, E 30 mg, B_1 1.5 mg, B_2 1.7 mg, B_3 20 mg, B_6 2 mg, B_{12} 6 mcg, C 60 mg, folic acid 0.4 mg w/tartrazine/Tab. Bot. 75s. *otc.*
Use: Mineral, vitamin supplement.

Theragran Hematinic. (Apothecon) Iron 66.7 IU, vitamins A 1400 IU, D 400 IU, E 5 IU, B_1 3.3 mg, B_2 3.3 mg, B_3 33.3 mg, B_5 11.7 mg, B_6 3.3 mg, B_{12} 50 mcg, C 100 mg, folic acid 0.33 mg, Ca, Cu, Mg/Tab. Bot. 90s. *Rx.*
Use: Mineral, vitamin supplement.

Theragran Liquid. (Bristol-Myers Squibb) Vitamins A 5000 IU, D 400 IU, B_1 10 mg, B_2 10 mg, B_3 100 mg, B_5 21.4 mg, B_6 4.1 mg, B_{12} 5 mcg, C 200 mg/5 ml. Liq. Bot. 120 ml. *otc.*
Use: Vitamin supplement.

Theragran-M. (Bristol-Myers Squibb) Ca 40 mg, iron 27 mg, vitamins A 5000 IU, D 400 IU, E 30 mg, B_1 3 mg, B_2 3.4 mg, B_3 20 mg, B_5 10 mg, B_6 3 mg, B_{12} 9 mcg, C 90 mg, folic acid 0.4 mg, Cl, Cr, Cu, I, K, Mg, Mn, Mo, P, Se, Zn 15 mg, biotin 30 mcg, lactose, sucrose/ Capl. Bot. 90s, 130s, 180s, 200s. *otc.*
Use: Mineral, vitamin supplement.

Theragran Stress Formula. (Bristol-Myers Squibb) Iron 27 mg, vitamins E 30 IU, B_1 15 mg, B_2 15 mg, B_3 100 mg, B_5 20 mg, B_6 25 mg, B_{12} 12 mcg, C 600 mg, folic acid 0.4 mg, biotin 45 mcg/ Tab. Bot. 75s. *otc.*
Use: Mineral, vitamin supplement.

Thera Hematinic. (Major) Iron 66.7 mg, A 8333 IU, D 133 IU, E 5 IU, B_1 3.3 mg, B_2 3.3 mg, B_3 33.3 mg, B_5 11.7 mg, B_6 3.3 mg, B_{12} 50 mcg, C 100 mg, folic acid 0.33 mg, Cu, Mg/Tab. Bot. 250s, 1000s. *otc.*
Use: Mineral, vitamin supplements.

Thera-Hist. (Major) Pseudoephedrine HCl 60 mg, chlorpheniramine maleate 4 mg, acetaminophen 500 mg, sucrose. Pow. Pks. 6. *otc.*
Use: Analgesic, antihistamine, decongestant.

Thera-Hist Syrup. (Major) Phenylpropanolamine HCl 12.5 mg, chlorpheniramine maleate 2 mg/5 ml. Syr. Bot. 120 ml. *otc.*
Use: Antihistamine, decongestant.

Thera H Tabs. (Major) Bot. 100s, 250s.
Use: Mineral, vitamin supplement.

Thera-M. (Various Mfr.) Vitamins A 5000 IU, B_1 3 mg, B_2 3.4 mg, B_3 20 mg, B_5 10 mg, B_6 3 mg, B_{12} 9 mcg, C 90 mg, D 400 IU, E 30 IU, iron 27 mg, folic acid 0.4 mg, biotin 30 mcg, P, Ca, Cu, Cr, Se, Mo, K, Cl, I, Mg, Mn, zinc 15 mg. Tab. Bot. 130s, 1000s. *otc.*
Use: Mineral, vitamin supplement.

Thera Multi-Vitamin. (Major) Vitamins A 10,000 IU, D 400 IU, B_1 10 mg, B_2 10 mg, B_3 100 mg, B_5 21.4 mg, B_6 4.1 mg, B_{12} 5 mcg, C 200 mg/5 ml. Liq. Bot. 118 ml. *otc.*
Use: Vitamin supplement.

Theramycin Z. (Medicis Dermatologics) Erythromycin 2%, SD alcohol 40-B 81%. Topical Soln. 60 ml. *Rx.*
Use: Dermatologic, acne.

Theraneed. (Hanlon) Vitamins A 16,000 IU, B_1 10 mg, B_2 10 mg, B_6 2 mg, C 300 mg, calcium pantothenate 10 mg, niacinamide 10 mg, B_{12} 10 mcg/Cap. Bot. 100s. *otc.*
Use: Mineral, vitamin supplement.

Therapals. (Faraday) Vitamins A 25,000 IU, D 400 IU, B_1 10 mg, B_2 5 mg, niacinamide 150 mg, B_6 0.5 mg, E 5 IU, C 150 mg, B_{12} 10 mcg, calcium 103 mg, cobalt 0.1 mg, copper 1 mg, potassium 0.15 mg, magnesium 6 mg, manganese 1 mg, molybdenum 0.2 mg, phosphorus 80 mg, potassium 5 mg, zinc 1.2 mg/Tab. Bot. 100s, 250s, 1000s. *otc.*
Use: Mineral, vitamin supplement.

Therapeutic B Complex with Vitamin C. (Upsher-Smith Labs) Vitamins B_1 15 mg, B_2 10.2 mg, B_3 50 mg, B_5 10 mg, B_6 5 mg, C 300 mg/Cap. Bot. UD 100s. *otc.*
Use: Vitamin supplement.

Therapeutic-H. (Zenith Goldline) Iron 66.7 mg, A 8333 IU, D 133 IU, E 5 IU, B_1 3.3 mg, B_2 3.3 mg, B_3 33.3 mg, B_5 11.7 mg, B_6 3.3 mg, B_{12} 50 mcg, C 100 mg, folic acid 0.33 mg, Cu, Mg/Tab. Bot. 100s. *otc.*
Use: Mineral, vitamin supplement.

Therapeutic-M. (Zenith Goldline) Iron 27 mg, vitamins A 5000 IU, D 400 IU, E 30 IU, B_1 3 mg, B_2 3.4 mg, B_3 20 mg, B_5 10 mg, B_6 3 mg, B_{12} 9 mcg, C 90 mg, folic acid 0.4 mg, Ca, Cl, Cr, Cu, I, K, Mg, Mn, Mo, P, Se, Zn 15 mg, biotin 30 mcg/Tab. Bot. 1000s. *otc.*
Use: Mineral, vitamin supplement.

Therapeutic Mineral Ice. (Bristol-Myers) Menthol 2%, ammonium hydroxide, carbomer 934, cupric sulfate, isopropyl alcohol, magnesium sulfate, thymol. Gel. Tube 105 g, 240 g, 480 g. *otc.*
Use: Liniment.

Therapeutic Tablets. (Zenith Goldline) Vitamins A 5000 IU, D 400 IU, E 30 IU, B_1 3 mg, B_2 3.4 mg, B_3 20 mg, B_5 10 mg, B_6 3 mg, B_{12} 9 mcg, C 90 mg, folic acid 0.4 mg, d-biotin 30 mcg/Tab. Bot. 100s, 130s. *otc.*
Use: Vitamin supplement.

Therapeutic V & M. (Whiteworth Towne) Vitamins A 10,000 IU, D 400 IU, B_1 10 mg, B_2 10 mg, B_6 5 mg, B_{12} 5 mcg, niacinamide 100 mg, calcium pantothenate 20 mg, C 200 mg, E 15 IU, iodine 0.15 mg, iron 12 mg, copper 2 mg, manganese 1 mg, magnesium 60 mg, zinc 1.5 mg/Tab. *otc.*
Use: Mineral, vitamin supplement.

Therapeutic Vitamin Formula w/Minerals. (Towne) Vitamins A palmitate 10,000 IU, D 400 IU, B_1 15 mg, B_2 10 mg, B_6 5 mg, B_{12} 12 mcg, C 200 mg, niacinamide 100 mg, calcium pantothenate 20 mg, E 15 IU, calcium 103 mg, iron 10 mg, manganese 1 mg, potassium 5 mg, zinc 1.5 mg, magnesium 6 mg/Cap. Bot. 30s, 60s, 100s, 250s. *otc.*
Use: Mineral, vitamin supplement.

Therapeutic Vitamin Formula w/Minerals. (Towne) Vitamins A palmitate 25,000 IU, D 1000 IU, B_1 10 mg, B_2 5 mg, B_6 1 mg, B_{12} 5 mcg, C 150 mg, niacinamide 100 mg, calcium 103 mg, phosphorus 80 mg, iron 10 mg, iodine 0.1 mg, manganese 1 mg, potassium 5 mg, copper 1 mg, zinc 1.4 mg, magnesium 5.5 mg/Cap. Bot. 100s, 1000s. *otc.*
Use: Mineral, vitamin supplement.

Theraphon. (Health for Life Brands) Vitamins A 25,000 IU, D 1000 IU, B_1 10 mg, B_2 5 mg, C 150 mg, niacinamide 150 mg/Cap. Bot. 100s, 1000s. *otc.*
Use: Vitamin supplement.

Theraplex T. (Medicis Dermatologics) Coal tar 1%, benzyl alcohol. Shampoo. Bot. 240 ml. *otc.*
Use: Antiseborrheic.

Theraplex Z. (Medicis Dermatologics) Pyrithione zinc 1%. Shampoo. Bot. 240 ml. *otc.*
Use: Antiseborrheic.

Theravee Hematinic Vitamin. (Vangard) Iron 66.7 mg, A 8333 IU, D 133 IU, E 5 IU, B_1 3.3 mg, B_2 3.3 mg, B_3 33.3 mg, B_5 11.7 mg, B_6 3.3 mg, B_{12} 50 mcg, C 100 mg, folic acid 0.33 mg, Cu, Mg/Tab. Bot. UD 100s. *otc.*
Use: Mineral, vitamin supplement.

Theravee-M. (Vangard) Iron 27 mg, vitamin A 5000 IU, D 400 IU, E 30 IU, B_1 3 mg, B_2 3.4 mg, B_3 30 mg, B_5 10 mg, B_6 3 mg, B_{12} 9 mcg, C 120 mg, folic acid 0.4 mg, Ca, Cl, Cr, Cu, K, I, Mg, Mn, Mo, Se, Zn 15 mcg, biotin 15 mcg, beta carotene 2500 IU/Tab. Bot. 100s, 1000s. UD 100s. *otc.*
Use: Mineral, vitamin supplement.

Theravee Vitamin. (Vangard) Vitamins A 5500 IU, D 400 IU, E 30 IU, B_1 3 mg, B_2 3.4 mg, B_3 30 mg, B_5 10 mg, B_6 3 mg, B_{12} 9 mcg, C 120 mg, folic acid 0.4 mg, biotin 15 mcg/Tab. Bot. 100s. UD 100s. *otc.*

Use: Vitamin supplement.

Theravim. (NBTY) Vitamins A 5000 IU, D 400 IU, E 30 IU, B_1 3 mg, B_2 3.4 mg, B_3 30 mg, B_5 10 mg, B_6 3 mg, B_{12} 9 mcg, C 90 mg, folic acid 0.4 mg, beta carotene 1250 IU, biotin 35 mcg/Tab. Bot. 130s. *otc.*
Use: Vitamin supplement.

Theravim-M. (NBTY) Iron 27 mg, vitamins A 5000 IU, D 400 IU, E 30 mg, B_1 3 mg, B_2 3.4 mg, B_3 20 mg, B_5 10 mg, B_6 3 mg, B_{12} 9 mcg, C 90 mg, folic acid 0.4 mg, Ca, Cl, Cr, Cu, I, K, Mg, Mn, Mo, P, Se, zinc 15 mg, biotin 30 mcg/Tab. Bot. 130s. *otc.*
Use: Mineral, vitamin supplement.

Theravite. (Alphalma USPD) Vitamins A 10,000 IU, D 400 IU, B_1 10 mg, B_2 10 mg, B_3 100 mg, B_5 21.4 mg, B_6 4.1 mg, B_{12} 5 mcg, C 200 mg/5 ml. Liq. Bot. 118 ml. *otc.*
Use: Vitamin supplement.

Therems. (Rugby) Vitamins A 5000 IU, D 400 IU, E 30 mg, B_1 3 mg, B_2 3.4 mg, B_3 30 mg, B_5 10 mg, B_6 3 mg, B_{12} 9 mcg, C 120 mg, folic acid 0.4 mg, beta carotene 1250 IU, biotin 15 mcg/ Tab. Bot. 130s, 1000s. *otc.*
Use: Vitamin supplement.

Therems-M. (Rugby) Iron 27 mg, vitamins A 5500 IU, D 400 IU, E 30 mg, B_1 3 mg, B_2 3.4 mg, B_3 20 mg, B_5 10 mg, B_6 3 mg, B_{12} 9 mcg, C 90 mg, folic acid 0.4 mg, Ca, Cl, Cr, Cu, I, K, Mg, Mn, Mo, P, Se, zinc 15 mg, biotin 30 mcg/Tab. Bot. 90s, 100s, 1000s. *otc.*
Use: Mineral, vitamin supplement.

Therevac. (Jones Medical Industries) Docusate potassium 283 mg, benzocaine 20 mg/Tube capsule w/soft soap in PEG 400 and glycerin base. Unit 4 ml, packages 4s, 12s, 50s. *otc.*
Use: Bowel evacuant.

Therevac Plus. (Jones Medical Industries) Docusate sodium 283 mg, benzocaine 20 mg in a base of soft soap, PEG 400, glycerin/Cap. 3.9 g Jar 30s. Disposable enema. *otc.*
Use: Laxative.

Therevac-SB. (Jones Medical Industries) Docusate sodium 283 mg in a base of soft soap, PEG 400, glycerin/Cap. 3.9 g Bot. 30s. Disposable enema. *otc.*
Use: Laxative.

Therex No. 1. (Halsey) Vit A 10,000 IU, D 400 IU, E 15 IU, C 200 mg, B_1 10 mg, B_2 10 mg, niacinamide 100 mg, B_6 5 mg, B_{12} 5 mcg, calcium pantothenate 20 mg/Tab. Bot. 100s. *otc.*
Use: Vitamin/mineral supplement.

Therex and Zinc. (Halsey).
Use: Dietary supplement.

Therex-M. (Halsey) Vitamins A 10,000 IU, D 400 IU, E 15 IU, C 200 mg, B_1 10 mg, B_2 10 mg, niacinamide 100 mg, B_6 5 mg, B_{12} 5 mcg, calcium pantothenate 20 mg, iodine 150 mcg, iron 12 mg, Mg 65 mg, Cu 2 mg, zinc 1.5 mg, Mn 1 mg/Tab. Bot. 100s. *otc.*
Use: Mineral, vitamin supplement.

Therex-Z. (Halsey) Vitamins A 10,000 IU, D 400 IU, E 15 IU, C 200 mg, B_1 10 mg, B_2 10 mg, niacinamide 100 mg, B_{12} 5 mcg, B_6 5 mg, Ca pantothenate 20 mg, iodine 150 mcg, Cu 2 mg, iron 12 mg, Zn 22.5 mg/Tab. Bot. 100s. *otc.*
Use: Mineral, vitamin supplement.

Therma-Kool. (Nortech) Compresses in following sizes: 3"×5", 4"×9", 8.5"×10.5".
Use: Cold, hot compress.

Thermazene. (Sherwood Medical) Silver sulfadiazine 1% in white pet. Cream. In 50, 400 and 1000 g. *Rx.*
Use: Burn therapy.

Thermodent. (Mentholatum) Strontium Cl. 10%. Tubes. *otc.*
Use: Dentrifice.

Theroal. (Vangard) Theophylline 24 mg, ephedrine HCl 24 mg, phenobarbital 8 mg/Tab. Bot. 100s, 1000s. *Rx.*
Use: Antiasthmatic combination.

Theroxide Wash. (Medicis Dermatologics) Benzoyl peroxide 10%. Liq. 120 ml. *Rx.*
Use: Dermatologic, acid.

ThexForte. (KM Lee) Vitamins B_1 25 mg, B_2 15 mg, B_3 100 mg, B_5 10 mg, B_6 5 mg, C 500 mg/Cap. Bot. 75s. *otc.*
Use: Vitamin supplement.

Thia. (Sigma-Tau Pharmaceuticals) Thiamine HCl 100 mg/ml. Vial 30 ml. *Rx.*
Use: Vitamin supplement.

•**thiabendazole.** (THIGH-uh-BEND-uh-zole) U.S.P. 23.
Use: Anthelmintic.
See: Mintezol, Tab., Susp. (Merck).

thiacetarsamide sodium. Sodium mercaptoacetate S,S-diester with p-carbamoyldithiobenzenearsonous acid.
Use: Antitrichomonal.

Thia-Dia-Mer-Sulfonamides. Sulfadiazine w/sulfamerazine & sulfathiazole.

thialbarbital.
See: Kemithal.

•**thiamine hydrochloride.** (THIGH-uh-min) U.S.P. 23.
Use: Enzyme co-factor vitamin.
See: Apatate (Kenwood Labs).

Betalin S, Amp., Elixir, Tab. (Eli Lilly).
Thia, Vial (Sigma-Tau Pharmaceuticals).

•**thiamine mononitrate.** (THIGH-uh-min) U.S.P. 23.
Use: Enzyme co-factor vitamin.
W/Sodium salicylate, colchicine.

•**thiamiprine.** (thigh-AM-ih-preen) USAN.
Use: Antineoplastic.

•**thiamphenicol.** (THIGH-am-FEN-ih-kahl) USAN.
Use: Anti-infective.

•**thiamylal.** (thigh-AM-ih-lahl) U.S.P. 23.
Use: Anesthetic (intravenous)

•**thiamylal sodium, for injection.** U.S.P. 23.
Use: Anesthetic (intravenous).
See: Surital Sodium, Prep. (Parke-Davis).

thiazesim.
Use: Antidepressant.

•**thiazesim hydrochloride.** (thigh-AZE-eh-sim) USAN.
Use: Antidepressant.

•**thiazinamium chloride.** (THIGH-ah-ZIN-am-ee-uhm) USAN.
Use: Antiallergic.

thiethylene thiophosphoramide.
See: Thiotepa.

•**thiethylperazine.** (THIGH-eth-ill-PURR-ah-zeem) USAN.
Use: Central nervous system depressant; antiemetic.

•**thiethylperazine malate.** (THIGH-eth-ill-PURR-ah-zeen MAL-ee-ate) U.S.P. 23.
Use: Antiemetic.

•**thiethylperazine maleate.** U.S.P. 23.
Use: Antiemetic.
See: Norzine, Inj., Supp., Tab. (Purdue Frederick).
Torecan, Amp., Supp., Tab. (Boehringer Ingelheim).

thihexinol methylbromide.
Use: Anticholinergic.

•**thimerfonate sodium.** (thigh-MER-foe-nate) USAN.
Use: Anti-infective, topical.

•**thimerosal.** (thigh-MER-oh-sal) U.S.P. 23.
Use: Anti-infective, topical; pharmaceutic aid (preservative).
See: Aeroaid, Aerosol (Aeroceuticals).
Merphol Tincture 1:1000, Liq. (Jones Medical Industries).
Mersol, Liq. (Century Pharm).
Merthiolate, Prep. (Eli Lilly).
W/Trifluridine.
See: Viroptic, Soln. (Monarch Pharm).

thiocarbanidin. Under study.
Use: Tuberculosis.

thiocyanate sodium. Sodium thiocyanate.
Use: Hypotensive.

thiodinone. Name used for Nifuratel.

thiodiphenylamine.
See: Phenothiazine.

thiofuradene.

thioglycerol.
W/Sod. citrate, phenol, benzyl alcohol.
See: Sulfo-ganic, Vial (Marcen).

•**thioguanine.** (THIGH-oh-GWAHN-een) U.S.P. 23.
Use: Antineoplastic.
See: Tabloid (GlaxoWellcome).

thiohexamide. N-(p-Methyl-mercaptophenylsulfonyl)N'-cyclohexylurea.
Use: Blood sugar-lowering compound.

thioisonicotinamide. Under study.
Use: Antituberculosis.

Thiola. (Mission Pharmacal). Tiopronin 100 mg. Tablets: In 100s. *Rx.*
Use: Anticholelithiasis.

•**thiopental sodium.** (thigh-oh-PEN-tahl) U.S.P. 23.
Use: Anesthetic (intravenous), anticonvulsant.
See: Pentothal Sodium, Amp. (Abbott Laboratories).

thiopental sodium. (IMS) Thiopental sodium 20 mg/ml or 25 mg/ml. Pow. for Inj. **20 mg/ml:** 400 mg *Min-I-Mix* vial w/ injector; **25 mg/ml:** 250 or 500 mg *Min-I-Mix* vials w/ injector; 500 mg, 1 g, 2.5 g, 5 g, 10 g kits. *Rx.*
Use: Anesthetic, general.

thiophosphoramide.
See: Thiotepa, Vial (ESI Lederle Generics).

Thioplex. (Immunex) Thiotepa 15 mg. Powd. for Inj. Vials. *Rx.*
Use: Antineoplastic.

thiopropazate hydrochloride.
Use: Anxiolytic.

thioproperazine mesylate.
Use: Central depressant; antiemetic.

•**thioridazine.** (THIGH-oh-RID-uh-zeen) U.S.P. 23.
Use: Antipsychotic, hypnotic, sedative.
See: Mellaril, Preps. (Novartis).

•**thioridazine hydrochloride.** (THIGH-oh-RID-ah-zeen) U.S.P. 23.
Use: Antipsychotic, hypnotic, sedative.
See: Mellaril, Tabs., Soln. (Novartis).

thioridazine hydrochloride concentrate. (Various Mfr.) Thioridazine HCl **30 mg/ml.** Bot. 120 ml. **100 mg/ml.** Bot 120 ml, 3.4 ml (UD 100s). *Rx.*

Use: Antipsychotic.

thioridazine hydrochloride intensol oral solution. (Roxane) Thioridazine HCl oral concentrated soln. 30 mg/ml or 100 mg/ml. Bot. 120 ml w/calibrated dropper. *Rx.*
Use: Antipsychotic.

thioridazine hydrochloride tablets. (Various Mfr.) 10 mg, 15 mg, 25 mg, 50 mg, 100 mg, 150 mg, 200 mg. Bot. 100s, 500s, 1000s, UD 100s. *Rx.*
Use: Antipsychotic.

•**thiosalan.** (THIGH-oh-sal-AN) USAN.
Use: Disinfectant.

thiosalicylic acid salt.

Thiosulfil Forte. (Wyeth-Ayerst) Sulfamethizole 500 mg. Tab. Bot. 100s. *Rx.*
Use: Anti-infective.

•**thiotepa.** (thigh-oh-TEP-uh) U.S.P. 23.
Use: Antineoplastic.
See: Thioplex, Pow. For Inj. (Immunex).

thiotepa. (thigh-oh-TEP-uh) (ESI Lederle Generics) Powder for reconstitution: Thiotepa powder 15 mg, sodium chloride 80 mg, sodium bicarbonate 50 mg/Vial. Vial 15 mg. *Rx.*
Use: Antineoplastic.
See: Thioplex, Powd. (Immunex).

•**thiothixene.** (THIGH-oh-THIX-een) U.S.P. 23.
Use: Antipsychotic.
See: Navane, Cap. (Roerig).
Navane Concentrate Solution (Roerig).

•**thiothixene hydrochloride.** (THIGH-oh-THIX-een) U.S.P. 23.
Use: Antipsychotic.
See: Navane Cap. (Pfizer).

thiothixene. (Various Mfr.) Thiothixene. **Tab.:** 1 mg, 2 mg, 5 mg, 10 mg, 20 mg. Bot. 100s, 500s, 1000s. **Conc.:** 5 mg/ml. Bot. 30 ml, 120 ml. *Rx.*
Use: Antipsycotic.

thiothixene hydrochloride intensol. (Roxane) Thiothixene HCl 5 mg/ml, EDTA. Alcohol free. Soln. Bot. 30 ml, 120 ml with dropper. *Rx.*
Use: Antipsychotic.

thiouracil. 2-Thiouracil.
Use: Treatment of hyperthyroidism, antianginal, congestive heart failure.

thioxanthenes.
See: Chlorprothixine (Taractan Roche).
Navane (Roerig).
Thiothixine (Various Mfr.).

thioxanthene derivative.
See: Taractan, Prep. (Roche Laboratories).

thiphenamil. F.D.A. S-[2-(Diethylamino)-ethyl]-diphenylthioacetate.

•**thiphenamil hydrochloride.** (thigh-FEN-ah-mill) USAN.
Use: Muscle relaxant.

•**thiphencillin potassium.** (thigh-fen-SILL-in) USAN.
Use: Anti-infective.

Thipyri-12. (Sigma-Tau Pharmaceuticals) Vitamins B_1 1000 mg, B_6 1000 mg, cyanocobalamin (B_{12}) 10,000 mcg, sod. chloride 0.5%, sod. bisulfite 0.1%, benzyl alcohol (as preservative) 0.9%. Univial 10 ml. *Rx.*
Use: Vitamin supplement.

•**thiram.** (THIGH-ram) USAN.
Use: Antifungal.

Thixo-Flur Topical Gel. (Colgate Oral) Acidulated phosphate sodium fluoride in gel base 1.2%. Bot. 32 oz. 8 oz., 4 oz.
Use: Dental caries agent.

•**thonzonium bromide.** (thahn-ZOE-nee-uhm) USAN. U.S.P. XXII.
Use: Detergent.
W/Colistin base, neomycin base, hydrocortisone acetate, polysorbate 80, acetic acid, sodium acetate.
See: Coly-Mycin-S, Otic, Liq. (Warner Chilcott).
W/Isoproterenol.
See: Nebair, Aerosol (Warner Chilcott).
W/Neomycin sulfate, gramicidin, thonzylamine HCl, phenylephrine HCl.
See: Biomydrin, Spray, Drops (Warner Chilcott).

•**thonzylamine hydrochloride.** USAN.
Use: Antihistamine.

Thorazine. (SmithKline Beecham Pharmaceuticals) Chlorpromazine HCl,
Tab.: 10, 25, 50, 100, 200 mg. Bot. 100s, 1000s. *Rx.*
Amp.: 25 mg w/ascorbic acid 2 mg, sodium bisulfite 1 mg, sodium sulfite 1 mg, NaCl 6 mg/1 ml, 1 ml, 2 ml. Vial 10 ml.
Spansule: 30, 75, 150 & 200 mg. Bot. 50s.
Syr.: 10 mg/5 ml. Bot. 120 ml.
Supp.: Chlorpromazine base, w/glycerin, glyceryl monopalmitate, glyceryl monostearate, hydrogenated coconut oil fatty acids, hydrogenated palm kernel oil fatty acids. 25, 100 mg Box 12s. **Conc.:** 30 mg/ml. Bot. 120 ml. 100 mg/ml Bot. 240 ml.
Use: Antiemetic, antipsychotic.

Thorets. (Buffington) Benzocaine lozenge. Dispens-A-Kits 500s. Sugar, lactose and salt free. *otc.*

Use: Sore throat relief.

Thor-Prom Tabs. (Major) Chlorpromazine 10 mg, 25 mg, 50 mg, or 100 mg Tab. Bot. 100s, 1000s; 200 mg/Tab. Bot. 250s, 1000s.
Use: Antiemetic, antipsychotic.

Thor Syrup. (Towne) Dextromethorphan HBr 90 mg, pyrilamine maleate 22.5 mg, phenylephrine HCl 10 mg, ephedrine sulfate 15 mg, sod. citrate 325 mg, ammon. chloride 650 mg, guaifenesin 50 mg/fl. oz. Bot. 4 oz. *otc.*
Use: Antitussive, antihistamine, decongestant, expectorant.

•**thozalinone.** (thoe-ZAL-ah-nohn) USAN.
Use: Antidepressant.

Threamine DM. (Various Mfr.) Phenylpropanolamine HCl 12.5 mg, chlorpheniramine maleate 2 mg, dextromethorphan HBr 10 mg/5 ml Syr. Bot. pt., gal. *otc.*
Use: Antihistamine, antitussive, decongestant.

Three-Amine TD. (Eon Labs Manufacturing) Phenylpropanolamine HBr 50 mg, pheniramine maleate 25 mg, pyrilamine maleate 25 mg/Time Rel. Cap. *otc.*
Use: Antihistamine, decongestant.

•**threonine.** (THREE-oh-neen) U.S.P. 23.
Use: Amino acid, antispasmodic. [Orphan drug]
See: Threostat.

threonine. (Various Mfr.) Threonine 500 mg. **Capsules:** In 60s and 100s. **Tablets:** In 100s and 250s. *otc.*
Use: Nutritional supplement.

Threostat. (Tyson and Associates) *Rx.*
Use: Antispasmodic.
See: Threonine.

Throat Discs. (SmithKline Beecham Pharmaceuticals) Capsicum, peppermint, mineral oil, sucrose. Box 60s. *otc.*
Use: Throat preparation.

Throat-Eze. (Faraday) Cetylpyridinium chloride 1:3000, cetyl dimethyl benzyl ammonium chloride 1:3000, benzocaine 10 mg/Wafer. Loz., foil wrapped. Vial 15. *otc.*
Use: Anesthetic, local.

Thrombate III.
See: Antithrombin III Human.

•**thrombin.** (THRAHM-bin) U.S.P. 23.
Thrombin, topical, mammalian origin.
Use: Hemostatic.
See: Thrombinar, Pow. (Jones Medical Industries).
Thrombin-JMI, Pow. (Jones Medical Industries).
Thrombogen, Pow. (Johnson & Johnson Consumer Products).
Thrombostat, Pow. (Parke-Davis).

Thrombinar. (Jones Medical Industries) Thrombin topical. 1000 units: 50% mannitol, 45% sodium chloride. 5000 units: 50% mannitol, 45% sodium chloride, sterile water for injection. 50,000 units: 50% mannitol, 45% sodium chloride. Pow. Vials. Preservative free. *Rx.*
Use: Hemostatic, topical.

Thrombin-JMI. (Jones Medical Industries) Pow. 10,000, 20,000 or 50,000 units. *Rx.*
Use: Hemostatic, topical.

Thrombogen. (Johnson & Johnson Consumer Products) Thrombin 1000 units. 5000 units: With isotonic saline diluent and transfer needle. 10,000 units or 20,000 units: With isotonic saline diluent, benzethonium chloride and transfer needle. *Rx.*
Use: Hemostatic, topical.

thrombolytic enzymes.
See: Abbokinase (Abbott Laboratories).
Abbokinase Open-Cath (Abbott Laboratories).
Eminase (SmithKline Beecham Pharmaceuticals).
Kabikinase (Pharmacia & Upjohn).
Streptase (Astra).

thromboplastin.
Use: Diagnostic aid (prothrombin estimation).

Thrombostat. (Parke-Davis) Prothrombin is activated by tissue thromboplastin in the presence of calcium chloride. **1000 U.S. (N.I.H.) units:** Vial 10 ml: **5000 U.S. units:** Vial 10 ml and 5 ml diluent. **10,000 U.S. units:** Vial 20 ml and 10 ml diluent. **20,000 U.S. units:** Vial 30 ml and 20 ml diluent. *Rx.*
Use: Hemostatic.

Thylox. (C.S. Dent) Medicated bar soap w/absorbable sulfur. Bar 3.4 oz. *otc.*
Use: Cleanser.

•**thymalfasin.** (thigh-MAL-fah-sin) USAN.
Formerly Thymosin α*1.*
Use: Antineoplastic; vaccine enhancement; hepatitis, infectious disease treatment.

•**thymol.** (THIGH-mole) N.F. 18.
Use: Antifungal; anti-infective; anesthetic, local; antitussive; decongestant; pharmaceutic aid (stabilizer).
See: Vicks Regular & Wild Cherry Medicated Cough Drops (Procter & Gamble).
Vicks Vaporub, Oint. (Procter & Gamble).

W/Combinations.
See: Listerine Antiseptic, Soln. (Warner Lambert).

thymol. (Various Mfr.) 0.25 lb, 1 lb.
Use:
Use: Antifungal; anti-infective; anesthetic, local; antitussive; decongestant; pharmaceutic aid (stabilizer).

thymol iodide.
Use: Antifungal; anti-infective.

•**thymopentin.** (THIGH-moe-PEN-tin) USAN. *Formerly Thymopoietin 32-36.*
Use: Immunoregulator.

thymosin alpha-1.
Use: Antiviral, hepatitis B. [Orphan drug]

thyodatil. Name used for Nifuratel.

Thypinone. (Abbott Diagnostics) Protirelin 500 mcg/1 ml Amp.
Use: Diagnostic aid, thyroid.

Thyrar. (Rhone-Poulenc Rorer) Bovine thyroid preparation 0.5 gr, 1 gr, 2 gr/ Tab. Bot. 100s. *Rx.*
Use: Antihypothyroid.

Thyrel-TRH. (Ferring Pharmaceuticals) Protirelin 0.5 mg/ml/Inj. 1 ml. *Rx.*
Use: Diagnostic aid.

Thyro-Block. (Wallace Laboratories) Potassium iodide 130 mg/Tab. In 14s. *Rx.*
Use: Antithyroid.

•**thyroid.** (THIGH-royd) U.S.P. 23.
Use: Hormone, thyroid.
See: Arco Thyroid, Tab. (Arco).
Armour Thyroid, Tab. (Rhone-Poulenc Rorer).
Delcoid, Tab. (Delco).
Marion Thyroid, Tab. (Hoechst Marion Roussel).
S-P-T., Cap. (Fleming).

thyroid combinations.
See: Henydin, Prep. (Arcum).

thyroid desiccated. (THIGH-royd DESS-ih-KATE-uhd)
Use: Hormone, thyroid.
See: Armour Thyroid (Rhone-Poulenc Rorer).
S-P-T (Fleming).
Thyrar (Rhone-Poulenc Rorer).
Thyroid Strong (Jones Medical Industries).
Thyroid USP (Various Mfr.).

thyroid diagnostic aids.
Use: Diagnostic aid.
See: Relefact TRH (Hoechst Marion Roussel).
Sodium Iodide I 123 (Mallinckrodt Diagnostics).
Thypinone (Abbott Laboratories).
Thytropar (Centeon).

thyroid hormones.
See: Liothyronine Sod.
Thyroxin (Various Mfr.).

thyroid preparations.
See: Proloid, Tab. (Parke-Davis).
Thyrar, Tab. (Rhone-Poulenc Rorer).
Thyroxin, Prep. (Var. Mfr.).

thyroid stimulating hormone (TSH).
Use: Adjunct in diagnosis of thyroid cancer. [Orphan drug]

Thyroid Strong. (Jones Medical Industries) Thyroid desiccated 30 mg, 60 mg, 120 mg/Tab. Bot. 100s, 1000s; 30 mg, 120 mg, 180 mg Tab. Bot. 100s; 60 mg/sugar coated. Tab. Bot. 100s, 1000s. *Rx.*
Use: Hormone, thyroid.

Thyrolar. (Forest Pharmaceutical) Liotrix. 0.25 gr/Tab. Bot. 100s; 0.5 gr, 1 gr, 2 gr, 3 gr/Tab. Bot. 100s, 1000s. *Rx.*
Use: Hormone, thyroid.

•**thyromedan hydrochloride.** (thigh-ROW-meh-dan) USAN.
Use: Thyromimetic.

thyropropic acid. 4-(4-Hydroxy-3-iodophenoxy)-3,5-diio-dohydrocinnamic acid. Triopron (Warner Chilcott).
Use: Anticholesteremic.

thyrotropic hormone. *Rx.*
Use: In vivo diagnostic aid.
See: Thytropar (Centeon).

thyrotropic principle of bovine anterior pituitary glands.
See: Thytropar, Vial (Centeon Labs.).

thyrotropin.
Use: Diagnostic aid.
See: Thytropar (Centeon).

thyrotropin-releasing hormone.
Use: Diagnostic aid.
See: Relefact TRH (Hoechst Marion Roussel).
Thypinone (Abbott Laboratories).

•**thyroxine I 125.** (thigh-ROX-een) USAN.
Use: Radiopharmaceutical.

•**thyroxine I 131.** USAN.
Use: Radiopharmaceutical.

thyrozyme-II A. (Abbott Diagnostics) T-4 diagnostic kit. 100 & 500 test units.
Use: Diagnostic aid, thyroid.

Thytropar. (Centeon) Thyrotropin from bovine anterior pituitary glands. Thyrotropin. Vial 10 IU.
Use: Thyroid agent.

•**tiacrilast.** (TIE-ah-KRILL-ast) USAN.
Use: Antiallergic.

•**tiacrilast sodium.** (TIE-ah-KRILL-ast) USAN.
Use: Antiallergic.

Tiagabine. (Abbott/Novo Nordisk)
Use: Antiepileptic.

•**tiagabine hydrochloride.** USAN.
Use: Anticonvulsant.
See: Gabitril, Tab. (Abbott)

Tiamate. (Hoechst Marion Roussel) Diltiazem maleate 120 mg, 180 mg, 240 mg, sucrose/ER Tab. Bot. UD 30s. *Rx.*
Use: Calcium channel blocker.

•**tiamenidine.** (TIE-ah-MEN-ih-DEEN) USAN.
Use: Antihypertensive.

•**tiamenidine hydrochloride.** (TIE-ah-MEN-ih-DEEN) USAN.
Use: Antihypertensive.

•**tiapamil hydrochloride.** (tie-APP-ah-mill) USAN.
Use: Antagonist (to calcium).

•**tiaramide hydrochloride.** (TIE-ar-ah-MIDE) USAN.
Use: Antiasthmatic.

Tiazac. (Forest Pharmaceutical) Diltiazem HCl 120, 180, 240, 300 or 360 mg/ER Cap. Bot. 30s, 90s, 1000s. *Rx.*
Use: Calcium channel blocker.

•**tiazofurin.** (TIE-AZE-oh-few-rin) USAN.
Use: Antineoplastic.

TI-Baby Natural. (Fischer) Titanium dioxide 5%. SPF 16. Lot. Bot. 120 ml. *otc.*
Use: Sunscreen.

•**tibenelast sodium.** (TIE-ben-ell-ast) USAN.
Use: Antiasthmatic; bronchodilator.

•**tibolone.** (TIH-bole-ohn) USAN.
Use: Menopausal symptoms suppressant.

•**tibric acid.** (TIE-brick) USAN.
Use: Antihyperlipoproteinemic.

•**tibrofan.** (TIE-broe-fan) USAN.
Use: Disinfectant.

•**ticabesone propionate.** (tie-CAB-eh-sone) USAN.
Use: Corticosteroid, topical.

Ticar. (SmithKline Beecham Pharmaceuticals) Ticarcillin disodium. 1 g, 3 g, 6 g/Vial in 10s. Piggyback Vials 3 g in 10s. Bulk Pharmacy Pkg. 20 g in 10s. Bulk Pharmacy Pkg. 30 g/Vial, 10s. ADD-Vantage 3 g Pkg. 10s. *Rx.*
Use: Anti-infective.

•**ticarbodine.** (tie-CAR-boe-deen) USAN.
Use: Anthelmintic.

ticarcillin and clavulanate potassium.
Use: Penicillin.
See: Timentin Preps. (SmithKline Beecham Pharmaceuticals).

•**ticarcillin cresyl sodium.** (tie-CAR-SIH-lin KREH-sill) USAN.
Use: Anti-infective.

•**ticarcillin disodium, sterile.** (tie-CAR-SIH-lin) U.S.P. 23.
Use: Anti-infective.
See: Ticar, inj. (SmithKline Beecham Pharmaceuticals).

ticarcillin disodium and clavulanate potassium, sterile.
Use: Anti-infective, inhibitor (β-lactamase).
See: Timentin, Inj. (SmithKline Beecham Pharmaceuticals).

•**ticarcillin monosodium.** (tie-CAR-SIH-lin) U.S.P. 23.
Use: Anti-infective.

TICE BCG Vaccine. (Organon Teknika) BCG. Intravesical 50 mg/2 ml amps. Freeze-dried suspension for reconstitution. *Rx.*
Use: Antineoplastic.

•**ticlatone.** (TIE-klah-tone) USAN.
Use: Anti-infective, antifungal.

Ticlid. (Syntex) Ticlopidine 250 mg/Tab. Bot. 30s, UD 100s. *Rx.*
Use: Antiplatelet.

•**ticlopidine hydrochloride.** (tie-KLOE-pih-DEEN) USAN.
Use: Inhibitor (platelet).
See: Ticlid, Tab. (Syntex).

•**ticolubant.** (tih-kahl-YOU-bant) USAN.
Use: Antipsoriatic.

Ticon. (Roberts Pharm) Trimethobenzamide HCl 100 mg per ml/Inj. Vial 20 ml. *Rx.*
Use: Antiemetic, antivertigo.

ticonazole.
Use: Antifungal, vaginal.
See: Vagistat-1, Oint. (Bristol-Myers Squibb).

•**ticrynafen.** (TIE-krin-ah-fen) USAN.
Use: Diuretic, uricosuric, antihypertensive.

Tidex. (Allison) Dextroamphetamine sulfate, 5 mg/Tab. Bot. 100s, 1000s. *c-II.*
Use: Antiobesity agent.

Tidexsol Tablets. (Sanofi) Acetaminophen. *otc.*
Use: Analgesic.

•**tifurac sodium.** (TIE-fyoor-ak) USAN.
Use: Analgesic.

Tigan. (Roberts Pharm) Trimethobenzamide hydrochloride. **Cap.** 100 mg Bot. 100s, 250 mg Bot. 100s. **Amp:** (100 mg/ml) 2 ml. Box 10s. Vial 20 ml **Supp:** 200 mg Box 10s, 50s. **Pediatric Supp:** 100 mg Box 10s. *Rx.*
Use: Antiemetic.

•**tigemonam dicholine.** (TIE-jem-OH-nam die-KOE-leen) USAN.
Use: Antimicrobial.

•**tigestol.** (tie-JESS-tole) USAN.
Use: Hormone, progestin.

Tigo. (Burlington) Polymyxin B sulfate 5000 units, zinc bacitracin 400 units, neomycin sulfate 5 mg/g Oint. Tube 0.5 oz. *otc.*
Use: Anti-infective, topical.

Tihist-DP. (Vita Elixir) d-methorphan HBr 10 mg, pyrilamine maleate 16 mg, sodium citrate 3.3 gr/5 ml. *otc.*
Use: Antitussive, antihistamine.

Tihist Nasal Drops. (Vita Elixir) Pyrilamine maleate 0.1%, phenylephrine HCl 0.25%, sodium bisulfite 0.2%, methylparaben 0.02%, propylparaben 0.01%/30 ml. *otc.*
Use: Antihistamine, decongestant.

Tija Tablets. (Vita Elixir) Oxytetracycline HCl 250 mg/Tab. *Rx.*
Use: Anti-infective, tetracycline.

Tija Syrup. (Vita Elixir) Oxytetracycline HCl 125 mg/5 ml. *Rx.*
Use: Anti-infective, tetracycline.

Tilade. (Medeva) Nedocromil sodium. 1.75 mg per actuation. Aerosol/Can. 16.2 g with mouthpiece. *Rx.*
Use: Respiratory, anti-inflammatory.

•**tiletamine hydrochloride.** (tie-LET-ah-meen) USAN.
Use: Anesthetic; anticonvulsant.

•**tilidine hydrochloride.** (TIH-lih-DEEN) USAN.
Use: Analgesic.

TI-lite. (Fischer) Ethylhexyl p-methoxycinnamate 7.5%, titanium dioxide 2%, cetyl alcohol, phenethyl alcohol, parabens, EDTA. Cream 60 g. *otc.*
Use: Sunscreen.

•**tilomisole.** (TILL-oh-mih-sahl) USAN.
Use: Immunoregulator.

•**tilorone hydrochloride.** (TIE-lore-ohn) USAN.
Use: Antiviral.

•**tiludronate disodium.** (tie-LOO-droe-nate) USAN.
Use: Paget's disease, osteoporosis.
See: Skelid, Tab. (Sanofi Winthrop).

Timed Reducing Aids-Caffeine Free. (Weeks & Leo) Phenylpropanolamine HCl 75 mg/T.R. Cap. Bot. 28s, 56s. *otc.*
Use: Dietary aid.

•**timefurone.** (tie-MEH-fyoor-OHN) USAN.
Use: Antiatherosclerotic.

Timentin. (SmithKline Beecham Pharmaceuticals) Ticarcillin disodium 3 g, clavulanic acid (as potassium salt) 0.1 g. Vials 3.1 g, Box 10s. Piggyback Vials 3.1 g, Box 10s. *Rx.*
Use: Anti-infective.

•**timobesone acetate.** (tie-MOE-beh-sone) USAN.
Use: Adrenocortical steroid, topical.

Timolide 10-25. (Merck) Timolol maleate 10 mg, hydrochlorothiazide 25 mg/Tab. Bot. 100s. *Rx.*
Use: Antihypertensive.

•**timolol.** (TI-moe-lahl) USAN.
Use: Antiadrenergic (β-receptor).
See: Betimol, Soln. (Ciba Vision).

•**timolol maleate.** (TI-moe-lahl) U.S.P. 23.
Use: Treatment of chronic open angle, aphakic and secondary glaucoma, antihypertensive, prevention of recurrent MI; antiadrenergic (β-receptor).
See: Blocadren, Tab. (Merck) Timoptic, Oph. (Merck).
Timoptic In Ocudose, Oph. (Merck).

timolol maleate. (TI-moe-lahl) (Various Mfr.) 0.25% or 0.5%. Ophth. Soln. Bot. 5 ml, 10 ml, 15 ml.
Use: Treatment of chronic open angle, aphakic and secondary glaucoma, antihypertensive, prevention of recurrent MI; antiadrenergic (β-receptor).

timolol maleate and hydrochlorothiazide tablets.
Use: Antihypertensive combination.
See: Timolide,Tab. (Merck).

timolol maleate ophthalmic solution. (Various) Timolol maleate 3.4 mg/0.25 ml and 6.8 mg/0.5 ml/Soln. Bot. 2.5 ml, 5 ml, 10 ml, 15 ml. *Rx.*
Use: Antiglaucoma agent.

Timoptic. (Merck) Timolol maleate 0.25% and 0.5% solution. Ocumeter Ophthalmic Dispenser 2.5 ml, 5 ml, 10 ml, 15 ml. *Rx.*
Use: Antiglaucoma agent.

Timoptic in Ocudose. (Merck) Timolol maleate 0.25% or 0.5%. Preservative free in sterile ocudose ophthalmic UD 60s. *Rx.*
Use: Antiglaucoma agent.

Timoptic-XE. (Merck) Timolol maleate 0.25% or 0.5%. Gel. Tube 2.5 ml, 5 ml. *Rx.*
Use: Antiglaucoma agent.

•**tinabinol.** (tie-NAB-ih-NOLE) USAN.
Use: Antihypertensive.

Tinactin. (Schering Plough) **Soln. 1%:** Tolnaftate (10 mg/ml) w/butylated hydroxytoluene, in nonaqueous homogeneous PEG 400. Plastic squeeze bot. 10 ml. **Cream 1%:** Tolnaftate (10 mg/g) in homogeneous, nonaqueous vehicle of PEG-400, propylene glycol, carboxypolymethylene, monoamylamine, titanium dioxide and butylated hydroxytolu-

ene. Tube 15 g, 30 g, UD 0.7 g. **Powder 1%:** Tolnaftate w/corn starch, talc. Plastic container 45 g, 90 g. **Powd. Aerosol 1%:** Tolnaftate w/butylated hydroxytoluene, talc, polyethylene-polypropylene glycol monobutyl ether, denatured alcohol and inert propellant of isobutane. Spray can 100 g. **Liq. Aerosol 1%:** Tolnaftate w/butylated hydroxytoluene, polyethylene-polyproplyene glycol monobutyl ether, 36% alcohol, and inert propellant of isobutane. Spray can 120 ml. *otc.*
Use: Antifungal.

Tinastat. (Vita Elixir) Sodium hyposulfite, benzethonium Cl/2 oz. *otc.*
Use: Keratolytic.

Tinaval Powder. (Pal-Pak) Tolnaftate 1%. Bot. 45 g. *otc.*
Use: Antifungal for jock itch, athlete's foot.

tine test, old tuberculin. (Wyeth Ayerst). Box of 25, 100 or 250 test applicators.
See: Tuberculin Tine Test (ESI Lederle Generics).

tine test, purified protein derivative. (Wyeth Ayerst). Box of 25 or 100 test applicators.
See: Tuberculin Tine Test (ESI Lederle Generics).

tin fluoride. Stannous Fluoride, U.S.P. 23.

•**tinidazole.** (tie-NIH-dah-zole) USAN.
Use: Antiprotozoal.
See: Fasigyn (Pfizer).

Tinset. (Janssen) Oxatomide.
Use: Antiallergic, antiasthmatic.

Tinver Lotion. (PBH Wesley Jessen) Sodium thiosulfate 25%, salicylic acid 1%, isopropyl alcohol 10%, propylene glycol, menthol, disodium edetate, colloidal alumina. Bot. 4 oz., 6 oz. *Rx.*
Use: Dermatologic.

•**tinzaparin sodium.** (tin-ZAP-ah-rin) USAN.
Use: Anticoagulant; antithrombotic.

•**tioconazole.** (TIE-oh-KOE-nah-zole) U.S.P. 23.
Use: Antifungal.
See: Vagistat (Fujisawa SmithKline)

•**tiodazosin.** (TIE-oh-DAY-zoe-sin) USAN.
Use: Antihypertensive.

•**tiodonium chloride.** (TIE-oh-doe-nee-uhm) USAN.
Use: Anti-infective.

•**tioperidone hydrochloride.** (tie-oh-PURR-ih-dohn) USAN.
Use: Antipsychotic.

•**tiopinac.** (tie-OH-pin-ACK) USAN.
Use: Anti-inflammatory, analgesic, antipyretic.

tiopronin.
Use: Homozygous cystinuria. [Orphan drug]
See: Thiola (Mission Pharmacal).

•**tiospirone hydrochloride.** (tie-OH-spih-rone) USAN.
Use: Antipsychotic.

•**tiotidine.** (TIE-OH-tih-deen) USAN.
Use: Antiulcerative.

•**tioxidazole.** (tie-OX-ih-DAH-zole) USAN.
Use: Anthelmintic.

•**tipentosin hydrochloride.** (TIE-pin-toe-SIN) USAN.
Use: Antihypertensive.

Tipramine Tabs. (Major) Imipramine 10 mg/Tab. Bot. 250s; 25 mg or 50 mg/ Tab. Bot. 250s, 1000s. *Rx.*
Use: Antidepressant.

•**tipredane.** (tie-PRED-ANE) USAN.
Use: Adrenocortical steroid, topical.

•**tiprenolol hydrochloride.** (tie-PREH-no-lole) USAN.
Use: Antiadrenergic (β-receptor).

•**tiprinast meglumine.** (TIE-prih-nast meh-GLUE-meen) USAN. A Bristol-Myers Squibb investigative drug.
Use: Antiallergic.

•**tipropidil hydrochloride.** (TIE-PRO-pih-dill) USAN.
Use: Vasodilator.

•**tiqueside.** (TIE-kweh-side) USAN.
Use: Antihyperlipidemic.

•**tiquinamide hydrochloride.** (tie-KWIN-ah-mide) USAN.
Use: Anticholinergic (gastric).

•**tirapazamine.** (tie-rah-PAZZ-ah-meen) USAN.
Use: Antineoplastic.

tiratricol.
Use: Antineoplastic. [Orphan drug]

•**tirilazad mesylate.** (tie-RIH-lah-zad MEH-sih-late) USAN.
Use: Inhibitor (lipid peroxidation).
See: Freedox (Pharmacia & Upjohn).

•**tirofiban hydrochloride.** (tie-rah-FIE-ban) USAN.
Use: Treatment of unstable angina.
See: Aggrastat, Inj. (Merck).

TI-Screen. (Pedinol) **Gel:** SPF 20+, ethylhexyl p-methoxycinnamate 7.5%, oxybenzone 5%, 2-ethylhexyl salicylate 5%, SD alcohol 40 71%. 120 g; **Lip Balm:** SPF 8+, ethylhexyl p-methoxycinnamate 7.5%, oxybenzone 5%, petrolatum. 4.5 g; **Lot.: SPF 8:** Ethylhexyl p-methoxycinnamate 6%, oxybenzone 2%. Bot. 120 ml; **SPF 15:** Ethyl-

hexyl p-methoxycinnamate 7.5%, oxybenzone 5%. Bot. 120 ml; **SPF 30:** Octyl methoxycinnamate 7.5%, octyl salicylate 5%, oxybenzone 6%, octocrylene 7.5%. Bot. 120 ml. *otc.*
Use: Sunscreen.

TI-Screen Natural. (Pedinol) Titanium dioxide 5%. Lot. Bot. 120 ml. *otc.*
Use: Sunscreen.

TI-Screen Sunless. (Pedinol) Octyl methoxycinnamate 7.5%, benzophene-3 3%, mineral oil, alcohols, PEG-100, parabens. SPF 17 or 23. Creme. 118 ml. *otc.*
Use: Sunscreen.

•**tisilfocon a.** (tih-sill-FOE-kahn) USAN.
Use: Contact lens material (hydrophobic).

Tisit. (Pfeiffer) Pyrethrins 0.3%, piperonyl butoxide technical 3%, petroleum distillate 1.2%, benzyl alcohol 2.4%. Shampoo. Bot. 118 ml. *otc.*
Use: Pediculicide.

TiSol. (Parnell) Benzyl alcohol 1%, menthol 0.04%, isotonic sodium chloride 0.9%, sorbitol, EDTA. Soln. Bot. 237 ml. *otc.*
Use: Throat preparation.

tissue fixative and wash solution. (Wampole Laboratories) A modified Michel's tissue fixative and buffered wash solution.
Use: Tissue specimen fixative.

tissue plasminogen activator, recombinant.
See: Activase (Genentech).

tissue respiratory factor (trf). (International Hormone) RSF, SRF, LYCD, PCO, Procytoxid marketed as 2000 units. Supplied as bulk liquid concentrate. *Rx.*
Use: Promotion of cellular oxidation.

Tis-U-Sol. (Baxter) Pentalyte irrigation containing NaCl 800 mg, KCl 40 mg, magnesium sulfate 20 mg, sodium phosphate 8.75 mg, and 6.25 mg monobasic potassium phosphate per 100 ml. Bot. 250 ml, 1000 ml. *Rx.*
Use: Irrigant.

Titan. (PBH Wesley Jessen) EDTA 2%, nonionic cleaner buffers, potassium sorbate 0.13%. Soln. Bot. 30 ml. *otc.*
Use: Contact lens care.

•**titanium dioxide,** (tie-TANE-ee-uhm die-OX-ide) U.S.P. 23.
Use: Solar ray protectant, topical.

titicum ripens.
W/Oxyquinoline sulfate, charcoal.
See: Triticoll, Tabs. (Western Research).

Titralac. (3M Pharm) Calcium carbonate 420 mg, saccharin, sodium 0.3 mg. Chew. Tab. Bot. 40s, 100s, 1000s. *otc.*
Use: Antacid.

Titralac Extra Strength Tablets. (3M Pharm) Calcium carbonate 750 mg, saccharin, sodium 0.6 mg. Chew. Tab. Bot. 100s. *otc.*
Use: Antacid.

Titralac Plus Liquid. (3M Personal Health Care) Calcium carbonate 500 mg, simethicone 20 mg, saccharin, sorbitol, sodium 0.15 mg. Bot. 360 ml. *otc.*
Use: Antacid.

Titralac Plus Tablets. (3M Pharm) Calcium carbonate 420 mg, simethicone 21 mg, saccharin, sodium 1.1 mg. Chew. Tab. Bot. 100s. *otc.*
Use: Antacid.

•**tixanox.** (TIX-ah-nox) USAN.
Use: Antiallergic.

•**tixocortol pivalate.** (tix-OH-kahr-tole PIH-vah-late) USAN.
Use: Anti-inflammatory, topical.

tizanidine hydrochloride. (tie-ZAN-ih-deen)
Use: Antispasmodic.
See: Zanaflex, Tab. (Athena Neurosciences).

•**tizanidine hydrochloride.** USAN.
Use: Antispasmodic. [Orphan drug]

T-Koff. (T.E. Williams) Phenylpropanolamine HCl 20 mg, phenylephrine HCl 20 mg, chlorpheniramine maleate 5 mg, codeine phosphate 10 mg/5 ml Syr. Bot. 480 ml Grape flavor. *c-v.*
Use: Antihistamine, antitussive, decongestant.

t-lymphotropic virus type III gp 160 antigens. *Rx.*
Use: Treatment for AIDS. [Orphan drug]
See: Vaxsyn HIV-1.

TMP-SMZ. *Rx.*
Use: Anti-infective.
See: Proloprim (GlaxoWellcome).
Trimethoprim (Various Mfr.).
Trimpex (Roche Laboratories).

TOBI. (PathoGenesis Corp) Tobramycin 300 mg, sodium chloride 11.25 g/5 ml. Soln for Inhalation. Single-use Amp. *Rx.*
Use: Cystic fibrosis.

Tobrades Suspension. (Alcon Laboratories) Dexamethasone 0.1%, tobramycin 0.3%, thimerisol 0.001%, alcohol 0.5%, propylene glycol, polyoxyethylene, polyoxypropylene. 2.5 ml, 5 ml. *Rx.*
Use: Anti-infective, corticosteroid.

TobraDex. (Alcon Laboratories). 0.3% tobramycin and 0.1% dexamethasone. Susp. Bot. 2.5 ml or 5 ml. *Rx.*
Use: Anti-infective, corticosteroid, ophthalmic.

TobraDex, Ointment. (Alcon Laboratories) Dexamethasone 0.1%, tobramycin 0.3%, chlorobutanol 0.5%, mineral oil, white petrolatum. Ophthalmic 3.5 g. *Rx.*
Use: Anti-infective, cortiocosteroid, ophthalmic.

•**tobramycin.** (TOE-bruh-MY-sin) U.S.P. 23. An antibiotic obtained from cultures of *Streptomyces tenebrarius.*
Use: Anti-infective, ophthalmic. [Orphan drug]
See: TOBI, Soln. (PathoGenesis).
Tobrex, Preps. (Alcon Laboratories).

tobramycin. (TOE-bruh-MY-sin) (Bausch & Lomb) Tobramycin 0.3%, benzalkonium Cl 0.01%, boric acid. Soln. 5 ml. *Rx.*
Use: Anti-infective, ophthalmic.

tobramycin and dexamethasone ophthalmic ointment.
Use: Anti-infective, ophthalmic.

tobramycin sulfate. (Various Mfr.) Tobramycin sulfate 40 mg/ml. Inj. Syringes: 1.5 ml, 2 ml. Vial 2 ml. Pediatric Inj. 10 mg/ml. Vial 2 ml. *Rx.*
Use: Aminoglycoside, anti-infective.

•**tobramycin sulfate.** (TOE-bruh-my-sin) U.S.P. 23.
Use: Anti-infective, aminoglycoside.
See: Nebcin, Amp., Hyporet. (Eli Lilly).

Tobrex Ophthalmic Ointment. (Alcon Laboratories) Tobramycin 0.3% in sterile ointment base. Tube 3.5 g. *Rx.*
Use: Anti-infective, ophthalmic.

Tobrex Solution. (Alcon Laboratories) Tobramycin 0.3%. ophthalmic solution. Bot. 5 ml Drop-Tainer. *Rx.*
Use: Anti-infective, ophthalmic.

•**tocainide.** (TOE-cane-ide) USAN.
Use: Antiarrhythmic, cardiovascular agent.
See: Tonocard, Tab. (Merck).

•**tocainide hydrochloride.** U.S.P. 23.
Use: Antiarrhythmic, cardiac depressant.

•**tocamphyl.** (toe-KAM-fill) USAN.
Use: Choleretic.
See: Gallogen, Tab. (SmithKline Beecham Pharmaceuticals).

tocopherol-dl-alpha. Vitamin E, U.S.P. 23.
Cap. & Tab.:
Denamone, Cap. (3 min., 10 min.) wheat germ oil (Vio-Bin).
Ecofrol, Cap. (O'Neal).
Eprolin, Gelseal (Eli Lilly).
Epsilan M, Cap. (Warren-Teed).
Oint.:
Myopone (Drug Prods.).
Sol.:
Aquasol E, Soln. (Rhone-Poulenc Rorer).

•**tocopherols excipient.** N.F. 18.
Use: Pharmaceutic aid (antioxidant).

•**tocophersolan.** (toe-KAHF-ehr-SO-lan) USAN.
Use: Vitamin supplement.

tocopheryl acetate-d-alpha. Vitamin E, U.S.P. 23.
See: Aquasol E, Prods. (Rhone-Poulenc Rorer).
Epsilan-M, Cap. (Warren-Teed).
Tocopher, Cap. (Quality Formulations).
Vitamins E. (Var. Mfr.).

tocopheryl acetates, conc. d-alpha. Vitamin E, U.S.P. 23.
Use: Treatment of habitual & threatened abortion.

tocopheryl acid succinated d-alpha. Vitamin E, U.S.P. 23.
See: E-Ferol Succinate, Tab., Cap. (Forest Pharmaceutical).
Vitamins E (Various Mfr.).

Tocosamine. (Trent) Sparteine sulfate 150 mg, sod. chl. 4.5 mg/ml. Amps. 1 ml. Box 12s, 100s. *Rx.*
Use: Oxytocic.

•**tofenacin hydrochloride.** (tah-FEN-ah-sin) USAN.
Use: Anticholinergic.

tofranazine. (Novartis) Combination of imipramine and promazine. Pending release.

Tofranil. (Novartis) Imipramine HCl. **Tab.** 10 mg Bot. 100s, 1000s; 25 mg & 50 mg. Bot. 100s, 1000s. UD 100s. Gy-Pak 100s, 1 unit (12×100); 6 units (72100). **Amps.** 25 mg/2 ml w/ascorbic acid 2 mg, sod. bisulfite 1 mg, sod. sulfite 1 mg and 2 ml amps. *Rx.*
Use: Antidepressant, antienuretic.

Tofranil-PM. (Novartis) Imipramine pamoate 75 mg, 100 mg, 125 mg or 150 mg/Cap. Bot. 30s, 100s. 75 mg/Cap. Bot. 1000s. UD 75 mg and 150 mg in 100s. *Rx.*
Use: Antidepressant.

Tolamide Tabs. (Major) Tolazamide 100 mg/Tab. Bot. 100s, 250s; 250 mg/Tab. 200s, 500s; 500 mg/Tab. Bot. 100s, 500s. *Rx.*
Use: Antidiabetic.

•**tolamolol.** (tahl-AIM-oh-lahl) USAN.
Use: Beta-adrenergic receptor blocker, coronary vasodilator, cardiovacular agent (antiarrhythmic).

•**tolazamide.** (tole-AZE-uh-mid) U.S.P. 23.
Use: Hypoglycemic, antidiabetic.
See: Tolinase, Tab. (Pharmacia & Upjohn).

tolazamide. (Various Mfr.) 100, 250 or 500 mg/Tab. 100s, 200s, 250s, 500s, 1000s, UD 100s. *Rx.*
Use: Antidiabetic.

•**tolazoline hydrochloride.** (tole-AZZ-oh-leen) U.S.P. 23.
Use: Antiadrenergic, antihypertensive, vasodilator (peripheral).
See: Priscoline, Inj. (Novartis).

•**tolbutamide.** (tole-BYOO-tuh-mide) U.S.P. 23.
Use: Hypoglycemic; antidiabetic.
See: Orinase, Tab. (Pharmacia & Upjohn).

tolbutamide. (Various Mfr.) 500 mg/Tab. 100s, 500s, 1000s, UD 100s. *Rx.*
Use: Antidiabetic.

•**tolbutamide sodium, sterile.** (tole-BYOO-tuh-mide) U.S.P. 23.
Use: Diagnostic aid (diabetes).
See: Orinase Diagnostic (Pharmacia & Upjohn).

•**tolcapone.** (TOLE-kah-pone) USAN. [Investigational]
See: Tasmar, Tab. (Roche).
Use: Antiparkinsonian.

•**tolciclate.** (tole-SIGH-klate) USAN.
Use: Antifungal.

Tolectin 200. (Ortho McNeil) Tolmetin sodium 200 mg/Tab. Bot. 100s. *Rx.*
Use: Analgesic, NSAID.

Tolectin 600. (Ortho McNeil) Tolmetin sodium 600 mg/Tab. Bot. 100s. *Rx.*
Use: Analgesic, NSAID.

Tolectin DS. (Ortho McNeil) Tolmetin sodium 400 mg/Cap Bot. 100s, 500s, UD 100s. *Rx.*
Use: Analgesic, NSAID.

Tolerex. (Procter & Gamble) Protein 20.6 g, carbohydrate 226.3 g, fat 1.45 g, sodium 468 mg, potassium 1172 mg, mOsm/Kg H_2O 550, cal/ml 1, vitamins A, B_1, B_2, B_3, B_5, B_6, B_{12}, C, D, E, K, folic acid, biotin, choline, Ca, P, I, Fe, Mg, Cu, Zn, Mn, Se, Mo, Cr. Assorted flavors Pow. Pkts. 80 g. *otc.*
Use: Mineral, vitamin supplement.

•**tolfamide.** (TAHL-fah-MIDE) USAN.
Use: Enzyme inhibitor (urease).

Tolfrinic. (B.F. Ascher) Ferrous fumarate 200 mg, Vitamins B_{12} 25 mcg, Vitamins C 100 mg/Tab. Bot. 100s. *otc.*
Use: Mineral, vitamin supplement.

•**tolgabide.** (TOLE-gah-bide) USAN.
Use: Antiepileptic (control of abnormal movements).

•**tolimidone.** (TAHL-IH-mih-dohn) USAN.
Use: Antiulcerative.

Tolinase. (Pharmacia & Upjohn) Tolazamide 100 mg (unit-of-use 100s), 250 mg (200s, 1000s, UD 100s, unit-of-use 100s), 500 mg (unit-of-use 100s)/Tab. *Rx.*
Use: Antidiabetic.

•**tolindate.** (TOLE-in-DATE) USAN.
Use: Antifungal.
See: Dalnate (Rhone-Poulenc Rorer).

•**tolmetin.** (TOLE-meh-tin) USAN.
Use: Anti-inflammatory.

•**tolmetin sodium.** (TOLE-meh-tin) U.S.P. 23.
Use: Anti-inflammatory.
See: Tolectin, Tab. (Ortho McNeil).
Tolectin DS, Cap. (Ortho McNeil).

tolmetin sodium. (Various Mfr.) Tolmetin sodium. **Tab.:** 200 mg, 600 mg. Bot. 100s, 500s, 1000s (600 mg only). **Cap.:** 400 mg. Bot. 100s, 500s, 1000s. *Rx.*
Use: Anti-inflammatory.

•**tolnaftate.** (tahl-NAFF-tate) U.S.P. 23.
Use: Antifungal.
See: Absorbine Prods. (W.F. Young).
Dr. Scholl's, Prods. (Schering-Plough).
Tinactin, Soln., Cream, Pow., Pow. Aer. (Schering Plough).

•**tolofocon a.** (TOE-low-FOE-kahn A) USAN.
Use: Contact lens material (hydrophobic).

tolonium chloride.

toloxychlorinal.
Use: Sedative.

•**tolpovidone I 131.** (tahl-POE-vih-dohn I 131) USAN.
Use: Diagnostic aid (hypoalbuminemia), radiopharmaceutical.
See: Raovin (Abbott Laboratories).

•**tolpyrramide.** (tahl-PIHR-ah-mid) USAN.
Use: Oral hypoglycemic; antidiabetic.

•**tolrestat.** (TOLE-ress-TAT) USAN.
Use: Inhibitor (aldose reductase).
See: Alredase (Wyeth Ayerst).

tolterodine tartrate.
Use: Urinary tract product.
See: Detrol, Tab. (Pharmacia & Upjohn).

•**tolu balsam.** (toe-LOO BALL-sam) U.S.P. 23. N.F. XVII.
Use: Pharmaceutic necessity for Com-

pound Benzoin Tincture, expectorant.
See: Vicks Regular & Wild Cherry Medicated Cough Drops (Procter & Gamble).

tolu balsam syrup. N.F. XVII. (Eli Lilly) Bot. 16 fl. oz.
Use: Vehicle.

tolu balsam tincture. N.F. XVII.
Use: Flavor.

toluidine blue o chloride.
See: Blutene Chloride.

Tolu-Sed (No Sugar). (Scherer) Codeine phosphate 10 mg, guaifenesin 100 mg/5 ml w/alcohol 10%. Bot. 4 oz., pt. *c-v.*
Use: Antitussive, expectorant.

Tolu-Sed DM (No Sugar). (Scherer) Dextromethorphan HBr 10 mg, guaifenesin 100 mg/5 ml w/alcohol 10%. Bot. 4 oz., pt. *otc.*
Use: Antitussive, expectorant.

•**tomelukast.** (tah-MELL-you-KAST) USAN.
Use: Antiasthmatic (leukotriene antagonist).

Tomocat. (Lafayette Pharm) CT barium sulfate 1.5% w/v. Case of 24 Bot.
Use: Mark alimentary tract during CT scans.

Tomocat 1000. (Lafayette Pharm) Barium sulfate suspension concentrate 5% w/v/Bot. for dilution to 1.5% w/v at time of use. Bot. 225 ml w/1000 ml dilution Bot. Case 24 Bot. and 2 Dilution Bot.
Use: Radiopaque medium used to mark the GI tract during CT scans.

•**tomoxetine hydrochloride.** (TOE-MOX-eh-teen) USAN.
Use: Antidepressant.

Tonavite-M Elixir. (Zenith Goldline) Bot. 12 oz., pt., gal.
Use: Dietary supplement.

•**tonazocine mesylate.** (tone-AZE-oh-SEEN) USAN.
Use: Analgesic.

Tono-B Pediatric. (Pal-Pak) Iron 5 mg, thiamine HCl 0.167 mg, riboflavin 0.133 mg/Tab. Bot. 1000s. *otc.*
Use: Mineral, vitamin supplement.

Tonocard. (Astra Merck) Tocainide HCl 400 mg and 600 mg/Tab. Bot. 100s. UD 100s. *Rx.*
Use: Antiarrhythmic.

Tonojug 2000. (Lafayette Pharm) Barium sulfate powder 1200 g for suspension to make 2000 ml. Bot. 2000 g Case: 8 Bot.
Use: Radiopaque contrast medium for use during x-ray examination of the GI tract.

Tonopaque Oral Barium. (Lafayette Pharm) Barium sulfate powder 180 g for suspension. Bot. 180 g Case 24s.
Use: Radiopaque contrast medium for use during x-ray examination of the GI tract.

Toothache Gel. (Roberts Pharm) Benzocaine, oil of cloves, benzyl alcohol, propylene glycol. Tube 15 g. *otc.*
Use: Anesthetic, local.

Toothache Relief-3 in 1. (C.S. Dent) Toothache gum, toothache drops, benzocaine lotion. *otc.*
Use: Analgesic, topical.

Topamax. (Ortho McNeil) Topiramate 25 mg, 100 mg, 200 mg, lactose/Tab. Bot. 60s. *Rx.*
Use: Anticonvulsant.

Top Brass ZP-11. (Revlon) Zinc pyrithione 0.5% in cream base.
Use: Antidandruff.

Top-Form. (Colgate Oral) Topical formfitting gel applicators. Disposable trays for topical fluoride office treatments, plus permanent trays for topical fluoride home self-treatments. Box 100s. *Rx.*
Use: Topical fluoride applications in home or office.

Topic. (Syntex) 5% benzyl alcohol in greaseless gel base containing camphor, menthol, w/30% isopropyl alcohol. Tube 2 oz. *otc.*
Use: Antipruritic.

topical anesthetics, miscellaneous.
See: Ethyl Chloride (Gebauer).
Flouri-Methane (Gebauer).
Fluro-Ethyl (Gebauer).

Topical Fluoride. (Pacemaker). Acidulated phosphate fluoride. Flavors: Orange, bubblegum, lime, raspberry, grape, cinnamon. Liq. Bot. 4 oz., pt.
Use: Corticosteroid, topical.

Topicort Cream. (Hoechst Marion Roussel) Desoximetasone 0.25% emollient cream consisting of isopropyl myristate, cetyl stearyl alcohol, white petrolatum, mineral oil, lanolin alcohol and purified water. Tubes 15 g, 60 g, 120 g. *Rx.*
Use: Corticosteroid, topical.

Topicort Gel. (Hoechst Marion Roussel) Desoximetasone 0.05% in gel base. 20% alcohol. Tube 15 g, 60 g. *Rx.*
Use: Corticosteroid, topical.

Topicort LP Cream. (Hoechst Marion Roussel) Desoximetasone 0.05%. Tubes 15 g, 60 g. *Rx.*
Use: Corticosteroid, topical.

Topicort Ointment. (Hoechst Marion Roussel) Desoximetasone 0.25% in

ointment base. Tube 15 g, 60 g. *Rx.*
Use: Corticosteroid, topical.

Topicycline. (Roberts Pharm) Tetracycline HCl 2.2 mg/ml w/sodium bisulfite, ethanol 40%. Bot. 70 ml w/diluent. *Rx.*
Use: Dermatologic, acne.

•**topiramate.** (toe-PIRE-ah-MATE) USAN.
Use: Anticonvulsant.
See: Topamax, Tab. (Ortho McNeil).

topocaine.
See: Surfacaine (Eli Lilly).

Toposar. (Pharmacia & Upjohn) Etoposide 20 mg, benzyl alcohol 30 mg, alcohol 30.5%/ml. Inj. 5 ml, 10 ml, 25 ml. *Rx.*
Use: Antineoplastic.

•**topotecan hydrochloride.** (toe-poe-TEE-kan) USAN.
Use: Antineoplastic (DNA topoisomerase I inhibitor).
See: Hycamtin, Pow. for inj. (SmithKline Beecham Pharmaceuticals).

Toprol XL. (Astra) Metoprolol succinate 47.5 mg, 95 mg or 190 mg/ER Tab. Bot. 100s. *Rx.*
Use: Antihypertensive.

•**topterone.** (TOP-ter-ohn) USAN.
Use: Antiandrogen.

TOPV.
Use: Immunization.
See: Orimune (ESI Lederle Generics).

•**toquizine.** (TOE-kwih-zeen) USAN.
Use: Anticholinergic.

Toradol. (Syntex) Ketorolac tromethamine 15 mg/ml and 30 mg/ ml. Injection. 15 mg/ml in 1 ml Tubex syringes, 30 mg/ml in 1 ml and 2 ml Tubex syringes. *Rx.*
Use: Analgesic, NSAID.

Toradol Tablets. (Syntex) Ketorolac tromethamine 10 mg/Tab. Bot. 100s, UD 100s. *Rx.*
Use: Analgesic, NSAID.

Torecan. (Boehringer Ingelheim) Thiethylperazine. **Tab.** 10 mg w/tartrazine. Bot. 100s. **Amp.** 10 mg/2 ml (w/sod. metabisulfite 0.5 mg, ascorbic acid 2 mg, sorbitol 40 mg, q.s. carbon dioxide). *Rx.*
Use: Antiemetic, antinauseant.

toremifene. (TORE-EM-ih-feen SIH-trate)
Use: Antineoplastic. [Orphan drug]
See: Estrinex.

•**toremifene citrate.** (TORE-EM-ih-feen SIH-trate) USAN.
Use: Antiestrogen; antineoplastic.
See: Fareston, Tab. (Schering-Plough).

Tornalate. (Dura Pharm) Bitolterol mesylate 0.2%, alcohol 25%, propylene glycol. Soln. for inhalation. Bot. 10 ml, 30 ml, 60 ml. *Rx.*
Use: Bronchodilator for bronchial asthma and reversible bronchospasms.

Tornalate Inhaler. (Dura Pharm) Bitolterol mesylate metered inhaler. Bot. 16.4 g w/oral inhaler. Refill 16.4 g. *Rx.*
Use: Bronchodilator for bronchial asthma and reversible bronchospasms.

Tornalate Tablets. (Sanofi) Bitolterol mesylate. *Rx.*
Use: Bronchodilator.

•**torsemide.** (TORE-suh-MIDE) USAN.
Use: Diuretic.
See: Demadex, Tab., Inj. (Boehringer Mannheim)

torula yeast, dried. Obtained by growing *Candida (torulopsis) utilis* yeast on wood pulp wastes (Nutritional Labs.) Conc. 100 lb. drums.
Use: Natural source of protein and Vitamin B-complex vitamins.

•**tosifen.** (TOE-sih-fen) USAN.
Use: Antianginal.

•**tosufloxacin.** (toe-SUE-FLOX-ah-sin) USAN.
Use: Anti-infective.

Totacillin. (SmithKline Beecham Pharmaceuticals) Ampicillin trihydrate equivalent to: **Cap.** 250 mg/Cap. Bot. 500s. 500 mg/Cap. Bot. 500s. **Susp.:** 125 mg/5 ml. Bot. 100 ml, 150 ml, 200 ml; 250 mg/5 ml. Bot. 100 ml, 200 ml. *Rx.*
Use: Anti-infective, penicillin.

Total. (Allergan) Polyvinyl alcohol, edetate disodium and benzalkonium chloride in a sterile, buffered, isotonic solution. Soln. Bot. 60 ml, 120 ml. *otc.*
Use: Contact lens care.

Total Eclipse Cooling Alcohol. (Novartis) Padimate O, oxybenzone, glyceryl PABA, alcohol 77%. SPF 15. Lot. Bot. 120 ml. *otc.*
Use: Sunscreen.

Total Eclipse Moisturizing. (Novartis) Padimate O, oxybenzone, octyl salicylate. Moisturizing base. SPF 15. Lot. Bot. 120 ml. *otc.*
Use: Sunscreen.

Total Eclipse Oil & Acne Prone Skin Sunscreen. (Eclipse) Padimate O, oxybenzone, glyceryl PABA, alcohol 77%. SPF 15. Lot. Bot. 120 ml. *otc.*
Use: Sunscreen.

Total Formula. (Vitaline) Iron 20 mg, vitamins A 10,000 IU, D 400 IU, E 30 IU, B_1 15 mg, B_2 15 mg, B_3 25 mg, B_5 25 mg, B_6 25 mg, B_{12} 25 mcg, C 100 mg, folic acid 0.4 mg, Ca, Cr, Cu, I, K, Mg, Mn, Mo, P, Se, Si, V, vitamin K, biotin 300 mcg, Zn 30 mg, choline, bioflavonoids, hesperidin, inositol, PABA, rutin/Tab. Bot. 90s, 100s. *otc.*
Use: Mineral, vitamin supplement.

Total Formula-2. (Vitaline) Iron 20 mg, vitamins A 10,000 IU, D 400 IU, E 30 IU, B_1 15 mg, B_2 15 mg, B_3 25 mg, B_5 25 mg, B_6 25 mg, B_{12} 25 mcg, C 100 mg, folic acid 0.4 mg, Ca, Cr, Cu, I, K, Mg, Mn, Mo, P, Se, Si, V, vitamin K, biotin 300 mcg, Zn 30 mg, choline, bioflavonoids, hesperidin, inositol, PABA, rutin/Tab. with boron. Bot. 60s. *otc.*
Use: Mineral, vitamin supplement.

Total Solution. (Allergan) Isotonic, buffered soln. of polyvinyl alcohol, benzalkonium chloride, EDTA. Soln. Bot. 60 ml, 120 ml. *otc.*
Use: Ophthalmic.

totaquine. Alkaloids from Cinchona bark, 7% to 12% quinine anhydrous, 70% to 80% total alkaloids (cinchonidine, cinchonine, quinidine & quinine).

totomycin hydrochloride. Tetracycline, U.S.P. 23.

Touro A & D. (Dartmouth Pharm) Chlorpheniramine maleate 4 mg, phenyltoloxamine citrate 50 mg, phenylephrine HCl 20 mg/SR Cap. Bot. 100s. *Rx.*
Use: Antihistamine, decongestant.

Touro EX. (Dartmouth Pharm) Guaifenesin 600 mg. SR Capl. Bot. 100s. *Rx.*
Use: Expectorant.

Touro LA. (Dartmouth Pharm) Pseudoephedrine HCl 120 mg, guaifenesin 500 mg/Cap. Bot. 100s. *Rx.*
Use: Decongestant, expectorant.

Toxo. (Wampole Laboratories) *Toxoplasma* antibody test system. Tests 120s.
Use: An IFA test system for the detection of antibodies to *Toxoplasma gondii.*

toxoid, diphtheria.
Use: Immunization.
See: Acel-Immune, Vial (Wyeth Ayerst).
ActHIB/DTP, Set of DTwP vial plus Hib Pow. for Inj. (Pasteur Merieux Connaught).
diphtheria and tetanus toxoids (pediatric strength).
diphtheria and tetanus toxoids with pertussis vaccine, Vial (Various Mfr.).
Infanrix (SKB).
tetanus and diphteria toxoids (adult strength), Vial.
Tetramune, Vial (Wyeth Ayerst).
Tri-Immunol, Vial (Wyeth Ayerst).
Tripedia, Vial (Pasteur Merieux Connaught).

toxoid, tetanus adsorbed.
Use: Immunization.

toxoid, tetanus. *Rx.*
Use: Immunization.
See: Acel-Immune, Vial (Wyeth Ayerst).
ActHIB/DTP, Set of DTwP vial plus Hib Pow. for Inj. (Pasteur Merieux Connaught).
diphtheria and tetanus toxoids (pediatric strength).
diphtheria and tetanus toxoids with pertussis vaccine, Vial (Various Mfr.).
Infanrix (SKB).
tetanus and diphteria toxoids (adult strength), Vial.
Tetramune, Vial (Wyeth Ayerst).
Tri-Immunol, Vial (Wyeth Ayerst).
Tripedia, Vial (Pasteur Merieux Connaught).

toxoplasmosis test.
Use: Diagnostic aid.
See: TPM Test (Wampole Laboratories).

t-PA.
Use: Tissue plasminogen activator.
See: Activase (Genentech).

T-Phyl. (Purdue Frederick) Theophylline 200 mg/Tab. Bot. 100s. *Rx.*
Use: Bronchodilator.

TPM-Test. (Wampole Laboratories) Indirect hemagglutination test for the qualitative and quantitative determination of antibodies to *Toxoplasma gondii* in serum. Kit 120s,
Use: Diagnostic aid, toxoplasmosis.

TPN Electrolytes. (Abbott Hospital Prods) Multiple electrolyte additive: 321 mg sodium chloride, 331 mg calcium chloride, 1491 mg potassium chloride, 508 mg magnesium chloride, 2420 mg sodium acetate; 20 ml in 50 ml fliptop or pintop vial or 20 ml Univ. Add. syr. *Rx.*
Use: Electrolyte supplement.

TPN Electrolytes II. (Abbott Laboratories) Na 15 mEq/L, K 18 mEq/L, Ca 4.5 mEq/L, Mg 5 mEq/L, Cl 35 mEq/L, acetate 7.5 mEq/L. In 20 ml fill in 50 ml fliptop and pintop vials and 20 ml fill syringes. *Rx.*
Use: Nutritional therapy, parenteral.

TPN Electrolytes III. (Abbott Laboratories) Na 25 Eq/L, K 40.6 mEq/L, Ca 5 mEq/L, Mg 8 mEq/L, Cl 33.5 mEq/L, acetate 40.6 mEq/L, gluconate 5 mEq/L. In 20 ml fill in 50 ml fliptop and pintop vials and 20 ml fill syringes. *Rx.*
Use: Nutritional therapy, parenteral.

•**tracazolate.** (track-AZE-oh-late) USAN.
Use: Sedative, hypnotic.

Trace. (Young Dental) Erythrosine conc. soln. Squeeze Bot. 30 ml, 60 ml Dispenser Packets 200s. *otc.*
Use: Diagnostic aid, disclose dental plaque.

Trace 28 Liquid. (Young Dental) D & C Red No. 28 in Aqueous Soln. Bot. 30 ml, 60 ml. *otc.*
Use: Diagnostic aid, disclose dental plaque.

Trace 28 Tablets. (Young Dental) D & C Red No. 28. Tablets. Box 30s, 180s, 700s. *otc.*
Use: Diagnostic aid, disclose dental plaque.

Tracelyte. (Fujisawa) A combination of electrolytes and trace elements additive. Vial 20 ml. *Rx.*
Use: Electrolyte, trace element supplement.

Tracelyte-II. (Fujisawa) A combination of electrolytes and trace elements additive. Vial 20 ml. *Rx.*
Use: Electrolyte, trace element supplement.

Tracelyte-II with Double Electrolytes. (Fujisawa) Combination of electrolytes and trace elements additive. Vial 40 ml. *Rx.*
Use: Electrolyte, trace element supplement.

Tracelyte with Double Electrolytes. (Fujisawa) A combination of electrolytes and trace elements additive. Vial 40 ml. *Rx.*
Use: Electrolyte, trace element supplement.

Traceplex. (Enzyme Process) Iron 30 mg, iodine 0.1 mg, copper 0.5 mg, magnesium 40 mg, zinc 10 mg, B_{12} 5 mcg/4 Tabs. Bot. 100s, 250s. *otc.*
Use: Mineral supplement.

Tracer bG. (Boehringer Mannheim) Reagent strips. Kit. 25s, 50s.
Use: Diagnostic aid.

Tracrium Injection. (GlaxoWellcome) Atracurium besylate 10 mg/ml Amp. 5 ml. Box 10s; 10 ml MDV. Box 10s. *Rx.*
Use: Muscle relaxant.

Trac Tabs 2X. (Hyrex) Atropine sulfate 0.06 mg, hyoscyamine sulfate 0.03 mg, methenamine 120 mg, methylene blue 6 mg, phenyl salicylate 30 mg, benzoic acid 7.5 mg/Tab. Bot. 100s, 1000s. *Rx.*
Use: Anti-infective, urinary.

•**tragacanth.** (TRAG-ah-kanth) N.F. 18.
Use: Pharmaceutic aid (suspending agent).

•**tralonide.** (TRAY-low-nide) USAN.
Use: Corticosteoid, topical.

•**tramadol hydrochloride.** (TRAM-uh-dole) USAN.
Use: Analgesic.
See: Ultram, Tab. (Ortho McNeil).

•**tramazoline hydrochloride.** (tram-AZE-oh-leen) USAN.
Use: Adrenergic.

trancin. Fluphenazine.
Use: Anxiolytic.

Trancopal. (Sanofi) Chlormezanone 100 mg w/saccharin/Cap. Bot. 100s. 200 mg/Cap. Bot. 100s, 1000s. *Rx.*
Use: Anxiolytic.

Trandate. (GlaxoWellcome) Labetalol HCl 100 mg. Tab. Bot. 100s, 500s, UD 100s. *Rx.*
Use: Antihypertensive.

Trandate Injection. (GlaxoWellcome) Labetalol HCl 5 mg/ml Amp. 1 ml. Box 1s. Vial 20 ml, 40 ml. Box 1s. Prefilled Syringes 4 ml, 8 ml. *Rx.*
Use: Antihypertensive.

Trandate Tablets. (GlaxoWellcome) Labetalol HCl 100 mg, 200 mg or 300 mg/Tab. Bot. 100s, 500s. UD 100s. *Rx.*
Use: Antihypertensive.

trandolapril.
Use: Antihypertensive.
See: Mavik, Tab. (Knoll Pharmaceuticals).
Tarka, ER Tab. (Knoll).

•**tranexamic acid.** (tran-ex-AM-ik) USAN.
Use: Hemostatic. [Orphan drug]
See: Cyklokapron, Tab., Inj. (Pharmacia & Upjohn).

•**tranilast.** (TRAN-ill-ast) USAN.
Use: Antiasthmatic.

tranquilizers.
See: A-poxide, Cap. (Abbott Laboratories).
Atarax, Prep. (Roerig).
Centrax, Cap. (Parke-Davis).
Compazine, Prep. (SmithKline Beecham Pharmaceuticals).
Equanil, Tab. (Wyeth Ayerst).
Fenarol, Tab. (Sanofi).
Haldol, Tab., Inj., Conc. Soln. (Ortho McNeil).
Harmonyl, Tab. (Abbott Laboratories).

Librium, Cap., Inj. (Roche Laboratories).
Loxitane, Prod. (ESI Lederle Generics).
Mellaril, Tab., Soln. (Novartis).
Meprobamate (Various Mfr.).
Miltown, Prep. (Wallace Laboratories).
Permitil, Prep. (Schering Plough).
Proketazine Maleate, Prep. (Wyeth Ayerst).
Prolixin, Prep. (Bristol-Myers Squibb).
Sparine HCl, Prep. (Wyeth Ayerst).
Stelazine, Prep. (SmithKline Beecham Pharmaceuticals).
Taractan, Prep. (Roche Laboratories).
Thorazine HCl, Prep. (SmithKline Beecham Pharmaceuticals).
Tindal, Tab. (Schering Plough).
Trancopal, Cap. (Sanofi).
Tranxene, Cap. (Abbott Laboratories).
Trilafon, Prep. (Schering Plough
Valium, Prep. (Roche Laboratories).
Vesprin, Prep. (Bristol-Myers Squibb).
Vistaril, Prep. (Pfizer).

Tranquils Capsules. (Halsey) Pyrilamine maleate 25 mg/Cap. Bot. 30s. *otc.*
Use: Sleep aid.

Tranquils Tablets. (Halsey) Acetaminophen 300 mg, pyrilamine maleate 25 mg/Tab. Bot. 30s. *otc.*
Use: Analgesic, sleep aid.

•**transcainide.** (trans-CANE-ide) USAN.
Use: Antiarrhythmic, cardiovascular agent.

Transclomiphene.

Transderm-Nitro. (Summit) Nitroglycerin 12.5 mg, 25 mg, 50 mg, 75 mg or 100 mg/patch. **12.5 mg, 25 mg, 50 mg:** Box 30s, UD 30s, 100s. **75 mg:** Box 30s. **100 mg:** Box 30s, UD 30s. *Rx.*
Use: Antianginal.

Transderm-Scop. (Novartis) Scopolamine 0.5 mg per 2-unit blister pkg. (programmed delivery over 3-day period).
Use: Antiemetic, antivertigo.

transforming growth factor-beta 2. (Celtrix)
Use: Immunomodulator. [Orphan drug]

Transthyretin EIA. (Abbott Diagnostics) Test kits 100s.
Use: Diagnostic aid.

Trans-Ver-Sal AdultPatch. (Doak Dermatologics) Salicylic acid 15%/Transdermal patch. 6 mm., 12 mm. In 40s. Securing tape and cleaning file. *otc.*
Use: Keratolytic.

Trans-Ver-Sal PediaPatch. (Doak Dermatologics) Salicylic acid 15%/Transdermal patch. 6 mm. In 20s. Securing tape and cleaning file. *otc.*
Use: Keratolytic.

Trans-Ver-Sal PlantarPatch. (Doak Dermatologics) Salicylic acid 15%, 20 mm patches, 25s. Securing tapes, cleaning file. *otc.*
Use: Dermatologic, wart therapy.

Tranxene Capsules. (Abbott Laboratories) Clorazepate dipotassium 3.75 mg, 7.5 mg or 15 mg/Cap. UD 100s. *c-IV.*
Use: Anxiolytic.

Tranxene-SD. (Abbott Laboratories) Clorazepate dipotassium 11.25 mg or 22.5 mg/Tab. Bot. 100s. *c-IV.*
Use: Anxiolytic.

Tranxene-SD Half Strength Tablets. (Abbott Laboratories) Clorazepate dipotassium 11.25 mg, 22.5 mg/Tab. Bot. 100s. *c-IV.*
Use: Anxiolytic.

Tranxene-T Tablets. (Abbott Laboratories) Clorazepate dipotassium tab. 3.75 mg, 7.5 mg or 15 mg/Tab. Bot. 100s, 500s, UD 100s. *c-IV.*
Use: Anxiolytic.

tranylcypromine sulfate. (tran-ill-SIP-row-meen) U.S.P. XXI..
Use: Antidepressant.
See: Parnate, Tab. (SmithKline Beecham Pharmaceuticals).

Trasicor. (Novartis) Oxprenolol HCl, B.A.N.

Trasylol. (Bayer Corp) Aprotinin 1.4 mg/ml. Inj. Vial 100 ml, 200 ml. *Rx.*
Use: Antihemophilic.

TraumaCal. (Bristol-Myers) Nutritionally complete formula for traumatized patients. Cans 8 oz. Vanilla flavor. *otc.*
Use: Specific for nitrogen and energy needs in a limited volume for multiple trauma and major burns.

T-Rau Tablet. (Tennessee Pharmaceutic) Rauwolfia serpentina 50 mg or 100 mg/Tab. Bot. 100s, 1000s. *Rx.*
Use: Hypotensive.

Travamulsion 10% Intravenous Fat Emulsion. 1.1 kcal/ml 270 mOsm/L. Bot. 500 ml. *Rx.*
Use: Nutritional supplement, parenteral.

Travamulsion 20% Intravenous Fat Emulsion. (Baxter) 2 kcal/ml 300 mOsm/L. Bot. 500 ml. *Rx.*
Use: Nutritional supplement, parenteral.

Travasol. (Baxter) Crystalline L-amino acids injection 5.5%, 8.5% (with or without electrolytes). IV Bot. 500 ml, 1000 ml, 2000 ml. *Rx.*
Use: Nutritional supplement, parenteral.

Travasol 3.5% M Injection with Electrolyte #45. (Baxter) Crystalline L-amino acids 3.5% Soln. Bot. IV 500 ml, 1000 ml. *Rx.*
Use: Nutritional supplement, parenteral.

Travasol 3.5% w/Electrolytes. (Clintec Nutrition) Amino acid concentration 3.5%, nitrogen 0.591 g/100 ml, 500 ml, 1000 ml. *Rx.*
Use: Nutritional supplement, parenteral.

Travasol 10%. (Baxter) Crystalline L-amino acids injection 10%. Bot. 200 ml, 500 ml, 1000 ml, 2000 ml. *Rx.*
Use: Nutritional supplement, parenteral.

Travasorb HN Peptide Diet. (Baxter) High-nitrogen defined peptide 333 kcal/Pkt. 6 pkt/Carton. *otc.*
Use: Nutritional supplement.

Travsorb MCT Liquid Diet. (Baxter) Digestible protein medium-chain triglyceride diet. 89 g packets. *otc.*
Use: Nutritional supplement.

Travasorb MCT Powder Diet. (Baxter) Digestible protein medium-chain triglyceride diet 400 kcal/Pkt. 6 pkt./Carton. *otc.*
Use: Nutritional supplement.

Travasorb Renal Diet. (Baxter) 467 kcal/Pkt. 6 pkt/Carton. 112 g packets. *otc.*
Use: Nutritional supplement.

Travasorb Standard Diet. (Baxter) Defined peptide diet, 333 kcal/pkt. 6 packets/Carton. *otc.*
Use: Nutritional supplement.

Travasorb STD. (Clintec Nutrition) Enzymatically hydrolyzed lactalbum 10 g, glucose oligosaccharides 63.3 g, MCT (fractioned coconut oil) 4.5 g, sunflower oil 4.5 g, sodium 307 mg, potassium 390 mg, mOsm/560 Kg, H_2O, cal 333.3/ml, vitamins A, B_1, B_2, B_3, B_5, B_6, B_{12}, C, D, E, K, Ca, Cl, Cu, Fe, I, Mg, Mn, P, Zn. Gluten free. Pow. Pkts. 83.3 g. *otc.*
Use: Nutritional supplement.

Travasorb Whole Protein Liquid Diet. (Baxter) Lactose free complete nutrition 250 kcal/Can. Cans 8 oz. *otc.*
Use: Nutritional supplement.

Travel Aids. (Faraday) Dimenhydrinate 50 mg/Tab. Bot. 30s. *otc.*
Use: Antiemetic, antivertigo.

Travel-Eze. (Health for Life Brands) Pyrilamine maleate 25 mg, hyoscine hydrobromide 0.325 mg/Tab. Pkg. 20s. *otc.*
Use: Antiemetic, antivertigo.

Travel Sickness. (Walgreens) Dimenhydrinate 50 mg/Tab. Bot. 24s. *otc.*
Use: Antiemetic, antivertigo.

Traveltabs. (Armenpharm) Dimenhydrinate 50 mg/Tab. Bot. 100s. *otc.*
Use: Antiemetic, antivertigo.

Travert. (Baxter) Invert sugar injection. 10% in water or saline. Plastic Bot. 500 ml, 1000 ml. *Rx.*
W/electrolyte No. 2 Bot. 500 ml, 1000 ml,
W/electrolyte No. 4 Bot. 250, 500 ml Soln. (10%).
Use: Fluid, electrolyte replacement.

5% Travert and Electrolyte No. 2. (Baxter) Invert sugar 50 g/L, calories 196 Cal/L, sodium 56 mEq/L, potassium 25 mEq/L, magnesium 6 mEq/L, chloride 56 mEq/L, phosphate 12.5 mEq/L, lactate 25 mEq/L, osmolarity 449 mOsm/L. 1000 ml. *Rx.*
Use: Nutritional supplement, parenteral.

10% Travert and Electrolyte No. 2. (Baxter) Invert sugar 100 g/L, calories 384 Cal/L, sodium 56 mEq/L, potassium 25 mEq/L, magnesium 6 mEq/L, chloride 56 mEq/L, phosphate 12.5 mEq/L, lactate 25 mEq/L, osmolarity 726 mOsm/L. 1000 ml. *Rx.*
Use: Nutritional supplement, parenteral.

•**trazodone hydrochloride.** (TRAY-zoe-dohn) U.S.P. 23.
Use: Antidepressant.
See: Desyrel, Tab. (Bristol-Myers).

•**trebenzomine hydrochloride.** (TRAY-BEN-zoe-meen) USAN.
Use: Antidepressant.

Trecator S.C. (Wyeth Ayerst) Ethionamide. 2-Ethyl thioisonicotinamide. 250 mg/Tab. Bot. 100s. *Rx.*
Use: Antituberculosis.

•**trecovirsen sodium.** (treh-koe-VEER-sin) USAN.
Use: Antiviral.

•**trefentanil hydrochloride.** (treh-FEN-tah-nill) USAN.
Use: Analgesic.

•**treloxinate.** (trell-OX-ih-nate) USAN.
Use: Antihyperlipoproteinemic.

Trental Tablets. (Hoechst Marion Roussel) Pentoxifylline 400 mg/Controlled Release Tab. Bot. 100s. UD 100s. *Rx.*
Use: Hemorrheologic.

Treo. (Biopharm Labs) *otc.* **SPF 8:** Octocrylene, octyl methoxycinnamate, benzophenone-3, octyl salicylate, isostearyl alcohol, diazolidinyl urea, propylparabens, citronella oil 0.05% (as insect repellant). Lot. Bot. 118 ml. **SPF 15:** Octocrylene, octyl methoxycinnamate, benzophenone-3, octyl salicylate, isostearyl alcohol, diazolidinyl urea,

propylparabens, citronella oil 0.05% (as insect repellant). Lot. Bot. 118 ml. **SPF 30:** Octocrylene, octyl methoxycinnamate, benzophenone-3, octyl salicylate, isostearyl alcohol, diazolidinyl urea, propylparabens, citronella oil 0.05% (as insect repellant). Lot. Bot. 118 ml.
Use: Sunscreen.

treosulfan.
Use: Antineoplastic. [Orphan drug]
See: Ovastat.

•**trepipam maleate.** (TREH-pih-pam MAL-ee-ate) USAN. *Formerly Trimopam Maleate.*
Use: Sedative, hypnotic.

•**trestolone acetate.** (TRESS-toe-lone) USAN.
Use: Antineoplastic, androgen.

trethocanoic acid.
Use: Anticholesteremic.

•**tretinoin.** (TREH-tih-NO-in) U.S.P. 23.
Use: Keratolytic. [Orphan drug]
See: Avita, Cream (DPT).
Retin-A, Cream, Gel, Soln. (Ortho McNeil).
Renova, Cream (Ortho McNeil).
Vesanoid, Cap. (Roche Laboratories).

tretinoin lf, iv. (Argus)
Use: Antineoplastic. [Orphan drug]

Trexan Cablets. (DuPont Merck Pharmaceuticals) Naltrexone HCl 50 mg/Tab. Bot. 50s. *Rx.*
Use: Opioid antagonist.

Triac. (Eon Labs Manufacturing) Triprolidine HCl 2.5 mg, pseudoephedrine HCl 60 mg/Tab. Bot. 100s, 1000s. *Rx.*
Use: Antihistamine, decongestant.

Triacet Cream. (Teva USA) Triamcinolone acetonide 0.1%. Tube 15 g, 80 g. *Rx.*
Use: Corticosteroid, topical.

•**triacetin.** (try-ah-SEE-tin) U.S.P. 23. *Formerly glyceryl triacetate.*
Use: Antifungal, topical.
See: Enzactin, Preps. (Wyeth Ayerst).
Fungacetin, Oint. (Blair Laboratories).

triacetyloleandomycin. (try-ASS-eh-till-oh-lee-AN-do-MY-sin) Troleandomycin. *Rx.*
Use: Anti-infective.

Triacin C. (Various Mfr.) Pseudoephedrine HCl 30 mg, triprolidine HCl 1.25 mg, codeine phosphate 10 mg/5 ml, alcohol 4.3%. Syr. Bot. pt., gal. *c-v.*
Use: Antihistamine, antitussive, decongestant.

Triact Liquid. (Sanofi) Aluminum, magnesium hydroxide, simethicone. *otc.*
Use: Antacid, antiflatulent.

Triact Tablets. (Sanofi) Aluminum, magnesium hydroxide, simethicone. *otc.*
Use: Antacid, antiflatulent.

Triad. (Forest Pharmaceutical) Butalbital 50 mg, acetaminophen 325 mg, caffeine 40 mg. Cap. Bot. 100s. *Rx.*
Use: Analgesic, hypnotic, sedative.

Triafed with Codeine Syrup. (Schein Pharmaceutical) Pseudoephedrine HCl 30 mg, triprolidine HCl 1.25 mg, codeine phosphate 10 mg. Bot. 473 ml. *c-v.*
Use: Antihistamine, antitussive, decongestant.

•**triafungin.** (TRY-ah-FUN-jin) USAN.
Use: Antifungal.

Triam-A. (Hyrex) Triamcinolone acetonide 40 mg/ml. Inj. Vial 5 ml. *Rx.*
Use: Corticosteroid.

•**triamcinolone.** (TRY-am-SIN-oh-lone) U.S.P. 23.
Use: Corticosteroid, topical.
See: Aristocort, Tab., Syr. (ESI Lederle Generics).
Aristoderm, Foam (ESI Lederle Generics).
Aristospan, Parenteral (ESI Lederle Generics).
SK-Triamcinolone, Tab. (SmithKline Beecham Pharmaceuticals).

•**triamcinolone acetonide.** (TRY-am-SIN-oh-lone ah-SEE-toe-nide) U.S.P. 23.
Use: Corticosteroid, topical, anti-inflammatory, topical.
See: Aristocort, Cream, Oint (Fujisawa).
Aristoderm Foam (ESI Lederle Generics).
Aristogel, Gel (ESI Lederle Generics).
Azmacort, Aer. (Rhone-Poulenc Rorer).
Delta-Tritex, Cream, Oint. (Dermol Pharmaceuticals).
Flutex, Cream, Oint. (Syosset Labs).
Kenalog Preps. (Westwood Squibb).
Kenonel, Cream (Marnel).
Nasacort, Spray (Rhone-Poulenc Rorer).
Nasacort AQ, Spray (Rhone-Poulenc Rorer).
Triacet, Cream (Teva USA).
Triderm, Cream (Del-Ray).
Tri-Kort, Inj. (Keene Pharmaceuticals).
W/Neomycin, gramicidin, Nystatin.
See: Mycolog, Preps. (Bristol-Myers Squibb).

triamcinolone acetonide. (Various Mfr.) **Cream: 0.025%, 0.1%:** Tube 15 g, 80 g, 454 g; **0.5%:** 15 g. **Lot.:** 0.025% or

0.1%. Bot. 60 ml. **Oint.: 0.025%, 0.1%:** Tube 15 g, 80 g, 454 g; **0.5%:** Tube 15 g. **Paste:** 0.1%.
Use: Corticosteroid, topical, anti-inflammatory, topical.

•**triamcinolone acetonide sodium phosphate.** (TRY-am-SIN-oh-lone ah-SEE-toe-nie) USAN.
Use: Costicosteroid, topical.

•**triamcinolone diacetate.** (try-am-SIN-oh-lone try-ASS-ah-tate) U.S.P. 23. Sterile Susp., Syrup, U.S.P. 23.
Use: Corticosteroid, topical.
See: Amcort, Inj. (Keene Pharmaceuticals).
Aristocort Diacetate Forte (ESI Lederle Generics).
Aristocort Diacetate Intralesional, Inj. (ESI Lederle Generics).
Kenacort, Syr. (Squibb Diagnostic).
Triam-Forte, Inj. (Hyrex).

•**triamcinolone hexacetonide.** (TRY-am-SIN-ole-ohn HEX-ah-SEE-tone-ide) U.S.P. 23.
Use: Costiscosteroid, topical.
See: Aristospan, Prep. (ESI Lederle Generics).

Triam Forte. (Hyrex) Triamcinolone diacetate 40 mg/ml. Vial 5 ml. *Rx.*
Use: Corticosteroid.

Triaminic. (Novartis) Pyrilamine maleate 25 mg, pheniramine maleate 25 mg, phenylpropanolamine HCl 50 mg/ Timed-release Tab. Bot. 100s, 250s. *otc.*
Use: Antihistamine, decongestant.
W/Dormethan, terpin hydrate.
See: Tussaminic, Tab. (Novartis).

Triaminic-12 Tablets. (Novartis) Phenylpropanolamine HCl 75 mg, chlorpheniramine maleate 12 mg/S.R. Tab. Pkg. 20s. *otc.*
Use: Antihistamine, decongestant.

Triaminic Allergy Tablets. (Novartis) Phenylpropanolamine HCl 25 mg, chlorpheniramine maleate 4 mg/Tab. Blister pk. 24s. *otc.*
Use: Antihistamine, decongestant.

Triaminic AM Decongestant Formula. (Novartis) Pseudoephedrine HCl 15 mg/5 ml, sorbitol, sucrose, orange flavor, alcohol and dye free. Syr. 118 ml, 237 ml. *otc.*
Use: Decongestant.

Triaminic AM Cough and Decongestant Formula. (Novartis) Pseudoephedrine HCl 15 mg, dextromethorphan HBr 7.5 mg/5 ml, sorbitol, sucrose, orange flavor. Alcohol and dye free. Liq. 118 ml, 237 ml. *otc.*
Use: Antitussive, decongestant.

Triaminic Chewable Tablets. (Novartis) Phenylpropanolamine HCl 6.25 mg, chlorpheniramine maleate 0.5 mg/Tab. Blister pkg. 24s. *otc.*
Use: Antihistamine, decongestant.

Triaminic Cold Syrup. (Novartis) Phenylpropanolamine HCl 12.5 mg, chlorpheniramine maleate 2 mg/5 ml. Bot. 4 oz., 8 oz. W/sorbitol. *otc.*
Use: Antihistamine, decongestant.

Triaminic Cold Tablets. (Novartis) Phenylpropanolamine HCl 12.5 mg, chlorpheniramine maleate 2 mg/Tab. Blister pkg. 24s. *otc.*
Use: Antihistamine, decongestant.

Triaminic-DM Syrup. (Novartis) Phenylpropanolamine HCl 6.25 mg, dextromethorphan HBr 5 mg, sorbitol, sucrose. Alcohol free. Bot. 120 ml, 240 ml. *otc.*
Use: Antitussive, decongestant.

Triaminic Expectorant. (Novartis) Phenylpropanolamine HCl 12.5 mg, guaifenesin 100 mg/5 ml w/alcohol 5%, saccharin, sorbitol. Bot. 4 oz., 8 oz. *otc.*
Use: Decongestant, expectorant.

Triaminic Expectorant w/Codeine. (Novartis) Phenylpropanolamine HCl 12.5 mg, codeine phosphate 10 mg, guaifenesin 100 mg/5 ml w/alcohol 5%, saccharin, sorbitol. Liq. Bot. pt. *otc.*
Use: Antitussive, decongestant, expectorant.

Triaminic Expectorant DH. (Novartis) Guaifenesin 100 mg, phenylpropanolamine HCl 12.5 mg, pheniramine maleate 6.25 mg, pyrilamine maleate 6.25 mg, hydrocodone bitartrate 1.67 mg/ 10 ml w/alcohol 5%, saccharin, sorbitol. Bot. pt. *c-III.*
Use: Antihistamine, antitussive, decongestant, expectorant.

Triaminic Nite Light Liquid. (Novartis). 15 mg pseudoephedrine, 1 mg chlorpheniramine maleate, 7.5 mg dextromethorphan HBr. 120 and 240 ml. *otc.*
Use: Antihistamine, antitussive, decongestant.

Triaminic Oral Infant Drops. (Novartis) Phenylpropanolamine HCl 20 mg, pheniramine maleate 10 mg, pyrilamine maleate 10 mg/ml. Dropper bot. 15 ml. *Rx.*
Use: Antihistamine, decongestant.

Triaminic Sore Throat Formula Liquid. (Novartis) Pseudoephedrine HCl 15 mg, dextromethorphan HBr 7.5 mg, acetaminophen 160 mg, EDTA, sucrose, al-

cohol free. Bot. 240 ml. *otc.*
Use: Antitussive, analgesic, decongestant.

Triaminic Syrup. (Novartis) Phenylpropanolamine HCl 6.25 mg, chlorpheniramine maleate 1 mg, sorbitol, sucrose, alcohol free. Bot. 120 ml, 240 ml. *otc.*
Use: Antihistamine, decongestant.

Triaminic TR Tablets. (Novartis) Phenylpropanolamine HCl 50 mg, pheniramine maleate 25 mg, pyrilamine maleate 25 mg/T.R. Tab. 100s, 250s. *otc.*
Use: Antihistamine, decongestant.

Triaminicin Cold, Allergy, Sinus Tablets. (Novartis) Phenylpropanolamine HCl 25 mg, acetaminophen 650 mg, chlorpheniramine maleate 4 mg/Tab. Pkg. 12s. *otc.*
Use: Analgesic, antihistamine, decongestant.

Triaminicol Multi Symptom Cold Syrup. (Novartis) Phenylpropanolamine HCl 12.5 mg, chlorpheniramine maleate 2 mg, dextromethorphan HBr 10 mg/5 ml. *otc.*
Use: Antihistamine, antitussive, decongestant.

Triaminicol Multi-Symptom Cough and Cold Tablet. (Novartis) Phenylpropanolamine HCl 12.5 mg, chlorpheniramine maleate 2 mg, dextromethorphan HBr 10 mg/Tab. Blister pkg. 24s. *otc.*
Use: Antihistamine, antitussive, decongestant.

Triaminicol Multi-Symptom Relief. (Novartis) Phenylpropanolamine HCl 6.25 mg, chlorpheniramine maleate 1 mg, dextromethorphan HBr 5 mg/5 ml. Liq. Bot. 120 ml. *otc.*
Use: Antihistamine, antitussive, decongestant.

triaminilone-16,17-acetonide.
See: Triamcinolone acetonide.

Triamolone 40. (Forest Pharmaceutical) Triamcinolone diacetate 40 mg/ml. Vial 5 ml. *Rx.*
Use: Corticosteroid.

Triamonide 40. (Forest Pharmaceutical) Triamcinolone acetonide 40 mg/ml. Vial 5 ml. *Rx.*
Use: Corticosteroid.

•**triampyzine sulfate.** (TRY-AM-pih-zeen SULL-fate) USAN.
Use: Anticholinergic.

•**triamterene.** (try-AM-tur-een) U.S.P. 23.
Use: Diuretic.
See: Dyrenium, Cap. (SmithKline Beecham Pharmaceuticals).

triamterene/hydrochlorothiazide. (Various Mfr.) **Cap.:** Triamterene 50 mg, hydrochlorothiazide 25 mg. Bot. 100s, 1000s. **Tab.:** Triamterene 37.5 mg, hydrochlorothiazide 25 mg. Bot. 100s, 500s, 1000s; Triamterene 75 mg, hydrochlorothiazide 50 mg. Bot. 100s, 250s, 500s, 1000s. *Rx.*
Use: Diuretic combination.

triamterene and hydrochlorothiazide capsules.
Use: Diuretic.
See: Dyazide, Cap. (SmithKline Beecham Pharmaceuticals).

Trianide. (Seatrace) Triamcinolone acetonide 40 mg/ml. Vial 5 ml. *Rx.*
Use: Corticosteroid.

Tri-Aqua. (Pfeiffer) Caffeine 100 mg, extracts of buchu, uva ursi, zea, triticum/ Tab. Bot. 50s, 100s. *otc.*
Use: Diuretic.

Tri-A-Vite F. (Major) F 0.5 mg, Vitamins A 1500 IU, D 400 IU, C 35 mg/ml Drops. Bot. 50 ml. *Rx.*
Use: Vitamin supplement.

Triaz. (Medicus Dermatologics) **Gel.:** Benzoyl peroxide 6%, 10%, EDTA. Tube 42.5 g. **Cleanser:** Benzoyl peroxide 10%, Menthol. 85.1 g. *Rx.*
Use: Antiacne.

•**triazolam.** (try-AZE-oh-lam) U.S.P. 23.
Use: Hypnotic, sedative.
See: Halcion, Tab. (Pharmacia & Upjohn).

triazolam. (Various Mfr.) Triazolam 0.125 mg, 0.25 mg. Tab. Bot. 10s, 100s, 500s, UD 100s. *c-IV.*
Use: Sedative.

Triban. (Great Southern) Trimethobenzamide HCl 200 mg, benzocaine 2%. Supp. Pkg. 10s, 50s. *Rx.*
Use: Antiemetic.

Triban, Pediatric. (Great Southern) Trimethobenzamide HCl 100 mg, benzocaine 2%. Supp. Pkg. 10s. *Rx.*
Use: Antiemetic.

•**tribenoside.** (try-BEN-oh-SIDE) USAN. Not available in U.S.
Use: Sclerosing agent.

Tri-Biocin. (Health for Life Brands) Bacitracin 400 units, polymyxin B sulfate 5000 units, neomycin 5 mg/g Tube 0.5 oz. *otc.*
Use: Antibiotic, topical.

Tribiotic Plus. (Thompson Medical) Polymyxin B sulfate 5000 units, neomycin sulfate (equivalent to 3.5 mg neomycin base), bacitracin 500 units, lidocaine 40 mg/g, lanolin, light mineral oil, petrolatum. Oint. Tube 28.35 g. *otc.*

Use: Anti-infective, topical.

tribromoethanol.
Use: Anesthetic (inhalation).

tribromomethane. Bromoform.

•**tribromsalan.** (try-BROME-sah-lan) USAN.
Use: Disinfectant.
See: Diaphene (or ASC-4) (Stecker).

tricalcium phosphate.
Use: Electrolytes, mineral supplement.
See: Posture (Whitehall Robins).

•**tricetamide.** (TRY-see-tam-id) USAN.
Use: Hypnotic, sedative.

Tri-Chlor. (Gordon Laboratories) Trichloroacetic acid 80%. Bot. 15 ml. *Rx.*
Use: Cauterizing agent.

trichloran.
See: Trichloroethylene.

•**trichlormethiazide.** (try-klor-meth-EYE-ah-zide) U.S.P. 23.
Use: Antihypertensive, diuretic.
See: Metahydrin, Tab. (Hoechst Marion Roussel).
Naqua, Tab. (Schering Plough).
W/Reserpine.
See: Naquival, Tab. (Schering Plough).

trichloroacetic acid. U.S.P. XXI. Acetic acid, trichloro.
Use: Topical, as a caustic.

trichlorobutyl alcohol.
See: Chlorobutanol.

trichlorocarbanilide.
W/Salicylic acid, sulfur.

•**trichloromonofluoromethane.** (try-klor-oh-mahn-oh-flure-oh-METH-ane) N.F. 18.
Use: Pharmaceutic aid (aerosol propellant).

tricholine citrate.
See: Choline citrate.

trichomonas test.
See: Isocult for *Trichomonas vaginalis.* (SmithKline Diagnostics).

Trichotine. (Schwarz Pharma) **Pow.:** Sodium lauryl sulf., sod. perborate, monohydrate silica. Pkg. 150 g, 360 g. **Liq.:** Sodium lauryl sulfate, sodium borate, SD alcohol 40 8%, SD alcohol 23-A, EDTA. Bot. 120 ml, 240 ml. *otc.*
Use: Feminine hygeine.

•**triciribine phosphate.** (TRY-SIH-bean FOSS-fate) USAN. *Formerly Phosphate Salt of Tricyclic Nucleoside.*
Use: Antineoplastic.

•**tricitrates oral solution.** (TRY-SIH-trates) U.S.P. 23.
Use: Alkalizer (systemic, urinary); antiurolithic (cystine calculi, uric acid calculi); buffer (neutralizing).

triclobisonium. Triburon, Oint. (Roche Laboratories).

triclobisonium chloride.
Use: Anti-infective, topical.

•**triclocarban.** (TRY-kloe-CAR-ban) USAN.
Use: Disinfectant.
See: Artra Beauty Ban (Schering Plough).
W/Clofulcarban.
See: Safeguard Bar Soap, (P & G).

•**triclofenol piperazine.** (TRY-kloe-FEE-nole pih-PURR-ah-zeen) USAN.
Use: Anthelmintic.

•**triclofos sodium.** (TRY-kloe-foss) USAN.
Use: Hypnotic, sedative.

•**triclonide.** (TRY-kloe-nide) USAN.
Use: Anti-inflammatory.

•**triclosan.** (TRY-kloe-san) USAN.
Use: Anti-infective; disinfectant.
See: Ambi 10, Bar (Kiwi Brands).
Clearasil Daily Face Wash (Procter & Gamble).
Clearasil Soap (Procter & Gamble).
Oxy ResiDon't, Liq. (SmithKline Beecham Pharmaceuticals).
Stridex Face Wash, Soln. (Stérling Health).

Tricodene Cough and Cold. (Pfeiffer) Pyrilamine maleate 12.5 mg, codeine phosphate 8.2 mg, menthol, honey, glucose, sucrose. Liq. Bot. 120 ml. *c-v.*
Use: Antihistamine, antitussive.

Tricodene Forte. (Pfeiffer) Phenylpropanolamine HCl 12.5 mg, chlorpheniramine maleate 2 mg, dextromethorphan HBr 10 mg/5 ml Liq. Bot. 120 ml. *otc.*
Use: Antihistamine, antitussive, decongestant.

Tricodene Liquid. (Pfeiffer) Chlorpheniramine maleate 0.5 mg, dextromethorphan HBr 10 mg, ammonium Cl 90 mg, sodium citrate, sorbitol, mannitol/5 ml Liq. Bot. 120 ml. *otc.*
Use: Antihistamine, antitussive, expectorant.

Tricodene NN. (Pfeiffer) Phenylpropanolamine HCl 12.5 mg, chlorpheniramine maleate 2 mg, dextromethorphan HBr 10 mg/5 ml. Syr. Bot. 120 ml. *otc.*
Use: Antihistamine, antitussive, decongestant.

Tricodene Pediatric Cough & Cold Liquid. (Pfeiffer) Phenylpropanolamine HCl 12.5 mg, Dextromethorphan HBr 10 mg/5 ml Liq. 120 ml. *otc.*
Use: Antitussive, decongestant.

Tricodene Sugar Free. (Pfeiffer) Chlor-

pheniramine maleate, dextromethorphan HBr 10 mg, menthol, saccharin, sorbitol, alcohol free. Liq. 120 ml. *otc.*
Use: Antihistamine, antitussive.

Tricodene Syrup. (Pfeiffer) Pyrilamine maleate 4.17 mg, codeine phosphate 8.1 mg, terpin hydrate, menthol/5 ml Syr. Bot. 120 ml. *c-v.*
Use: Antihistamine, antitussive.

Tricomine. (Major) Pseudoephedrine HCl 60 mg, carbinoxamine maleate 4 mg, dextromethorphan HBr 15 mg/5 ml, alcohol 5%. Expec. Bot. 120 ml. *otc.*
Use: Antihistamine, antitussive, decongestant.

Tricor. (Abbott) Fenofibrate 67 mg, lactose. Cap. Bot. 90s. *Rx.*
Use: Antihyperlipidemic.

Tricosal. (Invamed) Choline magnesium trisalicylate 500 mg, 750 mg, 1000 mg/ Tab. Bot. 100s, 500s. *Rx.*
Use: Salicylate.

tricylatate hydrochloride.

Triderm Cream. (Del-Ray) Triamcinolone acetonide 0.1%. Tube 30 g, 90 g. *Rx.[use]Use:Corticosteroid.*

Tridesilon Cream. (Bayer Corp) Desonide 0.05% in vehicle buffered to the pH range of normal skin w/glycerin, methyl paraben, sodium lauryl sulfate, aluminum sulfate, calcium acetate, cetyl stearyl alcohol, synthetic bees wax, white petrolatum, mineral oil. Tube 15 g, 60 g. *Rx.*
Use: Corticosteroid.

Tridesilon Otic. (Bayer Corp) Desonide 0.05%, acetic acid 2% in vehicle. Bot. 10 ml. *Rx.*
Use: Otic.

Tridex Tab., Timed Tridex Cap., Timed Tridex Jr. Cap. (Fellows) Changed to Daro Tab., Daro Timed Cap., Daro Jr. Timed Cap.

tridihexethyl chloride. U.S.P. XXII.
Use: Anticholinergic.
W/Phenobarbital.
See: Pathilon w/Phenobarbital Tab., Cap. (ESI Lederle Generics).

Tridil 0.5 mg/ml. (Faulding USA) Nitroglycerin 0.5 mg/ml w/alcohol 10%, water for injection, buffered with sodium phosphate. Amp. 10 ml. Box 20s. *Rx.*
Use: Vasodilator; antianginal, hypotensive.

Tridil 5 mg/ml. (Faulding USA) Nitroglycerin 5 mg/ml w/alcohol 30%, propylene glycol 30%, water for injection. Amp. 5 ml, 10 ml. Vial 5 ml, 10 ml, 20 ml. Box 20s. Special administration set w/10 ml Amp. *Rx.*
Use: Vasodilator; antianginal, hypotensive.

Tridione. (Abbott Laboratories) Trimethadione. (Troxidone). Cap. 300 mg, Bot. 100s. Dulcet Tab. 150 mg, Bot. 100s. *Rx.*
Use: Anticonvulsant.

Tridrate Bowel Evacuant Kit. (Mallinckrodt) Magnesium citrate soln. 300 ml, bisacodyl 5 mg/Tab. (3s), bisacodyl 10 mg/Supp. (1). Kit. *otc.*
Use: Laxative.

•**trientine hydrochloride.** (TRY-en-TEEN) U.S.P. 23.
Use: Chelating agent; Wilson's disease therapy adjunct. [Orphan drug]
See: Cuprid, Cap, (Merck).

triethanolamine.
See: Trolamine, N.F. 18.

triethanolamine polypeptide oleate condensate.
See: Cerumenex, Drops (Purdue Frederick).

triethanolamine salicylate.
See: Aspercreme, Cream (Thompson Medical).
Aspergel, Oint. (LaCrosse).
Myoflex, Cream (Warren-Teed).

triethanolamine trinitrate biphosphate. Trolnitrate Phosphate.

•**triethyl citrate.** N.F. 18.
Use: Pharmaceutic aid (plasticizer).

triethylenemelamine. Tretamine TEM. 2,4,6-Tris(1-aziridinyl)-5-triazine.
Use: Antineoplastic.

triethylenethiophosphoramide.
See: Thiotepa (ESI Lederle Generics).

Trifed-C. (Geneva Pharm) Pseudoephedrine HCl 30 mg, triprolidine HCl 1.25 mg, codeine phosphate 10 mg/5 ml, alcohol 4.3%. Syr. Bot. pt., gal. *c-v.*
Use: Antihistamine, antitussive, decongestant.

•**trifenagrel.** (try-FEN-ah-GRELL) USAN.
Use: Antithrombotic.

•**triflocin.** (try-FLOW-sin) USAN.
Use: Diuretic.

Tri-Flor-Vite with Fluoride. (Everett Laboratories) Fluoride 0.25 mg, vitamin A 1500 IU, D 400 IU, C 35 mg/ml/ Drop. 50 ml. *Rx.*
Use: Fluoride, vitamin supplement.

•**triflubazam.** (try-FLEW-bah-zam) USAN.
Use: Anxiolytic.

•**triflumidate.** (try-FLEW-mih-DATE) USAN.
Use: Anti-inflammatory.

•**trifluoperazine hydrochloride.** (try-flew-oh-PURR-uh-zeen) U.S.P. 23.

Use: Antipsychotic, anxiolytic, hypnotic, sedative.
See: Stelazine Inj., Liq., Tab. (SmithKline Beecham Pharmaceuticals).

trifluoperazine hydrochloride. (Various Mfr.) **Tab.:** 1 mg, 2 mg, 5 mg, 10 mg. Bot. 100s, 500s, 1000s, UD 100s. **Conc.:** 10 mg/ml. Bot. 60 ml. **Inj.:** 2 mg/ml. Vial 10 ml. *Rx.*
Use: Antipsycotic.

n-trifluoroacetyladriamycin-14-valerate. (Anthra Pharm)
Use: Antineoplastic. [Orphan drug]

trifluorothymidine. *Rx.*
Use: Ophthalmic.
See: Viroptic (GlaxoWellcome).

•**trifluperidol.** (TRY-flew-PURR-ih-dahl) USAN.
Use: Antipsychotic.

•**triflupromazine.** (try-flew-PRO-mah-zeen) U.S.P. 23.
Use: Antipsychotic, anxiolytic.

•**triflupromazine hydrochloride.** U.S.P. 23.
Use: Antipsychotic, anxiolytic.
See: Vesprin Prods. (Bristol-Myers).

•**trifluridine.** (try-FLEW-RIH-deen) USAN.
Use: Antiviral used to treat herpes simplex eye infections.
See: Viroptic Ophthalmic Soln., (GlaxoWellcome).

triglycerides, medium chain.
Use: Nutritional supplement.
See: MCT (Bristol-Myers).

triglyceride reagent strip. (Bayer Corp) Seralyzer reagent strip. Bot. 25s.
Use: Diagnostic aid, triglycerides.

Trihemic-600. (ESI Lederle Generics) Vitamins C 600 mg, B_{12} 25 mcg, intrinsic factor conc. 75 mg, folic acid 1 mg, Vitamins E 30 IU, ferrous fumarate 115 mg, dioctyl sod. succinate 50 mg/Tab. Bot. 30s, 500s. *Rx.*
Use: Mineral, vitamin supplement.

Trihexane. (Rugby) Trihexyphenidyl 2 mg/Tab. Bot. 100s, 1000s. *Rx.*
Use: Anticholinergic, antiparkinsonian.

Trihexidyl. (Schein Pharmaceutical) Trihexyphenidyl 2 mg/Tab. Bot. 100s, 1000s. *Rx.*
Use: Anticholinergic, antiparkinsonian.

Trihexy-2. (Geneva Pharm) Trihexyphenidyl 2 mg/Tab. Bot. 100s, 1000s. *Rx.*
Use: Anticholinergic, antiparkinsonian.

Trihexy-5. (Geneva Pharm) Trihexyphenidyl 5 mg/Tab. Bot. 100s, 1000s. *Rx.*
Use: Anticholinergic, antiparkinsonian.

•**trihexyphenidyl hydrochloride.** (try-hex-ee-FEN-in-dill) U.S.P. 23.
Use: Anticholinergic, antiparkinsonian.
See: Artane, Elixir & Tab. (ESI Lederle Generics).

TriHIBit. (Pasteur Merieux Connaught) Package containing lyophilized vials of ActHIB brand of Hib vaccine and vials of Tripedia brand of DTaP vaccine. *Rx.*
Use: Immunization.
See: ActHIB (Pasteur Merieux Conaught).
Tripedia (Pasteur Merieux Conaught).

Tri-Histin. (Recsei) **25 mg Tab.:** Pyrilamine maleate 10 mg, chlorpheniramine maleate 1 mg. **50 mg Tab.:** Pyrilamine maleate 20 mg, methapyrilene HCl 15 mg, chlorpheniramine maleate 2 mg. **100 mg S.A. Cap.:** Pyrilamine maleate 40 mg, pheniramine maleate 25 mg. **Expectorant:** Pyrilamine maleate 5 mg, chlorpheniramine maleate 0.5 mg, guaifenesin 20 mg, phenylpropanolamine 7.5 mg, phenylephrine HCl 2.5 mg, sod. citrate 100 mg/5 ml. Bot. pt. gal. **Liquid:** Pyrilamine maleate 5 mg, chlorpheniramine maleate 0.5 mg/5 ml. Bot. pt. gal. **Tab.:** Bot. 100s, 500s, 1000s. 50 mg Bot. 1000s. **Cap.:** Bot. 100s, 500s, 1000s. *otc, Rx.*
Use: Antihistamine combination.
W/Benzyl alcohol, chlorobutanol and isopropyl alcohol.
See: Derma-Pax, Liq. (Recsei).
W/Codeine phosphate, guaifenesin, phenylpropanolamine, phenylephrine HCl, sodium citrate.
See: Trihista-Cod., Liq. (Recsei).
W/Ephedrine HCl, aminophylline, mephobarbital.
See: Asmasan, Tab. (Recsei).

Tri-Hydroserpine. (Rugby) Hydrochlorothiazide 15 mg, reserpine 0.1 mg, hydralazine HCl 25 mg. Tab. Bot. 100s, 1000s. *Rx.*
Use: Antihypertensive combination.

Trihydroxyestrine. Trihydroxyestrin.

Trihydroxyethylamine. Triethanolamine.

Tri-Immunol. (Wyeth Ayerst) 12.5 LF units diphtheria, 5 LF units tetanus toxoids and 4 units pertussis vaccine combined, aluminum phosphate adsorbed purogenated. Vial 7.5 ml. *Rx.*
Use: Immunization.

triiodomethane.
See: Iodoform. (Various Mfr.).

Tri-K. (Century Pharm) Potassium acetate 0.5 g, potassium bicarbonate 0.5

g, potassium citrate 0.5 g/fl. oz. Saccharin. Bot. pt., gal. *Rx.*
Use: Electrolyte supplement.

•**trikates oral solution.** (TRY-kates) U.S.P. 23.
Use: Replenisher (electrolyte).

Tri-Kort. (Keene Pharmaceuticals) Triamcinalone acetonide suspension 40 mg/ml. Vial 5 ml. *Rx.*
Use: Corticosteroid, topical.

Trilafon. (Schering Plough) Perphenazine. **Tab.:** 2, 4, 8 & 16 mg. Bot. 100s, 500s. **Inj.:** 5 mg/ml, w/disodium citrate 24.6 mg, sod. bisulfite 2 mg, and water for injection/ml. Amp. 1 ml **Concentrate:** 16 mg/5 ml. Bot. 4 oz. w/dropper. *Rx.*
Use: Anxiolytic.

Tri-Levlen 21 Tablets. (Berlex). *Rx.*
Group 1: Levonorgestrel 0.05 mg, ethinyl estradiol 0.03 mg/Tab.
Group 2: Levonorgestrel 0.075 mg, ethinyl estradiol 0.04 mg/Tab.
Group 3: Levonorgestrel 0.125 mg, ethinyl estradiol 0.03 mg/Tab. Slidecase 21s. Box 3s.
Use: Contraceptive.

Tri-Levlen 28 Tablets. (Berlex). *Rx.*
Group 1: Levonorgestrel 0.05 mg, ethinyl estradiol 0.03 mg/Tab.
Group 2: Levonorgestrel 0.075 mg, ethinyl estradiol 0.04 mg/Tab.
Group 3: Levonorgestrel 0.125 mg, ethinyl estradiol 0.03 mg/Tab.
Group 4: Inert tablets. Slidecase 28s. Box 3s.
Use: Contraceptive.

Trilisate Liquid. (Purdue Frederick) Choline magnesium trisalicylate from choline salicylate 293 mg, magnesium salicylate 362 mg/ tsp. to provide 500 mg salicylate/tsp. Bot. 8 oz. *Rx.*
Use: Analgesic, NSAID.

Trilisate Tablets. (Purdue Frederick) Choline magnesium trisalicylate. **750 mg/Tab.** of salicylate from choline salicylate 400 mg and magnesium salicylate 544 mg Bot. 100s. 1000 mg/Tab. of salicylate from choline salicylate 587 mg, magnesium salicylate 725 mg Bot. 60s. *Rx.*
Use: Analgesic, NSAID.

Trilog. (Roberts Pharm) Triamcinolone acetonide 40 mg/ml. Vial 5 ml. *Rx.*
Use: Corticosteroid.

Trilone. (Century Pharm) Triamcinalone diacetate susp. Amp. 10 ml. *Rx.*
Use: Corticosteroid.

Trilone. (Roberts Pharm) Triamcinolone diacetate 40 mg/ml. Vial 5 ml. *Rx.*
Use: Corticosteroid.

•**trilostane.** (TRY-low-stane) USAN.
Use: Adrenocortical suppressant.

Trimahist Elixir. (Tennessee Pharmaceutic) Phenylephrine HCl 5 mg, prophenpyridamine maleate 12.5 mg, l-menthol 1 mg, alcohol 5%/5 ml. Bot. pt., gal. *Rx.*
Use: Antihistamine, decongestant .

Trimax Gel. (Sanofi) Aluminum, magnesium hydroxide, simethicone. *otc.*
Use: Antacid, antiflatulent.

Trimax Tablet. (Sanofi) Aluminum, magnesium hydroxide, simethicone. *otc.*
Use: Antacid, antiflatulent.

Trimazide. (Major) **Capsules:** Trimethobenzamide 250 mg/Cap. Bot. 100s. **Suppositories:** 100 mg and 200 mg/Supp. 10s. *Rx.*
Use: Antiemetic.

trimazinol.
Use: Anti-inflammatory.

•**trimazosin hydrochloride.** (try-MAY-zoe-sin) USAN.
Use: Antihypertensive.

•**trimegestone.** (try-meh-JESS-tone) USAN.
Use: Hormone, progestin.

trimetamide. Trimethamide.

•**trimethadione,** (try-meth-ah-DIE-ohn) U.S.P. 23.
Use: Anticonvulsant.
See: Tridione, Prep. (Abbott Laboratories).

trimethamide.
Use: Antihypertensive.

•**trimethaphan camsylate.** (try-METH-ah-fan KAM-sih-late) U.S.P. 23.
Use: Antihypertensive.

•**trimethobenzamide hydrochloride.** (try-meth-oh-BEN-zuh-mide) U.S.P. 23.
Use: Antiemetic.
See: Tegamide, Suppos. (G & W Laboratories).
Tigan, Preps. (SmithKline Beecham Pharmaceuticals).

trimethobenzamide hydrochloride and benzocaine suppositories.
Use: Antiemetic.
See: Pediatric Triban (Great Southern).
Triban (Great Southern).

•**trimethoprim.** (try-METH-oh-prim) U.S.P. 23.
Use: Anti-infective.
See: Proloprim, Tab. (GlaxoWellcome).
Trimpex, Tab. (Roche Laboratories).
W/Polymyxin B Sulfate.
See: Polytrim Ophth. Soln. (Allergan).
W/Sulfamethoxazole.

See: Bactrim, Oral Susp., Ped. Susp., Tab. (Roche Laboratories).
Septra, Tab. (GlaxoWellcome).
Septra DS, Tab. (GlaxoWellcome).

trimethoprim and sulfamethoxazole. (try-METH-oh-prim and suhl-fuh-meth-OX-uh-zole) (Various Mfr.) **Tab:** Trimethoprim 80 mg, sulfamethoxazole 400 mg/Tab. Bot. 100s, 500s. **Susp.:** Trimethoprim 40 mg, sulfamethoxazole 200 mg/5 ml. Bot. 150 ml, 200 ml, 480 ml. **Inj.:** Sulfamethoxazole 80 mg/ml, trimethoprim 16 mg/ml. 5 ml. *Rx.*
Use: Anti-infective combination.

trimethoprim and sulfamethoxazole DS. (Various Mfr.) Trimethoprim 160 mg, sulfamethoxazole 800 mg/Tab. Bot. 100s, 500s. *Rx.*
Use: Anti-infective combination.

•**trimethoprim sulfate.** (try-METH-oh-prim SULL-fate) USAN.
Use: Anti-infective.

trimethylene. Cyclopropane, U.S.P. 23.

•**trimetozine.** (try-MET-oh-zeen) USAN.
Use: Hypnotic, sedative.

•**trimetrexate.** (TRY-meh-TREK-sate) USAN.
Use: Antineoplastic.
See: Neutrexin, Vial (US Bioscience).

•**trimetrexate glucuronate.** (TRY-meh-TREK-sate glue-CURE-uh-nate) USAN.
Use: Antineoplastic. [Orphan drug]

Triminol. (Rugby) Phenylpropanolamine HCl 12.5 mg, chlorpheniramine maleate 2 mg, dextromethorphan HBr 10 mg/5 ml Syr. Bot. 120 ml. *otc.*
Use: Antihistamine, antitussive, decongestant.

•**trimipramine.** (TRY-MIH-prah-meen) USAN.
Use: Antidepressant.

•**trimipramine maleate.** (TRY-MIH-prah-meen) USAN.
Use: Antidepressant.
See: Surmontil (Wyeth Ayerst).

trimipramine maleate. (Various Mfr.) 25 mg, 50 mg or 100 mg. Cap. Bot. 100s, UD 100s.
Use: Antidepressant.

Trimixin. (Hance) Bacitracin 200 units, polymyxin B sulfate 4000 units, neomycin sulfate 3 mg/g Oint., Tube 0.5 oz. *otc.*
Use: Anti-infective, topical.

•**trimoprostil.** (TRY-moe-PRAHS-till) USAN.
Use: Gastric antisecretory.

Trimo-San. (Milex) Oxyquinoline sulfate 0.025%, boric acid 1%, sodium borate 0.7%, sodium lauryl sulfate 0.1%, glycerin, methylparaben. Jelly. 120 g w/ applicator, 120 g refill. *otc.*
Use: Vaginal agent.

Trimox. (Squibb Diagnostic) **Cap.:** Amoxicillin trihydrate 250 mg/Cap. Bot. 100s, 500s. **Oral Susp.:** 125 mg/5 ml. Bot. 80 ml, 100 ml, 150 ml, Unimatic Bot. 5 ml, Ctn. 4 × 25s; 250 mg/5 ml. Bot. 80 ml, 100 ml, 150 ml, Unimatic Bot. 5 ml, Ctn. 4 25s. *Rx.*
Use: Anti-infective, penicillin.

•**trimoxamine hydrochloride.** (TRY-MOX-am-een) USAN.
Use: Antihypertensive.

Trimpex. (Roche Laboratories) Tel-E-Dose 100s. *Rx.*
Use: Anti-infective, urinary.

Trim-Qwik. (Columbia) Powder-based meal food supplement. Can 10 oz. *otc.*
Use: Nutritional supplement.

Trimstat. (Laser) Phendimetrazine tartrate 35 mg/Tab. Bot. 100s, 1000s. *c-III.*
Use: Anorexiant.

Trim Sulf D/S. (Lexis) Sulfamethoxazole 800 mg, trimethoprim 160 mg/Tab. Bot. 100s, 500s. *Rx.*
Use: Anti-infective.

Trim Sulf S/S. (Lexis) Sulfamethoxazole 400 mg, trimethoprim 80 mg/Tab. Bot. 100s, 500s. *Rx.*
Use: Anti-infective.

Trim-Sulfa. *Rx.*
Use: Anti-infective.
See: Proloprim (GlaxoWellcome).
Trimethoprim (Various Mfr.).
Trimpex (Roche Laboratories).

Trinalin Repetabs. (Key Pharm) Azatadine maleate 1 mg, pseudoephedrine sulfate 120 mg/Tab. Bot 100s. *Rx.*
Use: Antihistamine, decongestant.

Trind. (Bristol-Myers) Phenylpropanolamine HCl 12.5 mg, chlorpheniramine maleate 2 mg/5 ml w/alcohol 5%, sorbitol. Bot. 5 oz. *otc.*
Use: Antihistamine, decongestant.

Tri-Nefrin Extra Strength. (Pfeiffer) Phenylpropanolamine HCl 25 mg, chlorpheniramine maleate 4 mg/Tab. in 24s. *otc.*
Use: Antihistamine, decongestant.

trinitrin tablets.
See: Nitroglycerin Tablets, U.S.P. 23.

trinitrophenol.
See: Picric Acid (Various Mfr.).

Tri-Norinyl. (Syntex) Norethindrone 1 mg with ethinyl estradiol 0.035 mg/Tab.

Norethindrone 0.5 mg with ethinyl estradiol 0.035 mg/Tab. 21 and 28 day. (7 inert tabs) Wallette. *Rx.*
Use: Contraceptive.

Trinotic. (Forest Pharmaceutical) Secobarbital 65 mg, amobarbital 40 mg, phenobarbital 25 mg/Tab. Bot. 1000s. *c-II.*
Use: Hypnotic.

Trinsicon. (UCB Pharmaceuticals) Liver-stomach concentrate 240 mg, iron 110 mg, vitamin C 75 mg, folic acid 0.5 mg, B_{12} 15 mcg. Cap. Bot. 60s, 500s, UD 100s. *Rx.*
Use: Nutritional supplement.

Trinsicon M. (UCB Pharmaceuticals) Formerly listed by Russ.

Triobead-125. (Abbott Diagnostics) T3 diagnostic kit. Test units 50s, 100s, 500s.
Use: T3 uptake radioassay for the measurement of thyroid function by indirectly determining the degree of saturation of serum thyroxine binding globulin (TBG).

triocil.
See: Hexetidine.

Triofed Syrup. (Alphalma USPD) Pseudoephedrine HCl 30 mg, triprolidine HCl 1.25 mg/5 ml Syr. Bot. 118 ml, 473 ml. *otc.*
Use: Antihistamine, decongestant.

•**triolein I 125.** (TRY-oh-leen) USAN.
Use: Radiopharmaceutical.

•**triolein I 131.** (TRY-oh-leen) USAN.
Use: Radiopharmaceutical.

Triostat. (SmithKline Beecham Pharmaceuticals) Liothyronine 10 mcg/ml, w/ ammonia 2.19 mg/ml, alcohol 6.8%. Vial 1 ml. *Rx.*
Use: Hormone, thyroid.

Triosulfon DMM. (CMC) Tab. Bot. 100s, 250s, 1000s.

Triotann. (Various Mfr.) Phenylephrine tannate 25 mg, chlorpheniramine tannate 8 mg, pyrilamine tannate 25 mg/ Tab. Bot. 100s, 500s. *Rx.*
Use: Antihistamine, decongestant.

Triotann Pediatric. (Various Mfr.) Phenylephrine tannate 5 mg, chlorpheniramine tannate 2 mg, pyrilamine tannate 12.5 mg, saccharin, sucrose. Susp. pt. *Rx.*
Use: Antihistamine, decongestant.

Tri-Otic. (Pharmics) Chloroxylenol 1 mg, pramoxine HCl 10 mg, hydrocortisone 10 mg/ml. Drops. Vial 10 ml. *Rx.*
Use: Otic.

trioxane.
See: Trioxymethylene (Various Mfr.).

•**trioxifene mesylate.** (TRY-OX-ih-feen) USAN.
Use: Antiestrogen.

•**trioxsalen.** (TRI-OX-sale-en) U.S.P. 23.
Use: Pigmenting and phototherapeutic agent.
See: Trisoralen, Tab. (Zeneca).

trioxymethylene. Name is incorrectly used to denote paraformaldehyde in some pharmaceuticals.
See: Paraformaldehyde (Various Mfr.).
W/Sod. oleate, triethanolamine, docusate sodium, stearic acid & aluminum silicate.
See: Cooper Creme (Whittaker).

Tri-Pain. (Ferndale Laboratories) Acetaminophen 162 mg, aspirin 162 mg, salicylamide 162 mg, caffeine 16.2 mg/ Tab. Bot. 100s. *otc.*
Use: Analgesic combination.

•**tripamide.** (TRIP-ah-mide) USAN.
Use: Antihypertensive, diuretic.

Tripedia. (Pasteur Merieux Connaught) Diphtheria 6.7 Lf units, tetanus 5 Lf units and acellular pertussis antigens 46.8 mcg/0.5 ml, aluminum potassium sulfate (alum), thimerosal, gelatin, polysorbate 80/Inj. 7.5 ml. *Rx.*
Use: Immunization.

•**tripelennamine citrate.** (trih-pell-EN-au-meen SIH-trate) U.S.P. 23.
Use: Antihistamine.

•**tripelennamine hydrochloride.** (trih-pell-EN-au-meen) U.S.P. 23.
Use: Antihistamine.
See: PBZ, Prods. (Novaratis).
Pyribenzamine hydrochloride, Preps. (Novartis).

Triphasil-21. (Wyeth Ayerst) Three drug phases in 21 day cycle: **Phase I:** 6 brown tab. Levonorgestrel 0.05 mg, ethinyl estradiol 0.03 mg/Tab. **Phase II:** 5 white tab. Levonorgestrel 0.075 mg, ethinyl estradiol 0.04 mg/Tab. **Phase III:** 10 yellow tab. Levonorgestrel 0.125 mg, ethinyl estradiol 0.03 mg/Tab. *Rx.*
Use: Contraceptive.

Triphasil-28. (Wyeth Ayerst) Three drug phases and one inert phase in 28 day cycle: **Phase I:** 6 brown tab. Levonorgestrel 0.05 mg, ethinyl estradiol 0.03 mg/Tab. **Phase II:** 5 white tab. Levonorgestrel 0.075/mg, ethinyl estradiol 0.04 mg Tab. **Phase III:** 10 yellow tab. Levonorgestrel 0.125 mg, ethinyl estradiol 0.03 mg/Tab. **Phase IV:** 7 inert green tablets. *Rx.*
Use: Contraceptive.

Tri-Phen-Chlor. (Rugby) Phenylpropanolamine HCl 20 mg, phenylephrine

HCl 5 mg, chlorpheniramine maleate 2.5 mg, phenyltoloxamine citrate 7.5 mg/5 ml Syr. Bot. 473 ml. *Rx.*
Use: Antihistamine, decongestant.

Tri-Phen-Chlor Tabs, Timed Released. (Rugby) Phenylpropanolamine HCl 40 mg, phenylephrine HCl 10 mg, chlorpheniramine maleate 5 mg, phenyltoloxamine citrate 15 mg. 100s. *Rx.*
Use: Antihistamine, decongestant.

Tri-Phen-Chlor Pediatric Drops. (Rugby) Phenylpropanolamine HCl 5 mg, phenylephrine HCl 1.25 mg, chlorpheniramine maleate 0.5 mg, phenyltoloxamine citrate 2 mg. Bot. w/drop 30 ml. *Rx.*
Use: Antihistamine, decongestant.

Tri-Phen-Chlor Pediatric Syrup. (Rugby) Phenylpropanolamine HCl 5 mg, phenylephrine HCl 1.25 mg, chlorpheniramine maleate 0.5 mg, phenyltoloxamine citrate 2 mg/5 ml. Syr. Bot. 118 ml, 473 ml, gal. *Rx.*
Use: Antihistamine, decongestant.

Tri-Phen-Mine Pediatric Drops. (Zenith Goldline) Phenylpropanolamine HCl 5 mg, phenylephrine HCl 1.25 mg, chlorpheniramine maleate 0.5 mg, phenyltoloxamine citrate 2 mg/ml. Drop. Bot. 30 ml. *Rx.*
Use: Antihistamine, decongestant.

Tri-Phen-Mine Pediatric Syrup. (Zenith Goldline) Phenylpropanolamine HCl 5 mg, phenylephrine HCl 1.25 mg, chlorpheniramine maleate 0.5 mg, phenyltoloxamine citrate 2 mg/5 ml. Syr. Bot. 473 ml. *Rx.*
Use: Antihistamine, decongestant.

Tri-Phen-Mine S.R. (Zenith Goldline) Chlorpheniramine maleate 5 mg, pyrilamine maleate 15 mg, phenylpropanolamine HCl 40 mg, phenylephrine HCl 10 mg/SR Tab. Bot. 100s. *Rx.*
Use: Antihistamine, decongestant.

Triphenyl. (Rugby) Phenylpropanolamine HCl 12.5 mg, Chlorpheniramine maleate 2 mg/5 ml, alcohol free. Syr. Bot. 118 ml. *otc.*
Use: Antihistamine, decongestant.

Triphenyl Expectorant. (Rugby) Phenylpropanolamine HCl 12.5 mg, guaifenesin 100 mg/5 ml, alcohol 5%. Expec. Bot. 120 ml, pt., gal. *otc.*
Use: Decongestant, expectorant.

triphenylmethane dyes.
See: Fuchsin.
Methylrosaniline Chloride.

Triphenyl T.D. (Rugby) Phenylpropanolamine HCl 50 mg, pyrilamine maleate 25 mg, pheniramine maleate 25 mg/ Tab. Bot. 100s, 1000s. *Rx.*
Use: Antihistamine, decongestant.

triphenyltetrazolium chloride. TTC.
See: Uroscreen (Pfizer).

tripiperazine dicititrate, hydrous.
See: Piperazine Citrate, U.S.P. 23.

triple antibiotic ophthalmics. (Various Mfr.) Polymyxin B sulfate 10,000 units/ g or ml, neomycin sulfate 3.5 mg/g or ml, bacitracin 400 units. Oint. 3.5 g. *Rx.*
Use: Anti-infective, ophthalmic.

triple antibiotic w/HC. (Various Mfr.) Hydrocortisone 1%, neomycin sulfate = neomycin base 0.35%, bacitracin zinc 400 units, polymyxin B sulfate/g 10,000.
Use: Anti-infective, corticosteroid, ophthalmic.

triple barbiturate elixir. (CMC) Phenobarbital 0.25 gr, butabarbital ⅛ gr, pentobarbital gr/5 ml. Bot. pt., gal. *c-II.*
Use: Sedative.

triple bromides, effervescent tablets. W/Phenobarbital.
See: Palagren, Liq. (Westerfield).

Triple Dye. (Kerr) Gentian violet, proflavine, hemisulfate, brilliant green in water. Dispensing Bot. 15 ml. Single Use Dispos-A-Swab 0.65 ml. Box 10s. Case 10×50 Box.
Use: Antiseptic.

Triple Dye. (Xttrium) Brilliant green 2.29 mg, proflavine hemisulfate 1.14 mg, gentian violet 2.29 mg/ml. Bot. 30 ml.
Use: Disinfectant.

Triple-Gen Suspension. (Zenith Goldline) Hydrocortisone 1%, neomycin sulfate 0.35%, polymyxin B sulfate 10,000 units/ml, benzalkonium chloride, cetyl alcohol, glyceryl monostearate, polyoxyl 40 stearate, propylene glycol, mineral oil. Bot. 7.5 ml. *Rx.*
Use: Anti-infective, corticosteroid, ophthalmic.

Triplen. (Henry Schein) Tripelennamine HCl 50 mg/Tab. Bot. 100s, 1000s. *Rx.*
Use: Antihistamine.

triple sulfa tablets. (Century; Stanlabs) Sulfadiazine 2.5 gr, sulfamerazine 2.5 gr, sulfamethazine 2.5 gr/Tab. Bot. 100s, 1000s. *Rx.*
Use: Anti-infective, sulfonamide.

•**triple sulfa vaginal cream.** U.S.P. 23.
Use: Anti-infective, vaginal.

triple sulfa vaginal tablets.
Use: Anti-infective, vaginal.

Triple Sulfoid. (Pal-Pak) Sulfadiazine 167 mg, sulfamerazine 167 mg, sulfamethazine 167 mg/5 ml or Tab. **Liq.:** Bot. pt., 2 oz. 12s. **Tab.:** Bot. 100s, 1000s. *Rx.*

Use: Anti-infective, sulfonamide.

triple sulfonamide. Dia-Mer-Thia Sulfonamides. Meth-Dia-Mer Sulfonamides.
Use: Anti-infective, sulfonamide.

Triple Vita. (Rosemont) Vitamins A 1500 IU, D 400 IU, C 35 mg/ml, alcohol free. Drops. Bot. 50 ml. *otc.*
Use: Vitamin supplement.

Triple Vita-Flor. (Rosemont) Fluoride 0.5 mg, vitamins A 1500 IU, D 400 IU, C 35 mg/ml, alcohol free. Drops. Bot. 50 ml. *Rx.*
Use: Dental caries agent, vitamin supplement.

Triple Vitamin ADC w/Fluoride. (Nilor Pharm) Fluoride 0.5 mg, vitamins A 1500 IU, D 400 IU, C 35 mg/ml. Drops. Bot. 50 ml. *Rx.*
Use: Mineral, vitamin supplement; dental caries agent.

Triple Vitamins w/Fluoride. (Major) Vitamin A 2500 IU, D 400 IU, C 60 mg, fluoride 1 mg, dextrose, sucrose/Chew. Tab. Bot. 100s. *Rx.*
Use: Vitamin supplement, dental caries agent.

Triplevite w/Fluoride. (Geneva Pharm) Fluoride 0.25 mg/ml, vitamins A 1500 IU, D 400 IU, C 35 mg, alcohol free. Drop. Bot. 50 ml. *Rx.*
Use: Dental caries agent, vitamin supplement.

Triplevite w/Fluoride. (Geneva Pharm) Fluoride 0.5 mg/ml, vitamins A 1500 IU, D 400 IU, C 35 mg/ml, alcohol free, cherry flavor. Drop. Bot. 50 ml. *Rx.*
Use: Dental caries agent, vitamin supplement.

Triple X. (Schmid) Pyrethrins 0.3%, piperonyl butoxide 3.0%, petroleum distillate 1.2%, benzyl alcohol 2.4%. Bot. 2 oz, 4 oz. *otc.*
Use: Pediculicide.

Tripodrine. (Schein Pharmaceutical) Pseudoephedrine HCl 60 mg, triprolidine HCl 2.5 mg/Tab. Bot. 100s, UD 100s. *Rx.*
Use: Antihistamine, decongestant.

Triposed Syrup. (Halsey) Triprolidine HCl 1.25 mg, pseudoephedrine HCl 30 mg/5 ml. Bot. 120 ml, 240 ml, 473 ml, gal. *otc.*
Use: Antihistamine, decongestant.

Triposed Tablets. (Halsey) Triprolidine HCl 2.5 mg, pseudoephedrine HCl 60 mg/Tab. Bot. 100s, 1000s. *otc.*
Use: Antihistamine, decongestant.

tripotassium citrate.
See: Potassium Citrate, U.S.P. 23.

•**triprolidine hydrochloride.** (try-PRO-lih-deen) U.S.P. 23.
Use: Antihistamine.

triprolidine hydrochloride and pseudoephedrine hydrochloride syrup. (Various Mfr.) Triprolidine HCl 1.25 mg, pseudoephedrine HCl 30 mg/5 ml. Syr. Bot. 118 ml, 237 ml. *Rx.*
Use: Antihistamine, decongestant.
See: Actifed, Syr. (GlaxoWellcome).

triprolidine hydrochloride and pseudoephedrine hydrochloride tablets. U.S.P. 23.
Use: Antihistamine, decongestant.
See: Actifed, Tab., (GlaxoWellcome).
Atridine, Tab. (Henry Schein).
Suda-Prol, Tab., Cap. (Quality Formulations).
Triphed, Tab. (Teva USA).

Triptifed. (Weeks & Leo) Triprolidine HCl 2.5 mg, pseudoephedrine HCl 60 mg/Tab. Bot. 36s, 100s. *Rx.*
Use: Antihistamine, decongestant.

Triptone Caplets. (Del Pharmaceuticals) Dimenhydrinate 50 mg/Tab. Bot. 12s. *otc.*
Use: Antiemetic, antivertigo.

•**triptorelin.** (TRIP-toe-RELL-in) USAN.
Use: Antineoplastic.

triptorelin pamoate.
Use: Antineoplastic. [Orphan drug]
See: Decapeptyl Injection (Organon Teknika).

trisaccharides a and b.
Use: Hemolytic disease of the newborn. [Orphan drug]

trisodium citrate concentration.
Use: Leukapheresis procedures. [Orphan drug]

Trisol. (Buffington) Borax, sodium Cl, boric acid. Irrigator Bot. oz, 4 oz. *otc.*
Use: Artificial tears.

Trisoralen. (Zeneca) Trioxsalen 5 mg/Tab. Tartrazine. Bot. 28s, 100s. *Rx.*
Use: Dermatologic.

Tri-Statin. (Rugby) Triamcinolone acetonide 0.1%, neomycin sulfate 0.25%, gramicidin 0.25 mg, nystatin 100,000 units/g Cream. In 15, 30, 60, 120 and 480 g. *Rx.*
Use: Anti-infective; corticosteroid, topical.

Tri-Statin II. (Rugby) Triamcinolone acetonide 0.1%, 100,000 units nystatin per g, white petrolatum, parabens. Cream. Tube 15 g, 30 g, 60 g, 120 g, 480 g. *Rx.*
Use: Antifungal, corticosteroid, topical.

Tristoject. (Merz) Triamcinolone diace-

tate 40 mg/ml. Vial 5 ml. *Rx.*
Use: Corticosteroid.
trisulfapyridmines.
Use: Anti-infective, sulfonamide.
See: Triple Sulfa No. 2 (Rugby).
•**trisulfapyrimidines oral susp..** (try-SOLL-fah-peer-IH-mih-deenz) U.S.P. 23.
Use: Anti-infective.
See: Meth-Dia-Mer Sulfonamides (Various Mfr.).
Neotrizine, Prep. (Eli Lilly).
Terfonyl, Liq., Tab. (Squibb Diagnostic).
Tritan. (Eon Labs Manufacturing) Phenylephrine tannate 25 mg, chlorpheniramine tannate 8 mg, pyrilamine tannate 25 mg/Tab. Bot. 100s, 250s, 1000s *Rx.*
Use: Antihistamine, decongestant.
Tritane. (Econo Med Pharmaceuticals) Brompheniramine maleate 2 mg, guaifenesin 100 mg, phenylephrine HCl 5 mg, phenylpropanolamine HCl 5 mg, alcohol 3.5%/5 ml. Bot. Gal. *Rx.*
Use: Antihistamine, decongestant, expectorant.
Tritane DC. (Econo Med Pharmaceuticals) Brompheniramine maleate 2 mg, guaifenesin 100 mg, phenylephrine HCl 5 mg, phenylpropanolamine HCl 5 mg, alcohol 3.5%, codeine phosphate 10 mg/5 ml. Bot. Gal. *c-v.*
Use: Antihistamine, antitussive, decongestant, expectorant.
Tri-Tannate. (Rugby) Phenylephrine tannate 25 mg, chlorpheniramine tannate 8 mg, pyrilamine tannate 25 mg. Tab. Bot. 100s, 250s. *Rx.*
Use: Antihistamine, decongestant.
Tri-Tannate Pediatric. (Rugby) Phenylephrine tannate 5 mg, chlorpheniramine tannate 2 mg, pyrilamine tannate 12.5 mg. Susp. Bot. 473 ml. *Rx.*
Use: Antihistamine, decongestant.
Tri-Tannate Plus Pediatric Suspension. (Rugby) Phenylephrine tannate 5 mg, ephedrine tannate 5 mg, chlorpheniramine tannate 4 mg, carbetapentane tannate 30 mg/5 ml. Bot. 480 ml. *Rx.*
Use: Antihistamine, antitussive, decongestant.
Tritec. (GlaxoWellcome) Ranitidine bismuth citrate 400 mg/Tab. Bot. 100s, UD 100s. *Rx.*
Use: In combination with clarithromycin to treat active duodenal ulcer associated with *H. pylori.*
•**tritiated water.** (TRISH-ee-at-ehd water) USAN.
Use: Radiopharmaceutical.
Tri-Tinic. (Vortech) Liver desic. 75 mg, stomach 75 mg, Vitamins B_{12} 15 mcg, Fe 110 mg, folic acid 1 mg, ascorbic acid 75 mg/Cap. Bot. 100s. *Rx.*
Use: Mineral, vitamin supplement.
Tritussin Cough Syrup. (Towne) Pyrilamine maleate 40 mg, pheniramine maleate 20 mg, citric acid 100 mg, codeine phosphate 58 mg/fl. oz. w/menthol and glycerin in flavored base. Bot. 4 oz. *c-v.*
Use: Antihistamine, antitussive, expectorant.
Triurisul. (Sheryl) Sulfacetamide 250 mg, sulfamethizole 250 mg, phenazopyridine HCl 50 mg/Tab. Bot. 100s. *Rx.*
Use: Analgesic; anti-infective, urinary.
Tri-Vert. (T.E. Williams) Dimenhydrinate 25 mg, niacin 50 mg, pentylenetetrazol 25 mg/Cap. Bot. 100s. *otc.*
Use: Motion sickness.
Tri-Vi-Flor 0.25 mg Drops. (Bristol-Myers Squibb) Fluoride 0.25 mg, Vitamins A 1500 IU, D 400 IU, C 35 mg/1 ml Drop. Bot. 50 ml. *Rx.*
Use: Dental caries agent, nutritional supplement.
Tri-Vi-Flor 0.25 mg with Iron Drops. (Bristol-Myers Squibb) Fluoride 0.25 mg, Vitamins A 1500 IU, D 400 IU, C 35 mg, iron 10 mg/1 ml Drop. Bot. 50 ml. *Rx.*
Use: Dental caries agent, nutritional supplement.
Tri-Vi-Flor 0.5 mg Drops. (Bristol-Myers Squibb) Fluoride 0.5 mg, Vitamins A 1500 IU, D 400 IU, C 35 mg/1 ml. Bot. 50 ml. *Rx.*
Use: Dental caries agent, nutritional supplement.
Tri-Vi-Flor 1.0 mg Tablets. (Bristol-Myers Squibb) Fluoride 1 mg, Vitamins A 2500 IU, D 400 IU, Vitamins C 60 mg, sucrose/Tab. Bot. 100s, 1000s. *Rx.*
Use: Dental caries agent, nutritional supplement.
Tri-Vi-Sol Drops. (Bristol-Myers Squibb) Vitamin A 1500 IU, D 400 IU, C 35 mg/1 ml Drops. Bot. 50 ml with calibrated "Safety-dropper." *otc.*
Use: Vitamin supplement.
Tri-Vi-Sol with Iron Drops. (Bristol-Myers Squibb) Vitamins A 1500 IU, C 35 mg, D 400 IU, iron 10 mg/ml. Bot. 50 ml. *otc.*
Use: Mineral, vitamin supplement.
Trivitamin Fluoride. (Schein Pharmaceutical) Drops: Fluoride 0.25 mg or

0.5 mg, vitamins A 1500 IU, D 400 IU, C 35 mg/ml. Bot. 50 ml. Chew. Tab.: Fluoride 0.5 mg, vitamins A 2500 IU, D 400 IU, C 60 mg, sucrose. Bot. 100s. *Rx.*
Use: Fluoride, vitamin supplement; dental caries agent.

Tri-Vitamin with Fluoride. (Rugby) Fluoride 0.5 mg, Vitamins A 1500 IU, D 400 IU, C 35 mg/ml Drops. Bot. 50 ml. *Rx.*
Use: Mineral, vitamin supplement.

Tri Vit w/Fluoride 0.25 mg. (Alphalma USPD) Fluoride 0.25 mg, vitamins A 1500 IU, D 400 IU, C 35 mg/ml. Drops. Bot. 50 ml. *Rx.*
Use: Mineral, vitamin supplement; dental caries agent.

Tri Vit w/Fluoride 0.5 mg. (Alphalma USPD) Fluoride 0.5 mg, vitamins A 1500 IU, D 400 IU, C 35 mg/ml. Drops. Bot. 50 ml. *Rx.*
Use: Mineral, vitamin supplement; dental caries agnet.

Tri-Vite. (Foy) Thiamine HCl 100 mg, pyridoxine HCl 100 mg, cyanocobalamine 1000 mcg/ml. Vial 10 ml. *Rx.*
Use: Vitamin supplement.

Trobicin. (Pharmacia & Upjohn) Spectinomycin HCl equivalent to spectinomycin activity: **2 g/Vial** w/ampule of diluent containing bacteriostatic water for injection 3.2 ml, benzyl alcohol 0.945% in ampule. **4 g/Vial** w/ampule of diluent containing bacteriostatic water for injection 6.2 ml, benzyl alcohol 0.945%. *Rx.*
Use: Anti-infective.

Trocaine. (Roberts Pharm) Benzocaine 10 mg. Lozenges. UD 4s, 500s. *otc.*
Use: Dietary aid.

Trocal. (Roberts Pharm) Dextromethorphan HBr 7.5 mg, guaifenesin 50 mg/Loz. In 500s. *otc.*
Use: Antitussive, expectorant.

•**troclosene potassium.** (TROE-kloe-seen) USAN.
Use: Anti-infective, topical.

•**troglitazone.** (TROE-glih-tazz-ohn) USAN.
Use: Antidiabetic.
See: Rezulin, Tab. (Parke-Davis).

•**trolamine.** (TROLE-ah-meen) N.F. 18. *Formerly Triethanolamine.*
Use: Pharmaceutic aid (alkalizing agent), analgesic.
W/Ortho-iodobenzoic.
See: Progonasyl (Saron).

•**troleandomycin.** (troe-lee-AN-doe-MY-sin) U.S.P. 23. *Formerly Triacetyloleandomycin.*
Use: Anti-infective.
See: Tao (Roerig).

tromal.
Use: Analgesic, antidepressant agent.

•**tromethamine.** (TROE-meth-ah-meen) U.S.P. 23.
Use: Alkalizer.

Tronolane Cream. (Ross Laboratories) Pramoxine HCl 1% in cream base. Tubes 30 g, 60 g. *otc.*
Use: Anorectal preparation.

Tronolane Suppositories. (Ross Laboratories) Zinc oxide 11%, hard fat 95%. Pkg. 10s, 20s. *otc.*
Use: Anorectal preparation.

Tronothane HCl. (Abbott Laboratories) Pramoxine HCl 1%, cetyl alcohol, glycerin, parabens. Cream. 28.4 g. *otc.*
Use: Anesthetic, local.

Tropamine +. (NeuroGenesis/Matrix) Vitamins D 250 mg, l-phenylalanine, l-tyrosine 150 mg, l-glutamine 50 mg, B_1 1.67 mg, B_2 2.5 mg, B_3 16.7 mg, B_5 15 mg, B_6 3.3 mg, B_{12} 5 mcg, folic acid 0.067 mg, C 100 mg, calcium 25 mg, chromium 0.01 mg, iron 1.5 mg, magnesium 25 mg, zinc 5 mg, yeast and preservative free. Cap. Bot. 42s, 180s. *otc.*
Use: Nutritional supplement.

•**tropanserin hydrochloride.** (trope-ANE-ser-IN) USAN.
Use: Seratonin receptor antagonist (specific in migraine).

TrophAmine Injection. (McGaw) Nitrogen 4.65 g, amino acids 30 g, protein 29 g/500 ml. Bot 500 ml IV infusion. *otc.*
Use: Nutritional supplement.

Troph-Iron. (SmithKline Beecham Pharmaceuticals) Vitamins B_{12} 25 mcg, B_1 10 mg, iron 20 mg/5 ml. Saccharin. Bot. 4 fl. oz. *otc.*
Use: Mineral, vitamin supplement.

Trophite (Iron. (Menley & James) Iron 60 mg, B_1 30 mg, B_{12} 75 mcg. Liq. Bot. 120 ml. *otc.*
Use: Mineral, vitamin supplement.

Tropicacyl. (Akorn) Tropicamide solution 0.5%. In 15 ml. 1% tropicamide. 2 ml, 15 ml. *Rx.*
Use: Cycloplegic, mydriatic.

Tropical Blend. (Schering Plough) A series of products is marketed under the Tropical Blend name including: Hawaii Blend Oil SPF 2 (Bot. 8 oz.); Hawaii Blend Lotion SPF 2 (Bot. 8 oz.); Rio Blend Oil SPF 2 (Bot. 8 oz.); Rio Blend Lotion SPF 2 (Bot. 8 oz.); Jamaica Blend Oil SPF 2 (Bot. 8 oz.); Jamaica

Blend Lotion SPF 2 (Bot. 8 oz.). All contain homosalate in various oil and lotion bases. *otc.*
Use: Sunscreen.

Tropical Blend Dark Tanning. (Schering Plough) **SPF 2:** Homosalate. **Oil:** Bot. 180 ml, 240 ml; **Lot.:** Bot. 240 ml. **SPF 4:** Ethylhexyl p-methoxycinnamate, oxybenzone. Bot. 240 ml; **Oil:** Padimate O, oxybenzone. Bot. 240 ml. *otc.*
Use: Sunscreen.

Tropical Blend Dry Oil. (Schering Plough) Homosalate, oxybenzone. Oil Bot. 180 ml. *otc.*
Use: Sunscreen.

Tropical Blend Tan Magnifier. (Schering Plough) Triethanolamine salicylate. Oil Bot. 240 ml. *otc.*
Use: Sunscreen.

Tropical Gold Dark Tanning Lotion. (Zenith Goldline) SPF 4. Ethylhexyl p-methoxycinnamate, oxybenzone, benzyl alcohol, parabens, aloe extract, jojoba oil, vitamin E, EDTA. PABA free. Waterproof. Lot. Bot. 240 ml. *otc.*
Use: Sunscreen.

Tropical Gold Dark Tanning Oil. (Zenith Goldline) SPF 2. Ethylhexyl p-methoxycinnamate, octyldimethyl PABA, mineral oil, coconut oil, cocoa butter, aloe, lanolin, eucalyptus oil, oils of plumeria, manako (mango), kuawa (guava), mikara (papaya), liliko (passion fruit), taro, kukui. Oil. Bot. 240 ml. *otc.*
Use: Sunscreen.

Tropical Gold Sport Sunblock. (Zenith Goldline) SPF 15. Ethylhexyl p-methoxycinnamate, oxybenzone, diazolidinyl urea, parabens, aloe extract, jojoba oil, vitamin E, EDTA. PABA free. Perspiration proof. Lot. Bot. 180 ml. *otc.*
Use: Sunblock.

Tropical Gold Sunblock. (Zenith Goldline) **SPF 15:** Ethylhexyl p-methoxycinnamate, oxybenzone, vegetable oil, benzyl alcohol, parabens, imidazolidinyl urea, vitamin E, aloe extract, jojoba oil, EDTA. PABA free. Waterproof. Lot. Bot. 118 ml. **SPF 17:** Ethylhexyl p-methoxycin- namate, 2-ethylhexyl salicylate, homosalate, oxybenzone, aloe extract, vitamin E, vegetable and jojoba oils, benzyl alcohol, imidazolidinyl urea, parabens, EDTA. PAPA free. Waterproof. Lot. Bot. 118 ml. **SPF 30:** Ethylhexyl p-methoxycinnamate, 2-ethylhexyl salicylate, homosalate, oxybenzone, aloe extract, vitamin E, vegetable and jojoba oils, benzyl alcohol, imidizolidinyl urea, parabens, EDTA. PABA free. Waterproof. 118 ml. *otc.*
Use: Sunblock.

Tropical Gold Sunscreen. (Zenith Goldline) SPF 8. Ethylhexyl p-methoxycinnamate, oxybenzone, benzyl alcohol, parabens, aloe extract, jojoba oil, vitamin E, EDTA. PABA free. Waterproof. Lot. Bot. 118 ml. *otc.*
Use: Sunscreen.

•**tropicamide.** (TROP-ik-ah-mid) U.S.P. 23.
Use: Anticholinergic (ophthalmic).
See: Mydriacyl, Drops. (Alcon Laboratories).
Opticyl, Soln. (Optopics).
Tropicacyl, Soln. (Akorn).

tropicamide. (Various Mfr.) 0.5%, 1%. Soln. Bot. 2 ml (0.5%), 15 ml.
Use: Anticholinergic (ophthalmic).

tropine benzohydryl ester methanesulfonate. (also named benztropine methane-sulfonate).

•**trospectomycin sulfate.** (TROE-speck-toe-MY-sin) USAN.
Use: Anti-infective.

•**trovafloxacin mesylate.** (TROE-vah-FLOX-ah-sin) USAN.
Use: Anti-infective.
See: Trovan, Tab. (Pfizer).

Trovan. (Pfizer) Trovafloxacin mesylate 100 mg, 200 mg. Tab. UD 40s. Alatrofloxacin mesylate 5 mg/ml. Ing. Vial. 40 mg (200 dose), 60 ml (300 dose). *Rx.*
Use: Anti-infective.

Trovit. (Sigma-Tau Pharmaceuticals) Vitamins B_2 0.3 mg, B_6 1 mg, choline Cl 25 mg, panthenol 2 mg, dl-methionine 10 mg, inositol 20 mg, niacinamide 50 mg, Vitamins B_{12} 10 mcg/ml. Vial 30 ml. *Rx.*
Use: Vitamin B supplement.

T.R.U.E. Test. (Glaxo Dermatology) Allergens incluse nickel sulfate, wool alcohols (lanolin), neomycin sulfate, potassium dichromate (chromium), caine mix (benzocaine, dibucaine, tetracaine), fragrance mix, colophony, epoxy resin, quinoline mix, balsam of peru, ethylenediamine, cobalt, p-tert-butylphenol formaldehyde, paraben mix, carba mix, black rubber mix, chloromethyl isothiazolinone, Quaternium-15, mercaptobenzothiazole, p-phenylenediamine, formaldehyde, mercapto mix, thimerosal and thiuram mix. Test in multipak cartons (5s). *Rx.*
Use: Diagnostic aid, allergic.

Truphylline. (G & W Laboratories) Aminophylline 250 mg/Supp. (equiv. to theophylline 198 mg) In UD 10s, 25s. *Rx.*
Use: Bronchodilator.

Trusopt. (Merck) Dorzolamide HCl 2%. Soln. Bot. 5 ml, 10 ml. *Rx.*
Use: Antiglaucoma.

Trynisin Cold Syrup. (Halsey) Bot. 4 oz., 8 oz.
Use: Antihistamine.

tryparsamide.

•**trypsin, crystallized.** (TRIP-sin) U.S.P. 23.
Use: Proteolytic enzyme.
W/Castor oil.
See: Granulex (Hickam).
W/Chymotrypsin.
See: Chymolase, Tab. (Warren-Teed).
Orenzyme, Tab. (Hoechst Marion Roussel).

tryptizol hydrochloride. Amitriptyline HCl, U.S.P 23.

•**tryptophan.** (TRIP-toe-FAN) U.S.P. 23.
Use: Amino acid.

Trysul. (Savage) Sulfathiazole 3.42%, sulfacetamide 2.86%, sulfabenzamide 3.7%, urea 0.64%. Tube 78 g. *Rx.*
Use: Anti-infective, vaginal.

T/Scalp. (Neutrogena) Hydrocortisone 1%. Liq. Greaseless. Bot. 60 ml, 105 ml. *otc.*
Use: Antipruritic, corticosteroid, topical.

T-Serp Tablet. (Tennessee Pharmaceutic) Reserpine alkaloid 0.25 mg/Tab. Bot. 100s, 1000s. *Rx.*
Use: Antihypertensive.

TSPA.
Use: Antineoplastic.
See: Thiotepa (ESI Lederle Generics).

T-Stat. (Westwood Squibb) Erythromycin 2% w/alcohol 71.2%. Bot. 60 ml; Pads, disposable premoistened 60s. *Rx.*
Use: Dermatologic, acne.

TTC. Triphenyltetrazolium Chloride.
See: Uroscreen, Tube (Pfizer).

tuaminoheptane sulfate. U.S.P. XX.
Use: Adrenergic.

•**tuberculin.** (too-BURR-kyoo-lin) U.S.P. 23.
Use: Diagnostic aid (dermal reactivity indicator).
See: Aplisol (Parke-Davis).
Aplitest (Parke-Davis).
Tubersol (Pasteur Merieux Connaught).

Tuberculin, Mono-Vacc Test. (Lincoln) Mono-Vacc test is a sterile, disposable multiple puncture scarifier with liquid Old Tuberculin on the points. Box 25 tests.
Use: Diagnostic aid.

Tuberculin, Old Monovacc Test. (ESI Lederle Generics) 5 TU activity test. Soln. of Old Tuberculin containing acacia 7%, lactose 8.5%. Test. Kits 25s, 100s, 250s.
Use: Diagnostic aid.

Tuberculin, Old, Tine Test. (ESI Lederle Generics) 5 TY activity per test. Soln. of Old Tuberculin, containing acacia 7%, lactose 8.5%. Test. Kits 25s, 100s, 250s.
Use: Diagnostic aid.

tuberculin purified protein derivative. (Bristol-Myers) (Pasteur Merieux Connaught) A concentrated solution for multiple puncture testing. Vial 1 ml.
Use: Diagnostic aid, tuberculosis.

tuberculin tests.
Use: Diagnostic aid.
See: Aplisol (Parke-Davis).
Aplitest (Parke-Davis).
Tine Test PPD (ESI Lederle Generics).
Tuberculin, Old Mono Vacc Test (Pasteur Merieux Connaught).
Tuberculin, Old, Tine Test (ESI Lederle Generics).
Tubersol (Bristol-Myers) (Pasteur Merieux Connaught).

tuberculin tine test. (ESI Lederle Generics) **Old Tuberculin (OT):** Each disposable test unit consists of a stainless steel disc, with four tines (or prongs) 2 millimeters long, attached to a plastic handle. The tines have been dip-dried with antigenic material. The entire unit is sterilized by ethylene oxide gas. The test has been standardized by comparative studies, utilizing 0.05 mg US Standard Old Tuberculin (5 International Units) or 0.0001 mg US Standard (5 International Units) by the Mantoux technique. The reliability appears to be comparable to the standard Mantoux. Tests in a jar 25s. Package 100s. Bin Package 250s. **Purified Protein Derivative (PPD):** Equivalent to or more potent than 5 TU PPD Mantoux test. Tests in a jar 25s. Package 100s.
Use: Diagnostic aid.

tuberculosis vaccine.
Use: Immunization.
See: TICE BCG (Organon Teknika).

Tuberlate. (Heun) Sod. p-aminosalicylate 12 gr, succinic acid 4 gr/Tab. Bot. 500s.
Use: Antituberculosis.

Tubersol. (Pasteur Merieux Connaught) Tuberculin purified protein derivative (Mantoux) 1 TU/0.1 ml: Vial 1 ml. 5 TU/0.1 ml: Vial 1 ml, 5 ml. 250 TU/0.1 ml: Vial 1 ml.
Use: Diagnostic aid, tuberculosis.

Tubex. (Wyeth Ayerst, Wyeth Ayerst) The following drugs are available in various Tubex sizes:
Ativan
Bicillin C-R
Bicillin C-R 900/300
Bicillin Long-Acting
Codeine Phosphate
Cyanocobalamin
Digoxin
Dimenhydrinate
Diphenhydramine HCl
Diphtheria and Tetanus Toxoids Adsorbed
(Pediatric Pharmaceuticals)
Epinephrine
Furosemide
Heparin Flush Kits
Heparin Lock Flush
Heparin Sodium Solution
Hydromorphone HCl
Hydroxyzine HCl
Influenza Virus Vaccine, Trivalent
Mepergan
Meperidine HCl
Morphine Sulfate
Naloxone Injection
Naloxone Injection, Neonatal
Oxytocin
Pentobarbital Sodium
Phenergan
Phenobarbital Sodium
Prochlorperazine Edisylate
Secobarbital Sodium
Sodium Chloride, Bacteriostatic
Sparine HCl
Tetanus and Diphtheria Toxoids Adsorbed (Adult)
Tetanus Immune Globulin (Human).
Tetanus Toxoid Alum. Phos. Ad.
Tetanus Toxoid, Fluid
Thiamine Hydrochloride
Wycillin

•**tubocurarine chloride.** (too-boe-cure-AHR-een) U.S.P. 23.
Use: Neuromuscular blocker.

tubocurarine chloride. (Eli Lilly) 3 mg/ml. Amp. 10 ml. (Abbott Laboratories) 3 mg/ml in 10 ml fliptop vials; 15 mg in 5 ml Abboject Syringe.
Use: Neuromuscular blocker.

tubocurarine chloride, dimethyl. Dimethyl ether of d-tubocurarine chloride.

tubocurarine chloride hydrochloride pentahydrate. Tubocurarine Chloride, U.S.P. 23.

tubocurarine iodide, dimethyl. Dimethyl ether of d-tubocurarine iodide.
Use: Muscle relaxant.
See: Metubine, Vial (Eli Lilly).

•**tubulozole hydrochloride.** (too-BYOO-lah-ZAHL) USAN.
Use: Antineoplastic (microtubule inhibitor).

Tucks. (Parke-Davis) Pads saturated with solution of witch hazel 50%, glycerin 10%, benzalkonium Cl 0.003%. Jar 40s, 100s. *otc.*
Use: Dermatologic, proctologic.

Tucks Clear Gel. (Warner Lambert Consumer Health Products) Hamamelis water 50%, glycerin 10%, benzyl alcohol, EDTA. Gel. Tube 19.8 g. *otc.*
Use: Anorectal preparation.

Tucks Take-Alongs. (Parke-Davis) Nonwoven wipes saturated with solution of witch hazel 50%, glycerine 10%, benzalkonium chloride 0.003%. Box 12s. *otc.*
Use: Anorectal preparation.

Tuinal. (Eli Lilly) Equal parts Seconal Sod. & Amytal Sod. Pulvule **100 mg** Bot. 100s; **200 mg** Bot. 100s. *c-II.*
Use: Hypnotic, sedative.

tumor necrosis factor-binding protein I and II. (Serono Labs) *Rx.*
Use: Treatment of AIDS. [Orphan drug]

Tums. (SmithKline Beecham Pharmaceuticals) Calcium carbonate 500 mg/Tab. Available in peppermint and assorted flavors in various package sizes. Rolls of 12 singles, 3-roll wraps. Bot. 75s, 150s. *otc.*
Use: Antacid.

Tums 500. (SmithKline Beecham Pharmaceuticals) Calcium carbonate 1250 mg (500 mg calcium), sucrose, sodium < 4 mg. Chew. Tab. Bot. 60s. *otc.*
Use: Antacid.

Tums E-X Extra Strength. (SmithKline Beecham Pharmaceuticals) Calcium carbonate 750 mg, wintergreen or fruit flavors. 12s, 48s, 96s. *otc.*
Use: Antacid.

Tums Plus. (SmithKline Beecham Pharmaceuticals) Calcium carbonate 500 mg, (elemental calcium 200 mg), simethicone 20 mg, sucrose, sodium ≤ 2 mg, assorted fruit and mint flavors. Tab. Bot. 48s. *otc.*
Use: Antacid.

Tur-Bi-Kal Nasal Drops. (Emerson) Phenylephrine HCl in a saline solution.

Dropper Bot. oz., 12s. *otc.*
Use: Decongestant.

Turbilixir. (Burlington) Chlorpheniramine maleate 2 mg, phenylephrine HCl 5 mg, phenylpropanolamine HCl 5 mg/5 ml. Bot. Pts., gal. *otc.*
Use: Antihistamine, decongestant.

Turbinaire.
See: Decadron Phosphate, Preps. (Merck).

Turbinaire Decadron Phosphate. (Merck) Each metered spray delivers dexamethasone sodium phosphate equivalent to ≈ dexamethasone 84 mcg (170 sprays per cartridge), alcohol 2%. Aerosol. 12.6 g w/adapter or 12.6 g refill. *Rx.*
Use: Corticosteroid, topical.

Turbispan Leisurecaps. (Burlington) Chlorpheniramine maleate 12 mg, 1-phenylephrine HCl 15 mg, phenylpropanolamine HCl 15 mg/Sus. Rel. Cap. Bot. 30s. *otc.*
Use: Antihistamine, decongestant.

Turgasept Aerosol. (Wyeth Ayerst) Ethyl alcohol 44.25%, essential oils 0.9%, n-alkyl (50% C-14, 40% C-12, 10% C-16) dimethyl benzylammonium Cl 0.33%, o-phenylphenol 0.25% w/propellant. Spray can 11.5 oz. in bouquet, fresh lemon, leather, citrus blossom scents.
Use: Deodorizer, disinfectant.

turpentine oil w/combinations.
See: Sloan's Liniment, Liq. (Warner Lambert).

Tusibron. (Kenwood/Bradley) Guaifenesin 100 mg/5 ml. 3.5% alcohol. Liq. Bot. 118 ml. *otc.*
Use: Expectorant.

Tusibron-DM. (Kenwood/Bradley) Guaifenesin 100 mg, dextromethorphan 15 mg/5 ml. Liq. Bot. 118 ml. *otc.*
Use: Antitussive, expectorant.

tusilan. Dextromethorphan HBr.

Tusquelin. (Circle) Dextromethorphan HBr 15 mg, chlorpheniramine maleate 2 mg, phenylpropanolamine 5 mg, phenylephrine HCl 5 mg, fl. ext. ipecac 0.17 min., potassium guaiacolsulfonate 44 mg/5 ml. Alcohol 5%. Syrup, pt. *Rx.*
Use: Antihistamine, antitussive, decongestant, expectorant.

Tussabar. (Tennessee Pharmaceutic) Acetaminophen 400 mg, salicylamide 500 mg, potassium guaiacolsulfonate 120 mg, pyrilamine maleate 30 mg, ammonium chloride 500 mg, sodium citrate 500 mg, phenylephrine HCl 30 mg/oz. Bot. pt., gal. *Rx.*
Use: Analgesic, antihistamine, decongestant, expectorant.

Tussabid. (ION Laboratories) Guaifenesin 200 mg, dextromethorphan HBr 30 mg/Cap. Bot. 24s, 100s. *otc.*
Use: Antihistamine, expectorant.

Tussafed Drops. (Everett Laboratories) Carbinoxamine maleate 2 mg, pseudoephedrine HCl 25 mg, dextromethorphan HBr 4 mg/1 ml. Bot. 30 ml with calibrated dropper. *Rx.*
Use: Antihistamine, antitussive, decongestant.

Tussafed Syrup. (Everett Laboratories) Dextromethorphan HBr 15 mg, pseudoephedrine HCl 60 mg, carbinoxamine maleate 4 mg/5 ml. Bot. 4 oz., 16 oz. *Rx.*
Use: Antihistamine, antitussive, decongestant.

Tussahist. (Defco) Codeine phosphate 10 mg, phenylpropanolamine HCl 12.5 mg, chlorpheniramine maleate 2 mg, pyrilamine maleate 7.5 mg, guaifenesin 100 mg/5 ml. Bot. 4 oz. pt, gal. *c-v.*
Use: Antihistamine, antitussive, decongestant, expectorant.

Tuss-Allergine Modified T.D. (Rugby) Phenylpropanolamine HCl 75 mg, caramiphen edisylate 40 mg/Cap. T.R. Bot. 100s. *Rx.*
Use: Antitussive, decongestant.

Tussafin Expectorant Liquid. (Rugby) Pseudoephedrine HCl 60 mg, hydrocodone bitartrate 5 mg, guaifenesin 200 mg, alcohol 2.5%. Bot. 480 ml. *c-III.*
Use: Antitussive, decongestant, expectorant.

Tussanil DH. (Misemer) Phenylpropanolamine HCl 25 mg, guaifenesin 100 mg, hydrocodone bitartrate 1.66 mg, salicylamide 300 mg/Tab. In 100s. *c-III.*
Use: Analgesic, antitussive, decongestant, expectorant.

Tussanil DH Syrup. (Misemer) Phenylephrine HCl 10 mg, chlorpheniramine maleate 4 mg, hydrocodone bitartrate 2.5 mg/5 ml w/alcohol 5%. Bot. pt. *c-III.*
Use: Antihistamine, antitussive, decongestant.

Tussanil Expectorant Syrup. (Misemer) Hydrocodone bitartrate 2.5 mg, phenylephrine HCl 10 mg, guaifenesin 100 mg/5 ml w/alcohol 5%. Bot. pt. *c-III.*
Use: Antitussive, decongestant, expectorant.

Tussanol. (Tyler) Pyrilamine maleate ¾ gr, codeine phosphate 1 gr, ammonium chloride 7.5 gr, sodium citrate 5 gr,

menthol gr/fl. oz. Bot. 4 fl. oz, pt, gal. *c-v.*
Use: Antihistamine, antitussive, expectorant.

Tussanol with Ephedrine. (Tyler) Ephedrine sulfate 2 gr, pyrilamine maleate 3/4 gr, codeine phosphate 1 gr, ammonium chloride 7.5 gr, sodium citrate 5 gr, menthol gr/30 ml. Bot. 16 fl. oz. *c-v.*
Use: Bronchodilator, antihistamine, antitussive, expectorant.

Tussar-2 Syrup. (Rhone-Poulenc Rorer) Codeine phosphate 10 mg, guaifenesin 100 mg, pseudoephedrine HCl 30 mg/5 ml, alcohol 2.5%. Bot. 473 ml. *c-v.*
Use: Antitussive, expectorant, decongestant.

Tussar DM. (Rhone-Poulenc Rorer) Dextromethorphan HBr 15 mg, chlorpheniramine maleate 2 mg, phenylephrine HCl 5 mg/5 ml w/methylparaben 0.1% Bot. 4 oz., pt. *Rx.*
Use: Antihistamine, antitussive, expectorant.

Tussar SF. (Rhone-Poulenc Rorer) Codeine phosphate 10 mg, guaifenesin 100 mg, pseudoephedrine HCl 30 mg/ 5 ml, alcohol 2.5%. Bot. 120 ml, 473 ml. *c-v.*
Use: Antitussive, decongestant, expectorant.

Tuss-DM. (Hyrex) Dextromethorphan HBr (10 mg), guaifenesin 200 mg, dye free. Tab. Bot. 100s, 1000s. *Rx.*
Use: Antitussive, expectorant.

Tussend. (Monarch Pharmaceuticals) Hydrocodone bitartrate 2.5 mg, chlorpheniramine maleate 2 mg/5 ml. 5% alcohol/Syrup. Bot. 480 ml, banana flavor. *c-III.*
Use: Antitussive, expectorant combination.

Tussex Cough. (Various Mfr.) Phenylephrine HCl 5 mg, dextromethorphan HBr 10 mg, guaifenesin 100 mg/5 ml Syr. Bot. 120 ml, gal. *Rx.*
Use: Antitussive, decongestant, expectorant.

Tuss-Genade Modified Caps. (Zenith Goldline) Phenylpropanolamine HCl 75 mg, caramiphen edisylate 40 mg. Bot. 100s, 1000s. *Rx.*
Use: Antitussive, decongestant.

Tussgen Expectorant. (Zenith Goldline) Bot. pt, gal.
Use: Expectorant.

Tussgen Liquid. (Zenith Goldline) Pseudoephedrine HCl 60 mg, hydrocodone bitartrate 5 mg/5 ml. Bot. 100s, 1000s. *c-III.*
Use: Antitussive, decongestant.

Tussidram. (Dram) Dextromethorphan 10 mg, phenylpropanolamine 12.5 mg, guaifenesin 50 mg, chlorpheniramine maleate 2 mg/5 ml. Bot. pt. *Rx.*
Use: Antihistamine, antitussive, decongestant, expectorant.

Tussigon. (Jones Medical Industries) Hydrocodone bitartrate 5 mg, homatropine methylbromide 1.5 mg/Tab. Bot. 100s, 500s. *c-III.*
Use: Anticholinergic, antispasmodic, antitussive.

Tussionex. (Medeva) Hydrocodone (as polistirex) 10 mg, chlorpheniramine 8 mg. Liq. Bot. 473 ml and 900 ml. *c-III.*
Use: Antihistamine, antitussive.

Tussi-Organidin DM NR. (Wallace Laboratories) Dextromethorphan HBr 10 mg, guaifenesin 100 mg/5 ml. Saccharin, sorbitol. Liq. Bot. 120 ml, pt, gal. *c-v.*
Use: Antitussive, expectorant.

Tussi-Organidin NR. (Wallace Laboratories) Codeine phosphate 10 mg, guaifenesin 100 mg/5 ml. Saccharin, sorbitol. Bot. 120 ml, pt, gal. *c-v.*
Use: Antitussive, expectorant.

Tussirex. (Scot-Tussin Pharmacal) Phenylephrine HCl 4.2 mg, pheniramine maleate 13.3 mg, codeine phosphate 10 mg, sodium citrate 83.3 mg, sodium salicylate 83.3 mg, caffeine citrate 25 mg/5 ml Syr. Bot. 120 and 240 ml, pt, gal. *c-v.*
Use: Antihistamine, antitussive, decongestant, expectorant.

Tussirex Sugar Free Liquid. (Scot-Tussin Pharmacal) Codeine phosphate 10 mg, pheniramine maleate 13.33 mg, phenylephrine HCl 4.17 mg, sodium citrate 83.33 mg, sodium salicylate 83.33 mg, caffeine citrate 25 mg/5 ml. Bot. 120 ml, pt. gal. *c-v.*
Use: Analgesic, antihistamine, antitussive, decongestant, expectorant.

Tuss-LA. (Hyrex) Pseudoephedrine HCl 120 mg, guaifenesin 500 mg/L.A. Tab. Bot. 100s. *Rx.*
Use: Decongestant, expectorant.

Tusso-DM. (Everett Laboratories) Dextromethorphan HBr 10 mg, iodianted glycerol 30 mg, alcohol free. Liq. Bot. 473 ml.
Use: Cough preparation.

Tussogest. (Major) Phenylpropanolamine HCl 75 mg, caramiphen edisylate 40 mg/Cap. T.R. Bot. 100s, 500s, 1000s. *Rx.*
Use: Antitussive, decongestant.

Tusstat. (Century Pharm) Diphenhydramine HCl 12.5 mg/5 ml, alcohol 5%. Syr. Bot. 118 ml, 473 ml, pt. gal. *Rx.*
Use: Antihistamine.

Tusstat Expectorant. (Century Pharm) Diphenhydramine HCl 80 mg, ammonium chloride 12 gr, sodium citrate 5 gr, menthol 1/10 gr, alcohol 5%/oz. Bot. 4 fl. oz, pt, gal. *Rx.*
Use: Antihistamine, expectorant.

•**tuvirumab.** (tuh-VIE-roo-mab) USAN.
Use: Monoclonal antibody (antiviral).

T-Vites. (Freeda Vitamins) Vitamins B_1 25 mg, B_2 25 mg, B_3 150 mg, B_5 25 mg, B_6 25 mg, C 100 mg, biotin 30 mcg, PABA, K, Mg, Mn carbonate 2 mg, Zn gluconate 20 mg/Tab. Bot. 100s. *otc.*
Use: Mineral, vitamin supplement.

tween 20, 40, 60, 80. (Zeneca) Polysorbates, N.F. 18.
Use: Surface active agents.

12-Hour Antihistamine Nasal Decongestant. (United Research Laboratories) Pseudoephedrine sulfate 120 mg, dexbrompheniramine maleate 6 mg, sugar, sucrose. SR Tab. Bot. 10s. *otc.*
Use: Decongestant.

12-Hour Cold Tablets. (Zenith Goldline) Dexbrompheniramine maleate 6 mg, pseudoephedrine sulfate 120 mg/SR Tab. Pkg. 10s, 20s. *otc.*
Use: Antihistamine, decongestant.

Twice-a-Day. (Major). Oxymetazoline 0.05%. Solution: In 15 and 30 ml. *otc.*
Use: Decongestant.

Twilite. (Pfeiffer) Diphenhydramine HCl 50 mg. Tab. 20s. *otc.*
Use: Sleep aid.

Twin-K Liquid. (Knoll Pharmaceuticals) Potassium ions 20 mEq./15 ml. Bot. pt. *Rx.*
Use: Treatment of hypokalemia.

2-Tone Disclosing Solution. (Young Dental) Dropper Bot. 2 oz.
Use: Disclosing solution.

2-24. (Walgreens) Belladonna alkaloids 0.2 mg, phenylpropanolamine HCl 50 mg, chlorpheniramine maleate 4 mg/Cap. Bot. 10s. *otc.*
Use: Anticholinergic, antispasmodic, decongestant, antihistamine.

TwoCal HN High Nitrogen Liquid Nutrition. (Ross Laboratories) High-nitrogen liquid nutrition (2 calories/ml). 1900 calories (1 quart) provide 100% US RDA for vitamins and minerals for adults and children over 4 yrs. Can 8 fl. oz. *otc.*
Use: Nutritional supplement.

•**tybamate.** (TIE-bam-ate) USAN.
Use: Anxiolytic.

Ty-Caplets. (Major) Acetaminophen 500 mg/Tab. Bot. 100s. *otc.*
Use: Analgesic.

Ty-Caps. (Major) Acetaminophen 500 mg/Cap. Bot. 100s, 1000s, UD 100s. *otc.*
Use: Analgesic.

Tycodene Sugar Free. (Pfeiffer) Chlorpheniramine maleate 2 mg, dextromethorphan HBr 10 mg, menthol, saccharin, sorbitol, alcohol free. Liq. Bot. 120 ml. *otc.*
Use: Antihistamine, antitussive.

Ty-Cold Tablets. (Major) 30 mg pseudoephedrine, 2 mg chlorpheniramine maleate, 15 mg dextromethorphan HBr, 325 mg acetaminophen. 24s. *otc.*
Use: Analgesic, antihistamine, antitussive, decongestant.

Tylenol Children's. (McNeil Consumer Products) Acetaminophen 160 mg/5 ml. Butylparaben, corn syrup, sorbitol. Alcohol free. Susp. Bot. 60 ml. *otc.*
Use: Analgesic.

Tylenol Children's Chewable Tablets. (McNeil Consumer Products) Acetaminophen 80 mg/Tab. Bot. 30s, 48s. Blisters 2s. Hospital pack 250 × 1. *otc.*
Use: Analgesic.

Tylenol Children's Elixir. (McNeil Consumer Products) Acetaminophen 160 mg/5 ml. Bot. 2 oz., 4 oz., pt. UD 100 × 5 ml, 100 × 10 ml. *otc.*
Use: Analgesic.

Tylenol Cold. (McNeil Consumer Products) Pseudoephedrine HCl 30 mg, chlorpheniramine maleate 2 mg, dextromethorphan HBr 15 mg, acetaminophen 325 mg, Tab. Cap. Bot. 24s, 50s. *otc.*
Use: Analgesic, antihistamine, antitussive, decongestant.

Tylenol Cold & Flu Medication. (McNeil Consumer Products) Pseudoephedrine HCl 60 mg, chlorpheniramine maleate 4 mg, dextromethorphan HBr, acetaminophen 650 mg, aspartame, sucrose, phenylalanine 11 mg, lemon flavor. Pow. Pks. 6s, 12s. *otc.*
Use: Analgesic, antihistamine, decongestant.

Tylenol Cold & Flu No Drowsiness. (McNeil Consumer Products) Acetaminophen 650 mg, pseudoephedrine HCl 60 mg, dextromethorphan HBr per packet 30 mg, aspartame (as phenylalanine 11 mg), sucrose, lemon flavor. Pow. 6s, 12s. *otc.*

Use: Analgesic, antihistamine, decongestant.

Tylenol Cold Liquid, Children's. (McNeil Consumer Products) Pseudoephedrine 15 mg, chlorpheniramine maleate 1 mg, acetaminophen 160 mg, sorbitol, sucrose, alcohol free, grape flavor. Liq. Bot. 120 ml. *otc.*
Use: Analgesic, antihistamine, decongestant.

Tylenol Cold Multisymptom Plus Cough, Children's. (McNeil Consumer Products) Acetaminophen 160 mg, dextromorphan HBr 5 mg, chlorpheniramine maleate 1 mg, pseudoephedrine 15 mg/5 ml. Liq. Bot. 120 ml. *otc.*
Use: Antihistamine, antitussive, decongestant.

Tylenol Cold Night Time. (McNeil Consumer Products) Pseudoephedrine HCl 10 mg, diphenhydramine HCl 8.3 mg, acetaminophen 108.3 mg/5 ml, alcohol 10%, sucrose, cherry flavor. Liq. Bot. 150 ml. *otc.*
Use: Analgesic, antihistamine, decongestant.

Tylenol Cold No Drowsiness Caplets & Gelcaps. (McNeil Consumer Products) Pseudoephedrine HCl 30 mg, dextromethorphan HBr 15 mg, acetaminophen 325 mg/Tab. **Capl.:** Bot. 24s, 50s. **Gel.:** 20s, 40s. *otc.*
Use: Analgesic, antitussive, decongestant.

Tylenol Cold Tablets, Children's. (McNeil Consumer Products) Pseudoephedrine HCl 7.5 mg, chlorpheniramine maleate 0.5 mg, acetaminophen 80 mg, aspartame, sucrose, phenylalanine 4 mg. Grape flavor. Chew. Tab. Bot. 24s. *otc.*
Use: Analgesic, antihistamine, decongestant.

Tylenol Cough. (McNeil Consumer Products) Dextromethorphan HBr, acetaminophen 250 mg, saccharin, sorbitol, sucrose. Liq. Bot. 120 ml. *otc.*
Use: Analgesic, antitussive.

Tylenol Cough w/Decongestant. (McNeil Consumer Products) Pseudoephedrine HCl 15 mg, dextromethorphan HBr 7.5 mg, acetaminophen 250 mg, alcohol 10%, saccharin, sobitol, sucrose. Liq. Bot. 120 ml, 240 ml. *otc.*
Use: Analgesic, antitussive, decongestant.

Tylenol Elixir, Children's. (McNeil Consumer Products) Acetaminophen 160 mg/5 ml. Elix. Bot. 60 mg, 120 ml. *otc.*
Use: Analgesic.

Tylenol Extended Relief. (McNeil Consumer Products) Acetaminophen 650 mg/ER Capl. 100s. *otc.*
Use: Analgesic.

Tylenol Extra Strength. (McNeil Consumer Products) Acetaminophen 500 mg/Tab. or Caplet. **Tab.:** Bot. 30s, 60s, 100s, 200s. **Caplets:** Bot. 24s, 50s, 100s, 175s. *otc.*
Use: Analgesic.

Tylenol Extra Strength Adult Liquid. (McNeil Consumer Products) Acetaminophen 1000 mg/30 ml w/alcohol 8.5%. Bot. 8 oz. Hosp. 8 oz. *otc.*
Use: Analgesic.

Tylenol Extra Strength Caplets. (McNeil Consumer Products) Acetaminophen 500 mg/Capl. Bot. 24s, 50s, 100s, 175s. *otc.*
Use: Analgesic.

Tylenol Extra Strength Gel-Cap. (McNeil Consumer Products) Acetaminophen 500 mg/Gelcap. Bot. 24s, 50s, 100s. *otc.*
Use: Analgesic.

Tylenol Extra Strength Geltabs. (McNeil Consumer Products) Acetaminophen 500 mg, parabens. Tab. Bot. 24s, 50s, 100s. *otc.*
Use: Analgesic.

Tylenol Flu Maximum Strength. (McNeil Consumer Products) Pseudoephedrine HCl 30 mg, dextromethorphan HBr 15 mg, acetaminophen 500 mg/Gelcap. Pkg. 10s, 20s. *otc.*
Use: Analgesic, antitussive, decongestant.

Tylenol Infant's Drops. (McNeil Consumer Products) Acetaminophen 80 mg/0.8 ml. Butylparaben, corn syrup, sorbitol. Alcohol free. Bot. w/dropper 7.5 ml, 15 ml. *otc.*
Use: Analgesic.

Tylenol Junior Strength. (McNeil Consumer Products) Acetaminophen 160 mg, aspartame (6 mg phenylalanine)/ Chew. tab. 24s. *otc.*
Use: Analgesic.

Tylenol Junior Strength Swallowable Tablets. (McNeil Consumer Products) 160 mg/Tab. Box. 30s. Hosp. 250 × 1. *otc.*
Use: Analgesic.

Tylenol Maximum-Strength Allergy Sinus. (McNeil Consumer Products) Pseudoephedrine HCl 30 mg, chlorpheniramine maleate 2 mg, acetaminophen 500 mg, Capl. Bot. 24s, 50s. Gelcap. Bot. 20s, 40s. *otc.*
Use: Analgesic, antihistamine, decongestant.

Tylenol Maximum Strength Sinus Medication. (McNeil Consumer Products) Acetaminophen 500 mg, pseudoephedrine HCl 30 mg/Tab. or Caplet. **Tab.:** Bot. 24s, 50s. **Caplet:** Bot. 24s, 50s. *otc.*
Use: Analgesic, decongestant.

Tylenol Multi-Symptom Hot Medication. (McNeil Consumer Products) Pseudoephedrine HCl 60 mg, chlorpheniramine maleate 4 mg, dextromethorphan HBr 30 mg, acetaminophen 650 mg. Powd. 6s. *otc.*
Use: Analgesic, antihistamine, antitussive, decongestant.

Tylenol No Drowsiness Cold. (McNeil Consumer Products) Pseudoephedrine HCl 30 g, dextromethorphan HBr 15 mg, acetaminophen 325 mg. Cap. Bot. 24s, 50s. *otc.*
Use: Analgesic, antitussive, decongestant.

Tylenol PM, Extra Strength. (McNeil Consumer Products) Acetaminophen 500 mg, diphenhydramine 25 mg. Tab. Cap. Bot. 24s, 50s. *otc.*
Use: Analgesic, antitussive.

Tylenol Regular Strength. (McNeil Consumer Products) Acetaminophen 325 mg/Tab. or Caplet. **Tab.:** Tin 12s. Vial 12s. Bot. 24s, 50s, 100s, 200s. **Caplet:** Bot. 24s, 50s. *otc.*
Use: Analgesic.

Tylenol Severe Allergy. (McNeil Consumer Products) Diphenhydramine HCl 12.5 mg, acetaminophen 500 mg/Capl. Pkg. 12s, 24s. *otc.*
Use: Analgesic, antihistamine.

Tylenol with Codeine. (Ortho McNeil) **Tab.:** Acetaminophen 300 mg with codeine phosphate. **No. 2:** codeine phosphate 15 mg. Bot. 100s, 500s. **No. 3:** Codeine phosphate 30 mg. Bot. 100s, 500s, 1000s, UD 100s. **No. 4:** Codeine phosphate 60 mg. Bot. 100s, 500s, UD 500s. *c-III.*
Use: Analgesic combination, narcotic.

Tylenol with Codeine Elixir. (Ortho McNeil) Acetaminophen 120 mg, codeine phosphate 12 mg/5 ml w/alcohol 7%. Bot. 480 ml. *c-v.*
Use: Analgesic combination, narcotic.

Tylosterone. (Eli Lilly) Diethylstilbestrol 0.25 mg, methyltestosterone 5 mg/Tab. Bot. 100s. *Rx.*
Use: Androgen, estrogen combination.

Tylox. (Ortho McNeil) Oxycodone HCl 5 mg, acetaminophen 500 mg/Cap. Bot. 100s UD 100s. *c-II.*
Use: Analgesic combination, narcotic.

•**tyloxapol.** (till-OX-ah-pahl) U.S.P. 23.
Use: Detergent, ophthalmic; cystic fibrosis. [Orphan drug].
See: Enuclene (Alcon Laboratories).

Tympagesic. (Pharmacia & Upjohn) Phenylephrine HCl 0.25%, antipyrine 5%, benzocaine 5%, in propylene glycol. Liq. Bot. w/dropper 13 ml. *Rx.*
Use: Antihistamine, otic.

Ty-Pap. (Major) **Elix.:** Acetaminophen 160 mg/5 ml. Bot. pt., gal. **Supp.:** Acetaminophen 120 mg, 650 mg In 12s. *otc.*
Use: Analgesic.

Typhim Vi. (Pasteur Merieux Connaught) Typhoid Vi polysaccharide vaccine 0.5 ml. Inj. Single-dose syringes and 25 ml, 50 ml vials. *Rx.*
Use: Immunization, typhoid.

•**typhoid vaccine,** (TIE-foyd) U.S.P. 23.
Use: Immunization.

typhoid vaccine. (Wyeth Ayerst) 8 units per ml (not > 1 billion organisms per ml). Heat-phenol treated vaccine. Vial 5 ml, 10 ml, 20 ml. Acetone-killed and dried vaccine. Pow. for Inj. 50-dose vial. *Rx.*
Use: Immunization.

typhoid vaccine capsule. *Rx.*
Use: Immnization.
See: Vivotif Berna (Berna Products).

typhoid vaccine polysaccharide. *Rx.*
Use: Immunization.
See: Typhim Vi (Pasteur Merieux Connaught).

Tyrex-2. (Ross Laboratories) Protein 30 g, fat 15.5 g, carbohydrates 30 g, Na 880 mg, K 1370 mg, Cal 410/100 g. With appropriate vitamins and minerals. Phenylalanine and tyrosine free. Pow. Can 325 g. *otc.*
Use: Nutritional supplement.

Tyrodone. (Major) Hydrocodone bitartrate 5 mg, pseudoephedrine HCl 60 mg/5 ml, alcohol 5%. Liq. Bot. 473 ml. *c-III.*
Use: Antitussive, decongestant.

Tyromex-1. (Ross Laboratories) Protein 15 g, fat 23.9 g, carbohydrates 46.3 g, linoleic acid 1800 mg, Fe 9 mg, Na 190 mg, K 675 mg, Cal 480/100 g. With appropriate vitamins and minerals. Phenylalanine, tyrosine and methionine free. Pow. Can 350 g. *otc.*
Use: Nutritional supplement.

•**tyropanoate sodium.** (TIE-row-PAN-oh-ate) U.S.P. 23.
Use: Diagnostic aid (radiopaque medium, cholecystographic).

See: Bilopaque (Sanofi).

tyropaque caps. (Sanofi) Tyropanoate sodium. *Rx.*
Use: Oral cholecystographic medium.

•**tyrosine.** (TIE-row-SEEN) U.S.P. 23. L-Tyrosine.
Use: Amino acid.

tyrosine hydroxylase inhibitor.
Use: Antihypertensive.
See: Demser (Merck).

Tyrosum Skin Cleanser. (Summers) Isopropanol 50%, polysorbate 80 2%, and acetone 10%. Bot. 120 ml, pt. Towelettes 24s, 50s. *otc.*
Use: Dermatologic, cleanser.

•**tyrothricin.** (tie-roe-THRYE-sin) U.S.P. 23. An antibiotic from *Bacillus brevis.* Tyrodac; Tyroderm.
Use: Antibacterial.

Ty-Tabs. (Major) Acetaminophen with codeine #2, #3, #4. Bot. 100s, 500s, 1000s. *c-III.*
Use: Analgesic combination, narcotic.

Ty-Tabs, Children's . (Major) Acetaminophen 80 mg/Tab. Bot. 30s, 100s. *otc.*
Use: Analgesic.

Ty-Tabs Extra Strength. (Major) Acetaminophen 500 mg/Tab. Bot. 100s, 1000s. *otc.*
Use: Analgesic.

Tyzine Nasal Solution. (Key Pharm) Tetrahydrozoline HCl 0.1%. Bot. pt., oz. *otc.*
Use: Decongestant.

Tyzine Nasal Spray. (Key Pharm) Tetrahydrozoline HCl 0.1%. Bot. 0.5 oz. *otc.*
Use: Decongestant.

Tyzine Pediatric Nasal Drops. (Key Pharm) Tetrahydrozoline HCl 0.05%. Bot. 0.5 oz. *otc.*
Use: Decongestant.

U

UAA. (Econo Med Pharmaceuticals) Methenamine 40.8 mg, phenyl salicylate 18.1 mg, methylene blue 5.4 mg, benzoic acid 4.5 mg, atropine sulfate 0.03 mg, hyoscyamine 0.03 mg/Tab. Bot. 100s, 1000s. *Rx.*
Use: Anti-infective, urinary.

UAD Cream. (Forest Pharmaceutical) Clioquinol 3%, hydrocortisone 1%, ceresin, glyceryl oleate, propylene glycol, parabens, mineral oil, pramoxine HCl. 15 g. *Rx.*
Use: Corticosteroid; anesthetic, local.

UAD Lotion. (Forest Pharmaceutical) Clioquinol 0.75%, hydrocortisone 0.25%, cetyl alcohol, glyceryl stearate, lanolin, parabens, mineral oil, pramoxine HCl, propylene glycol. 20 ml. *Rx.*
Use: Corticosteroid; anesthetic, local.

UAD Otic. (Forest Pharmaceutical) Hydrocortisone 1%, neomycin sulfate 5 mg, polymyxin B sulfate 10,000 units per ml, thimersol 0.01%, cetyl alcohol, propylene glycol, polysorbate 80. Susp. 10 ml w/dropper. *Rx.*
Use: Otic.

UBT. (Biomerica) For detection of blood in the urine.
Use: Diagnostic aid.

UCG-Beta Slide Monoclonal II. (Wampole Laboratories) Two-minute latex agglutination inhibition slide test for the qualitative detection of B-hCG/hCG (sensitivity 0.5 IU hCG/ml) in urine. Kit 50s, 100s, 300s.
Use: Diagnostic aid.

UCG-Beta Stat. (Wampole Laboratories) One-hour passive hemagglutination inhibition tube test for the qualitative detection and quantitative determination of B-hCG/hCG (sensitivity 0.2 IU hCG/ml) in urine. Kit 50s, 300s.
Use: Diagnostic aid.

UCG-Lyphotest. (Wampole Laboratories) One-hour passive hemagglutination inhibition tube test for the qualitative or quantitative determination of human chorionic gonadotropin (sensitivity 0.5-1 IU hCG/ml) in urine. Kit 10s, 50s, 300s.
Use: Diagnostic aid.

UCG-Slide Test. (Wampole Laboratories) Rapid latex agglutination inhibition slide test for the qualitative detection of human chorionic gonadotropin (Sensitivity: 2 IU hCG/ml) in urine. Kit 30s, 100s, 300s, 1000s.
Use: Diagnostic aid.

UCG-Test. (Wampole Laboratories) Two-hour hemagglutination inhibition tube test for the determination of human chorionic gonadotropin (sensitivity 0.5 IU hCG/ml undiluted specimen. 1.5 IU hCG/ml 1:3 diluted specimen) in urine and serum. Kit 10s, 25s, 100s, 300s.
Use: Diagnostic aid.

UCG-Titration Set. (Wampole Laboratories) A two-hour hemagglutination inhibition tube test for the determination of human chorionic gonadotropin (Sensitivity 1 IU hCG/ml) in urine or serum. Kit 45s.
Use: Diagnostic aid.

Uendex. Dextran sulfate, inhaled, aerosolized.
Use: Cystic fibrosis treatment.[Orphan drug]

Ulcerease. (Med Derm) Liquified phenol 0.6%, glycerin, sugar free/Liq. 180 ml. *otc.*
Use: Anesthetic, local.

Ulcerin P Tablets. (Sanofi Winthrop) Aluminum hydroxide. *otc.*
Use: Antacid.

Ulcerin Tablets. (Sanofi Winthrop) Aluminum hydroxide. *otc.*
Use: Antacid.

•**uldazepam.** (uhl-DAY-zeh-pam) USAN.
Use: Hypnotic, sedative.

Ulpax. (Roche Laboratories). Ablukast sodium.
Use: Antiasthmatic (leukotriene antagonist).

ULR-LA. (Geneva Pharm) Phenylpropanolamine HCl 75 mg, guaifenesin 400 mg. Tab. Bot. 100s. *Rx.*
Use: Decongestant, expectorant.

Ultane. (Abbott Laboratories) Volatile liquid for inhalation: sevoflurane. Bot. 250 ml. *Rx.*
Use: Anesthetic, general.

Ultiva. (GlaxoWellcome) Remifentanil HCl/Pow. for injection. Vial. 3 ml, 5 ml, 10 ml. *Rx.*
Use: Analgesic, narcotic.

Ultra B50. (NBTT) Vitamins B_1 50 mg, B_2 50 mg, B_3 50 mg, B_5 50 mg, B_6 50 mg, B_{12} 50 mcg, folic acid 0.1 mg, PABA 50 mg, inositol 50 mg, biotin 50 mcg, choline 50 mg, lecithin 50 mg/Tab. Bot. 60s, 180s. *otc.*
Use: Vitamin supplement.

Ultra B100. (NBTY) Vitamins B_1 100 mg, B_2 100 mg, B_3 100 mg, B_5 100 mg, B_6 100 mg, B_{12} 100 mcg, folic acid 0.1 mg, PABA 100 mg, inositol 100 mg, biotin 100 mcg, choline bitartrate 100 mg/

TR Tab. Bot. 50s. *otc.*
Use: Vitamin supplement.

Ultrabex. (Health for Life Brands) Vitamins B_1 20 mg, C 50 mg, B_2 2 mg, B_6 0.5 mg, niacinamide 35 mg, calcium pantothenate 0.5 mg, wheat germ oil 30 mg, B_{12} 20 mcg, liver desiccated 150 mg, iron 11.58 mg, calcium 29 mg, phosphorus 23 mg, dicalcium phosphate 100 mg, magnesium 1.11 mg, manganese 1.3 mg, potassium 2.24 mg, zinc 0.68 mg, choline 25 mg, inositol 25 mg, pepsin 32.5 mg, diastase 32.5 mg, hesperidin 25 mg, biotin 20 mcg, hydrolyzed yeast 81.25 mg, protein digest 47.04 mg, amino acids 34.21 mg/Cap. Bot. 50s, 100s, 1000s. *otc.*
Use: Mineral, vitamin supplement.

ULTRAbrom. (WE Pharm) Brompheniramine maleate 12 mg, pseudoephedrine HCl 120 mg/SR Cap. Bot. 100s. *Rx.*
Use: Antihistamine, decongestant.

ULTRAbrom PD. (WE Pharm) Brompheniramine maleate 6 mg, pseudoephedrine 60 mg/SR Cap. Bot. 100s. *Rx.*
Use: Antihistamine, decongestant.

Ultracal. (Bristol-Myers) Protein 44 g, carbohydrate 123 g, fat 45 g, Na 930 mg, K 1610 mg, mOsm 310 kg H_2O, cal. 1.06/ml, vitamins A, B_1, B_2, B_3, B_5, B_6, B_{12}, C, D, E, K, folic acid, choline, biotin, Ca, P, I, Fe, Mg, Cu, Zn, Mn, Cl, Se, Cr, Mo. Liq. Can. 8 oz. *otc.*
Use: Nutritional supplement.

Ultra Cap. (Weeks & Leo) Acetaminophen 300 mg, guaifenesin 100 mg, chlorpheniramine maleate 4 mg, phenylephrine HCl 10 mg, dextromethorphan HBr 6 mg/Cap. Vial 18s. *Rx.*
Use: Analgesic, antihistamine, antitussive, decongestant, expectorant.

Ultra-Care. (Allergan) **Disinfecting Soln.:** Hydrogen peroxide 3%, sodium stannate, sodium nitrate, phosphate buffer. Bot. 120 ml, 360 ml; **Neutralizer Tab.:** Catalase, hydroxypropyl methylcellulose, buffering agents. Pkg. 12s, 36s w/ cup. *otc.*
Use: Contact lens care.

Ultracortinol. (Novartis Pharmaceuticals) Agent to suppress overactive adrenal glands. Pending release.

Ultra Derm Bath Oil. (Baker/Cummins) Bot. 8 oz. *otc.*
Use: Emollient.

Ultra Derm Moisturizer. (Baker/Cummins) Bot. 8 oz. *otc.*
Use: Emollient.

Ultra Freeda. (Freeda Vitamins) Vitamins A 4166 IU, D 133 IU, E 66.7 mg, B_1 16.7 mg, B_2 16.7 mg, B_3 33 mg, B_5 33 mg, B_6 16.7 mg, B_{12} 33 mcg, C 333 mg, folic acid 0.27 mg, iron 2 mg, calcium 27 mg, zinc 1.1 mg, choline, inositol, bioflavonoids, PABA, biotin 100 mcg, Cr, I, K, Mg, Mn, Mo, Se. Tab. Bot. 90s, 180s, 270s. *otc.*
Use: Mineral, vitamin supplement.

Ultra Freeda Iron Free. (Freeda Vitamins) Vitamins A 4166 IU, D 133 IU, E 66.7_2 mg, B_1 16.7 mg, B_2 16.7 mg, B_3 33 mg, B_5 33 ng, B_6 16.7 mg, B_{12} 33 mcg, C 333 mg, FA 0.27 mg, Ca 27 mg, Zn 1.1 mg, choline, inositol, bioflavonoids, PABA, biotin 100 mcg, Cr, I, K, Mg, Mn, Mo, Se. Tab. Bot. 90s, 180s, 270s. *otc.*
Use: Mineral, vitamin supplement.

Ultragesic. (Stewart-Jackson) Acetaminophen 500 mg, hydrocodone bitartrate 5 mg/Cap. Bot. 100s. *c-III.*
Use: Analgesic combination, narcotic.

Ultralan. (Elan) Protein 60 g, fat 50 g, carbohydrates 202 g, Na 1.035 g, K 1.755 g/L. Lactose free. With appropriate vitamins and minerals. Liq. In 1000 ml New Pak systems with and without ColorCheck. *otc.*
Use: Nutritional supplement.

Ultralente insulin.
See: Iletin (Lilly).

Ultram. (Ortho McNeil) Tramadol HCl 50 mg/Tab. Bot. 100s, UD 100s. *Rx.*
Use: Analgesic.

Ultra Mide 25. (Baker/Cummins) Bot. 8 oz. *otc.*
Use: Emollient.

Ultrapred. (Horizon) Prednisolone acetate 1%. Susp. Bot. 5 ml. *Rx.*
Use: Corticosteroid, ophthalmic.

Ultrasone. (Gordon Laboratories) Ultrasound aid. Bot. qt, gal. Plastic Bot. 8 oz.
Use: Ultrasound contact cream.

Ultra Tears. (Alcon Laboratories) Hydroxypropyl methylcellulose 2910 1%, benzalkonium Cl 0.01%, NaCl. Bot. 15 ml. *otc.*
Use: Artificial tears.

Ultravate. (Westwood Squibb) Halobetasol propionate. *Rx.*
Use: Corticosteroid, topical.

Ultravist. (Berlex) **150 mgI/ml** (iopromide 311.7 mg, tromethamine 2.42 mg, EDTA 0.1 mg). Preservative free. Inj. Vial 50 ml. **240 mgI/ml** (iopromide 498.72 mg, tromethamine 2.42 mg,

EDTA 0.1 mg). Preservative free, Inj. Vial 50, 100, 200 ml. **300 mgI/ml** (iopromide 623.4 mg, tromethamine 2.42 mg, EDTA 0.1 mg). Preservative free. Inj. Vial 50, 100, 150 ml. **370 mgI/ml** (iopromide 768.86 mg, tromethamine 2.42 mg, EDTA 0.1 mg). Preservative free. Inj. Vial 50, 100, 150, 200 ml. *Rx.*
Use: Diagnostic aid.

Ultra Vitamin A & D. (NBTY) Vitamins A 25,000 IU, D 1000 IU. Tab. Bot. 100s. *otc.*
Use: Vitamin supplement.

Ultra Vita Time. (NBTY) Iron 6 mg, vitamins A 10,000 IU, D 400 IU, E 13 IU, B_1 25 mg, B_2 25 mg, B_3 50 mg, B_5 12.5 mg, B_6 15 mg, B_{12} 50 mcg, C 150 mg, folic acid 0.4 mg, B, Ca, Cr, Cu, I, K, Mg, Mn, Mo, P, Se, Zn 5 mg, biotin 1 mg, bioflavonoids, bone meal, PABA, choline bitartrate, betaine, inositol, lecithin, desiccated liver, rutin/Tab. Bot. 100s. *otc.*
Use: Mineral, vitamin supplement.

Ultrazyme Enzymatic Cleaner. (Allergan) Subtilisin A, effervescing, buffering and tableting agents for dilution in hydrogen peroxide 3%. Tab. Pkg. 5s, 10s, 15s, 20s. *otc.*
Use: Contact lens care.

Ultrum. (Towne) Vitamins A 5000 IU, E 30 IU, C 90 mg, folic acid 400 mcg, B_1 2.25 mg, B_2 2.6 mg, niacinamide 20 mg, B_6 3 mg, B_{12} 9 mcg, biotin 45 mcg, D 400 IU, pantothenic acid 10 mg, calcium 162 mg, phosphorus 125 mg, iodine 150 mcg, iron 27 mg, magnesium 100 mg, copper 3 mg, manganese 7.5 mg, potassium 7.5 mg, zinc 22.5 mg/Tab. Bot. 100s. *otc.*
Use: Mineral, vitamin supplement.

Ultrum with Selenium. (Towne) Vitamins A 5000 IU, E 30 IU, C 90 mg, folic acid 2.25 mg, B_1 2.25 mg, B_2 2.6 mg, niacinamide 20 mg, B_6 3 mg, B_{12} 9 mcg, D 400 IU, biotin 45 mcg, pantothenic acid 10 mg, calcium 162 mg, phosphorus 125 mg, iodine 150 mcg, iron 27 mg, magnesium 100 mg, copper 3 mg, manganese 7.5 mg, potassium 7.7 mg, chloride 7 mg, molybdenum 15 mcg, selenium 15 mcg, zinc 22.5 mg/Tab. Bot. 130s. *Rx.*
Use: Mineral, vitamin supplement.

Unasyn. (Roerig) Ampicillin sodium 1 g, sulbactam sodium 0.5 g, ampicillin sodium 2 g, sulbactam sodium 1 g. Pow. for inj. Vial, piggyback vial. *Rx.*
Use: Anti-infective, penicillin.

10-undecenoic acid. Undecylenic Acid, U.S.P. 23.
Use: Antifungal, topical.

10-undecenoic acid, zinc (2+) salt. Zinc Undecylenate, U.S.P. 23.
Use: Antifungal, topical.

undecoylium chloride-iodine. Virac, Preps. (Ruson).
Use: Anti-infective, topical.

•**undecylenic acid.** (un-deh-sill-EN-ik) U.S.P. 23.
Use: Antifungal, topical.
See: Desenex, Aer. Spray Pow., Cream, Foam, Oint., Pow., Fungoid AF, Sol. Preps (Novartis Pharmaceuticals).
W/Benzethonium Cl, benzalkonium Cl, tannic acid, isopropyl alcohol.
See: Tulvex, Liq. (Del Pharmaceuticals).
W/Dichlorophene.
See: Fungicidal Talc (Gordon Laboratories).
Onychomycetin, Liq. (Gordon Laboratories).
W/Salicylic acid.
See: Sal-Dex, Liq. (Scrip).
W/Salicylic acid, benzoic acid, sulfur, dichlorophene.
See: Fungicidal, Oint. (Gordon Laboratories).
W/Sodium propionate, sodium caprylate, propionic acid, salicylic acid, copper undecylenate.
See: Verdefam, Soln. (Texas).
W/Zinc undecylenate.
See: Cruex Cream, Spray Pow. (Novartis Pharmaceuticals) Desenex, Preps. (Novartis Pharmaceuticals).
Ting, Aerosol (Novartis Pharmaceuticals).

undecylenic acid salts. Calcium, copper, zinc.

Undelenic Ointment. (Gordon Laboratories) Undecylenic acid 5%, zinc undecylenate 20%. Jar oz, lb. *otc.*
Use: Antifungal, topical.

Undelenic Tincture. (Gordon Laboratories) Undecylenic acid 10%, chloroxylenol 0.5%. Brush Bot. oz. Bot. pt. *otc.*
Use: Antifungal, topical.

Unguentine Ointment "Original Formula". (Mentholatum) Phenol 1% in ointment base. Tube oz. *otc.*
Use: Dermatologic, counterirritant.

Unguentine Plus First Aid Cream. (Mentholatum) Parachlorometaxylenol 2%, lidocaine HCl 2%, phenol 0.5% in a moisturizing cream base. Tube ½ oz, 1 oz, 2 oz. *otc.*
Use: Dermatologic, counterirritant.

Unguentum Bossi. (Doak Dermatologics) Ammoniated mercury 5%, meth-

amine sulfosalicylate 2%, tar distillate "Doak" 5%, Doak oil 40%, petrolatum, sorbitol sesquioleate, cholesterol derivatives, beeswax. Cream. Tube 60 g, 480 g. *Rx.*
Use: Antipsoriatic.

Uni-Ace. (United Research Laboratories) Acetaminophen 100 mg per ml. Alcohol free. Liq. Bot. 15 ml with dropper. *otc.*
Use: Analgesic.

Unibase. (Parke-Davis) Water-absorbing oint. base. Jar lb. *Rx.*
Use: Pharmaceutical aid, ointment base.

Uni-Bent Cough. (United Research Laboratories) Diphenhydramine HCl 12.5 mg/5 ml, alcohol 5%. Syr. Bot 118 ml. *Rx.*
Use: Antihistamine.

Unicap Capsules. (Pharmacia & Upjohn) Vitamins A 5000 IU, D 400 IU, E 30 IU, B_1 1.5 mg, B_2 1.7 mg, B_3 20 mg, B_6 2 mg, B_{12} 6 mcg, C 60 mg, FA 0.4 mg/Cap. Bot. 120s. *otc.*
Use: Vitamin supplement.

Unicap Jr. Chewable. (Pharmacia & Upjohn) Vitamins A 5000 IU, D 400 IU, E 15 IU, C 60 mg, folic acid 400 mcg, B_1 1.5 mg, B_2 1.7 mg, B_3 20 mg, B_6 2 mg, B_{12} 6 mcg/Tab. Bot. 120s. *otc.*
Use: Vitamin supplement.

Unicap M. (Pharmacia & Upjohn) Iron 18 mg, vitamins A 5000 IU, D 400 IU, E 30 IU, B_1 1.5 mg, B_2 1.7 mg, B_3 20 mg, B_5 10 mg, B_6 2 mg, B_{12} 6 mcg, C 60 mg, folic acid 0.4 mg, Ca, Cu, I, K, Mn, P, Zn 15 mg, tartrazine/Tab. Bot. 120s. *otc.*
Use: Mineral, vitamin supplement.

Unicap Plus Iron. (Pharmacia & Upjohn) Vitamins A 5000 IU, D 400 IU, E 30 IU, C 60 mg, folic acid 0.4 mg, B_1 1.5 mg, B_2 1.7 mg, B_3 20 mg, B_5 10 mg, B_6 2 mg, B_{12} 6 mcg, iron 22.5 mg, Ca/Tab. Bot. 120s. *otc.*
Use: Mineral, vitamin supplement.

Unicap Sr. (Pharmacia & Upjohn) Iron 10 mg, vitamins A 5000 IU, D 200 IU, E 15 IU, B_1 1.2 mg, B_2 1.4 mg, B_3 16 mg, B_5 10 mg, B_6 2.2 mg, B_{12} 3 mcg, C 60 mg, folic acid 0.4 mg, Ca, Cu, I, K, Mg, Mn, P, Zn 15 mg/Tab. Bot. 120s. *otc.*
Use: Mineral, vitamin supplement.

Unicap T. (Pharmacia & Upjohn) Iron 18 mg, vitamins A 5000 IU, D 400 IU, E 30 IU, B_1 10 mg, B_2 20 mg, B_3 100 mg, B_5 25 mg, B_6 6 mg, B_{12} 18 mcg, C 500 mg, folic acid 0.4 mg, Cu, I, K, Mn, Se, Zn 15 mg, tartrazine/Tab. Bot. 60s. *otc.*
Use: Mineral, vitamin supplement.

Unicap Tablets. (Pharmacia & Upjohn) Vitamins A 5000 IU, D 400 IU, E 15 IU, B_1 1.5 mg, B_2 1.7 mg, B_3 20 mg, B_6 2 mg, B_{12} 6 mcg, C 60 mg, FA 0.4 mg/Tab. Bot. 120s. *otc.*
Use: Vitamin supplement.

Unicomplex-M. (Rugby) Iron 18 mg, vitamins A 5000 IU, D 400 IU, E 15 mg, B_1 1.5 mg, B_2 1.7 mg, B_3 20 mg, B_5 10 mg, B_6 2 mg, B_{12} 6 mcg, C 60 mg, folic acid 0.4 mg, Ca, Cu, I, K, Mn, Zn/Tab. Bot. 90s, 1000s. *otc.*
Use: Mineral, vitamin supplement.

Unicomplex-T with Minerals. (Rugby) Iron 10 mg, vitamins A 5000 IU, D 400 IU, E 15 mg, B_1 10 mg, B_2 10 mg, B_3 100 mg, B_5 20 mg, B_6 2 mg, B_{12} 4 mcg, C 300 mg, folic acid 0.4 mg, Ca, Cu, I, K, Mg, Mn/Tab. Bot. 60s. *otc.*
Use: Mineral, vitamin supplement.

Unicomplex - T & M. (Rugby) Iron 18 mg, vitamins A 5000 IU, D 400 IU, E 30 mg, B_1 10 mg, B_2 10 mg, B_3 100 mg, B_5 25 mg, B_6 6 mg, B_{12} 18 mcg, C 500 mg, FA 0.4 mg, Ca, Cu, I, K, Mn, Zn 15 mg/Tab. Bot. 60s. *otc.*
Use: Mineral, vitamin supplement.

Uni-Decon. (United Research Laboratories) Phenylpropanolamine HCl 40 mg, phenylephrine HCl 10 mg, chlorpheniramine maleate 5 mg, phenyltoloxamine citrate 15 mg/Tab. Bot. 100s, 500s and 1000s. *Rx.*
Use: Antihistamine, decongestant.

Uni-Dur. (Key Pharm) Theophylline 400 mg or 600 mg, sugar, lactose/ER Tab. Bot. 100s. *Rx.*
Use: Bronchodilator.

Unifiber. (Dow Hickam) Powdered cellulose 3 g per tbsp. < 4 calories per serving. Corn syrup solids, xanthan gum. Pow. Bot. 454 g. *otc.*
Use: Laxative.

•**unifocon a.** (you-nih-FOE-kahn A) USAN.
Use: Contact lens material (hydrophic).

Unilax. (B.F. Ascher) Docusate 230 mg, phenolphthalein 130 mg. Sorbitol. Cap. Bot. 15s, 20s, 60s. *otc.*
Use: Laxative.

Unipen. (Wyeth Ayerst) Sodium nafcillin. **Vial:** Vial 2 g, Piggyback Vial 2 g, Bulk vial 10 g. **Oral Soln.:** 250 mg/5 ml w/ alcohol 2%. Bot. to make 100 ml. *Rx.*
Use: Anti-infective, penicillin.

Uniphyl. (Purdue Frederick) Theophylline 200 mg, 400 mg, 600 mg/Controlled-release Tab. **200 mg:** Bot. 60s,

100s, UD 100s. **400 mg:** Bot. 60s, 100s, 500s, UD 100s. **600 mg:** Bot. 100s. *Rx.*
Use: Bronchodilator.

Uniretic. (Schwarz Pharma) Moexipril HCl 7.5 mg/hydrochlorothiazide 12.5 mg. Moexipril HCl 15 mg/hydrochlorothiazide 25 mg, lactose/Tab. Bot. 100s. *Rx.*
Use: Antihypertensive.

Unisol. (Alcon Laboratories) Buffered isotonic solution with sodium Cl, boric acid, sodium borate. Bot. 15 ml (25s), 120 ml (2s, 3s). *otc.*
Use: Contact lens care.

Unisol 4 Sterile Saline. (Alcon Laboratories) Buffered isotonic solution with sodium Cl, boric acid, sodium borate. Bot. 120 ml. *otc.*
Use: Contact lens care.

Unisol Plus. (Alcon Laboratories) Buffered isotonic solution w/ NaCl, boric acid, sodium borate. Aerosol 240 ml or 360 ml. *otc.*
Use: Contact lens care.

Unisom Nighttime Sleep-Aid. (Pfizer) Doxylamine succcinate 25 mg/Tab. Blister 8s, 16s, 32s, 48s.
Use: Sleep aid.

Unisom with Pain Relief. (Pfizer) Acetaminophen 650 mg, diphenhydramine HCl 50 mg/Tab. Blister 16s. *otc.*
Use: Analgesic, sleep aid.

Unituss HC. (United Research Laboratories) Hydrocodone bitartrate 2.5 mg, phenylephrine HCl 5 mg, chlorpheniramine maleate 2 mg/5 ml. Saccharin, sorbitol, sugar free. Syrup. Bot. 473 ml. *c-III.*
Use: Antihistamine, antitussive, decongestant.

Uni-Tussin DM. (United Research Laboratories) Dextromethorphan HBr 10 mg, guaifenesin 100 mg/5 ml. Syr. Bot. 118 ml. *otc.*
Use: Antitussive, expectorant.

Uni-Tussin Syrup. (United Research Laboratories) Dextromethorphan HBr 15 mg, guaifenesin 100 mg, alcohol 1.4%. Bot. 120 ml. *otc.*
Use: Antitussive, expectorant.

Univasc. (Schwarz Pharma) Moexipril HCl 7.5 mg or 15 mg, lactose/Tab. Bot. 100s, UD 90s. *Rx.*
Use: Antihypertensive.

unna's boot.
See: Zinc Gelatin, U.S.P. 23.

Unproco Capsules. (Solvay) Dextromethorphan HBr 30 mg, guaifenesin 200 mg/Cap. Bot. 100s. *otc.*
Use: Antitussive, expectorant.

Uplex. (Arcum) Vitamins A 5000 IU, D 400 IU, B_1 3 mg, B_2 3 mg, B_6 1 mg, B_{12} 2.5 mcg, nicotinamide 20 mg, calcium pantothenate 5 mg, C 50 mg/Cap. Bot. 100s, 1000s. *otc.*
Use: Mineral, vitamin supplement.

Uplex No. 2. (Arcum) Vitamins A palmitate 10,000 IU, D 400 IU, B_1 5 mg, B_2 5 mg, C 100 mg, B_6 2 mg, B_{12} 3 mcg, E 2.5 IU, niacinamide 25 mg, calcium pantothenate 5 mg/Cap. Bot. 100s, 1000s. *otc.*
Use: Mineral, vitamin supplement.

Urabeth Tabs. (Major) Bethanechol 5 mg, 10 mg, 25 mg or 50 mg/Tab. **5 mg:** Bot. 100s. **10 mg:** Bot. 250s. **25 mg:** Bot. 250s, 1000s. **50 mg:** Bot. 100s, UD 100s. *Rx.*
Use: Genitourinary.

Uracid. (Wesley Pharmacal) dl-Methionine 0.2 g/Cap. Bot. 100s, 1000s. *Rx.*
Use: Diaper rash preparation.

uradal.
See: Carbromal (Various Mfr.)

•**urea.** (you-REE-ah) U.S.P. 23.
Use: Topically for dry skin; diuretic.
See: Aquacare, Cream, Lot. (Allergan).
Aquacare-HP, Cream, Lot. (Allergan).
Artra Ashy Skin, Cream (Schering Plough).
Calmurid, Cream (Pharmacia & Upjohn).
Carmol, Cream (Ingram).
Carmol Ten, Lot. (Ingram).
Elaqua 10% or 20%, Cream (ICN Pharmaceuticals).
Gormel, Cream (Gordon Laboratories).
Nutraplus, Cream, Lot. (Galderma).
Rea-lo, Lot. (Whorton).

W/Benzocaine, benzyl alcohol, p-chloro-m-xylenol, propyleneglycol.
See: 20-Cain Burn Relief (Alto Pharmaceuticals Inc.).

W/Hydrocortisone acetate.
See: Carmol-HC, Cream (Ingram).

W/Glycerin.
See: Kerid Ear Drops, Liq. (Blair Laboratories).

W/Sulfur colloidal, red mercuric sulfide.
See: Teenac, Cream, Oint. (ICN Pharmaceuticals).

W/Zinc oxide, sulfur, salicylic acid, benzalkonium Cl, isopropyl alcohol.
See: Akne Drying Lotion

urea peroxide.
See: Cankaid (Becton Dickinson).
Gly-Oxide Liquid (Hoechst Marion Roussel).

Oragel Brace-aid Rinse (Del Pharmaceuticals).
Proxigel (Schwarz Pharma).

Ureacin-10 Lotion. (Pedinol) Urea 10%. Bot. 8 oz. *otc.*
Use: Emollient.

Ureacin-20 Creme. (Pedinol) Urea 20%. Jar 2.5 oz. *otc.*
Use: Emollient.

Ureaphil. (Abbott Hospital Prods) Sterile urea 40 g, citric acid 1 mg/150 ml. Bot. 150 ml. *Rx.*
Use: Diuretic.

Urecholine. (Merck) Bethanechol Cl. **Inj.:** 5 mg/ml Vial 1 ml, 6s. **Tab.:** 5 mg, 10 mg, 25 mg or 50 mg. Bot. 100s, UD 100s. *Rx.*
Use: Genitourinary.

•**uredepa.** (YOU-ree-DEH-pah) USAN.
Use: Antineoplastic.
See: Avinar (Centeon).

p-ureidobenzenearsonic acid.
See: Carbarsone, U.S.P. 23.

Urelief. (Rocky Mtn.) Methenamine 2 gr, salol 0.5 gr, methylene blue 1/10 gr, benzoic acid gr, hyoscyamine sulfate gr, atropine sulfate gr/Tab. Bot. 100s. *Rx.*
Use: Anti-infective, urinary.

Urese. (Roerig)
See: Benzthiazide.

urethan. Ethyl Carbamate, Ethyl Urethan, Urethane.
Use: Antineoplastic.

Urex Tablets. (3M Pharmaceuticals) Methenamine hippurate 1 g/Tab. Bot. 100s. *Rx.*
Use: Anti-infective, urinary.

U.R.I. (Sigma-Tau Pharmaceuticals) Atropine sulfate 0.2 mg, chlorpheniramine maleate 5 mg, phenylpropanolamine HCl 12.5 mg/ml. Vial 10 ml. *Rx.*
Use: Anticholinergic, antihistamine, antispasmodic, decongestant.

Uric Acid Reagent Strips. (Bayer Corp) Seralyzer reagent strip. For uric acid in serum or plasma. Bot. 25s.
Use: Diagnostic aid.

uricosuric agents.
See: Anturane, Tab., Cap. (Novartis Pharmaceuticals).
Benemid, Tab. (Merck).
ColBenemid, Tab. (Merck).

Uricult. (Orion Diagnostica) Urine culture test to detect bacteria and identify uropathogens. Bot. 10s.
Use: Diagnostic aid.

uridine, 2-deoxy-5-iodo-. Idoxuridine, U.S.P. 23.

uridine 5'-triphosphate. (Inspire Pharm)
Use: Cystic fibrosis; ciliany dyskinesia. [Orphan drug]

Uridium. (Ferndale Laboratories) Phenylazodiamine pyridine HCl 75 mg, sulfacetamide 250 mg/Tab. Bot. 30s, 100s, 1000s. (Ferndale Laboratories) 100s.
Use: Anti-infective, urinary.

Uridon Modified. (Rugby) Methenamine 40.8 mg, phenyl salicylate 18.1 mg, atropine sulfate 0.03 mg, hyoscyamine 0.03 mg, benzoic acid 4.5 mg, methylene blue 5.4 mg/Tab. Bot. 100s, 1000s. *Rx.*
Use: Anti-infective, urinary.

Urifon-Forte. (T.E. Williams) Sulfamethizole 450 mg, phenazopyridine HCl 50 mg/Cap. Bot. 100s, 1000s. *Rx.*
Use: Anti-infective, urinary.

Urigen. (Fellows) Calcium mandelate 0.2 g, methenamine 0.2 g, phenazopyridine HCl 50 mg, sodium phosphate 80 mg/Cap. Bot. 100s, 1000s. *Rx.*
Use: Anti-infective, urinary.

Urimar-T. (Marnel) Methenamine 81.6 mg, sodium biphosphate 40.8 mg, phenyl salicylate 36.2 mg, methylene blue 10.8 mg, hyoscyamine sulfate 0.12 mg. Tab. Bot. 100s. *Rx.*
Use: Anti-infective, urinary.

Urinary Antiseptic #2. (Various Mfr.) Atropine sulfate 0.03 mg, hyoscyamine 0.03 mg, methenamine 40.8 mg, methylene blue 5.4 mg, phenyl salicylate 18.1 mg, benzoic acid 4.5 mg/Tab. Bot. 100s, 1000s. *Rx.*
Use: Anti-infective, urinary.

Urinary Antiseptic #2 S.C.T. (Teva USA) Atropine sulfate 0.03 mg, hyoscyamine sulfate 0.03 mg, methenamine 40.8 mg, methylene blue 5.4 mg, phenyl salicylate 18.1 mg, benzoic acid 4.5 mg/Tab. Bot. 100s, 1000s. *Rx.*
Use: Anti-infective, urinary.

Urinary Antiseptic #3 S.C.T.. (Teva USA) Atropine sulfate 0.06 mg, hyoscyamine sulfate 0.03 mg, methenamine 120 mg, methylene blue 6 mg, phenyl salicylate 30 mg, benzoic acid 7.5 mg/Tab. Bot. 100s, 1000s. *Rx.*
Use: Anti-infective, urinary.

urine.
See: Diagnostic agents.

urine glucose tests.
See: Biotel Diabetes (Biotel).
Clinitest Tablets (Bayer Corp).
Chemstrip uG Strips (Boehringer Mannheim).
Clinistix Strips (Bayer Corp).
Dialstix Strips (Bayer Corp).

Test Tape (Eli Lilly).

urine sugar test.
See: Clinistix (Bayer Corp).

urine tests misc.
See: Nitrazine Paper (Apothecon).
Phenistix Reagent Strips (Bayer Corp).

Urin-Tek. (Bayer Corp) Tubes, plastic caps, adhesive labels, collection cups, and disposable tube holder. Package 100×5.

Urisan-P. (Sandia) Atropine sulfate 0.03 mg, hyoscyamine 0.03 mg, gelsemium 6.1 mg, methenamine 40.8 mg, salol 18.1 mg, benzoic acid 4.5 mg, methylene blue 5.4 mg, phenylazodiaminopyridine HCl 100 mg/Tab. Bot. 100s, 1000s. *Rx.*
Use: Anti-infective, urinary.

Urised. (PolyMedica) Atropine sulfate 0.03 mg, hyoscyamine 0.03 mg, methenamine 40.8 mg, methylene blue 5.4 mg, benzoic acid 4.5 mg, phenyl salicylate 18.1 mg/Tab. Bot. 100s, 500s. *Rx.*
Use: Anti-infective, urinary.

Urisedamine. (PolyMedica) Methenamine mandelate 500 mg, l-hyoscyamine 0.15 mg/Tab. Bot. 100s. *Rx.*
Use: Anti-infective, urinary.

Urispas. (SmithKline Beecham Pharmaceuticals) Flavoxate HCl 100 mg/Tab. Bot. 100s, UD 100s. *Rx.*
Use: Urinary antispasmodic.

Uristix. (Bayer Corp) Urine test for glucose and protein. Reagent strips. 100s.
Use: Diagnostic aid.

Uristix 4 Reagent Strips. (Bayer Corp) Urinalysis reagent strip test for glucose, protein, nitrite, leukocytes. Bot. 100s.
Use: Diagnostic aid.

Uristix Reagent Strips. (Bayer Corp) Urinalysis reagent strip test for protein and glucose. Bot. 100s.
Use: Diagnostic aid.

Uritin. (Global Source) Methenamine 40.8 mg, atropine sulfate 0.03 mg, hyoscyamine sulfate 0.03 mg, salol 18.1 mg, benzoic acid 4.5 mg, methylene blue 5.4 mg, gelsemium 6.1 mg/Tab. Bot. 1000s. *Rx.*
Use: Anti-infective, urinary.

Uritin Formula. (Various Mfr.) Atropine sulfate 0.03 mg, hyoscyamine 0.03 mg, methenamine 40.8 mg, methylene blue 5.4 mg, phenyl salicylate 18.1 mg, benzoic acid 4.5 mg/Tab. Bot. 1000s. *Rx.*
Use: Anti-infective, urinary.

Urobak. (Shionogi) Sulfamethoxazole 500 mg/Tab. Bot. 100s, 1000s. *Rx.*
Use: Anti-infective, sulfonamide.

Urobiotic. (Roerig) Oxytetracycline as the HCl equivalent to oxytetracycline 250 mg, sulfamethizole 250 mg, phenazopyridine HCl 50 mg/Cap. Bot. 50s, UD pack Box 100s. *Rx.*
Use: Anti-infective, urinary.

Urocit-K. (Mission Pharmacal) Potassium citrate **540 mg:** Tab. Bot. 100s; **10 mEq:** Tab. Bot. 100s. *Rx.*
Use: Genitourinary.

•**urofollitropin.** (YOUR-oh-fahl-ih-TROE-pin) USAN.
Use: Hormone (follicle-stimulating). Ovulation. [Orphan drug]
See: Fertinex, Pow. For Inj. (Serono).
Metrodin, Inj. (Serono Labs).

urogastrone. (Chiron Vision)
Use: Corneal transplant surgery. [Orphan drug]

Urogesic. (Edwards Pharmaceuticals) Phenazopyridine HCl 100 mg, hyoscyamine HBr 0.12 mg, atropine sulfate 0.08 mg, scopolamine HBr 0.003 mg/Tab. Bot. 100s, 500s. *Rx.*
Use: Analgesic, urinary.

Urogesic Blue. (Edwards Pharmaceuticals) Methenamine 81.6 mg, sodium biphosphate 40.8 mg, phenyl salicylate 36.2 mg, methylene blue 10.8 mg, hyoscyamine (as sulfate) 0.12 mg. Tab. Bot. 100s. *Rx.*
Use: Anti-infective, urinary.

urography agents.
See: Diodrast.
Iodohippurate Sodium, Inj.
Iodopyracet.
Iodopyracet Compound.
Methiodal, Inj.
Renografin (Bristol-Myers Squibb).
Renovist (Bristol-Myers Squibb).
Renovue (Bristol-Myers Squibb).
Sodium Acetrizoate, Inj.
Sodium Iodomethamate, Inj.

•**urokinase.** (YUR-oh-KIN-ace) USAN. Plasminogen activator isolated from human kidney tissue.
Use: Plasminogen activator.

Uro-KP-Neutral. (Star) Sodium (as dibasic sodium phosphate) 1361 mg, potassium 298.6 mg, phosphorus (as dibasic potassium phosphate) 1037 mg/6 Tab. Bot. 100s. *Rx.*
Use: Mineral supplement.

Urolene Blue. (Star) Methylene blue 65 mg/Tab. Bot. 100s, 1000s. *Rx.*

Use: Anti-infective, urinary.

Urologic Sol G. (Abbott Hospital Prods) Bot. 1000 ml.
Use: Irrigant, ophthalmic.
See: Thiosulfil, Preps. (Wyeth Ayerst).

Uro-Mag. (Blaine) Magnesium oxide 140 mg/Cap. Bot. 100s, 1000s. *otc.*
Use: Antacid.

uronal.
See: Barbital (Various Mfr.).

Uro-Phosphate. (ECR Pharmaceuticals) Sodium biphosphate 434.78 mg, methenamine 300 mg/Film Coated Tab. Bot. 100s. *Rx.*
Use: Anti-infective, urinary.

Uroplus DS. (Shionogi) Trimethoprim 160 mg, sulfamethoxazole 800 mg/Tab. Bot. 100s, 500s. *Rx.*
Use: Anti-infective.

Uroplus SS. (Shionogi) Trimethoprim 80 mg, sulfamethoxazole 800 mg/Tab. Bot. 100s, 500s. *Rx.*
Use: Anti-infective.

Uroquid-Acid No. 2. (Beach Pharmaceuticals) Methenamine mandelate 500 mg, sodium acid phosphate monohydrate 500 mg/Tab. Bot. 100s. *Rx.*
Use: Anti-infective, urinary.

urotropin new. Methenamine Anhydromethylene Citrate (Various Mfr.).

Urovist Cysto. (Berlex) Diatrizoate meglumine 300 mg, edetate calcium disodium 0.05 mg/ml. Dilution Bot. 500 ml w/300 ml Soln.
Use: Radiopaque agent.

Urovist Cysto Pediatric. (Berlex) Diatrizoate meglumine 300 mg, edetate calcium disodium 0.1 mg/ml. Dilution bot. 300 ml w/100 ml soln.
Use: Radiopaque agent.

Urovist Meglumine DIU/CT. (Berlex) Diatrizoate meglumine 300 mg, edetate calcium disodium 0.05 mg/ml. Bot. 300 ml, Ctn. 10s.
Use: Radiopaque agent.

Urovist Sodium 300. (Berlex) Diatrizoate sodium 500 mg, edetate calcium disodium 0.1 mg/ml. Vial 50 ml, Box 10s.
Use: Radiopaque agent.

Ursinus Inlay-Tabs. (Novartis) Pseudoephedrine HCl 30 mg, aspirin 325 mg/Tab. Bot. 24s. *otc.*
Use: Decongestant, analgesic.

URSO. (Novartis) Ursodiol.
Use: Management and treatment of primary biliary cirrhosis. [Orphan Drug]

ursodeoxycholic acid.
Use: Primary biliary cirrhosis. [Orphan drug]

•**ursodiol.** (ERR-so-DIE-ole) U.S.P. 23. Ursodeoxycholic acid.
Use: Anticholelithogenic, urolithic; management and treatment of primary biliary cirrhosis. [Orphan drug]
See: Actigall (Axcan Pharma).
URSO (Novartis).

uterine relaxant.
See: Ritodrine HCl, Inj. (Abbott Laboratories).
Yutopar, Inj. (Astra).

Utimox. (Parke-Davis) Amoxicillin trihydrate. **Cap.:** 250 mg Bot. 100s, 500s, UD 100s; 500 mg Bot. 100s, UD 100s; **Oral susp.:** 125 mg or 250 mg/5 ml Bot. 80 ml, 100 ml, 150 ml, 200 ml. *Rx.*
Use: Anti-infective, penicillin.

U-Tran. (Scruggs) Atropine sulfate 0.03 mg, hyoscyamine 0.03 mg, methenamine 40.8 mg, benzoic acid 4.5 mg, salol 18.1 mg, methylene blue 5.4 mg/Tab. Bot. 100s, 1000s. *Rx.*
Use: Anti-infective, urinary.

U-Tri Special Formula Ointment. (U-Tri) Oint. Jar 4 oz, 7 oz.
Use: Analgesic, topical.

Uvadex. (Therakos, Inc.)
Use: Sclerosis treatment; cardiac allograft rejection prevention. [Orphan drug]
See: 8-Methoxsalen.

uvaleral.
See: Bromisovalum.

Uvasal Powder. (Sanofi Winthrop) Sodium bicarbonate, tartaric acid. *otc.*
Use: Antacid.

uva ursi. Leaves. (Sherwood Labs.) Fluid extract. Bot. pt, gal.

Uviban. Sodium Actinoquinol.
Use: Treatment of flash burns (ophthalmic).

Uvinul MS-40. (General Aniline & Film)
See: Sulisobenzone.

V

vaccine, adenovirus. *Rx.*
Use: Immunization.
See: adenovirus vaccine (Wyeth Ayerst).

vaccine, anthrax. *Rx.*
Use: Immunization.
See: anthrax vaccine (Michigan Department of Public Health).

vaccine, BCG. *Rx.*
Use: Immunization.
See: TheraCys (Pasteur Merieux Connaught).
Tice BCG, Amp (Organon Teknika).

vaccine, cholera. *Rx.*
Use: Immunization.
See: cholera vaccine, Vial (Wyeth Ayerst).

vaccine, Haemophilus influenzae type B. *Rx.*
Use: Immunization.
See: ActHIB (Pasteur Merieux Connaught).
ActHIB/DTP, Set of DTwP vial plus Hib Pow. for Inj. (Pasteur Merieux Connaught).
HibTITER, Vial (Wyeth Ayerst).
OmniHIB, Pow. for Inj. (SmithKline Beecham Pharmaceuticals).
PedvaxHIB, Pow. for Inj. (Merck).
ProHIBIT, Vial, Syr. (Pasteur Merieux Connaught).
Tetramune, Vial (Wyeth Ayerst).

vaccine, hepatitis A. *Rx.*
Use: Immunization.
See: Havrix (SmithKline Beecham Pharmaceuticals).
Vaqta (Merck),

vaccine, hepatitis B. *Rx.*
Use: Immunization.
See: Engerix-B (SmithKline Beecham Pharmaceuticals).
Recombivax-HB (Merck).

vaccine, influenza A&B. *Rx.*
Use: Immunization.
See: Fluogen (Parke-Davis).
Flu-Shield (Wyeth Ayerst).
Fluvirin (Adams Labs).
Fluzone (Connaught).

vaccine, Japanese encephalitis. *Rx.*
Use: Immunization.
See: JE-Vax (Pasteur Merieux Connaught).

vaccine, measles. *Rx.*
Use: Immunization.
See: Attenuvax (Merck).
W/rubella vaccine.
See: M-R II (Merck).
W/mumps and rubella vaccines.
See: M-M-R II (Merck).

vaccine, meningococcal. *Rx.*
Use: Immunization.
See: Menomune A/C/Y/W-135, Pow. for Inj. (Pasteur Merieux Connaught).

vaccine, mumps. Mumps Virus Vaccine Live, U.S.P. 23.
Use: Immunization.
See: Mumpsvax (Merck).

vaccine, pertussis. Pertussis Vaccine.
Use: Immunization.
See: Acel-Imune, Vial (Wyeth Ayerst).
ActHIB/DTP, Set of DTwP vial plus Hib Pow. for Inj. (Pasteur Merieux Connaught).
diphtheria and tetanus toxoids with pertussis vaccine (Various Mfr.).
Infantrix (SKB).
Tetramune, Vial (Wyeth Ayerst).
Tri-Immunol, Vial (Wyeth Ayerst).
Tripedia, Vial (Pasteur Merieux Connaught).

vaccine, plague. *Rx.*
Use: Immunization.
See: plague vaccine (Greer Laboratories).

vaccine, pneumococcal. *Rx.*
Use: Immunization.
See: Pneumovax-23 (Merck).
Pnu-Imune 23 (Wyeth Ayerst).

vaccine, poliovirus. *Rx.*
Use: Immunization.
See: IPOL (Pasteur Merieux Connaught).
Orimune (Wyeth Ayerst).
Poliovirus vaccine, U.S.P. 23.

vaccine, rabies. Rabies Vaccine.
Use: Immunization.
See: Imovax Rabies (Pasteur Merieux Connaught).
RabAvert (Chiron).
Rabies vaccine adsorbed (Michigan Department of Public Health).

vaccine, smallpox. Smallpox Vaccine.
Use: Immunization.

vaccine, typhoid. *Rx.*
Use: Immunization.
See: Typhim Vi (Pasteur Merieux Connaught).
Typhoid vaccine (Wyeth Ayerst).
Vivotif Berna (Berna Products).

vaccine, varicella. *Rx.*
Use: Immunization.
See: Varivax (Merck).

vaccine, whooping cough. Pertussis Vaccine, U.S.P. 23.
Use: Immunization.
See: Acel-Imune, Vial (Wyeth Ayerst).
ActHIB/DTP, Set of DTwP vial plus

Hib Pow. for Inj. (Pasteur Merieux Connaught).
diphtheria and tetanus toxoids with pertussis vaccine (Various Mfr.).
Tetramune, Vial (Wyeth Ayerst).
Tri-Immunol, Vial (Wyeth Ayerst).
Tripedia, Vial (Pasteur Merieux Connaught).

vaccine, yellow fever. *Rx.*
Use: Immunization.
See: YF-Vax (Pasteur Merieux Connaught).

•**vaccinia immune globulin.** (vax-IN-ee-ah) U.S.P. 23. *Formerly Vaccinia Immune Human Globulin.*
Use: Immunization.

vaccinia immune globulin. (Baxter) Gamma globulin fraction of serum of healthy adults recently immunized w/ vaccinia virus 16.5%. Vial 5 ml. *Rx.*
Use: Immunization.

vacocin. Under study.
Use: Anti-infective.

Vademin-Z. (Roberts) Vitamin A 12,500 IU, D 50 IU, E 50 mg, B_1 10 mg, B_2 5 mg, B_3 25 mg, B_5 10 mg, B_6 2 mg, C 150 mg, zinc 2.6 mg, Mg, Mn/Cap. Bot. 60s. *otc.*
Use: Mineral, vitamin supplement.

Vagi-Gard Maximum Strength. (Lake) Benzocaine 20%, resorcinol 3%, methyl paraben, sodium sulfite, EDTA, mineral oil. Cream 45 g. *otc.*
Use: Vaginal agent.

Vagi-Gard Advanced Sensitive Formula. (Lake) Benzocaine 5%, resorcinol, methyl paraben, sodium sulfite, EDTA, mineral oil. Cream 45 g. *otc.*
Use: Vaginal agent.

Vaginex Creme. (Schmid) Tripelennamine HCl. In 30 g, 300 g. *otc.*
Use: Vaginal agent.

Vagisec Plus Suppositories. (Schmid) Polyoxyethylene nonylphenol 5.25 mg, sodium edetate 0.66 mg, docusate sodium 0.07 mg, aminoacridine HCl 6 mg. Box 28s. *Rx.*
Use: Vaginal agent.

Vagisil. (Combe) Benzocaine and resorcin with lanolin alcohol, parabens, trisodium HEDTA, mineral oil and sodium sulfite. Creme. 30, 60 g. *otc.*
Use: Vaginal agent.

Vagisil Powder. (Combe) Cornstarch, aloe, mineral oil, benzethonium chloride, magnesium stearate, silica, fragrance. Pow. 198 g, 312 g. *otc.*
Use: Vaginal agent.

Vagistat-1. (Bristol-Myers Squibb) Tioconazole 6.5%. Vaginal oint. Prefilled applicator 4.6 g. *otc.*
Use: Antifungal, vaginal.

Valacet. (Pal-Pak) Hyoscyamus 10.8 mg, aspirin 259.2 mg, caffeine anhydrous 16.2 mg, gelsemium extract 0.6 mg/Tab. or Cap. Bot. 100s, 1000s, 5000s. *Rx.*
Use: Analgesic, anticholinergic, antispasmodic.

•**valacyclovir hydrochloride.** (val-lay-SIGH-kloe-vihr) USAN.
Use: Antiviral.
See: Valtrex, Tab. (GlaxoWellcome).

Valergen. (Hyrex) Estradiol valerate 10 mg, 20 mg or 40 mg/ml. Vial 10 ml. *Rx.*
Use: Estrogen.

Valerian. (Eli Lilly) Tincture, alcohol 68%. Bot. 4 fl oz, 16 fl oz.
W/Phenobarbital, passiflora, hyoscyamus.
See: Aluro, Tab. (Foy).

Valertest. (Hyrex) **No. 1:** Estradiol valerate 4 mg, testosterone enanthate 90 mg/ml. Vial 10 ml. **No. 2:** Double strength. Vial 10 ml. Amp. 2 ml, 10s. *Rx.*
Use: Androgen, estrogen combination.

valethamate bromide.
Use: Anticholinergic.

•**valine.** (VAY-leen) U.S.P. 23.
Use: Amino acid.

valine, isoleucine and leucine.
Use: Hyperphenylalaninemia. [Orphan drug]
See: VIL (Leas Research).

Valisone. (Schering Plough) Betamethasone valerate. **Cream:** 1 mg/g Hydrophilic cream of water, mineral oil, petrolatum, polyethylene glycol 1000 monocetyl ether, cetostearyl alcohol, monobasic sodium phosphate, phosphoric acid, 4-chloro-m-cresol as preservative. Tube 15 g, 45 g, 110 g. Jar 430 g. **Oint.:** 1 mg/g base of liquid and white petrolatum and hydrogenated lanolin. Tube 15 g, 45 g. **Lot.:** 1 mg/g w/isopropyl alcohol 47.5%, water slightly thickened w/carboxy vinyl polymer, pH adjusted w/sodium hydroxide. Bot. 20 ml, 60 ml. **Reduced Strength Cream 0.01%:** Hydrophilic cream of water, mineral oil, petrolatum, polyethylene glycol 1000 monocetyl ether, cetostearyl alcohol, monobasic sodium phosphate, phosphoric acid, 4-chloro-m-cresol as preservative. Tube 15 g, 60 g. *Rx.*
Use: Corticosteroid, topical.

Valium Injection. (Roche Laboratories) Diazepam 5 mg/ml, propylene glycol 40%, ethyl alcohol 10%, sodium benzoate 5%, benzoic acid, benzyl alcohol 1.5%. Amp. 2 ml. Vial 10 ml. *Tel-E-Ject* (Disposable syringe) 2 ml. *c-IV.*
Use: Anxiolytic.

Valium Tablets. (Roche Laboratories) Diazepam 2 mg, 5 mg or 10 mg/Tab. Bot. 100s, 500s. UD 100s. *c-IV.*
Use: Anxiolytic.

vallergine.
See: Promethazine HCl, U.S.P. 23.

Valnac Cream. (NMC Labs) Betamethasone valerate 0.1%. Cream Tube 15 g, 45 g. *Rx.*
Use: Corticosteroid, topical.

Valnac Ointment. (NMC Labs) Betamethasone valerate 0.1%. Oint. Tube 15 g, 45 g. *Rx.*
Use: Corticosteroid, topical.

•**valnoctamide.** (val-NOCK-tah-mid) USAN.
Use: Anxiolytic.

valpipamate methylsulfate.
See: Pentapiperide Methylsulfate.

•**valproate sodium.** (VAL-pro-ate) USAN.
Use: Anticonvulsant.

•**valproic acid.** (VAL-pro-ik acid) U.S.P. 23
Use: Anticonvulsant, antimigraine.
See: Depakene, Cap., Liq. (Abbott Laboratories).
Depakote (Abbott Laboratories).
Myproic Acid Syr. (Rosemont).
valproic acid (Various Mfr.).

valproic acid. (Various Mfr.) **Cap.:** Valproic acid 250 mg. Bot. 100s, 250s, 500s. **Syrup:** 250 mg/5 ml. Cups. 50 ml, 480 ml, UD 5 ml. *Rx.*
Use: Anticonvulsant.

•**valsartan.** (VAL-sahr-tan) USAN.
Use: Antihypertensive.
See: Diovan, Cap. (Novartis Pharmaceutical).

Valtrex. (GlaxoWellcome) Valacyclovir HCl 500 mg/Capl. Bot. 42s, 60s, UD 100s. *Rx.*
Use: Antiviral.

Valuphed. (H.L. Moore) Pseudoephedrine HCl 60 mg, triprolidine HCl 2.5 mg/Tab. Pkg. 24s. *otc.*
Use: Antihistamine, decongestant.

Vamate. (Major) Hydroxyzine pamoate 50 mg/Cap. Bot. 100s, 250s, 500s, UD 100s. *Rx.*
Use: Anxiolytic.

Vanadryx TR. (Vangard) Dexbrompheniramine maleate 6 mg, psuedoephedrine sulfate 120 mg/Tab. Bot. 100s, 500s. *Rx.*
Use: Antihistamine, decongestant.

Vancenase AQ Nasal. (Schering Plough) Beclomethasone dipropionate monohydrate 0.042%, 0.084%, benzalkonium chloride. Bot. 25 g with metering atomizing pump and nasal adapter (0.042%), 19 g with metered pump (0.084%). *Rx.*
Use: Corticosteroid, nasal.

Vancenase Nasal Inhaler. (Schering Plough) Metered-dose aerosol unit containing beclomethasone dipropionate in propellants. Each actuation delivers 42 mcg. Canister 16.8 g w/nasal adapter. *Rx.*
Use: Corticosteroid, nasal.

Vancenase Pockethaler. (Schering Plough) Beclomethasone dipropionate contains ≈42 mcg/metered dose, Inhaler. In 7 g containers w/ adapter (200 metered doses).
Use: Corticosteroid, nasal.

Vanceril Inhaler. (Schering Plough) Metered-dose aerosol unit beclomethasone dipropionate in propellants. Each actuation delivers ≈42 mcg of beclomethasone dipropionate. Inhaler. Canister 6.7 g, 16.8 g (200 metered doses) w/oral adapter. Box 1s. *Rx.*
Use: Corticosteroid.

Vanceril Double Strength. (Schering Plough) Metered-dose aerosol unit beclomethasone dipropionate in propellants, Each actuation delivers ≈84 mcg of beclomethasone dipropionate. Inhaler. Canister 5.4 g (40 metered doses), 12.2 g (120 metered doses). Box 1s. *Rx.*
Use: Corticosteroid.

Vancocin IV. (Eli Lilly) Vancomycin HCl 500 mg/vial. 1s; 1 g/vial. 10s; ADD-Vantage 500 mg or 1 g/vial. 1s. *Rx.*
Use: Anti-infective.

Vancocin Capsules. (Eli Lilly) Vancomycin HCl 125 mg or 250 mg/Pulvule. Bot. 10s, 20s. *Rx.*
Use: Anti-infective.

Vancocin Oral. (Eli Lilly) Vancomycin HCl for oral soln. Traypak 1 g, Container 10 g. *Rx.*
Use: Anti-infective.

Vancoled Injection. (ESI Lederle Generics) Vancomycin HCl equivalent to vancomycin 500 mg/10 ml reconstituted soln. Vial 10 ml. *Rx.*
Use: Anti-infective.

•**vancomycin.** (van-koe-MY-sin) U.S.P. 23.

Use: Anti-infective.

•**vancomycin hydrochloride.** (van-koe-MY-sin) U.S.P. 23. An antibiotic from *Streptomyces orientalis.*
Use: (IV) Gram-positive (staph.) infection; anti-infective.
See: Vancocin, Prods. (Eli Lilly). Vancoled, Vial (ESI Lederle Generics).

vancomycin hydrochloride. (ESI Lederle Generics) Vancomycin (after reconstitution) 250 mg/ml. Pow. for Oral Soln. Bot. 1 g. *Rx.*
Use: Anti-infective.

Vancor Intravenous. (Pharmacia & Upjohn) Vancomycin HCl 500 mg or 1 g. Pow. for inj. Vials.
Use: Anti-infective.

Vanex Expectorant Liquid. (Jones Medical Industries) Pseudoephedrine HCl 30 mg, hydrocodone bitartrate 2.5 mg, guaifenesin 100 mg, alcohol 5%, glucose, saccharin, sorbitol, sucrose, tartrazine. Tropical fruit punch flavor. Liq. Bot. 473 ml. *c-III.*
Use: Antitussive, decongestant, expectorant.

Vanex Forte. (Jones Medical Industries) Phenylpropanolamine HCl 50 mg, phenylephrine HCl 10 mg, chlorpheniramine maleate 4 mg, pyrilamine maleate 25 mg, lactose, sugar. Cap. Bot. 100s. *Rx.*
Use: Antihistamine, decongestant.

Vanex Forte-R. (Schwarz Pharma) Phenylpropanolamine HCl 75 mg, chlorpheniramine maleate 12 mg/ER Cap. 100s. *Rx.*
Use: Antihistamine, decongestant.

Vanex-HD. (Jones Medical Industries) Phenylephrine HCl 5 mg, chlorpheniramine maleate 2 mg, hydrocodone bitartrate 1.67 mg. Liq. Bot. Pt. gal. *c-III.*
Use: Antitussive, decongestant.

Vanicream. (Pharmaceutical Specialties) Oil in water vanishing cream containing white petrolatum, cetearyl alcohol, ceteareth-20, sorbitol, propylene glycol, simethicone, glyceryl monostearate, polyethylene glycol monostearate, sorbic acid. Oint. lb. *otc.*
Use: Pharmaceutical aid, ointment base.

vanilla. N.F. XVII.
Use: Pharmaceutic aid (flavor).

vanillal.
See: Ethyl Vanillin.

•**vanillin.** (vah-NILL-in) N.F. 18. 4-Hydroxy-3-methoxy-benzaldehyde.
Use: Pharmaceutic aid (flavor).

vanirome.
See: Ethyl Vanillin.

Vanoxide. (Dermik Laboratories) Benzoyl peroxide 5%, cetyl alcohol, lanolin alcohol, parabens, EDTA, calcium phosphate 64%, silica 1%, mineral oil. Bot. 25 ml, 50 ml. *otc.*
Use: Dermatologic, acne.

Vanoxide-HC. (Dermik Laboratories) Hydrocortisone alcohol 0.5%, benzoyl peroxide 5%/25 g in lotion w/same ingredients as Vanoxide. Bot. 25 g. *Rx.*
Use: Dermatologic, acne.

Vanquish. (Bayer Corp) Aspirin 227 mg, acetaminophen 194 mg, caffeine 33 mg, dried aluminum hydroxide gel 25 mg, magnesium hydroxide 50 mg/Tab. Capsule shaped tablets. Bot. 30s, 60s, 100s. *otc.*
Use: Analgesic combination, antacid.

Vansil. (Pfizer) Oxamniquine 250 mg/Cap. Bot. 24s. *Rx.*
Use: Anthelmintic.

Vantin. (Pharmacia & Upjohn) Cefpodoxime proxetil, lactose. **Tab.:** 100, 200 mg. Bot. 20s, 100s, UD 100s; **Gran. for Susp.:** Sucrose, lemon creme flavor, 50 mg/5 ml, 100 mg/5 ml. Bot. 50, 75, 100 ml. Sucrose. *Rx.*
Use: Anti-infective.

•**vapiprost hydrochloride.** (VAP-ih-prahst) USAN.
Use: Antagonist (thromboxane A_2).

Vapocet Tablets. (Major) Hydrocodone 5 mg, acetaminophen 500 mg/Tab. Bot. 100s. *c-III.*
Use: Analgesic combination, narcotic.

Vaponefrin Solution. (Medeva) A 2.25% solution of bioassayed racemic epinephrine as HCl, chlorobutanol 0.5%. Vial 7.5 ml, 15 ml, 30 ml. *otc.*
Use: Bronchodilator.

Vaporizer in a Bottle. (Columbia) Wick dispensed medicated vapors.
Use: Cough, cold, sinus, hayfever preparation.

Vapor Lemon Sucrets. (SmithKline Beecham Pharmaceuticals) Dyclonine HCl 2 mg, corn syrup sucrose. Loz. Pkg. 18s. *otc.*
Use: Mouth and throat preparation.

VapoRub. (Procter & Gamble).
See: Vicks Vaporub (Procter & Gamble).

Vaposteam. (Procter & Gamble).
See: Vicks Vaposteam (Procter & Gamble).

•**vapreotide.** (vap-REE-oh-tide) USAN.

Use: Antineoplastic.

Vaqta. (Merck) **Adult:** Hepatitis A antigen 50 U/ml, Inj. Vial. Single-use (1s and 5s) Syringe single-use (1s and 5s). **Pediatric/Adolescent:** Hepatitis A antigen 25 U/0.5 ml, Inj. Vial. Single use (1s and 5s). Syringe. Single use (1s and 5s). *Rx.*
Use: Immunization, hepatitis A.

varicella virus vaccine.
Use: Immunization.
Use: Varivax, Inj. (Merck).

varicella-zoster IgG IFA test system. (Wampole Laboratories) Test for the qualitative or semi-qualitative detection of VZ IgG antibody in human serum. Test kit 100s.
Use. Diagnostic aid.

•**varicella-zoster immune globulin.** U.S.P. 23.
Use: Immunization.

varicella-zoster immune globulin, human. (Massachusetts Public Health Biologic Labs) Varicella-zoster virus antibody 125 units ≤ 2.5 ml. Vial, single dose.
Use: Immunization.

Vari-Flavors. (Ross Laboratories) Flavor packets to provide flavor variety for patients on liquid diets. Dextrose, artificial flavor, artificial color. Packet 1 g, Ctn. 24s. *Rx.*
Use: Flavoring.

Variplex-C. (NBTY) Vitamins B_1 15 mg, B_2 10 mg, B_3 100 mg, B_5 20 mg, B_6 5 mg, B_{12} 10 mcg, C 500 mg/Tab. Bot. 100s. *otc.*
Use: Vitamin supplement.

Varivax. (Merck) Varicella virus vaccine. 1350 PFU of Oka/Merck varicella virus (live). Inj. Single-dose vials (1s, 10s). *Rx.*
Use: Immunization.

Vascor. (Ortho McNeil) Bepridil HCl, 200 mg, 300 mg or 400 mg/Tab. Bot. 90s, UD 100s. *Rx.*
Use: Antianginal.

Vascoray. (Mallinckrodt Chemical) Iothalamate meglumine 52%, iothalamate sodium 26% (40% iodine). Vial 50 ml. Bot. 100 ml, 150 ml, 200 ml.
Use: Radiopaque agent.

Vascunitol. (Apco) Mannitol hexanitrate 0.5 gr/Tab. Bot. 100s. *Rx.*
Use: Vasodilator.

Vascused. (Apco) Mannitol hexanitrate 0.5 gr, phenobarbital 0.25 gr/Tab. Bot. 100s. *Rx.*
Use: Vasodilator.

Vaseline Dermatology Formula Cream. (Chesebrough-Pond's) Petrolatum, mineral oil, dimethicone. Jar 3 oz, 5.25 oz. *otc.*
Use: Emollient.

Vaseline Dermatology Formula Lotion. (Chesebrough-Pond's) Petrolatum, mineral oil, dimethicone. Bot. 5.5 oz, 11 oz, 16 oz. *otc.*
Use: Emollient.

Vaseline First Aid Carbolated Petroleum Jelly. (Chesebrough-Pond's) Petrolatum, chloroxylenol. Plastic Jar 1.75 oz, 3.75 oz. Plastic Tube 1 oz, 2.5 oz. *otc.*
Use: Medicated anti-infective.

Vaseline Intensive Care Active Sport. (Chesebrough-Pond's) Ethylhexyl p-methoxycinnamate, oxybenzone. PABA free. **SPF 8:** Lot. Bot. 120 ml; **SPF 15:** Lot. Bot. 120 ml. *otc.*
Use: Sunscreen.

Vaseline Intensive Care Baby SPF 15. (Chesebrough-Pond's) Titanium dioxide. PABA free. Waterproof. Lot. Bot. 120 ml. *otc.*
Use: Sunscreen.

Vaseline Intensive Care Baby SPF 30. (Chesebrough-Pond's) Ethylhexyl p-methoxycinnamate, oxybenzone, 2-ethylhexyl salicylate, titanium dioxide, C12-15 alkyl benzoate, glycerin, aloe vera gel, vitamin E, cetyl alcohol, parabens, EDTA. Lot. Bot. 118 ml. *otc.*
Use: Sunscreen.

Vaseline Intensive Care Blockout SPF 30. (Chesebrough-Pond's) Ethylhexyl p-methoxycinnamate, oxybenzone, 2-ethylhexyl salicylate, titanium dioxide. Waterproof. Lot. Bot. 120 ml. *otc.*
Use: Sunscreen.

Vaseline Intensive Care Blockout SPF 40+. (Chesebrough-Pond's) Padimate O, ethylhexyl p-methoxycinnamate, oxybenzone, 2-ethylhexyl salicylate, titanium dioxide. Waterproof. Lot. Bot. 120 ml. *otc.*
Use: Sunscreen.

Vaseline Intensive Care Moisturizing Sunscreen. (Chesebrough-Pond's) Ethylhexyl p-methoxycinnamate, oxybenzone, C12-15 alkyl octanoate, glycerin, aloe vera gel, cetyl alcohol, petrolatum, vitamin E, parabens, EDTA. **SPF8, SPF4:** Lot. Bot. 117 ml. *otc.*
Use: Sunscreen.

Vaseline Intensive Care No Burn No Bite SPF 8. (Chesebrough-Pond's) Ethylhexyl p-methoxycinnamate, oxybenzone. PABA free. Waterproof. Lot. Bot. 180 ml. *otc.*

Use: Sunscreen.

Vaseline Intensive Care Sport Sunblock. (Chesebrough-Pond's) Ethylhexyl p-methoxycinnamate, oxybenzone, C12-15 alkyl benzoate, aloe vera gel, vitamin E, EDTA. Lot. Bot. 118 ml. *otc.*
Use: Sunscreen.

Vaseline Intensive Care Sunblock. (Chesebrough-Pond's) Ethylhexyl p-methoxycinnamate, oxybenzone, 2-ethylhexyl salicylate. PABA free. Waterproof. **SPF 4:** Lot. Bot. 180 ml; **SPF 8:** Lot. Bot. 120 ml, 180 ml; **SPF 15:** Lot. Bot. 120 ml, 180 ml; **SPF 25:** Lot. Bot. 120 ml, 180 ml. *otc.*
Use: Sunscreen.

Vaseline Intensive Care Ultra Violet Daily Defense. (Chesebrough-Pond's) Ethylhexyl p-methoxycinnamate, oxybenzone, vitamin E, cetyl alcohol, acetylated lanolin, alcohol, parabens, EDTA. **SPF 15.** Lot. Bot. 118 ml. *otc.*
Use: Sunscreen.

Vaseline Pure Petroleum Jelly Skin Protectant. (Chesebrough-Pond's) White petrolatum. Tube 1 oz, 2.5 oz. Jar 1.75 oz, 3.75 oz, 7.75 oz, 13 oz. *otc.*
Use: Dermatologic, counterirritant.

Vaseretic. (Merck) Enalapril maleate 5 mg: Hydrochlorothiazide 12.5 mg, lactose. Unit-of-use 100s. 10 mg: Hydrochlorothiazide 25 mg/Tab. Bot. 100s. *Rx.*
Use: Antihypertensive.

Vasimid.
See: Tolazoline HCl, U.S.P. 23.

vasoactive intestinal polypeptide. (Research Triangle)
Use: Treatment of acute esophageal food impaction. [Orphan drug]

Vasocidin Ophthalmic Ointment. (Ciba Vision Ophthalmics) Prednisolone acetate 0.5%, sulfacetamide sodium 10%. Tube 3.5 g. *Rx.*
Use: Anti-infective; corticosteroid, ophthalmic.

Vasocidin Ophthalmic Solution. (Ciba Vision Ophthalmics) Prednisolone sodium phosphate 0.25%, sulfacetamide sodium 10%. Bot. 5 ml, 10 ml. *Rx.*
Use: Anti-infective; corticosteroid, ophthalmic.

VasoClear. (Ciba Vision Ophthalmics) Naphazoline HCl 0.02%. Bot. 15 ml. *otc.*
Use: Mydriatic, vasoconstrictor.

VasoClear A. (Ciba Vision Ophthalmics) Naphazoline HCl 0.02%. Bot. 15 ml. *otc.*
Use: Mydriatic, vasoconstrictor.

Vasocon-A Ophthalmic Solution. (Ciba Vision Ophthalmics) Naphazoline HCl 0.05%, antazoline phosphate 0.5%. Bot. 15 ml. *Rx.*
Use: Mydriatic, vasoconstrictor.

Vasocon Regular. (Ciba Vision Ophthalmics) Naphazoline HCl 0.1%. Bot. 15 ml. *Rx.*
Use: Mydriatic, vasoconstrictor.

Vasoderm. (Taro Pharm) Fluocinonide 0.05%, anhydrous glycerin base. Cream. Tube 15 g, 30 g, 60 g. *Rx.*
Use: Corticosteroid, topical.

Vasoderm-E. (Taro Pharm) Fluocinonide 0.05%, emollient mineral oil and white petrolatum base. Cream. Tube 15 g, 30 g, 60 g, 120 g. *Rx.*
Use: Corticosteroid, topical.

Vasodilan. (Bristol-Myers) Isoxsuprine HCl 10 mg or 20 mg/Tab. **10 mg:** Bot. 100s, 1000s, UD 100s. **20 mg:** Bot. 100s, 500s, 1000s, UD 100s. *Rx.*
Use: Vasodilator.

vasodilators.
See: Amyl Nitrite.
Apresoline, Tab., Amp. (Novartis Pharmaceutical).
Arlidin, Tab. (Rhone-Poulenc Rorer).
Cardilate, Tab. (GlaxoWellcome).
Cyclospasmol, Tab., Cap. (Wyeth).
Erythrityl Tetranitrate, Tab.
Glyceryl Trinitrate Preps.
Isordil, Tab. (Wyeth).
Kortrate, Cap. (T.E. Williams).
Mannitol Hexanitrate.
Metamine, Tab. (Pfizer).
Nisane, Elix. (T.E. Williams).
Nitroglycerin.
Pentritol, Cap., Tempule (Centeon).
Peritrate, Tab. (Parke-Davis).
Sodium Nitrate.
Sorbitrate, Tab. (Zeneca).
Vasodilan, Tab., Amp. (Bristol-Myers).

vasodilators, coronary.
See: Glyceryl Trinitrate, Preps. (Various Mfr.).
Isordil, Tab. (Wyeth).
Khellin (Various Mfr.).
Papaverine, Inj., Tab. (Various Mfr.).
Pentaerythritol Tetranitrate, Tab.
Peritrate, Tab. (Parke-Davis).
Roniacol Elix., Tab. (Roche Laboratories).
Sorbitrate, Tab. (Zeneca).

Vasoflo. (Roberts) Papaverine HCl 150 mg/Cap. Bot 100s. *Rx.*
Use: Vasodilator.

Vasolate. (Parmed) Pentaerythritol tetranitrate 30 mg/Cap. Bot. 100s, 1000s. *Rx.*

Use: Antianginal.

Vasolate-80. (Parmed) Pentaerythritol tetranitrate 80 mg/Cap. Bot. 100s, 1000s. *Rx.*
Use: Antianginal.

•**vasopressin.** (VAY-so-PRESS-in) U.S.P. 23. Beta-hypophamine. Posterior pituitary pressor hormone.
Use: Hormone (antidiuretic).
See: Pitressin, Amp. (Parke-Davis).

vasopressin. (American Regent) 20 pressor units/ml, chlorobutanol 0.5%/ Inj. Vial. 0.5 ml, 1 ml, 10 ml. *Rx.*
Use: Hormone.

Vasosulf. (Ciba Vision Ophthalmics) Sulfacetamide sodium 15%, phenylephrine HCl 0.125%. Bot. 5 ml, 15 ml. *Rx.*
Use: Anti-infective; decongestant, ophthalmic.

Vasotec. (Merck) Enalapril maleate 2.5 mg, 5 mg, 10 mg or 20 mg, lactose/ Tab. **2.5 mg:** Bot. 100s, 1000s, 10,000s, UD 100s, unit-of-use 90s, 180s. **5 mg; 10 mg:** 100s, 1000s, 4000s, 10,000s, UD 100s, unit-of-use 90s, 180s. **20 mg:** 100s, 1000s, 10,000s, UD 100s, unit-of-use 90s. *Rx.*
Use: Antihypertensive.

Vasotec I.V. (Merck) Enalaprilat 1.25 mg/ ml, benzyl alcohol 9 mg, Inj. Vial 1 ml, 2 ml. *Rx.*
Use: Antihypertensive.

Vasotus Liquid. (Sheryl) Codeine phosphate 1/6 gr, phenylephrine HCl, prophenpyridamine maleate. Liq. Bot. pt. *c-v.*
Use: Antihistamine, antitussive, decongestant.

Vasoxyl. (GlaxoWellcome) Methoxamine HCl 0.1%. Inj. 20 mg/ml. *Rx.*
Use: Vasoconstrictor.

Vaxsyn HIV-1. (MicroGeneSys) T-Lymphotropic Virtus Type III GP 160 Antigen.
Use: AIDS. [Orphan drug]

Vazosan. (Sandia) Papaverine HCl 150 mg/Tab. Bot. 100s, 1000s. *Rx.*
Use: Vasodilator.

VCF. (Apothecus) Contraceptive film: nonoxynol-9 28%, glycerin and polyvinyl alcohol. Pkg. 3s, 6s, 12s. *otc.*
Use: Contraceptive, spermicide.

V-Cillin K. (Eli Lilly) Penicillin V potassium 125 mg, 250 mg or 500 mg/Tab. **125 mg:** Bot. 100s. **250 mg:** Bot. 100s, 500s. **500 mg:** Bot. 24s, 100s, 500s. *Rx.*
Use: Anti-infective, penicillin.

V-Cillin K for Oral Solution. (Eli Lilly) Penicillin V potassium 125 mg or 250 mg/5 ml. **125 mg:** Bot. 100 ml, 150 ml, 200 ml, UD 5 ml. **250 mg:** Bot. 100 ml, 150 ml, 200 ml. *Rx.*
Use: Anti-infective, penicillin.

V-Dec-M. (Seatrace) Pseudoephedrine HCl 120 mg, guaifenesin 500 mg/SR Tab. Bot. 100s. *Rx.*
Use: Decongestant, expectorant.

VDRL Antigen. (Laboratory Diagnostics) VDRL antigen with buffered saline. Blood test in diagnosis of syphillis. **Vial:** Sufficient for 500 tests. **Amp.:** 10 × 0.5 ml sufficient for 500 tests.
Use: Diagnostic aid.

VDRL Slide Test. (Laboratory Diagnostics) VDRL antigen. Slide flocculation and spinal fluid test for syphilis. Vial 5 ml Complete kit, reactive control, nonreactive control, 5 ml.
Use: Diagnostic aid.

VE-400. (Western Research) Vitamin E 400 IU/Cap. Bot. 1008s. *otc.*
Use: Vitamin supplement.

Vectrin. (Warner Chilcott) Minocycline 50 mg, 100 mg. Cap. Bot. 50s (100 mg only), 100s, 1000s. *Rx.*
Use: Anti-infective.

•**vecuronium bromide.** (veh-CUE-row-nee-uhm) USAN.
Use: Neuromuscular blocker.

vecuronium. (Marsam) Vecuronium bromide 10 mg, 20 mg/Inj. Vial 10 ml (with and without diluent), 20 ml (without diluent).
Use: Neuromuscular blocker.

Veetids. (Bristol-Myers Squibb) Penicillin-V potassium. **Soln.:** 125 mg or 250 mg/ 5 ml Bot. 100 ml, 200 ml. **Tab.:** 250 mg or 500 mg. Bot. 100s, 1000s, Unimatic 100s. *Rx.*
Use: Anti-infective, penicillin.

Veetids '500'. (Bristol-Myers Squibb) Penicillin V potassium 500 mg/Tab. Bot. 100s, 1000s, UD 100s. *Rx.*
Use: Anti-infective, penicillin.

•**vegetable oil, hydrogenated,** N.F. 18.
Use: Pharmaceutic aid (tablet/capsule lubricant).

vehicle/n and vehicle/n mild. (Neutrogena) Topical vehicle system for compounding. Appliderm Applicator Bot. oz. *otc.*
Use: Pharmaceutical aid.

velacycline. N-Pyrrolidinomethyl tetracycline. *Rx.*
Use: Anti-infective, tetracycline.

Velban. (Eli Lilly) Extract from Vinca rosea Linn. Vinblastine sulfate, lyophi-

lized. Vial 10 mg. *Rx.*
Use: Antineoplastic.

•**velnacrine maleate.** (VELL-NAH-kreen) USAN.
Use: Inhibitor (cholinesterase).
See: Mentane (Hoechst Marion Roussel).

Velosef. (Bristol-Myers Squibb) Cephradine. **Pow. for Oral Susp.:** 125 mg or 250 mg/5 ml sucrose, fruit flavor. Bot. 100 ml.**Cap.:** 250 mg or 500 mg. **Pow. for Inj.:** (contains 6mEq (136 mg) sodium per g.) 250 mg, 500 mg, 1 g or 2 g Vial. Infusion Bot. 100 ml (2 g only) *Rx.*
Use: Anti-infective, cephalosporin.

Velosulin Human. (Novo Nordisk) Human insulin injection 100 IU/ml, Vial 10 ml. *otc.*
Use: Antidiabetic.

Velvachol. (Galderma) Hydrophilic ointment base petrolatum, mineral oil, cetyl alcohol, cholesterol, parabens, stearyl alcohol, purified water, sodium lauryl sulfate. Jar lb. *otc.*
Use: Pharmaceutical aid, ointment base.

venesetic.
See: Amobarbital Sodium, Preps. (Various Mfr.).

venethene. No mfr. listed.

venlafaxine.
Use: Antidepressant.
See: Effexor, Tab. (Wyeth Ayerst). Effexov XR, ER Cap. (Wyeth-Ayerst).

•**venlafaxine hydrochloride.** (VEN-lah-fax-EEN) USAN.
Use: Antidepressant.

Venoglobulin-I. (Alpha Therapeutics) Immune globulin IV (IGIV). Pow. for Inj. 500 mg. Vial 2.5 g, 5 g, 10 g. *Rx.*
Use: Immune globulin.

Venoglobulin-S. (Alpha Therapeutics) Immune globulin IV (human) 5%: Vial. 2.5 g, 5 g, 10 g. 10%: Vial 5 g, 10 g, 20 g. Solvent detergent treated. Inj. 50, 100, 200 ml w/sterile IV administration set. *Rx.*
Use: Immune globulin.

Venomil. (Bayer Corp) Freeze-dried venom or venom protein. Vials of 12 mcg or 120 mcg for honey bee, white-faced hornet, yellow hornet, yellow jacket or wasp. Vials of 36 mcg or 360 mcg for mixed vespids (white-faced hornet, yellow hornet, yellow jacket). Diagnostic 1 mcg/ml, Maintenance 100 mcg/ml. Individual patient kit. *Rx.*
Use: Antivenin.

Venstat. (Seatrace) Brompheniramine maleate 10 mg/ml. Vial 10 ml. *Rx.*
Use: Antihistamine.

Ventolin Inhalation Aerosol. (Glaxo-Wellcome) Albuterol 90 mcg/actuation. Aerosol canister 17 g containing 200 metered inhalations. Canister 17 g w/ oral adapter. Refill canister 17 g. *Rx.*
Use: Bronchodilator.

Ventolin Inhalation Solution. (Glaxo-Wellcome) Albuterol sulfate 5 mg/ml. Bot. 20 ml w/calibrated dropper. *Rx.*
Use: Bronchodilator.

Ventolin Nebules. (GlaxoWellcome) Albuterol sulfate 0.083%, sulfuric acid. Soln. for inhalation. In 3 ml unit dose nebules. *Rx.*
Use: Bronchodilator.

Ventolin Rotacaps. (GlaxoWellcome) Microfine albuterol 200 mg. Cap. for inhalation. Bot. UD 96s, Hosp. UD 24s. For use with the Rotahaler inhalation device. *Rx.*
Use: Bronchodilator.

Ventolin Syrup. (GlaxoWellcome) Albuterol sulfate 2 mg/5 ml. Bot. pt. *Rx.*
Use: Bronchodilator.

Ventolin Tablets. (GlaxoWellcome) Albuterol sulfate 2 mg or 4 mg/Tab. Bot. 100s, 500s. *Rx.*
Use: Bronchodilator.

VePesid. (Bristol-Myers/Bristol Oncology) Etoposide. **Vial:** 100 mg/Vial. **Cap.:** 50 mg/Cap. Bot. 20s. *Rx.*
Use: Antineoplastic.

Veracolate. (Numark Laboratories) Phenolphthalein 32.4 mg, cascara sagrada extract 75 mg, oleosorin capsicum 0.05 min/Tab. Bot. 100s. *otc.*
Use: Laxative.

•**veradoline hydrochloride.** (VEER-aid-OLE-een) USAN.
Use: Analgesic.

•**verapamil.** (veh-RAP-ah-mill) USAN.
Use: Vasodilator (coronary).

•**verapamil hydrochloride.** (veh-RAP-ah-mill) U.S.P. 23.
Use: Antianginal, antiarrhythmic, antihypertensive,.
See: Calan, Tab. (Searle).
Calan SR, Capl. (Searle).
Isoptin, Inj. (Knoll Pharmaceuticals).
Isoptin SR, Tab. (Knoll Pharmaceuticals).
Verelan, SR Cap. (ESI Lederle Generics).

verapamil hydrochloride. (Various Mfr.) Verapamil HCl **40 mg/Tab.:** Bot. 100s. **80 mg, 120 mg/Tab.:** 100s, 250s,

500s, 1000s, UD 100s. **180 mg, 240 mg/SR Tab.:** 100s and 500s. **5 mg/2 ml/Inj.:** 2 ml, 4 ml vials, amps and syringes and 4 ml fill in 5 ml vials. *Rx.*
Use: Antianginal, antiarrhythmic, antihypertensive.
See: Calan, Tab. (Searle).
Calan SR, Tab. (Searle).
Isopfin, Inj. (Knoll Pharmaceuticals).
Isoptin SR, Tab. (knoll Pharmaceuticals).
Verelan, SR Cap. (ESI Lederle Generics).

veratrum alba.
See: Protoveratrines A and B (Various Mfr.).

Verazeptol. (Femco) Chlorothymol, eucalyptol, menthol, phenol, boric acid, zinc sulfate. Pow. Bot. 3 oz, 6 oz, 10 oz. *otc.*
Use: Vaginal agent.

Verazinc. (Forest Pharmaceutical) Zinc sulfate 220 mg/Cap. Bot. 100s, 1000s. *otc.*
Use: Mineral supplement.

Verelan. (ESI Lederle Generics) Verapamil HCl 120, 180, 240, 360 mg/SR Cap. Bot. 100s. *Rx.*
Use: Calcium channel blocker.

Vergo Oint. (Daywell) Calcium pantothenate 8%, ascorbic acid 2%, starch. Tube 0.5 oz. *Rx.*
Use: Keratolytic.

Vergon. (Marnel) Meclizine HCl 30 mg. Cap. Bot. 100s. *otc.*
Use: Antiemetic, antivertigo.

•**verilopam hydrochloride.** (veh-RILL-OH-pam) USAN.
Use: Analgesic.

Verin. (Roberts) Aspirin (Acetylsalicylic Acid; ASA) 650 mg/TR Tab. Bot. 100s.
Use: Analgesic.

•**verlukast.** (ver-LOO-kast) USAN.
Use: Antiasthmatic (leukotriene antagonist).

Verluma. (NeoRx, DuPont Merck) Nofetumomab merpentan 10 mg for conjugation w/technetium-99m. Kit. *Rx.*
Use: Radioimmunoscintigraphy agent.

Vermox. (Janssen) Mebendazole 100 mg/Tab. Box 12s. *Rx.*
Use: Anthelmintic.

vernamycins. Under study.
Use: Anti-infective.

vernolepin. A sesquiterpene dilactone. Under study.
Use: Against Walker carcinosarcoma 256.

•**verofylline.** (VER-OH-fill-in) USAN.
Use: Antiasthmatic, bronchodilator.

veronal sodium.
See: Barbital Sodium (Various Mfr.).

Versacaps. (Seatrace) Pseudoephedrine HCl 60 mg, guaifenesin 300 mg/Cap. Bot. 100s. *Rx.*
Use: Decongestant, expectorant.

Versal. (Suppositoria) Bismuth subgallate, balsam peru, zinc oxide, benzyl benzoate/Supp. Box 12s, 100s, 1000s. *otc.*
Use: Anorectal preparation.

Versa-Quat. (Ulmer) Quaternary ammonium one-step cleaner-disinfectant-sanitizer-fungicide-virucide for general housekeeping. Bot. gal.
Use: Cleanser, disinfectant.

Versed. (Roche Laboratories) Midazolam HCl 1 mg or 5 mg/ml, sodium Cl 0.8%, disodium edetate 0.01%, benzyl alcohol 1%. **1 mg/ml:** Vial 2 ml, 5 ml, 10 ml. Box 10s. **5 mg/ml:** Vial 1 ml, 2 ml, 5 ml, 10 ml. Box 10s. Disposable Syringe 2 ml Box 10s. *c-IV.*
Use: Anesthetic, general.

versenate, calcium disodium.
See: Calcium Disodium Versenate, Amp. (3M).

versenate disodium.
See: Disodium Versenate, Amp. (3M).

•**versetamide.** (ver-SET-ah-mide) USAN.
Use: Pharmaceutic aid.

Versiclear. (Hope Pharmaceuticals) Sodium thiosulfate 25%, salicylic acid 1%, isopropyl alcohol 10%, propylene glycol, menthol, EDTA. Lot. 120 ml. *Rx.*
Use: Anti-infective, topical.

versidyne.
Use: Analgesic.

Verstran. (Parke-Davis) Prazepam.
Use: Anxiolytic.
See: Centrax, Tab. (Parke-Davis).

Vertab. (Forest Pharmaceutical) Dimenhydrinate 50 mg. Tab. Bot. 100s.
Use: Anticholinergic.

•**verteporfin.** (ver-teh-PORE-fin) USAN.
Use: Antineoplastic.

Verukan-20. (Syosset Labs) Salicylic acid 16.7%, lactic acid in flexible collodion 16.7%. Bot. 15 ml. *otc.*
Use: Keratolytic.

Verv Alertness Capsules. (APC) Caffeine 200 mg/Cap. Vial 15s. *otc.*
Use: CNS stimulant.

Vesanoid. (Roche Laboratories) Tretinoin 10 mg. Cap. Bot. 100s. *Rx.*
Use: Antineoplastic.

•**vesnarinone.** (VESS-nah-rih-NOHN) USAN.

Use: Cardiovascular agent.

Vesprin. (Apothecon) Triflupromazine HCl 10 mg/ml, 20 mg/ml, benzyl alcohol 1.5%. Multidose vial. *Rx.*
Use: Antiemetic, antipsychotic.

Vetuss HC. (Cypress) Hydrocodone bitartrate 1.7 mg, phenylephrine HCl 5 mg, phenylpropanolamine HCl 3.3 mg, pyrilamine maleate 3.3 mg, pheniramine maleate 3.3 mg/5 ml, alcohol 5%, strawberry flavor/Syrup. Bot. 473 ml. *c-III.*
Use: Antitussive combination.

Vexol. (Alcon Laboratories) Rimexolone 1%. Susp. Ophthalmic. Drop-Tainers. 5 ml, 10 ml. *Rx.*
Use: Corticosteroid, ophthalmic.

Viacaps. (Manne) Vitamins A (soluble) 45,000 IU, C 500 mg/Cap. Bot. 60s, 120s, 1000s. *otc.*
Use: Vitamin supplement.

Viagra. (Pfizer) Sildenafil Citrate 25 mg, 50 mg, 100 mg, lactose/Tab. 30s. *Rx.*
Use: Antiimpotence.

Vianain. (Genzyme) Ananain, comosain.
Use: Burn treatment. [Orphan drug]

Vi antigen. *Rx.*
Use: Immunization.
See: Typhim Vi (Pasteur Merieux Connaught).

vibesate. Polvinate 9.3%, molrosinol 3.1% with propellant.

Vibramycin. (Pfizer) Doxycycline. **Cap.:** 50 mg Bot. 50s, UD pak 100s, X-Pack (10 Cap.) 5s; 100 mg Bot. 50s, 500s; UD pak 100s, V-Pak (5 Cap) 5s, Nine-Pak 10s. **Pediatric Oral Susp.:** 25 mg/5 ml. Bot. 2 oz. **Syr.:** 50 mg/5 ml. Bot. oz, pt. *Rx.*
Use: Anti-infective, tetracycline.

Vibramycin IV. (Roerig) Doxycycline (as hyclate) 200 mg. Powder for Inj. Vial. *Rx.*
Use: Anti-infective, tetracycline.

Vibra-Tabs. (Pfizer) Doxycycline hyclate 100 mg/Tab. Bot. 50s, 500s, UD Pack 100s. *Rx.*
Use: Anti-infective, tetracycline.

Vicam IV. (Keene Pharmaceuticals) Vitamins B_1 50 mg, B_2 5 mg, B_{12} 1000 mcg, B_6 5 mg, dexpanthenol 6 mg, niacinamide 125 mg, C 50 mg/ml, benzyl alcohol 1% as preservative in water for injection. Vial multiple dose. *Rx.*
Use: Nutritional supplement, parenteral.

Vicam Injection. (Keene Pharmaceuticals) Vitamins B_1 50 mg, B_2 5 mg, B_3 125 mg, B_5 6 mg, B_6 5 mg, B_{12} 1000 mcg, C 50 mg/ml. Inj. Vial 10 ml. *Rx.*
Use: Vitamin supplement.

Vicks Children's Chloraseptic Lozenges. (Procter & Gamble) Benzocaine 5 mg, corn syrup, sucrose. Grape flavor. Loz. Pkg. 18s. *otc.*

Vicks Children's Chloraseptic Spray. (Procter & Gamble) Phenol 0.5%, saccharin, sorbitol. Alcohol free. Spray. Bot. 177 ml. *otc.*
Use: Anesthetic, antiseptic.

Vicks Children's NyQuil Nighttime Cold/Cough Liquid. (Procter & Gamble) Pseudoephedrine HCl 10 mg, dextromethorphan HBr 5 mg, chlorpheniramine maleate 0.67 mg/5 ml, alcohol free. Bot. 120 ml, 240 ml. *otc.*
Use: Antihistamine, antitussive, decongestant.

Vicks Chloraseptic Mouthrinse/Gargle. (Procter & Gamble) Phenol 1.4%, saccharin. Alcohol free. Liq. 355 ml. *otc.*
Use: Antiseptic.

Vicks Chloraseptic Sore Throat. (Procter & Gamble) Benzocaine 6 mg, menthol 10 mg. Loz. Pkg. 18s. *otc.*
Use: Anesthetic.

Vicks Cough Drops. (Procter & Gamble) Menthol. **Menthol flavor:** Benzyl alcohol, camphor, eucalyptus oil, tolu balsam, corn syrup, sucrose, thymol. **Cherry flavor:** Corn syrup, sucrose, citric acid. Box 14. Bag 40. *otc.*
Use: Mouth and throat preparation.

Vicks DayQuil Allergy Relief 4 Hour. (Procter & Gamble) Phenylpropanolamine HCl 25 mg, brompheniramine maleate 4 mg. Tab. Pkg. 24s. *otc.*
Use: Antitussive, decongestant.

Vicks DayQuil Allergy Relief 12 Hour. (Procter & Gamble) Phenylpropanolamine HCl 75 mg, brompheniramine maleate 12 mg/SR Tab. Pkg. 12s, 24s. *otc.*
Use: Antitussive, decongestant.

Vicks DayQuil Liquicaps. (Procter & Gamble) Dextromethorphan HBr 10 mg, pseudoephedrine HCl 30 mg, acetaminophen 250 mg, guaifenesin 100 mg. Softgel Cap. Pkg. 12s, 20s. *otc.*
Use: Analgesic, antitussive, decongestant, expectorant.

Vicks DayQuil Liquid. (Procter & Gamble) Pseudoephedrine HCl 60 mg, guaifenesin 200 mg, acetaminophen 650 mg, dextromethorphan HBr 20 mg/30 ml. Bot. 6 oz. *otc.*
Use: Analgesic, antitussive, decongestant, expectorant.

Vicks DayQuil Sinus Pressure & Pain

Relief. (Procter & Gamble) Pseudoephedrine HCl 30 mg, acetaminophen 500 mg. Cap. Pkg. 24s. *otc. otc.*
Use: Analgesic, decongestant.

Vicks Dry Hacking Cough. (Procter & Gamble) Dextromethorphan HBr 30 mg/10 ml, alcohol 10%, invert sugar. Liq. Bot. 4 oz, 8 oz w/Vicks AccuTip Dispenser. *otc.*
Use: Antitussive.

Vicks 44 Non-Drowsy Cold & Cough liquicaps. (Procter & Gamble) Dextromethorphan HBr 30 mg, pseudoephedrine HCl 60 mg. Cap. Pkg. 10s. *otc.*
Use: Antitussive, decongestant.

Vicks 44D Cough & Decongestant Liquid. (Procter & Gamble) Pseudoephedrine HCl 20 mg, dextromethorphan HBr 10 mg/5 ml, alcohol 10%, saccharin, sucrose. Bot. 120 ml, 240 ml. *otc.*
Use: Antitussive, decongestant.

Vicks 44D Cough & Head Congestion. (Procter & Gamble) Dextromethorphan 10 mg, pseudoephedrine HCl 20 mg/5 ml. Liq. Bot. 5 ml. *otc.*
Use: Antitussive, decongestant.

Vicks 44D Dry Hacking-Cough and Head Congestion, Pediatric. (Procter & Gamble) Dextromethorphan HBr 15 mg/15 ml, pseudephedrine HCl 3 mg, alcohol free, sorbitol, sucrose, cherry flavor. Liq. Bot. 120 ml with Vicks AccuTip Dispenser. *otc.*
Use: Antitussive, decongestant.

Vicks 44D Pediatric Cough & Decongestant Liquid. (Procter & Gamble) Pseudoephedrine HCl 10 mg, dextromethorphan HBr 5 mg/5 ml, alcohol free. Bot. 120 ml. *otc.*
Use: Antitussive, decongestant.

Vicks 44E Liquid. (Procter & Gamble) Dextromethorphan HBr 6.7 mg, guaifenesin 66.7 mg/5 ml. Bot. 118 ml, 236 ml. *otc.*
Use: Antitussive, expectorant.

Vicks 44E Pediatric Liquid. (Procter & Gamble) Dextromethorphan HBr 10 mg, guaifenesin 100 mg, sorbitol, sucrose. Alcohol free. Bot. 120 ml w/Vicks AccuTip Dispenser. *otc.*
Use: Antitussive, expectorant.

Vicks 44M Cough, Cold and Flu Liquid. (Procter & Gamble) Dextromethorphan HBr 30 mg, pseudoephedrine HCl 60 mg, chlorpheniramine maleate 4 mg, acetaminophen 650 mg/20 ml, alcohol 10%. Bot. 4 oz, 8 oz, with Vicks AccuTip Dispenser. *otc.*
Use: Analgesic, antihistamine, antitussive, decongestant.

Vicks 44M Cold, Flu & Cough Liquicaps. (Procter & Gamble) Dextromethorphan HBr 10 mg, pseudoephedrine HCl 30 mg, chlorpheniramine maleate 2 mg, acetaminophen 250 mg. Cap. Pkg. 12s. *otc.*
Use: Analgesic, antihistamine, antitussive, decongestant.

Vicks NyQuil LiquiCaps. (Procter & Gamble) Acetaminophen 250 mg, pseudoephedrine HCl 30 mg, dextromethorphan HBr 10 mg, doxylamine succinate 6.25 mg. Pkg. 12s, 20s. *otc.*
Use: Analgesic, antihistamine, antitussive, decongestant.

Vicks NyQuil Liquid Multi-Symptom Cold Flu Relief. (Procter & Gamble) Acetaminophen 1000 mg, doxylamine succinate 12.5 mg, pseudoephedrine HCl 60 mg, dextromethorphan HBr 30 mg/30 ml, alcohol 10%. Regular and cherry flavors. Regular contains FD&C Yellow No. 6. Bot. 6 oz, 10 oz, 14 oz. *otc.*
Use: Analgesic, antihistamine, antitussive, decongestant.

Vicks NyQuil Multi-Symptom Cold Flu Relief. (Procter & Gamble) Pseudoephedrine HCl 10 mg, doxylamine succinate 2.1 mg, dextromethorphan HBr 5 mg, acetaminophen 167 mg/5 ml. Liq. Alcohol 10%, sucrose, regular and cherry flavor. Bot. 180, 300 and 420 ml *otc.*
Use: Analgesic, antihistamine, antitussive, decongestant.

Vicks Sinex. (Procter & Gamble) Phenylephrine HCl 0.5%, camphor, menthol, eucalyptol, disodium EDTA. Nasal Spray. Plastic Squeeze Bot. 0.5 oz, 1 oz. *otc.*
Use: Decongestant.

Vicks Sinex 12-Hour. (Procter & Gamble) Oxymetazoline HCl 0.05%, camphor, menthol, eucalyptol, disodium EDTA. Nasal Spray. Plastic Squeeze Bot. 1 oz, 0.5 oz. *otc.*
Use: Decongestant.

Vicks Vapor Inhaler. (Procter & Gamble) l-Desoxyephedrine 50 mg, Special Vicks Vapors (menthol, camphor, bornyl acetate, lavender oil). Inhaler 0.007 oz (198 mg). *otc.*
Use: Decongestant.

Vicks VapoRub. (Procter & Gamble) Camphor 4.7%, menthol 2.6%, eucalyptus oil 1.2%, cedarleaf oil, nutmeg oil. **Ointment:** Mineral oil, petrolatum. **Cream:** EDTA, glycerin, imidazolidinyl

urea, cetyl alcohol, parabens, stearyl alcohol, spirits of turpentine, titanium dioxide. Cream. Jar 56.7 g. *otc.*
Use: Decongestant, vaporizing agent.

Vicks Vaposteam. (Procter & Gamble) Eucalyptus oil 1.5%, camphor 6.2%, menthol 3.2%, alcohol 74%, cedarleaf oil, nutmeg oil. Bot. 4 oz, 8 oz. *otc.*
Use: Antitussive, decongestant.

Vicks Vitamin C Drops. (Procter & Gamble) Vitamin C 60 mg as sodium ascorbate and ascorbic acid. Orange flavor. Bag. 14s, 30s. *otc.*
Use: Vitamin supplement.

Vicodin. (Knoll Pharmaceuticals) Hydrocodone bitartrate 5 mg, acetaminophen 500 mg/Tab. Bot. 100s, 500s, UD 100s. *c-iii.*
Use: Analgesic combination, narcotic.

Vicodin ES. (Knoll Pharmaceuticals) Hydrocodone bitartrate 7.5 mg, acetaminophen 750 mg/Tab. Bot. 100s, UD 100s. *c-iii.*
Use: Analgesic combination, narcotic.

Vicodin HP. (Knoll Pharmaceuticals) Hydrocodone bitartrate 10 mg, acetaminophen 660 mg/Tab. Bot. 100s, 500s. *c-iii.*
Use: Analgesic combination, narcotic.

Vicon-C. (UCB Pharmaceuticals) Vitamins B_1 20 mg, B_2 10 mg, B_3 100 mg, B_5 20 mg, B_6 5 mg, C 300 mg, Mg, zinc sulfate 80 mg/Cap. Bot. 60s, UD 100s. *otc.*
Use: Mineral, vitamin supplement.

Vicon Forte. (UCB Pharmaceuticals) Vitamins A 8000 IU, E 50 IU, C 150 mg, B_3 25 mg, B_1 10 mg, B_5 10 mg, B_2 5 mg, B_6 2 mg, B_{12} 10 mcg, folic acid 1 mg, zinc sulfate 18 mg, Mg, Mn, lactose/Cap. Bot. 60s, 500s, UD 100s. *Rx.*
Use: Mineral, vitamin supplement.

Vicon Plus. (UCB Pharmaceuticals) Vitamins A 4000 IU, E 50 IU, C 150 mg, B_3 25 mg, B_1 10 mg, B_5 10 mg, B_2 5 mg, zinc sulfate 18 mg, Mg, Mn, lactose, B_6 2 mg/Cap. Bot. 60s. *otc.*
Use: Mineral, vitamin supplement.

Victors. (Procter & Gamble) Special Vicks Medication (menthol, eucalyptus oil) in a soothing Vicks sugar base. Regular or Cherry flavor drops. Stick-Pack 10s, Bag 40s. *otc.*
Use: Anesthetic, local.

•**vidarabine,** (vih-DAR-ah-BEAN) U.S.P. 23.
Use: Antiviral.

•**vidarabine phosphate.** (vih-DAR-ah-BEAN) USAN.
Use: Antiviral.

•**vidarabine sodium phosphate.** (vih-DAR-ah-BEAN) USAN.
Use: Antiviral.

Vi-Daylin ADC Drops. (Ross Laboratories) Vitamins A 1500 IU, C 35 mg, D 400 IU/ml. Bot. 30 ml, 50 ml. Bot. 50 ml w/dropper. *otc.*
Use: Vitamin supplement.

Vi-Daylin ADC Vitamin + Iron Drops. (Ross Laboratories) Vitamins A 1500 IU, C 35 mg, D 400 IU, iron 10 mg/ml, methylparaben. Bot. 50 ml. *otc.*
Use: Mineral, vitamin supplement.

Vi-Daylin Chewable. (Ross Laboratories) Vitamins A 2500 IU, D 400 IU, E 15 IU, C 60 mg, folic acid 0.3 mg, B_1 1.05 mg, B_2 1.2 mg, niacin 13.5 mg, B_6 1.05 mg, B_{12} 4.5 mcg/Tab. Bot. 100s. *otc.*
Use: Vitamin supplement.

Vi-Daylin/F Chewable Multivitamin. (Ross Laboratories) Fluoride 1 mg, vitamins A 2500 IU, D 400 IU, E 15 mg, B_1 1.05 mg, B_2 1.2 mg, B_3 13.5 mg, B_6 1.05 mg, B_{12} 4.5 mcg, C 60 mg, folic acid 0.3 mg, sucrose, cherry flavor. Tab. Bot. 100s. *Rx.*
Use: Dental caries agent, mineral, vitamin supplement.

Vi-Daylin Chewable w/Fluoride. (Ross Laboratories) Fluoride 1 mg, vitamins B_1 1.05 mg, B_2 1.2 mg, niacinamide 13.5 mg, B_6 1.05 mg, C 60 mg, A 2500 IU, B_{12} 4.5 mcg, E 15 IU, folic acid 0.3 mg, D 400 IU/Tab. Bot. 100s. *Rx.*
Use: Dental caries agent; mineral, vitamin supplement.

Vi-Daylin Drops. (Ross Laboratories) Vitamins A 1500 IU, D 400 IU, E 5 IU, C 35 mg, B_1 0.5 mg, B_2 0.6 mg, niacin 8 mg, B_6 0.4 mg, B_{12} 1.5 mcg/ml. Bot. 50 ml. *otc.*
Use: Vitamin supplement.

Vi-Daylin/F ADC Vitamins Drops. (Ross Laboratories) Vitamins A 1500 IU, D 400 IU, C 35 mg, fluoride 0.25 mg/ml. Alcohol $\approx$ 0.3%, parabens. Bot. 50 ml. *Rx.*
Use: Dental caries agent, vitamin supplement.

Vi-Daylin/F ADC + Iron Drops. (Ross Laboratories) Vitamins A 1500 IU, C 35 mg, D 400 IU, iron 10 mg, fluoride 0.25 mg/ml, methylparaben. Bot. 50 ml. *Rx.*
Use: Dental caries agent; mineral, vitamin supplement.

Vi-Daylin/F Drops. (Ross Laboratories) Vitamins A 1500 IU, D 400 IU, E 5 IU,

C 35 mg, B_1 0.5 mg, B_2 0.6 mg, B_3 8 mg, B_6 0.4 mg, fluoride 0.25 mg/ml, methylparaben. Bot. 50 ml. *Rx.*
Use: Dental caries agent, vitamin supplement.

Vi-Daylin/F Multivitamin + Iron. (Ross Laboratories) **Drops:** Fluoride 0.25 mg, vitamins A 1500 IU, D 400 IU, E 4.1 mg, B_1 0.5 mg, B_2 0.6 mg, B_3 8 mg, B_6 0.4 mg, C 35 mg, iron 10 mg/ml, alcohol < 0.1%, methylparaben. Bot. 50 ml. **Chew. Tab.:** Fluoride 1 mg, vitamins A 2500 IU, D 400 IU, E 15 mg, B_1 1.05 mg, B_2 1.2 mg, B_3 13.5 mg, B_6 1.05 mg, B_{12} 4.5 mcg, C 60 mg, folic acid 0.3 mg, iron 12 mg. Bot. 100s. *Rx.*
Use: Dental caries agent; mineral, vitamin supplement.

Vi-Daylin Liquid. (Ross Laboratories) Vitamins A 2500 IU, B_1 1.05 mg, B_2 1.2 mg, B_6 1.05 mg, B_{12} 4.5 mcg, C 60 mg, D 400 IU, E 20.4 mg (as d-alpha tocopheryl acetate), niacin 13.5 mg/5 ml. Bot. 8 oz, pt. *otc.*
Use: Vitamin supplement.

Vi-Daylin Multivitamin Drops. (Ross Laboratories) Vitamins A 1500 IU, D 400 IU, E 5 mg, B_1 0.5 mg, B_2 0.6 mg, B_3 8 mg, B_6 0.4 mg, B_{12} 1.5 mcg, C 35 mg/ml, < 0.5% alcohol. Bot. 50 ml. *otc.*
Use: Vitamin supplement.

Vi-Daylin Multivitamin Liquid. (Ross Laboratories) Vitamins A 2500 IU, D 400 IU, E 15 mg, B_1 1.05 mg, B_2 1.2 mg, B_3 13.5 mg, B_6 1.05 mg, B_{12} 4.5 mcg, C 60 mg/5 ml, ≤ 0.5% alcohol. Bot. 240, 480 ml. *otc.*
Use: Vitamin supplement.

Vi-Daylin Multivitamin + Iron Drops. (Ross Laboratories) Iron 10 mg, vitamins A 1500 IU, D 400 IU, E 5 mg, B_1 0.5 mg, B_2 0.6 mg, B_3 8 mg, B_6 0.4 mg, C 35 mg, < 0.5% alcohol, methylparaben. Bot. 50 ml. *otc.*
Use: Mineral, vitamin supplement.

Vi-Daylin Multivitamin Plus Iron Chewable. (Ross Laboratories) Vitamins A 2500 IU, D 400 IU, E 15 IU, C 60 mg, folic acid 0.3 mg, B_1 1.05 mg, B_2 1.2 mg, B_3 13.5 mg, B_6 1.05 mg, B_{12} 4.5 mcg, iron 12 mg/Tab. Bot. 100s. *otc.*
Use: Mineral, vitamin supplement.

Vi-Daylin Multivitamin Plus Iron Liquid. (Ross Laboratories) Vitamins A 2500 IU, D 400 IU, C 60 mg, E 15 IU, B_1 1.05 mg, B_2 1.2 mg, B_3 13.5 mg, B_6 1.05 mg, B_{12} 4.5 mcg, iron 10 mg/tsp. ≤ 0.5% alcohol, glucose, sucrose, parabens. In 237 ml, 473 ml. *otc.*
Use: Mineral, vitamin supplement.

Videcon. (Vita Elixir) Vitamin D 50,000 units/Cap. *Rx.*
Use: Vitamin supplement.

Vi-Derm Soap. (Arthrins) Extract of Amaryllis 10%. Pkg. cake 1s. Bar 3.5 oz. *otc.*
Use: Dermatologic, cleanser.

•**vifilcon a.** (vie-FILL-kahn A) USAN.
Use: Contact lens material (hydrophilic).

•**vifilcon b.** (vie-FILL-kahn B) USAN.
Use: Contact lens material (hydrophilic).

Vifluorineed. (Hanlon) Vitamins A 5000 IU, D 400 IU, C 75 mg, B_1 2 mg, B_2 3 mg, niacinamide 20 mg, fluoride 1 mg/Chew. Tab. Bot. 100s. *Rx.*
Use: Mineral, vitamin supplement.

•**vigabatrin.** (vie-GAB-at RIN) USAN.
Use: Anticonvulsant (tardive dyskinesia).

Vigomar Forte. (Marlop Pharm) Iron 12 mg, vitamins A 10,000 IU, D 400 IU, E 15 IU, B_1 10 mg, B_2 10 mg, B_3 100 mg, B_5 20 mg, B_6 5 mg, B_{12} 5 mcg, C 200 mg, I, Mg, Mn, Cu, Zn 1.5 mg/Tab. Bot. 100s. *otc.*
Use: Mineral, vitamin supplement.

Vigortol. (Rugby) Vitamins B_1 0.8 mg, B_2 0.4 mg, B_3 8.3 mg, B_5 1.7 mg, B_6 0.2 mg, B_{12} 0.2 mcg, iron 0.3 mg, Zn 0.3 mg, choline, I, Mg, Mn, alcohol 18%, sugar, methylparaben. Liq. Bot. 473 ml. *otc.*
Use: Mineral, vitamin supplement.

VIL. (Leas Research)
Use: Hyperphenylalaninemia. [Orphan drug]

Vilex. (Dunhall Pharmaceuticals) Vitamin B_1 100 mg, riboflavin phosphate sodium 1 mg, B_6 10 mg, panthenol 5 mg, niacinamide 100 mg/ml. Amp. 30 ml. *Rx.*
Use: Vitamin supplement.

Viliva. (Vita Elixir) Ferrous fumarate 3 gr. *otc.*
Use: Mineral supplement.

•**viloxazine hydrochloride.** (vih-LOX-ah-zeen) USAN.
Use: Antidepressant.
See: Catatrol (Zeneca).

Viminate. (Various Mfr.) Vitamins B_1 2.5 mg, B_2 1.25 mg, B_3 25 mg, B_5 5 mg, B_6 0.5 mg, B_{12} 0.5 mcg, iron 7.5 mg, zinc 1 mg, choline, I, Mg, Mn/5 ml, alcohol 18%. Liq. Bot. 480. *otc.*
Use: Mineral, vitamin supplement.

Vi-Min-for-All. (Barth's) Vitamins A 3 mg, D 10 mcg, C 120 mg, B_1 35 mg, B_{12} 15 mcg, biotin, niacin 2.33 mg, E 30 IU, B_6, pantothenic acid, calcium 375 mg,

phosphorus 180 mg, iron 20 mg, iodine 0.1 mg, rutin 10 mg, hesperidin-lemon bioflavonoid complex 10 mg, choline, inositol 2.4 mg, copper 10 mcg, manganese 2 mg, zinc 110 mcg, silicone 210 mcg/Tab. Bot. 100s, 500s. *otc.*
Use: Mineral, vitamin supplement.

Vimms-38. (Health for Life Brands) Vitamins A 12,500 IU, D 1200 IU, B_1 15 mg, B_2 10 mg, C 75 mg, niacinamide 30 mg, calcium pantothenate 2 mg, B_6 0.5 mg, E 5 IU, Brewer's yeast 10 mg, B_{12} 15 mcg, iron 11.58 mg, desiccated liver 15 mg, choline bitartrate 30 mg, inositol 30 mg, calcium 59 mg, phosphorus 45 mg, zinc 0.68 mg, dicalcium phosphate 200 mg, manganese 1.11 mg, magnesium 1 mg, potassium 0.68 mg, pepsin 16.5 mg, diastase 16.5 mg, yeast 40.63 mg, protein digest 23.52 mg, amino acids 34.22 mg/Cap. Bot. 50s, 100s, 1000s. *otc.*
Use: Mineral, vitamin supplement.

Vinactane Sulfate. (Novartis Pharmaceutical) Viomycin Sulfate.

•**vinafocon a.** (VIE-nah-FOE-kahn A) USAN.
Use: Contact lens material (hydrophobic).

vinbarbital.
Use: Hypnotic, sedative.

vinbarbital sodium.
Use: Hypnotic, sedative.

•**vinblastine sulfate.** (vin-BLAST-een) U.S.P. 23. Vincaleukoblastine. Alkaloid extracted from *Vinca rosea* Linn.
Use: Antineoplastic.
See: Velban, Vial (Eli Lilly).

vinblastine sulfate. (Various Mfr.) Vinblastine sulfate 10 mg. Pow. for Inj. *Rx.*
Use: Mitotic inhibitor.

vinblastine sulfate. (Fujisawa) Vinblastine sulfate 1 mg/ml, 0.9% benzyl alcohol. Pow. for inj. 10 ml. *Rx.*
Use: Antineoplastic.

vincaleukoblastine, 22-oxo-sulfate (1:1) (salt). Vincristine Sulfate, U.S.P. 23.

Vincasar PFS. (Pharmacia & Upjohn) Vincristine sulfate 1 mg/ml. Vial 1 ml. *Rx.*
Use: Antineoplastic.

•**vincofos.** (VIN-koe-foss) USAN.
Use: Anthelmintic.

•**vincristine sulfate.** (vin-KRISS-teen) U.S.P. 23.
Use: Antineoplastic.
See: Oncovin, Amp. (Eli Lilly).
Vincasar PFS, Vial (Pharmacia & Upjohn).

•**vindesine.** (VIN-deh-seen) USAN.
Use: Antineoplastic.

•**vindesine sulfate.** (VIN-deh-seen) USAN.
Use: Antineoplastic.

•**vinepidine sulfate.** (VIN-eh-pih-DEEN) USAN.
Use: Antineoplastic.

•**vinglycinate sulfate.** (vin-GLIE-sin-ate) USAN.
Use: Antineoplastic.

•**vinleurosine sulfate.** (vin-LOO-row-seen) USAN. Sulfate salt of an alkaloid extracted from *Vinca rosea* Linn. Also see Vinblastine.
Use: Antineoplastic.

•**vinorelbine tartrate.** (vih-NORE-ell-bean) USAN. Sulfate salt of an alkaloid extracted from *Vinca Rosea* Linn.
Use: Antineoplastic.
See: Navelbine, Inj. (GlaxoWellcome).

•**vinpocetine.** (VIN-poe-SEH-teen) USAN.
Use: Antineoplastic.

•**vinrosidine sulfate.** (vin-ROW-sih-deen) USAN. Sulfate salt of an alkaloid extracted from *Vinca rosea* Linn.
See: Vinblastine.
Use: Antineoplastic.

vinylacetate-polyvinylpyrrolidone.
See: Ivy-Rid Spray (Roberts).

vinyl ether, U.S.P. XXI.
Use: Anesthetic, general.
See: Vinethene, Liq.

vinyzene. Bromchlorenone.
Use: Fungicide.

•**vinzolidine sulfate.** (VIN-ZOLE-ih-deen) USAN.
Use: Antineoplastic.

Vio-Bec. (Solvay) Vitamins B_1 25 mg, B_2 25 mg, niacinamide 100 mg, calcium pantothenate 40 mg, B_6 25 mg, C 500 mg/Cap. Bot. 100s. *otc.*
Use: Mineral, vitamin supplement.

Viodo HC. (NMC Labs) Iodochlorhydroxyquin 3%, hydrocortisone 1% in cream base. Tube 20 g. *otc.*
Use: Antifungal; corticosteroid, topical.

Vioform. (Novartis Pharmaceutical) Clioquinol. **Cream:** 3%. Tube oz. **Oint.:** 3% in petrolatum base. Tube oz. *otc.*
Use: Antifungal, topical.

Viogen-C. (Zenith Goldline) Vitamins B_1 20 mg, B_2 10 mg, B_3 100 mg, B_5 20 mg, B_6 5 mg, C 300 mg, Mg, zinc sulfate 50 mg, tartrazine/Cap. Bot. 100s. *otc.*
Use: Mineral, vitamin supplement.

Viokase. (Robins) **Tab.:** Lipase 8000 units, protease 30,000 units, amylase 30,000 units/Tab. Bot. 100s, 500s. **Pow.:** Lipase 16,800 units, protease 70,000 units, amylase 70,000 units/0.7 g (0.25 tsp.). *Rx.*
Use: Digestive enzyme.

Viosterol w/Halibut Liver Oil. Vitamins A 50,000 IU, D 10,000 IU/g. (Abbott Laboratories) Bot. 5 ml, 20 ml, 50 ml. Cap.: Vitamins A 5000 IU, D 1000 IU (Ives) Cap.: Vitamins A 5000 IU, D 1700 IU. *otc.*
Use: Vitamin supplement.

•**viprostol.** (vie-PRAHST-ole) USAN.
Use: Hypotensive, vasodilator.

Viquin Forte. (Zeneca) Hydrochloroquine 4%, padimate O 80 mg, dioxybenzone 30 mg, oxybenzone/g 20 mg, stearyl alcohol, cetearyl alcohol, EDTA, sodium metabisulfite/Cream. Tube 28.4 g. SPF 19. PABA-free. *Rx.*
Use: Dermatologic.

Vira-A Ophthalmic. (Monarch) Vidarabine 3%. Tube 3.5 g. *Rx.*
Use: Antiviral, ophthalmic.

Virac. (Ruson) Undecoylium Cl^-iodine. Iodine complexed with a cationic detergent. Surgical soln. Bot. 2 oz, 8 oz, 1 gal. *otc.*
Use: Antiseptic.

Viracept. (Agouron) Nelfinavir mesylate 250 mg/Tab. Bot. 270s. Nelfinavir mesylate 50 mg/g, aspartame (11.2 mg/g phenylanine), sucrose. Pow. Multidose bottles. 144 g Pow. w/ 1 g scoop. *Rx.*
Use: Antiviral.

Viracil. (Health for Life Brands) Phenylephrine HCl 5 mg, hesperidin 50 mg, thenylene HCl 12.5 mg, pyrilamine maleate 12.5 mg, vitamin C 50 mg, salicylamide 2.5 gr, caffeine 0.5 gr, sodium salicylate 1.25 gr/Cap. Bot. 16s, 36s. *otc.*
Use: Analgesic, antihistamine, decongestant, vitamin supplement.

Viractin. (J.B. Williams) Tetracaine 2%, hydrochloric acid, methylparaben. Cream 7.1 g. Tetracaine HCl 2%, parabens. Gel 7.1 g. *otc.*
Use: Anesthetic, local.

Viramisol. (Seatrace) Adenosine phosphate 25 mg/ml. Vial 10 ml. *otc.*
Use: Relief of varicose vein complications.

Viramune. (Roxane) Nevirapine 200 mg/Tab. Bot. *Rx.*
Use: Antiviral.

Viranol. (American Dermal) Salicylic acid in collodion gel w/lactic acid, camphor, pyroxylin, ethyl alcohol, ethyl acetate. Gel 8 g. *otc.*
Use: Dermatologic, wart therapy.

Virazole. (Zeneca) Ribavirin 6 g/Pow. for Aero. Reconst. Vial. 100 ml. Contains 20 mg/ml when reconstituted w/ 300 ml sterile water. *Rx.*
Use: Antiviral.

•**virginiamycin.** (vihr-JIH-nee-ah-MY-sin) USAN. An antibiotic produced by *Streptomyces virginie.*
Use: Anti-infective.

Viridium. (Vita Elixir) Phenylazodiaminopyridine HCl 100 mg/Tab.
Use: Genitourinary.

•**viridofulvin.** (vih-RID-oh-FULL-vin) USAN.
Use: Antifungal.

Virilon. (Star) Methyltestosterone 10 mg/SR Cap. Bot. 100s, 1000s. *c-III.*
Use: Androgen.

Virogen Herpes Slide Test. (Wampole Laboratories) Latex agglutination slide test for the detection of herpes simplex virus antigens directly from lesions or cell culture. Test kit 100s.
Use: Diagnostic aid.

Virogen Rotatest. (Wampole Laboratories) Latex agglutination slide test for the qualitative detection of rotavirus in fecal specimens. Test kit 50s.
Use: Diagnostic aid.

Virogen Rubella Microlatex Test. (Wampole Laboratories) Latex agglutination microlatex test for the detection of rubella virus antibody in serum. Test kit 500s, 5000s.
Use: Diagnostic aid.

Virogen Rubella Slide Test. (Wampole Laboratories) Latex agglutination slide test for the detection of rubella virus antibody in serum. Test kit 100s, 500s, 5000s.
Use: Diagnostic aid.

Virogen Rubella Slide Test with Fast Trak Slides. (Wampole Laboratories) Latex agglutination slide test for the detection of rubella virus antibody in serum.
Use: Diagnostic aid.

Viro-Med Tablets. (Whitehall Robins) Acetaminophen 500 mg, chlorpheniramine maleate 2 mg, pseudoephedrine HCl 30 mg, dextromethorphan HBr 15 mg/Tab. Bot. 20s, 48s. *otc.*
Use: Analgesic, antihistamine, antitussive, decongestant.

Viroptic Ophthalmic Solution. (Monarch Pharm) Trifluridine 1%, thimerosal 0.001% Bot. 7.5 ml. *Rx.*
Use: Antiviral, ophthalmic.

•**viroxime.** (vie-ROX-eem) USAN.
Use: Antiviral.

Virozyme Injection. (Marcen) Sodium nucleate 2.5%, phenol 0.5%, protein hydrolysate 2.5%, benzyl alcohol 0.2%. Vial 5 ml, 10 ml. *Rx.*
Use: Immunomodulator.

Virugon. Under study. Anhydro bis-(beta-hydroxyethyl) biguanide derivative.
Use: Treatment of influenza, mumps, measles, chicken pox and shingles.

viscarin w/iodine, boric acid, phenol, chlorophyll.

Viscoat Solution. (Alcon Laboratories) Sodium chondroitin sulfate 40 mg, sodium hyaluronate 30 mg, sodium dihydrogen phosphate hydrate 0.45 mg, disodium hydrogen phosphate 2 mg, sodium Cl 4.3 mg/ml. Syringe disposable 0.5 ml. *Rx.*
Use: Viscoelastic.

viscum album, extract. Visnico.
Use: Vasodilator.

Visine Allergy Relief. (Pfizer) Tetrahydrozoline HCl 0.05%. Bot. 15 ml, 30 ml. *otc.*
Use: Mydriatic, vasoconstrictor.

Visine Moisturizing. (Pfizer) Polyethylene glycol 400 1%, tetrahydrozoline HCl 0.05%. Drop Bot. 15 ml, 30 ml. *otc.*
Use: Mydriatic, vasoconstrictor.

Visine L.R. (Pfizer) Oxymetazoline HCl 0.025%. Soln. Bot. 15, 30 ml. *otc.*
Use: Mydriatic, vasoconstrictor.

Vision Care Enzymatic Cleaner. (Alcon Laboratories) Highly purified pork pancreatin to be diluted in saline solution. Tab. Pkg. 24s. *otc.*
Use: Contact lens care.

Visipaque. (Nycomed) Iodixanol 270 mg I/ml. EDTA. In 50 ml vials, 100 ml and 200 ml bottles, 150 ml fill/200 ml bottles, and 100 ml, 150 ml, 200 ml flexible containers. Iodixanol 320 mg I/ml, EDTA. 50 ml vials, 100 ml, 200 ml bottles, 150 ml/fill/200 ml bottles 100 ml, 150 ml, 200 ml flexible containers.
Use: Diagnostic aid.

Visken. (Novartis) Pindolol 5 mg or 10 mg/Tab. Bot. 100s. *Rx.*
Use: Antihypertensive.

Vistacon. (Roberts) Hydroxyzine HCl 50 mg/ml. Vial 10 ml. *Rx.*
Use: Anxiolytic.

Vistaril. (Pfizer) Hydroxyzine pamoate equivalent to hydroxyzine HCl. **Cap.:** 25 mg, 50 mg or 100 mg, sucrose. Bot. 100s, 500s, UD 100s. **Oral Susp.:** 25 mg/5 ml, sorbitol, lemon flavor. Bot. 120 ml, 480 ml, pt. *Rx.*
Use: Anxiolytic.

Vistaril I.M. (Roerig) Hydroxyzine HCl, brenzyl alcohol 0.9%. **25 mg/ml:** Vial 10 ml, Box 1s. **50 mg/ml:** Vial 10 ml, Box 1s.; Vial 1 ml, 2 ml, 10 ml. *Rx.*
Use: Anxiolytic.

Vistazine 50. (Keene Pharmaceuticals) Hydroxyzine HCl 50 mg/ml. Inj. Vial 10. *Rx.*
Use: Anxiolytic.

Vistide. (Gilead Sciences) Cidofovir 75 mg/ml/Inj. Amp. 5 ml. *Rx.*
Use: Antiviral.

Visual-Eyes. (Optopics) Sodium Cl, sodium phosphate mono- and dibasic, benzalkonium Cl, EDTA. Soln. Bot. 120 ml. *otc.*
Use: Irrigant, ophthalmic.

Vita-Bee with C Caplets. (Rugby) Vitamins B_1 15 mg, B_2 10.2 mg, B_3 50 mg, B_5 10 mg, B_6 5 mg, C 300 mg/TR Cap. Bot. 100s, 1000s. *otc.*
Use: Vitamin supplement.

Vitabix. (Spanner) Vitamins B_1 100 mg, B_2 2 mg, B_6 5 mg, B_{12} 30 mcg, niacinamide 100 mg, panthenol 10 mg/ml. Vial 10 ml. Multiple dose vial 30 ml. *Rx.*
Use: Vitamin supplement.

Vita-Bob Softgel Capsules. (Scot-Tussin Pharmacal) Vitamins A 5000 IU, D 400 IU, E 30 mg, B_1 1.5 mg, B_2 1.7 mg, B_3 20 mg, B_6 2 mg, B_{12} 6 mcg, C 60 mg, folic acid 0.4 mg/Cap. Bot. 100s. *otc.*
Use: Vitamin supplement.

Vita-C. (Freeda Vitamins) Ascorbic acid 4 g/tsp. Crystals 100 g, 500 g, 1000 g. *otc.*
Use: Vitamin supplement.

Vitacarn. (McGaw) L-carnitine 1 g/10 ml. UD Box 50s, 100s. *Rx.*
Use: L-carnitine supplement.

Vit-A-Drops. (Vision Pharm) Vitamin A 5000 IU, polysorbate 80. Bot. 10 ml, 15 ml. *otc.*
Use: Lubricant, ophthalmic.

Vitadye. (Zeneca) FD&C yellow No. 5, FD&C red No. 40, FD&C blue No. 1 dyes and dihydroxyacetone 5%. Bot. 0.5 oz, 2 oz. *otc.*
Use: Cosmetic for hyperpigmentation.

Vitafol. (Everett Laboratories) Iron 90 mg, B_3 39.9 mg, B_6 6 mg, B_{12} 25.02 mcg, folic acid 0.75 mg. Syr. Bot. 473 ml. *Rx.*

Use: Mineral, vitamin supplement.

Vitafol Caplets. (Everett Laboratories) Iron 65 mg, vitamins A 6000 IU, D 400 IU, E 30 mg, B_1 1.1 mg, B_2 1.8 mg, B_3 15 mg, B_6 2.5 mg, B_{12} 5 mcg, C 60 mg, folic acid 1 mg, calcium/Tab. Bot. 100s, 1000s. *Rx.*
Use: Mineral, vitamin supplement.

Vita-Iron Formula. (Barth's) Iron 120 mg, vitamins B_1 5 mg, B_2 10 mg, C 20 mg, niacin 2 mg, B_{12} 25 mcg, lysine, desiccated liver 200 mg, bromelain/Tab. Bot. 100s, 500s. *otc.*
Use: Mineral, vitamin supplement.

Vita-Kaps Filmtabs. (Abbott Laboratories) Vitamins A 5000 IU, D 400 IU, B_1 3 mg, B_2 2.5 mg, nicotinamide 20 mg, B_6 1 mg, C 50 mg, B_{12} 3 mcg/Filmtab. Bot. 100s, 1000s. *otc.*
Use: Vitamin supplement.

Vitakaps-M. (Abbott Laboratories) Vitamins A 5000 IU, D 400 IU, B_1 3 mg, B_2 2.5 mg, nicotinamide 20 mg, B_6 1 mg, B_{12} 3 mcg, C 50 mg, iron 10 mg, copper 1 mg, iodine 0.15 mg, manganese 1 mg, zinc 7.5 mg/Filmtab. Bot. 100s. *otc.*
Use: Mineral, vitamin supplement.

Vita-Kid Chewable Wafers. (Solgar) Vitamins A 10,000 IU, D 400 IU, E 10 mg, B_1 2 mg, B_2 2 mg, B_3 10 mg, B_6 2 mg, B_{12} 5 mcg, C 100 mg, FA 0.3 mg, orange flavor. Tab. Bot. 50s, 100s. *otc.*
Use: Vitamin Supplement.

Vitalax. (Vitalax) Candy base, gumdrop flavored. Pkg. 20s. *otc.*
Use: Laxative.

Vital B-50. (Zenith Goldline) Vitamins B_1 50 mg, B_2 50 mg, B_3 50 mg, B_5 50 mg, B_6 50 mg, B_{12} 50 mcg, folic acid 0.1 mg, biotin 50 mcg, PABA, choline bitartrate, inositol/TR Tab. Bot 60s. *otc.*
Use: Vitamin supplement.

Vitalets Tablets. (Freeda Vitamins) Iron 10 mg, vitamins A 5000 IU, D 400 IU, E 5 mg, B_1 2.5 mg, B_2 0.9 mg, B_3 20 mg, B_5 3 mg, B_6 2 mg, B_{12} 5 mcg, C 60 mg, biotin 25 mcg, Mn, Ca. Chew. Tab. Bot 100s, 250s. *otc.*
Use: Mineral, vitamin supplement.

VitalEyes. (Allergan) Vitamin A 10,000 IU, C 200 mg, E 100 IU, Zn 40 mg, Cu, Se, Mn/Cap. Bot. 60s. *otc.*
Use: Mineral, vitamin supplement.

Vital High Nitrogen. (Ross Laboratories) Amino acids, partially hydrolyzed whey, meat and soy, hydrolyzed cornstarch, sucrose, safflower oil, MCT mono and diglycerides, soy lecithin, vitamins A, B_1, B_2, B_3, B_5, B_6, B_{12}, C, D, E, K, folic acid, biotin, choline, Ca, P, Mg, Fe, Cu, Zn, Mn, I, Cl. Packet 80 g. *otc.*
Use: Nutritional supplement.

Vitalize SF. (Scot-Tussin Pharmacal) Iron 66 mg, B_1 30 mg, B_6 15 mg, B_{12} 75 mcg, L-lysine 300 mg. Liq. Bot. 120 ml. *otc.*
Use: Mineral, vitamin supplement.

Vitamel with Iron. (Eastwood) Drops 50 ml. Chew. Tab. Bot. 100s.
Use: Mineral, vitamin supplement.

•**vitamin A.** U.S.P. 23. *formerly Oleovitamin A.*
Use: Antixerophthalmic vitamin, emollient.
See: Aquasol A, Drops, Cap., Inj. (Astra USA)
Del-Vi-A, Cap. (Del-Ray).
Palmitate-A 5000, Tab. (Akorn).

vitamin A. (Various Mfr.) Cap. 10,000 IU: 100s, 250s and 1000s. *otc.*
25,000 IU: 100s, 250s, 500s and 1000s. *Rx.*
50,000 IU: 100s, 250s, 500s and 1000s. *Rx.*
Use: Antixerophthalmic vitamin, emollient.
See: Retinol, Cream (Nature's Bounty).

vitamin A acid.
See: tretinoin.

vitamin A, alphalin. (Eli Lilly) Vitamin A 50,000 IU/Gelseal. Bot. 100s. *Rx.*
Use: Vitamin supplement.

vitamin A, water miscible, or soluble. Water-miscible vitamin A.
Use: Vitamin supplement.

vitamin A w/ combinations.
See: Advanced Formula Zenate, Tab. (Solvay).
Advera, Liq. (Ross).
Bonamil Infant Formula with Iron, Conc., Liq. (Wyeth-Ayerst).
Boost, Liq. (Mead Johnson Nutritionals).
Choice dm, Liq. (Mead Johnson Pharmaceuticals).
Fosfree, Tab. (Mission).
Neocate One +, Liq. (SHS).
Nepro, Liq. (Ross).
Ocuvite Extra, Tab. (Storz).
Oncovite, Tab. (Mission).
Prenatal H.P., Tab. (Mission).
Prenatal Plus, Tab. (Zenith Goldline).
Prenatal Plus w/ Beta-Carotene, Tab. (Rugby).
Prenatal Rx, Tab. (Misson).
Prenatal Z Advanced Formula, Tab. (Ethex).
Stuartnatal Plus, Tab. (Wyeth-Ayerst).

Theregran AntiOxidant, Softgel (Bristol-Meyers Squibb).
Tri-Flor-Vite with Flouride, Drops (Everett).

vitamin Bc.
See: Folic Acid (Various Mfr.).

vitamin B_1. Thiamine HCl, U.S.P. 23.
Use: Vitamin supplement.

vitamin B_1 mononitrate. Thiamine mononitrate.
Use: Vitamin supplement.

vitamin B_1 w/pancreatin, ox bile extract pepsin, glutamic acid HCl.
See: Maso-Gestive, Tab. (Mason).

vitamin B_1 w/thyroid.
See: T & T, Tab. (Mason).

vitamin B_2. Riboflavin.
Use: Vitamin supplement.

vitamin B_3. Niacinamide, Nicotinamide.
Use: Vitamin supplement.

vitamin B_5. Calcium Pantothenate.
Use: Vitamin supplement.

vitamin B_6. Pyridoxine HCl.
Use: Vitamin supplement.
See: Hexa-Betalin, Tab. (Eli Lilly).
Hexavibex, Vial (Parke-Davis).

vitamin B_8.
See: Adenosine phosphate.

vitamin B_{12}. Cyanocobalamin. Cobalamine.
See:
Cap., Tab.:
Redisol (Merck).
Vial, Amp.:
Bedoce (Lincoln).
Berubigen (Pharmacia & Upjohn).
Betalin-12 (Eli Lilly).
Cabadon-M (Solvay).
Cobadoce Forte (Solvay).
Crysto-Gel (Solvay).
Cyano-Gel, Liq. (Maurry).
Dodex (Organon Teknika).
Redisol (Merck).
Rubramin (Bristol-Myers Squibb).
Ruvite 1000 (Savage).
Sigamine (Sigma-Tau Pharmaceuticals).
Sytobex-H (Parke-Davis).
Vi-Twel, Inj. (Berlex).
W/Ferrous sulfate, ascorbic acid, folic acid.
See: Intrin, Cap. (Merit).
W/Folic acid, niacinamide, liver.
See: Hepfomin 500, Inj. (Keene Pharmaceuticals).
W/Thiamine.
See: Cobalin, Vial (Ulmer).
Cyamine, Vial (Keene Pharmaceuticals).
W/Thiamine, vitamin B_6.
See: Orexin, Tab. (Zeneca).

vitamin B_{12}. (Various Mfr.) Cyanocobalamin crystalline 100 mcg/ml or 1000 mcg/ml. **100 mcg/ml:** Vials 30 ml. **1000 mcg/ml:** Multidose vials 10 ml or 30 ml. *Rx.*
Use: Vitamin supplement.

vitamin B_{12}. (Zenith Goldline) Cyanocobalamin crystalline 500 mcg or 1000 mcg. Tab. Bot. 100s. *otc.*
Use: Vitamin supplement.

vitamin B_{12} a & b.
See: Hydroxocobalamin (Various Mfr.).

vitamin B_{15}.
Use: Alleged to increase oxygen supply in blood. Not approved by FDA as a vitamin or drug. Illegal to sell Vitamin B_{15}.

vitamin B complex. Concentrated extract of dried brewer's yeast and extract of corn processed w/Clostridium acetobutylicum.
See: Becotin, Pulvules (Eli Lilly).
Betalin Complex, Amp. (Eli Lilly).
Savaplex, Vial (Savage).

Vitamin B complex 100. (McGuff) Vitamin B_1 100 mg, B_2 2 mg, B_3 100 mg, B_5 2 mg, B_6 2 mg/ml/Inj. Vial 10 ml, 30 ml. *Rx.*
Use: Vitamin supplement.

Vitamin B Complex No. 104. (Century Pharm) Vitamins B_1 100 mg, B_2 2 mg, B_6 2 mg, d-panthenol 10 mg, niacinamide 125 mg, benzyl alcohol 1%, gentisic acid ethanolamide 2.5%/Vial 30 ml. *Rx.*
Use: Vitamin supplement.

Vitamin B Complex, Betalin Complex, Elixir. (Eli Lilly) Vitamins B_1 2.7 mg, B_2 1.35 mg, B_{12} 3 mcg, B_6 0.555 mg, pantothenic acid 2.7 mg, niacinamide 6.75 mg, liver fraction 500 mg/5 ml, alcohol 17%. Bot. 16 oz. *otc.*
Use: Vitamin supplement.

Vitamin B Complex w/Vitamin C. (Century Pharm) Vitamins B_1 25 mg, B_2 5 mg, B_6 5 mg, niacinamide 50 mg, panthenol 5 mg, calcium 50 mg, propethylene glycol 300 10%, gentisic acid ethanolamide 2.5%, benzyl alcohol 2%/ Vial 30 ml. *Rx.*
Use: Mineral, vitamin supplement.

Vitamin B Complex, Betalin Complex Capsules. (Eli Lilly) Vitamins B_1 1 mg, B_2 2 mg, B_6 0.4 mg, pantothenic acid 3.333 mg, niacinamide 10 mg, B_{12} 1 mcg/Pulvule. Bot. 100s. *otc.*
Use: Vitamin supplement.
See: Advanced Formula Zenate, Tab. (Solvay).

Advera, Liq. (SHS).
B-C-Bid, Capl. (Roberts Pharm).
Bonamil Infant Formula with Iron, Conc. Liq., (Wyeth-Ayerst).
Boost, Liq. (Mead Johnson Nutritionals).
Choice dm, Liq. (Mead Johnson Nutritionals).
Fosfree, Tab. (Misson).
Neocate One +, Liq. (SHS).
Nephplex RX, Tab. (Nephro-Tec).
Nephron FA, Tab. (Nephro-Tec).
Nepro, Liq. (Ross).
Ocuvite Extra, Tab. (Storz).
Oncovite, Tab. (Mission).
Prenatal H.P., Tab. (Mission).
Prenatal Plus, Tab. (Zenith Goldline).
Prenatal Plus w/ Beta-Carotenc, Tab. (Rugby).
Prenatal Rx, Tab. (Mission).
Prenatal Z Advanced Formula, Tab. (Ethex).
Stuartnatal Plus, Tab. (Wyeth-Ayerst).
Vita-Feron, Tab. (Vitaline).

vitamin C.
See: Ascorbic Acid Preps.
One-A-Day Extras Vitamin C, Tab. (Bayer).

vitamin C, cevalin. (Eli Lilly) Ascorbic acid 250 mg or 500 mg/Tab. Bot. 100s. *otc.*
Use: Vitamin supplement.

vitamin C w/combinations.
See: Advanced Formula Zenate, Tab. (Solvay).
Advera, Liq. (Ross).
Allbee C-800, Prods. (Robins).
Allbee with C, Cap. (Robins).
Allbee-T, Tab. (Robins).
Antiox, Cap. (Merz).
Anti-therm, Tab. (Scrip).
B-C-Bid, Capl. (Roberts Pharm).
Bejectal w/Vitamin C (Abbott Laboratories).
Bonamil Infant Formula with Iron, Conc. Liq. (Wyeth-Ayerst).
Boost, Liq. (Mead Johnson Nutritionals).
Choice dm, Liq. (Mead Johnson Nutritionals).
Chromagen FA, Cap. (Savage).
Chromagen Forte, Cap. (Savage).
Colrex, Cap. (Solvay).
Fosfree, Tab. (Mission).
Neocate One +, Liq. (SHS).
Nephplex Rx, Tab. (Nephro-Tec).
Nephron FA, Tab. (Nephro-Tec).
Nepro, Liq. (Ross).
Nialexo-C, Tab. (Roberts).
Ocuvite Extra, Tab. (Storz).
Oncovite, Tab. (Mission).
Prenatal H.P., Tab. (Mission).
Prenatal Plus, Tab. (Zenithg Goldline).
Prenatal Plus w/ Beta-Carotene, Tab. (Rugby).
Prenatal Rx, Tab. (Mission).
Protegra Softgels, Cap. (ESI Lederle Generics).
Stuartnatal Plus, Tab. (Wyeth-Ayerst).
Theragran Antioxidant, Softgel (Bristol-Myers Squibb).
Thex, Cap. (Ingram).
Thex Forte, Cap. (Ingram).
Tri-Flor-Vite with Flouride, Drops (Everett).
Vicon-C, Cap. (GlaxoWellcome).
Vicon Forte, Cap. (GlaxoWellcome).
Vicon Plus, Cap. (GlaxoWellcome).
Vi-Zac, Cap. (GlaxoWellcome).
Z-BEC, Tab. (Robins).

vitamin D. Cholecalciferol.
Use: Vitamin D supplement.

Vitamin D. (Various) Ergocalciferol (D_2) 50,000 IU/Cap. Bot. 100s, 1000s. *Rx.*
Use: Vitamin supplement.

vitamin D, deltalin. (Eli Lilly) Vitamin D-2 50,000 units (1.25 mg)/Gelseal. Bot. 100s. *Rx.*
Use: Vitamin supplement.

vitamin D, synthetic.
See: Activated 7-Dehydro-cholesterol Calciferol.

vitamin D-1.
See: Dihydrotachysterol.

vitamin D-2. Activated ergasterol, Ergocalciferol.
See: Calciferol, Preps. (Various Mfr.).
Drisdol, Liq. (Sanofi Winthrop).
Viosterol (Various Mfr.).

vitamin D-3.
See: Activated 7-dehydrocholesterol.
Calciferol Prep. for related activity.

Vitamin D_3. (Freeda) Cholecalciferol (D_3) 1000 IU/Tab. Bot. 100s, 500s. *otc.*
Use: Vitamin supplement.

vitamin D-3-cholesterol. Compound of crystalline vitamin D-3 and cholesterol.

vitamin D-4.
See: Dihydrotachysterol, Preps. (Various Mfr.).

Vitamin D Oral Drops. (Cypress Pharm) Ergocalciferol (D_2) 8000 IU/ ml. Liq. 60 ml. *otc.*
Use: Vitamin supplement.

vitamin D w/combinations.
See: Advanced Formula Zenate, Tab. (Solvay).
Advera, Liq. (Ross).

Bonamil Infant Formula with Iron, Conc., Liq. (Wyeth-Ayerst).
Boost, Liq. (Mead Johnson Nutritionals).
Caltrate Plus, Tab. (Lederle).
Caltrate 600 + D, Tab. (Lederle).
Choice dm, Liq. (Mead Johnson Nutritionals).
Desert Pure Calcium, Tab. (Cal-White Mineral).
Fosfree, Tab. (Mission).
Neocate One +, Liq. (SHS).
Nepro, Liq. (Ross).
Oesto-Mins, Pow. (Tyson).
Oncovite, Tab. (Mission).
Prenatal Plus, Tab. (Zenith Goldline).
Prenatal Plus w/Beta-Carotene, Tab. (Rugby).
Prenatal Rx, Tab. (Mission).
Stuartnatal Plus, Tab. (Wyeth-Ayerst).
Tri-Flor-Vite with Flouride, Drops (Everett).

•**vitamin E.** U.S.P. 23.
Use: Vitamin E supplement.
See: Aquasol E (Rhone-Poulenc Rorer).
Eprolin, Gelseal (Eli Lilly).
E-Vites, Cap. (Quality Formulations).
Lactinol-E Creme (Pedinol).
One-A-Day Extras Vitamin E, Softgel cap. (Bayer).
Soft Sense, Lot. (Bausch & Lomb).
Tocopher, Prod. (Quality Formulations).
Tocopherol, Preps. (Various Mfr.).
Wheat Germ Oil (Various Mfr.).

vitamin E, eprolin. (Eli Lilly) Alpha-tocopherol 100 units/Gelseal. Bot. 100s.
Use: Vitamin supplement.

vitamin E w/combinations.
See: Advanced Formula Zenate, Tab. (Solvay).
Advera, Liq. (Ross).
Antiox, Cap. (Mayrand).
Bonamil Infant Formula with Iron, Conc., Liq. (Wyeth-Ayerst).
Boost, Liq. (Mead Johnson Nutritionals).
Choice dm, Liq. (Mead Johnson Nutritionals).
Neocate One +, Liq. (SHS).
Nepro, Liq. (Ross).
Ocuvite Extra, Tab. (Storz).
Oncovite, Tab. (Mission)
Prenatal Plus, Tab. (Zenith Goldline).
Prenatal Plus w/Beta-Carotene, Tab. (Rugby).
Stuartnatal Plus, Tab. (Wyeth-Ayerst).
Theragran AntiOxidant, Softgels (Bristol-Meyers Squibb).

vitamin E w/quinine sulfate, niacin.
See: Myodyne, Tab. (Paddock).

vitamin F.
See: Fats, Unsaturated.
Fatty Acids, Unsaturated.

vitamin G.
See: Riboflavin.

vitamin K.
See: Hykinone, Amp. (Abbott Laboratories).
Menadiol, Sodium Diphosphate, Preps. (Various Mfr.).
Menadione, Preps. (Various Mfr.).
Menadione Sodium Bisulfite, Preps. (Various Mfr.).

vitamin K-1.
See: Phytonadione, U.S.P. 23.

vitamin K-3.
See: Menadione, U.S.P. 23.

vitamin K oxide. Not available, but usually K-1 is desired.

vitamin K w/combinations.
See: Advera, Liq. (Ross).
Bonamil Infant Formula with Iron, Conc., Liq. (Wyeth-Ayerst).
Choice dm, Liq. (Mead Johnson Nutritionals).
Neocate One +, Liq. (SHS).

vitamin M.
See: Folic Acid, U.S.P. 23.

vitamin-mineral-supplement liquid. (Morton Grove) Vitamins B_1 0.83 mg, B_2 0.42 mg, B_3 8.3 mg, B_5 1.67 mg, B_6 0.17 mg, B_{12} 0.17 mcg, I, Fe 2.5 mg, Mg, Zn 0.3 mg, Mn, choline, alcohol 18%. Liq. 473 ml. *otc.*
Use: Mineral, vitamin supplement.

vitamin P. Citrin.
See: Bio-Flavonoid Compounds (Various Mfr.).
Hesperidin Preps. (Various Mfr.).
Quercetin (Various Mfr.).
Rutin, Preps. (Various Mfr.).

vitamin T. Sesame seed factor, termite factor.
Use: Claimed to aid proper blood coagulation and promote formation of blood platelets. Not approved by FDA as an active vitamin.

vitamin U. Present in cabbage juice.

vitamin, maintenance formula.
See: Stuart Formula, Tab., Liq. (Zeneca).
Vi-Magna, Cap. (ESI Lederle Generics).

vitamins: stress formula.
See: Cebefortis, Tab. (Pharmacia & Upjohn).
Folbesyn, Tab., Vial (ESI Lederle Generics).

Probec-T, Tab. (Zeneca).
Stresscaps, Cap. (ESI Lederle Generics).
Stresscaps With Iron (ESI Lederle Generics).
Stresscaps With Zinc (ESI Lederle Generics).
StressForm "605" w/ Iron, Tab. (NBTY).
Stress Formula with Iron, Tab. (NBTY).
Stresstabs-600 (ESI Lederle Generics).
Thera-combex Kap. (Parke-Davis).

vitamins w/antiobesity agents.
See: Fetamin, Tab. (Mission Pharmacal).
Obedrin, Cap. or Tab. (Massengill).

vitamins w/liver & lipotropic agents.
See: Heptuna, Cap. (Roerig).
Lederplex, Preps. (ESI Lederle Generics).
Livitamin, Preps. (SmithKline Beecham Pharmaceuticals).
Metheponex, Cap. (Rawl).
Methischol, Cap. (Rhone-Poulenc Rorer).

Vita Natal. (Scot-Tussin Pharmacal) Folic acid 1 mg/Tab. Bot. 100s. *Rx.*
Use: Vitamin supplement.

Vitaneed. (Biosearch Medical Products) P-beef, Ca and Na caseinates, CHO-maltodextrin. F-partially hydrogenated soy oil, mono and diglycerides, soy lecithin. Protein 35 g, CHO 125 g, fat 40 g, sodium 500 mg, potassium 1250 mg/L, 1 Cal/ml, 375 mOsm/kg H_2O. Liq. Ready-to-use 250 ml. *otc.*
Use: Nutritional supplement.

Vitaon. (Vita Elixir) Vitamin B_{12} 25 mcg, thiamine HCl 10 mg, ferric pyrophosphate 250 mg/5 ml. *otc.*
Use: Vitamin supplement.

Vita-Plus B12. (Scot-Tussin Pharmacal) Vitamin B_{12} 1000 mcg/ml. Inj. *Rx.*
Use: Vitamin supplement.

Vita-Plus E. (Scot-Tussin Pharmacal) Vitamin E 294 mg as d-alpha tocopheryl acetate/Cap. *otc.*
Use: Vitamin supplement.

Vita-Plus G Softgel. (Scot-Tussin Pharmacal) Vitamins A 5000 IU, D 400 IU, E 10 IU, B_1 5 mg, B_2 5 mg, B_3 15 mg, B_5 5 mg, B_6 1 mg, B_{12} 1 mcg, C 50 mg, iron 3.3 mg, Ca 145 mg, Zn 0.5 mg, K, Mg, Mn, P, I, Cu, choline, l-lysine, inositol/Cap. Bot. 100s. *otc.*
Use: Mineral, vitamin supplement.

Vita-Plus H Softgel. (Scot-Tussin Pharmacal) Iron 13.4 mg, vitamins A 5000 IU, D 400 IU, E 3 IU, B_1 3 mg, B_2 2.5 mg, B_3 20 mg, B_5 5 mg, B_6 1.5 mg, B_{12} 2.5 mcg, C 50 mg, Ca, K, Mg, Mn, P, Zn 1.4 mg/Cap. Bot. 100s. *otc.*
Use: Mineral, vitamin supplement.

Vita-Plus H Liquid Sugar Free. (Scot-Tussin Pharmacal) Vitamins B_1 30 mg, l-lysine monohydrochloride 300 mg, B_{12} 75 mcg, B_6 15 mg, iron pyrophosphate soluble 100 mg/5 ml. Bot. 4 oz, 8 oz, pt, gal. *otc.*
Use: Mineral, vitamin supplement.

Vita-PMS. (Bajamar Chemical) Vitamins A 2083 IU, E 16.7 IU, D_3 16.7 IU, folic acid 33 mcg, B_1 4.2 mg, B_2 4.2 mg, B_3 4.2 mg, B_5 4.2 mg, B_6 50 mg, B_{12} 10.4 mcg, biotin, C 250 mg, Ca, Mg, I, Fe, Cu, Zn 4.2 mg, Mn, K, Se, Cr, betaine/Tab. Bot. 100s. *otc.*
Use: Mineral, vitamin supplement.

Vita-PMS Plus. (Bajamar Chemical) Vitamins A 667 IU, E 16.7 IU, D_3 16.7 IU, folic acid 33 mcg, B_1 4.2 mg, B_2 4.2 mg, B_3 4.2 mg, B_5 4.2 mg, B_6 16.7 mg, B_{12} 10.4 mcg, biotin, C 250 mg, Mg, I, Ca, Fe, Cu, Zn 4.2 mg, Mn, K, Se, Cr, betaine/Tab. Bot. 100s. *otc.*
Use: Mineral, vitamin supplement.

Vita-Ray Creme. (Gordon Laboratories) Vitamins E 3000 IU, A 200,000 IU/oz w/ aloe 10%. Jar 0.5 oz, 2.5 oz. *otc.*
Use: Emollient.

Vitarex. (Taylor Pharmaceuticals) Vitamins A 10,000 IU, D 200 IU, B_1 15 mg, B_2 10 mg, B_6 5 mg, B_{12} 5 mcg, C 250 mg, B_3 100 mg, B_5 20 mg, E 15 mg, iron 15 mg, Ca, Cu, I, K, Mg, Mn, P, Zn 10 mg/Tab. Bot. 100s. *otc.*
Use: Mineral, vitamin supplement.

Vitazin. (Mesemer) Ascorbic acid 300 mg, niacinamide 100 mg, thiamine mononitrate 20 mg, d-calcium pantothenate 20 mg, riboflavin 10 mg, pyridoxine HCl 5 mg, magnesium sulfate 70 mg, zinc 25 mg/Cap. Bot. 100s. *otc.*
Use: Mineral, vitamin supplement.

Vita-Zoo. (Towne) Vitamins A 2500 IU, D 400 IU, E 15 IU, C 60 mg, folic acid 0.3 mg, B_1 1.05 mg, B_2 1.2 mg, niacin 13.5 mg, B_6 1.05 mg, B_{12} 4.5 mcg/Tab. Bot. 100s. *otc.*
Use: Vitamin supplement.

Vita-Zoo Plus Iron. (Towne) Vitamins A 2500 IU, D 400 IU, E 15 IU, C 60 mg, folic acid 0.3 mg, B_1 1.05 mg, B_2 1.2 mg, niacin 13.5 mg, B_6 1.05 mg, B_{12} 4.5 mcg, iron 15 mg/Tab. Bot. 100s. *otc.*
Use: Mineral, vitamin supplement.

Vitec. (Pharmaceutical Specialties) Dl-alpha tocopheryl acetate in a vanish-

ing cream base. Cream. 120 g. *otc.*
Use: Emollient.

Vitormains. (Roberts) Tab. Bot. 100s.
Use: Vitamin supplement.

Vitrasert. (Chiron Vision) Ganciclovir 4.5 mg (released over 5 to 8 months)/Intravitreal implant. Box. 1. *Rx.*
Use: Antiviral, cytomegalovirus.

Vivactil. (Merck) Protriptyline HCl 5 mg or 10 mg/Tab. **5 mg:** Bot. 100s. **10 mg:** Bot. 100s, UD 100s. *Rx.*
Use: Antidepressant.

Viva-Drops. (Vision Pharm) Polysorbate 80, sodium Cl, EDTA, retinyl palmitate, mannitol, sodium citrate, pyruvate. Soln. Bot. 10 ml, 15 ml. *otc.*
Use: Artificial tears.

Vivarin. (SmithKline Beecham Pharmaceuticals) Caffeine alkaloid 200 mg. Tab. Blister Pk. 16s, 40s, 80s. Capl. In 24s, 48s. *otc.*
Use: CNS stimulant.

Vivikon. (Zeneca) Vitamins B_1 5 mg, B_2 2 mg, B_6 10 mg, d-panthenol 5 mg, niacinamide 10 mg, procaine HCl 2%/ml. 100 ml. *otc.*
Use: Vitamin supplement.

Vivonex Flavor Packets. (Procter & Gamble) Non-nutritive flavoring for Vivonex diets when consumed orally. Orange-pineapple, lemon-lime, strawberry and vanilla. Pkg. 60s. *otc.*
Use: Flavoring.

Vivonex, Standard. (Procter & Gamble) Free amino acid/complete enteral nutrition. Six packets provide kilocalories 1800, available nitrogen 5.88 g as amino acids 37 g, fat 2.61 g, carbohydrate 407 g, and full day's balanced nutrition. Calorie:nitrogen ratio is 300:1. Unflavored pow. Packet 80 g, Pkg. 6s. *otc.*
Use: Nutritional supplement.

Vivonex T.E.N. (Procter & Gamble) Free amino acid, high nitrogen/high branched chain amino acid complete enteral nutrition. Ten packets provide kilocalories 3000, available nitrogen 17 g, amino acids 115 g, fat 8.33 g, carbohydrate 617 g and full day's balanced nutrition. Calorie:nitrogen ratio is 175:1. Unflavored pow. Packet 80 g, Pkg. 10s. *otc.*
Use: Nutritional supplement.

Vivotif Berna. (Berna Products) Typhoid vaccine (oral). *S. typhi* Ty21a (viable) 2 to 6 $\times 10^9$ colony forming units and *S. typhi* Ty21a[2] (non-viable) 5 to 50 $\times 10^9$ colony forming units/Cap. Single foil blister with 4 doses. *Rx.*
Use: Immunization.

Vi-Zac. (UCB Pharmaceuticals) Vitamins A 5000 IU, E 50 IU, C 500 mg, Zn 18 mg, lactose. Bot. 60s. *otc.*
Use: Mineral, vitamin supplement.

V-Lax. (Century Pharm) Psyllium mucilloid (hydrophilic) 50%, dextrose 50%. Pow. 0.25 lb, 1 lb. *otc.*
Use: Laxative.

Vlemasque. (Dermik Laboratories) Sulfurated lime topical solution 6% (Vleminck's Soln.), alcohol 7% in drying clay mask. Jar 4 oz. *otc.*
Use: Dermatologic, acne.

VM. (Last) Vitamins B_1 6 mg, B_2 4 mg, niacinamide 40 mg, iron 100 mg, calcium 188 mg, phosphorus 188 mg, manganese 4 mg, alcohol 12%. Bot. 16 oz. *otc.*
Use: Mineral, vitamin supplement.

V-M Capsules. (Pal-Pak) Vitamins A, D, B_1, B_2, B_6, C, niacinamide, Ca, Fe, calcium pantothenate, Mg, Mn, K, Zn, P/ Tab. Bot. 100s, 1000s. *otc.*
Use: Mineral, vitamin supplement.

•**volazocine.** (voe-LAY-zoe-SEEN) USAN. Under study.
Use: Analgesic.

Volidan. (British Drug House) Megestrol acetate. *Rx.*
Use: Hormone.

Volitane. (Trent) Parethoxycaine 0.2%, hexachlorophene 0.025%, dichlorophene 0.025%. Aerosol spray can 3 oz. *otc.*
Use: Counterirritant, antiseptic.

Volmax. (Muro) Albuterol sufate 4 mg or 8 mg/ER Tab. Bot. UD 100s, 500s. *Rx.*
Use: Bronchodilator.

Voltaren. (Novartis Pharmaceutical) Diclofenac sodium 25 mg, 50 mg, 75 mg, lactose, SR. Tab. **25 mg:** Bot. 60s, 100s, UD 100s; **50 mg, 75 mg:** Bot. 60s, 100s, 1000s, UD 100s. *Rx.*
Use: Analgesic, NSAID.

Voltaren-XR. (Novartis Pharmaceutical) Diclofenac sodium 100 mg, sucrose/ ER Tab. 100s, UD 100s. *Rx.*
Use: Analgesic, NSAID.

Voltaren, Ophthalmic Solution. (Ciba Vision Ophthalmics) Diclofenac sodium. 0.1%. Soln. Bot. 2.5, 5 ml w/ dropper. *Rx.*
Use: NSAID, ophthalmic.

vonedrine hydrochloride. Vonedrine (phenylpropylmethylamine) HCl. *otc.*
Use: Decongestant.

•**vorozole.** (VORE-oh-zole) USAN.
Use: Antineoplastic.

Vortel. Clorprenaline HCl.
Use: Bronchodilator.

VoSoL HC Otic Solution. (Wallace Laboratories) Propylene glycol diacetate 3%, acetic acid 2%, benzethonium Cl 0.02%, hydrocortisone 1%. Bot. 10 ml. *Rx.*
Use: Otic.

VoSoL Otic Solution. (Wallace Laboratories) Propylene glycol diacetate 3%, acetic acid 2%, benzethonium Cl 0.02%, sodium acetate 0.015%. Bot. 15 ml, 30 ml. *Rx.*
Use: Otic.

•**votumumab.** (vah-TOOM-uh-mab) USAN.
Use: Monoclonal antibody.

Voxsuprine Tabs. (Major) Isoxsuprine HCl 10 mg or 20 mg/Tab. Bot. 100s, 250s, 1000s, UD 100s. *Rx.*
Use: Vasodilator.

V-Tuss Expectorant. (Vangard) Hydrocodone bitartrate 5 mg, pseudoephedrine HCl 60 mg, guaifenesin 200 mg/ 5 ml, alcohol 12.5%. *c-III.*
Use: Antitussive, decongestant, expectorant.

Vumon. (Bristol-Myers Oncology/Immunology) Teniposide 10 mg/ml. Inj. Amp. 5 ml. *Rx.*
Use: Antineoplastic.

V.V.S. (Econo Med Pharmaceuticals) Sulfathiazole 3.42%, sulfacetamide 2.86%, sulfabenzamide 3.7%, urea 0.64%. Cream. Tube 90 g w/applicator. *Rx.*
Use: Anti-infective, vaginal.

Vytone Cream. (Dermik Laboratories) Hydrocortisone 1%, iodoquinol 1%, greaseless base. Cream. Bot. 30 g. *Rx.*
Use: Anti-infective; corticosteroid, topical.

VZIG. (Varicella-Zoster Immune Globulin) Human (American Red Cross, Northeast Region; Massachusetts Pub lic Health Biologic Laboratories) Globulin fraction of human plasma, primarily 1 G/10% to 18% in single dose vials containing 125 units varicella-zoster virus antibody in 2.5 mg or less. Inj.
Use: Immunization.

W

Wade Gesic Balm. (Wade) Menthol 3%, methyl salicylate 12%, petrolatum base. Tube oz, Jar lb. *otc.*
Use: Analgesic, topical.

Wade's Drops. Compound Benzoin Tincture.

Wakespan. (Weeks & Leo) Caffeine 250 mg/TR Cap. Vial 15s. *Rx.*
Use: CNS stimulant.

Wal-Finate Allergy Tabs. (Walgreens) Chlorpheniramine maleate 4 mg/Tab. Bot. 50s. *otc.*
Use: Antihistamine.

Wal-Finate Decongestant Tabs. (Walgreens) Chlorpheniramine maleate 4 mg, pseudoephedrine sulfate 60 mg/Tab. Bot. 50s. *otc.*
Use: Antihistamine, decongestant.

Wal-Formula Cough Syrup with D-Methorphan. (Walgreens) Dextromethorphan HBr 15 mg, doxylamine succinate 7.5 mg, sodium citrate 500 mg/10 ml. Bot. 6 oz, 8 oz. *otc.*
Use: Antihistamine, antitussive, expectorant.

Wal-Formula D Cough Syrup. (Walgreens) Dextromethorphan HBr 20 mg, phenylpropanolamine HCl 25 mg, guaifenesin 100 mg/10 ml, alcohol 10%. Bot. 6 oz, 8 oz. *otc.*
Use: Antitussive, decongestant, expectorant.

Wal-Formula M Cough Syrup. (Walgreens) Dextromethorphan HBr 30 mg, pseudoephedrine HCl 60 mg, guaifenesin 200 mg, acetaminophen 500 mg/20 ml Bot. 8 oz. *otc.*
Use: Analgesic, antitussive, decongestant, expectorant.

Wal-Frin Nasal Mist. (Walgreens) Phenylephrine HCl 0.5%, pheniramine maleate 0.2% Bot. 0.5 oz. *otc.*
Use: Antihistamine, decongestant.

Walgreen Artificial Tears. (Walgreens) Hydroxypropyl methylcellulose 0.5%. Bot. 0.5 oz. *otc.*
Use: Artificial tears.

Walgreen's Finest Iron Tablets. (Walgreens) Iron 30 mg/Tab. Bot. 100s. *otc.*
Use: Mineral supplement.

Walgreen's Finest Vit B_6. (Walgreens) Pyridoxine HCl 50 mg/Tab. Bot. 100s. *otc.*
Use: Vitamin supplement.

Walgreen Soda Mints. (Walgreens) Sodium bicarbonate 300 mg/Tab. Bot. 100s, 200s. *otc.*
Use: Antacid.

Wal-Minic. (Walgreens) Phenylpropanolamine HCl 12.5 mg, guaifenesin 100 mg/5 ml, alcohol 5%. Bot. 6 oz, 8 oz. *otc.*
Use: Decongestant, expectorant.

Wal-Minic Cold Relief Medicine. (Walgreens) Phenylpropanolamine HCl 12.5 mg, chlorpheniramine maleate 2 mg/5 ml Bot. 6 oz, 8 oz. *otc.*
Use: Antihistamine, decongestant.

Wal-Minic DM. (Walgreens) Phenylpropanolamine HCl 12.5 mg, dextromethorphan HBr 10 mg/5 ml Bot. 6 oz, 8 oz. *otc.*
Use: Antitussive, decongestant.

Wal-Phed Plus. (Walgreens) Pseudoephedrine HCl 60 mg, chlorpheniramine maleate 4 mg/Tab. Bot. 50s. *otc.*
Use: Antihistamine, decongestant.

Wal-Phed Syrup. (Walgreens) Pseudoephedrine HCl 30 mg/5 ml. Bot. 4 oz. *otc.*
Use: Decongestant.

Wal-Phed Tablets. (Walgreens) Pseudoephedrine HCl 30 mg/Tab. Bot. 50s, 100s. *otc.*
Use: Decongestant.

Wal-Tap Elixir. (Walgreens) Brompheniramine maleate 2 mg, phenylpropanolamine HCl 12.5 mg/5 ml. Bot. 4 oz. *otc.*
Use: Antihistamine, decongestant.

Wal-Tussin. (Walgreens) Guaifenesin 100 mg/5 ml. Bot. 4 oz. *otc.*
Use: Expectorant.

Wal-Tussin DM. (Walgreens) Guaifenesin 100 mg, dextromethorphan HBr 15 ml/5 ml. Bot. 4 oz, 8 oz. *otc.*
Use: Antitussive, expectorant.

Wampole One-Step hCG. (Wampole Laboratories) For in vitro detection of human chorionic gonadotropin in serum and urine. Test. In 3, 24, 96, 500 test kits.
Use: Diagnostic aid, pregnancy.

•**warfarin sodium,** (WORE-fuh-rin) U.S.P. 23.
Use: Anticoagulant.
See: Coumadin Sodium, Tab., Inj. (DuPont Merck Pharmaceuticals).

Wart Fix. (Last) Castor oil 100%. Bot. 0.3 fl oz. *otc.*
Use: Dermatologic, wart therapy.

Wart-Off. (Pfizer) Salicylic acid 17% in flexible collodion, alcohol 20.5%, ether 54.2%. Bot. 0.5 oz. *otc.*
Use: Keratolytic.

wasp vemon. *Rx.*
Use: Immunization.

Wellchol

See: Albay (Bayer Corp).
Pharmalgen (ALK Laboratories).
Venomil (Bayer Corp).

•**water for injection,** U.S.P. 23.
Use: Pharmaceutic aid (solvent).

•**water O 15 Injection.** U.S.P. 23.
Use: Diagnostic aid (radioactive, vascular disorders), radiopharmaceutical.

Water Babies Little Licks by Coppertone. (Schering Plough) SPF 30, ethylhexyl p-methoxycinnamate, oxybenzone, 2-ethylhexyl salicylate, cherry flavor. Tube 4.8 g. *otc.*
Use: Sunscreen.

Water Babies Sunblock Cream. (Schering Plough) SPF 25, ethylhexyl p-methoxycinnamate, 2-ethylhexyl salicylate, homosalate, oxybenzone, benzyl alcohol. PABA free, waterproof. Cream. Bot. 90 g. *otc.*
Use: Sunscreen.

Water Babies UVA/UVB Sunblock Lotion. (Schering Plough) SPF 30 ethylhexyl p-methoxycinnamate, 2-ethylhexyl salicylate, homosalate, oxybenzone, benzyl alcohol. PABA free, waterproof. Lot. Bot. 120 ml, 240 ml. *otc.*
Use: Sunscreen.

Water Babies UVA/UVB Sunblock Lotion. (Schering Plough) SPF 45, ethylhexyl p-methoxycinnamate, 2-ethylhexyl salicylate, otocrylene oxybenzone, benzyl alcohol. PABA free, waterproof. Lot. Bot. 120 ml. *otc.*
Use: Sunscreen.

Water Babies UVA/UVB Sunblock Lotion. (Schering Plough) Ethylhexyl-p-methoxycinnamate, oxybenzone in lotion base, SPF-15. Bot. 120 ml. *otc.*
Use: Sunscreen.

watermelon seed extract. Citrin (Table Rock).

watermelon seed extract. W/Phenobarbital, theobromine. Cithal (Table Rock).

•**water, purified,** U.S.P. 23.
Use: Pharmaceutic aid (solvent).

•**wax, carnauba,** N.F. 18.
Use: Pharmaceutic aid (tablet coating agent).

•**wax, emulsifying,** N.F. 18.
Use: Pharmaceutic aid (emulsifying, stiffening agent).

•**wax, microcrystalline,** N.F. 18.
Use: Pharmaceutic aid (stiffening, tablet coating agent).

•**wax, white,** N.F. 18.
Use: Pharmaceutic aid (stiffening agent).

•**wax, yellow,** N.F. 18.
Use: Pharmaceutic aid (stiffening agent).

Waxsol. Docusate Sodium, U.S.P. 23.

Wayds. (Wayne) Docusate sodium 100 mg/Cap. Bot. 100s. *otc.*
Use: Laxative.

Wayds-Plus Capsules. (Wayne) Docusate w/casanthranol. Bot. 50s. *otc.*
Use: Laxative.

Wayne-E Capsules. (Wayne) Vitamin E **100 IU or 200 IU/Cap.:** Bot. 1000s. **400 IU/Cap.:** Bot. 100s. *otc.*
Use: Vitamin supplement.

Wehless. (Roberts Pharm) Phendimetrazine tartrate 35 mg/Cap. Bot. 100s. *c-III.*
Use: Anorexiant.

Wehless-105 Timecelles. (Roberts Pharm) Phendimetrazine tartrate 105 mg/SA Cap. Bot. 100s. *c-III.*
Use: Anorexiant.

Wehydryl. (Roberts Pharm) Diphenhydramine HCl 50 mg/ml. Vial 10 ml. *Rx.*
Use: Antihistamine.

Welders Eye Lotion. (Weber) Tetracaine, potassium Cl, boric acid, camphor, glycerin, disodium edetate, benzalkonium Cl as preservatives. Bot. oz. *otc.*
Use: Burn therapy.

Wellbutrin. (GlaxoWellcome) Bupropion 75 mg or 100 mg/Tab. Bot. 100s. *Rx.*
Use: Antidepressant.

Wellbutrin SR. (GlaxoWellcome) Bupropion HCl 100 mg,150 mg/ER Tab. Bot. 60s.*Rx.*
Use: Antidepressant.

Wellcovorin. (GlaxoWellcome) Leucovorin 5 mg or 25 mg as calcium. **Tab.: 5 mg:** Bot. 20s, 100s, UD 50s. **25 mg:** Bot. 25s, UD 10s. **Pow. for Inj.:** 100 mg/vial as calcium. *Rx.*
Use: Hematopoietic. Colorectal cancer; osteosarcoma. [Oprhan drug].

Wellferon. (GlaxoWellcome) Interferon alfa-NL.
Use: Human papillomavirus in severe respiratory (laryngeal) papillomatosis. [Oprhan drug]

Wernet's Adhesive Cream. (Block Drug) Carboxymethylcellulose gum, ethylene oxide polymer, petrolatum in mineral oil base. Cream. Tube 1.5 oz. *otc.*
Use: Denture adhesive.

Wernet's Powder. (Block Drug) Karaya gum, ethylene oxide polymer. Bot. 0.63 oz, 1.75 oz, 3.55 oz. *otc.*
Use: Denture adhesive.

Wes-B/C. (Western Research) Vitamins

B_1 15 mg, B_2 10 mg, B_6 5 mg, niacinamide 50 mg, calcium pantothenate 10 mg, C 300 mg/Cap. Bot. 1000s. *otc.*
Use: Mineral, vitamin supplement.

Wesmatic Forte Tablets. (Wesley Pharmacal) Phenobarbital 1/8 gr, ephedrine sulfate 0.25 gr, chlorpheniramine maleate 2 mg, guaifenesin 100 mg/Tab. Bot. 100s, 1000s. *Rx.*
Use: Antihistamine, decongestant, expectorant, hypnotic, sedative.

Westcort Cream. (Westwood Squibb) Hydrocortisone valerate 0.2% in a hydrophilic base with white petrolatum. Tube 15 g, 45 g, 60 g, 120 g. *Rx.*
Use: Corticosteroid, topical.

Westcort Ointment. (Westwood Squibb) Hydrocortisone valerate 0.2% in hydrophilic base with white petrolatum, mineral oil. Tube 15 g, 45 g, 60 g. *Rx.*
Use: Corticosteroid, topical.

Westhroid. (Western Research) Thyroid 0.5 gr, 1 gr, 2 gr, 3 gr or 4 gr/Tab.; 5 gr/SC Tab. Handicount 28s (36 bags of 28s). *Rx.*
Use: Hormone, thyroid.

Westrim. (Western Research) Phenylpropanolamine HCl 37.5 mg/Tab. Bot. 100s. *otc.*
Use: Dietary aid, decongestant.

Westrim-LA 50. (Western Research) Phenylpropanolamine HCl 50 mg/TR Cap. Bot. 1000s. *otc.*
Use: Dietary aid, decongestant.

Westrim-LA 75. (Western Research) Phenylpropanolamine HCl 75 mg/TR Cap. Bot. 1000s. *otc.*
Use: Dietary aid, decongestant.

Wesvite. (Western Research) Vitamins B_1 10 mg, B_2 5 mg, B_6 2 mg, pantothenic acid 10 mg, niacinamide 30 mg, B_{12} 3 mcg, C 100 mg, E 5 IU, A 10,000 IU, D 400 IU, iron 15 mg, copper 1 mg, iodine 0.15 mg, manganese 1 mg, zinc 1.5 mg/Tab. Bot. 1000s. *otc.*
Use: Mineral, vitamin supplement.

Wet-N-Soak. (Allergan) Borate buffered. WSCP 0.006%, hydroxyethylcellulose. Soln. Bot. 15 ml. *otc.*
Use: Contact lens care.

Wet-N-Soak Plus. (Allergan). Polyvinyl alcohol, edetate disodium, benzalkonium Cl 0.003%. Soln. Bot. 120 ml, 180 ml. *otc.*
Use: Contact lens care.

Wetting Solution. (PBH Wesley Jessen) Polyvinyl alcohol, benzalkonium Cl 0.004%, EDTA 0.02%. Soln. Bot. 60 ml. *otc.*
Use: Contact lens care.

Wetting and Soaking. (PBH Wesley Jessen) Buffered, isotonic. Chlorhexidine gluconate 0.005%, EDTA 0.02%, NaCl, octylphenoxy (oxyethylene) ethanol, povidone, polyvinyl alcohol, propylene glycol, hydroxyethylcellulose. Soln. Bot. 120 ml. *otc.*
Use: Contact lens care.

Wetting and Soaking Solution. (Bausch & Lomb) Chlorhexidine gluconate 0.006%, EDTA 0.05%, cationic cellulose derivative polymer. Bot. 118 ml. *otc.*
Use: Contact lens care.

wheat germ oil. (Viobin) **Liq.:** Bot. 4 oz, 8 oz, pt, qt. **Cap.: 3 min.** Bot. 100s, 400s; **6 min.** Bot. 100s, 225s, 400s; **20 min.** Bot. 100s. *otc.*
Use: Vitamin supplement.

wheat germ oil. (Various Mfr.).
See: Natural Wheat Germ Oil, Cap., Oint. (Spirt).
Natural Viobin Wheat Germ Oil, Liq. (Spirt).
Tocopherol Preps. (Various Mfr.).
Use: Vitamin supplement.

Wheat Germ Oil Concentrate. (Thurston) Perles. 6 min. Bot. 100s. *otc.*
Use: Cardiovascular agent.

whey protein concentrate (bovine).
See: bovine whey protein concentrate.

WHF Lubricating Gel. (Lake) Chlorehexidine gluconate, methylparaben, glycerin/Gel. Tube 113.4 g. Ind. packets 3 g. *otc.*
Use: Vaginal dryness relief.

Whirl-Sol. (Sween) Moisturizing bath additive. Bot. 2 oz, 8 oz, 16 oz, 21 oz, gal, 5 gal, 30 gal, 55 gal. *otc.*
Use: Emollient.

white-faced hornet venom. *Rx.*
Use: Immunization.
See: Albay (Bayer Corp).
Pharmalgen (ALK Laboratories).
Venomil (Bayer Corp).

•**white lotion,** U.S.P. 23. Lotio Alba.
Use: Astringent.
See: Lotioblanc, Lot. (Arnar-Stone).

white precipitate.
See: Ammoniated Mercury, U.S.P. 23.

Whitfield's Ointment. (Various Mfr.) Benzoic acid 6%, salicylic acid 3%. *otc.*
Use: Antiinfective, topical.

whooping cough vaccine.
See: Acel-Imune, Vial (Wyeth Ayerst).
ActHIB/DTP, Set of DTwP vial plus Hib Pow. for Inj. (Connaught).
diphtheria and tetanus toxoids with

pertussis vaccine (Various Mfr.).
Infanrix (SKB).
Pertussis Vaccine, U.S.P. 23.
Tetramune, Vial (Wyeth Ayerst).
Tri-Immunol, Vial (Wyeth Ayerst).
Tripedia, Vial (Connaught).

Whorton's Calamine Lotion. (Whorton) Calamine, zinc oxide, glycerin (U.S.P. strength) in carboxymethylcellulose lotion vehicle. Bot. 4 oz, gal. *otc.*
Use: Dermatologic, counterirritant.

Wibi Lotion. (Galderma) Purified water, SD alcohol 40, glycerin, PEG-4, PEG-6-32 stearate, PEG-6-32, glycol stearate, carbomer 940, PEG-75, methylparaben, propylparaben, triethanolamine, menthol, fragrance. Bot. 8 oz, 16 oz. *otc.*
Use: Emollient.

widow spider species antivenin (latrodectus mactans). (Merck) Antivenin, Lactrodectus mactans, U.S.P. 23.
Use: Immunization.

Wigraine. (Organon Teknika) Ergotamine tartrate 1 mg, caffeine 100 mg/Tab. **Tab.:** Box 20s, 100s. *Rx.*
Use: Antimigraine.

wild cherry.
Use: Flavored vehicle.

Wilpowr. (Foy) Phentermine HCl 30 mg/Cap. Bot. 100s, 500s, 1000s.
Use: Anorexiant.

Wilpor-Clear. (Foy) Phentermine HCl 30 mg/Cap. Bot. 1000s. *c-IV.*
Use: Anorexiant.

WinRho SD. (Univax) RHo(D) immune globulin IV human. 600 IU or 1500 IU. Vial 2.5 ml (10s). *Rx.*
Use: Prevention of Rh isoimmunization; immune thrombocytopenic purpura.

Winstrol. (Sanofi Winthrop) Stanozolol 2 mg/Tab. Bot. 100s. *c-III.*
Use: Anabolic steroid.

Wintergreen Sucrets. (SmithKline Beecham Pharmaceuticals) Dyclonine HCl 0.1%, alcohol 10%, sorbitol. Spray. Bot. 90 ml. *otc.*
Use: Mouth and throat preparation.

•**witch hazel,** U.S.P. 23.
Use: Astringent.

witch hazel. (Various Mfr.) Hamamelis water (Witch Hazel). Bot. 120 ml, 240 ml, 280 ml, 480 ml, 960 ml, gal.
Use: Astringent.

Within. (Bayer Corp) Vitamins A 5000 IU, E 30 IU, C 60 mg, folic acid 0.4 mg, B_1 1.5 mg, B_2 1.7 mg, niacin 20 mg, B_6 2 mg, B_{12} 6 mcg, pantothenic acid 10 mg, D 400 IU, iron 27 mg, calcium 450 mg, zinc 15 mg/Tab. Bot. 60s, 100s. *otc.*
Use: Mineral, vitamin supplement.

WNS Suppositories. (Sanofi Winthrop) Sulfamylon HCl. *Rx.*
Use: Anorectal preparation.

Wonderful Dream. (Kondon) Phenylmercuric nitrate 1:5000, oils of tar, turpentine, olive and linseed, rosin, burgundy pitch, camphor, beeswax, mutton tallow. Salve. 34g. *otc.*
Use: Topical.

Wonder Ice. (Pedinol) Menthol in a specially formulated base. Gel. Tube 113 g. *otc.*
Use: Liniment.

Wondra. (Procter & Gamble) Petrolatum, lanolin acid, glycerin, stearyl alcohol, cyclomethicone, EDTA, hydrogenated vegetable glycerides phosphate, cetyl alcohol, isopropyl palmitate, stearic acid, PEG-100 stearate, carbomer-934, dimethicone, titanium dioxide, imidazolidinyl urea, parabens. Lot. Bot. 180 ml, 300 ml, 450 ml. *otc.*
Use: Emollient.

wood charcoal tablets. (Cowley) 5 gr or 10 gr/Tab. Bot. 1000s. *otc.*

wood creosote.
See: Creosote (Various Mfr.).

wool fat. Lanolin, Anhydrous.

Wyamine Sulfate Injection. (Wyeth Ayerst) Mephentermine sulfate 15 mg or 30 mg, methylparaben 1.8 mg, propylparaben 0.2 mg/ml. Vial 10 ml. Amp. 2 ml. *Rx.*
Use: Vasopressor.

Wyanoids Relief Factor. (Wyeth Ayerst) Cocoa butter 79%, shark liver oil 3%, corn oil, EDTA, parabens, tocopherol. Supp. 12s. *otc.*
Use: Anorectal preparation.

Wycillin. (Wyeth-Ayerst) Penicillin G procaine, aqueous (APPG) 600,000 u/dose. Inj. In 2 ml Tubex; 1,200,000 u/dose. Inj. In 2 ml Tubex; 2,400,000 u/dose. Inj. In 4 ml disp. syringe. With parabens, lecithin, povidone. *Rx.*
Use: Anti-infective.

Wydase Lyophilized. (Wyeth Ayerst) Purified bovine testicular hyaluronidase. Vial 150 units/ml or 1500 units/10 ml with lactose and thimerosal. *Rx.*
Use: Absorption facilitator; hypodermoclysis, urography.

Wydase Stabilized Solution. (Wyeth Ayerst) Purified bovine testicular hyaluronidase 150 units/ml in sterile saline

soln. with sodium Cl, EDTA, thimerosal. Vial 1 ml, 10 ml. *Rx.*
Use: Absorption facilitator; hypodermoclysis; urography.

Wygesic. (Wyeth Ayerst) Propoxyphene HCl 65 mg, acetaminophen 650 mg/ Tab. Bot. 100s, 500s, Redipak 100s. *C-IV.*
Use: Analgesic combination, narcotic.

Wymox. (Wyeth Ayerst) Amoxicillin as trihydrate. **Cap.:** 250 mg Bot. 100s, 500s; 500 mg Bot. 50s, 500s. **Oral Susp.:** 125 mg/5 ml Bot. to make 100 ml; 250 mg/5 ml Bot. to make 100 ml, 150 ml. *Rx.*
Use: Anti-infective, penicillin.

Wytensin. (Wyeth Ayerst) Guanabenz acetate. **4 mg/Tab.:** Bot. 100s, 500s, Redipak 100s. **8 mg/Tab.:** Bot. 100s. **16 mg/Tab.:** Bot. 100s. *Rx.*
Use: Antihypertensive.

X

Xalatan. (Pharmacia & Upjohn) Latanoprost 0.005% (50 mcg/ml), benzalkonium Cl 0.02%. Sol. In 2.5 ml fill dropper bottles.
Use: Agent for glaucoma.

•**xamoterol.** (ZAM-oh-ter-ole) USAN.
Use: Cardiovascular agent.

•**xamoterol fumarate.** (ZAM-oh-ter-ole) USAN.
Use: Cardiovascular agent.

Xanax. (Pharmacia & Upjohn) Alprazolam 0.25 mg, 0.5 mg, 1 mg or 2 mg. Tab. **0.25 mg, 0.5 mg, 2 mg:** 100s, 500s, UD 100s. Visipack 4 × 25s. **1 mg:** 30s, 90s, 100s, 500s, UD 100s. *c-iv.*
Use: Anxiolytic.

•**xanomeline.** (zah-NO-meh-leen) USAN.
Use: Cholinergic agonist (for Alzheimer's disease).

•**xanomeline tartrate.** (zah-NO-meh-leen) USAN.
Use: Cholinergic agonist (for Alzheimer's disease).

•**xanoxate sodium.** (ZAN-ox-ate) USAN.
Use: Bronchodilator.

•**xanthan gum,** N.F. 18.
Use: Pharmaceutic aid, suspending agent.

xanthine derivatives.
See: Caffeine.
Theobromine.
Theophylline.

•**xanthinol niacinate.** (ZAN-thih-nahl NYE-ah-SIN-ate) USAN.
Use: Vasodilator (peripheral).
See: Complamin (3M Pharm).

xanthiol hydrochloride.
Use: Antinauseant.
See: Daxid (Roerig).

xanthotoxin. Methoxsalen.

Xeloda. (Roche) Capecitabine 150 mg, 500 mg, lactose/Tab. Bot. 120s. *Rx.*
Use: Treatment of metastatic breast cancer.

•**xemilofiban hydrochloride.** (zem-ih-LOW-fih-ban) USAN.
Use: Treatment of unstable angina, prevention of post-recanalization reocclusion of coronary vessels.

•**xenalipin.** (ZEN-ah-LIH-pin) USAN.
Use: Hypolipidemic.

•**xenbucin.** (ZEN-BYOO-sin) USAN.
Use: Antihyperlipidemic.

•**xenon Xe 127,** (ZEE-nahn) U.S.P. 23.
Use: Diagnostic aid; medicinal gas; radiopharmaceutical.

•**xenon Xe 133,** U.S.P. 23.
Use: Radiopharmaceutical.

xenthiorate hydrochloride.

Xerac AC. (Person & Covey) Aluminum Cl hexahydrate 6.25% in anhydrous ethanol 96%. Bot 35 ml, 60 ml. *Rx.*
Use: Dermatologic, acne.

Xeroform Ointment 3%. (City, Consolidated) Pow. 0.25 lb, 1 lb. Jar 1 lb, 5 lb.

Xero-Lube. (Scherer) Monobasic potassium phosphate, dibasic potassium phosphate, magnesium Cl, potassium Cl, calcium Cl, sodium Cl, sodium fluoride, sorbitol soln., sodium carboxymethylcellulose, methylparaben. Bot. 6 oz. *otc.*
Use: Mouth and throat preparation.

•**xilobam.** (ZIE-low-bam) USAN.
Use: Muscle relaxant.

•**xipamide.** (ZIP-ah-mide) USAN.
Use: Antihypertensive, diuretic.

•**xorphanol mesylate.** (ZAHR-fan-ahl) USAN.
Use: Analgesic.

X-Prep Bowel Evacuant Kit-1. (Purdue Frederick) Kit contains Senokot S tab., X-Prep liquid, Rectolax supp. *otc.*
Use: Laxative.

X-Prep Bowel Evacuant Kit-2. (Purdue Frederick) Kit contains citralax granules, X-Prep liquid, Rectolax supp. *otc.*
Use: Laxative.

X-Prep Liquid. (Gray) Senna extract with alcohol 7%, sucrose 50 g. Bot. 2.5 oz. *otc.*
Use: Laxative.

X-Ray Contrast Media.
See: Iodine Products, Diagnostic.

X-Seb Plus. (Baker Norton) Pyrithionic zinc 1%, salicylic acid 2%. Shampoo. Bot. 120 ml. *otc.*
Use: Antiseborrheic.

X-Seb Shampoo. (Baker/Cummins) Salicylic acid 4%, coal tar soln. 10% in a blend of surface-active agents. Bot. 4 oz. *otc.*
Use: Antiseborrheic.

X-Seb T. (Baker/Cummins) Coal tar soln. 10%, salicylic acid 4%. Bot. 4 oz. *otc.*
Use: Antiseborrheic.

X-Sep T Plus. (Baker Norton) Coal tar solution 10%, salicylic acid, menthol 1%. Shampoo. Bot. 120 ml. *otc.*
Use: Antiseborrheic.

Xtracare. (Sween) Bot. 2 oz, 4 oz, 8 oz, 21 oz, gal. *otc.*
Use: Emollient.

Xtra-Vites. (Barth's) Vitamins A 10,000 IU, D 400 IU, C 150 mg, B_1 5 mg, B_2

1 mg, niacin 3.33 mg, pantothenic acid 183 mcg, B_6 250 mcg, B_{12} 215 mcg, E 15 IU, rutin 20 mg, citrus bioflavonoid complex 15 mg, choline 6.67 mg, inositol 10 mg, folic acid 50 mcg, biotin, aminobenzoic acid/Tab. Bot. 30s, 90s, 180s, 360s. *otc.*
Use: Vitamin supplement.

X-Trozine Capsules. (Rexar) Phendimetrazine tartrate 35 mg/Cap. Bot. 1000s. *c-III.*
Use: Anorexiant.

X-Trozine S.R. Capsules. (Rexar) Phendimetrazine tartrate 105 mg/SR Cap. Bot. 100s, 200s, 1000s. *c-III.*
Use: Anorexiant.

X-Trozine Tablets. (Rexar) Phendimetrazine tartrate 35 mg/Tab. Bot. 1000s. *c-III.*
Use: Anorexiant.

•**xylamidine tosylate.** (zie-LAM-ih-deen TAH-sill-ate) USAN.
Use: Serotonin inhibitor.

•**xylazine hydrochloride.** (ZIE-lih-zeen HIGH-droe-KLOR-ide) USAN.
Use: Analgesic.

•**xylitol,** (ZIE-lih-tahl) N.F. 18.
Use: Pharmaceutic aid.

Xylocaine Hydrochloride. (Astra) Lidocaine HCl. **Amp.:** (1%): 2 ml, 5 ml, 30 ml; w/epinephrine 1:200,000 30 ml. (1.5%): 20 ml; w/epinephrine 1:200,000 30 ml. (2%): 2 ml, 10 ml; w/epinephrine 1:200,000 20 ml. (4%): 5 ml. **Multidose Vial:** (0.5%): 50 ml; w/epinephrine 1:200,000 50 ml. (1%): 20 ml, 50 ml; w/epinephrine 1:100,000 20 ml, 50 ml. (2%): 20 ml, 50 ml; w/epinephrine 1:100,000 20 ml, 50 ml. **Single-dose Vial:** (1%): 30 ml. (1.5%) 20 ml; w/ epinephrine 1:200,000 10 ml, 30 ml. (2%) w/epinephrine 1:200,000 20 ml. *Rx.*
Use: Anesthetic, local.

Xylocaine Hydrochloride for Cardiac Arrhythmia. (Astra) **Intravenous:** Lidocaine 2%. Amp 5 ml, disp. syringe 5 ml. Continuous infusion 1 g/25 ml Vial; 2 g/50 ml Vial. Prefilled syringe 100 mg/5 ml, 12s. Continuous infusion prefilled syringe 1 g, 2 g. **Intramuscular:** Amp. 10%, 5 ml. *Rx.*
Use: Anesthetic, local.

Xylocaine Hydrochloride 4% Solution. (Astra) Topical use. Bot. 50 ml. *Rx.*
Use: Anesthetic, local.

Xylocaine Hydrochloride for Spinal Anesthesia. (Astra) Lidocaine HCl 1.5% or 5%, glucose 7.5%, sodium hydroxide to adjust pH. Specific gravity 1.028-1.034. Amp. 2 ml. Box 10s. *Rx.*
Use: Anesthetic, local.

Xylocaine Hydrochloride w/Dextrose. (Astra) Lidocaine HCl 1.5%, dextrose 7.5%. Inj. Amps. 2 ml. *Rx.*
Use: Anesthetic, local.

Xylocaine Hydrochloride w/Epinephrine. (Astra) Lidocaine HCl 2% w/epinephrine 1:200,000. Amps w/sodium metabisulfite 20 ml. Inj. Single dose vials w/sodium metabisulfite. 20 ml. *Rx.*
Use: Anesthetic, local.

Xylocaine Hydrochloride w/Glucose. (Astra) Lidocaine HCl 5%, glucose 7.5%. Inj. Amp. 2 ml. *Rx.*
Use: Anesthetic, local.

Xylocaine Jelly. (Astra) Lidocaine HCl 2% in sodium carboxymethylcellulose with parabens. Tube 5 ml and 30 ml. *Rx.*
Use: Anesthetic, local.

Xylocaine Ointment. (Astra) Lidocaine 2.5%, water soluble carbowaxes. 35 g *otc.*
Use: Anesthetic, local.

Xylocaine MPF Injection. (Astra) Lidocaine HCl. **0.5%** 50 ml. **1%** 2, 5, or 30 ml. **1.5%** 10 or 20 ml. **2%** 2, 5 or 10 ml. **4%** 5 ml. **1%** w/ epinephrine 1:200,000, sodium bisulfite. 5, 10 or 30 ml. **2%**w/ epinephrine, sodium bisulfite. 5, 10 or 20 ml. **5%**w/ glucose 7.5%. 2 ml. *Rx.*
Use: Anesthetic, local.

Xylocaine Viscous. (Astra) Lidocaine HCl 2%, sodium carboxymethylcellulose, parabens. Bot. 20 ml (25s), 100 ml, 450 ml and UD 20 ml. *Rx.*
Use: Anesthetic, local.

•**xylofilcon a.** (ZILE-oh-FILL-kahn A) USAN.
Use: Contact lens material (hydrophilic).

•**xylometazoline hydrochloride,** (zie-low-met-AZZ-oh-leen) U.S.P. 23.
Use: Adrenergic (vasoconstrictor).
See: Isohalent L.A., Liq. (Zeneca).
Long Acting Neo-Synephrine, Prods. (Winthrop Consumer Products).
Otrivin Spray (Novartis).
Rhinall L.A., Liq. (First Texas).
Sine-Off, Spray (Menley & James).
Vicks Sinex Long Acting, Nasal Spray (Procter & Gamble).

Xylo-Pfan. (Pharmacia & Upjohn) Xylose 25 g/Bot.
Use: Diagnostic aid.

Xylophan D-Xylose Tolerance Test. (Pfanstiehl) D-xylose 25 g/UD bot.
Use: Diagnostic aid.

•**xylose,** (ZIE-lohs) U.S.P. 23.
Use: Diagnostic aid. determination).

Y

Yager's Liniment. (Yager) Oil of turpentine and camphor w/clove oil fragrance, emulsifier, emollient, ammonium oleate (less than 0.5% free ammonia) penetrant base. *otc.*
Use: Rubefacient.

yatren.
See: Chiniofon, Tab.

YDP Lice Spray. (Youngs Drug) Synthetic pyrethroid in aerosol. Can 5 oz. *otc.*
Use: Pediculicide, inanimate objects.

yeast adenylic acid. An isomer of adenosine 5-monophosphate, has been found inactive.
See: Adenosine 5-Monophosphate, Preps. for active compounds.

yeast, dried.
Use: Protein and vitamin B Complex source.

yeast tablets, dried.
Use: Supplementary source of B complex vitamins.
See: Brewer's Yeast, Tab.

Yeast-Gard. (Lake Consumer Products) Pulsatilla 28x, *Candida albicans:* 28x. Supp. 10s w/applicator. *otc.*
Use: Vaginal agent.

Yeast-Gard Medicated Disposable Douche. (Lake Consumer Products) Povidone-iodine 0.3% when reconstituted. Soln. 180 ml twin-pack w/two 5.4 ml medicated douche concentrate packets. *otc.*
Use: Douche.

Yeast-Gard Medicated Disposable Douche Premix. (Lake Consumer Products) Octoxynol-9, lactic acid, sodium lactate, sodium benzoate, aloe vera. Soln. 180 ml twin-pack. *otc.*
Use: Douche.

Yeast-Gard Medicated Douche. (Lake Consumer Products) Povidone-iodine 10%. Soln. Concentrate. 240 ml. *otc.*
Use: Douche.

yeast, torula.
See: Torula Yeast.

yeast w/iron.
See: Natural Super Iron Yeast Powder (Spirt) Bot. 200s.

Yeast-X. (C.B. Fleet) **Supp.:** Pulsatilla 28x. Pkg. 12s w/applicator. *otc.*
Use: Vaginal agent.

Yelets. (Freeda Vitamins) Iron 20 mg, vitamins A 10,000 IU, D 400 IU, E 10 IU, B_1 10 mg, B_2 10 mg, B_3 25 mg, B_5 10 mg, B_6 10 mg, B_{12} 10 mcg, C 100 mg, folic acid 0.1 mg, PABA, lysine, glutamic acid, Ca, I, Mg, Mn, Se, Zn 4 mg/Tab. Bot. 100s, 250s. *otc.*
Use: Mineral, vitamin supplement.

yellow enzyme.
See: Riboflavin (Various Mfr.).

•**yellow fever vaccine.** U.S.P. 23.
Use: Immunization.
See: YF-Vax, Inj. (Pasteur Merieux Connaught).

yellow hornet venom.
See: Albay (Bayer Corp).
Pharmalgen (ALK Labs).
Venomil (Bayer Corp).
Use: Desensitizing agent.

yellow jacket venom.
See: Albay (Bayer Corp).
Pharmalgen (ALK Labs).
Venomil (Bayer Corp).
Use: Desensitizing agent.

yellow mercuric oxide 1%. (Various Mfr.) Oint. Tube 3.5, 3.75, 30 g. *otc.*
Use: Antiseptic.

yellow mercuric oxide 2%. (Various Mfr.) Oint. Tube 3.5, 3.75, 30 g. *otc.*
Use: Antiseptic.
See: Stye, Oint. (Del Pharmaceuticals).

yellow ointment.
Use: Pharmaceutic aid (ointment base).

yellow wax.
Use: Pharmaceutic aid (stiffening agent).

YF-Vax. (Pasteur Merieux Connaught) Yellow fever vaccine. Inj. Vial 1 dose, 5 dose, 20 dose with diluent. *Rx.*
Use: Immunization.

Yocon. (Palisades Pharm) Yohimbine HCl 5.4 mg/Tab. Bot. 100s, 1000s. *Rx.*
Use: Antiimpotence agent.

Yodora Deodorant Cream. (SmithKline Beecham Pharmaceuticals) Jar 2 oz. *otc.*
Use: Deodorant.

Yodoxin. (Glenwood) Iodoquinol 210 mg or 650 mg/Tab. Bot. 100s, 1000s. Pow. Bot. 25 g. *Rx.*
Use: Amebicide.

yohimbine hydrochloride. Indolalkylamine alkaloid. (Various Mfr.) 5.4 mg/Tab. Bot. 100s, 500s. *Rx.*
Note: Yohimbine has no FDA sanctioned indications.

W/Methyltestosterone, nux vomica extract.
See: Climactic, Tab. (Burgin-Arden)

Yohimex. (Kramer) Yohimbine HCl 5.4 mg/Tab. Bot. 100s. *Rx.*
Use: Antiimpotence agent.

Your Choice Non-Preserved Saline Solution. (Amcon Laboratories) Buffered, isotonic soln. w/ NaCl, boric acid, sodium borate. Bot. 360 ml. *otc.*
Use: Contact lens care.

Your Choice Sterile Preserved Saline Solution. (Amcon Laboratories) Isotonic. Sorbic acid 0.1%, EDTA, NaCl, boric buffer. Bot. 60 ml or 360 ml. *otc.*
Use: Contact lens care.

ytterbium Yb 169 pentetate injection. U.S.P. XXII.
Use: Radiopharmaceutical.

Yutopar. (Astra) Ritodrine HCl 10 mg/ml, Amp. 5 ml; 15 mg/ml, vial 10 ml, inj. syringe 10 ml. *Rx.*
Use: Uterine relaxant.

Z

•**zacopride hydrochloride.** (ZAK-oh-pride) USAN.
Use: Antiemetic, stimulant (peristaltic).

•**zafirlukast.** (zah-FEER-loo-kast) USAN.
Use: Antiasthmatic (leukotriene antagonist).
See: Accolate, Tab. (Zeneca).

Zagam. (Rhone-Poulenc Rorer) Sparfloxacin 200 mg/Tab. Bot. *Rx.*
Use: Fluoroquinolone.

•**zalcitabine.** (zal-SITE-ah-BEAN) USAN.
Use: Antiviral.

zalcitabine. (National Cancer Inst.)
Use: AIDS. [Orphan drug]
See: Hivid (Hoffman-La Roche)

•**zaleplon.** (ZAL-eh-plahn) USAN.
Use: Hypnotic, sedative.

•**zalospirone hydrochloride.** (zal-OH-spy-rone) USAN.
Use: Anxiolytic.

•**zaltidine hydrochloride.** (ZAHL-tih-deen) USAN.
Use: Antiulcerative.

Zanaflex. (Athena Neurosciences) Tizanidine HCl 4 mg, lactose/Tab. Bot. 150s *Rx.*
Use: Skeletal muscle relaxant.

•**zanamivir, .** (zan-AM-ih-veer) USAN.
Use: Antiviral; influenza virus neuraminidase inhibitor.

zankiren hydrochloride. (zan-KIE-ren) USAN.
Use: Antihypertensive.

Zanosar. (Pharmacia & Upjohn) Streptozocin 1 g. (100 mg/ml) Pow. For Inj. Vial. *Rx.*
Use: Antineoplastic.

•**zanoterone.** (zan-OH-ter-ohn) USAN.
Use: Antiandrogen.

Zantac EFFERdose Effervescent Granules and Tablets. (GlaxoWellcome) Ranitidine HCl 150 mg. **Granules:** 1.44 g packets (30s, 60s); **Tab:** Bot. 30s, 60s. *Rx.*
Use: Antiulcerative.

Zantac GELdose. (GlaxoWellcome) Ranitidine HCl 150 mg or 300 mg/Cap. **150 mg:** Bot. 60s, UD 60s; **300 mg:** Bot. 30s, UD 30s. *Rx.*
Use: Antiulcerative.

Zantac Injection. (GlaxoWellcome) Ranitidine 25 mg HCl/ml. Vial 2 ml, 10 ml, 40 ml, syringe 2 ml. *Rx.*
Use: Antiulcerative.

Zantac Injection Premixed. (GlaxoWellcome) Ranitidine 0.5 mg as HCl/ml. 100 ml single-dose plastic container. *Rx.*
Use: Antiulcerative.

Zantac 75. (GlaxoWellcome) Ranitidine 75 mg/Tab. In 4s, 10s, 20s. *otc.*
Use: Antiulcerative.

Zantac Syrup. (GlaxoWellcome) Ranitidine 15 mg as HCl/ml, alcohol 7.5%. Bot. 480 ml. *Rx.*
Use: Antiulcerative.

Zantac Tablets. (GlaxoWellcome) Ranitidine 150 mg or 300 mg as HCl/Tab. **150 mg:** Bot. 60s, 500s, UD 100s. **300 mg:** Bot. 30s, 250s, UD 100s. *Rx.*
Use: Antiulcerative.

Zantine. (Lexis) Dipyridamole 25 mg, 50 mg or 75 mg/Tab. Bot. 1000s. *Rx.*
Use: Coronary vasodilator.

Zantryl. (ION Laboratories) Phentermine HCl 30 mg/Cap. Bot. 100s. *c-iv.*
Use: Anorexiant.

Zarontin. (Parke-Davis) Ethosuximide. **Cap.:** 250 mg. Bot. 100s. **Syr.:** 250 mg/5 ml. Bot. pt. *Rx.*
Use: Anticonvulsant.

Zaroxolyn. (Medeva) Metolazone 2.5 mg, 5 mg or 10 mg/Tab. Bot. 100s, 500s, 1000s, UD 100s. *Rx.*
Use: Diuretic.

•**zatosetron maleate.** (ZAt-oh-SEH-trahn) USAN.
Use: Antimigraine.

Z-Bec. (Robins) Vitamins E 45 mg, C 600 mg, B_1 15 mg, B_2 10.2 mg, B_3 100 mg, B_6 10 mg, B_{12} 6 mcg, pantothenic acid 25 mg, zinc 22.5 mg/Tab. Bot. 60s, 100s, 500s. *otc.*
Use: Mineral, vitamin supplement.

ZBT Baby. (Glenwood) Talc, mineral oil, magnesium stearate, propylene glycol, BHT. Pow. 120 g. *otc.*
Use: Diaper rash preparation.

Zeasorb-AF. (Stiefel) Miconazole nitrate 2%. Pow. Can 2.5 oz. *otc.*
Use: Antifungal, topical.

Zeasorb Powder. (Stiefel) Talc, microporous cellulose, supersorb carbohydrate acrylic copolymer. Sifter-top Can 2.5 oz, 8 oz. *otc.*
Use: Dermatologic.

Zebeta. (ESI Lederle Generics) Bisoprolol fumarate. **5 mg:** Tab/Bot. 14s, 30s, 100s, 500s, 1000s, UD 10s, **10 mg:** Tab/Bot. 14s, 30s, 100s, 500s, 1000s, UD 10s. *Rx.*
Use: Beta-adrenergic blocker.

Ze Caps. (Everett Laboratories) Vitamin E 200 mg, zinc 9.6 mg as gluconate/Cap. Bot. 60s. *otc.*
Use: Mineral, vitamin supplement.

Zecnil. (UCB Pharm)

Zefazone. (Pharmacia & Upjohn) Cefmetazole sodium. **Pow. for Inj.:** 1 g or 2 g (2 mEq sodium/g). Vial. **Inj.:** 1 g/50 ml or 2 g/50 ml (2.7 mEq sodium/g) in frozen iso-osmotic, premixed soluition in single dose plastic container. *Rx.*
Use: Anti-infective.

•**zein.** (ZEE-in) N.F. 18.
Use: Pharmaceutic aid (coating agent).

Zemalo. (Alphalma USPD) Sulfur, zinc oxide, camphor, titanium oxide. Bot. 4 oz, pt, gal. *otc.*
Use: Dermatologic, counterirritant.

Zemplar. (Abbott) Paricaltol 5 mcg/ml Inj. Single-dose fliptop vials, 1 ml, 2 ml. *Rx.*
Use: Vitamin.

Zenapax. (Roche) Daclizumab 25 mg/5 ml, Preservative free. Inj. Vial. *Rx.*
Use: Prevent organ rejection.

Zenate. (Solvay)
Use: Mineral, vitamin supplement.
See: Advanced Formula Zenate, Tab. (Solvay)

•**zenazocine mesylate.** (zen-AZE-oh-seen MEH-sih-late) USAN.
Use: Analgesic.

Zendium. (Oral-B Laboratories) Sodium fluoride 0.22%. Tube 0.9 oz, 2.3 oz.
Use: Dental caries agent.

•**zeniplatin.** (zen-ih-PLAT-in) USAN.
Use: Antineoplastic.

Zentel. (SmithKline Beecham Pharmaceuticals) Albendazole.
Use: Anthelmintic.

Zephiran. (Sanofi Winthrop) **Aqueous soln.:** Benzalkonium Cl 1:750. Bot. 240 ml, gal. **Disinfectant concentrate:** 17% in 120 ml, gal. **Tincture:** 1:750 in gal. **Tincture spray:** 1:750 in 30 g, 180 g, gal. *otc.*
Use: Antiseptic, antimicrobial.

Zephiran Towelettes. (Sanofi Winthrop) Moist paper towels with soln. of zephiran Cl 1:750. Box 20s, 100s, 1000s. *otc.*
Use: Antiseptic, antimicrobial.

Zephrex Tablets. (Sanofi Winthrop) Pseudoephedrine HCl 60 mg, guaifenesin 400 mg/SR Tab. Bot. 100s. *Rx.*
Use: Decongestant, expectorant.

Zephrex-LA Tablets. (Sanofi Winthrop) Pseudoephedrine HCl 120 mg, guaifenesin 600 mg/Tab. Bot. 100s. *Rx.*
Use: Decongestant, expectorant.

Zepine. (Foy) Reserpine alkaloid 0.25 mg/Tab. Bot. 100s, 500s, 1000s. *Rx.*
Use: Antihypertensive.

•**zeranol.** (ZER-ah-nole) USAN.
Use: Anabolic.

Zerit. (Bristol-Myers Squibb) Stavudine 15 mg, 20 mg, 30 mg, 40 mg/Cap. Bot. 60s. Stavudine 1 mg/ml after reconstitution w/ 202 ml purified water, sucrose, parabens, dye free, fruit flavor. Pow. for Oral Sol. Bot. 200 ml. *Rx.*
Use: Antiviral.

Zestoretic. (Zeneca) Lisinopril 10 mg, hydrochlorothiazide 12.5 mg or lisinopril 20 mg, hydrochlorothiazide 12.5 mg or lisinopril 20 mg, hydrochlorothiazide 25 mg/Tab. Bot. 100s. *Rx.*
Use: Antihypertensive.

Zestril. (Zeneca) Lisinopril 5 mg, 10 mg, 20 mg, or 40 mg/Tab. Bot. 100s, UD 100s. *Rx.*
Use: Antihypertensive.

Zetar Emulsion. (Dermik Laboratories) Colloidal whole coal tar 30% (300 mg/ml) in polysorbates. Bot. 6 oz. *otc.*
Use: Antiseborrheic.

Zetar Shampoo. (Dermik Laboratories) Colloidal whole coal tar 1% in a shampoo. Bot. 6 oz. *otc.*
Use: Antiseborrheic.

Z-gen. (Zenith Goldline) Vitamins E 45 mg, B_1 15 mg, B_2 10.2 mg, B_3 100 mg, B_5 25 mg, B_6 10 mg, B_{12} 6 mcg, C 600 mg, zinc 22.5 mg/Tab. Bot. 60s, 100s. *otc.*
Use: Mineral, vitamin supplement.

Ziac. (ESI Lederle Generics) Bisoprolol fumarate 2.5 mg, 5 mg or 10 mg; hydrochlorothiazide 6.25 mg. Tab. **2.5 mg or 5 mg:** Bot. 30s, 100s. **10 mg:** Bot. 30s. *Rx.*
Use: Antihypertensive.

•**zidometacin.** (ZIE-doe-MEH-tah-sin) USAN.
Use: Anti-inflammatory.

•**zidovudine.** (zie-DOE-view-DEEN) USAN. *Formerly azidothymidine, AZT.*
Use: Antiviral.
See: Retrovir, Cap. (GlaxoWellcome).

zidovudine.
Use: AIDS. [Orphan drug]
See: Retrovir (GlaxoWellcome).

zidovudine.
Use: HIV infection.
W/ lamivdine
See: Combivir, Tab. (GlaxoWellcome).

•**zifrosilone.** (zih-FROE-sih-lone) USAN.
Use: Acetylcholinesterase inhibitor.

Ziks. (Nnodum) Methyl salicylate 12%, menthol 1%, capsaicin 0.025%, cetyl alcohol. Cream. 60 g. *otc.*
Use: Analgesic.

Zilactin-B Medicated. (Zila) Benzocaine

10%, alcohol 76%. Gel. Tube 7.5 g. *otc.*
Use: Anesthetic, local.

Zilactin-L. (Zila) Lidocaine 2.5%, alcohol 79.3%. Liq. Bot. 7.5 ml. *otc.*
Use: Anesthetic, local.

Zilactin Medicated Gel. (Zila) Tannic acid 7%, suspended in alcohol 80.8%. Tube 0.25 oz. *otc.*
Use: Cold sores.

ZilaDent. (Zila) Benzocaine 6%, alcohol 74.9%. Gel. Tube. 7.5 g and single packs. *otc.*
Use: Anesthetic, local.

•**zilantel.** (ZILL-an-tell) USAN.
Use: Anthelmintic.

•**zileuton.** (ZIE-loo-tone) USAN.
Use: Inhibitor (5-lipoxygenase).
See: Zyflo, Tab. (Abbott Laboratories).

zimco. (Sterwin) Vanillin.

•**zimeldine hydrochloride.** (zie-MELL-ih-deen) USAN. *Formerly Zimelidine Hydrochloride.*
Use: Antidepressant.

Zinacef. (GlaxoWellcome) Cefuroxime 750 mg, 1.5 g or 7.5 g as sodium Pow. For Inj. 750 mg, 1.5 g (as sodium)/Inj. **Pow. for Inj.:750 mg, 1.5 g:** Vials and infusion pack. **7.5 g:** Pharmacy bulk Pkg. **Inj.: 750 mg, 1.5 g, premixed:** 50 ml. *Rx.*
Use: Anti-infective, cephalosporin.

Zinc-220. (Alto Pharmaceuticals) Zinc sulfate 220 mg/Cap. Bot. 100s, 1000s, UD 100s. *otc.*
Use: Mineral supplement.

•**zinc acetate.** (zingk) U.S.P. 23. Acetic acid, zinc salt, dihydrate.
Use: Pharmaceutic necessity for Zinc-Eugenol Cement.

zinc acetate. (zingk)
Use: Wilson's disease. [Orphan Drug]
See: Benadryl Itch Relief, Children's, Cream, Spray (GlaxoWellcome).
Benadryl Itch Relief, Maximum Strength, Cream, Stick (GlaxoWellcome).
Benadryl Itch Relief, Spray (GlaxoWellcome).
Benadryl Itch Stopping Gel Maximum Strength, Gel (GlaxoWellcome).
Benadryl Itch Stopping Gel Children's Formula, Gel (GlaxoWellcome).
Galzin (Lemmon).

Zinca-Pak. (SoloPak) Zinc 1 mg or 5 mg/ml. Inj. **1 mg:** Vial 10 ml, 30 ml. **5 mg:** Vial 5 ml. *Rx.*
Use: Nutritional supplement, parenteral.

Zincate. (Paddock) Zinc sulfate 220 mg (elemental zinc 50 mg)/Cap. Bot. 100s, 1000s. *otc.*
Use: Mineral supplement.

zinc bacitracin. Bacitracin Zinc, U.S.P. 23.
Use: Anti-infective.

•**zinc carbonate.** U.S.P. 23.
Use: Antiseptic, topical; astringent.

•**zinc chloride.** U.S.P. 23.
Use: Astringent, dentin desensitizer.
W/Formaldehyde.
See: Forma ZConcentrate (Ingram).

•**zinc chloride Zn 65.** USAN.
Use: Radiopharmaceutical.

zinc citrate. (Zingk)
See: Zinc Lozenges (Goldline).

zinc-eugenol cement. U.S.P. XXI.
Use: Dental protectant.

Zincfrin. (Alcon Laboratories) Zinc sulfate 0.25%, phenylephrine HCl 0.12%. Soln. Droptainer 15 ml, 30 ml. *otc.*
Use: Astringent, decongestant, ophthalmic.

zinc gelatin. U.S.P. XXI. Impregnated gauge, U.S.P. 23.
Use: Topical protectant.

Zinc-Glenwood. (Glenwood) Zinc Sulfate 220 mg/Cap. Bot. 100s. *otc.*
Use: Mineral supplement.

•**zinc gluconate.** U.S.P. 23.
Use: Supplement (trace mineral).
See: Zinc Lozenges (Goldline).

zinchlorundesal. Zincundesal.

zinc insulin.
See: Insulin Zinc, Preps. (Various Mfr.).

Zincon Shampoo. (ESI Lederle Generics) Pyrithione zinc 1%, sodium methyl cocoyltaurate, sodium Cl, magnesium aluminum silicate, sodium cocoyl isethionate, glutaral, water w/pH adjusted. Bot. 4 oz, 8 oz. *otc.*
Use: Antiseborrheic.

Zinc Lozenges. (Zenith Goldline) Zinc citrate 23 mg, zinc gluconate, fructose, sorbitol/Lozenge. Bot. 30s. *otc.*
Use: Mineral supplement.

•**zinc oxide.** U.S.P. 23. Flowers of zinc.
Use: Astringent, topical protectant.
See: Calamine Preps.
W/Combinations.
See: Akne, Drying Lot. (Alto Pharmaceuticals).
Almophen, Oint. (Jones Medical Industries).
Anocaine, Supp. (Roberts Pharm).
Anugesic, Oint., Supp. (Parke-Davis).
Anusol, Oint., Supp. (Parke-Davis).
Anusol-HC, Supp. (Parke-Davis).
Aracain Rectal Oint., Supp. (Del Pharmaceuticals).
Blis-To-Sol, Pow. (Chattem).

Bonate, Supp. (Suppositoria).
Calamatum, Preps. (Blair Laboratories).
Cala-Zinc-Ol, Liq. (Emerson).
Caldesene, Oint. (Novartis Pharmaceuticals).
Caleate HC Cream, Oint. (Zeneca).
Caloxol, Oint. (Jones Medical Industries).
CZO, Lot. (Zeneca).
Dereq Medicone HC, Supp. (Medicone).
Dermatrol, Oint. (Gordon Laboratories).
Desitin, Oint. (Pfizer).
Diaprex, Oint. (Moss, Belle).
Doctient, Supp. (Suppositoria).
Elder Diaper Rash Oint. (Zeneca).
Epinephricaine, Oint. (Pharmacia & Upjohn).
Ergophene, Oint. (Pharmacia & Upjohn).
Hemocaine, Oint. (Roberts Pharm).
Hemorrhoidal Oint. (Towne).
Hydro Surco, Lot. (Alma).
Ladd's Paste (Paddock).
Lasan, Oint. (Stiefel).
Medicated Powder (Johnson & Johnson Consumer Products).
Medicated Foot Powder (Pharmacia & Upjohn).
Mexsana, Pow. (Schering Plough).
Nullo Foot Cream (DePree).
Pazo, Oint., Supp. (Bristol-Myers).
Petrozin Compound Oint. (Jones Medical Industries).
PZM Oint. (Wendt-Bristol).
Rectal Medicone HC, Supp. (Medicone).
RVPaque, Oint. (Zeneca).
Saratoga, Oint. (Blair Laboratories).
Schamberg, Lot. (Paddock).
Sebasorb, Lot. (Summer).
Taloin, Tube (Warren-Teed).
Ting, Cream, Pow. (Novartis Pharmaceuticals).
Unguentine Oint. "Original Formula" (Procter & Gamble).
Versal, Supp. (Suppositoria).
Wyanoids, Preps. (Wyeth Ayerst).
Xylocaine Supp. (Astra).
Zinc Boric Lotion, Liq. (Emerson).

zinc phenolsulfonate.
Use: Astringent.
W/Belladonna leaf extract, kaolin, pectin, sodium carboxymethylcellulose.
See: Gelcomul, Liq. (Del Pharmaceuticals).
W/Bismuth subgallate, kaolin, pectin, opium pow.
See: Diastay,Tab. (Zeneca).
W/Bismuth subsalicylate, salol, methyl salicylate.
See: Pepto-Bismol, Liq. (Procter & Gamble).
W/Kaolin, pectin.
See: Pectocel, Liq. (Eli Lilly).
W/Opium pow., bismuth subgallate, pectin, kaolin.
See: Bismuth, Pectin & Paregoric (Teva USA).

zinc pyrithione.
Use: Bactericide, fungicide, antiseborrheic.
See: Breck One, Shampoo (Breck).
Zincon, Shampoo (ESI Lederle Generics).
ZP-11, Liq. (Revlon).

•**zinc stearate.** U.S.P. 23. Octadecanoic acid, zinc salt.
Use: Dusting powder; pharmaceutic aid (tablet/capsule lubricant).
W/Combinations.
See: Ting, Cream, Pow. (Novartis Pharmaceuticals).

zinc sulfanilate. Zinc sulfanilate tetrahydrate. Nizin, Op-Isophrin-Z, Op-Isophrin-Z-M (Broemmel).
Use: Anti-infective.

•**zinc sulfate.** U.S.P. 23. Sulfuric acid, zinc salt (1:1), heptahydrate.
Use: Astringent, ophthalmic.
See: Eye-Sed, Soln. (Scherer).
Op-Thal-Zin Ophth. (Alcon Laboratories).
Scrip-Zinc, Cap. (Scrip).
Zinc-Glenwood, Cap. (Glenwood).
Zin-Cora, Cap. (Zeneca).
W/Boric acid, phenylephrine HCl.
See: Phenylzin Drops, Ophth. Soln. (Smith & Nephew United, Miller & Patch).
W/Calcium lactate.
See: Zinc-220, Cap. (Alto Pharmaceuticals).
W/Menthol, methyl salicylate, alum, boric acid, oxyquinoline citrate.
See: Maso pH Powder (Mason).
W/Phenylephrine HCl, polyvinyl alcohol.
See: Prefrin-Z, Liquifilm (Allergan).
W/Piperocaine HCl, boric acid, potassium Cl.
See: M-Z Drops (Smith & Nephew United, Miller & Patch).
W/Sodium Cl.
See: Bromidrosis Crystals (Gordon Laboratories).
W/Vitamins.
See: Neovicaps TR, Cap. (Scherer).
Vicon-C, Cap. (GlaxoWellcome).
Vicon Forte, Cap. (GlaxoWellcome).

Vicon Plus, Cap. (GlaxoWellcome).
Vi-Zac, Cap. (GlaxoWellcome).
Z-Bec, Tab. (Robins).

zinc sulfate. (Various Mfr.) Zinc 5 mg/ml (as sulfate 21.95 mg). Inj. Vial 5, 10 ml.
Use: Nutritional supplement, parenteral.

zinc sulfate. (Various Mfr.) Zinc 1 mg/ml (as sulfate 4.39 mg). Inj. Vial 10, 30 ml. *Rx.*
Use: Nutritional supplement, parenteral.

zinc sulfocarbolate.
W/Aluminum hydroxide, pectin, kaolin, bismuth subsalicylate, salol.
See: Wescola Antidiarrheal-Stomach Upset (Western Research).

zinc trace metal additive. (IMS) Zinc 4 mg/ml. Inj. Vial. 10 ml. *Rx.*
Use: Nutritional supplement, parenteral.

zincundesal.
See: Zinchlorundesal.

zinc-10-undecenoate.
See: Zinc Undecylenate, U.S.P. 23.

•**zinc undecylenate.** (zingk uhn-deh-SILL-en-ate) U.S.P. 23. (Various Mfr.).
Use: Antifungal.
See: Blis-To-Sol, Pow. (Chattem).
W/Benzocaine, hexachlorophene.
See: Fung-O-Spray (Scrip).
W/Benzocaine, undecylenic acid, menthol.
See: Decyl-Cream LBS (Scrip).
W/Caprylic acid, sodium propionate.
See: Deso-Cream (Quality Formulations).
Deso-Talc, Foot Pow. (Quality Formulations).
W/Undecylenic acid.
See: Cruex Cream, Spray Pow. (Novartis Pharmaceuticals).
Desenex, Prods. (Novartis Pharmaceuticals).
Ting, Aerosol (Novartis Pharmaceuticals).
Quinsana, Med. Oint. (Mennen).

Zincvit. (Kenwood Labs) Vitamin A 5000 IU, D_3 50 IU, E 50 IU, B_1 10 mg, B_2 5 mg, B_6 2 mg, C 300 mcg, B_3 25 mg, Zn 40 mg, Mg 9.7 mg, Mn 1.3 mg, folic acid 1 mg/Cap. Bot. 60s. *Rx.*
Use: Mineral, vitamin supplement.

Zinecard. (Pharmacia & Upjohn) Dexrazoxane 250 mg or 500 mg. Powd. for Inj. Lyophilized. Vial 25 ml (250 mg) or 50 ml (500 mg) of 0.167 Molar Sodium Lactate Injection. *Rx.*
Use: Antineoplastic, antidote. [Orphan drug]

•**zindotrine.** (ZIN-doe-TREEN) USAN.
Use: Bronchodilator.

•**zinoconazole hydrochloride.** (zih-no-KOE-nah-zole) USAN.
Use: Antifungal.

•**zinostatin.** (ZEE-no-STAT-in) USAN. *Formerly neocarzinostatin.*
Use: Antineoplastic.

•**zinterol hydrochloride.** (ZIN-ter-ole) USAN.
Use: Bronchodilator.

•**zinviroxime.** (zin-VIE-rox-eem) USAN.
Use: Antiviral.

•**ziprasidone hydrochloride.** (zih-PRAY-sih-dohn) USAN.
Use: Antipsychotic.

zirconium carbonate or oxide.
See: Dermaneed, Lot. (Hanlon).
W/Benzocaine, menthol, camphor.
See: Rhuli Cream, Oint. (ESI Lederle Generics).
W/Benzocaine, menthol, camphor, calamine, pyrilamine maleate.
See: Ivarest, Cream (Carbisulphoil).
W/Benzocaine, menthol, camphor, calamine, isopropyl alcohol.
See: Rhulispray, Aerosol (ESI Lederle Generics).
W/Parethoxycaine, calamine.
See: Zotox, Spray, Oint. (Del Pharmaceuticals).

Zithromax. (Pfizer) Azithromycin. **Tab.:** 250 mg, 600 mg. Lactose. In 30s, UD 50s (250 mg only), Z-Pak 3s 6s (250 mg only). **Pow. for Inj.:** 500 mg. 10 ml vials. **Pow. for Oral Susp.:** 100 mg/5ml. Sucrose. 300 mg Bot., 200 mg/5ml. Sucrose. 600, 900, 1200 mg. Bot., 1 g/packet. Sucrose. Single dose pack. 3s, 10s. *Rx.*
Use: Anti-infective, macrolide.

Zixoryn. (Farmacon) Flumecinal.
Use: Hyperbilirubinemia.

ZNG. (Western Research) Zinc gluconate 35 mg/Tab. Handicount 28s (36 bags of 28 tab.). *otc.*
Use: Mineral supplement.

ZNP Bar. (Stiefel) Zinc pyrithione 2%. Bar 4.2 oz. *otc.*
Use: Antiseborrheic.

ZN-Plus Protein. (Miller) Zinc in a zinc-protein complex made with isolated soy protein 15 mg/Tab. Bot. 100s. *otc.*
Use: Mineral supplement.

Zocor. (Merck) Simvastatin **5 mg Tab.** Bot. 60s, 90s, UD 100s. **10 mg Tab.** Bot. 60s, 90s, 1000s, 10,000s, UD 100s. **20 mg Tab.** Bot. 60s, 1000s, 10,000s, UD 100s. **40 mg Tab.** Bot. 60s. *Rx.*
Use: Antihyperlipidemic.

Zopenex

Zodeac-100. (Econo Med Pharmaceuticals) Iron 60 mg, vitamins A 8000 IU, D 400 IU, E 30 IU, B_1 1.7 mg, B_2 2 mg, B_3 20 mg, B_5 11 mg, B_6 4 mg, B_{12} 8 mcg, C 120 mg, folic acid 1 mg, biotin 300 mcg, Ca, Cu, I, Mg, Zn 15 mg/Tab. Bot. 100s. *Rx.*
Use: Mineral, vitamin supplement.

•**zofenopril calcium.** (zoe-FEN-oh-PRILL) USAN.
Use: Enzyme inhibitor (angiotensin-converting).

•**zofenoprilat arginine.** (zoe-FEN-oh-PRILL-at AHR-jih-neen) USAN.
Use: Antihypertensive.

Zofran. (GlaxoWellcome) Ondansetron HCl **Tab.:** 4 mg, 8 mg, lactose Bot. 30s, UD 100s, 1 x 3 UD pack. **Inj.:** 2 mg/ml in 2 ml, 20 ml vials, or 32 mg/50 ml (premixed) parabens (2 mg/ml); preservative free, with dextrose 2500 mg, citric acid 26 mg, sodium citrate 11.5 mg (32 mg/50 ml). 50 ml containers **Oral Sol.:** 4 mg/5 ml (5 mg as HCl), sorbitol, strawberry flavor. Bot. 50 ml. *Rx.*
Use: Antiemetic.

Zoladex. (Zeneca) Goserelin acetate 3.6 mg, 10.8 mg. Implant. Syringes. *Rx.*
Use: LHRH agonist.

•**zolamine hydrochloride.** (zoe-lah-meen) USAN.
Use: Antihistamine; anesthetic, topical.
W/Eucupin dihydrochloride.
See: Otodyne, Soln. (Schering Plough).

•**zolazepam hydrochloride.** (zole-AZE-eh-pam) USAN.
Use: Hypnotic, sedative.

•**zoledronate disodium.** (ZOE-leh-droe-nate) USAN.
Use: Bone resorption inhibitor; osteoporosis treatment and prevention.

•**zoledronate trisodium.** (ZOE-leh-droe-nate) USAN.
Use: Bone resorption inhibitor; osteoporosis treatment and prevention.

•**zoledronic acid.** (ZOE-leh-drah-nik) USAN.
Use: Calcium regulator; osteoporosis treatment and prevention.

•**zolertine hydrochloride.** (ZOE-ler-teen) USAN.
Use: Antiadrenergic, vasodilator.

•**zolimomab aritox.** (zah-LIM-ah-mab a-rih-TOX) USAN.
Use: Monoclonal antibody (antithrombotic).

•**zolmitriptan.** USAN,
Use: Antimigraine.

Zoloft. (Roerig) Sertraline 25 mg, 50 mg, 100 mg/Tab. Bot. 50s. *Rx.*
Use: Antidepressant.

•**zolpidem tartrate.** (ZOLE-pih-dem) USAN.
Use: Hypnotic, sedative.
See: Ambien.

•**zomepirac sodium.** (ZOE-mih-PEER-ack) USAN. U.S.P. XXI.
Use: Analgesic, anti-inflammatory.

•**zometapine.** (zoe-MET-ah-peen) USAN.
Use: Antidepressant.

Zomig. (Zeneca) Zolmitriptan 2.5 mg, 5 mg, lactose/Tab. Blister pack 6s (2.5 mg), 3s (5 mg). *Rx.*
Use: Antimigraine.

Zone-A Forte. (Forest Pharmaceutical) Hydrocortisone 2.5%, pramoxine HCl in a hydrophilic base containing stearic acid 1%, forlan-L, glycerin, triethanolamine, polyoxyl-40-stearate, diisopropyl adipate, povidone, silicone fluid-200. Paraben free. Lot. Bot. 60 ml. *Rx.*
Use: Corticosteroid; anesthetic, local.

Zone-A Lotion. (Forest Pharmaceutical) Hydrocortisone acetate 1%, pramoxine HCl 1%. Bot. 2 oz. *Rx.*
Use: Corticosteroid; anesthetic, local.

•**zoniclezole hydrochloride.** (zoe-NIH-klih-ZOLE) USAN.
Use: Anticonvulsant.

•**zonisamide.** (zoe-NISS-ah-MIDE) USAN.
Use: Anticonvulsant.

Zonite Liquid Douche Concentrate. (Menley & James) Benzalkonium Cl 0.1%, menthol, thymol, EDTA in buffered soln. Bot. 240 ml, 360 ml. *otc.*
Use: Vaginal agent.

•**zopolrestat.** (zoe-PAHL-reh-STAT) USAN.
Use: Antidiabetic, aldose reductase inhibitor.

•**zorbamycin.** (ZAHR-bah-MY-sin) USAN.
Use: Anti-infective.

ZORprin. (Knoll Pharmaceuticals) Aspirin 800 mg/SR Tab. Bot. 100s. *Rx.*
Use: Analgesic.

•**zorubicin hydrochloride.** (zoe-ROO-bih-sin) USAN.
Use: Antineoplastic.

Zostrix. (GenDerm) Capsaicin 0.025%. Cream 45 g. *Rx.*
Use: Analgesic, topical.

Zostrix-HP. (GenDerm) Formerly called Axsain, formerly marketed by Galen.

Zosyn. (ESI Lederle Generics) Piperacillin sodium/tazobactam sodium 2 g/0.25 g, 3 g/0.375 g, 4 g/0.5 g vials. *Rx.*
Use: Anti-infective, penicillins.

Zoto-HC. (Horizon) Chloroxylenol 1%, pramoxine HCl 10%, hydrocortisone 10%/ml in non-aqueous vehicle with 3% propylene glycol diacetate. Drops, otic. Vial 10 ml. *Rx.*
Use: Otic.

Zovia. (Watson) Ethinyl estradiol 35 mcg or 50 mcg, ethynodiol diacetate 1 mg/Tab. 21s, 28s (7 inert tabs in 28s). *Rx.*
Use: Contraceptive.

Zovirax Capsules. (GlaxoWellcome) Acyclovir 200 mg/Cap. Bot. 100s, UD 100s. *Rx.*
Use: Antiviral.

Zovirax Ointment 5%. (GlaxoWellcome) Acyclovir 50 mg/Gm. Tube 15 g. *Rx.*
Use: Antiviral, topical.

Zovirax Powder. (GlaxoWellcome) Acyclovir sodium 500 mg/vial or 1000 mg/vial. **500 mg:** Vial 10 ml. **1000 mg:** Vial 20 ml. *Rx.*
Use: Antiviral.

Zovirax Suspension. (GlaxoWellcome) Acyclovir 200 mg/5 ml. Susp. Bot. 473 ml. *Rx.*
Use: Antiviral.

Zovirax Tablets. (GlaxoWellcome) Acyclovir 400 mg or 800 mg/Tab. **400 mg:** Bot. 100s. **800 mg:** Bot. 100s, UD 100s, Shingles Relief Pak 35s. *Rx.*
Use: Antiviral.

Z-Pro-C. (Person & Covey) Zinc sulfate 200 mg (elemental zinc 45 mg), ascorbic acid 100 mg/Tab. Bot. 100s. *otc.*
Use: Mineral, vitamin supplement.

Z-Tec. (Seatrace) Iron equivalent 50 mg/ml from iron dextran complex. Vial 10 ml. *Rx.*
Use: Mineral supplement.

•**zucapsaicin.** (zoo-cap-SAY-sin) USAN.
Use: Analgesic, topical.

•**zuclomiphene.** (zoo-KLOE-mih-FEEN) USAN. *Formerly transclomiphene.*

Zurinol. (Major) Allopurinol. **100 mg/Tab.:** Bot. 100s, 500s, 1000s, UD 100s. **300 mg/Tab.:** Bot. 100s, 500s, UD 100s. *Rx.*
Use: Antigout agent.

Zyban. (GlaxoWellcome) Bupropion HCl 150 mg/SR Tab. In 60s. *Rx.*
Use: Smoking deterrent.

Zyderm I. (Collagen) Highly purified bovine dermal collagen 35 mg/ml implant. Sterile syringe 0.1 ml, 0.5 ml, 1 ml, 2 ml.
Use: Collagen implant.

Zyderm II. (Collagen) Highly purified bovine dermal collagen 65 mg/ml implant. Syringe 0.75 ml.
Use: Collagen implant.

Zydone. (DuPont Merck Pharmaceuticals) Hydrocodone bitartrate 5 mg, acetaminophen 500 mg/Cap. Bot. 100s. *c-III.*
Use: Analgesic combination, narcotic.

Zyflo. (Abbott Laboratories) Zileuton 600 mg/Tab. Bot. 120s. *Rx.*
Use: Antiasthmatic.

Zyloprim. (GlaxoWellcome) Allopurinol. **100 mg/Tab.:** Bot. 100s, 1000s, UD 100s; **300 mg/Tab.:** Bot. 30s, 100s, 500s, UD 100s. *Rx.*
Use: Antigout agent.

Zyloprim. (GlaxoWellcome) Allopurinol Sodium. Inj.
Use: Antineoplastic. [Orphan drug]

Zymacap. (Pharmacia & Upjohn) Vitamins A 5000 IU, D 400 IU, E 15 mg, C 90 mg, folic acid 400 mcg, B_1 2.25 mg, B_2 2.6 mg, niacin 30 mg, B_6 3 mg, B_{12} 9 mcg, pantothenic acid 15 mg/Cap. Bot. 90s, 240s. *otc.*
Use: Vitamin supplement.

Zymase. (Organon Teknika) Lipase 12,000 units, protease 24,000 units, amylase 24,000 units. Cap. Bot. 100s. *Rx.*
Use: Digestive enzyme.

Zyprexa. (Eli Lilly) Olanzapine 2.5 mg, 5 mg, 7.5 mg, 10 mg, lactose/Tab. Bot. 60s (except 2.5 mg), UD 100s. *Rx.*
Use: Antipsychotic.

Zyrkamine. (ILEX Oncology) Mitoguazone.
Use: Non-Hodgkin's lymphoma treatment. [Orphan drug]

Zyrtec. (Pfizer) Cetirizine 5 mg, 10 mg, lactose, povidone. Tab. Bot. 100s. Cetirizine 5 mg/ml, parabens, sugar, banana-grape flavor. Syrup. Bot. 120 ml and pt. *Rx.*
Use: Antihistamine.

Reference Information

Common Abbreviations

Word	Abbreviation	Meaning
ana	$\overline{aa}$, aa	of each
ante cibum	a.c.	before meals or food
ad	ad.	to, up to
aurio dextra	a.d.	right ear
ad libitum	ad lib	at pleasure
aurio laeva	a.l.	left ear
ante meridiem	A.M.	morning
aqua	aq.	water
aqua destillata	aq.dest	distilled water
aurio sinister	a.s.	left ear
aures utrae	a.u.	each ear
bis in die	b.i.d.	twice daily
bowel movement	b.m.	bowel movement
blood pressure	b.p.	blood pressure
cong	C.	a gallon
cum	c̄	with
capsula	caps	capsule
cubic centimeter	cc	cubic centimeter
compositus	comp	compound
dies	d.	day
dilue	dil	dilute
dispensa	disp.	dispense
divide	div	divide
dentur tales doses	d.t.d.	give of such a dose
elixir	el.	elixir
as directed	e.m.p.	as directed
et.	et	and
in water	ex aq	in water
fac, fiat, fiant	f., ft.	make, let be made
Food and Drug Administration	FDA	Food and Drug Administration
gramma	Gm., g.	gram
granum	gr	grain
gutta	gtt.	a drop
hora	h.	hour
hora somni	h.s., hor. som.	at bedtime
intramuscular	i.m., I.M.	intramuscular
intravenous	i.v.	intravenous
liquor	liq	a liquor, solution
microgram	mcg	microgram
milligram	mg	milligram
milliliter	ml	milliliter
misce	M.	mix
more dictor	m. dict.	as directed
mixtura	mixt.	a mixture
National Formulary	N.F.	National Formulary
numerus	no.	number
nocturnal	noc	in the night
non repetatur	non. rep.	do not repeat, no refills
octarius	O, Oct.	a pint
oculus dexter	o.d.	right eye
oculus laevus	o.l.	left eye
oculus sinister	o.s.	left eye
oculo uterque	o.u.	each eye

Word	Abbreviation	Meaning
post cibos	p.c., post. cib.	after meals
post meridiem	P.M.	afternoon or evening
per os	p.o.	by mouth
pro re nata	p.r.n.	as needed
pulvis	pulv.	a powder
quoque alternis die	q.a.d.	every other day
every day	q.d.	every day
quiaque hora	q.h.	every hour
quater in die	q.i.d.	four times a day
every other day	q.o.d.	every other day
quantum sufficiat	q.s.	a sufficient quantity
a sufficient quantity to make	q.s. ad.	a sufficient quantity to make
quam volueris	q.v.	as much as you wish
recipe	Rx	take, a recipe
repetatur	rep	let it be repeated
sine	s̄, s.	without
secundum artem	s.a.	according to art
sataratus	sat.	saturated
signa	Sig.	label, or let it be printed
solutio	sol.	solution
dissolve	solv.	dissolve
semis	$\overline{ss}$, ss	one-half
si opus sit	s.o.s.	if there is need
statim	stat.	at once, immediately
suppositorium	supp.	suppository
syrupus	syr.	syrup
tabella	tab.	tablet
such	tal.	such
such doses	tal. dos.	such doses
ter in die	t.i.d.	three times a day
tincture	tr., tinct.	tincture
tritura	trit.	triturate
teaspoonful	tsp	teaspoonful
unguentum	ung.	ointment
United States Adopted Names	USAN.	official adopted names
United States Pharmacopeia	U.S.P.	United States Pharmacopeia
ut dictum	ut. dict.	as directed
while awake	w.a.	while awake

NOTE: The listing of commonly used abbreviations is included as an aid in interpreting medical orders.

Common Systems of Weights and Measures*

METRIC SYSTEM

Metric Weight

1 microgram†	μg (mcg)	=	0.000001	g
1 milligram	mg	=	0.001	g
1 centigram	cg	=	0.01	g
1 decigram	dg	=	0.1	g
1 gram	g	=	1.0	g
1 dekagram	dag	=	10.0	g
1 hectogram	hg	=	100.0	g
1 kilogram	kg	=	1000.0	g

Metric Liquid Measure

1 microliter	μl	=	0.000001	l
1 milliliter	ml	=	0.001	l
1 centiliter	cl	=	0.01	l
1 deciliter	dl	=	0.1	l
1 liter	l	=	1.0	l
1 dekaliter	dal	=	10.0	l
1 hectoliter	hl	=	100.0	l
1 kiloliter	kl	=	1000.0	l

APOTHECARY SYSTEM

Apothecary Weight

1 grain‡	gr	=	1 gr		
1 scruple	℈	=	20 gr		
1 dram	ʒ	=	60 gr	=	3℈
1 ounce	℥	=	480 gr	=	8ʒ
1 pound	lb	=	5760 gr	=	12℥

Apothecary Liquid Measure

1 minim	♏	=	1♏		
1 fluidram	fʒ	=	60♏		
1 fluidounce	f℥	=	480♏	=	8 fʒ
1 pint	pt or O	=	7680♏	=	16 f℥
1 quart	qt	=	15630♏	=	32 f℥
1 gallon	gal or cong	=	61440♏	=	8 pt℥

AVOIRDUPOIS SYSTEM

Avoirdupois Weight

1 ounce	=	1 oz	=	437.5 grains (gr)		
1 pound	=	1 lb	=	16 ounces (oz)	=	7000 grains (gr)

* The listing of common systems of weights and measures is included to aid the practitioner in calculating dosages.

† The abbreviation μg or mcg is used for microgram in pharmacy rather than gamma (γ) as in biology.

‡ The grain in each of the above systems has the same value, and thus serves as a basis for the interconversion of the other units.

Approximate Practical Equivalents*

Weight Equivalents

1 grain	=	1 gr	=	64.8	milligrams
1 gram	=	1 g	=	15.432	grains
1 ounce avoirdupois	=	1 oz	=	28.35	grams
1 ounce apothecary	=	1 ℥	=	31.1	grams
1 pound avoirdupois	=	1 lb	=	454.0	grams
1 kilogram	=	1 kg	=	2.20	pounds avoirdupois (lb)

Measure Equivalents

1 milliliter	=	1 ml	=	16.23	minims (♏)
1 fluidram†	=	1 fʒ	=	3.4	ml
1 teaspoonful†	=	1 tsp	=	5.0	ml
1 tablespoonful	=	1 tbsp	=	15.0	ml
1 fluidounce	=	1 f℥	=	29.57	ml
1 wineglassful	=	2 f℥	=	60.0	ml
1 teacupful	=	4 f℥	=	120.0	ml
1 tumblerful	=	8 f℥	=	240.0	ml
1 pint	=	1 pt or O or Oct	=	473.0	ml
1 liter	=	1 l	=	33.8	fluidounces (f℥)
1 gallon	=	1 gal or C or Cong	=	3785.0	ml

* The listing of approximate practical equivalents is included to aid the practitioner in calculating and converting dosages among the various systems.

† On prescription a fluidram is assumed to contain a teaspoonful which is 5 ml.

International System of Units

The *Système international d 'unités* (International System of Units) or *SI* is a modernized version of the metric system. The primary goal of the conversion to SI units is to revise the present confused measurement system and to improve test-result communications.

The SI has 7 basic units from which other units are derived:

Base Units of SI		
Physical quantity	Base unit	SI symbol
length	meter	m
mass	kilogram	kg
time	second	s
amount of substance	mole	mol
thermodynamic temperature	kelvin	K
electric current	ampere	A
luminous intensity	candela	cd

Combinations of these base units can express any property although, for simplicity, special names are given to some of these derived units.

Representative Derived Units		
Derived unit	Name and symbol	Derivation from base units
area	square meter	m^2
volume	cubic meter	m^3
force	newton (N)	$kg{\bullet}m{\bullet}s^{-2}$
pressure	pascal (Pa)	$kg{\bullet}m^{-1}{\bullet}s^{-2}$ (N/m^2)
work, energy	joule (J)	$kg{\bullet}m^2{\bullet}s^{-2}$($N{\bullet}m$)
mass density	kilogram per cubic meter	kg/m^3
frequency	hertz (Hz)	1 cycle/s $^{-1}$
temperature degree	Celsius (°C)	°C = °K − 273.15
concentration		
mass	kilogram/liter	kg/L
substance	mole/liter	mol/L
molality	mole/kilogram	mol/kg
density	kilogram/liter	kg/L

Prefixes to the base unit are used in this system to form decimal multiples and submultiples. The preferred multiples and submultiples listed below change the quantity by increments of 10^3 or 10^{-3}. The exceptions to these recommended factors are within the middle rectangle.

Prefixes and Symbols for Decimal Multiples and Submultiples		
Factor	Prefix	Symbol
10^{18}	exa	E
10^{15}	peta	P
10^{12}	tera	T
10^9	giga	G
10^6	mega	M
10^3	kilo	k
10^2	hecto	h
10^1	deka	da
10^{-1}	deci	d
10^{-2}	centi	c
10^{-3}	milli	m
10^{-6}	micro	μ
10^{-9}	nano	n
10^{-12}	pico	p
10^{-15}	femto	f
10^{-18}	atto	a

To convert drug concentrations to or from SI units:

Conversion factor (CF) $= \frac{1000}{\text{mol wt}}$

Conversion *to* SI units: μg/ml x CF = μmol/L

Conversion *from* SI units: μmol/L ÷ CF = μg/ml

International System of Units

Normal Laboratory Values

In the following tables, normal reference values for commonly requested laboratory tests are listed in traditional units and in SI units. The tables are a guideline only. Values are method dependent and "normal values" may vary between laboratories.

Blood, Plasma or Serum		
	Reference Value	
Determination	Conventional Units	SI Units
Ammonia (NH_3) – diffusion	20-120 mcg/dl	12-70 mcmol/L
Amylase	35-118 IU/L	0.58-1.97 mckat/L
Antinuclear antibodies	negative at 1:10 dilution of serum	negative at 1:10 dilution of serum
Antithrombin III (AT III)	80-120 U/dl	800-1200 U/L
Bilirubin: Conjugated (direct)	≤ 0.2 mg/dl	≤ 4 mcmol/L
Total	0.1-1 mg/dl	2-18 mcmol/L
Calcitonin	< 100 pg/ml	< 100 ng/L
Calcium: Total	8.6-10.3 mg/dl	2.2-2.74 mmol/L
Ionized	4.4-5.1 mg/dl	1-1.3 mmol/L
Carbon dioxide content (plasma)	21-32 mmol/L	21-32 mmol/L
Carcinoembryonic antigen	< 3 ng/ml	< 3 mcg/L
Chloride	95-110 mEq/L	95-110 mmol/L
Coagulation screen:		
Bleeding time	3-9.5 min	180-570 sec
Prothrombin time	10-13 sec	10-13 sec
Partial thromboplastin time (activated)	22-37 sec	22-37 sec
Protein C	0.7-1.4 μ/ml	700-1400 U/ml
Protein S	0.7-1.4 μ/ml	700-1400 U/ml
Copper, total	70-160 mcg/dl	11-25 mcmol/L
Corticotropin (ACTH adrenocorticotropic hormone) – 0800 hr	< 60 pg/ml	< 13.2 pmol/L
Cortisol: 0800 hr	5-30 mcg/dl	138-810 nmol/L
1800 hr	2-15 mcg/dl	50-410 nmol/L
Creatine kinase: Female	20-170 IU/L	0.33-2.83 mckat/L
Male	30-220 IU/L	0.5-3.67 mckat/L
Creatine kinase isoenzymes, MB fraction	0-12 IU/L	0-0.2 mckat/L
Creatinine	0.5-1.7 mg/dl	44-150 mcmol/L
Fibrinogen (coagulation factor I)	150-360 mg/dl	1.5-3.6 g/L
Follicle stimulating hormone (FSH):		
Female	2-13 mIU/ml	2-13 IU/L
Midcycle	5-22 mIU/ml	5-22 IU/L
Male	1-8 mIU/ml	1-8 IU/L
Glucose, fasting	65-115 mg/dl	3.6-6.3 mmol/L
Haptoglobin	44-303 mg/dl	0.44-3.03 g/L
Hematologic tests:		
Hematocrit (Hct), female	36%-44.6%	0.36-0.446 fraction of 1
male	40.7%-50.3%	0.4-0.503 fraction of 1
Hemoglobin (Hb), female	12.1-15.3 g/dl	121-153 g/L
male	13.8-17.5 g/dl	138-175 g/L
Leukocyte count (WBC)	3800-9800/mcl	3.8-9.8 x 10^9/L
Erythrocyte count (RBC), female	3.5-5 × 10^6/mcl	3.5-5 x 10^{12}/L
male	4.3-5.9 × 10^6/mcl	4.3-5.9 x 10^{12}/L
Mean corpuscular volume (MCV)	80-97.6 mcm^3	80-97.6 fl
Mean corpuscular hemoglobin (MCH)	27-33 pg/cell	1.66-2.09 fmol/cell

Blood, Plasma or Serum		
	Reference Value	
Determination	Conventional Units	SI Units
Mean corpuscular hemoglobin concentrate (MCHC)	33-36 g/dl	20.3-22 mmol/L
Erythrocyte sedimentation rate (sedrate, ESR)	≤ 30 mm/hr	≤ 30 mm/hr
Erythrocyte enzymes: Glucose-6-phosphate dehydrogenase (G6PD)	250-5000 units/10^6 cells	250-5000 mcunits/cell
Ferritin	10-383 ng/ml	23-862 pmol/L
Folic acid: normal	> 3.1-12.4 ng/ml	7-28.1 nmol/L
Platelet count	150-450 × 10^3/mcl	150-450 × 10^9/L
Vitamin B_{12}	223-1132 pg/ml	165-835 pmol/L
Iron: Female	30-160 mcg/dl	5.4-31.3 mcmol/L
Male	45-160 mcg/dl	8.1-31.3 mcmol/L
Iron binding capacity	220-420 mcg/dl	39.4-75.2 mcmol/L
Lactate dehydrogenase	100-250 IU/L	1.67-4.17 mckat/L
Lactic acid (lactate)	6-19 mg/dl	0.7-2.1 mmol/L
Lead	≤ 50 mcg/dl	≤ 2.41 mcmol/L
Lipids:		
Total Cholesterol		
Desirable	< 200 mg/dl	< 5.2 mmol/L
Borderline-high	200-239 mg/dl	< 5.2-6.2 mmol/L
High	> 239 mg/dl	> 6.2 mmol/L
LDL		
Desirable	< 130 mg/dl	< 3.36 mmol/L
Borderline-high	130-159 mg/dl	3.36-4.11 mmol/L
High	> 159 mg/dl	> 4.11 mmol/L
HDL (low)	< 35 mg/dl	< 0.91 mmol/L
Triglycerides		
Desirable	< 200 mg/dl	< 2.26 mmol/L
Borderline-high	200-400 mg/dl	2.26-4.52 mmol/L
High	400-1000 mg/dl	4.52-11.3 mmol/L
Very high	> 1000 mg/dl	> 11.3 mmol/L
Magnesium	1.3-2.2 mEq/L	0.65-1.1 mmol/L
Osmolality	280-300 mOsm/kg	280-300 mmol/kg
Oxygen saturation (arterial)	94%-100%	0.94-1 fraction of 1
PCO_2, arterial	35-45 mm Hg	4.7-6 kPa
pH, arterial	7.35-7.45	7.35-7.45
PO_2, arterial: Breathing room air[1]	80-105 mm Hg	10.6-14 kPa
On 100% O_2	> 500 mm Hg	
Phosphatase (acid), total at 37°C	0.13-0.63 IU/L	2.2-10.5 IU/L or 2.2-10.5 mckat/L
Phosphatase alkaline[2]	20-130 IU/L	20-130 IU/L or 0.33-2.17 mckat/L
Phosphorus, inorganic,[3] (phosphate)	2.5-5 mg/dl	0.8-1.6 mmol/L
Potassium	3.5-5 mEq/L	3.5-5 mmol/L
Progesterone		
Female	0.1-1.5 ng/ml	0.32-4.8 nmol/L
Follicular phase	0.1-1.5 ng/ml	0.32-4.8 nmol/L
Luteal phase	2.5-28 ng/ml	8-89 nmol/L
Male	< 0.5 ng/ml	< 1.6 nmol/L
Prolactin	1.4-24.2 ng/ml	1.4-24.2 mcg/L
Prostate specific antigen	0-4 ng/ml	0-4 ng/ml

Blood, Plasma or Serum		
	Reference Value	
Determination	Conventional Units	SI Units
Protein: Total	6-8 g/dl	60-80 g/L
Albumin	3.6-5 g/dl	36-50 g/L
Globulin	2.3-3.5 g/dl	23-35 g/L
Rheumatoid factor	< 60 IU/ml	< 60 kIU/L
Sodium	135-147 mEq/L	135-147 mmol/L
Testosterone: Female	6-86 ng/dl	0.21-3 nmol/L
Male	270-1070 ng/dl	9.3-37 nmol/L
Thyroid Hormone Function Tests:		
Thyroid-stimulating hormone (TSH)	0.35-6.2 mcU/ml	0.35-6.2 mU/L
Thyroxine-binding globulin capacity	10-26 mcg/dl	100-260 mcg/L
Total triiodothyronine (T_3)	75-220 ng/dl	1.2-3.4 nmol/L
Total thyroxine by RIA (T_4)	4-11 mcg/dl	51-142 nmol/L
T_3 resin uptake	25%-38%	0.25-0.38 fraction of 1
Transaminase, AST (aspartate aminotransferase, SGOT)	11-47 IU/L	0.18-0.78 mckat/L
Transaminase, ALT (alanine aminotransferase, SGPT)	7-53 IU/L	0.12-0.88 mckat/L
Urea nitrogen (BUN)	8-25 mg/dl	2.9-8.9 mmol/L
Uric acid	3-8 mg/dl	179-476 mcmol/L
Vitamin A (retinol)	15-60 mcg/dl	0.52-2.09 mcmol/L
Zinc	50-150 mcg/dl	7.7-23 mcmol/L

[1] Age dependent
[2] Infants and adolescents up to 104 U/L
[3] Infants in the first year up to 6 mg/dl

Urine		
	Reference Value	
Determination	Conventional Units	SI Units
Calcium[1]	50-250 mcg/day	1.25-6.25 mmol/day
Catecholamines: Epinephrine	< 20 mcg/day	< 109 nmol/day
Norepinephrine	< 100 mcg/day	< 590 nmol/day
Copper[1]	15-60 mcg/day	0.24-0.95 mcmol/day
Creatinine: Female	0.6-1.5 g/day	5.3-13.3 mmol/day
Male	0.8-1.8 g/day	7.1-15.9 mmol/day
Phosphate[1]	0.9-1.3 g/day	29-42 mmol/day
Potassium[1]	25-100 mEq/day	25-100 mmol/day
Protein, quantitative	< 150 mg/day	< 0.15 g/day
Sodium[1]	100-250 mEq/day	100-250 mmol/day

[1] Diet dependent

Drug Levels†			
		Reference Value	
Drug Determination		Conventional Units	SI Units
Aminoglycosides	Amikacin		
	(trough)	1-8 mcg/ml	1.7-13.7 mcmol/L
	(peak)	20-30 mcg/ml	34-51 mcmol/L
	Gentamicin		
	(trough)	0.5-2 mcg/ml	1-4.2 mcmol/L
	(peak)	6-10 mcg/ml	12.5-20.9 mcmol/L
	Kanamycin		
	(trough)	5-10 mcg/ml	nd
	(peak)	20-25 mcg/ml	nd
	Netilmicin		
	(trough)	0.5-2 mcg/ml	nd
	(peak)	6-10 mcg/ml	nd
	Streptomycin		
	(trough)	< 5 mcg/ml	nd
	(peak)	5-20 mcg/ml	nd
	Tobramycin		
	(trough)	0.5-2 mcg/ml	1.1-4.3 mcmol/L
	(peak)	5-20 mcg/ml	12.8-21.8 mcmol/L
Antiarrhythmics	Amiodarone	0.5-2.5 mcg/ml	1.5-4 mcmol/L
	Bretylium	0.5-1.5 mcg/ml	nd
	Digitoxin	9-25 mcg/L	11.8-32.8 nmol/L
	Digoxin	0.8-2 ng/ml	0.9-2.5 nmol/L
	Disopyramide	2-8 mcg/ml	6-18 mcmol/L
	Flecainide	0.2-1 mcg/ml	nd
	Lidocaine	1.5-6 mcg/ml	4.5-21.5 mcmol/L
	Mexiletine	0.5-2 mcg/ml	nd
	Procainamide	4-8 mcg/ml	17-34 mcmol/ml
	Propranolol	50-200 ng/ml	190-770 nmol/L
	Quinidine	2-6 mcg/ml	4.6-9.2 mcmol/L
	Tocainide	4-10 mcg/ml	nd
	Verapamil	0.08-0.3 mcg/ml	nd
Anti-convulsants	Carbamazepine	4-12 mcg/ml	17-51 mcmol/L
	Phenobarbital	10-40 mcg/ml	43-172 mcmol/L
	Phenytoin	10-20 mcg/ml	40-80 mcmol/L
	Primidone	4-12 mcg/ml	18-55 mcmol/L
	Valproic acid	40-100 mcg/ml	280-700 mcmol/L
Antidepressants	Amitriptyline	110-250 ng/ml[3]	500-900 nmol/L
	Amoxapine	200-500 ng/ml	nd
	Bupropion	25-100 ng/ml	nd
	Clomipramine	80-100 ng/ml	nd
	Desipramine	115-300 ng/ml	nd
	Doxepin	110-250 ng/ml[3]	nd
	Imipramine	225-350 ng/ml[3]	nd
	Maprotiline	200-300 ng/ml	nd
	Nortriptyline	50-150 ng/ml	nd
	Protriptyline	70-250 ng/ml	nd
	Trazodone	800-1600 ng/ml	nd
Antipsychotics	Chlorpromazine	50-300 ng/ml	150-950 nmol/L
	Fluphenazine	0.13-2.8 ng/ml	nd
	Haloperidol	5-20 ng/ml	nd
	Perphenazine	0.8-1.2 ng/ml	nd
	Thiothixene	2-57 ng/ml	nd

Drug Levels†			
		Reference Value	
Drug Determination		Conventional Units	SI Units
Miscellaneous	Amantadine	300 ng/ml	nd
	Amrinone	3.7 mcg/ml	nd
	Chloramphenicol	10-20 mcg/ml	31-62 mcmol/L
	Cyclosporine[1]	250-800 ng/ml (whole blood, RIA)	nd
		50-300 ng/ml (plasma, RIA)	nd
	Ethanol[2]	0 mg/dl	0 mmol/L
	Hydralazine	100 ng/ml	nd
	Lithium	0.6-1.2 mEq/L	0.6-1.2 mmol/L
	Salicylate	100-300 mg/L	724-2172 mcmol/L
	Sulfonamide	5-15 mg/dl	nd
	Terbutaline	0.5-4.1 ng/ml	nd
	Theophylline	10-20 mcg/ml	55-110 mcmol/L
	Vancomycin		
	(trough)	5-15 ng/ml	nd
	(peak)	20-40 mcg/ml	nd

† The values given are generally accepted as desirable for treatment without toxicity for most patients. However, exceptions are not uncommon.

[1] 24 hour trough values [2] Toxic: 50-100 mg/dl (10.9-21.7 mmol/L) [3] Parent drug plus N-desmethyl metabolite

nd – No data available

Trademark Glossary

Many companies use trademarks to identify specific dosage forms or unique packaging materials. The following list is provided as a guide to the interpretation of these descriptions.

Abbo-Pac (Abbott)
Unit dose package

Accu-Pak (Ciba-Geigy)
Unit dose blister pack

Act-O-Vial (Pharmacia & Upjohn)
Vial system

ADD-Vantage (Abbott)
Sterile dissolution system for admixture

ADT (Upjohn)
Alternate day therapy

Arm-A-Med (Armour)
Single-dose plastic vial

Arm-A-Vial (Armour)
Single-dose plastic vial

Aspirol (Lilly)
Crushable ampule for inhalation

bidCAP (B-M Squibb)
Double strength capsule

Bristoject (B-M Squibb)
Unit dose syringe

Caplet (Various)
Capsule shaped tablet

Carpuject (Sanofi Winthrop)
Cartridge needle unit

Clinipak (Wyeth-Ayerst)
Unit dose package

ControlPak (Sandoz)
Unit dose rolls, tamper resistant

Detecto-Seal (Sanofi Winthrop)
Tamper resistant parenteral package

Dialpak (Ortho)
Compliance package

Dis-Co Pack (Wyeth-Ayerst)
Unit dose package

Disket (Lilly)
Dispersible tablet

Dispenserpak (GlaxoWellcome)
Unit-of-use package

Dispertab (Abbott)
Particles in tablet

Dispette (Wyeth-Ayerst)
Disposable pipette

Divide-Tab (Abbott)
Scored tablet

Dividose (Mead Johnson)
Tablet, bisected/trisected

Dosa-Trol Pack (B-M Squibb)
Unit-dose box packaging

Dosepak (Pharmacia & Upjohn)
Unit-of-use package

Dosette (Wyeth-Ayerst)
Single dose ampule or vial

Drop Dose (GlaxoWellcome)
Ophthalmic dropper dispenser

Drop-Tainer (Alcon)
Ophthalmic dropper dispenser

Dulcet (Abbott)
Chewable tablet

Dura-Tab (Berlex)
Sustained release tablet

Enseal (Lilly)
Enteric coated tablet

EN-tabs (Pharmacia & Upjohn)
Enteric coated tablet

Expidet (Wyeth-Ayerst)
Fast-dissolving doseform

Extencaps (Wyeth-Ayerst)
Continuous release capsules

Extentab (Wyeth-Ayerst)
Continuous release tablet

EZ Dial™ (Wyeth-Ayerst)
Dial dispenser

Fast-Trak (Wyeth-Ayerst)
Quick-loading hypodermic syringe

Filmlok (B-M Squibb)
Veneer coated tablet

Filmtab (Abbott)
Film coated tablet

Flo-Pack (GlaxoWellcome)
Vial for preparation of IV drips

Gelseal (Lilly)
Soft gelatin capsule

Gradumet (Abbott)
Controlled release tablet

Gy-Pak (Ciba-Geigy)
Unit-of-issue package

Gyrocap (Rhone-Poulenc Rorer)
Timed release capsule

Hyporet (Lilly)
Unit dose syringe

Identi-Dose (Lilly)
Unit dose package

Infatab (Parke-Davis)
Chewable pediatric tablet

Inject-all (B-M Squibb)
Prefilled disposable dilution syringe

Inlay-Tabs (Sandoz)
Inlaid tablets

Isoject (Pfizer)
Unit dose syringe

Kapseal (Parke-Davis)
Banded (sealed) capsule

Kronocap (Ferndale)
Sustained release capsule

Lederject (Wyeth-Ayerst)
Disposable syringe

Liquitab (Mission)
Chewable tablet

Memorette (Syntex)
Compliance package

Mini Pack™ (Wyeth-Ayerst)
Dial dispenser

Mix-O-Vial (Pharmacia & Upjohn)
Two compartment vial

Mono-Drop (Sanofi Winthrop)
Ophthalmic plastic dropper

Ocumeter (Merck & Co.)
Ophthalmic dropper dispenser

Perle (Forest)
Soft gelatin capsule

Pilpak (Wyeth-Ayerst)
Compliance pack

Plateau CAP (Marion Merrell Dow)
Controlled release capsule

Pulvule (Lilly)
Bullet-shaped capsule

Redipak (Wyeth-Ayerst)
Unit dose or unit-of-issue package

Redi Vial (Lilly)
Dual compartment vial

Repetabs (Schering)
Extended release tablet

Rescue Pak (GlaxoWellcome)
Unit dose packaging

Respihaler (Merck & Co.)
Aerosol for inhalation

SandoPak (Sandoz)
Unit dose blister package

Secule (Wyeth-Ayerst)
Single dose vial

Sequels (Wyeth-Ayerst)
Sustained release capsule or tablet

SigPak (Sandoz)
Unit-of-use package

Snap Tabs (Sandoz)
Tablet with facilitated bisect

Solvet (Lilly)
Soluble tablet

Spansule (SmithKline Beecham)
Sustained release capsule

Stat-Pak (Adria)
Unit dose package

Steri-Dose (Parke-Davis)
Unit dose syringe

Steri-Vial (Parke-Davis)
Ampule

Supprette (PolyMedica)
Suppository

Tabloid (GlaxoWellcome)
Branded tablet (with raised lettering)

Tamp-R-Tel (Wyeth-Ayerst)
Tubex, tamper resistant

Tel-E-Amp (Roche)
Single-dose amp

Tel-E-Dose (Roche)
Unit dose strip package

Tel-E-Ject (Roche)
Unit dose syringe

Tel-E-Pack (Roche)
Packaging system

Tel-E-Vial (Roche)
Single dose vial

Tembids (Wyeth-Ayerst)
Sustained action capsule

Tempule (Armour)
Timed release capsule or tablet

Thera-Ject (SmithKline Beecham)
Unit dose syringe

Tiltab (SmithKline Beecham)
Tablet shape

Timecap (Schwarz Pharma)
Sustained release capsule

Timecelle (Roberts Hauck)
Timed release capsule

Timespan (Roche)
Timed release tablet

Titradose (Wyeth-Ayerst)
Scored tablet

Traypak (Lilly)
Multivial carton

Tubex (Wyeth-Ayerst)
Cartridge-needle unit

Turbinaire (Adams)
Aerosol for nasal inhalation

UDIP (Marion Merrell Dow)
Unit dose identification pack

U-Ject (Pharmacia & Upjohn)
Disposable syringe

ULTRATAB (Warner Lambert Consumer)

Uni-Amp (Sanofi Winthrop)
Single-dose ampule

Unimatic (B-M Squibb)
Unit dose syringe

Uni-Nest (Sanofi Winthrop)
Ampule

UNI-Rx (Marion Merrell Dow)
Unit dose packages and containers

Unisert (Upsher-Smith)
Suppository

Vaporole (GlaxoWellcome)
Crushable ampule for inhalation

Visipak (Pharmacia & Upjohn)
Reverse numbered pack

Wyseals (Wyeth-Ayerst)
Film coated tablet

Medical Terminology Glossary

Abduction – the act of drawing away from a center.

Abstergent – a cleansing application or medicine.

Acaricide – an agent lethal to mites.

Achlorhydria – the absence of hydrochloric acid from gastric secretions.

Acidifier, systemic – a drug used to lower internal body pH in patients with systemic alkalosis.

Acidifier, urinary – a drug used to lower the pH of the urine.

Acidosis – an accumulation of acid in the body.

Acne – an inflammatory disease of the skin accompanied by the eruption of papules or pustules.

Addison's Disease – a condition caused by adrenal gland destruction.

Adduction – the act of drawing toward a center.

Adenitis – a gland or lymph node inflammation.

Adjuvant – an ingredient added to a prescription which complements or accentuates the action of the primary agent.

Adrenergic – a sypathomimetic drug that activates organs innervated by the sympathetic branch of the autonomic nervous system.

Adrenocorticotropic Hormone – an anterior pituitary hormone that stimulates and regulates secretion of the adrenocortical steroids.

Adrenocortical steroid, anti-inflammatory – an adrenal cortex hormone that participates in regulation of organic metabolism and inhibits the inflammatory response to stress; a glucocorticoid.

Adrenocortical steroid, salt regulating – an adrenal cortex hormone that maintains sodium-potassium electrolyte balance by stimulating and regulating sodium retention and potassium excretion by the kidneys.

Adsorbent – an agent that binds chemicals to its surface; it is useful in reducing the free availability of toxic chemicals.

Alkalizer, systemic – a drug that raises internal body pH in patients with systemic acidosis.

Allergen – a specific substance that causes an unwanted reaction in the body.

Amblyopia – pertaining to a dimness of vision.

Amebiasis – an infection with a pathogenic amoeba.

Amenorrhea – an abnormal discontinuation of the menses.

Amphiarthrosis – a joint in which the surfaces are connected by discs of fibrocartilage.

Anabolic – an agent that promotes conversion of simple substance into more complex compounds; a constructive process for the organism.

Analeptic – a potent central nervous system stimulant used to maintain vital functions during severe central nervous system depression.

Analgesic – a drug that selectively suppresses pain perception without inducing unconsciousness.

Ancyclostomiasis – the presence of hookworms in the intestine.

Androgen – a hormone that stimulates and maintains male secondary sex characteristics.

Anemia – a deficiency of red blood cells.

Anesthetic, general – a drug that eliminates pain perception by inducing unconsciousness.

Anesthetic, local – a drug that eliminates pain perception in a limited area by local action on sensory nerves; a topical anesthetic.

Angina pectoris – a sharp chest pain starting in the heart, often spreading down the left arm. A symptom of coronary disease.

Angiography – an X-ray of the blood vessels.

Anhydrotic – a drug that checks perspiration flow systemically; an antidiaphoretic.

Anodyne – a drug which acts on the sensory nervous system, either centrally or peripherally, to produce relief from pain.

Anorexiant – a drug that suppresses appetite, usually secondary to central stimulation of mood.

Anorexigenic – an agent promoting a dislike or aversion to food.

Antacid – a drug that neutralizes excess gastric acid locally.

Anthelmintic – a drug that kills or inhibits worm infestations such as pinworms and tapeworms (nematodes, cestodes, trematodes).

Antiadrenergic – a drug that prevents response to sympathetic nervous system stimulation and adrenergic drugs; a sympatholytic or sympathoplegic drug.

Antiamebic – a drug that kills or inhibits the pathogenic protozoan *Entamoeba histolytica,* the causative agent of amebic dysentery.

Antianemic – a drug that stimulates the production of erythrocytes in normal size, number and hemoglobin content; useful in treating anemias.

Antiasthmatic – an agent that relieves the symptoms of asthma.

Antibacterial – a drug that kills or inhibits pathogenic bacteria, the causative agents of many systemic gastrointestinal and superficial infections.

Antibiotic – an agent produced by or derived from living cells of molds, bacteria or other plants, which destroy or inhibit the growth of microbes.

Anticholesteremic – a drug that lowers blood cholesterol levels.

Anticholinergic – a drug that prevents response to parasympathetic nervous system stimulation and cholinergic drugs; a parasympatholytic or parasympathoplegic drug.

Anticoagulant – a drug that inhibits clotting of circulating blood or prevents clotting of collected blood.

Anticonvulsant – a drug that selectively prevents epileptic seizures; a central depressant used to arrest convulsions by inducing unconsciousness.

Antidepressant – a psychotherapeutic drug that induces mood elevation, useful in treating depressive neuroses and psychoses.

Antidiabetic – a drug used to prevent the development of diabetes.

Antidote – a drug that prevents or counteracts the effects of poisons or drug overdoses, by adsorption in the gastrointestinal tract (general antidotes) or by specific systemic action (specific antidotes).

Antieczematic – a topical drug that aids in the control of exudative inflammatory skin lesions.

Antiemetic – a drug that prevents vomiting, especially that of systemic origin.

Antifibrinolytic – an agent (drug) that inhibits liquifaction of fibrin.

Antifilarial – a drug that kills or inhibits pathogenic filarial worms of the superfamily *Filarioidea,* the causative agents of diseases such as loaiasis.

Antiflatulant – an agent inhibiting the excessive formation of gas in the stomach or intestines.

Antifungal – a drug that kills or inhibits pathogenic fungi, the causative agents of systemic, gastrointestinal and superficial infections.

Antihemophilic – a blood derivative containing the clotting factors absent in the hereditary disease hemophilia.

Antihistaminic – a drug that prevents response to histamine, including histamine released by allergic reactions.

Antihypercholesterolemic – a drug that lowers blood cholesterol levels, especially elevated levels sometimes associated with cardiovascular disease.

Antihypertensive – a drug that lowers blood pressure, especially diastolic blood pressure in hypertensive patients.

Antiinfective, local – a drug that kills a variety of pathogenic microorganisms and is suitable for sterilizing the skin or wounds.

Anti-inflammatory – a drug which counteracts or suppresses inflammation, and produces suppression of the pain, heat, redness and swelling of inflammation.

Antileishmanial – a drug that kills or inhibits pathogenic protozoa of the genus *Leishmania,* the causative agents of diseases such as kala-azar.

Antileprotic – an agent which fights leprosy, a generally chronic skin disease.

Antilipemic – an agent reducing the amount of circulating lipids.

Antimalarial – a drug that kills or inhibits the causative agents of malaria.

Antimetabolite – a substance that competes with or replaces a certain metabolite.

Antimethemoglobinemic – a drug that reduces nonfunctional methemoglobin (Fe^{+++}) to normal hemoglobin (Fe^{++}).

Antimycotic – an agent inhibiting the growth of fungi.

Antinauseant – a drug that suppresses nausea, especially that due to motion sickness.

Antineoplastic – a drug that is selectively toxic to rapidly multiplying cells and is useful in destroying malignant tumors.

Antioxidant – an agent used to reduce decay or transformation of a material from oxidation.

Antiperiodic – a drug that modifies or prevents the return of malarial fever; an antimalarial.

Antiperistaltic – a drug that inhibits intestinal motility, especially for the treatment of diarrhea.

Antipruritic – a drug that prevents or relieves itching.

Antipyretic – a drug employed to reduce fever temperature of the body; a febrifuge.

Antirheumatic – a drug that alleviates inflammatory symptoms of arthritis and related connective tissue diseases.

Antirickettsial – a drug that kills or inhibits pathogenic microorganisms of the genus *Rickettsia,* the causative agents of diseases such as typhus (e.g. Chloramphenicol USP).

Antischistosomal – a drug that kills or inhibits pathogenic flukes of the genus *Schistosoma,* the causative agents of schistosomiasis.

Antiseborrheic – a drug that aids in the control of seborrheic dermatitis ("dandruff").

Antiseptic – a substance that will inhibit the growth and development of microorganisms without necessarily destroying them.

Antisialagogue – a drug which diminishes the flow of saliva.

Antispasmodic – an agent used to quiet the spasms of voluntary and involuntary muscles; calmative or antihysteric.

Antisyphilitic – a remedy used in the treatment of syphilis.

Antitoxin – a biological drug containing antibodies against the toxic principles of a pathogenic microorganism, used for passive immunization against the associated disease.

Antitrichomonal – a drug that kills or inhibits the pathogenic protozoan *Trichomonas vaginalis,* the causative agent of trichomonal vaginitis.

Antitrypanosomal – a drug that kills or inhibits pathogenic protozoa of the genus *Trypanosoma,* the causative agents of diseases such as West African trypanosomiasis.

Antitussive – a drug that suppresses coughing.

Antivenin – a biological drug containing antibodies against the venom of a poisonous animal; an antidote for a venomous bite.

Anxiety – a feeling of apprehension, uncertainty and fear.

Aperient – a mild laxative.

Aphasia – the inability to use or understand written and spoken words, due to damage of cortical speech centers.

Aphonia – a whisper voice due to disease of the larynx or its innervation.

Apnea – the absence of breathing.

Areola – a pigmented ring on the skin.
Arsenical – having to do with arsenic.
Arteriosclerosis – a hardening of the arteries.
Arthritis – an inflammation of a joint.
Ascariasis – a condition caused by roundworms in the intestine.
Ascaricide – an agent that kills roundworms of the genus *Ascaris.*
Aspergillus – a fungi genus including many types of molds.
Astasia – the inability to stand up without help.
Asthma – a disease characterized by recurring breathing difficulty due to bronchial muscle constriction.
Astringent – a mild protein precipitant suitable for local application to toughen, shrink, blanch, wrinkle and harden tissue; diminish secretions and coagulate blood.
Ataractic – an agent having a quieting, tranquilizing effect.
Ataxia – incoordination, especially of gait.
Atheroma – a fatty granular degeneration of an artery wall.
Atrophy – a wasting away.
Avitaminosis – a disease caused by lack of one or more vitamins in the diet.
Axilla – armpit.
Bacteriostatic – an agent that inhibits the growth of bacteria.
Basedow's disease – a form of hyperthyroidism, also known as Grave's disease and Parry's disease.
Biliary Colic – a sharp pain in the upper right side of the abdomen due to a gallstone impaction.
Bilirubin – a bile pigment.
Biliuria – the presence of bile in the urine.
Blood Calcium Regulator – a drug that maintains the blood level of ionic calcium, especially by regulating its metabolic disposition elsewhere.
Blood Volume Supporter – an intravenous solution whose solutes are retained in the vascular system to supplement the osmotic activity of plasma proteins.
Bradycardia – a slow heart rate.
Bright's Disease – a disease of the kidneys, including the presence of edema and excessive urine protein formation.
Bromidrosis – foul smelling perspiration.
Bronchitis – an inflammation of the bronchi.
Bronchodilator – a drug which can dilate the lumina of air passages of the lungs.
Bruit – an arterial sound audible with a stethoscope.
Buerger's Disease – a thromboanglitis obliterans inflammation of the walls and surrounding rise of the veins and arteries.
Bursitis – an inflammation of the bursa.
Callus – a hard bonelike material developing around a fractured bone.
Calmative – a sedative.
Candidiasis – an infection by the yeastlike organism *Candida albicans.*
Carbonic Anhydrase Inhibitor – an enzyme inhibitor, the therapeutic effects of which are diuresis and reduced formation of intraocular fluid.
Carcinoma – a malignant growth.
Cardiac Depressant – a drug that depresses myocardial function so as to supress rhythmic irregularities characterized by fast rate; an antiarrhythmic.
Cardiac Stimulant – a drug that increases the contractile force of the myocardium, especially in weakened conditions such as congestive heart failure; a cardiotonic.
Cardiopathy – a disease of the heart.
Caries – decay of the teeth.
Carminative – an aromatic or pungent drug that mildly irritates the gastrointestinal tract and is useful in the treatment of flatulence and colic. Peppermint Water is a common carminative.
Caruncle – a small fleshy projection on the skin.
Cathartic – a drug that promotes defecation, usually by enhancing peristalsis or by softening and lubricating the feces.
Caudal – pertains to the distal end or tail.
Caustic – a topical drug that destroys tissue on contact and is suitable for removal of abnormal skin growths.
Central Depressant – a drug that reduces the functional state of the central nervous system and with increasing dosage induces sedation, hypnosis and general anesthesia; respiration is depressed.
Central Stimulant – a drug that increases the functional state of the central nervous system and with increasing dosage induces restlessness, insomnia, disorientation and convulsions; respiration is stimulated.
Cerebral – pertaining to the brain.
Cerumen – earwax.
Chloasma – skin discoloration.
Cholagogue – a drug that stimulates the empty ing of the gallbladder and the flow of bile into the duodenum.
Cholecystitis – an inflammation of the gallbladder.
Cholecystokinetic – an agent that promotes emptying of the gallbladder.
Cholelithiasis – the presence of calculi (stones) in the gallbladder.
Choleretic – a drug that increases the production and secretion of dilute bile by the liver.
Chorea – a disorder, usually of childhood, characterized by uncontrolled spasmotic muscle movements; sometimes referred to as St. Vitus' dance.
Chymotrypsin – a proteinase in the gastrointestinal tract; its proposed use has been the treatment of edema and inflammation.
Claudication – limping.
Climacteric – a time period in women just preceding termination of the reproductive processes.

Clonus – a spasm in which rigidity and relaxation succeed each other.
Coagulant – a drug that replaces a deficient blood factor necessary for coagulation; clotting factor.
Coccidiostat – a drug used in the treatment of coccidal (protozoal) infections in animals, especially birds; used in veterinary medicine.
Colitis – an inflammation of the colon.
Colloid – a disperse system of particles larger than those of true solutions but smaller than those of suspensions (1 to 100 millimicrons in size).
Collyrium – an eyewash.
Colostomy – the surgical formation of a more or less permanent opening into the colon.
Corticoid – a term applied to hormones of the adrenal cortex or any substance, natural or synthetic, having similar activity.
Corticosteroid – a steroid produced by the adrenal cortex.
Coryza – a headcold.
Counterirritant – an agent (irritant) which causes irritation of the part to which it is applied, and draws blood away from a deep seated area.
Cranial – pertaining to the skull.
Crepitation – the grating of a joint.
Cryptitis – an inflammation of a follicle or glandular tubule, usually in the rectum.
Cryptococcus – a genus of fungi which does not produce spores, but reproduces by budding.
Cryptorchidism – the failure of one or both testes to descend.
Cutaneous – pertaining to the skin.
Cyanosis – a blue or purple skin discoloration due to oxygen deficiency.
Cycloplegia – the loss of accommodation.
Cyclopegic – a drug which paralyzes accommodation of the eye.
Cystitis – an inflammation of the bladder.
Cystourethography – the examination by x-ray of the bladder and urethra.
Cytostasis – a slowing of the movement of blood cells at an inflamed area, sometimes causing capillary blockage.
Debridement – the cutting away of dead or excess skin from a wound.
Decongestant – a drug which reduces congestion caused by an accumulation of blood.
Decubitus – the patient's position in bed; the act of lying down.
Demulcent – an agent used generally internally to sooth and protect mucous membranes.
Dermatitis – an inflammation of the skin.
Dermatomycosis – lesions or eruptions caused by fungi on the skin.
Detergent – an emulsifying agent useful for cleansing wounds and ulcers as well as the skin.
Dextrocardia – when the heart is located on the right side of the chest.
Diagnostic Aid – a drug used to determine the functional state of a body organ or the presence of a disease.
Diaphoretic – a drug used to increase perspiration; a hydroticorsudorfice.
Diarrhea – an abnormal frequency and fluidity of stools.
Digestive Enzyme – an enzyme that promotes digestion by supplementing the naturally occurring counterpart.
Digitalization – the administration of digitalis to obtain a desired tissue level of drug.
Diplopia – double vision.
Disinfectant – an agent that destroys pathogenic microorganisms on contact and is suitable for sterilizing inanimate objects.
Distal – farthest from a point of reference.
Diuretic – a drug that promotes renal excretion of electrolytes and water, thereby increasing urine volume.
Dysarthria – difficulty in speech articulation.
Dysmenorrhea – pertaining to painful menstruation.
Dysphagia – difficulty in swallowing.
Dyspnea – difficult breathing.
Ecbolic – a drug used to stimulate the gravid uterus to the expulsion of the fetus, or to cause uterine contraction; an oxytocic.
Eclampsia – a toxic disorder occurring late in pregnancy involving hypertension, weight gain, edema and renal dysfunction.
Ectasia – pertaining to distension or stretching.
Ectopic – out of place; not in normal position.
Eczema – an inflammatory disease of the skin with infiltrations, watery discharge, scales and crust.
Effervescent – bubbling; sparkling; giving off gas bubbles.
Embolus – a blood clot in the blood stream lodged in a vessel, thus obstructing circulation.
Emetic – a drug that induces vomiting, either locally by gastrointestinal irritation or systemically by stimulation of receptors in the central nervous system.
Emollient – a topical drug, especially an oil or fat, used to soften the skin and make it more pliable.
Endometrium – the uterine mucous membrane.
Enteralgia – an intestinal pain.
Enterobiasis – a pinworm infestation.
Enuresis – involuntary urination, as in bedwetting.
Epidermis – the outermost layer of the skin.
Episiotomy – a surgical incision of the vulva when deemed necessary during childbirth.
Epistaxis – a nosebleed.
Erythema – redness.
Erythrocyte – a red blood cell.
Escharotic – corrosive.
Estrogen – a hormone that stimulates and maintains female secondary sex characteristics and functions in the menstrual cycle to promote uterine gland proliferation.
Etiology – the cause of a disease.

Euphoria – an exaggerated feeling of well being.
Eutonic – having normal muscular tone.
Exfoliation – a scaling of the skin.
Exophthalmos – a protrusion of the eyeballs.
Expectorant – a drug that increases secretion of respiratory tract fluid, thereby lowering its viscosity and cough-inducing irritancy and promoting its ejection.
Extension – the movement of a joint to move two body parts away from each other.
Exteroceptors – receptors on the exterior of the body.
Fasciculations – the visible twitching movements of muscle bundles.
Fibroid – a tumor of fibrous tissue, resembling fibers.
Filariasis – the condition of having round worm parasites reproducing in the body tissues.
Fistula – an abnormal opening leading from a body cavity to the outside of the body or to another cavity.
Flexion – the movement of a joint in which two moveable parts are brought toward each other.
Fungistatic – inhibiting the growth of fungi.
Furunculosis – a condition marked by the presence of boils.
Gallop Rhythm – a heart condition where three separate beats are heard instead of two.
Gastralgia – a stomach pain.
Gastritis – inflammation of the stomach lining.
Gastrocele – a hernial protrusion of the stomach.
Gastrodynia – pain in the stomach, a stomach ache.
Geriatrics – a branch of medicine which treats problems peculiar to old age.
Germicidal – an agent that is destructive to pathogenic microorganisms.
Gingivitis – an inflammation of the gums.
Glaucoma – a disease of the eye evidenced by an increase in intraocular pressure and resulting in hardness of the eye, atrophy of the retina and eventual blindness.
Glossitis – an inflammation of the tongue.
Glucocorticoid – a corticoid which increases gluconeogenesis, thereby raising the concentration of liver glycogen and blood sugar.
Glycosuria – an abnormal quantity of glucose in the urine.
Gout – a disorder which is characterized by a high uric acid level and sudden onset of recurrent arthritis.
Granulation – the formation of small round fleshy granules on a wound in the healing process.
Hematemesis – the vomiting of blood.
Hematinic – a drug that promotes hemoglobin formation by supplying a factor essential for its synthesis.
Hemiplegia – a condition in which one side of the body is paralyzed.
Hematopoietic – a drug that stimulates formation of blood cells, especially by supplying deficient vitamins.
Hemoptysis – expectoration of blood.
Histoplasmosis – a lung infection caused by the inhalation of fungus spores, often resulting in pneumonitis.
Hodgkin's Disease – a disease marked by chronic lymph enlargement sometimes including spleen and liver enlargement.
Hydrocholeresis – puffing out a thinner, more watery bile.
Hypercholesterolemia – the condition of having an abnormally large amount of cholesterol in the body cells.
Hemorrhage – copious bleeding.
Hemostatic – a locally acting drug that arrests hemorrhage by promoting clot formation or by serving as a mechanical matrix for a clot.
Hepatitis – an inflammation of the liver.
Hyperemia – an excess of blood in any part of the body.
Hyperesthesia – an increase in sensations.
Hyperglycemic – a drug that elevates blood glucose level, especially for the treatment of hypoglycemic states.
Hypertension – blood pressure above the normally accepted limits, high blood pressure.
Hypertriglyceridemia – an increased level of triglycerides in the blood.
Hypnotic – a central depressant which, with suitable dosage, induces sleep.
Hypodermoclysis – a subcutaneous injection with a solution.
Hypoesthesia – a diminished sensation of touch.
Hypoglycemic – a drug that promotes glucose metabolism and lowers blood glucose level, useful in the control of diabetes mellitus.
Hypokalemia – an abnormally small concentration of potassium ions in the blood.
Hyposensitize – to reduce the sensitivity to an agent, referring to allergies.
Hypotensive – a drug which diminishes tension or pressure, to lower blood pressure.
Ichthyosis – an inherited skin disease characterized by dryness and scales.
Idiopathic – denoting a disease of unknown cause.
Ileostomy – the establishment of an opening from the ileum to the outside of the body.
Immune Serum – a biological drug containing antibodies for a pathogenic microorganism, useful for passive immunization against the associated disease.
Immunizing Agent, active – an antigenic preparation (toxoid or vaccine) used to induce formation of specific antibodies against a pathogenic microorganism, which provides delayed but permanent protection against the associated disease.
Immunizing Agent, passive – a biological preparation (antitoxin, antivenin or immune serum) containing specific antibodies against a pathogenic microorganism, which provides immediate but temporary protection against the associated disease.

Impetigo – an inflammatory skin infection with isolated pustules.
Insulin – one of the hormones that regulate carbohydrate metabolism, used as replacement therapy in diabetes mellitus.
Inversion – a turning inward.
Irrigating solution – a solution for washing body surfaces or various body cavities.
Isoniazid – a compound effective in tuberculosis treatment.
Keratitis – an inflammation of the cornea.
Keratolytic – a topical drug that softens the superficial keratin-containing layer of the skin to promote exfoliation.
Lacrimal – pertaining to tears.
Laxative – a gentle purgative medicine; a mild cathartic.
Leishmaniasis – a number of types of infections transmitted by sand flies.
Leucocytopenia – a decrease in the number of white cells.
Leucocytosis – an increased white cell count.
Leukoderma – an absence of pigment from the skin.
Libido – sexual desire or creative energy.
Leucocyte – a white blood cell.
Lipoma – a fatty tumor.
Lipotropic – a drug, especially one supplementing a dietary factor, that prevents the abnormal accumulation of fat in the liver.
Lochia – a vaginal discharge of mucus, blood and tissue after childbirth.
Lues – a plague; specifically syphilis.
Macrocyte – a large red blood cell.
Malaise – a general feeling of illness.
Melasma – a darkening of the skin.
Melena – black feces or black vomit from altered blood in the higher GI tract.
Meninges – the membranes covering the brain and spinal cord.
Metastasis – the shifting of a disease or its symptoms from one part of the body to another.
Mastitis – an inflammation of the breast.
Miotics – agents which constrict the pupil of the eye; a myotic.
Moniliasis – an infection with any of the species of monilia types of fungi *(Candida)*.
Mucolytic – an agent that can destroy or dissolve mucous membrane secretions.
Myalgia – a pain in the muscles.
Myasthenia Gravis – a chronic progressive muscular weakness caused by myoneural conduction, usually spreading from the face and throat.
Myelocyte – an immature white blood cell in the bone marrow.
Myelogenous – originating in bone marrow.
Myoclonus – involuntary, sudden and rapid unpredictable jerks; faster than chorea.
Mydriatic – a drug that dilates the pupil of the eye, usually by anticholinergic or adrenergic mechanism.
Myoneural – pertaining to muscle and nerve.
Myopia – nearsightedness.
Narcotic – a drug that produces insensibility or stupor, a class of drug regulated by law.
Neonatal – pertaining to the first four weeks of life.
Neoplasm – an abnormal tissue growing more rapidly than usual showing a lack of structural organization.
Nephritis – an inflammation of the kidney.
Nephrosclerosis – a hardening of the kidney tissue.
Neuralgia – a pain extending along the course of one or more of the nerves.
Neurasthenia – nervous prostration.
Neuroglia – the supporting elements of the nervous system.
Neuroleptic – a substance that acts on the nervous system.
Neurosis – a functional disorder of the nervous system.
Nocturia – urination at night.
Normocytic – pertaining to anemia due to some defect in the blood-forming tissues.
Nuchal – the nape of the neck.
Nystagmus – a rhythmic oscillation of the eyes.
Oleaginous – oily or greasy.
Omphalitis – an inflammation of the navel in a newborn.
Onychomycosis – a ringworm or fungus infection of the nails.
Ophthalmic – pertaining to the eye.
Oral – pertaining to the mouth.
Orthopnea – a discomfort in breathing in any but the upright sitting or standing positions.
Ossification – a formation of, or conversion to, bone.
Osteomyelitis – an inflammation of the marrow of the bone.
Osteoporosis – a reduction in bone quantity; skeletal atrophy.
Otalgia – pain in the ear; an earache.
Otitis – inflammation of the ear.
Otomycosis – an ear infection caused by fungus.
Otorrhea – a discharge from the ear.
Oxytocic – a drug that selectively stimulates uterine motility and is useful in obstetrics, especially in the control of postpartum hemorrhage.
Palpitations – an awareness of one's heart action.
Paget's Disease – a disease characterized by lesions around the nipple and areola found in elderly women.
Pallor – the lack of the normal red color imparted to the skin by the blood of the superficial vessels.
Parasympatholytic – See Anticholinergic.
Parasympathomimetic – See Cholinergic.
Parenteral – pertaining to the administration of a drug by means other than through the alimen-

tary canal; subcutaneous, intramuscular or intravenous administration of drug.

Parkinsonism – a group of neurological disorders marked by hypokinesia, tremor, and muscular rigidity.

Paroxysm – a sudden recurrence or intensification of symptoms.

Pathogenic – giving origin to disease.

Pediatric – pertaining to children's diseases.

Pediculicide – an insecticide suitable for erradicating louse infestations in humans (pediculosis).

Pediculosis – an infestation with lice.

Pellagra – characterized by GI disturbances, mental disorders, and skin redness and scaling due to niacin deficiency.

Pernicious – particularly dangerous or harmful.

Phlebitis – an inflammation of a vein.

Pleurisy – an inflammation of the membrane surrounding the lungs and the thoracic cavity.

Pneumonia – an infection of the lungs.

Poikilocytosis – a condition in which pointed or irregularly shaped red blood cells are found in the blood.

Polydipsia – excessive thirst.

Posology – the science of dosage.

Posterior Pituitary Hormone(s) – a multifunctional hormone with oxytocic-milk ejection, and antidiuretic-vasopressor fractions.

Progestin – a hormone that functions in the menstrual cycle and during pregnancy to promote uterine gland secretion and to reduce uterine motility.

Pronation – the act of turning the palm downward or backward.

Prophylactic – a remedy that tends to prevent disease.

Protectant – a topical drug that remains on the skin and serves as a physical barrier to the environment.

Proteolytic Enzyme – an enzyme used to liquefy fibrinous or purulent exudates.

Psoriasis – an inflammatory skin disease accompanied with itching.

Psychotherapeutic – a drug that selectively affects the central nervous system to alter emotional state. See Antidepressant; Tranquilizer.

Ptosis – a drooping or sagging of the muscle.

Pulmonary – pertaining to the lungs.

Purulent – containing or forming pus.

Pyelitis – a local inflammation of renal and pelvic cells due to bacterial infection.

Pylorospasm – a spasmodic muscle contraction of the pyloric portion of the stomach.

Pyoderma – any skin discharge characterized by pus formation.

Radiopaque Medium – a diagnostic drug, opaque to X-rays, whose retention in a body organ or cavity makes X-ray visualization possible.

Raynaud's Phenomenon – spasms of the digital arteries with blanching and numbness of the fingers, usually with another disease.

Reflex Stimulant – a mild irritant suitable for application to the nasopharynx to induce reflex respiratory stimulation.

Rheumatoid – a condition resembling rheumatism.

Rhinitis – an inflammation of the mucous membrane of the nose.

Rubefacient – a topical drug that induces mild skin irritation with erythema, sometimes used to relieve the discomfort of deep-seated inflammation.

Rubeola – a synonym popularly used for both measles and rubella.

Saprophytic – getting nourishment from dead material.

Sarcoma – a malignant tumor derived from connective tissue.

Scabicide – an insecticide suitable for the erradication of itch mite infestations in humans (scabies).

Schistosomacide – an agent which destroys schistosomes; destructive to the trematodic parasites or flukes.

Schistosomiasis – an infection with *Schistosoma haematobium* involving the urinary tract and causing cystitis and hematuria.

Scintillation – a visual sensation manifested by an emission of sparks.

Sclerosing Agent – an irritant suitable for injection into varicose veins to induce their fibrosis and obliteration.

Scotomata – an area of varying size and shape within the visual field in which vision is absent or depressed.

Seborrhea – a condition arising from an excess secretion of sebum.

Sebum – the fatty secretions of sebaceous glands.

Sedative – a central depressant which, in suitable dosage, induces mild relaxation useful in treating tension.

Sinusitis – an inflammation of a sinus.

Skeletal Muscle Relaxant – a drug that inhibits contraction of voluntary muscles, usually by interfering with their innervation.

Smooth Muscle Relaxant – a drug that inhibits contraction of involuntary (eg, visceral) muscles, usually by action upon their contractile elements.

Sociopath – a psychopathic person who, due to his unaccepted attitudes, is badly adjusted to society.

Spasmolytic – an agent that relieves spasms and involuntary contraction of a muscle; an antispasmodic.

Sputum – mucous spit from the mouth.

Stenosis – the narrowing of the lumen of a blood vessel.

Stomachic – a drug which is used to stimulate the appetite and gastric secretion.

Stomatitis – an inflammation of the mouth.

Subcutaneous – under the skin.
Sudorific – causing perspiration.
Superacidity – an increase of the normal acidity of the gastric secretion; hyperacidity.
Supination – the act of turning the palm forward or upward.
Suppressant – a drug useful in the control, rather than the cure, of a disease.
Surfactant – a surface active agent that decreases the surface tension between two miscible liquids; used to prepare emulsions, act as a cleansing agent, etc.
Synarthrosis (fibrous joint) – a joint in which the bony elements are united by continuous fibrous tissue.
Syncope – fainting.
Synovia – clear fluid which lubricates the joints; joint oil.
Systole – the ventricular contraction phase of a heartbeat.
Tachycardia – a rapid contraction rate of the heart.
Taeniacide – an agent used to kill tapeworms.
Taeniafuge – agent to expel tapeworms.
Therapeutic – a treatment of disease.
Thoracic – pertaining to the chest.
Thyroid Hormone – a drug containing one or more of the iodinated amino acids that stimulate and regulate the metabolic rate and functional state of body tissues.
Thyroid Inhibitor – drug that reduces excessive thyroid hormone production, usually by blocking hormone synthesis.
Tics – a repetitive twitching of muscles, often in the face and upper trunk.
Tinea – a fungal infection of the skin.
Tonic – an agent used to stimulate the restoration of tone to muscle tissue.
Tonometry – the measurement of tension in some part of the body.
Topical – the local external application of a drug to a particular place.
Toxoid – a modified bacterial toxin, less toxic than the original form, used to induce active immunity to bacterial pathogens.
Tranquilizer – a psychotherapeutic drug that induces emotional repose without significant sedation, useful in treating certain neuroses and psychoses.
Tremors – involuntary rhythmic tremulous movements.
Trichomoniasis – an infestation with parasitic flagellate protozoa of the genus *Trichomonas.*
Trypanosomiasis – a disease caused by protozoan flagellates in the blood.
Uricosuric – drug that promotes renal uric acid excretion; used to treat gout.
Urolithiasis – a condition marked by the formation of stones in the urinary tract.
Urticaria – a rash of hives generally of systemic origin.
Vaccine – preparation of live attenuated or dead pathogenic microorganisms, used to induce active immunity.
Vasoconstrictor – an adrenergic drug used locally in the nose to constrict blood vessels and reduce tissue congestion.
Vasodilator – a drug that relaxes vascular smooth muscles, expecially for the purpose of improving peripheral or coronary blood flow.
Vasopressor – an adrenergic drug used systemically to constrict blood vessels and raise blood pressure.
Verruca – a wart.
Vertigo – illusion of movement.
Vesicant – an agent which, when applied to the skin causes blistering and the formation of vesicles, an epispastic.
Visceral – pertaining to the internal organs.
Vitamin – an organic chemical essential in small amounts for normal body metabolism, used therapeutically to supplement the naturally occurring counterpart in foods.

Container Requirements for U.S.P. 23 Drugs

The listing of container and storage requirements for U.S.P. drugs is included as an aid to the practitioner in storing and dispensing.

Legend:

A = Pressurized Container
C = Collapsible Tubes
CD = Cool, Dry Place
Co = Cold Place
F = Avoid Freezing
FR = Freezer Temp specified
G = Glass Specified
H = Reduced Moisture
He = Protect from Excessive Heat
In = Inert Atmosphere
LR = Light Resistant Container
Ox = Protect from Oxidation
OT = Ophthalmic Tube
P = Plastic Specified
R = Remote from Fire
S = Separate Ingredient Packaging Before Mixing
SC = Radioactive Shielding
S/M = Single Dose/Multi Dose
SP = Special Consideration
Sy = Syringes
T = Tight Container
TP = Tamper-Proof
U = Unit Dose
WC = Well Closed Container
WP = Well Filled Container
+ = Controlled Temperature

---

a = Tablets
b = Capsules
c = Solution
d = Syrup
e = Elixir
f = Cream
g = Ointment/Paste
h = Lotion
i = Suppository
j = Suspension
k = Ophthalmic
l = Aerosol
m = Vaginal
n = Lozenges
o = Powder
p = Enema
r = Inhalation
s = Nasal
t = Gel/Jelly
u = Granules
v = Otic
w = Intraocular Solution
x = Veterinary Use
y = Emulsion
z = Tincture
* = Effervescent
♦ = Sterile if Required

Drugs (Dosage Form)	WC	T	LR
Acebutolol HCl		X[o]	
Acepromazine Maleate	X[oa]		X[oa]
Acetaminophen	X[it]	X[abo]	X[o]
Acetaminophen Oral		X[ej*]	
Acetaminophen and Aspirin (tab)		X	
Acetaminophen, Aspirin and Caffeine	X[a]	X[b]	
Acetaminophen and Caffeine		X[ab]	
Acetaminophen and Codeine Phosphate		X[ab]	X[ab]
Acetaminophen and Codeine Phosphate Oral		X[cj]	X[cj]
Acetaminophen and Diphenhydramine Citrate (tab)		X	
Acetaminophen for Effervescent Oral Soln.		X	
Acetaminophen and Pseudoephedrine HCl		X[a]	
Acetohydroxamic Acid		X[ao+]	

Drugs (Dosage Form)	WC	T	LR
Acetazolamide	X[ao]		
Acetic Acid Otic Soln.		X	
Acetohexamide	X[ao]		
Acetohydroxamic Acid		X[ao+]	
Acetylcysteine (Soln.)		S/M(In)	
Acyclovir		X[og]	
Adenine	X[o]		
Air, Medical			
Alanine	X[o]		
Albendazole	X[o]		
Albendazole, Oral		X[j+]	
Albuterol	X[oa]		X[oa]
Albuterol Sulfate	X[o]		X[o]
Alclometasone Dipropionate		X[o]C[fg]	
Alcohol		R	
Alcohol, Dehydrated		R	
Alcohol, Rubbing		R	
Alfentanil HCl	X[o]		
Allopurinol	X[ao]		
Aloe	X		

Drugs (Dosage Form)	WC	T	LR
Alprazolam	X[o]	X[a]	X[a]
Alprostadil			X[+]
Alteplase	SP[+]		
Alum	X		
Amdinocilllin			X[o]
Alum, Ammonium	X		
Alum, Potassium	X		
Alumina & Magnesia	X[a]		
Alumina & Magnesia Oral			X[j+]
Alumina & Magnesium Carbonate Oral	X[a]		F[j+]
Alumina, Magnesia and Calcium Carbonate Oral	X[a]	F	
Alumina & Magnesium Carbonate and Magnesium Oxide (tab)		X	
Alumina & Magnesium Triscilicate Oral		X[j+a]	
Alumina, Magnesia, Calcium Carbonate, & Simethicone (tabs)	X		
Alumina, Magnesia & Simethicone Oral		F[j+]	
Aluminum Acetate Topical Soln.		X	
Aluminum Chloride		X[o]	
Aluminum Chlorhydrate	X[oc]		
Aluminum Chlorhydrex Polyethylene Glycol	X		
Aluminum Dichlorhydrate	X[oc]		
Aluminum Dichlorhydrex Polyethylene Glycol	X		
Aluminum Hydroxide Gel	X[ab]	X[j+]	
Aluminum Hydroxide Gel, Dried	X[ab]	X[o]	
Aluminum Phosphate Gel	F[a]	F[j+]	
Aluminum Sesquichlorhydrate	X[oc]		
Aluminum Sesquichlorhydrex Polyethylene Glycol	X		
Aluminum Subacetate Topical Soln.		X	
Aluminum Sulfate	X[o]		
Aluminum Sulfate and Calcium Acetate for Topical Solution		He[a]	
Aluminum Zirconium Octachlorohydrate	X[oc]		
Aluminum Zirconium Octachlorohydrex Gly	X[oc]		
Aluminum Zirconium Pentachlorohydrate	X[oc]		
Aluminum Zirconium Pentachlorohydrex Gly	X[oc]		
Aluminum Zirconium Tetrachlorohydrate	X[oc]		
Aluminum Zirconium Tetrachlorohydrex Gly	X[oc]		
Aluminum Zirconium Trichlorohydrate	X[oc]		
Aluminum Zirconium Trichlorohydrex Gly	X[oc]		
Amantadine HCl	X[o]	X[bd]	
Amcinonide	X[o]	X[fg]	
Amdinocillin		X[o]	
Amikacin	X[o]		
Amikacin Sulfate	X[o]		
Amiloride HCl	X[ao]		
Amiloride HCl & Hydrochlorothiazide (tab)	X		
Aminobenzoic Acid		X[tc]	X[tc]
Aminobenzoic Acid Topical		X[c]	X[c]
Aminobenzoate Potassium	X[ba]	X[c]	
Aminobenzoate Potassium Oral		X[c]	
Aminobenzoate Sodium	X[o]		
Aminocaproic Acid		X[ad]	
Aminoglutethimide	X[o]	X[a]	X[a]
Aminophylline	X[i+]	X[a]	
Aminophylline Delayed Release		X[a]	
Aminophylline, Oral		X[c]	
Aminosalicylate Sodium		X[ao+]	X[ao+]
Aminosalicylic Acid		X[ao+]	X[ao+]
Amitriptyline HCl	X[ao]		
Aromatic Ammonia Spirit		X[+]	X[+]
Ammonium Chloride	X[o]		
Ammonium Chloride Delayed Release (tab)		X	
Amobarbital Sodium		X[o]	
Ammonium Molybdate		X[o]	
Amodiaquine		X	
Amodiaquine HCl		X[oa]	
Amoxapine	X[a]	X[o]	
Amoxicillin		X[a]	X[abo+♦]
Amoxicillin Intramammary Infusion		Sy[x+]	
Amoxicillin Oral Susp.	M[x+]		
Amoxicillin for Oral Susp.		X[+]	

Drugs (Dosage Form)	WC	T	LR
Amoxicillin & Clavulanate Potassium		X[h+a]	
Amoxicillin & Clavulanate Potassium for Oral Susp.		X[+]	
Amphetamine Sulfate		X[ao]	
Amphotericin B	C[fgh]		
Ampicillin (all dosage forms)		X	
Ampicillin and Probenecid (cap)		X	
Ampicillin and Probenecid for Oral Susp.		U	
Ampicillin Boluses		X[x]	
Ampicillin Sodium		X[o◆]	
Ampicillin Soluble Powder		X[x]	
Amprolium (all dosage forms)		X	
Amrinone	X		X
Amyl Nitrite (inhalant)		UG[+]	UG[+]
Anileridine HCl		X[ao]	X[ao]
Antazoline Phosphate		X[o]	
Anthralin		X[fg+]	X[fg+]
Antimony Potassium Tartrate	X[o]		
Antimony Sodium Tartrate		X	
Antipyrine	X[o]		
Antipyrine & Benzocaine Otic Soln.		X	X
Antipyrine, Benzocaine and Phenylephrine HCl Otic Soln.		X	X
Apomorphine HCl		X[ao]	X[oa]
Apraclonidine HCl		X[o]	X[o]
Apraclonidine Ophthalmic		X[c]	X[c]
Arginine	X[o]		
Arginine HCl	X[o]		
Arsanilic Acid	X[o]		
Ascorbic Acid (tab)		X	X
Ascorbic Acid Oral		X[c]	X[c]
Ascorbate, Calcium		X[o]	X[o]
Aspirin	X[i+]	X[abo]	
Aspirin Boluses	X		
Aspirin, Buffered		X[a]	
Aspirin, Delayed Release		X[ab]	
Aspirin Effervescent Tablets for Oral Soln.		X	
Aspirin Extended-Release (tab)		X	

Drugs (Dosage Form)	WC	T	LR
Aspirin, Alumina and Magnesia (tab)		X	
Aspirin, Alumina, and Magnesium Oxide (tab)		X	
Aspirin, Caffeine and Dihydrocodeine Bitartrate (cap)		X	
Aspirin and Codeine Phosphate (tab)	X		X
Aspirin, Codeine Phosphate, Alumina and Magnesia (tab)	X		X
Aspirin, Codeine Phosphate and Caffeine	X[ab]		
Atenolol	X[oa]		
Atenolol and Chlorthalidone	X[a]		
Atropine		X[o]	X[o]
Atropine Sulfate	X[ao]		
Atropine Sulfate Ophthalmic	C[g]	X[c]	
Attapulgite Activated	X		
Activated Attapulgite, Colloidal	X		
Azaperone	X[o]		
Azatadine Maleate	X[ao]		
Azathioprine		X[a]	X[ao]
Azithromycin	X[b]	X[o]	
Azrithromycin for Oral		X[j]	
Azathioprine (tab)			X
Azlocillin Sodium		X[o◆]	
Aztreonam		X[o]	
Bacampicillin HCl		X[ao]	
Bacampicillin HCl for Oral Susp.		X	
Bacitracin		X[o+]	
Bacitracin (ointment)	X[g+]	COT[k+]	
Bacitracin and Polymixin B Sulfate Topical		A[l+]	
Bacitracin Methylene Disalicylate, Soluble	X[x]	X[ox]	
Bacitracin Zinc Soluble Powder		X[x]	
Bacitracin Zinc	X[g+]	X[o+]	
Bacitracin Zinc & Polymixin B Sulfate (ointment)	X	COT[k]	X
Baclofen	X[a]	X[o]	
Bandage, Adhesive	SP		
Bandage, Gauze	SP		
Barium Hydroxide Lime		X[o]	
Barium Sulfate	X[o]		

Drugs (Dosage Form)	WC	T	LR
Barium Sulfate for Suspension	X		
Beclomethasone Dipropionate	X		
Belladonna Extract		X[ao]	X[ao]
Belladonna Leaf	X[o]		X[o]
Belladonna Tincture		X[+]	X[+]
Bendroflumethiazide		X[ao]	
Benoxinate HCl	X[o]		
Benoxinate HCl Ophthalmic Soln.		X	
Benzethonium Chloride (Tincture)		X	X
Benzethonium Chloride Topical	X[c]	X[c]	
Benzocaine	X[tn]	X[fg+]	X[fg+]
Benzocaine Otic Soln.		X[+]	X[+]
Benzocaine Topical		x[cl+]	X[c+]
Benzocaine, Butamben, and Tetracaine HCl Topical	A[l+]	F[c+]	
Benzocaine, Butamben, and Tetracaine HCl		F[gt]	
Benzocaine and Menthol Topical		AH[e]	
Benzoic Acid	X[o]		
Benzoic & Salicylic Acid (ointment)	X[+]		
Benzoin (Resin)	X		
Benzoin Tincture Compound		X[+]	X[+]
Benzonatate		X[bo]	X[bo]
Hydrous Benzoyl Peroxide	SP		
Benzoyl Peroxide		X[ht]	
Benzthiazide		X[ao]	
Benztropine Mesylate	X[a]	X[o]	
Benzyl Benzoate		X[ho]	WP[o+]
Benzylpenicilloyl Polylysine Concentrate		X	
Beta Carotene		X[ob]	X[ob]
Betaine HCl	X		
Betamethasone	X[ad]	C[f]	
Betamethasone Acetate		X[o]	
Betamethasone Benzoate		X[ko]C[k]	
Betamethasone Dipropionate	XC[g]	X[hi]	C[f]
Betamethasone Dipropionate Topical		A[l+]	
Betamethasone Sodium Phosphate		X[o]	
Betamethasone Valerate	C[fg]	X[fgo]	X[h]
Betaxolol HCl		X[oa]	
Betaxolol HCl Ophthalmic		X[c]	
Bethanechol Chloride		X[oa]	
Biotin		X[o]	
Biperiden	X[o]		X[o]
Biperiden HCl	X[o]	X[a]	X[o]
Bisacodyl	X[aio+]		
Biscadoyl (Delayed Release)	RT[a]		
Bisacodyl Rectal Suspension	URT		
Milk of Bismuth	X[+]		
Bismuth Subcarbonate	X[o]		X[o]
Bismuth Subgallate		X[o]	X[o]
Bismuth Subnitrate	X[o]		
Bismuth Subsalicylate		X[o]	X[o]
Bleomycin Sulfate		X[o]	
Bretylium Tosylate	X[o]		
Bromocriptine Mesylate		X[ao+]	X[ao+]
Bromodiphenhydramine HCl		X[bo]	X[e]
Brompheniramine Maleate	X[e]	X[ao]	X[eo]
Brompheniramine Maleate and Pseudoephedrine Sulfate Syr.	X		X
Bumetanide		X[ao]	X[ao]
Buprenorphine HCl		X[o]	X[o]
Buspirone HCl		X[oa+]	X[oa+]
Busulfan	X[a]	X[o]	
Butabarbital		X[o]	
Butabarbital Sodium	X[ab]	X[eo]	
Butalbital	X[o]		
Butalbital, Acetaminophen, and Caffeine		X[ab]	
Butabital and Aspirin (tab)		X	
Butabital, Aspirin & Caffeine		X[ab]	
Butalbital, Aspirin, Caffeine and Codeine Phosphate		X[b]	X[b]
Butamben	X		
Butoconazole Nitrate	X[o]	C[f+]	X[o]
Butorphanol Tartrate		X[o]	
Caffeine, hydrous		X[o]	
Caffeine, anhydrous	X[o]		
Calamine	X[o]	X[h]	
Calamine, Phenolated		X[h]	
Calciferol		X[bo+]	X[bo+]
Calcium Acetate	X[a]	X[o]	
Calcium Ascorbate		X[o]	X[o]

Drugs (Dosage Form)	WC	T	LR
Calcium Carbonate	X[aon]		
Calcium Carbonate Oral		F[j]	
Calcium Carbonate & Magnesia (tab)	X		
Calcium & Magnesium Carbonates (tab)	X		
Calcium Carbonate, Magnesia & Simethicone (tab)	X		
Calcium Chloride		X[o]	
Calcium Citrate	X[o]		
Calcium Glubionate		X[d+]	
Calcium Gluceptate	X[o]		
Calcium Gluconate	X[ao]		
Calcium Hydroxide Topical Soln.		X	
Calcium Lactate	X[a]	X[o]	
Calcium Lactobionate	X[o]		
Calcium Levulinate	X[o]		
Calcium Pantothenate		X[ao]	
Calcium Pantothenate, Racemic		X[o]	
Calcium Phosphate, dibasic	X[ao]		
Calcium Polycarbophil		X[o]	
Calcium Saccharate	X[o]		
Calcium Undecylenate	X[o]		
Camphor		X[o]	
Camphor Spirit		X	
Candicidin	XT[g+]	X[m+]	
Capreomycin Sulfate		X[o]	
Capsaicin		CD	CD
Captopril		X[oa]	
Captopril and Hydrochlorothiazide		X[a]	
Carbachol		X[o]	
Carbachol Soln.		X[kw+]	
Carbamazepine		X[o]GH[a]	
Carbamazepine Oral		F[j+]	F[j+]
Carbamide Peroxide		X[o+]	X[o+]
Carbamide Peroxide Topical Soln.		X[+]	X[+]
Carbenicillin Disodium		X[o]	
Carbenicillin Indanyl Sodium		X[ao+]	
Carbidopa	X[o]		
Carbidopa & Levodopa	X[a]		X[a]
Carbinoxamine Maleate		X[ao]	X[ao]
Carbol-Fuchsin Topical Soln.		X	X
Carbon Dioxide	A		
Carbon Monoxide C-11	(S/M)A[+]		

Drugs (Dosage Form)	WC	T	LR
Carboprost Tromethamine	X[o+]		
Carboxymethylcellulose Sodium Paste	X[+]		
Carboxymethylcellulose Sodium		X[ao]	
Carisoprodol	X[a]	X[o]	
Carisoprodol and Aspirin (tab)	X		
Carisoprodol, Aspirin & Codeine Phosphate (tab)	X		
Carteolol HCl	X[o]	X[a]	
Carteolol HCl Soln.	X[k]		
Casanthranol		X[o+]	X[o+]
Cascara Sagrada Extract		X[+]	X[+]
Cascara Sagrada Fluid Extract		X[+]	X[+]
Cascara (tab)		X	
Cascara, Aromatic Fluid Extract		X[+]	X[+]
Castor Oil		X[by+]	
Castor Oil, Aromatic		X	
Cefaclor		X[bo]	
Cefaclor for Oral Susp.		X	
Cefadroxil		X[abo]	
Cefadroxil for Oral Susp.		X	
Cefamandol Naftate		X[o◆]	
Cefazolin		X[o]	
Cefazolin Sodium		X[o]	
Cefixime for Oral Suspension		X[j]	
Cefixime		X[ao]	
Cefmenoxime HCl		X[o◆]	
Cefonicid Sodium		X[o◆]	
Cefoperazone Sodium		X[o◆]	
Ceforanide		X[o◆]	
Cefotaxime Sodium		X[o◆]	
Cefotetan		X[o◆]	
Cefotetan DIsodium		X[o◆]	
Cefotiam HCl		X[o◆]	
Cefoxitin Sodium		X[o]	
Cefpiramide		X[o◆]	
Cefprozil		X[oa]	
Cefprozil for Oral Susp.		X[j]	
Ceftazidime		X[o◆]	
Ceftizoxime Sodium		X[o◆]	
Ceftriaxone Sodium		X[o◆]	
Cefuroxime Axetil	X[a]	X[o]	
Cefuroxime Sodium		X[o◆]	
Cellulose Sodium Phosphate	X		

Drugs (Dosage Form)	WC	T	LR
Cephalexin		X[abo]	
Cephalexin for Oral Susp.		X	
Cephalexin HCl		X[o]	
Cephalothin Sodium		X[o◆]	
Cephapirin Benzathine	X[o]		
Cephapirin Benzathine Intramammary Infusion	S[y+]		
Cephapirin Sod.		X[o◆]	
Cephapirin Sodium Intramammary Infusion	S[y+]		
Cephradine		X[ab◆]	
Cephradrine for Oral Susp.		X[j]	
Cetylpyridinium Chloride	X[no]	X[c]	
Cetylpyridinium Chloride Topical Solution		X[j]	
Charcoal, Activated	X		
Chloral Hydrate		X[bo]	X[d]
Chlorambucil	X[a]	X[o]	X[ao]
Chloramphenicol (all dosage forms)		X	
Chloramphenicol Ophthalmic		CTP[cg+]	
Chloramphenicol Palmitate		X[o]	
Chloramphenicol Palmitate Oral Susp.		X	X
Chloramphenicol and Hydrocortisone Acetate for Ophthalmic Susp.		X	
Chloramphenicol and Polymixin B Sulfate Ophthalmic Oint.		COT	
Chloramphenicol, Polymixin B Sulfate & Hydrocortisone Acetate Ophthalmic Oint.		COT	
Chloramphenicol & Polymixin B Sulfate Ophthalmic Oint.		COT	
Chloramphenicol & Prednisolone Ophthalmic Oint.		COT	
Chlordiazepoxide		X[ao]	X[ao]
Chlordiazepoxide & Amitriptyline HCl (tab)	X	X	
Chlordiazepoxide HCl		X[bo]	X[bo]
Chlordiazepoxide HCl and Clidinium Bromide (cap)		X	X

Drugs (Dosage Form)	WC	T	LR
Chlorphyllin Copper Complex Sodium		X[o]	X[o]
Chloroprocaine HCl	X[o]		
Chloroquine	X[o]		
Chloroquine Phosphate	X[ao]		
Chlorothiazide	X[ao]		
Chlorothiazide Oral Susp.		X	
Chloroxylenol	X[o]		
Chlorpheniramine Maleate		X[ado]	X[do]
Chlorpheniramine Maleate Extended Release (cap)		X	
Chlorpromazine	X[i]	X[o]	X[oi]
Chlorpromazine HCl	X[a]	X[do]	X[ao]
Chlorpromazine HCl Oral Concentrate		X	X
Chlorpromazine HCl (supp)	X[+]		X[+]
Chlorpropamide	X[ao]		
Chlorprothixene	X[ao]		X[ao]
Chlorprothixene Oral Susp.		X	X
Chlortetracycline Bisulfate		X[o]	X[o]
Chlortetracycline HCl	C[g]	X[bao◆]	C[g]X[ba]
Chlortetracycline and Sulfamethazine Bisulfates Soluble Pwd.		X[x]	X[x]
Chlortetracycline HCl Soluble Pwd.		X[x]	X[x]
Chlortetracycline HCl Ophthalmic Oint.		COT	
Chlorthalidone	X[ao]		
Chlorzoxazone		X[ao]	
Cholecalciferol		In[o+]	In[o+]
Cholestyramine Resin		X[o]	
Cholestyramine for Oral Susp.		X	
Chromic Chloride		X[o]	
Chymotrypsin		X[o+]	
Chymotrypsin for Ophthalmic Soln.		UG[+]	
Ciclopirox Olamine	X[o]C[f+]		
Ciclopirox Olamine Topical		X[j]	
Cimetidine		X[ao+]	X[ao+]
Cinoxacin	X[b]	X[o]	
Cinoxate		X[ho+]	X[ho+]
Ciprofloxacin	X[a]	X[o]	X[o]
Ciprofloxacin HCl	X[a]	X[o]	X[o]
Ciprofloxacin Soln.		RT[k]	X[k]
Ciprofloxacin Ophth.		X[c+]	X[c+]

Drugs (Dosage Form)	WC	T	LR
Cisplatin		X[o]	X[o]
Citric Acid		X[o]	
Clarithromycin		X[ao]	
Clarithromycin for Oral Susp.		X	
Clavulanate Potassium		X[o◆]	
Clemastine Fumarate	X[a]	X[o+]	X[o+]
Clidinium Bromide		X[bo]	X[bo]
Clindamycin HCl		X[bo]	
Clindamycin Palmitate HCl		X[o]	
Clindamycin Palmitate HCl for Oral Soln.		X	
Clindamycin Phosphate		X[ot◆]	
Clindamycin Phosphate Cream	X[m]		
Clindamycin Phosphate Topical		X[cj]	
Clioquinol	X[o]	C[fg]	C[fg]
Compound Clioquinol Topical		X[o]	
Clioquinol and Hydrocortisone		XC[fg]	X[fg]
Clocortolone Pivalate		X[o]C[f]	X[o]C[f]
Clofazimine	X[b]	X[o+]	X[o+]
Clofibrate	X[b]	X[o]	X[bo]
Clomiphene Citrate	X[ao]		X[a]
Clonazepam		X[ao+]	X[ao+]
Clonidine HCl	X[ao]		
Clonidine HCl & Chlorthalidone (tabs)	X		
Clorazepate Dipotassium		In[o]	In[o]
Clorsulon	X[o]		
Clotrimazole	X[mo+]	X[h+]	X[+]
Clotrimazole Topical		X[ct]	
Clotrimazole (cream)		C[+]	
Clotrimazole and Betamethasone Dipropionate (cream)		XC	
Cloxacillin Benzathine		X[ox◆]	
Cloxacillin Sodium		X[bo+◆]	
Cloxacillin Sodium for Oral Solution		X[c]	
Coal Tar		X[g]	
Coal Tar Topical		X[c]	
Cyanocobalamin Co-57	X[b]	X[c]	X[bc]
Cocaine		X[o]	X[o]
Cocaine HCl		X[o]	X[o]
Cocaine HCl Tablets for Topical Soln.	X		
Cod Liver Oil		In	
Codeine		X[o]	X[o]
Codeine Phosphate	X[a]	X[o]	X[ao]

Drugs (Dosage Form)	WC	T	LR
Codeine Sulfate	X[a]	X[o]	X[o]
Colchicine	X[a]	X[o]	X[ao]
Colestipol HCl		X[o]	
Colestipol HCl for Oral Susp.		XU	
Colistin Sulfate		X[o]	
Colistin Sulfate for Oral Susp.		X	X
Colistin & Neomycin Sulfates & Hydrocortisone Acetate Otic Susp.		X	
Collodion		X	
Collodion, Flexible		X[+]	
Colloidal Oatmeal	X		
Copper Gluconate	X[o]		
Cortisone Acetate	X[ao]		
Cotton, Purified	SP		
Cromolyn Sodium		X[o]	
Cromolyn Sodium Inhalation		S/M	
Cromolyn Sodium for Inhalation		X[+]	X[+]
Cromolyn Sodium Soln.		X[s]	X[s]
Cromolyn Sodium Ophthalmic		S/M[c]	S/M[c]
Croscarmellose Sodium		X	
Crotamiton		X[o]C[f]	C[f]X[o]
Cupric Chloride		X[o]	
Cupric Sulfate		X[o]	
Cyanocobalamin		X[o]	X[o]
Cyclacillin		X[ao]	
Cyclacillin for Oral Susp.		X	
Cyclizine HCl		X[ao]	X[ao]
Cyclobenzaprine HCl	X[ao]		
Cyclopentolate HCl		X[+]	
Cyclopentolate HCl Ophthalmic Soln.		X[+]	
Cyclophosphamide		X[ao+]	
Cyclopropane		A	
Cycloserine		X[bo]	
Cyclosporine		X[bo]	X[o]
Cyclosporine Oral Soln.		X	
Cyproheptadine HCl	X[ao]	X[d]	
Cysteine HCl	X[o]		
Cytarabine		X[o◆]	X[o◆]
Dacarbazine		X[o+]	X[o+]
Dactinomycin		X[o+]	X[o+]
Danazol	X[b]	X[o]	X[o]
Dapsone	X[ao]		X[ao]
Daunorubicin HCl		X[o+]	X[o+]
Decoquinate	PM[x]	X[o]	
Deferoxamine Mesylate		X[o]	
Dehydrocholic Acid	X[ao]		

Drugs (Dosage Form)	WC	T	LR
Demecarium Bromide		X[o]	X[o]
Demecarium Bromide Ophthalmic Soln.		X	X
Demeclocycline		X[o]	X[o]
Demeclocycline Oral Susp.		X	X
Demeclocycline HCl		X[abo]	X[abo]
Demeclocycline HCl & Nystatin		X[ab]	X[ab]
Desipramine HCl		X[ab]	
Deslanoside		X[o]	X[o]
Desoximetasone	C[ftg+]	C[ft+]	C[f]
Desoxycortisone Acetate	X[o]		X[o]
Dexamethasone	X[ao]	X[e]C[t+]	
Dexamethasone Topical	A[l+]		
Dexamethasone Ophth.		X[j]	
Dexamethasone Acetate	X[o]		
Dexamethasone Sodium Phosphate		C[f]X[rt]	C[k]
Dexamethasone Sodium Phosphate Inhalation	A[l+]		
Dexamethasone Sodium Phosphate Ophth.	C[k]	X[c]	X[c]
Dexbrompheniramine Maleate		X[o]	X[o]
Dexchlorpheniramine Maleate		X[ado]	X[do]
Dexpanthenol		X[o]	
Dexpanthenol Preparation		X	
Dextroamphetamine Sulfate	X[ao]	X[eb]	X[e]
Dextromethorphan		X[o]	
Dextromethorphan HBr		X[ao]	X[a]
Dextrose	X[o]		
Diatrizoate Meglumine	X[o]		
Diatrizoate Meglumine & Diatrizoate Sodium Solution		X	X
Diatrizoate Sodium	X[o]		
Diatrizoate Sodium Soln.		X	X
Diatrizoic Acid	X[o]		
Diazepam		X[abo]	X[abo]
Diazepam Extended-Release (cap)		X	X
Diazoxide	X[bo]		
Diazoxide Oral Susp.		X	X
Dibucaine		X[o]C[fg]	X[o]C[fg]
Dibucaine HCl		X[o]	X[o]
Dichloralphenazone	X[o]		
Dichlorphenamide	X[ao]		
Diclofenac Sodium		X	X
Diclofenac Sod. Delayed Release		X[a]	X[a]

Drugs (Dosage Form)	WC	T	LR
Dicloxacillin Sodium		X[bo]	
Dicloxacillin Sodium for Oral Susp.		X	
Dicyclomine HCl	X[abo]	X[d]	
Dienestrol	X[o]	C[f]	
Diethylcarbamazine Citrate		X[ao]	
Diethylpropion HCl	X[ao]		X[o]
Diethylstilbestrol	X[a]	X[o]	X[o]
Diethylstilbestrol Diphosphate		X[+]	
Diethyltoluamide		X[o]	
Diethyltoluamide Topical Soln.		X	
Diflorasone Diacetate		X[o]C[fg+]	C[fg+]
Diflunisal	X[ao]		
Digitalis		X[ab]	X[o]
Digitoxin	X[a]	X[o]	
Digoxin		X[aeo+]	
Dihydrocodeine Bitartrate		X[o]	
Dihydrostreptomycin Sulfate Boluses		X[x]	
Dihydroergotamine Mesylate		X[o]	X[o]
Dihydrotachysterol	X[ba]	In[o]	X[ba]
Dihydrotachysterol Oral Soln.		X	X
Dihydroxyaluminum Aminoacetate	X[abo]		
Dihydroxyaluminum Aminoacetate Magma	F[+]		
Dihydroxyaluminum Sodium Carbonate	X[a]	X[o]	
Diltiazem HCl		X[ao]	X[ab]
Diltiazem HCl Extended Release	X[ab]		
Dimenhydrinate	X[ao]	X[d]	
Dimercaprol		X[+]	
Dimethyl Sulfoxide		X[+]	X[+]
Dimethyl Sulfoxide		X[tx]	X[tx]
Dimethyl Sulfoxide Topical		X[cx]	X[cx]
Dinoprost Tromethamine		X[o]	
Diphenhydramine Citrate		X[o]	X[o]
Diphenhydramine HCl		X[bo]	X[eo]
Diphenhydramine and Pseudoephedrine (cap)		X	
Diphenoxylate HCl	X[o]		
Diphenoxylate HCl & Atropine Sulfate (tab)	X		X

Drugs (Dosage Form)	WC	T	LR
Diphenoxylate HCl and Atropine Sulfate Oral Soln.		X	X
Dipivefrin HCl		X[o]	X[o]
Dipivefrin HCl Ophth.		X[c]	X[c]
Dipyridamole		X[ao]	X[ao]
Disopyramide Phosphate	X[b]	X[o]	X[o]
Disopyramide Phosphate Extended-Release	X[b]		
Disulfiram		X[ao]	X[ao]
Dobutamine HCl		X[o+]	
Docusate Calcium	X[o]	X[b+]	
Docusate Potassium	X[o]	X[b+]	
Docusate Sodium	X[ao]	X[b+dc]	X[d]
Dopamine HCl		X[o]	
Doxapram		X[o]	
Doxepin HCl	X[bo]		
Doxepin HCl Oral Soln.		X	X
Doxorubicin HCl		X[o]	
Doxycycline		X[ob]	X[b]
Doxycycline for Oral Susp.		X	X
Doxycycline Calcium Oral Susp.		X	X
Doxycycline Hyclate		X[abo◆]	X[abo◆]
Doxycycline Hyclate Delayed-Release (cap)		X	X
Doxylamine Succinate	X[ao]	X[d]	X[ado]
Dronabinol	X[b+]	In[o+]	In[bo+]
Droperidol		In[o+]	In[o+]
Dusting Powder, Absorbable	X		
Dyclonine HCl Topical Soln.		X	X
Dyclonine HCl (gel)		P/G	G
Dydrogestrone	X[ao]		
Dydrogesterone (tab)	X		
Dyphylline		X[aeo]	
Dyphylline and Guaifenesin		X[ac]	
Echothiophate Iodide		X[o]	X[o]
Echothiophate Iodide for Ophthalmic Soln.		G[+]	
Econazole Nitrate	X[o]		X[o]
Edetate Calcium Disodium		X[o]	
Edrophonium Chloride	X[o]		
Elm	CD[o]		
Emetine HCl		X[o]	X[o]
Enalapril Maleate	X[ao]		
Enalapril Maleate and Hydrochlorothiazide	X[a]		

Drugs (Dosage Form)	WC	T	LR
Enalaprilat	X[o]		
Enflurane		X[o+]	X[o+]
Ephedrine		X[o+]	X[o+]
Ephedrine HCl	X[o]		X[o]
Ephedrine Sulfate	X[a]	X[bd]	X[bd]
Ephedrine Sulfate Nasal		X[c]	X[c]
Ephedrine Sulfate & Phenobarbital (cap)	X		
Epinephrine		X[o]	X[o]
Epinephrine Soln.		X[krs]	X[krs]
Epinephrine Inhalation Aerosol		X	X
Epinephrine Bitartrate	X[o]	X[k]	X[k]
Epinephrine Bitartrate Inhalation Aerosol	X	X	
Epinephryl Borate Ophthalmic Soln.		X	X
Epitetracycline HCl		X[o]	X[o]
Equilin		X[o]	X[o]
Ergocalciferol		In[o]X[ab]	In[o]X[ab]
Ergocalciferol Oral Soln.		X	X
Ergoloid Mesylates Oral Soln.		X[+]	X[+]
Ergoloid Mesylates		X[abo+]	X[abo+]
Ergonovine Maleate	X[a]	X[o]	X[o]
Ergotamine Tartrate	X[ao]		X[o]
Ergotamine Tartrate Inhalation Aerosol		A	A
Ergotamine Tartrate & Caffeine	X[a]	X[i+]	X[a]
Diluted Erythrityl Tetranitrate		X[+]	
Erythrityl Tetranitrate (tab)		X[+]	
Erythromycin		X[ao]	
Erythromycin Delayed-Release		X[ab]	
Erythromycin (oint)		CX[+]	
Erythromycin Ophthalmic		COT[g]	
Erythromycin Pledgets		X	
Erythromycin Topical		X[ct]	
Erythromycin and Benzoyl Peroxide Topical		SX[t]	
Erythromycin Estolate		X[abjo]	
Erythromycin Estolate Oral Susp.		X[+]	
Erythromycin Estolate for Oral Soln.		X	
Erythromycin Estolate & Sulfisoxazole Acetyl Oral		X[j]	
Erythromycin Ethylsuccinate		X[ao]	

Drugs (Dosage Form)	WC	T	LR
Erythromycin Ethylsuccinate Oral Susp.	X		
Erythromycin Ethylsuccinate for Oral Susp.		X	
Erythromycin Ethylsuccinate & Sulfisoxazole Acetyl for Oral Susp.	X		
Erythromycin Stearate		X[ao]	
Estradiol		X[ao]	X[ao]
Estradiol, Cream		C[m]	
Estradiol Cypionate		X[o]	X[o]
Estradiol Valerate		X[o]	X[o]
Estriol		X[o]	
Estrogens, Conjugated	X[ao]		
Estrogens, Esterified	X[a]	X[o]	
Estrone		X[o]	X[o]
Estropipate	X[a]	C[mf]X[o]	
Ethacrynic Acid	X[ao]		
Ethambutol HCl	X[ao]		
Ethchlorvynol		X[ba]P[o]	X[bao]
Ether		R[+]	R[+]
Ethinyl Estradiol	X[a]	X[o]	X[o]
Ethionamide		X[ao]	
Ethopropazine HCl	X[a]	X[o]	X[ao]
Ethosuximide		X[bo]	
Ethotoin		X[ao]	
Ethyl Chloride		R[+]	
Ethylene Diamine		WP,G	
Ethynodiol Diacetate	X[o]		
Ethynodiol Diacetate & Ethinyl Estradiol (tab)	X		
Ethynodiol Diacetate & Mestranol (tab)	X		
Etidronate Disodium		X[ao]	
Etoposide		X[bo]	X[bo]
Eucalyptol		X	
Eucatropine HCl		X[o]	X[o]
Eucatropine HCl Ophthalmic Soln.		X	
Eugenol	X	X	
Factor 1X Complex		X[+]	
Famotidine	X[ao]		X[ao]
Fenoprofen Calcium	X[abo]		
Fentanyl Citrate		X[o]	
Ferrous Fumarate		X[o]	X[a]
Ferrous Fumarate & Docusate Sodium Extended-Release (tabs)	X		
Ferrous Gluconate		X[abeo]	X[e]
Ferrous Sulfate		X[acdo]	X[c]
Ferrous Sulfate, Dried	X[o]		
Flecainide Acetate	X[ao]		X[a]
Floxuridine		X[o]	X[o]
Flucytosine		X[bo]	X[bo]
Fluhydrocortisone Acetate	X[ao]		X[o]
Flumethasone Pivalate		X[o]C[f]	X[o]
Flunisolide Nasal Soln.	X[+]	X[+]	
Flunixin Meglumine	X[oug]		
Fluocinolone Acetonide	X[o]	C[fg]	
Fluocinolone Acetate Topical Soln.		X	
Fluocinonide	X[o]C[fgt]		
Fluocinonide Topical		X[c]	
Fluorescein		X[o]	
Fluorescein Sodium		X[o]	
Fluorescein Sodium and Benoxinate HCl Ophthalmic		X[c]	X[c]
Fluorescein Sodium & Proparacaine HCl Ophthalmic		G+	G[+]
Fluorometholone		X[o]C[f]	X[o]
Fluorometholone Ophthalmic Susp.		X	
Fluorouracil		X[of+]	X[o]
Fluorouracil Topical		X[c+]	
Fluoxetine HCl		X	
Fluoxymesterone	X[ao]		X[ao]
Fluphenazine Decanoate	X[o]	X[o]	
Fluphenazine Enanthate	X[o]	X[o]	
Fluphenazine HCl Oral Soln.		X	X
Fluphenazine HCl		X[aeo]	X[eao]
Flurandrenolide		X[fgh]	X[fgh]
Flurandrenolide tape	X[+]		
Flurazepam HCl		X[bo]	X[bo]
Flurbiprofen	X[a]	X[o]	
Flurbiprofen Sodium		X[o]	
Flurbiprofen Sodium Ophthalmic Soln.		X	
Flutamide		X[ob]	X[ob]
Folic Acid	X[ao]		X[o]
Formaldehyde Soln.		X[+]	
Fructose		X[o]	
Basic Fuchsin	X[o]		
Furazolidone		X[j+o]	X[j+o]
Furosemide	X[a]	X[o+]	X[ao+]
Gallamine Triethiodide		X[o]	X[o]
Gauze (all)	X		
Gemfibrozil		X[ab]	
Gentamicin Sulfate		X[do]C[fg]	
Gentamicin Sulfate Ophthalmic	X[c+]	COT[g]	

Drugs (Dosage Form)	WC	T	LR
Gentamicin Sulfate and Betamethasone Acetate Soln.		X^{k}	
Gentamicin Sulfate and Betamethasone Valerate		CT^{2}	
Gentamicin Sulfate and Betamethasone Valerate Topical		X^{cv}	
Gentamicin and Prednisolone Acetate Ophthalmic	OT^{g+}	X^{j}	
Gentian Violet		$X^{c}C^{ft}$	
Gentian Violet Topical		X^{c}	
Glipizide		X^{o}	
Glucagon		InG^{+}	
Gluconolactone	X^{o}		
Glucose Enzymatic Test Strip	SP^{+}		
Glutaral Concentrate		X^{+}	X^{+}
Glutethimide	X^{abo}		
Glyburide	X^{a}	X^{o}	
Glycerin		X	
Glycerin Oral Soln.		X	
Glycerin Suppository	X^{+}		
Glycerin Ophthalmic Soln.		TPG/P	X
Glycopyrrolate		X^{ao}	
Gold Sodium Thiomalate	X^{o}	X^{o}	
Chorionic Gonadotropin	G^{+}		
Gramicidin		X^{o}	
Green Soap Tincture		X	
Griseofulvin		X^{abo}	
Griseofulvin Oral Susp.		X	
Griseofulvin, Ultramicrosize (tab)		X	
Guaifenesin		X^{abdo}	
Guaifenesin & Codeine Phosphate Syrup		X^{+}	X^{+}
Guaifenesin and Pseudoephedrin HCl		X^{b}	X^{b}
Guaifenesin, Pseudoephedrine HCl and Dextromethorphan HBr		X^{b}	X^{b}
Guanabenz Acetate		X^{ao}	X^{ao}
Guanadrel Sulfate	X^{o}	X^{a}	X^{a}
Guanfacine HCl		X^{oa}	X^{oa}
Gutta Percha	X^{o}		X^{o}
Halazone		X^{o}	X^{o}
Halazone Tablets for Solution		X	X
Halcinonide	X^{afgo}		
Haloperidol		X^{ao}	X^{ao}
Haloperidol Oral Soln.		X	X
Haloprogin		X^{+fo}	X^{fo}
Haloprogin Topical Soln.		X^{+}	X
Halothane		G^{+}	X^{+}
Helium		A	
Heparin Calcium		X^{o}	
Heparin Sodium		X^{o+}	
Hetacillin Potassium	X^{ao}		
Hetacillin Potassium Oral Susp.		X	
Hexachlorophen		X^{o}	X^{o}
Hexachlorophene Cleansing Emulsion		X	X
Hexachlorophene Liquid Soap		X	X
Hexylresorcinol		X^{no}	X^{o}
Histamine Phosphate		X^{o}	X^{o}
Histidine	X^{o}		
Homatropine HBr		X^{o}	X^{o}
Homatropine Hydrobromide Ophthalmic Soln.		X	
Homatropine Methylbromide		X^{ao}	X^{ao}
Hydralazine HCl		X^{ao}	X^{a}
Hydrochlorothiazide	X^{ao}		
Hydrocodone Bitartrate		X^{ao}	X^{ao}
Hydrocodone Bitartrate and Acetaminophen		X^{a}	X^{a}
Hydrocortisone	X^{ag}	X^{fhpt}	
Hydrocortisone Acetate	X^{fg}	X^{h}	
Hydrocortisone Acetate Ophthalmic		X^{gk}	
Hydrocortisone and Acetic Acid Otic Soln.		X	X
Hydrocortisone Butyrate	X^{fo}		
Hydrocortisone Hemisuccinate		X^{o}	
Hydrocortisone Sodium Phosphate		X^{o}	
Hydrocortisone Sodium Succinate		X^{o}	X^{o}
Hydrocortisone Valerate	X^{fo}		
Hydroflumethiazide		X^{ao}	
Hydrogen Peroxide Concentrate	SP^{+}		
Hydrogen Peroxide Topical Soln.		X^{+}	X^{+}
Hydromorphone HCl		X^{ao}	X^{ao}
Hydroquinone	X^{f}	X^{o}	X^{+o}
Hydroquinone Topical Soln.		X	X
Hydroxocobalamin		X^{o}	X^{o}
Hydroxyamphetamine HBr	X^{o}		X^{o}

Drugs (Dosage Form)	WC	T	LR
Hydroxyamphetamine HBr Ophthalmic Solution		X	X
Hydroxychloroquine Sulfate	X[o]	X[a]	X[ao]
Hydroxyprogesterone Caproate	X[o]		X[o]
Hydroxypropyl Cellulose Ocular System		U[+]	
Hydroxypropyl Methylcellulose (all grades)	X[o]		
Hydroxypropyl Methylcellulose Ophthalmic Soln.		X	
Hydroxyurea		X[bo]	
Hydroxyzine HCl		X[ado]	X[d]
Hydroxyzine Pamoate	X[b]	X[o]	
Hydroxyzine Pamoate Oral Susp.		X	X
Hyoscyamine	X[a]	X[o]	X[ao]
Hyoscyamine HBr		X[o]	X[o]
Hyoscyamine Sulfate		X[aeo+]	X[aeo+]
Hyoscyamine Sulfate Oral Soln.		X[+]	X[+]
Ibuprofen	X[a]	X[o]	
Ibuprofen Oral	X[j+]		
Ibuprofen and Pseudoephedrine HCl		X[a]	
Ichthammol	X	C[g+]	
Idarubicin HCl		X[o]	
Idoxuridine		X[o]	X[o]
Idoxuridine Ophthalmic	C[gt]	X[c]	X[c]
Ifosfamide		X[o+◆]	
Imipramine HCl		X[ao]	
Indapamide	X[oa]		
Indigotindisulfonate Sodium		X[o]	X[o]
Indium In 111 Oxyquinoline		U[c+]	
Indocyanine Green	X[o◆]		
Indomethacin	X[bi+o]		
Indomethacin Extended-Release (cap)	X		
Indomethacin Oral		X[j]	X[j]
Indomethacin Sodium	X[o◆]		X[o]
Insulin		X[+]	X
Insulin Human		X[+]	X
Inulin	X[o]		
Iocetamic Acid	X[o]	X[a]	
Iodine (all Soln. & Tinct.)		X[+]	X[+]
Iodide, Sodium, 1-123, 1-131	X[bc]		
Iodipamide	X[o]		
Iodoquinol	X[ao]		

Drugs (Dosage Form)	WC	T	LR
Iohexol	X[o]		X[o]
Iopamidol	X[o]		X[o]
Iopanoic Acid		X[ao]	X[ao]
Iophendylate		X	X
Iothalamic Acid	X[o]		
Ioversol	X		
Ioxaglic Acid	X[o]		
Ipecac		X[d+o]	
Ipodate Calcium		X[o]	
Ipodate Calcium for Oral Susp.	X		
Ipodate Sodium		X[ao]	
Isocarboxazid	X[ao]		X[a]
Isoetharine Inhalation Soln.		WF	Ox
Isoetharine HCl		X[o]	
Isoetharine Mesylate		X[o]	
Isoetharine Mesylate Inhalation Aerosol			X
Isoflurane		X[o]	X[o]
Isoflurophate		G[+]	
Isoflurophate Ophthalmic		C[g]	
Isoleucine	X[o]		
Isometheptene Mucate	X[o]		
Isometheptene Mucate Dichloralphenazone, and Acetaminophen	X[b]		
Isoniazid	X[a]	X[do]	X[ado]
Isopropamide Iodide	X[ao]		X[o]
Isopropyl Alcohol (all)		X[+]	
Isoproterenol Inhalation Soln.		WF	Ox
Isoproterenol HCl	X[a]	X[arlo]	X[arlo]
Isoproterenol HCl Inhalation		A[l]	
Isoproterenol HCl & Phenylephrine Bitartrate Inhalation Aerosol		X	X
Isoproterenol Sulfate		X[o]	X[o]
Isoproterenol Sulfate Inhalation		WF[cl]	Ox[cl]
Isosorbide Concentrate		X	X
Isosorbide Oral Soln.	X		
Isosorbide Dinitrate, Diluted		X	
Isosorbide Dinitrate (tab)	X		
Isosorbide Dinitrate Chewable (tab)	X		
Isosorbide Dinitrate Extended Release	X[ab]		
Isosorbide Dinitrate Sublingual (tab)	X		

Drugs (Dosage Form)	WC	T	LR
Isotretinoin		In[mo]	X[o]
Isoxsuprine HCl		X[ao]	
Isradipine	X		X
Juniper Tar		X[+]	X[+]
Kanamycin Sulfate		X[bo]	
Kaolin	X[o]		
Ketamine HCl	X[o]		
Ketoconazole	X[ao]		
Ketoprofen		X[o]	
Ketorolac Tromethamine	X[o]H[a+]		X[o]H[a+]
Krypton Ke 81m		SP[+]	
Labetalol HCl		X[oat]	X[oat]
Lactase	X[t]		
Lactic Acid		X	
Lactulose (soln/conc)		X[+]	
Lanolin	X[+]		
Modified Lanolin		X[+](Rust proof)	
Leucine	X[o]		
Leucovorin Calcium	X[a+o]		X[a+o]
Levamisole HCl	X[ao]		X[o]
Levmetamfetamine		X	X
Levobunolol HCl	X[o]		
Levobunolol HCl Ophthalmic Soln.		X	
Levocarnitine		X[ao]	
Levocarnitine Oral Soln.		X	
Levodopa		X[abo+]	X[abo+]
Levonordefrin	X[o]		
Levonorgestrel	X[ao]		X[ao]
Levonorgestrel and Ethinyl Estradiol (tab)	X		
Levorphanol Tartrate	X[ao]		
Levothyroxine Sodium		X[ao]	X[ao]
Levothyroxine Sodium Oral		X[o]	X[o]
Lidocaine	X[o]	X[gl]	
Lidocaine Topical		A[l]	
Lidocaine Oral Topical Soln.		X	
Lidocaine HCl Oral Topical Soln.		X	
Lidocaine Topical Soln.		X	
Lidocaine HCl	X[o]	X[t]	
Lime		X	
Lincomycin HCl		X[bdo◆]	
Lindane		X[fho]	
Lindane Shampoo		X	
Liothyronine Sodium		X[ao]	
Liotrix (tab)		X	
Lisinopril	X[oa]		
Lithium Carbonate	X[abo]		
Lithium Carbonate Extended-Release (tab)	X		

Drugs (Dosage Form)	WC	T	LR
Lithium Citrate		X[do]	
Lithium Hydroxide		X[o]	
Loperamide HCl	X[bao]		
Loracarbef	X[b]	X[o]	
Loracarbef for Oral Susp.		X	
Lorazepam		X[ao]	X[ao]
Lorazepam Oral Conc.	X		X
Lovastatin	X[a+]	In[o+]	X[a+]
Loxapine Succinate		X[o]	
Loxapine		X[bo]	
Lypressin Nasal Soln.		P	
Lysine Acetate	X[o]		
Lysine HCl	X[o]		
Mafenide Acetate		X[f+o]	X[f+o]
Magaldrate	X[ao]		
Magaldrate Oral Susp.		X	
Magaldrate & Simethicone (tab)	X		
Magaldrate & Simethicone Oral Susp.		X[+]	
Milk of Magnesia		F[+]	
Magnesia (tab)	X		
Magnesium Carbonate	X[o]		
Magnesium Carbonate & Sodium Bicarbonate for Oral Susp.		X	
Magnesium Chloride		X[o]	
Magnesium Citrate		X	
Magnesium Citrate Oral Soln.		SP[+]	
Magnesium Gluconate	X[ao]		
Magnesium Hydroxide		X[o]	
Magnesium Hydroxide Paste		X	
Magnesium Oxide	X[abo]		
Magnesium Salicylate		X[ao]	
Magnesium Sulfate	X[o]		
Magnesium Trisilicate	X[ao]		
Malathion		X[o]G[h]	X[o]
Maltitol		X[c]	
Manganese Chloride		X[o]	
Manganese Gluconate	X[o]		
Manganese Sulfate		X[o]	
Mannitol	X[o]		
Maprotiline HCl	X[a]	X[o]	
Mazindol		X[ao+]	
Mebendazole	X[ao]		
Mebrofenin		X[o]	
Mecamylamine HCl	X[a]	X[o]	
Mechlorethamine HCl		X	X
Meclizine HCl	X[a]	X[o]	

Drugs (Dosage Form)	WC	T	LR
Meclocycline Sulfosalicylate		X[fo+]	X[fo+]
Meclofenamate Sodium		X[bo+]	X[bo+]
Medroxyprogesterone Acetate	X[aj]	X[o]	X[o]
Mefenamic Acid		X[ob]	X[o]
Megestrol Acetate	X[ao]		X[o]
Meglumine	X[o]		
Melphalon	X[a]	G[o]	G[o]
Menadiol Sodium Diphosphate	X[a]	X[o+]	X[ao+]
Menadione	X[o]		X[o]
Menotropins		G[o+]	
Menthol	X[n]	X[+]	
Meperidine HCl	X[a]	X[d]	X[ad]
Mephentermine Sulfate	X[o]		X[o]
Mephenytoin	X[ao]		
Mephobarbital	X[ao]		
Mepivacaine HCl	X[o]		
Meprednisone		X[+]	X[+]
Meprobamate	X[a]	X[o]	
Meprobamate Oral Susp.		X	
Mercaptopurine	X[ao]		
Ammoniated Mercury	X[o]		X[o]
Mercury, Ammoniated (ointment)		C[k]	
Mesoridazine Besylate	SP[a]X[o]		X[ao]
Mesoridazine Besylate Oral Soln.		X[+]	X[+]
Mestranol	X[o]		X[o]
Metacresol		X[o]	X[o]
Metaproterenol Sulfate	X[a]	X[od]	X[oda]
Metaproterenol Sulfate Soln.	A[r]	WF[l]	Ox[l]
Metaraminol Bitartrate	X[o]		
Methacholine Chloride		X[o]	
Methacycline HCl		X[ao]	X[ao]
Methacycline HCl Oral Susp.		X	X
Methadone HCl	X[a]	X[o]	X[o]
Methadone HCl Oral Soln.		X[+]	X[+]
Methadone HCl Oral Concentrate		X[+]	X[+]
Methamphetamine HCl	X[a]	X[o]	X[oa]
Methazolamide	X[ao]		
Methdilazine		X[ao]	X[ao]
Methdilazine HCl		X[ado]	X[ado]
Methenamine	X[ao]	X[e]	
Methenamine & Monobasic Sodium Phosphate (tab)		X	
Methenamine Mandelate (tab)	X		
Methenamine Mandelate Delayed Release	X[a]		
Methenamine Mandelate for Oral Soln.	X[c]	X[j]	
Methicillin Sodium		X[+◆]	
Methimazole	X[ao]		X[ao]
Methionine	X[o]		
Methocarbamol		X[ao]	
Methohexital		X[o]	
Methotrexate	U[a]	X[o]	X[o]
Methoxsalen	X[o]	X[b]	X[bo]
Methotrimeprazine	X[o]		X[o]
Methoxsalen Topical Solution		X	X
Methoxyflurane		X[o+]	X[o+]
Methsuximide		X[bo+]	
Methylclothiazide	X[ao]		
Methylbenzethonium Chloride	X[e]	X[bo]C[g]	
Methylbenzethonium Chloride Topical		X[o]	
Methylcellulose	X[ao]		
Methylcellulose Ophth Soln.		X	
Methylcellulose Oral Soln.		X[+]	X[+]
Methyldopa	X[ao]		X[o]
Methyldopa Oral Susp.		X[+]	X[+]
Methyldopa and Chlorothiazide (tab)	X		
Methyldopa & Hydrochlorothiazide (tab)	X		
Methyldopate HCl	X[o]		
Methylene Blue	X[o]		
Methylergonovine Maleate		X[ao+]	X[ao+]
Methylphenidate HCl	X[o]	X[a]	
Methylphenidate HCl Extended-Release		X[a]	
Methylprednisolone		X[ao]	X[ao]
Methylprednisolone Acetate	X[p]	X[o]C[f]	X[fo]
Methylprednisolone Hemisuccinate		X[o]	
Methylprednisolone Sodium Succinate		X[o]	X[o]
Methyltestosterone	X[abo]		X[o]
Methysergide Maleate		X[ao]	X[o]
Metoclopramide Oral Soln.		F[+]	F[+]
Metoclopramide HCl		X[oa]	X[oa]
Metocurine Iodide		X[o]	

Drugs (Dosage Form)	WC	T	LR
Metolazone		X[oa]	X[oa]
Metoprolol Fumarate		X[o]	X[o]
Metoprolol Tartrate		X[oa]	X[oa]
Metoprolol Tartrate & Hydrochorothiazide (tab)		X	X
Metronidazole	X[ao]	CP[t+]	X[ao]
Metyrapone		X[ao+]	X[ao+]
Metyrosine (cap)	X		
Mezlocillin Sodium		X[◆]	
Mexiletine HCl		X[bo]	
Miconazole	X[o]		X[o]
Miconazole Nitrate		X[mi]C[f]	
Miconazole Nitrate Topical	X[o]		
Miconazole Nitrate Vaginal (Supp)		X[+]	
Mineral Oil		X[py]	
Mineral Oil, Light, Topical		X	
Minocycline HCl		X[abo◆]	X[abo]
Minocycline HCl Oral Susp.		X	X
Minoxidil	X[o]	X[a]	
Mitomycin		X[o]	X[o]
Mitotane		X[ao]	X[ao]
Mitoxantrone HCl		X[o]	
Molindone HCl		X[ao]	X[ao]
Monensin	X[x]		
Monensin, Granulated	X[x]		
Monensin, Premix	X[x]		
Monensin, Sodium	X[x]		
Monobenzone		X[fo+]	X[o+]
Moricizine HCl		X[oa]	
Morphine Sulfate		X[o]	X[o]
Mupirocin	XC[g]	X[o]	
Nadolol	X[o]	X[a]	
Nadolol and Bendroflumethiazide (tab)		X	
Nafcillin Sodium		X[bao]	X[a]
Nafcillin Sodium for Oral Soln.		X	
Naftifine HCl		X[oft]	
Nalidixic Acid		X[ao]	
Nalidixic Acid Oral Susp.		X	
Nalorphine HCl		X[o]	X[o]
Naloxone HCl		X[o]	X[o]
Nandrolone Decanoate		X[o]	X[o]
Nandrolone Phenpropionate		X[o]	X[o]
Naphazoline HCl		X[o]	X[o]
Naphazoline HCl Soln.		X[ks]	X[ks]
Naproxen	X[o]	X[o]	
Naproxen Oral		X[j+]	X[j+]
Naproxen Sodium	X[a]	X[o]	
Natamycin		X[o]	X[o]
Natamycin Ophthalmic Susp.		TP	
Neomycin Sulfate	X[gf+]	X[ao◆]	X[o◆]
Neomycin Sulfate Ophthalmic Oint.		COT[+]	
Neomycin Sulfate Oral Soln.		X[+]	X[+]
Neomycin Sulfate & Bacitracin		X[g+]	X[g+]
Neomycin Sulfate & Bacitracin Zinc	XC[g]		
Neomycin Sulfate & Dexamethasone Sodium Phosphate		X[f]	
Neomycin Sulfate & Dexamethasone Sodium Phosphate Ophthalmic	X[c+]	COT[g]	X[c+]
Neomycin Sulfate & Fluocinolone Acetonide		XC[f]	
Neomycin Sulfate & Fluorometholone	CX[g]		
Neomycin Sulfate & Flurandrenolide		CX[fgh]	X[fgh]
Neomycin Sulfate & Gramicidin	CX[g]		
Neomycin Sulfate & Hydrocortisone	CX[fg]		
Neomycin Sulfate & Hydrocortisone Otic Susp.	X	X	
Neomycin Sulfate & Hydrocortisone Acetate	CX[fgh]		
Neomycin Sulfate & Hydrocortisone Acetate Ophthalmic		X[i]COT[g]	
Neomycin Sulfate & Methylprednisolone Acetate		CX[f]	X[f]
Neomycin Sulfate & Prednisolone Acetate Ophthalmic		COTX[i]	
Neomycin Sulfate & Prednisolone Sodium Phosphate Ophthalmic Oint.		COT	
Neomycin Sulfate, Sulfacetamide Sodium and Prednisolone Acetate Ophthalmic		COT[g]	

Drugs (Dosage Form)	WC	T	LR
Neomycin Sulfate & Triamcinolone Acetonide		XCT[f]	
Neomycin Sulfate & Triamcinolone Acetonide Ophthalmic Oint.		COT	
Neomycin & Polymixin B Sulfates	X[g+]		
Neomycin & Polymixin B Sulfates Ophthalmic	COT[g+]		X[c+]
Neomycin & Polymixin B Sulfate & Bacitracin Zinc	CX[g]	CX[g]	X[g+]
Neomycin & Polymixin B Sulfate & Bacitracin Zinc & Hydrocortisone Acetate Ophthalmic Oint.		COT	
Neomycin & Polymixin B Sulfate & Bacitracin Zinc & Hydrocortisone Acetate Oint.	CX[+]		
Neomycin and Polymixin B Sulfates, Bacitracin and Lidocaine	X[g+]		
Neomycin & Polymixin B Sulfates, Bacitracin Zinc & Hydrocortisone Acetate Ointment	X[gk+]		
Neomycin & Polymixin B Sulfate & Hydrocortisone Otic Soln.		X	X
Neomycin & Polymixin B Sulfates & Dexamethasone Ophthalmic	COT[g]X[j]	X[j]	
Neomycin & Polymixin B Sulfate & Gramicidin	CX[f]		
Neomycin & Polymixin B Sulfate & Gramicidin Ophthalmic Soln.		X	
Neomycin & Polymixin B Sulfates, Gramicidin & Hydrocortisone Acetate Cream	X		
Neomycin & Polymixin B Sulfates & Hydrocortisone Susp.		TP[kv]	X[kv]
Neomycin & Polymixin B Sulfate & Hydrocortisone Soln.		TP[kv]	X[kv]
Neomycin & Polymixin B Sulfates & Hydrocortisone Acetate Ophthalmic Susp.		X	
Neomycin & Polymixin B Sulfates & Prednisolone Acetate Ophthalmic Susp.		X	
Neostigmine Bromide		X[ao]	
Neostigmine Methylsalicylate		X[o]	
Netilmicin Sulfate		X[o]	
Niacin	X[ao]		
Niacinamide		X[ao]	
Nicotine	InH[+]		H[+]
Nicotine Transdermal System	SPU		SPU
Nicotine Polacrilex		X	
Nicotine Polacrilex Gum	SPU		SPU
Nifedipine		X[bo+]	X[bo+]
Nitrofurantoin		X[abo]	X[abo]
Nitrofurantoin Oral Susp.		X	X
Nitrofurazone		X[fgo]	X[fgo]
Nitrofurazone Topical Soln.		X	X
Nitroglycerin, Diluted		X[+]	X[+]
Nitroglycerin		G[a+]	X[g]
Nitromersol		X[o]	X[o]
Nitromersol Topical Solution		X	X
Nitrous Oxide		A[+]	
Nizatidine		X[ob+]	X[ob+]
Nonoxynol 9		X[o]	
Norepinephrine Bitartrate		X[o]	X[o]
Norethindrone	X[ao]		
Norethindrone & Ethinyl Estradiol (tab)	X		
Norethindrone & Mestranol (tab)	X		
Norethindrone Acetate	X[ao]		
Norethindrone Acetate & Ethinyl Estradiol (tab)	X		
Norethynodrel	X[o]		
Norfloxacin	X[a]	X[o]	X[o]
Norgestrel	X[ao]		
Norgestrel & Ethinyl Estradiol (tab)	X		
Nortriptyline HCl		X[ao]	X[o]
Nortryptyline HCl Oral		X[c]	X[c]
Noscapine	X[o]		
Novobiocin Sod		X[bo]	X[b]
Nystatin	X[g+]	X[ah+n]	X[ah+n]
Nystatin Cream		XC[+]	
Nystatin Vaginal		X[ai+]	X[ai+]
Nystatin Oral Susp.		X	X
Nystatin for Oral Susp.		X	

Drugs (Dosage Form)	WC	T	LR
Nystatin, Neomycin Sulfate, Gramicidin & Triamcinolone Acetonide		X[fg]	
Nystatin, Neomycin Sulfate, Thiostrepton, and Triamcinolone Acetonide		X[fg]	
Nystatin & Triamcinolone Acetonide		X[fg]	
Ofloxacin	X[o]		X[o]
Ointment, White or Yellow	X		
Hydrophilic Ointment		X	
Oleovitamin A & D		X[b]In	X[b]In
Omeprazole	COH[o]		
Bland Lubricating Ophthalmic	OT[g]		
Opium Powder	X		
Opium Tincture		X[+]	X[+]
Orphenadrine Citrate		X[o]	X[o]
Oxacillin Sodium		X[bo+◆]	
Oxacillin Sodium for Oral Soln.		X[+]	
Oxamniquine	X[o]	X[b]	
Oxandrolone	X[o]	X[a]	X[ao]
Oxazepam	X[abo]		
Oxprenolol HCl	X[o]	X[a]	X[a]
Oxprenolol HCl Extended Release (tab)		X	X
Oxtriphylline	X[o]		
Oxtriphylline Oral		X[c]	
Oxtriphylline Delayed Release (tab)		X	
Oxtriphylline Extended Release (tab)		X	
Oxybenzone		X[o]	X[o]
Oxybutynin Chloride	X[o]	X[ad]	X[ad]
Oxycodone and Acetaminophen		X[ab]	X[ab]
Oxycodone and Aspirin (tab)		X	X
Oxycodone HCl		X[oa]	X[a]
Oxycodone HCl Oral Soln.		X	X
Oxycodone Terephthalate		X[o]	
Oxygen 93 Percent		A[+]	
Oxymetazoline HCl		X[o]	
Oxymetazoline HCl Soln.		X[ks]	
Oxymetholone	X[ao]		
Oxymorphone HCl	X[i+]	X[o]	X[o]
Oxyphenbutazone		X[ao]	
Oxytetracycline		X[ao◆]	X[ao]

Drugs (Dosage Form)	WC	T	LR
Oxytetracycline Calcium	X[o]	X[o]	
Oxytetracycline Calcium Oral Susp.		X	X
Oxytetracycline HCl		X[bo]	X[bo]
Oxytetracycline & Nystatin (cap)		X	X
Oxytetracycline and Nystatin for Oral Susp.		X[+]	X[+]
Oxytetracycline HCl & Hydrocortisone Ointment	X		X
Oxytetracycline HCl & Hydrocortisone Acetate Ophthalmic Susp.		X	X
Oxytetracycline & Phenazopyridine Hydrochlorides & Sulfamethizole (cap)		X	X
Oxytetracycline HCl & Polymixin B Sulfate	X[gom]		X[g]
Oxytetracycline HCl & Polymixin B Ophthalmic Oint.		COT	
Oxtriphylline		X[a]	
Oxytocin Nasal Soln.	SP		
Padimate O		X[ho]	X[ho]
Pancreatin		X[abo+]	
Pancrelipase		X[abo+]	
Pancrelipase Delayed-Release		X[b+]	
Panthenol		X[o]	
Papain		X[o]	X[o]
Papain Tablets for Topical Soln.		X[+]	X[+]
Papaverine HCl		X[ao]	X[o]
Parachlorophenol		X[o]	X[o]
Parachlorophenol, Camphorated		X	X
Paraldehyde		G,WF[+]	WF[+]
Paramethasone Acetate	X[a]	X[o]	
Paregoric		X[+]	X[+]
Paromomycin Sulfate		X[bdo]	
Pectin	X		
Penbutolol Sulfate	X[a]	X[oa]	X[oa]
Penicillamine		X[abo]	
Penicillin G Benzathine	X[ao◆]		
Penicillin G Benzathine Oral Susp.		X	
Penicillin G Potassium		X[ao◆]	
Penicillin G Potassium Tablets for Oral Soln.		X	

Drugs (Dosage Form)	WC	T	LR
Penicillin G Procaine, Neomycin & Polymixin B Sulfates & Hydrocortisone Acetate Topical Susp.	X		
Penicillin V		X[ao]	
Penicillin V for Oral Susp.		X	
Penicillin V Benzathine		X	
Penicillin V Benzathine Oral Susp.		X[+]	
Penicillin V Potassium		X[ao]	
Penicillin V Potassium for Oral Soln.		X	
Pentaerythritol Tetranitrate		X[ao+]	
Pentazocine		X[o]	X[o]
Pentazocine HCl		X[ao]	X[ao]
Pentazocine HCl & Aspirin (tab)		X	X
Pentazocine and Naloxone HCl (tab)		X	X
Pentetic Acid	X[o]		
Pentobarbital		X[aeo]	
Pentobarbital Sodium		X[bo]	
Peppermint Spirit		X	
Perflubron		X[o]	X[o]
Perphenazine	X[d]	X[ao]	X[dao]
Perphenazine Oral Soln.	X		X
Perphenazine & Amitriptyline HCl (tab)	X		
Petrolatum (all)	X		
Petrolatum, Hydrophilic	X		
Phenacemide	X[a]	X[o]	
Phenazopyridine HCl		X[ao]	
Phendimetrazine Tartrate	X[a]	X[bo]	
Phenelzine Sulfate		X[ao+]	X[ao+]
Phenmetrazine HCl		X[ao]	
Phenobarbital	X[ao]	X[e]	X[e]
Phenol		X	X
Phenol, Liquefied		G	G
Phenolphthalein (all)	X[o]	X[a]	
Phenoxybenzamine HCl	X[ob]		
Phentermine HCl		X[bao]	
Phentolamine Mesylate	X[o]		X[o]
Phenylalanine	X[o]		
Phenylbutazone		X[abo]	
Phenylbutazone Boluses	X[x]		
Phenylephrine HCl		X[o]	X[o]
Phenylephrine HCl Soln.		X[ks]	X[ks]
Phenylephrine HCl Nasal Jelly	X		
Phenylethyl Alcohol		X[+]	X[+]
Phenylpropanolamine HCl		X[o]	X[o]
Phenylpropanolamine HCl Extended-Release		X[ba]	X[ba]
Phenytoin	X[a]	X[o]	
Phenytoin Oral Susp.		X[+]	
Phenytoin Sodium		X[o]	
Phenytoin Sodium, Extended (cap)		X	
Phenytoin Sodium, Prompt (cap)		X	
Physostigmine		X[o]	X[o]
Physostigmine Salicylate		X[o]	X[o]
Physostigmine Salicylate Ophthalmic Solution		X	X
Physostigmine Sulfate		X[o]	X[o]
Physostigmine Sulfate Ophthalmic Ointment		COT	
Phytonadione	X[a]	X[o]	X[ao]
Pilocarpine		X[o]	X[o]
Pilocarpine HCl		X[o]	X[o]
Pilocarpine HCl Ophthalmic Soln.		X	
Pilocarpine Nitrate		X[o]	X[o]
Pilocarpine Nitrate Ophthalmic		X	X
Pimozide		X[oa]	X[ao]
Pindolol	X[ao]		X[ao]
Piperacillin	X[o◆]		
Piperacillin Sodium		X[o]	
Piperazine		X	X
Piperazine Citrate	X[o]	X[ad]	
Piroxicam		X[bo]	X[bo]
Plantago Seed	X		
Plicamycin		X	X
Podophyllum Resin		X[o]	X[o]
Podophyllum Resin Topical Soln.		X	X
Poloxelene		X	
Polycarbophil		X[o]	
PEG 3350 and Electrolytes for Oral Soln.		X	
Polymixin B Sulfate		X[o◆]	X[o◆]
Polymixin B Sulfate & Bacitracin Zinc Topical	X[o]	A[lt]	
Polymixin B Sulfate & Hydrocortisone Otic Soln.		X	X
Polythiazide		X[ao]	X[ao]
Polyvinyl Alcohol	X[o]		
Sulfurated Potash		SP	
Potassium Acetate		X[o]	
Potassium Bicarbonate	X[o]		

Drugs (Dosage Form)	WC	T	LR
Potassium Bicarbonate Effervescent Tabs for Oral Soln.		X[+]	
Potassium Bicarbonate & Potassium Chloride for Effervescent Oral Soln.		X[+oa]	
Potassium and Sodium Bicarbonate and Citric Acid Effervescent for Oral Solution (tab)		X	X
Potassium Bitartrate		X[o]	
Potassium Carbonate	X[o]		
Potassium Chloride	X[o]		
Potassium Chloride Oral Soln.		X	
Potassium Chloride for Oral Soln.		X	
Potassium Chloride Extended Release		X[ab+]	
Potassium Chloride, Potassium Bicarbonate, and Potassium Citrate Effervescent Tablets for Oral Soln.		X[+]	
Potassium Citrate		X[o]	
Potassium Citrate Extended-Release (tabs)		X	
Potassium Citrate & Citric Acid Oral Solution		X	
Potassium Gluconate		X[aeo]	X[e]
Potassium Gluconate & Potassium Chloride for Oral Soln.	X		
Potassium Gluconate & Potassium Chloride Oral		X	
Potassium Gluconate & Potassium Citrate Oral Soln.	X		
Potassium Gluconate, Potassium Citrate, & Ammonium Chloride Oral Soln.		X	
Potassium Guaiacolsulfonate	X[o]		X[o]
Potassium Iodide		X[o]	
Potassium Iodide Delayed Release		X[a]	
Potassium Iodide Oral Soln.		X	X
Potassium Nitrate		X[oc]	
Potassium Permanganate	X[o]		

Drugs (Dosage Form)	WC	T	LR
Dibasic Potassium Phosphate	X[o]		
Potassium Sodium Tartrate		X[o]	
Povidone		X[o]	
Povidone-Iodine		X	
Povidone-Iodine Topical Soln.		X[+]	
Povidone-Iodine Topical Aerosol Solution		A[+]	
Povidone-Iodine Oint.		X	
Povidone-Iodine Cleansing Soln.		X	
Pralidoxime Chloride	X[ao]		
Pramoxine HCl		X[ft]C[t]	
Prazepam		X[abo]	X[abo]
Praziquantel	X[o]	X[a]	X[o]
Prazosin HCl	X[b]	X[o]	X[bo]
Prednisolone	X[ao]	X[cfd]	X[d]
Prednisolone Acetate	X[o]		
Prednisolone Acetate Ophthalmic Susp.		X	
Prednisolone Hemisuccinate		X[o]	
Prednisolone Sodium Phosphate		X[o]	
Prednisolone Sodium Phosphate Ophthalmic Solution		X	X
Prednisolone Tebutate		In[+]	
Prednisone	X[ao]	X[d]	
Prednisone Oral Soln.		X	
Prilocaine HCl	X[o]		
Primaquine Phosphate	X[ao]		X[ao]
Primadone	X[a]		
Primadone Oral Susp.		X	X
Probenecid	X[ao]		
Probenecid & Colchicine (tab)	X		X
Probucol	X[ao]		X[ao]
Procaine HCl	X[o]		
Procainamide HCl		X[abo]	
Procainamide HCl Extended Release (tab)		X	
Procarbazine HCl		X[bo]	X[bo]
Prochlorperazine		X[co]	X[o]
Prochlorperazine Oral		X[c]	X[c]
Prochlorperazine Edisylate		X[o]	X[o]
Prochlorperazine Edisylate Oral Soln.		X	X
Prochlorperazine Maleate	X[a]	X[o]	X[ao]
Procyclidine HCl		X[ao+]	X[o+]

Drugs (Dosage Form)	WC	T	LR
Progesterone		X[o]	X[o]
Promazine HCl		X[ado]	X[ado]
Proline	X[o]		
Promazine HCl Oral Soln.		X	X
Promethazine HCl		X[adi+]	X[adi+]
Propafenone HCl		X[o]	X[o]
Propantheline Bromide	X[ao]		
Proparacaine HCl	X[o]		
Proparacaine HCl Ophthaimic Soln.		X	X
Propoxycaine HCl	X[o]		X[o]
Propoxyphene HCl		X[bo]	
Propoxyphene HCl & Acetaminophen (tab)		X	
Propoxyphene HCl, Aspirin, & Caffeine (cap)		X[+]	
Propoxyphene Napsylate		X[ao]	
Propoxyphene Napsylate Oral Susp.		X	X
Propoxyphene Napsylate & Acetaminophen (tab)		X[+]	
Propoxyphene Napsylate & Aspirin (tab)		X	
Propranolol HCl	X[ao]		
Propranolol HCl Extended-Release (cap)	X		
Propranolol HCl and Hydrochlorothiazide (tab)	X		
Propranolol HCl and Hydrochlorothiazide Extended-Release (cap)	X		
Propylene Glycol		X	
Propylhexedrine		X	
Propylhexedrine Inhalant		X[+]	
Propylthiouracil	X[ao]		
Protamine Sulfate		X[+]	X[+]
Protriptyline HCl	X[o]	X[a]	
Pseudoephedrine HCl		X[ado]	X[do]
Psyllium Hydrophilic Mucilloid for Oral Susp.		X	
Pumice	X[o]		
Pyrantel Pamoate	X[o]		X[o]
Pyrantel Pamoate Oral Suspension		X	X
Pyrazinamide	X[ao]		
Pyrethrum Extract		X	X
Pyridostigmine Bromide		X[ado]	X[d]
Pyridoxine HCl	X[a]	X[o]	X[ao]
Pyrilamine Maleate	X[a]	X[o]	X[o]

Drugs (Dosage Form)	WC	T	LR
Pyrimethamine		X[ao]	X[ao]
Pyroxylin			SP
Pyrvinium Pamoate		X[ao]	X[ao]
Pyrvinium Pamoate Oral Susp.		X	X
Quazepam	X[oa]		
Quinidine Gluconate	X[o]		X[o]
Quinidine Gluconate Extended-Release	X[a]		X[a]
Quinidine Sulfate	X[ao]	X[b]	X[abo]
Quinidine Sulfate Extended Release (tab)	X		X
Quinine Sulfate	X[ao]	X[b]	X[o]
Racepinephrine		X[o]	X[o]
Racepinephrine Soln.		X[r+]	X[r+]
Racepinephrine HCl		X[o]	X[o]
Ranitidine HCl		X[ao]	X[ao]
Ranitidine Oral Soln.		X[+]	X[+]
Rauwolfia Serpentina	SP	X[a]	X[a]
Purified Rayon	SP		
Rehydration Salts, Oral		SX[a+]	
Reserpine		X[aeo]	X[aeo]
Reserpine & Chlorothiazide (tab)		X	X
Reserpine, Hydralazine HCl & Hydrochlorothiazide (tab)		X	X
Reserpine & Hydrochlorothiazide (tab)		X	X
Resorcinol	X[o]		X[o]
Resorcinol, Compound Ointment		X[+]	
Resorcinol & Sulfur Lotion	X		
Resorcinol Monoacetate		X	X
Ribavirin		X[o]	
Ribavirin for Inhalation Soln.		H[+]	
Riboflavin		X[ao]	X[ao]
Riboflavin 5'-Phosphate Sodium		X[o]	X[o]
Rifampin		X[bo+]	X[bo+]
Rifampin & Isoniazid (cap)		X[+]	X[+]
Ritodrine HCl		X[ao+]	
Rose Water Ointment		X	X
Saccharin Calcium	X[o]		
Saccharin Sodium	X[ao]		
Saccharin Sodium Oral Solution		X	
Safflower Oil		X	X
Salicylamide	X[o]		
Salicylic Acid	X[o]		
Salicylic Acid Collodion		X[+]	

Drugs (Dosage Form)	WC	T	LR
Salicylic Acid Gel		XC[+]	
Salicylic Acid Plaster	X[+]		
Salicylic Acid Topical Foam		X	
Salsalate		X[oab]	
Sargramostim	U(FR)		
Scopolamine HBr		X[ao]	X[ao]
Scopolamine HBr Ophthalmic		X[c]C[g]	
Secobarbital		X[o]	
Secobarbital Elixir		X	
Secobarbital Sodium		X[bo]	
Secobarbital Sodium and Amobarbital Sodium	X[b]		
Selegiline HCl	X[oa]		X[oa]
Selenious Acid		X[o]	
Selenium Sulfide	X[o]		
Selenium Sulfide Lotion		X	
Senna Fluid Extract		X[+]	X[+]
Senna Syrup		X[+]	
Sennosides	X[ao]		
Serine	X[o]		
Silver Nitrate		X[o]	X[o]
Silver Nitrate Ophthalmic Soln.		X	X
Toughened Silver Nitrate		X	X
Simethicone	X[a]	X[yo]	
Simethicone Oral Susp.		X	X
Simvastatin	In[o]		
Sisomicin Sulfate		X[o]	
Sodium Acetate		X[o]	
Sodium Acetate Soln.		X	
Sodium Ascorbate		X[o]	X[o]
Sodium Bicarbonate	X[ao]		
Sodium Bicarbonate Oral Powder	X[o]		
Sodium Chloride	X[ao]◆		
Sodium Chloride Ophthalmic		X[c]C[k]	
Sodium Chloride Inhalation Soln.	S[r]		
Sodium Chloride Tablet for Soln.	X		
Sodium Chloride & Dextrose (tab)	X		
Sodium Citrate & Citric Acid Oral Soln.		X	
Sodium Fluoride	X[o]	X[a]	
Sodium Fluoride Oral Soln.		XP	
Sodium Fluoride & Phosphoric Acid		P[t]	
Sodium Fluoride and Phosphoric Acid Topical Soln.		P	
Sodium Gluconate	X[o]		
Sodium Hypochlorite Soln.		X[+]	X[+]
Sodium Iodide		X[o]	
Sodium Lactate Soln.		X	
Sodium Monofluorophosphate	X[o]		
Sodium Nitrate		X[o]	
Sodium Nitroprusside		X[o]	X[o]
Dibasic Sodium Phosphate		X[o]	
Monobasic Sodium Phosphate	X[o]		
Sodium Phosphate	X[P]		
Sodium Phosphates Oral Soln.		X	
Sodium Polystyrene Sulfonate	X[o]		
Sodium Polystyrene Sulfonate Susp.	X[+]		
Sodium Salicylate	X[ao]		X[o]
Sodium Sulfate Inj.		X[+]	
Sodium Thiosulfate		X[o]	
Sorbitol Soln.		X	
Soybean Oil		X[+]	X[+]
Spectinomycin HCl		X[o]◆	
Spironolactone (tab)	X[o]	X[a]	X[a]
Spironolactone and Hydrochlorothiazide		X[a]	X[o]
Stannous Fluoride	X[o]		
Stannous Fluoride Gel	X		
Stanozolol		X[ao]	X[ao]
Starch, Topical	X		
Storax	X[o]		
Succinyl Chloride	X[o]		
Sucralfate		X[ao]	
Sufentanil Citrate	X[o]		
Sulbactam Sodium		X◆	
Sulconazole Nitrate	X[o]		X[o]
Triple Sulfa Vaginal	X[a]C[f]		X[a]C[f]
Sulfabenzamide	X[o]		X[o]
Sulfacetamide	X[o]		X[o]
Sulfacetamide Sodium		X[o]	X[o]
Sulfacetamide Sodium Ophthalmic	COT[g]	X[c+]	X[c+]
Sulfacetamide Sodium & Prednisolone Acetate Ophthalmic		TP[j] CTP[g]	
Sulfachlorpyridazine	X[o]	X[o]	
Sulfadiazine	X[ao]	X[ao]	
Sulfadiazine, Silver	X[o]	C[f]	X[fo]

Drugs (Dosage Form)	WC	T	LR
Sulfadoxine	X[o]		X[o]
Sulfadoxine & Pyrimethamine (tab)	X		X
Sulfamerazine	X[ao]		X[o]
Sulfamethizole	X[ao]		X[o]
Sulfamethazine	X[o]		X[o]
Sulfamethazine Granulated	X[x]		
Sulfamethizole Oral Susp.		X	X
Sulfamethoxazole	X[ao]		X[ao]
Sulfamethoxazole Oral Susp.		X	X
Sulfamethoxazole & Trimethoprim	X[a]		X[a]
Sulfamethoxazole and Trimethoprim Oral Susp.		X	X
Sulfapyridine	X[ao]		X[ao]
Sulfaquinoxaline	X[o]		X[o]
Sulfaquinoxaline Oral		X[c]	X[c]
Sulfasalazine	X[a]	X[o]	X[o]
Sulfasalazine Delayed Release	X[a]		
Sulfathiazole	X[o]		X[o]
Sulfinpyrazone	X[ab]		
Sulfisoxazole (tab)	X		X
Sulfisoxazole Diolamine		X[o]	X[o]
Sulfisoxazole Acetyl Oral Suspension		X	X
Sulfisoxazole Diolamine Ophthalmic		C[g]X[c]	X[c]
Sulfur, Precipitated	X[o]		
Sulfur Ointment	X[+]		
Sulfur, Sublimed	X[o]		
Sulindac	X[ao]		
Suprofen	X[o]		
Suprofen Ophthalmic		X[c]	
Sutilains		X[+]	
Sutilains Ointment		CX[+]	
Surgical Suture, Absorbable	SP		
Surgical Suture, Nonabsorbable	SP		
Talc	X		
Tamoxifen Citrate	X[ao]		X[ao]
Tannic Acid		X[o]	X[o]
Tape, Adhesive	X[+]		
Temazepam	X[bo]		X[bo]
Terbutaline Sulfate	X[o+]	X[+]	X[o+]
Terbutaline Sulfate Inhalation		A[l+]	A[l+]
Terfenadine		X[oa]	X[oa]
Terpin Hydrate	X[o]		
Terpin Hydrate Elixir		X	
Terpin Hydrate & Codeine Elixir		X	
Terpin Hydrate & Dextromethorphan HBr Elixir		X	
Testolactone	X[ao]		
Testosterone	X[o]		
Testosterone Cypionate	X[o]		X[o]
Testosterone Enanthate	X[o+]		
Testosterone Propionate	X[o]		X[o]
Tetracaine Ophthalmic Oint.		C	
Tetracaine		X[o]C[f]	X[o]
Tetracaine & Menthol Oint.		C	
Tetracaine HCl		X[o]C[f]	X[o]
Tetracaine HCl Topical Soln.		X	X
Tetracaine HCl Ophthalmic Soln.		X	X
Tetracycline		X[o]	X[o]
Tetracycline Boluses		X[x]	
Tetracycline Oral Suspension		X	X
Tetracycline HCl (tablet/capsule/ophthalmic/suspension/topical/ solution)		X	X
Tetracycline HCl Ophthalmic	COT[g]		
Tetracycline HCl Soluble Pwd.		X[x]	
Tetracycline HCl for Topical Soln.		X	X
Tetracycline HCl and Novobiocin Sodium (tab)		X[x]	
Tetracycline Phosphate Complex and Novobiocin Sodium (cap)		X[x]	
Tetracycline HCl & Nystatin (cap)		X	X
Tetracycline Phosphate Complex		X[bo]	X[bo]
Tetrahydrozoline HCl		X[o]	
Tetrahydrozoline HCl Soln.		X[ks]	
Theophylline	X[abo]		
Theophylline Extended Release (cap)	X		
Theophylline, Ephedrine HCl & Phenobarbital (tab)	X		
Theophylline & Guaifenesin		X[b]	

Drugs (Dosage Form)	WC	T	LR
Theophylline Guaifenesin Oral Soln.	X		
Theophylline Sodium Glycinate	X^{a}	X^{e}	
Thiabendazole	X^{o}	X^{a}	
Thiabendazole Oral Susp.		X	
Thiamine HCl		X^{aeo}	X^{aeo}
Thiamine Mononitrate		X^{eo}	X^{eo}
Thiamylal	X^{o}		
Thiethylperazine Maleate		X^{aio+}	X^{aio+}
Thimerosal		X^{o}	X^{o}
Thimerosal Topical		X^{cl+}	X^{cl+}
Thimerosal Tincture		X^{+}	X^{+}
Thioguanine		X^{ao}	
Thiopental Sodium		X^{o}	
Thioridazine	X^{o}		X^{o}
Thioridazine Oral Susp.		X	X
Thioridazine HCl		X^{ao}	X^{ao}
Thioridazine HCl Oral Soln.		X^{+}	X^{+}
Thiostrepton		X^{o}	
Thiotepa		X^{o}	X^{o}
Thiothixene	X^{b}	X^{o}	X^{bo}
Thiothixine HCl		X^{o}	X^{o}
Thiothixene HCl Oral Solution		X	X
Threonine	X^{o}		
Thyroid		X^{ao}	
Ticarcillin Monosodium		X^{o}	
Timolol Maleate Ophthalmic Soln.		X	
Timolol Maleate	X^{ao}		X^{a}
Timolol Maleate & Hydrochlorothiazide (tab)	X		X
Tioconazole		X^{oaf}	
Titanium Dioxide	X^{o}		
Tobramycin		X^{o}	
Tobramycin Ophthalmic		$X^{c}COT^{g}$	
Tobramycin and Dexamethasone Ophthalmic		$X^{j}C^{g}$	
Tobramycin and Fluorometholone Acetate Ophthalmic		X^{c}	
Tobramycin Sulfate		X^{o}	
Tocainide HCl	X^{oa}		
Tolazamide	X^{o}	X^{a}	
Tolbutamide	X^{ao}		
Tolmetin Sodium	X^{ao}	X^{b}	
Tolnaftate		X^{fto}	
Tolnaftate Topical		X^{lco+}	
Tolu Balsam		X^{+}	
Trazodone HCl		X^{oa}	X^{oa}
Trenbolone Acetate		CO	
Tretinoin		$C^{f}X^{c}$	X^{cft}
Triacetin		X	
Triamcinolone	X^{ao}		
Triamcinolone Acetonide	X^{go}	X^{fh}	
Triamcinolone Acetonide Topical		X^{i+}	
Triamcinolone Acetonide Dental Paste		X	
Triamcinolone Diacetate	X^{o}	X^{d}	X^{d}
Triamcinolone Hexacetonide	X		
Triamterene		X^{hn}	X^{bo}
Triamterene and Hydrochlorothiazide		X^{ab}	X^{ab}
Triazolam		X^{ao}	X^{ao}
Trichlorfon	X^{+}		
Trichlormethiazide	X^{o}	X^{a}	
Tricitrates Oral Soln.		X	
Trientine HCl		X^{ao+}	In^{o}
Trifluoperazine HCl	X^{a}	X^{do}	X^{ado}
Triflupromazine		X^{o}	X^{o}
Triflupromazine Oral Suspension		X	X
Triflupromazine HCl (tab)	X		X
Trifluridine		X	X
Trihexyphenidyl HCl		X^{aeo}	
Trihexyphenidyl HCl Extended-Release (cap)		X	
Trikates Oral Soln.		X	X
Trimeprazine Tartrate	X^{a}	X^{do}	X^{ado}
Trimethadione		X^{abco+}	
Trimethaphan Camsylate		X^{+}	
Trimethobenzamide HCl	X^{bo}		
Trimethoprim		X^{ao}	X^{ao}
Trioxsalen	X^{ao}		X^{ao}
Tripelennamine Citrate	X^{a}	X^{e}	X^{ee}
Tripelennamine HCl	X^{ao}		X^{o}
Triprolidine HCl		X^{ado}	X^{ado}
Triprolidine & Pseudoephedrine Hydrochlorides		X^{ad}	X^{ad}
Trisulfapyrimidines (tab)	X		
Trisulfapyrimidines Oral Susp.		X^{+}	
Tromethamine		X^{o}	
Tropicamide		X^{o}	X^{o}
Tropicamide Ophthalmic Soln.		X^{+}	

Drugs (Dosage Form)	WC	T	LR
Trypsin, Crystallized		X[+]	
Tryptophan	X[o]		
Tubocurarine Chloride		X[o]	
Tylosine HHe[x]		X[x]	
Tylosine Granulated HHeSp[x]			
Tyloxapol		X[o]	
Tyropanoate Sodium		X[bo]	X[bo]
Tyrosine	X[o]		
Tyrothricin		X[o]	
Undecylenic Acid		X[o]	X[o]
Undecylenic Acid, Compound Ointment		X[+]	
Urea	X[o]		
Valine	X[o]		
Valproic Acid		GP[o]X[bd+]	
Vancomycin		X[o]	
Vancomycin HCl		X[bo]	
Vancomycin HCl for Oral Soln.		X	
Verapamil HCl		X[ao]	X[ao]
Verapamil HCl Extended Release		X[a]	X[a]
Vidarabine		X[◆]	
Vidarabine Ophthalmic Ointment		COT[+]	
Vinblastine Sulfate		X[+]	X[+]
Vincristine Sulfate		X[+]	X[+]
Vitamin A		X[bo+]	X[bo+]
Vitamin E		In[o]X	X
Vitamin E Preparation		In	X
Vitamins, Oil-Soluble		X[ab]	X[ab]
Warfarin Sodium	X[o]	X[a]	X[ao]
Water, Purified		X	
Water, Sterile Purified		X[◆]	
White Lotion		X	
Witch Hazel		X	
Xylometazoline HCl		X[o]	X[o]
Xylometazoline HCl Nasal Soln.		X	X
Xylose		X[+]	
Zidovudine		X[bo]	X[bo]
Zidovudine Oral		X[c]	X[c]
Zinc Acetate		X[o]	
Zinc Carbonate		X[o]	
Zinc Chloride		X[o]	
Zinc Gluconate	X[oa]		
Zinc Oxide	X[o]		
Zinc Oxide (oint/paste)	X[+]		
Zinc Oxide and Salicylic Acid Paste	X		
Zinc Stearate	X[o]		
Zinc Sulfate		X[o]	
Zinc Sulfate Ophthalmic Solution		X	
Zinc Undecylenate	X[o]		

Provided by Dr. Kenneth S. Alexander, Professor of Pharmacy, College of Pharmacy, University of Toledo.
The listing of container and storage requirements for Compendial drugs is included as an aid to the practitioner in storing and dispensing.

Container and Storage Requirements for Sterile U.S.P. 23 Drugs

The listing of container and storage requirements for U.S.P. drugs is included as an aid to the practitioner in storing and dispensing.

Legend:

A	=	Type I Glass	N	=	Intact Flexible Container Meeting the General Requirements
B	=	Type II Glass	O	=	Original Package
C	=	Type III Glass	P	=	Plastic
CP	=	Cool Place	PA	=	Does not adversely affect performance
CV	=	Controlled Volume	R	=	Refrigerator (2°-8°C)
D	=	Type II or III Glass Depending on Final Soln. pH	RT	=	Controlled Room Temperature
DF	=	Do Not Freeze	S	=	Single Dose
F	=	Freezer (-4°C)	SC	=	Radioactive Shielding
H	=	Protect From Heat	SS	=	Stated Size Limitation
He	=	Hermetic Container	Sy	=	Syringe
I	=	Containers for Sterile Solids as Described Under Injections	T	=	Avoid Toxic Substances
In	=	Inert Atmosphere	Ti	=	Tight Container
L	=	Protect from Light	TP	=	Tamper-Proof
LR	=	Light Resistant	Tr	=	Treated to Prevent Adsorption
M	=	Multiple Dose	U	=	Unspecified
Mo	=	Protect from Moisture	W	=	Transparent
			X	=	Colorless
			WC	=	Well Closed

Drugs	Container	Glass Type	Storage Conditions
Acepromazine Maleate Inj.	S,M	A	L
Acetazolamide for Inj.	I	C	
Acetic Acid Irrigation	S,P	A,B	
Acetylcholine for Ophthalmic Soln.	I		
Acetylcysteine and Isoproterenol HCl Inhal. Soln.	S,M	A	WC
Acetylcysteine Solution	S,M	A,P	O_2 excluded
Albumin, Human	S	U	RT
Alcohol in Dextrose Inj.	S	A,B	
Alcohol Inj., Dehydrated	S	A	In (head space)
Alfentanil Inj.	S,M	A	
Alphaprodine HCl Inj.	S,M	A	
Alprostadil Inj.	S	A	R
Alteplase for Inj.			R-RT/L
Amdinocillin for Inj.	I		
Amikacin Sulfate Inj.	S,M	A,C	
Aminoacetic Acid Irrigation	S	A,B	
Aminocaproic Acid Inj.	S,M	A	
Aminohippurate Sodium Inj.	S,M	A	
Aminophylline Inj.	S	A	CO_2 excluded
Amitriptyline HCl Inj.	S,M	A	
Ammonium Chloride Inj.	S,M	A,B	
Ammonium Molybdate Inj.	S,M	A,B	
Amobarbital Sodium for Inj.	I	D	
Amoxicillin for Injectable Suspension	I	I	
Amphotericin B for Inj.	I		R,L

Drugs	Container	Glass Type	Storage Conditions
Ampicillin and Sulbactam for Inj.	I		
Ampicillin for Inj.	I		
Ampicillin for Injectable Oil Suspension	S,M	A	
Ampicillin for Injectable Suspension	I		
Amrinone Inj.	S	A	L,RT
Anileridine Inj.	S,M	A	L
Anticoagulant Citrate Dextrose Solution	M	A,B	
Anticoagulant Citrate Phosphate Dextrose Adenine Solution	S,P	A,B	X,W
Anticoagulant Heparin Soln.	S,P	A,B	
Anticoagulant Sodium Citrate Soln.	S	A,B	
Antihemophilic Factor			R
Antihemophilic Factor, Cryoprecipitated			F (-18°C)
Antirabies Serum	U		R
Antivenin (Crotalidae) Polyvalent	S		H
Antivenin (Latrodectus mactans)	S		H
Antivenin (Micrurus fulvius)	S		H
Arginine HCl Inj.	S	B	
Ascorbic Acid Inj.	S	A,B	LR
Atenolol Inj.	S,M	A	CP,RT,LR,DF
Atropine Sulfate Inj.	S,M	A	
Aurothioglucose Injectable Oil Suspension	S,M	A	L
Aurothioglucose Suspension, Sterile	I		
Azaperone Inj.	S,M	A	L
Azathioprine Sodium for Inj.	I	C	RT
Azlocillin for Inj.	I		
Aztreonam	I		
Aztreonam for Inj.	I		F
Bacitracin for Inj., Sterile	I	D	R
Bacitracin Zinc, Sterile	I		CP
BCG Vaccine	U	A	R
Benztropine Mesylate Inj.	S,M	A	
Benzylpenicilloyl-Polylysine Inj.	S,M	A	R
Betamethasone Sodium Phosphate and Betamethasone Acetate Injectable Suspension	M	A	
Betamethasone Sodium Phosphate Inj.	S,M	A	
Bethanechol Chloride Inj.	S	A	
Biological Indicator for Dry Heat Sterilization, Paper Strip	O		L,H,Mo,PA
Biological Indicator for Ethylene Oxide Sterilization, Paper Strip	O		L,H,Mo,PA
Biological Indicator for Steam Sterilization, Paper Strip	O		L,H,Mo,PA
Biological Indicator for Steam Sterilization, Self-contained	O		L,H,Mo,PA
Biperiden Lactate Inj.	S	A	L
Bleomycin for Inj.	I	B	
Blood Grouping Serums (All)	U		R
Botulism Antitoxin	S		R
Bretylium Tosylate in Dextrose Inj.	S,M	A,B,P	
Bretylium Tosylate Injection	S	A	
Brompheniramine Maleate Inj.	S,M	A	L

Drugs	Container	Glass Type	Storage Conditions
Bumetanide Inj.	S,M	A	L
Bupivacaine and Epinephrine Inj.	S,M	A	L
Bupivacaine HCl Inj.	S,M	A	
Bupivacaine in Dextrose Inj.	S	A	
Butorphanol Tartrate Inj.	S,M	A	L
Caffeine and Sodium Benzoate Inj.	S	A	
Calcium Chloride Inj.	S	A	
Calcium Gluceptate Inj.	S	A,B	
Calcium Gluconate Inj.	S	A	
Calcium Levulinate Inj.	S	A	
Capreomycin for Inj.	I	B	R
Carbenicillin for Inj.	I	D	
Carboprost Tromethamine Inj.	S,M	A	R
Cefamandole Nafate for Inj.	I	D	
Cefamandole Nafate, Sterile	I		
Cefamandole Sodium for Inj.	I		
Cefamandole Sodium, Sterile	I		
Cefazolin Inj.	I		F
Cefmenoxime for Inj.	I		
Cefonicid for Inj.	I		
Cefoperazone for Inj.	I		
Cefoperazone Inj.	I		F
Ceforanide for Inj.	I		
Cefotaxime Sodium Inj.	S,M		F
Cefotetan Disodium	I		
Cefotetan for Injection	I		
Cefotetan Injection	I		F
Cefotiam for Inj.	I	C	
Cefotaxime for Inj.	I		
Cefoxitin Sodium Inj.	I		F
Cefpiramide for Inj.	I		
Ceftazidime for Inj.	I		L
Ceftazidime Inj.	I		F
Ceftazidime, Sterile	I		L
Ceftizoxime for Inj.	I		
Ceftizoxime Inj.	I		F
Ceftriaxone for Inj.	I		F
Ceftriaxone Inj.	I		F
Cefuroxime for Inj.	I		
Cellulose Oxidized (all)	I		L,R
Cefuroxime Inj.	I		F
Cephalothin for Inj.	I		
Cephalothin Inj.	I		F
Cephapirin for Inj.	I		
Cephradine for Inj.	I		
Chloramphenicol Inj.	S,M		
Chloramphenicol Sodium Succinate, Sterile	I	B	
Chloramphenicol, Sterile	I		
Chlordiazepoxide HCl, Sterile	I	B	L
Chloroprocaine HCl Inj.	S,M	A	
Chloroquine HCl Inj.	S	A	

Drugs	Container	Glass Type	Storage Conditions
Chlorothiazide Sodium for Inj.	I	C	
Chlorphenamine Maleate Inj.	S,M	A	L
Chlorpromazine HCl Inj.	S,M	A	L
Chlorprothixene Inj.	S		L
Chlortetracycline HCl	I		L
Cholera Vaccine	U		R
Chromate Cr51 Inj., Sodium	S,M		
Chromic Chloride Inj.	S,M	A,B	
Cilastatin Sod., Sterile	I	C	R
Ciprofloxacin Inj.	S,M	A	R,L
Cisplatin for Inj.	I		
Citric Acid, Magnesium Oxide Sodium Carbonate Irrigation	S	A,B	
Clavulanate Potassium	I		
Clindamycin for Inj.	I		
Clindamycin Inj.	S,M	A,P	
Cloxacillin Benzathine	U (tight)		
Cloxacilllin Benzathine Intramammary Infusion	Sy		
Cloxacillin Sodium	U (tight)		
Cloxacillin Sodium Intramammary Infusion	Sy		TP
Coccidioidin			R
Codeine Phosphate Inj.	S,M	A	L
Colchicine Inj.	S	A	L
Colistimethate for Inj.	I		
Colistimethate Sodium	I		
Corticotropin for Inj.	I	B	
Corticotropin Inj.	S,M	A	R
Corticotropin Inj., Repository	S,M	A	
Corticotropin Zinc Hydroxide Injectable Suspension	S,M	A	RT
Cortisone Acetate Injectable Suspension	S,M	A	
Cromolyn Sodium Inhalation	S (double-ended Ampul)	A,B,P	
Cupric Chloride Inj.	S,M	A,B	
Cupric Sulfate Inj.	S,M	A,B	
Cyanocobalamin Inj.	S,M	A	LR
Cyclizine Lactate Inj.	S	A	
Cyclophosphamide for Inj.	I	B	RT
Cyclosporine for Inj.	S,M		
Cysteine HCl Inj.	S,M	A	
Cytarabine	I		
Cytarabine for Inj.	I		
Dacarbazine for Inj.	S,M or I	A	L
Dactinomycin for Inj.	I	B	LR
Daunorubicin HCl for Inj.	I	B	LR
Deferoxamine Mesylate for Inj.	S,M	A	
Deslanoside Inj.	S	A	
Desoxycorticosterone Acetate Inj.	S,M	A,C	Lh.
Desoxycorticosterone Acetate Pellets	U (tight)		
Dexamethasone Acetate Injectable Suspension	S,M	A	
Dextrose and Sodium Chloride Inj.	S	A,B,P	

Drugs	Container	Glass Type	Storage Conditions
Dextrose Inj.	S	A,B,P	
Diatrizoate Meglumine and Diatrizoate Sodium Inj.	S	A,C	L
Diatrizoate Meglumine Inj.	S,M	A,C	L
Diatrizoate Sodium Inj.	S. M	A,C	L
Diazepam Inj.	S,M	A	L
Diazoxide Inj.	S	A	L
Dibucaine HCl Inj.	S,M	A	L
Dicyclomine HCl Inj.	S,M	A	
Diethylstilbestrol Diphosphate Inj.	S,M		
Diethylstilbestrol Inj.	S,M	A	LR
Digitoxin Inj.	S,M	A	L
Digoxin Inj.	S	A	LR, H
Dihydroergotamine Mesylate Inj.	S	A	Avoid heat
Dihydrostreptomycin Inj.	S,M		
Dimenhydrinate Inj.	S,M	A,C	
Dimercaprol Inj.	S,M	A,C	
Dimethyl Sulfoxide Irrigation	S		RT,L
Dinoprost Tromethamine Inj.	S,M	A	
Diphenhydramine HCl Inj.	S,M	A	L
Diphtheria and Tetanus Toxoids	U		R
Diphtheria and Tetanus Toxoids/Adsorbed	U		R
Diphtheria and Tetanus Toxoids and Pertussis Vaccine	U		R
Diphtheria and Tetanus Toxoids and Pertussis Vaccine Adsorbed	U		R
Diphtheria Antitoxin	U		R
Diphtheria Toxin for Schick Test	U		R
Diphtheria Toxoid	U		R
Diphtheria Toxoid Adsorbed	U		
Dobutamine Inj.	S,M	A	
Dobutamine for Inj.	I	B	RT
Dopamine HCl Inj.	S	A	
Dopamine HCl and Dextrose Inj.	S	A,B	
Doxapram HCl Inj.	S,M	A	
Doxorubicin HCl for Inj.	I	B	(not to exceed 250 ml if multidose)
Doxorubicin HCl Inj.	S,M	A	LR,R (not to exceed 100 ml if multidose)
Doxycycline for Inj.	I	B	L
Droperidol Inj.	S,M	A	L
Dyphylline Inj.	S,M	A	RT,L
Edetate Calcium Disodium Inj.	S	A	
Edetate Disodium Inj.	S	A	
Edrophonium Chloride Inj.	S,M	A	
Electrolytes and Dextrose Inj. (Type 1), Multiple	S	A,B,P	
Electrolytes and Dextrose Inj. (Type 2), Multiple	S	A,B,P	
Electrolytes and Dextrose Inj. (Type 3), Multiple	S	A,B,P	
Electrolytes and Dextrose Inj. (Type 4), Multiple	S	A,B,P	
Electrolytes and Invert Sugar Inj. (Type 1), Multiple	S	A,B,P	

Drugs	Container	Glass Type	Storage Conditions
Electrolytes and Invert Sugar Inj. (Type 2), Multiple	S	A,B,P	
Electrolytes and Invert Sugar Inj. (Type 3), Multiple	S	A,B,P	
Electrolytes Inj. (Type 1), Multiple	S	A,B,P	
Electrolytes Inj. (Type 2), Multiple	S	A,B,P	
Elements Inj., Trace	S,M	A,B	
Emetine HCl Inj.	S	A	LR
Ephedrine Sulfate Inj.	S,M	A	LR
Epinephrine Bitartrate for Ophthalmic Solution	I		
Epinephrine Inj.	S,M	A	LR
Epinephrine Injectable Oil Susp.	S	A,C	LR
Ergonovine Maleate Inj.	S	A	LR,R
Ergotamine Tartrate Inj.	S	A	LR
Erythromycin Ethylsuccinate Inj.	S,M	A	
Erythromycin Ethylsuccinate, Sterile	I		
Erythromycin Gluceptate, Sterile	I	D	
Erythromycin Lactobionate, Sterile	I		
Erythromycin Lactobionate for Inj.	I	D	
Estradiol Cypionate Inj.	S,M	A	LR
Estradiol Injectable Suspension	S,M	A	
Estradiol Pellets	U		
Estradiol Valerate Inj.	S,M	A,C	LR
Estrone Inj.	S,M	A	
Estrone Injectable Suspension	S,M	A	
Ethacrynate Sodium for Inj.	I	D	
Ethiodized Oil Inj.	S,M		LR
Fentanyl Citrate Inj.	S	A	L
Ferrous Citrate Fe 59 Inj.	S,M		
Floxuridine, Sterile	M	A	L (discard after 2 wks when reconstituted)
Fludeoxyglucose F 18 Inj.	S,M		SC
Flunixin Meglumine Injection	M		RT
Fluorescein Inj.	S	A	
Fluorescein Sodium Ophth. Strips	S,SS,U		
Fluoride F 18 Inj., Sodium	S,M		SC
Fluorodopa F 18 Inj.	S,M	SC	
Fluorouracil Inj.	S	A	RT,L
Fluphenazine Decanoate Inj.	S,M	A	L
Fluphenazine Enanthate Inj.	S,M	A,C	L
Fluphenazine HCl Inj.	S,M	A	L
Folic Acid Inj.	S,M	A	
Fructose and Sodium Chloride Inj.	S	A,B	
Fructose Inj.	S	A,B	
Furosemide Inj.	S,M	A	LR
Gadopentetate Dimeglumine Inj.	S	A	LR,RT
Gallamine Triethiodide Inj.	S,M	A	L
Gallium Citrate Ga 67 Inj.	S,M		
Gelatin Film, Absorbable	U		
Gelatin Sponge, Absorbable	U		
Gentamicin Sulfate Inj.	S,M	A	

Drugs	Container	Glass Type	Storage Conditions
Gentamicin Sulfate, Sterile	I		
Globulin, Immune	U		R
Globulin, Rho(D) Immune	U		R
Globulin Serum, Anti-Human	U		R
Glucagon for Inj.	I/S,M w/solvent		
Glycine Irrigation	S	A,B	
Glycopyrrolate Inj.	S,M	A	
Gold Sodium Thiomalate Inj.	S,M	A	L
Gonadotropin for Inj., Chorionic	I	D	
Guaifenesin for Inj.	S,M		RT
Haloperidol Inj.	S,M	A	L
Heparin Calcium Inj.	S,M	A	R
Heparin Lock Flush Solution	S,M	A	
Heparin Sodium Inj.	S,M	A	
Hepatitis B Immune Globulin	U		R
Hepatitis B Virus Vaccine Inactivated	U		R
Hetacillin Potassium Intramammary Infusion	Sy		
Histamine Phosphate Inj.	S,M	A	L
Histoplasmin	U		R
Hyaluronidase for Inj.	I	A,C	RT
Hyaluronidase Inj.	S,M	A	R
Hydralazine HCl Inj.	S,M	A	
Hydrocortisone Acetate Injectable Suspension	S,M	A	
Hydrocortisone Injectable Suspension	S,M	A	
Hydrocortisone Sodium Phosphate Inj.	I	C	
Hydrocortisone Sodium Succinate for Inj.	I	C	
Hydromorphone HCl Inj.	S,M	A	L
Hydroxocobalamin Inj.	S,M	A	L
Hydroxyprogesterone Caproate Inj.	S,M	A,C	
Hydroxyzine HCl Inj.	S,M		L
Hyoscyamine Sulfate Inj.	S,M	A	
Idarubicin HCl for Inj.	I		
Ifosfamide for Inj.	I		RT
Imipenem and Cilastatin Sodium for Inj.	I		RT
Imipenem and Cilastatin Sodium, Sterile	I		RT
Imipenem, Sterile	I		RT
Imipramine HCl Inj.	S	A	LR
Indigotindisulfonate Sodium Inj.	S	A	LR
Indium In 111 Chloride Solution	S		RT
Indium In 111 Pentetate Inj.	S		
Indium In 111 Satumomab Pendetide Inj.	S		SC,RT
Indocyanine Green for Inj.	I		
Indomethacin Sodium for Inj.	I		
Influenza Virus Vaccine	U		R
Insulin and Sodium Chloride Inj.	S	A,B	
Insulin Human Inj.	M		R
Insulin Inj.	M		R
Insulin Zinc Suspension	M		R
Insulin Zinc Suspension, Extended	M		R
Insulin Zinc Suspension, Prompt	M		R
Iobenguane I 123 Injection	S,M		SC,F

Drugs	Container	Glass Type	Storage Conditions
Iodinated I 125 Albumin Inj.	S,M		R
Iodinated I 131 Albumin Inj.	U		
Iodinated I 131 Albumin Aggreg. Inj.	S,M		R
Iodipamide Meglumine Inj.	S	A,C	
Iodohippurate Sodium 1123 Inj.	S,M		SC
Iodohippurate Sodium I 131 Inj.	S,M		
Iohexol Inj. (Intravascular/Intrathecal)	S	A	L
Iopamidol Inj. (Intravascular/Intrathecal)	S	A	L
Iophendylate Inj.	S	A	LR
Iothalamate Meglumine and Sodium Iothalamate Inj.	S	A	L
Iothalamate Meglumine Inj.	S	A	L
Iothalamate Sodium I-125 Inj.	S	A	L
Ioversol Inj.	S	A	L
Ioxaglate Meglumine and Ioxaglate Sodium Inj.	S	A	LR
Iron Dextran Inj.	S,M	A,B	
Iron Sorbitex Inj.	S	A	
Isoniazid Inj.	S,M	A	L
Isophane Insulin Suspension	M		R
Isoproterenol HCl Inj.	S	A	L
Isoxsuprine HCl Inj.	S,M	A	
Kanamycin Inj.	S,M	A,C	
Ketamine HCl Inj.	S,M	A	L,H
Ketorolac Tromethamine Inj.	S	A	LR,RT
Labetalol HCl Inj.	S,M (60 ml max)	A	R,RT,L
Leucovorin Calcium Inj.	S	A	LR
Levorphanol Tartrate Inj.	S,M	A	
Lidocaine and Epinephrine Inj.	S,M	A	LR
Lidocaine HCl and Dextrose Inj.	S	A,B	
Lidocaine HCl Inj.	S,M	A	
Lidocaine HCl, Sterile	I		
Lincomycin Inj.	S,M	A	
Lorazepam Inj.	S,M	A	L
Magnesium Sulfate in Dextrose Injection	S	A,G,P	
Magnesium Sulfate Inj.	S,M	A	
Manganese Chloride Inj.	S,M	A,B	
Manganese Sulfate Inj.	S,M	A,B	
Mannitol and Sodium Chloride Inj.	U	D	LR
Mannitol Inj.	S	A,B,P	
Measles and Mumps Virus Vaccine Live	S,M		LR,R
Measles and Rubella Virus Vaccine Live	S,M		LR,R
Measles, Mumps and Rubella Virus Vaccine Live	S,M		LR,R
Measles Virus Vaccine Live	S,M		LR,R
Mechlorethamine HCl for Inj	I	B	
Medroxyprogesterone Acetate Susp., Sterile	S,M	A	
Menadiol Sodium Diphosphate Inj.	S	A	LR
Menadione Inj.	S,M	A	
Meningococcal Polysaccharide Vaccine (Group A)	M		R
Meningococcal Polysaccharide Vaccine (Group C)	M		R
Meningococcal Polysaccharide Vaccine (Groups A and C combined)	M		R

Drugs	Container	Glass Type	Storage Conditions
Menotropins for Inj.	S,M	A	
Meperidine HCl Inj.	S,M	A	
Mephentermine Sulfate Inj.	S,M	A	
Mepivacaine HCl and Levonordefrin Inj.	S,M	A	
Mepivacaine HCl Inj.	S,M	A	
Meprobamate Inj.	S	A	
Mesoridazine Besylate Inj.	S	A	L
Metaraminol Bitartrate Inj.	S,M	A	L
Methadone HCl Inj.	S,M	A	LR
Methicillin for Inj.	I		L,RT
Methionine C II Inj.	S,M		SC
Methocarbamol Inj.	S	A	
Methohexital Sodium for Inj.	I	C	
Methotrexate for Inj.	I		L
Methotrexate Inj.	S,M	A	L
Methotrimeprazine Inj.	S,M	A	L
Methyldopate HCl Inj.	S	A	
Methylene Blue Inj.	S	A	
Methylergonovine Maleate Inj.	S	A	LR
Methylprednisolone Acetate Injectable Suspension	S,M	A	
Methylprednisolone Sodium Succinate for Inj.	I	C	
Metoclopramide Inj.	S,M	A	LR (no antioxidant)
Metocurine Iodide Inj.	S,M	A	
Metoprolol Tartrate Inj.	S	A,B	L
Metronidazole Inj.	S,P	A,B	L
Mezlocillin for Inj.	I		
Miconazole Inj.	S	A	RT
Minocycline HCl for Inj.	I		L
Mitomycin for Inj.	I	D	L
Mitoxantrone Inj.	S	A	
Morphine Sulfate Inj.	S	A	L
Morphine Sulfate Inj. (Preservative Free)	S	A	L
Morrhuate Sodium Inj.	S,M	A	
Moxalactam Disodium for Inj.	I		
Mumps Skin Test Antigen	U		R
Mumps Virus Vaccine Live	S,M		LR,R
Nafcillin Sodium for Inj.	I	D	
Nafcillin Sodium Inj.	I		F
Nafcillin Sodium, Sterile	I		
Nalorphine HCl Inj.	S,M	A	
Naloxone HCl Inj.	S,M	A	L
Nandrolone Decanoate Inj.	S,M	A	L
Nandrolone Phenpropionate Inj.	S,M	A	L
Neomycin and Polymyxin B Sulfates Soln. for Irrigation	U		
Neomycin for Inj.	I		I
Neostigmine Methylsulfate Inj.	S,M		L
Netilmicin Sulfate Inj.	S,M	A	
Niacinamide Inj.	S,M	A	
Niacin Inj.	S,M	A	
Ammonia N 13 Inj.	S,M		SC

Drugs	Container	Glass Type	Storage Conditions
Nitroglycerin Inj.	S,M	A,B	
Norepinephrine Bitartrate Inj.	S	A	LR
Novobiocin Sod. Intramammary Infusion	Sy		WC
Orphenadrine Citrate Inj.	S,M	A	L
Oxacillin for Inj.	I		RT
Oxacillin Inj.	I		F
Oxacillin Sodium	I		
Oxymorphone HCl Inj.	S,M	A	L
Oxytetracycline	I		L
Oxytetracycline for Inj.	I		L
Oxytetracycline HCl	I		L
Oxytetracycline Inj.	S,M		L
Oxytocin Inj.	S,M	A	(do not freeze)
Papaverine HCl Inj.	S,M	A	
Penicillin G Benzathine	I		
Penicillin G Benzathine and Penicillin G Procaine Injectable Susp.	S,M	A,C	
Penicillin G Benzathine Injectable Susp.	S,M	A,B	R
Penicillin G Potassium for Inj.	I	D	
Penicillin G Potassium Inj.	S		F
Penicillin G Procaine	I		
Penicillin G Procaine and Dihydrostreptomycin Sulfate Injectable Suspension	S,M (tight)		
Penicillin G Procaine, Dihydrostreptomycin Sulfate and Prednisolone Injectable Suspension	S,M (tight)		
Penicillin G Procaine, Dihydrostreptomycin Sulfate, Chlorpheniramine Maleate, and Dexamethasone Injectable Suspension	S,M (tight)		R
Penicillin G Procaine Dihydrostreptomycin Sulfate Intramammary Infusion	Sy (well closed)		
Penicillin G Procaine for Injectable Susp.	S,M	A,C	
Penicillin G Procaine Injectable Susp.	S,M	A,C	R
Penicillin G Procaine Intramammary Infusion	Sy (well closed)		
Penicillin G Procaine w/Aluminum Stearate Injectable Oil Suspension	S,M	A,C	
Penicillin G Sodium for Inj.	I		
Pentazocine Lactate Inj.	S,M	A	
Pentobarbital Sodium Inj.	S,M	A	
Perphenazine Inj.	S,M	A	L
Pertussis Immune Globulin	U		R
Pertussis Vaccine	U		R
Pertussis Vaccine Adsorbed	U		R
Phenobarbital Sodium Inj.	I	D	
Phenobarbital Sodium, Sterile	I	D	
Phentolamine Mesylate for Inj.	I	B	
Phenylbutazone Injection	S,M (vet. use)	A	L,R
Phenylephrine HCl Inj.	S,M	A	L
Phenytoin Sodium Inj.	S,M	A	RT
Phosphate P 32 Soln., Sodium	S,M		
Phosphate P 32 Susp., Chromic	S,M	Tr	
Physostigmine Salicylate Inj.	S	A	L
Phytonadione Inj.	S,M	A	L

Drugs	Container	Glass Type	Storage Conditions
Pilocarpine Ocular System	S		R
Piperacillin for Inj.	I		
Pituitary Inj., Posterior	S,M	A	
Plague Vaccine	U		R
Plasma Protein Fraction	U		(as labeled)
Platelet Concentrate	U	A,B	(as labeled)
Plicamycin for Inj.	I	D	L
Poliovirus Vaccine Inactivated	U		R
Poliovirus Vaccine Live Oral	S,M		F,R
Polymyxin B for Inj.	I		L
Potassium Acetate Inj.	S,M	A,B	
Potassium Chloride for Inj. Conc.	S,M	A,B	
Potassium Chloride in Dextrose and Sodium Chloride Inj.	S	A,B,P	
Potassium Chloride in Dextrose Inj.	S	A,B,P	
Potassium Chloride in Lactated Ringer's and Dextrose Inj.	S	A,B,P	
Potassium Chloride in Sodium Chloride Inj.	S	A,B,P	
Potassium Phosphates Inj.	S	A	
Pralidoxime Chloride, Sterile	I	B	
Prednisolone Acetate Injectable Susp.	S,M	A	
Prednisolone Sodium Phosphate Inj.	S,M	A	L
Prednisolone Sodium Succinate for Inj.	I	D	
Prednisolone Tebutate Injectable Susp.	S,M	A	
Prilocaine and Epinephrine Inj.	S,M	A	L
Prilocaine HCl Inj.	S,M	A	
Procainamide HCl Inj.	S,M	A	
Procaine HCl and Epinephrine Inj.	S,M	A,B	LR
Procaine HCl Inj.	S,M	A,B	
Procaine HCl, Sterile	I	D	
Procaine and Phenylephrine HCl Inj.	S,M	A	
Procaine and Tetracycline Hydrochlorides and Levonordefrin Inj.	S,M	A	
Prochlorperazine Edisylate Inj.	S,M	A	L
Progesterone Inj.	S,M	A,C	
Progesterone Injectable Susp.	S,M	A	
Progesterone Intrauterine Contraceptive Sys.	S		
Promazine HCl Inj.	S,M	A	L
Promethazine HCl Inj.	S,M	A	L
Propantheline Bromide, Sterile	S	D	
Propoxycaine and Procaine Hydrochlorides and Levonordefrin Inj.	S	A	
Propoxycaine and Procaine Hydrochlorides and Norepinephrine Bitartrate Inj.	S,M	A	
Propranolol HCl Inj.	S	A	LR
Propyliodone Injectable Oil Susp.	S		LR
Protamine Sulfate for Inj.	I	D	
Protamine Sulfate Inj.	S	A	R
Protein Hydrolysate Inj.	S	A,B	H
Pyridostigmine Bromide Inj.	S	A	L
Pyridoxine HCl Inj	S,M	A	L
Quinidine Gluconate Inj.	S,M	A	

Drugs	Container	Glass Type	Storage Conditions
Rabies Immune Globulin	U		R
Rabies Vaccine	U		R
Raclopeide C II Inj.	S,M		SC
Ranitidine Inj.	S,M	I	LR,RT
Ranitidine in Sodium Chloride Inj.	N	A,B	LR,R/RT
Reserpine Inj.	S	A	LR
Riboflavin Inj.	S,M	A	LR
Rifampin for Inj.	I		
Ringer's and Dextrose Inj.	S	A,B,P	
Ringer's and Dextrose Inj., Lactated	S	A,B,P	
Ringer's and Dextrose Inj., Half-Strength Lactated	S	A,B,P	
Ringer's and Dextrose Inj., Modified Lactated	S	A,B,P	
Ringer's Inj.	S	A,B,P	
Ringer's Inj., Lactated	S	A,B,P	
Ringer's Irrigation	S,SS	A,B,P	
Ritodrine HCl Inj.	S	A	RT
Rose Bengal Sodium I 131 Inj.	S,M		
Rubella and Mumps Virus Vaccine Live	S,M		LR,R
Rubella Virus Vaccine Live	S,M		LR,R
Rubidium Chloride Rb 82 Inj.			NA
Sargramostim for Inj.	He		R
Schick Test Control			R
Scopolamine Hydrobromide Inj.	S,M	A	L,R
Secobarbital Sodium Inj.	S,M	A	L,R
Secobarbital Sodium, Sterile	I	D	
Selenious Acid Inj.	S,M	A,B	
Sisomicin Sulfate Inj.	S,M	A	
Smallpox Vaccine	U		R
Sodium Acetate C II Inj.	S,M		SC
Sodium Acetate Inj.	S	A	
Sodium Bicarbonate Inj.	S	A	
Sodium Chloride Inhalation Soln.	S		
Sodium Chloride Inj.	S	A,B	
Sodium Chloride Inj., Bacteriostatic	S,M	A,B	
Sodium Chloride Irrigation	S,SS	A,B,P	
Sodium Lactate Inj.	S	A,B	
Sodium Nitrite Inj.	S	A	
Sodium Nitroprusside, Sterile	I	D	L
Sodium Pertechnetate Tc 99m Inj.	S,M		R
Sodium Phosphates Inj.	S,M	A	
Sodium Sulfate Inj.	S	A	
Sodium Thiosulfate Inj.	S	A	
Spectinomycin for Injectable Suspension	I		
Spectinomycin HCl, Sterile	I		
Streptomycin Sulfate Inj.	S,M	A	
Streptomycin Sulfate, Sterile	I	D	
Succinylcholine Chloride Inj.	S,M	A,B	R
Succinylcholine Chloride, Sterile	I	D	
Sufentanil Citrate Inj.	S,M	A	
Sugar Inj., Invert	S,P	A,B	
Sulfadiazine Sodium Inj.	S	A	LR

Drugs	Container	Glass Type	Storage Conditions
Sulfamethoxazole and Trimethoprim Inj.	S,M (50 mL)	A	L
Sulfisoxazole Diolamine Inj.	S,M	A	L
Technetium Tc 99m Albumin Aggregated Inj.	S,M		R
Technetium Tc 99m Albumin Colloid Inj.	S,M		R
Technetium Tc 99m Albumin Inj.	S,M		R
Technetium Tc 99m Bicisate Inj.	S,M		RT
Technetium Tc 99m Disofenin Inj.	S,M		In
Technetium Tc 99m Etidronate Inj.	S,M		
Technetium Tc 99m Exametazine Inj.	S,M		RT
Technetium Tc 99m Gluceptate Inj.	S,M		R
Technetium Tc 99m Lidofenin Inj.	S,M		R
Technetium Tc 99m Mebrofenin Inj.	S,M		RT
Technetium Tc 99m Medronate Inj.	S,M		
Technetium Tc 99m Oxidronate Inj.	S,M		
Technetium Tc 99m Pentetate Inj.	S,M		R
Technetium Tc 99m (Pyro- and Trimeta-) Phosphates Inj.	U		D
Technetium Tc 99m Pyrophos. Inj.	S,M		R
Technetium Tc 99m Succimer Inj.	S		RT,L
Technetium Tc 99m Sulfur Colloid Inj.	S,M		
Terbutaline Sulfate Inj.	S	A	L,RT
Testosterone Cypionate Inj.	S,M	A	L
Testosterone Enanthate Inj.	S,M	A	
Testosterone Injectable Susp.	S,M	A	
Testosterone Propionate Inj.	S,M	A	
Tetanus and Diphtheria Toxoids Adsorbed (for adult use)	U		R
Tetanus Antitoxin	U		R
Tetanus Immune Globulin	U		R
Tetanus Toxoid	U		R
Tetanus Toxoid Adsorbed	U		R
Tetracaine HCl in Dextrose Inj.	S,M (up to 100 ml)	A	R,L,RT (tray for 12 months)
Tetracaine HCl Inj.	S,M	A	R,L
Tetracaine HCl, Sterile	I	A	
Tetracycline HCl for Inj.	I	B	L
Tetracycline HCl, Sterile	I		L
Tetracycline Phosphate Complex for Inj.	I	B	L
Tetracycline Phosphate Complex, Sterile	I		L
Thallous Chloride Tl 201 Inj.	S,M		
Theophylline in Dextrose Inj.	S	A,B,P	
Thiamine HCl Inj.	S,M	A	L
Thiamylal Sodium for Inj.	I	C	
Thiethylperazine Maleate Inj.	S	A	L
Thiopental Sodium for Inj.	I	C	
Thiotepa for Inj.	I	D	R,L
Thiothixene HCl for Inj.	I		LR
Thiothixene HCl Inj.	S	A	L
Thrombin			R
Ticarcillin Disodium and Clavulanate Potassium Inj.	I		F

Drugs	Container	Glass Type	Storage Conditions
Ticarcillin Disodium and Clavulanate Potassium, Sterile	I		
Ticarcillin Disodium, Sterile	I	D	
Tilmicosin Injection	I		
Tobramycin Sulfate Inj.	S,M	A,P	
Tobramycin Sulfate, Sterile	I		
Tolbutamide Sodium, Sterile	I	D	
Triamcinolone Acetonide Injectable Susp.	S,M	A	L
Triamcinolone Diacetate Injectable Susp.	S,M	A	
Triamcinolone Hexacetonide Injectable Susp.	S,M	A	
Trifluoperazine HCl Inj.	M	A	L
Triflupromazine HCl Inj.	S,M	A	L
Trimethaphan Camsylate Inj.	S,M	A	R
Trimethobenzamide HCl Inj.	S,M	A	
Tromethamine for Inj.	S,M	A	C
Trypsin for Inhalation Aerosol, Crystallized	S	A	RT
Tuberculin			R
Tubocurarine Chloride	S,M		
Typhoid Vaccine	U		R
Urea, Sterile	I	D	
Vaccinia Immune Globulin	U		R
Vancomycin HCl for Inj.	I		
Varicella-Zoster Immune Globulin	U		R
Vasopressin Inj.	S,M	A	
Verapamil HCl Inj.	S	A	LR
Vidarabine Concentrate for Inj.	S,M	A	
Vinblastine Sulfate for Inj.	I	D	R
Vincristine Sulfate for Inj.	U		L,R
Vincristine Sulfate Inj.	U	U	L,R
Warfarin Sodium for Inj.	I	D	LR
Water 0-15 Inj.	S		SC
Water for Inhalation, Sterile	S		
Water for Inj.	SP		
Water for Inj., Sterile	S	A,B,P	SS
Water for Inj., Sterile Bacteriostatic	S,M, CV	A,B,P	
Water for Irrigation, Sterile	S	A,B	
Water, Sterile Purified	WC	U	
Xenon Xe 127	S (leakproof stoppers)		RT,SC
Xenon Xe 133	S (leakproof stoppers)		RT,SC
Xenon X3 133 Inj.	S (totally filled)		RT,SC
Yellow Fever Vaccine	U (nitrogen filled ampules)		R
Zidovudine Inj.	Ti		LR
Zinc Chloride Inj.	S,M	A,B	
Zinc Sulfate Inj.	S,M		

Provided by Dr. Kenneth S. Alexander, Professor of Pharmacy, College of Pharmacy, University of Toledo.

Oral Dosage Forms That Should Not Be Crushed or Chewed

This listing is included to alert the healthcare practitioner about oral dosage forms that should not be crushed or chewed and to serve as an aid in consulting with patients. Refer to the end of the table for a complete explanation of all alphabetical references.

Drug Product	Manufacturer	Dosage Form	Reason/Comments
Accutane	Roche	Capsule	Mucous membrane irritant
Actifed 12 Hour	Warner Lambert Consumer Health Products	Capsule	Slow release (i)
Acutrim	Novartis Consumer Health	Tablet	Slow release
Adalat	Bayer	Tablet	Slow release
Aerolate SR, JR, III	Fleming & Co.	Capsule	Slow release*(i)
Afrinol Repetabs	Schering-Plough	Tablet	Slow release
Allegra D	Hoechst Marion Roussel	Tablet	Slow release
Allerest 12 Hour	Novartis Consumer Health	Caplet	Slow release
Artane Sequels	Lederle	Capsule	Slow release*(i)
Arthritis Bayer TR	Bayer	Capsule	Slow release
ASA Enseals	Lilly	Tablet	Enteric-coated
Asbron G Inlay	Sandoz	Tablet	Multiple compressed tablet (i)
Atrohist Plus	Adams	Tablet	Slow release
Atrohist Sprinkle	Adams	Capsule	Slow release*
Azulfidine Entabs	Pharmacia & Upjohn	Tablet	Enteric-coated
Baros	Lafayette	Tablet	Effervescent tab (d)
Bayer Extra Strength Enteric 500	Sterling Health	Tablet	Slow release
Bayer Low Adult 81 mg Strength	Sterling Health	Tablet	Enteric-coated
Bayer Regular Strength 325 mg Caplet	Sterling Health	Tablet	Enteric-coated
Bayer Regular Strength EC Caplets	Sterling Health	Caplet	Enteric-coated
Betachron E-R	Inwood	Capsule	Slow release
Betapen-VK	Bristol	Tablet	Taste (c)
Biohist-LA	Wakefield	Tablet	Slow release (h)
Bisacodyl	(Various Mfr.)	Tablet	Enteric-coated (a)
Bisco-Lax	Raway	Tablet	Enteric-coated (a)
Bontril-SR	Carnrick	Capsule	Slow release
Breonesin	Sanofi Winthrop	Capsule	Liquid filled (b)
Brexin LA	Savage	Capsule	Slow release (i)
Bromfed	Muro	Capsule	Slow release (i)
Bromfed-PD	Muro	Capsule	Slow release (i)
Calan SR	Searle	Tablet	Slow release (h)
Cama Arthritis Pain Reliever	Sandoz Consumer	Tablet	Multiple compressed tablet
Carbiset-TR	Nutripharm	Tablet	Slow release
Cardizem	Hoechst Marion Roussel	Tablet	Slow release

Drug Product	Manufacturer	Dosage Form	Reason/Comments
Cardizem CD	Hoechst Marion Roussel	Capsule	Slow release*
Cardizem SR	Hoechst Marion Roussel	Capsule	Slow release*
Carter's Little Pills	Carter-Wallace	Tablet	Enteric-coated
Cefol Filmtab	Abbott	Tablet	Enteric-coated
Ceftin	GlaxoWellcome	Tablet	Taste (c) Use suspension for children
Charcoal Plus	Kramer	Tablet	Enteric-coated
Chloral Hydrate	(Various Mfr.)	Capsule	Liquid in capsule (i)
Chlorpheniramine Maleate Time Release	(Various Mfr.)	Capsule	Slow release
Chlor-Trimeton Repetab	Schering-Plough	Tablet	Slow release (i)
Choledyl SA	Parke-Davis	Tablet	Slow release (i)
Cipro	Bayer	Tablet	Taste (c)
Claritin-D	Schering-Plough	Tablet	Slow release
Codimal LA	Schwarz Pharma	Capsule	Slow release
Codimal LA Half	Schwarz Pharma	Capsule	Slow release
Colace	Roberts	Capsule	Taste (c)
Comhist LA	Roberts	Capsule	Slow release*
Compazine Spansule	SmithKline Beecham	Capsule	Slow release (i)
Congess SR, JR	Fleming & Co.	Capsule	Slow release
Constant T	Novartis	Tablet	Slow release*
Contac	SmithKline Beecham	Capsule	Slow release*
Cotazym-S	Organon	Capsule	Enteric-coated*
Covera-HS	Searle	Tablet	Slow release
Creon 10, 20	Solvay	Capsule	Enteric-coated*
Cystospaz-M	PolyMedica	Capsule	Slow release
Cytoxan	Bristol-Myers	Tablet	May be crushed but maker recommends injection.
Dallergy	Laser	Capsule	Slow release
Dallergy-D	Laser	Capsule	Slow release
Dallergy-JR	Laser	Capsule	Slow release
Deconamine SR	Kenwood	Capsule	Slow release (i)
Deconsal II	Adams	Tablet	Slow release
Deconsal Sprinkle	Adams	Capsule	Slow release*
Defen-LA	Horizon	Tablet	Slow release (h)
Demazin Repetabs	Schering-Plough	Tablet	Slow release (i)
Depakene	Abbott	Capsule	Slow release, mucous membrane irritant (i)
Depakote	Abbott	Capsule	Enteric-coated
Desoxyn Gradumets	Abbott	Tablet	Slow release
Desyrel	Apothecon	Tablet	Taste (c)
Dexatrim, Max. Strength	Thompson Medical	Tablet	Slow release
Dexedrine Spansule	SmithKline Beecham	Capsule	Slow release
Diamox Sequels	Lederle	Capsule	Slow release
Dilatrate SR	Schwarz Pharma	Capsule	Slow release
Dimetane Extentab	Robins	Tablet	Slow release (i)
Disobrom	Geneva Pharm.	Tablet	Slow release

Drug Product	Manufacturer	Dosage Form	Reason/Comments
Disophrol Chronotab	Schering-Plough	Tablet	Slow release
Dital	UAD	Capsule	Slow release
Donnatal Extentab	Robins	Tablet	Slow release (i)
Donnazyme	Robins	Tablet	Enteric-coated
Drisdol	Sanofi Winthrop	Capsule	Liquid filled (b)
Drixoral	Schering-Plough	Tablet	Slow release (i)
Drixoral Plus	Schering-Plough	Tablet	Slow release
Drixoral Sinus	Schering-Plough	Tablet	Slow release
Dulcolax	Boehringer Ingelheim	Tablet	Enteric-coated (a)
Dynabac	Bock Pharmacal	Tablet	Enteric-coated
Easprin	Parke-Davis	Tablet	Enteric-coated
Ecotrin	SmithKline Beecham	Tablet	Enteric-coated
E.E.S. 400	(Various Mfr.)	Tablet	Enteric-coated (i)
Efidac 24	Hogil Pharmaceutical	Tablet	Slow release
Elixophyllin SR	Forest	Capsule	Slow release*(i)
E-Mycin	Knoll Pharm.	Tablet	Enteric-coated
Endafed	UAD	Capsule	Slow release
Entex LA	Dura	Tablet	Slow release (i)
Entozyme	Robins	Tablet	Enteric-coated
Equanil	Wyeth-Ayerst	Tablet	Taste (c)
Ergostat	Parke-Davis	Tablet	Sublingual form (g)
Eryc	Parke-Davis	Capsule	Enteric-coated*
Ery-Tab	Abbott	Tablet	Enteric-coated
Erythrocin Stearate	Abbott	Tablet	Enteric-coated
Erythromycin Base	(Various Mfr.)	Tablet	Enteric-coated
Eskalith CR	SmithKline Beecham	Tablet	Slow release
Exgest LA	Carnrick	Tablet	Slow release
Fedahist Timecaps	Schwarz Pharma	Capsule	Slow release (i)
Feldene	Pfizer	Capsule	Mucous membrane irritant
Feocyte	Dunhall	Tablet	Slow release
Feosol	SmithKline Beecham	Tablet	Enteric-coated (i)
Feosol Spansule	SmithKline Beecham	Capsule	Slow release*(i)
Feratab	Upsher-Smith	Tablet	Enteric-coated (i)
Fergon	Sanofi Winthrop	Capsule	Slow release*
Fero-Grad-500	Abbott	Tablet	Slow release
Fero-Gradumet	Abbott	Tablet	Slow release
Ferralet SR	Mission	Tablet	Slow release
Festal 11	Hoechst Marion Roussel	Tablet	Enteric-coated
Feverall Sprinkle Caps	Ascent Pediatrics	Capsule	Taste*(j)
Flomax	Boehringer Ingelheim	Capsule	Slow release
Fumatinic	Laser	Capsule	Slow release
Gastrocrom	Medeva	Capsule	Dissolve in water (k)
Geocillin	Roerig	Tablet	Taste
Glucotrol XL	Pratt	Tablet	Slow release
Gris-PEG	Allergan	Tablet	Crushing may precipitate (l)
Guaifed	Muro	Capsule	Slow release
Guaifed-PD	Muro	Capsule	Slow release

Drug Product	Manufacturer	Dosage Form	Reason/Comments
Guaifenex LA	Ethex	Tablet	Slow release (h)
Guaifenex PSE 120	Ethex	Tablet	Slow release (h)
Guaimax-D	Schwarz Pharma	Tablet	Slow release
Humibid DM	Adams	Tablet	Slow release
Humibid DM Sprinkle	Adams	Capsule	Slow release*
Humibid LA	Adams	Tablet	Slow release
Humibid Sprinkle	Adams	Capsule	Slow release*
Hydergine LC	Sandoz	Capsule	Liquid in capsule (i)
Hydergine Sublingual	Sandoz	Tablet	Sublingual route (i)
Hytakerol	Sanofi Winthrop	Capsule	Liquid filled (b)(i)
Iberet	Abbott	Tablet	Slow release (i)
Iberet 500	Abbott	Tablet	Slow release (i)
ICaps Plus	LaHaye Labs	Tablet	Slow release
ICaps Time Release	LaHaye Labs	Tablet	Slow release
Ilotycin	Dista	Tablet	Enteric-coated
Imdur	Key	Tablet	Slow release (h)
Inderal LA	Wyeth-Ayerst	Capsule	Slow release
Inderide LA	Wyeth-Ayerst	Capsule	Slow release
Indocin SR	Merck	Capsule	Slow release*(i)
Ionamin	Medeva	Capsule	Slow release
Isoclor Timesule	Medeva	Capsule	Slow release (i)
Isoptin SR	Knoll Pharm.	Tablet	Slow release
Isordil Sublingual	Wyeth-Ayerst	Tablet	Sublingual form (g)
Isordil Tembid	Wyeth-Ayerst	Tablet	Slow release
Isosorbide Dinitrate SR	(Various Mfr.)	Tablet	Slow release
Isosorbide Dinitrate Sublingual	(Various Mfr.)	Tablet	Sublingual form (g)
Isuprel Glossets	Sanofi Winthrop	Tablet	Sublingual form (g)
K + 8	Alra	Tablet	Slow release (i)
K + 10	Alra	Tablet	Slow release (i)
Kaon Cl 6.7 mEq	Savage	Tablet	Slow release
Kaon Cl 8 mEq	Savage	Tablet	Slow release (i)
Kaon Cl-10	Savage	Tablet	Slow release (i)
K + Care E+	Alra	Tablet	Effervescent tablet (d)(i)
K-Lease	Adria	Capsule	Slow release*(i)
Klor-Con	Upsher-Smith	Tablet	Slow release (i)
Klor-Con/EF	Upsher-Smith	Tablet	Effervescent tablet (d)(i)
Klorvess	Sandoz	Tablet	Effervescent tablet (d)(i)
Klotrix	Mead Johnson	Tablet	Slow release (i)
K-Lyte	Mead Johnson	Tablet	Effervescent tablet (d)
K-Lyte/Cl 50	Mead Johnson	Tablet	Effervescent tablet (d)
K-Lyte DS	Mead Johnson	Tablet	Effervescent tablet (d)
K-Tab	Abbott	Tablet	Slow release (i)
Levsinex Timecaps	Schwarz Pharma	Capsule	Slow release
Lexxel	Astra Merck	Tablet	Slow release
Lithobid	Novartis	Tablet	Slow release (i)
Lodrane LD	ECR Pharmaceutical	Capsule	Slow release*
Mag-Tab SR	Niche	Tablet	Slow release

Drug Product	Manufacturer	Dosage Form	Reason/Comments
Meprospan	Wallace	Capsule	Slow release*
Mestinon Timespan	ICN	Tablet	Slow release (i)
Mi-Cebrin	Dista	Tablet	Enteric-coated
Mi-Cebrin T	Dista	Tablet	Enteric-coated
Micro K	Robins	Capsule	Slow release*(i)
Monafed	Monarch	Tablet	Slow release
Monafed DM	Monarch	Tablet	Slow release
Motrin	Pharmacia & Upjohn	Tablet	Taste (c)
MS Contin	Purdue Frederick	Tablet	Slow release (i)
MSC Triaminic	Sandoz	Tablet	Enteric-coated
Muco-Fen-LA	Wakefield	Tablet	Slow release (h)
Naldecon	Bristol	Tablet	Slow release (i)
Naprelan	Wyeth-Ayerst	Tablet	Slow release
Nasatab LA	ECR Pharmaceutical	Tablet	Slow release (h)
Niaspan	KOS	Tablet	Slow release
Nico-400	Jones Medical	Capsule	Slow release
Nicobid	Rhone-Poulenc Rorer	Capsule	Slow release
Nitro Bid	Hoechst Marion Roussel	Capsule	Slow release*
Nitrocine Timecaps	Schwarz Pharma	Capsule	Slow release
Nitroglyn	Kenwood	Capsule	Slow release*
Nitrong	Rhone-Poulenc Rorer	Tablet	Sublingual route (g)
Nitrostat	Parke-Davis	Tablet	Sublingual route (g)
Nitro-Time	Time-Cap Labs	Capsule	Slow release
Noctec	Apothecon	Capsule	Liquid in capsule (i)
Nolamine	Carnrick	Tablet	Slow release
Nolex LA	Carnrick	Tablet	Slow release
Norflex	3M Pharmaceuticals	Tablet	Slow release
Norpace CR	Searle	Capsule	Slow release
Novafed	Hoechst Marion Roussel	Capsule	Slow release
Novafed A	Hoechst Marion Roussel	Capsule	Slow release
Ondrox	Unimed	Tablet	Slow release
Optilets-500 Filmtab	Abbott	Tablet	Enteric-coated
Optilets-M-500 Filmtab	Abbott	Tablet	Enteric-coated
Oragrafin	Bracco DXS	Capsule	Liquid in capsule
Oramorph SR	Roxane	Tablet	Slow release (i)
Ornade Spansule	SmithKline Beecham	Capsule	Slow release
Oxycontin	Purdue Pharma	Tablet	Slow release
Pabalate	Robins	Tablet	Enteric-coated
Pabalate SF	Robins	Tablet	Enteric-coated
Pancrease	Ortho McNeil	Capsule	Enteric-coated*
Pancrease MT	Ortho McNeil	Capsule	Enteric-coated*
Panmycin	Pharmacia-Upjohn	Capsule	Taste
Papaverine Sustained Action	(Various Mfr.)	Capsule	Slow release
Pathilon Sequeles	Lederle	Capsule	Slow release*

Drug Product	Manufacturer	Dosage Form	Reason/Comments
Pavabid Plateau	Hoechst Marion Roussel	Capsule	Slow release*
PBZ-SR	Novartis Pharm	Tablet	Slow release (i)
Pentasa	Hoechst Marion Roussel	Tablet	Slow release
Perdiem	Rhone-Poulenc Rorer	Granules	Wax coated
Peritrate SA	Parke-Davis	Tablet	Slow release (h)
Permitil Chronotab	Schering	Tablet	Slow release (i)
Phazyme	Block	Tablet	Slow release
Phazyme 95	Block	Tablet	Slow release
Phenergan	Wyeth-Ayerst	Tablet	Taste (c)(i)
Phyllocontin	Purdue Frederick	Tablet	Slow release
Plendil	Astra Merck	Tablet	Slow release
Pneumomist	ECR Pharmaceutical	Tablet	Slow release (h)
Polaramine Repetabs	Schering-Plough	Tablet	Slow release (i)
Posicor	Roche	Tablet	Mucous membrane irritant
Prelu-2	Boehringer Ingelheim	Capsule	Slow release
Prevacid	TAP Pharmaceutical	Capsule	Slow release
Prilosec	Astra Merck	Capsule	Slow release
Pro-Banthine	Roberts	Tablet	Taste
Procainamide HCL SR	(Various Mfr.)	Tablet	Slow release
Procanbid	Parke-Davis	Tablet	Slow release
Procan SR	Parke-Davis	Tablet	Slow release
Procardia	Pfizer	Capsule	Delays absorption (b)(e)
Procardia XL	Pfizer	Tablet	Slow release, AUC is unaffected
Profen II	Wakefield	Tablet	Slow release (h)
Profen-LA	Wakefield	Tablet	Slow release (h)
Pronestyl SR	Apothecon	Tablet	Slow release
Propecia	Merck	Tablet	Pregnant women should exercise caution (m)
Proscar	Merck	Tablet	Pregnant women should exercise caution
Proventil Repetabs	Schering-Plough	Tablet	Slow release (i)
Prozac	Dista	Capsule	Slow release*
Quadra Hist	Schein	Tablet	Slow release
Quibron-T/SR	Bristol-Myers Squibb	Tablet	Slow release (i)
Quinaglute DuraTabs	Berlex	Tablet	Slow release
Quinalan Lanatabs	Lannett	Tablet	Slow release
Quinalan SR	Lannett	Tablet	Slow release
Quinidex Extentabs	Robins	Tablet	Slow release
Quin-Release	Major	Tablet	Slow release
Respa-1st	Respa	Tablet	Slow release (h)
Respa-DM	Respa	Tablet	Slow release (h)
Respa-GF	Respa	Tablet	Slow release (h)
Respahist	Respa	Capsule	Slow release*
Respaire SR	Laser	Capsule	Slow release
Respbid	Boehringer Ingelheim	Tablet	Slow release
Ritalin-SR	Novartis	Tablet	Slow release

Drug Product	Manufacturer	Dosage Form	Reason/Comments
Robimycin Robitab	Robins	Tablet	Enteric-coated
Rondec TR	Dura	Tablet	Slow release (i)
Roxanol SR	Roxane	Tablet	Slow release (i)
Ru-Tuss DE	Knoll Pharm.	Tablet	Slow release
Sinemet CR	DuPont Pharm	Tablet	Slow release (h)
Singlet	SmithKline Beecham	Tablet	Slow release
Slo-Bid Gyrocaps	Rhone-Poulenc Rorer	Capsule	Slow release*
Slo-Niacin	Upsher-Smith	Tablet	Slow release (h)
Slo-Phyllin GG	Rhone-Poulenc Rorer	Capsule	Slow release (i)
Slo-Phyllin Gyrocaps	Rhone-Poulenc Rorer	Capsule	Slow release*(i)
Slow FE	Novartis Consumer Health	Tablet	Slow release (i)
Slow FE with Folic Acid	Novartis Consumer Health	Tablet	Slow release
Slow-K	Summit	Tablet	Slow release (i)
Slow-Mag	Searle	Tablet	Slow release
Sorbitrate SA	Zeneca	Tablet	Slow release
Sorbitrate Sublingual	Zeneca	Tablet	Sublingual route
Sparine	Wyeth-Ayerst	Tablet	Taste (c)
S-P-T	Fleming	Capsule	Liquid gelatin thyroid suspension
Sudafed 12 hour	Warner Lambert Consumer Health Products	Capsule	Slow release (i)
Sudal 60/500	Atley	Tablet	Slow release
Sudal 120/600	Atley	Tablet	Slow release
Sudex	Atley	Tablet	Slow release (h)
Sular	Zeneca	Tablet	Slow release
Sustaire	Pfizer	Tablet	Slow release (i)
Syn-RX	Adams Lab	Tablet	Slow release
Syn-Rx DM	Adams Lab	Tablet	Slow release
Tavist-D	Hoechst	Tablet	Multiple compressed tablet
Teczam	Hoechst Marion Roussel	Tablet	Slow release
Tedral SA	Parke-Davis	Tablet	Slow release
Tegretol-XR	Novartis	Tablet	Slow release
Teldrin	SmithKline Beecham	Capsule	Slow release*
Tepanil Ten-Tab	3M Pharmaceuticals	Tablet	Slow release
Tessalon Perles	Forest	Capsule	Slow release
Theo-24	UCB Pharma	Tablet	Slow release (i)
Theobid Duracaps	UCB Pharma	Capsule	Slow release*(i)
Theobid Jr.	UCB Pharma	Capsule	Slow release*(i)
Theochron	Forest	Tablet	Slow release
Theoclear LA	Schwarz Pharma	Capsule	Slow release (i)
Theo-Dur	Key	Tablet	Slow release (i)
Theo-Dur Sprinkle	Key	Capsule	Slow release*(i)
Theolair SR	3M Pharmaceuticals	Tablet	Slow release (i)
Theo-Sav	Savage	Tablet	Slow release (h)
Theo-Time SR	Major	Tablet	Slow release

Drug Product	Manufacturer	Dosage Form	Reason/Comments
Theovent	Schering-Plough	Capsule	Slow release (i)
Theo-X	Carnrick	Tablet	Slow release
Therapy Bayer	Glenbrook	Caplet	Enteric-coated
Thorazine Spansule	SmithKline Beecham	Capsule	Slow release
Toprol XL	Astra	Tablet	Slow release (h)
Touro A & H	Dartmouth	Capsule	Slow release
Touro DM	Dartmouth	Tablet	Slow release
Touro EX	Dartmouth	Tablet	Slow release
Touro LA	Dartmouth	Tablet	Slow release
T-Phyl	Purdue Frederick	Tablet	Slow release
Trental	Hoechst Marion Roussel	Tablet	Slow release
Triaminic	Sandoz	Tablet	Enteric-coated (i)
Triaminic-12	Sandoz	Tablet	Slow release (i)
Triaminic TR	Sandoz	Tablet	Multiple compressed tablet (i)
Trilafon Repetabs	Schering-Plough	Tablet	Slow release (i)
Tri-Phen-Chlor Time Release	Rugby	Tablet	Slow release
Tri-Phen-Mine SR	Goldline	Tablet	Slow release
Triptone Caplets	Del Pharm	Tablet	Slow release
Tuss-LA	Hyrex	Tablet	Slow release
Tuss Ornade Spansule	SmithKline Beecham	Capsule	Slow release
Tylenol Extended Relief	McNeil Consumer Products	Capsule	Slow release
ULR-LA	Geneva Pharmaceutical	Tablet	Slow release
Uni-Dur	Key	Tablet	Slow release
Uniphyl	Purdue Frederick	Tablet	Slow release
Valrelease	Roche	Capsule	Slow release
Verelan	Lederle	Capsule	Slow release*
Volmax	Muro	Tablet	Slow release
Wellbutrin	GlaxoWellcome	Tablet	Anesthetize mucous membrane
Wyamycin S	Wyeth Ayerst	Tablet	Slow release
Wygesic	Wyeth-Ayerst	Tablet	Taste
ZORprin	Knoll Pharm.	Tablet	Slow release
Zyban	GlaxoWellcome	Tablet	Slow release
Zymase	Organon	Capsule	Enteric-coated

Revised by John F. Mitchell, PharmD, FASHP, from an article originally appearing in *Hospital Pharmacy*, 31:27-37, 1996.

* Capsule may be opened and the contents taken without crushing or chewing; soft food such as applesauce or pudding may facilitate administration; contents may generally be administered via nasogastric tube using an appropriate fluid provided entire contents are washed down the tube.

(a) Antacids or milk may prematurely dissolve the coating of the tablet.

(b) Capsule may be opened and the liquid contents removed for administration.

(c) The taste of this product in a liquid form would likely be unacceptable to the patient; administration via nasogastric tube should be acceptable.

(d) Effervescent tablets must be dissolved in the amount of diluent recommended by the manufacturer.

(e) If the liquid capsule is crushed or the contents expressed, the active ingredient will be, in part, absorbed sublingually.

(f) Acid contents of the stomach may prematurely activate the ingredients.

(g) Tablets are made to disintegrate under the tongue.

(h) Tablet is scored and may be broken in half without affecting release characteristics.

(i) Liquid dosage forms of the product are available; however, dose, frequency of administration, and manufacturers may differ from that of the solid dosage form.

(j) Capsule contents intended to be placed in a teaspoonful of water or soft food.

(k) Contents may be dissolved in water for administration.

(l) Crushing may result in precipitation of larger particles.

(m) Crushed or broken tablet should not be handled by women who are pregnant or who may become pregnant.

Drug Names That Look Alike and Sound Alike

Dispensing errors can be caused by drug names that look alike and sound alike. The list below contains several such combinations. Some similarities sound dangerously close while others may appear more obviously different. In both circumstances good communications skills are vital when dealing with these drugs.

This list has been prepared to sensitize health professionals and their support personnel for the need to properly communicate when writing, speaking, reading and hearing drug names.

Trade names are capitalized whereas other names are in lower case letters.

"Look-Alike, Sound-Alike Drugs" was originated and developed by Benjamin Teplitsky, retired Chief Pharmacist of Veterans Administration Hospitals in Albany, NY and Brooklyn, NY.

A

abciximab . . . . .arcitumomab
acetazolamide . . . . .acetohexamide
acetohexamide . . . . .acetazolamide
acetylcholine . . . . .acetylcysteine
acetylcysteine . . . . .acetylcholine
Acthar .Acthrel
Acthar .Acular
Acthrel . . . . .Acthar
Acular .Acthar
Adderall . . . . .Inderal
Adeflor M . . . . .Aldoclor
Adriamycin . . . . .Idamycin
Afrin . . . . .aspirin
Akineton. . . . . .Ecotrin
Albutein . . . . .albuterol
albuterol . . . . .atenolol
albuterol . . . . .Albutein
Alcaine . . . . .Alcare
Alcare .Alcaine
Aldactazide . . . . .Aldactone
Aldactone . . . . .Aldactazide
Aldoclor . . . . .Aldoril
Aldoclor . . . . .Adeflor M
Aldomet . . . . .Aldoril
Aldoril . . . . .Aldoclor
Aldoril . . . . .Aldomet
Alfenta . . . . .Sufenta
alfentanil . . . . .Anafranil
alfentanil . . . . .fentanyl
alfentanil . . . . .sufentanil
Alkeran . . . . .Leukeran
alprazolam . . . . .lorazepam
alprazolam . . . . .alprostadil
alprostadil . . . . .alprazolam
Altace .alteplase
Altace .Artane
alteplase . . . . .anistreplase
alteplase . . . . .Altace
Alupent . . . . .Atrovent
Ambenyl . . . . .Aventyl
Ambien . . . . .Amen
Amen .Ambien
Amicar . . . . .Amikin
Amikin . . . . .Amicar
amiloride . . . . .amiodarone
amiloride . . . . .amlodipine
aminophylline . . . . .amitriptyline
aminophylline . . . . .ampicillin
amiodarone . . . . .amiloride
amiodarone . . . . .amrinone
Amipaque . . . . .Omnipaque
amitriptyline . . . . .nortriptyline
amitriptyline . . . . .aminophylline
amlodipine . . . . .amiloride
amoxapine . . . . .amoxicillin
amoxicillin . . . . .amoxapine
ampicillin . . . . .aminophylline
amrinone . . . . .amiodarone
Anafranil . . . . .enalapril
Anafranil . . . . .nafarelin
Anafranil . . . . .alfentanil
Anaprox . . . . .Anaspaz
Anaspaz . . . . .Anaprox
Ancobon . . . . .Oncovin
anisindione . . . . .anisotropine
anisotropine . . . . .anisindione
anistreplase . . . . .alteplase
Antabuse . . . . .Anturane
Anturane . . . . .Artane

Anturane .... Antabuse
Anusol .... Aplisol
Anusol .... Aquasol
Aplisol .... Aplitest
Aplisol .... Anusol
Aplisol .... Atropisol
Aplitest .... Aplisol
Apresazide .... Apresoline
Apresoline .... Apresazide
Aquasol .... Anusol
arcitumomab .... abciximab
Aricept .... Ascriptin
Artane .... Altace
Artane .... Anturane
Asacol .... Os-Cal
Ascriptin .... Aricept
Asendin .... aspirin
aspirin .... Asendin
aspirin .... Afrin
Atarax .... Ativan
Atarax .... Marax
atenolol .... timolol
atenolol .... albuterol
Ativan .... Avitene
Ativan .... Atarax
Atropisol .... Aplisol
Atrovent .... Alupent
Aventyl .... Ambenyl
Aventyl .... Bentyl
Aventyl .... Serentil
Avitene .... Ativan
azatadine .... azathioprine
azathioprine .... azidothymidine
azathioprine .... Azulfidine
azathioprine .... azatadine
azidothymidine .... azathioprine
Azulfidine .... azathioprine

B

bacitracin .... Bactrim
bacitracin .... Bactroban
baclofen .... Bactroban
baclofen .... Beclovent
Bactine .... Bactrim
Bactine .... Banthine
Bactrim .... bacitracin
Bactrim .... Bactine
Bactroban .... bacitracin
Bactroban .... baclofen
Banthine .... Brethine
Banthine .... Bactine
Beclovent .... baclofen
Beminal .... Benemid
Benadryl .... Bentyl
Benadryl .... Benylin
Benadryl .... benazepril
benazepril .... Benadryl
Benemid .... Beminal
Benoxyl .... PerOxyl
Benoxyl .... Brevoxyl
Bentyl .... Aventyl
Bentyl .... Benadryl
Benylin .... Ventolin
Benylin .... Benadryl
benztropine .... bromocriptine
Bepridil .... Prepidil
Betadine .... betaine
Betagan .... Betagen
Betagen .... Betagan
betaine .... Betadine
Betoptic .... Betoptic S
Betoptic S .... Betoptic
Bicillin .... V-Cillin
Bicillin .... Wycillin
Brethaire .... Brethine
Brethaire .... Bretylol
Brethine .... Banthine
Brethine .... Brethaire
Bretylol .... Brevital
Bretylol .... Brethaire
Brevital .... Bretylol
Brevoxyl .... Benoxyl
brimonidine .... bromocriptine
bromocriptine .... benztropine
bromocriptine .... brimonidine
Bronkodyl .... Bronkosol
Bronkosol .... Bronkodyl
Bumex .... Buprenex
bupivacaine .... mepivacaine
Buprenex .... Bumex
bupropion .... buspirone
buspirone .... bupropion
butabarbital .... Butalbital
Butalbital .... butabarbital

C

Cafergot .... Carafate
Caladryl .... calamine

calamine .... Caladryl
calcifediol .... calcitriol
calciferol .... calcitriol
calcitonin .... calcitriol
calcitriol .... calcifediol
calcitriol .... calciferol
calcitriol .... calcitonin
calcium glubionate .... calcium gluconate
calcium gluconate .... calcium glubionate
Capastat .... Cepastat
Capitrol .... Captopril
Captopril .... Capitrol
Carafate .... Cafergot
Carbex .... Surbex
Carboplatin .... Cisplatin
Cardene .... Cardura
Cardene .... codeine
Cardene SR .... Cardizem SR
Cardizem SR .... Cardene SR
Cardura .... Coumadin
Cardura .... K-Dur
Cardura .... Cardene
Cardura .... Cordarone
Catapres .... Catarase
Catapres .... Cetapred
Catapres .... Combipres
Catarase .... Catapres
cefamandole .... cefmetazole
cefazolin .... cefprozil
cefmetazole .... cefamandole
Cefobid .... cefonicid
cefonicid .... Cefobid
Cefotan .... Ceftin
cefotaxime .... cefoxitin
cefotaxime .... cefuroxime
cefotetan .... cefoxitin
cefoxitin .... Cytoxan
cefoxitin .... cefotaxime
cefoxitin .... cefotetan
cefprozil .... cefazolin
ceftazidime .... ceftizoxime
Ceftin .... Cefotan
ceftizoxime .... ceftazidime
cefuroxime .... cefotaxime
cefuroxime .... deferoxamine
Cefzil .... Kefzol
Cepastat .... Capastat
cephapirin .... cephradine
cephradine .... cephapirin
Cerebyx .... Cerezyme
Ceredase .... Cerezyme
Cerezyme .... Cerebyx
Cerezyme .... Ceredase
Cetaphil .... Cetapred
Cetapred .... Cetaphil
Cetapred .... Catapres
Chenix .... Cystex
chlorambucil .... Chloromycetin
Chloromycetin .... chlorambucil
chloroxine .... Choloxin
chlorpromazine .... chlorpropamide
chlorpromazine .... clomipramine
chlorpropamide .... chlorpromazine
Choloxin .... chloroxine
Chorex .... Chymex
Chymex .... Chorex
Cidex .... Lidex
Ciloxan .... Cytoxan
Ciloxan .... cinoxacin
cimetidine .... simethicone
cinoxacin .... Ciloxan
Cisplatin .... Carboplatin
Citracal .... Citrucel
Citrucel .... Citracal
Clinoril .... Clozaril
clofazimine .... clozapine
clofibrate .... clorazepate
clomiphene .... clomipramine
clomiphene .... clonidine
clomipramine .... chlorpromazine
clomipramine .... clomiphene
clonidine .... quinidine
clonidine .... clomiphene
clorazepate .... clofibrate
clotrimazole .... co-trimoxazole
Cloxapen .... clozapine
clozapine .... clofazimine
clozapine .... Cloxapen
Clozaril .... Clinoril
co-trimoxazole .... clotrimazole
codeine .... Cardene
codeine .... Lodine
codeine .... Cordran
Combipres .... Catapres
Compazine .... Copaxone
Copaxone .... Compazine
Cordarone .... Cardura

Cordarone .... Cordran
Cordran .... codeine
Cordran .... Cordarone
Cort-Dome .... Cortone
Cortone .... Cort-Dome
Cortrosyn .... Cotazym
Cotazym .... Cortrosyn
Coumadin .... Kemadrin
Coumadin .... Cardura
Cozaar .... Zocor
cyclobenzaprine .... cycloserine
cyclobenzaprine .... cyproheptadine
cyclophosphamide .... cyclosporine
cycloserine .... cyclosporine
cycloserine .... cyclobenzaprine
cyclosporin .... Cyklokapron
cyclosporine .... cyclo phosphamide
cyclosporine .... cycloserine
Cyklokapron .... cyclosporin
cyproheptadine .... cyclobenzaprine
Cystex .... Chenix
Cytadren .... cytarabine
cytarabine .... vidarabine
cytarabine .... Cytadren
CytoGam .... Cytoxan
Cytosar U .... Cytovene
Cytosar U .... Cytoxan
Cytotec .... Cytoxan
Cytovene .... Cytosar U
Cytoxan .... Cytotec
Cytoxan .... Cytosar U
Cytoxan .... CytoGam
Cytoxan .... cefoxitin
Cytoxan .... Ciloxan

D

dacarbazine .... Dicarbosil
dacarbazine .... procarbazine
Dacriose .... Danocrine
dactinomycin .... daunorubicin
dactinomycin .... doxorubicin
Dalmane .... Dialume
Dalmane .... Demulen
Danocrine .... Dacriose
Dantrium .... Daraprim
dapsone .... Diprosone
Daranide .... Daraprim
Daraprim .... Dantrium
Daraprim .... Daranide
Daricon .... Darvon
Darvocet-N .... Darvon-N
Darvon .... Daricon
Darvon-N .... Darvocet-N
daunorubicin .... doxorubicin
daunorubicin .... dactinomycin
deferoxamine .... cefuroxime
Delsym .... Desyrel
Demerol .... Demulen
Demerol .... Dymelor
Demulen .... Dalmane
Demulen .... Demerol
Depo-Estradiol .... Depo-Testadiol
Depo-Medrol .... Solu-Medrol
Depo-Testadiol .... Depo-Estradiol
Dermatop .... Dimetapp
Desferal .... Disophrol
desipramine .... disopyramide
desipramine .... imipramine
desoximetasone .... dexamethasone
Desoxyn .... digitoxin
Desoxyn .... digoxin
Desyrel .... Zestril
Desyrel .... Delsym
dexamethasone .... desoximetasone
Dexedrine .... dextran
Dexedrine .... Excedrin
dextran .... Dexedrine
DiaBeta .... Zebeta
Dialume .... Dalmane
Diamox .... Trimox
diazepam .... diazoxide
diazepam .... Ditropan
diazoxide .... Dyazide
diazoxide .... diazepam
Dicarbosil .... dacarbazine
dichloroacetic acid .... trichloracetic acid
diclofenac .... Diflucan
diclofenac .... Duphalac
dicyclomine .... dyclonine
dicyclomine .... doxycycline
Diflucan .... diclofenac
digitoxin .... digoxin
digitoxin .... Desoxyn
digoxin .... doxepin
digoxin .... Desoxyn
digoxin .... digitoxin
Dilantin .... Dilaudid

Dilaudid	Dilantin
dimenhydrinate	diphenhydramine
Dimetane	Dimetapp
Dimetapp	Dermatop
Dimetapp	Dimetane
diphenhydramine	dimenhydrinate
Diprosone	dapsone
dipyridamole	disopyramide
Disophrol	Desferal
disopyramide	desipramine
disopyramide	dipyridamole
dithranol	Ditropan
Ditropan	diazepam
Ditropan	dithranol
dobutamine	dopamine
Donnagel	Donnatal
Donnatal	Donnagel
dopamine	Dopram
dopamine	dobutamine
Dopar	Dopram
Dopram	dopamine
Dopram	Dopar
doxacurium	doxapram
doxacurium	doxorubicin
doxapram	doxepin
doxapram	doxacurium
doxapram	doxazosin
doxapram	doxorubicin
doxazosin	doxapram
doxazosin	doxorubicin
doxazosin	doxepin
doxepin	doxazosin
doxepin	digoxin
doxepin	doxapram
doxepin	Doxidan
Doxil	Paxil
doxorubicin	doxapram
doxorubicin	dactinomycin
doxorubicin	daunorubicin
doxorubicin	doxacurium
doxorubicin	doxazosin
doxycycline	doxylamine
doxycycline	dicyclomine
doxylamine	doxycycline
dronabinol	droperidol
droperidol	dronabinol
Duphalac	diclofenac
Dyazide	diazoxide
dyclonine	dicyclomine
Dymelor	Demerol
Dynacin	DynaCirc
DynaCirc	Dynacin

E

Ecotrin	Edecrin
Ecotrin	Akineton
Edecrin	Ecotrin
Elavil	Equanil
Elavil	Mellaril
Eldepryl	enalapril
Emcyt	Eryc
enalapril	Anafranil
enalapril	Eldepryl
encainide	flecainide
Enduronyl Forte	Inderal 40 mg
enflurane	isoflurane
Entex	Tenex
ephedrine	epinephrine
epinephrine	ephedrine
Epogen	Neupogen
Equagesic	EquiGesic (Veterinary)
Equanil	Elavil
EquiGesic (Veterinary)	Equagesic
Eryc	Emcyt
Erythrocin	Ethmozine
Esimil	Estinyl
Esimil	Ismelin
Estinyl	Esimil
Estraderm	Testoderm
Ethmozine	Erythrocin
ethosuximide	methsuximide
etidocaine	etidronate
etidronate	etretinate
etidronate	etidocaine
etidronate	etomidate
etomidate	etidronate
etretinate	etidronate
Eurax	Serax
Eurax	Urex
Excedrin	Dexedrine

F

Factrel	Sectral
fentanyl	alfentanil
Feosol	Fer-in-Sol
Fer-in-Sol	Feosol
Feridex	Fertinex
Fertinex	Feridex

Fioricet ....Fiorinal
Fiorinal ....Florinef
Fiorinal ....Fioricet
flecainide ....encainide
Flexeril ....Floxin
Flexon ....Floxin
Florinef ....Fiorinal
Florvite ....Folvite
Floxin ....Flexeril
Floxin ....Flexon
Fludara ....FUDR
Flumadine ....flunisolide
Flumadine ....flutamide
flunisolide ....fluocinonide
flunisolide ....Flumadine
fluocinolone ....fluocinonide
fluocinonide ....flunisolide
fluocinonide ....fluocinolone
fluoxetine ....fluvastatin
flutamide ....Flumadine
fluvastatin ....fluoxetine
folic acid ....folinic acid
folinic acid ....folic acid
Folvite ....Florvite
fosinopril ....lisinopril
FUDR ....Fludara
Fulvicin ....Furacin
Furacin ....Fulvicin
furosemide ....Torsemide

G

Gantanol ....Gantrisin
Gantrisin ....Gantanol
Glaucon ....glucagon
glimepiride ....glipizide
glipizide ....glyburide
glipizide ....glimepiride
glucagon ....Glaucon
Glucotrol ....glyburide
glutethimide ....guanethidine
glyburide ....glipizide
glyburide ....Glucotrol
GoLYTELY ....NuLytely
gonadorelin ....gonadotropin
gonadorelin ....guanadrel
gonadotropin ....gonadorelin
guaifenesin ....guanfacine
guanabenz ....guanadrel
guanabenz ....guanfacine
guanadrel ....gonadorelin
guanadrel ....guanabenz
guanethidine ....guanidine
guanethidine ....glutethimide
guanfacine ....guanidine
guanfacine ....guaifenesin
guanfacine ....guanabenz
guanidine ....guanethidine
guanidine ....guanfacine

H

halcinonide ....Halcion
Halcion ....Haldol
Halcion ....Healon
Halcion ....halcinonide
Haldol ....Halog
Haldol ....Halcion
Halog ....Haldol
Halotestin ....Halotex
Halotestin ....halothane
Halotex ....Halotestin
halothane ....Halotestin
Healon ....Halcion
Heparin ....Hespan
Hespan ....Heparin
Humalog ....Humulin
Humulin ....Humalog
Hycodan ....Hycomine
Hycodan ....Vicodin
Hycomine ....Hycodan
hydralazine ....hydroxyzine
hydrochloro-thiazide ....hydroflumethia-zide
hydrocortisone ....hydroxychloro-quine
hydroflumethia-zide ....hydrochloro-thiazide
hydromorphone ....morphine
hydroxychloroquine ....hydrocortisone
hydroxyproges-terone ....medroxypro-ges terone
hydroxyurea ....hydroxyzine
hydroxyzine ....hydralazine
hydroxyzine ....hydroxyurea
Hygroton ....Regroton
HyperHep ....Hyperstat
Hyperstat ....Nitrostat
Hyperstat ....HyperHep
Hytone ....Vytone

I

Idamycin ....Adriamycin
Iletin ....Lente
Imipenem ....Omnipen
imipramine ....desipramine
Imodium ....Ionamin
Imuran ....Inderal
indapamide ....Iopidine
indapamide ....iodamide
indapamide ....iopamidol
Inderal ....Inderide
Inderal ....Isordil
Inderal ....Adderall
Inderal ....Imuran
Inderal 40 mg ....Enduronyl Forte
Inderide ....Inderal
interferon 2 ....interleukin 2
interferon alfa 2a ....interferon alfa 2b
interferon alfa 2b ....interferon alfa 2a
interleukin 2 ....interferon 2
Intropin ....Isoptin
iodamide ....indapamide
iodine ....Iopidine
iodine ....Lodine
iodapamide ....Iopidine
Ionamin ....Imodium
iopamidol ....indapamide
Iopidine ....Lodine
Iopidine ....indapamide
Iopidine ....iodine
Iopidine ....iodapamide
Ismelin ....Isuprel
Ismelin ....Esimil
isoflurane ....enflurane
Isoptin ....Intropin
Isopto Carbachol ....Isopto Carpine
Isopto Carpine ....Isopto Carbachol
Isordil ....Isuprel
Isordil ....Inderal
Isuprel ....Ismelin
Isuprel ....Isordil

K

K-Dur ....Cardura
K-Lor ....Kaochlor
K-Phos Neutral ....Neutra-Phos-K
Kaochlor ....K-Lor
Keflex ....Keflin
Keflin ....Keflex
Kefzol ....Cefzil
Kemadrin ....Coumadin
Klaron ....Klor-Con
Klor-Con ....Klaron

L

lactose ....lactulose
lactulose ....lactose
Lamictal ....Lomotil
Lamictal ....Lamisil
Lamisil ....Lamictal
lamivudine ....lamotrigine
lamotrigine ....lamivudine
Lanoxin ....Levsinex
Lasix ....Lidex
Lasix ....Luvox
Lente ....Iletin
Leukeran ....Leukine
Leukeran ....Alkeran
Leukine ....Leukeran
Leustatin ....lovastatin
Levatol ....Lipitor
Levbid ....Lithobid
levothyroxine ....liothyronine
Levsinex ....Lanoxin
Librax ....Librium
Librium ....Librax
Lidex ....Cidex
Lidex ....Lasix
Lioresal ....lisinopril
liothyronine ....levothyroxine
Lipitor ....Levatol
lisinopril ....fosinopril
lisinopril ....Lioresal
Lithobid ....Lithostat
Lithobid ....Lithotabs
Lithobid ....Levbid
Lithonate ....Lithostat
Lithostat ....Lithobid
Lithostat ....Lithonate
Lithostat ....Lithotabs
Lithotabs ....Lithostat
Lithotabs ....Lithobid
Livostin ....lovastatin
Lodine ....codeine
Lodine ....iodine
Lodine ....Iopidine
Lomotil ....Lamictal
Loniten ....Lotensin
Lopressor..................Lopurin

Lopurin	Lopressor
Lopurin	Lupron
Lorabid	Lortab
lorazepam	alprazolam
Lortab	Lorabid
Lotensin	Loniten
Lotensin	lovastatin
lovastatin	Lotensin
lovastatin	Leustatin
lovastatin	Livostin
Luminal	Tuinal
Lupron	Nuprin
Lupron	Lopurin
Luvox	Lasix

M

Maalox	Maolate
Maalox	Marax
magnesium sulfate	manganese sulfate
manganese sulfate	magnesium sulfate
Maolate	Maalox
Marax	Atarax
Marax	Maalox
Maxidex	Maxzide
Maxzide	Maxidex
Mazicon	Mivacron
Mebaral	Medrol
Mebaral	Mellaril
mecamylamine	mesalamine
Medrol	Mebaral
medroxyprogesterone	methyltestoster one
medroxyprogesterone	hydroxyprogesterone
medroxyprogesterone	methylprednisolone
Mellaril	Elavil
Mellaril	Mebaral
melphalan	Mephyton
Mephenytoin	Mephyton
Mephenytoin	phenytoin
mephobarbital	methocarbamol
Mephyton	melphalan
Mephyton	Mephenytoin
mepivacaine	bupivacaine
mesalamine	mecamylamine
Mesantoin	Mestinon
Mestinon	Mesantoin
Mestinon	Metatensin
metaproterenol	metoprolol
metaproterenol	metipranolol
Metatensin	Mestinon
methazolamide	metolazone
methenamine	methionine
methicillin	mezlocillin
methionine	methenamine
methocarbamol	mephobarbital
methsuximide	ethosuximide
methylprednisolone	medroxyproges terone
methyltestosterone	medroxyproges terone
metipranolol	metaproterenol
metolazone	metoprolol
metolazone	methazolamide
metoprolol	metaproterenol
metoprolol	metolazone
metyrapone	metyrosine
metyrosine	metyrapone
Mevacor	Mivacron
mezlocillin	methicillin
miconazole	Micronase
miconazole	Micronor
Micro-K	Micronase
Micronase	Micronor
Micronase	Micro-K
Micronase	miconazole
Micronor	miconazole
Micronor	Micronase
Midrin	Mydfrin
Milontin	Miltown
Milontin	Mylanta
Miltown	Milontin
Minocin	Mithracin
Minocin	niacin
Mithracin	Minocin
mithramycin	mitomycin
mitomycin	mithramycin
Mivacron	Mazicon
Mivacron	Mevacor
Moban	Mobidin
Mobidin	Moban
Modane	Mudrane
Monopril	Monurol
Monurol	Monopril
morphine	hydromorphone
Mudrane	Modane
Myambutol	Nembutal
Mycelex	Myoflex

Myciguent ....Mycitracin
Mycitracin ....Myciguent
Mydfrin ....Midrin
Mylanta ....Mynatal
Mylanta ....Milontin
Myleran ....Mylicon
Mylicon ....Myleran
Mynatal ....Mylanta
Myoflex ....Mycelex

N

nafarelin ....Anafranil
Naldecon ....Nalfon
Nalfon ....Naldecon
naloxone ....naltrexone
naltrexone ....naloxone
Narcan ....Norcuron
Navane ....Nubain
Navane ....Norvasc
Nembutal ....Myambutol
Nephro-Calci ....Nephrocaps
Nephrocaps ....Nephro-Calci
Neupogen ....Nutramigen
Neupogen ....Epogen
Neutra-Phos-K ....K-Phos Neutral
niacin ....Minocin
nicardipine ....nifedipine
Nicobid ....Nitro-Bid
Nicoderm ....Nitroderm
Nicorette ....Nordette
nifedipine ....nimodipine
nifedipine ....nicardipine
Nilstat ....Nitrostat
Nilstat ....Nystatin
nimodipine ....nifedipine
Nitro-Bid ....Nicobid
Nitroderm ....Nicoderm
nitroglycerin n..............itroprusside
nitroprussid ....nitroglycerin
Nitrostat ....Nystatin
Nitrostat ....Hyperstat
Nitrostat ....Nilstat
Norcuron ....Narcan
Nordette ....Nicorette
Norflex ....Noroxin
Norgesic #40 ....Norgesic Forte
Norgesic Forte ....Norgesic #40
Noroxin ....Norflex
nortriptyline ....amitriptyline
Norvasc ....Navane
Nubain ....Navane
NuLytely ....GoLYTELY
Nuprin ....Lupron
Nutramigen ....Neupogen
Nystatin ....Nilstat
Nystatin ....Nitrostat

O

OctreoScan ....OncoScint
Ocufen ....Ocuflox
Ocuflox ....Ocufen
olanzapine ....olsalazine
olsalazine ....olanzapine
Omnipaque ....Amipaque
Omnipen ....Unipon
Omnipen ....Imipenem
OncoScint ....OctreoScan
Oncovin ....Ancobon
Ophthaine ....Ophthetic
Ophthetic ....Ophthaine
Oretic ....Oreton
Oreton ....Oretic
Orexin ....Ornex
Orinase ....Ornade
Orinase ....Ornex
Ornade ....Orinase
Ornex ....Orexin
Ornex ....Orinase
Os-Cal ....Asacol
Otobiotic ....Urobiotic
oxaprozin ....oxazepam
oxazepam ....oxaprozin
oxymetazoline ....oxymetholone
oxymetholone ....oxymetazoline
oxymetholone ....oxymorphone
oxymorphone ....oxymetholone

P

paclitaxel ....paroxetine
paclitaxel ....Paxil
Panadol ....pindolol
pancuronium ....pipecuronium
Paraplatin ....Platinol
paregoric ....Percogesic
Parlodel ....pindolol
paroxetine ....paclitaxel
Patanol ....Platinol
Pathilon ....Pathocil
Pathocil ....Placidyl

Pathocil ....Pathilon
Pavabid ....Pavatine
Pavatine ....Pavabid
Pavulon ....Peptavlon
Paxil ....Doxil
Paxil ....paclitaxel
Paxil ....Taxol
Pediapred ....PediaProfen
Pediapred ....Pediazole
PediaProfen ....Pediapred
Pediazole ....Pediapred
Penetrex ....Pentrax
penicillamine ....penicillin
penicillin ....Polycillin
penicillin ....penicillamine
pentobarbital ....phenobarbital
pentosan ....pentostatin
pentostatin ....pentosan
Pentrax ....Permax
Pentrax ....Penetrex
Peptavlon ....Pavulon
Percocet ....Percodan
Percodan ....Percogesic
Percodan ....Periactin
Percodan ....Percocet
Percogesic ....paregoric
Percogesic ....Percodan
Periactin ....Persantine
Periactin ....Percodan
Permax ....Pentrax
Permax ....Pernox
Pernox ....Permax
PerOxyl ....Benoxyl
Persantine ....Periactin
phenobarbital ....pentobarbital
phentermine ....phentolamine
phentolamine ....phentermine
phenytoin ....Mephenytoin
Phos-Flur ....PhosLo
PhosChol ....PhosLo
PhosChol ....Phosphocol P32
PhosLo ....Phos-Flur
PhosLo ....PhosChol
Phosphocol P32 ....PhosChol
Phrenilin ....Trinalin
physostigmine ....Prostigmin
physostigmine ....pyridostigmine
pindolol ....Parlodel
pindolol ....Panadol
pindolol ....Plendil
pipecuronium ....pancuronium
Pitocin ....Pitressin
Pitressin ....Pitocin
Placidyl ....Pathocil
Platinol ....Paraplatin
Platinol ....Patanol
Plendil ....pindolol
Polocaine ....prilocaine
Polycillin ....penicillin
Ponstel ....Pronestyl
pralidoxime ....Pramoxine
pralidoxime ....pyridoxine
Pramoxine ....pralidoxime
Pravachol ....Prevacid
Pravachol ....propranolol
prednimustine ....prednisone
prednisolone ....prednisone
prednisone ....primidone
prednisone ....prednimustine
prednisone ....prednisolone
Premarin ....Primaxin
Prepidil ....Bepridil
Prevacid ....Pravachol
Prilocaine ....Prilosec
prilocaine ....Polocaine
Prilosec ....Prozac
Prilosec ....Prilocaine
Prilosec ....Prinivil
Primaxin ....Premarin
primidone ....prednisone
Prinivil ....Proventil
Prinivil ....Prilosec
ProAmatine ....protamine
Probenecid ....Procanbid
Procanbid ....Probenecid
procarbazine ....dacarbazine
Proloprim ....Protropin
promazine ....promethazine
promethazine ....promazine
Pronestyl ....Ponstel
propranolol ....Pravachol
Proscar ....Psorcon
Proscar ....ProSom
Proscar ....Prozac
ProSom ....Proscar
ProSom ....Prozac
ProSom ....Psorcon
Prostigmin ....physostigmine

protamine ....Protopam
protamine ....Protropin
protamine ....ProAmatine
Protopam ....protamine
Protopam ....Protropin
Protropin ....Protopam
Protropin ....Proloprim
Protropin ....protamine
Proventil ....Prinivil
Prozac ....Proscar
Prozac ....Prilosec
Prozac ....ProSom
Psorcon ....Proscar
Psorcon ....ProSom
Pyridium ....pyridoxine
pyridostigmine ....physostigmine
pyridoxine ....pralidoxime
pyridoxine ....Pyridium

Q

Quarzan ....quazepam
Quarzan ....Questran
quazepam ....Quarzan
Questran ....Quarzan
quinidine ....quinine
quinidine ....Quinora
quinidine ....clonidine
quinine ....quinidine
Quinora ....quinidine

R

ranitidine ....ritodrine
ranitidine ....rimantadine
Reglan ....Regonol
Regonol ....Reglan
Regonol ....Regroton
Regroton ....Regonol
Regroton ....Hygroton
reserpine ....Risperidone
Restoril ....Vistaril
Retrovir ....ritonavir
Revex ....ReVia
ReVia ....Revex
Ribavirin ....riboflavin
riboflavin ....Ribavirin
rifabutin ....rifampin
Rifadin ....Ritalin
Rifamate ....rifampin
rifampin ....rifabutin
rifampin ....Rifamate
rimantadine ....ranitidine
Risperidone ....reserpine
Ritalin ....Rifadin
ritodrine ....ranitidine
ritonavir ....Retrovir
Roxanol ....Roxicet
Roxicet ....Roxanol

S

salsalate ....sucralfate
salsalate ....sulfasalazine
Sandimmune ....Sandoglobulin
Sandimmune ....Sandostatin
Sandoglobulin ....Sandostatin
Sandoglobulin ....Sandimmune
Sandostatin ....Sandimmune
Sandostatin ....Sandoglobulin
saquinavir ....Sinequan
Sectral ....Factrel
Sectral ....Septra
selegiline ....Stelazine
Septa ....Septra
Septra ....Sectral
Septra ....Septa
Serax ....Xerac
Serax ....Eurax
Serentil ....Serevent
Serentil ....Aventyl
Serevent ....Serentil
simethicone ....cimetidine
Sinequan ....saquinavir
Slow FE ....Slow-K
Slow-K ....Slow FE
Solu-Medrol ....Depo-Medrol
somatrem ....somatropin
somatropin ....sumatriptan
somatropin ....somatrem
sotalol ....Stadol
Stadol ....sotalol
Stelazine ....selegiline
sucralfate ....salsalate
Sufenta ....Alfenta
Sufenta ....Survanta
sufentanil ....alfentanil
sulfadiazine ....sulfasalazine
sulfamethizole ....sulfameth-oxazole
sulfamethoxazole ....sulfamethizole
sulfasalazine ....sulfisoxazole
sulfasalazine ....salsalate

sulfasalazine . . . . .sulfadiazine
sulfisoxazole . . . . .sulfasalazine
sumatriptan . . . . .somatropin
Surbex . . . . .Surfak
Surbex . . . . .Carbex
Surfak . . . . .Surbex
Survanta . . . . .Sufenta

T

Taxol . . . . .Paxil
Tazicef . . . . .Tazidime
Tazidime . . . . .Tazicef
Tegopen . . . . .Tegretol
Tegopen . . . . .Tegrin
Tegretol . . . . .Toradol
Tegretol . . . . .Tegopen
Tegrin . . . . .Tegopen
Ten-K . . . . .Tenex
Tenex . . . . .Xanax
Tenex . . . . .Entex
Tenex . . . . .Ten-K
terbinafine . . . . .terbutaline
terbutaline . . . . .tolbutamide
terbutaline . . . . .terbinafine
terconazole . . . . .tioconazole
Testoderm . . . . .Estraderm
testolactone . . . . .testosterone
testosterone . . . . .testolactone
Theolair . . . . .Thyrolar
Thera-Flur . . . . .TheraFlu
TheraFlu . . . . .Thera-Flur
thiamine . . . . .Thorazine
thioridazine . . . . .Thorazine
Thorazine . . . . .thiamine
Thorazine . . . . .thioridazine
Thyrar . . . . .Thyrolar
Thyrolar . . . . .Theolair
Thyrolar . . . . .Thyrar
Ticar .Tigan
Tigan .Ticar
timolol . . . . .atenolol
Timoptic . . . . .Viroptic
tioconazole . . . . .terconazole
TobraDex . . . . .Tobrex
tobramycin . . . . .Trobicin
Tobrex . . . . .TobraDex
tolazamide . . . . .tolbutamide
tolbutamide . . . . .terbutaline
tolbutamide . . . . .tolazamide
tolnaftate . . . . .Tornalate
Topic .Topicort
Topicort . . . . .Topic
Toradol . . . . .Tegretol
Tornalate . . . . .tolnaftate
Torsemide . . . . .furosemide
Trandate . . . . .Trental
Trandate . . . . .Tridrate
Trental . . . . .Trandate
tretinoin . . . . .trientine
triamcinolone . . . . .Triaminicin
triamcinolone . . . . .Triaminicol
Triaminic . . . . .TriHemic
Triaminic . . . . .Triaminicin
Triaminicin . . . . .Triaminic
Triaminicin . . . . .triamcinolone
Triaminicol . . . . .triamcinolone
triamterene . . . . .trimipramine
trichloracetic acid . . . . dichloroacetic acid
Tridrate . . . . .Trandate
trientine . . . . .tretinoin
trifluoperazine . . . . .triflupromazine
triflupromazine . . . . .trifluoperazine
TriHemic . . . . .Triaminic
trimipramine . . . . .triamterene
Trimox . . . . .Tylox
Trimox . . . . .Diamox
Trinalin . . . . .Phrenilin
Trobicin . . . . .tobramycin
Tronolane . . . . .Tronothane
Tronothane . . . . .Tronolane
Tuinal . . . . .Tylenol
Tuinal . . . . .Luminal
Tylenol . . . . .Tylox
Tylenol . . . . .Tuinal
Tylox .Trimox
Tylox .Tylenol

U

Unicap . . . . .Unipen
Unipen . . . . .Urispas
Unipen . . . . .Omnipen
Unipen . . . . .Unicap
Urex . . . . .Eurax
Urised . . . . .Urispas
Urispas . . . . .Urised
Urispas . . . . .Unipen
Urobiotic . . . . .Otobiotic

V

V-Cillin ....Bicillin
Vancenase ....Vanceril
Vanceril ....Vansil
Vanceril ....Vancenase
Vansil ....Vanceril
Vantin ....Ventolin
Vasocidin ....Vasodilan
Vasodilan ....Vasocidin
Vasosulf ....Velosef
Velosef ....Vasosulf
Ventolin ....Benylin
Ventolin ....Vantin
VePesid ....Versed
Verelan ....Vivarin
Verelan ....Voltaren
Verelan ....Virilon
Versed ....VePesid
Vexol ....VoSol
Vicodin ....Hycodan
vidarabine ....cytarabine
vinblastine ....vincristine
vinblastine ....vinorelbine
vincristine ....vinblastine
vinorelbine ....vinblastine
Virilon ....Verelan
Viroptic ....Timoptic
Visine ....Visken
Visken ....Visine
Vistaril ....Restoril
Vivarin ....Verelan
Voltaren ....Verelan
VoSol ....Vexol
Vytone ....Hytone

W

Wellbutrin ....Wellcovorin
Wellbutrin ....Wellferon
Wellcovorin ....Wellferon
Wellcovorin ....Wellbutrin
Wellferon ....Wellbutrin
Wellferon ....Wellcovorin
Wyamine ....Wydase
Wycillin ....Bicillin
Wydase ....Wyamine

X

Xanax ....Zantac
Xanax ....Tenex
Xerac ....Serax

Z

Zantac ....Zofran
Zantac ....Xanax
Zarontin ....Zaroxolyn
Zaroxolyn ....Zarontin
Zebeta ....DiaBeta
Zestril ....Zostrix
Zestril ....Desyrel
Zocor ....Cozaar
Zofran ....Zantac
Zofran ....Zosyn
ZORprin ....Zyloprim
Zostrix ....Zovirax
Zostrix ....Zestril
Zosyn ....Zofran
Zovirax ....Zostrix
Zyloprim ....ZORprin
Zyprexa ....Zyrtec
Zyrtec ....Zyprexa

This list was compiled by Neil M. Davis MS, Pharm D, FASHP, President, Safe Medication Practices Consulting, Inc., 1143 Wright Drive, Huntingdon Valley, PA, 19006.

Recommended Childhood Immunization Schedule

In January 1995, the recommended childhood immunization schedule was published in *MMWR* following issuance by the Advisory Committee on Immunization Practices (ACIP), the American Academy of Pediatrics, and the American Academy of Family Physicians (*1*). This schedule was the first unified schedule developed through a collaborative process among the recommending groups, the pharmaceutical manufacturing industry, and the Food and Drug Administration. This collaborative process should assist in maintaining a common childhood vaccination schedule and enabling further simplification of the schedule.

OPV remains the recommended vaccine for routine polio vaccination in the United States. IPV is recommended for persons with compromised immune systems and their household contacts and is an acceptable alternative for other persons. ACIP is developing recommendations for expanded use of IPV in the United States.

Vaccine Recommendations Changes: *Hepatitis B, infant.* Because of the availability of different formulations of hepatitis B vaccine, doses are presented in micrograms rather than volumes. In addition, the footnote includes recommendations for vaccination of infants born to mothers whose hepatitis B surface antigen status is unknown.

Hepatitis, B adolescent. The three-dose series of hepatitis B vaccine should be initiated or completed for adolescents ages 11-12 years who have not previously received three doses of hepatitis B vaccine.

Poliovirus. Although oral poliovirus vaccine (OPV) is recommended for routine vaccination, inactivated poliovirus vaccine (IPV) is indicated for certain persons (ie, those with a compromised immune system and their household contacts) and continues to be an acceptable alternative for other persons. The schedule for IPV is included in the footnote.

Measles-mumps-rubella vaccine. The second dose of measles-mumps-rubella vaccine is routinely administered at age 4-6 years or at age 11-12 years; however, it may be administered at any visit if at least 1 month has elapsed since receipt of the first dose.

Var. Var was licensed in March 1995 and has been added to the schedule. This vaccine is recommended for all children at age 12-18 months. It may be adminstered to susceptible persons any time after age 12 months, and should be given at age 11-12 years to previously unvaccinated persons lacking a reliable history of chickenpox.

References

1. ACIP. Recommended childhood immunization schedule – United States, 1998. *MMWR* 1998; 47:8-12.

Recommended Childhood Vaccination Schedule* – United States, 1998

	Age										
Vaccine	Birth	1 Mo.	2 Mos.	4 Mos.	6 Mos.	12 Mos.	15 Mos.	18 Mos.	4-6 Yrs.	11-12 Yrs.	14-16 Yrs.
Hepatitis B†§		Hep B-1									
			Hep B-2				Hep B-3			Hep B§	
Diphtheria and tetanus toxoids and acellular pertussis¶			DTaP or DTwP	DTaP or DTwP	DTaP or DTwP		DTaP or DTwP		DTaP or DTwP	Td	
Haemophilus influenzae type b**			Hib	Hib	Hib		Hib				
Poliovirus††			Polio	Polio			Polio		Polio		
Measles-mumps-rubella§§							MMR		MMR	MMR	
Varicella-zoster virus¶¶							Var			Var	

[ ] Range of acceptable ages for vaccination

( ) Vaccines to be assessed and administered, if necessary

* This schedule indicates the recommended age for routine administration. Give catch-up immunizations whenever feasible. Combination vaccines may be used if at least one component of the vaccine is indicated, and none are contraindicated. Consult the manufacturers' package inserts for detailed recommendations. Bars indicate range of acceptable ages for vaccination. Ovals indicate catch-up vaccination opportunities.

† Give infants born to hepatitis B surface antigen (HBsAg)-negative mothers 2.5 mcg of Merck vaccine (*Recombivax HB*) or 10 mcg of SmithKline Beecham (SB) vaccine (*Engerix-B*). Give the second dose ≥ 1 month after the first dose. Give the third dose ≥ 2 months after the second, but not before 6 months of age.

Give infants born to HBsAg-positive mothers 0.5 ml HBIG within 12 hours of birth and either 5 mcg of *Recombivax HB* or 10 mcg of *Engerix-B* at a separate site. The second dose is recommended at age 1 to 2 months and the third dose at age 6 months. Draw blood at the time of delivery to determine the mother's HBsAg status; if positive, give the infant HBIG as soon as possible (by age 1 week). Base the dosage and timing of subsequent vaccine doses on the mother's HBsAg status.

§ Children and adolescents who have not been vaccinated against hepatitis B during infancy may begin the series during any childhood visit. Those who have not previously received three doses of hepatitis B vaccine should initiate or complete the series at age 11 to 12 years. Unvaccinated older adolescents should be vaccinated whenever possible. Give the second dose ≥ 1 month after the first dose, and give the third dose ≥ 4 months after the first dose and ≥ 2 months after the second dose.

¶ DTaP is the preferred vaccine for all doses in the vaccination series, including completion of the series in children who have received one or more doses of DTwP. DTwP is an acceptable alternative to DTaP. The fourth dose of DTwP or DTaP may be administered as early as 12 months of age, provided 6 months have elapsed since the third dose and the child is considered unlikely to return at age 15 to 18 months. Tetanus and diphtheria toxoids (Td), absorbed, for adult use, is recommended at age 11 to 12 years if ≥ 5 years have elapsed since the last dose of DTwP, DTaP or diphtheria and tetanus toxoids (DT). Subsequent routine Td boosters are recommended every 10 years.

** Three *Haemophilus influenzae* type b (Hib) conjugate vaccines are licensed for infant use. If PRP-OMP (*PedvaxHIB*, Merck) is administered at ages 2 and 4 months, a dose at age 6 months is not required.

†† Two poliovirus vaccines are currently licensed in the US: Inactivated poliovirus vaccine (IPV) and oral poliovirus vaccine (OPV). The following schedules are all acceptable to ACIP, AAP and AAFP, and parents and providers may choose among them: (1) IPV at ages 2 and 4 months and OPV at age 12 to 18 months and at age 4 to 6 years; (2) IPV at ages 2, 4 and 12 to 18 months and at age 4 to 6 years; and (3) OPV at ages 2, 4 and 6 to 18 months and at age 4 to 6 years. ACIP routinely recommends schedule 1. IPV is the only poliovirus vaccine recommended for immunocompromised people and their household contacts.

§§ The second dose of measles-mumps-rubella vaccine is routinely recommended at age 4 to 6 years but may be administered during any visit provided ≥ 1 month has elapsed since receipt of the first dose and that both doses are administered at or after age 12 months. Those who have not previously received the second dose should complete the schedule no later than the routine healthcare visit at age 11 to 12 years.

¶¶ Susceptible children may receive varicella vaccine (Var) during any visit after the first birthday. Vaccinate those who lack a reliable history of chickenpox at age 11 to 12 years. Give susceptible people aged ≥ 13 years two doses ≥ 1 month apart.

Source: Advisory Committee on Immunization Practices (ACIP), American Academy of Pediatrics (AAP) and American Academy of Family Physicians (AAFP).

Radio-Contrast Media

Generic Name	Dose Form	Trade Name	Manufacturer
Barium sulfate	Powder	Baroflave	Lannett
Barium sulfate	Powder	various	various
Barium sulfate	Suspension	E-Z-CAT	E-Z-EM
Barium sulfate	Suspension	E-Z-Paque	E-Z-EM
Barium sulfate	Suspension	Intropaque	Lafayette
Barium sulfate	Suspension	Novopaque	Picker
Barium sulfate	Suspension	Polibar-Plus	E-Z-EM
Barium sulfate	Suspension	Preview	Lafayette
Barium sulfate	Suspension	Redi-CAT	E-Z-Em
Barium sulfate	Suspension	Sol-O-Pake	E-Z-EM
Barium sulfate 1.5%	Suspension	Baro-Cat	Lafayette
Barium sulfate 1.5%	Suspension	PrepCat	Lafayette
Barium sulfate 46%	Granules	Baros	Lafayette
Barium sulfate 5%	Suspension	EneCat	Lafayette
Barium sulfate 5%	Suspension	TomoCat	Lafayette
Barium sulfate 50%	Suspension	Entrobar	Lafayette
Barium sulfate 60%	Suspension	Barosperse Liq.	Lafayette
Barium sulfate 85%	Suspension	HD 85	Lafayette
Barium sulfate 91%	Powder	Intropaque	Lafayette
Barium sulfate 92.5%	Powder	Barotrast	Armour
Barium sulfate 92%	Powder	Micropaque	Picker
Barium sulfate 95%	Powder	Barosperse	Lafayette
Barium sulfate 95%	Powder	E-Z-Paque	E-Z-EM
Barium sulfate 95%	Powder	Tonopaque	Lafayette
Barium sulfate 95%	Powder	Ultra-R	E-Z-EM
Barium sulfate 96%	Powder	Baroloid	Lafayette
Barium sulfate 96%	Powder	Mixture III	Picker
Barium sulfate 96%	Powder	Polibar	E-Z-EM
Barium sulfate 97%	Powder	Barodense	Lafayette
Barium sulfate 97%	Powder	Sol-O-Pake	E-Z-EM
Barium sulfate 97%	Suspension	Barobag	Lafayette
Barium sulfate 98%	Powder	Baricon	Lafayette
Barium sulfate 98%	Powder	HD 200 Plus	Lafayette
Barium sulfate 100%	Paste	Anatrast	Lafayette
Barium sulfate 100%	Suspension	Flo-Coat	Lafayette
Barium sulfate 100%	Suspension	Liquipake	Lafayette
Barium sulfate 150%	Suspension	Epi-C	Lafayette
Diatrizoate meglumine	Injection	Angiovist 282	Berlex
Diatrizoate meglumine	Injection	Cystografin	Squibb
Diatrizoate meglumine	Injection	Hypaque Meglumine 30%	Nycomed
Diatrizoate meglumine	Injection	Hypaque Meglumine 60%	Nycomed
Diatrizoate meglumine	Injection	Hypaque-Cysto	Nycomed
Diatrizoate meglumine	Injection	Hypaque-M 18%	Nycomed

Generic Name	Dose Form	Trade Name	Manufacturer
Diatrizoate meglumine	Injection	Hypaque-M 30%	Nycomed
Diatrizoate meglumine	Injection	Hypaque-M 60%	Nycomed
Diatrizoate meglumine	Injection	Reno-Dip	Squibb
Diatrizoate meglumine	Injection	Reno-M-60	Squibb
Diatrizoate meglumine	Injection	Urovist Cysto	Berlex
Diatrizoate meglumine	Injection	Urovist Meglumine DIU/CT	Berlex
Diatrizoate meglumine & Iodipamide meglumine	Injection	Sinografin	Squibb
Diatrizoate meglumine & sodium	Injection	Angiovist 292	Berlex
Diatrizoate meglumine & sodium	Injection	Angiovist 370	Berlex
Diatrizoate meglumine & sodium	Injection	Gastrografin	Squibb
Diatrizoate meglumine & sodium	Injection	Gastrovist	Berlex
Diatrizoate meglumine & sodium	Injection	Hypaque-76	Nycomed
Diatrizoate meglumine & sodium	Injection	Hypaque-M 75%	Nycomed
Diatrizoate meglumine & sodium	Injection	Hypaque-M 76%	Nycomed
Diatrizoate meglumine & sodium	Injection	MD-76	Mallinckrodt
Diatrizoate meglumine & sodium	Injection	MD-Gastroview	Mallinckrodt
Diatrizoate meglumine & sodium	Injection	Renografin-60	Squibb
Diatrizoate meglumine & sodium	Injection	Renografin-76	Squibb
Diatrizoate meglumine & sodium	Injection	Renovist	Squibb
Diatrizoate meglumine & sodium	Injection	Renovist II	Squibb
Diatrizoate sodium	Injection	Hypaque Oral (Canada)	Nycomed
Diatrizoate sodium	Injection	Hypaque Sodium 25%	Nycomed
Diatrizoate sodium	Injection	Hypaque Sodium 50%	Nycomed
Diatrizoate sodium	Injection	Hypaque Sodium Oral Powder	Nycomed
Diatrizoate sodium	Injection	Hypaque Sodium Oral Solution	Nycomed
Diatrizoate sodium	Injection	Urovist Sodium 300	Berlex
Ethiodized oil	Injection	Ethiodol	Savage
Iocetamic acid	Tablets	Cholebrine	Mallinckrodt
Iodamide meglumine	Injection	Renovue-65	Squibb
Iodipamide meglumine	Injection	Cholografin	Squibb
Iodixanol	Injection	Visipaque	Nycomed
Iohexol	Injection	Omnipaque	Nycomed
Iopamidol	Injection	Isovue-128	Squibb
Iopamidol	Injection	Isovue-200	Squibb

Generic Name	Dose Form	Trade Name	Manufacturer
Iopamidol	Injection	Isovue-300	Squibb
Iopamidol	Injection	Isovue-370	Squibb
Iopamidol	Injection	Isovue-M 200	Squibb
Iopamidol	Injection	Isovue-M 300	Squibb
Iopanoic acid	Tablet	Telepaque	Nycomed
Iopental		Imagopaque	Nycomed
Iopromide	Injection	Ultravist	Berlex
Iothalamate meglumine	Injection	Conray	Mallinckrodt
Iothalamate meglumine	Injection	Conray-30	Mallinckrodt
Iothalamate meglumine	Injection	Conray-43	Mallinckrodt
Iothalamate meglumine	Injection	Conray-60	Mallinckrodt
Iothalamate meglumine	Injection	Cysto-Conray	Mallinckrodt
Iothalamate meglumine	Injection	Cysto-Conray II	Mallinckrodt
Iothalamate meglumine & sodium	Injection	Vascoray	Mallinckrodt
Iothalamate sodium	Injection	Angio-Conray	Mallinckrodt
Iothalamate sodium	Injection	Conray-325	Mallinckrodt
Iothalamate sodium	Injection	Conray-400	Mallinckrodt
Ioversol	Injection	Optiray 160	Mallinckrodt
Ioversol	Injection	Optiray 240	Mallinckrodt
Ioversol	Injection	Optiray 320	Mallinckrodt
Ioversol	Injection	Optiray 350	Mallinckrodt
Ioxaglate meglumine & sodium	Injection	Hexabrix	Mallinckrodt
Ioxaglate meglumine & sodium	Injection	Hexabrix 200	Mallinckrodt
Ioxaglate meglumine & sodium	Injection	Hexabrix 320	Mallinckrodt
Ipodate calcium	Granules	Oragrafin	Squibb
Ipodate sodium	Capsules	Bilivist	Berlex
Ipodate sodium	Capsules	Oragrafin Sodi.	Squibb
Isosulfan blue	Injection	Lymphazurin	Hirsch Industries
Metrizamide	Powder for Inj	Amipaque	Nycomed
Polyvinyl chloride	Capsules	Sitzmarks	Konsyl Pharm
Propyliodone in peanut oil	Suspension	Dionosil Oily	Allen & Hanburys
Tyropanoate sodium	Capsules	Bilopaque	Nycomed
nd		Iopamiron	Berlex

nd = No data available.

Radio-Isotopes

Active Isotope	Generic Name	Dose Form or Packaging	Trade Name	Manufacturer
18-F	Fluorine F-18	Injection	nd	Medi-Physics
32-P	Chromic Phosphate P-32	Suspension	Phosphocol P32	Mallinckrodt
		Injection	Phosphotope	Squibb
		Oral Solution	Phosphotope	Squibb
32-P	Sodium Phosphate P-32	Capsules	nd	Mallinckrodt
		Oral Solution	nd	Mallinckrodt
51-Cr	Sodium Chromate Cr-51	Injection	Chromitope	Squibb
		Injection	nd	Mallinckrodt
57-Co	Cyanocobalamin Co-57	Capsules	nd	Mallinckrodt
		Kit	Rubratope-57	Squibb
57&58 Co	Cyanocobalamin Co-57 & Co-58	Kit	Dicopac Kit	Amersham
59-Fe	Ferrous Citrate Fe-59	Injection	nd	Mallinckrodt
60-Co	Cyanocobalamin Co-60	Capsules	Rubratope-60	Squibb
67-Ga	Gallium Citrate Ga-67	Injection	nd	DuPont-Merck
		Injection	nd	Mallinckrodt
		Injection	nd	Medi-Physics
		Injection	Neoscan	Medi-Physics
75-Se	Selenomethionine Se-75	Injection	Sethotope	Squibb
		Injection	nd	Mallinckrodt
		Injection	nd	Medi-Physics
81m-Kr	Krypton Kr-81m	Gas Generator	nd	Medi-Physics
82-Sr&Rb	Strontium Sr-82/Rubidium Rb-82	Generator	Cardiogen-82	Squibb
89-Sr	Strontium Chloride Sr-89	Injection	Metastron	Medi-Physics/ Amersham
99m-Tc	Technetium Tc-99m	Generator	nd	Cintichem
		Generator (fission)	nd	DuPont-Merck
		Generator (neutron)	nd	DuPont-Merck
		Generator	Ultra-TechneKow	Mallinckrodt
		Generator	Minitec II	Squibb
		Generator	Technetope II	Squibb
99m-Tc	Technetium-99m Albumin Aggegated	Kit	AN Stannous Ag.	Benedict Nuclear
		Kit	nd	CIS-US
		Kit	Pulmolite	DuPont-Merck
		Kit	TechneScan MAA	Mallinckrodt
		Kit	Lungaggregate Reagent	Medi-Physics
		Kit	nd	Merck
		Kit	Macrotec	Squibb
99m-Tc	Technetium-99m Albumin Colloid	Kit	Microlite	DuPont-Merck
99m-Tc	Technetium-99m Arcitumomab	Kit	CEA-Scan	Immuno-medics/ Mallinckrodt
99m-Tc	Technetium-99m Serum Albumin	Kit	nd	Medi-Physics

Active Isotope	Generic Name	Dose Form or Packaging	Trade Name	Manufacturer
99m-Tc	Technetium-99m Bicisate	Kit	Neurolite	DuPont-Merck
99m-Tc	Technetium-99m Disofenin	Kit	Hepatolite	DuPont-Merck
99m-Tc	Technetium-99m Etidronate	Kit		
		Kit	Tc-99m Diphos-phonate-Tin	Medi-Physics
		Kit	Tc-99m HEDSPA	Medi-Physics
		Kit	Stannous Diphosphonate	Medi-Physics
99m-Tc	Technetium-99m Exametazime	Kit	Ceretec	Amersham
99m-Tc	Technetium-99m Lidofenin	Kit	TechneScan HIDA	Merck
99m-Tc	Technetium-99m Mebrofenin	Kit	Choletec	Squibb
99m-Tc	Technetium-99m Medronate	Kit	Amer-Scan MDP	Amersham
		Kit	AN-MDP	CIS-US
		Kit	Osteolite	DuPont-Merck
		Kit	nd	Medi-Physics
		Kit	TechneScan MDP	Merck
		Kit	MDP-Squibb	Squibb
99m-Tc	Technetium-99m Mertiatide	Kit	TechneScan MAG3	Mallinckrodt
99m-Tc	Technetium-99m Oxidronate	Kit	Ostescan HDP	Mallinckrodt
99m-Tc	Technetium-99m Pentetate Sodium	Kit	AN-DTPA	CIS-US
		Kit	MPI DTPA Kit	Medi-Physics
		Kit	TechneScan DTPA	Merck
		Kit	Techneplex	Squibb
		Kit	Renotec-Iron	Squibb
			Ascorbate-DTPA	nd
99m-Tc	Tc-99m Pyro- & Trimeta- Phos-phates	Kit	AN-Pyrotec	CIS-US
		Kit	Pyrolite	DuPont-Merck
		Kit	TechneScan PYP	Mallinckrodt
		Kit	Tc-99m Poly-phosphate	Medi-Physics
		Kit	Phosphotec	Squibb
99m-Tc	Technetium-99m Red Blood Cell	Kit	RBC-Scan	Cadema Med.
		Kit	Ultratag	Mallinckrodt
99m-Tc	Technetium-99m Sestamibi	Kit	Cardiolite	DuPont-Merck
99m-Tc	Technetium-99m Sodium Gluceptate	Kit	Glucoscan	DuPont-Merck
		Kit	Technescan Gluceptate	Merck
99m-Tc	Technetium-99m Succimer	Kit	Tc-99m DMSA	Medi-Physics

Active Isotope	Generic Name	Dose Form or Packaging	Trade Name	Manufacturer
99m-Tc	Technetium-99m Sulfur Colloid	Injection	nd	CIS-US
		Injection	nd	Mallinckrodt
		Injection	nd	Medi-Physics
		Inj. & Kit	nd	Medi-Physics
		Kit	nd	CIS-US
		Kit	TSC	Medi-Physics
		Kit	TechneColl	Mallinckrodt
		Kit	Tesuloid	Squibb
99m-Tc	Technetium-99m Teboroxime	Kit	CardioTec	Squibb
99m-Tc	Sodium Pertechnetate Tc-99m	Injection	nd	CIS-US
		Injection	nd	Mallinckrodt
		Injection	nd	Medi-Physics
99m-Tc	Tc-99m Nofetumomab Merpentan	Kit	Verluma	NeoRx/ DuPont Merck
111-In	Indium-111 Capromab Pendetide	Kit	ProstaScint	Cytogen
111-In	Indium-111 Imciromab Pentetate	Kit	Myoscint	Centocor
111-In	Indium-111 Oxine	Solution	nd	Amersham
111-In	Indium-111 Oxyquinoline Sodium	Solution	nd	Amersham
111-In	Indium-111 Pentetate Disodium	Injection	In-111 DTPA	Medi-Physics
111-In	Indium-111 Pentetreotide	Injection	OctreoScan	Mallinckrodt
111-In	In-111 Satumomab Pentetide	Injection	OncoScint CR/OV	Cytogen
123-I	Sodium Iodide-123	Capsules	nd	Benedict Nuclear
		Capsules	nd	Mallinckrodt
		Capsules	nd	Medi-Physics
123-I	Iohippurate Sodium I-123	Injection	Nephroflow	Medi-Physics
123-I	Iofetamine HCl I-123	Injection	Spectamine	Medi-Physics
125-I	Iothalamate Sodium I-125	Injection	Glofil-125	Iso-Tex
125-I	Iodinated Albumin I-125	Injection	Jeanatope 125-I	Iso-Tex
		Injection	nd	Mallinckrodt
125-I	Iodinated Fibrinogen I-125	Injection	Ibrin	Amersham
127-Xe	Xenon Xe-127	Gas	nd	Mallinckrodt
131-I	Iodinated Albumin I-131	Injection	Megatope	Iso-Tex
131-I	Iodinated-131 Albumin Aggegated	Injection	Albumitope L-S	Squibb
131-I	Iodohippurate Sodium I-131	Injection	nd	CIS-US
		Injection	Hippuran	Mallinckrodt
		Injection	Hipputope	Squibb
131-I	Rose Bengal Sodium I-131	Injection	Robengatope	Squibb
131-I	Sodium Iodide I-131	Capsules	nd	CIS-US
		Capsules	nd	Mallinckrodt
		Capsules	nd	Squibb

Active Isotope	Generic Name	Dose Form or Packaging	Trade Name	Manufacturer
		Capsules	nd	Syncor
		Oral Solution	nd	CIS-US
		Oral Solution	nd	Mallinckrodt
		Oral Solution	nd	Squibb
		Oral Solution	nd	Syncor
133-Xe	Xenon Xe-133	Injection	nd	DuPont-Merck
		Gas	nd	DuPont-Merck
		Gas	nd	General Electric
		Gas	nd	Mallinckrodt
		Gas	nd	Medi-Physics
		Kit (V.S.S.)	nd	Medi-Physics
197-Hg	Chlormerodrin Hg-197	Injection	nd	Squibb
198-Au	Gold Au-198	Injection	Aureotope	Squibb
201-Tl	Thallous Chloride Tl-201	Injection	nd	DuPont-Merck
		Injection	nd	Mallinckrodt
		Injection	nd	Medi-Physics
		Injection	nd	Squibb

nd = No data available.

Agents for Imaging

Active Isotope	Generic Name	Dose Form	Trade Name	Manufacturer
Agents for MRI Imaging				
	Gadodiamide & caldiamide sodium	Injection	Omniscan	Sanofi Ny
	Gadopentetate dimeglumine	Injection	Magnevist	Berlex
	Gadoteridol & calteridol calcium	Injection	ProHance	Squibb
	Perflubron	Liquid	Imagent GI	Alliance
	Ferumoxides (investigational)		Feridex	Nycomed
Agents for PET Imaging				
13-N	Nitrogen	nd	nd	nd
15-O	Oxygen	nd	nd	nd
18-F	Fludeoxyglucose [2-fluoro(F-18)-2-deoxyglucose]	nd	nd	nd
82-Rb	Rubidium	nd	nd	nd
Agents for Ultrasonic Imaging				
	Perfluorodecalin & Perfluorotripropylamine		Fluosol-DA	nd
	Investigational		Levovist	Berlex
	Investigational		Cavisomes	Berlex

nd = No data available.

Pharmaceutical Company Labeler Code Index

LISTED IN NUMERICAL ORDER

00002
Eli Lilly and Co.

00003
Apothecon
Braccho Diagnostics
Bristol-Myers Squibb
ConvaTec

00004
Roche Laboratories

00005
ESI Lederle Generics
Lederle Laboratories

00006
Merck & Co.

00007
SmithKline Beecham Pharmaceuticals

00008
Wyeth-Ayerst Laboratories

00009
Pharmacia & Upjohn

00011
Becton Dickinson Microbiology Systems

00013
Pharmacia & Upjohn

00014
Searle

00015
Apothecon
Bristol-Myers Oncology
Mead Johnson

00017
Wampole Laboratories

00019
Mallinckrodt Medical, Inc.

00021
Schwarz Pharma

00023
Allergan Herbert
Allergan, Inc.

00024
Sanofi Winthrop Pharmaceuticals

00025
Searle

00026
Bayer Corporation (Biological Division and Pharmaceutical Division)
Bayer (Allergy)

00028
Novartis

00029
SmithKline Beecham Pharmaceuticals

00031
Whitehall Robins Laboratories
Wyeth-Ayerst

00032
Solvay

00033
Roche Laboratories
Syntex Laboratories

00034
Purdue Frederick Co.

00037
Wallace Laboratories

00039
Hoechst-Marion Roussel

00041
Oral-B Laboratories, Inc.

00043
Novartis Consumer

00044
Knoll Laboratories
Knoll Pharmaceuticals

00045
McNeil Consumer Products Co.
McNeil Pharmaceutical
Ortho McNeil Corp.

00047
Warner Chilcott Laboratories
Watson Laboratories

00048
Knoll Laboratories
Knoll Pharmaceuticals

00049
Roerig

00052
Organon, Inc.

00053
Centeon

00054
Roxane Laboratories, Inc.

00056
Du Pont Pharma

00062
Advanced Care Products
Ortho McNeil Corp.

00065
Alcon Laboratories, Inc.

00066
Dermik Laboratories, Inc.

00067
Novartis Consumer

00068
Hoechst-Marion Roussel

00069
Pfizer US Pharmaceutical Group

00070
Arcola Laboratories

00071
Parke-Davis
Warner Lambert Consumer Health Products

00072
Westwood Squibb Pharmaceuticals

00074
Abbott Diagnostics
Abbott Hospital Products
Abbott Laboratories

00075
Rhone-Poulenc Rorer Pharmaceuticals, Inc.

00076
Star Pharmaceuticals, Inc.

00077
PBH Wesley Jessen

00078
Novartis Pharmaceutical

00081
GlaxoWellcome
Monarch Products

00083
Novartis Pharmaceutical
Novartis Consumer

00085
Key Pharmaceuticals
Schering-Plough Corp.
Schering Plough Healthcare Products

00086
Carnrick Laboratories, Inc.

00299
Galderma Laboratories, Inc.

00300
Tap Pharmaceuticals

00304
J.J. Balan, Inc.

00310
Zeneca Pharmaceuticals

00314
Hyrex Pharmaceuticals

00316
Del-Ray Laboratory, Inc.

00317
Whorton Pharmaceuticals, Inc.

00327
Guardian Laboratories

00332
Teva Pharmaceuticals USA

00346
Ciba Vision Ophthalmics

00348
Medtech Laboratories, Inc.

00349
Parmed Pharmaceuticals, Inc.

00362
Novocol Chemical Mfr. Co.

00364
Schein Pharmaceutical, Inc.

00372
Scot-Tussin Pharmacal, Inc.

00374
Lyne Laboratories

00378
Mylan Pharmaceuticals

00386
Gebauer Co.

00394
Mericon Industries, Inc.

00395
Humco Holding Group, Inc.

00396
Milex Products, Inc.

00398
C & M Pharmacal, Inc.

00402
Steris Laboratories, Inc.

00406
Mallinckrodt Chemical

00407
Nycomed Inc.

00418
Taylor Pharmaceuticals

00421
Fielding Co.

00426
Morton Grove Pharmaceuticals

00433
Research Industries Corp.

00436
Century Pharmaceuticals, Inc.

00451
Muro Pharmaceutical, Inc.

00454
Lexis Laboratories

00456
Forest Pharmaceutical, Inc.

00463
C. O. Truxton, Inc.

00466
Block Drug

00469
Fujisawa USA, Inc.

00472
Alpharma

00482
Kenwood Laboratories

00485
Edwards Pharmaceuticals, Inc.

00486
Beach Pharmaceuticals

00487
Nephron Pharmaceuticals Corp.

00494
Foy Laboratories

00496
Ferndale Laboratories, Inc.

00501
Warner Lambert Consumer Health Products

00514
Dow Hickam, Inc.

00516
Glenwood, Inc.

00517
American Regent

00521
Chesebrough-Pond's, USA

00524
Knoll Laboratories
Knoll Pharmaceuticals

00527
Lannett, Inc.

00535
Forest Pharmaceuticals, Inc.

00536
Rugby Labs, Inc.
Eon Labs Manufacturing, Inc.

00537
Spencer Mead, Inc.

00539
American Urologicals, Inc.

00548
I.M.S., Ltd.

00551
Seatrace Pharmaceuticals

00555
Barr Laboratories, Inc.

00556
H.R. Cenci Labs, Inc.

00563
Bock Pharmacal Co.

00573
Whitehall Robins Laboratories

00574
Paddock Laboratories

00575
Zenith Goldline Laboratories, Inc.

00576
Medical Products Panamericana

00585
Medeva Pharmaceuticals

00586
Heather Drug, Inc.

00588
Keene Pharmaceuticals, Inc.

00590
DuPont Pharma

00597
Boehringer Ingelheim, Inc.

00598
Health for Life Brands, Inc.

00603
Qualitest Products, Inc.

00615
Vangard Labs, Inc.

00619
Walker Pharmacal Co.

00641
Elkins-Sinn, Inc.

00642
Everett Laboratories, Inc.

00659
Circle Pharmaceuticals, Inc.

00663
Pfizer US Pharmaceutical Group

00665
International Laboratories

00677
United Research Laboratories

00682
Marnel Pharmaceuticals, Inc.
Mikart, Inc.

00684
Primedics Laboratories

00686
Raway Pharmacal, Inc.

00689
Jones Pharma Inc.

00703
Gensia Laboratories, LTD.

00713
G & W Laboratories

00725
Circa Pharmaceuticals, Inc.

00729
Fidelity Halsom

00731
Alto Pharmaceuticals, Inc.

00741
Walker, Corp. and, Inc.

00744
Daywell Laboratories Corp.

00766
SmithKline Beecham Consumer Healthcare

00777
Dista Products Co.

00781
Geneva Pharmaceuticals

00785
Forest Pharmaceuticals

00813
Pharmics, Inc.

00814
Interstate Drug Exchange

00832
Morton Grove Pharmaceuticals
Rosemont Pharmaceutical Corp.

00837
Columbia Laboratories, Inc.

00839
H.L. Moore Drug Exchange, Inc.

00879
Halsey Drug Co.

00884
Pedinol Pharmacal, Inc.

00904
Major Pharmaceuticals

00905
SCS Pharmaceuticals

00917
Wesley Pharmacal, Inc.

00918
General Medical Corp.

00927
Pfeiffer Co.

00938
Davis and Geck

00944
Baxter Hyland

00961
Cook-Waite Laboratories, Inc.

00978
SmithKline Diagnostics

00998
Alcon Laboratories, Inc.
PolyMedica Pharmaceuticals

01020
Cumberland Packing Corp.

05745
Nastech Pharmaceutical, Inc.

08026
Smith & Nephew United

08884
Sherwood Medical

10019
Ohmeda Pharmaceuticals

10038
Ambix Laboratories, Inc.

10106
Mallinckrodt-Baker

10116
Bartor Pharmacal Co.

10118
Norstar Consumer Products

10119
Bausch & Lomb Personal Products Division

10157
Blistex, Inc.

10158
Block Drug, Inc.

10160
Bluco Inc./Med. Discnt. Outlet

10223
Cetylite Industries, Inc.

10310
Del Pharmaceuticals, Inc.

10331
E. E. Dickinson Co.

10337
Doak Dermatologics

10356
Beiersdorf, Inc.

10432
Freeda Vitamins, Inc.

10481
Gordon Laboratories

10486
C. S. Dent & Co. Division

10651
Lavoptik, Inc.

10706
Manne

10712
Marlyn, Inc.

10742
Mentholatum, Inc.

10797
Oakhurst Co.

10812
Neutrogena Corp.

10865
Parthenon, Inc.

10888
Advanced Nutritional Technology

10952
Recsei Laboratories

10956
Reese Pharmaceutical, Inc.

10961
Requa, Inc.

10974
Pegasus Medical, Inc.

11012
Schaffer Laboratories

11086
Summers Laboratories, Inc.

11089
McGregor Pharmaceuticals, Inc.

11290
Thompson Medical Co.

11370
Warner Lambert Co.

11414
Willen

11428
Wonderful Dream Salve Corp.

11444
W. F. Young, Inc.

11509
Combe, Inc.

11584
International Ethical Labs

11704
Survival Technology, Inc.

11793
Pasteur-Mérieux-Connaught

11808
ION Laboratories, Inc.

11845
Mason Distributors, Inc.

11940
Medco Lab, Inc.

11980
Allergan America

12071
Richie Pharmacal, Inc.

12120
Wisconsin Pharmacal Co.

12136
Bird Corp.

12165
Graham Field

12225
Quality Formulations, Inc.

12463
Jones Pharma Inc.

12496
Reckitt & Colman

12622
Olin Corp.

12758
Mason Pharmaceuticals, Inc.

12843
Bayer Corp. (Consumer Division)

12934
Nion Corp.

12939
Marlop Pharmaceuticals, Inc.

13723
Dr. Nordyke Footcare Products

14362
Mass. Public Health Bio. Lab.

16500
Bayer Corp. (Consumer Div)

16837
J & J Merck Consumer Pharm.

17022
Veratex Corp.

17156
MediPhysics, Inc., Amersham Healthcare

17204
Miller Pharmacal Group, Inc.

17314
Alza Corp.

17478
Akorn, Inc.

17808
Himmel Pharmaceuticals, Inc.

18393
Roche Laboratories
Syntex Laboratories

18686
InnoVisions, Inc.

19200
Reckitt & Coleman

19458
Eckerd Drug Co.

19810
Bristol-Myers Products

21406
Columbia Laboratories, Inc.

21659
Pharmaceutical Labs, Inc.

22200
Mennen Co.

22840
Greer Laboratories, Inc.

23317
NMC Laboratories

23558
Lee Pharmaceuticals

23731
Cytosol Laboratories

23900
Procter & Gamble Co.

24208
Bausch & Lomb Pharmaceuticals

25074
Penederm, Inc.

25077
Hudson Corp.

25332
Legere Pharmaceuticals, Inc.

25358
Donell DerMedex

25866
Vicks Pharmacy Products

28105
Hill Dermaceuticals, Inc.

28851
Kendall Health Care Products

30103
Randob Laboratories, Ltd.

30727
Merit Pharmaceuticals

31280
Becton Dickinson & Co.

31600
Kiwi Brands, Inc.

31795
Fibertone Co.

33130
Continental Quest Research

33984
Solgar, Inc.

34044
Continental Consumer Products

34567
Milex Products, Inc.

34999
Nutraloric

37000
Procter & Gamble Co.

38083
Campbell Laboratories

38130
Econo Med Pharmaceuticals

38137
Spectrum Chemical Mfg. Corp.

38245
Copley Pharmaceutical, Inc.

38697
ALK Laboratories

39506
Somerset Pharmaceuticals

39769
SoloPak Pharmaceuticals, Inc.

39822
Pharma Tek, Inc.

52152
Amide Pharmaceuticals, Inc.

52189
Invamed, Inc.

52238
Optopics Laboratories, Corp.

52268
Braintree Laboratories, Inc.

52311
Biosearch Medical Products

52489
Chemi-Tech Laboratories

52544
Watson Laboratories

52555
Martec Pharmaceutical, Inc.

52584
General Injectables & Vaccines

52604
Jones Medical

52747
US Pharmaceutical Corp.

52761
GenDerm Corp.

52836
Milance Laboratories, Inc.

53014
Medeva

53020
Trinity Technologies, Inc.

53118
Millgood Laboratories, Inc.

53124
Lederle-Praxis Biologicals

53159
Palisades Pharmaceuticals, Inc.

53169
Monarch Pharmaceuticals
Boehringer Mannheim Corp.

53191
Bio-Tech

53258
VHA Supply Co.

53335
Tyson & Associates, Inc.

53385
Standard Drug Co.

53489
Mutual Pharmaceutical, Inc.

53905
Chiron Therapeutics

53926
Amsco Scientific

53978
Med-Pro, Inc.

53983
Natren, Inc.

54022
Vitaline Corp.

54092
Roberts Pharmaceuticals

54129
Immuno U.S., Inc.

54198
Liquipharm

54323
Flanders, Inc.

54391
R & D Laboratories, Inc.

54396
Gynex Pharmaceuticals, Inc.

54429
Chase Laboratories

54482
Sigma-Tau Pharmaceuticals

54569
Allscrips

54627
ValMed, Inc.

54686
Ethitek Pharmaceuticals

54765
GynoPharma Laboratories

54799
Cynacon/OCuSOFT

54807
R.I.D., Inc.

54838
Silarx Pharmaceuticals, Inc.

54891
Vision Pharmaceuticals, Inc.

54921
IPR Pharmaceuticals, Inc.

54964
Murdock, Madaus, Schwabe

55298
3M Personal Healthcare Products

55299
Kingswood Laboratories, Inc.

55326
Curatek Pharm.

55390
Bedford Laboratories

55422
Pharmakon Laboratories, Inc.

55425
Dal-Med Pharmaceuticals

55499
Numark Laboratories, Inc.

55505
Kramer Laboratories, Inc.

55513
Amgen, Inc.

55515
Oclassen Pharmaceuticals, Inc.

55516
Dyna Pharm, Inc.

55559
Calgon Vestal Laboratories

55566
Ferring Laboratories, Inc.

55688
Speywood Pharmaceuticals, Inc.

55806
Effcon Labs, Inc.

55953
Novopharm USA, Inc.

55994
Dakryon Pharmaceuticals

56083
Stiefel

56091
Johnson & Johnson Medical

56146
Nexstar

57267
Novartis Pharmaceuticals

57317
Fujisawa USA, Inc.

57480
Medirex, Inc.

57506
American Drug Industries, Inc.

57664
Caraco Pharmaceutical Labs

57665
Enzon, Inc.

57706
Storz Ophthalmics

57782
Bausch & Lomb Pharmaceuticals

99207
Medicis Dermatologicals, Inc.

99766
Faulding USA

Pharmaceutical Manufacturer and Drug Distributor Listing

LISTED IN ALPHABETICAL ORDER

00089, 55298, 55326
3M Personal Healthcare Products
3M Center
Building 275-5W-05
St. Paul, MN 55133
612-733-1110

00089
3M Pharmaceutical
3M Center
Building 275-3W-01
St. Paul, MN 55133
612-736-4930

12463
Abana Pharmaceuticals, Inc.
See Jones Medical

00074
Abbott Diagnostics
Customer Support Center
Dept. 94P
Abbott Park, IL 60064
800-323-9100

00074
Abbott Hospital Products
1 Abbott Park Road
Abbott Park, IL 60064-3500
847-937-6100

00074
Abbott Laboratories
1 Abbott Park Road
Abbott Park, IL 60064-3500
847-937-6100

Able Laboratories, Inc.
6 Hollywood Ct.
South Plainfield, NJ 07080
908-754-2253

Academic Pharmaceuticals, Inc.
25720 Saunders Road North
Lake Forest, IL 60045

Acme United Corp.
75 Kings Highway Cutoff
Fairfield, CT 06430
203-332-7330

53014
Adams Laboratories
14801 Sovereign Road
Ft. Worth, TX 76155-2645
817-545-7791

Adria Laboratories
See Pharmacia & Upjohn

00062
Advanced Care Products
Route 202
P.O. Box 610
Raritan, NJ 08869
800--582-6097

10888
Advanced Nutritional Technology
6988 Sierra Court
Dublin, CA 94568
510-828-2128

Advanced Vision Research
7 Alfred Street,
Suite 330
Woburn, MA 01801
617-932-8327

Agouron Pharmaceuticals
10350 North Torrey Pines
La Jolla, CA 92037-1020
619-622-3000

A.H. Robins Consumer Products
See Wyeth-Ayerst

00031
A.H. Robins, Inc.
See Wyeth-Ayerst

17478
Akorn, Inc.
100 Tri-State International, Suite 100
Lincolnshire, IL 60069
847-236-3800

41383
AKPharma, Inc.
P.O. Box 111
Pleasantville, NJ 08232
609-645-5100

A.L. Labs
See Alpharma

00065, 00998
Alcon Laboratories, Inc.
6201 South Freeway
Ft. Worth, TX 76134
817-551-8057

ALK Laboratories, Inc.
27 Village Lane
Walllingford, CT 06492
203-949-2727

38697
ALK Laboratories
2840 Eighth Street
Berkeley, CA 94710-2707
510-843-6846

00173
Allen & Hanburys
See GlaxoWellcome

Allercreme
See Carme, Inc.

11980
Allergan America
See Allergan, Inc.

00023
Allergan Inc.
2525 DuPont Drive
Irvine, CA 92715-9534
800-433-8871

Allermed
7203 Convoy Ct.
San Diego, CA 92111
619-292-1060

Alliance Pharmaceuticals
3040 Science Park Road
San Diego, CA 92121
619-558-4300

54569
Allscrips
1033 Butterfield Road
Vernon Hills, IL 60061
708-680-3515

Alpha 1 Biomedicals, Inc.
6903 Rockledge Drive
Bethesda, MD 20817
301-564-4400

49669
Alpha Therapeutic Corp.
5555 Valley Blvd.
Los Angeles, CA 90032
213-225-2221

00472
Alpharma
See Alpharma USPD

Alpharma USPD
7205 Windsor Blvd.
Baltimore, MD 21244-2654
800-638-9096

51641
Alra Laboratories, Inc.
3850 Clearview Court
Gurnee, IL 60031
708-244-9440

Altana Incorporated
60 Baylis Road
Melville, NY 11747
516-454-7677

00731
Alto Pharmaceuticals, Inc.
P.O. Box 1910
Land O'Lakes, FL 34639-1910
813-949-7464

72959
Alva/Amco Pharmacal Cos. Inc.
6625 Avondale Ave.
Chicago, IL 60631
773-792-0200

17314
Alza Corp.
950 Page Mill Road
Palo Alto, CA 94303-0802
650-494-5000

10038
Ambix Laboratories, Inc.
210 Orchard Street
East Rutherford, NJ 07073
201-939-2200

89709, 90605
Amcon Laboratories
40 N. Rock Hill Road
St. Louis, MO 63119
314-961-5758

Americal Pharmaceutical, Inc.
See Akorn, Inc.

51201
American Dermal Corp.
51 Apple Tree Lane
P.O. Box 900
Plumsteadville, PA 18949-0900
610-454-8000

57506
American Drug Industries, Inc.
5810 S. Perry Ave.
Chicago, IL 60621
312-667-7070

American Lecithin Company
115 Hurley Road, Unit 2B
Oxford, CT 06478
800-364-4416

00517
American Regent
1 Luitpold Drive
Shirley, NY 11967
516-924-4000

00539
American Urologicals, Inc.
10031 Pines Blvd., Suite 216
Pembroke Pines, FL 33024
954-438-5070

55513
Amgen, Inc.
One Amgen Center Drive
Thousand Oaks, CA 91320-1789
805-447-3505

52152
Amide Pharmaceuticals, Inc.
101 E. Main Street
Little Falls, NJ 07424
201-890-1440

53926
Amsco Scientific
See Steris Laboratories

Amswiss Scientific, Inc.
2170 Broadway
Suite 1200
New York, NY 10024

Anaquest
See Ohmeda Pharmaceuticals

Andrew Jergens
2535 Spring Grove
Cincinnati, OH 45214
513-421-1400

Andrulis Pharmaceutical Corp.
11800 Baltimore Ave.
Beltsville, MD 20705
301-419-2400

Anthra Pharmaceuticals, Inc.
19 Carson Road
Princeton, NJ 08540

Antibodies, Inc.
P.O. Box 1560
Davis, CA 95617
916-758-4400

48028
Aplicare Inc.
P.O. Box 237
Prichard, WV 25555
304-486-5656

Apotex USA
1776 Broadway
Suite 1900
New York, NY 10019
800-700-3092

Apothecary Products, Inc.
11531 Rupp Drive
Burnsville, MN 55337-1295
612-890-1940

00003, 00015
Apothecon
P.O. Box 4500
Princeton, NJ 08543-4500
800-321-1335

48723
Apothecus, Inc.
20 Audrey Avenue
Oyster Bay, NY 11771
516-624-8200

Applied Biotech
10237 Flanders Ct.
San Diego, CA 92121
619-587-6771

Applied Genetics
205 Buffalo Ave.
Freeport, NY 11520
516-868-9026

Applied Medical Research
308 15th Avenue North
Nashville, TN 37203
615-327-0676

Approved Drug
See Health for Life Brands, Inc.

00275
Arco Pharmaceuticals, Inc.
90 Orville Drive
Bohemia, NY 11716
516-567-9500

00070
Arcola Laboratories
500 Arcola Road
Collegeville, PA 19426
610-454-8000

Argus Pharmaceuticals, Inc.
3400 Research Forest Drive
The Woodlands, TX 77381

Armour Pharmaceutical
See Centeon

48558
Arther, Inc.
P.O. Box 1455
W. Caldwell, NJ 07007
201-226-5288

61113
Astra Merck
725 Chesterbrook Blvd.
Wayne, PA 19087-5677
800-236-9933

00186
Astra USA, Inc.
50 Otis Street
Westborough, MA 01581
508-366-1100

59075
Athena Neurosciences, Inc.
800 Gateway Blvd.
South San Francisco, CA 94080
415-877-0900

59702
Atley Pharmaceuticals, Inc.
14433 N. Washington Highway
Ashland, VA 23005
804-752-8400

Autoimmune, Inc.
128 Spring Street
Lexington, MA 02173
617-860-0710

00225
B. F. Ascher and Co.
15501 W. 109th St.
Lenexa, KS 66219
913-888-1880

44184
Bajamar Chemical, Inc.
9609 Dielman Rock Island
St. Louis, MO 63132
314-997-3414

58174
Baker Cummins Dermatologicals
4400 Biscayne Blvd.
Miami, FL 33137
800-735-2315

00575, 11414
Baker Norton Pharmaceuticals
4400 Biscayne Blvd.
Miami, FL 33137
800-735-2315

00304
J.J. Balan, Inc.
5725 Foster Ave.
Brooklyn, NY 11234
718-251-8663

00555
Barr Laboratories, Inc.
2 Quaker Road
Pomona, NY 01970
914-362-1100

10116
Bartor Pharmacal Co.
70 High Street
Rye, NY 10580
914-967-4219

58887
Basel Pharmaceuticals
See Novartis

10119
Bausch & Lomb Personal Products Division
1400 N. Goodman Street
P.O. Box 450
Rochester, NY 14692-0450
716-338-6000

24208, 57782
Bausch & Lomb Pharmaceuticals
8500 Hidden River Pkwy.
Tampa, FL 33637
813-975-7700

Baxter Healthcare
1 Baxter Parkway DF4-1W
Deerfield, IL 60015
847-270-5700

00944
Baxter Hyland
550 North Brand Blvd.
Glendale, CA 91203
818-956-3200

00118
Bayer Corp. (Allergy Div.)
P.O. Box 3145
Spokane, WA 99220
509-489-5656

00026, 00161, 00192
Bayer Corp. (Biological and Pharmaceutical Div.)
400 Morgan Lane
West Haven, CT 06516
203-812-2373

12843, 16500
Bayer Corp. (Consumer Div.)
36 Columbia Road
Morristown, NJ 07962-1910
800-331-4536

00193
Bayer Corp. (Diagnostic Div.)
430 South Beiger Street
Mishawaka, IN 46544-2004
219-262-7926

BDI Pharmaceuticals, Inc.
P.O. Box 78610
Indianapolis, IN 46278-0610
317-228-5008

00486
Beach Pharmaceuticals
5220 South Manhattan Avenue
Tampa, FL 33681
800-322-8210

31280
Becton Dickinson & Co.
One Becton Drive
Franklin Lakes, NJ 07417-1881
201-847-6800

00011
Becton Dickinson Microbiology Systems
7 Loveton Circle
Sparks, MD 21152
410-316-4000

55390
Bedford Laboratories
300 Northfield Road
Bedford, OH 44146
216-232-3320

Behringwerke Aktiengesellschaft
500 Arcola Road
P.O. Box 1200
Collegeville, PA 19426-0107

10356
Beiersdorf, Inc.
P.O. Box 5529
S. Norwalk, CT 06856-5529
203-853-8008

50419
Berlex Laboratories, Inc.
15049 San Pable Avenue
Richmond, CA 94804-0099
201-694-4100

58337
Berna Products Corp.
4216 Ponce De Leon Blvd.
Coral Gables, FL 33146
305-443-2900

Best Generics
See Goldline Laboratories, Inc.

00283
Beutlich, Inc.
1541 Shields Dr.
Waukegan, IL 60085
847-473-1100

Biocare International, Inc.
2643 Grand Avenue
Bellmore, NY 11710
516-781-5800

00332
Biocraft Laboratories, Inc.
See Teva Pharmaceuticals

Biocryst Pharmaceuticals, Inc.
2190 Parkway Lake Drive
Birmingham, AL 35244

59527
BioDevelopment Corp.
8180 Greensboro Drive
Suite 1000
McLean, VA 22102
703-506-0290

Biofilm, Inc.
3121 Scott Street
Vista, CA 92083-8323
760-727-9030

Biogen
14 Cambridge Center
Cambridge, MA 02142
617-679-2000

BioGenex Laboratories
4600 Norris Canyon Road
Suite 400
San Ramon, CA 94583
510-275-0550

Bioline Labs, Inc.
See Zenith Goldline

Biomedical Frontiers, Inc.
1095 10th Ave. S.E.
Minneapolis, MN 55414
612-378-0228

Biomerica, Inc.
1533 Monrovia Ave.
Newport Beach, CA 92663
714-645-2111

Biomune Systems, Inc.
2401 South Foothill Drive
Salt Lake City, UT 84109
801-466-3441

Biopure Corp.
1100 Hurley
Cambridge, MA 02111
617-234-6500

52311
Biosearch Medical Products
P.O. Box 1700
Somerville, NJ 08876
908-722-5000

53191
Bio-Tech
P.O. Box 1992
Fayetteville, AR 72702
501-443-9148

Bio-Technology General Corp.
70 Wood Ave. South
Iselin, NJ 08830
908-632-8800

BIRA Corp.
2525 Quicksilver
McDonald, PA 15057
412-796-1820

50289
Birchwood Laboratories, Inc.
7900 Fuller Road
Eden Prairie, MN 53344
800-328-6156

12136
Bird Corp.
1100 Bird Center Drive
Palm Springs, CA 92262
619-778-7200

00165
Blaine, Inc.
1465 Jamike Lane
Erlanger, KY 41018-1878
606-283-9437

00154
Blair Laboratories
100 Connecticut Ave.
Norwalk, CT 06850-3590
203-853-0123

50486
Blairex Labs, Inc.
P.O. Box 2127
Columbus, IN 47202-2127
812-378-1864

10157
Blistex, Inc.
1800 Swift Drive
Oak Brook, IL 60523
630-571-2870

10158
Block Drug, Inc.
257 Cornelison Ave.
Jersey City, NJ 07302
201-434-3000

10160
Bluco Inc./Med. Discnt. Outlet
14849 W. McNichols
Detroit, MI 48235
313-273-0322

00563
Bock Pharmacal Co.
P.O. Box 419056
St. Louis, MO 63141-9056
314-579-0770

00597
Boehringer Ingelheim, Inc.
900 Ridgebury Road
Ridgefield, CT 06877
203-798-9988

53169
Boehringer Mannheim Corp.
101 Orchard Ridge Drive
Gaithersburg, MD 20878
800-621-3784

50924
Boehringer Mannheim Diags.
9115 Hague Road
P.O. Box 50100
Indianapolis, IN 46250-0100
800-428-5074

44437
Bolan Pharmaceutical, Inc.
P.O. Box 230
Hurst, TX 76053
817-284-8878

Boots Pharmaceuticals, Inc.
See Knoll Laboratories

00222
Boyle and Co. Pharm.
1613 Chelsea Rd.
San Marino, CA 91108
818-441-0284

00003
Bracco Diagnostics
P.O. Box 5225
Princeton, NJ 08543
609-514-2200

Bradley Pharmaceutical
See Kenwood Laboratories

52268
Braintree Laboratories, Inc.
60 Columbian
P.O. Box 361
Braintree, MA 02185-0929
617-843-2202

51991
Breckenridge Pharmaceutical, Inc
P.O. Box 206
Boca Raton, FL 33429
561-367-8512

72363
Brimms, Inc.
425 Fillmore Ave.
Tonawanda, NY 14150
716-694-7100

Bristol Laboratories
See Bristol-Myers Squibb

Bristol-Myers Oncology
P.O. Box 4500
Princeton, NJ 08543
609-897-2000

19810
Bristol-Myers Products
225 High Ridge Road
Stanford, CT 06905
800-468-7746

00003, 00087
Bristol-Myers Squibb
P.O. Box 4500
Princeton, NJ 08543-4000
609-897-2000

Britannia Pharmaceuticals
Forum Hs Brighton Road Redhill
Surrey, UK RH 1 6YS

Burroughs Wellcome Co.
See GlaxoWellcome

00398
C & M Pharmacal, Inc.
1721 Maplelane Avenue
Hazel Park, MI 48030-1215
248-548-7846

00132
C. B. Fleet, Inc.
4615 Murray Place
Lynchburg, VA 24506
804-528-4000

00463
C. O. Truxton, Inc.
P.O. Box 1594
Camden, NJ 08101
609-365-4118

10486
C. S. Dent & Co. Division
317 E. Eighth Street
Cincinnati, OH 45202
513-241-1677

55559
Calgon Vestal Laboratories
5035 Manchester Road
St. Louis, MO 63110
314-535-1810

California Department Health Service
2151 Berkeley Way
Berkeley, CA 94704

00147
Camall, Inc.
P.O. Box 307
Romeo, MI 48065-0307
313-752-9683

Cambridge Neuroscience, Inc.
1 Kendall Square
Building 700
Cambridge, MA 02139
617-225-0600

38083
Campbell Laboratories
P.O. Box 639
Deerfield Beach, FL 33443
305-570-9834

Can-Am Care Corp.
Cimetra Industrial Park
Chazy, NY 12921
800-461-7448

Cangene Corp.
104 Chancellor Matheson Road
Winnipeg, CANADA R3T 2N2
204-989-6850

Capmed USA
P.O. Box 14
Bryn Mawr, PA 19010

59046
Caprice-Greystoke
1259 Activity Drive
Vista, CA 92083
619-598-9300

57664
Caraco Pharmaceutical Labs
1150 Elijah McCoy Drive
Detroit, MI 48202
313-871-8400

Care Technologies, Inc.
55 Holly Hill Lane
Greenwich, CT 06830

Carme, Inc.
84 Galli
Novato, CA 94949
415-382-4000

Carnation
800 North Brand Blvd.
Glendale, CA 91203
800-628-2229

00086
Carnrick Laboratories, Inc.
65 Horse Hill Road
Cedar Knolls, NJ 07927
973-267-2670

46287
Carolina Medical Products
P.O. Box 147
Farmville, NC 27828
919-753-7111

Carrington Labs
1300 E. Rochelle Blvd.
Irving, TX 75062
972-518-1300

00164
Carter Wallace
Half Acre Road
P.O. Box 1001
Cranbury, NJ 08512-0181
609-655-6000

Cavitation-Control Technology
55 Knollwood Road
Farmington, CT 06032
203-673-0507

Celgene Corp.
7 Powder Horn Drive
Warren, NJ 07059
908-271-1001

Cell Pathways, Inc.
1700 Broadway
Suite 2000
Denver, CO 80290

Cell Technology
1668 Valtec Lane
Boulder, CO 80301
303-790-0587

Cellegy Pharmaceuticals, Inc.
371 Bel Marin Keys
Suite 210
Novato, CA 94949

Celtrix Pharmaceuticals, Inc.
3055 Patrick Henry Drive
Santa Clara, CA 95054

00053
Centeon
1020 First Avenue
King of Prussia, PA 19406-1310
215-386-2066

00268
Center Laboratories
35 Channel Drive
Port Washington, NY 11050
516-767-1800

Centers for Disease Control
1600 Clifton Road
Mail Stop D-09
Atlanta, GA 30333
404-639-3670

Centocor, Inc.
200 Great Valley Pkwy.
Malvern, PA 19355
610-651-6000

00131
Central Pharmaceuticals, Inc.
See Schwarz Pharma

00436
Century Pharmaceuticals, Inc.
10377 Hague Road
Indianapolis, IN 46256-3399
317-849-4210

Cephalon, Inc.
145 Brandywine Pkwy.
West Chester, PA 19380
215-344-0200

00173
Cerenex Pharmaceuticals
See GlaxoWellcome

10223
Cetylite Industries, Inc.
9051 River Road
P.O. Box 90006
Pennsauken, NJ 08110
609-665-6111

54429
Chase Laboratories
280 Chestnut Street
Newark, NJ 07105-1598
201-589-8181

49447
Chattem Consumer Products
1715 W. 38th Street
Chattanooga, TN 37409
615-821-4571

Chembiomed, Ltd.
P.O. Box 8050
Edmonton, CANADA AB T6H4NP

52489
Chemi-Tech Laboratories
74-80 Marine Street
Farmingdale, NY 11735

00521
Chesebrough-Pond's, USA
33 Benedict Place
Greenwich, CT 06830
203-661-2000

Chiesi Pharmaceuticals, Inc.
150 Danbury Road
Ridgefield, CT 06877

53905
Chiron Therapeutics
4560 Horton Street
Emeryville, CA 94608
800-244-7668

Chiron Vision
500 Iolab Drive
Claremont, CA 91711
909-624-2020

Chugai-Upjohn, Inc.
6133 North River Road
Suite 800
Rosemont, IL 60018

00067, 00083
Ciba Self-Medication, Inc.
See Novartis

00346
Ciba Vision Ophthalmics
11460 Johns Creek Pkwy.
Duluth, GA 30136
404-418-4101

00083
Ciba-Geigy Pharmaceuticals
See Novartis

00677, 00725, 71114
Circa Pharmaceuticals, Inc.
33 Ralph Ave.
Copiague, NY 11726-0030
516-842-8383

00659
Circle Pharmaceuticals, Inc.
6320 B Rucker Road
Indianapolis, IN 46220
317-475-1921

City Chemical Corp.
132 W. 22nd Street
New York, NY 10011
201-653-6900

45802
Clay-Park Labs, Inc.
1700 Bathgate Ave.
Bronyx, NY 10457
212-901-2800

Clintec Nutrition
Three Pkwy. North
Suite 500
Deerfield, IL 60015
708-317-2800

Cocensys, Inc.
213 Technology Drive
Irvine, CA 92718
714-453-0131

Colgate Oral Pharmaceuticals
1 Colgate Way
Canton, MA 02021
617-821-2880

Collagen Corp.
2500 Faber Place
Palo Alto, CA 94303
415-856-0200

00837, 21406
Columbia Laboratories, Inc.
2665 South Bayshore Drive
Miami, FL 33133
305-860-1670

11509
Combe, Inc.
1101 Westchester Ave.
White Plains, NY 10604
914-694-5454

11793, 49281, 50361
Connaught Labs
See Pasteur Mérieux Connaught

00223
Consolidated Midland Corp.
20 Main St.
Brewster, NY 10509
914-279-6108

34044
Continental Consumer Products
770 Forest
Suite B
Birmingham, MI 48009
800-542-5903

33130
Continental Quest Research
220 W. Carmel Drive
Carmel, IN 46032
800-451-5773

00003
ConvaTec
P.O. Box 5254
Princeton, NJ 08543-5254
908-359-9200

00961
Cook-Waite Laboratories, Inc.
90 Park Ave.
New York, NY 10016
212-907-2000

Cooper Biomedical, Inc.
One Technology Court
Malvern, PA 19355
215-219-6300

Cooper Development Co.
455 East Middlefield Road
Mountain View, CA 94043
415-969-9030

59426
CooperVision
10 Faraday
Irvine, CA 92618
714-597-8130

38245
Copley Pharmaceutical, Inc.
25 John Road
Canton, MA 02021
617-821-6111

Cord Labs
See Geneva Pharmaceuticals

Coulter Corp.
11800 S.W. 147 Ave.
P.O. Box 169015
Miami, FL 33116
305-380-3800

50752
Creighton Products Corp.
59 Route 10
East Hanover, NJ 07936-1080
201-503-6099

CTRC Research Foundation
11812 Becket Street
Potomac, MD 20854

01020
Cumberland Packing Corp.
35 Old Ridgefield Road
P.O. Box 7688
Willton, CT 06897
800-206-9454

55326
Curatek Pharmaceuticals
See 3M Pharmaceuticals

Cutter Biologicals
See Bayer Corp. (Biological and Pharmaceutical Div.)

Cyclin Pharmaceuticals Inc.
429 Gammon Place
Madison, WI 53715
608-833-8462

54799
Cynacon/OCuSOFT
P.O. Box 429
Richmond, TX 77406-0429
800-233-5469

Cytel Corp.
3525 John Hopkins Court
San Diego, CA 92121
619-552-3000

Cytogen
600 College Road East
Princeton, NJ 08540
609-987-8200

23731
Cytosol Laboratories
55 Messina Drive
Braintree, MA 02184

CytRx
150 Technology Pkwy.
Norcross, GA 30092
404-368-9500

55994
Dakryon Pharmaceuticals
2579 S. Loop
Suite 8
Lubbock, TX 79423-1400
806-745-2872

55425
Dal-Med Pharmaceuticals
5701 N. Pine Island Road
Tamarac, FL 33321
800-543-9151

Danbury Pharmacal
See Schein Pharmaceutical, Inc.

00689
Daniels Pharmaceuticals, Inc.
See Jones Medical

Dapat Pharmaceuticals, Inc.
5040 Linbar Drive,
Suite 102
Nashville, TN 37211
615-833-2616

Darby Pharmaceuticals, Inc.
100 Banks Ave.
Rockville Centre, NY 11570

58869
Dartmouth Pharmaceuticals
19 Whaler's Way
North Dartmouth, MA 02747
508-636-5553

00938
Davis and Geck
See Sherwood Davis & Geck

52041
Dayton Laboratories, Inc.
3307 NW 74th Ave.
Miami, FL 33122
305-594-0988

00744
Daywell Laboratories Corp.
78 Unquowa Place
Fairfield, CT 06430
203-255-3154

Degussa Corp.
65 Challenger Road
Ridgefield Park, NJ 07660
201-641-6100

10310
Del Pharmaceuticals, Inc.
163 East Bethpage
Plainview, NY 11803
516-293-7070

48532
Delmont Laboratories, Inc.
P.O. Box 269
Swarthmore, PA 19081
215-543-3365

00316
Del-Ray Laboratory, Inc.
22 20th Ave. N.W.
Birmingham, AL 35215
205-853-8247

00295
Denison Laboratories, Inc.
60 Dunnell Lane
P.O. Box 1305
Pawtucket, RI 02862
401-723-5500

00066
Dermik Laboratories, Inc.
500 Arcola Road
P.O. Box 1200
Collegeville, PA 19426
610-454-8000

50744
Dermol Pharmaceuticals, Inc.
3807 Roswell Road
Marietta, GA 30062
404-977-7779

49502
Dey Laboratories, Inc.
2751 Napa Valley Corporate Dr.
Napa, CA 94558
707-224-3200

Discovery Experimental & Development, Inc.
29949 SR 54 West
Wesley Chapel, FL 33543
813-973-7200

00777
Dista Products Co.
See Lilly

10337
Doak Dermatologics
383 Route 46 West
Fairfield, NJ 07004-2402
201-882-1505

25358
Donell DerMedex
342 Madison Ave.
Suite 1422
New York, NY 10173
212-697-3800

00514
Dow Hickam, Inc.
P.O. Box 2006
Sugarland, TX 77487
713-240-1000

13723
Dr. Nordyke Footcare Products
1650 Palma Drive
Suite 102
Ventura, CA 93003
805-650-8333

00094
Du Pont Merck Pharmaceutical
4301 Lancaster Pike
Wilmington, DE 19805
302-892-7050

00056, 00590
Du Pont Pharma
P.O. Box 800723
Wilmington, DE 19880
800-474-2762

51479
Dura Pharmaceuticals
5880 Pacific Center Blvd.
San Diego, CA 92121-4202
619-457-2553

51285
Duramed Pharmaceuticals
5040 Lester Road
Cincinnati, OH 45213
513-731-9900

Durex Consumer Products
3585 Engineering Drive
Suite 200
Norcross, GA 30092
770-582-2222

55516
Dyna Pharm, Inc.
P.O. Box 2141
Del Mar, CA 92014-2141
619-792-9523

10331
E. E. Dickinson Co.
2 Enterprise Drive
Shelton, CT 06484
203-929-1197

00168
E. Fougera and Co.
60 Baylis Road
Melville, NY 11747
516-454-6996

Eagle Vision, Inc.
6263 Poplar Ave.
Suite 650
Memphis, TN 38119
901-767-3937

Eastman Kodak Co.
10 Indigo Creek Drive
Rochester, NY 14650-0862
800-526-8811

Eaton Medical Corp.
2288 Dunn Ave.
Memphis, TN 38114
901-744-8024

19458
Eckerd Drug Co.
P.O. Box 4689
Clearwater, FL 34618
813-397-7461

38130
Econo Med Pharmaceuticals
4305 Sartin Road
Burlington, NC 27217-7522
919-226-1091

00095, 59010
ECR Pharmaceuticals
3981 Deep Rock Road
Richmond, VA 23233
804-527-1950

00485
Edwards Pharmaceuticals, Inc.
111 Mulberry Street
Ripley, MS 38663
601-837-8182

55806
Effcon Labs, Inc.
1800 Sandy Plains Pkwy.
Marietta, GA 30066
404-428-7011

Elan Corp.
1300 Gould Drive
Gainesville, GA 30504
404-534-8239

Elder
See Zeneca

00002, 59075
Eli Lilly and Co.
Lilly Corp. Center
Indianapolis, IN 46285
317-276-2000

00641
Elkins-Sinn, Inc.
See Wyeth Ayerst

EM Industries, Inc.
5 Skyline Drive
Hawthorne, NY 10532
914-592-4660

60951
Endo Laboratories
P.O. Box 80390
Wilmington, DE 19880
800-462-4467

57665
Enzon, Inc.
40 Kingsbridge Road
Piscataway, NJ 08854-3998
908-980-4500

00185, 00536
Eon Labs Manufacturing, Inc.
227-15 North Conduit Ave.
Laurelton, NY 11413
718-276-8600

Epitope Inc.
8505 SW Creekside Place
Beaverton, OR 97008
503-641-6115

E.R. Squibb & Sons, Inc.
See Bristol-Myers Squibb

Escalon Ophthalmics, Inc.
182 Tamarack Circle
Skillman, NJ 08558
609-497-9141

00005, 59911
ESI Lederle Generics
P.O. Box 8299
Philadelphia, PA 19101
610-688-4400

58177
Ethex Corp.
10888 Metro Court
St. Louis, MO 63043-2413
314-567-3307

Ethicon, Inc.
Route 22 West
P.O. Box 151
Somerville, NJ 08876-0151
908-218-0707

54686
Ethitek Pharmaceuticals
7701 North Austin
Skokie, IL 60077
708-675-6611

00642
Everett Laboratories, Inc.
29 Spring Street
West Orange, NJ 07052
973-324-0200

Evreka
600 Montgomery Street
San Francisco, CA 94111
415-627-2040

Falcon Ophthalmics, Inc.
6201 S. Freeway
Fort Worth, TX 76134
800-343-2133

Farmacon, Inc.
90 Grove Street
Suite 109
Ridgefield, CT 06877-4118
203-431-9989

99766
Faulding USA
200 Elmora Ave.
Elizabeth, NJ 07207
800-526-6978

00496
Ferndale Laboratories, Inc.
780 W. Eight Mile Road
Ferndale, MI 48220-1218
313-548-0900

55566
Ferring Laboratories, Inc.
400 Rella Blvd.
Suite 201
Suffern, NY 10901
914-368-7900

31795
Fibertone Co.
14851 N. Scottsdale Road
Scottsdale, AZ 85254
800-462-7596

00729
Fidelity Halsom
1330 Farr Drive at Stanley
Dayton, OH 45404
800-356-3065

Fidia Pharmaceutical
1401 I Street N.W.
Washington, DC 20005
202-371-9898

00421
Fielding Co.
94 Weldon Pkwy.
Maryland Heights, MO 63043
314-567-5462

51687
Fischer Pharmaceuticals, Inc.
165 Gibraltar Court
Sunnyvale, CA 94089
408-747-1760

Fiske Industries
339 N. Main Street
New City, NY 10956
914-634-5099

Fisons Consumer Health
See Ciba Self-Medication, Inc.

00585
Fisons Corp.
See Medeva Pharmaceuticals

54323
Flanders, Inc.
P.O. Box 39143
Charleston, SC 29407-9143
803-571-3363

00256
Fleming & Co.
1600 Fenpark Drive
Fenton, MO 63026-2918
314-343-8200

00288
Fluoritab Corp.
P.O. Box 507
Temperance, MI 48182-0507
313-847-3985

00258, 00456, 00535, 00785
Forest Pharmaceutical, Inc.
13622 Lakefront Drive
St. Louis, MO 63045
314-344-8870

00494
Foy Laboratories
906 Penn Ave.
Wyomissing, PA 19610
215-678-9460

Free Radical Sciences, Inc.
245 First Street
Cambridge, MA 02142
617-374-1200

10432
Freeda Vitamins, Inc.
36 E. 41st Street
New York, NY 10017-6203
212-685-4980

Fuisz Technologies, Ltd.
3810 Concorde Pkwy.
Suite 100
Chantilly, VA 22021
703-803-3260

00469, 57317
Fujisawa USA, Inc.
3 Parkway North Center
Deerfield, IL 60015-2548
708-317-0600

00713
G & W Laboratories
111 Coolidge Street
South Plainfield, NJ 07080
908-753-2000

Galagen, Inc.
4001 Lexington Ave. North
Arden Hills, MN 55126-2998
612-481-2105

00299
Galderma Laboratories, Inc.
P.O. Box 331329
Ft. Worth, TX 76163
817-263-2600

00254
Gambro, Inc.
1185 Oak Street
Lakewood, CO 80215
800-525-2623

57844
Gate Pharmaceuticals
650 Cathill Road
Sellersville, PA 18960
800-292-4283

00386
Gebauer Co.
9410 St. Catherine Ave.
Cleveland, OH 44104
216-271-5252

00028
Geigy Pharmaceuticals
See Novartis

Gencon
6116 N. Central Expy. 200
Dallas, TX 75206
214-373-4665

52761
GenDerm Corp.
See Medicis

50242
Genentech, Inc.
460 Point San Bruno Blvd.
South San Francisco, CA 94080
415-225-1000

50272
General Generics, Inc.
P.O. Box 510
Oxford, MS 38655
601-234-0130

52584
General Injectables & Vaccines
U.S. Hwy. 52
Bastian, VA 24314
703-688-4121

00918
General Medical Corp.
8741 Landmark Road
Richmond, VA 23261
804-264-7500

Genetic Therapy, Inc.
938 Copper Road
Gaithersburg, MD 20878
301-590-2626

00781
Geneva Pharmaceuticals
2599 W. Midway Blvd.
P.O. Box 469
Broomfield, CO 80038-0469
800-525-8747

Gen-King
See Kinray

00703
Gensia Laboratories, LTD.
19 Hughes
Irvine, CA 92718-1902
800-331-0124

58468
Genzyme Corp.
One Kendall Square
Cambridge, MA 02139
617-252-7500

Geriatric Pharmaceutical Corp.
See Roberts Pharmaceuticals

Gilead Sciences, Inc.
353 Lakeside Drive
Forsten City, CA 94404

59366
Glades Pharmaceuticals
255 Alhambra Center
Suite 1000
Coral Gables, FL 33134
800-452-3371

00081, 00173
GlaxoWellcome
Five Moore Drive
Research Triangle Pk., NC 27709
919-248-2100

00516
Glenwood, Inc.
83 N. Summit Street
Tenafly, NJ 07670
201-569-0050

Global Source
3001 N. 29th Ave.
Hollywood, FL 33020
305-921-0006

Glycomed, Inc.
860 Atlantic Ave.
Alameda, CA 94501
510-523-5555

00182
Goldline Laboratories, Inc.
See Zenith Goldline Pharmaceuticals

74684
Goody's Manufacturing Corp.
436 Salt Street
Winston Salem, NC 27108
910-723-1831

10481
Gordon Laboratories
6801 Ludlow Street
Upper Darby, PA 19082-1694
215-734-2011

12165
Graham Field
400 Rabro Drive East
Hauppauge, NY 11788
516-582-5900

00152
Gray Pharmaceutical Co.
100 Connecticut Ave.
Norwalk, CT 06856
203-853-0123

51301
Great Southern Laboratories
10863 Rockley Road
Houston, TX 77099
713-530-3077

Green Turtle Bay Vitamin Co.
P.O. Box 642
Summit, NJ 07902
908-277-2240

59762
Greenstone
Moors Bridge Road
Portage, MI 49002
800-447-3360

22840
Greer Laboratories, Inc.
P.O. Box 800
Lenoir, NC 28645-0800
704-754-5327

00327
Guardian Laboratories
230 Marcus Blvd.
Hauppauge, NY 11788
516-273-0900

54396
Gynex Pharmaceuticals, Inc.
1175 Corporate Woods Pkwy.
Vernon Hills, IL 60061
708-913-1144

54765
GynoPharma Laboratories
50 Division Street
Somerville, NJ 08876
908-725-3100

00879
Halsey Drug Co.
1827 Pacific Street
Brooklyn, NY 11233
718-467-7500

Hannan Ophthalmic Marketing Services, Inc.
163 Meetinghouse Road
Duxbury, MA 02332

51432
Harber Pharmaceutical Co.
350 Meadowlands Pkwy.
Secaucus, NJ 07094
201-348-3700

HDC Corporation
2109 O'Toole Ave.
San Jose, CA 95131
408-954-1909

Health & Medical Techniques
See Graham Field

50383
Health Care Products
369 Bayview Ave.
Amityville, NY 11701
516-789-8455

00598
Health for Life Brands, Inc.
1643 E. Genesee Street
Syracuse, NY 13210
315-478-6303

51662
Healthfirst Corp.
22316 70th Ave. W.
Mountlake Terrace, WA 98043
206-771-5733

59512
Healthline Laboratories, Inc.
835 Potts Ave.
Green Bay, WI 54304
414-497-3322

00586
Heather Drug, Inc.
1 Fellowship Road
Cherry Hill, NJ 08003
609-424-3663

Helena Laboratories
P.O. Box 752
Beaumont, TX 77704-0752
409-842-3714

HEM Research
1617 John F. Kennedy Blvd.
Philadelphia, PA 19103
215-988-0080

Hemacare Corp.
4954 Van Nuys Blvd.
Sherman Oaks, CA 91403
818-986-3883

Herald Pharmacal Inc.
6503 Warwick Rd.
Richmond, VA 23225
804-524-3112

Herbert Laboratories
See Allergan Inc.

48017
Hermal Pharmaceutical Labs
163 Delaware Ave.
Delmar, NY 12054
518-475-0175

28105
Hill Dermaceuticals, Inc.
P.O. Box 149283
Orlando, FL 32814-9283
407-896-8280

17808
Himmel Pharmaceuticals, Inc.
P.O. Box 5479
Lake Worth, FL 33466-5479
407-585-0070

50673
Hirsch Industries, Inc.
4912 West Broad Street
Richmond, VA 23230-0964
804-355-4500

Hiscia
CH-4144, Arlesheim Kirshweg
Switzerland
4106172-2323

00839
H.L. Moore Drug Exchange, Inc.
389 John Downey Drive
New Britain, CT 06050
203-826-3600

00039, 00068, 00088
Hoechst-Marion Roussel
P.O. Box 9627
Kansas City, MO 64134
908-231-2000

58573
Hogil Pharmaceutical Corp.
1 Byram Brook Place
Armonk, NY 10504
914-273-9666

47992
Holles Laboratories, Inc.
30 Forest Notch
Cohasset, MA 02025-1198
617-383-0741

Hollister-Stier
See Bayer Corp. (Allergy Div.)

Home Diagnostics, Inc. (HDI)
51 James Way
Eatontown, NJ 07724
908-542-7788

Hope Pharmaceuticals
2961 W. MacArthur Blvd.
Santa Ana, CA 92704
714-556-4673

59630
Horizon Pharmaceutical Corp.
1125 Northmeadow Pkwy.
Roswell, GA 30076
404-442-9707

59229
Horus Therapeutics, Inc.
2320 Brighton-Henrietta Town
Rochester, NY 14623
716-292-4820

00196
Houba, Inc.
P.O. Box 190
Culver, IN 46511
219-842-3305

00556
H.R. Cenci Labs, Inc.
1420 E. Street
P.O. Box 12524
Fresno, CA 93778-2524
209-237-3346

58407
Huckaby Pharmacal, Inc.
104 E. Main Street
LaGrange, KY 40031
502-222-4700

25077
Hudson Corp.
90 Orville Drive
Bohemia, NY 11716
516-567-9500

00395
Humco Holding Group, Inc.
P.O. Box 2550
Texarkana, TX 75504
903-793-3174

Hybritech
P.O. Box 269006
San Diego, CA 92196-9006
619-455-6700

Hyland Therapeutics
See Baxter Hyland

Hynson, Westcott & Dunning
See Becton Dickinson Microbiology Systems

00314
Hyrex Pharmaceuticals
P.O. Box 18385
Memphis, TN 38181-0385
901-794-9050

Iatric Corp.
2330 S. Industrial Park Drive
Tempe, AZ 85282-1893
602-966-7248

ICI Pharmaceuticals
See Zeneca Pharmaceuticals

00163, 00187
ICN Pharmaceuticals, Inc.
3300 Hyland Avenue
Costa Mesa, CA 92626
714-545-0100
800-556-1937

51244
I.C.P. Pharmaceuticals
P.O. Box 294
Cudahy, WI 53110
414-521-4647

IDEC Pharmaceuticals
11099 N. Torrey Pines Road #160
La Jolla, CA 92037
619-458-0600

Immucell Corp.
56 Evergreen Drive
Portland, ME 04103
207-878-2770

00205, 58406
Immunex Corp.
51 University Street
Seattle, WA 98101
206-587-0430

Immuno Clinical Research Corp.
155 East 56th Street
New York, NY 10022
212-759-3521

54129
Immuno U.S., Inc.
1200 Parkdale Road
Rochester, MI 48307-1744
313-652-7872

Immunobiology Research Inst.
Route 22 East
P.O. Box 999
Annandale, NJ 08801-0999
908-730-1700

ImmunoGen
148 Sidney Street
Cambridge, MA 02139
617-661-9312

Immunomedics
300 American Road
Morris Plains, NJ 07950
973-605-8200

Immunotherapeutics
3505 Riverview Circle
Morehead, MN 56560
701-232-9575

Imreg
144 Elk Place
Suite 1400
New Orleans, LA 70112
504-523-2875
504-523-6201

00548
I.M.S., Ltd.
1886 Santa Anita Ave.
South El Monte, CA 91733
818-913-4660

Infusaid, Inc.
1400 Providence Highway
Norwood, MA 02062
617-769-8330
800-523-8446

18686
InnoVisions, Inc.
6065 Frantz Road
Suite 202
Dublin, OH 43017
614-766-5477

Interchem Corp.
120 Route 17 North
Suite 115
Paramus, NJ 07652
800-261-7332
201-261-7333

Interfalk U.S., Inc.
25 Margaret
Plattsburgh, NY 12901

Interferon Sciences
783 Jersey Ave.
New Brunswick, NJ 08901
732-249-3250

11584
International Ethical Labs
Reparto Metropolitano
Rio Piedras, PR 00921
787-765-3510

00665
International Laboratories
901 Sawyer Road
Marietta, GA 30062
404-578-5583

Interneuron Pharmaceuticals
1 Ledgemont Center
99 Hayden Ave.
Lexington, MA 02173
781-861-8444

Interpro
P.O. Box 1823
Haverhill, MA 01831
508-373-2438

00814
Interstate Drug Exchange
1500 New Horizons Blvd.
Amityville, NY 11701-1130
516-957-8300

Intramed
102 Tremont Way
Augusta, GA 30907

52189
Invamed, Inc.
2400 Route 130N
Dayton, NJ 08810
732-274-1040

Inveresk Research
4470 Redwood Hwy.
San Rafael, CA 94903
415-491-6460

00258
Inwood Laboratories
300 Prospect Street
Inwood, NY 11696
516-371-1155

Iolab Pharmaceuticals
See Ciba Vision Ophthalmics

61646
Iomed
7425 Pebble Drive
Fort Worth, TX 76118
817-589-7257

11808
ION Laboratories, Inc.
7431 Pebble Drive
Ft. Worth, TX 76118
817-589-7257

IOP, Inc.
3100 Airway Ave.
Suite 106
Costa Mesa, CA 92626
714-549-1185

54921
IPR Pharmaceuticals, Inc.
P.O. Box 6000
Carolina, PR 00984
800-477-6385

50914
Iso Tex Diagnostics, Inc.
1511 County Road 129
Friendswood, TX 77546
281-482-1231

16837
J & J Merck Consumer Pharm.
Camp Hill Road
Ft. Washington, PA 19034
215-233-7000

88395
J. R. Carlson Laboratories
15 College Drive
Arlington Heights, IL 60004-1985
708-255-1600

49938
Jacobus Pharmaceutical Co.
37 Cleveland Lane
Princeton, NJ 08540
609-921-7447

50458
Janssen Pharmaceutical, Inc.
P.O. Box 200
Titusville, NJ 08560-0200
609-730-2000

JMI-Canton Pharmaceuticals
See Jones Medical Industries

00137
Johnson & Johnson
Grandview Road
Skillman, NJ 08558-9418
908-524-0400

56091
Johnson & Johnson Medical
P.O. Box 130
Arlington, TX 76004-0130
800-433-5009

00252, 52604, 00689, 12463
Jones Medical Industries
P.O. Box 46903
St. Louis, MO 63146-6903
314-576-6100

10106
J.T. Baker, Inc.
See Mallinckrodt-Baker

KabiVitrum, Inc.
See Pharmacia & Upjohn

Kanetta
90 Park Ave.
New York, NY 10016
212-907-2690

00588
Keene Pharmaceuticals, Inc.
P.O. Box 7
Keene, TX 76059-0007
817-645-8083

28851
Kendall Health Care Products
15 Hampshire Street
Mansfield, MA 02048
508-261-8000

Kendall-McGaw Labs, Inc.
See McGaw, Inc.

00482
Kenwood Laboratories
383 Rt. 46 W.
Fairfield, NJ 07006-2402
201-882-1505

00085
Key Pharmaceuticals
2000 Galloping Hill Road
Kenilworth, NJ 07033
908-298-4000

60793
King Pharmaceuticals Inc.
501 Fifth Street
Bristol, TN 37620
615-989-6232

55299
Kingswood Laboratories, Inc.
10375 Hague Road
Indianapolis, IN 46256
317-849-9513

Kinray
152-35 10th Ave.
Whitestone, NY 11357
718-767-1234

58223
Kirkman Sales, Inc.
P.O. Box 1009
Wilsonville, OR 97070-1009
503-694-1600

31600
Kiwi Brands, Inc.
447 Old Swede Road
Douglassville, PA 19518-1239
215-385-9322

KLI Corp.
1119 Third Ave. S.W.
Carmel, IN 46032
317-846-7452

00044, 00048, 00524
Knoll Laboratories
3000 Continental Drive North
Mt. Olive, NJ 07828-1234
973-426-2600

00044, 00048, 00524
Knoll Pharmaceuticals
3000 Continental Drive North
Mt. Olive, NJ 07828-1234
973-331-7633

Kodak Dental
343 State Street
Rochester, NY 14650

00224
Konsyl Pharmaceuticals
4200 South Hulen
Suite 513
Ft. Worth, TX 76109
817-763-8011

55505
Kramer Laboratories, Inc.
8778 S.W. 8th Street
Miami, FL 33174-9990
305-223-1287

La Haye Laboratories, Inc.
2205 152nd Ave. N.E.
Redmond, WA 98052
206-644-2020

Lacrimedics, Inc.
190 North Arrowhead Avenue
Suite B
Rialto, CA 92376

41383
Lactaid, Inc.
7050 Camp Hill Road
Ft. Washington, PA 19034
215-233-7000

59081
Lafayette Pharmaceuticals, Inc.
P.O. Box 4499
Lafayette, IN 47903-4499
317-447-3129

Lake Pharmaceutical, Inc.
625 Forest Edge Dr.
Vernon Hills, IL 60061
847-793-0230

00527
Lannett, Inc.
9000 State Road
Philadelphia, PA 19136
215-333-9000

00277
Laser, Inc.
2200 W. 97th Place
P.O. Box 905
Crown Point, IN 46307
219-663-1165

10651
Lavoptik, Inc.
661 Western Ave.
St. Paul, MN 55103
612-489-1351

00005
Lederle Laboratories
North Middletown Road
Pearl River, NY 10965-1299
914-732-5000

53124
Lederle-Praxis Biologicals
North Middletown Road
Pearl River, NY 10965
914-272-7000

23558
Lee Pharmaceuticals
1444 Santa Anita Blvd.
South Elmonte, CA 91733
800-950-5337

Leeming
See Pfizer US Pharmaceutical Group

25332
Legere Pharmaceuticals, Inc.
7326 E. Evans Road
Scottsdale, AZ 85260
602-991-4033

19200
Lehn & Fink
See Reckitt & Coleman

Leiner Health Products
901 East 233rd Street
Carson, CA 90745

Leiras Pharmaceuticals, Inc.
2345 Waukegan Road
Suite N-135
Bonnockburn, IL 60015

00093, 00332
Lemmon Co.
See Teva Pharmaceuticals

Lenti-Chemico Pharmaceuticals
500 Frank W. Burr Blvd.
Teaneck, NJ 07666
201-836-1196

00454
Lexis Laboratories
P.O. Box 202887
Austin, TX 78720
512-328-8484

Lifescan
1000 Gibraltar
Milpitas, CA 95035-6312
408-263-9789

Ligand Pharmaceuticals, Inc.
9393 Towne Centre Drive
San Diego, CA 92121
619-535-3900

00002, 59075
Eli Lilly and Co.
Lilly Corp. Center
Indianapolis, IN 46285
317-276-2000

Lincoln Diagnostics
P.O. Box 1128
Decatur, IL 62525
217-877-2531

60799
Liposome Co.
One Research Way
Princeton, NJ 08540
609-452-7060

54198
Liquipharm
10716 McCune Avenue
Los Angeles, Ca 90034
310-558-3344

Loch Pharmaceuticals
See Bedford Laboratories

00273
Lorvic Corp.
See Young Dental

59417
Lotus Biochemical
7335 Lee Highway
P.O. Box 3586
Radford, VA 24143-3586
703-633-3500

LTR Pharmaceuticals, Inc.
145 Sakonnet Blvd.
Narragansett, RI 02882

LuChem Pharmaceuticals, Inc.
See H.N. Norton Co.

00374
Lyne Laboratories
260 Tosca Drive
Stoughton, MA 02072
800-525-0450

00466
Macsil, Inc.
P.O. Box 29276
Philadelphia, PA 19125-0976
215-739-7300

00904
Major Pharmaceuticals
1640 W. Fulton
Chicago, IL 60612
312-666-9600

10106
Mallinckrodt-Baker
222 Red School Lane
Phillipsburg, NJ 08865
908-859-2151

00406
Mallinckrodt Chemical
16305 Swingley Ridge Drive
Chesterfield, MO 63017
314-654-2000

00019
Mallinckrodt Medical, Inc.
675 McDonnell Blvd.
P.O. Box 5840
St. Louis, MO 63134
314-654-2000

10706
Manne
P.O. Box 825
Johns Island, SC 29457
800-517-0228

Marlin Industries
P.O. Box 560
Grover City, CA 93483-0560
800-423-5926

12939
Marlop Pharmaceuticals, Inc.
5704 Mosholu Ave.
P.O. Box 536
Bronx, NY 10471
800-345-7192

10712
Marlyn, Inc.
14851 N. Scottsdale Road
Scottsdale, AZ 85254
800-462-7596

00682
Marnel Pharmaceuticals, Inc.
206 Luke Drive
Lafayette, LA 70506
318-232-1396

00209
Marsam Pharmaceuticals, Inc.
P.O. Box 1022
Cherry Hill, NJ 08034
609-424-5600

52555
Martec Pharmaceutical, Inc.
P.O. Box 33510
Kansas City, MO 64120-3510
816-241-4144

11845
Mason Distributors, Inc.
5105 N.W. 159th Street
Hialeah, FL 33014-6370
305-624-5557

12758
Mason Pharmaceuticals, Inc.
4425 Jamboree
Suite 250
Newport Beach, CA 92660
714-851-6860

14362
Mass. Public Health Bio. Lab.
305 South Street
Jamaica Plains, MA 02130
617-522-3700

Matrix Laboratories
1430 O'Brian Drive
Suite G
Menlo Park, CA 94025
415-326-6100

00259
Mayrand, Inc.
915 Bridge Street
Winston Salem, NC 27101
910-765-4252

00264
McGaw, Inc.
P.O. Box 19791
Irvine, CA 92713-9791
714-660-2000

11089
McGregor Pharmaceuticals, Inc.
8420 Ulmenton Road
Suite 305
Largo, FL 34641
813-530-4361

49072
McGuff, Inc.
3617 W. MacArthur Blvd.
Suite 507
Santa Ana, CA 92704
800-854-7220

50185
McHenry Laboratories, Inc.
118 N. Wells, Lee Building
Edna, TX 77957
512-782-5438

00045
McNeil Consumer Products Co.
Camp Hill Road
Mail Stop 278
Ft. Washington, PA 19034-2292
215-233-7000

MCR American Pharmaceuticals
120 Summit Parkway,
Suite 101
Birmingham, AL 35209
205-942-6415

58607
ME Pharmaceuticals, Inc.
2800 Southeast Pkwy.
Richmond, IN 47375
800-637-4276

Mead Johnson Laboratories
See Bristol-Myers Squibb

00087
Mead Johnson Nutritionals
2404 Pennsylvania Street
Evansville, IN 47721
812-426-6000

Mead Johnson Oncology
See Bristol-Myers Oncology

Mead Johnson Pharmaceuticals
See Bristol-Myers Squibb

Medac GmbH c/o Princeton Regulatory Assoc.
65 South Main Street
Pennington, NJ 08534
609-951-9596

Medarex
1545 Rte. 22E
P.O. Box 953
Annandale, NJ 08801
908-713-6001

MedChem
232 W. Cummings Park
Woburn, MA 01801
800-451-4716

Medclone, Inc.
2435 Military Avenue
Los Angeles, CA 90064

11940
Medco Lab, Inc.
P.O. Box 864
Sioux City, IA 51102-0864
712-255-8770

Medco Research, Inc.
P.O. Box 13886
Research Triangle Park, NC 27709
919-549-8117

45565
Med-Derm Pharmaceuticals
P.O. Box 5193
Kingsport, TN 37663
615-477-3991

Medea Research Laboratories
200 Wilson Street
Port Jefferson, NY 11776
516-331-7718

00585
Medeva Pharmaceuticals
755 Jefferson Road
Rochester, NY 14623-0000
888-963-3382

Medi Aid Corp.
8250 S. Akron Street
Suite 205
Englewood, CO 80155
303-790-1655

00576
Medical Products Panamericana
647 West Flagler Street
Miami, FL 33130
305-545-6524

99207
Medicis Dermatologicals, Inc.
4343 East Camelback Road
Suite 250
Phoenix, AZ 85018-2700
602-808-3853

60574
Medimmune, Inc.
35 West Watkins Mill Road
Gaithersburg, MD 20878
301-417-0770

Medimorphics
245 East 6th Street
St. Paul, MN 55101
612-224-2800

17156
MediPhysics, Inc., Amersham Healthcare
2636 S. Clearbrook Drive
Arlington Heights, IL 60005
800-322-6334

Medi-Plex Pharm., Inc.
See ECR Pharmaceuticals

57480
Medirex, Inc.
20 Chapin Road
Pine Brook, NJ 07058
201-227-4774

61563
Medisan
400 Lanidex Plaza
Parsippany, NJ 07054
201-515-5300

MediSense, Inc.
266 Second Street
Waltham, MA 02154

53978
Med-Pro, Inc.
210 E. 4th Street
Lexington, NE 68850
308-324-4571

00348, 75137
Medtech Laboratories, Inc.
3510 N. Lake Creek
P.O. Box 1108
Jackson, WY 83011-1108
307-733-1680

58281
Medtronic
800 53rd Ave. N.E.
Minneapolis, MN 55421
612-572-5000

87900
Menley & James Labs, Inc.
100 Tournament Drive
Horsham, PA 19044
215-441-6500

22200
Mennen Co.
See Colgate Palmolive

10742
Mentholatum, Inc.
1360 Niagara Street
Buffalo, NY 14213
716-882-7660

00006
Merck & Co.
P.O. Box 4
West Point, PA 19486
215-652-5000

00394
Mericon Industries, Inc.
8819 N. Pioneer Road
Peoria, IL 61615
309-693-2150

Merieux Institute, Inc.
See Pasteur Mérieux Connaught

30727
Merit Pharmaceuticals
2611 San Fernando Road
Los Angeles, CA 90065
213-227-4831

Michigan Department of Health
P.O. Box 30035
Lansing, MI 48909
517-335-8000

00682, 46672
Mikart
1750 Chattahoochee Avenue
Atlanta, GA 30318
404-351-4510

52836
Milance Laboratories, Inc.
P.O. Box 368
Millington, NJ 07946
908-580-1591

Miles, Inc.
See Bayer Corp. (Consumer Div.)

Miles, Inc.
See Bayer Corp. (Diagnostic Div.)

00396, 34567
Milex Products, Inc.
5915 Northwest Hwy.
Chicago, IL 60631-1032
312-631-6484

17204
Miller Pharmacal Group, Inc.
350 Randy Road, Unit #2
Carol Stream, IL 60188
630-871-9557

53118
Millgood Laboratories, Inc.
250 D Arizona Ave.
P.O. Box 170159
Atlanta, GA 30317
404-377-6538

00276
Misemer Pharmaceuticals, Inc.
4553 S. Campbell
Springfield, MO 65810-5918
417-881-0660

00178
Mission Pharmacal Co.
1325 East Durango Blvd.
San Antonio, TX 78278-6099
800-531-3333

53169
Monarch Pharmaceuticals
355 Beecham Street
Bristol, TN 37620
800-776-3637

Montgomery Medical Ventures
600 Montgomery Street
San Francisco, CA 94111

00426, 00832, 60432
Morton Grove Pharmaceuticals
6451 West Main Street
Morton Grove, IL 60053
708-967-5600

Morton Salt
100 N. Riverside Plaza
Chicago, IL 60606-1597
312-807-2000

MSD
See Merck & Co.

Mt. Vernon Foods, Inc.
13246 Wooster Road
Mt. Vernon, OH 43050
800-932-5525

54964
Murdock, Madaus, Schwabe
1400 Mountain Springs Pkwy.
Springvale, UT 84663
801-489-1500

00451
Muro Pharmaceutical, Inc.
890 East Street
Tewksbury, MA 01876-9987
508-851-5981

00150
Murray Drug Corp.
415 S. 4th Street
Murray, KY 42071
502-753-6654

53489
Mutual Pharmaceutical, Inc.
1100 Orthodox Street
Philadelphia, PA 19124
215-288-6500

00378
Mylan Pharmaceuticals
P.O. Box 4310
Morgantown, WV 26505
304-599-2595

05973
Nabi
5800 Park of Commerce Blvd.
Northwest
Boca Raton, FL 33487
305-625-5303

05745
Nastech Pharmaceutical, Inc.
45 Davids Drive
Hauppauge, NY 11788
516-273-0101

National Patent Medical
P.O. Box 419
Dayville, CT 06241
800-243-1172

53983
Natren, Inc.
3105 Willow Lane
Westlake Village, CA 91361

Natures Bounty, Inc.
See NBTY, Inc.

74312
NBTY, Inc.
105 Orville Drive
Bohemia, NY 11716
516-567-9500

72559
NCI Medical Foods
5801 Ayala Ave.
Irwindale, CA 91706
818-812-3393

Neorx Corp.
410 West Harrison
Seattle, WA 98119
206-281-7001

00487
Nephron Pharmaceuticals Corp.
4121 S.W. 34th Street
Orlando, FL 32811-6458
407-246-1389

Nephro-Tech, Inc.
P.O. Box 14703
Lenexa, KS 66285
913-894-6646

NeuroGenesis/Matrix Tech., Inc.
100 Louisiana
Suite 600
Houston, TX 77002
800-345-8912

10812, 70501
Neutrogena Corp.
5760 W. 96th Street
Los Angeles, CA 90045-5595
310-642-1150

Neutron Technology Corp.
877 Main Street
Boise, ID 83702
208-345-3460

New World Trading Corp.
P.O. Box 952
DeBary, FL 32713
407-668-7520

Newport Pharmaceuticals
140 Columbia
Laguna Hills, CA 92656-1459
714-362-1330

56146
Nexstar
2860 Wilderness Place
Boulder, CO 80301
303-444-5893

59016
Niche Pharmaceuticals, Inc.
200 N. Oak Street
P.O. Box 449
Roanoke, TX 76262
807-491-2770

12934
Nion Corp.
15501 First Street
Irwindale, CA 91706
818-969-1932

23317
NMC Laboratories
70-36 83rd Street
Glendale, NY 11385
718-326-1500

51801
Nomax, Inc.
40 North Rock Hill Road
St. Louis, MO 63119
314-961-2500

Norcliff Thayer
See SmithKline Beecham Consumer Healthcare

10118
Norstar Consumer Products
206 Pegasus Ave.
Northvale, NJ 07647
201-784-8155

North American Biologicals, Inc.
16500 N.W. 15th Ave.
Miami, FL 33169
305-625-5303

Novaferon Labs
2658 Patton Road
Roseville, MN 55713

00028, 00067, 00083, 58887
Novartis
556 Morris Ave.
Summit, NJ 07901
908-277-5000

00043
Novartis Consumer
59 Route 10
East Hanover, NJ 07936
201-503-7500

00212
Novartis Nutrition Corp.
5320 W. 23rd Street
Minneapolis, MN 55440
800-999-9978

00078
Novartis Pharmaceuticals
59 Route 10
East Hanover, NJ 07936
201-503-7500

Noven
11960 S.W. 144th Street
Miami, FL 33186
305-253-5099

00362
Novocol Chemical Mfr. Co.
P.O. Box 11926
Wilmington, DE 19850
302-328-1102

00169
Novo/Nordisk Pharm., Inc.
100 Overlook Center
Suite 200
Princeton, NJ 08540
800-727-6500

55953
Novopharm USA, Inc.
165 E. Commerce
Suite 100
Schaumberg, IL 60173-5326
708-882-4200

NPDC-AS101, Inc.
783 Jersey Avenue
New Brunswick, NJ 08901
716-636-9096

55499
Numark Laboratories, Inc.
P.O. Box 6321
Edison, NJ 08818
800-338-8079

34999
Nutraloric
350 N. Lantana, Unit G1
Camarillo, CA 93010
805-388-2811

NutraMax
9 Blackburn Drive
Gloucester, MA 01930
508-283-1800

Nutricia, Inc.
See Mt. Vernon Foods, Inc.

51081
Nutripharm Laboratories, Inc.
Salem Industrial Park
Building 5
Lebanon, NJ 08833
908-534-6267

00407
Nycomed Inc.
101 Carnegie Center
Princeton, NJ 08540-6231
609-514-6438

10797
Oakhurst Co.
3000 Hempstead Turnpike
Levittown, NY 11756
516-731-5380

55515
Oclassen Pharmaceuticals, Inc.
100 Pelican Way
San Rafael, CA 94901
415-258-4500

O'Connor, Inc.
See Columbia Laboratories, Inc.

51944
Ocumed, Inc.
119 Harrison Ave.
Roseland, NJ 07068
201-226-2330

Ohm Laboratories, Inc.
P.O. Box 7397
N. Brunswick, NJ 08902
908-297-3030

10019
Ohmeda Pharmaceuticals
110 Allen Road
Liberty Corner, NJ 07938
908-647-9200

12622
Olin Corp.
120 Long Ridge Road
Stamford, CT 06904-1355
203-356-2000

Omex International, Inc.
6001 Savoy
Suite 110
Houston, TX 77036
713-975-8325

Oncotherapeutics, Inc.
1002 East Park Blvd.
Cranbury, NJ 08512
609-655-5300

ONY, Inc.
1576 Sweet Home Road
Amherst, NY 14228
716-636-9096

Ophidian Pharmaceuticals, Inc.
2800 S. Fish Hatchery Road
Madison, WI 53711
608-271-0878

O.P.R. Development, LP
1501 Wakarusa Drive
Lawrence, KS 66047
913-749-0034

Optikem International, Inc.
2172 S. Jason Street
Denver, CO 80223
303-936-1137

50520
Optimox Corp.
2720 Monterey
Suite 406
Torrance, CA 90503
310-618-9370

52238
Optopics Laboratories, Corp.
32 Main Street
P.O. Box 210
Fairton, NJ 08320-0210
508-283-1800

00041
Oral-B Laboratories, Inc.
1 Lagoon Drive
Redwood City, CA 94065
415-961-8130

00052
Organon, Inc.
375 Mt. Pleasant Ave.
West Orange, NJ 07052
201-325-4500

Organon Teknika Corp.
100 Akzo Ave.
Durham, NC 27704
919-620-2000

Orion Diagnostica
71 Veronica Ave.
P.O. Box 218
Somerset, NJ 08875-0218
908-246-3366

Orphan Medical
13911 Ridgedale Drive
Minnetonka, MN 55305
612-513-6900

59676
Ortho Biotech, Inc.
Route 202 South
Raritan, NJ 08869-0602
908-325-7504

00062
Ortho McNeil Pharmaceutical
Route 202 South
Raritan, NJ 08869-0602
908-218-6000

59148
Otsuka America Pharmaceutical
2440 Research Blvd.
Rockville, MD 98101
206-682-5300

Owen/Galderma
See Galderma Laboratories, Inc.

Oxis International
6040 N. Cutter Circle
Suite 317
Portland, OR 97212
503-283-3911

00217
Oxypure
P.O. Box 100
Gravette, AR 72736
501-787-5232

00574
Paddock Laboratories
3940 Quebec Avenue
North Minneapolis, MN 55427
612-546-4676

53159
Palisades Pharmaceuticals, Inc.
64 N. Summit Street
Tenafly, NJ 07670
201-569-8502

Pan America Labs
P.O. Box 8950
Mandeville, LA 70470-8950
504-893-4097

49884
Par Pharmaceuticals
One Ram Ridge Road
Spring Valley, NY 10977
914-425-7100

00071
Parke-Davis
201 Tabor Road
Morris Plains, NJ 07950
800-223-0432

00349
Parmed Pharmaceuticals, Inc.
4220 Hyde Park Blvd.
Niagara Falls, NY 14305
716-284-5666

50930
Parnell Pharmaceuticals, Inc.
Larkspur Landing Circle
Larkspur, CA 94939
415-461-4900

10865
Parthenon, Inc.
3311 W. 2400 South
Salt Lake City, UT 84119
801-972-5184

00418
Pasadena Research Labs
See Taylor Pharmaceuticals

11793, 49281, 50361
Pasteur Mérieux Connaught Labs
Route 611
P.O. Box 187
Swiftwater, PA 18370-0187
717-839-7187

00077
PBH Wesley Jessen
7976 Engineer Road
San Diego, CA 92111
619-614-7600

Pediatric Pharmaceuticals
718 Bradford Ave.
Westfield, NJ 07090
908-225-0989

00884
Pedinol Pharmacal, Inc.
30 Banfi Plaza North
Farmingdale, NY 11735
516-293-9500

10974
Pegasus Medical, Inc.
1 Technology Drive
Building 1C
Suite 525
Irvine, CA 92718-2325
714-753-9055

Pennex Pharmaceutical, Inc.
See Morton Grove Pharmaceuticals

Permeable Technologies, Inc.
712 Ginesi Drive
Morganville, NJ 07751
908-972-8585

00096
Person and Covey, Inc.
616 Allen Ave.
P.O. Box 25018
Glendale, CA 91221-5018
818-240-1030

00927
Pfeiffer Co.
43-45 N. Washington
P.O. Box 100
Wilkes-Barre, PA 18701
717-026 0000

Pfipharmecs
See Pfizer US Pharmaceutical Group

00069, 00663, 74300
Pfizer US Pharmaceutical Group
235 E. 42nd Street
New York, NY 10017-5755
800-438-1985

39822
Pharma Tek, Inc.
P.O. Box 1920
Huntington, NY 11743-0568
516-757-5522

58197
Pharmacel Laboratory, Inc.
203 South Coolidge Ave.
Tampa, FL 33609
813-289-2750

00121
Pharmaceutical Associates, Inc.
P.O. Box 128
Conestee, SC 29636
803-277-7282

Pharmaceutical Basics, Inc.
See Rosemont Pharmaceutical

51655
Pharmaceutical Corp.
12348 Hancock Street
Carmel, IN 46032
317-573-8000

21659
Pharmaceutical Labs, Inc.
1229 W. Corporate Drive
Arlington, TX 76006
817-633-1461

45334
Pharmaceutical Specialties, Inc.
P.O. Box 6298
Rochester, MN 55903
507-288-8500

Pharmachemie USA, Inc.
P.O. Box 145
Oradell, NJ 07049
201-265-1942

00013, 00016
Pharmacia & Upjohn
7000 Portage Road
Kalamazoo, MI 49001-6529
616-833-8244

PharmaControl
661 Palisade Ave.
P.O. Box 931
Englewood Cliffs, NJ 07632
201-567-9004

Pharmafair
See Bausch & Lomb Pharmaceuticals

55422
Pharmakon Laboratories, Inc.
6050 Jet Port Industrial Blvd.
Tampa, FL 33634
813-886-3216

Pharmaquest Corp.
See Inveresk Research

Pharmatec
County Road 2054
P.O. Box 730
Alachua, FL 32615
904-462-1210

Pharmavene, Inc.
35 West Watkins Mill Road
Gaithersburg, MD 20878
301-417-0033

Pharmedic Co.
28101 Ballard Road
Suite F
Lake Forest, IL 60045
708-549-8600

00813
Pharmics, Inc.
P.O. Box 27554
Salt Lake City, UT 84127
801-972-4138

Plexus Pharmaceuticals, Inc.
8122 Datapoint Drive
Suite 600
San Antonio, TX 78229

Plough, Inc.
See Schering-Plough Healthcare Products

00998
PolyMedica Pharmaceuticals
2 Constitution Way
Woburn, MA 01801
617-933-2020

47144
Polymer Technology Corp.
100 Research Drive
Wilmington, MA 01887
800-343-1445

Polymer Technology International
1595 N.W. Gilman Blvd.
Suite 17
Issaquah, WA 98027
206-391-2650

Porton Product Limited
See Speywood Pharmaceuticals, Inc.

Poythress
See ECR Pharmaceuticals

59012
Pratt Pharmaceuticals
235 E. 42nd Street
New York, NY 10017-5755
800-438-1985

Precision-Cosmet
See Chiron Vision

Premier, Inc.
See Advanced Polymer Systems

00684
Primedics Laboratories
15524 S. Broadway
Gardenia, CA 90248
213-770-3005

Princeton Pharm. Products
See Bristol-Myers Squibb

23900, 37000, 76660
Procter & Gamble Co.
1 Procter & Gamble Plaza
Cincinnati, OH 45202
513-983-1100

00149
Procter & Gamble Pharm.
P.O. Box 191
Norwich, NY 13815-0191
607-335-2111

00034
Purdue Frederick Co.
100 Connecticut Ave.
Norwalk, CT 06850-3590
203-853-0123

00228
Purepac Pharmaceutical Co.
200 Elmora Ave.
Elizabeth, NJ 07207
908-527-9100

QLT Phototherapeutics, Inc.
401 North Middletown Road
Pearl River, NY 10965

00603
Qualitest Products, Inc.
1236 Jordan Road
Huntsville, AL 35811
205-859-4011

12225
Quality Formulations, Inc.
P.O. Box 827
Zachary, LA 70791-0827
504-654-6880

Quidel Corp.
10165 McKellar Court
San Diego, CA 92121
619-552-1100

54391
R & D Laboratories, Inc.
4640 Admiralty Way,
Suite 710
Marina Del Rey, CA 90292
310-305-8053

R & R Registrations
P.O. Box 262079
San Diego, CA 92196-2069
619-586-0751

00196
Rachelle Laboratories, Inc.
See Houba Inc.

30103
Randob Laboratories, Ltd.
P.O. Box 440
Cornwall, NY 12518
914-699-3131

00686
Raway Pharmacal, Inc.
15 Granit Road
Accord, NY 12404-0047
914-626-8133

12496, 19200
Reckitt & Colman
1901 Huguenot Road
Suite 110
Richmond, VA 23235
804-379-1090

10952
Recsei Laboratories
330 S. Kellogg
Building M
Goleta, CA 93117-3875
805-964-2912

48028
Redi-Products Labs, Inc.
See Aplicare Inc.

00021
Reed & Carnrick
See Schwarz Pharma

10956
Reese Pharmaceutical Inc.
10617 Frank Ave.
Cleveland, OH 44106
216-231-6441

Regeneron Pharmaceuticals
777 Old Saw Mill River Road
Tarrytown, NY 10591-6707
914-347-7000

Reid Rowell
See Solvay

Remel, Inc.
12076 Santa Fe Drive
Lenexa, KS 66215

10961
Requa, Inc.
1 Seneca Place
P.O. Box 4008
Greenwich, CT 06830
203-869-2445

00433
Research Industries Corp.
6864 S. 300 West
Midvale, UT 84047
801-562-0200

Research Triangle Pharmaceuticals
4364 S. Alston Ave.
Durham, NC 27713
919-544-4029

60575
Respa Pharmaceuticals, Inc.
P.O. Box 88222
Carol Stream, IL 60188
708-462-9986

00122
Rexall Group
4031 N.E. 12th Terrace
Ft. Lauderdale, FL 33334
800-255-7399

Rexar Pharmaceuticals
See Richwood Pharmaceutical

RH Pharmaceuticals, Inc.
See Cangene Corp.

Rhone-Poulenc Rorer Consumer, Inc.
See Novartis

00075
Rhone-Poulenc Rorer Pharmaceuticals, Inc.
500 Arcola Road
P.O. Box 1200
Collegeville, PA 19426
610-454-8110

Ribi Immunochem Research
553 Old Corvallis Road
Hamilton, MT 59840-3131
406-363-6214

Richardson-Vicks, Inc.
See Procter & Gamble Co.

12071
Richie Pharmacal, Inc.
197 State Ave.
P.O. Box 460
Glasgow, KY 42141
800-626-0250

58521
Richwood Pharmaceutical, Inc.
See Shire Richwood Pharmaceutical, Inc.

54807
R.I.D., Inc.
609 North Mednik Avenue
Los Angeles, CA 90022-1320
213-268-0635

54092
Roberts Pharmaceuticals
4 Industrial Way West
Eatontown, NJ 07724
908-389-1182

A.H. Robins Consumer Products
See Wyeth-Ayerst

00031
A.H. Robins, Inc.
See Wyeth-Ayerst

Roche Diagnostic Systems, Inc.
1080 U.S. Highway 202
Somerville, NJ 08876-3771
908-253-7200

00004, 00033, 00140, 18393, 42987
Roche Laboratories
340 Kingsland Street
Nutley, NJ 07110-1199
800-526-6367

00049
Roerig
See Pfizer

00832
Rosemont Pharmaceutical Corp.
301 South Cherokee Street
Denver, CO 80223
303-733-7207

00074
Ross Laboratories
6480 Busch Blvd.
Columbus, OH 43229
614-624-3333

00054
Roxane Laboratories, Inc.
P.O. Box 16532
Columbus, OH 43216-6532
614-276-4000

51875
Royce Laboratories, Inc.
16600 N.W. 54 Ave.
Miami, FL 33014
305-624-1500

00536
Rugby Labs, Inc.
898 Orlando Ave.
West Hempstead, NY 11552
516-536-8565

Russ Pharmaceuticals
See UCB Pharmaceuticals

46500
Rydelle Laboratories
1525 Howe Street
Racine, WI 53403-5011
414-631-2000

00263
Rystan, Inc.
P.O. Box 214
Little Falls, NJ 07424-0214
201-256-3737

51353
Sanitube Co.
19 Concord Street
S. Norwalk, CT 06854
203-853-7856

00024
Sanofi Winthrop Pharmaceuticals
90 Park Ave.
New York, NY 10016
800-446-6267

00281
Savage Laboratories
60 Baylis Road
Melville, NY 11747-2006
800-231-0206

Scandinavian Natural Health & Beauty Products
13 N. 7th St.
Perkasie, PA 18944
215-453-2505

58914
Scandipharm, Inc.
22 Inverness Center Pkwy.
Suite 310
Birmingham, AL 35242
800-950-8085

11012
Schaffer Laboratories
1058 North Allen Ave.
Pasadena, CA 91104
818-798-8644

00364
Schein Pharmaceutical, Inc.
100 Campus Drive
Florham Park, NJ 07932
914-278-3724

00274
Scherer Laboratories, Inc.
16200 N. Dallas Pkwy.
Suite 165
Dallas, TX 75248
800-858-9888

00085
Schering-Plough Corp.
2000 Galloping Hill Road
Kenilworth, NJ 07033-0530
908-298-4000

00085
Schering-Plough Healthcare Products
110 Allen Road
Liberty Corner, NJ 07938
908-298-4000

Schiapparelli Searle
See SCS Pharmaceuticals

Schiff Products
P.O. Box 26708
Salt Lake City, UT 84126
801-975-1166

00234
Schmid Products Co.
See Durex Consumer Products

Scholl, Inc.
See Schering-Plough Healthcare Products

00021, 00091, 00131
Schwarz Pharma
5600 W. County Line
Mequon, WI 53092
800-558-5114

Scios Nova, Inc.
2450 Bayshore Pkwy.
Mountain View, CA 94043
415-966-1550

00372
Scot-Tussin Pharmacal, Inc.
50 Clemence Street
P.O. Box 8217
Cranston, RI 02920-0217
800-638-7268

00905
SCS Pharmaceuticals
P.O. Box 5110
Chicago, IL 60680
800-323-1603

00014, 00025
Searle
Box 5110
Chicago, IL 60680-5110
847-982-7000

00551
Seatrace Pharmaceuticals
P.O. Box 363
Gadsden, AL 35902-0363
205-442-5023

Sequus Pharmaceuticals, Inc.
960 Hamilton Court
Menlo Park, CA 94025
415-833-7207

50694
Seres Laboratories
3331 Industrial Drive
P.O. Box 470
Santa Rosa, CA 95401
707-526-4526

44087
Serono Laboratories, Inc.
100 Longwater Circle
Norwell, MA 02061
617-982-9000

97692
S.G. Labs, Inc.
500 North Broadway
Jericho, NY 11753
516-822-2900

49731
Sherman Pharmaceuticals, Inc.
P.O. Box 1377
Mandeville, LA 70470-1377
504-893-0007

08884
Sherwood Davis & Geck
1915 Olive Street
St. Louis, MO 63103
314-621-7788

45809
Shionogi USA
3848 Carson Street
Suite 206
Torrance, CA 90503
310-540-1161

58521
Shire Richwood Pharmaceutical, Inc.
P.O. Box 6497
Florence, KY 41022
800-974-4700

50111
Sidmak Laboratories, Inc.
P.O. Box 371
East Hanover, NJ 07936
201-386-5566

54482
Sigma-Tau Pharmaceuticals, Inc.
800 S. Frederick Avenue
Gaithersburg, MD 20877-4150
301-948-1041

54838
Silarx Pharmaceuticals, Inc.
19 West Street
Spring Valley, NY 10977
914-352-4020

08026
Smith & Nephew United
11775 Starkey Road
Largo, FL 34643
800-876-1261

00766
SmithKline Beecham Consumer Healthcare
1500 Littleton
Parsippany, NJ 07054-3884
800-245-1040
201-631-8700

00007, 00029, 00108, 00128
SmithKline Beecham Pharmaceuticals
One Franklin Plaza,
P.O. Box 7929
Philadelphia, PA 19103
215-751-4000

00978
SmithKline Diagnostics
225 Baypoint Pkwy.
San Jose, CA 95134-1622
800-877-6242

Sola/Barnes-Hind
See PBH Wesley Jessen

33984
Solgar, Inc.
410 Ocean Ave.
Lynbrook, NY 11563
516-599-2442

39769
SoloPak Pharmaceuticals, Inc.
1845 Tonne Road
Elk Grove Village, IL 60007-5125
847-806-0080

00032
Solvay Pharmaceuticals
901 Sawyer Road
Marietta, GA 30062-2224
770-578-9000

39506
Somerset Pharmaceuticals
5215 West Laurel Street
Tampa, FL 33607
813-223-7677

Sparta Pharmaceuticals
P.O. Box 13288
Research Triangle Park, NC 27709
919-361-3461

Spectra Pharmaceuticals
See Cooper Pharmaceuticals

38137
Spectrum Chemical Mfg. Corp.
14422 S. San Pedro Street
Gardena, CA 90248-9985
800-772-8786

00537
Spencer Mead, Inc.
100 Banks Ave.
Rockville Center, NY 11570
800-645-3737

55688
Speywood Pharmaceuticals, Inc.
27 Maple Street
Milford, MA 01757-2658
508-478-8900

Sphinx Pharmaceutical Corp.
P.O. Box 52330
Durham, NC 27717
919-489-0909

Squibb Diagnostic Division
See Bracco Diagnostics

Stanback Co.
P.O. Box 1669
Salisbury, NC 28145-1669
704-633-9231

53385
Standard Drug Co.
P.O. Box 710
Riverton, IL 62561
217-629-9884

00076
Star Pharmaceuticals, Inc.
1990 N.W. 44th Street
Pompano Beach, FL 33064-1278
305-971-9704

51318
Stellar Pharmacal Corp.
1990 N.W. 44th Street
Pompano Beach, FL 33064
800-845-7827

00402
Steris Laboratories, Inc.
620 N. 51st Ave.
Phoenix, AZ 85043
602-278-1400

Sterling Health
See Bayer Corp. (Consumer Div.)

Sterling Winthrop
See Sanofi Winthrop Pharmaceuticals

00145
Stiefel Laboratories, Inc.
255 Alhambra Circle
Coral Gables, FL 33134
800-327-3858

89223
Stockhausen, Inc.
2408 Doyle Street
Greensboro, NC 27406
800-334-0242

41701
Stolle
6954 Cornell Road
Cincinnati, OH 45242
513-489-4235

57706
Storz Ophthalmics
3365 Tree Court Industrial
St. Louis, MO 63122-6694
314-225- 5051

58980
Stratus Pharmaceuticals, Inc.
P.O. Box 4632
Miami, FL 33265
800-442-7882

Stuart Pharmaceuticals
See Zeneca Pharmaceuticals

Sublingual Products International
See Pharmaceutical Labs, Inc.

11086
Summers Laboratories, Inc.
103 G.P. Clement Drive
Collegeville, PA 19426
610-454-1471

57267
Summit Pharmaceuticals
See Novartis Pharmaceuticals

11704
Survival Technology, Inc.
2275 Research Blvd.
Rockville, MD 20850
301-926-1800

Syncom Pharmaceuticals, Inc.
155 Passaic Ave.
Fairfield, NJ 07004

Synergen, Inc.
See Amgen

00033, 18393, 42987
Syntex Laboratories
3401 Hillview Ave.
Palo Alto, CA 94304
415-855-5050

Syntex-Synergen Neuroscience
1885 33rd Street
Boulder, CO 80301
303-442-1926

Syva Co.
929 Queensbridge
St. Louis, MO 63021
314-391-5374

Tag Pharmaceuticals
P.O. Box 904
Sellersville, PA 18960
215-723-5544

Tambrands, Inc.
777 Westchester Ave.
White Plains, NY 10604
914-696-6060

Tanning Research Labs, Inc.
1190 U.S. 1 North
Ormond Beach, FL 32174
904-677-9559

00300
Tap Pharmaceuticals
2355 Waukegan Road
Deerfield, IL 60015
800-621-1020

51672
Taro Pharmaceuticals USA, Inc.
Six Skyline Drive
Hawthorne, NY 10532-9998
914-345-9001

00418
Taylor Pharmaceuticals
P.O. Box 5136
San Clemente, CA 92674-5136
714-492-4030

83926
Tec Laboratories, Inc.
615 Water Ave. S.E.
P.O. Box 1958
Albany, OR 97321-0512
503-926-4577

Telluride Pharm. Corp.
146 Flanders Drive
Hillsborough, NJ 08876-4656
908-359-1375

00093, 00332
Teva Pharmaceuticals USA
650 Cathill Road
Sellersville, PA 18960

49158
Thames Pharmacal, Inc.
2100 Fifth Ave.
Ronkonkoma, NY 11779-6906
516-737-1155

Therakos, Inc.
201 Brandywine Pkwy.
West Chester, PA 19380
610-430-7900

Therapeutic Antibodies, Inc.
1500 21st Ave.
Suite 310
Nashville, TN 37212
615-327-1027

11290
Thompson Medical Co.
222 Lakeview Ave.
West Palm Beach, FL 33401
407-820-9900

T/I Pharmaceuticals, Inc.
See Fischer Pharmaceuticals

49483
Time-Cap Labs, Inc.
7 Michael Avenue
Farmingdale, NY 11735
516-753-9090

TNI Pharmaceuticals
5105 N. Pearl Street
Schiller Park, IL 60176
708-678-3067

93312
Trask Industries, Inc.
163 Farrell Street
Somerset, NJ 08873
908-214-9267

Triage Pharmaceuticals
See Health for Life Brands, Inc.

Triangle Labs, Inc.
1000 Robins Road
Lynchburg, VA 24504-3558
804-845-7073

53020
Trinity Technologies, Inc.
28510 Hayes
Roseville, MI 48066
313-778-5630

79511
Triton Consumer Products, Inc.
561 West Golf
Arlington Heights, IL 60005
708-228-7650

Tsumura Medical
1000 Valley Park Drive
Shakopee, MN 55379
612-496-4700

Tweezerman
55 Sea Cliff Ave.
Glen Cove, NY 11542-3695
516-676-7772

53335
Tyson & Associates, Inc.
12832 Chadron Ave.
Hawthorne, CA 90250-5525
310-675-1080

UAD Laboratories, Inc.
See Forest Pharmaceutical, Inc.

59640
UBI Corp.
2920 N.W. Boca Raton Blvd.
Boca Raton, FL 33431
407-367-1252

UCB Pharmaceuticals, Inc.
P.O. Box 4410
Hampton, VA 23664-0410
804-851-4618

62592
Ucyclyd Pharma, Inc.
10819 Gilroy Road,
Suite 100
Hunt Valley, MD 21031
410-584-0001

51079
UDL Laboratories, Inc.
P.O. Box 10319
Rockford, IL 61131-3019
815-282-1201

Ueno Fine Chemicals Industry
31 Koraibashi
Osaka 541, Japan
06-203-0761

00127
Ulmer Pharmacal Co.
2440 Fernbrook Lane
Plymouth, MN 55447-9987
612-559-0601

41785
Unimed
2150 E. Lake Cook Road
Buffalo Grove, IL 60089
800-541-3492

00677
United Research Laboratories
3600 Marshall Lane
P.O. Box 8546
Bensalem, PA 19020-8546
215-638-2626

48663
Unitek Corp.
2724 South Peck Road
Monrovia, CA 91016
818-445-7960

Univax Biologics
12280 Wilkins Ave.
Rockville, MD 20852
301-770-3099

00009
Upjohn Co.
See Pharmacia & Upjohn

00245
Upsher-Smith Labs, Inc.
14905 23rd Ave. N.
Minneapolis, MN 55447
612-473-4412

58178
US Bioscience
100 Front Street
Suite 400
West Conshohocken, PA 19428
800-447-3969

US Packaging Corp. Medical
506 Clay Street
LaPorte, IN 46350
219-362-9782

52747
US Pharmaceutical Corp.
2401-C Mellon Court
Decatur, GA 30035
(770) 987-4745

54627
ValMed, Inc.
203 Southwest Cutoff
Northboro, MA 01532
800-477-0487

00615
Vangard Labs, Inc.
P.O. Box 1268
Glasgow, KY 42142-1268
502-651-6188

17022
Veratex Corp.
1304 E. Maple Road
P.O. Box 4031
Troy, MI 48007
810-619-0800

Vertex Pharmaceuticals, Inc.
40 Allston Street
Cambridge, MA 02139-4211
617-576-3111

53258
VHA Supply Co.
300 Decker Drive
P.O. Box 160909
Irving, TX 75016
214-650-4444

23900
Vicks Health Care Products
See Procter & Gamble Co

25866
Vicks Pharmacy Products
See Procter & Gamble Products

Vintage Pharmaceuticals, Inc.
3241 Woodpark Blvd.
Charlotte, NC 28256
704-596-0516

Viratek
3300 Hyland Ave.
Costa Mesa, CA 92627
714-540-1866

54891
Vision Pharmaceuticals, Inc.
P.O. Box 400
Mitchell, SD 57301-0400
605-996-3356

54022
Vitaline Corp.
385 Williamson Way
Ashland, OR 97520
503-482-9231

Vita-Rx Corp.
P.O. Box 8229
Columbus, GA 31908
706-568-1881

00298
Vortech Pharmaceuticals
6851 Chase Road
Dearborn, MI 48126
313-584-4088

11444
W. F. Young, Inc.
111 Lyman Street
Springfield, MA 01102
413-737-0201

59310
Wakefield Pharmaceuticals, Inc.
1050 Cambridge Square
Suite C
Alpharetta, GA 30201
404-664-1661

00741
Walker, Corp. and, Inc.
P.O. Box 1320
Syracuse, NY 13201
315-463-4511

00619
Walker Pharmacal Co.
4200 Laclede Ave.
St. Louis, MO 63108
314-533-9600

00037
Wallace Laboratories
Halfacre Road
Cranbury, NJ 08512
609-655-6000

00017
Wampole Laboratories
Half Acre Road
P.O. Box 1001
Cranbury, NJ 08515-0181
609-655-6000

00047
Warner Chilcott Laboratories
182 Tabor Road
Morris Plains, NJ 07950
800-521-8813

00071, 00081, 00501, 11370
Warner Lambert Consumer Health Products
201 Tabor Road
Morris Plains, NJ 07950
201-540-2000

59930
Warrick Pharmaceuticals, Corp.
1095 Morris Ave.
Union, NJ 07083
908-629-3600

00047, 52544
Watson Laboratories
311 Bonnie Circle Drive
Corona, CA 91720
909-270-1400

59196
WE Pharmaceuticals, Inc.
P.O. Box 1142
Ramona, CA 92065
619-788-9155

Wendt Laboratories
P.O. Box 128
Belle Plaine, MN 56011
800-328-5890

00917
Wesley Pharmacal, Inc.
114 Railroad Drive
Ivyland, PA 18974
215-953-1680

59591
West Point Pharma
P.O. Box 4
West Point, PA 19486-0004
212-652-2121

50893
Westport Pharmaceuticals, Inc.
1 Turkey Hill Road S.
Westport, CT 06880
203-226-0622

00143
West-Ward, Inc.
465 Industrial Way W.
Eatontown, NJ 07724
908-542-1191

00003, 00072
Westwood Squibb Pharmaceuticals
100 Forest Ave.
Buffalo, NY 14213
609-897-2000

50474
Whitby Pharmaceuticals, Inc.
See UCB Pharmaceuticals, Inc.

00031, 00573
Whitehall Robins Laboratories
Five Giralda Farms
Madison, NJ 07940-0871
201-660-5500

00317
Whorton Pharmaceuticals, Inc.
4202 Gary Ave.
Fairfield, AL 35064
205-786-2584

Willen Pharmaceuticals
See Baker Norton Pharmaceuticals

Winthrop Consumer
See Bayer Corp. (Consumer Div.)

Winthrop Pharmaceuticals
See Sanofi Winthrop Pharmaceuticals

12120
Wisconsin Pharmacal Co.
1 Repel Road
Jackson, WI 53037
414-677-4121

11428
Wonderful Dream Salve Corp.
18546 Old Homestead
Harper Woods, MI 48225
313-521-4233

Woodward Laboratories, Inc.
10357 Los Alamitos Blvd.
Los Alamitos, CA 90720
310-598-0800

WTD, Inc.
8819 N. Pioneer Road
Peoria, IL 61615
309-693-2150

00008, 00031
Wyeth-Ayerst Laboratories
P.O. Box 8299
Philadelphia, PA 19101
610-688-4400

50962
Xactdose, Inc.
722 Progressive Lane
South Beloit, IL 61080
815-624-8523

Xoma
2910 Seventh Street
Berkeley, CA 94710
510-644-1170

00116
Xttrium Laboratories, Inc.
415 West Pershing Road
Chicago, IL 60609
312-268-5800

64855
Young Again Products
43 Randolph Road
Suite 125
Silver Spring, MD 20904
301-622-1073

00273, 60077
Young Dental
13705 Shoreline Court E.
Earth City, MO 63045
314-344-0010

Young Pharmaceutical
1840 Berlin Turnpike
Wethersfield, CT 06109
203-529-7919

00163, 00187, 00310
Zeneca Pharmaceuticals
1800 Concord Pike
Wilmington, DE 19897
302-886-3000

00172, 00182
Zenith Goldline Pharmaceuticals
1900 W. Commercial Blvd.
Ft. Lauderdale, FL 33309
305-491-4002

51284
Zila Pharmaceuticals, Inc.
5227 N. 7th Street
Phoenix, AZ 85014-2817
602-266-6700

Zymogenetics, Inc.
1201 Eastlake Ave. E.
Seattle, WA 98102
206-547-8080

ISBN 1-57439-041-4